Cancer Inhibitors from Chinese Natural Medicines

Cancer Inhibitors from Chinese Natural Medicines

Jun-Ping Xu

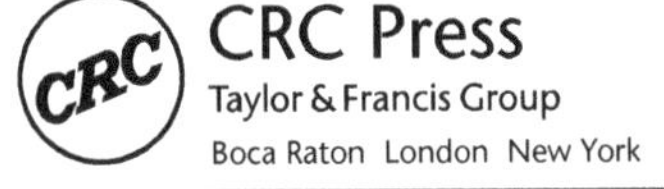

CRC Press is an imprint of the
Taylor & Francis Group, an **informa** business

CRC Press
Taylor & Francis Group
6000 Broken Sound Parkway NW, Suite 300
Boca Raton, FL 33487-2742

First issued in paperback 2021

Version Date: 20160802

ISBN 13: 978-1-03-209739-8 (pbk)
ISBN 13: 978-1-4987-8764-2 (hbk)

Library of Congress Cataloging-in-Publication Data

Names: Xu, Jun-Ping.
Title: Cancer inhibitors from Chinese natural medicines / Jun-Ping Xu.
Description: Boca Raton, FL : CRC Press, 2017. | Includes bibliographical references and index.
Identifiers: LCCN 2016032439 | ISBN 9781498787642 (hardcover : alk. paper)
Subjects: LCSH: Cancer--Prevention. | Medicine, Chinese. | Herbs--Therapeutic use.
Classification: LCC RC268 .X8 2017 | DDC 616.99/405--dc23
LC record available at https://lccn.loc.gov/2016032439

Visit the Taylor & Francis Web site at
http://www.taylorandfrancis.com

and the CRC Press Web site at
http://www.crcpress.com

This book is dedicated to Prof. P.R. Pettit, director of the Cancer Research Institute at Arizona State University, and to Prof. H. Itokawa, supervisor of my PhD program at Tokyo University of Pharmacy and Life Sciences, for their outstanding accomplishments in the discovery and development of novel anticancer agents from natural sources and herbs; to my wife, Wendy, and son, Alex, for their full understanding and strong support; to the memories of my parents, Mr. Bingheng Xu and Mrs. Tingying Li, for their deep love; and to my uncle-in-law, Dr. Mike Y.H. Wu, for his earnest encouragements.

Contents

Preface

The risk of cancer is significantly increasing nowadays, which is a serious social and health problem threatening human beings. Hence numerous scientists continuously endeavor on this imperative issue of conquering the malignant disease and declining the incidence of cancer. Because over 60% of currently used anticancer agents are derived from natural sources directly or indirectly, the discovery and development of new effective and safe cancer inhibitors from folk medicines still are important research subjects. In recent decades a large quantity of natural products isolated from Chinese natural medicines have been found to have remarkable bioactivities in the inhibition of cancer cell proliferation, induction of apoptotic death, lessening of metastasis, blockage of angiogenesis in the tumor tissues, and enhancement of present chemo- and radiotherapies. All these remarkable achievements not only afford scientific reasons for utilizing Chinese herbs to augment conventional therapies but also provide various important information for new drug design and development and new therapy strategies to improve the quality of cancer treatment and prevention. The greatest successful example of the discovery and development of novel drugs from Chinese natural medicines is artemisinin, a powerful antimalaria drug from a Chinese herb, *Artemisia apiacea*. The drug was complimented by the World Health Organization for saving millions of patients who suffered from the malarial disease, and the discoverer, Dr. Du Niuniu, was awarded the Nobel Prize for medicine in 2015. This fact strongly inspires scientists to dig into the treasure of Chinese natural medicines. There is an enormous and untapped potential in natural herbs that are beneficial to human health.

The overview of cancer inhibitors from Chinese natural medicines could roughly be classified into five types: (1) inhibitors with powerful cytotoxicity similar to those of current chemotherapeutic agents but displaying toxicity and side effects; (2) inhibitors that exert marked anticancer effects but are lower than (1)-type inhibitors and have minor toxicity or nontoxicity; (3) inhibitors with moderate effects on cancer cells and also have immunoregulative and/or antioxidant properties; (4) inhibitors that are weakly effective against cancer cells but are capable of stimulating the functional immune system and antioxidative system; and (5) inhibitors that normally do not directly affect cancer cells but remarkably enhance the cytotoxicity of the functional immune factors of the host to attack the cancer cells. Based on research results, the multiple types of cancer inhibitors are known to be often involved in single herbs that play diverse roles in cancer therapies. For the improvement of life quality and life duration, different inhibitor-containing herbs, in many cases, are effectively combined in the prescriptions of Chinese medicine by doctors in China to treat cancer patients.

This book primarily is focused on the interface of chemistry/biology and molecular biology, and comprehensively summarizes recent cutting-edge research advances in the field of cancer inhibitors (including extracts and compounds) from Chinese natural medicines. To underline how Chinese natural medicines research continues to make predominant contributions in the domain of the discovery and development of novel cancer inhibitors, this book highlights the scientific evidences of 238 Chinese herbs in eight major aspects: (1) advanced discoveries of cancer inhibitors from Chinese natural medicines; (2) *in vitro* and *in vivo* inhibitory effects against different types of cancer cells, such as their antiproliferative, antigrowth, antimetastatic, antitumorigenic, and antioxidant properties; (3) modern exploration of suppressive mechanisms; (4) synergetic activities in the combination of current cancer therapies with the inhibitors; (5) reversal advantage of the inhibitors against drug resistance; (6) structural modification to derive more important molecules for drug development; (7) formulation researches on nanocapsules/microparticles, immunotoxin/antibody–drug conjugate, and metal complex; and (8) clinical trials and practices of herb extracts and/or promising inhibitors derived from Chinese Natural Medicines (CNM).

Consequently, this book brings readers comprehensive and illuminating insights into cancer inhibitors from Chinese natural medicines. The 238 Chinese herbs have been categorized into 14 chapters in the book according to their main functions in Chinese medicine. For most of the selected herbs, the research data have been collected up to October 2015, from the latest challenges in the anticancer approaches. A large number of abbreviations are used in the book for the convenient description of the mechanisms and others, thus an Index of Acronyms was provided for the entire explanation. Also, numerous Asian journals are cited in the Reference sections of this book. Many of the journal names are quoted with a phonetic transcription of Chinese, Japanese, or Korean. Readers can use Google to search their corresponding English translation, and Google may sometimes bring you to the website of the journal you are searching for.

Finally, I desire that this reference book should provide readers not only abundant information on anticancer chemical biology and molecular biology but also elicit great ideas for utilizing the potential drug candidates and/or adjuvants to challenge the cancer disease in both therapy/prevention and drug development.

Jun-Ping Xu

Author

Jun-Ping Xu, a research professor at the School of Molecular Science at Arizona State University, USA, received his undergraduate training in pharmaceutical science at Shanghai University of Traditional Chinese Medicine, China, and pursued advanced professional studies at Shanghai Institute for Drug Control, China. He started his academic career on Chinese natural medicines at Shanghai Institute of Pharmaceutical Industry, China, and then studied abroad in Japan. After he earned his PhD degree at Tokyo University of Pharmacy, Japan, he returned to Shanghai to join Professor Rensheng Xu's group at the Shanghai Institute of Materia Medica (SIMM), Chinese Academy of Science, to research biologically active and functional agents from Chinese herbs. During two years at SIMM, he submitted nine papers to well-known international science journals and one review. In 1991 he came to the United States to join the Cancer Research Institute at Arizona State University as a postdoctoral research fellow, working with the director, Professor George R. Pettit, on the discovery and development of novel cancer inhibitors from marine organisms and microorganisms. He has published over 100 scientific papers related to these interests. From 2008 to 2013, he taught a class on the history of Chinese medicine to introduce the origination and development of Chinese medicine and basic concepts of the Chinese medicine theoretical system and practice skills, as well as ancient Chinese philosophy, for university students in the Chinese flagship program.

List of Herbs

1

Anticancer Activities of Exogenous Pathogenic Factor-Eliminating Herbs

CONTENTS

1 Niu Bang Zi 牛蒡子

Great burdock seed

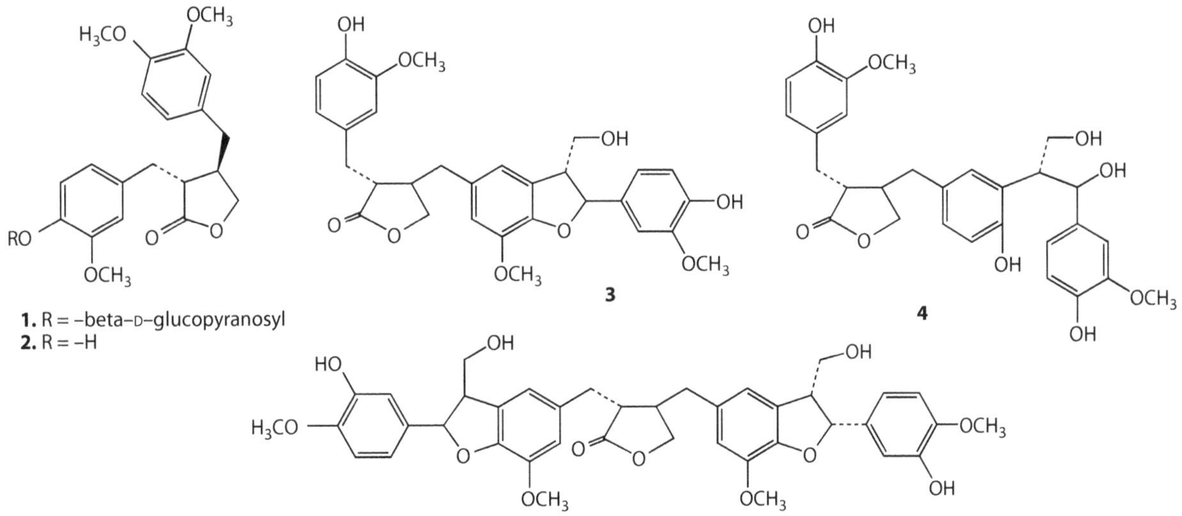

1. R = –beta–D–glucopyranosyl
2. R = –H

Herb Origination

The herb Niu Bang Zi (great burdock seed) is the dried ripe seeds of a Compositae plant *Arctium lappa*. This plant is native to the broad temperate regions from Scandinavia to the Mediterranean and from the British Isles through Russia and the Middle East to China and Japan, and it is naturalized almost everywhere in the world now. Besides the seeds, the leaves, the stems, and the roots of the plant were also used as folk medicines in China.

Antitumor Activities and Constituents

The methanolic extract of Niu Bang Zi displayed obvious inhibitory effects against human prostate cancer cells *in vitro*, and its 70% ethanolic extract exerted potent antiproliferative activity against B cell hybridoma MA60 cells.[1,2] The *in vitro* assay revealed the antiproliferative effect of its dichloromethane extract on various human cancer cell lines, especially K562 leukemia, MCF-7 breast cancer, and 786-0 renal cancer cell lines.[3] NI-07, a product derived from *A. lappa*, could significantly repress the viability of breast cancer cell lines (HCC1419, MCF-7, MDA-MB-231, MDA-MB-468, and SKBR-3) after a 48 h treatment, but it had no cytotoxicity in normal mammary epithelial HME50HT cells and normal mammary fibroblast CCD-1074sk cells.[4] In addition, its hydroethanolic extracts exerted marked free radical-scavenging activity.[3]

The major antineoplastic components discovered from these extracts were identified as dibenzylbutyrolactone lignans. Arctiin (**1**) and arctigenin (**2**) are the most potent inhibitors against the proliferation of cancer cells among these lignans. Both displayed strong cytotoxicity against human HepG2 hepatoma cells but little toxicity toward normal Chang liver cells.[5]

Arctiin

Arctiin (**1**) was reported to have the abilities to influence sex hormone metabolism and to inhibit protein synthesis and steroid biosynthesis.[6] The antigrowth effect of arctiin (**1**) was found to partly correlate with the downregulation of cyclin-D1 expression in various types of human neoplastic cell lines, including on PC3 prostate cancer, osteosarcoma, melanoma, and cancers in lung, colorectal, kidney, cervical, and breast.[7] In the initiation or the postinitiation period of mammary carcinogenesis caused by 2-amino-1-methyl-6-phenylimidazo[4,5-b]pyridine in female rats, arctiin (**1**) markedly reduced the incidence of mammary carcinoma, implying that arctiin (**1**) possesses chemopreventive potential on the carcinogenesis in the breast, particularly in the mammary gland.[8] Moreover, during an anaerobic incubation with a human intestinal bacteria, arctiin (**1**) could be transferred to six bioactive metabolites. Among them, one metabolite termed (2R,3R)-2-(3′-hydroxybenzyl)-3-(3″,4″-dihydroxybenzyl)butyrolactone at a concentration of 10 μM displayed the most potent suppressive activity against the estradiol-mediated proliferation of human MCF-7 breast cancer cells *in vitro*.[9]

Arctigenin

The potent antiproliferative effect of arctigenin (**2**) was observed in two kinds of human HL-60 and K562 leukemia cells (IC_{50}: 0.1 μg/mL) and mouse MH60 hybridoma cells (IC_{50}: 1.0 μM), which activity closely correlated with the induction of apoptosis evidenced with DNA fragmentation and DNA laddering, downregulation of B cell lymphoma 2 (Bcl-2) expression, upregulation of Bcl-2-associated X (Bax), cleave of poly(adenosine diphosphate [ADP]-ribose) polymerase (PARP), and activation of caspase-3.[2,10] Also, arctigenin (**2**) was the most effective lignan toward M1 myeloid leukemia cells, while sesquilignans and diligenans derived from Niu Bang Zi were less effective. Arctigenin (**2**) also induced a differentiation of M1 myeloid leukemia cells in mice and activated phagocyte to the leukemia cells at a concentration of 0.5 μM.[11] Comparing the three lignan structures with the activities revealed that the esterification of arctigenin (**2**) augmented the differentiation of leukemic cells, but its aliphatic esters were more dynamic in the induction of the M1 cells to differentiation than its aromatic esters. Especially, the *n*-docanoate of arctigenin was the most active derivative that induced more than half of the M1 cells into the phagocytic cells at a concentration of 2 μM.[12] But the lignoid analogue was inactive toward the HL-60 cells *in vitro*.[11]

Moreover, arctigenin (**2**) at a concentration of 0.01 μg/mL was 100% preferential cytotoxic to nutrient-deprived cancer cells but not active under a nutrient-rich condition.[13] Arctigenin (**2**) showed the cytotoxic effect on A549 (lung), HepG2 (liver), and KATO III (gastric) cancer cell lines accompanied with the promotion of apoptosis. The ED_{50} values were 4.5 μg/mL in HepG2 cells, 5.4 μg/mL in A549 cells, and 11.0 μg/mL in KATO III cells. Its antiproliferative effect was also shown in A431 epidermoid cancer cells (ED_{50}: 49.8 μg/mL) and VMRC-LCP lung squamous cell cancer cells (ED_{50}: 62 μg/mL).[14] The growth inhibition of arctigenin (**2**) was also observed in several tested pancreatic carcinoma cell lines *in vitro* and in nude mice implanted with human PANC-1 pancreatic neoplasm.[13] 3′-*O*-Demethylarctigenin, an anaerobic microbiological metabolite of arctigenin, demonstrated the cytotoxicity in the PANC-1 cells but is less active than arctigenin (**2**).[15] The mechanism of antipancreatic cancer effect was revealed to be related to the blocking of the nutrient supplement and the activation of Akt by glucose starvation.[13] In human OVCAR3 and SKOV3 ovarian cancer cell lines, arctigenin (**2**) treatment resulted in a dose-dependent inhibition of the proliferation and the induction of caspase-3-dependent apoptosis, associating with the blocking of inducible nitric oxide synthase/nitric oxide/signal transducer and activator of transcription 3 (STAT3)/survivin signaling.[16] Through a reactive oxygen species (ROS)/p38 mitogen-activated protein kinases (MAPK) pathway and the epigenetic inhibition of Bcl-2 by the upregulation of histone H3K9 trimethylation, arctigenin (**2**) stimulated the apoptosis of human MDA-MB-231 breast cancer cells and consequently restrained the cell growth *in vitro* and *in vivo*.[17] However, it was inactive to human HeLa (cervix), SKBR-3 (breast), PC-14, and RERF-LC-KJ (lung) cancer cell lines, ACC-MESO-4 malignant pleural mesothelioma cells and several normal cell lines.[14] Similarly, by selectively blocking the expression of unfolded protein response (UPR) target genes such as phosphorylated-PERK, ATF4, CHOP, and GRP78 and enhancing eIF2α phosphorylation during glucose deprivation, arctigenin (**2**) preferentially obstructed the viability of human HT-29 colon cancer xenografts *in vivo*, and the UPR suppression led to apoptosis via a caspase-activated mitochondrial pathway.[18] In addition, arctigenin (**2**) was able to inhibit both constitutively activated and IL-6-induced STAT3 phosphorylation and subsequent nuclear translocation in the cancer cells. Therefore, arctigenin (**2**) could dramatically promote cisplatin-induced cell death in the cancer cells by enhancing the sensitivity of tumor cells to cisplatin primarily via STAT3 suppression.[19]

According to the evidence, arctigenin (**2**) was considered as a potential drug lead for structure modification to develop safer and more potent agents.[20] From the arctigenin, α-[3-(β-chloroethyl methylaminomethyl)-4-hydroxy-5-methoxybenzyl-β-(3,4-dimethoxybenzyl)-butyrolactone was synthesized. It acted as a mustard inhibitor to exert the tumoricidal activity against Amytal ascites sarcoma, solid sarcoma 37 cells, and Nemeth–Kellner ascites lymphoma, but it was not effective in Ehrlich ascites cancer and solid sarcoma 180 cell lines. In this molecule, both monofunctional mustard and γ-lactone moieties were largely related to the antitumor activity. But the antitumor mustard showed a curare-like acute toxicity (LD_{50} of 36 mg/kg by intraperitoneal (i.p.) administration) to markedly reduce the bone marrow cellularity and the peripheral leukocyte concentration.[21]

Lappaols

Lappaols C (**3**), A (**4**), and F (**5**) separated from the ethanolic extract of Niu Bang Zi displayed a moderate suppressive effect against the proliferation of human LNCaP prostate cancer cells *in vitro* with IC_{50} values of 8, 16, and 40 μg/mL, respectively.[1] In the *in vitro* experiments, lappaol F (**5**) time and dose dependently obstructed the growth of neoplastic cell lines of various tissue types, such as colon (HT-29, RKO, and HCT-116), breast (MCF-7, MDA-MB-231, and MDA-MB-468), cervix (HeLa), prostate (DU145), lung (A549), leukemia (K562, HL-60, and Jurkat), osteosarcoma (U2OS), and melanoma (A375 and SK-Mel-103), but exhibited minimal cytotoxic effect on MCF10A noncancerous breast epithelial cells under a similar condition (3 days) or a prolonged treatment (6 days). Its EC_{50} values were 13.3, 16.8, and 25.2 μmol/L for the MCF-7, MDA-MB-231, and RKO cell lines, respectively. During the inhibition, lappaol F (**5**) induced G1 and G2 cell cycle arrest via the activation of p21 and p27 and the reduction of cyclin-B1 and cyclin-dependent kinase 1 (CDK1), where p21 protein played a crucial role in lappaol F-mediated regulation of CDK1 and cyclin-B1 and G2 arrests. Its antigrowth activity was further demonstrated in nude mice implanted with xenograft HeLa tumor.[22] According to these data, lappaol F (**5**) could be considered to have a developing potential as a therapeutic agent/adjuvant for the cancer therapy.

Furthermore, in cotreatment with the cytotoxic doxorubicin, lappaols C (**3**), F (**5**), arctiin (**1**) and matairesinol not only exerted synergistic effects in Caco-2 colorectal adenocarcinoma cells but also displayed synergistic activity in P-glycoprotein (gp) overexpressed CEM/ADR 5000 cells to amplify the retention of P-gp substrate rhodamine 123 in the cells, indicating that these lignans were capable of obstructing the P-gp activity.[23] The finding provided an important insight into the potential chemosensitizing activity of the lignans, which might have a strong potential to be developed for the improvement of anticancer chemotherapies.

Other Compounds

L-Asparagine isolated from the burdock root was found to have an antimetastatic activity. It was able to augment the antimetastatic activity of cyclophosphane and also to partially reduce the toxicity caused by cyclophosphane on the organism without lessening its antitumor and antimetastatic activities.[24]

Other Bioactivities

Various parts of this burdock are widely used in the popular medicine for hypertension, gout, hepatitis, and other inflammatory disorders. Pharmacological studies indicated that the burdock roots have antiinflammatory, free radical-scavenging, and hepatoprotective activities, and the seeds (Niu Bang Zi) showed hypotensive, antikidney disease, antibacterial, and antivirus effects. Particularly, the Niu Bang Zi extract inhibited the HIV virus, and the lignin components in the herb displayed potent Ca^{2+} antagonistic activity.[25]

References

1. Ming, D. S. et al. 2004. Isolation and characterization of compounds with anti-prostate cancer activity from *Arctium lappa* L. using bioactivity-guided fractionation. *Pharm. Biol.* 42: 44–8.
2. Moritani, S. et al. 1996. Cytotoxic components of Bardanae fructus (Goboshi). *Biolog. Pharm. Bull.* 19: 1515–7.
3. Predes, F. S. et al. 2011. Antioxidative and in vitro antiproliferative activity of *Arctium lappa* root extracts. *BMC Complem. Alternat. Med.* 11: 25.
4. Gollahon, L. S. et al. 2011. The natural product NI-07, is effective against breast cancer cells while showing no cytotoxicity to normal cells. *Open Breast Cancer J.* 3: 31–44.
5. Matsumoto, T. et al. 2006. Antiproliferative and apoptotic effects of butyrolactone lignans from *Arctium lappa* on leukemic cells. *Planta Med.* 72: 276–8.
6. Zeng, Y. et al. 2005. Lack of significant modifying effect of arctiin on prostate carcinogenesis in probasin/SV40 T antigen transgenic rats. *Cancer Lett.* 222: 145–51.
7. Matsuzaki, Y. et al. 2008. Arctiin induces cell growth inhibition through the down-regulation of cyclin D1 expression. *Oncol. Reports* 19: 721–7.
8. Hirose, M. et al. 2000. Effects of arctiin on PhIP-induced mammary, colon and pancreatic carcinogenesis in female Sprague–Dawley rats and MeIQx-induced hepatocarcinogenesis in male F344 rats. *Cancer Lett.* 155: 79–88.
9. Xie, L. H. et al. 2003. Transformation of arctiin to estrogenic and antiestrogenic substances by human intestinal bacteria. *Chem. Pharm. Bull.* 51: 378–84.
10. Wang, L. et al. 2008. Induction of apoptosis of the human leukemia cells by arctigenin and its mechanism of action. *Yaoxue Xuebao* 43: 542–7.
11. Umehara, K. et al. 1993. Studies on differentiation-inducers from *Arctium fructus. Chem. Pharm. Bull.* 41: 1774–9.
12. Umehara, K. et al. 1996. Studies on differentiation inducers: VI. Lignan derivatives from *Arctium fructus. Chem. Pharm. Bull.* 44: 2300–4.
13. Awale, S. et al. 2006. Identification of arctigenin as an antitumor agent having the ability to eliminate the tolerance of cancer cells to nutrient starvation. *Cancer Res.* 66: 1751–7.
14. Susanti, S. et al. 2012. Tumor specific cytotoxicity of arctigenin isolated from herbal plant *Arctium lappa* L. *J. Nat. Med.* 66: 614–21.
15. Tezuka, Y. et al. 2013. Anti-austeric activity of phenolic constituents of seeds of *Arctium lappa. Nat. Prod. Commun.* 8: 463–6.
16. Huang, K. et al. 2014. Arctigenin promotes apoptosis in ovarian cancer cells via the iNOS/NO/STAT3/survivin signalling. *Basic Clinical Pharmacol. Toxicol.* 115: 507–11.
17. Hsieh, C. J. et al. 2014. Arctigenin, a dietary phytoestrogen, induces apoptosis of estrogen receptor-negative breast cancer cells through the ROS/p38 MAPK pathway and epigenetic regulation. *Free Radical Biol. Med.* 67: 159–70.
18. Kim, J. Y. et al. 2010. Arctigenin blocks the unfolded protein response and shows therapeutic antitumor activity. *J. Cell. Physiol.* 224: 33–40.
19. Yao, X. Y. et al. 2011. Arctigenin enhances chemosensitivity of cancer cells to cisplatin through inhibition of the STAT3 signaling pathway. *J. Cellular Biochem.* 112: 2837–2849.
20. Chen, G. R. et al. 2013. (-)-Arctigenin as a lead compound for anticancer agent. *Nat. Prod. Res.* 27: 2251–5.
21. Dombradi, G. A. et al. 1970. Tumor-growth inhibiting substances of plant origin: II. Experimental animal tumor-pharmacology of arctigenin-mustard. *Chemother* (Basel, Switzerland). 15: 250–65.
22. Sun, Q. et al. 2014. Lappaol F, a novel anticancer agent isolated from plant *Arctium lappa* L. *Mol. Cancer Therap.* 13: 49–59.
23. Su, S. et al. 2015. Natural lignans from *Arctium lappa* modulate P-glycoprotein efflux function in multidrug resistant cancer cells. *Phytomed.* 22: 301–7.
24. Urazova, L. N. et al. 2011. Efficacy of natural L-asparagine in the complex therapy for malignant tumors in experimental studies. *Experim. Oncol.* 33: 90–3.
25. Anonymous. 1989. In vitro screening of traditional medicines for anti-HIV activity: Memorandum from a WHO meeting. *Bull. World Health Organ (WHO)* 67: 613–8.

2 Chai Hu 柴胡

Chinese thorowax

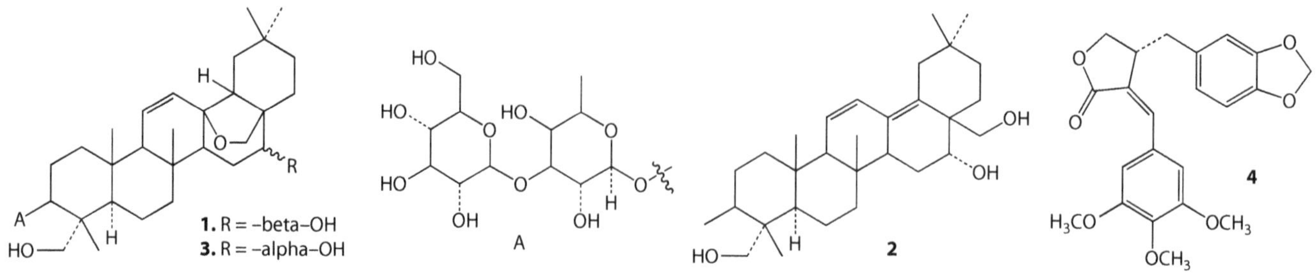

Herb Origination

The herb Chai Hu (Chinese thorowax) originates from the roots of two Umbelliferae plants *Bupleurum scorzonerifolium* and *Bupleurum chinense*, which are perennial plants extensively distributed in China. The major producing areas of the former origin are in the northern China, while the later one is mainly in the provinces of Hubei, Jiangsu, and Sichuan. Their roots are normally collected in spring and autumn and dried in the sun for uses in the medical practice. The herb has been a staple of traditional Chinese medicine for over 2000 years and was documented in the first Chinese materia medica entitled *Shennong Ben Cao Jing*.

Antitumor Activity and Constituents

The aqueous extract of Chai Hu (*B. chinense*) hindered the proliferation and the mitochondria metabolism activity of human SMMC-7721 hepatoma cells in an *in vitro* assay.[1] When the extract is injected into mice by i.p. administration in a dose of 33.3 mg/kg for 9 days, the entity sarcoma 180 was suppressed by 87.21% *in vivo*.[1] Also, the extract treatment could accumulate intracellular vincristine in human BEL-7402 hepatoma cells, indicating multidrug resistance (MDR)-reversing activity. The anti-MDR mechanism was correlated with the blockade of a calcium channel and the elevation of free calcium concentration in the BEL-7402 cells.[2,3] AE-BS, which is an acetone extract of *Bupleurum scorzonerifolium*, showed a dose-dependent antiproliferative effect on human A549 non-small cell lung cancer cells. The exposure of AE-BS (60 μg/mL) for 3 days restrained the A549 cell proliferation by 33% with IC_{50} value of 59 μg/mL (24 h); that data was much lower than the IC_{50} value of 150 μg/mL in WI38 human normal lung fibroblast cells by AE-BS.[4] The inhibitory effect of AE-BS was also proved in an *in vivo* model with A549 xenograft tumors.[4,5] The proliferative suppression of the lung cancer cells was found to be associated with elicitation of G2/M cell arrest and apoptotic death via the inhibition of telomerase activity, activation of caspase-3 and caspase-9, and induction of tubulin polymerization.[4,5]

Based upon the molecular biological studies, the constituents such as some saikosaponins (saikosides) as well as a lignan were discovered in response of the antitumor property of Chai Hu.[6]

Saikosaponins

Three saponins, i.e., saikosaponins a (**1**), b2 (**2**), and d (**3**), have been reported having different selective anticancer property. The treatment with saikosaponin a (**1**) inhibited the proliferation and the viability of human MDA-MB-231 and MCF-7 breast carcinoma cell lines in a dose-dependent manner and obviously promoted sub-G1 population of cell cycles and apoptosis. The apoptosis in the MDA-MB-231 cells was elicited by increases of Bax/Bcl-2 ratio and c-Myc level and activation of caspase-3 in a p53/p21 independent pathway, whereas in the MCF-7, the cells were correlated with an augmented c-Myc level and a p53/p21 dependent pathway.[7] Also, saikosaponin a (**1**) elicited the death of a HuH-7 human hepatoma cells with a significance of sub-G1 peak in a DNA histogram, implying that the HuH-7 cell death *is* not only from apoptosis but also from typical necrosis.[8] The treatment with 20 μg/mL of saikosponin a (**1**) moderately restrained the growth of HepG2 and PLC/PKF hepatoma cell lines, which IC_{50} value was 50 μg/mL in HepG2 cells, whereas saikusponins b2 and c exhibited a weak effect on the PLC/PKF cells.[9] Similarly, the antiproliferative effect of saikosaponin b2 (**2**) on B16 melanoma cells was accompanied with the induction of the G1 phase accumulation and the G1 increase-dependent apoptosis. The downregulation of PKC activity might also be involved in the suppression of B16 cells.[10]

The antitumor effect of saikosaponin d (SSd) (**3**) was observed in different hepatoma cell lines (HepG2, Hep3B, SMMC-7721, and 2.2.15), where SSd (**3**) blocked the cell cycle progression at G1 phase by augmenting p21/WAF1 and p53 expressions, induced the apoptotic death by enhancing Fas/Fas ligand (FasL) and Bax protein, and restrained the cell survival signaling by lessening NF-κB level/activity and Bcl-xL expression, thereby retarding the proliferation of HepG2 and Hep3B hepatoma cell lines in a concentration-dependent manner.[11] At 10 mg/L concentration with a 48 h treatment time, SSd (**3**) reached the maximum inhibitory response to the HepG2 cells.[12] Also, SSd (**3**) was able to reverse the malignant phenotype of HepG2 cells and to elicit the HepG2 cells to differentiation by the upregulation of p27 mRNA expression.[13] The PLC/PRF hepatoma cells were completely killed by SSd (**3**) at a concentration of 100 μg/mL (IC_{50}: 20 μg/mL).[9] In a combination with radiation, SSd (**3**) could enhance the effects of radiation to induce G0/G1 arrest and apoptotic death of SMMC-7721 hepatoma cells by upregulating p53 and Bax expressions and reducing Bcl-2 expression under oxia and hypoxia, implying that SSd is a promising radiosensitizer.[14] SSd (**3**), despite showing no antihepatitis B virus (HBV) activity, still restrained the proliferation of HBV-infected hepatoma 2.2.15 cells in a dose-dependent fashion between 5 and 20 μg/mL, with IC_{50} value of 12.1 μg/mL, but saikosaponin c exhibited anti-HBV and inhibitory effects against the 2.2.15 cells.[15]

Moreover, through a mechanism, i.e., the enhancement of p53 and p21/WAF1 activities and Fas/FasL apoptotic system, SSd (**3**) promoted the apoptosis and the G1 cell arrest and inhibited the proliferation of A549 nonsmall cell lung cancer cells.[16] The inhibitory effect was also observed in three SSd (**3**)-treated human anaplastic thyroid cancer cell lines (ARO, 8305C, and SW1736), where the enhanced apoptosis and G1 phase cell cycle arrest were associated with the activation of p53, p21, and Bax expressions and the reduction of CDK2 and cyclin-D1 activities and Bcl-2 expression. Moreover, in the xenograft tumorigenesis model, the marked weight and volume reduction of thyroid carcinomas was reached after the SSd (**3**) treatment *in vivo*.[17] Also, tumor necrosis factor α (TNFα)-mediated cell death in HeLa and HepG2 cancer cell lines could be significantly potentiated by SSd (**3**) via the suppression of TNFα-induced NF-κB activation and abolishment of TNFα-induced tumor cell invasion. SSd (**3**) was also capable of promoting the apoptosis of HeLa cells via eliciting mitochondrial membrane potential loss and of repressing the angiogenesis of human umbilical vein endothelial cells.[18] In addition, the induction of autophagy was probably found to be involved in the anticancer mechanisms of SSd (**3**) as well.[19]

The antileukemia potential of SSd (**3**) was demonstrated *in vitro* against HL-60 human promyelocytic leukemia and K562 human erythroleukemia cell lines. The elicitation of apoptosis and G0/G1 cell arrest in HL-60 cells was associated with the increase of glucocorticoid receptor mRNA expression and the blocking of M-thymidine incorporation after treatment with 10 μg/mL SSd (**3**) for 48 h.[20–22] Moreover, the saikosides (saikosaponins) at a noncytotoxic dose of 5.0 mg/L was able to reverse the MDR and to amplify the adriamycin (Adm) accumulation in K562/Adm cells, thereby promoting the apoptosis and the G0/G1 cell cycle arrest and obstructing the proliferation of K562/Adm cells.[23]

Taken together, the research results substantiated that SSd (**3**) as well as saikosaponins are potential agents for chemotherapy and chemoprevention of hepatoma, lung cancer, cervical cancer, leukemia, and undifferentiated thyroid carcinoma. The findings also recommended that saikosides have a significant potential to be developed as an adjuvant to combine with TNFα to remedy cancer patients.

Lignans and Flavones

Several γ-butyrolactone type of lignans such as chaihulactone, isochaihulactone, and chaihulactone analogues were isolated from the root of *B. scorzonerifolium*. Isochaihulactone (**4**) showed a moderate to weak degree of cytotoxicity on a variety of human tumor cell lines such as H520 lung squamous cancer, OVCAR3 ovarian cancer, Denver Brain Tumor Research Group glioblastoma, MCF-7 breast cancer, HepG2 hepatoma, HT-29 colon cancer, H1299 p53-null and p16-deficient nonsmall cell lung cancer, A549 lung cancer, A549-T12 paclitaxel-resistant lung cancer with mutant Ka-1 tubulin, KB oral epidermoid cancer, and KB-TAX50 P-gp overexpressive oral carcinoma, *in vitro*. Interestingly, the inhibitory effect on the drug-resistant A549-T12 cells (IC_{50}: 9.4 μM) was greater than all the tested nondrug-resistant cancer cell lines (IC_{50}: 12.1–49.7 μM). During the suppression, isochaihulactone (**4**) also elicited G2/M cell cycle arrest and apoptosis and blocked tubulin polymerization in a time- and concentration-dependent manner, through a mechanism correlated with the increase of p21/WAF1 levels, the downregulation of checkpoint proteins cyclin-B1/cdc2 and mobility of cdc25C, and the activation of caspase-9 and caspase-3.[24] By the similar mechanism plus the activation of NAG-1 via a Jun amino-terminal kinases (JNK) signaling, isochaihulactone (**4**) triggered the cell cycle arrest at G2/M phase and the apoptosis in human LNCaP prostate cancer cells.[25] When isochaihulacton (**4**) is combined with paclitaxel, an enhanced synergistic antitumor activity could be achieved against human lung cancer cells via NAG-1 activation and ERK1/2 signaling pathway.[26] Moreover, the antigrowth effect of isochaihulactone (**4**) on the A549 nonsmall cell lung cancer was further proved in a nude mice xenograft model, with doses of 30 and 50 mg/kg.[27] These described findings highlighted that isochaihulactone (**4**) is a promising anticancer agent with a potential for clinic application in future investigation.

Other Bioactivities

The herb Chai Hu (Chinese thorowax) is commonly prescribed in traditional medicine for treatment of inflammatory and infectious diseases in China, Korea, and Japan since ancient times. The bupleurum's root is an important ingredient in a famous East Asian medicine prescription called Xiao-chai-hu-tang/Sho-saiko-to. Pharmacological studies have proven that Chai Hu has analgesic, antipyretic, immunomodulatory, antiinflammatory, hepatoprotective, antibacterial, and antipathogen activities. Clinical studies have advised that Chai Hu may be effective in the treatment of hepatitis. Recently, the isolated eugenin and saikochromone showed potent immunosuppressive activities toward PMA^+ anti-CD28-costimulated T cells without a significant cytotoxic effect on T lymphocyte cells' survival.[24]

References

1. Song, J. G. et al. 2011. Effects of the extracts from BCDC on human hepatoma SMMC-7721 cells and mice implanted S180 tumor. *J. Shandong TCM Univ.* 25: 299–301.
2. Zhu, J. Q. et al. 2005. Effects of the extracts from BCDC on cellular VCR concentration of human hepatoma BEL-7402 cells. *Beihua Daxue Xuebao, Ziran Kexueban* 6: 62–4.
3. Han, X. H. et al. 2006. Effects of the extracts from BCDC on intracellular free calcium concentration and VCR accumulation of human hepatoma BEL-7402 cells. *Zhongliu* (4): 314–7.
4. Cheng, Y. L. et al. 2003. Acetone extract of Bupleurum scorzonerifolium inhibits proliferation of A549 human lung cancer cells via inducing apoptosis and suppressing telomerase activity. *Life Sci.* 73: 2383–94.
5. Cheng, Y. L. et al. 2005. Anti-proliferative activity of *Bupleurum scrozonerifolium* in A549 human lung cancer cells in vitro and in vivo. *Cancer Lett.* (Amsterdam, Netherlands) 222: 183–93.

6. Wang, Y. L. et al. 2006. Progress in research on antitumor activity of saikosaponin and its mechanims. *J. Chin. Integrative Med.* 4: 98–100.
7. Chen, J. C. et al. 2003. Saikosaponin-A induces apoptotic mechanism in human breast MDA MB-231 and MCF-7 cancer cells. *Am. J. Chin. Med.* 31: 363–77.
8. Qian, L. et al. 1995. Saikosaponin A-induced cell death of a human hepatoma cell line (HuH-7): The significance of the "sub-G1 peak" in a DNA histogram. *Pathol. Intl.* 45: 207–14.
9. Motoo, Y. et al. 1994. Antitumor effects of saikosaponins, baicalin and baicalein on human hepatoma cell lines. *Cancer Lett.* 86: 91–5.
10. Zong, Z. et al. 1996. Saikosaponin b2-induced apoptosis of cultured B16 melanoma cell line through down-regulation of PKC activity. *Biochem. Biophys Res. Commun.* 219: 480–5.
11. Hsu, Y. L. et al. 2004. Involvement of p53, nuclear factor κB and Fas/Fas ligand in induction of apoptosis and cell cycle arrest by saikosaponin-d in human hepatoma cell lines. *Cancer Lett.* 213: 213–21.
12. Zhang, G. P. et al. 2009. The influence of saikosaponin-d on the proliferation and cell cycle of human HepG2 hepatoma cells. *J. Guangdong Med. College* 27: 603–5.
13. Zhu, B. H. et al. 2011. Effect of Saikosaponins-d on reversing malignant phenotype of HepG2 cells in vitro. *Chin. J. Hepatol.* 19: 764–7.
14. Wang, B. F. et al. 2013. Saikosaponin-d increases the radiosensitivity of smmc-7721 hepatocellular carcinoma cells by adjusting the G0/G1 and G2/M checkpoints of the cell cycle. *BMC Complem. Altern. Med.* 13: 263.
15. Chiang, L. C. et al. 2003. Cytotoxicity and anti-hepatitis B virus activities of saikosaponins from Bupleurum species. *Planta Med.* 69: 705–9.
16. Hsu, Y. L. et al. 2004. The proliferative inhibition and apoptotic mechanism of Saikosaponin D in human non-small cell lung cancer A549 cells. *Life Sci.* 75: 1231–42.
17. Liu, R. Y. 2014. Saikosaponin-d inhibits proliferation of human undifferentiated thyroid carcinoma cells through induction of apoptosis and cell cycle arrest. *Europ. Review for Med. Pharmacol. Sci.* 18: 2435–43.
18. Wong, V. K. W. et al. 2013. Saikosaponin-d enhances the anticancer potency of TNFα via overcoming its undesirable response of activating NF-κB signalling in cancer cells. *Evidence-Based Complem. Alternative Med.* 2013, Article ID 745295.
19. Law, B. Y. K. et al. 2014. Autophagic effects of chaihu (dried roots of *Bupleurum chinense DC* or *Bupleurum scorzonerae-folium* WILD). *Chin. Med.* 9: 21.
20. Chen, J. P. et al. 2001. The inhibitory effect of saikosaponin-d on the proliferation of HL-60 cells. *Beijing Daxue Xuebao, Sci. Edit.* 2: 486–8.
21. Bu, S. Z. et al. (a) 1999. Effect of Saikosaponin-d on up-regulating GR mRNA expression and inhibiting cell growth in human leukemia cells. *Chin. J. Hematol.* 20: 354–6; (b) 2000. *Zhongguo Zhongxiyi Jiehe Zazhi* (5): 350–2.
22. Xia, W. et al. 2002. The inhibitory effect of saikosaponin-d (SSd) on the proliferation of K562 cells. *Beijing Daxue Xuebao, Sci. Edit.* 3: 113–5.
23. Ge, X. D. et al. 2012. Reverse effects of saikoside on multidrug resistance of human leukemic cell line K562/ADM in vitro. *Zhongguo Bingli Shengli Zazhi* 28: 76–80.
24. Chang, W. L. et al. 2003. Immunosuppressive flavones and lignans from *Bupleurum scorzonerifolium*. *Phytochem.* 64: 1375–9.
25. Chiu, S. C. et al. 2011. Activation of NAG-1 via JNK signaling revealed an isochaihu-lactone-triggered cell death in human LNCaP prostate cancer cells. *BMC Cancer* 11: 146.
26. Yu, Y. L. et al. 2012. Synergistic anti tumor activity of isochaihulactone and paclitaxel on human lung cancer cells. *J. Cell. Physiol.* 227: 213–22.
27. Chen, Y. L. et al. 2006. In vitro and in vivo studies of a novel potential anticancer agent of isochaihulactone on human lung cancer A549 cells. *Biochem. Pharmacol.* 72: 308–19.

3 Shi Hu Sui 石胡荽

Spreading sneezeweed

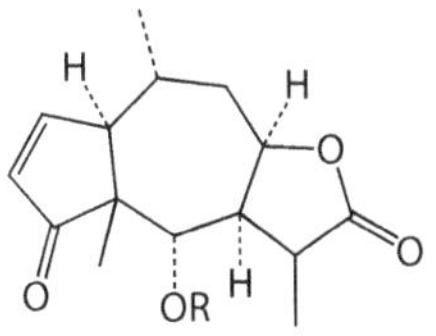

1. R = -A
2. R = -H
5. R = -B

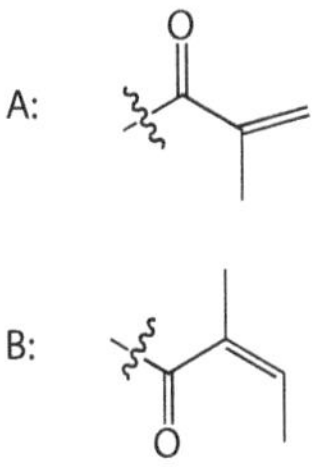

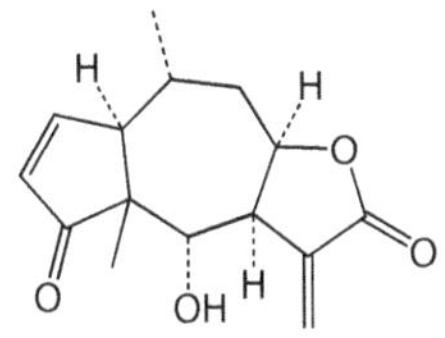

A:

B:

3 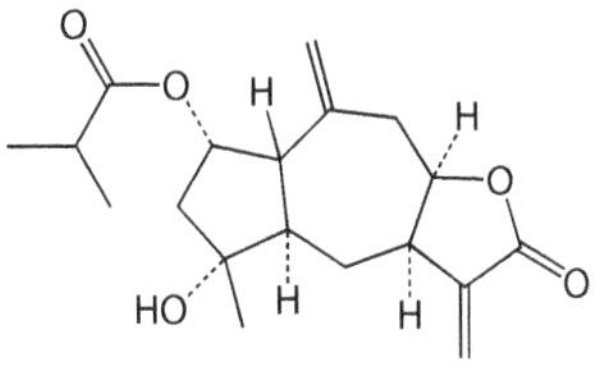 **4** 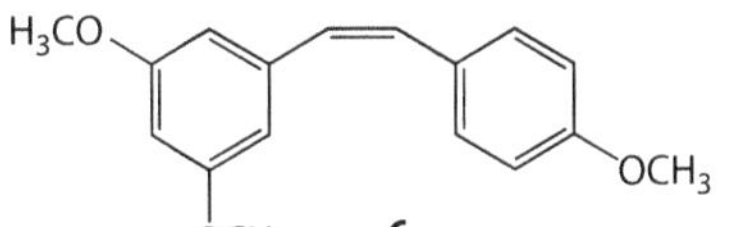 **6**

Herb Origination

The herb Shi Hu Sui (spreading sneezeweed) is a whole plant of *Centipeda minima* (Compositae). The annual herbal plant is broadly distributed throughout tropical Africa, eastern Asia, the Oceania continent, and the Pacific islands. For Chinese folk medicinal practice, the herb is normally collected during flowering and fruiting periods between September and November and dried in the shade, but it is also used in any season through fresh collection.

Antitumor Activities

In vitro experiments demonstrated the extracts of *C. minima* possess antineoplastic property. Its acetone extract of Shi Hu Sui leaves could cause 89.18% death of human PC3 prostate cancer cells.[1] Its 95% ethanolic extract promoted human CNE-1 nasopharyngeal carcinoma cells to apoptosis and suppressed the proliferation of CNE-1 cells in time- and concentration-dependent manners with IC_{50} values of 30 μg/mL (48 h) and 25 μg/mL (72 h), but it weakly affected normal human Hs68 skin cells.[2] Its partitioned fractions of petroleum ether and ethyl acetate at each concentration of 400 μg/mL could obstruct the proliferation of mouse LA795 lung adenocarcinoma cells by less than 90% *in vitro*.[2,3]

The investigation of Shi Hu Sui volatile oils, which were prepared by steam distillation (SD) and supercritical fluid extraction (SFE), showed that the CNE cells were more susceptible to the SFE oil than to the SD oil in the antiproliferative effects. The IC_{50} values of the SFE oil were 8.7 (in 48 h) and 5.2 μg/mL (in 72 h). A mechanistic investigation revealed that the CNE cell death enhanced by SFE oil was correlated with apoptosis induction via reduced Bcl-2 protein expression, dysfunction of mitochondria, release of cytochrome c into the cytosol, activated caspase-9, and subsequently cleaved caspase-3 and caspase-7.[4]

Antitumor Constituents and Activities

Sesquiterpene Lactones

The major constituents in the herb were approved to be a group of sesquiterpene lactones, minimolides A, E, F, G, and H, arnicolide D (**1**), plenolin (**2**), florilenalin-2α-*O*-isobutyrate, helenalin (**3**), and 2β-(isobutyryloxy)florilenalin (**4**), which displayed the inhibitory effect against the CNE cell proliferation (IC_{50}: 1.1–20.3 μM). Helenalin (**3**), which has both α-methylene-γ-lactone and α,β-unsaturated cyclopentenone moieties, exhibited stronger inhibitory activity (IC_{50}: 1.1 μM) than cisplatin (a chemotherapeutic agent) on the CNE cells together with the induction of apoptosis and G2/M cell cycle arrest. The IC_{50} values of arnicolide D (**1**), 2β-(isobutyryloxy) florilenalin (**4**), and florilenalin-2α-*O*-isobutyrate in the CNE cells were 6.6, 3.1, and 2.7 μM, respectively.[5–8] The treatment with arnicolide D (**1**) and isobutyroylplenolin amplified the intracellular ROS levels and diminished the NF-κB levels, resulting in a cell cycle arrest in Gl phase and the apoptosis of human HT-29 colon cancer cells. The cytotoxic activity of arnicolide D (**1**) and isobutyroylplenolin was stronger than that of cisplatin on the HT-29 cells and lower than that of cisplatin on normal cells.[9] The CNE cell apoptosis triggered by 2β-(isobutyryloxy)florilenalin (**4**) was found to be associated with the depletion of mitochondrial membrane potential, the downregulation of Bcl-2 family proteins, the release of cytochrome c to cytosol, and the cleavage of caspases.[8] Plenolin (**2**) also restrained the proliferation of human PC3 prostate cancer cells *in vitro*. The treatment with helenalin (**3**), brevilin A, and arnicolide C in each concentration of 100 μg/mL resulted in marked inhibitory rates of 94.1%, 79.1%, and 68.1% against the growth of LA795 mouse lung cancer cells, respectively.[3]

Moreover, brevilin (= angeloylplenolin, **5**), a sesquiterpene lactone isolated from Shi Hu Sui, has been known to have an antitumor activity against human colorectal, liver, stomach, lung, and skin carcinoma cells. *In vitro* models showed that it was effective in the inhibition of several human neoplastic cell lines such as MKN-45 (stomach), HL-60 (leukemia), LoVo (colon), A431 (epidermoid), 95D (lung), A375 (skin), and BEL-7402 (liver) cells with moderate to weak degree. Its best suppressive effect in the assay was observed in the HL-60 and MKN-45 cell lines with IC_{50} values of 13.6 and 19.4 μmol/L, respectively.[10] The moderate antiproliferative effect of 6-*O*-angeloylplenolin (**5**) was observed in four human tumor cell lines, A549 lung cancer, SGC-7901 gastric cancer, Kasumi-1 acute myeloid leukemia, and K562 erythroleukemia (IC_{50}: 7.1–7.9 μM).[11] Through mitochondrial/caspase and NF-κB pathways, 6-*O*-angeloylplenolin (**5**) promoted the apoptosis of human HL-60 promyelocytic leukemia cells and obstructed the growth of multiple myeloma cells concomitantly with induction mitotic arrest and cyclin-B1 increase.[12] The treatment with 6-*O*-angeloylplenolin (**5**) also exhibited the cytotoxicity on three types of myeloma cell lines (dexamethasone-sensitive MM.1S cells, dexamethasone-resistant U266 cells, and drug-sensitive

RPMI 8226 cells) and concurrently triggered these myeloma cells to apoptosis *in vitro* in the presence of cleaved caspase-3 and PARP.[12,13] In a mouse model, the antineoplastic activity of 6-*O*-angeloylenolin (**5**) was confirmed *in vivo* to obviously suppress the growth of Lewis lung carcinoma cells.[11]

Overall, the results suggested that the active sesquiterpene lactones deserve more extensive investigation for their potential anticancer application, and the scientific evidences also support the herb being used in Chinese herb prescriptions for clinical cancer therapy and prevention.

Polyphenols and Flavonoids

(Z)-3,5,4′-Trimethoxystilbene (**6**) is a resveratrol analogue naturally present in *C. minima* as well as other different plants (*Virola cuspidata*, *V. elongata*, *Schoenus nigricans*, and *Rheum undulatum*). After being treated with 0.4 μM (Z)-3,5,4′-trimethoxystilbene (**6**), the growth of human Caco-2 colon carcinoma cell line was completely arrested, and the tubulin polymerization in the Caco-2 cells was obstructed in a dose-dependent manner.[14] (Z)-3,5,4′-Trimethoxystilbene (**6**) was proven to be more efficient in the growth inhibition and the induction of DNA damage and cell cycle arrest of human DU145 prostate carcinoma cells, compared to resveratrol.[15] Among the polyphenols isolated from Shi Hu Sui, two flavonoids assigned as 3-methoxyquercetin and quercetin exerted the moderate inhibition against the proliferation of human SGC-7901 gastric cancer cells *in vitro*. (IC_{50}: 47.5 and 26.5 μg/mL, respectively), whereas centipedephenol and 10-hydroxy-8,9-dioxyisopropylidenethymol had a weak inhibitory effect.[10]

Triterpenes and Steroids

Several triterpene and steroid components isolated from the herb also showed an antitumor effect. In the *in vitro* assay, taraxasterol and lupeol moderately restrained the proliferation of SGC-7901 gastric cancer cells, and 5α,8α-epidioxy-(22E,20S,24R)-ergosta-6,22-dien-3β-ol only had a certain inhibitory activity.[10]

Other Bioactivities

The herb Shi Hu Sui (spreading sneezeweed) has been used in Chinese medicine for the treatments of rhinitis, sinusitis, acute pleural effusion, rheumatic lumbar, muscle paralysis, pain, and swelling. Pharmacological studies evidenced Shi Hu Shi possessing antiinflammatory, antiallergen, antiprotozoal, antiasthma, antimicrobial, and antibacterial properties.

References

1. Pradeep, V. et al. 2012. Phytochemical screening, antimicrobial and anti-proliferative properties of *Centipeda minima* (Asteraceae) on prostate epithelial cancer cells. *J. Pharmacy Res.* 5: 4804–7.
2. Guo, Y. Q. et al. 2013. Proliferation inhibition and apoptosis induction of *Centipeda minima* extracts on human nasopharyngeal carcinoma cell CNE-1. *Shenwu Jiagong Guochen* 11: 65–70.
3. Pu, S. C. 2013. Studies on antitumor constituents of *Centipeda minima*. *J. Anhui Agricult. Sci.* 36: 13833–4.
4. Su, M. X. et al. 2010. Antiproliferative effects of volatile oils from *Centipeda minima* on human nasopharyngeal cancer CNE cells. *Nat. Prod. Commun.* 5: 151–6.
5. Wu, P. et al. 2012. Supercritical fluid extraction assisted isolation of sesquiterpene lactones with antiproliferative effects from *Centipeda minima*. *Phytochem.* 76: 133–40.
6. Li, Y. L. et al. 2010. Preparation method and antitumor application of sesquiterpene lactones extracted from *Centipeda minima*. *Faming Zhuanli Shenqing* CN 101732383 A 20100616.
7. Wu, P. et al. 2012. Two new sesquiterpene lactones from the supercritical fluid extract of *Centipeda minima*. *J. Asian Nat. Prod. Res.* 14: 515–20.
8. Su, M. X. et al. 2009. 2β-(isobutyryloxy)florilenalin, a sesquiterpene lactone isolated from the medicinal plant *Centipeda minima*, induces apoptosis in human nasopharyngeal carcinoma CNE cells. *Mol.* 14: 2135–46.
9. Huang, X. D. et al. 2014. Cytotoxic activity of two natural sesquiterpene lactones, isobutyroylplenolin and arnicolide D, on human colon cancer cell line HT-29. *Nat. Prod. Res.* 28: 914–6.
10. Wu, H. Z. et al. 2007. New formulations of brevilin for cancer therapy. *Faming Zhuanli Shenqing* CN 1907277 A 20070207.
11. Li, C. L. et al. 2008. 6-O-Angeloylenolin induces apoptosis through a mitochondrial/caspase and NF-κB pathway in human leukemia HL60 cells. *Biomed. Pharmacother.* 62: 401–9.
12. Liu, Y. et al. 2013. Small compound 6-*O*-angeloylplenolin induces caspase-dependent apoptosis in human multiple myeloma cells. *Oncol. Lett.* 6: 556–8.
13. Ding, L. F. et al. 2009. Two new terpene glucosides and antitumor agents from *Centipeda minima*. *J. Asian Nat. Prod. Res.* 11: 732–5.
14. Chabert, P. et al. 2006. Anti-mitotic properties of resveratrol analog (Z)-3,5,4′-trimethoxy-stilbene. *BioFactors.* 27: 37–46.
15. Malfa, G. et al. 2010. Chemotherapeutic effects of Resveratrol and its analogue 3,5,4′-*trans*-trimethoxystilbene on DU145 cells. *Trends Cancer Res.* 6: 45–54.

4 Sheng Ma 昇麻

Black cohosh

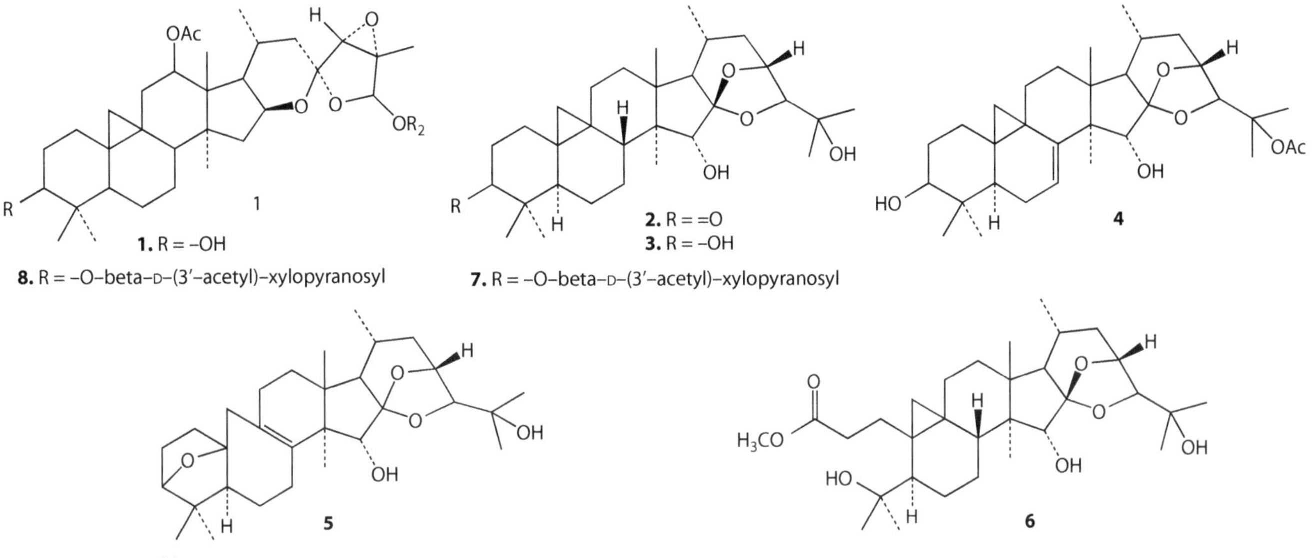

1. R = -OH
8. R = -O-beta-D-(3′-acetyl)-xylopyranosyl

2. R = =O
3. R = -OH
7. R = -O-beta-D-(3′-acetyl)-xylopyranosyl

4

5

6

(a)

9. R = -O-alpha-L-(3′-acetyl)-arabinopyranosyl
11. R = -O-beta-D-xylopyranosyl

10. R = -O-beta-D-xylopyranosyl

14

15

12. R = -O-beta-D-xylopyranosyl

13. R = -O-beta-D-xylopyranosyl

16. R_1 = $-OCH_3$, R_2 = -OH
17. R_1 = -OH, R_2 = $-OCH_3$

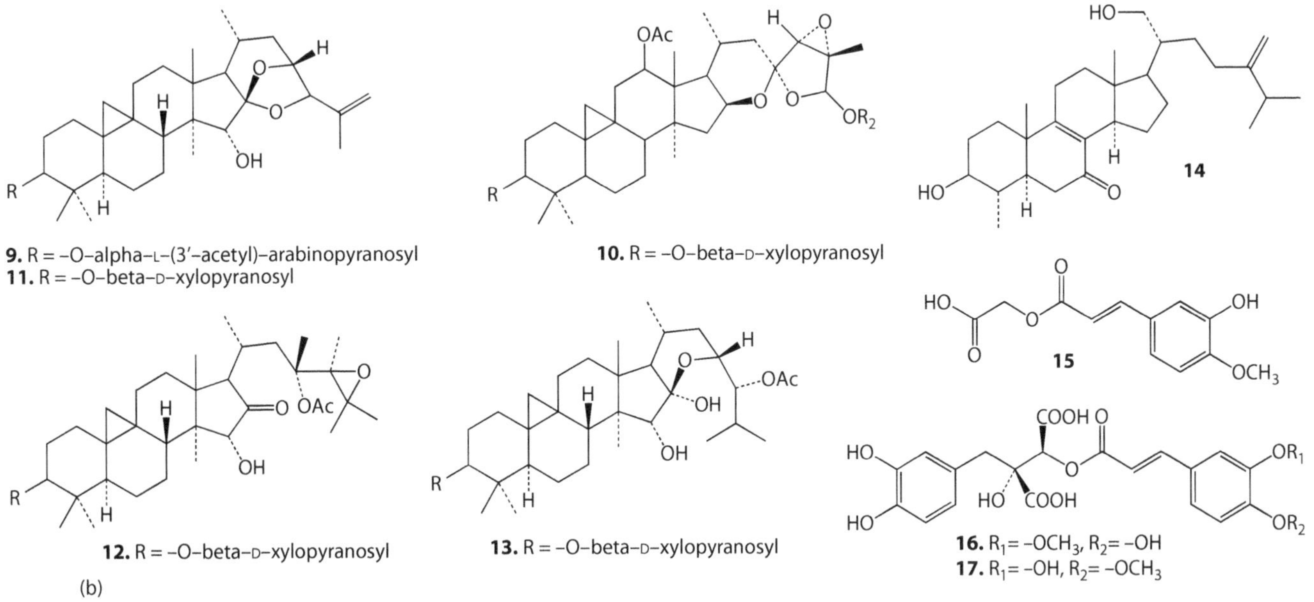

(b)

Herb Origination

The herb Sheng Ma has three plant origins, i.e., *Cimicifuga foetida*, *C. dahurica*, and *C. heracleifolia* (Ranunculaceae). Their rhizomes are traditionally used for medicinal purposes for over 2000 years. Sheng Ma is one of the famous herbs documented in the Chinese first materia medica entitled *Shennong Ben Cao Jing*. The rhizomes are collected in autumn and dried in the sun for medicinal practices. The aerial part of these plants was discarded as a waste by-product in China, but phytochemical studies in recent years demonstrated that both the rhizomes and the aerial part of the species are rich in similar constituents.

Antitumor Constituents and Activities

An ethyl acetate fraction (EAF) prepared from the aerial part of *C. foetida* demonstrated moderate to weak cytotoxic activity on a small panel of hepatocytes *in vitro*, which IC_{50} values were 21, 43, and 80 μg/mL on human hepatoma HepG2 cells, drug-resistant R-HepG2 cells, and primary cultured normal mouse hepatocytes, respectively. The data implied that EAF has a relative selectivity to exert the antihepatoma effect. In a concentration of 25 μg/mL, EAF induced the hepatoma cell cycle arrest at G0/G1 stage, but in a concentration of 50 μg/mL, it triggered G2/M cell arrest. When the concentration was raised to 100 μg/mL, the apoptosis of hepatoma cells was enhanced via increase of the Bax/Bcl-2 ratio, activation of downstream effector caspase-3, and cleavage of poly(ADP-ribose) polymerase (PARP).[1] The *in vivo* antihepatoma activity of EAF was proved in mice implanted with H22 liver tumor, and the growth inhibitory rate could reach to 63.32% in a dose of 200 mg/kg intragastric feeding (i.g.).[1]

The antitumor active constituents were summarized as follows. The scientific evidences not only provided a solid support for using Sheng Ma in the herb prescriptions for cancer treatment but also recommended that its bioactive triterpenoids are promising candidates that deserve further development for cancer prevention and chemotherapy.

Total Triterpenoid Glycosides

The total triterpenoid glycosides prepared from different sources of Sheng Ma were demonstrated to be the most important constituents in the herb, having a marked pharmaceutical potential for the cancer chemotherapy. TGCF, the total glycosides isolated from the roots of *C. foetida*, exerted the growth inhibitory effect against human HepG2 hepatoma cells *in vitro* (IC_{50}: 76.16 mg/L) and arrested the cell cycle progression at G2/M stage time-dependently at a concentration of 50 mg/L. *In vivo* antihepatoma activity of TGCF were demonstrated in a transplant hepatoma H22 mouse model and a human BEL-7402 hepatoma xenograft nude mice model at a dose of 0.8 g/kg.[2] The antitumor activity of TGCD which is the total glycosides from *C. dahurica* roots was observed in a panel of human tumor cell lines. The IC_{50} values TGCD ranged from 20.3 to 32.7 μg/mL in A549 (lung), HepG2 (liver), HL-60 (leukemia), Eca-109 (esophagus), and MDA-MB-231 (breast) neoplastic cell lines. The oral administration of TGCD in doses of 100 and 200 mg/kg remarkably retarded the growth of sarcoma 180 cells in mice by 42.8% and 54.6% and hindered the growth of A549 lung adenocarcinoma cells in nude mice with treatment group/control group (T/C) values of 58.1% and 52.2%, respectively. The *in vitro* and *in vivo* antitumor effects of TGCD was revealed to correlate with the apoptotic induction.[3]

TGA was the total glycosides extracted from the aerial part of *C. dahurica*, which contains 29 cimigenol-type glycosides. The cytotoxicity of TGA was evaluated in HepG2 cells and primary normal mouse hepatocytes. At the same concentrations, TGA demonstrated the same degree of activities against the HepG2 cells as the EAF in the antiproliferation, the apoptotic induction, and the G0/G1 and G2/M cell cycle elicitation. The administration of TGA in a daily dose of 200 mg/kg by i.g. for 10 days significantly suppressed the growth of H22 hepatoma in mice with slight loss of body weight. On normal mouse hepatocytes, TGA showed a bidirectional property, i.e., the proliferation was promoted at a lower concentration but inhibited at a higher concentration (IC_{50}: 105 μg/mL). The evidences indicated that TGA may possess selective cytotoxicity to the hepatoma cells.[4]

9,19-Cycloartane Triterpenes

The *Cimicifuga* genus plants are rich in 9,19-cycloartane triterpenes and glycosides, which are responsible for most of the bioactivities in Sheng Ma. Several of the triterpenes displayed obvious to weak inhibitory effects on the proliferation of carcinoma cell lines *in vitro*. Among them, the impressive molecules are acetylacteol (**1**) and actrin-3-one (**2**), which both showed marked antiproliferative effect on HepG2 hepatoma cells (IC_{50}: 2.56 and 5.51 μM, respectively),[5] while cimigenol (**3**) was effective in SMMC-7721 hepatoma cells (IC_{50}: 7.87 μM) and A549 lung adenocarcinoma cells (IC_{50}: 12.16 μM).[6] Relatively, HL-60 promyelocytic leukemia cells were sensitive to 25-*O*-acetyl-7/8-en-cimigenol (**4**) with IC_{50} value of 10.5 μM,[7] and SW480 colon cancer cells were sensitive to 25-*O*-acetyl-7/8-en-cimigenol (**4**) and acerinol (**5**) with similar IC_{50} data of 13.8 μM.[7,8] The relatively higher suppressive effect on MCF-7 breast cancer cells was exerted by cimigenol-1/2-en-3-one (IC_{50}: 15.1 μM).[7] Likewise, a seco-9,19-cyclolanostane triterpene assigned as methyl 3,4-seco-4-hydroxy-3-cimigenolate (**6**), which was isolated from the roots of *C. heracleifolia*, interestingly displayed a potent inhibitory effect as cisplatin (an anticancer drug) against HL-60 leukemia cells (IC_{50}: 0.83 μM) and more potent activities against the A549 cells (IC_{50}: 2.59 μM) and the SMMC-7721 cells (IC_{50}: 1.41 μM).[8] Its anticancer activity was greater than the 9,19-cycloartane triterpenes and their glycosides derived from the plant sources of Sheng Ma.

Importantly, acerinol (**5**) could reverse ATP binding cassette subfamily B member 1 (ABCB1)-mediated MDR in HepG2/Adm and MCF-7/Adm cells and significantly augment the cytotoxicity of chemotherapeutic drugs (such as doxorubicin, paclitaxel, and vincristine) by modulating the function of ABCB1,[9] indicating that acerinol (**5**) has a potential for developing to a new MDR reversal agent.

9,19-Cycloartane Triterpenoid Glycosides

Quite a number of 9,19-cycloartane triterpenoid glycosides discovered from the related plants displayed a marked to moderate inhibitory activity against tumor cell lines in the *in vitro* models. Structural analysis showed that most of the active glycosides have a cimigenol skeleton in the aglycone moiety, and some have 25-anhydrocimigenol or acteol types of skeletons. Only two kinds of monosaccharides such as β-D-xylopyranose and α-L-arabinopyranose had a hydroxyl group at C-3 of the aglycones. The potent antitumor active glycosides are often coupled with one or two acetyl group(s) or one butenoyl group at the aglycone moiety and/or the monosaccharide moiety. According to the reported data, it is recognized that the glycosides were sensitive to HepG2 hepatoma and HL-60 leukemia cell lines in many cases. Among them, the most potent glycosides were 25,3′-*O*-diacetylcimigenol-3-*O*-β-D-xyloside (**7**), 25,4′-*O*-diacetylcimigenol-3-β-D-xyloside, 25-*O*-acetylcimigenol-3-*O*-[4′-*O*-(E)-2-butenoyl]-β-D-xyloside, and 3′-*O*-acetyl-23-epi-26-deoxyactein (**8**) on the HepG2 cells with respective IC_{50} values of 0.71, 2.8, 1.29, and 1.41 μM,[5,10] whereas cimigenol-3-*O*-[3′,4′-*O*-diacetyl]-α-L-arabinoside, 25-anhydrocimigenol-3-*O*-[3′-*O*-acetyl]-α-L-arabinoside, cimigenol-3-*O*-[2′-*O*-(E)-2-butenoyl]-α-L-arabinoside, 25-*O*-acetylcimigenol-3-*O*-[2′-*O*-acetyl]-α-L-arabinoside, and 25-*O*-acetylcimigenol-3-*O*-[3′-*O*-acetyl]-α-L-arabinoside on the HL-60 cells with IC_{50} values ranging from 4.1 to 5.99 μM.[7,8] 25,3′-*O*-Diacetylcimigenol-3-*O*-β-D-xyloside (**7**) and 25,4′-*O*-diacetylcimigenol-3-*O*-β-D-xyloside were also more effective in suppressing SMMC-7721 hepatoma cells (IC_{50}: 5.5 and 6.3 μM, respectively), compared to the other glycosides.[10] Also, 24-*O*-acetylcimigenol-3-*O*-β-D-xyloside(**9**),23-*O*-acetylcimigenol-3-*O*-β-D-xyloside (**10**), and 25-*O*-acetylcimigenol-3-*O*-β-D-xyloside demonstrated moderate antihepatoma activity on the drug-resistant R-HepG2 cells (IC_{50} 11.96–15.07 μg/mL), which cytotoxic effect was found to correlate with the induction of apoptosis and G2/M cell cycle arrest via reduction of cdc2 protein and cyclooxygenase-2 protein expressions.[11]

Likewise, these glycosides were inhibitors on the other types of carcinomas in colon, breast, lung, pancreas, and/or others. Particularly, 25-anhydrocimigenol-3-*O*-[3′-*O*-acetyl]-α-L-arabinoside (**11**), 7,8-didehydro-25-anhydrocimigenol-3-*O*-β-D-xyloside, and 7,8-didehydro-25-*O*-acetylcimigenol-3-*O*-α-L-arabinoside exerted more potent cytotoxicities than cisplatin against SMMC-7721, A549, MCF-7, and SW480 human tumor cell lines (IC_{50}: 5.02–11.40 μM).[8] Cimigenol-3-*O*-xyloside, 25-acetyl-7,8-didehydrocimigenol-3-*O*-xyloside, 7,8-didehydrocimigenol-3-*O*-xyloside, and actein were effective in the inhibition of ER negative Her2 overexpressing human breast cancer MDA-MB-453 cells (IC_{50}: 5.7, 3.2, 7.2, and 9 μg/mL, respectively),[12] which effect was parallel with the induction of a stress response and apoptosis in the breast cancer cells.[12] The *in vitro* assay also exhibited weak cytotoxicity of 24-epi-7,8-didehydrocimigenol-3-*O*-β-D-xyloside and 23-*O*-acetylshengmanol-3-*O*-β-D-xyloside on SNU638 and AGS gastric cancer cell lines in addition to the inhibition of *Helicobacter pylori*.[13] The AGS cell cycle arrest was elicited by cimiside E (**12**) in S phase at a lower concentration (30 μM) but in G2/M phase at higher concentrations (60 and 90 μM), and the apoptotic AGS cells were triggered through the induction of caspase cascade by both extrinsic and intrinsic pathways.[14] The findings implied that the glycosides may be used for the treatment and prevention of gastric injury and carcinogenesis.

Structure–Activity Relationships

The large numbers of 9,19-cycloartane triterpenes and glycosides with the suppressive data are helpful for scientists to explore the relationships between the structure and the biological property. Based upon the analyses of their bioassay information, the preliminary structure–activity relationships have been proposed, i.e., (1) the activity of triterpenoid aglycones were cimigenol > 25-anhydrocimigenol and acteol, (2) the C-23(R) and C-24(S) configurations in the triterpenoids were necessary for antitumor activity, and (3) the substituent of a hydroxyl group at C-25 of aglycone with hydrophobic groups (like acetoxy and methoxyl) and the attachment of groups like acetyl or butenoyl to the saccharide moiety could improve the inhibitory activities.[7,15,16]

Sterol

From the aerial parts of *C. foetida*, a 4α-methyl sterol designated as cimisterol A (**13**) was isolated, which exhibited a broad spectrum of cytotoxic activities against six tested human neoplastic cell lines such as HL-60, Jurkat and K562 (leukemia), U937 (lymphoma), HepG2 (hepatoma), and SGC-7091 (gastric cancer) cells, having IC_{50} values of 7.23, 2.89, 6.88, 3.38, 4.21, and 4.89 μM, respectively.[17]

Caffeic Acid Derivatives

From the *n*-butanol extract of *C. heracleifolia* rhizomes, three cytotoxic caffeic acid derivatives were isolated and were elucidated as carboxymethyl isoferulate (**14**), cimicifugic acid A (**15**), and cimicifugic acid B (**16**). At concentrations ranging from 2.5 to 40 μM, the three compounds displayed a moderate inhibitory effect against the proliferation of human HCT-116 colon cancer cells in a dose-dependent manner, which effect was associated with the augmented expression of cleaved PARP, a critical apoptosis marker. Their IC_{50} values were 18.74, 15.38, and 12.42 μM, respectively, in the HCT-116 cells.[18] Also, caffeic acid showed a more potent suppressive effect on AGS gastric cancer cells (IC_{50}: 23.30 μg/mL) than on SNU638 cells.[13] In addition, ferulic acid and caffeic acid were the potent antioxidant agents in the free radical-scavenging test and were the inhibitors of *Helicobacter pylori* that causes common chronic inflammation in the stomach.[13]

Other Active Compounds

During the biological investigation of the rhizomes of *C. foetida*, two active minor compounds were isolated. As one of the chromones of *Cimicifuga* species, norcimifugin exhibited its marked inhibitory activity on human HepG2 hepatoma cell line (IC_{50}: 5.55 μM).[5] One indole alkaloid designated as (E)-3-(3′-methylbutylidene)-2-indolinone was cytotoxic on human HL-60 leukemia cells with IC_{50} of 19.57 μM.[6]

Other Bioactivities

The herb Sheng Ma as a common traditional Chinese medicine has been employed for cooling, detoxification, analgesic, and antipyretic remedies since ancient times. Pharmacological approaches have proven that Sheng Ma possesses antipyretic, analgesic, cooling, antiinflammatory, hepatoprotective, spasm-relieving, and immuno-moderating properties. However, overdose of black cohosh may cause toxic reactions in liver and its traditional doses are 0.5 to 3 g/day. It is unsuitable for women who are or may become pregnant due to the potentials of inhibition of embryo implantation and abortifacient effects.[19,20] In addition, a close plant *Cimicifuga racemose*, commonly called black cohosh, is a Native American medicine, which is used for effectively treating the symptoms associated with menopause for women in Western countries.

References

1. Tian, Z. et al. 2007. Cimicifuga foetida extract inhibits proliferation of hepatocellular cells via induction of cell cycle arrest and apoptosis. *J. Ethnopharmacol.* 114: 227–33.
2. Zheng, Y. Q. et al. 2013. Antitumor activity of total glycoside of *Cimicifuga foetida L.* and its effect on tumor cell cycle. *J. Yunnan College TCM* 36(4): 17–20.
3. Cao, L. et al. 2008. Experimental study on antitumor effects of total glycoside *Cimicifuga dahurica Maxin. Chin. J. Inform. TCM.* 15: 31–3.
4. Tian, Z. et al. 2007. Antitumor activity and mechanisms of action of total glycosides from aerial part of *Cimicifuga dahurica* targeted against hepatoma. *BMC Cancer* 7: 237.
5. Nian, Y. et al. 2010. Cytotoxic chemical constituents from the roots of *Cimicifuga foetida. J. Nat. Prod.* 73: 93–8.
6. Lu, L. et al. 2012. Studies on the constituents of *Cimicifuga foetida* collected in Guizhou province and their cytotoxic activities. *Chem. Pharm. Bull.* 60: 571–7.

7. Nian, Y. et al. 2013. Cytotoxic cycloartane triterpenes of the traditional Chinese medicine "shengma" (*Cimicifuga dahurica*). *Planta Med.* 79: 60–9.
8. Nian, Y. et al. 2012. Cytotoxic cycloartane triterpenes from the roots of *Cimicifuga heracleifolia*. *Tetrahedron* 68: 6521–7.
9. Liu, D. L. et al. 2014. Acerinol, a cyclolanstane triterpenoid from *Cimicifuga acerina*, reverses ABCB1-mediated multidrug resistance in HepG2/ADM and MCF-7/ADR cells. *Eur. J. Pharmacol.* 733: 34–4.
10. Chen, J. Y. et al. 2014. Cycloartane triterpenoids and their glycosides from the rhizomes of *Cimicifuga foetida*. *J. Nat. Prod.* 77: 1997–2005.
11. Tian, Z. et al. 2005. Cytotoxicity of three cycloartane triterpenoids from *Cimicifuga dahurica*. *Cancer Lett.* 226: 65–75.
12. Einbond, L. S. et al. 2008. Growth inhibitory activity of extracts and compounds from Cimicifuga species on human breast cancer cells. *Phytomed.* 15: 504–11.
13. Kim, M. J. et al. 2011. Protective effect of *Cimicifuga heracleifolia* ethanol extract and its constituents against gastric injury. *J. Health Sci.* 57: 289–92.
14. Guo, L. Y. et al. 2009. Cimiside E arrests cell cycle and induces cell apoptosis in gastric cancer cells. *Archiv. Pharmacal Res.* 32: 1385–92.
15. Nian, Y. et al. 2011. Cycloartane triterpenoids from the aerial parts of *Cimicifuga foetida Linnaeus*. *Phytochem.* 72: 1473–81.
16. Sun, L. R. et al. 2007. Cimicifoetisides A and B, two cytotoxic cycloartane triterpenoid glycosides from the rhizomes of *Cimicifuga foetida*, inhibit proliferation of cancer cells. *Beilstein J. Org. Chem.* 3: 3.
17. Nian, Y. et al. 2012. A cytotoxic 4α-methyl steroid from the aerial parts of *Cimicifuga foetida L. Fitoterapia* 83: 293–7.
18. Yim, S. H. et al. 2012. Cytotoxic caffeic acid derivatives from the rhizomes of *Cimicifuga heracleifolia*. *Archiv. Pharm. Res.* 35: 1559–65.
19. Mahady, G. B. et al. 2008. United States Pharmacopeia review of the black cohosh case reports of hepatotoxicity. *Menopause* 15(4 Pt 1): 628–38.
20. Ernst, E. et al. 2002. Herbal medicinal products during pregnancy: Are they safe? *BJOG.* 109: 227–35.

5 Ge 葛

Kudzu

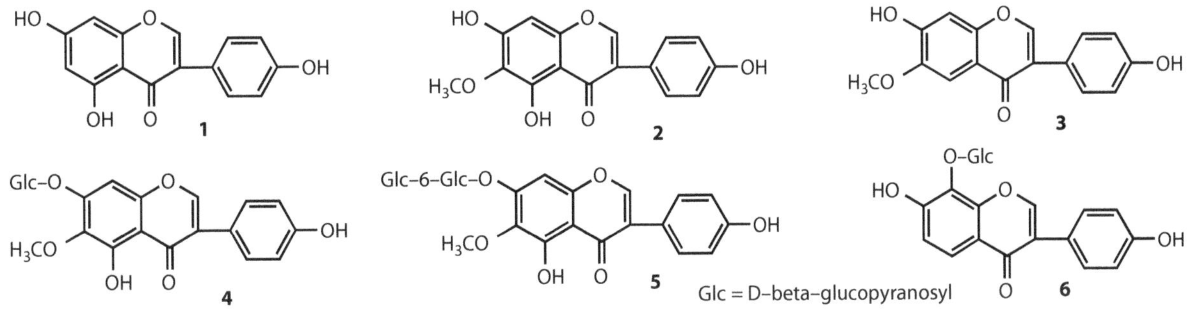

Glc = D-beta-glucopyranosyl

Herb Origination

The origin of herbal plant Ge (kudzu) is two climbing, coiling, and trailing vines *Pueraria lobata* and *P. thomsonii* (Leguminosae). Both plants are native to southeast China and southern Japan. In the late 1800s, it was brought to the United States from Japan and is widely naturalized in the eastern United States and the southern part of the North American continent. Its roots and flowers are separately used in China as two traditional medicines called Ge Gen and Ge Hua, respectively. The roots (Ge Gen) are usually collected in winter and dried in the sun, while the flowers (Ge Hua) are collected before autumn.

Antitumor Constituents and Activity

The *in vitro* anticancer effect of Ge Gen was demonstrated in murine B16-F10 melanoma, human MK-1 gastric adenocarcinoma, and HeLa cervical cancer cell lines.[1] The Ge Gen extract showed a strong inhibitory activity against the proliferation of hepatoma cells, associating with the marked induction of cell cycle arrest and apoptotic death. It also could synergistically enhance the cytotoxicity of mitomycin C against the hepatoma cells.[2] Its ethanolic extract significantly restrained the proliferation of five breast cancer cell lines (MCF-7, ZR-75-1, MDA-MB-231, SKBR-3, and Hs578T) *in vitro*. In addition to the antitumor effect, the Ge Gen extract was capable of promoting the production and the activation of immune-related cytokines such as peritoneum macrophages and TNF in a serum after oral administration to mice or intravenous injection to rabbits, indicating that the extract exerts positive immuno-regulating function to indirectly potentiate the cancer-suppressive potential.[3]

Isoflavonoids

Antiproliferative Effect

An active component assigned as S86019 as well as total flavonoids derived from Ge Gen notably demonstrated the antigrowth effect on human HL-60 acute promyelocytic leukemia cells in time- and dose-dependent fashions at 14–22 μg/mL concentrations, together with the induction of cell cycle arrest at G1 phase and apoptotic death.[4,5] Genistein, (**1**) along with six isoflavonoids such as tectorigenin (**2**), glycitein (**3**), tectoridin (**4**), glycitin, 6″-*O*-xylosyltectoridin (**5**) and 6″-*O*-xylosylglycitin, was isolated from Ge Hua and/or Ge Gen. Genistein (**1**) and tectorigenin (**2**) showed the antiproliferative effects against various human cancer cell lines, but glycitein (**3**) had lower cytotoxicity, and its glycosides were inactive. The results implied that both the isoflavone skeleton and 5-hydroxyl group are crucial for the cytotoxic properties. Moreover, tectorigenin (**2**) and glycitein (**3**) were able to cause apoptotic DNA changes in the HL-60 cells.[6] Tectorigenin (**2**) exerted a significant inhibition against the proliferation of human SMMC-7721 hepatoma cells *in vitro* in association with the induction of early apoptosis.[7]

Another valuable isoflavonoid discovered from the plant Ge was puerarin (**6**), which demonstrated marked suppressive property against the proliferation of four acute myeloid leukemia (AML) cells (HL-60, NB4, Kasumi-1, and U937) and a human H446 small cell lung cancer cells *in vitro*.[8–10] The intensity of the antileukemia activity in the AML cell lines from high to low was as follows: NB4 > Kasumi-1 > U937 > HL-60. By increasing the puerarin (**6**) concentration, the NB4 cell apoptosis and the cell cycle arrest were enhanced.[8,9] Concurrently, the mRNA expressions of progressive multifocal leukoencephalopathy/retinoic acid receptor alpha, Bcl-2, and survivin were lessened, and the protein expressions of JNK, FasL, caspase-3 and caspase-8 were augmented in the apoptotic process.[8] Moreover, after the treatment of H446 cells with puerarin (**6**), the expressions of PCNA, CDK2, CDK4, and cyclin-D1 were markedly lessened, and the expression levels of Fas and p27 were enlarged. These interactions evoked by puerarin (**6**) were found to be involved in the anticancer mechanisms.[10] Despite tectoridin (**4**) only having lower antitumor property, tectoridin (**4**) and 6″-*O*-xylosyltectoridin (**5**) could be metabolized to tectorigenin (**2**) by most human intestinal bacteria, indicating that tectoridin (**4**) and 6″-*O*-xylosyltectoridin (**5**) may be used as prodrugs of tectorigenin (**2**).[11]

Consequently, all the results advocated that the isoflavonoids of *P. lobata* and *P. thomsonii* possess a moderate anticancer property and supported the usage of the herbs and the isoflavonoids in cancer therapy and prevention.

Synergistic Effect

The treatment of HL-60 leukemia cells with combined S86019 (10 μg/mL) and anticancer drugs, BC-4 (5 μg/mL), arabinosylcytosine (Ara-C) (0.06 μg/mL), or cisplatin (cDDP)

(0.2 μg/mL), respectively, obviously augmented the antileukemia effects. The cotreatment with S86019 and BC-4 or Ara-C also significantly augmented the HL-60 cell differentiation to mature granulocytes by 90%.[12] When flavone extract is combined with arsenic trioxide, the proliferation and induction of early apoptosis of Kasumi-1 AML cells were effectively obstructed but no significant effect on HL-60 promyelocytic leukemia cells.[13]

Antiinvasive Effect

Glycitein (**3**) is an inhibitor of cancer cell invasion and migration. For suppressing the invasion of human U87MG astroglioma cells, glycitein (**3**) acted as a transcription factor to lessen the expressions of matrix metallopeptidase (MMP)-3 and MMP-9 and to reduce the DNA binding and NF-κB and AP-1 transcriptional activities.[14]

MDR Reversal Effect

Tectorigenin (**2**) and pueratin (**6**) demonstrated the reversal ability against the MDR of chemotherapeutic agents. In three drug-resistant ovarian cancer cell lines (MPSCITR, A2780TR, and SKOV3TR) and their naive counterparts, tectorigenin (**2**) sensitized the MDR ovarian cancer cells to paclitaxel and synergistically enhanced the growth inhibitory and apoptotic effects of paclitaxel via the inactivation of Akt/IκB kinase (IκK)/IκB/NF-κB signaling pathway and the activation of caspases.[15] Through restraining MDR1 expression and diminishing cAMP-responsive element transcriptional expression and NF-κB activity, pueratin (**6**) amplified the intracellular accumulation of adriamycin and its cytotoxic effect in MCF-7/Adm human MDR breast cancer cells, resulting in the effective MDR reversal effect.[16] In addition, the Puerariae radix flavonoids could elicit the apoptosis of retinoic acid-resistant NB4-R1 acute promyelocytic leukemia cells through a TNFα-activated MAPK signaling pathway together with the increase of JNK1 and JNK2/3 and the decrease of ERK1/2 and p38MAPK, leading to the proliferative inhibition of NB4-R1 cells.[17]

Differentiation Effect

Tectorigenin (**2**) and glycitein (**3**) were able to promote the differentiation of HL-60 leukemia cells to granulocytes and monocytes/macrophages and to cause apoptotic DNA changes in the leukemia cells. During the action, tectorigenin (**2**) retarded the autophosphorylation of epidermal growth factor receptor, but the activity was less than that of genistein (**3**).[6] S86.019 also efficaciously differentiated the original promyelocyte of HL-60 cells to ripped myelocyte, metamyelocyte, and ripped stab nucleus.[4,5]

Spinasterol

From the herb extract, a cytotoxic component assigned as spinasterol was isolated, which exerted dose- and time-dependent suppressive effects *in vitro* against the proliferative of two breast cancer cells (MCF-7, MDA-MB-231), A2774 ovarian cancer cells, and HeLa cervical cancer cells. In addition, the spinasterol also exerted an estrogenic activity similar to 17β-estradiol and activated both estrogen receptor-α and estrogen receptor-β.[18]

Nanoformulation

For the improvement of the low oral bioavailability and the inhibitory effect on advanced hepatocarcinoma, a puerarin (**6**) nanosuspension (Pue-NS) was developed by a high pressure homogenization technique, which was composed of puerarin (**6**) and poloxamer 188 with 218.5 nm particle size and −18.8 mV zeta potential. In an *in vitro* assay, Pue-NS effectively restrained the proliferation of HepG2 cells (IC_{50}: 3.39 μg/mL for Pue-NS versus 5.73 μg/mL for puerarin only), implying that the nanoformulation is a promising approach for drug delivery in cancer treatment.[19]

Other Bioactivities

The herb Ge Gen (kudzu roots) has been used in traditional Chinese medicine mostly in the treatment of gastroenteritis, diabetes, deafness, tinnitus, and vertigo and in the prevention of excessive consumption and alcoholic cravings. Ge Hua (kudzu flowers) is a useful Chinese herb to alleviate symptoms such as intoxication and hepatic and gastrointestinal tract lesion induced by alcohol. Pharmacological approaches have identified that Ge Gen has extensive medicinal benefits including hypotensive, microcircule-promotive, antiarrhythmic, antithrombosis, antihypoxemia, coronary and cerebral vasodilative, antioxidative, hypoglycemic, antiplatelet aggregation, hypolipidemic, antiallergies, antimyocardial ischemia, antispasmodic, and immunostimulative properties, while Ge Hua mainly displays antialcohol and hepatoprotective effects.[20]

References

1. Chen, X. L. et al. 2001. Effects of *Pueraria lobata* extract on the proliferation and cell cycle of liver tumor cells. *J. Guangdong Med. College* 17: 183–184.
2. Nagao, T. et al. 2004. Anti-proliferative phenolic constituents in plants and structure-activity relationships. *Foods Food Ingredients J. Jpn.* 209: 3–12.
3. Du, D. J. et al. 1995. Influerences of *Radix Pueraria* on tumor necrosis factor production and macrophage function. *Zhongyao Yaoli yu Linchuang* 11: 16–9.
4. Jiao, L. et al. 1990. Differentiation and cell cycle progression-inducing effect of Pueraria active ingredient S86019 on HL-60 cells. *Zhonghua Xueyexue Zazhi* 11: 83–6.
5. Yuan, H. B. et al. 2007. Effect of Kudzu flavonoids extracts on proliferation and apoptosis of HL-60 cells. *Zhongliu Fangzhi Yanjiu* 34: 671–4, 736.
6. Lee, K. T. et al. 2001. Tectorigenin, an isoflavone of *Pueraria thunbergiana* BENTH, induces differentiation and apoptosis in human promyelocytic leukemia HL-60 cells. *Biolog. Pharm. Bull.* 24: 1117–21.
7. Wang, X. L. et al. 2010. Effect of tectorigenin of flower on proliferation of hepatocarcinoma SMMC-7721 cells in vitro. *J. Chin. New Drugs.* 19: 168–71.
8. Shao, H. M. et al. 2010. Inhibitory effect of flavonoids of puerarin on proliferation of different human acute myeloid leukemia cell lines in vitro. *Zhongguo Shiyan Xueyexue Zazhi* 18: 296–9.

9. Tang, Y. H. et al. 2010. Apoptosis of NB4 cells induced by flavonoids of puerarin in vitro. *Zhongguo Shiyan Xueyexue Zazhi* 18: 326–9.
10. Zhang, L. et al. 2008. Effect of CP and SP on tumor associated protein expression level in H446 cells of human small cell lung cancer. *Shandong Yiyao* 48: 20–2.
11. Bae, E. A. et al. 1999. Metabolism of 6″-*O*-xylosyltectoridin and tectoridin by human intestinal bacteria and their hypoglycemic and in vitro cytotoxic activities. *Biolog. Pharm. Bull.* 22: 1314–8.
12. Jing, Y. K. et al. 1993. Combination induction of cell differentiation of HL-60 cells by daidzein (S86019) and BC-4 or Ara-C. *Yaoxue Xuebao* 28: 11–16.
13. Tang, Y. H. et al. 2011. Effects of co-treatment with *Pueraria lobata* flavones and arsenic trioxide on proliferation and apoptosis of Kasumi-1 cells and HL-60 cells. *Shanghai Jiaotong Daxue Xuebao, Yixueban* 31: 1564–7.
14. Lee, E. J. et al. 2010. Glycitein inhibits glioma cell invasion through down-regulation of MMP-3 and MMP-9 gene expression. *Chemico-Biol. Interact.* 185: 18–24.
15. Yang, Y.-I. et al. 2012. Tectorigenin sensitizes paclitaxel-resistant human ovarian cancer cells through downregulation of the Akt and NF-κB pathway. *Carcinogen.* 33: 2488–98.
16. Hien, T. et al. 2010. Molecular mechanism of suppression of MDR1 by puerarin from *Pueraria lobata* via NF-κB pathway and cAMP-responsive element transcriptional activity-dependent up-regulation of AMP-activated protein kinase in breast cancer MCF-7/adr cells. *Mol. Nutri. Food Res.* 54: 918–28.
17. Ji, O. et al., 2013. *Puerariae radix* flavonoids on proliferation and apoptosis of retinoic acid-resistant acute promyelocytic leukemia cell line NB4-R1. *Zhonghua Xueyexue Zazhi* 34: 455–7.
18. Jeon, G. et al. 2005. Antitumor activity of spinasterol isolated from Pueraria roots. *Experim. Mol. Med.* 37: 111–20.
19. Lu, W. L. et al. 2015. In vitro antitumor efficacy of Puerarin nanosuspension against human HepG2 cells. *Advanced Materials Res.* (Durnten-Zurich, Switzerland). 1083(Advanced Measurement and Test IV): 27–31.
20. Zhou, Y. X. et al. 2014. Puerarin: A review of pharmacological effects. *Phytother. Res.* 28: 961–75.

2

Anticancer Potentials of Antipyretic Herbs

CONTENTS

6 Chuan Xin Lian 穿心蓮

Green chirayta

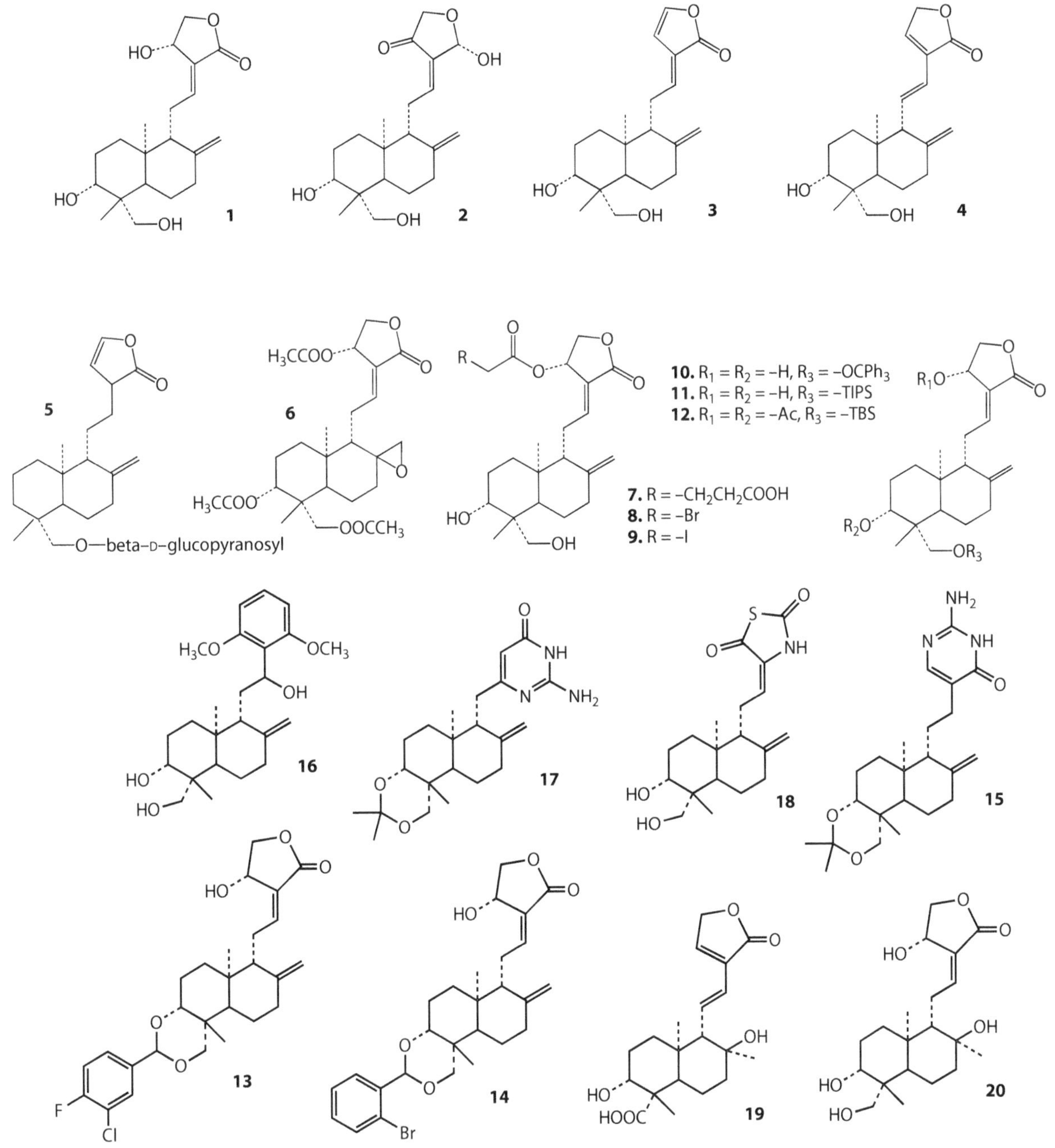
1
2
3
4
5
6
10. R1 = R2 = -H, R3 = -OCPh3
11. R1 = R2 = -H, R3 = -TIPS
12. R1 = R2 = -Ac, R3 = -TBS
7. R = -CH2CH2COOH
8. R = -Br
9. R = -I
O—beta-D-glucopyranosyl
16
17
18
15
13
14
19
20

Herb Origination

The herb Chuan Xin Lian (Green chirayta) is the dried whole plant of *Andrographis paniculata* (Acanthaceae). This herbaceous plant is indigenous to South Asian countries like India and China, and the herb is mainly cultivated in southern Chinese provinces. The best season for the collection of the herb is in autumn when its flowers are in full bloom, and the collected herbs are dried in the sunlight for folk medicinal practice.

Antitumor Activities and Constituents

The *A. paniculata* plant extract is known to possess a variety of pharmacological activities. The methanolic extract from its leaves showed significant cytotoxicity against human KB oral carcinoma and murine P388 leukemia cells, and a dichloromethane fraction derived from the extract appreciably obstructed the proliferation of human HT-29 colon cancer cells and augmented the proliferation of human peripheral blood lymphocytes at low concentrations.[1,2] The ethanolic extract of

Chuan Xin Lian was inhibitory to human HL-60 AML cells (IC_{50}: 14 μg/mL, in 24 h) *in vitro*.[1] From various parts of the plant, particularly from the leaves, *ent*-labdane-type diterpenoid lactones were discovered as the major constituents. The representative diterpenoid was assigned as andrographolide (**1**), whose content was 1.375% (w/w) in the aerial parts of the plant, and it implicated toward the pharmacological activity of the herb. Therefore, the diterpenoid lactone has received extensive attention from research groups.

Andrographolide and Analogs

The investigations highlighted that Chuan Xin Lian and andrographolide (**1**) possess a dual property, i.e., inhibitory effects acting both directly and indirectly against the cancer cells. The mechanisms in the suppression of cancer growth and carcinogenesis were revealed to be mediated by multiple interactions such as (1) lessening of Janus tyrosine kinases signal transducers and transcription activators and constraint of phosphatidylinositol 3-kinase and NF-κB signaling pathways; (2) suppression of cyclins, CDKs, metalloproteinases (MMPs), tumor growth factors, and heat shock protein (HSP) 90; (3) induction of tumor suppressor proteins p53 and p21; and (4) reduction of nitric oxide, lipid mediators, adhesion molecules, cytokines, and chemokines, thereby leading to the suppression of cancer cell growth, survival, metastasis, and angiogenesis.[3] By incessant efforts, the antineoplastic activities of Chuan Xin Lian extract and andrographolide (**1**) with multiple characteristics have been established and described as follows.

Cytotoxic and Antiproliferative Effects

In *in vitro* assays, andrographolide (**1**) exerted the highest degree of cytotoxicity on diverse human neoplastic cell lines such as MCF-7 (breast), KB (nasopharynx), HCT-116 (colon), HL-60 (leukemic), and murine P388 leukemia cells.[1–7] Compared to other diterpenes, andrographolide (**1**) and isoandrographolide (**2**) displayed superior antiproliferative effects with GI_{50} values of 9.33 and 6.30 μM in HL-60 cells, and 6.5 and 5.1 μg/mL in KB cells, respectively.[8,9] Andrographolide (**1**) and its analogs, isoandrographolide (**2**), 14-deoxy-14,15-didehydroandrographolide (**3**), and 14-deoxy-11,14-didehydroandrographolide (**4**), exerted cytotoxic effect against human Jurkat T cell leukemia, PC3 prostate cancer, and Colo 205 colon cancer cell lines, wherein the IC_{50} values of 14-deoxy-14,15-didehydroandrographolide ranged from 0.05 to 0.07 mM.[10]

Andrographolide (**1**) was also found to exhibit the growth inhibition and the cytotoxic activity against PC3 and DU145 hormone-independent and LNCaP hormone-dependent prostate cancer cell lines *in vitro*, whereas 14-deoxy-11,12-didehydroandrographolide was cytotoxic to T-47D breast cancer cells.[11,12] Moreover, a number of analogs, which were synthesized by the modification of andrographolide at the hydroxyl groups, displayed much higher cytotoxic activities than the parent molecule on a panel of cell lines including KB (human oral tumor), Col-2 (human colon cancer), LU-1 (human lung cancer), MCF-7 (human breast cancer), P388 (murine leukemia), and ASK (rat glioma). A 19-*O*-triphenylmethyl ether analog exerted higher cytotoxicity than ellipticine (an anticancer drug).[13]

The anticancer activity of andrographolide (**1**) was further substantiated in mouse models *in vivo* with B16-F10 melanoma syngenic and HT-29 colon carcinoma xenograft.[7] The antiviability effect of andrographolide (**1**) was shown in both androgen-stimulated and castration-resistant human prostate cancer cells *in vivo*, and no significant toxicity was shown on normal immortalized prostate epithelial cells. The effect was found to be correlated to the inhibition of IL-6 expression at both mRNA and protein levels and the inhibition of both IL-6 autocrine loop- and paracrine loop-induced cell signalings including STAT3 and extracellular signal-related kinase (ERK) phosphorylation.[14] By blocking IL-6 expression and IL-6-mediated signaling, the treatment with andrographolide (**1**) obviously restrained the proliferation of castration-resistant human DU145 prostate carcinoma cells that expressed a constitutive IL-6 autocrine loop.[14]

Apoptosis- and Cell Cycle Arrest-Inducing Effects

The antiproliferative effect of andrographolide (**1**) was closely related to its ability in the increases of apoptosis and cell cycle arrest. Andrographolide (**1**) promoted the apoptosis of human cancer cell lines such as TD-47 (breast), PC3 (prostate), SMMC-7721 (liver), and Tb (tongue) cells *in vitro* in concentration- and time-dependent manners via the activation of caspase-3 and p53, the upregulation of Bax, and the downregulation of Bcl-2.[15,16] The apoptotic mechanism in human Hep3B hepatoma cells was revealed mainly through a JNK signaling pathway, i.e., activation of mitogen-activated protein kinases (MAPKs) including p38 kinase, c-Jun N-terminal kinase and ERK1/2, but it had no marked effect on apoptosis-related proteins such as caspase-3 and Bcl-xL.[17,18] The apoptosis of HL-60 leukemia cells induced by andrographolide (**1**) was progressed by a mitochondria-dependent intrinsic pathway, i.e., up-expression of Bax, down-expression of Bcl-2, induction of BH3 interacting-domain (BID) cleavage and mitochondrial translocation, release of cytochrome c from mitochondria, and activation of caspase-9, caspase-8, and caspase-3.[6,7,19] The treatment with andrographolide (**1**) also elicited the apoptotic death of a series different types of lymphoma cell lines such as Burkitt p53-mutated lymphoma Ramos cells, mantle cell lymphoma (MCL) Granta cells, diffuse large B-cell lymphoma (DLBCL) SUDHL4 cells, and follicular lymphoma (FL) HF-1 cells, as well as the primary cells from patients with FL, DLBCL, or MCL, in a dose- and a time-dependent fashion. Likewise, andrographolide (**1**) prominently promoted ROS production, and then ROS triggered the cleavage of PARP and the activation of caspase-3, caspase-8, and caspase-9, leading to the apoptosis of lymphoma cells.[20]

The antiproliferation effect of andrographolide (**1**) in human LoVo colorectal cancer cells was found to be also associated with G1-S cell cycle arrested at ≤30 μM concentration, whose arrest event was elicited by the increase of the expression of p53, p21, and p16 and the decrease of the activity of cyclin-D1/CDK4 and/or cyclin-A/CDK2 as well as retinoblastoma (Rb) phosphorylation.[21] Similarly, through cycle inhibitory protein p27 activation and CDK4 reduction, the cell cycle of HL-60 leukemia cells was arrested at the G0/G1 stage after being treated with andrographolide (**1**) for 36 h.[4] The induction of G2/M cell arrest in PC3 prostate cancer cells was accompanied by the decline of the CDK1 level without affecting the levels of CDK4 and cyclin-D1, then the events led to the predominantly apoptotic mode of cell death in association with the enhancement of executioner caspase-9 and Bax proteins and activation of caspase-8.[11]

In addition, 14-deoxy-11,12-didehydroandrographolide exerted the cytotoxicity on T-47D breast cancer cells by regulating cell cycle inhibitory genes and eliciting cell death by both apoptosis and autophage.[12] In parallel with the downexpression of p34/CDC2 kinase and the decrease of cyclin-B and mos-associated proteins, 14-deoxy-14,15-didehydroandrographolide (**3**) arrested the cell cycle progression of Jurkat leukemia at the G2/M phase, but isoandrographolide (**2**) and 14-deoxy-11,14-didehydroandrographolide (**4**) disturbed the Jurkat cells at the G0/G1 phase.[10,15]

Differentiation-Inducing Activity

Besides the andrographolide-like diterpenoids as well as their dimers and glycosides that displayed notable growth inhibitory and phagocytosis activities, the *ent*-labdane-type diterpenoids and the methanolic extract of Chuan Xin Lian also showed a capability for promoting the differentiation of mouse M1 myeloid leukemia cells. In the treatment, the M1 leukemia cells were generally differentiated to phagocytes.[22]

Antiangiogenic Activity

The intraperitoneal (i.p.) administration of andrographolide (**1**) markedly inhibited B16F-10 melanoma cell-induced capillary formation in mice, implying that the anticancer effect was closely correlated to the antiangiogenic activity. The *in vitro* and *in vivo* antiangiogenic effects were associated with regulating the production of various pro- and antiangiogenic factors such as (1) decrease of proinflammatory cytokines (IL-1β, IL-6, TNFα, and granulocyte macrophage colony-stimulating factor [GM-CSF]), nitric oxide, and vascular endothelial growth factor (VEGF) and (2) increase of antiangiogenic factors such as IL-2 and TIMP-1.[23] Moreover, the antiangiogenic effect of andrographolide (**1**) in human A549 NSCLC cells was found to be correlated with the inhibition of hypoxia-inducible factor (HIF)-1α expression and HIF-1α transformed VEGF expression and then to obstruct the cell growth of A549 carcinoma.[24]

Antiadhesion and Antiepidermal Growth Factor Receptor Effect

The treatment of andrographolide (**1**) obstructed the adhesion of cancer cells to vascular endothelial cells in human gastric cancer cell lines (SGC7901, MGC803, BGC823), whose effect was mainly achieved by expressing a high level of sialyl Lewis (X) antibody (Ab) to human vascular endothelial cells by blocking E-selectin expression.[25] Also, andrographolide (**1**) largely diminished epidermal growth factor receptor (EGFR) and transferrin receptor (TfR) trafficking on the surface of human A431 epidermoid tumor cells by blocking the receptor movement from the late endosomes to lysosomes. These findings suggested that the antiadhesion and anti-EGFR effects at least partially contributed to the anticancer mechanisms of andrographolide (**1**).[26]

Antiinvasive and Antimigratory Activity

Andrographolide (**1**) at noncytotoxic concentrations inhibited the invasive and migratory abilities of human A549 (lung), LoVo (colorectal), and HT-29 (colon) cancer cell lines and murine CT26 colon cancer cells in a dose-dependent manner. The inhibition on invasion and migration was mediated by the decrease of matrix MMP-2 activity in both CT26 and HT-29 colon tumor cells.[27] Likewise, in the A549 cells and the LoVo cells, the antiinvasive and antimigratory effects were achieved by a different mechanism, i.e., the down-expression of MMP-7 and the reduction of MMP-7-mediated cellular events including the blockage of PI3K/Akt signaling pathway and the decline of the nuclear protein level and the DNA-binding level of AP-1.[24,28,29] The findings indicated that the andrographolide (**1**) might be a potential agent of prevention of cancer metastasis.

Chemosensitizing and Synergistic Activities

The extract and some diterpenes derived from Chuan Xin Lian are natural chemosensitizer for the antitumor effect. By combining with andrographolide (**1**), the sensitivity of cancer cells was augmented to doxorubicin (DOX), and the DOX-induced cell death was dramatically enhanced. The chemosensitizing effect was achieved by restraining the constitutively activated and IL-6-induced STAT3 phosphorylation and subsequently reducing the nuclear translocation, as well as inhibiting the Janus-activated kinase (JAK)1/2 and the interaction between gp130 and STAT3.[30] The pretreatment of andrographolide (**1**) significantly stimulated the TNF-related apoptosis-inducing ligand (TRAIL)-induced apoptosis in various human carcinoma cell lines and also obviously sensitized the TRAIL-resistant cancer cells to apoptosis. The reversal of TRAIL-resistance by andrographolide (**1**) was found to be accomplished by death receptor-4 (DR4) transcriptional regulation and p53 activation.[31] Andrographolide (**1**) was also able to sensitize cisplatin-induced human tumor cell killing independent of p53.[32] Additionally, a diterpene glucoside designated as neoandrographolide (**5**) acted as a chemosensitizer as well, which could enhance the cytotoxicity of etoposide on S-Jurkat cells and X-linked inhibitor of apoptosis protein (XIAP)-overexpressing Jurkat cells.[33]

Moreover, with the increase of the functions of p53 and caspase-8 and the significant changes of Bax conformation, andrographolide (**1**) synergistically potentiated the cytotoxic and apoptosis-inducing effects of 5-fluorouracil (5-FU) against the growth of human SMMC-7721 hepatoma cells.[34] *In vivo* treatment with the ethanolic extract of Chuan Xin Lian notably augmented the both chemo- and radiotherapeutic effects in association with elevating the levels of serum TNFα, IL-2, and GM-CSF and enhancing the total whole body hyperthermia count, but myeloid leukemia these were declined by cyclophosphamide (CTX) and radiation in animal models.[35,36] The evidences toughly suggested a potential strategy of using Chua Xin Lian extract/andrographolide (**1**) in combination with chemotherapy and radiotherapy to overcome drug resistance and to promote the efficacy of cancer treatment.

Antichemotoxic and Chemopreventive Effects

The protective effect of andrographolide (**1**) and Chuan Xin Lian extract was verified by *in vivo* investigations. The i.p. administration of the extract (10 mg) or the andrographolide (**1**) (0.5 mg) remarkably retarded CTX-caused urothelial toxicity, urinary protein level, and urinary urea N_2 level in animal models. A decreased level of glutathione (GSH) in liver and bladder and lowered levels of IL-2 and interferon (IFN) γ after CTX administration could be elevated by Chuan Xin Lian extract and andrographolide (**1**).[37] The oral administration of the 80% alcoholic extract of Chuan Xin Lian in doses of 50–100 mg/kg per day for 14 days resulted in significant decreases in lactate dehydrogenase activity and malondialdehyde (MDA) formation and noticeable increases in the levels of cytochrome P450 and its reductase, cytochrome b5 reductase, S-transferase, superoxide dismutase, DT-diaphorase, and acid-soluble sulphydryl content. All the interactions led to antichemotoxic and chemopreventive activities.[38]

Likewise, andrographolide (**1**) was able to block the NF-κB binding to DNA and to reduce the aberrant NF-κB activation, exerting potential antiinflammatory properties and effective prevention benefit for retarding chemical-induced carcinogenesis.[39–41] By reducing oxidative stress and obviously activating superoxide dismutase, GSH S-transferase, and catalase, the aqueous extract of Chuan Xin Lian was able to potentiate the antioxidant defense system in the liver of lymphoma-bearing mice.[42] Also, andrographolide (**1**) could repress the hexachlorocyclohexane (BHC)-induced live neoplastic nodule formation and emphasize the recovery of BHC-damaged liver *in vivo*. At the same time, a group of enzymes (such as γ-glutamyl transpeptidase, serum glutamate pyruvate transaminase, serum glutamate oxalate transaminase, alkaline phosphatase, and acid phosphatase) were significantly inhibited.[43] Therefore, the results proved that Chuan Xin Lian extract and andrographolide (**1**) have the marked preventive potential toward the chemotoxicity, the radiotoxicity, as well as the carcinogenicity.

Immunostimulatory Activity

The immunostimulatory activity of the most of andrographolide analogs and Chuan Xin Lian extract were evidenced by promoting the proliferation of cytotoxic lymphocytes through the enhanced secretion of IL-2 and IFNγ by T cells.[41] *In vitro* and *in vivo* assays demonstrated that andrographolide (**1**) also elicited TNFα production and CD marker expression and amplified the cytotoxicity of lymphocytes against diverse cancer cells.[3,7,41,44] All the immunopotentiating effects can exert the tumor-killing effect indirectly.

Flavanones

Four flavanones, assigned as (2S) 5-hydroxy-7,8-dimethoxyflavanone, (2S) 5,2′-dihydroxy-7,8-dimethoxyflavanone, 5-hydroxy-7,8-dimethoxyflavanone, and 5-hydroxy-2′,7,8-trimethoxyflavone, were isolated from the herb. All these flavanones displayed moderate to weak suppressive effects against two human tumor cell lines (Jurkat and Colo 205) *in vitro*.[10]

Structure–Activity Relationship

Preliminary studies on structure–activity relationship (SAR) revealed that the presence of α-alkylidene-γ-butyro-lactone moiety of andrographolide is crucial for exhibiting cytotoxicity. Indeed, the two double bonds of C-12/13 and C-8/17 and the C-14 hydroxyl group were reported being also critically responsible for the antitumor potencies of andrographolide (**1**). The C-12/13 double bond possibly contributed the ability to promote the alkylation of biological nucleophiles such as enzyme through Michael addition to the exo-alkene of α-alkylidene-γ-butyrolactone moiety.

Compared to andrographolide (**1**), isoandrographolide (**2**) exerted greater inhibitory effects on human MCF-7, HCT-116, and HL-60 cancer cell lines.[5] The IC_{50} values of andrographolide (**1**) and isoandrographolide (**2**) were 28.34 and 7.15 μmol/L in the HL-60 cells and the inhibitory rates were 61.2% and 64.4% in mice implanted with H22 murine hepatoma in a dose of 100 mg/kg (subcutaneous), respectively.[45] The results indicated that the isolactone unit in isoandrographolide (**2**) might boost up better antitumor activity than the lactone unit in andrographolide (**1**). The reduction of the C-12/13 olefin bond led to the loss of the activity and the removal of C-14 hydroxyl to yield a conjugated diene system in C-12/13 and/or C-14/15 that would diminish the activity. When an exocyclic C-12/13 olefin bond and an allylic hydroxyl group at C-14 were attempted to be introduced to the butyrolactone moiety, the esterification of C-14 allylic alcohol significantly augmented the supressive activity against the growth of six human cancer cell lines such as H522 (lung), MCF-7 (breast), SW-620 (colon), UACC62 (skin), DU145 (prostate), and PA1 (ovary) cells (GI_{50}: 2.0–6.5 μM).[46,47] The acylation of three hydroxyl groups (C-3, C-14, and C-19) in andrographolide (**1**) could simultaneously or selectively improve the cytotoxicity, implying that the enhancement of their lipid solubility by either introducing a substituted benzylidene moiety, acylated groups, or both has a major effect in improving the cytotoxicity and the selectivity of andrographolide analogs.[46–48] Accordingly, the SAR analysis clearly provided the important clues for the design and the development of more bioavailaible derivatives of andrographolide.

Structural Modification

The promising agent andrographolide (**1**) has poor oral bioavailability due to its rapid biotransformation and efflux by P-gp.[49] Thus, the extensive libraries of andrographolide analogs have been established mainly by structurally modifying the α,β-unsaturated γ-butyrolactone moiety, the two double bonds C-8/17 and C-12/13, and the three hydroxyls at C-3 (secondary), C-14 (allylic), and C-19 (primary). Many of the synthetic analogs exhibit superior anticancer activity over the natural andrographolides (**1**). One of the most potent derivatives assigned as DRF-3188 showed greatly improved anticancer and immunostimulatory acitivities *in vivo*. Similar to andrographolides (**1**), DRF-3188 blocked the tumor cell cycle at G0/G1 stage through the activation of a cell cycle inhibitor p27 and the concomitant decrease of CDK4 level, indicating that both agents exerted the anticancer effect by an alike mechanism.[41,50] 3,14,19-Triacetyl-8,17-epoxyandrographolide (**6**) exerted the enhanced inhibitory effect against ADR-resistant MCF breast carcinoma cells *in vitro* (GI_{50}: 5.5 μM).[47,51] In the National Cancer Institute (NCI) screening with 60 human cancer cell lines derived from nine cancer types, 3,19-isopropylideneandrographolide showed selective suppression on leukemia and colon carcinoma cells, whereas 14-acetylandrographolide was selective toward leukemia, ovarian, and renal cancer cells.[52]

In a family of C-14-ester analogs of andrographolide, two of the analogs, K1 (**7**) and K2, exhibited better potency in the suppression of human leukemic cells (U937, THP1, and K562) and normal cells (NIH3T3 and L132). Three of the derivatives termed K3 (**8**), K4 (**9**), and K5 exerted obvious cytotoxicity with IC_{50} values of 8–12 μM in HEK-293 kidney cancer cells and

6.0–8.4 μM in MCF-7 cells and low toxicity toward normal cells (VERO and MCF-10A). The apoptosis of HEK-293 cells was found to be mediated by a p53-dependent, capase-3 activated and NF-κB-dereased mechanism.[53,54]

A number of C-19-substituted andrographolide analogs were synthesized by the introduction of silyl ether or triphenylmethyl ether group into the C-19 of the andrographolide and led to the increase in the cytotoxicity against the KB, COL-2, MCF-7, LU-1, P388, and ASK cancer cell lines. The derivatives of 19-*O*-triphenylmethyl ether (**10**), 3,14-diactyl-19-*O*-tertbutyldimethylsilyl ether (**11**), and 19-*O*-triisopropylsilyl ether (**12**) showed markedly enhanced (>sixfold) cytotoxicity against the test cell lines (IC_{50}: 0.34–3.62 μM) compared to andrographolide (IC_{50}: 2.25–27.37 μM), whose effects were greater than or similar to an anticancer drug ellipticine (IC_{50}: 1.62–3.56 μM), suggesting that these C-19-substituted analogs may serve as a potential structure lead for the development of new anticancer drugs.[55] A group of benzylidene derivatives of andrographolide showed potent inhibitory effect on MCF-7 (breast) and HCT-116 (colon) cancer cell lines in nanomolar to micromolar concentrations. Among them, SRJ09 (**13**) and SRJ23 (**14**) demonstrated greater cytotoxicity and selectivity than andrographolide (**1**) in the NCI screenings.[56]

By the selective oxidative degradation of the C12/13 olefin bond, andrographolide (**1**) was converted to a key intermediate with an aldehyde functional group. From the key intermediate, a group of structurally diverse labdane diterpenes were semi-synthesized. All the labdane derivatives were evaluated for their *in vitro* cytotoxicity by using NCI standard protocol (a panel of 60 human cancer cell lines derived from nine cancer types). Derivative 15 exerted potent cytotoxicity (GI_{50}: 0.01 μM) against MCF-7 breast cancer cells, while derivatives 16, 17, and 18 selectively exerted the inhibitory activity on DU145 prostate cancer cells *in vitro* (GI_{50}: 0.17, 0.20, and 0.78 μM, respectively).[57]

Additionally, by the bioconversion of andrographolide (**1**) with *Aspergillus ochraceus*, a metabolite assigned as 8β-hydroxy-8(17)-dihydro-14-deoxy-11,12-didehydroandrographolide 19-oic acid (**19**), displayed the improved (three- to fourfold) cytotoxicity on the MCF-7 (breast) and HCT116 (colon) cancer cell lines and two metabolites, 8β-hydroxy-8(17)-dihydroandrographolide (**20**) and 14-deoxy-11,12-didehydroandrographolide 19-oic acid, exerted 1.5–2.3-fold enhanced activity on the HL-60 leukemia cells.[58]

Other Bioactivities

The herb Chuan Xin Lian (Green chirayta) has a wide range of medicinal applications in China, India, and other Southeast Asian regions for treatment of cold, fever, laryngitis, diarrhea, and several infectious diseases ranging from malaria to dysentery. Pharmacological study results exhibited that the herb possesses a wide spectrum of biological properties, such as antiinflammatory, antimyocardial ischemia, antithrombotic, antioxidant, leukocytic ability-enhancing, antiplatelet aggregation, hepatoprotective, hypoglycemic, hypotensive, antipyretic, antidiabetic, sedative, antifilarial, antifertile, antimalarial, choleretic, nematocidal, antiparasitic, anti-HIV, anti-spasmodic, protozoacidal, and antibacterial effects. The herb also is a potent scavenger of a variety of ROS, including superoxide anion, hydroxyl radical, singlet oxygen, peroxynitrite, and nitric oxide.

References

1. Siripong, P. et al. 1992. Cytotoxic diterpenoid constituents from *Andrographis paniculata* Nees, leaves. *J. Sci. Soc. Thailand* 18: 187–94.
2. Kumar, R. A. et al. 2004. Anticancer and immunostimulatory compounds from *Andrographis paniculata*. *J. Ethnopharmacol.* 92: 291–5.
3. Lim, J. C. W. et al. 2012. Andrographolide and its analogues: Versatile bioactive molecules for combating inflammation and cancer. *Clin. Experim. Pharmacol. Physiol.* 39: 300–10.
4. Cheung, H. Y. et al. 2005. Andrographolide isolated from *Andrographis paniculata* induces cell cycle arrest and mitochondrial-mediated apoptosis in human leukemic HL-60 cells. *Planta Med.* 71: 1106–11.
5. Jada, S. R. et al. 2006. Semisynthesis and cytotoxic activities of Andrographolide analogues. *J. Enzyme Inhib. Med. Chem.* 21: 145–55.
6. Kim, T. G. et al. 2005. Morphological and biochemical changes of andrographolide-induced cell death in human prostatic adenocarcinoma PC3 cells. *In Vivo* 19: 551–7.
7. Rajagopal, S. et al. 2003. Andrographolide, a potential cancer therapeutic agent isolated from *Andrographis paniculata*. *J. Experim. Therap. Oncol.* 3: 147–58.
8. Chen, L. X. et al. 2008. ent-Labdane diterpenoid lactone stereoisomers from *Andrographis paniculata*. *J. Nat. Prods.* 71: 852–5.
9. Li, W. K. et al. 2007. Secondary metabolites from *Andrographis paniculata*. *Chem. Pharm. Bull.* 55: 455–8.
10. Madamanchi, G. et al. 2008. Cytotoxic constituents from *Andrographis paniculata* induce cell cycle arrest in Jurkat cells. *Phytother. Res.* 22: 1336–41.
11. Wong, H. C. et al. 2011. Andrographolide induces cell cycle arrest and apoptosis in PC-3 prostate cancer cells. *Afri. J. Pharmacy Pharmacol.* 5: 225–33.
12. Tan, M. L. et al. 2012. Identification of genes involved in the regulation of 14-deoxy-11,12-didehydro-andrographolide-induced toxicity in T-47D mammary cells. *Food Chem. Toxicol.* 50: 431–44.
13. Sirion, U. et al. 2012. New substituted C-19-andrographolide analogues with potent cytotoxic activities. *Bioorg. Med. Chem. Lett.* 22: 49–52.
14. Chun, J. Y. et al. 2010. Andrographolide, an herbal medicine, inhibits interleukin-6 expression and suppresses prostate cancer cell growth. *Genes Cancer* 1: 868–876.
15. Zhao, F. et al. 2008. Antitumor activities of andrographolide, a diterpene from *Andrographis paniculata*, by inducing apoptosis and inhibiting VEGF level. *J. Asian Nat. Prods. Res.* 10: 467–73.
16. Sukardiman, H. et al. 2007. Apoptosis inducing effect of andrographolide on TD-47 human breast cancer cell line. *Afri. J. Trad. Complem. Altern. Med.* 4: 345–51.
17. Ji, L. L. et al. 2007. Andrographolide inhibits human hepatoma-derived Hep3B cell growth through the activation of c-Jun N-terminal kinase. *Planta Med.* 73: 1397–401.
18. Ji, L. L. et al. 2011. Critical roles of cellular glutathione homeostasis and JNK activation in andrographolide-mediated apoptotic cell death in human hepatoma cells. *Mol. Carcinogenesis* 50: 580–91.
19. Zhou, J. et al. 2006. Critical role of pro-apoptotic Bcl-2 family members in andrographolide-induced apoptosis in human cancer cells. *Biochem. Pharmacol.* 72: 132–44.

20. Yang, S. et al. 2010. Mitochondrial-mediated apoptosis in lymphoma cells by the diterpenoid lactone andrographolide, the active component of *Andrographis paniculata*. *Clin. Cancer Res.* 16: 4755–68.
21. Shi, M. et al. 2008. Inhibition of cell-cycle progression in human colorectal carcinoma Lovo cells by andrographolide. *Chemico-biol. Interactions* 174: 201–10.
22. Matsuda, T. et al. 1991. Studies on the cell differentiation inducers of *Andrographis paniculata*. *Tennen Yuki Kagobutsu Toronkai Koen Yoshishu* 33rd, 433–40.
23. Sheeja, K. et al. 2007. Antiangiogenic activity of *Andrographis paniculata* extract and andrographolide. *Intl. Immunopharmacol.* 7: 211–21.
24. Lin, H. et al. 2011. Andrographolide down-regulates hypoxia-inducible factor-1α in human non-small cell lung cancer A549 cells. *Toxicol. Applied Pharmacol.* 250: 336–45.
25. Jiang, C. G. et al. 2007. Andrographolide inhibits the adhesion of gastric cancer cells to endothelial cells by blocking E-selectin expression. *Anticancer Res.* 27: 2439–47.
26. Tan, Y. et al. 2010. Andrographolide regulates epidermal growth factor receptor and transferrin receptor trafficking in epidermoid carcinoma (A431) cells. *British J. Pharmacol.* 159: 1497–510.
27. Chao, H. P. et al. 2010. Andrographolide exhibits anti-invasive activity against colon cancer cells via inhibition of MMP2 activity. *Planta Med.* 76: 1827–133.
28. Lee, Y. C. et al. 2010. Inhibitory effects of andrographolide on migration and invasion in human non-small cell lung cancer A549 cells via down-regulation of PI3K/Akt signaling pathway. *Eur. J. Pharmacol.* 632: 23–32.
29. Shi, M. D. et al. 2009. Andrographolide could inhibit human colorectal carcinoma Lovo cells migration and invasion via down-regulation of MMP-7 expression. *Chemico-Biol. Interactions* 180: 344–52.
30. Zhou, J. et al. 2010. Inhibition of the JAK-STAT3 pathway by andrographolide enhances chemosensitivity of cancer cells to doxorubicin. *Biochem. Pharmacol.* 79: 1242–50.
31. Zhou, J. et al. 2008. Andrographolide sensitizes cancer cells to TRAIL-induced apoptosis via p53-mediated death receptor 4 up-regulation. *Mol. Cancer Therap.* 7: 2170–80.
32. Zhou, J. et al. 2012. Andrographolide sensitizes cisplatin-induced apoptosis via suppression of autophagosome-lysosome fusion in human cancer cells. *Autophagy* 8: 338–49.
33. Pfisterer, P. H. et al. 2011. Neoandrographolide from *Andrographis paniculata* as a potential natural chemosensitizer. *Planta Med.* 76: 1698–700.
34. Yang, L. et al. 2009. Andrographolide enhances 5-fluorouracil-induced apoptosis via caspase-8-dependent mitochondrial pathway involving p53 participation in hepatocellular carcinoma (SMMC-7721) cells. *Cancer Lett.* 276: 180–8.
35. Sheeja, K. et al. 2009. Ameliorating effects of *Andrographis paniculata* extract against cyclopho-sphamide-induced toxicity in mice. *Asian Pacific J. Cancer Prevention* 7: 609–14.
36. Sheeja, K. et al. 2008. Effect of *Andrographis paniculata* as an adjuvant in combined chemo-radio and whole body hyperthermia treatment—A preliminary study. *Immunopharmacol. Immunotoxicol.* 30: 181–94.
37. Sheeja, K. et al. 2006. Protective effect of *Andrographis paniculata* and andrographolide on cyclophosphamide-induced urothelial toxicity. *Integrative Cancer Therapies* 5: 244–51.
38. Singh, R. P. et al. 2011 Modulatory influence of *Andrographis paniculata* on mouse hepatic and extrahepatic carcinogen metabolizing enzymes and antioxidant status. *Phytother. Res.* 15: 382–90.
39. Wang, L. J. et al. 2011. Andrographolide inhibits oral squamous cell carcinogenesis through NF-κB inactivation. *J. Dental Res.* 90: 1246–54.
40. Sheeja, K. et al. 2007. Activation of cytotoxic T lymphocyte responses and attenuation of tumor growth in vivo by *Andrographis paniculata* extract and andrographolide. *Immunopharmacol. Immunotoxicol.* 29: 81–93.
41. Kumar, A. R. et al. 2004. Anticancer and immunomodulatory potential of DRF-3188, an analogue of andrographolide. In Tan, B. K. H. et al. (eds.) *Novel Compounds from Natural Products in the New Millennium*, 205–16. Discovery Research, Vernon, BC.
42. Verma, N. et al. 2008. Antioxidant action of *Andrographis paniculata* on lymphoma. *Mol. Biol. Reports* 35: 535–40.
43. Trivedi, N. P. et al. 2009. Potency of andrographolide as an antitumor compound in BHC-induced liver damage. *Integr. Cancer Therapies* 8: 177–89.
44. Hidalgo, M. A. et al. 2005. Andrographolide interferes with binding of NF-κB to DNA in HL-60-derived neutrophilic cells. *Brit. J. Pharmacol.* 144: 680–6.
45. Han, G. et al. 2008. Synthesis and antitumor structure-activity relationship of diterpene lactones of *Andrographis paniculata* Nees. *Zhongguo Yaoxue Zazhi* 43: 790–4.
46. Nanduri, S. et al. (a) 2003. Synthesis and evaluation of novel ester analogs of andrographolide as potent anticancer agents; Synthesis and SAR studies of C12-substituted andrographolide analogs as novel anticancer agents. *Abstracts of Papers, 225th ACS National Meeting, New Orleans, LO, U.S.A., March 23–27, 2003*, MEDI-093 and MEDI-094; (b) 2001. Process for the preparation of andrographolide derivs. and pharmaceutical compositions containing them for use as novel anticancer agents. *PCT Int. Appl.* WO 2001085710 A1 20011115; 2001. Preparation of andrographolide derivatives for pharmaceutical use in the treatment of a variety of disorders, such as cancer and HIV infection. *PCT Int. Appl.* WO 2001085709 A2 20011115; 2001. Preparation and anti-tumor activity of andrographolide derivs. *PCT Int. Appl.* WO 2001057026 A1 20010809.
47. Lim, J. C. W. et al. 2012. Andrographolide and its analogues: Versatile bioactive molecules for combating inflammation and cancer. *Clin. Experim. Pharmacol. Physiol.* 39: 300–10.
48. Taki, T. et al. 1988. Isolation of andrographolide and its deoxy derivative from *Andrographis paniculata* as antitumor agents and pharmaceutical compositions containing them. *Jpn. Kokai Tokkyo Koho* JP 63088124 A 19880419.
49. Ye, L. et al. 2011. Poor oral bioavailability of a promising anticancer agent andrographolide is due to extensive metabolism and efflux by P-glycoprotein. *J. Pharma. Sci.* 100: 5007–17.
50. Satyanarayana, C. et al. 2004. DRF 3188 a novel semisynthetic analog of andrographolide: Cellular response to MCF7 breast cancer cells. *BMC Cancer* 4: 26.
51. Nanduri, S. et al. 2004. Synthesis and structure-activity relationships of andrographolide analogues as novel cytotoxic agents. *Bioorg. Med. Chem. Lett.* 14: 4711–7.
52. Jada, S. R. et al. 2007. Semisynthesis and in vitro anticancer activities of andrographolide analogues. *Phytochem.* 68: 904–12.

53. Bimolendu, D. et al. 2010. Synthesis, cytotoxicity, and structure-activity relationship (SAR) studies of andrographolide analogues as anticancer agent. *Bioorg. Med. Chem. Lett.* 20: 6947–50.
54. Preet, R. et al. 2014. Synthesis and biological evaluation of andrographolide analogues as anticancer agents. *Eur. J. Med. Chem.* 85: 95–106.
55. Sirion, U. et al. 2012. New substituted C-19-andrographolide analogues with potent cytotoxic activities. *Bioorg Med Chem Lett.* 22: 49–52.
56. Jada, S. R. et al. 2008. Benzylidene derivatives of andrographolide inhibit growth of breast and colon cancer cells in vitro by inducing G1 arrest and apoptosis. *Brit. J. Pharmacol.* 155: 641–54.
57. Nanduri, S. et al. 2004. Novel routes for the generation of structurally diverse labdane diterpenes from andrographolide. *Tetrahedron Lett.* 45: 4883–6.
58. He, X. J. et al. 2011. Novel bioconversion products of andrographolide by *Aspergillus ochraceus* and their cytotoxic activities against human tumor cell lines. *J. Mol. Catal. B Enzym.* 68: 89–93.

7 She Gan 射干

Blackberry lily or Leopard lily

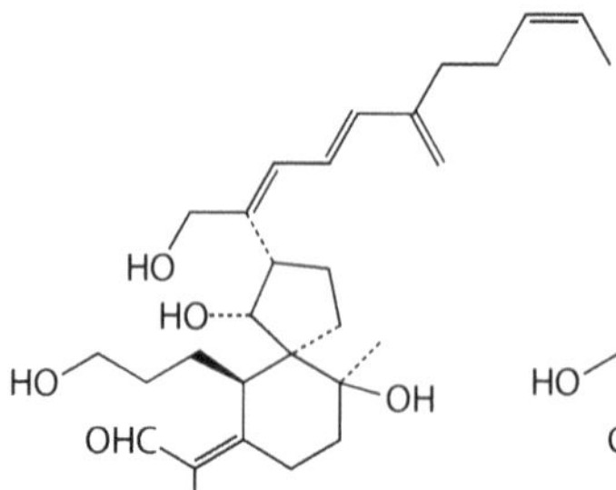

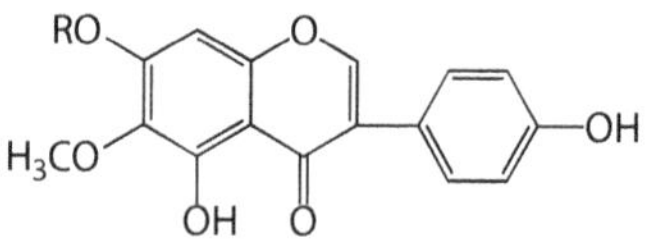

5. R = -H
6. R = -beta-D-glucopyranosyl

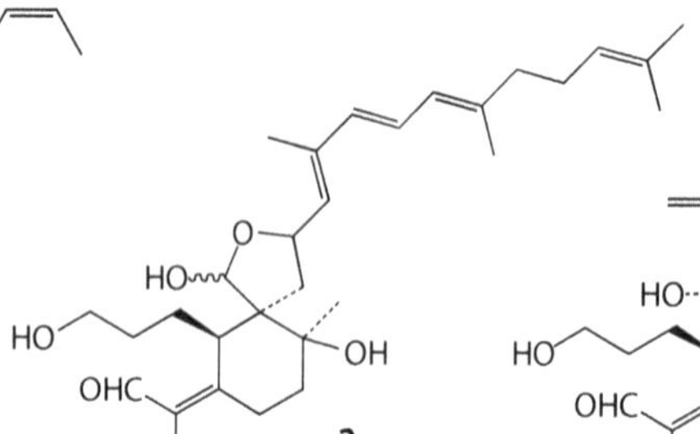

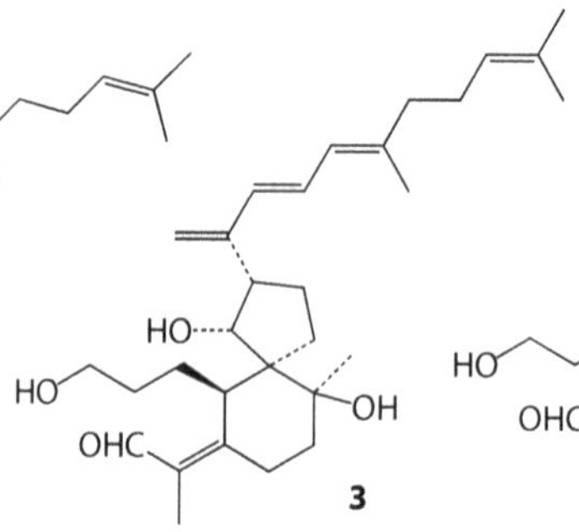

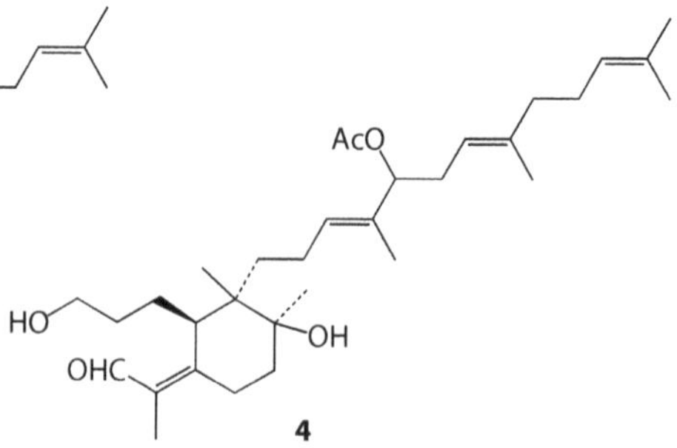

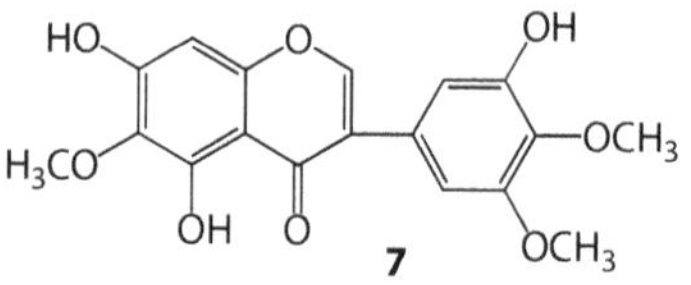

Herb Origination

The herb She Gan (Blackberry lily) is the dried rhizomes of an Iridaceae plant *Belamcanda chinensis*. The herbaceous plant is native to East Asia, especially China. The best season for the collection of the herb is during autumn, although it can be collected in spring. She Gan was documented in *Shennong Ben Cao Jing*, the first Chinese materia medica, which denoted that She Gan has been used as a Chinese folk medicine for over a thousand years. Blackberry lily is often cultivated in gardens of the world because of the attractive foliage and flowers.

Antitumor Activity

In a mouse model with sarcoma 180, the treatment with She Gan extract exerted 44.74% inhibition against the tumor growth.[1] She Gan extract is fed to male nude mice implanted with human LNCaP prostate carcinoma cells and markedly restrained the growth of tumor cells *in vivo*.[2] She Gan extract also demonstrated the inhibitory effect against the proliferation of malignant testicular germ cell tumor cell lines (TCam-2 and NTera-2), together with downregulating the expressions of stem cell factors (NANOG and POU5F1) in the tumor cells.[3] The ethyl acetate extract of She Gan exhibited a great suppressive effect against human neoplastic cell lines such as MGC-803 (stomach), PC3 (prostate), Bcap-37, and MCF-7 (breast) tumors *in vitro*.[4] The methanolic extract of She Gan was found to inhibit the adhesion activity of human HL-60 leukemia cells through the stimulation of the cell morphological changes.[2] These findings provided solid evidences to support the application of She Gan in Chinese medical prescription for cancer therapy.

Antitumor Constituents and Activity

Several types of constituents have been discovered from the phytochemical investigations of the herb. But, its triterpenoid and isoflavonoid components were reported to be mainly responsible for the antitumor activity of She Gan.

Triterpenoids

Four common triterpenes assigned as ursolic acid, betulin, betulonic acid, and betulone were isolated from the ethyl acetate extract of She Gan. These all displayed obvious antiproliferative effect against MGC-803, Bcap-37, MCF-7, and PC3 neoplastic cell line *in vitro*, and the inhibitory rates ranged between 43.7% and 68.1%.[1] A group of unusual iridal-type triterpenoids were also isolated from She Gan. Of the triterpenoids, 28-deacetylbelamcandal (**1**), (6R,10S,11R)-2-ξ-hydroxy-(13R)-oxaspiroirid-16-enal (**2**), (6R,10S,11S,14S,26R)-26-hydroxy-15-methylidenespiroirid-16-enal (**3**), and 16-*O*-acetylisoiridogermanal (**4**) were proven to be active substances that restrained the cell adhesion of HL-60 leukemia by 100% in the concentrations of 0.5, 1.3, 2.5, and 5 μM, respectively, whereas iridotectoral-A was inactive within the concentration range (10–40 μM).[2]

Flavonoids

Among the isolated flavonoids from the herb, kampferol showed relatively better cytotoxicity on PC3, MGC-803, Bcap-37, and MCF-7 human tumor cell lines, while the flavonoids such as quercetin, 4′,5,6-trihydroxy-7-methoxyisoflavone, tectorigenin, tectoridin, irisflorentin, irilin-A, iridin, irigenin, iristectorigenin-A, as well as two organic acids (shikimic acid and gallic acid) only had a weak effect on the cancer cells (<29.4% inhibition).[1] The isoflavones referring to irigenin, tectorigenin, irisflorentin, iridin, and tectoridin had a marked inhibitory effect on the growth of A549 lung cancer, LoVo colon cancer, 6T-CEM, and HL-60 leukemia cell lines.[5] The i.p. administration of tectorigenin (**5**) or tectoridin (**6**) at a dose of 30 mg/kg to mice bearing sarcoma 180 for 10 days notably suppressed the tumor weight by 44.2% and 24.8%, respectively. Tectorigenin (**5**), when subcutaneously injected at the same dosage for 20 days to the tumor-bearing mice, markedly restrained the volume of murine Lewis lung carcinoma by 30.8%.[6]

Importantly, tectorigenin (**5**), tectoridin (**6**), irigenin (**7**), and other isolated isoflavonoids, which act as phytoestrogens, could exert antiproliferative effects against different hormone-correlated cancer cells. The proliferation of RWPE-1, LNCaP, and PC3 prostate cancer cell lines could be inhibited by tectorigenin (**5**) and irigenin (**7**) in a dose-dependent manner in association with a cell cycle arrest at the G1 phase via the induction of p21 (WAF1) or p27 protein expression.[7] After the LNCaP cells were treated, tectorigenin (**5**) and other isoflavones declined the expression of androgen and its coactivator PDEF, diminished human telomerase reverse transcriptase (hTERT), and insulin-like growth factor 1 (IGF-1) receptor gene expressions, reduced prostate-specific antigen (PSA) secretion, and restrained NKX3.1 expression and telomerase activity, thereby demonstrating the antiprostate cancer potential. Through the upregulation of TIMP-3 gene expression, tectorigenin (**5**) and other isoflavones also inhibited the invasion of LNCaP tissue.[3,8] Similarly, tectorigenin (**5**) and other isoflavonoids repressed the proliferation of malignant testicular germ cell tumor cells (TGCT) in concomitant with the downregulation of stem cell factors (NANOG and POU5F1), indicating that the anti-TGCT effect may be triggered by a histone-independent mechanisms.[9] Due to the potent estrogenic effects mainly via both estrogen receptor (ER)-dependent genomic pathway and GPR30-dependent nongenomic pathway, tectoridin (**6**) limited the proliferation of human MCF-7 breast cancer cells.[10] In addition, tectorigenin (**5**) and tectoridin (**6**) also showed antiangiogenesis property in the studies due to lessened vessel formation in both chick embryo chorioallantoic membrane assay and in mouse Matrigel plug assay.[6] Therefore, the isoflavonoids are the interesting agents for treating hormone-involved male prostate cancer and female carcinomas of breast, uterus, and ovaries.[11]

Other Medical Uses

Due to having multiple biological properties such as analgesic, depurative, expectorant, febrifuge, antiinflammatory, purgative, pectoral, stomachic, antibacterial, and antifungal effects, She Gan is generally prescribed in Chinese herb remedies to treat acute laryngitis, acute tonsillitis, mumps, edema of glottis, and cough with profuse sputum, and it is also used as a poultice for dermatitis, rheumatism, and goiters. Additionally, as a Nepal folk medicine, its root juice is used to treat liver complaints and to additively improve appetite. The juice also can be used to abort a fetus during the first trimester of pregnancy. Therefore, the root is contraindicated during pregnancy.

References

1. Chen, Q. et al. 2013. The in vivo antitumor effect of *Belamcanda chinensis* extract. *Baifang Yaoxue* (5): 72.
2. Takahashi, K. et al. 2000. Iridals from *Iris tectorum* and *Belamcanda chinensis*. *Phytochem*. 53: 925–9.
3. Thelen, P. et al. 2005. Tectorigenin and other phytochemicals extracted from leopard lily *Belamcanda chinensis* affect new and established targets for therapies in prostate cancer. *Carcinogenesis* 26: 1360–7.
4. Liu, M. C. et al. 2012. Chemical constituents of the ethyl acetate extract of *Belamcanda chinensis* roots and their antitumor activities. *Mol.* 17: 6156–69.
5. Chen, H. S. et al. 2010. Application of isoflavones in the preparation of antitumor drug or food. *China Patents* CN 101797247 A 20100811.
6. Jung, S. H. et al. 2003. Anti-angiogenic and antitumor activities of isoflavonoids from the rhizomes of *Belamcanda chinensis*. *Planta Med.* 69: 617–22.
7. Morrissey, C. et al. 2004. Phytoestrogens derived from *Belamcanda chinensis* have an antiproliferative effect on prostate cancer cells in vitro. *J. Urol.* (Hagerstown, MD, United States) 172(6, Pt.1): 2426–33.
8. Thelen, P. et al. 2007. Phytoestrogens from *Belamcanda chinensis* regulate the expression of steroid receptors and related cofactors in LNCaP prostate cancer cells. *BJU Intl.* 100: 199–203.
9. Hasibeder, A. et al. 2013. Phytoestrogens regulate the proliferation and expression of stem cell factors in cell lines of malignant testicular germ cell tumors. *Intl. J. Oncol.* 43: 1385–94.
10. Kang, K. S. et al. 2009. Tectoridin, a poor ligand of estrogen receptor-α, exerts its estrogenic effects via an ERK-dependent pathway. *Mol. Cells* 27: 351–7.
11. Jung, S. H. et al. 2007. Tectoridin from Belamcanda extracts for treating female cancers or diseases associated with female hormone. *Repub. Korea* KR 740184 B1 20070718.

8 Ya Dan Zi 鸦膽子

Java brucea seed

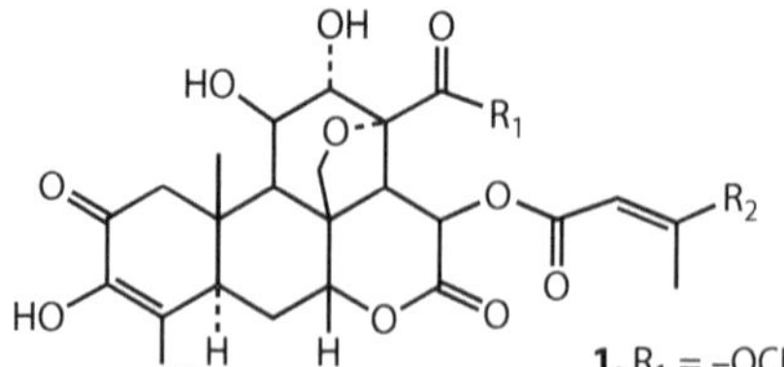

1. $R_1 = -OCH_3$ $R_2 = -CH_3$
2. $R_1 = -OCH_3$ $R_2 = -CH(CH_3)_2$
7. $R_1 = -OH$ $R_2 = -CH_3$

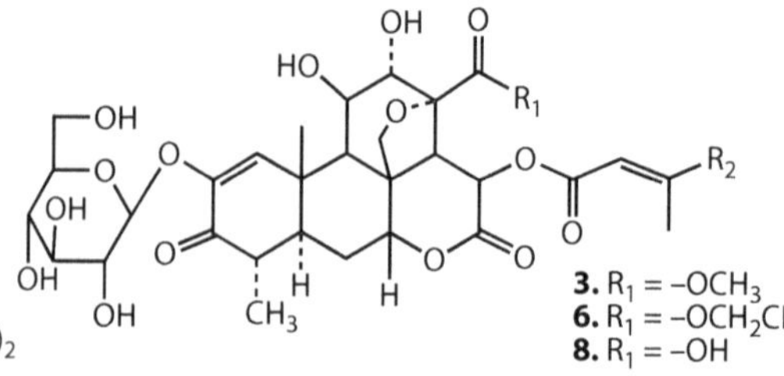

3. $R_1 = -OCH_3$ $R_2 = -CH_3$
6. $R_1 = -OCH_2CH_2CH_3$ $R_2 = -CH_3$
8. $R_1 = -OH$ $R_2 = -CH(CH_3)_2$

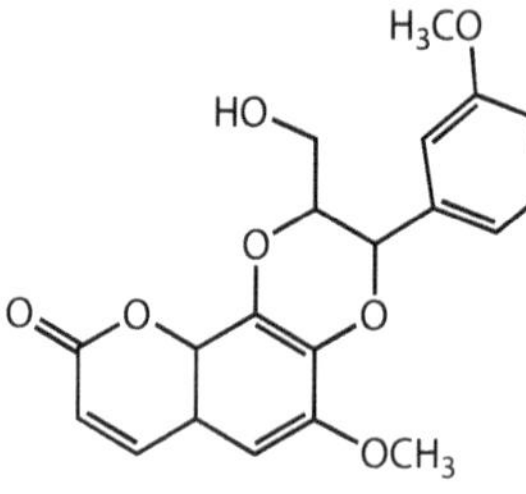

4 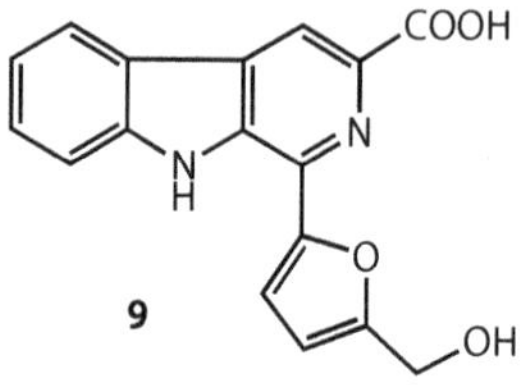 **9** 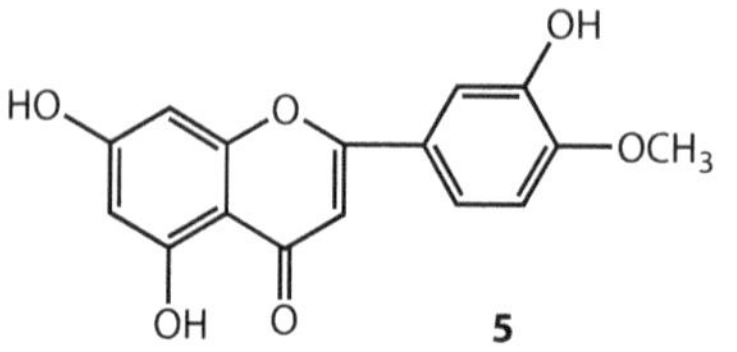 **5** 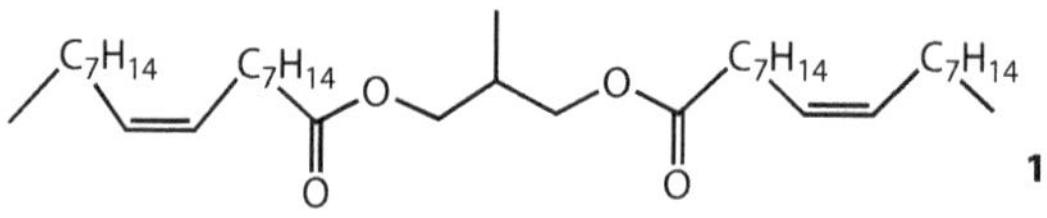 **10**

Herb Origination

The herb Ya Dan Zi (Java brucea seed) is the dried seeds of a Simaroubaceae plant *Brucea javanica*. This plant is an evergreen shrub originally from Southeast Asia and northern Australia. As a Chinese medicine, its seeds are typically harvested in late autumn and winter when its fruit is ripe and turns black.

Antitumor Activities

Seed Oil

Ya Dan Zi is the oil-rich seeds showing a potent inhibitory property against the growth of cancer cells. The seed oil and its oil emulsion demonstrated the suppressive effect on Ehrlich ascites carcinoma, ascites hepatoma, and T24 bladder cancer and HeLa cervix cancer cell lines, *in vitro*. The *in vivo* experiments confirmed that the emulsion was effective in murine models against Ehrlich ascites cancer, sarcoma 37, and sarcoma 180 by local administration.[1–3] The suppressive potency of the emulsion by intravenous injection to mice bearing bladder carcinoma was comparable to that of mitomycin C.[4] The i.p. administration of the emulsion to the tumor-bearing murine animals obviously obstructed the growth of both ascites and entity hepatoma cells and W256 sarcoma cells, but it showed to be invalid to sarcoma 180, Ehrlich ascites cancer, and U14 cervical carcinoma.[5]

Mixing a 5% Ya Dan Zi emulsion with Ehrlich ascites cells *in vitro* would kill 80% of the cells in 1 h and 100% in 4 h,[5] which tumoricidal effect was by means of attacking the biomembrane structure, markedly destroying the cancer cell structure, and inducing the cell membrane damage and mitochondrion vacuolization.[6] The antitumor effect of the oil emulsion on HeLa cells was mainly correlated with the induction of apoptosis and the S cell cycle arrest.[3] By treatment with the oil emulsion *in vitro*, the P388 leukemia cell cycle was depressed at S, G2, and G0 phases.[7] The apoptotic mechanism of the oil in T24 bladder cancer cell was accompanied by the notable suppression of the NF-κB and COX-2 expressions and up-expression of caspase-3 and caspase-9.[2] The oil at 5.0 mg/mL concentration could also resist the VEGF mRNA expression and secretion in human A549 lung carcinoma and esophageal cancer cells.[8,9] All the events must involve in the antitumor mechanism of the Ya Dan Zi oil and the oil products. If combined with radiotherapy, the emulsion treatment exhibited better short-time curative effect, higher survival rate, lighter side reactions, and obviously lower serum VEGF.[9]

Moreover, the oil emulsion at 0.025 mg/mL concentration was also able to markedly reverse the MDR in various human drug-resistant cancer cell lines such as K562/A02 erythroleukemia, MCF-7/Adm breast cancer, and KB/vincristine (VCR) nasopharyngeal carcinoma.[10] Ya Dan Zi oil is useful for the treatment of melanoma and papilloma by skin irritation. The local administration of the oil on skin tumors could cause degeneration and necrosis of tumor cells.[11] DNA topoisomerase (Topo)-II-mediated kDNA degeneration was markedly inhibited by the oil emulsion at 0.31 mg/mL concentration, and the Topo-II activity was totally suppressed at a dose of 2.5 mg/mL. However, the oil emulsion showed no direct influence on DNA and on DNA Topo-I mediated pBR322 relaxation.[11] In addition, the oleic acid-type components in the Ya Dan Zi oil was able to restrain the incorporation of thymidine into the DNA of Ehrlich ascites tumor cells (EACs), resulting in the blockage of DNA synthesis in a concentration-dependent manner.[12]

Aqueous Extracts

The aqueous extract of Ya Dan Zi showed a moderate inhibitory effect on human KB nasopharyngeal cells (IC_{50}: 16.85 μg/mL), whose effect was lower than its chloroform fraction (IC_{50}: 0.55 μg/mL).[8] In an *in vitro* assay, the aqueous extract was cytotoxic to other human cancer cell lines, such as MCF-7 (breast), LNCaP (prostate), HT1080 (fibrosarcoma), and A431 (epidermoid) cells and less active to normal cells. The aqueous extract also effectively restrained the growth of four cervical cancer cell lines (HeLa, CaSki, SiHa, C33A). More evidences indicated that the Ya Dan Zi extract is able to elicit the tumor cell apoptosis through both p53-dependent and. p53-independent pathways.[13] The warmed water extract of *B. javanica* (BJE) could strongly stimulate the apoptosis of all four tested human tumor cell lines, A549 (lung), Hep3B (liver), MDA-MB-231 (breast), and SLMT-1 (esophageal squamous) cells. The cell apoptosis caused by the BJE in MDA-MB-231 cells was probably through a mitochondrial-dependent pathway associated with caspase-3 activation.[14]

Antitumor Constituents and Activities

Many quassinoids have been separated from Ya Dan Zi, and most of them demonstrated remarkable tumoricidal activity. The isolated quassinoids were designated as brusatols, bruceantins, bruceolides, bruceins, bruceantinosides, bruceosides, javanicolides, yadanziolides, and yadanziosides. Of them, brusatol (**1**) and bruceosides were considered as the most significant antitumor components in the herb.[15–20]

Quassinoids

Brusatol (**1**) and bruceine-B demonstrated significant inhibitory activities against a panel of human HL-60 (leukemic), SMMC-7721 (liver), A549 (lung), and MCF-7 (breast) cancer cell lines *in vitro*.[21] Bruceine-B, bruceine-E, bruceine-H, and dehydrobrusatol exerted cytotoxicity against HepG2 (liver), HCT-8 (colon), BGC-823 (stomach), SKOV3 (ovary), and A549 (lung) human neoplastic cell lines (IC_{50}: 0.12–9.3 μM), while javanicolide-H and javanicolide-E selectively obstructed the growth of BGC-823, A549, and SKOV3 cells (IC_{50}: 0.52, 0.95, 0.23 μM and IC_{50}: 1.43, 6.36, 1.49 μM, respectively).[22]

The apoptosis-inducing and antiproliferative properties of bruceine-D are present in three pancreatic cancer cell lines (PANC-1, SW1990, and CAPAN-1), associating with the activation of p38-MAPK signaling pathway, but it had a modest cytotoxic effect on nontumorigenic Hs68 cells.[23] The most potent *in vitro* antipancreatic cancer effect was achieved by brusatol (**1**) with IC_{50} values of 0.36 μM in the PANC-1 and 0.10 μM in the SW1990 cells.[24] Bruceantin (**2**) exerted powerful cytotoxicity toward human KB nasopharyngeal carcinoma cells *in vitro* (ED_{50}: 0.008 μg/mL)[25] and significant inhibitory effects on human MCF-7 (breast), LNCaP (prostate), and Lu1 (lung) neoplastic cell lines.[26] Interestingly, in the presence of (−)-hydnocarpin (a flavonolignan in Ya Dan Zi), the cytotoxicity of bruceantin (**2**) could be augmented against the MCF-7 cells by 10-fold.[26] Daily i.p. injection of bruceantin (**3**) or bruceoside-A in a dose range of 0.25–1.0 mg/kg *in vivo* obstructed the growth of mouse P388 lymphocytic leukemia cells markedly and prolonged the life span of the tested mice.[16,17] In an i.p. dose of 0.125 mg/kg per day, brusatol (**1**) obviously suppressed the growth of P388 leukemia cells *in vivo* with a T/C value of 158.[27]

Moreover, the treatment with brusatol (**1**) and bruceantin also obviously elicit the differentiation of eight leukemia-related cell lines including HL-60, K562, NB4, U937, BV173, K562, SUPB13, and S4-11 cells, concomitant with the downregulation of c-Myc expression. Bruceine-D in a concentration of 0.1 μg/mL obviously accelerated the HL-60 cell differentiation by 43.1%, whereas brusatol (**1**) induced the differentiation of various leukemic cells in 5–25 ng/mL concentration range.[26,28] The activation and the translocation of NF-κB into the nucleus caused by brusatol (**1**) are also probably responsible for the differentiation of HL-60 cells.[29] Therefore, the biological phytochemistry clearly demonstrated that the quassinoid components are primarily responsible for the antitumor activity of the seed oil, which may be developed as drug leads in cancer preclinical investigation.

Quassinoid Glucosides

The antigrowth effect was also notably shown in the quassinoid glucosides derived from the herb. Bruceoside-A (**3**) and bruceoside-B demonstrated the antigrowth effect against Walker sarcoma, Ehrlich ascites carcinoma, and leukemic cell lines. The selective cytotoxicity in leukemia and solid tumor cell lines of the lung, the colon, the central nervous system (CNS), the ovary, and the skin were accomplished in presence of bruceosides D–F (log GI_{50}: from −4.14 to −5.72).[30,31] The inhibition of bruceoside-D on P388 leukemia and colon HCT carcinoma cell lines was moderate, but its remarkable cytotoxicity was shown on KB nasopharynx, RPMI melanoma, A549 lung cancer, and TE-671 brain tumor cell lines *in vitro* (ED_{50}: <0.1–0.29 μg/mL).[32] The *in vitro* antiproliferative effect of yadanziosides was observed in the P388 cells, and the *in vivo* inhibitory activities were further substantiated by yadanzioside-K, yadanzioside-I, and yadanzioside-L in mice implanted with P388 leukemia.[19]

Other Types of Components

A lignan component cleomiscosin-A (**4**) isolated from Ya Dan Zi could repress the growth of P388 leukemia cells *in vitro* (ED_{50}: 0.4 μg/mL).[20] Chrysoeriol (**5**), a flavonoid type NF-κB inhibitor derived from the herb, selectively suppressed HL-60 leukemia cells with greater potency. It also showed an ability to upregulate the nuclear factor of activated T cells transcriptional pathway via the amplification of intracellular ROS, indicating that the chrysoeriol (**5**) can serve as a potential chemotherapeutic modifier for the treatment of leukemia.[33]

Anticarcinogenic Constituents

Besides the anticancer effects, the quassinoids and other components derived from the herb also play effective roles in anticarcinogenesis, antimutagenesis, and antitumor promotion. Bruceoside-D, its butanol ester (**6**), and two other quassinoids, desmethylbrusatol (**7**) and desmethylbruceantinoside-A (**8**), exerted the inhibitory effects against 12-*O*-tetradecanoylphorbol-13-acetate (TPA)-promoted Epstein–Barr virus early antigen (EBV-EA) activation.[34] Two quassionoids, yadanziolide-S and brucein-D, and two nonquassinoids, flazine (**9**) and glycerol 1,3-bisoleate (**10**), exerted the suppressive effect against mouse mammary preneoplastic lesions induced by a mutagen 7,12-dimethylbenz[a]anthracene. The most active compound in this assay was flazine (**9**), which showed a 75% inhibitory rate in a concentration of 4 μg/mL.[35] In addition, glycerol 1,3-bisoleate (**10**) is a marked inhibitor of

COX-2, whose anti-COX-2 activity might be correlated with the anticarcinogenic effect.[35]

Clinical Trials

1. Ninety-eight patients suffering from lung cancer with brain metastasis were treated with Ya Dan Zi oil. Daily infusion by intravenous drip (20–30 mL) of the 10% emulsion in physiological saline ≈250 L for 30 continuous days resulted in the best curative effect. Ninety percent of the patients exhibited symptoms promoting the effect, and the average lifetime was 8.27 months after the treatment. Among them, 26.9% of the patients survived over one year. This treatment was beneficial with low side effects and no toxicity in long-term use.[36]
2. Twenty-five patients bearing bladder cancer (including 15 cases that were replaced after surgical operation) were treated with 10% Ya Dan Zi oil emulsion. Thirteen of them were orally administered with 50 mL of the emulsion three times per day for 15 successive days with one to four cycles. In the final phase, 10 cases were cured, but three cases were invalid. The other 10 cases were administered with 50 mL of the emulsion by perfusion into bladder in one to two times per week for 5–10 continuous weeks × 1–10 cycles, resulting in 100% cured patients. The two remaining cases that were in the late phase of cancer metastasis showed no significant effect after the treatment with 10% emulsion. In the course of the treatments, no toxicity and side effects were found.[37]
3. Seventy-two advanced cancer patients with medium or abundant malignant ascites have been treated by the seed oil (50 mL) combined with hydroxycamptothecin (20 mg) after draining the ascites with an i.p. catheter. The i.p. drug administration was repeated for two to three times in one week after the first treatment. The chemotherapy was feasible and effective for the inhibition of the malignant ascites. The result was 20% completely effective and 50% partially effective. But some side effects such as neutropenia and thrombocytopenia were induced during the treatment.[38]
4. Fifty-seven patients with primary superficial bladder cancer received perfusion of 60 mL 10% Ya Dan Zi oil, and eight perfusions were regularly carried out per week and per patient after operation. The clinical trial result showed that the perfusion of 10% Ya Dan Zi oil is safer and more effective in preventing superficial bladder tumor relapse and worth popularizing due to lower relapse rate (14.04%, 8/57) and side effect (12.28%) compared to the treatment with mitomycin-C or bacillus Calmette-Guérin (BCG).[39]
5. Seventy-two lung cancer patients with malignant pleural effusion were randomly divided into the therapy group and the control group, 36 cases in each group. The patients in the therapy group were administered by recombinant human interleukin-2 by intrathoracic perfusion and, at the same time, treated with *B. javanica* oil emulsion through intravenous drip, but the patients in the control group were administered with recombinant human interleukin-2 only. The resulting total effective rate of the therapy group is significantly higher, indicating that this combinational treatment significantly improved the therapy effect.[40]

Other Bioactivities

The oil of Ya Dan Zi (Java brucea seed) has been used for centuries to treat dysentery and malaria. It is also made into an ointment to treat skin problems such as corns and warts. The antimalaria and amebicide properties of the oil have been proven by pharmaceutical experiments. Importantly, the oil is able to enhance the phagocytosis of abdominal macrophage and to promote the proliferation of marrow hematopoietic stem cells after being damaged by ^{60}Co-irritation.

References

1. Su, X. R. et al. 1981. Studies on antitumor effect of oil from *Brucea javanica* 10: Pharmaco-kinetics of 3H-labeled oleic acid, the active principle in the oil from *Brucea javanica. Zhongcaoyao* 12: 21–4.
2. Lou, G. G. et al. 2010. *Brucea javanica* oil induces apoptosis in T24 bladder cancer cells via upregulation of caspase-3, caspase-9, and inhibition of NF-κB and COX-2 expressions. *Am. J. Chin. Med.* 38: 613–24.
3. Yin, X. J. et al. 2008. Inhibitory effect of *Brucea javanica* oil emulsion against cervical cancer cell line Hela and its mechanism. *Zhongguo Zhongliu Shengwu Zhiliao Zazhi* 15: 393–5.
4. Wang, H. et al. 2001. Effects of *Brucea javanica* oil emulsion intravesical instillation for treatment of bladder carcinoma in mice. *Disi Junyi Daxue Xuebao* 22: 1886–1891.
5. Wang, N. Q. et al. (a) 1980. Antitumor activity of *Brucea javanica* and cyclic AMP content in the cancer cells. *Zhongyi Zazhi.* 21: 631; (b) 1999. *Chinese Materia Medica.* Vol. 5, 5–3833, 9–11. Shanghai Science and Technology Press, Shanghai, China.
6. Yang, Z. B. et al. 1986. Effects of emulsions of seed oil of *Brucea javanica* and emulsions of oleic acid on the ultrastructure of tumor cells. *J. Shenyang Pharm. Univ.* 3: 1–7.
7. Li, M. et al. (a) 1984. Studies on the antitumor action of *Brucea javanica*: Studies on the effects of oleic acid which prevents the incorporation of 3H-TdR into the Ehrlich ascitic cancer cell for synthesizing DNA. *Shenyang Yaoxueyuan Xuebao* 1: 40–3; (b) 1984. Cytokinetic effect of an intravenous emulsion of *Brucea javanica* seed oil on Ehrlich ascites carcinoma cells. *J. Shenyang Pharm. Univ.* 1: 161–5.
8. Xu, X. et al. 2008. Effects of *Brucea javanica* oil on expression of vascular endothelial growth factor in A549 cell line. *Zhongguo Zhongyao Zazhi* 33: 2517–20.
9. Liao, J. R. 2012. The effect of *Brucea javanica* emulsion on serum VEGF and curative efficiency of patients with esophageal carcinoma. *Zhongguo Laonianxue Zazhi* 32: 4535–6.
10. Zhang, J. Z. et al. (a) 1965. Experimental observation in skin cancer treatment with *Brucea javanica. Zhonghua Pifuke Zazhi.* 11: 328; (b) 1999. *Chinese Materia Medica.* Vol. 5, 5–3833. Shanghai Science and Technology Press, Shanghai, China.
11. Tang, T. et al. 2001. Reversal of multidrug resistance and inhibition of DNA topoisomerase II by emulsion of seed oil of *Brucea javanica. Zhongguo Yaolixue Tongbao* 17: 534–9.

12. Anderson, M. M. et al. 1990. In vivo cytotoxicity of antiplasmosidal tests for selection of potential antimalarials from *Brucea javanica* fruits. *Planta Med.* 56: 649.
13. Gao, H. et al. 2011. Tumor cell selective cytotoxicity and apoptosis induction by an herbal preparation from *Brucea javanica. N. A. J. Med. Sci.* 4: 62–6.
14. Lau, F. Y. et al. 2005. Antiproliferative and apoptosis-inducing activity of *Brucea javanica* extract on human carcinoma cells. *Intl. J. Mol. Med.* 16: 1157–62.
15. Kim, I. H. et al. 2004. New quassinoids, javanicolides C and D and javanicosides B-F, from seeds of *Brucea javanica. J. Nat. Prods.* 67: 863–8.
16. Hall, I. H. et al. 1979. Antitumor agents XXXIV: Mechanism of action of bruceoside a and brusatol on nucleic acid metabolism of P-388 lymphocytic leukemia cells. *J. Pharm. Sci.* 68: 883–7.
17. Sakaki, T. et al. (a) 1986. Yadanzioside P, a new antileukemic quassinoid glycoside from *Brucea javanica* (L.) Merr with the 3-*O*-(β-D-glucopyranosyl) bruceantin structure. *Chem. Pharm. Bull.* 34: 4447–50; (b) 1986. Two new quassinoid glycosides, yadanziosides N and O isolated from seeds of *Brucea javanica* (L.) Merr. *Tetrahedron Lett.* 27: 593–6; (c) 1986. Structures of yadanziosides K, M, N, and O, new quassinoid glycosides from *Brucea javanica* (L.) Merr. *Bull. Chem. Soc. JP* 59: 3541–6.
18. Yang, Z. Q. et al. (a) 1997. Chemical studies of the active antitumor constituents from the fruit of *Brucea javanica* (L.) Merr (II). *Shenyang Yaoxueyuan Xuebao* 14: 46–7; (b) 1996. Chemical studies of the active antitumor components from the fruits of *Brucea javanica* (L.) *Tianran Chenwu yu Kaifa* 8: 35–9.
19. Takahashi, T. et al. (a) 1986. Antitumor quassinoids from *Brucea javanica. Jpn. Kokai Tokkyo Koho* JP 61197590 A 19860901; (b) 1986. Yadanziosides from *Brucea javanica* as antitumor and antiviral agents. *Jpn. Kokai Tokkyo Koho* JP 61065895 A 19860404; (c) 1986. New quassinoids from *Brucea javanica. Jpn. Kokai Tokkyo Koho* JP 61065896 A 19860404.
20. Yoshimura, S. et al. 1985. Isolation and structures of antileukemic bitter principles from Ya-dan-zi (*Brucea javanica* (L.) Merr. *Tennen Yuki Kagobutsu Toronkai Koen Yoshishu* 27: 513–20.
21. Liu, J. Q. et al. 2011. One new pregnane glycoside from the seeds of cultivated *Brucea javanica. Archiv. Pharm. Res.* 34: 1297–300.
22. Liu, J. H. et al. 2012. Bioactive quassinoids from the seeds of *Brucea javanica. J. Nat. Prod.* 75: 683–8
23. Lau, S. T. et al. 2009. Brucein D induces apoptosis in pancreatic adenocarcinoma cell line PANC-1 through the activation of p38-mitogen activated protein kinase. *Cancer Lett.* 281: 42–52.
24. Zhao, M. et al. 2011. Seven quassinoids from *Fructus bruceae* with cytotoxic effects on pancreatic adenocarcinoma cell lines. *Phytother. Res.* 25: 1796–800.
25. Anderson, M. M. et al. 1991. In vitro cytotoxicity of a series of quassinoids from *Brucea javanica* fruits against KB cells. *Planta Med.* 57: 62–4.
26. Pan, L. et al. 2009. Bioactivity-guided isolation of cytotoxic constituents of *Brucea javanica* collected in Vietnam. *Bioorg. Med. Chem.* 17: 2219–24.
27. Lee, K. et al. 1984. Brusatol and cleomiscosin-A, antileukemic principles from *Brucea javanica. J. Nat. Prod.* 47: 551–2.
28. Wang, R. et al. 2006. Traditional medicines used in differentiation therapy of myeloid leukemia. *Asian J. Traditional Med.* 1: 37–44.
29. Cuendet, M. et al. 2004. Brusatol-induced HL-60 cell differentiation involves NF-κB activation. *Cancer Lett.* 206: 43–50.
30. Li, X. et al. 1980. Studies on the anticancer principles in the seed of Yadanzi (*Brucea javanica*): III. Isolation and structural elucidation of bruceoside A. *Zhongcaoyao* 11: 530–2.
31. Ohnishi, S. et al. 1995. Bruceosides D, E, and F, three new cytotoxic quassinoid glucosides from *Brucea javanica. J. Nat. Prods.* 58: 1032–8.
32. Fukamiya, N. et al. 1992. Antitumor agents, 127. Bruceoside C, a new cytotoxic quassinoid glucoside, and related compounds from *Brucea javanica. J. Nat. Prod.* 55: 468–75.
33. Kim, J. A. et al. 2010. NF-κB inhibitors from *Brucea javanica* exhibiting intracellular effects on reactive oxygen species. *Anticancer Res.* 30: 3295–300.
34. Rahman, S. et al. 1999. Three new quassinoid derivatives and related compounds as antitumor promoters from *Brucea javanica. Bull. Chem. Soc. JP* 72: 751–6.
35. Su, B. N. et al. 2002. Bioactive constituents of the seeds of *Brucea javanica. Planta Med.* 68: 730–3.
36. Su, S. Y. et al. 1989. Treatment of lung cancer with brain metastasis using an intravenous drip of a 10% emulsion of *Brucea javanica* seminal oil. *Shiyong Zhongliuxue Zazhi* 3: 33.
37. Gao, W. et al. 1991. Inhibition of Javanica oil emulsion against bladder cancer in animal experiments and clinical applications. *Linchuan Miniao Waike Zazhi* 6: 129–31.
38. Pan, D. J. et al. 2007. Study on efficacy and safety of intraperitoneal catheter drainage combined with hydroxycamptothecin and seed oil of *Brucea javanica* in patients with malignant ascites. *Xiandai Zhongxiyi Jiehe Zazhi* 16: 4101–2.
39. Wang, F. L. et al. 2011. Prospective clinical studies at the efficacy of *Brucea javanica* oil, mitomycin and BCG for preventing postoperative relapse of superficial bladder cancer through perfusion. *Chinese-German J. Clinical Oncol.* 10: 228–31.
40. Jiang, A. Y. et al. 2012. Clinical observation of *Brucea javanica* injection combined with recombinant human interleukin-2 in treatment of lung cancer malignant pleural effusion. *Jianyan Yixue Yu Linchuang* 9: 2077–8.

9 Lin Mao Jiu 鱗毛蕨

Dryopteris ferns

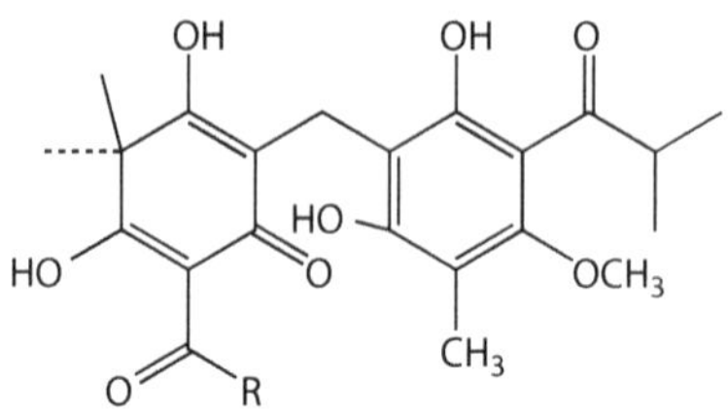

1. R = $-CH(CH_3)_2$
3. R = $-CH_2CH_3$

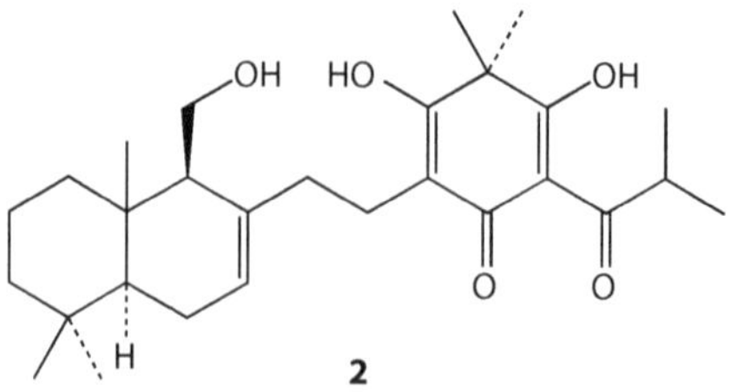

2

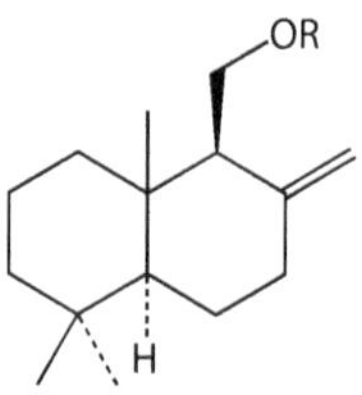

4. R = –H
5. R = –Ac

Herb Origination

There are several herbs originated from the plants of the Dryopteris genus in traditional Chinese medicine. Of them, Guang Zhong (貫衆 or *Dryopteris crassirhizoma*) is one of the most common ferns used in Chinese medicine, which was documented in the Chinese *Pharmacopedia* (1995 Edition). Its distribution is mainly in the northeast of Asia, and its rhizomes are collected in autumn and dried in the sun for folk medical application. *Dryopteris fragrans* termed *Xiang Lin Mao Jue* (香鱗毛蕨) in China is an herb in the north areas, which was reported to have an obvious cancer inhibitory property in recent years. It is primarily distributed in the cold north temperate zone, including Asia, Europe, and North America.

Antitumor Activities and Constituents

The ethanolic extract of *D. crassirhizoma* at a concentration of 100 μg/mL markedly suppressed the proliferation of human prostate carcinoma PC3 and PC3-MM2 cell lines and showed no cytotoxicity to normal spleen cells. It could effectively induce cell cycle arrest and apoptosis in the PC3-MM2 cells through extrinsic and intrinsic pathways, including the activation of caspase-3, caspase-8, caspase-9, BID, and PARP.[1] When combined with TRAIL, the extract exerted an additive effect in the inhibition of prostate cancer cells.[1] The treatment with the extract also resulted in the inhibitory effect against the viability of mouse neuroblastoma cells (Neuro-2) and against the growth of lung cancer cells with apoptosis promotion.[2,3]

Phloroglucinol Derivatives

Characteristic phloroglucinols are the bioactive constituents in most species of *Dryopteris*, exerting the anticancer activity on various transplantable neoplasms. A group of phloroglucinol derivatives, such as norflavaspidic acids, flavaspidic acids, albaspidins, deaspidins, paraaspidins and filixic acids, have been reported as the bioactive constituents of *D. crassirhizoma* that is largely responsible for the antitumor, antitumor-promoting, and antioxidant activities. In an *in vitro* assay, these phloroglucinol derivatives were able to restrain the tumor cell respiration and elicited the mitochondrial degeneration and swelling of P388 mouse leukemia cells.[4] Three phloroglucinol derivatives, aspidin-BB (**1**), dryofragin (**2**), and aspidin-PB (**3**), are the major ichthyotoxic agents isolated from *D. fragrans*, exhibiting strong antitumor activity against sarcoma 180, Lewis lung carcinoma, and HepA hepatoma cells *in vivo* with high security.[5] Aspidin-BB (**1**) also moderately inhibited the proliferation of eight human neoplastic cells such as HO-8910 (ovary), MCF-7 (breast), HeLa (cervix), PC3 (prostate), HCT-8 (colon), A549 (lung), HepG2 (liver), and CEM (T-lymphoblasts) cells *in vitro* (IC_{50}: 15.02–35.55 μM, in 72 h). Meanwhile, aspidin-BB (**1**) provoked the S phase arrest of HO-8910 cells through the upregulation of pRb, E2F1, CDK2, cyclin-E, and cyclin-A proteins, and it enhanced the apoptosis of HO-8910 cells through (1) the downregulation of Bcl-2 expression and increase of Bax expression to disintegrate the outer mitochondrial membrane, (2i) the release of cytochrome c to activate caspase-3, and (3) the cleavage of PARP in the nucleus.[6]

Similarly, dryofragin (**2**) could restrain the growth of human MCF-7 breast cancer cells (IC_{50}: 27.26 μM, 72 h) in time- and concentration-dependent manners and elicit the apoptosis via a ROS-mediated mitochondria-dependent pathway.[7,8] Aspidin-PB (**3**) was effective in the suppression of MCF-7 breast cancer cells and HepG2 hepatoma cells in a time- and a dose-dependent manner with IC_{50} value of 10.59 μM (72 h) in the HepG2 cells.[9,10] Aspidin-PB (**3**) was able to induce the apoptotic death of HepG2 cells. Block of PI3K/Akt/GSK3β signal pathway was found being a major apoptotic mechanism by aspidin-PB (**3**) in the HepG2 cells.[10] Aspidinol showed a moderate antiproliferative effect against A549 (lung) and MCF-7 (breast) human cancer cell lines (IC_{50}: 12.59 and 10.58 μM, respectively).[11]

Moreover, of the isolates from a whole plant of *D. fragrans*, five phloroglucinols (dryofragin, aspidin-AB, aspidin-BB, aspidin-PB, and aspidinol) exhibited a potent inhibitory effect against the activation of EBV-EA induced by a tumor promoter TPA, indicating these compounds possessing antitumor-promoting property. Aspidin-BB (**1**), as a stronger inhibitor on the EBV-EA activation, obviously retarded a two-stage carcinogenesis on mouse skin *in vivo*.[12] Two dimeric phlorophenones assigned as desaspidin and aspidin were the most active among the tested phloroglucinols. Both displayed a significant inhibitory effect on 7,12-dimethylbenz[a]anthracene (DMBA)-TPA that caused tumor promotion and two-stage mouse skin carcinogenesis *in vivo*.[13]

The summarization evidenced that the phloroglucinols are potential candidates for cancer prevention and treatment due to their broad antitumor spectrum, fewer side effects, high safety/reliability, and easy preparation.

Sesquiterpenoids

Two sesquiterpenoids, assigned as albicanol (**4**) and albicanyl acetate (**5**), were isolated from *D. fragrans*. Both showed a marked antitumor-promoting effect against the activation of EBV-EA induced by TPA. Albicanol (**4**) also significantly retarded the two-stage carcinogenesis on mouse skin *in vivo*[12] and moderately inhibited SMMC-7721 (liver), HeLa (cervix), PANC-1 (pancreas), and MCF-7 (breast) human cancer cell lines *in vitro*.[11,14]

Coumarins and Lignans

Three coumarines, assigned as esculetin, isoscopoletin, dryofracoumarin-A and two lignans assigned as *trans*- and *cis*-3-(3,4-dimethoxyphenyl)-4-[(E)-3,4-dimethoxystyryl]cyclohex-1-ene, were isolated from *D. fragrans*, showing a moderate antiproliferative effect against A549 (lung), MCF-7 (breast), and/or HepG2 (liver) human cancer cell lines *in vitro*. The IC_{50} values of esculetin and isoscopoletin were 2.73–10.15 μM and 4.76–8.58 μM in the tested three cell lines, whereas of dryofracoumarin-A was 6.56–10.14 μM in the A549 and MCF-7 cells. The highest inhibition on the MCF-7 and A549 cell lines was showed by esculetin (IC_{50}: 2.73 and 3.82 μM, respectively), and on the HepG2 cells was isoscopoletin (IC_{50}: 4.76 μM).[11]

Other Bioactivities

Some herbs of *Dryopteris* have been used as vermifuge, astringent, vulnerary, antiinflammatory, and antibacterial agents and internally used in the treatment of hemorrhage, uterine bleeding, and mumps. *Dryopteris fragrans* is used in the northeastern regions of China as an herb to remedy various skin diseases and arthritis, especially for the treatment of psoriasis and arthritis. The flavonoid component of *Dryopteris* is an inhibitor of acetylcholinesterase, and the isolated kaempferol glycosides are the inhibitors of HIV reverse transcriptase-associated DNA polymerase and ribonuclease-H activities.

References

1. Chang, S. H. et al. 2010. *Dryopteris crassirhizoma* has anticancer effects through both extrinsic and intrinsic apoptotic pathways and G0/G1 phase arrest in human prostate cancer cells. *J. Ethnopharmacol.* 130: 248–54.
2. Mazzio, E. A. et al. 2009. In vitro screening for the tumoricidal properties of international medicinal herbs. *Phytother. Res.* 23: 385–98.
3. Hwang, S. Y. et al. 2012. Crassirhizomae Rhizoma extracts for treating lung cancer. *Repub. Korean Kongkae Taeho Kongbo* KR 2012109780 A 20121009.
4. Xue, W. J. et al. 1987. Antitumor component of *Dryopteris crassirhizoma* on ultrastructure and cell respiration of P388 cells. *Chin. Pharmacol. Bull.* 3: 291–3.
5. Shen, Z. B. et al. 2007. Application of phloroglucinol compounds extracted from *Dryopteris fragrans* in preparation of antitumor agent. *Faming Zhuanli Shenqing* CN 101066261 A 20071107.
6. Sun, Y. et al. 2013. Aspidin BB, a phloroglucinol derivative, induces cell cycle arrest and apoptosis in human ovarian HO-8910 cells. *Chemico-Biol. Interactions* 204: 88–97.
7. Zhang, Y. et al. 2012. Dryofragin, a phloroglucinol derivative, induces apoptosis in human breast cancer MCF-7 cells through ROS-mediated mitochondrial pathway. *Chemico-Biol. Interactions* 199: 129–36.
8. Fu, Y. J. et al. 2013. Application of dryofragin from *Dryopteris fragrans* for producing antineoplastic drugs. *Faming Zhuanli Shenqing* CN 103371990 A 20131030.
9. Fu, Y. J. et al. 2013. Application of *Dryopteris fragrans*-derived aspidin PB in preparing antitumor drugs. *Faming Zhuanli Shenqing* CN 103191087 A 20130710.
10. Sun, Y. et al. 2013. Aspidin PB, a phloroglucinol derivative, induces apoptosis in human hepatocarcinoma HepG2 cells by modulating PI3K/Akt/GSK3β pathway. *Chemico-Biol. Interactions* 201: 1–8.
11. Zhao, D. D. et al. 2014. Compounds from *Dryopteris fragrans* (L.) *Schott* with cytotoxic activity. *Mol.* 19: 3345–55.
12. Ito, H. et al. 2000. Ichthyotoxic phloroglucinol derivatives from *Dryopteris fragrans* and their antitumor promoting activity. *Chem. Pharm. Bull.* 48: 1190–1195.
13. Kapadia, G. et al. 1996. Antitumor promoting activity of *Dryopteris phlorophenone* derivatives. *Cancer Lett.* 105: 161–5.
14. Wu, L. S. et al. 2013. Cytotoxic metabolites from *Perenniporia tephropora*, an endophytic fungus from *Taxus chinensis* var. *mairei*. *Applied Microbiol. Biotechnol.* 97: 305–15.

10 Yu Xin Cao 魚腥草

Fishwort or Lizard tail

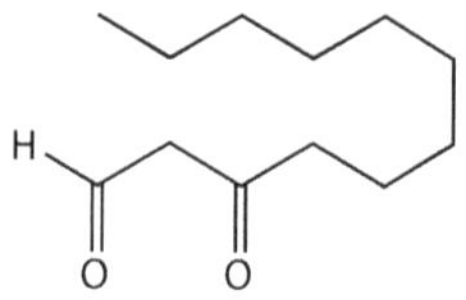

Herb Origination

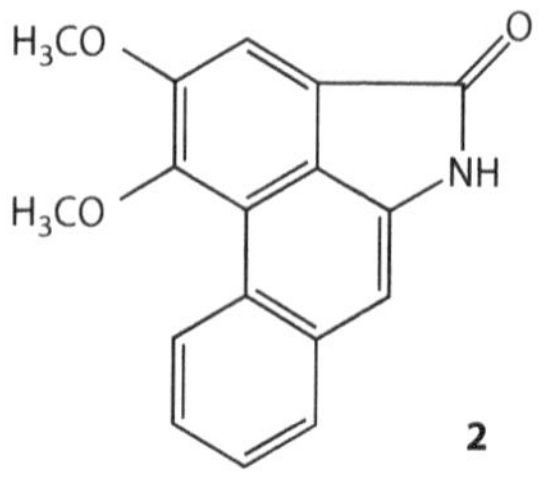

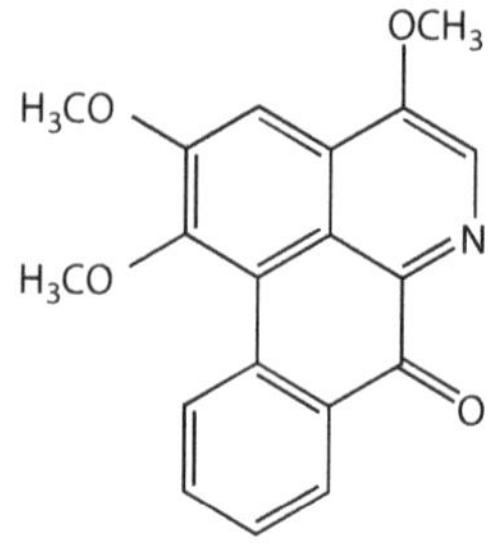

The herb Yu Xin Cao (Fishwort) originates from an herbaceous Saururaceae plant *Houttuynia cordata*. This perennial plant has a broad native range, from Nepal and India, through southern China and Indochina to Korea and Japan, and south via Thailand and Vietnam to Java of Indonesia. It has been introduced to Australia, New Zealand, some Pacific islands, and south of North America. The plant grows in moist and shady places, but it is frequently considered a weed. The whole plant is used fresh as an herb or an edible wild vegetable, and it also is collected in summer and autumn and dried in the sun for medical practice.

Antitumor Constituents and Activities

Yu Xin Cao has been prescribed in herbal formulae for the treatment of malignant diseases, showing anticancer and immunoimproving benefits. *In vitro* and *in vivo* experiments revealed that Yu Xin Cao is one of the contributors for cancer therapies. Its ethanolic extract (HCT-E) could restrain the cell viability and the proliferation of various human carcinoma cell lines such as A549 (lung), HT-29 (colon), HL-60, Jurkat, and U937 (leukemia) and primary colorectal cancer cells derived from patients, as well as murine L1210 leukemia cells.[1–5] The antileukemia activity of HCT-E was also established in a mouse model implanted with L1210 cells with very meager toxicity on normal lymphocytes. The injection of HCT-E on an acupuncture point could prevent the increase of the mass weight of B16 melanoma in mice.[6] Six fractions derived from HCT-E by a column chromatography were cytotoxic to human Molt-4 lymphoblastic leukemia cells in a dose-dependent manner, and its fraction-4 exerted the inhibitory and apoptotic effects on the Molt-4 cells through an endoplasmic reticulum (ER) stress pathway.[7] A methanolic extract derived from *H. cordata* root in a concentration of 100 μg/mL displayed marked protective effects against hydrogen peroxide-induced DNA damage in the HepG2 cells, indicating that the plant root extract acted as an antioxidant to exert the anticarcinogenic properties.[8] When orally administrated, its methanolic extract (HCT-M) suppressed the growth of L1210 cells and prolonged the life duration by 47.8%.[9] Hot water extracts prepared from *H. cordata* (HCWE) restrained the proliferation of five leukemia cell lines (L1210, U937, K562, Raji, and P3HR1) *in vitro*.[10] The effective components, which were volatile oil, ethyl acetate fraction, and ethanol fraction, have been patented for the antitumor activity against human neoplastic cell lines such as HepG2 hepatoma, A549 lung carcinoma, MCF-7 breast adenocarcinoma, and Raji lymphoma.[11]

The investigations disclosed that the antitumor effect of Yu Xin Cao mostly correlated with the induction of apoptotic death and/or cell cycle arrest. The apoptosis-eliciting mechanisms were found to be through distinctive pathways dependent on the different tumor cells, for instance, (1) through the augmentation of Fas/CD95 protein level and the activation of p27 and caspase-8 and caspase-3 then led the A549 cells to apoptosis[1]; (2) through a mitochondrial-dependent pathway, i.e., the decline of Bax/Bcl-2 ratio, the increase of ROS generation, the loss of mitochondria membrane potential, the release of cytochrome c, Apaf-1, and apoptosis-inducing factor (AIF) from the mitochondria, and the increase of caspase-9 and caspase-3 activities, promoting HT-29 cell apoptotic death[2]; and (3) through the harm of mitochondrial membrane potential, the release of cytochrome c, the activation of procaspase-9 and caspase-3, and the cleavage of PARP, stimulated by HL-60 cell apoptosis.[4] Other evidences showed that the cell cycle G_0/G_1 arrest of A549 cells caused by HCT-E was related to the enhancement of p27 activity and the reduction of the functions of cyclin-D1, cyclin-A, CDK-4, and CDK-2.[1]

Additionally, the fermentation of Yu Xin Cao was reported to be able to potentiate antitumor potency, and the fermented herb ethanolic extract exerted a greater effect than the nonfermented extract in the inhibition of human leukemia cells. This fermented extract was more cytotoxic to HL-60 cells than to Molt-4 cells and was more active to elicit the leukemia cell apoptosis via oxidative stress-provoked mitochondrial pathway.[12]

Antitumor Activities

Houttuynin

Houttuynin (**1**) is a unique and bioactive constituent derived from fresh *H. cordata*, but it is unstable. For this reason, houttuynin is normally converted to a stable sodium houttuyfonate, which is designated as houttuyninum. An *in vitro* experiment showed that houttuyninum dose dependently inhibited the phosphorylation of HER2/neu tyrosine kinase, which in turn retarded both pathways of ERK1/2 and PI3K/AKT, resulting in the inhibitory effect against the growth of HER2/neu overexpressed MDA-MB-453 breast cancer cells, but there was no such effect on EGFR-overexpressed MDA-MB-468 breast cancer cells. Similarly, the administration of houttuyninum to nude mice significantly diminished the phosphorylated HER2 levels in breast cancer xenograft and reduced the volume of BT474 human breast and N87 human gastric cancer xenografts, whose both breast cancers showed overexpressed HER2/neu. The discoveries demonstrated the therapeutic value of houttuyninum in the treatment of malignant tumor diseases, especially with overexpression of HER2/neu.[13]

Flavonoids

The total flavonoid component extracted from the leaves of *H. cordata* exhibited a cytotoxic activity on sarcoma 180 cells and exerted great inhibition against the growth of ascites sarcoma 180 in a mouse model.[14] Also, the flavonoids suppressed the proliferation of human HL-60 leukemia cells and mouse B16BL6 melanoma cells and enhanced the cell apoptotic death in an *in vitro* assay. Its IC_{50} values were 0.122 μg/mL in B16-BL6 cells and 0.410 μg/mL in HL-60 cells.[15] Therefore, these results recommended that the Yu Xin Cao flavonoids may be a potential supplement in cancer prevention and therapy.

Alkaloids

The bioassay-guided fractionation of the Yu Xin Cao (aerial part) methanolic extract led to the isolation of six bioactive alkaloids identified as aristolactam-B (**2**), piperolactam-A, aristolactam-A, cepharadione-B, norcepharadione-B, and splendidine (**3**). The alkaloids (except for norcepharadione-B) exhibited marked to moderate cytotoxicity against XF498 (brain), A549 (lung), SKOV-3 (ovary), SK-MEL-2 (skin), and HCT-15 (colon) human carcinoma cell lines *in vitro* (IC_{50}: 0.84–47.5 μg/mL). Of these active alkaloids, splendidine (**3**) and aristolactam-B (**2**) were two greater inhibitors against the proliferation of all five tested carcinoma cell lines (IC_{50}: 1.4–5.8 μg/mL and 0.84–23.2 μg/mL, respectively). The strongest cytotoxicity in the assay was achieved by aristolactam-B (**2**) on XF498 cells (IC_{50}: 0.84 μg/mL).[16] The results provided positive evidences to support both splendidine (**3**) and aristolactam-B (**2**) going to *in vivo* investigation for further development.

Other Bioactivities

The herb Yu Xin Cao is commonly used as an antiinflammatory, antiallergic, antibacterial, and antiviral herbal medicine in China and other Asian countries. Hence, Yu Xin Cao injection is often used to relieve abnormal lung symptoms, infectious disease, refractory hemoptysis, and malignant pleural effusion in China. Pharmacological studies have proven that Yu Xin Cao possesses analgesic, antioxidant, heat-relieving, diuretic, immunoregulating, antisensitive, asthma-relieving, cough-relieving, antiobesity, antihypertensive, and antimicrobial properties. Yu Xin Cao injection exerted a direct inhibitory activity against pseudorabies, herpes virus, severe acute respiratory syndrome, and pneumonia *in vitro*.[17]

References

1. Chen, Y. F. et al. 2013. *Houttuynia cordata Thunb* extract modulates G_0/G_1 arrest and Fas/CD95-mediated death receptor apoptotic cell death in human lung cancer A549 cells. *J. Biomed. Sci.* 20: 18.
2. Tang, Y. J. et al. 2009. *Houttuynia cordata Thunb* extract induces apoptosis through mitochondrial-dependent pathway in HT-29 human colon adenocarcinoma cells. *Oncol. Reports* 22: 1051–6.
3. Pawinwongchai, J. et al. 2011. Antileukemic activity of *Houttuynia cordata Thunb* extracts in Jurkat and U937 human leukemic cells. *J. Chem. Pharm. Res.* 3: 204–12.
4. Kwon, K. B. et al. 2003. Herba houttuyniae extract induces apoptotic death of human promyelocytic leukemia cells via caspase activation accompanied by dissipation of mitochondrial membrane potential and cytochrome c release. *Experim. Mol. Med.* 35: 91–7.
5. Lai, K. C. et al. 2010. *Houttuynia cordata Thunb* extract inhibits cell growth and induces apoptosis in human primary colorectal cancer cells. *Anticancer Res.* 30: 3549–56.
6. Bae, W. et al. 2001. Experimental study on the effect of houttuyniae herbal accupuncture on the growth of melanoma B16 in mice. *Korean Acupuncture Moxibustion J.* 18: 186–201.
7. Prommaban, A. et al. 2012. *Houttuynia cordata Thunb* fraction induces human leukemic Molt-4 cell apoptosis through the endoplasmic reticulum stress pathway. *Asian Pac. J. Cancer Prev.* 13: 1977–81.
8. Hah, D. S. et al. 2007. Evaluation of protective effects of *Houttuynia cordata* on H_2O_2-induced oxidative DNA damage using an alkaline comet assay in human HepG2 cells. *J. Toxicol. Public Health* 23: 25–31.
9. Ha, H. K. et al. 2004. Anticancer effect of *Houttuynia cordata* extract on cancered ICR mouse and L1210 cells with changes of SOD and GPx activities. *Yakhak Hoechi* 48: 219–25.
10. Chang, J. S. et al. 2001. Antileukemic activity of *Bidens pilosa* L. var.*fminor (Blume) Sherff* and *Houttuynia cordata Thunb. Am. J. Chin. Med.* 29: 303–12.
11. Zhang, Z. L. et al. 2013. Extraction of *Houttuynia cordata* effective fractions with antitumor activity. *Faming Zhuanli Shenqing* CN 103055006 A 20130424.
12. Banjerdpongchai, R. et al. 2011. Ethanolic extract of fermented *Houttuynia cordata Thunb* induces human leukemic HL-60 and Molt-4 cell apoptosis via oxidative stress and a mitochondrial pathway. *Asian Pac. J. Cancer Prev.* 12: 2871–4.
13. Zhou, N. N. et al. 2012. Houttuyninum, an active constituent of Chinese herbal medicine, inhibits phosphorylation of HER2/neu receptor tyrosine kinase and the tumor growth of HER2/neu-overexpressing cancer cells. *Life Sci.* 90: 770–5.
14. Hoang, T. H. et al. 2003. Antineoplastic activity of flavonoid components extracted from leaves of *Houttuynia cordata Thunb* in Vietnam. *Tap Chi Duoc Hoc* (10): 9–10.
15. Fan, H. W. et al. 2008. Experimental investigation for antitumor activity of flavonoid from the *Houttuynia cordata Thunb* in vitro. *Zhongguo Yiyuan Yaoxue Zazhi* 28: 528–31.
16. Kim, S. K. et al. 2001. Cytotoxic alkaloids from *Houttuynia cordata. Archiv. Pharm. Res.* 24: 518–21.
17. Fu, J. G. et al. 1013. *Houttuynia cordata Thunb*: A review of phytochemistry and pharmacology and quality control. *Chin. Med.* 4: 101–23.

11 Jin Yin Hua 金銀花

Honeysuckle flower

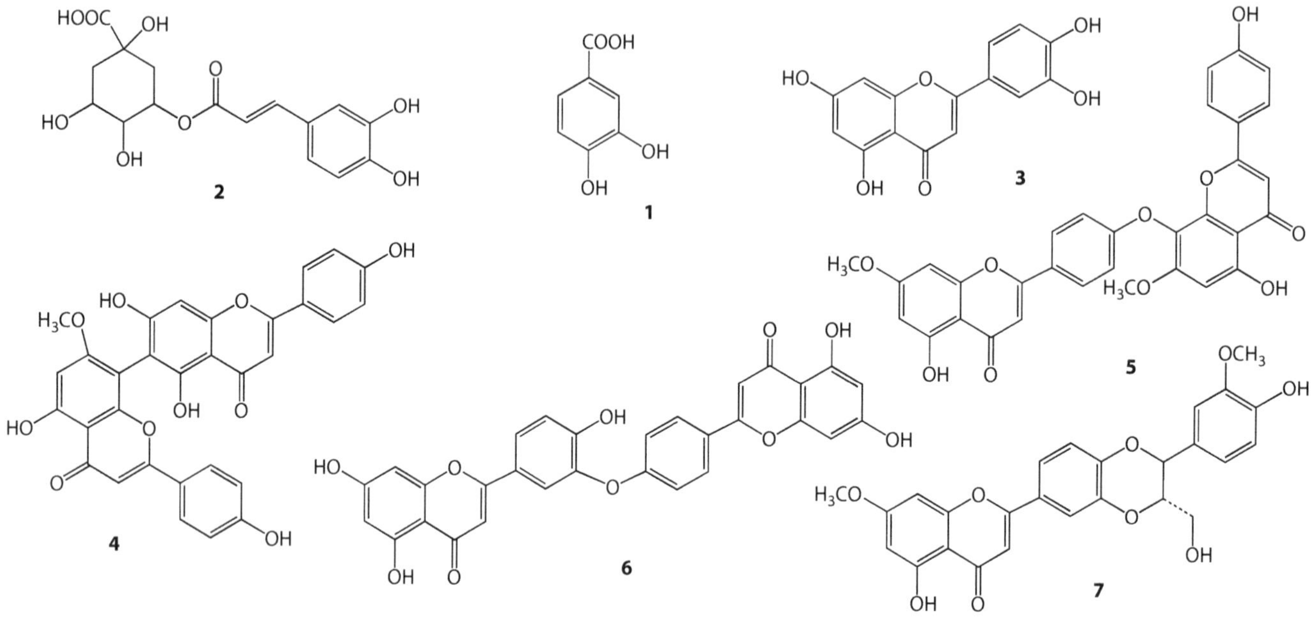

Herb Origination

The herb Jin Yin Hua (Honeysuckle flower) originated from the flower buds of four Caprifoliaceae plants, *Lonicera japonica*, *Lonicera confusa*, *Lonicera fulvotomentosa*, and *Lonicera hypoglauca*. The flower buds must be collected in the early summer before flowering to obtain a higher quality of the herb and dried in the shade for folk medical use.

Antitumor Activities and Constituents

The water and alcoholic extracts of Jin Yin Hua demonstrated a marked cytotoxic effect against the growth of mouse sarcoma 180, Ehrlich ascites cancer cells, and several human carcinoma cells including HepG2 hapetoma *in vitro*.[1,2] Ninety-five percent ethanolic extract of Jin Yin Hua at a concentration range of 50–150 μg/mL with 0.4–1.2 J/cm^2 light dose displayed significant photocytotoxicity on human CH27 lung squamous cancer cells. The photodynamic therapeutic effect (PDT) of Jin Yin Hua extract in CH27 cells was accompanied by the induction of caspase-3-independent apoptotic death via the activation of AIF and p38-associated pathway, as well as the distribution of HSP27.[3]

Volatile Components

The volatiles of Jin Yin Hua cultivated in Egypt contain a major constituent assigned as linalool and others (such as 4-terpineol, nerolidol, *cis*-jasmone, *cis*-3-hexenyl tiglate, *trans*-linalool oxide and methyl palmitate). Both of its floral absolute volatiles (FAV) and hydrodistilled/hexane-extracted volatiles (HHV) have capabilities to inhibit the proliferation of human tumor cells *in vitro*. HHV displayed cytotoxicity against HepG2 hepatoma cells (IC_{50}: 7.58 μg/mL), while FAV had a notable cytotoxic effect toward U251 glioma cells (IC_{50}: 7.92 μg/mL). The antitumor activity on the U251 cell lines was comparable to that of an anticancer drug cisplatin (IC_{50}: 8.66 μg/mL).[4]

Polyphenolic Components

The major antitumor constituents in Jin Yin Hua should be a group of polyphenolic components. The polyphenolic extract inhibited the viability of HepG2 hepatoma cells dose dependent concomitant with the induction of the cell cycle arrest at G2/M transition and apoptosis. After the treatment with the polyphenolic extract, the expressions of CDK1, CDC25C, cyclin-B1, PARP, and procaspase-3 and procaspase-9 were reduced; PI3K/Akt was inhibited, and the MAPKs were activated for the antihepatoma effect.[5] Two phenols, protocatechuic acid (**1**) and chlorogenic acid (**2**) isolated from Jin Yin Hua, could effectively kill HepG2 hepatoma cells at a concentration of 100 μmol/L. Protocatechuic acid (**1**) also promoted the JNK-dependent apoptosis of the HepG2 cells during its suppressive action.[6]

Flavonoids

From the extracts, a group of bioactive flavonoids were separated and subjected to bioassays. Many flavonoids derived from Jin Yin Hua were proven to possess anticancer, antioxidant, and prooxidant properties. Its anticancer activity might correlate to its behavior as either an antioxidant or a prooxidant. Luteolin (**3**), an active flavonoid in Jin Yin Hua, exerted inhibitory effects against the growth of carcinoma cell lines. Luteolin (**3**) at a concentration of 100 μmol/L was effective in the suppression of human HepG2 hepatoma cells.[6] By the activation of antioxidant enzymes such as superoxide dismutase and catalase, luteolin (**3**) induced the apoptosis of human lung carcinoma CH27 cells; however, the mechanism did not relate to the production of ROS and the disruption of the mitochondrial membrane potential.[7] In addition, luteolin (**3**) exhibited a significant ability to block the activations of NF-κB, ERK1/2, and JNK1/2 and to suppress the expressions of TNFα, IL-8, IL-6, GM-CSF, and COX-2, via the decline of intracellular Ca^{2+} levels. By the mechanism-related interactions, luteolin (**3**) exerted an obvious inhibition against inflammation and carcinogenesis.[8]

Biflavonoids

Three biflavonoids, 7″-methylagathisflavone (**4**), 7,7″-dimethyllanaraflavone (**5**), and ochnaflavone (**6**), were isolated from the caulis of a Jin Yin Hua plant to have noticeable antiproliferative benefits against a small panel of human tumor cell lines. The inhibitory activity of 7″-methylagathisflavone (**4**) was shown against HT-29 (colon), NCl-H460 (lung), MCF-7 (breast), OVCAR-3 (ovary), and RXF-393 (renal) human cancer cell lines (IC_{50}: 4.38–5.58 μg/mL), whereas 7,7″-dimethyllanaraflavone (**5**) displayed a weak suppressive effect against the proliferation of NCI-H460, MCF-7, and OVCAR-3 cell lines (IC_{50}: 1.77–3.59 mg/mL).[9] In the *in vitro* treatment of human HCT-15 colon cancer cells, ochnaflavone (**6**) inhibited the proliferation together with induction of G2/M cell cycle arrest and apoptotic death (IC_{50}: 4.1 μM). The mechanism was found to correlate with the modulation of cell cycle-regulating protein expression (including CDC2-Tyr15, cyclin-A, cyclin-B1, and cyclin-E); the activation of caspase-3, caspase-8, and caspase-9; and the cleavage of PARP.[10] The marked antiproliferative activities of ochnaflavone (**6**) were also confirmed in the treatment of blood cancers such as leukemia and lymphoma.[11]

Lignan

Hydnocarpin (**7**), a lignin isolated from the aerial parts of the *L. japonica* plant, was found as a potential inhibitor for Wnt/β-catenin signalings. Hydnocarpin (**7**) demonstrated a moderate antiproliferative activity against human SW480 colon cancer cells (IC_{50}: 20.3 μM), which effect was mediated by black of Wnt/β-catenin-mediated signaling pathway. Also, the increase of axin interaction might be additionally involved in the inhibitory effect.[12]

Polysaccharides

A polysaccharide component isolated from Jin Yin Hua was evaluated in an *in vivo* model with sarcoma 180, resulting in 23.95% and 30.02% tumor growth inhibitions in its middle and high doses, respectively. The antitumor property was found to be related to the regulation of Bcl-2/Bax-involved apoptosis pathway and the promotion of TNFα. In a high dose of polysaccharides, the immune function could be concurrently improved.[13]

Other Bioactivities

The herb Jin Yin Hua (Honeysuckle flower) is a commonly used folk medicinal herb in East Asian countries for clinical treatment of fever, influenza, boils, carbuncle, sore throat, dysentery, urinary disorders, pneumonia, breast infections, and many other infections. Pharmacological studies showed the herb Jin Yin Hua possesses multiple biological functions such as antioxidant, anti-inflammatory, antiatherogenic, hypolipidemic, hepatoprotective, antipyretic, antihypertensive, antifungal, antiviral, and antibacterial properties besides anticancer. Jin Yin Hua is also able to potentiate the ability of leukocyte.

References

1. The First Hospital of Chinese Army 245 (a) 1973. *Technol. News* (3): 41; (b) 1999. *Chinese Materia Medica*. Vol. 7, 7–6568, 533, Shanghai Science and Technology Press, Shanghai, China.
2. Phan, M. G. et al. 2002. Phytochemical investigation and study on cytotoxic and antimicrobial activities of *Lonicera japonica Thunb*, Caprifoliaceae, of Vietnam. *Tap Chi Hoa Hoc* 40: 103–7.
3. Leung, H. W. C. et al. 2008. P38-associated pathway involvement in apoptosis induced by photo-dynamic therapy with *Lonicera japonica* in human lung squamous carcinoma CH27 cells. *Food Chem. Toxicol.* 46: 3389–400.
4. El-Kashoury, E. A. et al. 2007. Antitumor volatile constituents from the flowers of *Lonicera japonica Thunb* cultivated in Egypt. *Egyp. J. Biomed. Sci.* 23: 135–45.
5. Park, H. S. et al. 2012. Polyphenolic extract isolated from Korean *Lonicera japonica Thunb* induce G2/M cell cycle arrest and apoptosis in HepG2 cells: Involvements of PI3K/Akt and MAPKs. *Food Chem. Toxicol.* 50: 2407–16.
6. Yip, E. C. H. et al. 2006. Protocatechuic acid induces cell death in HepG2 hepatocellular carcinoma cells through a c-Jun N-terminal kinase-dependent mechanism. *Cell Biol. Toxicol.* 22: 293–302.
7. Leung, W. C. et al. 2006. Antioxidant enzymes activity involvement in luteolin-induced human lung squamous carcinoma CH27 cell apoptosis. *Eur. J. Pharmacol.* 534: 12–8.
8. Kang, O. H. et al. 2010. Luteolin isolated from the flowers of *Lonicera japonica* suppresses inflammatory mediator release by blocking NF-κB and MAPKs activation pathways in HMC-1 cells. *Mol.* 15: 385–98.
9. Pradhan, D. et al. 2009. Anticancer activity of biflavonoids from *Lonicera japonica* and *Benincasa hispida* on human cancer cell lines. *J. Pharmacy Res.* 2: 983–5.
10. Kang, Y. J. et al. 2009. Ochnaflavone, a natural biflavonoid, induces cell cycle arrest and apoptosis in HCT-15 human colon cancer cells. *Biomol. Therap.* 17: 282–7.
11. Kang, S. S. et al. 1996. Anticancer agents of biflavonoids from *Ginkgo biloba* and *Lonicera japonica*. *Repub. Korea* KR 93-1152, 19930129.
12. Lee, M. A. et al. 2013. Anti-proliferative activity of hydnocarpin, a natural lignan, is associated with the suppression of Wnt/β-catenin signaling pathway in colon cancer cells. *Bioorg. Med. Chem. Lett.* 23: 5511–4.
13. Liu, Y. G. et al. 2012. Inhibitory effect and mechanism of polysaccharide from *Lonicera japonica* on mice bearing S180 sarcoma. *Zhongliuxue Zazhi* 18: 584–7.

12 Bei Dou Gen 北豆根

Asian moonseed

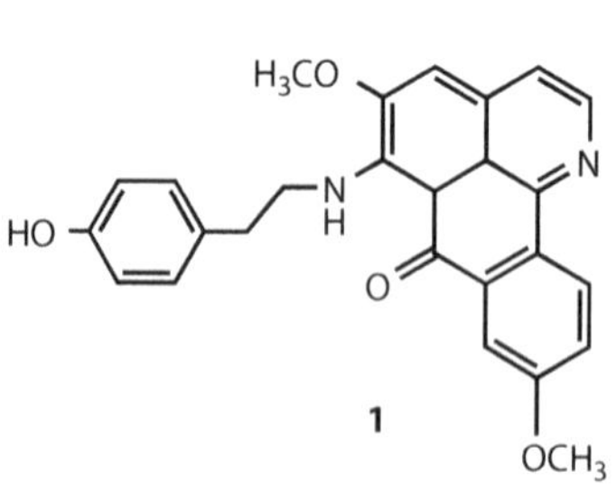

Herb Origination

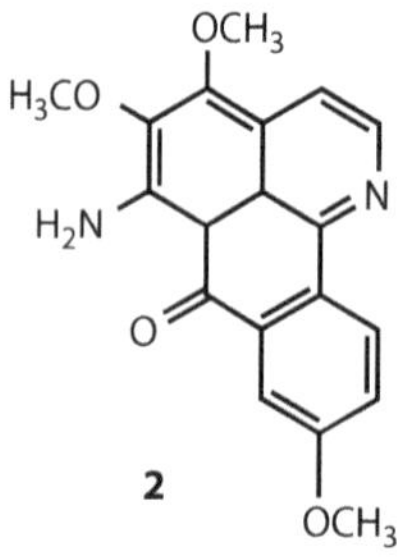

The herb Bei Dou Gen (Asian moonseed) is the dried rhizomes of a Menispermaceae plant *Menispermum dauricum*. The plant is largely distributed in the north and east regions of China, Korea, Japan, and south of far east of Russia. The rhizomes are generally collected in spring and autumn and dried in the sunlight for Chinese medical treatment.

Antitumor Constituents and Activities

Alkaloids

The ethanolic extract of Bei Dou Gen and its phenolic alkaloid components (phenolic alkaloids of *Menispermum dauricum* [PAMD]) demonstrated a marked antineoplastic activity.[1] The *in vitro* treatment with PAMD obviously restrained the proliferation of human PC3 (prostate) and BT5637 (bladder) cancer cell lines (IC_{50}: 7.51 and 9.93 μg/mL, respectively). In a concentration of 5 μg/mL, the inhibitory rates of PAMD on the PC3 and BT5637 cells were 42.38% and 43.53%, respectively.[2] The treatment with 10–160 μg/mL of PAMD for 24 and 48 h suppressed the proliferation of MGC-803 gastric cancer cells; 20–80 μg/mL of PAMD for 24 and 48 h elicited the MGC-803 cells at S stage arrest and apoptosis and significantly inhibited the expressions of EGFR and HER-2.[3] PAMD, by subcutaneous heterotopic transplantation, remarkably restrained the growth of human BXPC-3 pancreatic carcinoma in nude mice with 34.91–52.83% inhibitory ratio, whose effect was found to correlate with the induction of (1) tumor cell apoptosis by affecting the expression of genes related to apoptosis such as the downregulation of DPC4 and K-ras expressions, (2) antiangiogenesis via the reduction of basic fibroblast growth factor (bFGF) and VEGF expression levels to block the signal transmission of TGTβ, (3) antimetastasis by decreasing MMP-2 and MMP-3 contents in the BXPC-3 tumor tissues, and (4) reduction of the contents of inducible NO synthase (iNOS), IL-1, and TNFα in the peripheral blood of BXPC-3 tumor-bearing mice,[4–11] indicating that PAMD contributed multiple activities on the pancreatic cancer, such as growth/proliferative inhibition, apoptosis-induction, abd angiogenesis- and metastasis-suppression as well as immunomodulation. Likewise, PAMD treatment was able to elicit G0/G1 cell cycle arrest and apoptosis of human K562 leukecythemia cells, thereby exerting the antileukemia effect.[12] PAMD also demonstrated an obvious antiproliferative effect against human SGC-7901 gastric carcinoma cells in a time- and a concentration-dependent manner (IC_{50}: 7.47 μg/mL in 24 h and 16.43 μg/mL in 48 h).[13]

Two oxoisoaporphine alkaloids, daurioxoisoporphine-A (**1**) and daurioxoisoporphine-B (**2**), were isolated from the ethanolic extract. They obviously suppressed the growth of human MCF-7 breast carcinoma cells *in vitro* with IC_{50} values of 3.0 and 6.2 μM, respectively, whose effects were more potent than that of etoposide (a therapeutic agent) by two to four times. But their antigrowth activities were less than those of etoposide in human HL-60 leukemia and A549 lung cancer cell lines and mouse P388 leukemia cells *in vitro*. The IC_{50} values of daurioxoisoporphine-A (**1**) and daurioxoisoporphine-B (**2**) were 8.8 and 9.6 μM in the A549 cells, respectively.[14]

Polysaccharides

Three antitumor active polysaccharibe components were purified from the rhizomes of *M. dauricum*. Water-soluble *Menispermum dauricum* polysaccharide (WMDP) is a homogeneous and water-soluble polysaccharide (average molecular weight: 3.5×10^4 Da), which was composed of xylose, glucose, galactose, rhamnose, arabinose, and mannose in a ratio of 1.05:2.45:2.13:1.29:1.63:1.45. In an *in vitro* model, WMDP obviously inhibited the proliferation and the DNA synthesis of human SKOV3 ovarian carcinoma cells in a concentration-dependent manner. The apoptotic death of the SKOV3 cells was promoted by WMDP through ROS productive stimulation, NF-κB inactivation, and GSH depletion.[15] MDP-A1 and MDP-A2 were two other acidic polysaccharides isolated from the herb and their apparent molecular weights were 9.1×10^4 Da and 5.8×10^4 Da, respectively. Both contain galactose, glucose, mannose, arabinose, glucuronic acid, and galacturonic acid but with different molar ratios. MDP-A1 and MDP-A2 were able to inhibit the proliferation of SKOV3 cells *in vitro* and *in vivo* in a bell-shaped concentration-dependent manner. The treatment with either MDP-A1 or MDP-A2 also significantly promoted the activities of caspase-3 and caspase-8, thereby significantly amplifying the number of apoptotic cells.[16] Consequently, the scientific data established that the Bei Dou Gen polysaccharides may serve as a supplement for cancer treatment and prevention.

Other Bioactivities

The principal component in Bei Dou Gen is dauricine, whose biological activities were proven by pharmacological studies to display hypertensive, antiarrhythmia, antithrombotic, antiinflammatory, antithrombocyte-agglutinative, analgesic, cough-relieving and expectorant, muscle-relaxing, antibacterial, and local paralytic effects.

References

1. Chen, C. F. et al. 1992. Mouse lymphocytic leukemia P388 for screening antitumor agents from crude plant extracts and fermentation broth. *Zhonghua Yaoxue Zazhi* 44: 381–8.
2. Su, Y. M. et al. 2007. Effects of PAMD on the proliferation of human tumor cells PC-3 and BT5637. *Harbin Yike Daxue Xuebao* 41: 129–31.
3. Liu, H. Y. et al. 2014. Influences of *Menispermum dauricum* phenolic alkaloids on EGFR and HER-2 expressions and proliferation of human gastric cancer MGC-803 cells. *Zhongyaocai* 37: 1654–7.

4. Yin, R. et al. 2009. Effect of PAMD on BXPC-3 tumor-bearing mice cell apoptosis gene p53 expression. *Zhongyiyao Xuebao* 37: 35–7.
5. Wen, X. Y. et al. 2009. Inhibitory effect of phenolic alkaloids of *Menispermum dauricum* on the bxpc-3 tumor and its effect on iNOS content in tumor-bearing mice. *Zhongguo Yaofang* 20: 1370–2.
6. Jiao, G. Y. et al. 2009. The inhibitive effect of PAMD on BXPC-3 tumor model and study the effect of content of IL-1 in peripheral blood of tumor-bearing mice. *Xibei Yaoxue Zazhi* 24: 194–5.
7. Su, Y. M. et al. (a) 2010. Effects of phenolic alkaloids from menispermum dauricum on tumor inhibitory and expression of VEGF in BXPC-3 nude mice. *J. Chendu Med. College* 5: 25–7; (b) 2009. Effects of phenolic alkaloids from *Menispermum dauricum* on tumor inhibitory and expression of bFGF in BxPC-3 nude mice. *J. Chendu Med. College* 4: 245–7.
8. Su, Y. M. et al. (a) 2010. The influence of PAMD on the content of MMP-2 in BXPC-3 tumour tissues. *J. Chendu Med. College* 5: 113–5; (b) 2010. The influence of PAMD on the content of MMP-9 in BXPC-3 tumour tissues. *Acta Chin. Med. Pharmacol.* 38: 33–4.
9. Wang, J. M. et al. 2010. Effects of PAMD on the DPC4 expression in BXPC-3 tumour tissues. *Acta Chin. Med. Pharmacol.* 38: 27–9.
10. Feng, D. Z. et al. 2010. Bats gregory examined on major metropolises in the pancreas tissue alkaline K-ras protein expression. *Inform. on Tradit. Chin. Med.* 27: 112–4.
11. Men, D. et al. 2010. Effects of phenolic alkaloids from menispermum dauricum on tumor inhibitory and TNFα content in peripheral blood in BXPC-3 nude mice. *Inform. on Tradit. Chin. Med.* 27: 29–31.
12. Su, Y. M. et al. 2008. Effect of PAMD on the proliferation of K562 and BXPC-3 cells. *J. Gansu College TCM.* 25: 1–4.
13. Zhang, H. F. et al. 2013. Experimental study of phenolic alkaloids of *Menispermum dauricum* on proliferation of human gastric cancer cell line SGC-7901. *Practice Oncol. J.* 27: 116–9.
14. Yu, B. W. et al. 2001. Cytotoxic oxoisoaporphine alkaloids from *Menispermum dauricum. J. Nat. Prod.* 64: 968–70.
15. Lin, M. et al. 2013. Characterization and antitumor activities of a polysaccharide from the rhizoma of *Menispermum dauricum. Intl. J. Biol. Macromol.* 53: 72–6.
16. Lin, M. et al. 2013. Anti-ovarian cancer potential of two acidic polysaccharides from the rhizoma of *Menispermum dauricum. Carbohydrate Polymers* 92: 2212–7.

13 She She Cao 蛇舌草

Spreading hedyotis

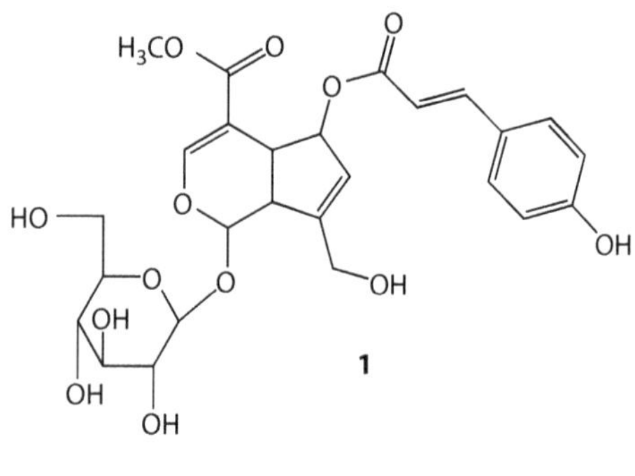

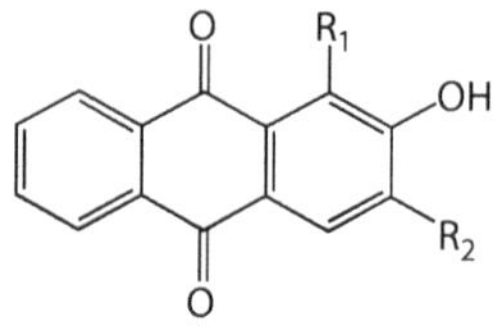

3. $R_1 = -OCH_3, R_2 = -H$
4. $R_1 = -H, R_2 = -CH_3$

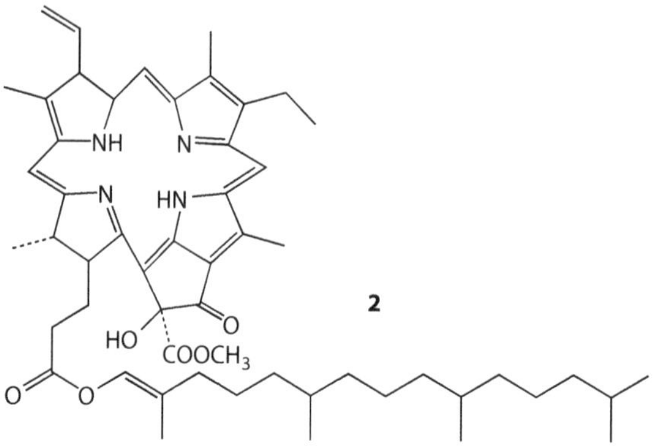

Herb Origination

The herb She She Cao (Spreading hedyotis) is the whole plant of a Rubiaceae plant *Oldenlandia diffusa* (= *Hedyotis diffusa*). This herbaceous plant is broadly distributed in the southern area of China in moist fields, as well as South Japan, South Korea, and Southern Asian countries. The herb is normally collected in summer and autumn and dried in the sun for Chinese folk medicinal use. The herb is applied fresh as well.

Antitumor Activities

She She Cao is one of the herbs most commonly used in Chinese folk medicine for treating carcinogenesis and carcinoma in patients.[1] Pharmacological approaches demonstrated that the aqueous extract of She She Cao markedly suppressed the proliferation of all seven human carcinoma cells (A549, C-33A, MCF-7, Ln-Cap, Tsu-Pr1, MDA-MB-453, DU-145) *in vitro* (IC_{50}: 7–25 mg (raw material)/mL, in 48 h).[2] The oral gavage of the aqueous extract to tumor-bearing mice in a daily dose of 5 g/kg (raw material/body weight) for ~12 days effectively increased the apoptosis of mouse B16-F10 melanoma cells and retarded the lung metastasis of B16-F10 cells by 70%, whereas oral feeding of the She She Cao extract (4 mg/day, per mouse) significantly obstructed the cell growth of murine renal cell cancer (Renca) in mice, where both treatments showed no noticeable adverse effects.[2,3] The extract of She She Cao also exerted the anticancer property against murine H22 hepatoma implanted in mice, whose effect was found to be achieved mostly by inducing the expression of HSP70 and enhancing the immunegenicity.[4,5] In association with enhancing p53 expression as a result of an increased binding of ERα/Sp1 complex to the p53 promoter region, the extract markedly restrained the anchorage-dependent and -independent cell growths and induced the apoptosis of ERα-positive MCF-7 breast cancer cells.[6] The treatment of HL-60 promyelocytic leukemia cells with its ethanolic extract augmented superoxide production and caspase-2 and caspase-3 activations, leading to the promotion of HL-60 cells to apoptotic death effectively.[7] Moreover, a water extract of She She Cao remarkably inhibited HepG2 hepatoma cell proliferation *in vitro* and *in vivo* in a dose-dependent manner concomitant with the induction of the cell cycle arrest at G0/G1 phase.[8] The water extract also remarkably potentiated the antihepatoma efficiency of 5-FU at low dose by downregulating both mRNA and protein levels of cyclin-E, CDK2, and E2F1, without overt toxicity.[8]

Additionally, the She She Cao was found to be exerting the significant inhibitory effect toward mutagenesis and tumorigenesis provoked by oncogens such as aflatoxin-B1 (AFB1) and/or benzo[a]pyrene (BAP) and exercising a protective effect against radiation-induced hematopoietic damage.[9–11] More investigations further revealed that the She She Cao extract is capable of systemically stimulating the immune function to kill or engulf the tumor by augmenting the phagocytosis of macrophage and the proliferation of spleen cells, potentiating the activity of NK cells and the cytotoxicity of T lymphocyte, promoting the productions of monocytes' cytokine and B cells' Ab and increasing the production of Ab-mediated spleen secretory cells.[2,12,13] All the positive evidences provided the scientific support for using She She Cao in Chinese herb prescriptions as a safe adjuvant chemotherapy.

Antitumor Constituents and Activities

For searching the cancer growth inhibitory molecules from She She Cao, the continuous phytochemical researches have been extensively executed with *in vitro* and *in vivo* bioassays. Various types of bioactive constituents with moderate antitumor and anticarcinogenic activities were discovered from She She Cao. The scientific evidences as summarized in this section have provided a deeper insight into the anticancer and immunoregulating functions of She She Cao and have also elucidated the efficiency of clinically employed She She Cao as a chemotherapeutic supplement.

Iridoids and Pheophytins

From its active extract, 6-*O*-(E)-p-coumaroyl scandoside methyl ester (**1**) and 10(S)-hydroxypheophytin-a (**2**) were discovered exerting the moderate suppressive effect against the proliferation of human PC3 prostate cancer cells (androgen-independent) *in vitro*. 10(S)-hydroxypheophytin-a (**2**) was active in the proliferative inhibition of human LNCaP prostate neoplasm cells (androgen-sensitive).[14]

Anthraquinones

1-Methoxy-2-hydroxyanthraquinone (**3**) and 2-hydroxy-3-methylanthraquinone (**4**), which are both modest inhibitors of Src tyrosine kinase, were isolated from the She She Cao extract. The two anthraquinones could accelerate the cancer cell apoptosis through a mitochondrial pathway and arrest the cell growth through the inhibition of protein tyrosine kinases v-src and pp60 src activities *in vitro* in human cancer cell lines such as SPC-1-A (lung), Bcap37 (breast), and HepG2 (liver). 2-Hydroxy-3-methylanthraquinone (**4**) showed to be more active as an antagonist of Src kinase and has a higher potency to amplify the carcinoma cell growth arrest and apoptosis,[15] and it also could potently obstruct the proliferation of many types of neoplastic cells. The marked apoptosis and the cell cycle arrest provoked by 2-hydroxy-2-methylanthraquinone (**4**) were figured out to be mediated by a Ca^{2+}/calpain/caspase-4 pathway, i.e., (1) rising intracellular calcium levels, (2) promoting JNK phosphorylation and calpain activation, (3) decreasing mitochondrial membrane potential, (4) releasing cytochrome c from mitochondria to cytosol, and (5) inducing cleavage of caspase-4, caspase-9 and caspase-7, thereby enforcing the antiproliferative activity against the cancer cells including human MCF-7 breast cancer cells.[16] 2-Hydroxy-3-methylanthraquinone (**4**) was also able to enhance the caspase-3-dependent apoptosis of U937 lymphoma cells, at least in part, through the activation of p38MAPK and the downregulation of p-ERK1/2.[17]

Flavonoids

Flavonoids isolated from She She Cao were effective in the growth inhibition against SMMC-7721 and BEL-7402, MCF-7 (breast), BGC-823 (stomach), Colo-205 (colon), Hep2, A549 (lung), CNE1 (nasopharynx), A375, and B16 (skin) cancer cell lines *in vitro* and against mouse H22 liver tumor, sarcoma 180, HepA hepatoma, and Ehrlich tumor *in vivo*, whose effect was found to be associated with the blockage of tumor cell proliferation cycle and the promotion of tumor cell apoptosis through both intracellular and extracellular signal transduction pathways. During the *in vivo* antigrowth action, the total flavonoids also simultaneously regulated the immune circumstances, such as markedly elevating the thymus index and the splenic lymphocyte transformation rate and increasing levels of TNFα and IFNγ in the serum.[18–22]

Triterpenoids

Oleanolic acid and ursolic acid, whose two common triterpenoids in the phytochemistry was isolated from the herb, were found possessing both moderate chemotherapeutic and chemopreventive activities against human SMMC-7721 hepatoma cells and human BGC823 gastric carcinoma cells, and the IC_{50} value was 36.88 μmol/L for ursolic acid in BGC823 cells at 24 h.[23,24] The antiproliferative effect was corresponding to the induction of apoptosis and the blockage of the cell cycle at G2/M phase in the BGC823 cells.[23] In the *in vitro* models, ursolic acid was also effective in the inhibition of other human carcinoma cell lines, such as Colo 205 (colon), Hep3B (liver), H460 (lung), A2780, and SKOV3 (ovary) cells,[25,26] which respective IC_{50} values were 50 and 65 μM in the SKOV3 and A2780 cells. In parallel with the antitumor effect, ursolic acid promoted the cell apoptosis via the activations of caspase-9 and caspase-3, the cleavage of PARP, and the phosphorylations of glycogen synthase kinase (GSK-3β) and ERK in the SKOV3 cells.[26,27]

Most importantly, ursolic acid was found to effectively retard the proliferation of DOX-resistant human R-HepG2 hepatoma cells (IC_{50}: 20 μM, at 48 h). The MDR reversal effect was not dependent on the expression and the activity of the P-gp, but the apoptosis of R-HepG2 cells was notably inducted by both extrinsic and intrinsic apoptotic pathways and caspase-independent AIF signaling pathway, including (1) increase of Bak expression and externalization of externalizing phosphatidyl serine, (2) reduction of mitochondrial membrane potential and release of AIF and cytochrome c from the mitochondria to the cytosol, and (3) activation of caspase cascade. A further *in vivo* study confirmed the growth inhibition on the R-HepG2 cells in the ursolic acid-treated nude mice (30 mg/kg/day, intravenous), with negligible body weights loss and damages toward the heart, the spleen, and the liver.[25,28] Similarly, the ursolic acid and the oleanolic acid not only obstructed the growth of MCF-7 breast cancer cells with enhanced p53 expression but also reduced the growth of tamoxifen-resistant breast cancer cells and effectively reversed the resistance of breast cancer cells to the antiestrogen treatment.[6] The findings revealed the potential of ursolic acid and oleanolic acid as adjunctive agents for the chemotherapeutic treatment of neoplasm and some multidrug resistant carcinomas.

Sterol

Stigmasterol derived from She She Cao demonstrated some modest/marginal inhibitive effect as well against the proliferation of human hepatoma cell lines (SMMC-7721 and BEL-7402) *in vitro* and against the growth of murine H22 hepatoma cells in mice, whose effect was concomitant with the promotion of apoptosis and the blockage of tumor cell multiplication cycle.[29]

Polysaccharides

Polysaccharides prepared from She She Cao displayed remarkable growth-inhibiting and apoptosis-inducing effects on tested human HL-60 promyelocytic leukemia, Bel-7402 hepatoma, HeLa cervical cancer cell lines, and mouse B16BL6 melanoma cell line *in vitro*.[30,31] After treatment with the polysaccharides in concentrations from 1 to 4 mg/mL, the growth of RPMI 8226 multiple myeloma cells were suppressed in a dose- and a time-dependent manner, and the highest inhibition rate reached to 92.3%. Concurrently, the apoptotic cells were elicited after 24 h of exposure with concentrations of 1–3 mg/mL, associating with the activation of caspase-8, caspase-9, and caspase-3 and the inhibition of p-AKT and NF-κB expressions.[32] An *in vivo* experiment further confirmed the direct antineoplastic property of She She Cao polysaccharides. When polysaccharides are administered to an animal model at a dose of 30 mg/kg intragastrically for 10 days, the growth inhibitory rates were showed as 36.09% in mice implanted with sarcoma 180 and as 49.68% in mice bearing H22 hepatoma, with no distinct side effect on the thymus and the spleen.[33]

Other Bioactivities

The herb She She Cao (Spreading hedyotis) is extensively used in modern Chinese herb practice for the treatment of viral infections (especially hepatitis), urethral infection, tonsillitis, inflammation, sore throat, appendicitis, and arthritis, in addition to malignant tumors in the liver, the lung, and the stomach. Pharmacological studies have proven that She She Cao possesses antiinflammatory, antioxidative, hepatoprotective, immunostimulatory, neuroprotective, and antibacterial properties.

References

1. Xu, B. J. et al. 2005. Chemical constituents and pharmacological activities of *Hedyotis diffusa*. *Nat. Prod. Sci.* 11: 1–9.
2. Wong, B. Y. et al. 1996. *Oldenlandia diffusa* and *Scutellaria barbata* augment macrophage oxidative burst and inhibit tumor growth. *Cancer Biother. Radiopharm.* 11: 51–6.
3. Gupta, S. L. et al. 2004. Anticancer activities of *Oldenlandia diffusa*. *J. Herb Pharmacother.* 4: 21–33.
4. Hu, L. et al. 2009. Effect of Herba *Hedyotis diffusae* on expression of heat shock protein 70 and P16 in mice with hepatoma cell-transplanted tumor. *Zhongyao Xinyao Yu Linchuang Yaoli* 20: 18–20.
5. Li, J. et al. 2009. Study on inhibiting action of Hedyotis on mice with hepatocarcinoma H22. *Zhongguo Zhongyiyao Keji* 16: 28–9.
6. Gu, G. W. et al. 2012. *Oldenlandia diffusa* extracts exert anti-proliferative and apoptotic effects on human breast cancer cells through ERα/Sp1-mediated p53 activation. *J. Cell. Physiol.* 227: 3363–72.
7. Yadav, S. K. et al. 2006. Evidence *for Oldenlandia diffusa*-evoked cancer cell apoptosis through superoxide burst and caspase activation. *Zhongguo Zhongxiyi Jiehe Zazhi* 4: 485–9.
8. Chen, X. Z. et al. 2012. Water extract of *Hedyotis diffusa Willd* suppresses proliferation of human HepG2 cells and potentiates the anticancer efficacy of low-dose 5-fluorouracil by inhibiting the CDK2-E2F1 pathway. *Oncol. Reports* 28: 742–8.
9. Zhang, C. L. et al. 2002. Study on antagonizing mutagenesis to B(a)P of Chinese herbal medicine and green tea. *Zhongguo Gonggong Weisheng* 18: 393–4.
10. Yang, J. et al. 1997. The possible use of Peh-Hue-Juwa-Chi-Cao as an antitumor agent and radioprotector after therapeutic irradiation. *Phytother. Res.* 11: 6–10.
11. Wong, B. Y. et al. 1993. Inhibition of dexamethasone-induced cytochrome P450-mediated mutagenicity and metabolism of aflatoxin B1 by Chinese medicinal herbs. *Eur. J. Cancer Prev.* 2: 351–6.
12. Qin, F. H. et al. 1990. The immunoenhancing activity of *Oldenlandia diffusa* in mice. *Shanghai Mianyixue Zazhi* 10: 321.
13. Shan, B. E. et al. 2001. Immunomodulatory activity and antitumor activity of *Oldenlandia diffusa* in vitro. *Zhongguo Zhongxiyi Jiehe Zazhi* 21: 370–4.
14. Li, M. et al. 2010. Authentication of the antitumor herb Baihuasheshecao with bioactive marker compounds and molecular sequences. *Food Chem.* 119: 1239–1245.
15. Shi, Y. et al. 2008. Apoptosis-inducing effects of two anthraquinones from *Hedyotis diffusa Willd. Biol. Pharm. Bull.* 31: 1075–8.
16. Liu, Z. et al. 2010. Methylanthraquinone from *Hedyotis diffusa Willd* induces Ca^{2+}-mediated apoptosis in human breast cancer cells. *Toxicol. in Vitro* 24: 142–7.
17. Wang, N. et al. 2013. 2-Hydroxy-3-methylanthraquinone from *Hedyotis diffusa Willd* induces apoptosis in human leukemic U937 cells through modulation of MAPK pathways. *Archiv. Pharm. Res.* 36: 752–8.
18. Zhang, S. et al. 2007. Inhibitory effect of flavonoids from *Hedyotis diffusa Willd* on hepatoma cells in vitro and vivo and its influence on transplanted H22 tumor cells' proliferation cycle, apoptosis and immune circumstances in mice. *Shijie Huaren Xiaohua Zazhi* 15: 1347–52.
19. Zhang, S. et al. 2007. Target gene regulation involved in the inhibitory effect of flavonoids from *Hedyotis diffusa Willd* on human hepatoma cell line SMMC-7721. *Shijie Huaren Xiaohua Zazhi* 15: 1060–6.
20. Wang, Y. L. et al. 2014. Antitumor effect of total flavones of *Oldenlandia diffusa Willd. Anhui Yike Daxue Xuebao* 49: 1622–5.
21. Yang, X. et al. 2011. Effects of FOD on the proliferation and apoptosis of melanoma A375 and B16 cells. *J. Diagn. Ther. Dermato-venereol.* 18: 359–62.
22. Deng, X. Q. et al. 2011. Effects of the total flavones of *oldenlandia diffusa willd* on proliferation and apoptosis of nasopharyngeal carcinoma cell line CNE1. *New Chinese Med.* 42: 571–3.
23. Zhao, X. Y. et al. 2010. Effects and mechanisms of ursolic acid on inducing apoptosis of human gastric carcinoma BGC823 cells. *Zhongguo Aizheng Zazhi* 20: 101–4.
24. Wu, P. et al. 2009. Oleanolic acid isolated from *Oldenlandia diffusa* exhibits a unique growth inhibitory effect against ras-transformed fibroblasts. *Life Sci.* 85: 113–21.
25. Yang, L. et al. 2010. Ursolic acid induces doxorubicin-resistant HepG2 cell death via the release of apoptosis-inducing factor. *Cancer Lett.* 298: 128–38.
26. Lee, H. Z. et al. 2011. Clarification of the phenotypic characteristics and antitumor activity *of Hedyotis diffusa. Am. J. Chin. Med.* 39: 201–13.
27. Song, Y. H. et al. 2012. Ursolic acid from *Oldenlandia diffusa* induces apoptosis via activation of caspases and phosphorylation of glycogen synthase kinase 3 beta in SKOV3 ovarian cancer cells. *Biol. Pharm. Bull.* 35: 1022–8.
28. Zhang, D. M. et al. 2007. Antiproliferative effect of ursolic acid on multidrug resistant hepatoma cells R-HepG2 by apoptosis induction. *Cancer Biol. Therapy* 6: 1381–9.
29. Zhang, S. et al. 2008. Inhibitive effect of stigmasterol from *Hedyotis diffusa Willd* on hepatoma cells in vitro and vivo and its influence on transplanted H22 tumor cell's multiplication cycle, apoptosis. *Xiandai Shengwu-yixue Jinzhan* 8: 2016–7, 2009.
30. Fan, H. W. et al. 2009. Antitumor effect of *Oldenlandia diffusa* on HL60 and B16BL6 cell lines in vitro. *Zhongguo Yiyuan Yaoxue Zazhi* 29: 1754–7.
31. Yang, P. M. et al. 2010. Antitumor effect *of Hedyotis diffusa* polysaccharides on S180 and H22 experimental tumor. *Xibei Yaoxue Zazhi* 25: 33–4.
32. Lin, S. Y. et al. 2013. Apoptosis of multiple myeloid cells induced by polysaccharides extracts from *Hedyotis diffusa* and its mechanism. *Zhonghua Xueyexue Zazhi* 34: 337–40.
33. Yang, P. M. et al. 2010. Antitumor effect of *Hedyotis diffusa* polysaccharides on S180 and H22 experimental tumor. *Xibei Yaoxue Zazhi* 25: 33–4.

14 Chong Lou 重樓

Rhizoma paridis

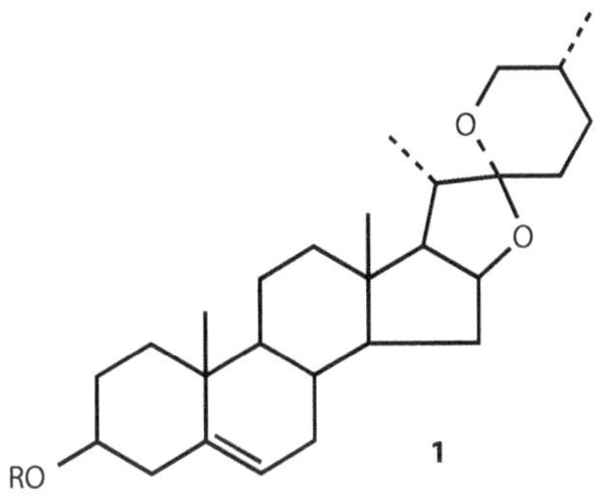

R = –Glu(*p*)–[(2–1)–Rham(*p*)]–(4–1)–Ara(*f*)

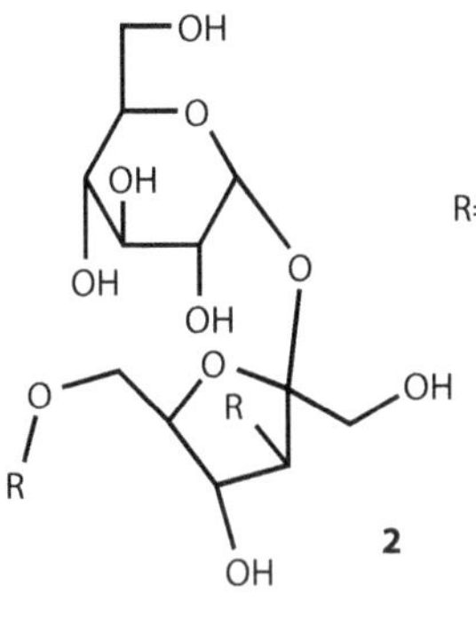

Herb Origination

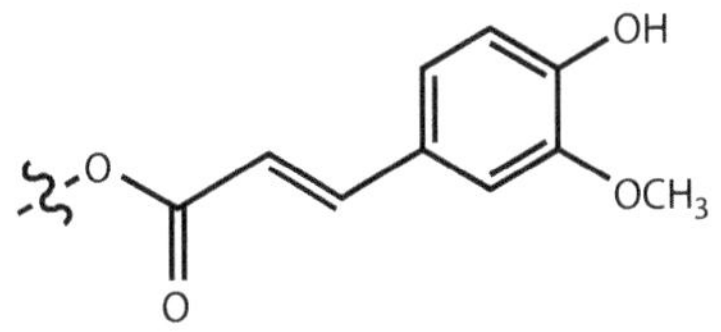

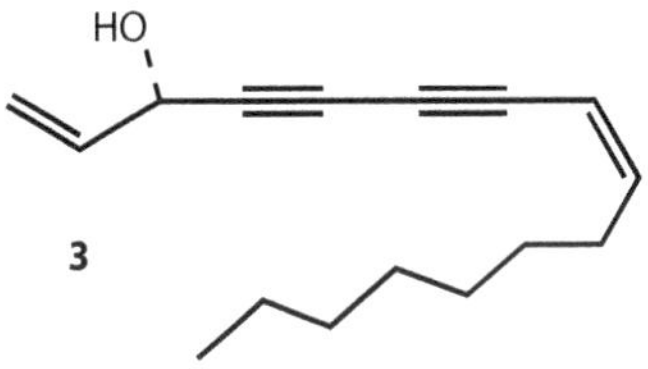

The herb Chong Lou is the dried rhizome of three Liliaceae plants *Paris polyphylla* and its two varieties, *Paris polyphylla* var. *chinensis* (PPC) and *P. polyphylla* var. *yunnanensis* (PPY). These plants are distributed throughout the Asiatic countries, especially in the southeastern regions. The *P. polyphylla* grows in a variety of gardens throughout the world. In China, the rhizomes are collected in September and October and dried in the sun or by oven for medicinal uses.

Antitumor Activities and Constituents

The herb Chong Lou is currently being used in hospitals together with some other natural herbs and in conjunction with conventional drugs in the treatment of lung and breast carcinomas in China. In lab investigations, its methanolic extract demonstrated remarkable *in vitro* and *in vivo* antineoplastic properties, which effectively inhibited the growth of human HeLa cervical cancer cells and mouse fibroblast L929 cells.[1] By increasing the expressions of Bad and connexin-26 and decreasing the expression of Bcl-2, the extract obviously promoted apoptosis and inhibited the proliferation of human Eca109 esophageal carcinoma cell line.[2] The i.p. injection of the extract to tumor-bearing mice exhibited a marked suppressive effect against Ehrlich ascite cancer *in vivo*.[3] The extract also showed modest antimutagenic activity against benzo(a) pyrene and picrolonic acid-induced mutation.[4]

Steroidal Saponins

Steroidal saponins have been identified to be major principals in Chong Lou, whose antitumor property was proven by *in vitro* and *in vivo* experimental systems. The saponins showed an antigrowth effect on mouse U14 cervical cancer cells *in vitro* and *in vivo* and prolonged the survival time of mice, together with an increased serum IFNγ level and a reduced serum IL-4 level in the tumor-bearing mice, implying that the antitumor activity was partially mediated by the saponins and improved the body's immune system.[5] Oral (a dose of 350 mg/kg) or i.p. (a dose of 5–10 mg/kg) administration of the total saponins to mice markedly inhibited the growth of H22 entity hepatoma cells *in vivo* in association by (1) resisting the incorporation of thymine and uracil into the cells and blocking the synthesis of DNA and RNA[6] and (2) repressing the fatty acid oxidant pathway and the gluconeogenesis pathway, which participated in the energy supply for the body.[7] PPC saponin treatment (5.0 and 7.5 mg/kg) markedly inhibited the volume and weight of Lewis tumor in C57BL/6 mice, whose inhibitory rates reached to 40.32% and 54.94%, respectively. The saponins simultaneously augmented the indexes of the spleen, and the thymus remarkably and lessened the levels of inflammatory cytokines including TNFα, IL-8, and IL-10 in the serum.[8] In T739 mice injected with mouse LA795 lung adenocarcinoma cells, the PPY saponins clearly inhibited the tumor growth and metastases *in vivo* by upregulating the expression of TIMP-2 and downregulating the levels of MMP-2 and MMP-9.[9]

In *in vitro* assays, the treatment of human gastric carcinoma cells with the saponins showed a potent antitumor activity concomitantly with blocking the cell cycle progression and increasing the apoptotic rate via the significant down-expression of EphA2 and survivin and up-expression of caspase-3.[10] At concentrations of 10 or 20 μg/mL, the saponins showed more potent inhibitory effects on MNN-45 cell line than on MGC80-3 cell line, but the effects on the two gastric cancer cells were different, i.e., the MNK-45 cells were arrested in G_0/G_1 phase, and the MGC80-3 cells in the S phase after the treatments.[11] For A549 lung cancer cells, the saponins (0.25, 0.50, and 0.75 mg/mL) elicited nuclear changes with DNA condensation and fragmentations of chromatin and promoted apoptosis. Also, the antigrowth effect of PPC saponins on the A549 cells was associated with the amelioration of inflammation responses, such as a significant inhibition of proinflammatory cytokines (MCP-1, IL-6, TGF-β1) and repression of cell adhesion molecule (ICAM-1), as well as the attenuation of intracellular ROS.[8] The PPC saponins display the marked cytotoxicity on human HL-60 promyelocytic leukemia cells *in vitro* as well.[12]

These results recommended that the total saponins implied a potential therapeutic effect in cancer treatment, especially for carcinomas of the lung, the stomach, and the liver. From the total saponin components, many individual steroidal saponins have been separated, displaying the cancer inhibitory activity. The most interesting saponin in the herb is polyphyllin-D (**1**) whose antitumor property has been widely investigated *in vitro* and *in vivo*.

Polyphyllin-D

Polyphyllin-D (= polyphyllin-I, **1**) (PD) is one of the major saponins in the Rhizoma Paridis, whose anticancer activity was established in many types of neoplastic cell lines such as nonsmall cell lung cancer (NSCLC) (A549, SK-MES-1, H460), breast cancer (MCF-7, MDA-MB-231), lung cancer (LA795), hepatoma (HepG2), osteosarcoma (MG-63, Saos-2 and U-2OS), gastric cancer (SGC7901), ovarian cancer (SKOV3 and Ho8910PM), pancreatic cancer (BxPC3), cervical cancer (HeLa), and glioma (U87) *in vitro* and/or *in vivo*. The IC_{50} values of PD (**1**) were 5 and 2.5 μM in human MCF-7 and MDA-MB-231 breast cancer cells, 1.24–2.40 μg/mL in NSCLC cells, and 0.2–1.4 μM in ovarian cancer cells. The most potent cytotoxicity of PD (**1**) was present on HepG2, SGC7901, and BxPC3 cell lines (IC_{50}s <0.01 μg/mL).[13] The antiviability and antigrowth effects of PD (**1**) were demonstrated by *in vivo* studies with marked apoptotic promotion and no significant toxicity in the heart and the liver to the host. The daily intravenous injection of PD (2.73 mg/kg) to nude mice implanted with MCF-7 cells for 10 days diminished the tumor weight and size by 50%.[14] Either i.p. or per os (p.o.) administration of PD (**1**) to mice bearing SKOV3 tumor markedly obstructed the growth of human ovarian carcinoma cells by 66% and 52%, respectively, in a xenograft mouse model.[15] The oral administration of PD or diosgenin (PD's aglycone) to mice suppressed the growth LA795 metastatic lung adenocarcinoma cells by 29.44% and 33.94%, respectively, and caused typical apoptosis dose dependently.[16]

The proapoptotic mechanisms of PD (**1**) were revealed to characteristically vary from the different types of carcinomas, such as being associated with (1) a caspase-9-expressed mitochondrial pathway in the MCF-7 and MDA-MS-231 cells,[14] (2) a ER stress-promoted and caspase-activated mitochondrial pathway with p53 activation in the NCI-H460 cells,[17] (3) a ROS-increased mitochondrial pathway in the HeLa cells,[18] (4) a c-Jun NH2-terminal kinase pathway in the U87 and HO-8910PM cells,[19,20] (5) mitochondrial and MAPK kinase pathways with dramatic G2/M phase cell arrest in the SKOV3 cells,[15] and (6) activation of unfolded protein response/ER stress signaling cascade with the inactivation of NF-κB induction of S cell arrest via the downregulation of c-Myc, cyclin-B1, cyclin-D1, and CDK1 in the MG-63, Saos-2, and U-2 OS cells.[21] Moreover, PD (**1**) was also able to lessen the migration and the invasion of the MG-63, Saos-2, and U-2 OS osteosarcoma cells and to restrain the expressions of HIF-1α and VEGF mRNAs in Lewis lung tumor (LLC) cells.[21,22] The down-expression of PIK3C2B and Wnt5A and the up-expression of caspase-9, c-Jun, and p-c-Jun by PD (**1**) jointly inhibited the metastasis of HO-8910PM cells.[20]

The *in vitro* exploration further showed that PD (**1**) could exert a well radiosensitization effect on the A549 cells concomitant with reduced survivin activity and increased p21 protein activity, leading the A549 cells to G2/M cell cycle arrest and apoptosis additively.[23,24] PD (**1**) also was capable of sensitizing 12 ovarian cancer cell lines to cisplatin-induced growth arrest.[25] Through a mitochondrial apoptotic pathway and the disruption of MMP, PD (**1**) elicited the G2/M cell arrest and apoptosis of K562/A02 cells, leading to the antiproliferative effect on drug-resistant human chronic myeloid leukemia.[26] Likewise, PD (**1**) was effective in the suppression of both drug-resistant R-HepG2 cells and drug-sensitive hepatoma HepG2 cells. The drug resistance reversal effect by PD (**1**) was mediated by the induction of a mitochondrial apoptotic pathway including generation of H_2O_2 and the depolarization of the mitochondrial transmembrane potential and the release of AIF and cytochrome c then elicited the apoptotic death of R-HepG2 cells overexpressing P-gp, where PD (**1**) also triggered the phosphatidylserine externalization and the DNA fragmentation in R-HepG2 cells.[27,28] In addition, the oral bioavailability of PD (**1**) could be augmented from 0.62 to 3.52% and 3.79%, and the efflux ratio of polyphyllin I (PPI) could be diminished from 12.5 to 2.96 and 2.22 in rats implanted with Caco-2 colon cancer during the cotreatment with verapamil and cyclosporine A, respectively, indicating that the inhibition of P-gp can enhance its bioavailability.[29]

All these findings provided novel insights that the PD (**1**) may have a potential to serve as a candidate in the treatments of selective neoplastic diseases, especially breast cancer, lung cancer, hepatoma, and it also has an ability to reverse MDR. However, the toxicity of PD (**1**) on human erythrocytes was reported to cause hemolysis and erythroptosis/eryptosis and induce the erythrocyte apoptotic death through Ca^{2+} rise and membrane permeabilization.[30]

Formosanin-C

Similar to polyphyllin-D (**1**), formosanin-C (FC) is another major active component in the saponins of *P. polyphylla* as well as a close plant *P. formosana*. FC exhibited almost the same inhibitory effect as PD (**1**) did obviously against LA795 and A549 NSCLC cells (IC_{50}: 1.16–2.17 μg/mL), HeLa cervical cancer cells (IC_{50}: 3.19–4.03 μg/mL), and Caco-2 colon cancer cells (IC_{50}: 7.33–9.37 μg/mL), moderately against HL-60 leukemia cells, A498 renal carcinoma cells, and A431 melanoma cells (IC_{50}: 10.47–21.37 μg/mL), and reasonably against HepG2 and Bel7402 hepatoma cells and KB oral cancer cells (IC_{50}: 21.06–53.68 μg/mL).[31] FC treatment caused caspase-2 activation and mitochondria dysfunction leading to the death of human HT29 colorectal cancer cells.[32] By strongly blocking MMP-2 and MMP-9 activities, FC showed much more effective inhibitions against the growth and the pulmonary metastasis in mice bearing LA795 cells compared to cisplatin,[33] implying that FC may provide a potential therapeutic modality for the treatment of lung tumors.

Moreover, the presence of FC at lower concentrations in mouse L929 fibroblast cells significantly enhanced the blastogenic response of human peripheral blood cells to phytohemagglutinin, significantly increased the lymphocytes, and augmented the responsiveness of the granulocyte/macrophage colony-forming cells to the L929 cells.[34] The i.p. injection of 2.5 mg/kg of FC markedly induced IFN production and enhanced natural killer cell activity. With the i.p. treatment with 1–2.5 mg/kg of FC, the growth of transplanted MH134 mouse hepatoma cells was retarded, and the activity of 5-FU was potentiated against the hepatoma.[35] These results pointed out that the enhancement of immune functions must be partially contributed for the antitumor activity of FC.

Other Active Steroidal Saponins

Up to now, numerous steroidal glycosidies have been discovered from the isolation of the herb. Besides PD (**1**) and FC, several other same types of saponins were reported possessing the moderate to weak cytotoxicity on the *in vitro*-cultured neoplastic cells.[33–38] After being treated with the three saponins (**A**, **B**, and **C**) in a concentration of 10 μg/mL, the inhibitory ratios were 94.69%, 82.58%, and 82.64% on HeLa cells and 90.34%, 87.42%, and 57.61% on L929 cells, respectively. While after being treated with a 30 μg/mL concentration, the inhibitory rates against the HeLa and L929 cells were raised to 95–99%.[36,39]

The saponins (**A**, **B**, and **D**) also showed significant effects as inhibitors of P-gp-mediated drug efflux in drug-resistant K562/R7 cells. At concentrations of 20 and 10 μM, Paris saponin-H (**A**) exerted the highest ability to restrain the P-gp activity, leading to 108% and 77% inhibitions against the K562/R7 cells, respectively.[40] Paris saponin-H (**A**) was able to inhibit the cancer cell migration via the downregulation of the expression of MMP-1, MMP-3, and MMP-14, whereas Paris saponin-VII (**E**) slightly restrained the metastasis via the decrease of the expression of MMP-9 and MMP-14.[38–40] In addition, a mixture of the saponins including PD, FC, dioscin, Paris saponin-H and Paris saponin-VII, and saponin (**F**) could suppress the migration of LA795 murine lung cancer cells in a noncytotoxic dose, both *in vitro* and *in vivo*.[39,41] More steroidal saponins were separated from the rhizomes of PPY. Of them, (3β,25R)-spirost-5-en-3-ol glycosides (**G–K**) and (3β,17α,25R)-spirost-5-en-3,17-diol glycosides (**L–Q**) established more potent inhibitory effects (IC_{50}: 1.5–11.1 μM) than cisplatin (IC_{50}: 23.73 μM) against human nasopharyngeal carcinoma epithelial cells concomitant with the induction of apoptosis and cell cycle arrest.[42–44] Moreover, pairs saponin-I (1 μg/mL) combined with radiation could markedly obstruct the proliferation and the clonogenesis of human PANC-1 pancreatic cancer cells, whose radiosensitization promoted a higher apoptotic rate and G2/M cell cycle arrest in the PANC-1 cells.[45]

Structure and Activity Relationship

Structurally, the Rhizoma Paridis saponins can be divided into two groups: diosgenyl saponins and pennogenyl saponins, according to their aglycones having or not 17α-hydroxyl. Both types of saponins suppressed the metastasis of B16 melanoma cells *in vivo*, but the different saponins exhibited different levels of inhibition on the MMPs. The results indicated that the 17α-OH amplified the sensitivity of diosgenyl saponins to the membrane-bound protease to stimulate proMMP-2 activation, leading to the decrease of the antimetastatic activity. The antimetastatic effect in the B16 cells by diosgenyl saponins was also largely mediated by the down-expression of collagenases, gelatinases, and stromelysin.[46]

A group of steroidal glycosides were also evaluated for cytotoxicity against human HL-60 promyelocytic leukemia cells. The obtained data were used for the analysis of the structure and the activity relationship, revealing that the spirostanol framework and the 3-*O*-glycoside moiety may play important roles in the cytotoxicity of steroidal saponins, and the number, different locations, and variety of glycosides has a strong influence on their anticancer activity. The results indicated that (1) the spirostanol saponins were highly cytotoxic, but the furostanol saponins showed no such toxic activity; (2) the substitution of hydroxyl group at C-12 or C-17 of the aglycon caused a reduction of the activity; (3) two hydroxyl groups at C-5 and C-6 and no 5-ene in the aglycone exhibited no such activity; (4) the attachment of an α-L-rhamnopyranosyl at C-2 of the inner glucopyranosyl moiety led to a remarkable increase of the activity; (5) the addition of a β-D-glucopyranosyl at C-3 of the inner glucopyranosyl moiety slightly lessened its activity; (6) when an α-L-arabinofuranosyl or two α-L-rhamnopyranosyls were added to the C-4 of the inner glucopyranosyl, its cytotoxicity was markedly amplified; and (7) the attachment of an α-L-rhamnopyranosyl or a β-D-glucopyranosyl at C-5 of the arabinofuranosyl moiety led to a slight reduction in its toxicity.[47] The analytical data in the structure and activity relationship afforded some important clues for the structural modification and the drug design.

Other Types of Active Components

A phenylpropanoid glycoside assigned as 2-feruloyl-*O*-α-glucopyranosyl-(1′-2)-3,6-*O*-feruloyl-β-fructofuranoside (**2**) was isolated from the PPY roots. An *in vitro* assay showed that it has a cytotoxic effect in a dose-dependent manner against the mouse LA795 lung adenocarcinoma cell line.[48] Falcarindiol (**3**), a polyacetylene prepared from the herb, was found to also have an anticarcinoma activity. It was reported to have the ability to effectively repress the growth of three neoplastic cells (MK-1, SW620, B16) but exerted a marginal cytotoxic effect on human HeLa cervical cancer cells and mouse L929 fibroblast cells.[36] From the PPY extract, two hydroxy fatty acids were isolated and elucidated as (8R*,9R*,10S*,6Z)-trihydroxyoctadec-6-enoic acid and methyl (9S,10 R, 11S)-trihydroxy-12(Z)-octadecenoate (**X**). The fatty acid **X** showed antiproliferative effect on CNE nasopharyngeal cancer epithelial cells (IC_{50}: 20.77 μmol/L).[48]

Other Bioactivities

The herb Chong Lou has been used in traditional Chinese herbs for many years in the treatment of insect bites, poisonous snakebites, boils, ulcers, diphtheria, and epidemic Japanese B encephalitis. The herb was shown to have analgesic, antitussive, antiphlogistic, antipyretic, depurative, febrifuge, antispasmodic, and narcotic activities by pharmacological studies.

References

1. Kosuge, T. et al. 1985. Studies on antitumor activities and antitumor principles of Chinese herbs: I. *Yakugaku Zasshi* 105: 791–5.
2. Li, F. R. et al. 2012. *Paris polyphylla Smith* extract induces apoptosis and activates cancer suppressor gene connexin26 expression. *Asian Pacific J. Cancer prev.* 13: 205–9.
3. Wang, Q. et al. (a) 1987. Research on cytotoxicity of Paris polyphlla Sm. var. against L-929 cells. *Zhongcaoyao.* 18: 526; (b) 1999. *Chinese Materia Medica.* Vol. 8, 8–133. Shanghai Science and Technology Press, Shanghai, China.
4. Lee, H. et al. 1988. Antimutagenic activity of extracts from anticancer drugs in Chinese medicine. *Mutation Res.* 204: 229–34.

5. Chen, G. L. et al. 2013. Effect of Paris saponin on antitumor and immune function in U14 tumor-bearing mice. *Afrcan J. Tradit. Complem. Altern. Med.* 10: 503–7.
6. Shi, X. F. et al. 1992. The antitumor activity of total saponins from *Paris polyphylla* in mice bearing H22 hepatoma. *Zhongyaocai* 15: 33–6.
7. Man, S. L. et al. 2014. Antitumor pathway of Rhizoma Paridis saponins based on the metabolic regulatory network alterations in H22 hepatocarcinoma mice. *Steroids* 84: 17–21.
8. Li, Y. et al. 2013. The anti-lung cancer activities of steroidal saponins of *P. polyphylla Smith* var. *chinensis Hara* through enhanced immuno-stimulation in experimental Lewis tumor-bearing C57BL/6 mice and induction of apoptosis in the A549 cell line. *Mol.* 18: 12916–36.
9. Man, S. L. et al. 2009. Antitumor and antimetastatic activities of Rhizoma Paridis saponins. *Steroids* 74: 1051–6.
10. Jia, K. et al. 2011. Effects of total saponins of *Paris polyphylla* root on growth of gastric carcinoma cell line MGC-803 in vitro. *Zhongguo Shenghua Yaowu Zazhi* 32: 284–6, 290.
11. Bao, Y. L. et al. 2012. Effects of *Paris polyphylla* total saponins on growth of gastric carcinoma cell lines MNK-45 and MGC80-3. *Anhui Zhongyi Xueyuan Xuebao* 31: 51–5.
12. Mimaki, Y. et al. 2000. Steroidal saponins from the rhizomes of *Paris polyphylla* var. *chinensis* and their cytotoxic activity on HL-60 cells. *Nat. Prod. Lett.* 14: 357–64.
13. Huang, Y. et al. 2007. Separation and identification of steroidal compounds with cytotoxic activity against human gastric cancer cell lines in vitro from the rhizomes of *Paris polyphylla* var. *chinensis. Chem. Nat. Compds.* 43: 672–7.
14. Lee, M. S. et al. 2005. Effects of polyphyllin D, a steroidal saponin in *Paris polyphylla*, in growth inhibition of human breast cancer cells and in xenograft. *Cancer Biol. Ther.* 4: 1248–54.
15. Xiao, X. et al. 2009. The antitumoral effect of Paris saponin I associated with the induction of apoptosis through the mitochondrial pathway. *Mol. Cancer Therap.* 8: 1179–88.
16. Yan, L. L. et al. (a) 2009. Antitumor activity of steroid saponins extracted from *Paris polyphylla* var. *yunnanensis* against lung adenocarcinoma cells in vitro and in vivo. *Zhongcaoyao* 40: 424–8; (b) 2009. In vitro and in vivo anticancer activity of steroid saponins of *Paris polyphylla* var. *yunnanensis. Experim. Oncol.* 31: 27–32.
17. Siu, F. M. et al. 2008. Proteomic and transcriptomic study on the action of a cytotoxic saponin (Polyphyllin D): Induction of endoplasmic reticulum stress and mitochondria-mediated apoptotic pathways. *Proteomics* 8: 3105–17.
18. Cheng, H. et al. 2013. Effect and mechanism of polyphyllin I on human cervical cancer cell HeLa in vitro. *Zhongyaocai.* 36: 1815–9.
19. Yu, Q. et al. 2014. Polyphyllin D induces apoptosis in U87 human glioma cells through the c-Jun NH2-terminal kinase pathway. *J. Med. Food* 17: 1036–42.
20. Gu, L. et al. 2013. Polyphyllin I inhibits proliferation and metastasis of ovarian cancer cell line HO-8910PM in vitro. *J. Tradit. Chin. Med.* 33: 325–33.
21. Chang, J. L. et al. 2015. Molecular mechanisms of Polyphyllin I-induced apoptosis and reversal of the epithelial-mesenchymal transition in human osteosarcoma cells. *J. Ethnopharmacol.* 170: 117–27.
22. Ma, D. D. et al. 2009. Polyphyllin D exerts potent antitumour effects on Lewis cancer cells under hypoxic conditions. *J. Intl. Med. Res.* (3): 631–40.
23. Kong, M. J. et al. 2010. Effects of polyphyllin I on growth inhibition of human non-small lung cancer cells and in xenograft. *Acta Biochimica et Biophysica Sinica* 42: 827–33.
24. Zhao, P. J. et al. 2012. In vitro study of radiosensitization of saponin I on lung adenocarcinoma A549 cell line. *Zhongliuxue Zazhi* 18: 108–10.
25. Al Sawah, E. et al. 2015. The Chinese herb polyphyllin D sensitizes ovarian cancer cells to cisplatin-induced growth arrest. *J. Cancer Res. Clin. Oncol.* 141: 237–42.
26. Wu, L. et al. 2014. Polyphyllin D induces apoptosis in K562/A02 cells through G2/M phase arrest. *J. Pharmacy Pharmacol.* 66: 713–21.
27. Cheung, N. Y. et al. 2005. Polyphyllin D is a potent apoptosis inducer in drug-resistant HepG2 cells. *Cancer Lett.* 217: 203–11.
28. Lee, R. K. Y. et al. 2009. Polyphyllin D—A potential anticancer agent to kill hepato-carcinoma cells with multi-drug resistance. *Current Chem. Biol.* 3: 409–19.
29. Zhu, H. et al. 2015. Study on the pharmacokinetics profiles of Polyphyllin I and its bioavailability enhancement through co-administration with P-glycoprotein inhibitors by LC-MS/MS method. *J. Pharm. Biomed. Anal.* 107: 119–24.
30. Gao, M. H. et al. 2012. Polyphyllin D induces apoptosis in human erythrocytes through Ca^{2+} rise and membrane permeabilization. *Archiv. Toxicol.* 86: 741–52.
31. Yan, L. L. et al. 2008. Cytotoxicity of *Paris polyphylla* root saponins on 10 kinds of tumor cell strains and their structure-activity relationship research. *Zhongguo Zhongyao Zazhi* 33: 2057–60.
32. Lee, J. C. et al. 2009. Formosanin C-induced apoptosis requires activation of caspase-2 and change of mitochondrial membrane potential. *Cancer Sci.* 100: 503–13.
33. Man, S. L. et al. 2011. Formosanin C-inhibited pulmonary metastasis through repression of matrix metalloproteinases on mouse lung adenocarcinoma. *Cancer Biol. Ther.* 11: 592–8.
34. Wu, R. T. et al. 1990. Formosanin-C, an immunomodulator with antitumor activity. *Intl. J. Immuno-pharmacol.* 12: 777–86.
35. Zhang, Y. N. et al. 2005. Two new steroid saponins from *Paris polyphylla. Heterocycles* 65: 1197–203.
36. Wang, Y. et al. 2006. Antitumor constituents from *Paris polyphylla. Asian J. Tradit. Med.* 1: 7–10.
37. Zhang, L. T. et al. 2007. Antitumor activities of extracts and chemical components of *Paris polyphylla Smith* var. *yunnanensis (Franch.)* Hand.-Mazz. *Zhongcaoyao* 38: 422–4.
38. Zhu, L. C. et al. 2011. In vitro antitumor activity and antifungal activity of pennogenin steroidal saponins from *Paris polyphylla* var. *yunnanensis. Iranian J. Pharm. Res.* 10: 279–86.
39. A: Paris saponin-H; B: Polyphyllin-V = Paris saponon-V; C: dioscin; D: gracillin; E: Paris saponon-VII; F: Pennogenin-3-*O*-L-α-rhamno-pyranosyl (1-4)-[L-α-rhamnopyranosyl (1-2)]-D-β-glucopyranoside; G: (3β,25R)-Spirost-5-en-3-ol 3-*O*-α-L-rhamnopyranosyl-(1-2)-β-D-glucopyranoside; H: (3β,25R)-Spirost-5-en-3-ol 3-*O*-α-L-rhamno-pyranosyl-(1-4)-α-L-rhamnopyranosyl-(1-4)-[α-L-rhamnopyranosyl-(1-2)]-β-D glucopyranoside; I: (3β,25R)-Spirost-5-en-3-ol-3-*O*-β-D-apio-furanosyl-(1-3)-[α-L-rhamnopyranosyl-(1-2)]-β-D-glucopyranoside; J: (3β,25R)-Spirost-5-en-3-ol-3-*O*-α-L-arabinofuransyl-(1-4)-[α-L-rhamnopyranosyl-(1-2)]-β-D-glucopyranoside; K: (3β,25R)-Spirost-5-en-3-ol-3-*O*-β-D-glucopyranosyl-(1-3)-[α-L-rhamnopyranosyl-(1-2)]-β-D-glucopyranoside; L: (3β,17α,25R)-

Spirost-5-ene-3,17-diol 3-*O*-α-L-rhamnopyranosyl-(1-2)-β-D-glucopyranoside, M: (3β,17α,25R)-Spirost-5-ene-3,17-diol 3-*O*-α-L-arabinofuranosyl-(1-4)-[α-L-rhamnopyranosyl-(1-2)]-β-D-glucopyranoside; N: (3β,17α, 25R)-Spirost-5-ene-3,17-diol-3-*O*-β-D-apiofuranosyl-(1-3)-[α-L-rhamno pyranosyl-(1-2)]-β-D-glucopyranoside; O: (3β,17α, 25R)-Spirost-5-ene-3,17-diol-3-*O*-β-D-gluco-pyranosyl-(1-5)-α-L-arabinofuranosyl-(1-4)-[α-L-rhamnopyranosyl-(1-2)]-β-D-glucopyranoside; P: (3β,25R)-Spirost-5-en-3-ol-3-*O*-β-D-glucopyranosyl-(1-4)-α-L-rhamnopyranosyl-(1-4)-[α-L-rhamnopyranosyl-(1-2)]-β-D-glucopyranoside; and Q: (3β, 17α, 25R)-Spirost 5-ene-3,17-diol-3-*O*-α-L-rhamnopyranosyl-(1-4)-α-L-rhamnopyranosyl-(1-4)-[α-L-rhamnopyranosyl-(1-2)]-β-D-glucopyranoside.

40. Nguyen, V. T. B. et al. 2009. Selective modulation of P-glycoprotein activity by steroidal saponines from *Paris polyphylla*. *Fitoterapia* 80: 39–42.
41. Man, S. L. et al. 2011. Paridis saponins inhibiting carcinoma growth and metastasis in vitro and in vivo. *Archiv. Pharm. Res*. 34: 43–50.
42. Wu, X. et al. 2012. New steroidal saponins and sterol glycosides from *Paris polyphylla* var. *yunnanensis*. *Planta Med*. 78: 1667–75.
43. Wu, X. et al. 2012. Steroidal saponins from *Paris polyphylla* var. *yunnanensis*. *Phytochem*. 81: 133–43.
44. Jiang, H. et al. 2014. Radiosensitivity of Pairs saponin I on pancreatic carcinoma cell line PANC-1 in vitro. *Zhongliuxue Zazhi* 20: 483–7.
45. Man, S. L. et al. 2011. Inhibition of matrix metalloproteinases related to metastasis by diosgenyl and pennogenyl saponins. *J. Ethno-pharmacol*. 137: 1221–7.
46. Zhao, Y. et al. 2009. Steroidal saponins from the rhizome of *Paris polyphylla* and their cytotoxic activities. *Planta Med*. 75: 356–63.
47. Yan, L. L. et al. 2008. A new phenylpropanoid glycosides from *Paris polyphylla* var. *yunnanensis*. *Fitoterapia* 79: 306–7.
48. Wu, X. et al. 2014. Identification of two hydroxy fatty acids from *Paris polyphylla* var. *yunnanensis* and their antiproliferative activities against nasopharyngeal carcinoma cells. *Guangdong Yaoxueyuan Xuebao* 30: 698–701.

15 Mu Tou Hui 墓頭回

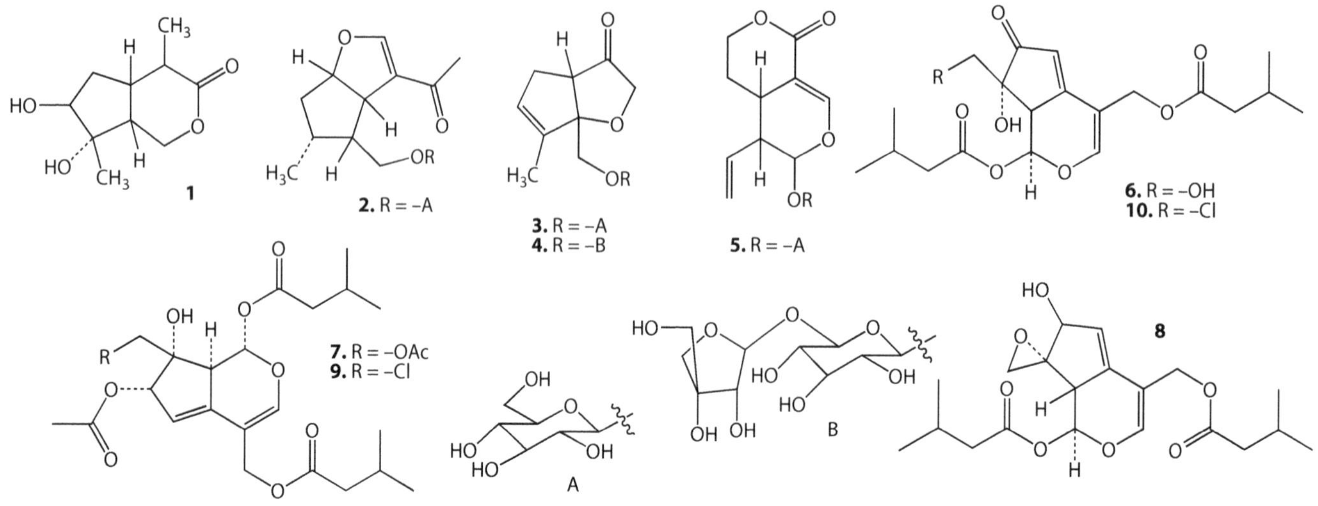

Herb Origination

The herb Mu Tou Hui originated from two Valerianaceae plants, *Patrinia heterophylla* and *P. rupestris* subsp. *scabra* (= *Patrinia scabra*). The former plant is wildly distributed in most of China and the latter plant is in the northeast and north regions of China as well as Mongolia and Siberia. Their roots are normally collected in autumn and dried in the sun for the application in Chinese folk medicine.

Antitumor Activities

In Chinese clinics, Mu Tou Hui (mainly *P. heterophylla*) is normally used in the prescription with other herbs to treat patients suffering from leukemia and malignant tumors in the stomach, the liver, the cervix, etc. Early investigations showed that the *in vitro* treatment with the extract of *P. heterophylla* destructively acted on EACs in its concentration of over 0.5 mg/mL. The administration of the extract to EAC-bearing mice by either oral, i.p., or subcutaneous resulted in a remarkable inhibitory effect on EAC solid tumor, and the inhibitory rates reached to 78–82% by i.p. and 64% by subcutaneous.[1] The i.p. administration of the extract in doses of 40 and 60 mg/kg exhibited a marked suppressive effect on the growth of hepatoma H22 cells in mice with inhibitory rates of 46.3% and 57.2%, respectively.[2] Also, the local injection of 5% of the extract (0.2 mL) into the EAC tumor notably suppressed the tumor growth. Similarly, its 50% water extract injected in a dose of 0.1 mL/10 g into sarcoma 180 (S180) exhibited 62.5% inhibitory effect *in vivo*. The i.p. administration not only directly killed S180 ascites cells but also enhanced the phagocytic activity and the cytotoxicity of macrophages in mice.[1] The water extract was also reported to be sensitive to acute leukemia cells but less sensitive to chronic myeloid leukemia cells.[3] The *in vitro* assay with a panel of human cancer cell lines was used to test an extract of *P. heterophylla* (PHEB). Human PC3 prostate adenocarcinoma was the most responsive cell line to PHEB in the growth inhibition (IC_{50}: 9.21 μg/mL), and HepG2 hepatoma and K562 leukemia were the most resistant (IC_{50}: 24.7 and 36.03 μg/mL, respectively) cell lines to PHEB. Together with the promotion of early apoptosis, PHEB concentration and time dependent restrained the proliferation of PC3 cells and K562 cells.[2–4] All four solvent-partitioned fractions (petroleum ether, chloroform, ethyl acetate, and n-butanol) were moderately cytotoxic to human HL-60 myeloid leukemia cells, but the chloroform fraction was the strongest one (IC_{50}: 17.91 μg/mL) on the HL-60 cells. The chloroform fraction was also moderately cytotoxic to human HepG2 hepatoma cells (IC_{50}: 19.57 μg/mL) and human SGC-7901 gastric adenocarcinoma cells (IC_{50}: 44.04 μg/mL) *in vitro*.[5]

An extract was prepared from another source of the herb *P. rupestris*, which contains 21.4% polysaccharide and 41.8% saponin. The *in vivo* treatment with the extract could increase the life prolongation rate of S180-bearing mice and induce the cell apoptosis by decreasing the mitochondrial membrane potential and increasing the free radical level in S180 cells.[6] Giving the ethanolic extract of *P. rupestris* to tumor-bearing mice by intragastric (i.g.) route also obviously augmented the functions of macrophages in phagocytosis and cytotoxicity.[7]

Antitumor Constituents and Activities

According to bioorganic chemical researches, the herb has been revealed to have the presence of various types of molecules such as triterpenoids, iridoids, steroils, flavonoids, coumarins, organic acids, volatile oils, and polysaccharides. Of these components, some iridoids, triterpenoids, flavonoids, coumarins, and polysaccharides were reported to have anticarcinoma related potentials.

Iridoids

A group of iridoid glucosides have been isolated from an ethanolic extract of the roots of *P. scabra* (= *P. rupestris*). Moreover, isopatriscabrol (**1**) showed a modest inhibitory effect against human HeLa cervical cancer cells (IC_{50}: 24.5 μM); other six iridoid glucosides elucidated as patriridoside-D (**2**), patriridoside-G (**3**), patriridoside-H (**4**), patriridoside-I, patrinioside, and sweroside

(**5**) showed moderate cytotoxic activities against human MNK-45 gastric cancer cells *in vitro* (respective IC_{50}: 15.6, 8.7, 9.4, 30.9, 23.8, and 11.2 μM).[8] A iridoid aglycone assigned as PS-1 (**6**) was separated from the *P. scabra*, exhibiting an antiproliferative effect on two human DU-145 and PC3 prostate cancer cell lines.[9] The treatment with PS-1 (**6**) and isopatriscabrol (**1**) in a concentration of 10 mg/mL restrained the proliferation of mouse C26 colon cancer cells by 60.44% and 53.34%, respectively, *in vitro*. Oral administration of PS-1 (**6**) and isopatriscabrol (**1**) in doses of 200 or 800 mg/kg per day to C26 tumor-bearing mice for 10 days reduced the tumor weight by 27.4% and 41.4%, respectively.[10] Additionally, the *in vivo* treatment with total iridoid components concurrently enlarged the thymus and spleen indexes, amplified the spleen lymphocyte production and the serum hemolysin level, and augmented the macrophage phagocytosis and the lymphocyte activity. The notable effects on the immune system function importantly contribute to the *in vivo* antitumor effect.[11]

From the herb (*P. heterophylla*), eight active iridoid esters have been isolated and evaluated *in vitro* with human neoplastic cell lines. All these displayed the antiproliferative effect against SGC-7901 (stomach) and PC3 (prostate) cancer cells, and the activity of isovaltrate acetoxyhydrin (**7**) and deacetylisovaltrate (**8**) was greater than those of others. Deacetylisovaltrate (**8**) showed the relatively strongest inhibitory effect on the two cell lines among the four iridoids (respective IC_{50}: 0.842 and 2.55 μmol/L), whose molecule contains an epoxy group. The epoxy group in deacetylisovaltrate (**8**) may modify the cysteine residue of proteins (such as STAT3, Jaks, NF-κB, Keapl), thereby exerting some additive antitumor activity.[12,13] In the investigation for the cancer suppressive mechanism, isovaltrate acetoxyhydrin (**7**) triggered the apoptosis and the cell cycle G2/M phase arrest of the SGC-7901 cells via the up-expression of cyclin-B1 and Bax, the down-expression of Bcl-2, the depolarization of mitochondrial membranes, and the activition of caspase-3 and caspase-9 signaling pathways.[14] Also, patriheterdoid-A, isovaltrate chlorohydrin (**9**), patrirupin-A (**10**), and 1β, 3α-diethyloxy-7-hydroxymethyl-4-(3-methylbutyryloxymethyl)-cyclopenta-4α,7α-diene[c]pyran-6-onewere were weakly active in the inhibition of MCF-7 breast cancer cells, and the IC_{50} values were 9.24–13.5 mol/L for the iridoids (**9** and **10**).[13]

In addition, PHEBB was the iridoid ester mixture prepared from *P. heterophylla* (PHEB), which was composed of desacetylisovaltratum (65%) and isovaltrate acetoxyhydrin (25%). An *in vitro* assay showed that PHEBB markedly restrained the proliferation of SGC-7901 (gastric), KB (oral), and Colo205 (colon) human cancer cell lines (respective IC_{50}: 2.27, 3.80, 5.49 μg/mL). In a mouse tumor model, the i.p. injection with PHEBB at a dose of 60 mg/kg resulted in a 45.5% inhibition on sarcoma 180 and 54.2% on H22 hepatoma. Concurrently, PHEBB also obviously stimulated the cell apoptosis and obstructed the microvessel growth and density in the tumor tissue.[15]

Triterpenes

A total triterpenes derived from *P. heterophylla* was known to be capable of suppressing the growth of human K562 leukemia cell line. A proteomic analysis revealed that the total triterpenes could stimulate four proteins (aldolase-A, glyceraldehyde-3-phosphate dehydrogenase, flavin reductase, and Hb subunit) and down-regulate four proteins (HSP90α, moesin, eukaryotic translation initiation factor-5A, tublin), whose data provided valuable insights into the antitumor mechanism of the total triterpenes against the K562 cells.[16] Six triterpenoids and one triperpene glycoside were isolated from the roots of *P. heterophylla*. The *in vitro* assay displayed that oleanic acid, ursolic acid, hederagenin, as well as oleanic acid 3-*O*-α-L-arabinopyranoside exerted an obvious inhibitory effect on the proliferation of HepG2 (liver), SGC-7901 (stomach), and HL-60 (leukemic) human cancer cell lines (IC_{50}: 4.58–18.07 μg/mL). Hederagenin demonstrated greater inhibitory activity on the HL-60 myeloid leukemia cells in the *in vitro* assay.[5]

Total Glycosides

Tripterygium glycosides tablet (TGT) is a tablet of total glycosides derived from *P. heterophyllya* roots, which have been tested in a nude mice model implanted with HT-29 colon cancer cells. The administration of the tablets to mice for eight weeks reduced the tumor weight and promoted the HT-29 cells to apoptotic death via the enlargement of Bax/Bcl-2 expression rate and caspase-3 activity.[17] The TGTs have been subjected to clinical trials to treat patients with colon carcinoma combined with surgery and/or chemotherapy, resulting in additive therapeutic effect.[18,19]

Lignans

Several lignans, such as lariciresinol, isolariciresinol, syringaresinol, nortracheloside, and other lignin glycosides, have been separated from the *P. scabra* roots. The total lignin components demonstrated the marked anticarcinoma activity against human K562 erythroleukemia cells *in vitro* with 99.38% maximal inhibitory rate (IC_{50}: 21.16 μg/mL, in 96 h). Concurrently, the total lignins elicited the apoptosis and suppressed the growth of K562 cells in concentration- and time-dependent manners.[20] Patrineolignan-A (**11**) and patrineolignan-B (**12**), whose two norlignans were isolated from the roots of *P. scabra*, exerted the potent antiproliferative effect on HeLa (cervix) and MNK-45 (stomach) human cancer cell lines.[21] Moreover, three lignans were discovered having an anticancer activity from the roots of *P. heterophylla*. Nortrachelogenin (**13**), (+)-pinoresinol (**14**) and (+)-lariciresinol (**15**) displayed a remarkable inhibition against the proliferation of PC3 (prostate), SGC (gastric), and NB-4 (leukemic) human tumor cell lines *in vitro*.[22]

Polysaccharides

PHB-P, PHB-P1, and PHB-P2 are polysaccharide components derived from the roots of *P. heterophylla* or *P. scabra*. The treatment of HeLa cervical cancer cells with PHB-P (50 μg/mL) and of U14 cervical cancer cells with PHB-P2 (40 mg/mL) resulted in the induction of G0/G1 cell cycle arrest and apoptosis in association with the down-expression of Bcl-2 and the activation of p53 and Bax, thereby exerting the antigrowth effect against HeLa cells (IC_{50}: 52 μg/mL) and U14 cells *in vitro*.[23,24] By the similar induction of apoptosis and cell cycle arrest, PHB-P1 treatment in doses of 30 and 60 mg/kg and PHB-P2 in doses of 40 and 80 mg/mL notably reduced the tumor weight of mice implanted with U14 cervix cancer cells.[24,25] The polysaccharides were also proven to have a remarkable capability to significantly potentiate the host immune system, such as to augment the immune organ weight and the lymphocyte activity and to enhance the macrophage function, the serum hemolysin production, etc.[26]

Clinical Trial

1. The TGTs have been clinically trialed to treat 50 patients with colon carcinoma combined with surgery and chemotherapy. The integrated treatment (surgery + chemotherapy + TGT) significantly amplified the lifetime and the living quality of patients. The resulted survival rates were 79% for one year, 61% for two years, and 40% for three years, whose data were better than 58%, 37%, and 8%, respectively, for the treatment (surgery + chemotherapy) without TGT. The clinical trial also showed that the one-year survival rates could reach 83% for patients in B and C stages, but only 62% of one-year survival rates for patients in the D stage after being treated with the TGT combined with surgery and chemotherapy.[18] Due to TGT significantly diminishing the level of carcinoembryonic antigen and enhancing the immune function T cells and the cytotoxicity of NK cells, the TGT additive treatment noticeably augmented the physical condition of patients and improved clinical symptoms.[18]
2. One hundred thirty-two colorectal cancer patients were randomly divided into three groups: those treated with chemotherapy alone, TGT alone, or a combination of chemotherapy and TGT, respectively. The two treatments (TGT alone and chemotherapy plus TGT) resulted in a greatly improved life quality. The short-term effective and survival time rates in the group with TGT integrated chemotherapy were significantly upgraded; the immunological function was markedly enhanced; and the toxicity of chemotherapy was decreased.[19]

Consequently, the two clinic trials evidenced that the TGT (total glycosides) is a potential agent for augmenting the efficacy of chemotherapy, especially in the treatment of colorectal carcinomas.[19]

Other Medical Uses

The herb Mu Tou Hui has been used as a folklore medicine in Asia for several hundred years in the treatment of abscesses, hepatitis, tonsillitis, ulcers, malaria, anthracia, stasis, typhoid, leukorrhea, metrorrhagia, and metrostaxis.

References

1. State Chinese Medicine Administration Bureau of China. 1999. *Chinese Materia Medica*. Vol. 7, 567–70. Shanghai Science and Technology Press, Shanghai, China.
2. Yang, B. et al. 2011. Preliminary evaluation of antitumor effect and induction apoptosis in PC-3 cells of extract from *Patrinia heterophylla*. *Braz. J. Pharmacogn. Revista*. 21: 471–6.
3. Sun, W. L. et al. 1990. MTT study on cytotoxic effect of Mutouhui on leukemia. *J. Gansu College TCM* 7: 34–6.
4. Cheng, W. D. et al. 2007. Inductive effect of diversifolious patrinia root extract on K562 cells apoptosis. *J. Beijing Univ. TCM* 30: 51–3.
5. Ding, L. et al. 2007. Studies on the chemical constituents of *Patrinia heterophylla Bunge* and their antitumor activities. *J. Northwest Normal Univ.* 43: 62–5.
6. Wang, X. X. et al. 2008. Antitumor effects and mechanisms of *Patrinia rupestris (Pall.) Juss.* subsp. *scabra (Bunge)* H. J. Wang extract. *Zhongcaoyao* 39: 572–4.
7. Ma, Q. H. et al. 2010. Advanced studies on chemical components and pharmacological effects of *Patrinia scabra*. *China Pharmacist* 13: 879–81.
8. Li, N. et al. 2012. Cytotoxic iridoids from the roots of *Patrinia scabra*. *J. Nat. Prod.* 75: 1723–8.
9. Mao, J. Q. et al. 2007. Effects of the iridoid aglycones from *Patrinia scabra* on colon cancer. *J. Pharm. Practice* 25: 10–2.
10. Li, T. J. et al. 2004. Antitumor effects of the iridoid aglycones from *Patrinia scabra*. *Pharm. J. Chin. People's Liberation Army* 20: 101–2.
11. Chu, Z. Y. et al. 2008. Effect of iridoid aglycones from *Patrinia scabra* on mouse immune function. *Zhongyaocai* 31: 882–6.
12. Yang, B. et al. 2013. Two new cytotoxic iridoid esters from the rhizomes and roots of *Patrinia heterophylla*. *Nat. Prod. Res.* 27: 2105–10.
13. Yang, B. et al. 2014. A new cytotoxic iridoid from the rhizomes and roots of *Patrinia heterophylla*. *Chem. Nat. Compds.* 50: 661–4.
14. Yang, B. et al. 2013. Induction of cytotoxicity and apoptosis in human gastric cancer cell SGC-7901 by isovaltrate acetoxyhydrin isolated from *Patrinia heterophylla Bunge* involves a mitochondrial pathway and G2/M phase cell cycle arrest. *Asian Pacific J. Cancer Prev.* 14: 6481–6.
15. Yang, B. et al. 2013. Antitumor effect of iridoid ester fraction from Patriniae radix and its mechanism. *Chin. Tradit. Herbal Drugs* 44: 2884–8.
16. Wei, D. F. et al. 2012. Proteomic analysis of the effect of triterpenes from *Patrinia heterophylla* on leukemia K562 cells. *J. Ethnopharmacol.* 144: 576–83.
17. Chen, J. X. et al. 2007. Effects of Yiye Baijiang Zonggan tablets on apoptosis of human colon cancer HT-29 cells. *Chin. J. Hospital Pharmacy* 27: 159–61.
18. Chen, J. X. et al. 1999. Study on the Mutouhui glycosides tablets in clinical treatment of colon cancer. *Zhongcaoyao* 30: 528–9.
19. Wang, H. Z. et al. 2001. A clinical study on the effect of *radix Patriniae heterophylla* glucoside tablets on colorectal cancer. *Chin. J. Clin. Oncol. Rehabilitat.* 8: 37–9.
20. Chen, R. et al. 2007. Growth-inhibiting effect of lignanoids from *Patrinia scabra* on K562 cells. *J. Sichuan TCM* 25: 14–6.
21. Di, L. et al. 2013. Two new neolignans from *Patrinia scabra* with potent cytotoxic activity against HeLa and MNK-45 cells. *Archev. Pharm. Res.* 36: 1198–203.
22. Chen, X. Y. et al. 2013. Study on lignans constituents of *Patrinia heterophylla* root and cytotoxic activity. *Zhonghua Zhongyiyao Xuekan* 31: 2168–70.
23. Lu, W. Z. et al. 2009. Polysaccharide from *Patrinia heterophylla Bunge* inhibits HeLa cell proliferation through induction of apoptosis and cell cycle arrest. *Science* 40: 161–6.
24. Lu, W. Z. et al. 2009. Antitumor activity of polysaccharides isolated from *Patrinia scabra Bunge* on U14 cervical carcinoma bearing mice. *Am. J. Chin. Med.* 37: 933–44.
25. Lu, W. Z. et al. 2010. Antitumor activity of polysaccharides isolated from *Patrinia heterophylla*. *Pharm. Biol.* (London) 48: 1012–7.
26. Tang, Q. X. et al. 1998. Inference of Mutouhui on mouse immune functions. *Chin. J. Basic Med. in TCM* (4): 27–8.

16 Bai Jiang Cao 敗醬草

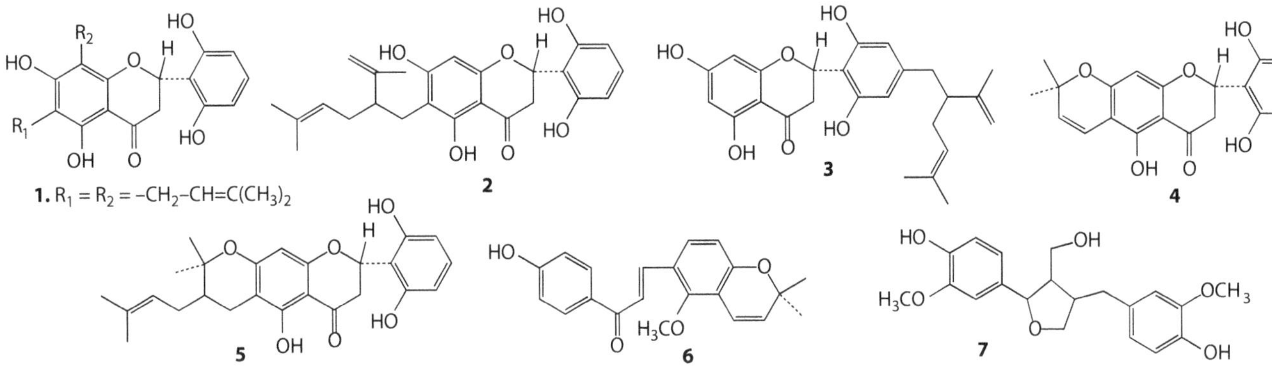

1. $R_1 = R_2 = -CH_2-CH=C(CH_3)_2$

Herb Origination

The herb Bai Jiang Cao has two plant origins, *Patrinia scabiosaefolia* and *Patrinia villosa* (Valerianaceae). The two Patrinia plants are similarly distributed in the northeast, north, east, and south regions as well as a part of the southwest areas of China. The whole plant is collected in summer and autumn for wide-growing plant, but the best collection time for the cultured plant is before blooming. The collected whole plant is dried in the sun for the employment in Chinese folk medicine.

Antitumor Activity

The herb Bai Jiang Cao is a well-known oriental folk medicine for the clinical treatment of various malignancies including gastrointestinal cancers. The bioactivity-related phytochemical investigations provided many scientific evidences to show the antitumor potential of Bai Jiang Cao.

Extract from P. scabiosaefolia

In the treatment of a panel of human cancer cell lines including MCF-7 (breast), A375 (skin), HepG2 (liver), A549 (lung), and PC3 (prostate) cells for 48 h *in vitro*, its ethyl acetate extract (EAE-PS) exerted a marginal inhibitory effect against these cell proliferations. The most responsive cell line to the EAE-PS was the MCF-7 breast cancer cells (IC_{50}: 112.3 μg/mL), while the most resistant one was PC3 prostate cancer cells. In the assay, EAE-PS multiplied the apoptosis of MCF-7 cells by 14.5-fold after 36 h of treatment, whose apoptosis was found being elicited by activating a caspase-independent mitochondrial cell death pathway.[1] Through the inhibition of the STAT3 pathway and the down-expression of cyclin-D1 and Bcl-2, its ethanol extract (EEPS) showed apoptotic induction and proliferative suppression against human U266 multiple myeloma cells.[2] Both *in vitro* and *in vivo* models confirmed that the EEPS was able to restrain the growth of mouse colorectal cancer cells and human HT-29 colon cancer cells in association with the promotion of cell apoptosis without apparent adverse side effects. More data revealed that the augmentation of mitochondrial-dependent pathway might be one of the apoptotic mechanisms by EEPS, where EEPs limited the expression of antiapoptotic Bcl-2 and enhanced the proapoptotic Bax expression at both transcriptional and translational levels, leading to mitochondrial membrane potential loss and caspase-9 and caspase-3 activations in the HT-29 cells.[3] Moreover, EEPS treatment also suppressed the expression of VEGF-A in the HT-29 cells and attenuated the intratumoral microvessel density in the tumor tissues. EEPS was also able to obstruct several key processes of the proliferation, migration, angiogenesis, and tube formation of human umbilical vein endothelial cells (HUVECs). These evidences confirmed that the antiangiogenic property of EEPS might largely contribute to its *in vivo* anticolon cancer effect.[4]

Extract from P. villosa

Two human cancer cell lines (HeLa and MCF-7) showed sensibility to the crude extract of *P. villosa*. The extract was fractionated by a macroporous resin column, and its 80% ethanolic eluate demonstrated a marked suppressive activity against the proliferation of HeLa (cervix), EJ (bladder), MCF-7 (breast), and HCT-8 (colon) human cancer cell lines *in vitro*. The IC_{50} values were 11.90 μg/mL in HeLa cells, 12.55 μg/mL in MCF-7 cells, 15.61 μg/mL in HCT-8 cells, and 65.32 μg/mL in EJ cells. The 80% ethanolic eluate was chemically examined to contain 61.81% of total saponins and 8.69% of total flavonoids, whose constituents could be considered as the active components of *P. villosa* for the antitumor effect.[5] Its ethyl acetate fraction exhibited an antioxidant activity and a moderate to weak degree of cytotoxic effect on A549 (lung), HepG2 and SSMC-7721 (liver), and HeLa (cervix) human neoplastic cell lines *in vitro*. The oral administration of the fraction (120 mg/kg) for 10 days reduced the tumor weight of sarcoma 180 in mice.[6]

Antitumor Constituents and Activities

Triterpenoid Saponins

The *P. villosa* saponins (SPV) were demonstrated to have an inhibitory activity against the proliferation of human HeLa cervical cancer cells in a dosage-dependent manner, associated with the promotion of caspase-3-activated apoptosis.[7] SPV also exerted dose-dependent antiproliferative effect against mouse B16 melanoma, mouse L1210 leukemia, and human MCF-7 breast cancer cell lines *in vitro* concomitant with the inhibition of CDK4 and cyclin-D1 expressions and the arrest of the cell cycle at G0/G1 stage.[8] The antitumor effect of SPV was further demonstrated in a mouse model transplanted with U14 cervical carcinoma cells, where SPV in doses of 50 and 100 mg/kg effectively reduced the weight of the U14 tumor by 35.1% and 57.1%, respectively.[9] Also, the i.g. administration with SPV in doses of 250 and 500 mg/kg for 15 days suppressed the U14 solid tumor by 46.60% and 52.15% and prolonged the life duration of mice bearing U14 ascites tumor by 71.42% and 46.10%, respectively.[10] The antitumor effect was found to be mediated by inducing apoptosis and inhibiting the expressions of proliferating cell nuclear antigen (PCNA), mutant P53, and Bcl-2 protein besides causing G0/G1 cell arrest.[9] Ursolic acid, a triterpenoid isolated from *P. villosa* extract, showed an obvious suppressive effect on breast cancer cells (IC_{50}: 15.0 μg/mL), whose ursolic acid is often an aglycone of saponins in the plant.[11] The administration of ursolic acid by i.p. (25 or 50 mg/kg/day) or orally (100 or 150 mg/kg/day) for two weeks markedly restrained the proliferation and the tumor weight of H22 hepatoma xenograft mice, whose ant-hepatoma activity was also contributed by the ursolic acid-enhanced immune functions such as the improvement of TNF-α level and IL-12 concentration in serum, the increase of white blood cell count, thymus index, and spleen index, and the promotion of lymphocytes, including $CD4^+$, $CD8^+$ T cell infiltration in tumor tissue.[12,13]

Similarly, the triterpenoid saponins from *P. scabiosaefolia* roots are the important antitumor constituents. Several saponins were separated and then hydrolyzed in an alkaline condition to remove the glycosidic chain at C-28 carboxyl group of the aglycones. The i.p. administration of five isolated secondary saponins (P24b, P25b, P26b, P27b, and P29b) to the tumor-bearing mice in a daily dose of 5 mg/kg for 10 days notably reduced the tumor weight in mice implanted with SMMC-7721 hepatoma cells, whose respective suppressive rates were 55.7%, 54.2%, 71.9%, 69.3%, and 58.9%, and the activities of P26b and P27b were comparable to a positive control (CTX, 68.2%). Among the five secondary saponins, P26b demonstrated the relatively strongest suppression (IC_{50}: 3.2 μg/mL) against human SMMC-7721 hepatoma cells *in vitro* and *in vivo*.[14,15]

Flavonoids

In vitro experiments exhibited that the total flavonoids (FPV) derived from *P. villosa* was effective in the inhibition of four neoplastic cell lines (L1210, B16, MCF-7, and HeLa), associated with the inhibition of CDK4 and cyclin-D1 expressions and the induction of G0/G1 cell arrest. Of these cell lines, mouse L1210 leukemia cells were more sensitive to the FPV.[8] Bioassay-combined phytochemical research led to six separate antitumor flavonoids from the FPV. These were all active in the inhibition of A549 (lung), Bel-7402 (liver), SGC-7901 (stomach), HT-29 (colon), A498 (kidney), and K562 (leukemia) human cancer cell lines, especially being more sensitive to A549, Bel-7402, and K562 cell lines (IC_{50}: 1.64–12.25 μg/mL) compared to HT-29, SGC-7901, MCF-7, and A498 cell lines (IC_{50}: 4.08–49.52 μg/mL). (2S)-5,7,2′,6′-Tetrahydroxy-6,8-di-(γ,γ-dimethylallyl) flavanone (**1**), (2S)-5,7,2′,6′-tetrahydroxy-6-lavandulylated flavanone (**2**), and (2S)-5,7,2′,6′-tetrahydroxy-4′-lavandulylated flavanone (**3**) showed a greater suppressive effect on the seven human cancer cell lines (IC_{50}: 1.64–10.20 μg/mL), particularly on K562 leukemia cells (IC_{50}: 1.64–3.04 μg/mL). Other flavonoids assigned as licoagrochalcone-B (**6**), (2S)-5,2′,6′-trihydroxy-2″,2″-dimethyl-pyrano-[5″,6″:6,7]flavanone (**4**), and (2S,3″S)-5,2′,6′-trihydroxy-3″-γ,γ-dimethylallyl-2″,2″-dimethyl-3″,4″-dihydropyrano[5″,6″:6,7] flavan-one (**5**) were relatively sensitive to A549, K562, and Bel-7402 cell lines (IC_{50}: 6.58–13.20 μg/mL).[16]

Lignan

Lariciresinol (**7**) was a bioactive lignan isolated from *P. villosa*, which exerted a marked suppressive effect against the proliferation of four tested cell lines such as human PC3 prostate cancer, NB4 acute promyelocytic leukemia, KB nasopharyngeal epidermoid cancer cell lines, and mouse B16 melanoma cells *in vitro*. The respective IC_{50} values were 0.32, 0.59, 3.92, and 2.17 μg/mL. The anticancer effect of lariciresinol (**7**) was closely related to apoptosis induction.[17]

Other Medical Uses

The herb Bai Jiang Cao, a well-known Chinese medicinal herb, has been widely used to clinically treat various types of diseases such as carbuncles, diarrhea, blood stasis, acute appendicitis, hepatapostema, pancreatitis, pneumonia, hepatitis, tonsillitis, parotitis, neurasthenia insomnia, snakebite, etc.[18]

References

1. Chiu, L. C. M. et al. 2006. Ethyl acetate extract of *Patrinia scabiosaefolia* downregulates anti-apoptotic Bcl-2/Bcl-xL expression, and induces apoptosis in human breast carcinoma MCF-7 cells independent of caspase-9 activation. *J. Ethnopharmacol.* 105: 263–8.
2. Peng, J. et al. 2011. *Patrinia scabiosaefolia* extract suppresses proliferation and promotes apoptosis by inhibiting the STAT3 pathway in human multiple myeloma cells. *Mol. Med. Reports* 4: 313–8.
3. Liu, L. Y. et al. 2013. *Patrinia scabiosaefolia* induces mitochondrial-dependent apoptosis in a mouse model of colorectal cancer. *Oncol. Reports* 30: 897–903.
4. Chen, L. W. et al. 2013. *Patrinia scabiosaefolia* inhibits colorectal cancer growth through suppression of tumor angiogenesis. *Oncol. Reports* 30: 1439–43.
5. Song, T. et al. 2012. Antitumor effect of extracts of *Patrinia villosa Juss. Shizhen Guoyi Guoyao* 23: 2410–2.
6. Lei, J. C. et al. 2015. Antioxidant and antitumour activities of extracts from *Patrinia villosa* and its active constituents. *J. Functional Foods* 16: 289–94.
7. Zhang, T. et al. 2012. Caspase-3 participates in *Patrinia villosa* saponin-induced HeLa apoptosis. *Zhongguo Laonianxue Zazhi* 32: 2321–3.
8. Guo, L. X. et al. 2013. Antitumor effects and mechanisms of total saponin and total flavonoid extracts from *Patrinia villosa Juss. Afri. J. Pharm. Pharmacol.* 7: 165–71.
9. Zhang, T. et al. 2008. Antitumor effects of saponin extract from *Patrinia villosa Juss* on mice bearing U14 cervical cancer. *Phytother. Res.* 22: 640–5.
10. Wang, L. L. 2011. Study on antitumor effects of the saponin from *Patrinia villosa* on mice cerivical cancer. *Inlt. J. Trad. Chin. Med.* 33: 1083–5.
11. Huang, L. et al. 2007. Studies on chemical constituents of *Patrinia villosa. Zhongyaocai* 30: 415–7.

12. Yao, H. B. et al. 2013. Inhibitory effects of ursolic acid on tumor growth in hepatocarcinoma 22-bearing mice. *Carcinog. Teratog. Mutag.* 25: 1–6.
13. Fang, X. H. et al. 2013. Antitumor and immune effects of ursolic acid on H22 xenograft growth in mice. *J. Chin. Oncol.* 19: 199–201.
14. Liu, J. Y. et al. 2012. Triterpenoid saponin compounds with antitumor effect. *Faming Zhuanli Shenqing* CN 102627683 A 20120808.
15. P24b: 3-*O*-β-D-xylopyranosyl (1-3)-α-L-rhamnopyranosyl (1-2)-α-L-arabinopyranosyl oleanolic acid; P25b: 3-*O*-D-xylopyranosyl (1-3)-α-L-rhamno-pyranosyl (1-2)-β-D-xylopyranosyl oleanolic acid; P26b: 3-*O*-β-D-glucopyranosyl (1-4)-β- D-xylopyranosyl (1-3)-α-L-rhamnopyranosyl (1-2)-β-D-xylopyranosyl oleanolic acid; P27b: 3-*O*-β-D-glucopyranosyl (1-4)-β-D-xylopyranosyl (1-3)-α-L-rhamno-pyranosyl (1-2)-α-L-arabinopyranosyl oleanolic acid; and P29b: 3-*O*-β-D-xylopyranose (1-3)-α-L-rhamnopyranosyl (1-2)-α-L-arabinopyranosyl hederagenin.
16. Peng, J. Y. et al. 2006. Preparative isolation of four new and two known flavonoids from the leaf of *Patrinia villosa Juss* by counter-current chromatography and evaluation of their anticancer activities in vitro. *J. Chromatog. A* 1115: 103–11.
17. Ding, Y. X. et al. 2012. Studies on antitumor activity in vitro of lariciresinol from *Patrinia villosa Juss. Zhonghua Zhongyiyao Xuekan* 30: 420–2.
18. Kim, J. S. et al. 2013. Chemical constituents of plants from the genus *Patrinia. Nat. Prod. Sci.* 19: 77–119.

17 Ma Chi Xian 馬齒莧

Common Purslane or Verdolaga

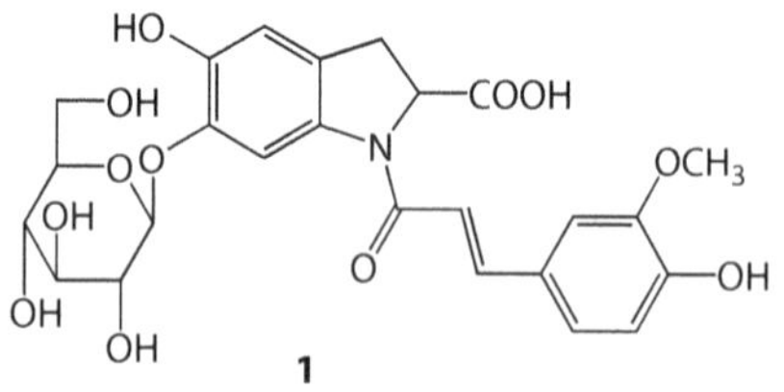

Herb Origination

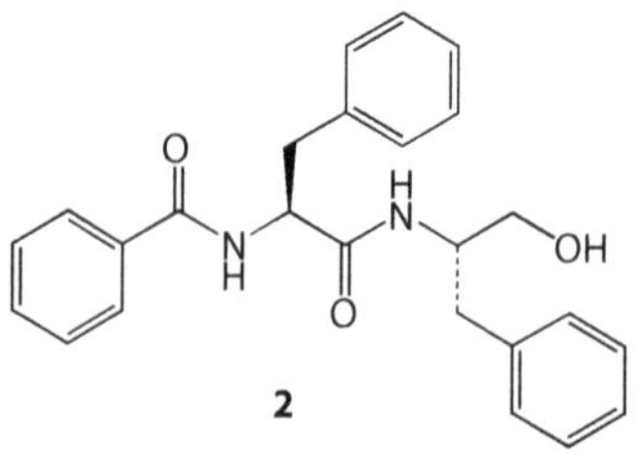

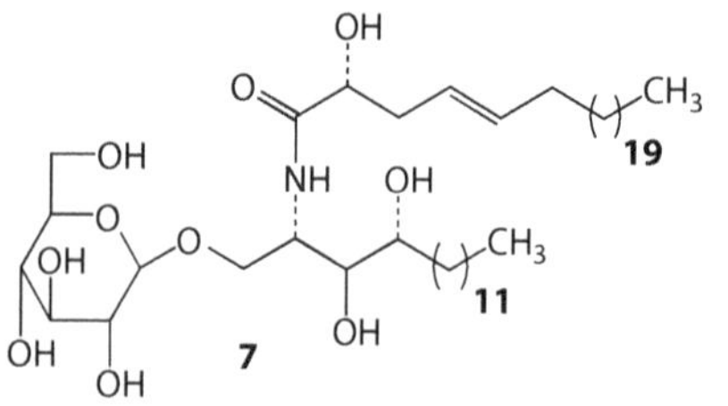

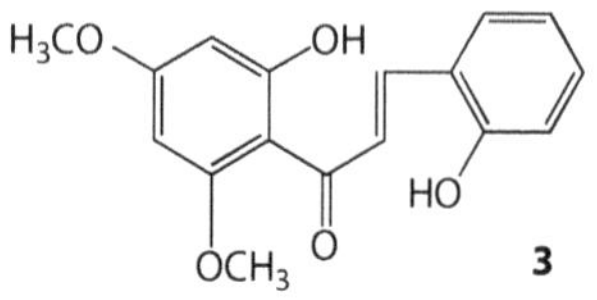

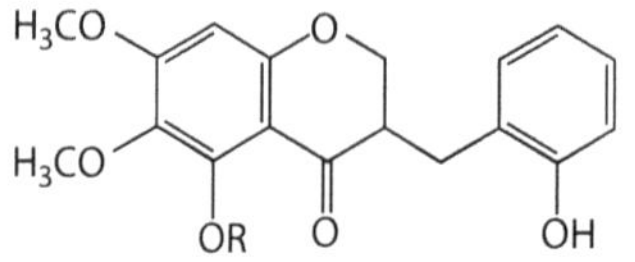

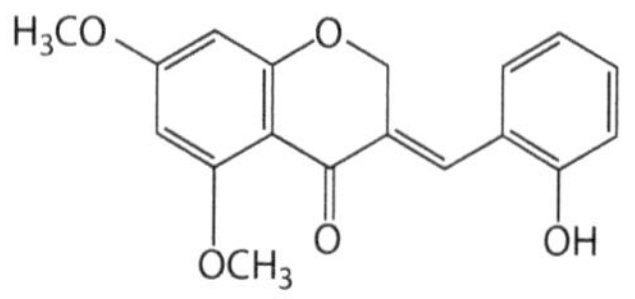

The herb Ma Chi Xian (common Purslane) is an annual succulent *Portulaca oleracea* L. (Portulacaceae), whose plant has an extensive distribution extending from North Africa through the Middle East to world tropical and temperate zones. The purslane is considered a weed in many places, but it is eaten throughout much of Europe, the middle east, Asia, and Mexico as a wild vegetable.

Antitumor Activities and Constituents

In pharmacological investigations, Ma Chi Xian exhibited multiple bioactivities including anticarcinogenesis and anticancer. Its methanolic extract was effective to human Calu-6 pulmonary cancer cells (IC_5: <25.0 µg/mL) but not active to human SNU-601 gastric cancer cells *in vitro*.[1] Its 75% ethanolic extract showed a selective cytotoxic effect against human Colo 320 HSR colon adenocarcinoma and KATO-III gastric cancer cells *in vitro* in concentration- and time-dependent manners and no such activity on normal fibroblast cell lines such as L929 and WI38. The extract at 0.6 mg/mL concentration could kill KATO-III gastric cancer cells by 74% in 24 h, 92% in 48 h, and 100% in 72 h. In nude mice inoculated with Colo 320 HSR cells, the treatment with 5 mg of the extract per day for 10 days markedly depressed the colon cancer size and growth *in vivo*.[2]

Many kinds of constituents were identified from Ma Chi Xian, including organic acids, flavonoids, terpenoids, coumarins, alkanoids, polysaccharides, as well as volatile oil. Some of them demonstrated different degrees of antitumor activity in the bioassays.

Alkaloids

An alkaloid fraction prepared from Ma Chi Xian in an *in vitro* assay exerted an obvious antiproliferative effect against A549 (lung), HeLa (cervix), and HEp-2 (larynx) human cancer cell lines.[3] Two alkaloids assigned as oleracein-B (**1**) and aurantiamide (**2**) were reported to have marked suppressive activity against the proliferation of human K562 leukemia cells and human A549 lung adenocarcinoma cells *in vitro*.[4] Additionally, oleracein-A, oleracein-B, and oleracein-E showed an antioxidant effect, whose lipid peroxidant-reducing and radical-scavenging functions are related to the anticarcinogenic effect.[5] Four other types of alkaloids assigned as N-*trans*-feruloyltyramine, (7′R)-N-feruloylnormetanephrine, (3R)-3,5-bis(3-methoxy-4-hydroxyphenyl)-2,3-dihydro-2(1H)-pyridinone, and 1,5-dimethyl-6-phenyl-1,2-dihydro-1,2,4-triazin-3(2H)-one, which were isolated from its air-dried aerial parts, exhibited a moderate suppressive effect against A549 lung adenocarcinoma cells (IC_{50}: 21.76–37.20 µmol/L) but weak activity on K562 leukemia cells.[6]

Flavonoids

Its flavonoid component showed marked cytotoxicity on human malignant fetal rhabdomyoma RD cells *in vitro*. In a mouse model transplanted with sarcinoma 180, the flavonoid component obstructed the tumor weight by 38%, whose effect was greater than the other components.[3] From the aerial parts of fresh plant *P. oleracea*, four homoisoflavonoids and other flavonoids were separated. Portulacanone-B, portulacanone-D and 2,2′-dihydroxy-4′,6′-dimethoxychalcone (**3**) showed *in vitro* cytotoxic effect toward four human cancer cell lines. Especially, 2,2′-dihydroxy-4′,6′-dimethoxychalcone (**3**) was found to be inhibitory to SGC-7901 gastric cancer cells (IC_{50}: 1.6 µg/mL), which was 8.1-fold more potent than an antitumor drug mitomicin (IC_{50}: 13.0 µg/mL). This chalcone (**3**) also moderately restrained human K562 erythroleukemia cells (IC_{50}: 24.6 µg/mL).[6] Portulacanone-B (**4**) displayed a moderate suppressive effect against SGC-7901 (gastric) and HCL-H460 (lung) human carcinoma cell lines (IC_{50}: 16.2 and 17.8 µg/mL, respectively), whereas portulacanone-D (**5**) was cytotoxic to NCI-H460 (lung) and SF-268 (CNS) human cancer cell lines (IC_{50}: 14.3 and 15.0 µg/mL, respectively).[7] The antiproliferative effect of portulacanone-C (**6**) was only shown in the NCL-H460 cells *in vitro* (IC_{50}: 20.1 µg/mL).[7] In addition, the flavonoid component, as proven by animal experiments, effectively prevented renal damage caused by an antitumor drug cisplatin and advantaged no toxic and no adverse effects.[3,8]

Triterpenoids

Among the tritepenoids isolated from Ma Chi Xian, friedelan-4α-methyl-3β-ol at 100 μmol concentration reached a 50% inhibitory rate on HeLa cervical carcinoma cell line.[9] (2α,3α)-3-{[4-O-(β-D-glucopyranosyl)-β-D-xylopyranosyl]oxy}-2,23-dihydroxy-30-methoxy-30-oxoolean-12-en-28-oic acid and (2α,3α)-2,23,30-trihydroxy-3-[(β-D-xylopyranosyl)oxy]olean-12-en-28-oic acid only showed a weak cytotoxic activity on HepG2 hepatoma cells *in vitro*.[9]

Cerebroside

Portulacerebroside-A (PCA, **7**), in an *in vitro* assay, markedly restrained the viability of human HCCLM3 hepatoma cells in time- and dose-dependent manners, simultaneously elicited chromatin aggregation and fragmented nuclei, and augmented the percentage of apoptotic cells, whose PCA (**7**)-induced apoptosis was associated with the activation of a p38 MAPK- and JNK-triggered mitochondrial death pathway including the disruption of mitochondrial membrane penetrability, the release of mitochondrial cytochrome c and AIF to cytosol, and the activation of caspase-9 and caspase-3.[10] The PCA (**7**) treatment significantly inhibited cell viability, markedly induced apoptosis, reduced HeLa cells adhesion, and decreased the migration and the invasion of HeLa cells.[11] The findings suggested the potential therapeutic and preventive effects of PCA (**7**) on hepatoma and cervical cancer.

Betacyanins

Combinational experiments confirmed that betacyanin components extracted from *P. oleracea* could enhance the therapeutic effect of CTX in the cancer treatment and also attenuate the side effects of CTX in mice implanted with sarcoma 180. During the 10-day treatment, the different doses of betacyanins not only augmented the tumor inhibition rate of CTX, but also notably improved the indexes of the spleen and the thymus and the levels of immunoglobulin G and immunoglobulin M; enlarged the number of bone marrow karyocytes, white blood cells (WBC), and platelets; and alleviated CTX-induced increase of alanine aminotransferase (ALT) and blood urea nitrogen (BUN). The immunopotentiating functions help the host to resist the toxicity of chemotherapy and to restore the damaged immune system.[12]

Glycolipids

A glycolipid component was prepared from *P. oleracea* and identified as 6-*O*-[(2E,6S)-2,6-dimethyl-6-hydroxy-2,7-octadienoyl]-(α~β)-D-glucopyranose, which displayed a good anticarcinoma effect and showed a potential of being a health food supplement for preventing and treating neoplasm.[13] In addition, the fatty acid components from Ma Chi Xian also showed a certain activity in the suppression of HEp-2 larynx carcinoma cells *in vitro*.[3]

Polysaccharides

Polysaccharides were purified from MaChi Xian as antitumor components. The polysaccharides dose dependently restrained the proliferation of human hepatoma SMMC-7721 cells *in vitro* and inhibited the growth of ascites type of sarcoma 180 by 52.72% together with the amplified T lymphocyte amount in a mouse model.[14] An isolated unique polysaccharide (POP) exerted a significant inhibitory effect against the growth of sarcoma 180 transplanted in mice, associated with its immunostimulating properties, such as increases in the numbers of WBC and $CD4^+$ T lymphocytes, elevation of the ratio of $CD4^+/CD8^+$, and decline of the levels of serum aspartate transanimase (AST), ALT, BUN, and creatinine.[15] PHP was a polysaccharide extracted from *P. oleracea*, which at a high-dose administration obviously restrained both solid and ascites types of U14 cervical cancer in mice by 43.76% and 47.73%, respectively and improved the survival time and the living quality of the tumor-bearing mice with very little acute side effects. It also showed significantly inhibitory potential against lung metastases of U14 cervical cancer cells, whose effect was better than CTX.[16] POL-P3b, a water-soluble polysaccharide purified from the herb, exhibited an antiproliferative effect against *in vitro* HeLa cervix cancer cells and triggered sub-G1 phase cell cycle arrest, DNA damage, and intrinsic apoptosis of HeLa cells. Its antineoplastic and apoptosis-promoting effects of POL-P3b were also showed in U14 cervical tumor-bearing mice.[17] POP1 is a water-soluble antitumor polysaccharide from *P. oleracea*. When introduced sulfated groups into C-6 and C-2 positions of POP1 to give four sulfated derivatives (POP1-sl, POP1-s2, POP1-s3, and POP1-s4), these derivatives had different degrees of substitution ranging from 1.01 to 1.81, and different average molecular masses (m.w.) ranging from 41.4 to 48.5 kDa. In an *in vitro* experiment, these sulfated derivatives were markedly cytotoxic to HepG2 cells and HeLa cells *in vitro*, implying that the sulfated modification can augment the cytotoxic activity of POP1 on the tumor cells.[18]

Moreover, polysaccharides of Ma Chi Xian not only enhanced the body weight, the peripheral WBC count, the thymus and spleen indexes and remarkably promoted splenocytes proliferation and serum cytokines (IL-2, IL-4, and TNFα) genesis, but also provided a remarkable protection against oxidative injury by enhancing superoxide dismutase (SOD), catalase (CAT), GSH-Px activities in rats implanted with gastric cancer induced by N-methyl-N′-nitro-N-nitrosoguanidine, whose enhancement of antioxidants and immune response might be responsible for the anticancer effect.[19]

Other Bioactivities

As a Chinese folk medicine and edible wild vegetable, Ma Chi Xian (common Purslane) has been used as diuretic, antiseptic, antiscorbutic, febrifuge, antispasmodic, and vermifuge drugs with a long history. Pharmacological approaches confirmed that Ma Chi Xian possesses antiinflammatory, antioxidant, hypoglycemic, hypolipidemic, antiaging, antiatherosclerosis, antiviral and antibacterial activities. Also, Ma Chi Xian is rich in SL3 fatty acid and vitamin A like substances that are healthful supplements. The aqueous extract was found to have marked protective property against cisplatin-induced hepatotoxicity.[20]

References

1. Chon, S.-U. et al. 2008. Characteristics of the leaf parts of some traditional Korean salad plants used for food. *J. Sci. Food Agricul.* 88: 1963–8.

2. Ham, S. S. et al. 1998. Specific inhibition of tumor cell growth by *Portulaca oleracea PCT/CA* 1997/000873 WO 1998024457 A1.
3. Li, Y. P. et al. 2009. Screening antitumor effect of active constituents from *Portulaca oleracea* L. in vitro and in vivo. *Shizhen Guoyi Guoyao* 20: 2726–8.
4. Zhao, Q. C. et al. 2013. Application of *Portulaca oleracea* alkaloid monomer compounds in manufacture of antitumor drugs. *Faming Zhuanli Shenqing* CN 103110655 A 20130522.
5. Yang, Z. J. et al. 2009. Phenolic alkaloids as a new class of antioxidants in *Portulaca oleracea. Phytother. Res.* 23: 1032–5.
6. Zhou, Y. X. et al. 2015. *Portulaca oleracea* L.: A review of phytochemistry and pharmacological effects. *Biomed Res Intl.* 2015: 925631.
7. Yan, J. et al. 2012. Homoisoflavonoids from the medicinal plant *Portulaca oleracea. Phytochem.* 80: 37–41.
8. Xie, S. Y. et al. 2011. Recent progress on chemical constituents of *Portulaca oleracea* L. and their pharmacological effects. *Xiandai Yaowu yu Linchuang* 26: 212–5.
9. Xin, H. L. et al. 2008. Two novel triterpenoids *from Portulaca oleracea L. Helv. Chim. Acta* 91: 2075–80.
10. Zheng, G. Y. et al. 2014. Portulacerebroside A induces apoptosis via activation of the mitochondrial death pathway in human liver cancer HCCLM3 cells. *Phytochem. Lett.* 7: 77–84.
11. Zheng, G. Y. et al. 2014. Effects of portulacerebroside A on apoptosis, migration and invasion of human cervical cancer HeLa cells. *Zhongliu Fangzhi Yanjiu* 41: 388–391.
12. Yang, G. Q. et al. 2010. Antitumor effects of betacyanins extracted from *Portulaca oleracea L. Shizhen Guoyi Guoyao* 21: 388–90.
13. Wu, B. 2012. Glycolipids compound from *Portulaca oleracea*, its preparation process and application in preparing the medical preparations or health food for preventing and treating neoplasm. *Faming Zhuanli Shenqing* CN 102516324 A 20120627.
14. Cui, M. et al. 2002. Antineoplastic activity of polysaccharide from *Portulaca oleracea. J. Shandong Norm. Univ.* 17: 73–6.
15. Shen, H. et al. 2013. Purification and characterization of an antitumor polysaccharide from *Portulaca oleracea* L. *Carbohydrate Polymers* 93: 395–400.
16. Zhao, R. 2013. Anti-uterine cervix cancer study of polysaccharide from *Portulace oleracea* L. on aged tumor-bearing mice. *Zhongguo Laonianxue Zazhi* 33: 4480–2.
17. Zhao, R. et al. 2013. Antitumor activity of *Portulaca oleracea* L. polysaccharides against cervical carcinoma in vitro and in vivo. *Carbohydrate Polymers* 96: 376–83.
18. Chen, T. et al. 2010. Sulfated modification and cytotoxicity of *Portulaca oleracea* L. polysaccharides. *Glycoconjugate J.* 27: 635–42.
19. Li, Y. Q. et al. 2014. Evaluation of antioxidant and immuno-enhancing activities of Purslane polysaccharides in gastric cancer rats. *Intl. J. Biol. Macromol.* 68: 113–6.
20. Sudhakar, D. et al. 2010. *Portulaca oleracea* L. extract ameliorates the cisplatin-induced toxicity in chick embryonic liver. *Indian J. Biochem. Biophys.* 47: 185–9.

18 Bai Tou Weng 白頭翁

Chinese pulsatilla anemone

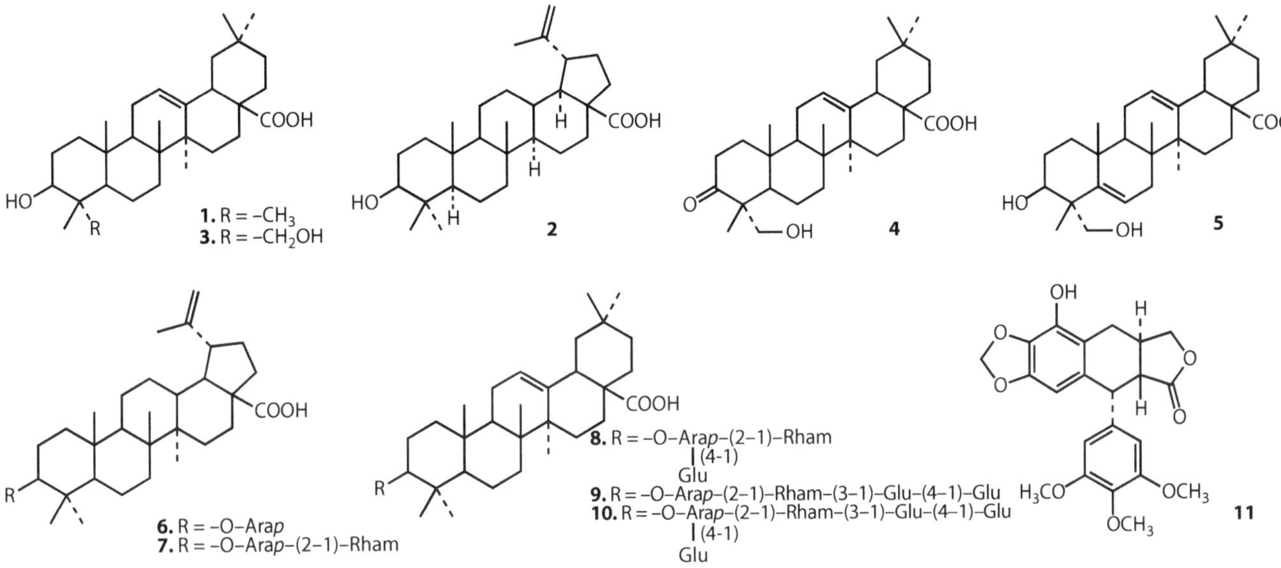

1. R = $-CH_3$
3. R = $-CH_2OH$

2

4

5

6. R = -O-Ara*p*
7. R = -O-Ara*p*-(2–1)-Rham

8. R = -O-Ara*p*-(2–1)-Rham
| (4-1)
Glu
9. R = -O-Ara*p*-(2–1)-Rham-(3–1)-Glu-(4–1)-Glu
10. R = -O-Ara*p*-(2–1)-Rham-(3–1)-Glu-(4–1)-Glu
| (4-1)
Glu

11

Herb Origination

The herb Bai Tou Weng (Chinese pulsatilla) originates from six Pulsatilla genus plants (Ranunculaceae), but *Pulsatilla chinensis* (= *Anemone chinensis*) is the most popular source for this herb. *P. chinensis* is native to the north of China and the east of Siberia, and its root is normally collected between March and April or September and October. Bai Tou Weng is one of the 50 fundamental herbs applied in traditional Chinese medicine. The earliest record of Bai Tou Weng was in the first Chinese materia medica titled as *Shennong Ben Cao Jing*.

Antitumor Activities

Both the alcohol and water extracts of Chinese pulsatilla root demonstrated obvious anticancer and anticarcinogenic properties, but the activity of alcoholic extract (PAE) was normally better than that of its water extract (PWE). In *in vitro* experiments, PAE markedly repressed the proliferation of K562 (leukemic), BGC823 (gastric), Bcap-37 (breast), and CoC1 (ovary) human cancer cell lines, but both PAE and PWE had weak inhibition against SMMC-7721 (liver), HeLa (cervix), and MKN-45 (gastric) human cancer cell lines. Two bioactive fractions A and B derived from the PAE displayed a much improved antiproliferative effect on eight types of human tumor cell lines, such as K562, Bcap-37, SK and CoC1 (ovary), MCF-7 (breast), Col-26 (colon), PANC-1 and BxPC-3 (pancreas), HeLa (cervix), and 9L (gliosarcoma) cells, *in vitro*, and the IC_{50} values were 1.2–5.6 μg/mL on the cancer cell lines except of the HeLa and 9L cells. The strongest inhibitory effect of both fractions was showed in the 9L cells (IC_{50}: 0.27–0.34 μg/mL).[1–3] Moreover, a light petroleum fraction (PEF) derived from PAE showed a marked antiproliferative effect against human HL-60 promyelocytic leukemia cells *in vitro* with its IC_{50} value of 14 μg/mL.[4]

In vivo investigations also confirmed the antiproliferative effect of Bai Tou Weng extracts. The oral administration of its decoction to tumor-bearing murine animals for 10 continuous days resulted in the tumor growth suppressive effects against sarcoma 180, hepatoma HepA, Ehrlich ascites tumor, and Lewis lung cancer.[5] When PAE was orally administrated to mice implanted with H22 hepatoma in doses of 10 and 20 g/kg for 10 days, its tumor weight and the tumor microvessel density could be significantly reduced, indicating that the antiangiogenic effect must be related to the *in vivo* antitumor activity.[6] At a dose of 20 mg/kg per day, PEF restrained the growth of sarcoma 180 cells by 36.7% in mice, but the tumor inhibitory response was unusual in a reverse dose-dependent manner.[4] The extracts of radix Pulsatillae also noticeably attenuated the incidences of colon carcinogenesis caused by dimethylhydrazine (an oncogene) in mice by 63%, whose effect is largely related to its abilities in protecting SOD and GSH-Px activities, scavenging free radicals, and repressing colon mucous cell proliferation.[7]

Antitumor Constituents and Activities

Triterpene Acids

The major anticarcinoma constituents in the herb were found to be a group of triterpene acids, which also exist in the herb as sapogenins composed of triterpenoid saponins. Pulsatillic acid (**1**) displayed cytotoxicity on human large cell lung carcinoma, murine P388 leukemia, and Lewis lung carcinoma (IC_{50}: 1.9, 4.8, and 5.9 μg/mL, respectively).[8] Betulinic acid (**2**), 23-hydroxybetulinic acid (**3**, 23-HBA), and 3-oxo-23-hydroxybetulinic acid (23-HBA) (**4**) exerted moderate cytotoxicity on murine B16 melanoma cells (IC_{50}: 22.5–32 μg/mL), whereas lupeol and betulin exhibited the weak cytotoxicity (IC_{50}: >100 μg/mL). The treatment with these derivatives of betulinic acid (**2**) rapidly augmented the production of ROS and directly dissipated the mitochondrial membrane potential, leading the B16 cells to apoptosis.[9] 23-HBA (**3**) at a low concentration (10–20 μg/mL) also elicited the differentiation of the melanoma cells besides the antiproliferation *in vitro* and *in vivo*.[10] The moderate inhibition on human tumor cells including HeLa (cervx), SMMC-7721 (liver), and HL-60 (leukemia) was achieved by betulinic acid (**2**), 23-HBA (**3**) hederagonic acid (**5**), hederagenin, pulsatilla triterpenic acids A to C, ursolic acid, and oleanolic acid. Among the triterpenes, hederagenin, and hederagonic acid (**5**) relatively exerted the most marked inhibitory effect (IC_{50}: 11.88–15.24 μg/mL), and the IC_{50}: of other triterpenes ranged from 19.53 μg/mL to 31.22 μg/mL.[11]

Moreover, 23-HBA (**3**) as the major bioactive constituent in the herb also significantly improved the sensitivity of various cancer cell lines to DOX (a chemotherapeutic drug), by increasing the intratumor DOX content and inhibiting the DOX-induced upregulation of P-gp in tumor cells *in vitro* and *in vivo*.[12] When HBA (**3**) was radioiodinated with ^{125}I, the produced ^{125}I-23-HBA exerted a greater cytotoxic effect after being intratumorally injected to HepA hepatoma-bearing mice.[13] 23-*O*-(1,4′-bipiperidine-1-carbonyl) betulinic acid (BBA) is a synthetic derivative of HBA, which could reverse P-gp-mediated MDR and reverse MDR protein 7 (MRP7)-mediated MDR, leading to the enhancement of the sensitivity of MRP7-transfected HEK293 cells to paclitaxel, docetaxel, and vinblastine.[14] The findings suggest that HBA and BBA have the potential to be used in combination with chemotherapeutic agents to augment the response to chemotherapy.

Saponins

The total saponins derived from *P. chinensis* roots inhibited the proliferation of human Bel-7402 hepatom, HT-29 colon cancer, and K562 leukemia cell lines *in vitro* with the promotion of apoptosis. The *in vitro* antiproliferative rates were 76.0–97.6% on the HT-29 cells after being treated with the saponins at doses of 5–20 μg/mL.[15–17] The *in vivo* anticancer effect of the saponins was confirmed in nude mice transplanted with the Bel-7402 hepatoma. The administration of the total saponins by oral in doses of 100 or 200 mg/kg per day for 19 days markedly diminished the tumor mass and stimulated the apoptosis of Bel-7402 hepatoma cells *in vivo* without toxic/side effects,[15] whose antigrowth mechanism was found to be related with regulating energy metabolism through an HIF-1α pathway.[18] From the total saponins, several saponins were separated and were proven to have anticancer properties by *in vitro* and/or *in vivo* assays.

In parallel with G2/M cell cycle arrest and apoptotic induction, pulchinenoside-B4 significantly restrained the proliferation of HepG2 hepatoma cells by 71.5%.[19] Pulsatilloside-A (**6**) and ulsatilloside-B (**8**) displayed an obvious antigrowth effect against two human cancer cell lines *in vitro*, and the IC_{50} values were 3.3 and 7.3 μM in K562 leukemia cells and 6.8 and 8.4 μM in HeLa cervical cancer cells, respectively. Their aglycone betulinic acid (**2**) and its derivative 23 HBA (**3**) showed little lower inhibitory effect on the two cell lines with IC_{50} values of 12.3–13.2 μM in the K562 cells and 8.6–11.2 μM in the HeLa cells.[20] Simultaneously, 23-HBA (**3**) promoted S cell cycle arrest and cell apoptosis of the K562 leukemia via intrinsic pathway.[17] In cell culture, Pulsatilla saponin-A markedly inhibited the growth of human SMCC-7721 hepatoma, BXPC3, and SW1990 pancreatic cancer cell lines. Its cancer inhibitory activities were further proven in mouse xenograft tumor models with Bel-7402 hepatoma and SW1990 pancreatic cancer. The suppressive effect of Pulsatilla saponin-A was associated with the induction of G2 arrest, DNA damage, and apoptosis in the cancer cell lines.[21] Similarly, the anticancer effect of Pulsatilla saponin-D was demonstrated on the SMMC-7721 cells *in vitro* and on mouse H22 hepatoma *in vivo*.[22] Other eight saponins with oleanolic acid or hederagenin as their aglycones exerted moderate cytotoxicity against HL-60 human promyelocytic leukemia cells (IC_{50}: 2.3–7.8 μg/mL), while the aglycones (oleanolic acid and hederagenin) gave the respective IC_{50} values of 4.4 and 7.1 μg/mL. Among the tested saponins, the oleanolic saponins (**8–10**) demonstrated the stronger growth inhibition on the HL-60 cells (IC_{50}: 2.3–2.7 μg/mL).[23] Furthermore, alkali hydrolyzate of total saponins dose dependently obstructed the proliferation and the colony formation of human U251 glioma cells and triggered the U21 cells to apoptosis.[24] More investigations revealed that the cancer inhibitory potency could be potentiated by the C-3 glycosidation at the aglycone but would be significantly attenuated if the glycosidation was at the C-28 ester.[15–24]

Lignans

From the herb, the antitumor activities of two types of lignans assigned as (+)-pinoresinol and β-peltatin (**11**) were separated and evaluated. β-Peltatin (**11**) was the most potent cytotoxic to the HL-60 cells with an IC_{50} value of 0.0052 μg/mL, while (+)-pinoresinol showed no such activity.[23]

Polysaccharides

The inhibitory effect of *P. chinensis* polysaccharides (PCPS) was evaluated in both *in vivo* and *in vitro* models with glioma. PCPS exerted a significant antiproliferative effect against C6 glioma cell line *in vitro* and a remarkable inhibitory effect against the growth of C6 glioma *in vivo* with the prolongation of life survival. Simultaneously, the treatment also elevated the indexes of the thymus and the spleen in mice and relieved the damages in the liver and the kidney by diminishing the levels of AST, MDA, ALT and urea and enhancing the activities of SOD and CAT in the plasma of tumor-bearing mice.[25] The findings suggested that the PCPS may be considered as a possible supplement to improve cancer chemotherapy and chemoprevention. PCPw, a water-soluble polysaccharide purified from the herb, showed the antitumor activity in mice with transplantable mouse 4T1 breast tumor. After 10 days of PCPw (50, 100, and 200 mg/kg) treatment once daily, the oral administration of PCPw to mice notably retarded the growth of transplantable 4T1 tumor *in vivo* and concurrently improved both cellular and humoral immune responses.[26]

Glycoprotein

PcG-A, a glycoprotein isolated from the dried root of *P. chinensis*, is an immunostimulator. *In vitro* experiments substantiated that PcG-A could significantly augment phagocyticactivity and nitric oxide (NO) release of peritoneal macrophages. It also had some

positive effects on IL-l secretion, whose specific activities in the enhancement of macrophage immune functions should have a close correlation to the anticancer and anti-arcinogenic activities.[27]

Formulations

For the improvement of oral bioavailability, the saponins of *P. chinensis* were prepared to four different types of formulations, such as PRS-Na (salt form), hydroxypropyl-β-cyclodextrin inclusion complex (PRS-HPβCD), PRS-O/W (oil-in-water emulsion), and PRS-silica (micronization). The formulation techniques obviously improved the solubility of saponins and enhanced the oral bioavailability of saponins to varying degrees, as PRS-HPβCD > PRS-silica > PRS-O/W > PRS-Na. In particular, PRS-HPβCD was the most effective way to promote the absorption and the bioavailability of the saponins by > 20 times.[28] Based upon the research results, the formulations afforded valuable information for further development of *P. chinensis* saponins.

Other Bioactivities

The herb Bai Tou Weng (Chinese pulsatilla roots) has therapeutic effects on diseases of the urinary system, the digestive system, the cardiovascular system, and the hematopoietic system. Pharmacological studies corroborated that Bai Tou Weng possesses antiprotozoan, detoxification, antiviral, and antibacterial effects besides antitumor effects, and it is also able to improve human body immunity and to inhibit IL-6 secretion of macrophage.

References

1. Yuan, Y. et al. 1999. Antitumor activity of Chinese pulsatilla (*Pulsatilla chinensis*) in vitro. *Zhongcaoyao* 30: 441–3.
2. Zhu, J. T. et al. 2007. Study on antitumor effect of *Pulsatilla chinensis (Bunge) Regel* extracts in vitro. *Aibian, Jibian, Tubian* 19: 67–9.
3. Feng, X. Z. et al. 2011. Study of apoptosis in gastric cancer cells induced by Chinese Pulsatilla root. *China Modern Doctor* 49, 1–2.
4. Zhang, M. et al. 2008. The antitumor effect of the light petroleum extract from *Pulsatilla chinensis Regel*. *Nat. Prod. Commun.* 3: 819–22.
5. Zhuang, X. H. et al. 1999. Antitumor activity of Chinese pulsatilla (*Pulsatilla chinensis*) in. vivo. *Shiyong Zhongliu Zazhi* 14: 94–6.
6. Zhu, L. J. et al. 2011. The antiangiogenic effect of alcohol extract of radix Pulsatillae on a xenograft model of transplanted hepatocellular carcinoma. *Xiandai Zhongliu Yixue* 12: 2382–5.
7. Zhang, R. H. et al. 1999. The preventive and therapeutic effect of radix Pulsatillae on mice colorectal cancer induced by dimethylhydrazine. *Zhongyao yaoli yu Linchuang* 15: 33–5.
8. Ye, W. C. et al. 1996. Triterpenoids from *Pulsatilla chinensis*. *Phytochem*. 42: 799–802.
9. Liu, W. K. et al. 2004. Apoptotic activity of betulinic acid derivatives on murine melanoma B16 cell line. *Eur. J. Pharmacol.* 498: 71–8.
10. Ye, Y. Y. et al. 2001. The differentiation induced by 23-Hydroxybetulinic acid on B16 cells. *Zhongguo Shenghua Yaowu Zazhi* 22: 163–6.
11. Shu, Z. et al. 2011. Three new triterpenoids from *Pulsatilla chinensis (Bunge) Regel* and their cytotoxic activities. *Heterocycles* 83: 2365–72.
12. Zheng, Y. T. et al. 2010. 23-Hydroxybetulinic acid from *Pulsatilla chinensis (Bunge) Regel* synergizes the antitumor activities of doxorubicin in vitro and in vivo. *J. Ethnopharmacol.* 128: 615–22.
13. Yang, M. et al. 2010. Potential of radioiodinated anticancer compounds of traditional Chinese medicine for cancer therapy. *J. Radioanal. Nuclear Chem.* 283: 189–91.
14. Chen, J. J. et al. 2013. BBA, a synthetic derivative of 23-hydroxybutulinic acid, reverses multidrug resistance by inhibiting the efflux activity of MRP7 (ABCC10). *PLoS One* 8: e74573.
15. Xu, Q. M. et al. 2012. Antitumor activity of *Pulsatilla chinensis (Bunge) Regel* saponins in human liver tumor 7402 cells in vitro and in vivo. *Phytomed.* 19: 293–300.
16. Luo, Y. Y. et al. 2013. Effects of *Pulsatilla chinensis* saponins on proliferation and apoptosis of HT29 cells. *Zhongyao Yaoli Yu Linchuang* 29: 52–56.
17. Liu, M. et al. 2015. Cytotoxicity of the compounds isolated from *Pulsatilla chinensis* saponins and apoptosis induced by 23-hydroxybetulinic acid. *Pharm. Biol.* (London, UK) 53: 1–9.
18. Luo, Y. Y. et al. 2014. Regulation of saponins from *Pulsatilla chinensis* on energy metabolism of Bel-7402 xenograft in nude mice. *Zhongcaoyao* 45: 973–7.
19. Wang, H. X. et al. 2011. Effect of pulchinenoside B4 on the proliferation and apoptosis of human liver cancer cell line HepG2 in vitro. *J. Shanghai Jiaotong Univ.* (*Med. Edit.*) 31: 1481–5.
20. Ye, W. C. et al. 2002. New lupane glycosides from *Pulsatilla chinensis*. *Planta Med.* 68: 183–6.
21. Liu, Q. et al. 2014. Pulsatilla saponin A, an active molecule from *Pulsatilla chinensis*, induces cancer cell death and inhibits tumor growth in mouse xenograft models. *J. Surgical Res.* 188: 387–95.
22. Xu, K. et al. 2014. Effect of pulsatilla saponin d on hepatocarcinoma in vivo and in vitro. *Zhongchengyao* 36: 240–4.
23. Mimaki, Y. et al. 1999. Triterpene saponins and lignans from the roots of *Pulsatilla chinensis* and their cytotoxic activity against HL-60 cells. *J. Nat. Prod.* 62: 1279–83.
24. Peng, C. P. et al. 2014. Anti-glioma effect and mechanism of alkali hydrolysate of total saponins from *Pulsatilla chinensis* on human glioma U251 cells. *Zhongyao Xinyao Yu Linchuang Yaoli* 25: 254–9.
25. Zhou, F. G. et al. 2012. Inhibitory effect of *Pulsatilla chinensis* polysaccharides on glioma. *Intl. J. Biol. Macromol.* 50: 1322–6.
26. Liu, T. et al. 2013. Immunopontentiating and antitumor activities of a polysaccharide from *Pulsatilla chinensis (Bunge) Regel*. *Intl. J. Biol. Macromol.* 54: 225–9.
27. Dai, L. et al. 2000. The immuno-enhancing effect of PcG-A-a glycoprotein isolated from dried root of *Pulsatilla chinensis (Bunge) Regel*. *Zhongguo Shenghua Yaowu Zazhi* 21: 230–1.
28. Huang, J. et al. 2015. Comparative pharmacokinetic profiles of five poorly soluble pulchinenosides in different formulations from *Pulsatilla chinensis* saponins extracts for enhanced bioavailability. *Biomed. Chromatogr.* 29: 1885–92.

19 Ban Zhi Lian 半枝蓮

Barbat skullcap

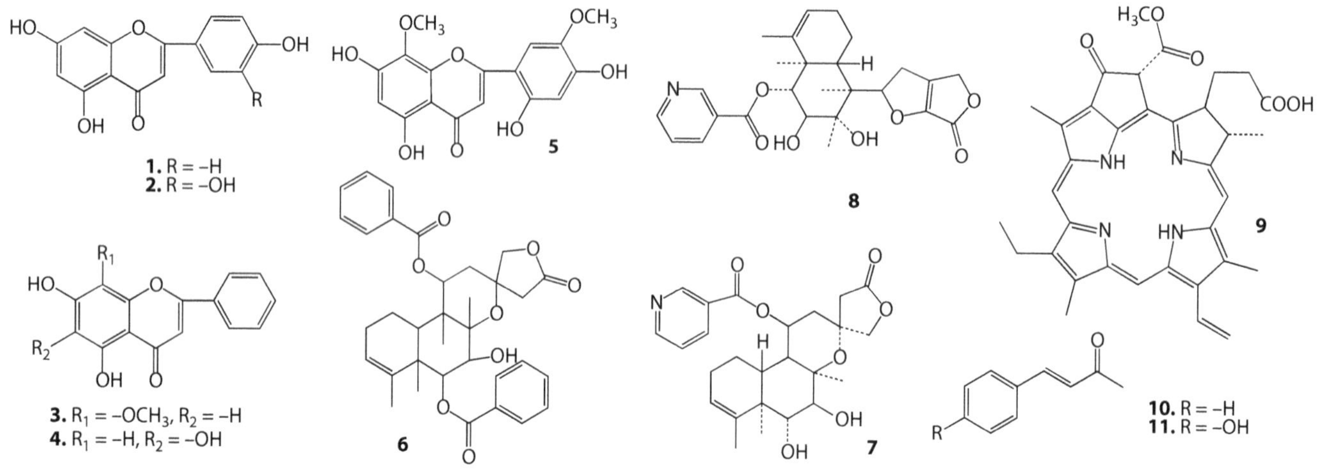

1. R = -H
2. R = -OH
3. R_1 = $-OCH_3$, R_2 = -H
4. R_1 = -H, R_2 = -OH

5 6 7 8 9

10. R = -H
11. R = -OH

Herb Origination

The herb Ban Zhi Lian (Barbat skullcap) originated from a Lamiaceae plant *Scutellaria barbata*. The perennial plant is natively distributed throughout southern China and some middle Chinese provinces, as well as Korea. The whole plant is usually collected in May, July, and September, and dried in the sun for traditional Chinese medicinal practice.

Antitumor Activities

The herb Ban Zhi Lian has long been used in China for the clinical treatment of various solid carcinomas in organs such as colorectal, lung, liver, breast, ovary, and digestive system, as well as chorioepithelioma. A preliminary investigation revealed that the juice prepared from its fresh fruits and the herb aqueous extract were capable of inhibiting the proliferation and inducing the apoptosis of a variety of cancer cells, including MDA-MB231 and MCF-7 (breast), A549 and LU (lung), Lovo (colon), HepG2 and Hep3B (liver), SLMT-1 (esophageal), LNCaP (prostate), KB (epidermoid), and KG-1 (leukemic), as well as ovarian cancer cell lines, *in vitro*,[1–3] and the aqueous extract also restrained the proliferation of uterine myometrial and leiomyomal cells.[4–12] A Ban Zhi Lian decoction exerted marked growth inhibitory and chemopreventive activities against human HeLa cervical carbinoma cells *in vivo* (IC_{50}: 16–70 μg/mL, in 48 h). Among them, the chloroform fraction showed the strongest cytotoxicity on the tumor cell lines and lower cytotoxicity on normal liver cells. The fraction at a dose of 60 mg/kg/day significantly inhibited the proliferation of Bel-7402 hepatoma cells *in vivo* and improved the life span of mice bearing ascites carcinoma.[13] The chloroform fraction also induced apoptosis and inhibited proliferation of human colon cancer cell lines (SW620, HT-29, and HCT-8) *in vitro*.[14] The methylene chloride fraction efficiently inhibited the proliferation of human U937 histiocytic lymphoma cells (IC_{50}: ≤10 μM) and promoted the apoptosis through a mitochondria-mediated signaling pathway, i.e., upregulation of Bax and downregulation of Bcl-2, decrease of IGF-I expression, release of cytochrome c from mitochondria, cleavage of PARP, activation of caspase-9 and caspase-3, as well as the increase of the sub-G1 DNA contents in the cell cycle progression.[15–17] The *in vivo* anticancer effect of a Ban Zhi Lian extract was further substantiated in a mouse model implanted with H22 hepatoma cells.[18] In addition, the ethanolic extract could significantly synergize the antitumor effects of a low dose 5-FU both *in vivo* and *in vitro* and concurrently enhance the apoptosis-inducing effect of a low dose 5-FU in both HCT-8 colon cancer cells and Bel-7402 hepatoma cells.[19]

Likewise, the Ban Zhi Lian extracts efficiently obstructed the angiogenesis in the tissues of HeLa cervical cancer and LoVo and HT-29 colon cancers as well, whose effect was associated with the inhibition of endothelial cell migration and tube formation, via the suppression of VEGF-A and Akt kinase.[20–22] In a colorectal cancer mouse xenograft model, the ethanolic extract potently obstructed the angiogenesis via the blockage of the Sonic hedgehog pathway and the decline of VEGF-A expression besides stimulating the apoptosis of colon cancer cells, leading to the effective reduction of tumor size without affecting the body weight gain in mice.[23] Also, by repressing the cytochrome P450IA-mediated metabolism of carcinogens (BAP and AFB1) and blocking the BAP bound to the DNA, the extracts exerted a marked antimutagenic effect.[24] Consequently, these investigations provided the scientific evidences to support the use of Ban Zhi Lian as a safe and effective herb in cancer chemoprevention and antitumor therapy.

BZL101

BZL101 (Bezielle) is a product derived from the aqueous extract of Ban Zhi Lian that is shown to have chemopreventive and growth inhibitory properties on a variety of human cancer cells. Its anticancer activity has been demonstrated in two human breast cancer cell lines (MCF-7 and MDA-MB-231) and two human prostate cancer cell lines (LNCaP and PC3).[25]

Different types of cancer cell lines may have different sensitivity and mechanism to the same extract. The antigrowth effect of BZL101 mainly accompanied by the G1-cell cycle arrest with the corresponding decline of estrogen receptor-α (ERα) transcript expressions, ablation of cyclin-D1, CDK2, and CDK4, and blockage of growth factor stimulatory pathways in early-stage estrogen-sensitive MCF-7 breast cancer cells. Similarly, BZL101 induced the growth arrests in G2/M-phase and suppressed the expressions of cyclin-B1, CDK1, and androgen receptor (AR) in early-stage androgen-sensitive LNCaP prostate cancer cells. After the BZL101 treatment, an S phase arrest with corresponding ablations in cyclin-A2 and CDK2 expression were confirmed in late-stage estrogen-insensitive breast MDA-MB-231 cells and androgen-insensitive prostate cancer PC3 cells.[25] By regulating the mediator proteins (p27Kip1, p21Cip1, and Jab1) and stimulating the ROS production and the PARP hyperactivation, BZL101 triggered the cell death and the G2 cycle arrest in ER^+-BT474 cells and ER–SKBR3 cells, leading to the anti-breast-cancer effect. In addition, the BZL101 treatment was capable of restraining the glucose metabolism and glycolysis and decreasing the fatty acid synthase (FAS) in the breast cancer cells, then causing the depletion of ATP and nicotinamide adenine dinucleotide and the blockage of the major energy-producing pathways.[26] The anticancer effect of BZL101 was further confirmed in a murine breast cancer xenograft model. Oral and i.p. administrations of BZL101 restrained the breast tumor formation without any toxicity.[27] Based upon the evidences, the cytotoxicity of BZL101 was revealed to primarily correlate with the inhibition of metabolic pathways that are preferentially activated in tumor cells.

Clinical Trials of BZL101

Two phase I clinical trials of BZL101 have been practiced for patients with metastatic breast cancer and advanced breast cancer, respectively.[8,28] Both trials demonstrated encouraging clinical potential and favorable tolerability profile in the heavily pretreated population. The results suggested that the BZL101 may be valuable for the potential development of BZL-based therapeutic strategies on human reproductive cancers. Currently, BZL101 is in phase II clinical trial in patients with advanced breast cancer.[29,30]

Antitumor Constituents and Activities

According to the phytochemical investigation, flavonoids and diterpenoids were known as the major constituents in Ban Zhi Lian. Both components were found to be principally responsible for the biological activities of the herb, including moderate anticancer and anticarcinogenic activities. Despite no sharp cancer inhibitors discovered from the herb, the scientific evidences offered solid support for the uses in cancer therapy and prevention.

Flavonoids

In the *in vitro* assay, the total flavonoids of *S. barbata* (TF-SB) significantly inhibited the proliferation and the invasion and induced the apoptosis of human highly metastatic MHCC97H hepatoma cells in a dose-dependent manner, whose proapoptosis was mediated by a mitochondrial pathway, and its antiinvasive effect was correlated with the decrease of MMP-2 and MMP-9 expressions and the increase of TIMP-1 and TIMP-2 expressions.[31,32] Both *in vitro* and *in vivo* experiments demonstrated that TF-SB dose dependently inhibited the proliferation and the migration of HUVECs and simultaneously blocked HUVEC angiogenesis via the downregulation of VEGF activity.[33] These results evidenced that TF-SB may serve as potential antiproliferative, antimetastatic, and antiangiogenic agents against hepatoma.[34] Several antitumor active flavonoids such as apigenin (**1**), luteolin (**2**), wogonin (**3**), baicalein (**4**), viscidulin-III (**5**), and 2′,3′,5,7-tetrahydroxyflavone were isolated from Ban Zhi Lian, showing a moderate inhibition on various tumor cell lines (IC_{50}: 9.5–23 μM).[35] The major flavonoids apigenin (**1**) and luteolin (**2**) dose and time dependently elicited the apoptosis of human HL-60 promyelocytic leukemia and SGC-7901 gastric cancer cell lines, associated with the up-expression of Bad and Bax, the down-expression of Bcl-2 and Bcl-xL, the disruption of mitochondrial membrane potential, the release of cytochrome c, the cleavage of PARP, and the activation of caspase-9 and caspase-3.[36,37] Apigenin (**1**) induced p53 expression, which is related to cell cycle arrest and apoptosis in neuroblastoma cells, and it also exerted an antioxidant defense against N-nitrosodiethylamine-caused oxidative stress, lipid peroxidation, and DNA damage in animal models bearing hepatoma.[38–40] Luteolin (**2**), wogonin (**3**), hispidulin, as well as phytol also showed a cytotoxic effect on human Bel-7402 hepatoma cells *in vitro* with IC_{50} values of 8–20 μg/mL.[9]

Both *in vivo* and *in vitro* experiments proved that the STAT3/Fas signaling pathway was suppressed for the apoptosis of human hepatoma cells induced by luteolin (**2**). Besides a mitochondrial pathway for inducing apoptosis, luteolin (**2**) also completely inhibited the catalytic activity of eukaryotic DNA Topo-I at a concentration of 40 μM.[34,41] The pretreatment with luteolin (**2**) greatly suppressed NF-κB-targeted antiapoptotic genes and sensitized TNFα-induced apoptosis in HeLa (cervix), Colo205, and HCT-116 (colorectal) human cancer cell lines.[42] In addition, apigenin (**1**) and luteolin (**2**) obviously inhibited VEGF-induced angiogenesis *in vivo* and *in vitro*.[43,44] These findings evidenced that both apigenin (**1**) and luteolin (**2**) as well as the total flavonoids have great value for chemoprevention and chemotherapy as adjutant supplements.

In addition, three flavonoids, i.e., protoapigenone, scutellarein, and scutellarin, which were separated from *S. barbata*, were reported to have an obvious ability to sensitize cisplatin (an anticancer drug) to human ovarian cancer cells, leading to the synergistical potentiation of the cytotoxicity of conventional antitumor drugs.[45]

Diterpenoids

Ban Zhi Lian is rich in *neo*-clerodane- and *ent*-clerodane-diterpenoids. Most of diterpenoids isolated from the herb, such as barbatins, scutehenanines, and scutelinquanines, demonstrated an impressive anticancer effect *in vitro*. The diterpenoids exerted a similar degree of cytotoxic effect against HONE-1 (nasopharyngeal), KB (oral epidermoid), and HT-29 (colorectal) human cancer cell lines *in vitro* (IC_{50}: 2.0–8.5 μM), whose effects were comparable to those of a clinic anticancer agent cisplatin but lower than those of etoposide.[46–51] A *neo*-clerodane diterpenoid, 8,13-epoxy-3-en-7-hydroxy-6,11-*O*-dibenzoyl-15,16-clerodan-olide (**6**), moderately restrained the proliferation of LU (lung), LNCaP (prostate), MCF7 (breast), and KB (oral) of human carcinoma cell lines (IC_{50}: 2.15–8.3 μM).[49]

The *neo*-clerodane diterpenoids designated as scutebatas and scutebarbatine-B were separated from the herb. Scutebatas-H–O demonstrated a moderate cytotoxicity against HL-60 (leukemic), A549 (lung), SMMC-7721 (liver), MCF-7 (breast), and SW480 (colon) human neoplastic cell lines (IC_{50}: 12.6–31.4 μM), whereas scutebata-A and scutebata-H showed a selective cytotoxic effect against human breast cancer cell lines (SK-BR-3 and MCF-7), respectively.[52] Also, scutebarbatine-B, scutebata-E, scutebata-P, and scutebata-O showed a weak inhibition against K562 and HL-60 leukemia cell lines.[53,54]

Diterpenoid Alkaloids

A purified alkaloid extract derived from Ban Zhi Lian was reported to inhibit the proliferation of HepG2 (liver) and CNE-1 (nasopharyngeal) human cancer cell lines by provoking the cell apoptosis and cell cycle arrest.[55] The isolation of Ban Zhi Lian led to the discovery of a group of *nor*-diterpenoid alkaloids named scutebarbatines. Scutebarbatine-A exerted a significant antitumor effect on human A549 lung cancer cells *in vivo* and *in vitro* via mitochondria-mediated apoptosis.[56] Scutebarbatines-C–N and several derivatives (**7** and **8**) from scutebarbatine-G and scutebarbatine-H showed a marked cytotoxic effect against human KB oral epidermoid cancer, HT-29 colorectal cancer, and HONE-1 nasopharyngeal cancer cell lines *in vitro*, and the IC_{50} values ranged between 2.0 and 8.5 μM.[57,58] However, scutebarbatine-F was not cytotoxic to the HL-60 leukemia, MCF-7 breast cancer, and LLC cell lines *in vitro*.[53]

Pheophorbide-a

Pheophorbide-a (**9**) is a different type of anticancer agent as a photosensitzier derived from Ban Zhi Lian. It could induce the apoptosis of human Hep3B hepatoma cells at a concentration of 40 μg/mL and no toxicity to normal human WRL-68 liver cells, where the sub-G1 cell cycle arrest and the apoptosis of Hep3B cells were elicited by pheophorbide-a (**9**).[59] Pheophorbide-a (**9**)-mediated photodynamic therapy (Pa-PDT) was developed to obviously potentiate the inhibitory effect against the growth of Hep3B cells (IC_{50}: 1.5 μM). The Pa-PDT treatment led to the depolarization of the mitochondrial membrane potential and the release of cytochrome c from the mitochondria to the cytosol, the activation of caspase cascade, finally enforcing the target tumor cells to apoptosis and/or necrosis. In a nude mice model, Pa-PDT treatment for 14 days remarkably diminished the hepatoma size by 57%.[60] Pheophorbide-a (**9**) activated by a light-emitting diode also elicited significant cytotoxic and apoptotic effects in ovarian cancer cells.[61]

Phenylbutenones

Phenylbutenone (**10**) and E-1-(4′-hydroxyphenyl)-but-1-en-3-one (**11**) isolated from Ban Zhi Lian exhibited weak to moderate cytotoxicity on human K562 erythroleukemia cells (IC_{50}: 60 μM and 7 μg/mL, respectively).[46]

Polysaccharides

The polysaccharide components prepared from Ban Zhi Lian displayed a definite inhibitory effect on sarcoma 180 cells and ascites hepatoma cells *in vivo* or *in vitro*. One of the polysaccharides was composed of xylose, rhamnose, fucose, mannose, arabinose, glucose, and galactose, in a molar ratio of 0.09:0.22:0.26:0.51:1.0:1.82:209.[62,63] Crude *S. barbata* polysaccharides (SPS or SBPS) exhibited a significant capacity in the promotion of immunocompetence (such as improve T cell percentage, enhance IL-2, TNFα and INFγ activities, augment uninucleate phagocyte function, and increase Ca^{2+} of spleen cells) besides the antigrowth effect on sarcoma 180 cells. Due to the notable immunoregulation, the SBPS demonstrated efficiency-enhancing and toxicity-reducing effects in cytoxan-combined chemotherapies.[64,65] In a mouse model transplanted with C26 murine colon adenocarcinoma, SPS treatment restrained the development of C26 tumor and enhanced the cell apoptosis by the activation of caspase-9 and caspase-3.[66] Moreover, PSB, a polysaccharide extract from *S. barbata* exerted an antitumor growth activity on human 95-D lung cancer *in vitro* and *in vivo* by directly repressing the c-Met signaling pathway and also showed a marked suppression against the invasion and the migration of 95-D cells in a dose-dependent manner in a 50–200 μg/mL concentration range, whose antivasive and antimigrative effects were associated with the down-expression of c-MET and the up-expression of E-cadherin (E-CAD).[67,68]

Other Bioactivities

The herb Ban Zhi Lian (Barbat skullcap) has been used in traditional Chinese medicine as a nervous restorative drug for alleviating anxiety, migraines, and depression. Pharmacological data showed that Ban Zhi Lian is also a helpful herb for antiinflammatory, expectorant, antispasmodic, immunomodulation and antibacterial activities.

References

1. Chui, C. H. et al. 2005. Activities of fresh juice of *Scutellaria barbata* and warmed water extract of radix Sophorae Tonkinensis on anti-proliferation and apoptosis of human cancer cell lines. *Intl. J. Mol. Med.* 16: 337–41.
2. Powell, C. B. et al. 2003. Aqueous extract of herba *Scutellaria barbatae*, a Chinese herb used for ovarian cancer, induces apoptosis of ovarian cancer cell lines. *Gynecologic Oncol.* 91: 332–40.
3. Goh, D. et al. 2005. Inhibitory effects of a chemically standardized extract from *Scutellaria barbata* in human colon cancer cell lines, Lovo. *J. Agricult. Food Chem.* 53: 8197–8204.
4. Lee, T. K. et al. 2004. Inhibitory effects of *Scutellaria barbata D. Don* on human uterine leiomyomal smooth muscle cell proliferation through cell cycle analysis. *Intl. Immumopharmcol.* 4: 447–54.
5. Lee, T. Y. et al. 2004. Differential inhibition of *Scutellaria barbata D. Don* (Lamiaceae) on HCG-promoted proliferation of cultured uterine leiomyomal and myometrial smooth muscle cells. *Immunopharmacol. Immunotoxicol.* 26: 329–42.
6. Suh, S. J. et al. 2007. Chemoprevention of *Scutellaria barbata* on human cancer cells and tumorigenesis in skin cancer. *Phytother. Res.* 21: 135–41.

7. Wong, B. Y. et al. 2009. Chinese medicinal herb *Scutellaria barbata* modulates apoptosis and cell survival in murine and human prostate cancer cells and tumor development in TRAMP mice. *Eur. J. Cancer Prev.* 18: 331–41.
8. Yin, X. et al. 2004. Anticancer activity and mechanism of *Scutellaria barbata* extract on human lung cancer cell line A549. *Life Sci.* 75: 2233–44.
9. Lin, J. M. et al. 2006. Inhibition activity of *Scutellariae barbata* extracts against human hepatocellular carcinoma cells. *Nanfang Yiye Daxue Xuebao* 26: 591–3,
10. Wei, L. H. et al. 2011. *Scutellaria barbata D. Don* induces apoptosis of human colon carcinoma cell through activation of the mitochondrion-dependent pathway. *J. Med. Plants Res.* 5: 1962–1970.
11. Ye, R. et al. 2011. Effect of ethanol extract of *Scutellaria barbata D. Don* on the proliferation in human colon cancer HT-29 cells. *Jiepouxue Zazhi* 34: 324–6, 335.
12. Lin, J. M. et al. 2014. *Scutellaria barbata D Don* inhibits colorectal cancer growth via suppression of multiple signaling pathways. Integrative *Cancer Therapies* 13: 240–248.
13. Yu, J. Q. et al. 2007. Antitumor activity of chloroform fraction of *Scutellaria barbata* and its active constituents. *Phytother. Res.* 21: 817–22.
14. Zhang, L. et al. 2014. Chloroform fraction of *Scutellaria barbata D. Don* promotes apoptosis and suppresses proliferation in human colon cancer cells. *Mol. Med. Reports* 9: 701–6.
15. Cha, Y. Y. et al. 2004. Methylene chloride fraction of *Scutellaria ba*rbata induces apoptosis in human U937 leukemia cells via the mitochondrial signaling pathway. *Clin. Chim. Acta* 348: 41–8.
16. Lee, T. Y. et al. 2006. Pharmacological activity in growth inhibition and apoptosis of cultured human leiomyomal cells of tropical plant *Scutellaria barbata D. Don* (Lamiaceae). *Envir. Toxicol. Pharmacol.* 21: 70–9.
17. Kim, D. I. et al. 2005. Regulation of IGF-I production and proliferation of human leiomyomal smooth muscle cells by *Scutellaria barbata D. Don* in vitro: Isolation of flavonoids of apigenin and luteolin as acting compounds. *Toxicol. Applied Pharmacol.* 205: 213–24.
18. Dai, Z. J. et al. 2011. In vitro and in vivo antitumor activity of *Scutellaria barbate* extract on murine liver cancer. *Mol.* 16: 4389–400.
19. Xu, H. L. et al. 2013. *Scutellaria barbata D. Don* extract synergizes the antitumor effects of low dose 5-fluorouracil through induction of apoptosis and metabolism. *Phytomed.* 20: 897–903.
20. Zhang, N. N. et al. 2005. Inhibitory effect of *Scutellaria barbata D. Don* on tumor angiogenesis and its mechanism. *Aizheng* 24: 1459–63.
21. Zhao, Z. H. et al. 2012. Antitumor and anti-angiogenic activities of *Scutellaria barbata* extracts in vitro are partially mediated by inhibition of Akt/protein kinase B. *Mol. Med. Reports* 5: 788–92.
22. Wei, L. H. et al. 2011. Inhibition of tumor angiogenesis by *Scutellaria barbata D. Don* via suppressing proliferation, migration and tube formation of endothelial cells and downregulation of the expression of VEGF-A in cancer cells. *J. Med. Plants Res.* 5: 3260–8.
23. Wei, L. H. et al. 2012. *Scutellaria barbata D. Don* inhibits tumor angiogenesis via suppression of Hedgehog pathway in a mouse model of colorectal cancer. *Intl. J. Mol. Sci.* 13: 9419–30.
24. Wong, B. Y. Y. et al. 1993. Modulation of cytochrome P-450IA1-mediated mutagenicity, DNA binding and metabolism of benzo[a]pyrene by Chinese medicinal herbs. *Cancer Lett.* 68: 75–82; *Eur. J. Cancer Prev.* 2: 351.
25. Marconett, C. N. et al. 2010. BZL101, a phytochemical extract from the *Scutellaria barbata* plant, disrupts proliferation of human breast and prostate cancer cells through distinct mechanisms dependent on the cancer cell phenotype. *Cancer Biol. Ther.* 10: 397–405.
26. Klawitter, J. et al. 2011. Bezielle (BZL101)-induced oxidative stress damage followed by redistribution of metabolic fluxes in breast cancer cells: A combined proteomic and metabolomic study. *Intl. J. Cancer* 129: 2945–2957.
27. Perez, A. T. et al. 2008. A phase I trial of *Scutellaria barbata* (BZL101) for metastatic breast cancer. *J. Clin. Oncol.* 2008, ASCO Annual Meeting Proceedings (Post-Meeting Edit.). 26(15S), (May 20 Suppl; abstr 1099).
28. Rugo, H. et al. 2007. Phase I trial and antitumor effects of BZL101 for patients with advanced breast cancer. *Breast Cancer Res. Treat.* 105: 17–28.
29. Fong, S. et al. 2008. Molecular mechanisms underlying selective cytotoxic activity of BZL101, an extract of *Scutellaria barbata*, towards breast cancer cells. *Cancer Biol. Ther.* 7: 577–86.
30. Perez, A. T. et al. 2010. A phase 1B dose escalation trial of Scutellaria barbata (BZL101) for patients with metastatic breast cancer. *Breast Cancer Res. Treat.* 120: 111–18.
31. Dai, Z. J. et al. 2013. Anti-angiogenic effect of the total flavonoids in *Scutellaria barbata D. Don. BMC Complement. Altern. Med.* 13: 150.
32. Gao, J. et al. 2014. Induction of apoptosis by total flavonoids from *Scutellaria barbata D. Don* in human hepatocarcinoma MHCC97-H cells via the mitochondrial pathway. *Tumor Biol.* 35: 2549–59.
33. Dai, Z. J. et al. 2013. Total flavonoids of *Scutellaria barbata* inhibit invasion of hepatocarcinoma via MMP/TIMP in vitro. *Mol.* 18: 934–50.
34. Selvendiran, K. et al. 2006. Luteolin promotes degradation in signal transducer and activator of transcription 3 in human hepatoma cells: An implication for the antitumor potential of flavonoids. *Cancer Res.* 66: 4826–34.
35. Sonoda, M. et al. 2004. Cytotoxic activities of flavonoids from two Scutellaria plants in Chinese medicine. *J. Ethnopharmcol.* 91: 65–8.
36. Wu, K. et al. 2005. Inhibitory effects of apigenin on the growth of gastric carcinoma SGC-7901 cells. *World J. Gastroenterol.* 11: 4461–4.
37. Cheng, A. C. et al. 2005. Induction of apoptosis by luteolin through cleavage of Bcl-2 family in human leukemia HL-60 cells. *Eur. J. Pharmacol.* 509: 1–10.
38. Zheng, P. W. et al. 2005. Apigenin induced apoptosis through p53-dependent pathway in human cervical carcinoma cells. *Life Sci.* 76: 1367–79.
39. Singh, J. P. V. et al. 2005. Apigenin inhibits oxidative stress-induced macromolecular damage in N-nitrosodiethyl-amine (NDEA)-induced hepatocellular carcinogenesis in Wistar albino rats. *Mol. Carcinogenesis* 44: 11–20.
40. Singh, J. P. V. et al. 2004. Protective role of apigenin on the status of lipid peroxidation and antioxidant defense against hepatocarcinogenesis in Wistar albino rats. *Phytomed.* 11: 309–14.

41. Chowdhury, A. R. et al. 2002. Luteolin, an emerging anticancer flavonoid, poisons eukaryotic DNA topoisomerase I. *Biochem. J.* 366: 653–61.
42. Shi, R. X. et al. 2004. Luteolin sensitizes tumor necrosis factor-α-induced apoptosis in human tumor cells. *Oncogene* 23: 7712–21.
43. Liu, L. Z. et al. 2005. Apigenin inhibits expression of vascular endothelial growth factor and angiogenesis in human lung cancer cells: Implication of chemoprevention of lung cancer. *Mol. Pharmacol.* 68: 635–43.
44. Bagli, E. et al. 2004. Luteolin inhibits vascular endothelial growth factor-induced angiogenesis: Inhibition of endothelial cell survival and proliferation by targeting phosphatidylinositol 3′-kinase activity. *Cancer Res.* 64: 7936–46.
45. Li, J. et al. 2014. Sensitisation of ovarian cancer cells to cisplatin by flavonoids from *Scutellaria barbata*. *Nat. Prod. Res.* 28: 683–9.
46. Ducki, S. et al. 1996. Isolation of E-1-(4′-hydroxyphenyl)-but-1-en-2-one from *Scutellaria barbata*. *Planta Med.* 62: 185–6.
47. Dai, S. J. et al. 2007. Bioactive *ent*-clerodane diterpenoids from *Scutellaria barbata*. *Planta Med.* 73: 1217–20.
48. Dat, S. J. et al. (a) 2010. New *neo*-clerodane diterpenoids from *Scutellaria barbata* with cytotoxic activities. *Fiterapia* 81: 737–741; (b) 2006. *neo*-Clerodane diterpenoids from *Scutellaria barbata* with cytotoxic activities. *Phytochem.* 67: 1326–30.
49. Zhu, F. et al. 2010. Cytotoxic neoclerodane diterpenoid alkaloids from *Scutellaria barbata*. *J. Nat. Prod.* 73: 233–6.
50. Qu, G. W. et al. 2010. Two new cytotoxic ent-clerodane diterpenoids from *Scutellaria barbata*. *J. Asian Nat. Prod. Res.* 12: 859–64.
51. Nie, X. P. et al. 2010. Scutelinquanines A-C three new cytotoxic *neo*-clerodane diterpenoid from *Scutellaria barbata*. *Phytochem. Lett.* 3: 190–3.
52. Zhu, F. et al. 2011. Neoclerodane diterpenoids from *Scutellaria barbata*. *Planta Med.* 77: 1536–41.
53. Lee, H. K. et al. 2010. Two novel neo-clerodane diterpenoids from *Scutellaria barbata*. *Bioorg. Med. Chem. Lett.* 20: 288–90.
54. Li, Y. Y. et al. 2013. Bioassay-guided isolation of neo-clerodane diterpenoids from *Scutellaria barbata*. *J. Asian Nat. Prod. Res.* 15: 941–9.
55. Wang, T. S. et al. (a) 2011. Purified alkaloid extract of *Scutellaria barbata* inhibits proliferation of hepatoma HepG-2 cells by inducing apoptosis and cell cycle arrest at G2/M phase. *Afri. J. Pharmacy Pharmacol.* 5: 1046–53; (b) 2011. Purified alkaloid extract of Scutellaria barbata inhibits proliferation of nasopharyngeal carcinoma CNE-1 cells by inducing apoptosis and cell cycle arrest at S phase. *J. Med. Plants Res.* 5: 3687–96.
56. Yang, X. K. et al. 2014. In vitro and in vivo antitumor activity of scutebarbatine a on human lung carcinoma A549 cell lines. *Mol.* 19: 8740–51.
57. Dai, S. J. et al. (a) 2009. Two-new norditerpenoid alkaloids from *Scutellaria barbata* with cytotoxic activities. *J. Asian Nat. Prod. Res.* 11: 451–60; (b) 2008. New norclerodane diterpenoid alkaloids from *Scutellaria barbata* with cytotoxic activities. *Chem. Pharm. Bull.* 56: 207–9; (c) 2011. New norditerpenoid alkaloids from *Scutellaria barbata* with cytotoxic activities. *Nat. Prod. Res.* 25: 1019–24; (d) 2011. New norditerpenoid alkaloids from *Scutellaria barbata* with cytotoxic activities. *Nat. Prod. Res.* 15: 1–6; (e) 2007. New *neo*-clerodane diterpenoid alkaloids from *Scutellaria barbata* with cytotoxic activities. *Chem. Pharm. Bull.* 55: 1218–21; (f) 2006. Four new *neo*-clerodane diterpenoid alkaloids from *Scutellaria barbata* with cytotoxic activities. *Chem. Pharm. Bull.* 54: 869–72.
58. Wang, F. et al. 2010. Scutebarbatines W-Z, new neo-clerodane diterpenoids from *Scutellaria barbata* and structure revision of a series of 13-spiro neo-clerodanes. *Chem. Pharm. Bull.* 58: 1267–70.
59. Chan, J. Y. et al. 2006. Pheophorbide a, a major antitumor component purified from *Scutellaria barbata*, induces apoptosis in human hepato-cellular carcinoma cells. *Planta Med.* 72: 28–33.
60. Tang, P. M. et al. 2006. Pheophorbide a, an active compound isolated from *Scutellaria barbata*, possesses photodynamic activities by inducing apoptosis in human hepatocellular carcinoma. *Cancer Biol. Therapy* 5: 1111–6.
61. Liu, L. et al. 2011. LED-activated pheophorbide a in ovarian cancer cells: Cytotoxicity and apoptosis induction. *Laser Physics* 21: 423–6.
62. Meng, Y. F. et al. 1992. Study on polysaccharide from *Scutellaria Barbata*. *J. Lanzhou Univ., Sci. Edition* 28: 112.
63. Meng, Y. F. et al. 1993. SPS4 fraction of Polysaccharide from *Scutellaria Barbata*. *Shengwu Huaxue Zazhi* 9: 224–8.
64. Song, G. C. et al. 2010. Experiments on efficiency enhancing and toxicity reducing of *Scutellaria barbata* polysaccharides on cytoxan and its immunology mechanism. *Acta Chin. Med. Pharm.* 28: 48–50.
65. Zhang, X. J. et al. 2008. Experiment research of effect of *Scutellaria Barbata D. Don* polysaccharides on antitumor and immune regulation in entrails. *Asia-Pacific Tradit. Med.* 4: 54–56.
66. Ye, H. et al. 2012. Effect of *Scutellaria barbata* polysaccharides on caspase-3,8,9 activity in C26 tumor bearing mice. *Zhongguo Laonianxue Zazhi* 32: 5152–3.
67. Yang, X. K. et al. 2013. Inhibitory effect of polysaccharides from *Scutellaria barbata D. Don* on invasion and metastasis of 95-D cells lines via regulation of C-MET and E-CAD expressions. *Tropical J. Pharm. Res.* 12: 517–22.
68. Yang, X. K. et al. 2014. Antitumor effect of polysaccharides from *Scutellaria barbata D. Don* on the 95-D xenograft model via inhibition of the C-Met pathway. *J. Pharmacol. Sci. (Tokyo, Jpn)* 125: 255–63.

20 Tu Fu Ling 土茯苓

Sarsaparilla

Herb Origination

The herb Tu Fu Ling (Sarsaparilla) originates from a Smilacaceae plant *Smilax glabra*. The distribution of this scandent subshrub is mostly in southeastern Asia including southern China. Its rhizomes are normally collected in summer and autumn and dried in the sun for folk medicinal application. But the rhizome collected in the late autumn shows better quality.

Antitumor Activities and Constituents

The alcoholic extract of Tu Fu Ling effectively suppressed the proliferation of human HepG2 and Hep3B hepatoma cell lines together with the induction of apoptosis and cell cycle arrest at either S phase or S/G2 stages. The apoptosis was elicited by intracellular [Ca^{2+}] elevation, and the ROS increase initiated cascade alterations such as mitochondrial transmembrane depolarization, release of cytochrome c, cleavage of PARP, and activation of caspase-3. The activation of p38, JNK, and ERK mitogen-activated protein kinase signaling also involved in the mitochondria caspase-dependent apoptotic pathway in the hepatoma cell lines after the extract treatment.[1] Moreover, the extract was able to dose dependently inhibit the growth of MCF-7 (breast), HT-29 (colon), and BGC-823 (gastric) human cancer cell lines and murine JCT-26 cervical cancer cells *in vitro. In vivo* tests confirmed the antineoplastic and apoptosis-inducing activities of the extract against human HT-29 colon carcinoma and murine H22 hepatoma.[2,3] A supernatant of the water-soluble extract (SW) from Sarsaparilla was shown to markedly inhibit the growth of a broad spectrum of cancer cell lines *in vitro* and *in vivo*. Concomitantly, the SW destroyed the induced oxidative stress and a MAPK1 pathway, intracellular-reduced glutathione/oxidized glutathione (GSH/GSSG) balance, then activated the ERK1/2 pathway, whose interactions contributed to the SW-induced S phase arrest, apoptosis, autophagy, and resultant growth-suppressive effect. LC/MS-IT-TOF analysis identified flavonoids, alkaloids, and phenylpropanoids as the major bioactive components of the SW.[4]

The anticarcinogenic property of Tu Fu Ling was also observed in an animal model. The diet mixed with Tu Fu Ling (377.7 mg) that was fed to rats for two weeks notably reduced AFB1-induced liver carcinogenesis, but it showed no obvious inhibition against N-butyl-N-(4-hydroxybutyl) nitrosamine (BBN) caused bladder carcinogenesis in female mice.[5] Several clinical trials with the herb prescriptions containing Tu Fu Ling had been performed in China, which were effective in the treatment of 50 cases of primary bronchogenic lung cancer and 28 cases of esophageal/cardiac cancer. The therapies notably attenuated the symptoms and prolonged the living duration of patients.[6]

Glycoprotein

A fetuin-binding glycoprotein referred as SGPF2 was isolated from the herb, whose molecular mass was established as about 58 kDa with a major protein subunit of 26 kDa. Five subfractions (SGPF1a–SGPF1e) of nonfetuin-binding glycoproteins were also separated, all of which contained the major band at 26 kDa. The isolated proteins of 26 kDa have similar N-terminal amino acid sequences, implying that they are probably the isoforms putatively originated from a multigene family with different binding affinity and ionic strength. These glycoproteins showed the abilities to inhibit the proliferation of MCF-7 breast cancer cells and to cause the cell apoptosis and sub-G1 phase arrest.[5]

Proteins

From fractionation of fresh *Smilax glabra* rhizomes, a protein designated as smilaxin (molecular weight: 30 kDa) was obtained, which has a novel N-terminal amino acid sequence. Its antitumor activity mainly present in the inhibition of thymidine uptake by MBL2 and PU5 tumor cell lines but not in the uptake by sarcoma 180 and L1210 leukemia cell lines. However, smilaxin was found to possess a capacity to stimulate the uptake of thymidine by murine splenocytes, peritoneal macrophages, and bone marrow cells and to augment the production of NO by peritoneal macrophages. These evidences suggested that smilaxin is a DNA/RNA inhibitor in the cancer cells and a stimulator in the immune system.[7]

Other Bioactivities

Pharmacological studies have demonstrated that Tu Fu Ling can play an important role in bioactivities such as antiatherosclerosis, antithrombosis, analgesic, antiinflammation, diuresis, and detoxification besides antineoplasm. The Tu Fu Ling glycoprotein SGPF2 exhibited a great antiviral activity against respiratory syncytial virus and Herpes simplex virus type 1 (HSV-1), whereas five glycoproteins (SGPF1a–SGPF1e) could attenuate the activity of HIV-1-reverse transcriptase.[6,8] Tu Fu Ling is capable of lowering the melanogenesis on pimples and rough skin due to its remarkable melanin inhibition, showing beauty and whitening effects.[8]

References

1. Sa, F. et al. 2008. Anti-proliferative and pro-apoptotic effect of *Smilax glabra Roxb* extract on hepatoma cell lines. *Chemico-Biol. Interactions* 171: 1–14.
2. Gao, Y. J. et al. 2011. Mitochondrial apoptosis contributes to the anticancer effect of *Smilax glabra Roxb. Toxicol. Lett.* 207: 112–20.
3. Li G. X. 1992. *Chinese Medicine and Clinical Pharmacology and Toxicology*. Tianjin Publication of Technology and Translation, Tianjin, China, p. 42.
4. She, T. T. et al. 2015. Sarsaparilla (*Smilax glabra* rhizome) extract inhibits cancer cell growth by S phase arrest, apoptosis, and autophagy via redox-dependent ERK1/2 pathway. *Cancer Prevent. Res.* 8: 464–474.
5. Ooi, L. S. M. et al. 2008. Antiviral and anti-proliferative glycoproteins from the rhizome of *Smilax glabra Roxb* (Liliaceae). *Am. J. Chin. Med.* 36: 185–95.
6. Du, Z. M. et al. 2000. The progress of Smilax pharmacological effects and clinical applications. *Primary J. Chin. Mat. Med.* 14: 57–9.

7. Chu, K. T. et al. 2006. Smilaxin, a novel protein with immunostimulatory, antiproliferative, and HIV-1-reverse transcriptase inhibitory activities from fresh Smilax glabra rhizomes. *Biochem. Biophys. Res. Commun.* 340: 118–24.
8. Kubota, R. et al. 2010. Skin-whitening agents in *Smilax glabra. Pacifichem 2010: International Chemical Congress of Pacific Basin Societies*, Honolulu, HI, December 15–20, AGRO-172.

21 Shan Dou Gen 山豆根

Vietnamese sophora root

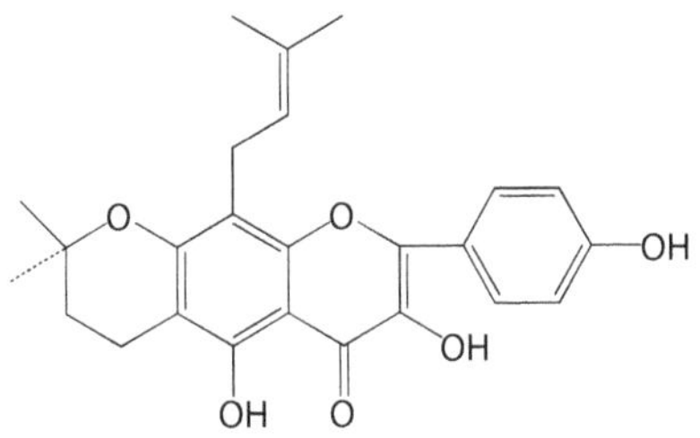

1 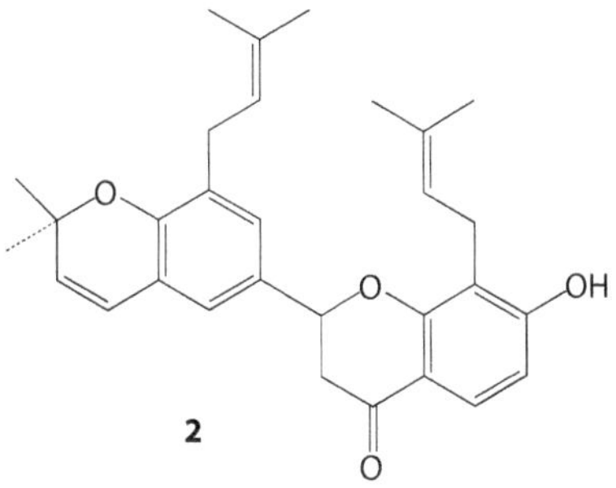 2 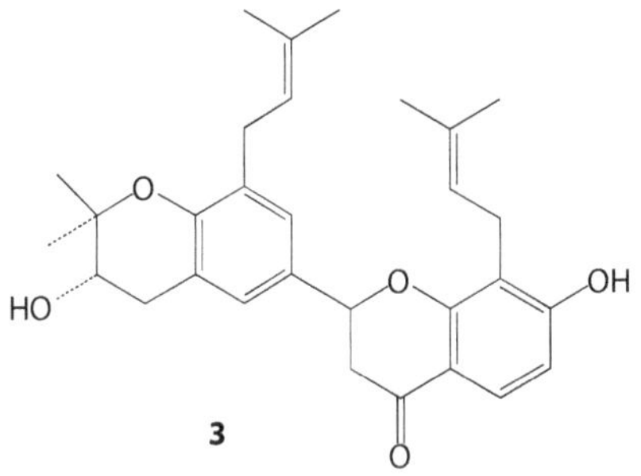 3

Herb Origination

The herb Shan Dou Gen stems from the root and the rhizome of a Leguminosae plant *Sophorae tonkinensis*. This small bush is mainly distributed in southern China and Vietnam. As a traditional Chinese medicine, the rhizome-like roots are usually collected in the autumn and dried in the sunlight for medicinal practice. The first document of Shan Dou Gen was shown in *Kaibao Ben Cao* (AD 973), an official Pharmacopeia in the Song dynasty of China.

Antitumor Activity and Constituents

The warmed water extract of radix of *S. tonkinensis* (RSTE) has been subjected to a test for the antiproliferative and apoptotic potentials on a small panel of cancer cell lines *in vitro*, including HepG2 and Hep3B hepatoma, MDA-MB231 breast cancer, A549 lung cancer, and KG-1 acute myelogenous leukemia. RSTE restrained the growth of cancer cells and promoted the cells to apoptosis. Despite the significant activation of caspase-3 and DNA fragmentation, RSTE elicited the cell apoptosis and then obstructed the proliferation of HepG2 cells.[1] The aqueous extract (STAE) of the herb showed the antigrowth effect against human Eca-109 esophageal squamous carcinoma cells *in vitro*.[2] The STAE was further investigated in animal models implanted with mouse lymphoma cell lines (MPC-11 or MOPC-315). Daily fed STAE for three days provoked the lymphoma cell apoptosis and concurrently augmented the expressions of immune modulators such as IL-2, IFNγ, TNFα mRNA, and protein of spleen cells, thereby potentiating the antilymphoma activity *in vivo*.[3] Through silica gel chromatography eluted with methanol and dichloromethane (1:50), an antitumor effective extract was prepared from the ethyl acetate fraction of *S. tonkinensis*, whose extract could inhibit the growth of human U251 glioma cells.[4] In addition, an injection was prepared with a Chinese herb combination in which Shan Dou Gen is used as a major component. An *in vivo* test showed that the injection was effective in the inhibition of mouse B16 melanoma and Lewis lung carcinoma and the prolongation of the mouse life duration.[2]

Alkaloids

According to phytochemistry studies, the anticarcinoma constituents in the herb should be a group of quinolizidine alkaloids such as matrine, matrine N-oxide, oxymatrine, sophocarpine, sophocarpine N-oxide, cytosine, sophoranol and sophoramine,[5] whose cancer suppressive property of these major alkaloids have also been discussed in Section Ku Shen. The total alkaloid of *S. tonkinensis* has been used to make the soft capsules for cancer treatment in China, whose soft capsules contain matrine no less than 80%.[6]

Flavonoids

A flavonol elucidated as tonkinensisol (**1**) was isolated from the herb, displaying the moderate cytotoxic effect against the proliferation of human HL-60 leukemia cells *in vitro* (IC_{50}: 36.48 μg/mL).[6] The isopentenyl flavanones isolated from the herb, such as sophoranochromene (**2**) and 2-(3-hydroxy-2,2-dimethyl-8-prenyl-6-chromanyl)-7-hydroxy-8-prenyl-4-chromanone (**3**), were used as the cancer inhibitors to formulate drugs for treating lung cancers, prostatic cancers, nasopharyngeal cancers, and large intestine cancers.[8]

Other Bioactivities

The herb Shan Dou Gen (Vietnamese sophora root) used in Chinese folk medicines has received a great deal of attention traditionally for its antiinflammatory, antioxidation, antiarrhythmia, antiasthmatic, antiulcerative, immunomoderating, and antiinfectious properties besides antineoplasm. But the herb has certain toxic side effects, whose toxic components in the Shan Dou Gen were believed to be matrine and oxymatrine. Therefore, the clinical practice of Shan Dou Gen must be processed under a safety toxicological precaution.

References

1. Chui, C. H. et al. 2005. Activities of fresh juice of *Scutellaria barbata* and warmed water extract of radix Sophorae tonkinensis on anti-proliferation and apoptosis of human cancer cell lines. *Intl. J. Mol. Med.* 16: 337–41.

2. Tan, C. M. et al. 2009. Biological active ingredient and pharmacological effects of radix Sophorae Tonkinensis. *J. Guangxi Agricul. Sci.* 40: 1494–7.
3. Chu, C. Y. et al. 2009. Anti-lymphoma and immunomodulatory functions of the aqueous extract of *Sophora tonkinensis* in mice. *J. Hungkuag* 56: 98–107.
4. Yu, J. N. et al. 2013. Manufacture and applications of *Sophora tonkinensis* antitumor effective ingredient extract. *Faming Zhuanli Shenqing* CN 103006761 A 20130403.
5. He, X. Y. et al. 2011. Research advance in chemical constituent and pharmacology of *Sophorae tonkinensis*. *J. Zhongnan Univ.* 9: 525–8.
6. Zhou, Y. W. 2007. Antitumor soft capsules containing total alkaloids of Sophora. *Faming Zhuanli Shenqing* CN 101077349 A 20071128.
7. Chen, D. F. et al. 2011. Use of isopentenyl flavanones isolated from *Sophora tonkinensis* roots for preparing antitumor drugs. *Faming Zhuanli Shenqing* CN 102100692 A 20110622.

22 Qing Dai 青黛

Natural Indigo

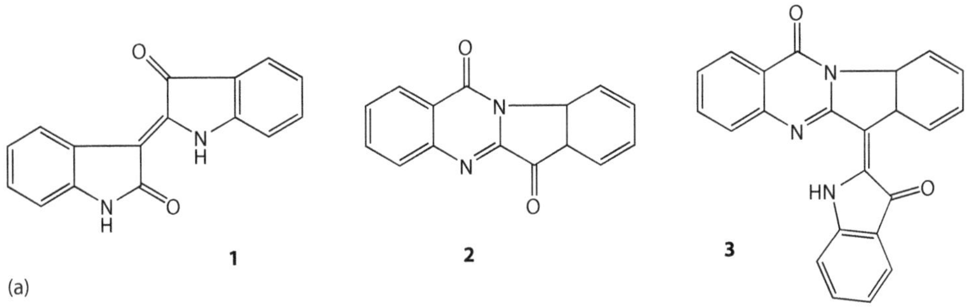

(a)

1 **2** **3**

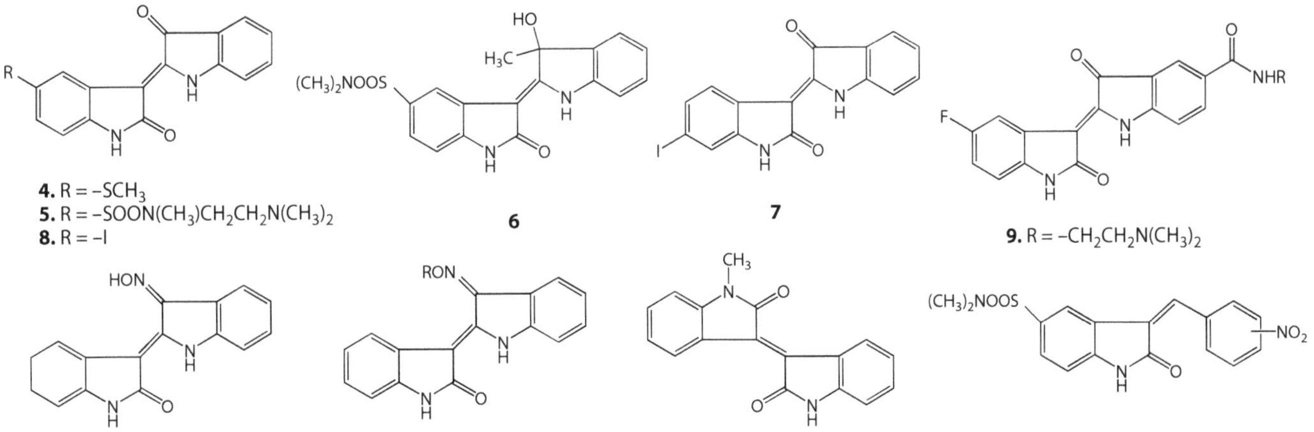

4. R = $-SCH_3$
5. R = $-SOON(CH_3)CH_2CH_2N(CH_3)_2$
8. R = $-I$

6 **7**

9. R = $-CH_2CH_2N(CH_3)_2$

10 **11.** R = $-CH_2CH(OH)-CH_2OH$ **12** **13**

(b)

Herb Origination

Qing Dai (natural Indigo) is the distinctive blue dye mainly made from a variety of specific plant leaves or stems throughout history. In China, the most natural Indigo was produced from four different family plants, i.e., *Isatis indigotica* (Cruciferae), *Indigofera tinctoria* (Leguminosae), *Baphicacanthus cusia* (Acanthaceae), and *Polygonum tinctoria* (Polygonaceae).

Antitumor Constituents and Activity

Qing Dai normally contains two major components, indigo (5–8%) and indirubin (0.05–0.4%). Their quantities depend on the original sources as well as the plants' growing places and harvest times.[1] Indirubin (**1**) exerts potent biological properties related to antineoplasm, especially antileukemia, and anticarcinogenesis.

Indirubin

In earlier investigations, the oral, the subcutaneous, or the i.p. administration of indirubin (**1**) in 200 mg/kg dose per day for 6–10 successive days could effectively suppress W256 entity sarcoma by 47–58% and prolong the survival time of rat bearing W256 ascites sarcoma. If the daily oral dose was increased to 500 mg/kg for 9–10 days, indirubin (**1**) could significantly inhibit the cell growth of Lewis lung cancer, breast adenocarcinoma, and sarcoma 180 in mice,[2,3] where indirubin (**1**) interfered with the DNA by intercalating into a DNA double helix and interacted with the phosphate groups of DNA in the tumor cells[2] but showed no action on the protein synthesis and no damages to the chromosome DNA and the macronucleic acids except a slight inhibition on RNA synthesis.[4–7] Also, indirubin (**1**) acted as a marked inducer of quinone reductase (QR) *in vivo*, being able to enhance the activities of chemotherapeutic agents, promote antioxidative functions, and prevent carcinogenesis.[8] The antitumor properties of indirubin (**1**) have indeed been paid attention for extensive investigations.

Indirubin and Leukemia

Although there is no significant *in vivo* activity against three lymphocytic leukemia models (L7112, P388, and L1210),[5] indirubin (**1**) and its analog, meisoindigo, are currently used in the clinical treatment of chronic myelogenous leukemia (CML) in China. Both agents can induce cell apoptosis and hematological remission in patients with chronic phase CML as effective as hydroxyurea and busulfan.[9,10] The treatment with indirubin (**1**) rapidly decreased the amount of peripheral leukocyte in the marrow of CML patients and showed no influences on matured neutral granulocytes, erythrocytes, lymphocytes, and monocytes, but the activity of the DNA polymerase in the peripheral leukocytes of CML patients was notably suppressed by indirubin (**1**) together with the decrease of electric density at the surface of the chronic granulocyte leukemia cells and the reduction of mobility in the membrane of the leukocytes. Moreover, the *in vitro* investigation also revealed that the inhibitory effect of indirubin (**1**) on the growth of human K562 chronic myelogenous leukemia cells and human HL-60 promyelocyte leukemia cells was related to the suppression of CDKs or Src kinase.[11] All these interactions closely contributed to the chemotherapeutic activity of indirubin (**1**) for the treatment of leukemia diseases.[5,12,13]

Indirubin and Other Carcinomas

Indirubin (**1**) was further verified to be effective in the inhibition of other types of cancer cell lines such as lymphoma, gallbladder carcinoma, hepatoma, uterine cervix carcinoma, gastric cancer, and hilar cholangiocarcinoma *in vitro*.[11] At its concentrations of 1–10 μM, indirubin (**1**) dose and time dependently inhibited the proliferation of ScaBER bladder cancer cells concomitant with the down-expression of Oct-4, Sox-2, and Nanog genes.[14] Indirubin (**1**) and its analogs that acted as GSK-3 inhibitors could repress the invasion of glioma cells and glioma-initiating cell-enriched neurospheres *in vitro* and *in vivo*. After being treated by indirubins, the survival of glioma-bearing mice was lengthened and the blood vessel density was substantially attenuated. The *in vivo* studies also revealed that β-catenin signaling plays an important role in mediating the antiinvasive effects.[15]

Indirubin and NF-κB Activation

Indirubin (**1**) dose and time dependent restrained TNF-induced NF-κB activation and IκB phosphorylation and degradation by blocking the IκB kinase activation and phosphorylation and blocking the p65 nuclear translocation. At the same time, indirubin (**1**) diminished the expressions of NF-κB-regulated gene products such as those involved in antiapoptosis (Bcl-2, Bcl-xL, IAP1, IAP2, and TRAF1), proliferation (cyclin-D1 and c-Myc), and invasion (COX-2 and MMP-9), thereby eliciting the cancer cells to apoptosis and obstructed the cancer cell proliferation and the cytokine-induced cellular invasion. These observations confirmed that the anticancer and antiinflammatory activities of indirubin (**1**) were mediated in part through the inhibition of the NF-κB pathway.[16]

Indirubin and Kinases

Indirubin (**1**) is a potent inhibitor of CDKs and a powerful low nanomolar inhibitor of an evolutionarily related kinase, GSK-3β. By high-affinity binding into the enzymes of ATP binding site by van der Waals interactions and hydrogen bonds, indirubin (**1**) exerted the potent inhibitory potential toward CDKs, wherein it competed with the ATP for binding to the catalytic site of CDKs.[17–22] Due to the inhibition of CDKs, indirubin (**1**) was effective in blocking the tumor cell cycle progression, whose events might display the main mechanism underlying the cytotoxicity against neoplasm.

Indirubin and Cell Differentiation

More investigations showed that the neutrophilic differentiation of HL-60 myelocytic leukemia cells could be promoted by indirubin (**1**) by restraining the CDK2-dependent phosphorylation of retinoblastoma protein and activating the transcription factor PU.1. Qing Dai (*Indigo naturalis*) at a dose of 100 μg/mL elicited the obvious monocytic differentiation of human erythroleukemia cells, besides the induction of 59.28% proliferative inhibition and 18.4% apoptosis increase *in vitro*.[23,24]

Indirubin and Angiogenesis

Indirubin (**1**) exerted the inhibitory effect on the growth and the angiogenesis of prostate cancer in a xenograft mouse model. The suppressive effect of indirubin (**1**) against prostate tumor cell growth, endothelial cell migration, and tube formation was found to be attributed to the blockage of the angiogenesis in tumor. The antiangiogenic activity directly correlated with the blockage of the VEGF receptor 2-mediated JAK/STAT3 signaling pathway.[25]

Indirubin and Immune Effects

Based on both clinic treatments in patients and experiments in animal models, indirubin (**1**) was found to possess remarkable immunoregulating functions. After the treatment with indirubin (**1**), the depressed cellular immunity (including the phagocytic function of macrophage) and humoral immunity induced by the malignant tumor could be restored to normal levels.[5]

Tryptanthrin and Qingdainone

Besides indirubin (**1**) and its analogs, Qing Dai also contains two minor cancer inhibitors, tryptanthrin (**2**) and qingdainone (**3**). Both were effective in the inhibition of B16 melanoma cells *in vitro*, and qingdainone (**3**) was therapeutically active against Lewis lung carcinoma in mice.[26] Tryptanthrin (**2**) exerted potent cytocidal effects on various leukemia and solid tumors *in vitro* accompanied by the induction of cell apoptosis.[27] After the treatment with low concentrations of tryptanthrin (**2**), the activity of α-naphthyl butyrate esterase was markedly increased and the expression of cell differentiation markers were enhanced in human HL-60 (promyelocytic) and U937 (monocytic) leukemia cell lines, indicating the leukemia cell differentiation to monocytes/macrophages. After treated with tryptanthrin (**2**) at higher concentrations, the leukemia cells occurred to cytoplasmic vacuolation and mitochondrial destruction and then died via a caspase-3-activated and Fas-induced apoptosis.[27] Moreover, an isomer assigned as tryptanthrin-B demonstrated cytotoxicity on human BEL-7402 hepatocellular carcinoma and A2780 ovarian cancer cell lines (respective IC_{50}: 8.2 and 7.8 μg/mL). The treatment with tryptanthrin-B also caused leukemia cell differentiation and dramatically declined the activity of telomerase *in vitro*.[28]

Besides leukemia, tryptanthrin (**2**) strongly inhibited the growth of fibroblast cells in association with the potent inhibition of hepatocyte growth factor production and expression.[29] The oral administration of tryptanthrin (**2**) in a dose of 50 mg/kg (five days per week) for 7 or 30 weeks significantly reduced the formation of cancer precursor and atypical crypt foci induced by azoxymethane *in vivo* and declined the incidence of intestinal tumors in rats.[30] Administering the tryptanthrin (**2**) in an effective dose also enhanced the immune response in a subject for the treatment of neoplasm and a subject to an antigen.[31] However, tryptanthrin (**2**) markedly restrained the expression of iNOS and had no effect on the cyclooxygenase-2.[32]

Structural Modification

For the optimization of the therapeutic activity with less side effects, the various molecular modifications based on the drug lead have been reported, wherein three reactions (monooximation, substitution, and glycosidation) are mostly used in the structural modification of indirubin. The valuable derivatives demonstrated the broad spectrum of cancer inhibition and provides a comprehensive foundation for the development of novel anticancer agents.[33–40]

Indirubin Derivatives

By the substitution at the benzene rings of indirubin, a series of novel derivatives such as thioether-substituted indirubin (**4**), sulfonyl indirubin (**5**), aryl indirubin (**6**), and iodides of indirubin (**7** and **8**) were developed showing a promoted inhibitory effect against the growth of carcinoma cells and against the activities of CDK/cyclin.[41–49] Four halogen-substituted derivatives exerted a higher inhibitory effect against L7212 leukemia in mice and W256 sarcoma in rats than indirubin (**1**), with the prolongation of life span.49 A derivative, 5′-methoxyindirubin, exhibited the cell death-increasing effect on three human neuroblastoma cell lines (IMR-32, SK-N-SH, and NB-39) but no inhibition on normal cells (normal human dermal fibroblasts and HUVEC).[50] A group of synthesized derivatives, e.g., (**9**), was evaluated *in vitro* by using SGC7901 (stomach), HCT116 (colon), SKBR-3 (breast), A549 (lung), and HL-60 (leukemic) human cancer cell lines. Most of the derivatives with improved water solubility displayed more potent inhibitory effects than sunitinib (an anticancer drug).[51] Likewise, the indirubin analogs with 5-nitro, halide, and bulky groups containing acyl amino substitution usually demonstrated a higher antiproliferative effect and a potent CDK2 inhibition.[20] MLS-2438, a 7-bromo-3′-hydrophilic indirubin, demonstrated an anticancer activity and induced the apoptosis of human melanoma cells (A2058, A375, G361, and MeWo) *in vitro* associated with the inhibition of STAT3 and Akt signaling pathways. The antimelanoma activity of MLS-2438 was further proven in a mouse xenograft model of MeWo melanoma with low toxicity.[52] N1-(n-butyl)-7-azaisoindigo is a synthesized 7-azaisoindigo derivative, which showed an obvious inhibition effect on cancer cell proliferation, especially on A549 human lung cancer cells *in vitro* in a dose- and a time-dependent way and on human hepatoma xenograft *in vivo* with low inhibition on CDK2/cyclin-D, increase of GSH and decrease of MDA, whose antiheptoma rate was 61.85%, comparable to that of 5-FU and superior to indirubin.[53]

Meisoindigo and Its Analogs

Meisoindigo (Natura-α, **12**), an indirubin analog, has been employed in China for the treatment of CML. *In vitro* cell line studies have shown that the agent elicited the apoptosis and the myeloid differentiation of AML. It also served as an effective therapeutic agent for the inhibition of both androgen-sensitive and androgen-refractory human prostate cancer cell growths and invasions *in vitro* and *in vivo* with minimal side effects.[54] The potential of meisoindigo (**12**) was further confirmed in the treatment of human colorectal cancer in HT-29 xenograft nude mice model at a dose of 100 mg/kg. Its antiproliferative effect paralleled with the induction of the cell cycle arrest at G2/M phase and the cell apoptosis.[55] Meisoindigo (**12**) was evaluated in acute promyelocytic leukemia cells, AML cells, and myelomonocytic leukemia cells (NB4, NB4.007/6, HL-60, and U937) comprising both retinoic acid-sensitive and retinoic acid-resistant cells *in vitro*. Meisoindigo effectively inhibited the growth/proliferation of these four cell types at micromolar levels in association with the induction of apoptosis but independent of cell cycle arrest.[56]

An SAR investigation of meisoindigo (**12**) revealed that a phenalkyl side chain onto the lactam NH should be a bioactive center contributing to the antileukemia activity on the K562 cells. When the phenyl ring was substituted with a basic heterocycle, the solubility was significantly improved and the inhibitory profile was acceptably retained. Thus, a derivative designated as (E)-1-(2-(4-methylpiperazin-1-yl)-ethyl)-[3,3′-biindolinylidene]-2,2′-dione exerted more potent inhibitory effects than meisoindigo (**12**) against a panel of malignant tumor cells and also showed at least 40 times greater solubility than meisoindigo. This promising derivative markedly prolonged the life period of nude mice with the K562 leukemia-induced xenografts.[57]

Azaindirubins

A series of azaindirubins have been synthesized by coupling of 7-azaisatin, 7-azaoxindol, 7-azaindoxyl acetate, and their non-aza counterparts, respectively, to aza- and diaza-bisindoles. Among them, 7,7′-diazaindirubin exhibited a substantially enhanced growth inhibitory effect in the NCI 60 cell line panel and displayed the antiproliferative activity preferential in LXFL529L (large cell lung), MCF-7 (breast), and HT-29 (colon) human cancer cell lines (respective IC_{50}: 0.06, 0.5, and 2.0 μM), where a key mechanism was revealed that primarily CK2 inhibition by 7,7′-diazaindirubin was causally related to the growth inhibition of human tumor cells. Additionally, 7-azaindirubin and 7′-azaindirubin were moderately active in suppressing the LXFL529L and MCF-7 cell lines (IC_{50}: 2.9–5.0 μM).[58]

Indirubin-3′-monoxime

Indirubin-3′-monoxime (**10**, I3M) is a potent inhibitor of CDKs, which has been assayed in various types of human neoplastic cells *in vitro*. It displayed a great capacity to obstruct the proliferation of many malignant tumor cell lines such as HL-60, JM1, K562, RS4-11, and MV4-11(leukemic); Jurkat and CEM-T (T lymphoid); IM9 and Reh6 (B lymphoid), EC-1 and Kyse70 (esophagus); RENCA, CAKI-1, CAKI-2, and A498 (kidney); HT-29 and NCT-116 (colon); HEp-2 (larynx); HepG2 (liver); MCF-7 (breast); HeLa (cervix); Cal-27 and HSC-3 (oral); and LA-N-1, SH-SY5Y, and SK-N-DZ (brain) cells.[48,59–68] The anticancer effects of I3M (**10**) have been found to closely correlate to the induction of cell cycle progression arrest and apoptosis via multiple pathways selectively, such as (1) suppression of CDK/cyclin; (2) reduction of STAT3 signaling, downregulation of Bcl-2, Bcl-xL, Mcl-1, and survivin, and upregulation of Bax and caspases; (3) activation of p53 or p21 and inhibition of FLT3; and (4) decrease of Notch1 transcriptional activity.[59–72] Mechanistic studies in LA-N-1 human neuroblastoma cells showed that I3M (1) specifically decreased the expression of the mitochondrial regulators ERRγ and PGC-1β and caused mitochondrial dysfunction through the elevation of ROS levels, resulting to growth inhibition, and (2) amplified the level of CDK inhibitor p27Kip1 and reduced the levels of CDK2 and cyclin E in LA-N-1 cells, leading to cell cycle arrest at the G0/G1 phase.[73]

The antileukemia effect and mechanism of I3M was found to be associated with the promotion of both autophagic and apoptotic death and G2/M cell cycle arrest in JM1 human acute lymphoblastic leukemia (ALL) cells and K562 human chronic myelogenous leukemia cells.[74] In HeLa cervical cancer cells, I3M (**10**) induced apoptosis mainly through an extrinsic pathway and next through an intrinsic pathway, via the enhanced surface expression of DR4 and DR5 and induced type II response mediated by Bid and Bax and activated caspase-8, caspase-9 and caspase-3, which correlated with the increase of p53 and its transcriptional activity.[68] Besides the dose-dependent promotion of G2/M cell arrest and apoptosis, I3M was also able to suppress the migration and the invasion in Cal-27 oral cancer cells by inhibiting focal adhesion kinase expression, urokinase-type plasminogen inhibitor, and MMP-9.[75]

Moreover, in a cotreatment, I3M (**10**) obviously augmented the inhibitory rate of nedaplatin against human EC-1 esophageal cancer cells.[76] I3M (**10**) also showed the reversal of paclitaxel resistance in NCI-H520/TAX25 lung adenocarcinoma cell subline. The decrease in both mRNA expression and protein level of survivin, Oct-4, and Sox-2 might be the molecular mechanism for the reversal of pacilitaxel resistance.[77] The ability of I3M (**10**) also presented to significantly obstruct the proliferation, the migration, and the tube formation in HUVEC cells via the inhibition of VEGFR-2 signaling pathway, leading to restrain the angiogenesis in the tumor development.[78,79]

Moreover, in transitional human tumor cell lines such as RT4, RT112, TCCSUP, and T24 (bladder) and HBL-100 (breast) cells, I3M (**13**) caused a reversible growth arrest,[62–64] whose growth inhibition by I3M (**10**) was mediated by apoptosis-independent upregulation of survivin with no obvious changes in CDK expression.[70] In addition, an *in vivo* test established the anticancer and apoptosis-inducing effects against BAP-induced lung carcinogenesis.[80] All the research results proposed that the I3M (**10**) has a therapeutic potential as a novel drug candidate for treating cancers.

Indirubin-3′-monoxime Derivatives

Anticancer I3M Derivatives

A series of indirubin-3′-monoxime derivatives are the most developed anticancer agents in a structural modification. The introduction of bromine to C-6 of the indirubin-3′-monoxime (**10**) could augment the cytotoxic effect against AML cells and malignant lymphoid cells.[60,61] 5- and 5′-Substituted indirubin-oxime derivatives and 5-fluoroindirubin-3′-oxime exerted more potent cytotoxic effects against the AML cells compared to its parent molecule.[81] 5′-Nitroindirubin-oxime significantly promoted the cell cycle arrest and the apoptosis by (1) reducing Cdc2/cyclin-B activity and increasing mitochondria-dependent activation of caspase cascade in human KB oral cancer cells, (2) blocking Notch-1 signaling in human salivary gland adenocarcinoma cells, and (3) down-expressing polo-like kinase-1 and/or peptidyl-prolyl *cis/trans* isomerase in human lung cancer cells.[82–86] 5-Nitro-5′-hydroxyindirubin-3′-oxime and 5-nitro-5′-fluoroindirubin-3′-oxime were potent CDK2 inhibitors, which demonstrated an antiproliferative effect against seven human cancer cell lines (HCT116, HT1080, SNU638, K562, KB, MCF-7, and A549) with IC_{50} values of 0.2–3.3 μM.[87] Additionally, the significant antigrowth and apoptotic effects of 5′-nitroindirubin-oxime, 5′-trimethylacetaminoindirubin-oxime, and 5′-fluoroindirubin-oxime were also showed in rat solid carcinoma models with RK3E-ras rat kidney epithelial cells harboring k-ras gene.[88,89]

E564, E728, and E804 (**11**), other indirubin-3′-monoxime analogs, potently blocked the constitutive STAT3 signaling in human breast and prostate tumor cell lines.[90,91] E804 (**11**) was the most potent in the series of derivatives in blocking STAT5 signaling in human K562 CML cells and CD34-positive primary CML cells from patients, leading to the apoptosis of these CML cells.[92] 5-Diphenylacetamidoindirubin-3′-oxime (LDD398) was a mitochondria-targeting antileukemic agent. The treatment with LDD398 resulted in caspase activation, cell death, and growth arrest at the G2/M phases in six leukemia cell lines (Kasumi-1, HL-60, THP-1, AML-2, U937, and K562) with IC_{50} values of 1.82–2.91 μM, where LDD398 quickly collapsed the mitochondrial membrane potential, accompanied by cytochrome c release into the cytosol and a consequent depletion of ATP.[93] Indirubin 3′-(*O*-oxiran-2-ylmethyl) oxime (Epox/Ind), in an *in vitro* assay, exerted the antiproliferative effect against HepG2 hepatoma cells (IC_{50}: 1.7 μM), whose data were comparable to that of cisplatin (4.0 μM). Also, Epox/Ind was found to be metabolized by a HepG2 cell lysate into E804.[94]

Antiangiogenic I3M Derivatives

E804 (**11**) exerted potent antiangiogenic effects, which was evidenced by a significant suppression on the proliferation, migration, tube formation, as well as vascular endothelial growth factor in HUVEC cells. The antiangiogenic potency of E804 (**11**) was more significant than other indirubin-3′-oximes.[95,96] Therefore, by intratumor injections of E804 (**11**), the growth of colon cancer CT-26 allografts was obstructed by repressing the phosphorylation of VEGF receptor-2, AKT, and extracellular signal-regulated kinases in syngeneic mice.[97] According to the remarkable antigrowth and angiosuppressive activities, indirubin-3′-oximes, especially E804, may be considered as potential drug candidates for cancer chemotherapy. More studies displayed that a self-nanoemulsifying drug delivery system (SNEDDS) amplified the bioavailability of E804 by 984.23%, suggesting that the developed SNEDDS may be used as a possible formulation for E804 to improve its solubility and oral bioavailability.[98]

Antimetastatic I3M Derivatives

In the treatment of head and neck cancer cells with 5′-nitroindirubinoxime, the metastasis of carcinoma cells was inhibited by blocking the integrin β1/FAK/Akt pathway.[85] E804 (**11**) was the most potent in this series of derivatives in blocking STAT5 signaling in human K562 CML cells, imatinib-resistant human KCL-22 CML cells (expressing T315I mutant Bcr-Abl), and CD34-positive primary CML cells from patients, leading to apoptosis of these CML cells. Through abolishing survivin expression and inhibiting STAT signaling pathway, E804 (**11**) at a subtoxic dose was able to sensitize a drug-resistant leukemia MV4-11-R cells to ABT-869 treatment, resulting in potent *in vivo* efficacy in the MV4-11-R xenograft model.[92] Moreover, E804 (**11**) also displayed potent angiosuppressive effects, which significantly decreased the proliferation, migration and tube formation of vascular endothelial growth factor in human umbilical vein endothelial cells (HUVECs). The antiangiogenic potency of E804 (**11**) was more significant than indirubin-3′-oxime.[95,96] By intratumor injections of E804 (**11**), the growth of colon cancer CT-26 allografts was accompanied with obstructed the phosphorylation of VEGF receptor-2, AKT and extracellular signal regulated kinase to be supressed in syngeneic mice.[97] Due to the marked antigrowth and angiosuppressive activities, E804 was considered as a potential candidate for antitumor chemotherapies. 6-Bromoindirubin-3′-oxime (6BIO) was a promising antimetastatic agent, which suppressed the adhesion, the migration, and the invasion of a variety of metastatic cancer cell lines (T24, HuH-7, MDA-MB-231, and 4T1 cells) *in vitro* and reduced the formation of lung metastasis *in vivo* with aggressive 4T1 murin breast neoplastic model. The antimetastatic mechanism of 6BIO was revealed to be associated with the down-expression of CTEN and MMP-2 by blocking Jak/STAT, GSK3b, PDK1 signaling pathways.[99]

Drug-Resistant Reversal I3M Derivatives

5′-OH-5-nitro-Indirubin oxime efficiently reduced the viabilities of K562 human CML cells (IC_{50}: 0.67 μM) and imatinib-resistant K562 cells (IC_{50}: 0.71–0.86 μM) *in vitro* and *in vivo*, accompanied by the inhibition of Rb protein phosphorylation.[100] Similarly, LDD398 was effective in the inhibition of imatinib-resistant K562/GR and AML-2/IDAC leukemia cells (respective IC_{50}: 3.65 and 2.36 μM).[93] Besides the suppression of MCF7 and/or HepG2 cells, 7-methoxyindirubin 3′-oxime as well as 5-methoxyindirubin could suppress endogenous MDR1 transcription without any inhibitory effect on NF-Y expression, leading to the enlargement of the sensitivity of DOX on MCF7 cells.[101]

Indirubin-N′-glycosides

The glycosidation of indirubin is one of the approaches for the improvement of the antitumor activity of indirubin in a structural modification. Three indirubin-N′-glycosides showed the significant antiproliferative activity against human cancer cell lines selectively. The medium to high-degree antiproliferative activity was observed in all tested cancer cell lines in the treatment with indirubin-N′-mannoside, while the greatest inhibitory effect and selectivity were observed against human MCF-7 breast cancer cells by two indirubin-N′-(α or β)-rhamnosides (respective IC_{50}: 0.67 and 0.76 μM), whose data were comparable to that of etoposide.[102] A synthesized thia-analog, indirubin-N′-β-L-rhamnoside, was effective in the promotion of apoptosis and the inhibition of melanoma cells, whose antimelanoma effect was attributed to the reduction of transcription factor c-Jun and JNK phosphorylation.[103]

PHII-7

Besides PHII-7 (**13**), an indirubin derivative, achieved its cytotoxicity on K562 leukemia and MCF-7 breast cancer cell lines by intracellular ROS-increased apoptosis induction; it also demonstrated an important capacity in reversing drug resistance by significantly downregulating the P-gp expression and decreasing the P-gp efflux pump function. Thus, PHII-7 (**13**) contributed to both apoptosis and cell cycle arrest in K562/A02 and MCF-7/Adm drug-resistant cells. The elicitation of JNK phosphorylation and the downexpression of prooncogene c-fos were also involved in the inhibition of PHII-7, respectively, on the proliferation of K562/A02 and MCF-7/Adm drug-resistant cells.[104–107] Likewise, PHII-7 (**13**) was able to noticeably reserve the sensitivity of chemotherapy in drug-resistant tumor cells and augment the cytotoxic effect of adriamycin in human MCF-7/Adm drug-resistant breast cancer cells.[108]

Toxicity and Side Effects

Indirubin (**1**) may be safe to humans at its clinical doses (150–200 mg, per day). Only slight liver toxicities were noted when humans received 2240 mg/day (equivalent 100 mg/kg in dogs). The common side effects of indirubin (**1**) in the clinical trials are gastrointestinal irritations such as nausea, vomiting, abdominal pain, diarrhea, and blood stool. Due to the slight bone marrow suppression, thrombocytopenia will occure in the treatment with indirubin (**1**).[109] In murine animal models, oral doses of 20–200 mg/kg of indirubin (**1**) to dogs for six months or a dose of 200 mg/kg to rats for one month caused decreases in RNA and pathology changes in the liver's ultrastructure, resulting in dose-dependent toxicity to the liver.[109]

Some Indirubin Derivatives and Prostate Cancer

Some indirubin derivatives are known as potent inhibitors of CDK and GSK-3β, which may be effective against various cancers. But *in vitro* experiments showed that indirubin-3′-oxime and 6-bromoindirubin-3′-oxime increased the proliferation of androgen-dependent human LNCaP prostate cancer cells and activated the expression of PSA at low concentrations of 0.03–1.0 μM. If their concentration was raised to >1 μM, the apoptosis of LNCaP cells would occur. The findings suggested that the indirubin derivatives in a cancer treatment context must be used within an appropriate therapeutic dose range, especially for AR-dependent prostate cancer.[110]

Other Medical Uses

The novel family of indirubin analogs, which are VEGF receptor inhibitors as described as earlier, may also be useful in several noncancer ailments including Alzheimer's disease, diabetes, and autoimmune diseases, besides the cancer therapeutic potential.[21,76]

References

1. Deng, B. L. 1986. Direct colometric method for determination of indigo and indirubin in Qingdai. *Chin. Tradit. Herb. Drugs* 17: 163–4.
2. Ji, X. J. et al. 1981. Studies on the antineoplastic effect and toxicity of synthetic indirubin. *Yaoxue Xuebao* 16: 146–8.
3. Wang, Y. S. 1983. *Pharmacology and Application of Chinese Materia Medica*. 597–604, Beijing: People's Health Publisher, Beijing, China.
4. Ye, B. X. et al. 2005. Electrochemical and spectroscopic study of the interaction of indirubin with DNA. *Electroanal.* 17: 1523–8.
5. Wu, G. Y. et al. (a) 1980. *Zhonghua Yixue Zazhi.* 60: 451; (b) 1999. *Chinese Materia Medica* Vol. 7, 7-6454, 447. Shanghai Science and Technology Press, Shanghai, China.

6. Du, D. J. et al. (a) 1981. *Zhongcaoyao*. 12: 22; (b) 1999. *Chinese Materia Medica*. Vol. 7, 7–6454, 447. Shanghai Science and Technology Press, Shanghai, China.
7. Wang, Y. S. et al. 1983. *Pharmacology and Applications of Chinese Materia Medica*. 597–604, Beijing, People's Health Publication, Shanghai, China.
8. Yamamodo, N. et al. 2003. Indirubin as quinone reductase inducer for modulating functions of organs. *Jpn. Kokai Tokkyo Koho JP* 2001–227149.
9. Xiao, Z. J. et al. 2002. Indirubin and meisoindigo in the treatment of chronic myelogenous leukemia in China. *Leuk. Lymph*. 43: 1763–8.
10. Liu, X. M. et al. 1996. Induction of differentiation and down-regulation of c-myb gene expression in ML-1 human myeloblastic leukemia cells by the clinically effective anti-leukemia agent meisoindigo. *Biochem. Pharmacol*. 51: 1545–51.
11. Wu, Q. W. et al. 2008. Inhibitory effect of indirubin on growth of some cancer cells and its mechanism. *Tianjin Zhongyiyao* 25: 55–8.
12. Gan, W. J. et al. 1987. Studies on the mechanism of indirubin by treatment of chronic myelocytic leukemia. *Shengwu Huaxue Zazhi* 3: 225–30.
13. Wang, X. Q. et al. 1984. Effect of indirubin on the surface of chronic leukemia cells. *Tianjin Yiyao* 12: 707–10.
14. Cao, J. et al. 2008. Effect of indirubin on proliferation of bladder cancer cell line ScaBer and its mechanism. *Shandong Yiyao* 48: 61–2.
15. Williams, S. P. et al. 2011. Indirubins decrease glioma invasion by blocking migratory phenotypes in both the tumor and stromal endothelial cell compartments. *Cancer Res*. 71: 5374–80.
16. Sethi, G. et al. 2006. Indirubin enhances tumor necrosis factor-induced apoptosis through modulation of nuclear factor-κB signaling pathway. *J. Biol. Chem*. 281: 23425–35.
17. Eisenbrand, G. et al. 2004. Molecular mechanisms of indirubin and its derivatives: Novel anticancer molecules with their origin in traditional Chinese phytomedicine. *J. Cancer Res. Clinical Oncol*. 130: 627–35.
18. Carson, D. A. et al. 2004. Therapeutic inhibition of protein kinases and a cellular ATP synthetic pathway in cancer cells. *PCT Int. Appl*. WO 2003-US24439 20030801.
19. Hoessel, R. et al. 1999. Indirubin, the active constituent of a Chinese antileukemia medicine, inhibits cyclin-dependent kinases. *Nat. Cell Biol*. 1: 60–7.
20. Moon, M. J. et al. 2006. Synthesis and structure-activity relationships of novel indirubin derivatives as potent anti-proliferative agents with CDK2 inhibitory activities. *Bioorg. Med. Chem*. 14: 237–46.
21. Leclerc, S. et al. 2001. Indirubins inhibit glycogen synthase kinase-3β and CDK5/P25, two protein kinases involved in abnormal tau phosphorylation in Alzheimer's disease: A property common to most cyclin-dependent kinase inhibitors. *J. Biol. Chem*. 276: 251–60.
22. Knockaert, M. et al. 2004. Independent actions on cyclin-dependent kinases and aryl hydrocarbon receptor mediate the antiproliferative effects of indirubins. *Oncogene* 23: 4400–12.
23. Suzuki, K. et al. 2005. Indirubin, a Chinese anti-leukaemia drug, promotes neutrophilic differentiation of human myelocytic leukaemia HL-60 cells. *British J. Haematol*. 130: 681–90.
24. Jiang, P. J. et al. 2011. Effects of active ingredient of indigo naturalis on proliferation, apoptosis and differentiation of human erythro-leukemia (HEL) cell line. *Zhongguo Shenghua Yaowu Zazhi* 32: 190–3.
25. Zhang, X. L. et al. 2011. Indirubin inhibits tumor growth by antitumor angiogenesis via blocking VEGFR2-mediated JAK/STAT3 signaling in endothelial cells. *Intl. J. Cancer* 129: 2502–11.
26. Zou, J. C. et al. 1985. Minor constituents of Qing Dai, a traditional Chinese medicine: I. Isolation, structure determination and synthesis of tryptanthrin and qingdainone. *Yaoxue Xuebao* 20: 45–51.
27. Kimoto, T. et al. 2011. Cell differentiation and apoptosis of monocytic and promyelocytic leukemia cells (U937 and HL-60) by tryptanthrin, an active ingredient of *Polygonum tinctorium Lour. Pathol. Intl*. 51: 315–25.
28. Liang, Y. H. et al. 2000. Studies on in vitro anticancer activity of tryptanthrin-B. *Zhongcaoyao* 31: 531–3.
29. Motoki, T. et al. 2005. Inhibition of hepatocyte growth factor induction in human dermal fibroblasts by tryptanthrin. *Biol. Pharm. Bull*. 28: 260–6.
30. Koya-Miyata, S. et al. 2001. Prevention of azoxymethane-induced intestinal tumors by a crude ethyl acetate-extract and tryptanthrin extracted from *Polygonum tinctorium Lour. Anticancer Res*. 21: 3295–300.
31. Valiante, N. 2004. Use of tryptanthrin compounds for immune potentiation. (Chiron Corporation, USA). *PCT Int. Appl*. WO 2004-US1637 20040121.
32. Ishihara, T. et al. 2000. Tryptanthrin inhibits nitric oxide and prostaglandin E2 synthesis by murine macrophages. *Eur. J. Pharmacol*. 407: 197–204.
33. Marko, D. et al. 2001. Inhibition of cyclin-dependent kinase 1 (CDK1) by indirubin derivatives in human tumor cells. *British J. Cancer* 84: 283–9.
34. Tian, F. A. et al. (a) 1995. Structural and antileukemic studies of indirubin derivatives. *J. Chem. Res. in Chin. Univ*. 11: 75–8; (b) 1996. Studies on the structure and properties of N1′-methy-lindirubin monooxime. *Gaodeng Xuexiao Huaxue Xuebao* 17: 69–72; (c) 1994. Studies on the structure and properties of indirubin monooxime methyl ether. *Zhongguo Yaowu Huaxue Zazhi* 4: 101–4.
35. Duensing, S. et al. 2004. Cyclin-dependent kinase inhibitor indirubin-3′-oxime selectively inhibits human papillomavirus type 16 E7-induced numerical centrosome anomalies. *Oncogene* 23: 8206–15.
36. Eisenbrand, G. et al. 2000. Use of cell membrane penetrating indigoid bisindole derivatives. *PCT Intl. Appl*. 30 pp. WO 2000-EP3210 20000411.
37. Jautelat, R. et al. 2002. Preparation of soluble CDK-inhibitory indirubin derivatives for treatment of cancer, AIDS and neurodegenerative diseases. *PCT Intl. Appl*. 92 pp. WO 2002-EP6132 20020605.
38. Damiens, E. et al. 2000. Chemical inhibitors of cyclin-dependent kinases: Preclinical and clinical studies. *Pathol. Biol*. 48: 340–51.
39. Jautelat, R. et al. 2002. Preparation of indirubin derivatives having an increased solubility and their use as inhibitors of cyclin-dependent kinases. *PCT Intl. Appl*. 75 pp. WO 2002-EP2983 20020318.

40. Jautelat, R. et al. 2005. From the insoluble dye indirubin towards highly active, soluble CDK2-inhibitors. *ChemBioChem* 6: 531–40.
41. Eisenbrand, G. et al. 2001. Use of indirubin derivatives as enzyme inhibitors in pharmaceutical compositions. *PCT Intl. Appl.* 49 pp. WO 2000-FR3264 20001123.
42. Kosmopoulou, M. N. et al. 2004. Binding of the potential antitumour agent indirubin-5-sulphonate at the inhibitor site of rabbit muscle glycogen phosphorylase b: Comparison with ligand binding to pCDK2-cyclin A complex. *Eur. J. Biochem.* 271: 2280–90.
43. Davies, T. G. et al. 2001. Inhibitor binding to active and inactive CDK2 the crystal structure of CDK2-cyclin A/indirubin-5-sulphonate. *Structure* 9: 389–97.
44. Zhang, N. et al. 2005. Molecular models of cyclin-dependent kinase 4 complexed with indirubin and its analogues. *Huaxue Xuebao* 63(9): 809–13.
45. Prien, O. et al. 2002. Production of sulphur-containing indirubin derivatives and their use in the treatment of cancer, cardiovascular and neurodegenerative diseases and viral infections. *PCT Intl. Appl.* 54 pp. WO 2001-EP12007 20011017.
46. Prien, O. et al. 2002. The production of aryl-substituted indirubin derivatives and their use as inhibitors of cyclin-dependent kinases. *PCT Intl. Appl.* 49 pp. WO 2001-EP12339 20011022.
47. Eisenbrand, G. et al. 2000. Preparation of indigoid bisindole indirubin derivatives for pharmaceutical use in the treatment of solid cancers. *PCT Intl. Appl.* 50 pp. WO 2000-EP3285 20000412.
48. Du, D. J. et al. 1993. Antitumor activities of 5′-iodoindirubin. *Recent Adv. Chem. Mol. Biol. Cancer Res., Int. Symp.*, Meeting Date 1991, 345–50.
49. Gu, Y. C. et al. 1989. Synthesis of some halogenated indirubin derivatives. *Yaoxue Xuebao* 24: 629–32.
50. Saito, H. et al. 2011. Synthesis of methoxy- and bromo-substituted indirubins and their activities on apoptosis induction in human neuroblastoma cells. *Bioorg. Med. Chem. Lett.* 21: 5370–3.
51. Wang, T. C. et al. 2010. Design, synthesis and antiproliferative studies of a novel series of indirubin derivatives. *Chin. Chem. Lett.* 21: 1407–10.
52. Liu, L. et al. 2012. A novel 7-bromoindirubin with potent anticancer activity suppresses survival of human melanoma cells associated with inhibition of STAT3 and Akt signaling. *Cancer Biol. Ther.* 13: 1255–61.
53. Li, X. et al. 2013. Study on antitumor effect of a newly synthesized 7-azaisoindigo in vitro and in vivo. *Zhongguo Xibao Shengwuxue Xuebao* 35: 334–40.
54. Li, Y. R. et al. 2011. Natura-alpha targets forkhead Box M1 and inhibits androgen-dependent and -independent prostate cancer growth and invasion. *Clin. Cancer Res.* 17: 4414–24.
55. Zuo, M. X. et al. 2008. The antitumor activity of meisoindigo against human colorectal cancer HT-29 cells in vitro and in vivo. *J. Chemother.* (Firenze, Italy) 20: 728–33.
56. Huang, M. et al. 2014. Evaluation of meisoindigo, an indirubin derivative: In vitro antileukemic activity and in vivo pharmacokinetics. *Intl. J. Oncol.* 45: 1724–34.
57. Wee, X. K. et al. 2012. Exploring the anticancer activity of functionalized isoindigos: Synthesis, drug-like potential, mode of action and effect on tumor-induced xenografts. *ChemMedChem* 7: 777–91.
58. Cheng, X. L. et al. 2014. 7,7′-Diazaindirubin-A small molecule inhibitor of casein kinase 2 in vitro and in cells. *Bioorg. Med. Chem.* 22: 247–55.
59. Cuong, N. M. et al. 2010. Inhibitory effects of indirubin derivatives on the growth of HL-60 leukemia cells. *Nat. Prod. Commun.* 5: 103–6.
60. Chebel, A. et al. 2009. Indirubin derivatives inhibit malignant lymphoid cell proliferation. *Leukemia Lymphoma* 50: 2049–60.
61. Han, S. Y. et al. 2010. Effects of indirubin derivatives on the FLT3 activity and growth of acute myeloid leukemia cell lines. *Drug Develop. Res.* 71: 221–7.
62. Paulkumar, K. et al. 2010. Anticancer effect of indirubin-3′-monoxime for human laryngeal carcinoma. *Intl. J. Cancer Res.* 6: 27–34.
63. Kameswaran, T. R. et al. 2009. Indirubin-3-monooxime induced cell cycle arrest and apoptosis in Hep-2 human laryngeal carcinoma cells. *Biomed. Pharmacother.* 63: 146–54.
64. Chen, X. B. et al. 2009. Effect of indirubin-3′-monoxime on cell proliferation, cell cycle and survivin expression in human esophageal cancer EC-1 cell line. *J. Zhengzhou Univ. (Med. Edit.)* 44: 465–8.
65. Chen, X. B. et al. 2009. Effects of indirubin-3′-monoxime on proliferation and cell cycle of human EC-1 and Kyse70 esophageal cancer cells. *Zhongliu* 29: 350–3.
66. Chen, X. B. et al. 2009. Effect of indirubin-3′-monoxime on proliferation and apoptosis of human HT-29 cells. *Zhongguo Aizheng Zazhi* 19: 503–7.
67. Perabo, F. G. E. et al. 2011. Antiproliferative and apoptosis inducing effects of indirubin-3′-monoxime in renal cell cancer cells. *Urologic Oncol.* 29: 815–20.
68. Shi, J. et al. 2008. Critical role of Bid and Bax in indirubin-3′-monoxime-induced apoptosis in human cancer cells. *Biochem. Pharmacol.* 75: 1729–42.
69. Damiens, E. et al. 2001. Anti-mitotic properties of indirubin-3′-monoxime, a CDK/GSK-3 inhibitor: Induction of endoeplication following prophase arrest. *Oncogene* 20: 3786–97.
70. Perabo, F. G. E. et al. 2006. Indirubin-3′-monoxime, a CDK inhibitor induces growth inhibition and apoptosis-independent upregulation of survivin in transitional cell cancer. *Anticancer Res.* 26: 2129–36.
71. Liu, X. L. et al. 2008. Inhibitory effect of indirubin formaldoxime on bladder transitional cell carcinoma T24 cell proliferation in vitro. *Shandong Yiyao* 48: 62–3.
72. Lee, M. J. et al. 2008. Indirubin-3′-monoxime, a derivative of a Chinese antileukemia medicine, inhibits Notch1 signaling. *Cancer Lett.* 265: 215–25.
73. Liao X. M. et al. 2013. Indirubin-3'-oxime induces mitochondrial dysfunction and triggers growth inhibition and cell cycle arrest in human neuroblastoma cells. *Oncol. Reports* 29: 371–9.
74. Lee, M. Y. et al. 2013. Indirubin-3′-monoxime promotes autophagic and apoptotic death in JM1 human acute lymphoblastic leukemia cells and K562 human chronic myelogenous leukemia cells. *Oncol. Rep.* 29: 2072–8.
75. Lo, W. Y. et al. 2013. An indirubin derivative, indirubin-3′-monoxime suppresses oral cancer tumorigenesis through the downregulation of surviving. *PLoS One* 8: e70198.

76. Kim, J. Y. et al. 2011. Indirubin-3′-monoxime, a derivative of a Chinese antileukemia medicine, inhibits angiogenesis. *J. Cell. Biochem.* 112: 1384–91.
77. Luo, S. X. et al. 2013. Molecular mechanism of indirubin-3′-monoxime and Matrine in the reversal of paclitaxel resistance in NCI-H520/TAX25 cell line. *Chin. Med. J.* (Beijing, China, Eng. Edit.) 126: 925–9.
78. Chen, X. B. et al. 2009. Antitumor effect of indirubin-3′-monoxime combined with nedaplatin on human esophageal cancer cell line EC-1. *Zhongliu Fangzhi Yanjiu* 36: 914–6.
79. Siemeister, G. et al. 2002. Therapeutic use of selective indirubin derivatives as VEGF receptor inhibitors. *PCT Intl. Appl.* WO 2002-EP5029 20020507.
80. Ravichandran, K. et al. 2010. Effect of indirubin-3-monoxime against lung cancer as evaluated by histological and transmission electron microscopic studies. *Microscopy Res. Tech.* 73: 1053–8.
81. Choi, S. J. et al. 2010. Indirubin derivatives as potent FLT3 inhibitors with anti-proliferative activity of acute myeloid leukemic cells. *Bioorg. Med. Chem. Lett.* 20: 2033–7.
82. Yoon, J. H. et al. 2010. 5′-Nitro-indirubinoxime induces G1 cell cycle arrest and apoptosis in salivary gland adenocarcinoma cells through the inhibition of Notch-1 signaling. *Biochimica et Biophysica Acta* 1800: 352–8.
83. Kim, S.-A. et al. 2009. 5′-Nitro-indirubinoxime induces G2/M cell cycle arrest and apoptosis in human KB oral carcinoma cells. *Cancer Lett.* 274: 72–7.
84. Yoon, H.-E. et al. 2012. Inhibition of Plk1 and Pin1 by 5′-nitro-indirubinoxime suppresses human lung cancer cells. *Cancer Lett.* 316: 97–104.
85. Khanal, P. et al. 2011. 5′-Nitro-indirubinoxime inhibits epidermal growth factor- and phorbol ester-induced AP-1 activity and cell transformation through inhibition of phosphorylation of Pin1. *Mol. Carcinogenesis* 50: 961–71.
86. Kim, S.-A. et al. 2012. 5′-Nitro-indirubinoxime, an indirubin derivative, suppresses metastatic ability of human head and neck cancer cells through the inhibition of Integrin β1/FAK/Akt signaling. *Cancer Lett.* 306: 197–204.
87. Choi, S. J. et al. 2010. 5,5′-Substituted Indirubin-3′-oxime derivatives as potent cyclin-dependent kinase inhibitors with anticancer activity. *J. Med. Chem.* 53: 3696–706.
88. Lee, J. W. et al. 2005. Induction of apoptosis by a novel indirubin-5-nitro-3′-monoxime, a CDK inhibitor, in human lung cancer cells. *Bioorg. Med. Chem. Lett.* 5: 3948–52.
89. Kim, S. A. et al. 2007. Antitumor activity of novel indirubin derivatives in rat tumor model. *Clin. Cancer Res.* 13: 253–9.
90. Nam, S. et al. 2005. Indirubin derivatives inhibit Stat3 signaling and induce apoptosis in human cancer cells. *Proceedings of the National Academy of Sciences of the United States of America* 102: 5998–6003.
91. Jakobs, S. et al. 2005. Molecular targets of indirubins. *Intl. J. Clin. Pharmacol. Therap.* 43: 592–4.
92. Zhou, J. B. et al. 2009. Enhanced activation of STAT pathways and overexpression of survivin confer resistance to FLT3 inhibitors and could be therapeutic targets in AML. *Blood* 113: 4052–62.
93. Song, J. H. et al. 2015. 5-diphenylacetamido-indirubin-3′-oxime as a novel mitochondria-targeting agent with anti-leukemic activities. *Mol. Carcinogenesis* Ahead of Print.
94. Ichimaru, Y. et al. 2015. Indirubin 3′-(O-oxiran-2-ylmethyl) oxime: A novel anticancer agent. *Bioorg. Med. Chem. Lett.* 25: 1403–6.
95. Nam, S. et al. 2012. Indirubin derivatives induce apoptosis of chronic myelogenous leukemia cells involving inhibition of Stat5 signaling. *Mol. Oncol.* 6: 276–83.
96. Shim, E. Y. et al. 2012. Indirubin derivative E804 inhibits angiogenesis. *BMC cancer* 12: 164.
97. Chan, Y. et al. 2012. An indirubin derivative, E804, exhibits potent angiosuppressive activity. *Biochem. Pharmacol.* 83: 598–607.
98. Heshmati, N. et al. (a) 2013. Enhancement of oral bioavailability of E804 by self-nanoemulsifying drug delivery system (SNEDDS) in rats. *J. Pharm. Sci.* 102: 3792–9; (b) 2014. In vitro and in vivo evaluations of the performance of an indirubin derivative, formulated in four different self-emulsifying drug delivery systems. *J. Pharmacy Pharmacol.* 66: 1567–75.
99. Braig, S. et al. 2013. Indirubin derivative 6BIO suppresses metastasis. *Cancer Res.* 73: 6004–12.
100. Kim, W. S. et al. 2013. 5′-OH-5-nitroindirubin oxime (AGM130), an Indirubin derivative, induces apoptosis of Imatinib-resistant chronic myeloid leukemia cells. *Leukemia Res.* 37: 427–33.
101. Tanaka, T. et al. 2014. Indirubin derivatives alter DNA binding activity of the transcription factor NF-Y and inhibit MDR1 gene promoter. *Eur. J. Pharmacol.* 741: 83–9.
102. Libnow, S. et al. 2008. Synthesis of indirubin-N′-glycosides and their anti-proliferative activity against human cancer cell lines. *Bioorg. Med. Chem.* 16: 5570–83.
103. Kunz, M. et al. 2010. Synthesis of thia-analogous indirubin N-glycosides and their influence on melanoma cell growth and apoptosis. *ChemMedChem* 5: 534–9.
104. Shi, R. Z. et al. 2012. The cytotoxicity of indirubin derivative PHII-7 against human breast cancer MCF-7 cells and its mechanisms. *Zhongguo Zhongxiyi Jiehe Zazhi* 32: 1521–5.
105. Peng, H. W. et al. 2012. PhII-7 induces apoptosis on k562 and k562/a02 by increasing ros production. *Zhongguo Yaolixue Tongbao* 28: 911–6.
106. Peng, H. W. et al. 2013. PHII-7 inhibits cell growth and induces apoptosis in leukemia cell line K562 as well as its MDR-counterpart K562/A02 through producing reactive oxygen species. *Eur. J. Pharmacol.* 718: 459–68.
107. Shi, R. 2012. Indirubin derivative PHII-7 suppresses the proliferation of resistant human breast cancer MCF-7/Adr cells via inhibiting c-fos expression. *Zhongyao Yaoli Yu Linchuang* 28: 39–42.
108. Shi, R. Z. et al. 2011. A novel indirubin derivative PHII-7 potentiates adriamycin cytotoxicity via inhibiting P-glycoprotein expression in human breast cancer MCF-7/ADR cells. *Eur. J. Pharmacol.* 669: 38–44.
109. Wen, Z. J. et al. 1988. Effects of indirubin on the histology and histochemistry of canine and rat livers. *Zhongyao Tongbao* 13: 306–7.
110. Rivest, P. et al. 2011. Proliferative and androgenic effects of indirubin derivatives in LNCaP human prostate cancer cells at sub-apoptotic concentrations. *Chemico-Biol. Interactions* 189: 177–85.

23 Xiang Si Zi 相思子

Rosary pea

Herb Origination

The herb Xiang Si Zi (Rosary pea) is the dried seed of *Abrus precatorius* L. (Leguminosae). The tree is native to India, Indonesia, and other parts of tropical Asia. Now, the tree widely grows in tropical and subtropical climates including southern China, Florida, tropical Africa, and the West Indies. In China, the seeds are usually collected when its fruits have ripened and are dried in the sun for Chinese folk medical use.

Antitumor Constituents and Activity

Abrins

Anticancer Activity

The major component in Rosary pea is a galactose-specific and highly toxic abrin (a lectin-type phytoprotein). It displayed potent cytotoxic and tumoricidal effects to various cancer cells *in vitro* and *in vivo*, being stronger than diphtherotoxin and ricin.[1] When treated at a sublethal dose of 7.5 μg/kg every alternate day for 10 days *in vivo*, both intralesional and i.p. injections of the abrin were effective in lessening the tumor mass development caused by EAC or Dalton's ascites lymphoma (DAL). The i.p. injection lengthened the life duration of mice bearing ascites tumor, but it was ineffective in prophylactic administration.[2] If the mice were treated by subcutaneous injection or oral administration of the lectins (200 ng) for four days before being inoculated with sarcoma 180 cells, 50% of the mice were free of metastases, 33% had first degree metastases, and 17% had third degree metastases after three weeks.[3] If combined with CTX, a low dose of abrin achieves a marked synchronal antitumor effect.[4] Moreover, the abrin was also capable of enhancing the cellular immune responses in both normal and tumor-bearing animal models. The proliferation of lymphocytes (splenocytes and thymocytes) was remarkably potentiated, and the NK cell activity and Ab-dependent cellular cytotoxicity were also significantly enhanced in the presence of abrin.[5]

The abrin was further separated to give abrin-A (molecular weight: ≈65000) and abrin-B (molecular weight: ≈67000). Both lectins appeared to have two glycoprotein subunits with similar tryptic maps, where the two subunit chains were connected by a disulfide bond.[6] The injection of abrin-A (1 ng) to mice implanted with Meth-A fibrosarcoma suppressed the tumor growth by 90%.[7] Both abrin-A and abrin-B inhibited the growth of mouse sarcoma 180 and EAC *in vivo* at their sublethal doses.[8] However, abrin-A at a concentration of 5 μg/mL could adhere to sarcoma 180 cells and EAC cells, but the similar effect required 150 μg/mL for abrin-B. The result evidenced that abrin-A had a higher affinity for binding to tumor cells than abrin-B, implying that the different binding sites largely influenced their anticancer potencies.[8]

Abrin-P2, another purified abrin from Xiang Si Zi, could obstruct the proliferation of human HepG2 hepatoma cells *in vitro* and *in vivo* (IC_{50}: 5.172 ×10^{-3} μg/mL, in 48 h). The anti-hepatoma effect was related to the elicitation of S cell arrest and cell apoptosis and inactivation of telomerase. I.g. giving abrin-P2 to mice in a dose of 100 μg/kg for 10 days restrained the growth of H22 hepatoma cells by 62.47% with low inference on the thymus and the spleen. Its LD_{50} value in the oral administration was 6.77 mg/kg in mice.[9]

Immunotoxins

Abrin-A was used to conjugate with monoclonal Ab AF20. The produced immunotoxin displayed a specificity in inhibiting human pancreatic carcinoma cells.[10] The recombinant-A chain of abrin was conjugated with antibodies to target the human gonadotropin-releasing hormone receptor. The conjugated immunotoxin mAb F1G4-rABRa-A obstructed the protein synthesis specifically on cells expressing the gonadotropin-releasing hormone receptor, whose intracellular trafficking pathway is distinct from that by abrin.[11]

Agglutinins

Amyloid-ß Oligomer-Binding Peptide

Amyloid-ß oligomer-binding peptide (ABP) is a peptide fraction (molecular weight: 600–1500 Da) derived from Abrus abrin. In an *in vitro* assay, the inhibitory effect of ABP was shown in several tumor cell lines (including Dalton's lymphoma and HeLa cervical cancer) but no any cytotoxicity to normal cell lines in a dose of 1 μg/mL. ABP at a dose of 100 μg/kg (body weight) restrained the growth of DAL cells by 89.7% and amplified the life span of a mice model by 104.6% without acute toxicity.[12,13] An analysis of the antigrowth mechanism revealed that ABP elicited the apoptosis of DAL cells with nuclear fragmentation and condensation by reducing the ratio of Bcl-2/Bax and augmenting the release of cytochrome c and caspase-3 activity. In addition, the LD_{50} (50% lethal dose) value of ABP was 2.25 mg/kg (body weight) in mice.[13]

Abrus Agglutinin

Abrus agglutinin (AAG) prepared from the seeds is a heterotetrameric gal-β-(1-3) NAc gal-specific lectin-type protein. AAG acted as a cancer inhibitor and immunostimulator in its native and heat-denatured conditions. The treatment with AAG diminished the tumor size and prolonged the survival time significantly in a murine DAL model. Even at a concentration as low as ~1 ng/mL, AAG still showed an ability to enhance the peritoneal macrophage and spleen-derived NK cells *in vitro*, exerting their cytotoxicity against the DAL cells. The findings revealed that the anticancer activity of AAG at a nontoxic dose was primarily elicited by the stimulation of the innate immune system and Th1-type immunoregulation.[14] The anticancer effect of AGG was also shown against human hepatoma cells *in vitro* and *in vivo*, where AGG dose and time dependently induced the apoptosis of HepG2 cells by a caspases-activated pathway with NF-κB/Hsp90-inactivation.[15] The agglutinin may be a potential alternative natural remedy in the treatment of hepatocellular carcinoma and ascites lymphoma.

Abrus Agglutinin Peptide

AAGP is an Abrus agglutinin peptide fraction (500–3000 Da). At low concentrations of 1–10 kg/mL, AAGP exerted selective antiproliferative activity on several cancer cell lines *in vitro* but no cytotoxicity on normal cells even in a 100 μg/mL concentration. The antigrowth mechanism in human HeLa cervical cancer cells was closely associated with the induction of nuclear fragmentation and apoptosis of HeLa cells via the increase of ROS generation, the decrease of Bcl-2/Bax ratio, and the activation of mitochondrial permeability transition and caspase-3.[16]

10KDAGP

An agglutinin-derived peptide termed 10KDAGP was prepared from *A. precatorius*. It induced ROS-dependent mitochondrial apoptosis of human HeLa cervical cancer cells through different pathways in the cellular system such as JNK and Akt/P38/P53 as well as autophagy. An *in vivo* model with HeLa cancer proved that the 10kDAGP treatment killed the cancer cells mediated by the activation of JNK.[17]

Triterpenoids

Six triterpenoids, assigned as abruslactone-A, abrusogenin, abrusgenic acid, subprogenin-D, triptotriterpenic acid-B, and abrusoside-C, were isolated from the leaves and the stems of *A. precatorius*. Among them, abruslactone-A and abrusogenin demonstrated a moderate cytotoxic effect on SW1990 (pancreas), HeLa (cervix), Du-145 (prostate), and MCF-7 (breast) human cancer cell lines, *in vitro*.[18]

Other Bioactivities

The highly poisonous Xiang Si Zi (Rosary pea) seeds possess abortifacient, aphrodisiac, anodyne, diuretic, emetic, expectorant, febrifuge and hemostat, laxative, purgative, sedative, refrigerant, and antimicrobial activities that have been proven by pharmacological studies. Its powdered seeds are able to disturb the uterine functions and to prevent conception in women. Its seed oil was reported to have the ability to promote the growth of human hair. Its roots can be used for the treatment of gonorrhea, jaundice, and hemoglobinuric bile.[19]

References

1. Hwang, K. M. et al. 1984. Selective antitumor effect on L10 hepatocarcinoma cells of a potent immuno-conjugate composed of a chain of abrin and a monoclonal antibody to a hepatoma-associated antigen. *Cancer Res.* 44: 4579–86.
2. Ramnath, V. et al. 2002. Antitumor effect of abrin on transplanted tumors in mice. *Ind. J. Phys. Pharmco.* 46: 69–77.
3. Tung, T. C. et al. 1989. Agglutinins and lectins for oral administration for the inhibition of neoplasm metastasis formation. *Ger. Offen.* Application: DE 88–3825186 19880725.
4. Olesnes, S. et al. 1982. Toxic lectins and related proteins. *Molecular Action of Toxins and Virus* (Cohen, P. et al. eds). 51–106. Elsevier Biomedical Press, Amsterdam.
5. Ramnath, V. et al. 2006. Effect of abrin on cell-mediated immune responses in mice. *Immunopharmacol. Immunotoxicol.* 28: 259–68.
6. Li, L. Q. et al. 2004. Advance in research on anticancer of abrin. *Yaowu Shengwu Jishu* 11: 339–43.
7. Eisai Co. Ltd. Japan, 1984. Immune adjuvant formulations containing abrin A. *Jpn. Tokkyo Koho* JP 59205326 A 19841120.
8. Lin, J. W. et al. 1978. Isolation of antitumor proteins abrin-A and abrin-B from *Abrus precatorious. Int. J. Peptide Protein Res.* 12: 311–7.
9. Qin, D. D. et al. 2011. Investigation of the antihepatoma effect of abrin P2 and its influence on telomerase activity. *Zhongguo Yaolixue Tongbao* 27: 1666–71.
10. Sato, N. et al. 1993. Monoclonal antibody reactive with human pancreas cancer tissue. Eur. Pat. Appl: EP 92–113367, 19920805.
11. Gadadhar, S. et al. 2013. Abrin immunotoxin: Targeted cytotoxicity and intracellular trafficking pathway. *PLoS One* 8: e58304.
12. Bhutia, S. K. et al. 2009. Abrus abrin derived peptides induce apoptosis by targeting mitochondria in HeLa cells. *Cell Biol. Internat.* 33: 720–7.
13. Bhutia, S. K. et al. 2009. Inhibitory effect of abrus abrin-derived peptide fraction against Dalton's lymphoma ascites model. *Phytomed.* 16: 377–85.
14. Ghosh, D. et al. 2007. Immunomodulatory and antitumor activities of native and heat denatured Abrus agglutinin. *Immunobiol.* 212: 589–99.
15. Mukhopadhyay, S. et al. 2014. Abrus agglutinin suppresses human hepatocellular carcinoma in vitro and in vivo by inducing caspase-mediated cell death. *Acta Pharmacol. Sinica* 35: 814–24.
16. Bhutia, S. K. et al. 2008. Induction of mitochondria-dependent apoptosis by Abrus agglutinin derived peptides in human cervical cancer cells. *Toxicol. in Vitro* 22: 344–51.
17. Behera, B. et al. 2014. Abrus precatorius agglutinin-derived peptides induce ROS-dependent mitochondrial apoptosis through JNK and Akt/P38/P53 pathways in HeLa cells. *Chemico-Biological Interactions* 222: 97–105.
18. Xiao, Z. H. et al. 2012. A new triterpenoid saponin from *Abrus precatorius Linn. Mol.* 17: 295–302.
19. Zhang, P. et al. 2014. Progress of chemical constituents and pharmacological effects in *Abrus precatorius. Guangdong Yaoxueyuan Xuebao* 30: 654–8.

24 Mao Ren Shen 猫人参

Cat ginseng

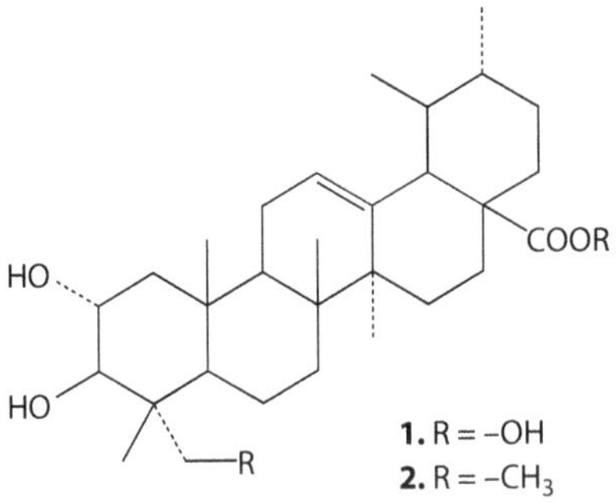

1. R = -OH
2. R = $-CH_3$
3 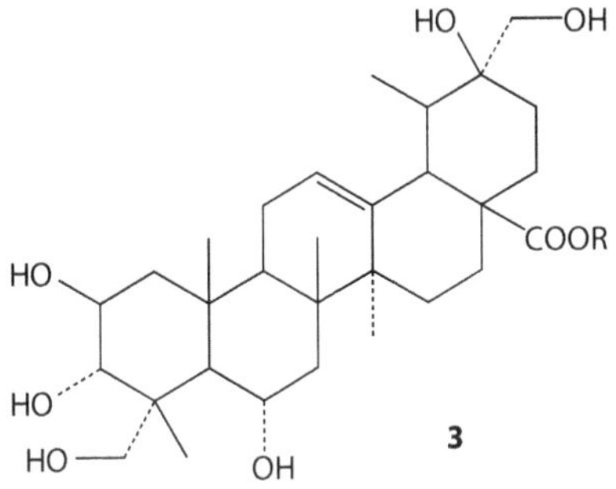
R = -D-beta-glucopyranose
4 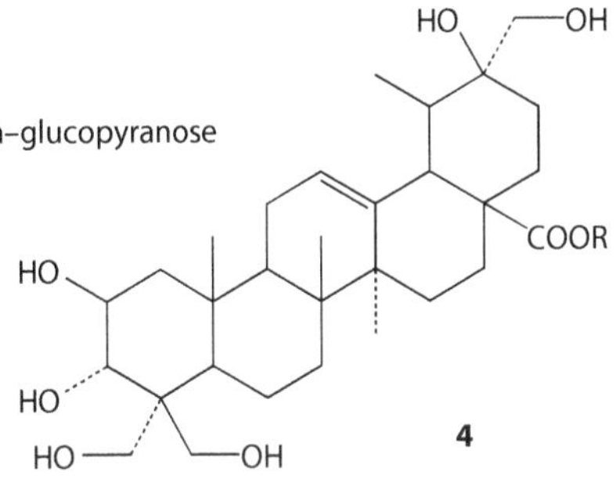

Herb Origination

The herb Mao Ren Shen (Cat ginseng) is a popular folk medicine in southeast China. The name stems from the function attracting cats to use the plant as a stimulant and a healer for wounds. The herb's origin is two Actinidiaceae plants *Actinidia macrosperma* and *A. valvata*. Both plants are deciduous scandent shrub mainly growing in alley forests. Their roots and stems are collected in late summer and autumn and dried in the sun for use in treating various ailments. Due to lack of resource of *A. macrosperma*, its close plant *A. valvata* has been employed as Cat ginseng in most cases.

Antitumor Activities

Mao Ren Shen was useful in eastern China for the treatment of cancers in the lung, the liver, and the digestive system. The investigations provided more positive evidences to support the anticancer effect. An injection prepared from *A. valvata* roots exhibited antitumor efficacy on three liver cancer cell lines (H22, CBRH-7919, and SMMC-7721) *in vitro*.[1] Its extracts of hexane, dichloromethane ($CHCl_3$), and methanol (MeOH) were moderately effective in the inhibition of human SMMC-7721 hepatoma cell line (IC_{50}: 51–77 μg/mL), whereas its ethyl acetate (EtOAc) and aqueous extracts showed a lower antihepatoma effect (IC_{50}: 192–212 μg/mL). Some fractions derived from the active extracts exerted the growth inhibition against transplanted H22 hepatoma in mice together with induction of apoptosis and G0/G1 cell cycle arrest.[2] Similarly, the hexane, EtOAc, and $CHCl_3$ extracts from *A. macrosperma* roots displayed dose-dependent cytotoxicity, but its MeOH and aqueous extracts had weak activities in the *in vitro* test.[3] The Cat ginseng-treated serum could suppress the EGFR expression in human A549 lung carcinoma cells.[4] Moreover, the aqueous extract of *A. macrosperma* also significantly enhanced the overall immune functions *in vivo* (especially at 100 and 250 mg/kg) and markedly exerted free radical-scavenging and lipid peroxidation-decreasing activities.[3,5] The antioxidant potency of *A. macrosperma* extracts was in order as MeOH extract > EtOAc extract > water extract > $CHCl_3$ extract > hexane extract.[3] Apparently, based on the anticarcinogenesis-related immunoregulatory and antioxidant activities, Mao Ren Shen potentiated the inhibitory activity against the growth of cancer cells and markedly diminished the toxicity/side effects of cancer chemo- and radiotherapies.

Antitumor Constituents and Activities

The major constituents in the Cat ginseng are triterpenoids and triterpene saponins, which were scientifically responsible for the bioliogical activities of the herb including cancer suppression and immuno-stimulation.

Saponins

The total saponins isolated from Mao Ren Shen were used to treat six human hepatoma cell lines (BEL-7402, HepG2, PLC, SMMC-7721, MHCC-97-H, and MHCC-97-L) *in vitro*. At 1.5 mg/mL concentration, the saponins obstructed the proliferation of BEL-7402 cells by 61.08%, 74.12%, and 84.55% at 24, 48, and 72 h, respectively, and inhibited the proliferation of MHCC-97-H cells by 36% at 24 h. However, at the same concentration, the inhibitory rates were below 30% at 24 h on PLC, SMMC-7721, and HepG2 cell lines. Moreover, the saponins at the 200 μg/mL concentration obviously restrained the adhesion, the invasion, the migration, and the mobility of BEL-7402 and MHCC-97-H cells *in vitro*.[6] Mao Ren Shen saponins were further tested in a mouse model transplanted with H22 hepatoma cells, resulting in the inhibitory rate of 43.5–53.2%. Simultaneously, the expression of VEGF in the transplanted tumor was obstructed in the treatment, implying the antiangiogenesis involved in the antihepatoma mechanisms.[7]

Triterpenoids

The $CHCl_3$ fraction of *A. valvata* roots is a rich source of triterpenoids that also exist as aglycones of the saponins. Of the separated triterpenoids, asiatic acid (**1**) and corosolic acid (**2**) showed a certain cytotoxic effect against human LoVo colon cancer and HepG2 hepaoma cell lines,[8] and two polyoxygenated triterpenoids assigned as (2β,3α,6α)-2,3,6,20,23,30-hexahydroxyurs-12-en-28-oic acid (**3**) and (2β,3α)-2,3,20,23,24,30-hexahydroxyurs-12-en-28-oic acid *O*-β-D-glucopyranosyl ester (**4**) displayed a moderate inhibitory effect against both SMMC-7721 and BEL-7402 hepatoma cell lines.[9] In association with up-expressing the Bax and depolarizing the mitochondrial transmembrane, corosolic acid (**2**) at a 35 μmol/L concentration notably induced the apoptotic and suppressive effects against the SMCC-7721 cells.[10] Additionally, the leaves of *A. valvata* are also rich in corosolic acid (**2**), maslinic acid, ursolic acid, etc. The separated triterpenoids from the leaves, such as corosolic acid (**2**), 2α,3β,24-trihydroxyurs-12-en-28-oic acid, 2α,3α,24-trihydroxyurs-12-en-28-oic acid, and 2α,3α,19α,24-tetrahydroxyurs-12-en-28-oic acid, showed the inhibitory effect against a small panel of human neoplastic cell lines including hepatoma (PLC, Hep3B, HepG2, Bel7402), cervical cancer (HeLa), colon cancer (SW480), and breast cancer (MCF-7) cells, *in vitro*.[11]

Polysaccharides

A polysaccharide component was extracted from the herb and was demonstrated playing important roles in tumor cell suppression and immunity regulation. Thus, it may be developed as a supplement for cancer prevention and therapy by oral administration, injection, fluid infusion, percutaneous absorption, and mucosa absorption dosage pattern.[12]

Clinical Trials

Several clinical trials have confirmed that Mai Ren Shan has a significant ability to improve appetite, to alleviate weakness, and to stabilize WBC counts, NK cells, IL-2 level, and CD4/CD8 ratio in cancer patients receiving chemotherapy or radiotherapy.[13,14]

Other Bioactivities

The herb Mao Ren Shen (Cat ginseng) has been extensively employed to treat various ailments such as leprosy, abscess, rheumatism, arthritis inflammation, jaundice, and abnormal leucorrhea. A pharmacological study proved that cat ginseng possesses antioxidant, hypoglycemic, antiinflammatory, immunopotentiating, antibacterial, and antifungal properties.[15] Abrin is the principal toxic component in Xiang Si Zi. The respective LDs of abrin-A and abrin-B were 10 and 25 μg/kg (body weight) for mice recorded within 48 h.

References

1. Wan, X. Y. et al. 2004. Experimental study on Antihepatocarcinoma effect of Maorenshen injection in vitro. *J. Zhejiang TCM Coll.* 28: 45–7.
2. Zhang, Y. N. et al. 2006. Inhibition effect of active fraction from *Actinidia valvata* on growth of transplanted mouse tumor cells and preliminary study of its mechanism. *Zhongguo Zhongyao Zazhi* 31: 918–20.
3. Lu, Y. et al. 2012. *Actinidia macrosperma* C. F. Liang (a wild kiwi): Preliminary study of its antioxidant and cytotoxic activities. *Evidence-Based Complem. Altern. Med.* Vol. 2012, Article ID 180262.
4. Guo, H. F. et al. 2010. Cats ginseng containing serum inhibit the EGFR expression in human lung adenocarcinoma A549 cell line. *Jiangxi Zhongyiyao* 12: 29–30.
5. Lu, Y. et al. 2007. Immunomodulatory activity of aqueous extract of *Actinidia macrosperma. Asia Pacific J. Clin. Nutri.* 16 (Suppl. 1): 261–5.
6. Zheng, G. Y. et al. 2012. Total saponin from root of *Actinidia valvata Dunn* prevents the metastasis of human hepatocellular carcinoma cells. *Chin. J. Integr. Med.* 18: 197–202.
7. Yi, T. J. et al. 2009. Inhibitory effects of total saponin from *Actinidia valvata* on murine transplanted tumor. *Zhonghua Zhongyiyao Xuekan* 27: 1642–3.
8. Xu, Y. X. et al. 2011. Antitumor constituents from the roots of *Actinidia valvata. Dier Junyi Daxue Xuebao* 32: 749–53.
9. Xin, H. L. et al. 2008. Two new polyoxygenated triterpenoids from *Actinidia valvata. Helv. Chim. Acta* 91: 575–580.
10. Li, H. Y. et al. 2011. Preliminary study on the growth inhibition of SMCC-7721 cells by corosolic acid. *Shandong Yiyao* 52: 44–6.
11. Xin, H. L. et al. 2010. Four triterpenoids with cytotoxic activity from the leaves of *Actinidia valvata. Zhongguo Tianran Yaowu* 8: 260–3.
12. Lou, W. M. 2004. Method for extracting anticarcinogenesis polysaccharide composite AVDS from *A. valvatad* and its use as medicament. *Faming Zhuanli Shenqing Gongkai Shuomingshu* CN 1524869 A 20040901.
13. Zhou, X. Z. 2000. Tang Fu'an talk about lung cancer treatment variation. *J. Zhejiang TCM College* 24: 45–6.
14. Lai, P. F. et al. 2002. The research progress of TCM Cat Ginseng in Zhejiang province location. *J. Zhejiang TCM College* 26: 77–8.
15. Lu, Y. et al. 2007. Composition and antimicrobial activity of the essential oil of *Actinidia macrosperma* from China. *Nat. Prod. Res.* 21: 227–33.

25 Ye Gu 野菰

Ghost flower

Herb Origination

The herb Ye Gu (Ghost flower) is the whole plant of *Aeginetia indica* L. (Orobanchaceae). The herb is a parasitic plant widely distributed throughout tropical and subtropical Asia, from India and Sri Lanka to China, Korea, and Japan. The main part of this plant used in Chinese folk medicine is its pulpous stalk, which is usually collected from spring to summer and dried in the sun. The herb Ye Gu also can be used fresh.

Antitumor Activities and Constituents

The extract from Ye Gu seeds had not exerted a direct cytotoxicity against Meth-A fibrosarcoma cells *in vitro*, but IL-2, IFNγ, TNF, and IL-6 as well as thymocytes were significantly produced when the cells were stimulated by the Ye Gu seed extract. The test also revealed that the CD4$^+$ T cells were the main producers of IL-2 and TNF upon the motivation with the extract *in vitro*, and both CD4$^+$ and CD8$^+$ T cells secreted IFN. Moreover, the extract was mitogenic to T-enriched splenic lymphocytes as well as B-enriched splenic lymphocytes *in vitro*. The i.p. injection of the extract in a dose of 2.5 mg/kg (every two days) after a one-week treatment established antigenicity in mice bearing Meth-A fibrosarcoma and prolonged the survival period. As a result of the extract treatment, the mice survived after the first tumor inoculation showed an ability to overcome the second inoculation with homologous Meth-A without additional administration of the extract. All the treated mice were completely recovered from the tumor without any side effects. Therefore, the stimulated cytokine production and the lymphocyte proliferation should be the key contributors in the induction of cancer inhibitory effects. These findings highlighted that the extract is capable of stimulating antigen-specific concomitant immunity and enhancing potent antitumor immunity.[1,2]

Polysaccharides and Proteins

The Ye Gu seed extract contains biologically active polysaccharides and proteins. The polysaccharides could induce B cell mitogenic and thymocyte costimulatory effects *in vitro*, and the proteins, especially AILb-A (50–60 kDa), having noncarbohydrate epitopes could mediate the antitumor activity *in vivo*.[3] AILb-A is capable of inducing a Th1-type T cell response, markedly increasing multiple Th1 cytokines levels (such as IFNγ, TNFα, IL-2, IL-6, IL-12, IL-18, and GN-CS) and improving killer cell activity of human peripheral blood mononuclear cells, finally exerting a marked inhibitory effect in tumor-bearing mice.[4–6] Further studies revealed that IL-18 played a most significant role for IFNγ- and killer cell-promoting abilities of AILb-A. The AILb-A-augmented antitumor immune responses (such as cytokine production, MAP kinase phosphorylation, killer cell activation, dendritic cell maturation, and nuclear translocation of IFN-regulatory factor-3) were found to be also strongly mediated by toll-like receptor-4. However, the antitumor effect of AILb-A was relatively less in athymic nude mice.[7,8] The findings strongly suggested that AILb-A may be a potential immunotherapeutic agent for cancer patients.

References

1. Chai, J. G. et al. 1992. An extract of seeds from *Aeginetia indica* L., a parasitic plant, induces potent antigen-specific antitumor immunity in Meth A-bearing BALB/c mice. *Cancer Immunol. Immunother.* 35: 181–5.
2. Chai, J. G. et al. 1994. Seed extract of *Aeginetia indica* L. induces cytokine production and lymphocyte proliferation in vitro. *Immunopharmacol.* 27: 13–21.
3. Chai, J. G. et al. 1995. Dissociation between the mitogenic effect and antitumor activity of seed extract from *Aeginetia indica* L. *Immunopharmacol.* 30: 209–15.
4. Ohe, G. et al. 2001. Thl-cytokine induction and antitumor effect of 55 kDa protein isolated from *Aeginetia indica* L., a parasitic plant. *Cancer Immunol. Immunother.* 50: 251–9.
5. Ohe, G. et al. 2001. Purification and characterization of anticancer immunity-inducing molecule from *Aeginetia indica* L., a parasitic plant. *Shikoku Shigakkai Zasshi* 14: 89–110.
6. Okamoto, M. et al. 2000. Purification and characterization of cytokine-inducing protein of seed extract from *Aeginetia indica* L., a parasitic plant. *Immunopharmacol.* 49: 377–89.
7. Nishikawa, H. 2003. Analysis of molecular mechanism for antitumor immunity induced by 55 kDa protein derived from *Aeginetia indica*, a parasitic plant: Involvement of toll-like receptor 4. *Shikoku Shigakkai Zasshi* 16: 347–67.
8. Okamoto, M. et al. 2004. Toll-like receptor 4 mediates the antitumor host response induced by a 55-kilodalton protein isolated from *Aeginetia indica* L., a parasitic plant. *Clin. Diagn. Lab. Immunol.* 11: 483–95.

26 Fan Li Zhi 番荔枝

Sugar apple or Custard apple

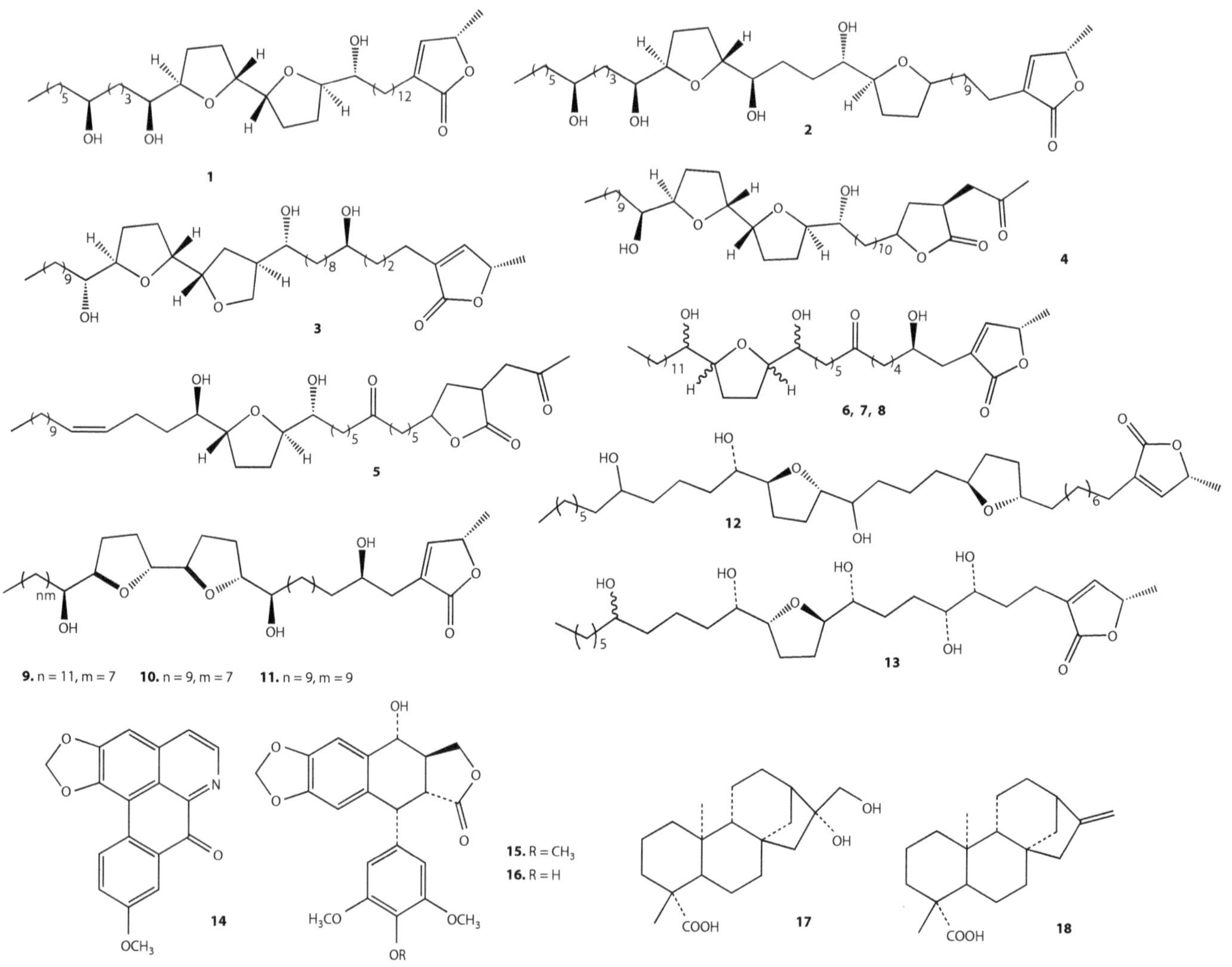

1, 2, 3, 4, 5, 6, 7, 8, 9. n = 11, m = 7 10. n = 9, m = 7 11. n = 9, m = 9, 12, 13, 14, 15. R = CH_3 16. R = H, 17, 18

Herb Origination

The herb Fan Li Zhi (Sugar apple) originated from *Annona squamosa* L., an Annonaceae plant, which initially grew in tropical areas of the American continent such as southern Mexico, West Indies, Bahamas, and Bermuda, as well as in Asian tropical regions including India and Pakistan. Now, the plants are cultivated in Southern China. The fruits, roots, and leaves of Fan Li Zhi are used as folk medicines in China. The herb collection is normally between summer and autumn. In addition, the fruits are popular in tropical markets, having a delicious whitish pulp.

Antitumor Activities and Constituents

The cytotoxicity of aqueous and organic solvent extracts of Fan Li Zhi seeds was shown in rat AK-5 histiocytic tumor, human MCF-7 breast cancer, and K562 erythroleukemia cell lines *in vitro*. Both extracts notably elicited the tumor cells to apoptosis with nuclear condensation and DNA fragmentation via the increase of ROS generation, the downregulation of antiapoptotic genes Bcl-2 and Bcl-xL, and the activation of caspase-3, whose events also correlated with the decreased levels of intracellular GSH and intracellular GSH. Although the two extracts failed in the *in vitro* assay with human Colo 205 colon carcinoma cell line, the aqueous extract exerted a significant antitumor activity *in vivo* in a rat model with the AK-5 tumor.[1,2] In addition, an ethanolic extract derived from the flowers of *A. squamosal* exerted a anticancer activity against the MCF-7 cells *in vitro* (IC_{50}: 6.87 μg/mL).[3]

Acetogenins

The bioactive constituents have been found in several portions of Fan Li Zhi plant such as stems, branches, fruit, and seeds. Acetogenin-type bistetrahydrofurans are characteristic agents discovered from the plant, which are abundant in the seeds and the stem bark, demonstrating a broad spectrum of bioactivities such as potent cytotoxic, antitumor, antiparasitic, pesticidal and immunosuppresive activities. In the *in vitro* assays, the total acetogenins moderately obstructed the proliferation of Bel-7402 (liver) and A549 (lung) human cancer cell lines and elicited the cell apoptosis and/or cell cycle arrest.[4,5] At concentrations of 10^{-4}–10^{0} μg/mL, three fractions of acetogenins were cytotoxic to KB and CNE2 (nasopharyngeal), Bel-7402 (liver), and MCF-7 (breast) cancer cell lines. The respective IC_{50} values were 0.46, 0.00031, 0.078, and 1.72 μg/mL for fraction-A and 0.24, 0.0043, 0.043, and 2.97 μg/mL for fraction-B.[6] Moreover, the growth of two multidrug resistant cell lines and human normal endothelial cell line (ECV304) was restrained by the three fractions. The IC_{50} values of fraction A were 0.32 μg/mL in MCF-7/Adr cells, 0.027 μg/mL in KVB200 cells, and 0.39 μg/mL in ECV304 cells, indicating the potent activities in MDR reversal and antiagiogenesis. The antigrowth activity of the fractions was also investigated in an animal model with sarcoma 180 at a dose of 30 μg/kg, whose average *in vivo* inhibitory rate for fraction A was 52.8% in mice.[6]

Squamocin (**1**) and squamostatin-A (**2**) isolated from the seeds displayed a cytotoxic effect against murine L1210 leukemia cells *in vitro* (respective ED_{50}: 0.58 and 0.5 μg/mL). Squamostolide, an acetogenin obtained from the seeds, demonstrated the growth inhibition against human Bel-7402 hepatoma and CNE2 nasopharyngeal cell lines *in vitro*.[7,8] More annonaceous acetogenins with anticancer activities *in vitro* and/or *in vivo* have been discovered from the seeds of *A. squamosal*, such as squamostatin-E, desacetyluvaricin, annosquacins A–D, annosquatin-A, bullatacin, and annosquatin-B.[9–11] However, more powerful acetogenins were isolated from other parts of Fan Li Zhi, whose ED_{50} values reached a range of 10^{-3}–10^{-4} μg/mL.[12,13]

The bioactivity-directed separation of the stem bark of Fan Li Zhi led to the discovery of more acetogenins. Bullacin-B (**3**), bullatacinone (**4**), and tetrahydrosquamone showed the selective cytotoxicity to human MCF-7 breast cancer cells. Bullacin-B (**3**) was cytotoxic in a panel of six human tumor cell lines, and its potency on the breast cancer cells was nearly a million times stronger than that of adriamycin.[14,15] Mosinone-A (**5**), mosin-B (**6**) and mosin-C (**7**), and annoreticin-9-one (**8**) showed no inhibitory activities toward MCF-7, HT-29, and A498 carcinoma cell lines but exhibited a selective cytotoxic effect against some human cancer cell lines. Their respective ED_{50} values were 0.0022, 0.00025, 0.00012, and 0.00024 μg/mL in PACA-2 pancreatic cancer cells, and the respective ED_{50} values of mosinone-A (**5**), mosin-B (**6**), and annoreticin-9-one (**8**) were 0.032, 0.35, and 0.096 μg/mL in PC3 prostate cancer cells, whose activities were 10–100 times more potent than that of adriamycin (an anticancer drug).[16–18] Squamotacin (**9**), molvizarin (**10**), and bullatacin (**11**), which were acetogenins with *threo/trans/threo/trans/erythro* relative configuration isolated from the bark of a Sugar apple, exerted a potent inhibitory effect against the growth of PACA-2 (pancreas), A498 (kidney), PC3 (prostate), A549 (lung), and/or HT-29 (colon) neoplastic cell lines (ED_{50}: 10^{-1} to $<10^{-9}$ μg/mL). Especially, the strongest cytotoxic effects were demonstrated in the PC3 cells (ED_{50}: 10^{-8} to $<10^{-9}$ μg/mL) by squamotacin (**9**) and molvizarin (**10**), and in the PACA-2 cells (ED_{50}: $<10^{-9}$ μg/mL) by bullatacin (**11**).[19] Moreover, squamotacin (**9**), molvizarin (**10**), and bullatacin (11) exerted a moderate cytotoxicity toward MCF-7 cells, whereas mosin-B (**6**) and mosin-C (**7**), and annoreticin-9-one (**8**) were effective in inhibiting A549 cells (ED_{50}: 10^{-1} μg/mL).[16–18]

Because Fan Li Zhi is a rich source of acetogenins, more novel acetogenins were continuously isolated in recent years, and many of them possess a remarkable anticancer effect as similar potencies to formerly reported acetogenins. Squamostanin-A (**12**) and squamostanins-B were potently effective in the antiproliferation of MCF-7, HCT, A549, and PC3 human cancer cell lines (ED_{50}: 10^{-2}–10^{-4} μg/mL).[20,21] Squadiolin-A (**13**) and squadiolin-B showed potent inhibition against HepG2 hepatoma cells (IC_{50}: 10^{-2}–10^{-3} μM) and significant cytotoxicity against human MDA-MB-231 breast cancer cells (IC_{50}: 10^{-1} μM). The cytotoxicity of squafosacin-B was present in HepG2 and Hep3B, MCF-7, and A549 human cancer cell lines *in vitro* (IC_{50}: 10^{-1} μM).[22]

Alkaloid and Lignans

A tumor inhibitory isoquinoline alkaloid designated as oxoxylopine (**14**) was found from unripe Fan Li Zhi fruits.[23] From the branches of Fan Li Zhi grown in the Philippines, two strong anticancer lignans, podophyllotoxin (**15**) and 4′-demethyl-podophyllotoxin (**16**), were separated. The high degree of cytotoxicity of the lignans was present in human lung and colon neoplastic cell lines *in vitro*.[24]

Diterpenoids

By the bioactivity-directed separation, two kaurane-type diterpenes, 16α,17-dihydroxy-*ent*-kauran-19-oic acid (**17**) and (–)-*ent*-kaur-16-en-19-oic acid (**18**), were separated from the Fan Li Zhi fruit pericarp. Both of the diterpenoids (16α,17-dihydroxy-*ent*-kauran-19-oic acid (**17**) and (–)-*ent*-kaur-16-en-19-oic acid (**18**) were cytotoxic to *in vitro* cultures of Dalton's lymphoma cells and HeLa cervical cancer cells.[25] Also, from the stem bark of the plant, a group of *ent*-kaurane diterpenoids were isolated. Seven of them showed promising antiproliferative activities against 95-D (lung) and A2780 (ovary) human cancer cell lines (IC_{50}: 0.38–34.66 μM). (15α)-15,16-Epoxy-17-hydroxy-*ent*-kauran-19-oic acid and 16,17-dihydroxy-*ent*-kauran-19-al were the most potent diterpenoids on the A2780 cells (respective IC_{50}: 0.89 and 0.38 μM), and 16,17-dihydroxy-*ent*-kauran-19-oic acid methyl ester (**19**) and *ent*-kaur-16-en-19-oic acid (**18**) were the most cytotoix agents on the 95-D cells (respective IC_{50}: 1.63 and 7.78 μM).[26]

Fatty Acids

Two cytotoxic fatty acid derivatives were isolated from the seeds of *A. squamosal*, which both were moderately effective in the inhibition of MCF-7 (breast), HeLa (cervix), PC3 (prostate), HT-29 (colon), ACHN (renal) human cancer cell lines, and B16 mouse melanoma cells (IC_{50}: 4.66–36.32 μg/mL). (Z)-2-hydroxy-3-(octadec-9-enoyloxy) propanoic acid and hexadecanoic acid-2,3-dihydroxy propyl ester showed potential cytotoxicity against HeLa cells (respective IC_{50}: 5.45 and 9.16 μg/mL) and MCF-7 (respective IC_{50}: 4.66 and 12.05 μg/mL) cells.[27]

Other Bioactivities and Application

The seeds of Fan Li Zhi (Sugar apple tree) demonstrated amazing medical qualities, like antiovulatory, antibed, abortifacient, and insecticide effects. Pharmacological studies have established that the major active component, annonaceous acetogenins, possesses remarkable biological activities such as antiparasitic, pesticidal and immunosuppresive properties. Importantly, the plant was recently found to be effective in the treatment of diabetes.

References

1. Pardhasaradhi, B. V. V. et al. 2004 Antitumour activity of *Annona squamosa* seed extracts is through the generation of free radicals and induction of apoptosis. *Ind. J. Biochem. Biophys.* 14: 167–2.
2. Pardhasaradhi, B. V. V. et al. 2005. Differential cytotoxic effects of *Annona squamosa* seed extracts on human tumor cell lines: Role of reactive oxygen species and glutathione. *J. Biosci.* 30: 237–44.
3. Sumithra, P. et al. 2014. Anticancer activity of *Annona squamosa* and *Manilkara zapota* flower extract against MCF-7 cell line. *Pharmacia Sinica* 5: 98–104.
4. Yang, R. M. et al. 2015. Anticancer effect of total annonaceous acetogenins on hepatocarcinoma. *Chin. J. Integrative Med.* 21: 682–8.
5. Liu, L. F. et al. 2012. Experimental study on apoptosis induced by annonaceous acetogenins in human pulmonary carcinoma cell A549 and its molecular mechanism. *Xiandai Zhongxiyi Jiehe Zazhi* 21: 3785–9, 3793.
6. Xie, B. F. et al. 2007. Comparative experiments on antitumor activities and acute toxicity of Anuoning and its fractions. *Zhongcaoyao* 38: 1199–202.
7. Xie, H. H. et al. 2003. A new cytotoxic acetogenin from the seeds of *Annona squamosa. Chinese Chem. Lett.* 14: 588–90.
8. Yu, J. G. et al. 2005. Chemical constituents from the seeds of *Annona squamosa. Yaoxue Xuebao* 40: 153–8.
9. Yu, J. Z. et al. 2012. The suppression effects of desacetyluvaricin on hepatocellular carcinoma and its possible mechanism. *Pharmacogn. Magazine* 8: 225–30.
10. Chen, Y. et al. 2012. Six cytotoxic annonaceous acetogenins from *Annona squamosa* seeds. *Food Chem.* 135: 960–6.
11. Chen, Y. et al. 2012. Antitumor effects of bistetrahydrofuran annonaceous acetogenins in vivo. *Zhongcaoyao* 43: 139–42.
12. Fujimoto, Y. et al. 1988. Squamocin, a new cytotoxic bistetrahydrofuran containing acetogenin from *Annona squamosa. Chem. Pharm. Bull.* 36: 4802–6.
13. Ikegawa, N. et al. 1991. Anticancer bis(tetrahydrofuran) compounds from *Annona squamosa* seeds and pharmaceutical compositions containing them. *Jpn Kokai Tokkyo Koho* 6 pp. JP 03041076 A 19910221.
14. Hopp, D. C. et al. 1998. Three new bioactive bis-adjacent THF-ring acetogenins from the bark of *Annona squamosa. Bioorg. Med. Chem.* 6: 569–75.
15. Li, X. H. et al. 1990. Bullatacin, bullatacinone, and squamone, a new bioactive acetogenin, from the bark of *Annona squamosa. J. Nat. Prod.* 53: 81–6.
16. Hopp, D. C. et al. 1997. Novel monotetrahydrofuran ring acetogenins, from the bark of *Annona squamosa*, showing cytotoxic selectivities for the human pancreatic cell line, PACA-2. *J. Nat. Prods.* 60: 581–6.
17. Hopp, D. C. et al. 1998. Mono-THF ring annonaceous acetogenins from *Annona squamosa. Phytochem.* 47: 803–9.
18. Hopp, D. C. et al. 1999. Using countercurrent chromatography to assist in the purification of new Annonaceous acetogenins from *Annona squamosa. Phytichem. Analy.* 10: 339–47.
19. Hopp, D. C. et al. 1996. Squamotacin: An annonaceous acetogenin with cytotoxic selectivity for the human prostate tumor cell line (PC3). *J. Nat. Prod.* 59: 97–9.
20. Yang, H. J. et al. 2009. Two new cytotoxic acetogenins from *Annona squamosa. J. Asian Nat. Prods. Res.* 11: 250–6.
21. Yang, H. J. et al. 2009. New nonadjacent bis-THF ring acetogenins from the seeds of *Annona squamosa. Fitoterapia* 80: 177–81.
22. Liaw, C. C. et al. 2008. Monotetrahydrofuran annonaceous acetogenins from *Annona squamosa* as cytotoxic agents and calcium ion chelators. *J. Nat. Prods.* 71: 764–71.
23. Wu, Y. C. et al. 1994. Bioactive alkaloids from *Annona squamosa. Chin. Pharm. J.* (Taiwan) 46: 439–46.
24. Hatano, H. et al. 2003. Cytotoxic constituents in the branches of *Annona squamosa* grown in Philippines. *Yakuruto Institute Kenkyu Hokokushu* 22: 5–9.
25. Joy, B. et al. 2008. Antitumor constituents from *Annona squamosa* fruit pericarp. *Med. Chem. Res.* 17: 345–55.
26. Zhou, C. X. et al. 2013. Cytotoxic diterpenoids from the stem bark of *Annona squamosa* L. *Helv. Chim. Acta* 96: 656–62.
27. Chandrababu, N. R. et al. 2012. Fatty acid derivatives from seeds *of Annona squamosa* Linn. *J. Chem. Pharm. Res.* 4: 4558–61.

27 Deng Long Cao 燈籠草

Cape gooseberry or Golden berry

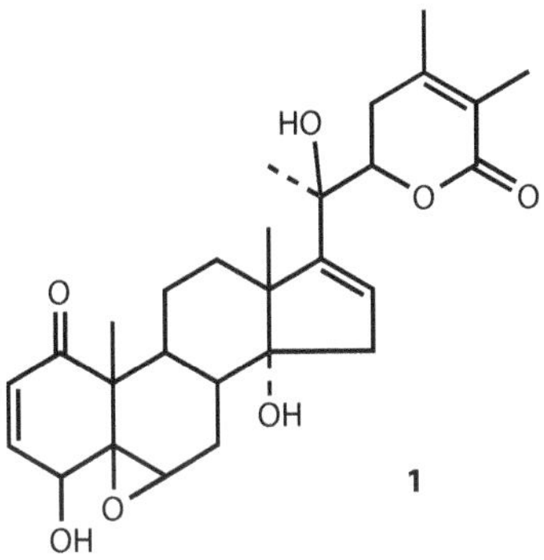

1

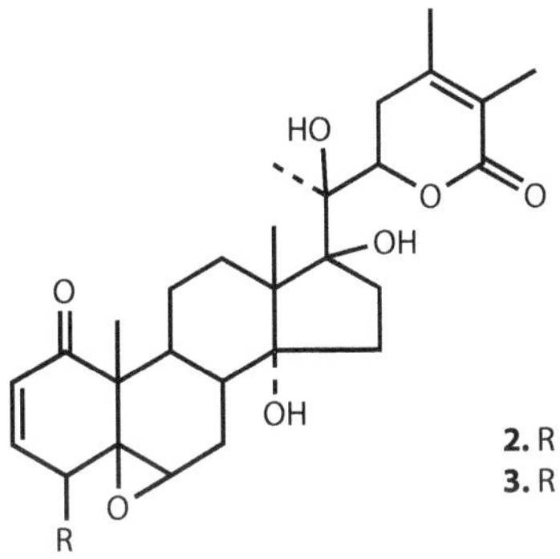

2. R = -OH
3. R = -H

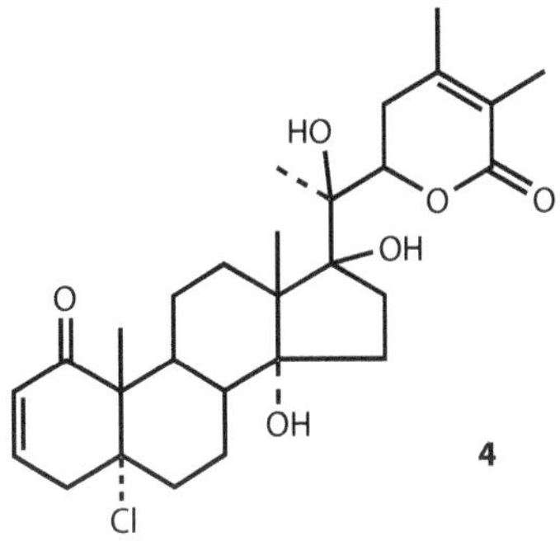

4

Herb Origination

The herb Deng Long Cao (Golden berry) originated from the whole plant of *Physalis peruviana* L. (Solanaceae), which is indigenous to Peru and Chile, and it is widely introduced into cultivation in other tropical and subtropical areas. This herbal plant is mainly cultivated in Southern China, and the whole plant is normally collected in summer and autumn and dried in the sun for the medical application in China. The herb can also be used fresh annually.

Antitumor Activities and Constituents

The extracts prepared from different parts of Deng Long Cao could prolong the life duration in EAC tumor-bearing murine animals by 70% for its leaf extract, 60% for its calyx extract, 30% for its stem extract, and 10% for its root extract.[1] *In vitro* assays demonstrated that the ethanolic extracts of the leaves and the stems exerted cytotoxicity in HT-29 (colon), PC3 (prostate), and K562 (leukemic) human tumor cell lines. The IC_{50} values of leave and stem extracts were 0.35 and 0.37 μg/mL for HT-29; 0.87 and 1.01 μg/mL for PC3 cells; and 0.02 and 0.03 μg/mL for K562 cells, respectively.[2] SCEPP-5 is a supercritical carbon dioxide extract of Deng Long Cao, which contains high contents of total flavonoids and phenols, demonstrating a potent inhibitory effect on the proliferation of human H661 lung cancer cells with the elicitation of cell cycle S arrest and apoptosis through a p53 signaling transduction pathway and modification of Bax and XIAP proteins.[3]

Withanolids

Seventeen withanolides were separated from the fruit-bearing aerial parts of Deng Long Cao. An *in vitro* assay showed that four withanolides assigned as phyperunolide-A (**1**), 4β-hydroxywithanolide-E (**2**), withanolide-E (**3**), and withanolide-C (**4**) demonstrated marked cytotoxicity on HepG2 and Hep3B (liver), MDA-MB-231 and MCF-7 (breast), and A549 (lung) human neoplastic cell lines (IC_{50}: 0.06–4.03 μg/mL).[4] Withanolide-C (**4**), which has an unusual 5-chloride, exerted the most potent antigrowth activity on the tested cell lines (IC_{50}: 0.06–0.80 μg/mL). Its cytotoxicity was almost five times more potent on the HepG2 hepatoma cells and similar but a little less on the Hep3B hepatoma cells and A549 lung cancer cells compared to DOX.[4] The suppressive effect of 4β-hydroxywithanolide-E (**2**) was also shown on human H1299 lung cancer cells *in vitro* (IC_{50}: 0.6 μg/mL, at 24 h), and a complete G2/M arrest and apoptosis of H1299 cells were elicited in a treatment with 5 μg/mL of 4β-hydroxywithanolide-E (**2**) for 24 h.[5,6] In human MCF-7 breast cancer cells, 4β-hydroxywithanolide-E (**2**) promoted the ROS production and triggered the cell apoptosis through an ataxia telangiectasia-mutated protein (ATM)-dependent DNA damage signaling pathway.[7] Withanolide-E (**3**) was able to sensitize renal carcinoma cells to TRAIL-mediated apoptosis by increasing cFLIP degradation, whose effect and lack of toxicity were also confirmed in animal studies.[8] Accordingly, the evidences suggested that the four withanolides have the development potential for improving the chemotherapeutic treatment of hepatoma and lung cancer. Besides, as a preliminary SAR rule, the presence of 5β,6β-epoxy-2-en-1-ones moiety in the withanolide structures is important for the cytotoxicity.[4]

Other Medical Uses

The herb Deng Long Cao (Golden berry) is widely used as a medicinal herb in China for treating hepatitis, malaria, asthma, dermatitis, and rheumatism besides carcinoma and leukemia. Scientific investigations exhibited that its constituents, possibly polyphenols and/or carotenoids, possess antioxidant, antiinflammatory, antihypertension, and antidiabetes activities. A 95% ethanolic extract of Deng Long Cao displayed a marked antioxidant property, including strong superoxide anion-scavenging and inhibitory effects on xanthine oxidase activity.[9]

References

1. Zaki, A. Y. et al. 1987. Study of withanolides, physalins, antitumor and antimicrobial activity of *Physalisperuviana* L. *Egyp. J. Pharm. Sci.* 28: 235–45.
2. Quispe-Mauricio, A. et al. 2009. Cytotoxic effect of physalis peruviana in cell culture of colorectal and prostate cancer and chronic myeloid leukemia. *Revistade gastroenterologia del Peru* 29: 239–46.
3. Wu, S. J. et al. 2009. Supercritical carbon dioxide extract of *Physalis peruviana* induced cell cycle arrest and apoptosis in human lung cancer H661 cells. *Food Chem. Toxicol.* 47: 1132–8.

4. Lan, Y. H. et al. 2009. New cytotoxic withanolides from *Physalis peruviana. Food Chem.* 116: 462–9.
5. Yen, C. Y. et al. 2010. 4β-Hydroxywithanolide E from *Physalis peruviana* (golden berry) inhibits growth of human lung cancer cells through DNA damage, apoptosis and G2/M arrest. *BMC Cancer* 10: 46.
6. Sakurai, K. et al. 1976. Isolation of 4β-hydroxywithanolide E, a new withanolide from *Physalis peruviana* L. *Chem. Pharm. Bull.* 24: 1403–5.
7. You, B. J. et al. 2014. Non-homologous end joining pathway is the major route of protection against 4β-hydroxy-withanolide E-induced DNA damage in MCF-7 cells. *Food Chem. Toxicol.* 65: 205–12.
8. Henrich, C. J. et al. 2015. Withanolide E sensitizes renal carcinoma cells to TRAIL-induced apoptosis by increasing cFLIP degradation. *Cell Death Disease* 6: e1666.
9. Wu, S. J. et al. 2005. Antioxidant activities of *Physalis peruviana. Biol. Pharm. Bull.* 28: 963–6.

28 Dong Ling Cao 冬凌草

Blushred rabdosi or rubescens

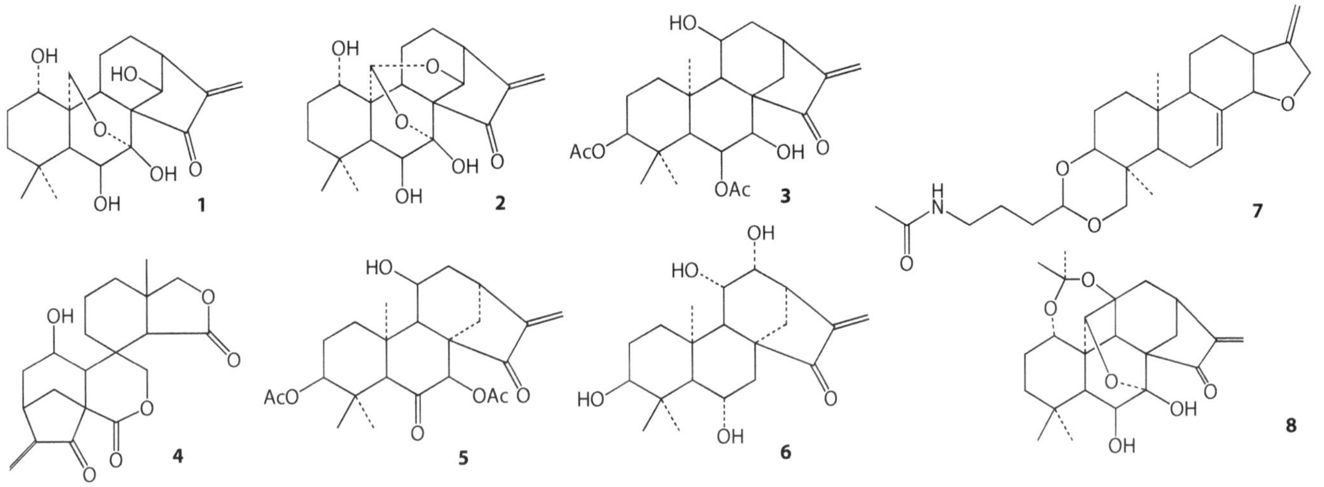

(a)

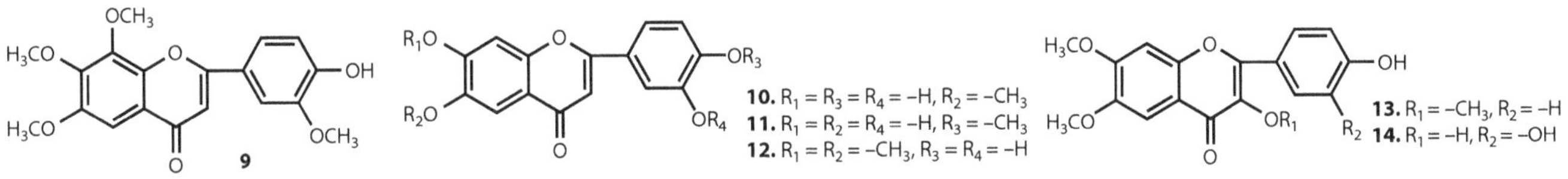

10. $R_1 = R_3 = R_4 = -H$, $R_2 = -CH_3$
11. $R_1 = R_2 = R_4 = -H$, $R_3 = -CH_3$
12. $R_1 = R_2 = -CH_3$, $R_3 = R_4 = -H$

13. $R_1 = -CH_3$, $R_2 = -H$
14. $R_1 = -H$, $R_2 = -OH$

(b)

Herb Origination

The herb Dong Ling Cao is the dried whole plant of *Rabdosia rubescens* (= *Isodon rubescens*) (Labiatae). This perennial plant is broadly distributed in many Chinese provinces; it especially grows close to the drainage areas of the Yellow River and the Yangtze River. The whole plants are generally collected in autumn and dried in the sun for Chinese medicinal purpose.

Antitumor Activities and Constituents

Dong Ling Cao with multiple biological properties has been a folk remedy for cancers in China. Its water extracts and alcoholic extracts displayed a significant cytotoxicity on HeLa (cervix), A2780 (ovary), MDA-MB231 (breast), CaEs-17, and Eca-109 (esophagus) human cancer cell lines *in vitro* but no effect on drug-resistant A2780/CP70 cells.[1,2] Either oral or injection administration of the two extracts to murine animals resulted in the anticancer effect on sarcoma 180, Ehrlich ascites cancer, U14 cervical cancer, and Walker 256 sarcoma.[3] The *in vitro* treatment with the extract suppressed the growth of CaEs-17 esophageal cancer cells by 57.5% and potently inhibited the proliferation of HUVECs *in vitro*, implying that the extracts may restrain the angiogenesis. *In vivo* experiments demonstrated that the extracts decreased the tumor vessel density and reduced breast cancer xenograft size in mice.[4]

Diterpenoids

The anticancer components in Dong Ling Cao were proven to be a group of *ent*-kaurane diterpenoids. Over 50 *ent*-kaurane diterpenoids have been discovered from the leaves and the stems of Dong Ling Cao and its varieties. Oridonin (**1**) and ponicidin (**2**) are the two major diterpenoids largely responsible for the anticancer activity of the herb.

Oridonin

Oridonin (**1**) displayed a broad spectrum of antitumor activities in both *in vitro* and *in vivo* models. It effectively suppressed the proliferation of a wide variety of cell lines derived from non-small cell lung cancer (NSCL, NCI-H520, NCI-H460, NCI-H1299), prostate cancer (LNCaP, DU-145, and PC3), breast cancer (MCF-7, MDA-MB 231), ovarian cancer (A2780, PTX10), multiple myeloma (U266, RPMI8226, MM), leukemia (K562, NB4), and glioblastoma multiform (GBM) (U118, U138) with ED_{50} values ranging from 1.8 to 7.5 μg/mL or IC_{50} values between 5.8 and 11.72 μM.[5–7] Oridonin (**1**) was also significantly sensitive to the inhibition of other types of human cancer cell lines: CaEs-17 and EC-1 (esophagus), MGc80-3 and MKN45 (stomach), A375-S2 and A431 (skin), U87 (brain), SW620 and SW680 (colon), A549 (lung), HepG2 and HuH-6 (liver), HeLa (cervix), U937 and HL-60 (leukemia), fresh acute promyelocytic leukemia cells (obtained from patients), as well as murine L929 fibrosarcoma cells, whose tumoricidal activity occurred in dose- and time-dependent manners.[7–13] In recent years, the antiproliferative, antigrowth, and apoptosis-inducing effects of oridonin (**1**) were extensively demonstrated in SW1990 (pancreas) cancer cells, SNU-5 (gastric), A549 and NCI-H292 (lung), SGC996 and NOZ (gallbladder), HCT-116 and LoVo (colon) carcinoma cell lines, and NPM1c$^+$ AML OCI-AML3 cells.[14–19]

The anticancer effect had been demonstrated by *in vivo* experiments in animal models. With i.p. doses of 10–15 mg/kg, oridonin (**1**) obstructed the growth of ascites sarcoma 180, Ehrlich ascites carcinoma, L1210 leukemia, reticulum cell sarcoma, and hepatoma. When oridonin (**1**) was i.p. administered daily in doses of 20 or 30 mg/kg to mice bearing Ehrlich ascites cancer for seven days, the T/C values obtained in 30 days were 173–199% and 205%, respectively. However, it had no such activity against L615 leukemia and L1 ascites lymphatic sarcoma.[20–24] The i.p. administration of oridonin (**1**) also resulted in an effective suppressive effect against the growth of SGC996 and NOZ gallbladder cancers, HCT-116 and Lovo colon cancers, A549 and NCI-H292 lung cancers, and SNU-5 gastric cancer in xenograft nude mice models.[16–18] Moreover, the combinational treatment with imatinib and oridonin (**1**) synergistically augmented the inhibitory effect on Ph^+ ALL cells by blocking LYN/mTOR and STAT5 signaling pathways.[25] When mouse sarcoma 180 cells were treated with cisplatin plus oridonin (**1**) (0.5 and 1 μg/mL), the growth inhibitory activity was augmented to 3.4 and 6.7 times, respectively, compared to the cisplatin alone.[26] According to remarkable scientific evidences, oridonin (**1**) has been paid extensive attention as a drug lead for the development in cancer therapy.

Ponicidin

Ponicidin (**2**) is another major diterpenoid with an anticancer property isolated from Dong Ling Cao. Ponicidin (**2**) displayed a not so broad anticancer spectrum as oridonin (**1**) did but selectively exerted the inhibitory effect on L615 leukemia, HL-60 promyelocytic leukemia, and two monocytic leukemia U937 and THP-1 cells, associated with the promotion of apoptosis and cell cycle arrest.[27–32] The findings suggested that ponicidin (**2**) may serve as a potential therapeutic agent particularly for the treatment of leukemia. Similar to oridonin (**1**), poniciden (**2**) also exerted tumoricidal effects against BEL-7402 (liver) and Eca-109 (esophagus) human cancer cell lines and obviously inhibited the cancer colony formation. When increasing the concentration, the diterpenoids could kill the cancer cells at S phase or just before S phase.[33,34] *In vivo* experiments on mice further proved the antineoplastic activity of ponicidin (**2**), but it was less active against S37 entire sarcoma.[24]

Other Diterpenoids

Most of the isolated *ent*-diterpenoids demonstrated a significant cytotoxicity on various types of human and murine cancer cell lines. Lasiokaurin (a 7,20-epoxy-*ent*-kauranoids) was cytotoxic to U937 lymphoma cells (IC_{50}: 0.62 μM), and ludongnin-F was effective in the inhibition of HeLa cervical cancer and CA hepatoma cell lines (IC_{50}: 0.70 and 0.09 μg/mL, respectively) *in vitro*. Similar to oridonin (**1**) and poniciden (**2**), melissoidesin-G (**3**), ludongnin-A (**4**) and ludongnin-F, xindongnin-A (**5**) and xindongnin-B (**6**), rubescensin-K (**7**), lushanrubescensin-J, guidongnin-A, lasiokaurin, angustifolin, dawoensin-A, sculponeatin-J, and 6-epi-angustifolin displayed a significant suppressive effect against human K562 erythroleukemia cells (IC_{50}: 0.10–0.93 μg/mL), which were more active than cisplatin (IC_{50}: 1.44 μg/mL).[35–42] In an *in vitro* assay, rabdosin-A and isodocarpin markedly retarded the proliferation of four tested human cancer cells, and their activities (IC_{50}: 2.15–3.76 μM) were superior than those of cisplatin (IC_{50}: 8.86–16.65 μM) in SMMC-7721 (liver), A549 (lung), MCF-7 (breast), and SW480 (colon) human cancer cells, but cisplatin showed little better effect in HL-60 leukemia cells (IC_{50}: 1.81 μM) than the two diterpenoids (IC_{50}: 2.11 and 3.02 μM). In the *in vitro* assay, epinodosin and enmein exerted a moderate to weak inhibitory effect on the five cancer cell lines.[43] In association with the promotion of apoptosis by inducing the cell cycle arrest and activating the mitochondria pathway, Jaridonin potently lessened the viabilities of esophageal cancer cell lines (EC-109, EC9706, and EC-1) and inhibited the growth of human HeLa (cervix), Spc-1 (lung), and HT-29 (colon) cancer cell lines.[44,45] Even in a nanomolar range, henryin selectively obstructed the proliferation of human HCT-116 colorectal cancer cells *in vitro*.[46] Based upon the results and the structure–bioactivity relationship analysis, the existence of α-exo-methylene-cyclopentanone was known to be crucial for the antitumor activity.[43]

Other 15 human cancer cell lines were used in the assay for the examination of these *ent*-kaurane diterpenoids. The most potent antileukemia (HL-60) diterpenoids were identified as flexicanlin-A, phyllostachysin-F, (20S)-11β,14β-dihydroxy-20-ethoxy-7α,20-epoxy-*ent*-kaur-16-en-15-one (**X**), and (20S)-11β,14β-dihydroxy-7α,20-epoxy-20-methoxy-*ent*-kaur-16-en-15-one (**Y**) (IC_{50}: 0.64–0.95 μM).[47] For suppressing human NB4 acute promyelocytic leukemia cells, effusanin-E, isodonal, exidonin, and acetylexidonin were the most effective diterpenoids derived from the herb (IC_{50}: 2.72–4.03 μM).[47] Phyllostachysin-F, isolushinin-D, and the diterpenoids (20S)-11β,14β-dihydroxy-20-ethoxy-7α,20-epoxy-*ent*-kaur-16-en-15-one (**X**) and (20S)-11β,14β-dihydroxy-7α,20-epoxy-20-methoxy-*ent*-kaur-16-en-15-one (**Y**) also exerted the highest anti-growth effect against SMMC-7721 (liver), A549 (lung), and SK-BR-3 (breast) carcinoma cell lines (IC_{50}: 3.3–6.4 μM), whereas phyllostachysin-F, flexicanlin-A, and the diterpenoid (20S)-11β,14β-dihydroxy-20-ethoxy-7α,20-epoxy-*ent*-kaur-16-en-15-one (**X**) exerted the top suppression against PANC-1 pancreatic cancer cells (IC_{50}: 4.5–5.7 μM). According to the IC_{50} data, these diterpenoids are known to be more cytotoxic than oridonin (**1**) on five cell lines (NB4, SMMC-7721, A549, SKBR-3, and PANC-1).[48] Moreover, some other Dong Ling Cao *ent*-kauranoids presented the moderate cytotoxicity on other human tumor cell lines, such as Bcap37 (breast), CNE (nasopharynx), BGC823 (stomach), BIU87 (bladder), and SHSY5Y (brain) cells.[35–48] These *in vitro* evidences afforded strong scientific support for the application of Dong Ling Cao in cancer treatment, but their potential effectiveness in *in vivo* and clinics need further investigation.

Besides, an acetonide derivative (**8**) of lasiodonin made by a structural modification displayed more a potently enhanced inhibitory effect against the growth of carcinoma cell lines (K562, BIU87, HeLa, CNE, Bcap37, BGC823, and CA). Its IC_{50} values ranged from 0.01 to 0.70 μg/mL, showing greater antitumor potential than cisplatin.[40]

Flavonoids

Eight flavonoids were isolated from the aerial parts of Dong Ling Cao. The highest inhibitory effect presented in human HL-60 leukemia cells was by 5,4′-dihydroxy-6,7,8,3′-tetramethoxyflavone

(**9**), whose IC_{50} value of 7.55 μM was comparable to DOX (IC_{50}: 4.64 μM). Other five flavonoids such as pedalitin (**10**), nodifloretin (**11**), cirsiliol (**12**), penduletin (**13**), and quercetin (**14**) displayed moderate antigrowth effect against the HL-60 cells *in vitro*. The moderate or weak inhibitory effect of penduletin (**10**) was shown in the assay used in Colo205 (colon) and MCF-7 (breast) human cancer cell lines. The preliminary analysis of the bioactivity–structure relationship by using the HL-60 cells shows that a methoxy group at C-8 seems important to selective inhibition.[49] In addition, several antioxidative flavonoids as well as triterpenoids have also been identified from Dong Ling Cao.[24]

Polysaccharides

Polysaccharides prepared from Dong Ling Cao were found to have a direct cytotoxic effect against Ehrlich ascites carcinoma *in vitro* and against the growth of sarcoma 180 *in vivo* with 35% inhibitory rate. The polysaccharides were also able to enhance the proliferation of mouse splenocytes. These results established that the antitumor effect of the polysaccharides might be also contributed by their immunostimulating activity.[50]

Mechanism Exploration

Due to the remarkable anticancer spectrum and activity of Dong Ling Cao diterpenoids, especially oridonin (**1**), the mechanisms have been extensively explored. The cancer growth inhibitory mechanisms were revealed to closely associate with the six events summarized as follows.

Inhibition of DNA and RNA Synthesis

Oridonin (**1**) was capable of obstructing the incorporation of thymidine into DNA, uterine into RNA, and luecine into protein and obstructing the syntheses of DNA, RNA, and protein in a variety of tumor cells, where the anti-DNA synthesis was more prominent than the blockage of the syntheses of RNA and protein.[51–54] Also, oridonin (**1**) showed inhibitory effects toward DNA polymerase-II and interaction with DNA bases in a variety of cancer cells *in vitro*.[6,47] The synergistic inhibitory effect of cisplatin plus oridonin on sarcoma 180 cells was attributed to the formation of DNA interstrand cross-link and DNA–protein cross-link.[26] The DNA damage caused by the oridonin treatment in MCF-7 breast cancer cells could provoke p53-mediated cell cycle arrest and apoptosis.[55]

Arrest of Cell Cycle

Oridonin (**1**) and ponicidin (**2**) are nonspecific inhibitors of the cell cycle. Both could arrest tumor cell cycles at several phases through characteristic pathways in diffirent types of cancer cell lines.[22] By diminishing the levels of cyclin-B1, cdc2, transcription factor E2F, and Rb phosphorylation, the cell cycle progression of MCF-7 breast cancer was arrested at S/G2M and G1/S stages after being treated with oridonin (**1**) or ponicidin (**2**).[56] In the inhibition of LNCaP and NCI-H520 prostate cancer cells by oridonin, p53 protein played a central role in the G0/G1 cell cycle arrest.[5] Oridonin induced a G1 phase arrest in AR-positive LNCaP prostate cancer cells (wild-type p53) and blocked the cell cycle at G2 and M phases in AR-negative DU-145 prostate cancer cells (mutated p53).[6] Also, the treatment with oridonin (**1**) elicited a G2/M phase arrest as well as a differentiation in murine K1735M2 melanoma cells.[57] Oridonin (**1**) also elicited the G2/M cell arrest of HuH-6 hepatoblastoma cells and MCF-7 breast cancer cells and disturbed the cell cycle of MDA-MB-231 breast cancer at sub-G1 phase.[58,59] Furthermore, through the increase of p53 and p21waf1/Cip1 activities, Jaridonin caused a G2/M arrest in the cell cycle progression of EC-1 esophageal cancer cells.[44] Henryin enhanced the G1/S phase arrest of HCT116 colon cancer cells via the down-expression of cyclin D1 and c-Myc and the inhibition of aberrant Wnt/β-catenin signaling.[46]

Induction of Apoptosis

The induction of apoptosis is one of the major mechanisms caused by oridonin (1) in many tumor cell lines. Generally, the apoptosis increase was revealed to follow a mitochondrial apoptotic pathway, i.e., the decrease of Bcl-2 and Bcl-xL expressions and increase of Bax activity, the loss of the mitochondrial membrane potential, and the release of cytochrome c into cytosol, upregulation of p53, and ERK, degradation of PARP, substantial activation of AIF and caspase-3.[53–69] HeLa cell apoptosis induced by oridonin was also mediated by a PI3K/Akt pathway besides the caspase-dependent apoptosis.[70] The apoptosis of human HEp2 laryngeal cancer cells was triggered by oridonin via both intrinsic and extrinsic apoptotic pathways.[71] The ER stress and ASK1-JNK1 signaling pathways was found to be involved in the oridonin (**1**)-induced apoptosis of hepatoblastoma HuH-6 cells.[58] The apoptotic mechanism in leukemia K562, NB4, and HL-60 cells was also related to lessening the telomerase activity, which played another important role in the acceleration of leukemia cell death.[51,60–62]

Usually, the multiple pathways should involve in the apoptosis induction by oridonin (**1**) in many cases. Oridonin treatment augmented phagocytosis through the activation of TNFα and IL-1β, and the activated macrophages markedly promoted the apoptosis of U937 histocytic lymphoma cells.[63] In p53-deficient HEp-2 cells, the apoptosis and G_2/M phase arrest elicited by oridonin were mediated by p21/WAF1-dependent and p53-independent manners, where the generation of ROS was found to be a critical mediator in the apoptosis promotion.[57] The generation of ROS and hydroxyl radical (•OH) stimulated by oridonin also played a pivotal role in the induction of apoptosis and autophagy of A431 melanoma cells.[59] Through the blockage of JNK/MAPK and the enhancement of oxidative stress, the oridonin-induced the A431 cell apoptosis could be enhanced by tyrphostin AG1478 (a selective EGFR inhibitor).[72] More multiple pathways were found to participate in the oridonin (**1**)-induced the apoptotic death of cancer cells, such as the apoptosis of SW1990 pancreatic tumor cells via p53- and caspase-dependent induction of p38 MAPK,[14] of SNU-5 gastric cancer via direct regulation of c-Met signaling pathway,[15] of A549 and NCI-H292 lung cancer cell lines via the inhibition of mTORC1 function and Mtor signaling,[16] of SGC996 and NOZ gallbladder cancer cells via the caspase-dependent mitochondrial pathway and the inhibition of NF-κB nuclear translocation,[17] of HCT-116 and LoVo colon carcinoma cells via the inhibition of microRNA-32 expression,[18] of NPM1c^{+} AML

OCI-AML3 cells via the increase of p53 and p14arf expressions and the induction of caspase-3 activation and NPM1c+ protein nuclear translocation,[19] and of A375-S2 melanoma cells partially via the repression of p53-involved IGF-1R signaling.[73]

Similarly, the apoptotic mechanism of ponicidin (**2**) in A549 and GLC-82 lung cancer cells was revealed to be mediated by a mitochondrial apoptotic pathway.[64] In leukemia HL-60 cells, the upregulation of p16 and p21 expressions and the activation of caspase-3 may be the important events for ponicidin (**2**) to elicit the apoptosis and the G0/G1 phase arrest.[74] By amplifying the ROS production and the annexin V-positive staining cells and augmenting p53, p21wqf1/Cip1, and Bax expressions, Jaridonin triggered the mitochondria-mediated and caspase-activated apoptosis of esophageal tumor EC-1 cells.[44] All the research findings provided indeed gave insight into the characteristic roads of oridonin and its analogue in the promotion of apoptotic death.

Antimigration and Antiinvasion

Oridonin also showed an ability to significantly suppress the migration and the invasion of breast cancer cells by decreasing MMP-2 and MMP-9 expressions and inhibiting Integrin-β1 and FAK expressions in metastatic human MDA-MB-231 breast cancer cells besides the induction of apoptosis via the reduction of Bcl-2/Bax ratio, caspase-8, NF-κB (p65), IKK, IKKβ, phospho-mTOR and the up-expression of cleaved PARP, Fas, and PPARγ in a time-dependent manner.[75]

Inhibition of NF-κB

The diterpenoids such as oridonin (**1**), ponicidin (**2**), xindongnin-A and xindongnin-B were found to be potent and selective NF-κB inhibitors, whose targets are to block the transcription of NF-κB and to decline the expressions of its downstream targets such as COX2 and inducible NO synthase. The diterpenoids directly interfered with the DNA-binding activity of NF-κB.[76] Oridonin (**1**) also blocked the NF-κB activity in Jurkat cells as well as RAW264.7 murine macrophages. By the suppression of NF-κB-DNA-binding activity, oridonin (**1**) lessened the survival of freshly isolated adult T cell leukemia, non-Hodgkin's lymphoma, ALL, chronic lymphocytic leukemia, and multiple myeloma cells from patients, but it had no effect on normal lymphoid cells from healthy volunteers.[5] These results implied that the cell proliferation in lymphoid malignancies obstructed by Dong Ling Cao diterpenoids is partially attributed to the blockage of NF-κB signal pathways.

FAS Suppression

The suppression of FAS was revealed to be involved in the antiviability effect of oridonin (**1**) against human colorectal cancer cell lines (SW680 and SW620), where oridonin effectively obstructed the FAS and SREBP1 expressions and reduced the transcriptional activity of the FAS promoter region containing the SREBP1 binding site in the colorectal cancer cell lines, where the FAS inhibition was associated to the lessening of the cellular palmitate and the stearic acid. These findings revealed a new molecular mechanism for the oridonin (**1**) and afforded a scientific basis for the therapeutic support of oridonin in the treatment of colorectal cancer.[77]

Clinical Practice

Four hundred forty-eight patients with esophageal carcinoma had been treated with Dong Ling Cao alone or Dong Ling Cao combined with chemotherapy. For early-stage esophageal cancer patients, the treatment with Dong Ling Cao extract resulted in a control of the tumor progression and marked prolongation of the survival time. The average life duration in the treatment was 83 months calculated from diagnosis to death. Its extract is also able to synergistically enhance the effect of chemotherapy on advanced esophageal cancer patients. The combinational treatment with Dong Ling Cao and pingyangmycin- or bleomycin (BLM)-based chemotherapy demonstrated a significantly better clinical efficacy for the esophageal cancer patients in the middle-late stage. But there was no significant difference in the side effects between the combined chemotherapy and the Dong Ling Cao chemotherapy alone.[78] In comparison to the *in vivo* test result, the inhibitory rate of the cotreatment with oridonin (**1**) and BLM reached 83% in a mouse model with sarcoma 180, whose effect was significantly higher than that of oridonin (52%) or BLM (44%) alone,[79] showing that the results from clinical trials in patients were consistent with those obtained from *in vivo* investigations.

Side Effects

Little toxicity and side effects such as mild abdominal symptoms, diarrhea, and skin itching have been noted in the Dong Ling Cao treatment, but none of them were serious. For safely using Dong Ling Cao, the recommended dosages are 90–120 g of the fresh herb (this corresponds, roughly, to 30–40 g of dried herb) and 30 g of the dried herb.

Nanoformulation

In order to promote the delivery of oridonin (**1**) specifically to tumor cells, an oridonin nanoliposomes injection (O-NL) and an oridonin nanosuspension were prepared. The O-NL dramatically augmented the cytotoxicity on HepG2 cells and MGC-803 cells *in vitro*, and the maximum inhibitory rates were elevated to 75.6% and 80.0% from 42.1% and 22.1% at 96 h, respectively. The *in vivo* suppressive ratio against murine H22 hepatoma was raised by oridonin to 78.4% from 25.4% at an intravenous dose of 16.8 mg/kg per day.[27] Similarly, the oridonin nanosuspension could notably enhance the cytotoxicity against K562 leukemia cells and PANC-1 pancreatic cancer cells *in vitro*, and it exhibited a higher decrease of tumor volume and weight in mice bearing solid sarcoma 180 at a dose of 20 mg/kg.[28,29] ORI-PLA-NPs is an oridonin-loaded atactic poly(D,L-lactic acid) nanoparticle. When a peptide Arg-Gly-Asp (RGD) was used to modify the ORI-PLA-NPs by surface cross-linking, a complex ORI-PLA-RGD-NP was generated. In an *in vivo* mouse model with H22 hepatoma, ORI-PLA-RGD-NPs displayed a greater anticarcinoma efficacy than ORI-PLA-NPs and oridonin, as reflected by the tumor growth decrease and the survival time extension.[30] Therefore, these results demonstrated that the nanoencapsulation is a promising approach for improving the tumor-targeting efficiency and subsequent antitumor efficiency of oridonin.

Other Medical Uses

Historically, Don Ling Cao (Blushred rabdosi) was a rarely used therapeutic herb in the Chinese medicine system, although it can cleanse toxins and relieve swelling and pain. Dong Ling Cao has been used in the remedies for insect bites, snakebites, and inflamed tonsils. Today, the herb is promoted for the treatment of cancers, especially esophagus neoplasm. This herbal product is available as capsules in Chinese clinics.

References

1. Henan Institute of Medicinal Sciences. (a) 1974. *Zhongliu Fangzhi Yanjiu* (2): 82; (b) 1999. *Chinese Materia Medica*, Vol. 7, 7–6171, 151–2. Shanghai Science and Technology Press, Shanghai, China.
2. Yu, J. J. et al. 1995. Preliminary-study of the effect of selected Chinese natural drugs on human ovarian cancer cells. *Oncol. Reports* 2: 571–6.
3. Henan Institute of Medicinal Sciences. (a) 1975. Studies on the antitumor activity of and other pharmacological effects. *J. Henan Med. Univ.* (2): 9–16; (b) 1999. *Chinese Materia Medica*, Vol. 7, 7–6171, 151–2. Shanghai Science and Technology Press, Shanghai, China.
4. Sartippour, M. R. et al. 2005. *Rabdosia rubescens* inhibits breast cancer growth and angiogenesis. *Intl. J. Oncol.* 26: 1–128.
5. Ikezoe, T. et al. (a) 2003. Oridonin induces growth inhibition and apoptosis of a variety of human cancer cells. *Intl. J. Oncol.* 23: 1187–94; (b) 2005. Oridonin, a diterpenoid purified from *Rabdosia rubescens*, inhibits the proliferation of cells from lymphoid malignancies in association with blockade of the NF-κB signal pathways. *Mol. Cancer Therapeutics* 4: 578–86.
6. Chen, S. et al. 2005. The cytostatic and cytotoxic effects of oridonin (Rubescenin), a diterpenoid from *Rabdosia rubescens*, on tumor cells of different lineage. *Intl. J. Oncol.* 26: 579–88.
7. Xie, R. J. et al. 2011. Two new diterpenoids and other constituents from *Isodon rubescens. Fitoterapia* 82: 726–30.
8. Li, X. T. et al. 1985. Comparing the sensitivity of rubescensin A in eight human cancer cell lines. *Yaoxue Xuebao.* 20: 243.
9. Huang, J. et al. 2005. A comparison of the signal pathways between the TNFα- and oridonin-induced murine L929 fibrosarcoma cell death. *Acta Medica Okayama* 59: 261–70.
10. Liu, J. J. et al. 2005. Apoptotic effect of oridonin on NB4 cells and its mechanism. *Leukemia & Lymphoma* 46: 593–7.
11. Ji, Z. et al. 2011. Oridonin-induced apoptosis in SW620 human colorectal adenocarcinoma cells. *Oncol. Lett.* 2: 1303–7.
12. Wang, H. et al. 2010. Oridonin induces G2/M cell cycle arrest and apoptosis through MAPK and p53 signaling pathways in HepG2 cells. *Oncol. Reports* 24: 647–51.
13. He, X. J. et al. 2009. Empirical study of oridonin-induced gastric cancer cells MKN45 apoptosis. *Zhonghua Weichang Waike Zazhi* 12: 607–10.
14. Bu, H. Q. et al. 2014. Oridonin induces apoptosis in SW1990 pancreatic cancer cells via p53- and caspase-dependent induction of p38 MAPK. *Oncol. Reports* 31: 975–82.
15. Liu, H. et al. 2014. Antitumor activity of oridonin on SNU-5 subcutaneous xenograft model via regulation of c-Met pathway. *Tumor Biol.* 35: 9139–46.
16. Wang, Y. Y. et al. 2014. Oridonin inhibits Mtor signaling and the growth of lung cancer tumors. *Anti-cancer Drugs* 25: 1192–200.
17. Bao, R. F. et al. 2014. Oridonin induces apoptosis and cell cycle arrest of gallbladder cancer cells via the mitochondrial pathway. *BMC Cancer* 14: 217/1–217/13.
18. Yang, J. et al. 2015. Oridonin triggers apoptosis in colorectal carcinoma cells and suppression of microRNA-32 expression augments oridonin-mediated apoptotic effects. *Biomed. Pharmacother.* 72: 125–34.
19. Li, F. F. et al. 2014. Oridonin induces NPM mutant protein translocation and apoptosis in NPM1c+ acute myeloid leukemia cells in vitro. *Acta Pharmacol. Sinica* 35: 806–813.
20. Henan Institute of Medicinal Sciences. 1978. Now antitumor agent Rubescenine A. *Kexue Tongbao* 23: 53.
21. Zhang, T. M. et al. 1980. Rubescenine B, Another antitumor constituent in *Rabdosia rubescen. Kexue Tongbao* 25: 1051.
22. Wang, M. Y. et al. 1985. Dynamic influence of oridonin on mouse L1210 cells. *Zhongguo Yaoli Xuebao* 6: 195.
23. Fujita, T. et al. 1988. Cytotoxic and antitumor activities of Rabdosia diterpenoids. *Planta Med.* 54: 414–6.
24. Bai, N. S. et al. 2002. Chemistry and potential bioactivity of *Rabdosia rubescen. Abst. of 223rd ACS Nat. Meeting, Orlando, FL, USA*, April 7–11, 2002, AGFD-093.
25. Guo, Y. et al. 2012. Oridonin in combination with imatinib exerts synergetic anti-leukemia effects in Ph+ acute lymphoblastic leukemia cells in vitro by inhibiting activation of LYN/mTOR signaling pathway. *Cancer Biol. Ther.* 13: 1244–54.
26. Gao, Z. G. et al. 1993. Cytotoxicity of oridonin and cisplatin on mouse sarcoma 180 cells and their DNA cross-linking. *Zhongguo Yaoli Xuebao* 14: 561–4.
27. Wang, C. J. et al. 2008. Study on in vitro cytotoxicity and in vivo antitumor effect of nanoliposomes containing oridonin. *Asian J. Pharmacodyn. Pharmacokinet.* 8: 324–8.
28. Lou, H. Y. et al. 2009. In vitro and in vivo antitumor activity of oridonin nanosuspension. *Intl. J. Pharm.* 379: 181–6.
29. Qi, X. L. et al. 2012. Oridonin nanosuspension was more effective than free oridonin on G2/M cell cycle arrest and apoptosis in the human pancreatic cancer PANC-1 cell line. *Intl. J. Nanomed.* 7: 1793–804.
30. Xu, J. et al. 2012. RGD-modified poly(D,L-lactic acid) nanoparticles enhance tumor targeting of oridonin. *Intl. J. Nanomed.* 7: 211–9.
31. Liu, J. J. et al. 2008. Ponicidin inhibits monocytic leukemia cell growth by induction of apoptosis. *Intl. J. Mol. Sci.* 9: 2265–77.
32. Bai, N. et al. 2010. Ent-kaurane diterpenoids from *Rabdosia rubescens* and their cytotoxic effects on human cancer cell lines. *Planta Med.* 76: 140–5.
33. Zhang, J. F. et al. 2006. Antiproliferation effects of oridonin on the hepatocellular carcinoma Bel-7402 cells and its mechanism. *Zhonghua Zhongliu Fangzhi Zazhi* 13: 1131–3.
34. Lin, B. L. et al. 2000. Molecular pharmacology and clinic treatment strategy of antitumor oridonins. *Guangdong Yaoxue* 10: 8–10.
35. Han, Q. B. et al. 2004. (a) New ent-abietanoids from *Isodon rubescens. Helv. Chim. Acta* 87: 1007–15; (b) Rubescensins S and T: Seco-ent-kaurane diterpenoids from *Isodon rubescens* var. *taihangensis. Helv. Chim. Acta* 87: 1119–24.

36. Han, Q. B. et al. 2004. (a) Cytotoxic ent-kaurane diterpenoids from *Isodon rubescens* var. *rubescens. Planta Med.* 70: 269–271; (b) A novel cytotoxic oxetane ent-kauranoid from *Isodon japonicas. Planta Med.* 70: 581–4.
37. Han, Q. B. et al. 2003. Ent-kaurane diterpenoids from *Isodon rubescens* var. *lushanensis. Chem. Pharm. Bull.* 51: 790–3.
38. Han, Q. B. et al. 2003. Cytotoxic constituents of *Isodon rubescens* var. *lushiensis. J. Nat. Prod.* 66: 1391–4.
39. Han, Q. B. et al. 2005. An asymmetric ent-kauranoid dimer from *Isodon rubescens* var. *lushanensis. Tetrahedron Lett.* 46: 5373–5.
40. Han, Q. B. et al. 2005. Ent-kauranoids from *Isodon rubescens* var. *taihangensis. J. Asian Nat. Prods. Res.* 7: 31–6.
41. Zhang, H. B. et al. 2010. Two novel diterpenoids from *Isodon rubescens* var. *lushanensis. Tetrahedron Lett.* 51: 4225–8.
42. Zhang, H. B. et al. 2010. Four new ent-kauranoids from *Isodon rubescens* var. *lushanensis* and data reassignment of dayecrystal B. *Chem. Pharm. Bull.* 58: 56–60.
43. Liu, X. et al. 2012. Enmein-type diterpenoids from the aerial parts of *Isodon rubescens* and their cytotoxicity. *Fitoterapia* 83: 1451–5.
44. Ma, Y. C. et al. 2013. Jaridonin, a novel ent-kaurene diterpenoid from *Isodon rubescens*, inducing apoptosis via production of reactive oxygen species in esophageal cancer cells. *Current Cancer Drug Targets* 13: 611–24.
45. Ma, Y. C. et al. 2013. Bioactivity and mechanism of jaridonin, a novel ent-kaurne diterpenoid compound, on tumor cells growth in vitro. *Zhongguo Yaoxue Zazhi* 48: 1266–70.
46. Li, X. Y. et al. 2013. Henryin, an ent-kaurane diterpenoid, inhibits Wnt signaling through interference with β-catenin/TCF4 interaction in colorectal cancer cells. *PLoS One* 8: e68525.
47. Gao, X. M. et al. 2011. Antiproliferative diterpenoids from the leaves of *Isodon rubescens. Planta Med.* 77: 169–74.
48. Luo, X. et al. 2010. Cytotoxic ent-kaurane diterpenoids from *Isodon rubescens* var. *lushiensis. J. Nat. Prods.* 73: 1112–6.
49. Bai, N. S. et al. 2010. Flavonoids from *Rabdosia rubescens* exert anti-inflammatory and growth inhibitory effect against human leukemia HL-60 cells. *Food Chem.* 122: 831–5.
50. Wang, Y. F. et al. 2002. Antitumor and immunological activities of polysaccharides from *Rabdosia rubescens. Zhongguo Bingli Shengli Zazhi* 18: 1341.
51. Wang, M. Y. et al. (a) 1985. The effect of oridonin on the incorporation of ^{3}HTdR, ^{3}H UR and ^{3}H leucine into the ECA cells in vitro. *J. Henan Med. College* 20: 15–8; (b) 1999. *Chinese Materia Medica* Vol. 7, 7–6171, 152. Shanghai Science and Technology Press, Shanghai, China.
52. Wang, M. Y. et al. 1987. Study on the influence of oridonin on the synthesis of DNA, RNA and protein in L1210 cells. *Zhongguo Yaoli Xuebao* 8: 164–5.
53. Li, Y. et al. 1987. (a) Fluence of oridonin on nucleotide metabolism of mouse tumor cells. *Zhongguo Yaoli Xuebao* 8: 271–9; 1988. (b) Influence of oridonin on DNA synthesis in vitro with no cells. *Zhongguo Yaoli Xuebao* 9: 465–7.
54. Li, X. T. et al. 1986. Characteristic of oridonin in killing in vitro tumor cells. *Zhongguo Yaoli Xuebao* 7: 361–3.
55. Cui, Q. et al. 2007. P53-mediated cell cycle arrest and apoptosis through a caspase-3-independent, but caspase-9-dependent pathway in oridonin-treated MCF-7 human breast cancer cells. *Acta Pharmacol. Sinica* 28: 1057–66.
56. Hsieh, T. C. et al. 2005. Differential control of growth, cell cycle progression, and expression of NF-κB in human breast cancer cells MCF-7, MCF-10A, and MDA-MB-231 by ponicidin and oridonin, diterpenoids from the Chinese herb *Rabdosia rubescens. Biochem. Biophys. Res. Commun.* 337: 224–31.
57. Ren, K. K. et al. 2006. The effects of oridonin on cell growth, cell cycle, cell migration and differentiation in melanoma cells. *J. Ethno-pharmacol.* 103: 176–80.
58. Cai, D. T. et al. 2013. ER stress and ASK1-JNK activation contribute to oridonin-induced apoptosis and growth inhibition in cultured human hepatoblastoma HuH-6 cells. *Mol. Cell. Biochem.* 379: 161–9.
59. Yu, Y. et al. 2012. Hydroxyl radical (•OH) played a pivotal role in oridonin-induced apoptosis and autophagy in human epidermoid carcinoma A431 cells. *Biol. Pharm. Bull.* 35: 2148–59.
60. Liu, J. J. et al. 2005. Oridonin-induced apoptosis in leukemia K562 cells and its mechanism *Neoplasma* 52: 225–30.
61. Liu, J. J. et al. 2004. (a) Antiproliferation effects of oridonin on HL-60 cells. *Annals of Hematol.* 83: 691–695; (b) Antiproliferation effect of oridonin on HL-60 cells and its mechanism. *China Med. Sci. J.* 19: 134–7.
62. Liu, Y. Q. et al. 2005. Oridonin enhances phagocytosis of UV-irradiated apoptotic U937 cells. *Biol. Pharm. Bull.* 28: 461–7.
63. Liu, J. J. et al. 2005. Antiproliferation effects of ponicidin on human myeloid leukemia cells in vitro. *Oncol. Rep.* 13: 653–8.
64. Liu, J. J. et al. 2004. Anti-proliferative effects of oridonin on SPC-A-1 cells and its mechanism of action. *J. Intl. Med. Res.* 32: 617–25.
65. Liu, J. J. et al. 2004. Oridonin-induced apoptosis of Jurkat cells and its mechanism. *Comparative Clin. Pathol.* 13: 65–9.
66. Zhang, C. L. et al. 2004. Oridonin induces a caspase-independent but mitochondria- and MAPK dependent cell death in the murine fibro-sarcoma cell line L929. *Biol. Pharm. Bull.* 27: 1527–31.
67. Zhang, C. L. et al. 2004. Cytochrome *c* release from oridonin-treated apoptotic A375-S2 cells is dependent on p53 and extracellular signal-regulated kinase activation. *J. Pharmacol. Sci.* 96: 155–63.
68. Liu, J. J. et al. 2004. Inhibitory effect of oridonin on the proliferation of NB4 cells and its mechanism. *Chin.-Germ. J. Clin. Oncol.* 3: 51–4.
69. Kang, N. et al. 2010. Induction of G2/M phase arrest and apoptosis by Oridonin in human laryngeal carcinoma cells. *J. Nat. Prod.* 73: 1058–63.
70. Hu, H. Z. et al. 2007. Oridonin induces apoptosis via PI3K/Akt pathway in cervical carcinoma HeLa cell line. *Acta Pharmacol. Sin.* 28: 1819–26.
71. Kang, N. et al. 2010. Inhibition of EGFR signaling augments oridonin-induced apoptosis in human laryngeal cancer cells via enhancing oxidative stress coincident with activation of both the intrinsic and extrinsic apoptotic pathways. *Cancer Lett.* 294: 147–58.
72. Yu, Y. et al. 2012. The tyrphostin AG1478 augments oridonin-induced A431 cell apoptosis by blockage of JNK MAPK and enhancement of oxidative stress. *Free Radical Res.* 46: 1393–405.
73. Wang, H. J. et al. 2008. Oridonin induces human melanoma A375-S2 cell death partially through inhibiting insulin-like growth factor 1 receptor signaling. *J. Asian Nat. Prod. Res.* 10: 777–88.
74. Liu, X. D. et al. 2010. Anti-proliferation effect of Ponicidin on leukemia HL-60 cells. *J. Clin. Rehabilitative Tissue Engineering Res.* 14: 5062–6.
75. Wang, S. P. et al. 2013. Oridonin induces apoptosis, inhibits migration and invasion on highly-metastatic human breast cancer cells. *Am. J. Chin. Med.* 41: 177–96.

76. Leung, C. H. et al. 2005. Novel mechanism of inhibition of nuclear factor-κB DNA-binding activity by diterpenoids isolated from *Isodon rubescens*. *Mol. Pharmacol.* 68: 286–97.
77. Kwan, H. Y. et al. 2013. The anticancer effect of oridonin is mediated by fatty acid synthase suppression in human colorectal cancer cells. *J. Gastroenterol.* 48: 182–92.
78. Wang, R. et al. 2007. Clinical efficacy for the treatment of esophageal cancer with *Rabdosia rubescens* alone and combining with chemotherapy. *Life Sci. J.* 4: 22–5.
79. Zhang, T. M. et al. 1986. Antitumor effects of different combinations of oridonin, bleomycin A5 and nitrocaphane. *Acta Pharmacol. Sinica* 7: 457–60.

29 Long Kui 龍葵

Black nightshade

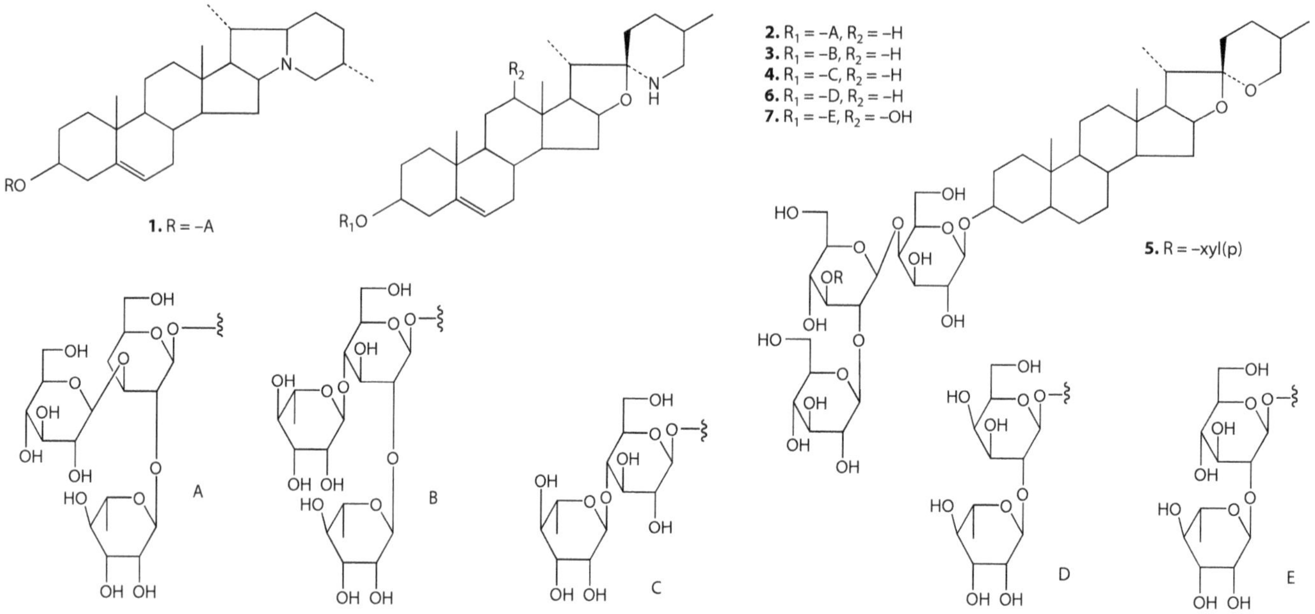

1. R = -A

2. R_1 = -A, R_2 = -H
3. R_1 = -B, R_2 = -H
4. R_1 = -C, R_2 = -H
6. R_1 = -D, R_2 = -H
7. R_1 = -E, R_2 = -OH

5. R = -xyl(p)

A B C D E

Herb Origination

The herb Long Kui (Black nightshade) has a long history for its medicinal usage, dating back to the ancient Tang dynasty in China. The herb was documented at an official pharmacopeia entitled *Xinxiu Ben Cao* in AD 659. The origin of Long Kui is a whole plant of *Solanum nigrum* L. (Solanaceae). This annual plant is native to Eurasia, and it was introduced into the Americas, Australasia, and South Africa. In China, the whole plant is normally collected in summer and autumn and dried in the sun for the medicinal utilization, and the herb can also be used fresh.

Antitumor Activities

Long Kui has been often used in Chinese traditional medicine as a remedy for the treatment of carcinomas in the digestive system and as an antiinflammatory and hepatoprotective herb. In an *in vitro* investigation, its alcoholic extract arrested the cell cycle at G0/G1 phase and augmented the cell apoptosis of multiple U266 myeloma despite showing low cytotoxicity against the U266 cells.[1] Its aqueous extract induced cytotoxicity on HepG2 hepatoma cells dose dependently but much less to normal hepatic cell lines (Chang liver and WRL-68). The antihepatoma activity was found to be mediated by two distinct cell death-inducing pathways (apoptosis and autophagocytosis). In higher doses (2 and 5 mg/mL), the HepG2 cell apoptosis was induced by the extract through the increases of p-JNK and Bax expressions, the mitochondrial release of cytochrome c, and the activation of caspases, while in the lower doses (~1.0 mg/mL), the cell autophagocytosis was elicted with morphological and ultrastructural changes such as increases of specific markers of autophagy and enhancement of autophagic vacuoles and LC3-I and LC3-II proteins.[2] The marked cytotoxic effect of a Long Kui leaf aqueous extract on human AU565 breast neoplastic cells was also similarly mediated by the two different mechanisms (apoptosis and autophagy) depending on its exposure concentrations.[3] At a middle dose, its n-butanolic extract exerted the antitumor rate of 44.36% being comparable to that of 5-FU (46.74%) against H22 hepatom in mice, whose effect was associated with significant increases in the indexes of the thymus and the spleen and improvement of the immune function.[4]

Besides reducing the weight of murine B16-F1 melanoma by >50%, the aqueous extract was also effective in suppressing the invasion, the migration, and the lung metastasis of melanoma cells *in vitro* and *in vivo*, associated with the diminishment of serum MMP-9 and Akt activities and the reduction of PKCα, Ras, and NF-κB protein expressions.[5] Moreover, Long Kui was also found to enhance NO production by rIFN-γ-primed macrophages and to activate of NF-κB, which both play a critical role in antimetastatic effects.[6] Consequently, the application of Long Kui for cancer treatment and prevention has been scientifically established, and the results indeed attracted researchers for further investigation in searching valuable drug candidates from Long Kui.

In addition, the ethanolic extract derived from ripe Long Kui fruits could obviously accelerate the apoptosis of human MCF-7 breast carcinoma cells and strongly suppressed the proliferative capacity of the MCF-7 cells. The fruit extract could also scavenge free hydroxyl radicals and 2,2-diphenyl-1-picrylhydrazyl (DPPH) radicals rather than superoxide anions, showing a potential value for antioxidant and cancer chemoprevention.[7]

Antitumor Constituents and Activities

Biology-coordinated phytochemical approaches revealed that the herb Long Kui contains five types of the anticancer principles, such as steroidal alkaloid saponins, steroidal saponins, polyphenols, glycoproteins, and polysaccharides.

Steroidal Alkaloid Saponins and Steroidal Saponins

SNL-A, a total alkaloid derived from Long Kui, inhibited the proliferation of human HeLa cervical cancer cells and induced the cell apoptosis *in vitro* and *in vivo* but showed much lower toxicity to human normal lymphocytes.[8] Several cytotoxic steroidal alkaloid saponins assigned as solanine (**1**), solasonine (**2**), solamargine (**3**) and β2-solamargine (**4**), as well as degalactotigonin (**5**) have been discovered from the herb. Solanine (**1**) was a poison occurring primary gastrointestinal and neurological disorders, but it exerted anticancer and proapoptotic effects on three types of human digestive system tumors such as SGC-7901 (stomach), HepG2 (liver), and LS-174 (colon) lines *in vitro*, and the IC_{50} values were 14.47 μg/mL in the HepG2 cells and >50 μg/mL in the LS-174 and SGC-7901 cells, whose inhibition on the HepG2 cells was concomitant with the significant induction of G2/M cell cycle arrest and decrease of Bcl-2 expression.[9] Also, solanine (**1**) was able to inhibit the invasion of human PC3 prostate cancer cell by suppressing epithelial-mesenchymal transition and MMP expression, reducing ERK and PI3K/Akt signaling pathways, and moderating miR-21 and miR-138.[10,11] *In vivo* models, solanine (**1**) displayed a remarkable growth inhibitory effect against mouse sarcoma 180 and H22 hepatoma, whose antigrowth mechanism has been revealed to follow multipathways: (1) inhibiting protein synthesis declining the RNA/DNA ratio; (2) reducing the tumor cell membrane fluidity and membrane protein level; (3) lessening the sialic acid level and blocking the cell membrane to force the cell to be broken; (4) reducing Na^+-K^+-ATPase and Ca^{2+}-Mg^{2+}-ATPase activities on tumor cell membrane and hindering the cell abnormal proliferation; and (5) escalating the cell apoptotic death by raising the Ca^{2+} level, down-expressing Bcl-2, losing the mitochondrial membrane potential, releasing cytochrome c to cytosol, and activating caspase-3.[10,11] The inhibition of β-catenin expression by solanine (**1**) might be partially involved in the regulation of signaling in apoptosis MGC-803 gastric cancer cells.[12] In addition, the solanine (**1**) also exerted an immunopotentiating function to indirectly fight the tumor growth.[10,11]

The cytotoxicity of solamargine (**3**), β2-solamargine (**4**), and degalactotigonin (**5**) were investigated in HT-29 and HCT-15 (colon), LNCaP and PC3 (prostate), and T47D and MDA-MB-231 (breast) human solid tumor cell lines. Solamargine (**3**) significantly obstructed the proliferation of all the cell lines (IC_{50}: 1–3 μM), being the most potent anticancer agent among the saponins, and it also inhibited the proliferation of SMMC-7721 (liver), K562 (leukemic), and MGC-803 (stomach) cancer cell lines.[13–16] Especially, its cytotoxicity on the PC3 cells was stronger than that of etoposide by six times.[10,11] The marked antigrowth activity was also proven in mouse models implanted with Ehrlich ascites carcinoma or H22 hepatoma in an intravenous dose of 2.4 mg/kg of solamargine (**3**).[17] The growth of NSCLC cells was inhibited by solamargine (**3**) in a time- and a dose-dependent manner, concomitant with the promotion of apoptosis-inducing effects through p38 MAPK-mediated suppression of phosphorylation and protein expression of STAT3, followed by inducing STAT3 downstream effector p21.[18] The mechanism investigation further revealed that the cytotoxic activity of solamargine (**3**) on K562 leukemia cells was involved in a lysosomal–mitochondrial death pathway, i.e., the induction of an early lysosomal rupture and intracellular calcium increase, subsequent damage of mitochondrial, decrease of membrane potential, and release of cytochrome c, besides down-expression of Bcl-2, up-expression of Bax, and activation of caspase-3 and caspase-9.[14]

Moreover, β2-solamargine (**4**) showed a moderate cytotoxicity against the T47D and LNCaP cell lines but not active to the HT-29 cells,[13] whereas degalactotigonin (**5**) was markedly cytotoxic to NCI-H460 (colon), HepG2 (liver), MCF-7 (breast), and SF-268 (brain) human tumor cell lines (IC_{50}: 0.25–4.49 μM)[19] and was moderately active in the inhibition of HT-29, HCT-15, LNCaP, PC3, T47D, and MDA-MB-231 tumor cell lines.[13] Also, β1-solasonine (**6**), solasonine (**2**), and solanigroside-P (**7**) exerted cytotoxicity to MGC-803 gastric cancer cells.[15] Solasonine (**2**), solamargine (**3**), and desgalactotigonin (**5**) at a concentration of 15 μg/mL showed remarkable inhibitory rates of 100%, 97.9%, and 100% *in vitro* against human JTC-26 cervical carcinoma cells, respectively.[20]

Furthermore, the analysis of the relationship of structure–cytotoxicity revealed that a hydroxyl group on the steroidal backbone or the sugar moieties with α-L-rhamnopyranosyl at C′-2 might be important for the alkaloid saponins exerting the growth inhibitory and apoptosis-inducing effects on the gastric cancer cells.[16]

Polyphanolic Extract

Long Kui polyphanolic extract (SNPE) was especially effective in the suppression of hepatoma *in vitro* and *in vitro*. The oral administration of SNPE in doses of 1–2 μg/mL to tumor-bearing nude mice extensively reduced the weight and the volume of human HepG2 hepatoma by 90–100% in association with the induction of G2/M cell cycle arrest and cell apoptosis via the decline of CDC25A, CDC25B, and CDC25C levels and the activation of caspase-3, caspase-8, and caspase-9.[21] The treatment of SNPE also restrained TPA-induced migration and invasion of HepG2 cells by obviously inhibiting p38 and ERK phosphorylation and reducing TPA-elicited PKCα expression.[22]

Additionally, a polyphenolic extract (SNP) derived from ripe Long Kui berries, in the *in vitro* assay, obviously accelerated the G2/M cell cycle arrest and the apoptosis of various types of human prostate carcinoma cells (CA-HPV-10, LNCaP, 22Rv1, DU145, and PC3) without affecting normal prostate epithelial cells (PZ-HPV-7); therefore, the SNP treatment (5–20 μg/mL) notably exerted the cytotoxicity to deteriorate the prostate tumor cell viability.[23] The findings recommended that the polyphanolic components derived from Long Kui has further developing potential as a promising agent for chemotherapy and prevention of prostate cancer and hepatoma as well as hepatic diseases.

Lunasin

Lunasin, a cancer chemopreventive peptide (4.8 kDa), which contains a sequence with 43-amino acids, was initially derived from soybean and was also isolated from autoclaved Long Kui. Lunasin has been reported to suppress carcinogen-induced carcinogenesis in mammalian and skin cells in mouse models, associated with the attenuation of IL-6 (a proinflammatory mediator) levels. During the carcinogenesis inhibition, lunasin displayed a prominent ability to protect the DNA from the oxidative damage induced by hydroxyl radical and Fe^{2+} ion by chelating Fe^{2+} and blocking the fenton reaction between Fe^{2+} and H_2O_2.[24] Lunasin was also demonstrated to restrain core histone H3 and H4 acetylation, histone acetyltransferase activity, and Rb phosphorylation.[25] The evidences indicated that the consumption of Long Kui and lunasin may play an imperative role in chemoprevention, especially in blocking oxidative carcinogenesis.

Glycoprotein

From the isolation of Long Kui, a cytotoxic SNL glycoprotein (150 kDa) was isolated, which consists of 69.74% carbohydrate content and 30.26% protein content. The protein unit in SNL contains more than 50% hydrophobic amino acids such as glycine and proline.[26] The treatment of human cancer cells with the SNL glycoprotein for 4 h exerted the significant cytotoxic and apoptosis-inducing effects against Hep3B (liver), HT-29 and HCT-116 (colon), HeLa (cervix), and MCF-7 (breast) cancer cell lines at concentrations of 40–80 μg/mL. The SNL glycolprotein also markedly obstructed a tumor-promoter TPA-induced protein kinase C (PKC) translocation, NF-κB activity, and NF-κB/DNA-binding activity in the MCF-7, HT-29, and HCT-116 cells, implying that the cytotoxicity and the apoptosis induced in breast cancer cells and colon cancer cells were mediated by the inhibition of PKCα and NF-κB activities and NO production.[27–30]

More investigations revealed that SNL glycoprotein-provoked cancer cell apoptosis was involved in two signaling pathways. In mitochondria-mediated apoptotic pathway, the SNL glycoprotein stimulated the production of intracellular ROS, regulation of Bcl-2 and Bax expressions, release of mitochondrial cytochrome c, cleavage of poly(ADP-ribose) polymerase, and subsequently activations of caspases. Likewise, in NF-κB-mediated apoptotic pathway, SNL glycoprotein dose-dependently blocked DNA-binding activity of NF-κB and/or AP-1, reduced the activity of iNOS and the production of inducible NO, and then transferred the cell death signals from cytochrome c to caspase 3 by inhibiting the NF-κB and iNOS activation in the tumor cells.[28–34] Therefore, SNL glycoprotein may be speculated as a potential candidate in the field of developing anticancer drugs and prevention agents.

In addition, glycoprotein-A (molecular weight: 3.0×10^4) and glycoprotein-B (molecular weight: 2.5×10^4) were separated from a polysaccharide–protein complex of the Long Kui fruit, showing weak cytotoxicity on the MCF-7 breast cancer cells *in vivo*.[35]

Polysaccharides

The antitumor activity of Long Kui aqueous extract was also mainly contributed by its polysaccharides. Different doses of the polysaccharides not only obviously inhibited the growth of mouse H22 hepatoma cells and improved the survival time of tumor-bearing mice but also potentiated the immune system such as elevation of lymphocyte proliferation, IL-2 level, and calcium ion concentration in the lymphocytes.[36]

SNL-P is a polysaccharide from the herb, exerting a significant growth inhibition on U14 ascites cervical cancer *in vitro* and *in vivo*. The SNL-P treated U14 cells were arrested in G2/M cell cycle, resulting in a massive necrosis of tumor tissues with the up-expression of Bax, the down-expression of Bcl-2 and mutant p53 then triggering the cell apoptosis. Concurrently, the SNL-P treatment reduced TNFα and IL-4 levels and augmented IFNγ level in blood serum, as well as increased the number of $CD4^+$ T lymphocyte subsets and decreased the number of $CD8^+$ T lymphocyte subsets in the peripheral blood.[33–40] In parallel, SNL-P markedly lessened the membrane microviscosity and enhanced the membrane fluidity of red cells in H22 and S180 tumor-bearing mice whose effects improved and restored the functions of erythrocyte membrane.[39–42] In addition, a bioactive fraction-la was prepared from SNL-P, which has the abilities to protect the thymus tissue and to promote more thymus lymphocytes, leading to the antigrowth effect on the U14 tumor in mice.[43] All the resulted data evidenced that the antitumor activity of SNL-P was contributed by the enhancement of immune responses in the host rather than by directly attacking the cancer cells.

From the fractionation of Long Kui aqueous extract, SNLWP and SNLAP were prepared as water-extractable and alkali-extractable polysaccharides, respectively. Further separation of the SNLWP and the SNLAP afforded three polysaccharide subfractions (SNLWP-1, SNLAP-1, and SNLAP-2). The major sugar components in SNLWP-1 were galactose and arabinose, while both SNLAP-1 and SNLAP-2 were rich in xylose, galactose, and arabinose. All the three polysaccharide subfractions showed noticeable immunostimulating anticancer property *in vivo*.[44]

Nanoformulation

The silver nanoparticles were synthesized using *Solanum nigrum* and *Cardiospermum halicacabum*, which showed the cytotoxic effect on human MG-63 osteosarcoma cell line *in vitro*. The nanoformulation may be useful for the potentiaton of therapeutic properties and drug delivery.[45]

Other Bioactivities

The herb Long Kui (Black nightshade) is a widely used plant in oriental medicine as a diuretic and an antipyretic drug. Pharmacological studies have appreciably demonstrated the medicinal potentials of Long Kui, such as antioxidant, hepatoprotective, antiinflammatory, anticonvulsant, antiulcerogenic, and immunoenhancing properties. Moreover, the herb can potentiate the activities of liver mitochondrial succinate dehydrogenase and cytochrome oxidase. SNL glycoprotein also has a strong scavenging activity against free lipid peroxyl radicals, and it can markedly reduce the plasma lipoprotein levels and obviously strengthen the activities of detoxicant enzymes.[22]

References

1. Wang, W. et al. 2005. An in vitro study of cytotoxic and antineoplastic effect of *Solanum nigrum* L. extract on U266. *Beijing Xaxue Xuebao, Yixueban*, 37: 240–4.
2. Lin, H. M. et al. 2007. Induction of autophagy and apoptosis by the extract of *Solanum nigrum* Linn in HepG2 cells. *J. Agricul. Food Chem.* 55: 3620–8.

3. Huang, H. C. et al. 2010. Chemical composition of *Solanum nigrum* Linn extract and induction of autophagy by leaf water extract and its major flavonoids in AU565 breast cancer cells. *J. Agricul. Food Chem.* 58: 8699–708.
4. Chen, P. F. et al. 2013. Inhibition effect of butanol extract of *Solanum nigrum* on cancer of mice bearing H22 hepatic cancer and impact on immunologic function. *Zhongguo Zhongyiyao Keji* 20: 141–2.
5. Wang, H. et al. 2010. *Solanum nigrum* Linn water extract inhibits metastasis in mouse melanoma cells in vitro and in vivo. *J. Agricul. Food Chem.* 58: 11913–23.
6. An, H. J. et al. 2005. *Solanum nigrum* produces nitric oxide via NF-κB activation in mouse peritoneal macrophages. *Eur. J. Cancer Prev.* 14: 345–50.
7. Son, Y. O. et al. 2003. Ripe fruit of *Solanum nigrum* L. inhibits cell growth and induces apoptosis in MCF-7 cells. *Food Chem. Toxicol.* 41: 1421–8.
8. Li, J. et al. 2008. Antitumor effects of total alkaloids isolated from *Solanum nigrum* in vitro and in vivo. *Pharmazie* 63: 534–8.
9. Ji, Y. B. et al. 2008. Induction of apoptosis in HepG2 cells by solanine and Bcl-2 protein. *J. Ethnopharmacol.* 115: 194–202.
10. Shen, K. H. et al. 2014. α-Solanine inhibits invasion of human prostate cancer cell by suppressing epithelial-mesenchymal transition and MMPs expression. *Mol.* 19: 11896–914.
11. Gui, X. L. et al. 2009. A review to antitumor mechanism of Solanine. *Chin. J. Inform. Tradit. Chin. Med.* 16(z1): 80–2.
12. Zhang, W. D. et al. 2013. Effect of *Solanum nigrum* on the expression of E-cadherin in human gastric carcinoma cells of MGC-803 tumor-bearing mice. *Anhui Nongye Kexue* 41: 11965–6.
13. Hu, K. et al. 1999. Antineoplastic agents. III: Steroidal glycosides from *Solanum nigrum. Planta Med.* 65: 35–8.
14. Sun, L. M. et al. 2010. A lysosomal-mitochondrial death pathway is induced by solamargine in human K562 leukemia cells. *Toxicol. in Vitro* 24: 1504–11.
15. Ding, X. et al. 2012. Induction of apoptosis in human hepatoma SMMC-7721 cells by solamargine from *Solanum nigrum* L. *J. Ethno-pharmacol.* 139: 599–604.
16. Ding, X. et al. 2013. Purification, antitumor activity in vitro of steroidal glycoalkaloids from black nightshade (*Solanum nigrum* L.) *Food Chem.* 141: 1181–6.
17. Tang, Z. H. et al. 2011. Extraction, purification technology and antineoplastic effects of solamargine. *Zhongguo Zhongyao Zazhi* 36: 2192–5.
18. Zhou, Y. et al. 2014. Targeting signal transducer and activator of transcription 3 contributes to the solamargine-inhibited growth and -induced apoptosis of human lung cancer cells. *Tumor Biol.* 35: 8169–78.
19. Zhou, X. L. et al. 2006. Steroidal saponins from *Solanum nigrum. J. Nat Prods.* 69: 1158–63.
20. Saijo, R. et al. 1982. Studies on the constituents of Solanum plants II. *Yakugaku Zasshi* 102: 300–5.
21. Wang, H. C. et al. 2011. *Solanum nigrum* L. polyphenolic extract inhibits hepatocarcinoma cell growth by inducing G2/M phase arrest and apoptosis. *J. Sci. Food Agricult.* 91: 178–85.
22. Yang, M. Y. et al. 2010. Polyphenol-rich extracts from *Solanum nigrum* attenuated PKC α-mediated migration and invasion of hepatocellular carcinoma cells. *J. Agricult. Food Chem.* 58: 5806–14.
23. Nawab, A. et al. 2012. Selective cell cycle arrest and induction of apoptosis in human prostate cancer cells by a polyphenol-rich extract of *Solanum nigrum. Intl. J. Mol. Med.* 29: 277–84.
24. Jeong, J. B. et al. 2010. Lunasin peptide purified from *Solanum nigrum* L. protects DNA from oxidative damage by suppressing the generation of hydroxyl radical via blocking fenton reaction. *Cancer Lett.* 293: 58–64.
25. Jeong, J. B. et al. 2007. Cancer-preventive peptide lunasin from *Solanum nigrum* L. inhibits acetylation of core histones H3 and H4 and phosphorylation of retinoblastoma protein (Rb). *J. Agricul. Food Chem.* 55: 10707–13.
26. Lee, S. J. et al. 2006. 150 kDa glycoprotein isolated from *Solanum nigrum* L. stimulates caspase-3 activation and reduces inducible nitric oxide production in HCT-116 cells. *Toxicol. in Vitro* 20: 1088–97.
27. Heo, K. S. et al. 2005. Glycoprotein isolated from *Solanum nigrum* L. modulates the apoptotic-related signals in TPA-stimulated MCF-7 cells. *J. Med. Food* 8: 69–77.
28. Lim, K. T. et al. 2005. Glycoprotein isolated from *Solanum nigrum* L. kills HT-29 cells through apoptosis. *J. Med. Food* 8: 215–26
29. Lee, S. J. et al. 2004. A 150-kDa glycoprotein isolated from *Solanum nigrum* L. has cytotoxic and apoptotic effects by inhibiting the effects of PKCα, nuclear factor-κB and inducible nitric oxide in HCT-116 cells. *Cancer Chemother. Pharmacol.* 54: 562–72.
30. Lee, S. J. et al. 2005. Glycine- and proline-rich glycoprotein isolated from *Solanum nigrum* L. activates caspase-3 through cytochrome c in HT-29 cells. *Oncol. Reports* 14: 789–96.
31. Lee, S. J. et al. 2006. Apoptosis induced by glycoprotein (150-kDa) isolated from *Solanum nigrum* L. is not related to intracellular ROS in HCT-116 cells. *Cancer Chemoth. Pharmacol.* 57: 507–16.
32. Lee, S. J. et al. 2008. Cell death signal by glycine- and proline-rich plant glycoprotein is transferred from cytochrome c and nuclear factor κB to caspase 3 in Hep3B cells. *J. Nutri. Biochem.* 19: 166–74.
33. Oh, P. S. et al. 2007. HeLa cells treated with phytoglycoprotein (150 kDa) were killed by activation of caspase 3 via inhibitory activities of NF-κB and AP-1. *J. Biomed. Sci.* 14: 223–32.
34. Heo, K. S. et al. 2004. Glycoprotein isolated from *Solanum nigrum* L. inhibits the DNA-binding activities of NF-κB and AP-1, and increases the production of nitric oxide in TPA-stimulated MCF-7 cells. *Toxicol. in Vitro* 18: 755–63.
35. Ji, Y. B. et al. 2011. Material basis of cytotoxicity in polysaccharide from *Solanum nigrum. Zhongcaoyao* 42: 2275–8.
36. Chen, H. et al. 2013. Study on the effect of polysaccharides from *Solanum nigrum Linne* on cellular immune function in tumour-bearing mice. *Afri. J. Tradit. Complem. Altern. Med.* 10: 41–6.
37. Li, J. et al. 2007. Antitumor activity of crude polysaccharides isolated from *Solanum nigrum* on U14 cervical carcinoma bearing mice. *Phytotherapy Res.* 21: 832–40.
38. Li, J. et al. 2009. Antitumor and immunomodulating effects of polysaccharides isolated from *Solanum nigrum Linne. Phytother. Res.* 23: 1524–1530.
39. Li, J. et al. 2008. Study on antitumor activity and immunomodulating effect of polysaccharides isolated from *Solanum nigrum Linne. Anhui Nongye Kexue* 36: 14589–90, 14632.

40. Li, J. et al. 2008. Aqueous extract of *Solanum nigrum* inhibit growth of cervical carcinoma (U14) via modulating immune response of tumor bearing mice and inducing apoptosis of tumor cells. *Fitoterapia* 79: 548–56.
41. Yuan, H. L. et al. 2011. Effects of *Solanum nigrum* polysaccharide on functioning of erythrocyte membrane of H22 tumor-bearing mice. *J. Harbin Business Univ.*, (*Sci. Etid.*) 27: 7–11.
42. Gao, S. Y. et al. 2011. Enhancement of erythrocyte immunity in S180 or H22-bearing mice by *Solanum nigrum* polysaccharide through increasing quantity and activity of red cell CR1. *Zhongguo Yaoxue Zazhi* 46: 1405–11
43. Li, J. et al. 2010. Protective effects of fraction 1a of polysaccharides isolated from *Solanum nigrum Linne* on thymus in tumor-bearing mice. *J. Ethnopharmacol.* 129: 350–6.
44. Ding, X. et al. 2012. Purification, antitumour and immunomodulatory activity of water-extractable and alkali-extractable polysaccharides from *Solanum nigrum L. Food Chem.* 131: 677–84.
45. Chauhan, R. et al. 2015. Cytotoxic effect on human osteosarcoma cell line MG-63 and antimicrobial activity on clinical pathogens by plant mediated silver nanoparticles. *World J. Pharm. Res.* 4: 1012–27.

30 Ma Bian Cao 馬鞭草

Common Vervain

2. $R_1 = R_3 = R_5 = -H, R_2 = -Caffeoyl, R_4 = R_6 = -Ac$
3. $R_1 = R_2 = R_4 = -H, R_3 = -Caffeoyl, R_5 = R_6 = -Ac$
4. $R_1 = -OH, R_2 = -feruloyl, R_3 = R_6 = -Ac, R_4 = R_5 = -H$
5. $R_1 = -OH, R_2 = -feruloyl, R_5 = R_6 = -Ac, R_5 = R_6 = -H$

Herb Origination

The herb Ma Bian Cao (common Vervain) is the dried aerial part of a Verbenaceae plant *Verbena officinalis* L., which is a perennial plant native to Europe, and it has spread over the world from temperate zones to tropical regions. In China, the herbage is broadly distributed in eastern, southern, and southwestern provinces as well as part of the northwestern areas. Generally, the herb is collected in its blooming season from June to August and then dried in the sun for application in Chinese folk medicine.

Antitumor Activities

Despite showing no effect on human SMMC-7721 hepatoma cells *in vitro*, the oral administration of the alcoholic and aqueous extracts to tumor-bearing mice in the same dose of 32 g/kg for 10 days inhibited the growth of mouse H22 hepatoma cells by 32.5% and 40.3%, respectively.[1] When the aqueous extract is combined with cisplatin (an antitumor agent), the antihepatoma rate was amplified to 44.8%.[2] However, the treatment caused the decline of the spleen index and the IL-2 activity and the reduction of the mouse growth weight but no damage on the immune system.[1,3] Both *in vitro* and *in vivo* experiments showed that the alcoholic extract at a small dose was able to improve the anti-growth effect of paclitaxel synergistically against murine sarcoma 180 cells.[4] Remarkably, the alcoholic extract showed a specificity to human JAR choriocarcinoma cells. In the *in vitro* tests, the extract induced G2/M cell cycle arrest and apoptosis of the JAR cells via augmented proapoptotic gene Bax and lessened anti-apoptotic gene Bcl-2, as well as diminished EGFR expression, thereby obviously obstructing the proliferation of JAR cells.[5,6] A C fraction, which was derived from the alcohol extract, in a concentration of 40 mg/mL, suppressed the JAR cells by 65% after being treated for 72 h.[7]

Antitumor Constituents and Activities

Flavonoids

4′-Methylether-scutellarein (**1**, 4′-MS) is the major antitumor constituent isolated from Ma Bian Cao, which played a role in the inhibitory effect against the JAR choriocarcinoma cells. Similarly, through an endogenous signal transduction pathway, i.e., the downregulation of survivin and the direct activation of Bax, cytochrome c, caspase-3, caspase-9, and p38 MAPK, 20 or 40 μg/mL of 4′-MS (**1**) elicited the G2/M cell cycle arrest and apoptosis of the JAR cells.[8,9] Moreover, 4′-MS (**1**) was also capable of reversing the MDR of human JAR/VP16 choriocarcinoma cells. Exposure to 20 μg/mL of 4′-MS (**1**) significantly sensitized the JAR VP16 cells to the chemotherapeutic drugs, etoposide (VP16), methotrexate (MTX), and actinomycin-D (ACTD), and their drug resistances were reduced to up to 5.02-, 3.67-, and 2.48-folds, showing the reversal ratios of 81.19%, 76.89%, and 64.08%, respectively. During the MDR-reversal effect, the expression levels of some apoptosis-promoting genes (i.e., Apaf-1, ASC, ATM, Bad, Bak, Bax, and BimL) were amplified, and those of some apoptosis-suppressing genes (i.e., Bcl-2, BFL1, NAIP, and p63) were attenuated. Significantly, the expressions of some multidrug-resistant genes (i.e., MDR1, MRP1, MRP2, MRP6, AHR, COMT, FGF2, and P-gp) were notably lessened, sequentially enlarging the intracellular concentration of the drugs in the drug-resistant tumor cells.[10–12] The evidences recommend that 4′-methylether-scutellarein (**1**) is a potential drug lead for the development of a new therapeutic agent specifically toward choriocarcinoma.

Phenylethanoid Glycosides

Bioassay-guided fractionation led to the isolation of 12 phenylethanoid glycosides with an antiproliferative activity. Of them, 2‴,4‴-diacetyl-*O*-verbascoside (**2**), 3‴,4‴-diacetyl-*O*-isoverbascoside (**3**), 4‴,6″-acetyl-*O*-betonyoside-A (**4**), and 3‴,4‴-diacetyl-*O*-betonyoside-A (**5**) exhibited a potent antiproliferative activity against DHD/K12/PROb rat colonic epithelial cells and HCT-116 human colon adenocarcinoma cells, whose activities were similar to that of vinblastine sulfate (IC_{50}: 1.28 μg/mL). 6″-acetyl-*O*-verbascoside, 4‴-acetyl-*O*-verbascoside, and 4‴-acetyl-*O*-isoverbascoside were active to both cell lines (IC_{50}: 8.16–10.80 μg/mL in 72 h).[13]

Triterpenoids

Five triterpenoid constituents were isolated from Ma Bian Cao. Of the triterpenes, 4-*epi*-barbinervic acid (**6**) was reported to have an obvious antiproliferative activity against human Bel-7402 hepatoma cell line *in vitro*.[14]

Essential Oil

Citral (**7**), a key component of lemon-scented essential oils extracted from *Verbena officinalis* as well as other herbal plants, such as lemon grass (*Cymbopogon citratus*) and melissa (*Melissa officinalis*), is used as a food additive and as a fragrance in cosmetics. The growth of MCF-7 breast carcinoma cells could be restrained by citral (**7**) (IC_{50}: 0.18 μM, 48 h) with the induction of G2/M cell cycle arrest and apoptosis.[15] The inhibitory effect of citral (**7**) on acute promyelocytic leukemia NB4 cell line was revealed to be correlated with the promotion of apoptotic death, whose mechanism was found to be through a mitochondrial pathway, i.e., the downregulation of Bcl-2 mRNA level and NF-κB protein level, the upexpression of Bax, the reduction of mitochondrial membrane potential, and the direct procaspase-3 activation.[16] In the treatment with the essential oil or the citral (**7**), the apoptosis was induced in granulocytes collected from both CML patients and healthy donors and in lymphocytes collected from both chronic lymphocytic leukemia (CLL) patients and normal blood donors, but the percentage of apoptotic cells was significantly greater in CLL and CML patients.[17–19] The evidences indicate that citral may be a possible lead molecule to develop new therapeutic agents for CLL and CML. The antitumor activity of citral (**7**) was also demonstrated in assays using other types of human cancer cell lines *in vitro*. *In vivo* experiments also proved that citral (**7**) markedly blocked hamster buccal pouch carcinogenesis caused by DMBA and mammalian cell mutagenesis caused by cyclophos-phamide. More evidences proved that the chemopreventive potential of citral (**7**) is most likely due to its antilipid peroxidative, antioxidant, and potent free radical-scavenging activities and its modulating effect on the detoxification cascade.[20,21]

Other Bioactivities

The herb Ma Bian Cao (common Vervain) has been used in Chinese folk medicine for a long time for its multiple biological activities such as antimicrobial, antiinflammatory, neuroprotective, hepatoprotective, gastroprotective, analgesic, hypnotic/sedative, and antioxidant. In pharmacological investigations, the Ma Bian Cao extracts displayed analgesic, antioxidant, antirheumatic, nerve growth factor-potentiating, antifungal, and antibacterial properties.

References

1. Cao, Z. R. et al. 2008. Experimental study of effect on tumor-inhibition in mice. *J. Hebei Med. College for Continu. Edu.* 25: 8–9.
2. Li, X. R. et al. 2011. Antitumor activity of *Verbena officinalis* on mouse hepatoma and its influence on IL-2 activity. *Hebei Med. J.* 33: 234–5.
3. Kou, W. Z. et al. 2013. Study on in-vivo antitumor activity of *Verbena officinalis* extract. *Afri. J. Trad. Complem. Altern. Med.* 10: 512–7.
4. Xu, H.-E. et al. 2008. Synergistic antitumor effect of alcohol extract of *Verbena officinalis* and paclitaxel. *Acta Univ. Med. Nanjing* 28: 1275–8.
5. Xu, S. et al. 2000. Effects of alcohol extract of *Verbena officinalis* on proliferation and EGFR expression of choriocarcinoma JAR cells. *J. China Pharm. Univ.* 31: 281–4.
6. Wang, J. J. et al. 2004. Blockage in G2/M phase and induction apoptosis on human choriocarcinoma JAR cells by *Verbena officinalis* C. *Nanjing Yike Daxue* 24: 598–601.
7. Zhang, L. P. et al. 2005. Inhibitory effects of the Part C in alcohol extract of *Verbena officinalis* on human choriocarcinoma JAR cell line. *Zhongguo Zhongliu Linchuang* 24: 470–4.
8. Feng, B. et al. 2008. Inhibitory effect of 4′-methylether-scutellarein on human choriocarcinoma JAR cells and its possible mechanism. *Zhongguo Zhongliu Shengwu Zhiliao Zazhi* 15: 444–50.
9. Yang, Z. S. et al. 2011. Signal transduction mechanism of induced apoptotic effects of 4′-methylether-scutellarein on human choriocarcinoma JAR cells. *Zhongyao Yaoli Yu Linchuang* 27: 20–3.
10. Zhu, L. Q. et al. 2007. Reversal of multidrug resistance in drug-resistant human choriocarcinoma cell line JAR/VP16 by effective component of *Verbena officinalis* L. *Nanjing Yike Daxue Xuebao* 27: 419–23, C2.
11. Xu, S. et al. 2006. Reversal effect of 4′-methylether-scutellarein on multidrug resistance of human choriocarcinoma JAR/VP16 cell line. *Shengwu Huaxue Yu Shengwu Wuli Jinzhan* 33: 1061–73.
12. Zhu, L. Q. et al. 2009. Reverse mechanism of 4′-methylether-scutellarein on multidrug resistant human choriocarcinoma cell line. *Nanjing Yike Daxue Xuebao* 29: 1215–9.
13. Encalada, M. A. et al. 2015. Antiproliferative effect of phenylethanoid glycosides from *Verbena officinalis* L. on colon cancer cell lines. *LWT-Food Sci. Technol.* 63: 1016–22.
14. Shu, J. C. et al. 2013. A new triterpenoid from *Verbena officinalis* L. *Nat. Prod. Res.* 27: 1293–7.
15. Chaouki, W. et al. 2009. Citral inhibits cell proliferation and induces apoptosis and cell cycle arrest in MCF-7 cells. *Fundam. Clinic Pharmacol.* 23: 549–56.
16. Xia, H. L. et al. 2013. The in vitro study of apoptosis in NB4 cell induced by citral. *Cytotechnol*. 65: 49–57.
17. De Martino, L. et al. 2009. *Verbena officinalis* essential oil and its component citral as apoptotic-inducing agent in chronic lymphocytic leukemia. *Intl. J. Immunopathol. Pharmacol.* 22: 1097–104.
18. De Martino, L. et al. 2008. *Verbena officinalis* essential oil and citral as apoptotic inductors in leukocytes of healthy subjects and chronic myeloid leukemia patients. *Pharmacologyonline* (2): 170–5.
19. De Martino, L. et al. 2011. Active caspase-3 detection to evaluate apoptosis induced by *Verbena officinalis* essential oil and citral in chronic lymphocytic leukaemia cells. *Revista Brasileira de Farmacognosia* 21: 869–73.
20. Rajasekaran, D. et al. 2011. Evaluation of chemo-preventive efficacy of citral in 7,12-dimethylbenz(a)anthracene (DMBA) induced hamster buccal pouch carcinogenesis. *Intl. J. Res. in Phytochem. Pharmacol.* 1: 136–43.
21. Rabbani, S. I. 2004. Studies on antimutagenic effects of citral in mice. *J. Food, Agricult. Envir.* 2: 62–4.

31 Zhi Mu 知母

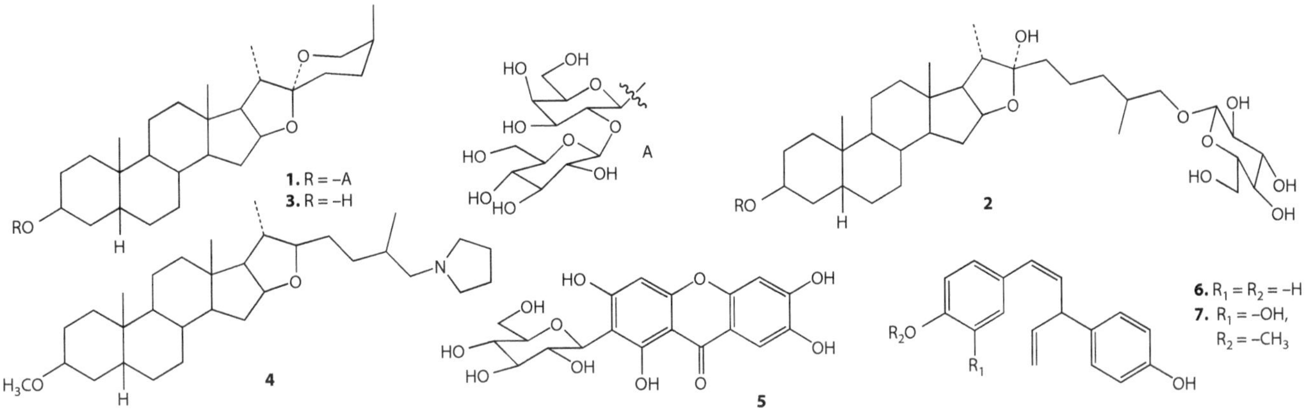

1. R = -A
3. R = -H

A

2

4

5

6. $R_1 = R_2 = -H$
7. $R_1 = -OH$, $R_2 = -CH_3$

Herb Origination

The herb Zhi Mu is the dried rhizomes of a Liliaceae plant *Anemarrhena asphodeloides*, whose perennial herbal is native to the sandy hillsides in northern China. Its distribution is extended to Korea and Japan from east of the Gansu province of China. Spring and autumn are the best seasons for collection of a high quality of the herb Zhi Mu. The ethnomedical uses of Zhi Mu has been recorded in China, Korea, and Japan for thousands of years. Especially, Zhi Mu was documented in the first Chinese herbal classic entitled *Shennong Ben Cao Jing*, which has been used in Chinese medicine for over two thousand years.

Antitumor Constituents and Activities

Phytochemical researches revealed the presence of several types of constituents, steroids, steroidal saponins, xanthones, alkaloids, flavonoids, phenypropanoids, and others in Zhi Mu. The major constituents were identified as neomangiferin, mangiferin, timosaponin-BII, anemarrhenasaponin-I, and timosaponin-AIII, whose compounds were largely obligated to the biological activities of the herb. The antitumor activity of Zhi Mu was known to be primarily contributed by several isolated steroidal saponins, especially timosaponin-AIII.

Steroidal Saponins

Anticancer Effects

Timosaponin-AIII (**1**) was isolated from the EtOAc soluble fraction of its methanol extract in a bioassay-guided fractionation, exerting an extensive antiproliferative activity against two panels of human tumor cell lines *in vitro*. Its ED_{50} values were 1.55–3.06 μg/mL in A549 (lung), SK-MEL-2 (skin), SKOV-3 (ovary), XF498 (brain), and HCT-15 (colon) cancer cell lines, and the IC_{50} values were 1.8–13.0 μg/mL in HL-60 and K562 (leukemic), DLD-1 and HCT-15 (colon), SKOV-3 (ovary), MCF-7 (breast), and A549 (lung) cancer cell lines.[1,2] The broad spectrum of anticancer activity was also proven in HeLa, HepG2, Bel-7402, HT-29, MDA-MB-468, HCT116, HT1080, T475-S2, and U937 tumor cell lines *in vitro*, and the IC_{50} value was 6.97 μM (24 h) in the T475-S2 melanoma cells. More studies revealed that timosaponin-AIII (**1**) at a concentration of 6 μM induced the apoptosis and autophagy of T475-S2 cells, whose inhibitory effects against the T475-S2 cells were stronger than paclitaxel and 5-FU.[3,4] The promotion of apoptosis and autophagy was also observed in some selected cancer cell lines after being treated with timosaponin-AIII (**1**).[5,6] In addition, timosaponin-BII (**2**), another steroidal glycoside separated from Zhi Mu, was reported to have the inhibitory activity against the proliferation of HL-60 (leukemic), HeLa (cervix), HepG2 and Bel-7402 (liver), HT-29 (colon), and MDA-MB-468 (breast) human carcinoma cell lines with an IC_{50} value of 15.5 μg/mL in the HL-60 cells.[4,7]

Induction of Apoptosis and Cell Cycle Arrest

The apoptosis-enhancing effect was found to be mediated by (1) induction of ROS-overproduced mitochondrial dysfunction and reduction of mitochondrial membrane potential and (2) release of cytochrome c and activation of caspase-3, whereas the autophagy was caused by (1) suppression of mTOR and induction of ER stress and (2) elicitation of early autophagic vacuole formation, GFP-LC3 translocation, and LC3-II increase in the absence of caspase-3 cleavage.[5,6] Consequently, timosaponin-AIII (**1**) was revealed not only to promote the caspase-dependent and p53-independent apoptosis but also to induce AMPKα/mTOR-dependent and XIAP degradation-involved autophagy–lysosomal pathway. According to multiple death-promoting mechanisms, timosaponin-AIII (**1**) exerted a potent cytotoxic effect on human hepatocellular carcinoma cells (HCC) without severe hepatic toxicity.[8] Moreover, the inhibition on HCT-15 colorectal cancer cells by timosaponin-AIII (**1**) was accompanied with the arrest of the cell cycle in G0/G1 and G2/M phases and the induction of apoptosis, via (1) the downregulation of cyclin-A, cyclin-B1, CDK2, CDK4, proliferating cell nuclear antigen, and c-Myc and (2) the down-expression of Bcl-xL and Bcl-2, the augmentation of DNA fragmentation and cleaved PARP, and the activation of caspases.[7] The *in vivo* antitumor activity of timosaponin-AIII (**1**) was proven in nude mice xenograft models implanted with human HCT-15 colon cancer and human hepatoma, respectively.[8,9] Based on *in vitro* and *in vivo* results, the possibility of further developing timosaponin-TAIII as a cancer therapeutic agent is worth considering.

Steroids

Sarsasapogenin (**3**) is a sapogenin isolated from the herb and is also the aglycon of timosaponin-AIII (**1**). *In vitro* studies with human HepG2 hepatoma and HeLa cervical cancer cell lines showed that sarsasapogenin (**3**) induced distinct dose- and time-dependent diminutions of cell viability and elicited the promotion of cell apoptosis with the arrest of the cell cycle in G2/M phase, and the IC_{50} value was 42.4 μg/mL (48 h) in HepG2 cells.[10,11] The apoptosis of HeLa cells promoted by sarsasapogenin (**3**) was triggered by both ROS-mediated mitochondrial dysfunction and ER stress-induced cell death.[11] However, sarsasapogenin (**3**) did not display the growth inhibition on human tumor cell lines (A549, SKOV-3, SK-MEL-2, XF498, and HCT-15) *in vitro*.[1] Compared to timosaponin-AIII (**3**), the sarsasaponin disclosed a lower cytotoxicity with no induction of autophagy, signifying that the saccharide moiety in timosaponin-AIII is indispensable to the higher antitumor effect.[6] A range of the sarsasapogenin derivatives have been synthesized by a simple and facile synthetic route. Most of the derivatives showed excellent selective cytotoxicity toward the cancer cell lines. In particular, a derivative, (22R,25S)-3β-methoxy-26-pyrrolidinylamino-5β-furostan (**4**), displayed the inhibitory activity against A375-S2 (IC_{50}: 0.56 μM) and HT1080 (IC_{50}: 0.72 μM) cells, being approximately 13–49-fold more potent than timosaponin TA-III (**1**) and 5-FU. Meanwhile, compared to TA-III and 5-FU, it exerted a higher cytotoxicity against the other cancer cells (HeLa, MCF-7, HepG2, HCT-116, A549, A375-S2, HT1080, HL-60, U937). The cytotoxicity data also disclosed that the substituent at the C-3 and C-26 positions has a great influence on the selective antitumor activity.[12]

Xanthone

Mangiferin (**5**), a glucosylxanthone isolated from *A. asphodeloides*, demonstrated an obvious suppressive effect against the proliferation of human MDA-MB-231 breast cancer cells *in vitro*. When treated with mangiferin (**5**) in a 1 μmol/L concentration for 24 h, the inhibitory rate was 20.55% on the MDA-MB-231 cells.[13] By obstructing the binding of NF-κB and AP-1 to the MMP-9 promoter and hindering the phosphorylation of Akt and MAP kinases, mangiferin (**5**) suppressed the invasiveness of human glioma cells.[14] The results suggested that the specific inhibitory activity of mangiferin (**5**) on MMP-9 may be pharmacologically valuable for the treatment of invasive gliomas.[14] Another active xanthone was tetraacetate norathyriol, which was effective in the inhibition of HT-29, Bel-7402, MDA-MB-468, and HeLa human cancer cell lines.[4]

Norlignan

The phytochemical investigation of Zhi Mu chloroform extract lead to the isolation of a norlignan component assigned as *cis*-hinokiresinol (**6**). It showed cytotoxicity against seven human tumor cell lines (i.e., SKOV3, A549, HCT-15, DLD1, MCF-7, HL-60, and K562) and mouse P388 cell line *in vitro*. The IC_{50} values were 3.5 and 4.6 μg/mL in HL-60 and K562 leukemia cells, 6.9 and 9.6 μg/mL in DLD1 and HCT15 colon cancer cells, 12.0 and 15.0 μg/mL in A549 lung and MCF-7 breast cancer cells, and 34.0 and 26.0 μg/mL in SKOV-3 ovarian carcinoma and P388 leukemia cells, respectively.[2] Prominently, *cis*-hinokiresinol (**6**) was able to selectively restrain the endothelial cell proliferation compared to cancer cells, especially having an obvious inhibition on bFGF- and/or VEGF-induced growth of endothelial cells. By the hinokiresinol treatment, the endothelial cell migration and the tube formation were obstructed, and the vessel growth induced by VEGF was diminished in a mouse corneal neovascularization model. The evidences implied the potential of *cis*-hinokiresinol (**6**) as a drug lead for the development of a novel antiangiogenic agent.[15] Another isolated bioactive norlignan was (-)-(3R)-3″-hydroxy-4″-*O*-methylnyasol (**7**), which inhibited the proliferation of HeLa and MCF-7 cancer cells with IC_{50} values of 0.64 and 1.3 μM, respectively.[16]

Other Bioactivities

Based upon the pharmacological investigation, the herb Zhi Mu was confirmed possessing multiple properties such as antivirus, antiinflammation, antisenescence, antidementia, antiepilepsy, antihyperthyroidism, antiosteoporosis, and antiskin aging/damage. Studies further showed that the major constituents, steroidal saponins, possess a broad range of pharmacological activities such as improving senile dementia, preventing cerebral ischemia, anticoagulated blood, antiinflammation, antiosteoporosis, antioxidant, lowering blood pressure, lowering blood sugar, and lowering blood fat.[17] Mangiferin (**5**), another major constituent in the herb, was found to have abilities to significantly prevent the progression of diabetic nephropathy and to improve renal function.[1]

References

1. Lee, S. H. et al. 1995. Antitumor agent from the rhizome of *Anemarrhena asphodeloides*. *Kor. J. Pharmacogn.* 26: 47–50.
2. Park, S. Y. et al. 1994. Isolation of cytotoxic compounds from *Anemarrhena asphodeloides*. *Soul Taehakkyo Yakhak Nonmunjip* 19: 61–73.
3. Song, S. J. et al. 2014. Application of timosaponin AIII in *Anemarrhena asphodeloides* to the preparation of antitumor drugs. *Faming Zhuanli Shenqing* CN 103599122 A 20140226.
4. Guo, J. et al. 2015. Cytotoxic activities of chemical constituents from rhizomes of *Anemarrhena asphodeloides* and their analogues. *Archiv. Pharm. Res.* 38: 598–603.
5. King, F. W. et al. 2009. Timosaponin AIII is preferentially cytotoxic to tumor cells through inhibition of mTOR and induction of ER stress. *PLoS One* 4: e7283.
6. Sy, L. K. et al. 2008. Timosaponin A-III induces autophagy preceding mitochondria-mediated apoptosis in HeLa cancer cells. *Cancer Res.* 68: 10229–37.
7. Cheng, S. H. et al. 2009. Total synthesis of a furostan saponin, timosaponin BII. *Org. Biomol. Chem.* 7: 3112–8.
8. Wang, N. et al. 2013. A novel mechanism of XIAP degradation induced by timosaponin AIII in hepatocellular carcinoma. *Biochimica et Biophysica Acta, Mol. Cell Res.* 1833: 2890–9.
9. Kang, Y. J. et al. 2011. Cytotoxic and antineoplastic activity of timosaponin A-III for human colon cancer cells. *J. Nat. Prod.* 74: 701–6.
10. Bao, W. N. et al. 2007. The apoptotic effect of sarsasapogenin from *Anemarrhena asphodeloides* on HepG2 human hepatoma cells. *Cell Biol. Internat.* 31: 887–92.

11. Shen, S. Y. et al. 2013. Sarsasapogenin induces apoptosis via the reactive oxygen species-mediated mitochondrial pathway and ER stress pathway in HeLa cells. *Biochem. Biophys. Res. Commun.* 441: 519–24.
12. Yin, Y. et al. 2015. Synthesis and biological evaluation of novel sarsasapogenin derivatives as potential antitumor agents. *Steroids* 93: 25–31.
13. Wu, T. M. et al. 2011. Microwave-assisted extraction of mangiferin with antitumor activities from *Anemarrhena asphodeloides* bge. *Nanjing Zhongyiyao Daxue Xuebao* 27: 260–2.
14. Jung, J. S. et al. 2012. Selective inhibition of MMP-9 gene expression by mangiferin in PMA-stimulated human astroglioma cells: Involvement of PI3K/Akt and MAPK signaling pathways. *Pharmacol. Res.* 66: 95–103.
15. Jeong, S. J. et al. 2003. cis-Hinokiresinol, a norlignan from *Anemarrhena asphodeloides*, inhibits angiogenic response in vitro and in vivo. *Biol Pharm Bull.* 26: 1721–4.
16. Miyamoto, T. et al. 2014. Novel compound containing nyasol compound, and antitumor agent containing same. *PCT Int. Appl.* WO 2014136786 A1 20140912.
17. Cai, F. et al. 2011. Advances in the pharmacological studies on timosaponins and their sapogenins. *Yaoxue Shijian Zazhi* 29: 331–5.
18. Wang, Y. L. et al. 2014. The genus *Anemarrhena* Bunge: A review on ethnopharmacology, phytochemistry and pharmacology. *J. Ethnopharmacol.* 153: 42–60.

32 Zhu Sha Geng 朱砂根

Coral Ardisa root

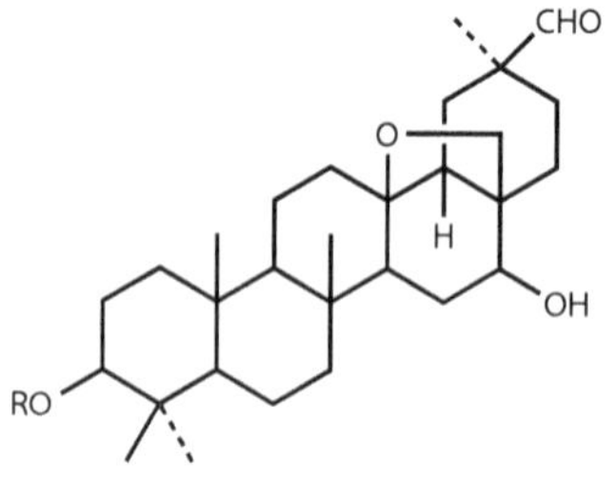

1. R = -Ara-(4-1)-Glc-(2-1)-Xyl
-(2-1)-Glc
2. R = -Ara-(4-1)-Glc-(2-1)-Rham
-(2-1)-Glc 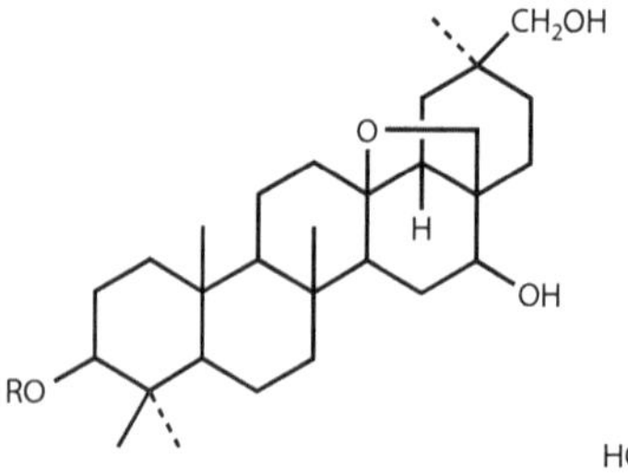
3. R = -Ara-(4-1)-Glc
-(2-1)-Xyl 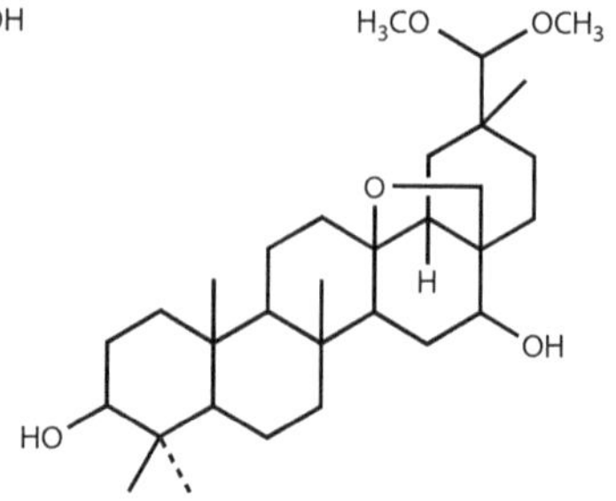
4. R = -Ara-(4-1)-Glc-(2-1)-Glc
5. R = -Ara-(4-1)-Glc
-(2-1)-Rham

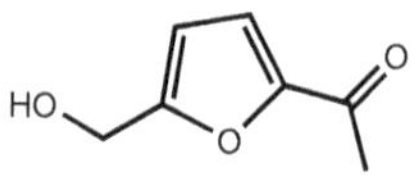

Herb Origination

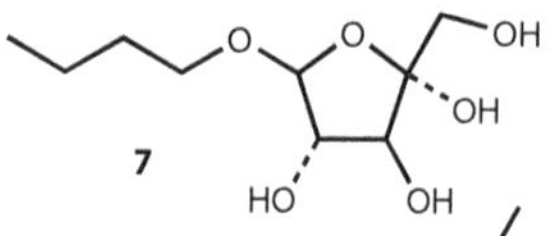

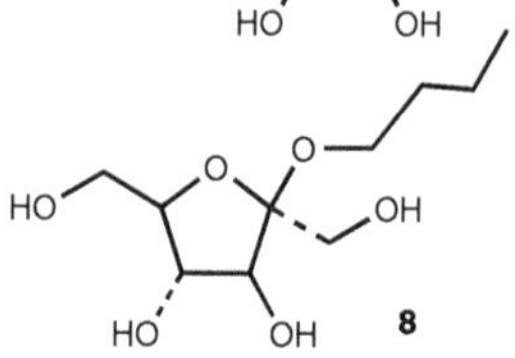

The herb Zhu Sha Geng (Coral Ardisa root) originated from two species of Myrsinaceae plants, *Ardisia crenate* and its variant *bicolor*. The two evergreen shrubs are native to East Asia. In China, the distributional region of these two plants is closely in southern area of the Yangtze River, as well as in Taiwan, Hainan, and the southeast area of Tibet. The roots are normally collected in autumn and dried in the sun, but it can be used fresh annually.

Antitumor Activities and Constituents

Saponins

The Zhu Sha Geng extract contains rich triterpenoid saponin components. The inhibition of the total saponins were showed toward murine tumors (U14 cervical cancer, sarcoma 180, H22 hepatoma, and Lewis lung tumor).[1,2] Ardisiacrispin-A (**1**) and ardisiacrispin-B (**2**), ardisicrenoside-B (**3**), ardisicrenoside-I (**4**), and ardisicrenoside-J (**5**) presented a moderate cytotoxicity in a group of human cancer cell lines such as MCF-7 (breast), NCI-H460 (lung), SF-268 (brain), HepG2 (liver), and HepG2R (MDR-liver) cells (IC_{50}: 2.36–23.58 μM) but no effect on human normal kidney HEK 293 cells *in vitro*.[3,4] The IC_{50} values of ardisiacrispin-B (**2**) ranged between 1.59 and 2.05 μg/mL in HCT-8 (ileocecal), BGC-823 (stomach), Bel-7402 (liver), A549 (lung), A2780 (ovary), and KETR3 (renal) human tumor cell lines.[5] A mixture of ardisiacrispin-A (**1**) and ardisiacrispin-B (**2**) with a fixed proportion (2:1) was derived from the herb, demonstrating an *in vitro* growth inhibitory effect on seven human tumor cell lines such as Bel-7402 (liver), KB (nasopharynx), SKOV-3 (ovary), HeLa (cervix), BGC-823 (stomach), MCF-7 (breast), and HL-60 (leukemia) cells, where the Bel-7402 cells were the most sensitive cell line to the mixture (IC_{50}: 0.9 μg/mL). The antiproliferatory effect on the Bel-7402 cells at concentrations of 1–10 μg/mL was associated with the induction of apoptosis and microtubule disassembly.[6,7] Ardisicrenoside-A and ardisicrenoside-M demonstrated a selective inhibition against human NCI-H460 NSCLC cells (IC_{50}: 14.51 and 13.36 μM), and ardisicrenoside-N exerted the cytotoxic effect against MCI-7 and NCI-H460 cancer cells at 11.0 and 22.1 μM concentrations *in vitro*, respectively.[3,4] Also, other saponins assigned as primulanin, cyclaminorin, and cyclamiritin-A also exerted the significant inhibitory effect against human ovarian cancer A2780 cells *in vitro* (IC_{50}: 2.48, 1.51, and 6.40 μg/mL, respectively).[5] The findings clearly disclosed that the triterpenoid saponins are the important cancer inhibitors in the Zhu Sha Geng (Coral Ardisa root), but their anticancer activities need *in vivo* assessment.

Other Constituents

Interestingly, eight other nontriterpenoid constituents, 5-hydro xymethyl-2-furfural, ethyl-β-D-fructopyranoside, n-butyl-β-D-fructofuranoside, n-butyl-α-D-fructofuranoside, methyl-α-D-fructofuranoside, asperulosidic acid, syringic acid, and bergenin as well as ardisiacrispin-B (**2**), have been reported to have positive antitumor metastatic activities. Among them, the significant antimetastatic constituents were demonstrated by 5-hydroxymethyl-2-furfural (**6**), n-butyl-α-D-fructofuranoside (**7**) and ardisiacrispin-B (**2**). At a concentration of 0.8 mg/L, the metastatic inhibitory ratio of n-butyl-α-D-fructofuranoside (**7**) reached to 93.8% in an assay with human MDA-MB-231 breast carcinoma cells.[8] n-Butyl-β-D-fructofuranoside (**8**) was effective in the inhibition of human Bel-7402 hepatoma cells and the induction of cell cycle arrest at G0/G1 phase and apoptosis through the down-expression of Bcl-2 and the up-expression of Bax and p53 activities.[9]

Other Bioactivities

The herb Zhu Sha Geng (Coral Ardisa root) and its saponin constituents exhibited antifertile, antiearly pregnancy, and uterus-stimulating effects in pharmacological experiments.

References

1. Bian, B. L. et al. 2000. Total triterpenoid saponin in Coral Ardisa root or other plants in same family and preparing process thereof. *Faming Zhuanli Shenqing Gongkai Shuomingshu* 5 pp., CN 1999–105451 19990408.

2. Newell, A. M. B. et al. 2010. Comparative in vitro bioactivities of tea extracts from six species of Ardisia and their effect on growth inhibition of HepG2 cells. *J. Ethnopharmacol.* 130: 536–44.
3. Liu, D. L. et al. 2011. Three new triterpenoid saponins from *Ardisia crenata*. *Helv. Chim. Acta* 94: 693–702.
4. Liu, D. L. et al. 2011. A new triterpenoid saponin from the roots of *Ardisia crenata*. *Chin. Chem. Lett.* 22: 957–60.
5. Zheng, Z. F. et al. 2008. Cytotoxic triterpenoid saponins from the roots of *Ardisia crenata*. *J. Asian Nat. Prods. Res.* 10: 833–9.
6. Li, M. et al. 2008. Pro-apoptotic and microtubule-disassembly effects of ardisiacrispin (A+B), triterpenoid saponins from *Ardisia crenata* on human hepatoma Bel-7402 cells. *J. Asian Nat. Prods. Res.* 10: 729–36.
7. Wei, S. Y. et al. 2007. Study on inhibitory effects and mechanism of ardisiacrispin (A+B) on human promyeloleukemic HL-60 cells. *Chin. Pharm. Bull.* 23: 31–5.
8. Wang, X. et al. 2011. Studies on antitumor metastatic constituents from *Ardisia crenata*. *Zhongguo Zhongyao Zazhi* 36: 881–5.
9. Lu, P. et al. 2014. Antiproliferative effects of n-butyl-β-D-fructofuranoside from Kangaisan on Bel-7402 cells. *Ind. J. Pharmacol.* 46: 69–75.

33 Qing Hao 青蒿

Sweet wormwood

1. R = -O-O-
3. R = -O-

(a)

9. R = -O-O-
10. R = -O-

9. R = $-COCH-(C_3H_7)_2$
10. R = $-COCH_3$
11. R = $-COCH_2CH_2CH_3$
12. R = $-CH_2CH-(CH_3)_2$
13. R = $-COC-(CH_3)_3$

(b)

Herb Origination

The herb Qing Hao (Sweet wormwood) is the dried aerial part of a Compositae plant *Artemisia annua* L. The hardy perennial plant is native to temperate Asia, but it is naturalized throughout the world. The herb is normally collected in the autumn just before its flower is in blossom and dried in the shade for folk medicinal practice.

Antitumor Constituents and Activities

According to medicinal documents in China, the herb has been used for the treatment of malaria for over a thousand years. In 1972, in China, a group of sesquiterpene lactone endoperoxides in Qin Hao was finally elucidated as artemisinin (**1**) and its analogs. Besides its antimalarial activity, Qing Hao and its major bioactive principle artemisinin (**1**) were also effective in the growth inhibition of tumor cells.

Sesquiterpene Lactone Endoperoxides

In the *in vitro* assays, artemisinin (**1**) displayed a significant cytotoxicity to many human and murine tumor cell lines such as A549 and ASTC-a-1 (lung), SMMC-7721 and HepG2 (liver), LNCaP (prostate), MCF-7 (breast), HeLa (cervix), HT-29 (colon), and P388 (leukemia) cells. Because cancer cells uptake a relatively larger amount of iron than normal cells, artemisinin (**1**) and its analogs react with iron to form free radicals that kill cells and augment the apoptotic death of the cancer cells.[1–5] The *in vivo* anticancer effect of artemisinin (**1**) and artemisitene (**2**) was proven in murine animal models implanted with Ehrlich ascites carcinoma or fibrosarcoma.[4] The anticancer mechanism of artemisinin (**1**) was found to be correlated with eliciting caspase-dependent but Bax/Bak-independent apoptosis (such as in ASTC-a-1 cells) and eliciting cell cycle arrest by the downregulation of CDK protein and transcript level (such as in SMMC-7721 and LNCaP cells).[1–3] In MCF-7 cells, artemisinin (**1**) effectively blocked the estrogen-dependent cell cycle progression and proliferation by ablating the estrogenic induction of endogenous progesterone receptor transcripts and reducing the ERα protein level and transcripts without altering the ERβ activity.[6] Concurrently, artemisinin (**1**) also selectively declined the cell cycle related to the transcript and reduced the protein levels of CDK-2 and CDK-4 and cyclin-E, cyclin-D1, and E2F1 transcription factors.[7] The effective antigrowth effect in MCF-7 cells was further proved by *in vivo* xenografts in nude mice.[7] In addition, the combination with holotransferrin notably sensitized the antigrowth and apoptotic effects of artemisinin (**1**) on the SMMC-7721 cells.[8]

By inducing the TIMP2 expression and reducing the MMP-2 level, artemisinin (**1**) also significantly suppressed the invasion and metastasis of HepG2 hepatoma cells *in vitro* and *in vivo*, where the E-cadherin activity was enhanced and the Cdc42 was activated, leading to a greater inhibition on cell–cell adhesion and metastasis.[9] Additionally, feeding artemisinin (**1**) markedly obstructed the breast carcinogenesis caused by DMBA in rats, resulting in an obvious attenuation of lower incidence and smaller size of breast tumor.[10] Because deoxy-artemisinin (**3**) presented the much reduced antitumor effect, the endoperoxide group in artemisinin (**1**) was revealed to play a critical role in the cytotoxicity to cancer cells.[4]

Artemisinin–Transferrin Conjugate

The levels of TfRs are usually overexpressed in the cancer cells for Fe-uptake. A conjugate was prepared by covalently tagging artemisinin (**1**) to N-glycoside chains of the transferrin. The produced conjugate was able to enhance the selectivity and the cytotoxic activity of artemisinin (**1**) toward the cancer cells. The conjugate of artemisinin–transferrin killed human DU-145 prostate cancer cells *in vitro* via the promotion of apoptotic mitochondrial pathway.[11] In a rat model implanted with highly metastatic MTLn3 breast cancer, the daily intravenous injections of the conjugate significantly retarded the growth rate of breast tumor cells without obvious side effects.[12] HAIYPRH is a peptide targeted by the TfR, which binds to a cavity on the surface of the TfR. After artemisinin (**1**) was covalently conjugated to the peptide, the HAIYPRH-enabled artemisinin (**1**) was cointernalized with receptor-bound transferrin and the iron was released from the transferrin-activated artemisinin to generate toxic radical species and then to destroy the neoplastic cells. Thus, the conjugate exerted a potent inhibitory effect against Molt-4 leukemia cells with a significantly improved selectivity of cancer cells and normal cells.[13]

Other Terpenoids

Drimartol-A (**4**) and (Z)-7-acetoxy-methyl-11-methyl-3-methylenedodeca-1,6,10-triene were isolated from the cell culture of Qin Hao hairy roots. Both sesquiterpenes exerted a moderate cytotoxicity against HO8910 (ovary), 95-D (lung), QGY (liver), and HeLa (cervix) human neoplastic cell lines.[14,15] Also, (Z)-7-acetoxymethyl-11-methyl-3-methylenedodeca-1,6,10-triene was effective in the inhibition of HeLa cervical cancer cells (IC_{50}: 20.12 μmol/L).[16] The antiproliferative effect on 95-D lung carcinoma cell by drimartol-A (**4**) was revealed to be associated with the induction of G2 cell cycle arrest and apoptosis of the 95-D cells through a mitochondrial-dependent pathway.[14]

Phenols and Flavonoids

The contents of the total phenols and the flavonoids in the Qin Hao leaves were about twofold higher than those in the Qin Hao stems. In an *in vitro* assay, phenol- and flavonoid-rich ethanolic extracts of the leaves displayed a marked antigrowth activity against four human cancer cells, and the growth inhibitory rates were 76.26% and 52.59% on MCF-7 and MDA-MB-231 breast cancer cells at a 0.25 mg/mL concentration and 61.07% and 57.24% on HeLa cervix cancer cells and AGS gastric cancer cells at a 0.5 mg/mL concentration, respectively.[17,18] The ethanolic extract also displayed significant antioxidant, DPPH radical-scavenging, and tyrosinase-inhibiting activities.[17,18] A flavonoid ingredient assigned as quercetagetin 6,7,3′,4′-tetramethyl ether (**5**) was separated from the Qin Hao, showing an obvious cytotoxic activity against a group of tumor cell lines, A549, HT-29, MCF-7, KB, and P388, *in vitro*.[19]

Coumarins

Three alkyl *trans*-p-coumarates derived from Qin Hao were potent inhibitors of human Topos, which both restrained the growth of human HCT-116 colon cancer cells. Among the three compounds, docosyl *trans*-p-coumarate (**6**) was the strongest inhibitor on the colon cancer cells and the Topo-II activity, where docosyl *trans*-p-coumarate (**6**) arrested the cell cycle at G2/M phases and induced the apoptosis in p53(+/+)-HCT116 cells, but it was inactive on the cell cycle of p53(-/-) HCT116 colon cancer cells.[20]

Polysaccharides

The antitumor effect of the polysaccharide components (HQG) prepared from Qin Hao was demonstrated in mice implanted with tumor cells (S180, EAC, or Heps). The growth inhibitory rates of HQG at an intravenous dose of 100 mg/kg (every two days for eight days) were 46.41% for S180, 51.19% in EAC cells, and 56.75% in Heps cells with low acute toxicity.[21] HQG exerted inhibitory effects against the cell growth and the mitochondrial membrane potential in human 7402 hepatoma cells *in vitro*. In an *in vivo* model, HQG not only retarded the growth of H22 hepatoma cells and facilitated the cell apoptosis, but also improved immunodefense such as the enhancement of $CD4^+$ and $CD8^+$ T lymphocytes subpopulation and the increase of IFNγ and IL-4 secretion in the spleen lymphocytes of the host.[22]

Essential Oil

The essential oil of Qing Hao was also an interesting source of carcinoma inhibitor for it can induce the apoptosis of human SMMC-7721 hepatoma cells *in vitro*. The treatment of the SMMC-7721 cells with the essential oil in a 100 μg/mL concentration for 24 h elicited a series of apoptosis-related morphological changes such as DNA ladder pattern, exhibition of sub-G1 peak, fragmentation of nuclear chromatin, and condensation of cytoplasm.[23]

Structure Modification

For the optimization of the anticancer property with a lower side effect, the structural modification of artemisinin (**1**) has been extensively explored. Artesunate (ART) (**7**) and dihydroartemisinin (**8**) are two of the most important semisynthetic derivatives developed from artemisinin (**1**). Both derivatives were considered as potential therapeutic candidates for further improvement to treat cancer patients in clinics.

Artesunate

ART (**7**) displayed a wider range of cytotoxic effects on a large panel of human cancer cells in NCI, United States. The most potent inhibitory activity of ART (**7**) was established on leukemia and colon cancer cell lines (GI_{50}: 1.11 and 2.13 μM, respectively), while NSCLC cells showed the lowest sensitivity toward ART (GI_{50}: 25.62 μM). Intermediate GI_{50} values were observed for the carcinoma of skin, breast, ovarian, prostate, CNS, and kidney.[24] The *in vitro* and *in vivo* tests demonstrated that ART (**7**) was effective in the inhibition of the growth of osteosarcoma (HOS), pancreatic carcinoma (BxPC-3, CFPAC-1, and Panc-1), and colorectal carcinoma. But the cytotoxic mechanisms in the three types of human cancer were found to be quite different,[25–27] whose effect was achieved by ART (**7**) mainly through (1) the induction of oncosis-like cell death for human pancreatic cancer cells,[27] (2) a hyperactive Wnt/β-catenin signaling pathway for human colorectal cancer cells,[27] and (3) an intrinsic apoptotic pathway for human osteosarcoma cells.[25] ART (**7**) also exerted the evident cytotoxicity to human SMMC-7721 hepatoma cells *in vitro* (IC_{50}: 2.07–2.48 μg/mL). In the treatment with ART (**7**) at an oral dose of 300 mg/kg per day for seven days, the growth of murine H22 hepatoma cells was obviously suppressed by 46.6–49.1%, and the survival of the tested mice was prolonged by 45%.[28] By disturbing the cell cycle progression and accelerating the apoptotic death, ART (**7**) obstructed the cell growth of mouse SP2/0 myeloma, human HEC-1B endometrial cancer, human A431 epidermal squamous cancer, human MCF-7 breast cancer, and human HeLa cervical carcinoma.[29–33] The apoptotic mechanism of ART (**7**) in the three breast carcinoma cell lines (MCF-7, T47D, and MDA-MB-231) was triggered by a hierarchical signaling from the lysosomes to the mitochondria and a production of iron-catalyzed lysosomal ROS.[34] Also, ART (**7**) could synergistically potentiate the antitumor activity of 5-FU in the *in vivo* study.[28] However, the drug resistance was elicited in the ART (**7**)-treated highly metastatic MDA-MB-231 cells.[35]

Moreover, ART (**7**) is a powerful inducer of oxidative DNA damage. It provoked a DNA damage response with phosphorylation of ATM, ATR, Chk1, and Chk and induced oxidative DNA lesions and DNA double strand breaks, which are all involved in the mechanism for triggering tumor cell death. After the ART treatment, the oxidative DNA damage was dose dependently observed in human LN-229 glioblastoma cells in parallel with the cell death executed by apoptosis and necrosis.[36,37] Similarly, through the induction of oxidative DNA damage, ART (**7**) exerted the inhibitory effect against the growth of xenografted Kaposi's sarcoma in mice.[37] Prominently, ART (**7**) displayed potential antiinvasive, antimetastatic, and antiangiogenic activities. The angiogenic ability of K562 CML cells and RPMI8226 multiple myeloma cells was effectively restrained by ART (**7**) in time- and dose-dependent patterns, associated with the decrease of the VEGF level and the expression and the blockage of ERK1/2 activation and Ang-1 expression.[38,39] The antiangiogenic effect of ART was also proven in nude mice implanted with human HO-8910 ovarian cancer, where the microvessel density and the cell growth were markedly diminished by the ART treatment with no apparent toxicity. Also, the inhibition of VEGF expression and KDR/flk-1 expression was acted in both carcinoma cells and endothelial cells, and the activities of NF-κB and IKKα (a NF-κB activator) were obviously repressed during the treatment.[40–42] ART (**7**) showed a significant ability to impair the Matrigel invasion and the metastasis in six NSCLC cells by means of specifically obstructing MMP-2 and MMP-7 and transcription of urokinase plasminogen activator (u-PA).[43] Moreover, ART (**7**) synergized with DOX to elicit a ROS-mediated apoptotic death in DOX-resistant T leukemia cells.[44] But the drug cross-resistant action had been found in ART (**7**) in the experiments by using a CEM leukemia cell subline, which also showed the resistance to either anticancer agents, DOX, VCR, and methotrexate.[23]

Consequently, these established data clearly suggested that ART (**7**) is a promising drug candidate and an adjunct to standard chemotherapeutic agents for further development.

Dihydroartemisinin

Dihydroartemisinin (DHA) (**8**), another semisynthetic derivative of artemisinin, displayed a promising anticancer activity with low toxicity. DHA (**8**) was markedly effective in the viability diminution of three types of human lung adenocarcinoma cells (SPC-A-1, PC-14, and ASTC-a-1) and four types of human hepatoma cells (BEL-7402, HepG2, PLC/PRF/5, and Hep3B) *in vitro* with apoptosis promotion.[45–48] But the studies further revealed that the apoptotic signaling in the three lung carcinoma cells was progressed in the different pathways. DHA (**8**)-induced apoptotic signaling pathway in the PC-14 cells was mainly triggered by Ca^{2+} increase and p38 activation, while the raised calcium level and the reduced survivin were related to the enhancement of the SPC-A-1 cell-programmed death.[47,48] The ASTC-a-1 cell apoptosis was provoked by DHA mainly by promoting a ROS-mediated caspase-8/Bid activation and a caspase-3-dependent mitochondrial pathway.[48] The significant antigrowth effect of DHA (**8**) in the HCC *in vitro* and *in vivo* was clearly correlated to its ability in the elicitation of cell cycle arrest and apoptosis. The activation of p21 protein and the inhibition of cyclin-B and CDC25C mainly contributed to the DHA-induced G2/M arrest and the caspase-dependent mitochondrial pathway in the HCC.[45] Furthermore, the i.p. injection of DHA to nude mouse models resulted in a significant inhibition of HCC xenograft hepatomas.[48] DHA (**8**) also exerted the anticancer activity on human U937 leukemic monocyte lymphoma *in vitro* and *in vivo*. A pronounced increase in apoptotic death and a clear decrease in cell growth were observed in both transformed and primary U937 cells after the DHA treatment, whose effect is mechanistically involved in the inactivation of MEK/ERK, the downregulation of Mcl-1, the release of cytochrome c, and the activation of caspases, but no such events happened in normal peripheral blood mononuclear cells.[49,50] Recently, DHA (**8**) has been investigated in lung cancer cells and leukemia cells. By markedly inducing the apoptosis, DHA potently killed human Molt-4 lymphoblastoid leukemia cells. When 20 μM of DHA (**8**) was combined with sodium butyrate, all Molt-4 cells were destroyed at a 24 h time point but showed a lower effect on normal human lymphocytes.[51,52]

Likewise, the proliferation of four human osteosarcoma cell lines could be blocked by the DHA (**8**) treatment via the induction of apoptosis and cell cycle arrest, but p53 wild-type osteosarcoma cells were more sensitive to DHA (**8**).[53] By the DHA (**8**) treatment, the proliferation, the adhesion, the invasion, and the migration of human HO8910PM ovarian cancer cells were markedly suppressed *in vitro* and *in vivo* in association with downregulating the expressions of pFAK, MMP-2, and Von Willebrand factor as well as diminishing macrophage infiltration.[54] Interestingly, DHA (**8**) was also found to have a potent ability in influencing the lymphatic endothelial cell behavior. At its 10 μg/mL concentration, DHA (**8**) significantly elicited the apoptosis and inhibited the migration and tube-like formation of the lymphatic endothelial cells, indicating that DHA (**8**) is a potential inhibitor on the lymph angiogenesis.[55] In addition, both DHA (**8**) and ART (**7**) were also able to synergize the β-ray radiosensitization on two human U87 and CHG-5 glioma cells, whose inhibitory activity was greater than the parent molecule, artemisinin (**1**) for five to seven times.[56]

Taken together, the investigations have provided the extensive evidences to support DHA (**8**) as a potential drug candidate for clinical development in the treatment of neoplasm.

Other Derivatives

Two semisynthesized dimers of dihydroartemisinin (**9** and **10**) displayed a specific cytotoxicity on Ehrlich ascites cancer and HeLa cervical cancer cells *in vitro*. The inhibitory potencies were about 100 times more potent than that of artemisinin (**1**). The IC_{50} values ranged between 10^{-1}–10^{-2} µg/mL against the proliferation of human carcinomas in the colon, the skin, the prostate, the breast, the ovary, the lung, the brain, and the kidney as well as leukemia, *in vitro*.[4] Other four derivatives originated from the modification of artemisinin-B exhibited remarkable suppressive effects against the growth of P388 leukemia and SGC-7901 gastric cancer cell lines, whose inhibitory rates reached to 82–100%.[57,58] Eight artemisinin derivatives (AD1-AD8) have been synthesized and evaluated by using *in vitro* models of liver and colon cancer cell lines. After being treated with the derivatives for 6 and 72 h periods, it was revealed that AD5 (**9**) exerted a greater antiproliferative effect (IC_{50}: 1–5 µM) on all tested HepG2 hepatoma, SK-HEP-1 hepatoma, and LS174T colon cancer cell lines but showed low acute toxicity, whereas AD2 (**10**), AD3 (**11**), AD4 (**12**), and AD6 (**13**) selectively repressed the proliferation of SK-HEP-1 hepatoma cells (IC_{50}: 2–10 µM).[59]

Clinical Trials

Sixty patients with advanced NSCLC had been treated with NP (a chemotherapy regimen of vinorelbine and cisplatin), combined with ART (**7**) (120 mg, once a day by intravenous administration), leading to the elevation of short-term survival rate and prolonged life duration of the patients.[60] One patient with stage IV metastatic uveal melanoma experienced a stabilization of the disease after the combinational therapy with dacarbazine and ART (**7**), followed by objective regressions of splenic and lung metastases and positive survival time.[61]

Other Bioactivities and Side Effects

Qing Hao (Sweet wormwood) is an herb traditionally used in Chinese medicine for exerting antipyretic, antiinflammatory, antiviral, antimalarial, antiparasitic, immunomodulating, and antibacterial effects. The herb and its major component artemisinin (**1**) are nontoxic at therapeutic doses. Only very few side effects have been reported in the clinical treatments. However, artemisinin (**1**) and artemisitene (**2**) also showed cytotoxicity on murine bone marrow CFU-GM. The SAR studies revealed that the endoperoxide group also plays a role in the cytotoxicity to the CFU-GM cells.[4] High doses of artemisinin (**1**) might suppress hematopoiesis and cause cardiac, renal, and hepatic toxicities in monkey models.[54]

References

1. Wang, G. L. et al. 2005. Investigation on the molecular mechanisms of anti-hepatocarcinoma herbs of traditional Chinese medicine by cell cycle microarray. *Zhongguo Zhongyao Zazhi* 30: 50–4.
2. Xiao, F. L. et al. 2011. Artemisinin induces caspase-8/9-mediated and Bax/Bak-independent apoptosis in human lung adenocarcinoma (ASTC-a-1) cells. *J. X-Ray Sci. Technol.* 19: 545–55.
3. Willoughby, J. A. et al. 2009. Artemisinin blocks prostate cancer growth and cell cycle progression by disrupting Sp1 interactions with the cyclin-dependent kinase-4 (CDK4) promoter and inhibiting CDK4 gene expression. *J. Biol. Chem.* 284: 2203–13.
4. Beekman, A. C. et al. 1998. Artemisinin-derived sesquiterpene lactones as potential antitumor compounds, cytotoxic action against bone marrow and tumor cells. *Planta Med.* 64: 615–9.
5. Jung, M. et al. 2004. Recent advances in artemisinin and its derivatives as antimalarial and antitumor agents. *Curr. Med. Chem.* 11: 1265–84.
6. Sundar, S. N. et al. 2008. Artemisinin selectively decreases functional levels of estrogen receptor-alpha and ablates estrogen-induced proliferation in human breast cancer cells. *Carcinogenesis* 29: 2252–8.
7. Tin, A. S. et al. 2012. Antiproliferative effects of artemisinin on human breast cancer cells requires the downregulated expression of the E2F1 transcription factor and loss of E2F1-target cell cycle genes. *Anti-Cancer Drugs* 23: 370–9.
8. Deng, X. R. et al. 2013. Holotransferrin enhances selective anticancer activity of artemisinin against human hepatocellular carcinoma cells. *J. Huazhong Univ. Sci. Tech., Med. Sci.* 33: 862–5.
9. Tan, W. F. et al. 2011. Artemisinin inhibits in vitro and in vivo invasion and metastasis of human hepatocellular carcinoma cells. *Phytomed.* 18: 158–62.
10. Lai, H. et al. 2006. Oral artemisinin prevents and delays the development of 7,12-dimethylbenz [a] anthracene (DMBA)-induced breast cancer in the rat. *Cancer Lett.* 231: 43–8.
11. Nakase, I. et al. 2009. Transferrin receptor-dependent cytotoxicity of artemisinin-transferrin conjugates on prostate cancer cells and induction of apoptosis. *Cancer Lett.* 274: 290–8.
12. Lai, H. et al. 2009. Artemisinin-transferrin conjugate retards growth of breast tumors in the rat. *Anticancer Res.* 29: 3807–10.
13. Oh, S. et al. 2009. Synthesis and anticancer activity of covalent conjugates of artemisinin and a transferrin-receptor targeting peptide. *Cancer Lett.* 274: 33–9.
14. Zhai, D. D. et al. 2010. Inhibition of tumor cell proliferation and induction of apoptosis in 95-D lung cancer cells by drimartol A from hairy root cultures of Artemisia annua. *Latin Am. J. Pharmacy* 29: 1159–65.
15. Zhai, D. D. et al. 2010. Inhibition of tumor cell proliferation and induction of apoptosis in human lung carcinoma 95-D cells by a new sesquiterpene from hairy root cultures of Artemisia annua. *Phytomed.* 17: 856–61.
16. Zhai, D. D. et al. 2010. A new sesquiterpene from hairy root culture of *Artemisia annua*. *Chin. Chem. Lett.* 21: 590–2.
17. Ryu, J. et al. 2011. Nutritional properties and biological activities of *Artemisia annua*. *Han'guk Sikp'um Yongyang Kwahak Hoechi* 40: 163–70.

18. Ryu, J. et al. 2011. Antioxidant and anticancer activities of *Artemisia annua* L. and determination of functional compounds. *Han'guk Sikp'um Yongyang Kwahak Hoechi* 40: 509–16.
19. Zheng, G. Q. et al. 1994. Cytotoxic terpenoids and flavonoids from *Artemisia annua*. *Planta Med.* 60: 54–7.
20. Mizushina, Y. et al. 2010. Inhibitory effects of docosyl p-coumarate on DNA topoiso-merase activity and human cancer cell growth. *Intl. J. Oncol.* 37: 993–1000.
21. Xue, M. et al. 2008. Experimental study on antitumor effect of polysaccharides from *Artemisia annua* L. *Shizhen Guoyi Guoyao* 19: 937–8.
22. Chen, J. Y. et al. 2014. Antitumour effects of polysaccharides isolated from *Artemisia annua* L. by inducing cell apoptosis and immunomodulatory anti-hepatoma effects of polysaccharides. *Afri. J. Tradit. Complem. Altern. Med.* 11: 15–22.
23. Li, Y. et al. 2004. Induction of apoptosis of cultured hepatocarcinoma cell by essential oil of *Artemisia annua* L. *Sichuan Daxue Xuebao. Yixue Ban* 35: 337–9.
24. Efferth, T. et al. 2001. The anti-malarial artesunate is also active against cancer. *Intl. J. Oncol.* 18: 767–73.
25. Xu, Q. et al. 2011. Artesunate inhibits growth and induces apoptosis in human osteosarcoma HOS cell line in vitro and in vivo. *J. Zhejiang Univ. (Sci. B)* 12: 247–55.
26. Du, J. H. et al. 2010. Artesunate induces oncosis-like cell death in vitro and has antitumor activity against pancreatic cancer xenografts in vivo. *Cancer Chemother. Pharmacol.* 65: 895–902.
27. Li, L. N. et al. 2007. Artesunate attenuates the growth of human colorectal carcinoma and inhibits hyperactive Wnt/β-catenin pathway. *Intl. J. Cancer* 121: 1360–5.
28. Wang, Q. et al. 2001. Experimental studies of antitumor effect of artesunate on liver cancer. *Zhongguo Zhongyao Zazhi* 26: 707–8, 720.
29. Li, S. H. et al. 2009. Effect of artesunate on inhibiting proliferation and inducing apoptosis of SP2/0 myeloma cells through affecting NF-κB p65. *Intl. J. Hematol.* 90: 513–21.
30. Li, S. H. et al. 2007. Strong suppression of SP2/0 myeloma cell proliferation and enhanced apoptosis by artesunate. *Zhongchengyao* 29: 434–5.
31. Wang, L. J. et al. 2010. Effect of artesunate on human endometrial carcinoma HEC-1B cells. *J. Med. Colleges of PLA* 25: 143–51.
32. Jiang, Z. Y. et al. 2009. Artesunate inhibits proliferation and apoptosis of epidermal squamous cell line A431. *Di-San Junyi Daxue Xuebao* 31: 615–8.
33. Wu, X. Y. et al. 2007. Experimental study of artesunate on antitumor effect of Hela cells. *Zhongguo Yaoye* 16: 6–7.
34. Hamacher-Brady, A. et al. 2011. Artesunate activates mitochondrial apoptosis in breast cancer cells via iron-catalyzed lysosomal reactive oxygen species production. *J. Biol. Chem.* 286: 6587–601.
35. Bachmeier, B. et al. 2011. Development of resistance towards artesunate in MDA-MB-231 human breast cancer cells. *PLoS One* 6: e20550.
36. Berdelle, N. et al. 2011. Artesunate induces oxidative DNA damage, sustained DNA double-strand breaks, and the ATM/ATR damage response in cancer cells. *Mol. Cancer Therap.* 10: 2224–33.
37. Li, P. C. H. et al. 2008. Artesunate derived from traditional Chinese medicine induces DNA damage and repair. *Cancer Res.* 68: 4347–51.
38. Zhou, H. J. et al. 2007. Artesunate inhibits angiogenesis and downregulates vascular endothelial growth factor expression in chronic myeloid leukemia K562 cells. *Vascular Pharmacol.* 47: 131–8.
39. Chen, H. et al. 2010. Artesunate inhibiting angiogenesis induced by human myeloma RPMI8226 cells. *Intl. J. Hematol.* 92: 587–97.
40. Chen, H. H. et al. 2004. Inhibitory effects of artesunate on angiogenesis and on expressions of vascular endothelial growth factor and VEGF receptor KDR/flk-1. *Pharmacol.* 71: 1–9.
41. Yance, D. R. Jr. 2006. Targeting angiogenesis with integrative cancer therapies. *Integrative Cancer Therapies* 5: 9–29.
42. Wang, W. Q. et al. 2011. Effects of artesunate on inhibition of NF-κB activity in K562 cells. *Zhonghua Zhongyiyao Xuekan* 29: 1655–7.
43. Rasheed, S. A. K. et al. 2010. First evidence that the antimalarial drug artesunate inhibits invasion and in vivo metastasis in lung cancer by targeting essential extracellular proteases. *Intl. J. Cancer* 127: 1475–85.
44. Efferth, T. et al. 2007. Artesunate induces ROS-mediated apoptosis in doxorubicin-resistant T leukemia cells. *PLoS One* 2: e693.
45. Mu, D. G. et al. 2008. The role of calcium, P38 MAPK in dihydroartemisinin-induced apoptosis of lung cancer PC-14 cells. *Cancer Chemother. Pharmacol.* 61: 639–45.
46. Lu, J. J. et al. 2012. Dihydroartemisinin-induced inhibition of proliferation in BEL-7402 cells: An analysis of the mitochondrial proteome. *Mol. Med. Reports* 6: 429–33.
47. Zhang, C. Z. Y. et al. 2012. Dihydroartemisinin exhibits antitumor activity toward hepatocellular carcinoma in vitro and in vivo. *Biochem. Pharmacol.* 83: 1278–89.
48. Lu, Y. Y. et al. 2010. Single-cell analysis of dihydroartemisinin-induced apoptosis through reactive oxygen species-mediated caspase-8 activation and mitochondrial pathway in ASTC-a-1 cells using fluorescence imaging techniques. *J. Biomed. Optics* 15: 046028/1–046028/16.
49. Gao, N. et al. 2011. Interruption of the MEK/ERK signaling cascade promotes dihydroartemisinin-induced apoptosis in vitro and in vivo. *Apoptosis* 16: 511–23.
50. Wang, J. et al. 2007. Induction of apoptosis and inhibition of cell migration and tube-like formation by dihydroartemisinin in murine lymphatic endothelial cells. *Pharmacol.* 80: 207–18.
51. Singh, N. P. et al. 2004. (a) Artemisinin induces apoptosis in human cancer cells. *Anticancer Res.* 24: 2277–80; 2005. (b) Synergistic cytotoxicity of artemisinin and sodium butyrate on human cancer cells. *Anticancer Res.* 25: 4325–31; 2011. (c) Cytotoxicity of ethanolic extracts of Artemisia annua to Molt-4 human leukemia cells. *Planta Med.* 77: 1788–93.
52. Chan, H. W. et al. 2013. Cytotoxicity of dihydroartemisinin toward molt-4 cells attenuated by N-tertbutyl-alpha-phenylnitrone and deferoxamine. *Anticancer Res.* 33: 4389–94.
53. Ji, Y. et al. 2011. Antitumor effects of dihydroartemisinin on human osteosarcoma. *Mol. Cell. Biochem.* 351: 99–108.
54. Wu, B. C. et al. 2012. Dihydroartiminisin inhibits the growth and metastasis of epithelial ovarian cancer. *Oncol. Reports* 27: 101–8.
55. Mu, D. G. et al. 2007. Calcium and survivin are involved in the induction of apoptosis by dihydroartemisinin in human lung

cancer SPC-A-1 cells. *Methods and Findings in Experimental and Clinical Pharmacol.* 29: 33–8.

56. Dong, J. Q. et al. 2010. Artesunate enhances radiosensitivity of human glioma cell line CHG-5 to β-ray. *Di-San Junyi Daxue Xuebao* 32: 588–92.
57. Sun, W. C. et al. 1992. Antitumor activities of 4 derivatives of artemisic acid and artemisinin B in vitro. *Zhongguo Yaoli Xuebao* 13: 541–3.
58. Woerdenbag, H. J. et al. 1994. Progress in the research of artemisinin-related antimalarials. *Pharmacy World Sci.* 16: 169–80.
59. Blazquez, A. G. et al. 2013. Novel artemisinin derivatives with potential usefulness against liver/colon cancer and viral hepatitis. *Bioorg. Med. Chem.* 21: 4432–41.
60. Zhang, Z. Y. et al. 2008. Artesunate combined with vinorelbine plus cisplatin in treatment of advanced non-small cell lung cancer: A randomized controlled trial. *Zhongxiyi Jiehe Xuebao* 6: 134–8.
61. Berger, T. G. et al. 2005. Artesunate in the treatment of metastatic uveal melanoma-first experiences. *Oncol. Reports* 14: 1599–603.

34 Huang Qin 黄芩

Baikal skullcap

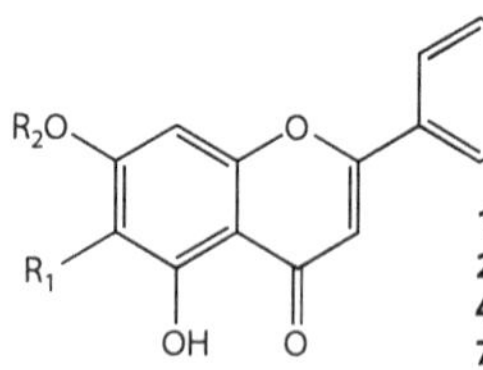

1. R_1 = –OH, R_2 = –glucose
2. R_1 = –OH, R_2 = –H
4. R_1 = –OCH_3, R_2 = –H
7. R_1 = R_2 = –H

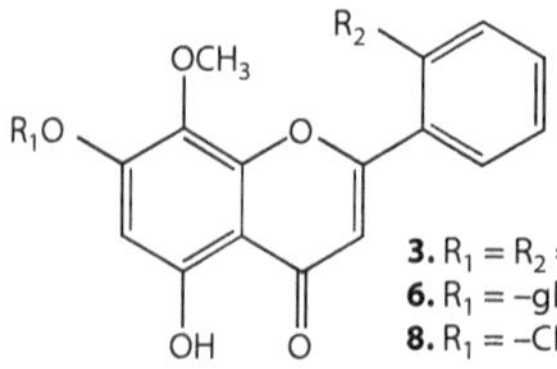

3. R_1 = R_2 = –H
6. R_1 = –glucose, R_2 = –H
8. R_1 = –CH_3, R_2 = –OH

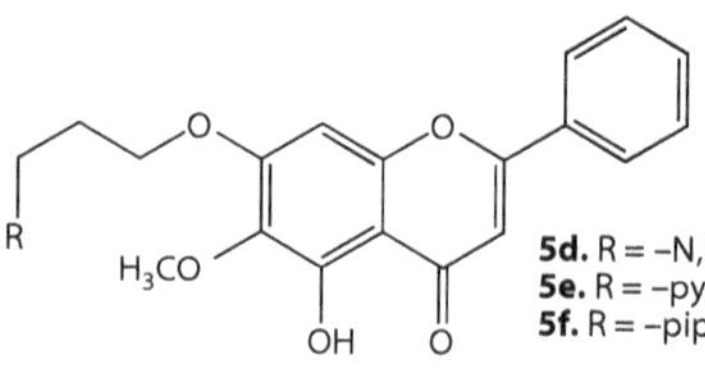

5d. R = –N,N-diethylamine
5e. R = –pyrrolidine
5f. R = –piperidine

Herb Origination

The herb Huang Qin (Baikal skullcap), one of the 50 fundamental herbs historically employed in traditional Chinese medicine, has long been used as an official and traditional medicine in the northeast Asian region. The herb usually refers to the dried roots of a Labiatae plant *Scutellaria baicalensis*. The perennial plant is native to Mongolia, North China, Siberia, and Korea. Three other similar plants *S. viscidula*, *S. amoena*, and *S. likiangensis* are also the source for producing the herb in China, but Baikal skullcap (*S. baicalensis*) is the most common origin.

Antitumor Activities

The Huang Qin extract is clinically used in Chinese medicine as an adjuvant to the chemotherapy of cancer patients. An *in vitro* assay demonstrated that its water extract dose dependently restrained the proliferation of various types of human cancer cell lines such as HepG2 (liver), MCF-7 (breast), KM-12 and HCT-15 (colon), KB and SCC-15 (squamous), LNCaP (androgen-dependent prostate), and PC3 (androgen-independent prostate) cells. However, the inhibition was low, and the IC_{50} ranged between 0.15 and 1.5 mg/mL.[1–4] The anticancer effect was reported to be associated with the suppression of cyclins/CDKs and COX-2/PGE2 pathways and the downregulation of ETS1, Cdc25B, p63, ERK1/2, EGFR, XIAP, HIF-2α, and Cdc25C in treatment. Its ethanolic extract was effective in the inhibition of three human lung cancer cell lines (A549, SK-LU-1, and SK-MES-1) with moderate to weak potencies (IC_{50}: 57.2–102.1 μg/mL) but showed no such effect in normal human lung fibroblasts.[3] The extract treatment induced cell cycle arrest and apoptosis of the lung cancer cell lines through the upregulation of p53 and Bax, exerting an antiproliferative effect.[5] The water extract exerted a 50% reduction of prostate carcinoma volume in a mouse model after a seven-week treatment period.[3] *Scutellaria baicalensis* water extract (SBWE), a water extract of the herb, also promoted a strong protective effect against MMP-2-mediated motility/metastasis and retarded the proliferation in the A549 cells through the downregulation of cyclin-D1, indicating that the herb is useful for the chemotherapy of lung cancer.[6]

The herb dimethyl sulfoxide (DMSO) extract was sensitive to hematopoietic cancer cell lines such as NCI-H929 myeloma, Nalm-6 lymphocytic leukemia, Daudi lymphoma, and HL-60 myeloid leukemia. The DMSO extract treatment in a dose of 50 μg/mL for 48 h elicited the hematopoietic cancer cells to early apoptosis and retarded the cell clonal growth, associated with mitochondrial damage, depressed Bcl family of genes, increased level of CDK inhibitor p27(KIP1), and decreased level of c-myc oncogene, and showed the ED_{50} data from 4.57 to 12.3 μg/mL.[7] Also, the proliferation of human THP-1 monocytic leukemia and HOS osteogenic sarcoma cells was obstructed *in vitro* by its methanolic extract treatment.[8] In an *in vivo* model, the oral administration of the Scutellariae radix extract at a daily dose of 10 mg per mouse for 10 days resulted in a significant inhibition of tumor growth of MBT-2 bladder cancer cells in mice.[9]

Moreover, the herb can be used to improve the clinical efficacy of chemotherapy and to reduce the drug toxicity. The cotreatment with the extract (300 μg/mL) obviously enlarged the inhibition rate of cisplatin (5 μg/mL) from 15.8 to 37.3% and promoted the apoptotic rate from 15.1 to 42.2% against human SKOV-3 ovarian cancer cells.[10] In the combination with CTX, the extract not only enhanced the antimetastatic effect in mice grafted with Lewis lung carcinoma but also modulated the cytotoxicities of NK cells and peritoneal macrophages.[11] If the extract is integrated with 1,3-bis(2-chloroethyl)-1-nitrosourea (BCNU), the inhibitory effect of BCNU could be enhanced against the growth of primary, recurrent, and drug-resistant malignant glioma cells, which were derived from three patients with glioblasfomas multiforme.[12] Also, the methanolic extract of Scutellariae radix significantly induced a QR activity in murine Hepa1c1c7 hepatoma cells in a dose-dependent manner.[13] In a clinical test, the administration of 88 patients with lung cancer during anticarcinoma chemotherapy with the herb preparation displayed hemopoiesis stimulation, intensification of bone marrow erythro- and granulocytopoiesis, and increase in the content of circulating precursors of the type of erythroid and granulomonocytic colony-forming units.[14] By inducing the cell cycle arrest at G2/M stage and activating ERK-dependent apoptosis via Bax and caspase pathway, its ethanolic extract plays a central role in inhibiting the liver fibrogenesis.[15] The evidences indicated that the extract is a readily available chemopreventive medicine against liver carcinogenesis.

Therefore, the investigations suggested that Huang Qin should be developed as an adjuvant in the combination with chemotherapy to clinical trials against various malignancies. In addition, a methanolic extract of the plant leaves displayed a dose-dependent antigrowth effect against human LoVo colon carcinoma cells.[16] The leaf extracts of the four close plants *S. angulosa*, *S. integrifolia*, *S. ocmulgee*, and *S. scandens* were also found to have the marked anticancer activities.[17]

Antitumor Constituents and Activities

The anticancer activity of *S. baicalensis* was mostly contributed by four major flavonoid constituents, i.e., baicalin (**1**), baicalein (**2**), wogonin (**3**), and oroxylin-A (**4**). The total flavonoid fraction (TFSB) demonstrated a moderate antiproliferation activity against murine sarcoma 180, HepA22 ascites hepatoma and human Bcap-37 breast cancer, HCT-116 and HT-29 colorectal cancer cell lines *in vitro*. The TFSB induced S and G2/M cell cycle arrests and apoptotic death of the HCT116 and HT-29 cells.[18,19] The *in vivo* antitumor activity of TFSB was shown in mouse models implanted with sarcoma 180, HepA22 hepatoma, or U14 cervical cancer,[19] where TFSB concomitantly enhanced G0/G1 cell cycle arrest and apoptosis of U14 cervical cancer cells.[20]

Despite holding similar molecules, the four major flavonoids, baicalin (**1**), baicalein (**2**), wogonin (**3**), and oroxylin-A (**4**), showed not quite the same characteristics in cancer suppression. Each of them has been investigated in the continuous efforts.

Baicalin

The content of baicalin (**1**) in Huang Qin highly reached to 21%. Structurally, baicalin (**1**) is a monoglucuronide of baicalein (**2**); thus, it can be converted to baicalein (**2**) by β-glucuronidase. *In vitro* and *in vivo* investigations have evidenced the apoptosis induction-related anticancer activity of baicalin. The treatment of four human prostate cancer cell lines (DU-145, PC3, LNCaP, and CA-HPV-10) with baicalin (**1**) for two to four days suppressed the proliferation of these prostate cancer cells *in vitro*. Relatively, the response of baicalin (**1**) was most sensitive to the DU-145 cells and was most resistant to the LNCaP cells. At a concentration of 150 μM, baicalin (**1**) restrained 50% of the DU-145 cells.[21] By activating an intrinsic (mitochondrial) pathway and regulating a PI3K/serine/threonine kinase signaling pathway, the exposure of baicaline (**1**) (10 μM) for 48 h obviously promoted the apoptosis and markedly suppressed the proliferation and colony formation of CA46 Burkitt lymphoma cells.[22] Baicalin (**1**) also demonstrated a cytotoxic effect on human HL-60 promyelocytic leukemia cells and concurrently elicited the HL-60 cells to apoptosis via multiple pathways, i.e., (1) augmented the levels of ROS and Ca^{2+} and decreased the levels of Grp78 and Bcl-2; (2) promoted the levels of Gadd153 and Bax; (3) reduced mitochondrial membrane potential and elicited the release of cytochrome c and activated caspase-3 and caspase-12.[23] The treatment with baicalin-enriched extract reduced the viability of peripheral blood leukocytes (PBLs) obtained from patients with ALL but showed no impact on healthy leukocytes. In the assays, the extract stimulated the cell apoptosis of B-type human leukemia line (NALM-6) and PBLs in marrow cells of ALL children, accompanied with the up-expression of annexin-V. By increasing IFNγ production in PBLs and decreasing TNFα and IL-10 production, the baicalin extract exerted immune system modulation in ALL patients and also protected PBLs and marrow cells to vesicular stomatitis virus infection.[24]

Likewise, the growth-inhibiting and apoptosis-inducing effects of baicalin (**1**) were also observed in a highly metastatic human Mc3 mucoepidermoid cancer cells *in vitro* and *in vivo*.[25] Baicalin (**1**) at a 1 μg/mL concentration significantly diminished the percentage of survival of two human KU-1 and EJ-1 bladder neoplastic cell lines and a murine MBT-2 bladder carcinoma cell line *in vitro*. The IC_{50} values of baicalin (**1**) were 3.4 μg/mL in the KU-1 cells, 4.4 μg/mL in the EJ-1 cells, and 0.93 μg/mL in the MBT-2 cells.[9] The daily i.p. administration of baicalin (**1**) in doses of 15–60 mg/kg for 21 days markedly inhibited the growth of gallbladder cancer cell xenografts in nude mice and prolonged the survival time of tested mice, whose effect was closely related to the induction of the cell apoptosis via a mitochondrial-mediated pathway, i.e., downregulation of Bcl-2, upregulation of Bax, inhibition of NF-κB nuclear translocation, and activation of caspase-3 and caspase-9 expression.[25] Moreover, oral administrations of baicalin (**1**) in a dose of 200 mg/kg per day promoted the apoptosis and inhibited the growth of C6 glioma cells, then prolonged the life of tumor-bearing mice. Its apoptotic mechanism in the C6 cells is probably correlated with the downregulation of mutant p53 activity.[25] Baicalin (**1**) also acted as a preventive agent to hinder the carcinogenesis in liver, whose effect was mediated by its time- and dose-dependent potentiations of QR mRNA levels in Hepa 1c1c7 cells.[15] However, baicalin (**1**) showed a low response to human HCT-116 and HT-29 colorectal cancer cells and human PaCa pancreas cancer cells *in vitro*[18] and even increased the growth of human MCF-7 breast cancer cells in its certain concentrations.[26]

Baicalein

In Vitro *Antitumor and Apoptosis-Inducing Effects*

The antiproliferative effect of baicalein (**2**) was shown in a variety of human tumor cell lines including pancreatic cancer (PaCa), esophageal cancer (EC-109), lung cancer (H460), leukemia (HL-60), myeloma (RPMI8226, U266, NOP2, AMO1, ILKM2), and hepatoma, as well as mouse U14 cervical cancer cells and canine osteosarcoma cell lines (HMPOS, D17, and OS 2.4).[27–42] The significant antigrowth effects were accompanied with the induction of cell cycle arrest and/or apoptotic death, whose mechanism was extensively associated with characteristic multiple pathways in different cancer cell lines, i.e., (1) enhanced caspase-dependent pathway in the PaCa cells via the suppression of antiapoptotic Mcl-1 protein, the release of cytochrome c from mitochondria, and the activation of caspase-3 and caspase-7[27]; (2) induced ROS-mediated mitochondrial dysfunction pathway in the HL-60 cells[33]; (3) inhibited 12-lipoxygenase activity in RPMI8226 cells and H460 cells and blocked IκBα degradation followed by down-expressing XIAP and IL-6 in three other myeloma cells[28,29,38]; (4) mediated by an intrinsic pathway and a PI3K/Akt pathway in EC-109 cells[29]; (5) elicited p53-dependent activation of Akt in the HT-29 cells[40]; and (6) repressed MEK-ERK signaling, activated caspases, and decreased ezrin, VEGF, and MMP-9 expressions in hepatoma cells.[32,33] However, the growth-suppressive potency of baicalein (**2**) was much lower in the hematopoietic cancer cell lines (such as HL-60, THP-1, Daudi, and NCI-H929) compared to that of baicalin (**1**).[7]

In Vivo *Antigrowth Effects*

The antineoplastic activity of baicalein (**2**) was further proven by using animal models *in vivo*. Per os administration of baicalein in a dose of 20 mg/kg per day for two weeks significantly diminished the growth of prostate cancer xenografts in nude mice by 55%.[42] Orally given baicalein (**2**) to mice implanted with U14 cervical cancer obstructed the tumor growth by 58.98%.[33] Baicalein (**2**) also exerted the marked antigrowth effect on human HT-29 colon cancer xenografts and human hepatoma xenografts in nude mice.[31,40] Similarly, the treatment with baicalein (**2**) concentration dependently obstructed the cell growth and induced the apoptotic death of HCT116 colon carcinoma cells.[43] In NSCLC cells, baicalein (**2**) significantly elicited the growth-inhibiting and cell apoptotic effects in time- and dose-dependent manners, whose mechanism was closely correlated with the increases in the expression and reciprocal interplay of RUNX3 and FOXO3a through a cross-talk of AMPKα and MEK/ERK1/2 signaling pathways.[44] More tests also evidenced that baicalein (**2**) prevented inflammation-associated and AOM/DSS-induced colon carcinogenesis in mice through the activation of PPARγ and the suppression of NF-κB activity.[43]

Inhibition on Tumor Cell Invasion

The continuing studies revealed that baicalein (**2**) was able to restrain the cell adhesion to fibronectin-coated substrate, to obstruct the cell migration and the invasion through the Matrigel, to inhibit the expression and the secretion of MMP-2 and MMP-9, and to block MAPK signaling pathway in human MDA-MB-231 breast cancer cells. The evidences implied that baicalein (**2**) may serve a potential activity for the suppression of breast cancer metastasis.[37] Within its noncytotoxic concentrations (2.5–40 μM), baicalein (**2**) displayed dose- and time-dependent suppressions on the expressions of total ezrin and phosezrin in A431 melanoma cells, whose events lead to the inhibition of tumor cell motility, invasion, and metastasis. When the A431 cells were treated with 20 μM baicalein, the cell motility and invasion was restrained by 73–80%.[41] The antiinvasive and antimetastatic mechanisms of baicalein (**2**) in AGS gastric cancer, ovarian cancer, U87MG, and U251MG glioma were associated with (1) suppression of the p38 signaling pathway, (2) lessening MMP-2 and MMP-9 expression levels, (3) inhibition of p38 MAPK-dependent NF-κB signaling pathway (such as in cells), and/or (4) inactivation of TGF-β/Smad4 signaling pathway (such as in AGS cells).[45–48] The suppression of pulmonary tumor metastasis by baicalein (**2**) was also found to be achieved by blocking agonist- and tumor cell-induced platelet aggregation via cAMP-mediated vasodilator-stimulated phosphoprotein (VASP) phosphorylation along with impaired MAPKs and PI3K-Akt activation in C6 rat glioma tumor cells *in vitro* and in CT26 colon cancer cells *in vivo*.[49] Both baicalein (**2**) and baicalin (**1**) were effective in reducing TGF-β1-mediated epithelial-mesenchymal transition (EMT), anchorage-independent growth, and cell migration of human breast cancer cell line (MDA-MB-231) and breast epithelial cell line (MCF10A).[50] Taken together, these features indicate that baicalein is a potential therapeutic drug for the prevention of cancer metastasis.

Antiangiogenic Effects

Baicalein (**2**) and baicalin (**1**) demonstrated an obvious antiangiogenesis potential. Both flavonoids exerted dual antigrowth (at low dose) and apoptogenic (at high dose) effects on HUVECs. In association with a dose-dependent decrease of MMP-2 activity, baicalein (**2**) and baicalin (**1**) exerted the inhibitory effects against the migration and the differentiation of endothelial cells into branching networks of tubular structures. The *in vivo* and *in vitro* assays showed that baicalein (**2**) was more potent than baicalin (**1**) in the antiangiogenic effect.[35,36]

Reduction of Anticancer Drug Toxicity and MDR

Baicalein (**2**) can minimize the toxicity and the side effect caused by chemotherapy. The adjunct treatment of 25 μM baicalein significantly reduced the cardiotoxicity caused by DOX through the attenuation of ROS generation and JNK phosphorylation in cardiomyocytes but did not interfere with its antiproliferative effect in MCF-7 cells. The results highlighted that the cotreatment with baicalein elicited antiapoptotic protection against DOX-induced cardiotoxicity besides the augmentation of the anticancer efficacy.[51] Through the inhibition of glycolysis via the regulation of the PTEN/Akt/HIF-1α signaling pathway, baicalein (**2**) could reverse hypoxia-caused 5-FU resistance in AGS gastric cancer cells.[52] In addition, when its structure is modified with O-alkylation and O-acylation at positions of 5-OH, 6-OH, and 7-OH in the baicalein, the reversal of MDR could be potentiated, and the activity of P-gp-170 could be repressed in the baicalein treatment singly or in combination.[53]

Wogonin

Wogonin (**3**) is one of the important and major antineoplastic flavonoids in the herb, which displayed notable inhibition against the proliferation of hematopoietic cancer cell lines and solid tumor cell lines *in vitro* and *in vivo*.

Anticancer Effects In Vitro *and* In Vivo

The moderate anticancer property of wogonin (**3**) was shown in a variety of solid tumor cell lines such as glioma (U251 and U87), GBM, breast carcinoma (MCF-7, T47D, MDA-MB-231, and SK-BR-3), hepatoma (HepG2, SMMC-7721, SK-HEP-1, and Bel-7402), colon crcinoma (HT-29), NSCLC (A549), prostate cancer (LNCaP and PC3), gallbladder cancer (GBC-SD, KU-1, EJ-1, and MBT-2), osteosarcoma (LM8 and U-2OS), melanoma (B16) and sarcoma 180, *in vitro*, but it was less effective in the inhibition of B16 melanoma cells compared to baicalein (**2**). It showed no such inhibition in human normal TIG-1 fetal lung diploid cells, Lo2 hepatocytes, and primary astrocytes.[54–61] The concentrations of wogonin to achieve a 50% inhibition were 42 μM in LNCaP cells, 50 μM in PC3 cells, 80 μM in S180 cells, 48 μg/mL in EJ-1 cells, and 100 μg/mL in KU-1 cells.[55] The treatment of 40 mg/kg wogonin (**3**) reduced the weight of sarcoma 180 in mice by 53.01%.[62] Compared to LNCaP androgen receptor-positive prostate cancer cells, PC3 AR-negative prostate cancer cells were less sensitive to wogonin (**3**), baicalein (**2**), neobaicalein, and skullcapflavone.[63]

By reducing the N-acetyl-transferase (NAT)-1 level and repressing the telomerase via the decrease of c-Myc, wogonin (**3**) obstructed the growth of human HL-60 promyelocytic leukemia cells.[64,65] The treatment of human NB4 promyelocytic leukemia cells with 50 μM wogonin (**3**) for a period of five days obviously inhibited the proliferation by 55–60%. Interestingly, the treatment showed only little effect on the induction of NB4 cell apoptosis but efficiently promoted the granulocytic differentiation of NB4 cells by upregulating the expression of PLSCR1 gene.[66] The antigrowth effect of wogonin (**3**) in human THP-1 monocytic leukemia cells was correlated with the wogonin-stimulated G2/M cell cycle arrest and apoptosis.[8] Wogonin (**3**) in concentrations of 70.4–352.0 μM was effective in the proapoptosis of human RPMI8226 myeloma cells by a Akt-modulated and Bax- and Bcl-2-related intrinsic apoptotic pathway.[67] These evidences provide more important insights into the mechanisms underlying the clinical use of wogonin (**3**) as a potential agent to improve hematopoietic neoplasm therapy.

The treatment with 75 μM wogonin (**3**) for 48 h demonstrated an obvious cytotoxic effect on SK-N-BE2 and IMR-32 malignant neuroblastoma cell lines, whose effect was mediated by the induction of mitochondrial dysfunction, apoptosis, and ER stress via the modulation of an IRE1α-dependent pathway, i.e., (1) up-expression of IRE1α and TRAF2 and increase of ASK1 and JNK phosphorylation; (2) up-expression of ER stress-related proteins (GRP78/Bip and GRP94/gp96) and activation of caspase-12 and caspase-4; as well as (3) alteration of expressions of Bcl-2 family (Bcl-2, Bax, and Bid), release of cytochrome c, activation of caspase-3, caspase-8, caspase-9, and PARP-1.[68]

Moreover, several *in vivo* experiments provided more evidences for the anticancer potential of wogonin (**3**). P.o. injection with wogonin markedly inhibited the growth of T47D estrogen receptor-positive and MDA-MB-231 estrogen receptor-negative cancer xenografts by up to 88% without any toxicity, implying that wogonin (**3**) was an effective agent for obstructing both hormone-dependent and hormone-independent prostate cancer and breast carcinoma.[55] Also, daily administration of wogonin (**3**) twice in doses of 25 or 50 mg/kg to mice retarded the growth LM8 osteo-sarcoma.[56]

Induction of Tumor Cell Cycle Arrest and Apoptotic Death

Apparently, the bioability of wogonin (**3**) in the promotion of cell cycle arrest and apoptotic death is correlated with its anticancer potency in most of the cases. After the treatment with wogonin (**3**), a G2/M arrest was observed in THP-1 monocytic leukemia and PC3 prostate cancer cell lines,[55] and a G1 phase arrest happened in MCF-7 breast cancer, LNCaP prostate cancer, and gliosblatoma multiform cell lines.[53,57,58] The cell cycle progression of B16 melanoma was blocked by wogonin (**3**) at the G0/G1 stage.[57] Extensive explorations focused on the apoptosis induced by wogonin have provided many interesting insights to view the characteristic mechanisms in the different types of neoplastic cells. For instance, wogonin (**3**)-provoked human U251 and U87 glioma cell apoptosis was mediated by ROS generation, ER stress activation, caspase-9 and caspase-3 activations as well as upregulation of cleaved PARP expression.[59] By upregulating p53 and p21 expressions, activating AMPK pathway, and decreasing the activity/expression of lipogenic enzymes, wogonin (**3**) enhanced the apoptosis of GBM cells.[57] H_2O_2-dependent and Ca^{2+} overload-triggered mitochondrial pathway played a critical role in the increase of HepG2 hepatoma cells by the apoptosis by wogonin.[61] The downregulation of the COX-2 gene expression by inhibiting c-Jun expression and AP-1 activation is involved in wogonin-induced apoptosis of A549 lung epithelial carcinoma cells.[69] The proapoptotic effect of wogonin in MCF-7 breast cancer was correlated to ROS generation, activation of ERK, and caspase-3, caspase-8, and caspase-9, and blockage of PI3K/Akt/survivin and p38 MAPK signal pathways.[60,61] Accompanied by the blockage of PI3K/Akt signaling as well as the down-expression of Bcl-2 and the up-expression of Bax, wogonin (**3**) promoted the apoptosis of HT-29 colon cancer cells.[70] In association with the increase of ROS production and intracellular Ca^{2+} and the elevation of the levels of Bad, Bax, cytochrome-c, cleaved caspase-9, cleaved caspase-3, Endo-G, AIF, Fas/CD95, caspase-8, GADD153, GRP78, ATF-6α, calpain-1, calpain-2, and caspase-4, wogonin (**3**) finally forced the osteosarcoma U-2 OS cells to apoptosis.[71] Similar to baicalin (**1**) and baicalein (**2**), wogonin (**3**) could also enhance the growth inhibition and apoptosis of human SCL-1 cutaneous squamous cell carcinoma cell line cells.[72]

Moreover, the apoptosis of breast cancer cells by wogonin (**3**) was indeed influenced by the hormone status. In ER-positive T47D and MCF-7 cells, the ERα expression was markedly obstructed by wogonin in both steady-state mRNA and total protein levels, whereas in ER-negative SK-BR-3 cells, the expression/activity of c-ErbB2 was suppressed by wogonin.[55] The breast cancer cell apoptosis-enhancing effect was also additionally associated with the upregulation of PARP and caspase-3 cleavages as well as proapoptotic Bax and the downregulation of Akt-dependent canonical Wnt signaling pathway and p27kip pathway.[55] Furthermore, if wogonin (**3**) was combined with other natural flavones such as apigenin, chrysin, and luteolin, which are inhibitors of CDK9, the cotreatment directly binded to CDK9 and preferentially obstructed CDK9, leading to the inhibition of RNA synthesis and the rapid down-expression of Mcl-1 (an anti-apoptotic protein), subsequently stimulating the apoptosis of cancer cells. The finding not only affords a new and safe strategy for cancer chemotherapy but also suggests CDK9 may be used as a therapeutic target in oncology.[73]

Inhibition on Lymphangiogenesis, Angiogenesis, and Metastasis

Wogonin (**3**) is an inhibitor of VEGF, which could obstruct VEGF-stimulated migration and tube formation of HUVECs, restrain tyrosine phosphorylation of VEGF receptor-2, then significantly reduce VEGF-triggered phosphorylated forms of ERK, AKT, and p38.[70] By these events, wogonin exerted an inhibition against the angiogenesis and the growth of human gastric cancer cells in nude mice.[70] Similarly, through the reduction of VEGF-C-induced VEGFR-3 phosphorylation and inhibition of COX-2 expression and IL-1β production in TAMs, wogonin (10–100 μM) exerted the antigrowth and antimetastatic effects and restrained VEGF-C-induced lymphangiogenesis against LM8 highly metastatic osteosarcoma in mice.[56] The mobility and the invasion of human GBC-SD gallbladder cancer cells could be obviously inhibited by wogonin (**3**) at doses of 1–10 μM, but it did not elicit apoptosis. The effect was found to correlate with wogonin-induced events such as the upregulation of a metastasis suppressor maspin and the suppression of MMP-2 and MMP-9 expressions and ERK1/2 phosphorylation.[74] In addition, wogonin (**3**) effectively repressed lipopolysaccharide (LPS) plus TPA-induced migration and invasion of glioma C6 cells *in vitro* and *in vivo*.[75] Wogonin (**3**) was also able to diminish LPS-induced vascular permeability by suppressing the MLCK/MLC pathway, suggesting a therapeutic potential of wogonin for the diseases related with the development of both inflammatory and tumor.[76]

Synergistic Antitumor and Toxicity-Reducing Effects

By impairing the P-gp function and calcein excretion, wogonin (**3**) amplified the intracellular content of etoposide in the neoplastic cells and potentiated the proapoptotic or cytotoxic activities of etoposide toward the cancer cell lines (Jurkat, HL-60, A549, and NCI-H226), but it had no such effect on other anticancer agents (such as 5-FU and cisplatin) on the cancer cells.[77–79] Wogonin (**3**) was also able to sensitize cisplatin-induced apoptosis of both

A549 cells and HeLa cells via robustly induced H_2O_2 accumulation in the cancer cells[80] and to greatly augment TRAIL-induced suppression against the growth of A549 cells, whose synergic effect was further proven in nude mice xenografted with A549 NSCLC.[81] In addtion, wogonin was able to restrain IL-6-induced AKR1C1/1C2 expression and to attenuate drug resistance in H23 NSCLC cells, and it also sensitized the resistant malignant T cells (CEM and Jurkat) to TNFα- and TRAIL-induced apoptosis.[82,83] Through the down-expression of MRP1 by inhibiting a Nrf2/ARE signaling pathway, wogonin (**3**) reversed the MDR of human myelogenous leukemia K562/A02 cells.[84]

Besides improving the efficacy of cytotoxic drugs, wogonin (**3**) also attenuated the side effects caused by chemotherapeutic agents in cotreatment.[82,83] Wogonin (**3**) was also reported to have an ability to prevent the various anticancer agents induced by the apoptotic death of normal cells such as bone marrow cells and thymocytes.[77–79]

Collectively, these findings revealed that wogonin (**3**) has the potential to be a chemopreventive and a therapeutic agent for malignant therapy and suggested that wogonin may be a useful chemotherapeutic adjuvant to improve the pharmacological actions of clinical anticancer drugs and to ameliorate their adverse effects.

Oroxylin-A

Anticancer and Apoptosis-Inducing Effects

Oroxylin-A (**4**) showed the effective anticancer activities against several human carcinoma cells with weak toxicities *in vivo* and *in vitro*. After treatment with oroxylin-A (**4**), the growth inhibition on human HeLa cervical carcinoma cells were observed *in vitro* (IC_{50}: 19.4 μM, in 48 h), and the significant decrease of tumor volumes and tumor weight were shown *in vivo*. During the inhibition, oroxylin-A (**4**) obviously promoted the apoptosis of HeLa cells by both extrinsic and intrinsic pathways.[85] The oral administration of oroxylin-A (**4**) also demonstrated the chemopreventive efficacy against human HCT-116 colon cancer in nude mice. Its proapoptotic effect in the HCT-116 cells was found to be associated with the increase of Nrf-2 expression and Nrf2 translocation into the nucleus and the elevation of intracellular ROS levels, as well as the down-expression of Bcl-2, the up-expression of Bax, and the activation of caspase-3 and caspase-9.[86] Also, the activation of a permeability transition pore (PTP)-independent and mitochondrial apoptosis-induced channel (MAC)-related mitochondrial pathway played a key role in the oroxylin-A (**4**)-induced HCT-116 cell apoptosis, and the regulation of UCP2 played a key role in a mitochondrial apoptotic pathway induced by oroxylin-A (**4**) in Caco cells.[87,88] In HepG2 and K562 cancer cell lines, oroxylin-A (**4**) obviously augmented the expression of p53 protein by reducing MDM2 expression and interfering MDM2-modulated proteasome-related p53 degradation.[89]

Reverse of Drug Resistance

Oroxylin-A (**4**) was effective in inhibiting P-gp-mediated drug efflux *in vitro* and *in vivo*. By markedly down-expressing Integrin-β1 and the related pathway, oroxylin-A (**4**) dramatically enhanced the apoptosis provoked by paclitaxel in a CAM-DR model of HepG2 cells to reverse the cell adhesion mediated drug resistance (CAM-DR) resistant.[90] Moreover, oroxylin-A (**4**) markedly increased the cellular accumulation of paclitaxel in a P-gp overexpressed and drug-resistant MCF-7/Adm cells concomitant with the induction of G2/M cell cycle arrest via Chk2/P53/NF-κB signaling pathway including the decrease of NF-κB binding activity and the increase of p-Chk2 (Thr68) expression; however, there was no such effect in the cells lacking P-gp expression. Thus, the cotreatment of oroxylin-A (30 mg/kg) significantly augmented the oral effect of paclitaxel (15 mg/kg) in rats.[91,92] These results disclosed the developing potential of oroxylin-A (**4**) in improving the cellular availability of P-gp substrates and safely reversing the drug resistance of chemotherapeutic drugs.

Inhibition on Cancer Cell Invasion and Metastasis

Oroxylin-A (**4**) is also capable of repressing the tumor cell adhesion, invasion, and migration in a concentration-dependent manner. *In vitro* and *in vivo* assays substantiated the suppressive effects of oroxylin-A (**4**) against the invasion and the migration of human MDA-MB-231 breast cancer cells, whose mechanism was revealed to be associated with the obstruction of the expressions of MMP-9 and MMP-2 and increased the expression of TIMP-2, as well as repressed PKCδ translocation and ERK1/2 phosphorylation and restrained AP-1 binding ability.[70] The oroxylin-A (**4**) treatment also obstructed the lung metastasis of B16-F10 melanoma cells[93] and inhibited the hypoxia-induced migration and invasion of MCF-7 (breast), DU145 (prostate), and HepG2 (liver) cancer cell lines.[94] The antimigrative and antiinvasive effects of oroxylin-A (**4**) in the MCF-7 cells were mediated by inhibiting the hypoxia-induced Notch pathway to block N1ICD translocating to the nucleus and binding to the epithelial–mesenchymal transition-related transcription factor Snail.[94] According to these positive evidences, oroxylin-A (**4**) has been proposed for further development as a potential candidate for the treatment of primary cancer, metastatic cancer, and drug-resistant cancer.

Structure Modification

For optimizing the tumor inhibitory molecule, the structure of oroxylin-A (**4**) has been modified by introduction of a nitrogen-containing hydrophilic and heterocyclic ring to its 7-OH position via a varying length of carbon chain. The three synthesized series of derivatives were screened by using human tumor cell lines (HepG2, HCT116, and BCG-823). The resulted antiproliferative activities showed three derivatives, **5d**, **5e**, and **5f**, displaying a significantly potentiated antigrowth activity against the neoplastic cell lines. The IC_{50} values were 2.4–6.6 μM in HepG2 hepatoma cells, 1.4–5.1 μM in HCT116 colon cancer cells, and 6.3–9.5 μM in BCG-823 gastric cancer cells, whose IC_{50} data were lower than that of oroxylin-A (**4**) by 5–13 times. According to the actions observed in the tests, **5f** was more likely considered as a necrosis-inducing agent or both apoptosis/necrosis inducers in the tested cancer cell lines.[95] Hence, the derivative **5f** has been used to explore its anticancer mechanism.

Other Active Flavonoids

Several structurally similar flavonoids were also isolated from the herb, exerting similar bioactivities. Wogonoside (**6**) demonstrated the growth inhibition on human MDA-MB-231 breast cancer cells in time- and dose-dependent manners, whose effect was correlated with the autophagy induced by wogonoside via a MAPK-mTOR pathway, i.e., (1) promoting the expressions of LC3-II and Beclin-1 and (2) reducing the activation of mTOR and p70-S6 kinase (p70S6K) by regulating the expression of ERK1/2 and p38 involved in MAPK signaling.[96] Wogonoside (**6**) exerted a cytotoxicity on human glioblastoma cells in association with the induction of autophagy and apoptosis via (1) enhanced autophagic flux as reflected by the increases of acidic vesicular organelles (AVO) formation, p62 degradation, and LC3 turnover; (2) p38/MAPK signaling pathway; (3) PI3K/AKT/mTOR/p70S6K signaling pathway; and (4) ROS participation.[97]

Chrysin (**7**), similar to wogonin (**3**), could restrain IL-6-induced AKR1C1 and AKR1C2 overexpression and reduce the drug resistance in human NSCLC cells, leading to the reversal of the cellular resistance to cisplatin and adriamycin.[82] In addition, skullcapflavone-I (**8**) has been subjected to treat rat hepatic stellate cells (T-HSC/Cl-6). The exposure of **8** in a 20 μM concentration for 24 h significantly and selectively induced the cell apoptosis via the activation of caspase-3 and caspase-9 and showed no change in hepatocyte viability,[98] evidencing that skullcapflavone-I (**8**) is a potentially useful agent for the prevention of liver fibrosis and carcinogenesis.

Other Bioactivities

The herb Huang Qin (Scutellaria radix) is one of the most popular medicines with multiple purposes employed in China traditionally for the treatment of inflammation, hypertension, cardiovascular diseases, and bacterial and viral infections. Accumulating pharmacological evidences demonstrate that Scutellaria radix has antiinflammatory, antioxidant, antihypersensitivity, antihyperlipidemia, hemopoietic, hepatoprotective, antipyretic, antimutagenic, antiallergic, antifungal, and antimicrobial properties.

References

1. Ye, F. et al. 2002. Anticancer activity of *Scutellaria baicalensis* and its potential mechanism. *J. Altern. Complem. Med.* (NY) 8: 567–72.
2. Zhang, D. Y. et al. 2003. Inhibition of cancer cell proliferation and prostaglandin E2 synthesis by *Scutellaria baicalensis*. *Cancer Res.* 63: 4037–43.
3. Ye, F. et al. 2007. Molecular mechanism of anti-prostate cancer activity of *Scutellaria baicalensis* extract. *Nutr. Cancer* 57: 100–10.
4. Ye, F. et al. 2009. The effect of *Scutellaria baicalensis* on the signaling network in hepatocellular carcinoma cells. *Nutr. Cancer* 61: 530–7.
5. Gao, J. Y. et al. 2011. The ethanol extract of *Scutellaria baicalensis* and the active compounds induce cell cycle arrest and apoptosis including upregulation of p53 and Bax in human lung cancer cells. *Toxicol. Applied Pharmacol.* 254: 221–8.
6. Park, K. I. et al. 2011. Korean *Scutellaria baicalensis* water extract inhibits cell cycle G1/S transition by suppressing cyclin D1 expression and matrix-metalloproteinase-2 activity in human lung cancer cells. *J. Ethnopharmacol.* 133: 634–41.
7. Kumagai, T. et al. 2007. *Scutellaria baicalensis*, a herbal medicine: Anti-proliferative and apoptotic activity against acute lymphocytic leukemia, lymphoma and myeloma cell lines. *Leukemia Res.* 31: 523–30.
8. Himeji, M. et al. 2007. Difference of growth-inhibitory effect of *Scutellaria baicalensis*-producing flavonoid wogonin among human cancer cells and normal diploid cells. *Cancer Lett.* (Amsterdam, Netherlands) 245: 269–74.
9. Ikemoto, S. et al. 2000. Antitumor effects of Scutellariae radix and its components baicalein, baicalin, and wogonin on bladder cancer cell lines. *Urol.* 55: 951–5.
10. Li, T. T. et al. 2011. Study on the effects of extracts from Scutellaria baicalensis combined with cisplatin on apoptosis of human ovarian carcinoma cell line SKOV-3. *Zhongguo Fuyou Baojian* 26: 1529–32.
11. Kaplya, O. A. et al. 2004. Effect of baikal skullcap extract administered alone or in combination with cyclophosphamide on natural cytotoxicity system in mice with Lewis lung carcinoma. *Bull. Experim. Biol. Med.* 137: 471–4.
12. Scheck, A. C. et al. 2006. Anticancer activity of extracts derived from the mature roots of *Scutellaria baicalensis* on human malignant brain tumor cells. *BMC Complem. Altern. Med.* 6: 27.
13. Park, H. J. et al. 1998. Induction of quinone reductase by a methanol extract of *Scutellaria baicalensis* and its flavonoids in murine Hepa 1c1c7 cells. *Eur. J. Cancer Prevent.* 7: 465–71.
14. Gol'dberg, V. E. et al. 1997. Dry extract of *Scutellaria baicalensis* as a hemostimulant in antineoplastic chemotherapy in patents with lung cancer. *Eksperimental'naia i klinicheskaia farmakologiia* 60: 28–30.
15. Pan, T. L. et al. 2012. Inhibitory effects of *Scutellaria baicalensis* extract on hepatic stellate cells through inducing G2/M cell cycle arrest and activating ERK-dependent apoptosis via Bax and caspase pathway. *J. Ethnopharmacol.* 139: 829–37.
16. Goh, D. et al. 2005. Inhibitory effects of a chemically standardized extract from *Scutellaria barbata* in human colon cancer cell lines, Lovo. *J. Agric. Food Chem.* 53: 8197–204.
17. Parajuli, P. et al. 2009. In vitro antitumor mechanisms of various Scutellaria extracts and constituent flavonoids. *Planta Med.* 75: 41–8.
18. Wang, C. Z. et al. 2013. Hydrophobic flavonoids from *Scutellaria baicalensis* induce colorectal cancer cell apoptosis through a mitochondrial-mediated pathway. *Intj. J. Oncol.* 42: 1018–26.
19. Sheng, J. et al. 2008. Inhibitory effects of total flavonoids of *Scutellaria baicalensis* georgi on S180, Hep-A-22 and Bcap-37 tumor cells *J. Jilin Univ. (Med. edit.)* 34: 401–4.
20. Peng, Y. et al. 2011. Antitumor activity of *Scutellaria baicalensis* Georgi total flavonoids on mice bearing U14 cervical carcinoma. *Afri. J. Biotechnol.* 10: 19167–75.
21. Chan, F. L. et al. 2000. Induction of apoptosis in prostate cancer cell lines by a flavonoid, baicalin. *Cancer Lett.* 160: 219–28.
22. Huang, Y. et al. 2012. Downregulation of the PI3K/Akt signaling pathway and induction of apoptosis in CA46 Burkitt lymphoma cells by baicalin. *J. Experim. Clin. Cancer Res.* 31: 48.
23. Lu, H. F. et al. 2007. ROS mediates baicalin-induced apoptosis in human promyelocytic leukemia HL-60 cells through the expression of the Gadd153 and mitochondrial-dependent pathway. *Anticancer Res.* 27: 117–26.
24. Orzechowska, B. et al. 2014. Baicalin from the extract of *Scutellaria baicalensis* affects the innate immunity and apoptosis in leukocytes of children with acute lymphocytic leukemia. *Intl. Immunopharmacol.* 23: 558–67.

25. Shu, Y. J. et al. 2014. Baicalin induces apoptosis of gallbladder carcinoma cells in vitro via a mitochondrial-mediated pathway and suppresses tumor growth in vivo. *Anti-Cancer Agents in Med. Chem.* 14: 1136–45.
26. Wang, C. Z. et al. 2010. Selective fraction of *Scutellaria baicalensis* and its chemopreventive effects on MCF-7 human breast cancer cells. *Phytomed.* 17: 63–8.
27. Takahashi, H. et al. 2011. Baicalein, a component of *Scutellaria baicalensis*, induces apoptosis by Mcl-1 down-regulation in human pancreatic cancer cells. *Biochimica et Biophysica Acta* 1813: 1465–74.
28. Li, Q. B. et al. 2006. Role of baicalein in the regulation of proliferation and apoptosis in human myeloma RPMI8226 cells. *Chin. Med. J.* (Beijing, China, Eng. edit.) 119: 948–52.
29. Liu, S. Q. et al. 2010. Inhibitory effect of baicalein on IL-6-mediated signaling cascades in human myeloma cells. *Eur. J. Haematol.* 84: 137–44.
30. Zhang, H. B. et al. 2013. Baicalein induces apoptosis in esophageal squamous cell carcinoma cells through modulation of the PI3K/Akt pathway. *Oncol. Lett.* 5: 722–8.
31. Liang, R. R. et al. 2012. Preferential inhibition of hepatocellular carcinoma by the flavonoid Baicalein through blocking MEK-ERK. *Intl. J. Oncol.* 41: 969–78.
32. Xiao, X. L. et al. 2012. Effect of baicalein on the in vitro migration and invasion of human hepatocellular carcinoma cell line SMMC-7721. *Zhongguo Zhongliu Linchuang* 39: 305–9.
33. Peng, Y. et al. 2011. Antitumor activity of baicalein on the mice bearing U14 cervical cancer. *Afri. J. Biotechnol.* 10: 14169–76.
34. Wang, J. W. et al. 2004. Baicalein induces apoptosis through ROS-mediated mitochondrial dysfunction pathway in HL-60 cells. *Intl. J. Mol. Med.* 14: 627–32.
35. Hsu, S. L. et al. 2001. Baicalein induces a dual growth arrest by modulating multiple cell cycle regulatory molecules. *Eur. J. Pharmacol.* 425: 165–71.
36. Liu, J. J. et al. 2003. Baicalein and baicalin are potent inhibitors of angiogenesis: Inhibition of endothelial cell proliferation, migration and differentiation. *Intl. J. Cancer* 106: 559–65.
37. Wang, L. et al. 2010. Flavonoid baicalein suppresses adhesion, migration and invasion of MDA-MB-231 human breast cancer cells. *Cancer Lett.* 297: 42–8.
38. Leung, H. W. C. et al. 2007. Inhibition of 12-lipoxygenase during baicalein-induced human lung nonsmall carcinoma H460 cell apoptosis. *Food Chem. Toxicol.* 45: 403–11.
39. Helmerick, E. C. et al. 2014. The effects of baicalein on canine osteosarcoma cell proliferation and death. *Veterinary Comp. Oncol.* 12: 299–309.
40. Kim, S. J. et al. 2012. Antitumor actions of baicalein and wogonin in HT-29 human colorectal cancer cells. *Mol. Med. Reports* 6: 1443–9.
41. Wu, B. et al. 2011. Baicalein mediates inhibition of migration and invasiveness of skin carcinoma through Ezrin in A431 cells. *BMC Cancer* 11: 527.
42. Bonham, M. et al. 2005. Characterization of chemical constituents in *Scutellaria baicalensis* with antiandrogenic and growth-inhibitory activities toward prostate carcinoma. *Clin. Cancer Res.* 11: 3905–14.
43. Kim, D. W. et al. 2013. Baicalein, an active component of *Scutellaria baicalensis* Georgi, induces apoptosis in human colon cancer cells and prevents AOM/DSS-induced colon cancer in mice. *Intl. J. Oncol.* 43: 1652–8.
44. Zheng, F. et al. 2015. Baicalein increases the expression and reciprocal interplay of RUNX3 and FOXO3a through crosstalk of AMPKα and MEK/ERK1/2 signaling pathways in human non-small cell lung cancer cells. *J. Exper. Clinical Cancer Res.* 34: 1–24.
45. Yan, X. et al. 2015. Baicalein inhibits the invasion of gastric cancer cells by suppressing the activity of the p38 signaling pathway. *Oncol. Reports* 33: 737–43.
46. Chen, F. L. et al. 2014. Baicalein inhibits migration and invasion of gastric cancer cells through suppression of the TGF-β signaling pathway. *Mol. Med. Reports* 10: 1999–2003.
47. Yan, H. et al. 2015. Baicalein inhibits MMP-2 expression in human ovarian cancer cells by suppressing the p38 MAPK-dependent NF-κB signaling pathway. *Anti-Cancer Drugs* 26: 649–56.
48. Zhang, Z. N. et al. 2014. Baicalein reduces the invasion of glioma cells via reducing the activity of p38 signaling pathway. *PLoS One* 9: e90318/1-e90318/8.
49. Kim, S. D. et al. 2014. Baicalein inhibits agonist- and tumor cell-induced platelet aggregation while suppressing pulmonary tumor metastasis via cAMP-mediated VASP phosphorylation along with impaired MAPKs and PI3K-Akt activation. *Biochem. Pharmacol.* (Amsterdam, Netherlands) 92: 251–65.
50. Chung, H. S. et al. 2015. Baicalin and baicalein inhibit transforming growth factor-β1-mediated epithelial-mesenchymal transition in human breast epithelial cells. *Biochem. Biophys. Res. Commun.* 458: 707–13.
51. Chang, W. T. et al. 2011. Baicalein protects against doxorubicin-induced cardiotoxicity by attenuation of mitochondrial oxidant injury and JNK activation. *J. Cell. Biochem.* 112: 2873–81.
52. Chen, F. L. et al. 2015. Baicalein reverses hypoxia-induced 5-FU resistance in gastric cancer AGS cells through suppression of glycolysis and the PTEN/Akt/HIF- 1α signaling pathway. *Oncol. Reports* 33: 457–63.
53. Wang, J. F. et al. 2011. Synthesis of ring A-modified baicalein derivatives. *Helvetica Chim. Acta* 94: 2221–30.
54. Watanabe, K. 1996. Inhibitory effects of baicalein and wogonin on the growth of B16 melanoma cells. *Acta Medica Kinki Univ.* 21: 377–85.
55. Chung, H. Y. et al. 2008. Anticancer effects of wogonin in both estrogen receptor-positive and -negative human breast cancer cell lines in vitro and in nude mice xenografts. *Intl. J. Cancer* 122: 816–22.
56. Kimura, Y. et al. 2013. Antitumor and anti-metastatic actions of wogonin isolated from Scutellaria baicalensis roots through anti-lymphangiogenesis. *Phytomed.* 20: 328–36.
57. Lee, D. H. et al. 2012. Wogonin induces apoptosis by activating the AMPK and p53 signaling pathways in human glioblastoma cells. *Cell. Signalling* 24: 2216–25.
58. Wei, L. B. et al. 2010. Different apoptotic effects of wogonin via induction of H2O2 generation and Ca(2+) overload in malignant hepatoma and normal hepatic cells. *J. Cell. Biochem.* 111: 1629–41.
59. Tsai, C. F. et al. 2012. Wogonin induces reactive oxygen species production and cell apoptosis in human glioma cancer cells. *Intl. J. Mol. Sci.* 13: 9877–92.
60. Huang, K. F. et al. 2012. Wogonin induces apoptosis and down-regulates survivin in human breast cancer MCF-7 cells by modulating PI3K-AKT pathway. *Intl. Immunopharmacol.* 12: 334–41.

61. Yu, J. S. et al. 2011. Wogonin induces apoptosis by activation of ERK and p38 MAPKs signaling pathways and generation of reactive oxygen species in human breast cancer cells. *Mol. Cells* 31: 327–35.
62. Wang, W. et al. 2006. The anticancer activities of wogonin in murine sarcoma S180 both in vitro and in vivo. *Biol. Pharm. Bull.* 29: 1132–7.
63. Bonham, M. et al. 2005. Characterization of chemical constituents in *Scutellaria baicalensis* with antiandrogenic and growth-inhibitory activities toward prostate carcinoma. *Clin. Cancer Res.* 11: 3905–14.
64. Huang, S. T. et al. 2010. Wogonin, an active compound in Scutellaria baicalensis, induces apoptosis and reduces telomerase activity in the HL-60 leukemia cells. *Phytomed.* 17: 47–54.
65. Yu, C. S. et al. 2005. Wogonin inhibits N-acetyltransferase activity and gene expression in human leukemia HL-60 cells. *Anticancer Res.* 25: 127–32.
66. Zhang, K. et al. 2008. Wogonin induces the granulocytic differentiation of human NB4 promyelocytic leukemia cells and upregulates phospholipid scramblase 1 gene expression. *Cancer Sci.* 99: 689–95.
67. Zhang, M. et al. 2013. Wogonin induces apoptosis in RPMI 8226, a human myeloma cell line, by downregulating phospho-Akt and overexpressing Bax. *Life Sci.* 92: 55–62.
68. Ge, W. L. et al. 2015. Wogonin induced mitochondrial dysfunction and endoplasmic reticulum stress in human malignant neuroblastoma cells via IRE1α-dependent pathway. *J. Mol. Neurosci.* 56: 652–62.
69. Chen, L. G. et al. 2008. Wogonin, a bioactive flavonoid in herbal tea, inhibits inflammatory cyclooxygenase-2 gene expression in human lung epithelial cancer cells. *Mol. Nutr. Food Res.* 52: 1349–57.
70. Lu, N. et al. 2008. Wogonin suppresses tumor growth in vivo and VEGF-induced angiogenesis through inhibiting tyrosine phosphorylation of VEGFR2. *Life Sci.* 82: 956–63.
71. Lin, C. C. et al. 2011. Wogonin triggers apoptosis in human osteosarcoma U-2 OS cells through the endoplasmic reticulum stress, mitochondrial dysfunction and caspase-3-dependent signaling pathways. *Intl. J. Oncol.* 39: 217–24.
72. Liu, M. et al. 2014. Three Scutellaria baicalensis extracts induce the apoptosis of a human cutaneous squamous cell carcinoma cell line SCL-1: An experimental study. *Zhonghua Pifuke Zazhi* 47: 650–3.
73. Polier, G. et al. 2011. Wogonin and related natural flavones are inhibitors of CDK9 that induce apoptosis in cancer cells by transcriptional suppression of Mcl-1. *Cell Death & Disease* 2: e182.
74. Dong, P. et al. 2011. Wogonin, an active ingredient of Chinese herb medicine Scutellaria baicalensis, inhibits the mobility and invasion of human gallbladder carcinoma GBC-SD cells by inducing the expression of maspin. *J. Ethnopharmacol.* 137: 1373–80.
75. Shen, S. C. et al. 2006. Lipopolysaccharide plus 12-o-tetradecanoylphorbol 13-acetate induction of migration and invasion of glioma cells in vitro and in vivo: Differential inhibitory effects of flavonoids. *Neurosci.* 140: 477–89.
76. Huang, Y. J. et al. 2015. Wogonin inhibits LPS-induced vascular permeability via suppressing MLCK/MLC pathway. *Vascular Pharmcol.* 72: 43–52.
77. Lee, E. et al. 2007. Wogonin, a plant flavone, potentiates etoposide-induced apoptosis in cancer cells. *Annals of the New York Academy of Sciences* (2007), 1095 (Signal Transduction Pathways, Part C), 521–6.
78. Lee, E. et al. 2009. Inhibition of P-glycoprotein by wogonin is involved with the potentiation of etoposide-induced apoptosis in cancer cells. *Annals of the New York Academy of Sciences* 1171 (Natural compounds and their role in apoptotic cell signaling pathways), 132–6.
79. Enomoto, R. et al. 2011. Wogonin potentiates the antitumor action of etoposide and ameliorates its adverse effects. *Cancer Chemother. Pharmacol.* 67: 1063–72.
80. He, F. et al. 2012. Wogonin potentiates cisplatin-induced cancer cell apoptosis through accumulation of intracellular reactive oxygen species. *Oncol. Reports* 28: 601–5.
81. Yang, L. et al. 2013. Wogonin enhances antitumor activity of tumor necrosis factor-related apoptosis-inducing ligand in vivo through ROS-mediated downregulation of cFLIP(L) and IAP proteins. *Apoptosis* 18: 618–26.
82. Wang, H. W. et al. 2007. Reversal of inflammation-associated dihydrodiol dehydrogenases (AKR1C1 and AKR1C2) overexpression and drug resistance in nonsmall cell lung cancer cells by wogonin and chrysin. *Intl. J. Cancer* 120: 2019–27.
83. Fas, S. C. et al. 2006. Wogonin sensitizes resistant malignant cells to TNFα- and TRAIL-induced apoptosis. *Blood* 108: 3700–6.
84. Xu, X. F. et al. 2014. Wogonin reverses multi-drug resistance of human myelogenous leukemia K562/A02 cells via downregulation of MRP1 expression by inhibiting Nrf2/ARE signaling pathway. *Biochem. Pharmacol.* (Amsterdam, Netherlands) 92: 220–34.
85. Li, H. N. et al. 2009. Apoptosis induction of oroxylin A in human cervical cancer HeLa cell line in vitro and in vivo. *Toxicol.* 257: 80–5.
86. Hu, R. et al. 2012. The role of Nrf2 and apoptotic signaling pathways in oroxylin A-mediated responses in HCT-116 colorectal adenocarcinoma cells and xenograft tumors. *Anti-Cancer Drugs* 23: 651–8.
87. Liu, W. et al. 2009. MAC-related mitochondrial pathway in oroxylin-A-induced apoptosis in human hepatocellular carcinoma HepG2 cells. *Cancer Lett.* 284: 198–207.
88. Qiao, C. et al. 2015. UCP2-related mitochondrial pathway participates in oroxylin A-induced apoptosis in human colon cancer cells. *J. Cellular Physiol.* 230: 1054–63.
89. Mu, R. et al. 2009. Involvement of p53 in oroxylin A-induced apoptosis in cancer cells. *Mol. Carcinogen.* 48: 1159–69.
90. Zhu, B. B. et al. 2012. Oroxylin A reverses CAM-DR of HepG2 cells by suppressing Integrinβ1 and its related pathway. *Toxicol. Applied Pharmacol.* 259: 387–94.
91. Go, W. J. et al. 2009. Evaluation of the flavonoid oroxylin A as an inhibitor of P-glycoprotein-mediated cellular efflux. *J. Nat. Prod.* 72: 1616–9.
92. Zhu, L. T. et al. 2013. Oroxylin A reverses P-glycoprotein-mediated multidrug resistance of MCF7/ADR cells by G2/M arrest. *Toxicol. Lett.* 219: 107–15.
93. Lu, Z. J. et al. 2012. Oroxylin A inhibits matrix metalloproteinase-2/9 expression and activation by up-regulating tissue inhibitor of metallo-proteinase-2 and suppressing the ERK1/2 signaling pathway. *Toxicol. Lett.* 209: 211–20.
94. Cheng, Y. et al. 2014. Oroxylin A inhibits hypoxia-induced invasion and migration of MCF-7 cells by suppressing the Notch pathway. *Anti-Cancer Drugs* 25: 778–89.

95. Fu, W. et al. 2012. Synthesis and biological evaluation of 7-O-modified oroxylin A derivatives. *Bioorg. Med. Chem. Lett.* 22: 1118–21.
96. Sun, Y. J. et al. 2013. Wogonoside induces autophagy in MDA-MB-231 cells by regulating MAPK-mTOR pathway. *Food Chem. Toxicol.* 51: 53–60.
97. Zhang, L. et al. 2014. Wogonoside induces autophagy-related apoptosis in human glioblastoma cells. *Oncol. Reports* 32: 1179–87.
98. Park, E. J. et al. 2005. Skullcapflavone I from *Scutellaria baicalensis* induces apoptosis in activated rat hepatic stellate cells. *Planta Med.* 71: 885–7.

35 Tian Hua Fen 天花粉

Snakegourd root powder

Herb Origination

Tian Hua Fen (Snakegourd root powder) originated from the dried root tubers of three Cucurbitaceae plants *Trichosanthes kirilowii*, *T. rosthornii*, and *T. japonica*. The root tuber is traditionally collected in spring and autumn and peeled and dried in the sun.

Antitumor Activity

The extracts of *T. kirilowii* tuber have been eluated by *in vitro* assays for the cancer inhibitory activity. *Trichosanthes kirilowii* extract (TKE), a methanolic extract of Tian Hua Fen, time dependently inhibited the growth of human HepG2 hepatoma cells at a ≈25 µg/mL concentration, concomitant with the induction of G2/M cell arrest and block of tubulin polymerization.[1] An extract of snakegourd root tubers demonstrated moderate antigrowth and apoptosis-inducing effects against human HeLa cervical cancer cells (IC_{50}: 33.4 mg/L, in 48 h), whose activity was four times more potent than that of trichosanthin (TCS), which is a major component in Tian Hua Fen.[2] Tianhua, an extract of the root powder, elicited the cell cycle arrest and the apoptosis of human A549 lung cancer cells, thereby restraining the proliferation, migration, and metastasis of A549 cells *in vitro* and *in vivo*. But, oral feeding with Tianhua to mice only resulted in an initial inhibition of the A549 cell growth *in vivo*.[3] Moreover, an aqueous extract of *T. kirilowii* tuber exerted strong angiogenetic activity in both models of bovine aortic endothelial cells and chick embryo chorioallantoic membrane.[4] The scientific data indicated that Tian Hua Fen may prevent or delay the tumorigenic process.[4]

Antitumor Constituents and Activities

Trichosanthin

TCS is a type I ribosome-inactivating protein (RIP-I) as a major component in the Gua Lou root powder, which has been used as an abortifacient for 1500 years in China due to its high toxicity on trophoblasts. Over the past 30 years, many reports have revealed that TCS is cytotoxic to a variety of tumor cell lines *in vitro* and *in vivo*.

Anticancer Activity

TCS exhibited suppressive effects against the proliferation of chorioepithelioma, A549 lung cancer, HT-29 colon cancer, and HDS osteosarcoma and WISH amnion cell lines *in vitro* (IC_{50}: 3.3–16, 18.3, 42.1, 41.4, and 70 µg/mL, respectively).[5,6] TCS is also capable of directly killing colon carcinoma cells, hepatoma cells, differentiated gastric cancer cells, and *ras*-positive Wef tumor cells but has weak inhibition on lung adenocarcinoma cells and *ras*-negative Def cancer cells.[7,8] The i.p. injection of TCS (0.2 mg, per mouse) potentiated the adherent ability of erythocytes with immunocomplex and obstructed the cancer cell growth and the ascetic production, which led to the obvious prolongation of the life span in mice bearing Ehrlich ascites cancer or ascites hepatoma.[9–11] TCS also suppressed the growth of a murine malignant tumor (MBI-2) *in vivo* and *in vitro*[20] but exerted a relatively lower inhibition on entity hepatoma cells.[9–11]

Cell Cycle Arrest and Apoptosis-Inducing Activity

During cancer growth inhibition, TCS augmented the cell cycle arrest and apoptosis of tumor cells and induced the necrosis of tumor cells by damaging the cellular ultrastructure, deforming the ER and mitochondria, and blocking the protein synthesis.[7,8] By eliciting the apoptotic death of CNE2 cells through the downregulation of Notch signaling, the proliferation and the soft agar colony formation of human CNE2 nasopharyngeal carcinoma cells were obstructed by the TCS treatment *in vitro*.[12] Either in estrogen-dependent MCF-7 cells or estrogen-independent MDA-MB-231 cells, TCS manifested antiproliferative and proapoptotic effects on the breast cancer cell lines, whose apoptotic mechanism was found to correlate with the activation of both caspase-8- and caspase-9-regulated pathways and, subsequently, the activation of caspase-3 and the cleavage of PARP.[13] By the potent apoptosis-inducing effect, the volume and the weight of the breast cancer were significantly reduced in TCS-treated nude mice-xenografted MDA-MB-231 breast cancer cells.[12] Through the activation of JNP/MARK pathways, TCS at a low concentration elicited the apoptosis and the cell cycle arrest of HEp-2 and AMC-HN-8 human laryngeal epidermoid carcinoma cells, thereby inhibiting the viability of the HEp-2 and AMC-HN-8 cells, independently of necrosis.[14] TCS of 5.0 µg/mL markedly inhibited the cell viability of CMT-93 mouse colorectal cancer and induced the cell apoptosis in association with the downexpression of pAkt 473 and pAkt 308 and the up-expression of γ-H2AX, Bid, Bax, and Bad.[15] When the concentration and time was enlarged, the proapoptosis and proliferative inhibition were induced by TCS in A549 human lung cancer cells via the changes in the cytoskeleton microtubule structure.[16]

Specific Effect

Due to the TCS affinity receptor on syncytiotrophoblast cells and Jar cells, TCS could activate the G-protein on the membrane of TCS-sensitive cells and apparently exert a specific cytotoxic effect toward trophoblastic cells by directly attacking the ribosome of the targeted tumor cells, resulting in TCS selectively inhibiting the growth of human choriocarcinoma cells and mouse melanoma cells in a time-dependent manner.[17–20] TCS triggered choriocarcinoma cells to apoptosis also by enhancing caspase-3 activity and release of cytochrome c from mitochondria and eliciting cell cycle phase distribution and macromolecule synthesis in the choriocarcinoma cells.[21,22] The antigrowth effect was further evidenced in a nude mice model against xenografts of choriocarcinoma. When given at a dose of 0.375 mg/kg per day, TCS prolonged the mean survival of the tested nude mice and caused no effect on the body weight.[23]

Synergetic Effect

More investigations further revealed that the antitumor activity of TCS was mainly contributed from the actions of its N-terminal sequences.[24] Also, the additive effect of TCS with chemotherapeutic drugs was further corroborated.[25] TCS synergistically enhanced imatinib-induced K562 leukemia cell growth arrest via the downregulation of p210Bcr-Abl and its downstream signals such as PKC, procaspase-3, Hsp90, NF-κB, and phosphorylated tyrosine kinase (PTK).[26] The antiviability effect of TCS in HeLa cervical carcinoma cells was markedly enhanced in a combination with EGTA-AM (a specific calcium chelator), where the elicited [Ca^{2+}] sequestration markedly disrupted the special microtubule ring structure, leading the HeLa cells to apoptotic death.[27] Therefore, the observations evidenced that TCS may help reduce the dose of conventional anticancer agents needed for given patients, thus decreasing the toxic side effects besides the enhancement of chemotherapies.

Polysaccharides

A polysaccharide fraction derived from the rhizome of *T. kirilowii* was composed of glucose, galactose, fructose, mannose, xylose, and a small amount of protein, showing marked antitumor and immunopotentiating activities.[28] The polysaccharides in 5–20 mmol/L concentrations inhibited the proliferation of MCF-7 (breast) and HeLa (cervix) human carcinoma cell lines and promoted the proliferation of peripheral blood mononuclear cells and circulating leukocytes *in vitro*.[29,30] The apoptosis of MCF-7 cells enhanced by the polysaccharides was found to be associated with the activation of intracellular caspase-3 and caspase-8.[31] Other immunoenhancing evidence confirmed that the lowered Ab-forming activity could be recovered by the polysaccharides in a mouse model. [29,30]

Lectins

Three isoforms of lectin were purified from the rhizomes of *T. kirilowii*, which possesses an ability to bind galactose. These lectin isomers were found to be able to kill some neoplastic cells like melanocytoma cells.[32]

Glycoproteins

Two glycoproteins termed karasurin-A and karasurin-B, were purified from fresh root tubers of *T. japonicum*. The two glycoproteins showed no differences in their molecular weight (ca. 28,000), amino acid composition, and neutral sugar content, but they have the similar part of amino acid sequence. The karasurins exhibited the same potencies of the suppressive effect toward the growth of BeWo choriocarcinoma cells.[33]

Immunotoxin Formulation

When the TCS was conjugated to anti-CEA monoclonal Ab, the formed immunotoxin showed a potent specific inhibitive effect against human colon cancer cells *in vitro* and *in vivo* with nude mice, and the antigrowth rates were 76–80% and 68–72%, respectively. This immunotoxin could extend the lifetime of the mice bearing the tumor without significant toxic and side effects.[34] An immunotoxin created by the linkage of TCS with Ng76 monoclonal Ab exerted a strong cytotoxicity *in vitro* against human M21 melanoma cell growth with an IC_{50} value of 5.6×10^{-10} mol/L.[35] If TCS was modified with 2-iminothiolane and then conjugated to Hepama-1 (a monoclonal Ab directed on human hepatoma), the hepatoma cytotoxicity of the immunotoxin was 500-fold higher than that of free trichosanthin but was approximately 600-fold less cytotoxic to HeLa cervical cancer cells, implying that the immunotoxin is a potent and specific antihepatoma agent that may be a considerable potential drug for the treatment of hepatoma selectively.[36]

Clinic Trials

Tian Hua Fen (Snakegourd root powder) can be applied in the treatment of patients suffering from chorioepithelioma and malignant hydatidiform mole. Except for cases of late-phase and cancer metastasis, TCS exhibited remarkable results in curing malignant hydatidiform mole by >95% and chorioepithelioma by 50–60%. If combined with surgical operation or radiotherapy, TCS would significantly promote the cure rate in the remedy for choriocarcinoma. The best administrational method is venoclysis by which the side effects showed to be lower. Due to the repeated drug resistance problem in using TCS, the dose should be progressively increased. A maximal dose at once can be reached to up to 16–20 mg, but the total daily dose ought to be about 40 mg.[31]

Other Bioactivities

The herb Tian Hua Fen (Snakegourd root powder) as well as trichosanthin have various pharmacological properties including abortifacient, anti-HIV, and immunoregulatory functions and antivirus besides antitumor. Trichosanthin also has protective effects against infectious brain injury induced by HSV-1 in mice. The *T. kirilowii* tuber has been prescribed in China for patients with diabetes, rigorous coughing, breast abscesses, and cancer-related symptoms. However, TCS has a marked antigenicity so that it can cause allergic reactions. The dose must be circumspect because the serious allergy is fatal. The common side effects caused by TCS are fever, headache, skin rash, sore throat, and stiff neck.[7]

References

1. Woo, S. J. et al. 2008. Trichosanthes kirilowii tuber extract induces G2/M phase arrest via inhibition of tubulin polymerization in HepG2cells. *J. Ethnopharmacol.* 115: 209–16.
2. Dou, C. M. et al. 2004. Effect of extracts of trichosanthes root tubers on HepA-H cells and HeLa cells. *World J. Gastroenterol.* 10: 2091–4.
3. Li, C. T. et al. 2010. The mechanisms of action of Tianhua® on antitumor activity in lung cancer cells. *Pharm. Biol.* 48: 1302–9.
4. Wang, S. S. et al. 2004. Angiogenesis and anti-angiogenesis activity of Chinese medicinal herbal extracts. *Life Sci.* 74: 2467–78.
5. Wang, Y. F. et al. 1989. Effect of trichosanthin protein and polysaccharide on choriocarcinoma cells in vitro. *Zhongliu* 9: 106–8.
6. Geng, B. et al. 1991. The in vitro inhibition of trichosanthin on human carcinoma cell lines. *Shiyong Zhongliu Zazhi* 6: 110–2.
7. Wu, Y. X. et al. (a) 1993. *Zhonghua Xiaohua Zazhi* 13: 263; (b) 1999. *Chinese Materia Medica* Vol. 5, 5–4663, 588. Shanghai Science and Technology Press, Shanghai, China.

8. Li, M. et al. 2010. Possible mechanisms of trichosanthin-induced apoptosis of tumor cells. *Anatomical Record* 293: 986–92.
9. Guo, F. et al. 1989. The effect of trichosanthin on mouse Ehrlich ascites carcinoma and the influence on the immune function of erythrocyte. *Zhongxiyi Jiehe Zazhi* 9: 418–20.
10. Liu, X. P. et al. 1991. Effect of trichosanthin on immune function of erythrocytes in tumor-bearing mice. *Zhongguo Yaolixue Tongbao* 7: 74.
11. Guo, F. et al. 1980. Treatment of trichosanthin on experimental ascites hepatoma and its immunemediating mechanism. *Acad. J. 2nd Military Med. Univ.*1: 9.
12. Liu, F. Y. et al. 2012. Trichosanthin down-regulates Notch signaling and inhibits proliferation of the nasopharyngeal carcinoma cell line CNE2 in vitro. *Fitoterapia* 83: 838–42.
13. Fang, E. F. et al. 2012. Trichosanthin inhibits breast cancer cell proliferation in both cell lines and nude mice by promotion of apoptosis. *PLoS One* 7: e41592.
14. Zhang, D. et al. 2015. Low concentrations of trichosanthin induce apoptosis and cell cycle arrest via c-Jun N-terminal protein kinase/mitogen-activated protein kinase activation. *Mol. Med. Reports* 11: 349–56.
15. Zhou, L. et al. 2014. Effects of trichosanthin on apoptosis and proliferation of colorectal cancer cell line CMT-93. *J. Shanghai Jiaotong Univ. (Med. Edit.)* 34: 257–62.
16. Zhuang, J. et al. 2014. Effect of trichosanthin on apoptosis and cytoskeleton microtubule structure reconfiguration in lung cancer A549 cells. *Zhongguo Zhongliu Linchuang* 41: 693–696.
17. Wu, Z. H. et al. 1999. Activation of G protein on the membrane of TCS-sensitive cells. *Shiyan Shengwu Xuebao* 32: 151–6.
18. Shaw, P. C. et al. 2005. Recent advances in trichosanthin, a ribosome-inactivating protein with multiple pharmacological properties. *Toxicon* 45: 683–89.
19. Tsao, S. W. et al. 1986. Selective killing of choriocarcinoma cells in vitro by trichosanthin, a plant protein purified from root tubers of the Chinese medicinal herb Trichosanthes kirilowii. *Toxicon* 24: 831–40.
20. Mi, S. L. et al. 2005. Trichomislin, a novel ribosome-inactivating protein, induces apoptosis that involves mitochondria and caspase-3. *Archiv. Biochem. Biophysics* 434: 258–65.
21. Dai, R. X. et al. 1993. The specific damage mechanism of trichomislin on trophoblastic cells. *Shiyan Shengwu Xuebao* 26: 411–28.
22. Wong, Y. F. et al. (a) 1990. Effects of trichosanthin on cell growth, cell cycle phase distribution and macromolecule synthesis in human choriocarcinoma cells. *Med. Sci. Res.* 18: 383–4; (b) 1990. Evaluation of trichosanthin against xenografts of human chorio-carcinoma. *Med. Sci. Res.* 18: 95–6.
23. Leung, K. N. et al. 1986. The immunomodulatory and antitumor activities of trichosanthin-an abortifacient protein isolated from tian-hua-fen (*Trichosanthes kirilowii*). *Asian Pac. J. Allergy Immunol.* 4: 111–20.
24. Takemoto, D. J. et al. 1998. Effect of trichosanthin an antileukemia protein on normal mouse spleen cells. *Anticancer Res.* 18: 357–61.
25. Wong, Y. F. et al. 1989. Effects of the combination of trichosanthin with Adriamycin and cisplatin on cultured tumor cells. *Med. Sci. Res.* 17: 167–9.
26. Zhang, K. Z. et al. 2007. Trichosanthin down-regulated p210Bcr-Abl and enhanced imatinib-induced growth arrest in chronic myelogenous leukemia cell line K562. *Cancer Chemother. Pharmacol.* 60: 581–7.
27. Wang, P. et al. 2009. Increase in cytosolic calcium maintains plasma membrane integrity through the formation of microtubule ring structure in apoptotic cervical cancer cells induced by trichosanthin. *Cell Biol. Internat.* 33: 1149–54.
28. Toyokawa, S. et al. 1991. Presence of protein polymorphism in karasurin, an abortifacient and antitumor protein, identified with physicochemical properties. *Chem. Pharm. Bull.* 39: 2132–4.
29. Chung, Y. B. et al. 1990. Studies on antitumor and immunopotentiating activities of polysaccharides from Trichosanthes rhizome. *Archiv. Pharm. Res.* 13: 285–8.
30. Zhao, G. Z. et al. 2011. Effect of Trichosanthes kirilowii polysaccharides on peripheral blood mononuclear cell proliferation and cell proliferation inhibition of breast cancer and cervical carcinoma. *Shizhen Guoyi Guoyao* 22: 2140–2.
31. Cao, L. L. et al. 2012. Effects of snakegourd root polysaccharide on apoptosis of MCF-7 cells. *Zhejiang Daxue Xuebao, Yixueban* 41: 527–34.
32. Sun, J. Z. et al. 1994. Purification of three isoforms of Trichosanthes kirilowii lectin and study on their biological properties. *Shengwu HuaXue Zazhi* 10: 727–32.
33. Huang, Y. L. et al. (a) 1987. Clinical treatment of 19 cases of malignant alimentary lobe tumor with Trichosanthin. *Chin. J. Integrated Tradit. Western Med.* 7: 154; (b) 1999. *Chinese Materia Medica* Vol. 5. Shanghai Science Technology Express, Shanghai China, 5–4663, pp. 588.
34. Gao, H. L. et al. 1992. The anticancer studies of trichosanthin conjugated with anti-CEA monoclonal antibody. *Zhongguo Mianyixue Zazhi* 8: 300–3.
35. Zhang, R. P. et al. 1993. The in vitro inhibition of trichosanthin on melanoma cells. *Zhongguo Mianyixue Zazhi* 9: 348–51.

36 Teng Li 藤梨

Kiwi

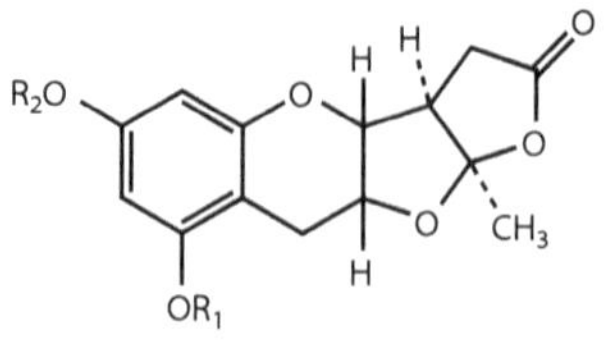

1. $R_1 = R_2 = -H$
2. $R_1 = -H, R_2 = -CH_3$
3. $R_1 = R_2 = -CH_3$
4. $R_1 = -H, R_2 = -Ac$

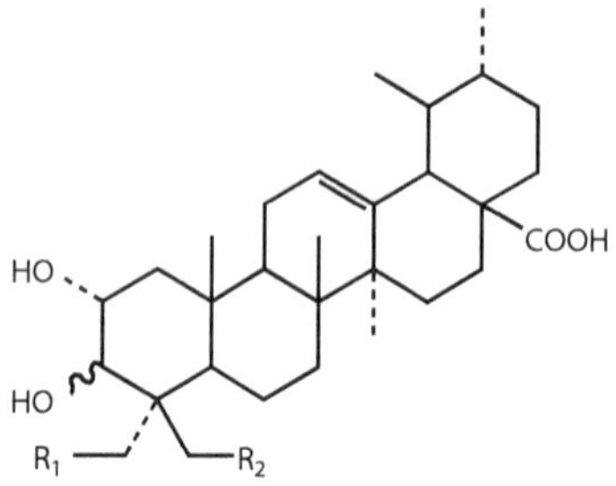

6. $R_1 = R_2 = H$, 3-beta-OH
7. $R_1 = -H, R_2 = -OH$, 3-alpha-OH
9. $R_1 = -OH, R_2 = -H$, 3-alpha-OH

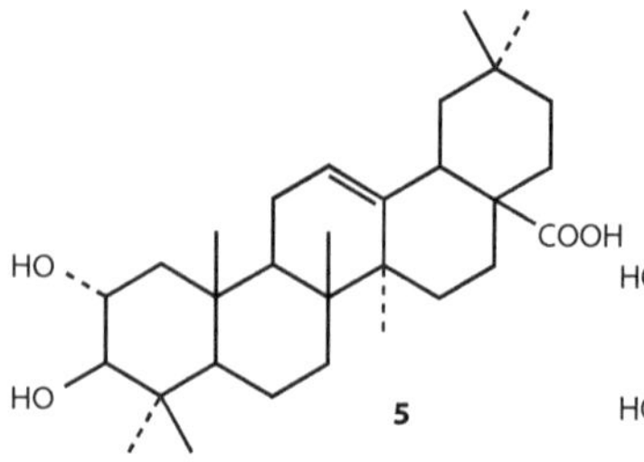

Herb Origination

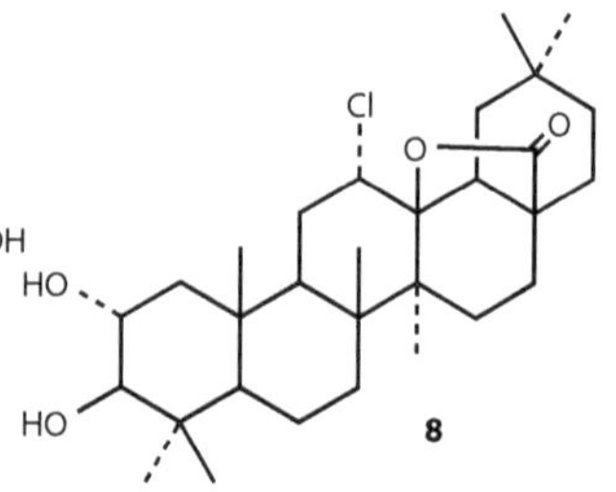

The herb Teng Li (Kiwi) is the fruit of an Actinidiaceae tree *Actinidia chinensis*. The plant is native to the Yangtze River valley of China as well as the Zhejiang province on the coast of eastern China. At the turn of the twentieth century, the kiwi seeds were first brought out of China by missionaries to New Zealand. Early nurserymen recognized the potential of the kiwifruit, and then it was developed as a commercial fruit in the world. The fresh and dried fruits, roots, and stems (>10 years old) of kiwi are used as a Chinese folk medicine.

Anticancer Activities

Modern studies revealed that kiwifruits displayed an antimutagenic activity against picrolonic acid or BAP-induced mutation.[1] Its juice could inhibit the nitrosamine formation and block the mutagenicity of α-tert-butane-*O*-benzoquinone.[2,3] *In vivo* experiments displayed that the juice was able to obstruct the production of nitritoproline in rats, pregnant mice, healthy persons, pregnant women, and patients with chronic atrophic gastritis.[4,5] The various extracts derived from its fruits and roots were demonstrated containing selective cytotoxic components against several types of human solid tumor cells (such as oral, esophagus, gastric, colon, and lung).[6–10] An EtOAc extract from *A. chinensis* could restrain the proliferation of human A549 lung cancer cells in its concentrations of 40–160 μg/mL, whose effect was correlated with the inhibition on DNA synthesis and reduction of Ki-67 antigen expressions.[11]

Anticancer Constituents and Activities

Flavonoids

From the roots of the kiwi plant (*A. chinensis*), 12 phenolic constituents and four pairs of isomeric flavonoids were isolated. The four phenolic compounds designated as planchols-A–D (**1–4**) possess a novel skeleton, demonstrating a marked inhibition on murine P388 leukemia cells and human A549 lung adenocarcinoma cells *in vitro*. The IC_{50} values were 2.5–5.05 μM in the P388 cells and 1.44–4.5 μM in the A549 cells. The preliminary SAR analysis showed that the hydroxyl groups in planchols-A–D (**1–4**) are essential for the inhibitory effect due to the reduced cytotoxicity when the hydroxyl group was substituted by methoxylation or acetylation.[12]

Triterpenoids

A group of triterpenoids were isolated from the roots of *A. chinensis*. Of them, 2α,3β-dihydroxyolean-12-en-28-oic acid (DHOA) (**5**), 2α,3β-dihydroxyurs-12-en-28-oic acid (DHUA) (**6**), and 2α,3α,24-trihydroxyurs-12-en-28-oic acid (**7**) showed a moderate inhibition on human LoVo colon cancer cells (IC_{50}: 6.0, 2.9 and 13.9 μg/mL, respectively), and DHUA (**6**) restrained the growth of human HepG2 hepatoma cells (IC_{50}: 9.2 μg/mL) *in vitro*.[13] 12α-Chloro-2α,3β,13β,23-tetrahydroxyolean-28-oic acid-13-lactone (**8**), 2α,3α,23-trihydroxyurs-12-en-28-oic acid (**9**), and three triterpenoids (DHOA (**5**), DHUA (**6**), and 2α,3α,24-trihydroxyurs-12-en-28-oic acid (**7**)) were also effective in the inhibition of human A549 pulmonic cancer cells with IC_{50} values between 30.4 and 34.6 μg/mL, whereas pseudotaraxasterol and triterpenoids 12α-chloro-2α,3β,13β,23-tetrahydroxyolean-28-oic acid-13-lactone (**8**), 2α,3α,23-trihydroxyurs-12-en-28-oic acid (**9**) showed the similar level of suppression on the LoVo cell line (IC_{50}: 31.1–31.6 μg/mL). Except for DHUA (**6**), the triterpenoids displayed a moderate cytotoxic effect on the HepG2 cells (IC_{50}: 25.5–35.7 μg/mL).[13] 2α,3α,23-Trihydroxy-12-en-28-ursolic acid induced the apoptosis of HeLa cells, associated with the activation of caspase-3 and caspase-7 and the inactivation of NF-κB.[14] Moreover, a HUVEC assay exhibited DHUA (**6**), 2α,3α,23-trihydroxyurs-12-en-28-oic acid (**9**), 2α,3α,24-trihydroxyolean-12-en-28-oic acid, and asiatic acid having an antiangiogenic potential.[15] The novel potential antiangiogenic agents are worthy of further translational research.

Polysaccharides

The anticancer polysaccharides such as ACPS-R, ACPS, and FP2 were prepared from the kiwi roots or fruits of *A. chinensis* by different research groups, displaying a potent *in vivo* suppressive effect against the growth of carcinoma cells. The i.p. injection of ACPS-R at doses of 75–125 mg/kg to tumor-bearing mice resulted in noticeable inhibitory rates, > 88.8% on ascitic hepatoma and Ehrlich ascites cancer, and > 49.6% on solid hepatoma. The life span of mice bearing EAC or P388 was significantly lengthened, and the percentage of EAC-free mice was increased by the ACPS-R treatment. ACPS-R was also capable of potentiating the cytotoxicity of an anticancer drug 5-FU in a cotreatment.[16] Also, the growth suppression of ACPS-R was apparently observed in a clinic cancer trail.[16]

By vena caudalis (v.c.) injection, ACPS demonstrated an obvious effect of restraining B16 melanoma *in vivo* and promoting the spleen index of tumor-bearing mice, whose antitumor rates were 40.90–48.67% in the middle and high doses against B16 melanoma. The chemotherapeutic potency was correlated with its abilities in distributing cell cycle at G1/S phase and regulating immunization.[17] *Actinidia chinensis* polysaccharides (ACP) induced the apoptosis of gastric cancer cells via the down-expression of Mcl-1, Bcl-2, and Bcl-xl and the up-expression of Bak and Bax *in vitro* and *in vivo*.[18] An injection derived from the kiwi root polysaccharide obstructed the growth of H22 hepatoma cells by 68.5% in its best dose *in vivo*, and also retarded the growth of gastric cancer and partly improved the immune function in mice, whose anticancer effect was found to be associated with a lower expression of PCNA and/or p53 and a toxic effect on the mitochondria.[19]

FP2 is a kiwifruit-derived polysaccharide, which is principally composed of D-glucose, D-mannose, and D-galactose. In a dosage of 150 mg/kg, FP2 evidently decreased the weight of sarcoma 180 in mice and reached the inhibitory rate to 54.2%.[20]

Enzyme

An enzyme called actinidine was prepared from the kiwifruits, which was claimed as an inhibitor of tumor proliferation and metastasis for the removal of albuminoids, e.g., skin-aging spot and wart. It was considered useful for anticarcinogenesis and prevention of Alzheimer's disease as a supplement.[21]

Other Bioactivities

Kiwifruits are rich in vitamin C and nutritional substances, and it also displays blood lipid-reductive, hepatoprotective, antiinflammatory, antianoxemia, and antiaging effects. Seventy percent of methanolic extract of kiwifruits was reported having significant anti-HIV, anti-free radical, and peroxide-eliminating activities. The polysaccharide called ACPS-R, in addition, demonstrated antiinflammatory, analgesic, anti-virus, and phagocytosis-enhancing effects.

References

1. Lee, H. et al. 1988. Antimutagenic activity of extracts from anticancer drugs in Chinese medicine. *Mutation Res.* 204: 229–34.
2. Mizuno, M. et al. 1988. Desmutagenic effects of sulfhydryl compounds on a mutagen formed from butylated hydroxyanisole reacted with sodium nitrite. *Agricul. Biol. Chem.* 52: 2843–9.
3. Song, P. J. et al. 1984. Cancer preventive effect of *Actinidia sinensis* Planch fruit juice: II. Detection of the blocking of N-nitrosamine formation in simulated human gastric juice in vitro by the ames test. *Yingyang Xuebao* 6: 241–6.
4. Song, P. J. et al. 1988. The block of N-nitritoproline synthesis in rats and health persons. *Yingyang Xuebao* 10: 50; 1984. 6: 109.
5. Xu, Y. et al. 1988. Anticancer effects of *Actinidia chinensis*. *Yingyang Xuebao* 10: 130; 10: 230.
6. Motohashi, N. et al. 2002. Cancer prevention and therapy with kiwifruit in Chinese folklore medicine: A study of kiwifruit extracts. *J. Ethnopharm.* 81: 357–364.
7. Cao, S. F. et al. 2007. The inhibitory effect of a ethyl acetate extract from Teng-Li roots against the growth of human cells. *J. Shanxi Med. Univ.* 38: 413–6.
8. Wei, P. F. et al. 2005. Studies on the extract of Teng-Li roots induces gastric cancer cell apoptosis. *J. Shaanxi TCM Univ.* 28: 52.
9. Sun, X. F. et al. 2006. Studies on the inhibition of Teng-Li roots extract against human lung adenocarcinoma A539 cells. *Shandong Yiyao* 46: 40–1.
10. Hu, B. et al. 2013. Root of *Actinidia chinensis* Planch induces anoikis in colon carcinoma RKO cells. *Zhongguo Shiyan Fangjixue Zazhi* 19: 242–5.
11. Du, Q. C. et al. 2011. Effects of ethyl acetate extracts of *Actinidia chinensis* on proliferation of lung cancer A549 cells. *Zhongguo Laonianxue Zazhi* 31: 4180–3.
12. Chang, J. et al. 2005. Cytotoxic phenolic constituents from the root of *Actinidia chinensis*. *Planta Med.* 71: 955–9.
13. Xu, Y. X. et al. 2010. Two new triterpenoids from the roots of *Actinidia chinensis*. *Fitoterapia* 81: 920–4.
14. Cheng, Q. L. et al. 2014. Apoptosis of cervical carcinoma HeLa cells induced by ursane triterpene compound A from roots of *Actinidia chinensis* Planch. and primary research on its action mechanisms. *Shizhen Guoyi Guoyao* 25: 2094–5.
15. Zhu, W. J. et al. 2013. Antiangiogenic triterpenes isolated from Chinese herbal medicine *Actinidia chinensis* Planch. *Anti-Cancer Agents in Med. Chem.* 13: 195–8.
16. Lin, P. F. et al. 1988. Antitumor effect of *Actinidia chinensis* polysaccharide on murine tumor. *Zhonghua Zhongliu Zazhi* 10: 441–4.
17. Shi, S. L. et al. 2009. Antitumor effect and its mechanism of *Actinidia chinensis* polysaccharide on B16-bearing mice. *Zhonghua Zhongyiyao Zazhi* 24: 777–9.
18. Shen, L. et al. 2014. Effect of *Actinidia chinensis* polysaccharide on apoptosis of MFC and their orthotopic transplanted tumor of gastric cancer. *Zhongcaoyao* 45: 673–8.
19. Zhang, G. J. et al. (a) 2013. Influence of *Actinidia chinensis* polysaccharide on expression of PCNA and p53 in orthotopic transplanted cancer of gastric tumor in 615 mice. *Zhonghua Zhongyiyao Zazhi* 28: 2538–41; (b) 2012. Mechanism study of kiwifruit root polysaccharide antitumor injection on tumor in vivo. *Zhonghua Zhongyiyao Zazhi* 27: 2177–9.
20. Lu, D. et al. 2005. Studies on purification and antitumor activity of fruit polysaccharide isolated from *Actinidia chinensis* Planch. *Shipin Kexue* (Beijing, China) 26: 213–5.
21. Tanaka, K. 2001. Actinidine as tumor proliferation and metastasis-inhibiting enzyme for removal of albuminoids. *Jpn. Kokai Tokkyo Koho* JP 99-332014 A 20010605.

37 Mao Dong Gua 毛冬瓜

Herb Origination

Mao Dong Gua is an herbal vine plant *Actinidia eriantha* (Actinidiaceae). This medical tree is distributed in southern China areas. Its roots have been used as a Chinese folk medicine in southeast China. The Mao Dong Gua roots can be annually collected and dried in the sun for medical practice. In addition, its leaves are also used as a Chinese herb in both fresh collection and dried material.

Antitumor Activities and Constituents

The Mao Dong Gua root is always used for the treatment of patients suffering from gastric carcinoma, breast cancer, or nasopharyngeal cancer in southeast China. In *in vitro* experiments, its decoction and both chloroform ($CHCl_3$) and EtOAc partition fractions, which were prepared from methanol extract and 80% methanol extract (by microwave) of the roots, demonstrated an antigrowth effect against SGC7901 (stomach), CNE2 (nasopharynx), MCF-7 (breast), and/or SMMC-7721 (liver) human neoplastic cell lines.[1,2] The EtOAc fraction at a concentration of 100 μg/mL induced the apoptosis of SGC-7901 cells and exerted a significant inhibitory effect on the proliferation of SGC-7901 cells with inhibitory rate of 92% (IC_{50}: 35 μg/mL, 72 h).[1] The $CHCl_3$ fraction dose dependently restrained the proliferation of human Bel-7402 hepatoma cells *in vitro* and inhibit the growth of mouse H22 hepatoma cells by 37.34% *in vivo* at a dose of 75 mg/kg.[3] The $CHCl_3$ fraction showed a superior activity in the SMMC-7721 hepatoma cells than the EtOAc fraction. However, the $CHCl_3$ fraction also showed to be toxic to normal L-02 hepatocytes, while the EtOAc fraction had no such effect.[2] In the *in vitro* test, the aqueous extract obviously restrained the proliferation and the cell invasion in human M21 melanoma cells, whose mechanisms might be related to reducing PD-L1 and PD-L2 mRNA and protein expression in the M21 cells.[4]

Polysaccharides

Up to now, no small molecules with antitumor activity have been reported from the *A. eriantha* roots, but the total polysaccharide *Actinidia eriantha* polysaccharide (AEP) was separated and four polysaccharides termed AEPA, AEPB, AEPC, and AEPD (average molecular weight: 1.43×10^6, 2.06×10^6, 1.73×10^6, and 1.13×10^6 Da, respectively) were purified from the AEP, which were found to contain similar neutral monosaccharide composition of galactose, fucose, arabinose, mannose, glucose, xylose as well as uronic acid, in which the molar ratios of galactose, fucose, arabinose, xylose, mannose, and glucose were 14.16:5.76:9.95:1.00:3.60:2.77 for AEPC and 13.59:5.51:8.29:1.00:3.49:3.99 for AEPD. The AEP and the purified polysaccharides were demonstrated to not only have a significant inhibition against the growth of mouse sarcoma 180 cells but also remarkably promote splenocyte proliferation, NK cell and cytotoxic T lymphocyte CTL activity, IL-2, and IFNγ production from splenocytes and elevate serum antigen-specific Ab levels in tumor-bearing mice. Among the purified polysaccharides, AEPC and AEPD exerted the higher *in vivo* antitumor and immunoenhancing activities.[4–7] More evidences confirmed that the AEPs strongly amplified both cellular and humoral immune responses and elicited a balanced Th1/Th2 response. The discoveries suggested that the AEPs may be efficacious and safe adjuvants suitable for cancer prevention and therapy.[5–8]

References

1. Lin, S. H. et al. 2013. Comparision of the antitumor activities between different parts of *Actinidia eriantha*. *J. Fujian TCM Univ.* 23: 46–7.
2. Wang, X. M. et al. 2011. Inhibiting effect of *Actinidia eriantha* Benth on liver cancer line SMMC-7721. *J. Zhejiang Sci-Tech Univ.* 28: 606–10.
3. Guo, H. H. et al. 2013. Study on antineoplastic activity of chloroform extraction of *Actinidia eriantha* Benth. *J. Zhejiang Institute of Sci.-Tech.* 30: 758–61.
4. Wang, S. Y. et al. 2013. Research on effect and potential mechanism of extractive of radix *Actinidiae erianthae* on proliferation inhibition in human melanoma M21 cells. *Liaoning Zhongyi Zazhi* 40: 2101–4.
5. Xu, H. S. et al. 2009. Antitumor and immunomodulatory activity of polysaccharides from the roots of *Actinidia eriantha*. *J. Ethnopharmacol.* 125: 310–7.
6. Sun, H. X. et al. 2009. *Actinidia eriantha* polysaccharides, its preparation process and application as antitumor agents or immunomodulants. *Faming Zhuanli Shenqing* CN 101518556 A 20090902.
7. Xu, H. S. et al. 2009. Chemical composition and antitumor activity of different polysaccharides from the roots of *Actinidia eriantha*. *Carbohydrate Polymers* 78: 316–22.
8. Sun, H. X. et al. 2009. Novel polysaccharide adjuvant from the roots of *Actinidia eriantha* with dual Th1 and Th2 potentiating activity. *Vaccine* 27: 3984–91.

38 Yin Chen 茵陳

Wormwood

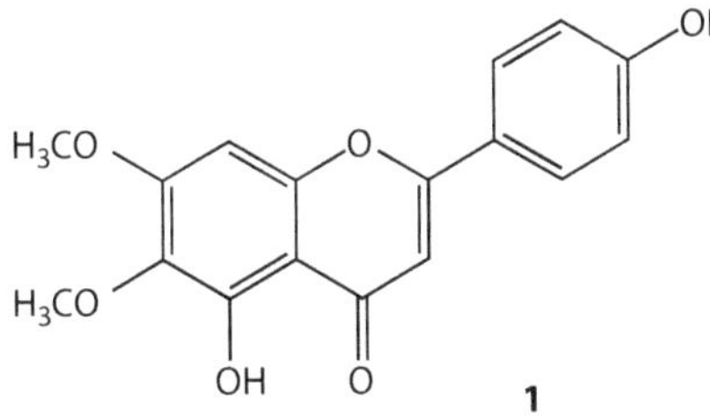

1 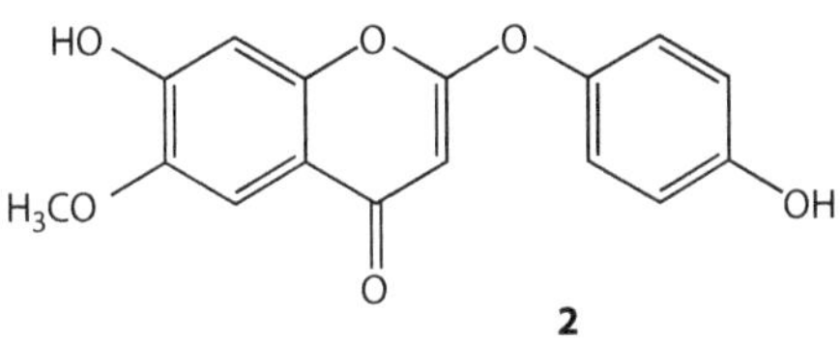 2 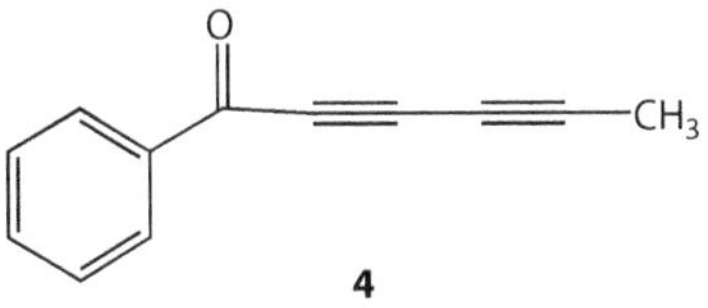 4

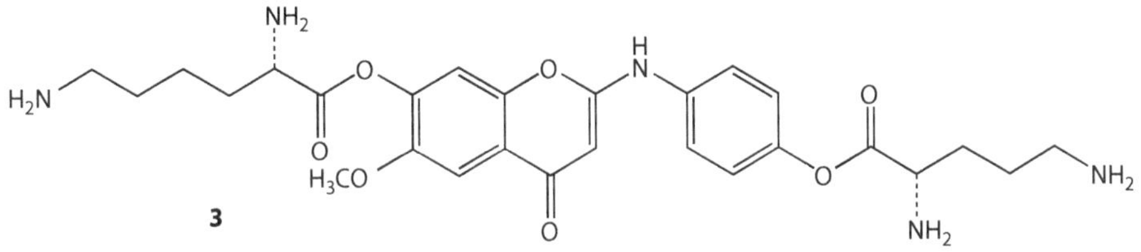

3 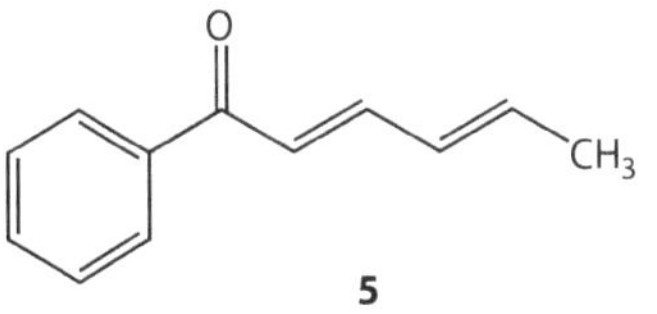 5

Herb Origination

The herb Yin Chen (Wormwood) was documented in *Shennong Ben Cao Jing*, the first Chinese classic of materia medica. The herb originated from two Compositae plants *Artemisia scoparia* (Zhu Mao Hao) and *A. capillaries* (Yin Chen Hao). Their aerial parts are collected in spring and autumn and dried in the sun for traditional Chinese medicinal use. The major producers of the herb in China are the provinces of Shaanxi, Shanxi, and Anhui.

Anticarcinogenetic Constituents and Activity

The two plants, Zhu Mao Hao (*A. scoparia*) and Yin Chen Hao (*A. capillaries*) are the major sources of the herb Yin Chen, but the bioactive components contained in these plants are not quite the same and present some different inhibitory activities on carcinogenesis and cancer cell proliferation.

*Agents from Zhu Mao Hao (*A. scopariae*)*

The Zhu Mao Hao could inhibit AFB1-induced carcinogenesis by decreasing the per mill rate of micronucleus of marrow cells and lessening the percentage of chromosomal aberration in mice, as well as reducing some sister chromatid exchanges per cells in a dose-dependent manner.[1] The herb could obstruct the interferential action of viral oncoprotein E6 and the binding between E6 and E6-associated RB protein (E6AP), an E3 ubiquitin protein ligase. This result indicated that the herb is able to block cervical carcinogenesis infected with human papillomavirus (HPV). 3,5-Di-*O*-caffeoylquinic acid (DCQA), a bioactive ingredient isolated from Zhu Mao Hao, inhibited the binding of E6 and E6AP and exerted a antiproliferative effect on human cervical cancer cell lines (SiHa and CaSKi) in a dose-response manner, indicating that DCQA may be a potential drug for the clinical treatment of cervical cancers infected with HPV.[2]

*Agents from Yin Chen Hao (*A. capillaries*)*

A chloroform fraction of Yin Chen Hao was prominently effective in reducing the mouse epidermal carcinogenetic incidence induced by 7,12-dimethylbenz[a]anthracene and inhibiting mouse L1210 leukemia cancer *in vivo*. The major bioactive constituents in the chloroform fraction were found to be camphor, 1-borneol, coumarin, and achillin by GC-MS elucidation.[3] Two flavonoids assigned as cirsimaritin (**1**) and capillarisin (**2**) were separated from Yin Chen Hao, exhibiting a dose-dependent cytocidal activity against the proliferation of human HeLa cervical cancer cells and murine Ehrlich tumor cells *in vitro*. The IC_{50} values were 3.2 and 3.4 μg/mL in HeLa cells and 0.54 and 0.03 μg/mL in the Ehrlich cells, respectively.[4] The oral administration of a fraction mainly containing capillarisin (**2**) to tumor-bearing mice markedly obstructed the growth of Meth-A fibrosarcoma *in vivo*.[5]

Capillarisin (**2**) as well as an essential oil prepared from the herb could suppress the proliferation of human KB nasopharyngeal cancer cells and induce cell apoptosis via p38/NF-κB and JNK/Bcl-2-mediated pathways.[6] The proliferation of HepG2 and HUH7 human hepatoma cells was moderately inhibited by capillarisin (**2**) *in vitro* (IC_{50}: <50 μg/mL).[6] In human multiple myeloma cells, capillarisin (**2**) specifically obstructed both constitutive and inducible STAT3 activations via the induction of SHP-1, SHP-2 tyrosine phosphatases, and potentiated bortezomib-induced apoptosis.[7] Capillarisin (**2**) was also found to markedly restrain the invasion of human MCF-7 breast cancer cells, associated with a specific inhibition on NF-κB-dependent MMP-9 transcriptional activity via p38 MAPK and JNK signaling pathways.[8] The investigations evidenced that capillarisin (**2**) may have a potential in the negative regulation of the growth, metastasis, and chemoresistance of cancer cells. Moreover, a semisynthesized capillarisin derivative termed 5-hydroxy-7-L-lysinyloxy-2-(4′-L-lysinyloxyanilino)-6-methoxychromone (Capi-N-Lys, **3**) displayed a more potent cytotoxicity against Meth-A fibrosarcoma cells compared to capillarisin (**2**).[9] A water-soluble form of Capi-N-lys (**3**), i.e., its tetrahydrochloride, significantly inhibited the growth of the Meth-A tumor cells in mice and augmented the Meth-A-induced delayed-type hypersensitivity and immune response in mice.[9]

Scoparone (**3**), a major constituent in *A. capillaries*, suppressed the proliferation of DU145 prostate cancer cells *in vitro* and *in vivo* concomitant with the induction of G1 cell cycle arrest by inhibiting the transcription of STAT3 target genes (such as cyclin D1, c-Myc, survivin, Bcl-2, and Socs3) and repressing both constitutive and IL-6-induced transcriptional activity of STAT3.[10] In addition, the essential oil of *A. capillaris* flower and capillin (**4**) isolated from the oil potently obstructed the growth of human leukemia HL-60 cells (IC_{50}: 1.1 and 3.9 μg/mL, respectively). The capillin (**4**) concurrently induced the apoptosis of HL-60 cells via a mitochondrial apoptotic pathway and the activation of c-Jun N-terminal kinase signaling.[11]

WACP, a water-soluble arabinogalactan fraction purified from the *A. capillaris*, whose molecular weight was about 5.8×10^4 Da, consists of arabinose and galactose in a ratio of 4:2. The anticancer potential of WACP was shown in the antiproliferative and apoptosis-inducing activities on human CNE-2 nasopharyngeal carcinoma cells. The apoptosis triggered by WACP was mediated by a mitochondrial apoptotic pathway, including the loss of mitochondrial membrane potential, release of cytochrome c, and activation of caspase-3 and caspase-9.[12]

Other Bioactivities

The herb Yin Chen (Wormwood) has been utilized in Chinese herbal medicine for over 2000 years, whose herb was demonstrated to possess analgesic, antipyretic, antiinflammatory, hepatoprotective, coronary-dilatory, hypotensive, hypolipemic, choleretic, and antimicrobial properties by pharmacological studies. An isolated vicenin-2 (a 6,8-di-*C*-glucoside of apigenin) is strong inhibitor of α-glucosidase, showing antidiabetic potential.[13]

References

1. Hong, Z. F. et al. 1996. Effect of herba *Artemisiae scopariae* on cytogenetic damage induced by aflatoxin B1. *Zhongyi Zazhi (Eng. edit.)* 16: 51–4.
2. Baek, T. et al. 2004. Effects of 3,5-di-*O*-caffeoylquinic acid from *Artemisia scoparia* Waldstein et Kitamura on the function of HPV16 oncoproteins. *Saengyak Hakhoechi* 35: 368–74.
3. Kim, Y. S. et al. 2008. Inhibition of 7,12-dimethylbenz[a]anthracene-induced mouse skin carcinogenesis by *Artemisia capillaris*. *J. Food Sci.* 73: T16-T20.
4. Jiang, J. Y. et al. 1992. Studies on the antitumor principles of Herba *Artemisiae capillaris*. *J. China Pharm. Univ.* 23: 283–6.
5. Cha, J. et al. 2009. Essential oil of *Artemisia capillaris* induces apoptosis in KB cells via mitochondrial stress and caspase activation mediated by MAPK-stimulated signaling pathway. *J. Food Sci.* 74: T75-T81.
6. Yang, C. C. et al. 2007. Supercritical fluids extraction of capillarisin from *Artemisia capillaris* and its inhibition of in vitro growth of hepatoma cells. *J. Supercritical Fluids* 42: 96–103.
7. Lee, J. H. et al. 2014. Capillarisin inhibits constitutive and inducible STAT3 activation through induction of SHP-1 and SHP-2 tyrosine phosphatases. *Cancer Lett.* (NY, U.S.) 345: 140–148.
8. Lee, S. O. et al. 2008. Suppression of PMA-induced tumor cell invasion by capillarisin via the inhibition of NF-κB-dependent MMP-9 expression. *Biochem. Biophys. Res. Commun.* 366: 1019–24.
9. Eda, S. et al. 1990. Preparation of chromone derivatives as anticancer agents. *Jpn. Kokai Tokkyo Koho* 10 pp. JP 88–322066 19881222.
10. Kim, J. K. et al. 2013. Scoparone exerts antitumor activity against DU145 prostate cancer cells via inhibition of STAT3 activity. *PLoS One* 8: e80391/1-e80391/13, 13 pp.
11. Masuda, Y. et al. 2015. Capillin, a major constituent of *Artemisia capillaris* Thunb flower essential oil, induces apoptosis through the mitochondrial pathway in human leukemia HL-60 cells. *Phytomed.* 22: 545–552.
12. Feng, G. F. et al. 2013. Antiproliferative potential of *Artemisia capillaris* polysaccharide against human nasopharyngeal carcinoma cells. *Carbohydrate Polymers* 92: 1040–5.
13. Islam, N. et al. 2014. Vicenin 2 isolated from *Artemisia capillaris* exhibited potent anti-glycation properties. *Food Chem. Toxicol.* 69: 55–62.

39 Yan Huang Lian 巖黃連

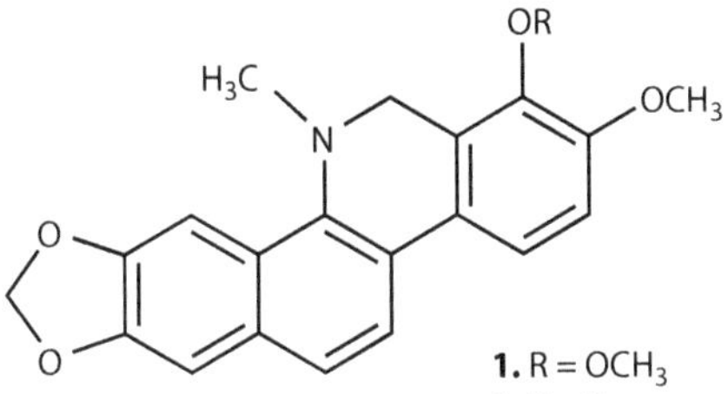

1. R = OCH_3
2. R = H

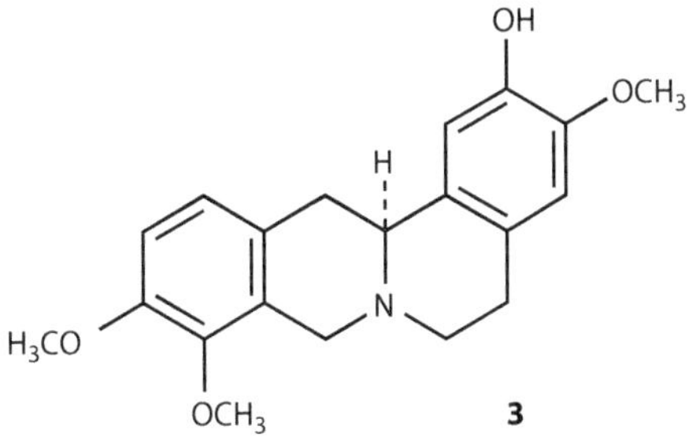

Herb Origination

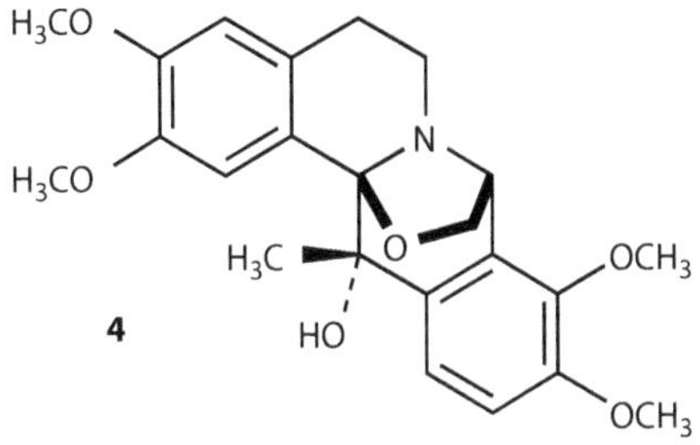

The herb Yan Huang Lian is the dried whole plant of *Corydalis saxicola* (Papaveraceae). The elegant perennial plant normally inhabits southern China, and the herb is normally collected after autumn and dried in the sun for folk medicinal use.

Antitumor Constituents and Activities

The alkaloid components isolated from Yan Huang Lian demonstrated a noticeable inhibitory effect against the cell growth of murine sarcoma 180 and Walker entity sarcoma 256 for 99.4% and 100%, respectively.[1] The major antitumor alkaloids in Yan Huang Lian were assigned as chelerythrine (**1**), tetrahydrocolumbamine (**2**), berberine and protopine (see Bai Qu Cai).[2] The i.p. or oral administration of the total alkaloids in doses of ~200 mg/kg to mice bearing carcinoma for 10 continuous days was significantly effective toward sarcoma 180, Walker sarcoma 256, and Ehrlich entity tumor. The cell growth of three ascites-type carcinomas (sarcoma 180, Ehrlich, and MCA-induced ascites carcinoma [HAC]) was notably inhibited by the alkaloids *in vivo*. The cell metabolism was also obstructed and the life duration of tumor-bearing mice was extended by 136–389% in dose- and time-dependent fashions.[1,3]

The PKC isoenzyme signaling pathway was known to play a key role in tumor cell proliferation, differentiation, and apoptosis. When the gastric carcinoma cells were incubated with chelerythrine (**1**), a PKC inhibitor, the cell growth was restrained through the induction of apoptosis and cell cycle quiescence at G0/G1 phase. Simultaneously, the protein levels of p53, p21waf/cip1, c-Myc, and Bax were augmented.[4] Chelerythrine (**1**) also displayed the cytotoxic effect in nine human neoplastic cell lines and exerted a significant *in vivo* tumor growth delay in nude mice bearing p53-deficient squamous cell carcinoma. Even a radio-resistant and chemo-resistant squamous cell cancer cells could rapidly undergo apoptosis after being treated with chelerythrine (**1**).[5,6] Moreover, in combination with chemotherapeutic agents, chelerythrine (**1**) was extremely cytotoxic to the solid tumors with direct DNA damage.[7] Benzo(c)phenan-thridine NK109 (**3**), a synthetic analog, showed more potent *in vitro* and *in vivo* anticarcinoma effects compared to chelerythrine (**1**) and sanguinarine.[8]

Seventeen alkaloids including tetrahydrocolumbamine (**2**) were isolated from several other plants of the *Corydalis* genus. The alkaloids could obstruct the activation of the Epstain–Barr virus early antigen individually, which was the evidence of the anticarcinogenic effect. Among the alkaloids, the most active alkaloid was solidaline (**4**) found in the *C. solida* plant.[9] Also, (–)-scoulerine and (–)-pallidine specifically inhibited the Topo activity and stabilized the enzyme-DNA complex. The strong anti-Topo-I effect might be attributed to an important role played by the quaternary ammonium ion in these molecules, whose activity is apparently involved in the antitumor mechanisms of Yan Huang Lian.[10–12]

Other Bioactivities

The herb Yan Huang Lian has long been used in traditional Chinese medicine to treat liver diseases such as hepatitis, jaundice, ascites, cirrhosis, and hepatoma. The pharmacological screening of this herb has demonstrated a wide spectrum of biological activities, including sedative, analgesic, antibacterial, antiviral, detumescence, antipyretic properties, as well as potential hepatoprotective activity against hepatitis virus B and A.

Its total alkaloid components could also enhance splenocytes proliferation, mixed lymphocyte reaction of allogenic spleen cells, IFN-γ production, and IL-2 production of splenocytes.[10] The three isolated protoberberine-type alkaloids (dehydrocavidine, dehydroapocavidine, and dehydroisoapocavidine) from the herb demonstrated antihepatitis B virus (HBV) activity. In a test, the alkaloids inhibited both HBsAg and HBeAg but no cytotoxicity against 2.2.15 cells (a kind of HBV-producing human hepatoblastoma cell line) *in vitro*.[11] However, chelerythrine (**1**) also causes minimal toxicity *in vivo*.[5]

References

1. Zhao, Y. et al. 1979. In vivo study on antitumor activity of *Corydalis saxicola*. *Guangxi Zhongyiyao* (3): 27.
2. Ke, M. M. et al. 1982. Studies on the active principles of *Corydalis saxicola* Bunting. *Zhiwu Xuebao* 24: 289–91.
3. Tan, Y. Z. et al. 1979. Inhibition *of Corydalis saxicola* on cancer cell lines. *Guangxi Zhongyiyao* (3): 31.
4. Zhu, G. H. et al. 1999. Pharmacological inhibition of protein kinase C activity could induce apoptosis in gastric cancer cells by differential regulation of apoptosis-related genes. *Digestive Dis. Sci.* 44: 2020–26.
5. Chmura, S. J. et al. 2000. In vitro and in vivo activity of protein kinase C inhibitor chelerythrine chloride induces tumor cell toxicity and growth delay in vivo. *Clin. Cancer Res.* 6: 737–42.
6. Herbert, J. M. et al. 1990. Chelerythrine is a potent and specific inhibitor of protein kinase C. *Biochem. Biophys. Res. Commun.* 172: 993–9.

7. Weichselbaum, R. R. et al. (a) 2002. *PCT Intl. Appl.* 47 pp, WO2001-US25021; (b) 1998. *PCT Intl. Appl.* 74 pp, WO1998-US5842.
8. Nakanishi, T. et al. 1999. Structural considerations of NK109, an antitumor benzo[c] phenanthridine alkaloid. *J. Nat. Prods.* 62: 864–7.
9. Ito, C. et al. 2001. Chemopreventive activity of isoquinoline alkaloids from Corydalis plants. *Planta Med.* 67: 473–5.
10. Tong, K. et al. 1995. Effects of total alkaloid from *Corydalis saxicola* on mouse immune function. *Mianyi Yixue Zazhi* 11: 238–41.
11. Li, H. L. et al. 2008. Alkaloids from *Corydalis saxicola* and their anti-hepatitis B virus activity. *Chem. Biodiver.* 5: 777–83.
12. Cheng, X. et al. 2008. DNA topoisomerase I inhibitory alkaloids from *Corydalis saxicola. Chem. Biodiver.* 5: 1335–44.

40 Xue Dan 雪膽

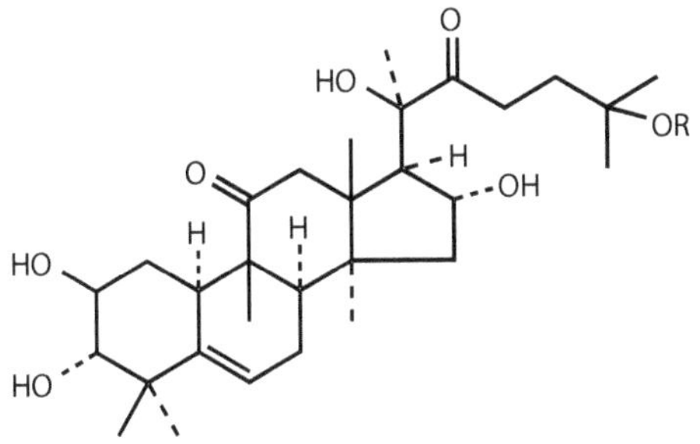

1. R = –H
2. R = –Ac

Herb Origination

The herb Xue Dan is the dried rhizome roots of a Cucurbitaceae plant *Hemsleya amabilis*, whose plant is native to the partial areas between Yunnan and Sichuan provinces in China. The plant is one of the sources of a Chinese herb termed Luo Guo Di (罗锅底).

Antitumor Activities and Constituents

The treatment with Xue Dan extract significantly inhibited the cell growth and the colony formation of tumor at low concentrations in three different types of human cancer cell lines such as U87 astrocytoma, MDA-MB-231 breast cancer, and Jurkat leukemia, *in vitro*, whose effect was correlated to apoptosis promotion with varied sensitivities. Relatively, the Jurkat cells were less sensitive to the treatments, while the U87 cells were more sensitive. Even at low concentrations, the extract could still induce the apoptosis of U87 astrocytoma cells.[1]

A group of anticancer cucurbitacins were discovered from the separation of Xue Dan roots. 23,24-Dihydro-cucurbitacin-F (DHCF) (1) obstructed the growth of DU-145, PC3, and LNCaP (prostate), A549 (lung), HT-29 (colon) human cancer cell lines, and P388 mouse leukemia cells, but it was invalid to KB, 3T3, and Meth-A cells *in vitro*.[2,3] The antiprostate cancer mechanism of DHCF was figured out to correlate with the promotion of G2/M cell cycle arrest and apoptosis via the induction of actin aggregation and formation of cofilinactin rod besides the upregulation of p21 (Cipl) and the downregulation of cyclin-A.[4] Cucurbitacin-IIa (= hemslecin-A) (**2**), the main ingredient of *H. amabilis*, showed a dose-dependent inhibitory effect on both proliferations and viability of human A549 NSCLC cells and murine primary splenocytes, but the inhibition on A549 cells was obviously higher.[5] The treatment with hemslecin (**2**) at a concentration of 100 mg/mL resulted in 43% and 52% cell death of human PC3 and CWR22Rv-1 prostate cancer cells, respectively, and 63% cell death of human NCI-H1299 lung carcinoma cells. Its *in vivo* antineoplastic activity had been proven in mouse models implanted with H22 mouse hepatoma cells or LLC cells.[6] Also, hemslecin A (**2**), 23,24-dihydro-cucurbitacin-B, 23,24-dihydro-cucurbitacin-E, and DHCF (**1**) exerted the cytotoxicity on human HeLa cervical cancer *in vitro*, where the IC_{50} values were 0.389 μM for hemslecin A (**2**) and 2.97–3.87 μM for other three. 3-Epi-isomer of the cucurbitacin showed less inhibition on the HeLa cells (IC_{50}: 7.45 μM).[7]

The cell cycle arrest and apoptosis-increasing mechanism of cucurtabicin-IIa (**2**) was revealed to be associated with (1) inducing the irreversible clustering of filamentous actin, (2) disrupting the actin cytoskeleton and mitosis, (3) reducing the expressions of cell cycle-regulated inhibitor of apoptosis protein and survivin, (4) markedly increasing the cleavage of PARP and activating caspases, and then (5) directing the cancer cells to mitotic blockage-induced cell death. Therefore, the actin–cytoskeletal signaling pathway was revealed to be a common target of cucurtabicins in the inhibition toward the growth and the viability of cancer cells.[6]

Other Medical Uses

The herb Xue Dan has long been utilized in China to treat bacillary dysentery, gastroenteritis, and infectious diseases besides the malignant tumor.

References

1. Wu, J. et al. 2002. Anticancer activity of *Hemsleya amabilis* extract. *Life Sci.* 71: 2161–70.
2. Frei, B. et al. 1998. Phytochemical and biological investigation of *Begonia heracleifolia*. *Planta Med.* 64: 385–6.
3. Delporte, C. et al. 2002. Pharmacotoxicological study of *Kageneckia oblonga*, Rosaceae. *Z. Naturforsch C.* 57: 100–8.
4. Ren, S. et al. 2012. Antiproliferative effect of 23,24-dihydrocucurbitacin F on human prostate cancer cells through induction of actin aggregation and cofilin-actin rod formation. *Cancer Chemother. Pharmacol.* 70: 415–24.
5. Gao, S. et al. 2012. Inhibitory effect of cucurbitacin IIa on proliferation of human non-small cell lung cancer A549 cells. *Zhongguo Shengwu Zhipinxue Zazhi* 25: 69–71.
6. Boykin, C. et al. 2011. Cucurbitacin IIa: Novel class of anticancer drug inducing non-reversible actin aggregation and inhibiting survivin independent of JAK2/STAT3 phosphorylation. *British J. Cancer* 104: 781–9.
7. Chen, X. B. et al. 2014. Cytotoxic cucurbitane triterpenoids isolated from the rhizomes of *Hemsleya amabilis*. *Fitoterapia* 94: 88–93.

41 Ma Lin Zi 馬蘭子

Chinese Iris seed

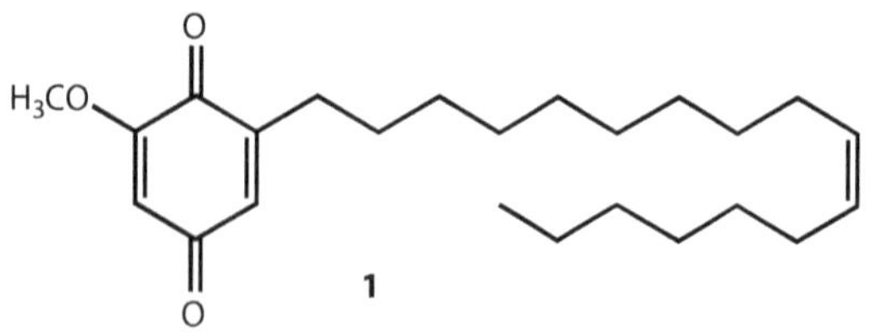

Herb Origination

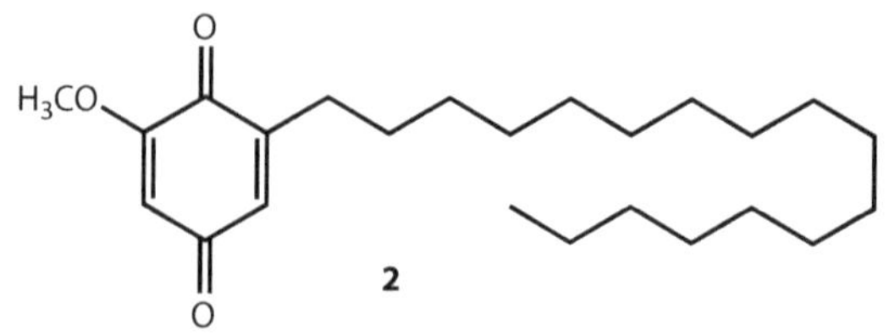

The herb Ma Lin Zi is the dried seed of an Iridaceae plant *Iris lactea* var. *chinensis*. This perennial herbaceous plant is broadly distributed in China, except in the southern region, as well as Korea and Japan. The seeds are collected in August and September when its fruits are ripe. Moreover, the root, the leaves, and the flowers of the plant are used in traditional Chinese medicines separately.

Antitumor Constituents and Activities

Pallasone A (= irisquinone) (**1**) and pallasone B (= dihydroirisquinone) (2) are the major antineoplastic constituents isolated from Ma Lin Zi where the contents of pallasoneA (**1**) and pallasone B (**2**) were 83–86% and 9–12%. Nine types of human tumor cells, including GLC-82 pulmonary cancer, BEL-7402 hepatoma, BCG-823 gastric adenocarcinoma, LA-N-5 neuroblastoma, TJ-905 astroglioma and MG-63 osteosarcoma, HL-60 and K562 leukemia, and K562/AO2 adriamycin-resistant cells, were used to evaluate their cytotoxic activity. The IC_{50} values of pallasone A (**1**) on the nine human cancer cell lines were <10 μg/mL in a 72 h exposure, whose data were similar with those of 5-FU. The most significant inhibitory effect of pallasone A (**1**) showed on BEL-7420 cells (IC_{50}: 2.5 μg/mL, at 48 h), K562 cells (IC_{50}: 2.79 μg/mL), and K562/AO2 cells (IC_{50}: 3.09 μg/mL, at 72 h).[1,2] Pallasone A (**1**) also exerted a moderate antiproliferative effect on different types of nasopharyngeal cancer cell lines (CNE-2, Sune-1, and Fadu) *in vitro* with an IC50 value range of 18.8–22.4 μmol/L. During the antitumor actions, pallasone A (**1**) augmented the CNE-2 cell apoptotic death and promoted the cell cycle arrest and the apoptosis of K562 cells at a concentration of 3.0 μg/mL.[1] The antitumor activity was also probably attributed to the ability of pallasone A (**1**) to damage cancer cell nuclei and the inhibition of the cell mitosis.[4,5] *In vivo* experiments demonstrated that i.p. injection (3–7 mg/kg) and oral administration (180–200 mg/kg) of pallason A (**1**) restrained U14 tumor, lymphosarcoma, and solid hepatoma by 30.4–55.5% in mice. The survival time of mice with ascites hepatoma and Ehrlich ascites tumor was extended by 158% and 83%, respectively, by the i.p. injection (5 mg/kg) of pallasone A (**1**). The prolongation of the life span was 67% for melanoma B16 and 170% for sarcoma 180 in mouse models injected with pallasone A (**1**) by i.p. at doses 4–10 mg/kg. Moreover, the pallasone A (**1**) treatment was also able to stimulate the cell-mediated immunity of normal and cancer-bearing mice.[5,6] In addition, pallasone B (**2**) in the assay displayed a significant suppressive effect on mouse leukemia P388 and L1210 cells and the inhibitory effect against EACs and U14 tumor cells.[4,7]

Importantly, pallasone A (**1**) was capable of retarding the growth of both drug-sensitive cancer cells and multidrug-resistant cancer cells with similar IC_{50} values, such as in K562 cells and K562/AO2 cells, but it has no inference on P-gp.[2,8] Also, pallasone A (**1**) at a low cytotoxic concentration dose independently enhanced the sensitivity of A549/DDP cells (a cisplatin-resistant human lung adenocarcinoma cells) to cisplatin by 7.9–8.9-fold. The MDR reversal effect on the A549/DDP cells might be relative to the intracellular GSH system, i.e., significantly the diminution of GSH content and GSTπ expression and the reduction of MRP protein expression.[9,10]

Radiosensitizing Activity

Pallasone A (= Iq7611) (**1**) is a radiosensitizer, which can selectively augment the radiosensitivity of neoplastic cells, especially hypoxic tumor cells. The radiosensitizing effect of pallasone A (**1**) was primarily demonstrated in HeLa cervical cancer cells *in vitro* with sensitizing-enhancement ratio (SER) as 1.68, and in MA737 breast tumor and U14 cervical cancer, *in vivo* with the SER of 1.33. Pallasone A (**1**) was also effective in the enhancement of the radiosensitivity of human mucoadenointestinal tumor in nude mice and of sarcoma 180 in mice but no such effect on normal cells.[11–13] The mechanism of its radiosensitization was revealed to correlate with (1) the decrease of respiration and oxygen consumption in the tumor cells (such as P388 cells); (2) the reduction of GSH content in tumor cells, leading the tumor cells lacking protection against radiation (such as HeLa cells); (3) the increase of the tumor cell cycle arrest at radiosensitive G1 phase; (4) the induction of mitochondrial damage (such as in EAC cells); and (5) the inhibition of the tumor cell rejoining and repair of DNA single-strand breaks caused by radiation.[13–16] Likewise, pallasone B (= Iq7612) (**2**) showed the similar radiosensitivity against the HeLa cells *in vitro*.[11]

Clinic Application

Numerous clinical trials have been performed in China by using the treatments combined with radiotherapies and pallasone A (**1**). The results clearly substantiated that the radiosensitizing effect of pallasone A (**1**) is helpful to improve the current radiotherapy, particularly for treatments of lung carcinoma, esophageal cancer, nasopharyngeal cancer, head and neck cancer, and other malignant tumors, with no obvious side-effects.[17–22] Pallasone A (**1**) was also effective in the inhibition of osteoblastic metastasis and cervical lymph nodes metastasis from nasopharyngeal cancer cells in the clinic trials.[2,24] An irisquinone capsule (containing both pallasone A and pallasone B) is now utilized in China clinics as a radiosensitive medicine for the anticancer therapies.

Other Medical Uses

The herb Ma Lin Zi (Chinese Iris seed) is traditionally used in China for the treatment of acute hepatitis A, dysentery, throat swelling and pain, bone tuberculosis, epistaxis, birth control, and so on.

References

1. Zhang, F. G. et al. 2010. In vitro anticancer effect of pallasone A and its induced apoptosis on leukemic K562 cells. *Zhongguo Yaoxue Zazhi* (Beijing, China) 45: 1716–9.
2. Li, D. H. et al. 2002. New application of 6-methoxy-2δ-10′-*cis*-heptadecenyl-1,4-benzoquinone. *Faming Zhuanli Shenqing Gongkai Shuomingshu* CN 1362061 A 20020807.
3. Cai, L. et al. 2000. Pallasone A induces the apoptosis of nasopharyngeal cancer. *Guangdong Yaoxue* (1): 6–7.
4. Tao, D. W. et al. 1991. Synthesis of pallasone B. *Zhongguo Yiyao Gongye Zazhi* 22: 57.
5. Wu, Z. X. et al. 1980. Pharmacological study of anticancer drug irisquinone. *Huanue Xuebao* 38: 156–9.
6. Tientsin City Institute of Pharmacology. 1980. Pharmacological study on the anticancer drug pallasone-A. *Yaoxue Tongbao* 15: 41.
7. Song, L. R. et al. 2001. *The Dictionary of Modern Chinese Herbal Medicines*. People's Medical Publish House Co., Beijing China, Part-I, 274.
8. Fu, L. W. et al. 2001. Irisquinone cytotoxicity to multidrug-resistant cancer cells. *Zhongguo Yaolixue Tongbao* 17: 234–6.
9. Liang, L. et al. 2001. The effect of irisquinone on the glutathione system and MRP expression of cisplatin-resistant human lung adeno-carcinoma cell line (A549DDP). *Chin. J. Cancer Res.* 13: 171–5.
10. Li, D. H. et al. 1981. Antitumor action and toxicity of 6-methoxy-2-delta 10′-*cis*-heptadecenyl-1,4-benzoquinone. *Zhongguo Yaoli Xuebao* 2: 131–4.
11. Zhu, L. et al. 1987. The radiosensitizing effect of lq7611 on Hela cells in vitro. *Chin. J. Clin. Oncol.*14: 69–70; 95.
12. Liang, J. P. et al. 2000. Heavy ion radiosensitization effect of irisquinone and its derivatives on S180 sarcoma borne in mouse. *Fushe Yanjiu Yu Fushe Gongyi Xuebao* 18: 45–51.
13. Wang, X. W. et al. 1999. Irisquinone: Antineoplastic, radiosensitizer. *Drugs of the Future* 24: 613–7.
14. Wang, S. X. et al. 1987. The effect of Iq 7611 on P388 cell's respiration. *Chin. J. Clin. Oncol.* 14: 88–9.
15. Li, M. R. et al. 1987. The inference of Iq7611 on the GSH content in human cervical cancer cells in vitro. *Chin. J. Clin. Oncol.* 14: 92–3.
16. Li, D. H. et al. 1987. Studies on the radiosensitivity of Iq7911. *Zhongguo Zhongliu Linchuang* 14: 67–68.
17. Yuan, L. et al. 1999. Treatment of esophageal cancer patients in combination of irisquinones with radiotherapy. *Chin. J. Clin. Oncol.* 26: 58–9.
18. Li, D. H. et al. 1999. Irisquinone, a new type of radiosensitive agent for anticancer treatment. *Chin. J. Clin. Oncol.* 26: 73–4.
19. Zhang, L. et al. 1999. Clinical study on the radiosensitive effect of irisquinones. *Aizheng* 18: 52–5.
20. Chan, J. et al. 2003. Prospective study of radiosensitizing activity of irisquinone in combination treatment of malignant neoplasms. *Chin. J. Clin. Oncol.* 30: 328–30.
21. Zhou, Y. Q. et al. 2001. Clinical study on NPC radiosensitization of irrisquinones. *J. Nanjing Med. Univ.* 21: 328–30.
22. Qiao, N. A. et al. 1998. Treatment of advanced cervical cancer patients with irrisquinone and radiotherapy. *Current Advances in Obstetrics Gynecol.* 1: 83–4.
23. Wu, T. G. et al. 2005. Effect of combined irisquinone and radiotherapy on cervical lymph nodes metastasis from nasopharyngeal cancer. *Jiceng Yixue Luntan* 9: 673–4.
24. Fan, W. et al. 1998. The inferences of irisquinone on 153Sm-EDTMP treated osteoblastic metastasis of nasopharyngeal cancer. *J. Zhongshan Med. Univ.* 2: 142–3.

42 Xiao Fan Hun 小返魂

Niruri or Stonebreaker

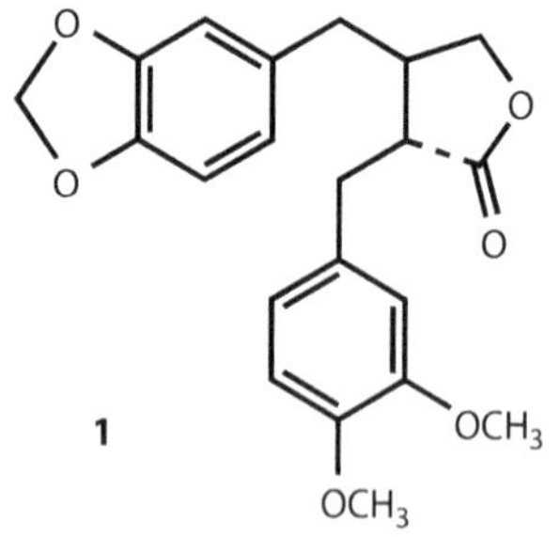

Herb Origination

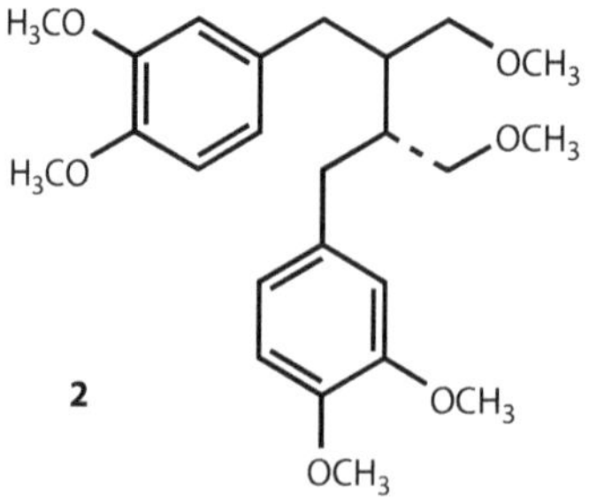

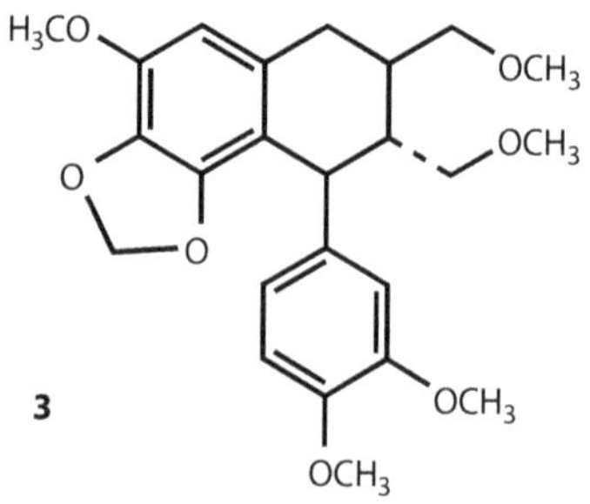

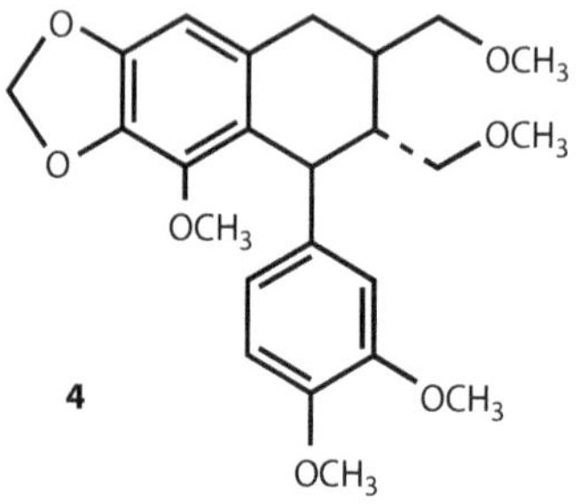

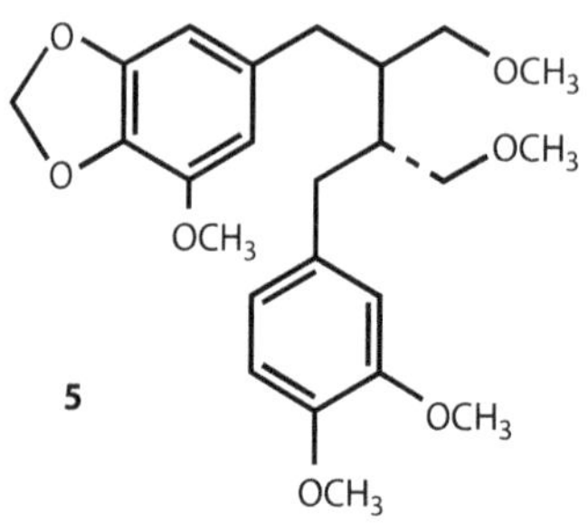

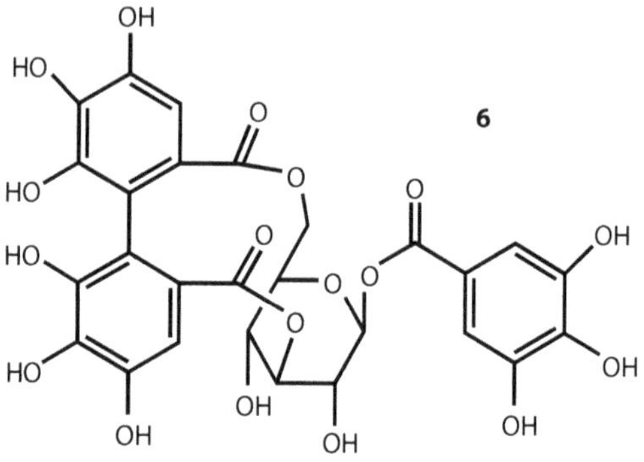

The herb Xiao Fan Hun (Niruri) is the dried entire plants of *Phyllanthus niruri* and *P. amarus* (Euphorbiaceae). The *P. niruri* plant grows in tropical areas like the rainforests of southern China, southern India, the Amazon, and the Bahamas, while *P. amarus* grows in drier climates in China and also in Brazil, India, Florida and Texas in the United States. In China, the herb is normally collected in summer and autumn and dried in the sun for the folk medicinal use.

Anticarcinogenic Activities

An aqueous extract of Xiao Fan Hun was a potent inhibitor of hepatocarcinogenesis. The treatment with the extract completely obstructed the initiation and the development of liver cancer induced by N-nitrosodiethylamine (NDEA) in rats; concurrently, the extract significantly lessened the levels of cytochrome P450 enzymes (such as glutamyl-S-transferase, γ-glutamyl *trans*-peptidase, reduced GSH, and aniline-4-hydroxylase) and protected the liver from any damages caused by NDEA. The results indicated that the antitumoragenic activity was partially attributed to the abilities in suppressing cytochrome P450 enzymes and scavenging oxidative free radicals.[1,2] The anticarcinogenic effect was also demonstrated in the inhibition of sarcoma development triggered by 20-methylcholanthrene with an obvious survival extension in mice and in the prevention of DNA single-strand breaks in liver caused by dimethylnitrosamine (DMN) in a hamster.[3,4] A two-stage skin carcinogenesis caused by 7,12-dimethylbenz[a]anthracene and croton oil was markedly restrained by Xiao Fan Hun alcoholic extract, resulting in an obvious decrease in tumor incidence, tumor yield, tumor burden, and cumulative number of papillomas.[5] More evidences indicated that the anticarcinogenic activity of Xiao Fan Hun might be related to the suppression of the metabolic activation of a carcinogen and the inhibition of cell cycle regulators and DNA repair.[3,4]

Its methanolic extract demonstrated a moderate to weak inhibition on MeWo melanoma cells and PC3 prostate cancer cells (IC_{50}: 50–150 μg/mL) but no important effect on normal human skin (CCD-1127Sk) and prostate (RWPE-1) cells, whose inhibitory effect was accompanied with the promotion of apoptosis and the induction of cell cycle arrest at Go/G1 phase for PC3 cells and at S phase for MeWo cells.[6] Given the extract to mice by p.o. obviously diminished the solid tumor volume and prolonged the life span of mice transplanted Dalton's lymphoma ascites or Ehrlich ascites carcinoma.[3] The methanolic extract prepared from the aerial parts of *P. amarus* was effective in the inhibition of human A2780 ovarian cancer cells *in vitro* (IC_{50}: 31.2 μg/mL), whereas the methanolic extract prepared from the hairy root cultures of *P. amarus* displayed a dose- and a time-dependent cytotoxicity against human MCF-7 breast adenocarcinoma cells *in vitro*.[7,8] By increasing the levels of intracellular ROS and lessening the mitochondrial membrane potential, the extract led the MCF-7 cells to apoptotic death.[8] In addition, SDEPN, a spray-dried extract of *P. niruri*, demonstrated a marked cytotoxic effect on human HepG2 and Huh-7 hepatoma cell lines *in vitro* with induced caspase-3-activated apoptosis, and also a protective effect on human normal HaCaT keratinocytes.[9]

Besides the anticancer activity, the Xiao Fan Hun extract synergistically enhanced the cytotoxicity of chemotherapeutic drugs and reduced the drug-caused toxicities. Its 75% methanolic extract appreciably attenuated the toxic side effects of CTX, such as the reduction of myelosuppression, the improvement of WBC count and bone marrow cellularity, the enhancement of GHS and GST systems, and the inhibition of phase I enzyme.[10] Therefore, the combination of Xiao Fan Huan extract with chemotherapies was encouraged for further investigation and clinical treatment against the malignant tumor.[10]

Antitumor Constituents and Activities

Lignans

Lignans are the major anticarcinoma constituents in Xiao Fan Hun. Three isolated lignans assigned as dibenzylbutyrolactone (**1**), phyllanthin (**2**), and hypophyllanthin (**3**) showed the inhibitory effect against cancer cell lines *in vitro*.[11–13] The treatment with a mixture of phyllanthin and hypophyllanthin (1:1) by oral administration at the doses of ~100 mg/kg enlarged the survival duration and the normal peritoneal cell count in mice bearing Ehrlich ascites.[12] The moderate anticancer activity of phyllanthin (**2**) and hypophyllanthin (**3**) was demonstrated in MCF-7 and MDA-MB-231 human breast cancer cell lines *in vitro* and N-methyl-N-nitrosourea-induced mammary carcinogensis *in vivo*.[13]

The two other lignans in Xiao Fan Hun, nirtetralin (**4**) and niranthin (**5**), exerted cytotoxic effects at a concentration of 43 μg/mL against human K562 leukemia cells with 61–62% the cell death.[14] Moreover, the lignans (nirtetralin (**4**) and niranthin (**5**)) are moderate inhibitors of P-gp. At the concentration of 43 μg/mL, nirtetralin (**4**) and niranthin (**5**) could suppress the growth of Lucena-1 cells (a VCR-resistant and P-gp-overexpressing subline) by 29.4% and 30.2%, respectively. The cotreatment with the two lignans significantly stimulated the apoptosis of Lucena-1 cells induced by 5 μM daunorubicin but not K562 cells.[14] Therefore, the results implied that nirtetralin (**4**) and niranthin (**5**) are potential agents for reversing the MDR and for synergizing the efficacy of chemotherapeutics.

Tannins

Corilagin (**6**) is a tannin isolated from the herb as a major active component, which has been discovered in many herbs as an antiinflammatory agent. *In vitro* experiment showed that corilagin (**6**) inhibited the proliferation of human SKOV-3ip and Hey ovarian cancer cell lines (IC_{50}: 2728 μM) but had much lower toxicity on normal ovarian surface epithelium cells. The anti-ovarian cancer effect was mediated by the blockage of TGFβ/AKT/ERK/Smad signaling pathways, concurrently, the induction of G2/M cell cycle arrest and apoptosis of ovarian cancer cells. The *in vivo* antigrowth effect was proven in nude mice transplanted with SKOV-3ip xenografts after the i.p. injection of corilagin (**6**) in a dose of 15 mg/kg for four weeks (three times per week).[15]

Nanoformulation

In order to increase the bioavailability of *P. niruri* extract, its stable nanoparticles were prepared with the average size of 150 ± 50 nm. The nanoparticles showed a concentration- and a time-dependent cytotoxicity on prostate cancer cells with a significant decrease in clonogenity, being a valuable candidate for prostate cancer therapy.[16]

Other Bioactivities

The herb Xiao Fan Hun (Niruri), especially from *P. niruri*, has a long history in herbal medicine systems worldwide, which has shown a promising activity in treating a wide range of human diseases including hepatitis, diabetes, kidney stones, etc. The studies and preclinical trials confirmed its medicinal properties such as antihepatotoxic, hepatoprotective, analgesic, antispasmodic, antidiabetic, antiparasitic, antihypertensive, antimalarial, anticholesterol, antilithic, antiviral, anti-HIV, and antibacterial. Additionally, the aqueous extract of Xiao Fan Hun is effective in the treatment of acute and chronic hepatitis B and healthy carriers of HBV, whose anti-HBV activity was mainly found to correlate with the inhibition of HBsAg secretion and DNA polymerase activity.[17] Also, the aqueous extract showed an anti-HIV reverse transcriptase and hypoglycemic effects.

References

1. Joy, K. L. et al. 1988. Inhibition by *Phyllanthus amarus* of hepatocarcinogenesis induced by N-nitrosodiethylamine. *J. Clin. Biochem. Nutri.* 24: 133–9.
2. Jeena, K. J. et al. 1999. Effect of *Emblica officinalis*, *Phyllanthus amarus* and *Picrorrhiza kurroa* on N-nitrosodiethylamine induced hepatocarcinogenesis. *Cancer Lett.* 136: 11–6.
3. Rajeshkumar, N. V. et al. 2002. Antitumor and anticarcinogenic activity of *Phyllanthus amarus* extract. *J. Ethnopharmacol.* 81: 17–22.
4. Sripanidkulchai, B. et al. 2002. Antimutagenic and anticarcinogenic effects of *Phyllanthus amarus*. *Phytomed.* 9: 26–32.
5. Sharma, P. et al. 2009. Antitumor activity of *Phyllanthus niruri* (a medicinal plant) on chemical-induced skin carcinogenesis in mice. *Asian Pacific J. Cancer Prev.* 10: 1089–94.
6. De Fernandes, A. et al. 2012. A dry extract of *Phyllanthus niruri* protects normal cells and induces apoptosis in human liver carcinoma cells. *Experim. Biol. Med.* 237: 1281–8.
7. Kumar, K. B. H. et al. 2005. Chemoprotective activity of an extract of *Phyllanthus amarus* against cyclophosphamide induced toxicity in mice. *Phytomed.* 12: 494–500.
8. Tang, Y. Q. et al. 2010. *Phyllanthus* spp. induces selective growth inhibition of PC3 and MeWo human cancer cells through modulation of cell cycle and induction of apoptosis. *PLoS One* 5: e12644.
9. Ajaiyeoba, E. et al. 2006. Cytotoxicity evaluation and isolation of a chroman derivative from *Phyllanthus amarus* aerial part extract. *Pharm. Biol.* 44: 668–71.
10. Gauri, A. et al. 2010. Hairy root extract of *Phyllanthus amarus* induces apoptotic cell death in human breast cancer cells. *Innovative Food Sci. Emerging Technol.* 11: 526–32.
11. Satyanarayana, P. et al. 1991. Isolation, structure and synthesis of new diarylbutane lignans from *Phyllanthus niruri*: Synthesis of 5'-desmethoxy niranthin and an antitumor extractive. *Tetrahedron* 47: 8931–40.

12. Islam, A. et al. 2008. Antitumor effect of phyllanthin and hypophyllanthin from *Phyllanthus amarus* against Ehrlich ascites carcinoma in mice. *Pharmacol. Online* (2): 796–807.
13. Parvathaneni, M. et al. 2014. Investigation of anticancer potential of hypophyllanthin and phyllanthin against breast cancer by in vitro and in vivo methods. *Asian Pacific J. Tropical Disease* 4(Suppl. 1): S71–S76.
14. Leite, D. F. P. et al. 2006. The cytotoxic effect and the multidrug resistance reversing action of lignans from *Phyllanthus amarus*. *Planta Med.* 72: 1353–8.
15. Jia, L. Q. et al. 2013. A potential antitumor herbal medicine, Corilagin, inhibits ovarian cancer cell growth through blocking the TGFβ signaling pathways. *BMC Complem. & Altern. Med.* 13: 33.
16. Unni, R. T. et al. 2014. Enhanced delivery of *Phyllanthus niruri* nanoparticles for prostate cancer therapy. *J. Bionanosci.* 8: 101–107.
17. Jayaram, S. et al. 1996. Inhibition of HBsAg secretion from Alexander cell line by *Phyllanthus amarus*. *Ind. J. Pathol. Microbiol.* 39: 211–5.

43 Ye Xia Zhu 葉下珠

Chamberbitter or Leaf flower

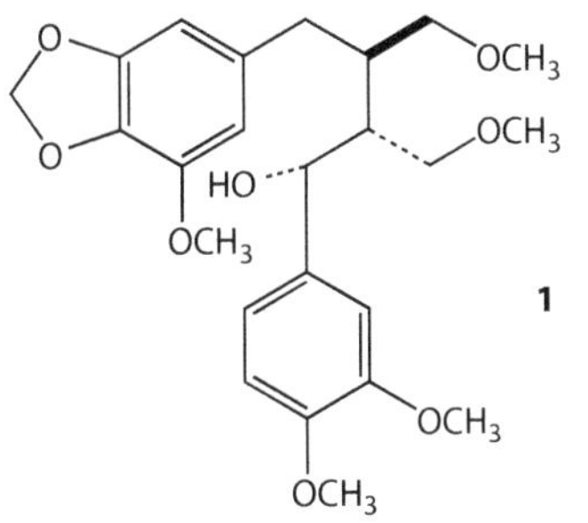

Herb Origination

The herb Ye Xia Zhu (Chamberbitter) originates from a Euphorbiaceae plant *Phyllanthus urinaria* L. This annual herbaceous plant is native to the Asian tropical region, but it has become a pantropical weed widely distributed in all tropical regions of the world. In China, the whole plant is generally collected in summer and autumn and dried in the sun for folk medical practice. The herb also can be used fresh after collection.

Antitumor Activity and Constituent

In China and Thailand, *P. urinaria* is traditionally used as an adjuvant and/or an alternative medicine for neoplastic patients. The water extract of Ye Xia Zhu demonstrated its antiproliferative and antiviability effects against various cancer cell lines such as Lewis lung carcinoma, PC3 prostate cancer, HepG2 hepatoma, K562 leukemia, HL-60 and Molt-3 leukemia, HT1080 fibrosarcoma, NPC-BM1 nasopharyngeal cancer, and 143B osteosarcoma *in vitro*, but it had no cytotoxic effect on human normal cells including liver cells and vascular endothelial cells under the same tested conditions. The *in vivo* cancer suppressive effect was proven in mice implanted with Lewis lung carcinoma. The anticancer effect was accompanied by the induction of apoptosis through mitochondria-associated intrinsic and/or extrinsic pathways with the downregulation of telomerase[1–10]; for instance, the extract promoted the apoptosis and obstructed the proliferation of human 143B osteosarcoma cells via an apoptotic extrinsic pathway, i.e., amplified both intracellular and mitochondrial ROS-modulated mitochondrial fission/fusion proteins, downregulation of Bcl-2 and upregulation of Bid, tBid and Bax, and activation of caspase.[6,7] The apoptosis of Lewis lung carcinoma cells triggered by the extract was associated with the downregulation of Bcl-2 gene expression but not with p53, p21, and Bax expressions.[8] Besides the gene expressions of Fas receptor/ligand enhancement, the activation of ceramide synthase was critical for the induction of HL-60 cell apoptosis.[9] In the treatment of the NPC-BM1 cells, the extract diminished a telomerase activity with the decrease of hTERT, hTP1, and c-Myc mRNA expressions,[10] whereas in PC3 cells, the expressions of six pathway reporters (Wnt, hypoxia, Myc/Max, NF-κB, MAPK/ERK, and MAPK/JNK) were notably declined and multiple signaling cascades (pan-Ras, c-Raf, RSK, Elk1, c-Jun, JNK1/2, p38 MAPK, c-Myc, DSH, β-catenin, Akt, HIF-1α, GSK3β, NF-κB p50 and p52, Bcl-2, Bax, and VEGF) were affected after the treatment, leading to the apoptosis induction of the PC3 cells and the reduction of cell adhesion, metastasis, angiogenesis, and glycogenesis.[11]

Furthermore, the studies using an *in vitro* matrix-induced tube formation of HUVECs confirmed the antiangiogenesis potential of *P. urinaria* extract, whose effect should be partly mediated by the inhibition of MMP-2 activity and MMP-2 secretion through zinc chelation.[1,2] Also, the extract was able to restrain the invasion and the migration of human Saos-2 osteosarcoma cells, human A549 lung cancer cells, and murine LLC cells, whose antimetastasis-related activity was associated with (1) transcriptional suppression of the activity of u-PA and decrease of the expression levels of MMP-2/MMP-9, (2) blocking ERK and Akt signaling and hypoxia pathways, and (3) repression of the DNA-binding activity and nuclear translocation of NF-κB and AP-1.[2,12–14] Considering the fact that Ye Xia Zhu has been used for a long time without any clinical side effects reported, these investigations provided the scientific evidences to support the safe application of Ye Xia Zhu as an adjunctive medicine to combine with chemotherapy and chemoprevention for the treatment of this deadly disease.

From biological assays integrated with conventional solvent fractionation, an inhibitor elucidated as 7′-hydroxy-3′,4′,5,9,9′-pentamethoxy-3,4-methylene dioxylignan (**1**) was separated, whose lignan was capable of suppressing the telomerase activity and activating c-Myc and caspase-3/caspase-8, thereby inducting the apoptosis and inhibition of four specific cancer cell lines such as HEp2 (larynx), HeLa (cervix), MCF-7 (breast), and EL-1 monocytes *in vitro*. Its IC_{50} value was 4.46 μM in HEp2 cells while that of an ethyl acetate fraction from the herb was 10 μM.[15]

Other Bioactivities

The herb Ye Xia Zhu (Chamberbitter) is broadly used as a folk medicine in most Asian countries in the tropical region. It demonstrated several proven pharmacological properties, including antioxidant, antihepatotoxic, hepatoprotective, antihypertension, antiinflammatory, antidiarrheal, immunoenhancing, antiviral, and antibacterial activities.[16,17] Ye Xia Zhu was also shown to have an important anti-HBV activity. It can significantly obstruct the activities of HBV-DNA and DNA polymerase and attenuate the expressions of HBsAg and HBeAg.[18,19] The herbal extract was capable of inhibiting hepatitis C virus replication in the experiments as well.[20]

References

1. Huang, S. T. et al. 2006. Antitumor and anti-angiogenic effects of *Phyllanthus urinaria* in mice bearing Lewis lung cancer. *Intl. Immunopharmacol.* 6: 870–9.
2. Huang, S. T. et al. 2010. Anticancer effects of *Phyllanthus urinaria* and relevant mechanisms. *Changgung Med. J.* 33: 477–87.
3. Lu, Y. H. et al. 2007. In vitro inhibitory effect of *Phyllanthus urinaria* compound on proliferation of human liver cancer cell HepG2 and its apoptosis induction. *Zhongyao Xinyao Yu Linchuang Yaoli* 18: 183–6.
4. Huang, S. T. et al. 2004. Aqueous extract of *Phyllanthus urinaria* induces apoptosis in human cancer cells. *Am. J. Chin. Med.* 32: 175–83.

5. Chudapongse, N. et al. 2010. Effects of *Phyllanthus urinaria* extract on HepG2 cell viability and oxidative phosphorylation by isolated rat liver mitochondria. *J. Ethnopharmacol.* 130: 315–9.
6. Wu, H. Y. et al. 2012. *Phyllanthus urinaria* induces apoptosis in human osteosarcoma 143B cells via activation of Fas/FasL- and mitochondria-mediated pathways. *Evidence-based Complem. Altern. Med.*: eCAM 2012: 925824.
7. Huang, S. T. et al. 2014. *Phyllanthus urinaria* induces mitochondrial dysfunction in human osteosarcoma 143B cells associated with modulation of mitochondrial fission/fusion proteins. *Mitochondrion* 17: 22–33.
8. Huang, S. T. et al. 2003. *Phyllanthus urinaria* triggers the apoptosis and Bcl-2 down-regulation in Lewis lung carcinoma cells. *Life Sci.* 72: 1705–16.
9. Huang, S. T. et al. 2004. *Phyllanthus urinaria* induces the Fas receptor/ligand expression and ceramide-mediated apoptosis in HL-60 cells. *Life Sci.* 75: 339–51.
10. Huang, S. T. et al. 2006. *Phyllanthus urinaria* increases apoptosis and reduces telomerase activity in human nasopharyngeal carcinoma cells. *Forschende Komplementarmedizin* 16: 34–40.
11. Tang, Y. Q. et al. 2013. Phyllanthus suppresses prostate cancer cell, PC3, proliferation and induces apoptosis through multiple signalling pathways (MAPKs, PI3K/Akt, NFκB, and Hypoxia). *Evidence-based Complem. Altern. Med.* 2013: 609581.
12. Tseng, H. H. et al. 2012. Antimetastatic potentials of *Phyllanthus urinaria* L. on A549 and Lewis lung carcinoma cells via repression of matrix-degrading proteases. *Integrative Cancer Therapies* 11: 267–78.
13. Lu, K. H. et al. 2013. *Phyllanthus urinaria* suppresses human osteosarcoma cell invasion and migration by transcriptionally. *Food Chem. Toxicol.* 52: 193–9.
14. Lee, S. H. et al. 2013. Inhibition of Raf-MEK-ERK and Hypoxia pathways by Phyllanthus prevents metastasis in human lung (A549) cancer cell line. *BMC Complem. Altern. Med.* 13: 271/1–271/20.
15. Giridharan, P. et al. 2002. Novel substituted methylenedioxy lignan suppresses proliferation of cancer cells by inhibiting telomerase and activation of c-myc and caspases leading to apoptosis. *British J. Cancer* 87: 98–105.
16. Wei, L. S. et al. 2012. Characterization of antioxidant, antimicrobial, anticancer property and chemical composition of Phyllanthus urinaria Linn. leaf extract. *Pharmacol. Online* 2: 36–40.
17. Ahmed, B. et al. 2008. Pharmacological and phytochemical review on Phyllanthus species. *Nat. Prod.* (An Indian J.) 4: 5–21.
18. Yang, C. M. et al. 2005. Acetone, ethanol and methanol extracts of *Phyllanthus urinaria* inhibit HSV-2 infection in vitro. *Antiviral Res.* 67: 24–30.
19. Yang, C. M. et al. 2007. Hippomanin A from acetone extract of *Phyllanthus urinaria* inhibited HSV-2 but not HSV-1 infection. *Phytother. Res.* 21: 1182–6.
20. Ravikumar, Y. S. et al. 2011. Inhibition of hepatitis C virus replication by herbal extract: *Phyllanthus amarus* as potent natural source. *Virus Res.* 158: 89–97.

44 Ban Bian Qi 半邊旗

Semi-pinnated brake

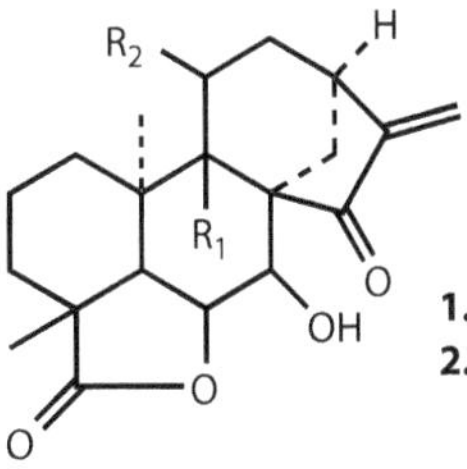

1. R_1 = -H, R_2 = -OH
2. R_1 = -OH, R_2 = -H
3 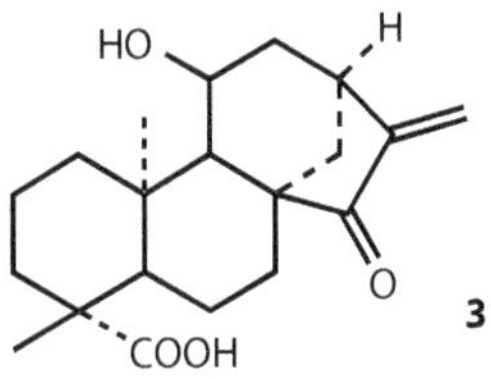

Herb Origination

The herb Ban Bian Qi (Semi-pinnated brake) is the whole plant or the rhizome of *Pteris semipinnata* L. (Pteridaceae). The plant is widely distributed in southern China as well as Southern Japan and Southern Asian region. The plant can be collected any season and used as fresh and dried herb in Chinese medicine.

Antitumor Constituents and Activities

Both water and ethanolic extracts of the herb obviously obstructed the proliferation of human K562 erythroleukemia and HL-60 promyelocytic leukemia cell lines *in vitro* in a dose-dependent manner and reduced the division index of HL-60 cells. The anti-growth activity of Ban Bian Qi was observed in mouse models bearing sarcoma 180 or HepA hepatoma treated with a dose of 5 mg/g of the herb. When combined with low dose of 5-FU, the aqueous extract in one-tenth of its common dose could increase the tumoricidal rate of 5-FU and did not reduce the numbers of leukocyte in the blood of tumor-bearing mice.[1]

Kaurane-Type Diterpenoids

Three anticancer kaurane-type diterpenoids elucidated as PsL-A (**1**), PsL-6F (**2**) and PsL-5F (**3**) were discovered from the ethanolic extract. The diterpenoids presented notable inhibitory effect against the growth of human HL-60 leukemia cells *in vitro* with IC_{50} values of 0.09 μmol/L for PsL-A (**1**) and 52.5 μmol/L for PsL-5F (**3**).[2–4] The treatment with PsL-6F (**2**) time- and dose-dependently enhanced the typical apoptosis of HL-60 cells and elicited the HL-60 cell necrosis when the dose rose to 29 μM for 3 h. Simultaneously, the expression levels of Bcl-2 and PKC were lessened and the cytosolic free calcium concentration ($[Ca^{2+}]i$) was amplified.[5–7] Furthermore, PsL-6F (**2**) synergistically augmented the cytotoxicity of a well-recognized antitumor agent genistein to the HL-60 cells.[8]

These diterpenoids also displayed a significant *in vitro* cytotoxic effects against five human solid tumor cell lines such as HepG2 and BEL-7402 (liver), SPC-A-1 (lung), CNE-2Z (low differentiated nasopharynx), and MGC-803 (gastric) cells.[2–4] PsL-6F (**2**) was the most active one among the agents on the five cell lines (IC_{50}: 0.1–0.6 μg/mL in 72 h).[2–4] The remarkable antiproliferative effect on the SPC-A-1 cells by PsL-6F (**2**) was accompanied with the induction of the G2/M cell cycle arrest and resistance of the synthesis of DNA, RNA, and protein.[9] In the inhibition of lung adenocarcinoma cells *in vitro*, PsL-A (**1**) repressed the expression of c-Myc and slightly reduced the TPK activity in the membrane.[10] In addition, PsL-A (**1**) and PsL-6F (**2**) are inhibitors of DNA Topo-I and Topo-II, whose anti-Topo activity might be partially related to their antitumor effect.[6]

PsL-5F (**3**) is the most important cancer inhibitor discovered from the herb, which has been truly investigated for the development of chemotherapeutic agent. The broad anticancer activity of PsL-5F (**3**) was showed in a panel of human tumor cell lines, such as erythroleukemia (K562), colon cancer (HT-29 and SW620), NCSLC (SPC-A-I, A549, NCI-H460, and PGCL3), hepatoma (HepG2 and Bel-7402), gastric cancer (MKN-45 and MKN-28), pancreatic cancer (AsPC-1), prostate cancer (PC3), nasopharyngeal cancer (CNE-2Z), undifferentiated thyroid carcinoma (FRO), and highly metastatic ovarian cancer (HO-8910PM) cells, *in vitro*.[11–26] The inhibitory rates of PsL-5F (**3**) were 73.18% on the growth of HO-8910PM cells after the treatment with 200 μmol/L of PsL-5F (**3**) for 24 h,[11] and its IC_{50} values were 1.02 μg/mL in NCI-H460 cells (in 72 h), 11.22 μg/mL in BEL-7402 cells (in 72 h), and 0.968 mg/mL in SW620 cells (in 48 h).[22,27,28] The cytotoxicity of PsL-5F (**3**) against MKN-45 (gastric cancer cell line bearing wild-type p53) cells was more potent than that against MKN-28 cells (gastric cancer cells with p53-mutation).[29] PsL-5F (**3**) also presented the inhibitory effect in NCI-H23 and CRL-2066 lung cancer cells *in vitro*.[30] By the induction of G2 phase cell arrest and apoptosis, PsL-5F concentration and time dependently inhibited the proliferation of Hep3B (liver), A549 (lung), and MDA-MB-231 (breast) human cancer cell lines.[31,32] The apoptosis of the MDA-MB-231 triple-negative breast cancer cells was stimulated by the PsL-5F treatment.[33] Additionally, the obvious suppression of diethylnitrosamine-induced mouse hepatoma by PsL-5F (**3**) was evidenced by the lessening of the tumor foci number and the tumor volume and the induction of the cell apoptosis.[34]

Moreover, with the PsL-5F (**3**) treatment, the migration, invasion, or adhesion was restrained in human highly metastatic ovarian cancer HO-8910PM cells and lung carcinoma NCI-H446 cells.[35–37] In a xenograft model with MDA-MB-231 breast cancer, 5F significantly reduced the volume of primate MDA-MB-231 cells and lessened the number of metastatic nodules in the lung without a toxic effect on the liver or the kidney, whose mechanism was largely related to the deduction of VEGF expression levels and its main receptor kinase domain insert containing receptor (KDR) in the tumor tissue.[38] Moreover, PsL-5F (**3**) was able to notably potentiate the cytotoxicity of chemotherapeutic agents (such as viscristine, cisplatin, and 5-FU) on HL-60 and K562 leukemia cells and/or CNE-2Z nasopharyngeal carcinoma cells in the cotreatments[14,39] and showed a synergistic effect with 3-isobutyl-1-methylxanthine (IBMX) against C26 colon cancer cells.[40] Additionally, giving PsL-5F (**3**) to mice for 18 weeks markedly obstructed a cigarette smoking carcinogen 4-methylnitrosamino-1-3-pyridylbutanone-induced mouse lung tumor formation and proliferation with minimal side effects.[32]

Likewise, the PsL-5F sodium solution markedly enhanced the solubility and the drug absorption, which was effective in the anti-growth of NCI-H460 cells and Bel-7402 cells (IC_{50}: 7.0 and 21 μg/mL, 72 h, respectively), but the activity was lower than that in the original molecule.[40] A glycoside of PsL-5F termed 11β-hydroxy-15-oxo-*ent*-kaur-16-en-19-oic acid 19-β-D-glucoside was less active to the CNE-2Z cells and A549 cells *in vitro*. However, the monoglucoside can be transformed to PsL-5F (**3**) by the metabolism in the human body.[41]

According to the positive experimental results, the PsL diterpenoids, especially PsL-5F (**3**), were considered to have a prospective potential as a novel anticancer drug candidate. Preliminary studies on the relationship of structure–activity suggested that the α,β-methylene cyclopentanone moiety in the molecule was the key center for the antitumor activity, and the site and the number of the hydroxyl groups also markedly affected the cytotoxic activity.[4]

Mechanism Exploration

The antiproliferative activity of PsL-5F (**3**) against the various neoplastic cells was found to strongly correlate with its ability in the induction of apoptosis,[42] whose mechanisms were summarized to selectively show the characteristic apoptosis promotion in different types of cancer cell lines, such as (1) down-expressing Bcl-2, up-expressing Bax, c-Fos, and c-Jun and activating p53 and caspase-3[12]; (2) reducing the membrane potential in p53-dependent manner and arresting the cell cycle progression[31]; (3) augmenting p38 and iNOS levels and diminishing NF-κB activity and p65 and p50 expressions (such as in HT-29, HepG2, NCI-H460, and CNE-2Z cells)[15,21,38,39,43]; (4) raising MAPK abnormal activation (such as in K562 cells)[13]; (5) amplifying ERK, JNK, and MAPK expressions (such as in FRO, NCI-H23, and CRL-2066 cells)[16,26,36]; (6) enlarging FAK, GDF15, and Nrld1 expressions (such in HO-8910PM cells)[11,17,18]; (7) amplifying p53-upregulated modulator of apoptosis (PUMA) expression (such as in PC3 and AsPC-1 cells)[20,22]; (8) elevating both levels of cyto-c and AIF in cytosol and declining VEGF level (such as in HepG2 cells)[21,23]; (9) rapidly increasing ROS level to trigger the cell apoptosis (such as in FRO and AsPC-1 cells)[16,20]; (10) repressing tumor cell tubulin polymerization and tubulin deploymerization[44]; (11) downregulating PCNA expression (such as in Bel-7402, NCI-H23, and CRL-2066 cells)[32]; (12) declining the level of Ezrin expression (such as in SW620 cells)[29]; (13) enhancing Fas expression (such as in keloid fibroblasts)[45]; and (14) activating adenylate cyclase and elevating cAMP content (such as in C26 cells).[40]

Importantly, the significant inhibition was observed on the invasion and the migration of NCI-H446 lung carcinoma cells after being treated by PsL-5 (**3**), whose effect was associated with the prominent diminution of MMP-9 and u-PA expressions.[36] PsL-5F (**3**) was notably effective in suppressing the metastasis of a highly metastatic HO-8910PM ovarian cancer cells with accelerated apoptosis. Its antiinvasive, antiadhesive, and antimetastatic mechanism was associated with a marked up-expression of Nrld1 and a noticeable down-expression of VEGF and NF-κB (p65).[34,40] Also, PsL-5F (**3**) evidently blocked the HO-8910PM cell cycle progression at G2/M phase by augmenting the active level of FAK and reducing NF-κB (p65) expression.[46]

Microformulation

For improving the bioavailability and the water solubility, PsL-5F has been prepared to a microemulsion, whose optimal formulation contained 45% water, 10% castor oil as the oil phase, 15% cremophor EL as the surfactant, and 30% as a cosurfactant mixture of 1,2-propanediol and polyethylene glycol (PEG)-400 (2:1, wt./wt.). Its bioavailability was markedly upgraded by 616.15% without hepatotoxicity in mice.[43]

Other Medical Uses

The herb Ban Bian Qi (Semi-pinnated brake) has been widely utilized as a Chinese folk medicine to treat toothache, diarrhea, jaundices, and viper bites.

References

1. Liao, C. et al. 1996. Studies on the antitumor activity and the acute toxicity of *Pteris semipinnata*. *Zhongyaocai* 19: 29–32.
2. Zhang, X. et al. 1997. The active constituents and antitumor action of *Pteris semipinnata*. *Zhongguo Yaoxue Zazhi* 32: 37–8.
3. Zhang, X. et al. 1999. Study on diterpenoid constituents and anticancer action of *Pteris semipinnata*. *Zhongguo Yaoxue Zazhi* 34: 512–4.
4. Li, J. H. et al. 1998. Comparison of the cytotoxicity of 5 constituents from *Pteris semipinnata* L. in vitro and analysis of their structure activity relationships. *Yaoxue Xuebao* 33: 641–4.
5. He, C. W. et al. 2002. Apoptosis in HL-60 cells induced by compound 6F isolated from *Pteris semipinnata*. *Zhongliu Fangzhi Zazhi* 9: 11–4.
6. He, C. W. et al. 2002. Role of calcium ion in the cytotoxicity and DNA fragment induction in HL-60 cells by 6F isolated from *Pteris semipinnata* L. *Zhongguo Bingli Shengli Zazhi* 18: 1025–8.
7. He, C. W. et al. 2003. Inhibitory effect of Compound 6F isolated from *Pteris semipinnata* L. on activity of protein kinase C in HL-60 cells. *Zhongguo Yaolixue Yu Dulixue Zazhi* 17: 81–6.
8. Li, J. H. et al. 1999. Effects of antitumor compounds isolated from *Pteris semipinnata* L on DNA topoisomerases and cell cycle of HL-60 cells. *Zhongguo Yaoli Xuebao* 20: 541–5.
9. Li, J. H. et al. 1999. Effect of compound 6F isolated from *Pteris semipinnata* on cell cycle and synthesis of DNA, RNA and protein of lung adenocarcinoma cell. *Zhongguo Yaolixue Tongbao* 15: 49–51.
10. Li, J. H. et al. 2001. Effect of active compounds isolated from *Pteris semipinnata* L. on DNA topoisomerases and tyrosine protein kinase and expression of c-myc in lung adenocarcinoma cells. *Chin. J. Cancer Res.* 13: 105–9.
11. He, T. P. et al. 2005. Effects of 5F from *Pteri semipinnata* L. on expression of NF-κB and FAK proteins in HO-8910PM cells. *Zhongliu Fangzhi Zazhi* 12: 565–8.
12. Wang, J. B. et al. 2002. Effects of a diterpenoid compound 5F isolated from *Pteris semipinnata* L. on the expressions of several oncogenes of K562 cells. *Zhongguo Yaolixue Tongbao* 18: 418–21.
13. Wang, J. B. et al. 2002. Effects of a diterpenoid compound 5F isolated from *Pteris semipinnata* L. on the activity and expression of mitogen activated protein kinase in K562 cells. *Zhongguo Yaolixue Tongbao* 18: 294–7.

14. Lan, L. B. et al. 2003. Purification of 5F from *Pteris semipinnata* and its enhanced cytotoxicity in vitro. *Zhongguo Yaolixue Tongbao* 19: 804–7.
15. Chen, G. G. et al. 2004. Over-expression of Bcl-2 against *Pteris semipinnata* L-induced apoptosis of human colon cancer cells via a NF-κB-related pathway. *Apoptosis* 9: 619–27.
16. Liu, Z. M. et al. 2009. Influences of *Pteris semipinnata* L. 5F on apoptosis and ROS level of undifferentiated thyroid carcinoma FRO cells. *Di-San Junyi Daxue Xuebao* 31: 1410–2.
17. He, T. P. et al. 2008. Effects of 5F from *Pteris semipinnata* and emodin on expression of GDF15 in HO-8910PM cell line. *Zhongyaocai* 31: 1845–8.
18. He, T. P. et al. 2009. Effect of 5F from *Pteris semipinnata* on expression of Nrld1 in HO-8910PM cell line. *Zhongguo Zhongyao Zazhi* 34: 1268–71.
19. Liu, Y. et al. 2009. Inhibitory effects of 5F from *Pteris semiinnata* L. on proliferation of non-small cell lung cancer NCI-H460 cells. *Zhongliu Fangzhi Yanjiu* 36: 9–12.
20. Zhang, K. J. et al. 2009. Effect and mechanism of 5F on the cell growth of pancreatic carcinoma. *J. Hainan Med. College* 15: 999–1002.
21. Liu, Y. et al. 2010. Effects of 5F on IκKβ, IκB, p65 and p50 mRNA expressions of non-small lung cancer NCI-H460 cells. *Zhongcaoyao* 41: 435–9.
22. Yang, B. et al. 2010. Mechanisms of inhibition on human pancreatic cancer PC-3 cell line by a diterpenoid compound 5F isolated from *Pteris semipinnata* L. treatment. *Zhonghua Zhongyiyao Zazhi* 25: 355–8.
23. Li, L. et al. 2010. Apoptosis effect and mechanism of 5f from *Pteris semipinnata* on HepG2 cells. *Zhongyaocai* 33: 77–80.
24. Li, L. et al. 2010. Apoptosis in HepG2 cells induced by *Pteris semipinnata* extract 5F involves p53 activation and VEGF inhibition. *Zhongcaoyao* 41: 241–5.
25. Wu, F. F. et al. 2009. Inhibition of proliferation by 5F from *Pteris semipinnata* L. in different kinds of non-small cell lung cancer lines. *Shandong Yiyao* 49: 6–8.
26. Liu, Z. M. et al. 2009. Influences of *Pteris semipinnata* L. 5F on apoptosis and ROS level of undifferentiated thyroid carcinoma FRO cells. *Di-San Junyi Daxue Xuebao* 31: 1410–2.
27. Chen, J. F. et al. 2011. Effect of *Pteris semipinnata* L. extract on ezrin expression and activity in human colon adenocarcinoma SW620 cells. *Huanan Guofang Yixue Zazhi* 25: 298–300, 304.
28. Wu, K. F. et al. 2010. Inhibitory effect of 5F from *Pteris semipinnata* extract on proliferation and proliferating cell nuclear antigen expression of hepatocellular carcinoma BEL-7402 cells. *Zhongguo Xiandai Yixue Zazhi* 20: 3687–90.
29. Liu, Z. M. et al. 2005. Cell death induced by *Pteris semipinnata* L. is associated with p53 and oxidant stress in gastric cancer cells. *FEBS Lett.* 579: 1477–87.
30. Li, M. Y. et al. 2010. Anticancer efficacy of 5F in NNK-induced lung cancer development of A/J mice and human lung cancer cells. *J. Mol. Med.* (Heidelberg, Germany) 88: 1265–76.
31. Ye, H. et al. 2012. Effects of 5F on cytotoxicity, apoptosis and cell cycle in human liver cancer cells. *Shizhen Guoyi Guoyao* 23: 1342–44.
32. Li, L. et al. 2012. Ent-11α-hydroxy-15-oxo-kaur-16-en-19-oic-acid inhibits growth of human lung cancer A549 cells by arresting cell cycle and triggering apoptosis. *Chin. J. Cancer Res.* 24: 109–15.
33. Wu, J. K. et al. 2014. A preliminary study on inhibitory effect of ent-11α-hydroxy-15-oxo-aur-16-en-19-olic acid from *Pteris semiinnata* L. on triple-negative human breast cancer cells and its mechanisms. *Zhonghua Shiyan Waike Zazhi* 31: 2414–6.
34. Chen, G. G. et al. 2012. *ent*-11α-Hydroxy-15-oxo-kaur-16-en-19-oic acid inhibits hepatocellular carcinoma in vitro and in vivo via stabilizing IkBα. *Investigational New Drugs* 30: 2210–8.
35. He, T. P. et al. 2005. Effect of 5F from *Pteris semipinnata* L. on invasion and metastasis of highly metastatic ovarian carcinoma HO-8,910PM cells in vitro. *Zhongguo Yaolixue Tongbao* 21: 540–4.
36. He, T. P. et al. 2009. Effect of 5F from *Pteris semipinnata* on expression of Nrld1 in HO-8910PM cell line. *Zhongguo Zhongyao Zazhi* 34: 1268–71.
37. Chen, J. et al. 2012. Effect of *Pteris semipinnata* active ingredient 5F on cytotoxicity, invasion, migration and expressions of MMP-9 and uPA of human small cell lung cancer NCI H446. *Di-San Junyi Daxue Xuebao* 34: 361–3.
38. He, Z. H. et al. 2014. Inhibitory effect of the diterperoid compound 5F isolated from *Pteris semipinnata* L. on breast cancer growth and metastasis in vivo. *J. Chin. Pharm. Univ.* 45: 92–6.
39. Wu, K. F. et al. 2013. *Ent*-11α-hydroxy-15-oxo-kaur-16-en-19-oic-acid induces apoptosis and cell cycle arrest in CNE-2Z nasopharyngeal carcinoma cells. *Oncol. Reports* 29: 2101–8.
40. Ye, H. et al. 2012. Effects of 5F isolated from *Pteris semipinnata* and cAMP levels in C26 colon cancer cells. *Liaoning Zhongyi Zazhi* 39: 2150–2.
41. Wu, K. F. et al. 2010. Preparation of 5F-Na solution and its inhibitory effect on cancer cells in vitro. *Zhongguo Yaofang* 21: 4419–21.
42. Lu, Y. N. et al. 2012. Characterization and evaluation of an oral microemulsion containing the antitumor diterpenoid compound ent-11α-hydroxy-15-oxo-kaur-16-en-19-oic-acid. *Intl. J. Nanomed.* 8: 1879–86.
43. Li, M. Y. et al. 2012. *Ent*-11α-hydroxy-15-oxo-kaur-16-en-19-oic-acid induces apoptosis of human malignant cancer cells. *Current Drug Targets* 13: 1730–7.
44. Liu, Y. et al. 2005. Effect of 5F isolated from *Pteris semipinnata* L. on tubulin polymerization in vitro. *Zhongguo Yaolixue Tongbao* 21: 447–9.
45. Cai, K. R. et al. 2004. Effects of 5F from *Pteris semipinnata* L on apoptosis and expression of Fas in keloid fibroblasts. *Huazhong Keji Daxue Xuebao, Yixueban* 33: 416–8.
46. He, T. P. et al. 2005. Study on the effect and its mechanisms of 5F from *Pteris semipinnata* L. on the cell cycle of highly metastatic ovarian carcinoma HO-8910PM cells. *Zhongyaocai* 28: 672–6.

45 Xi Huang Cao 溪黄草

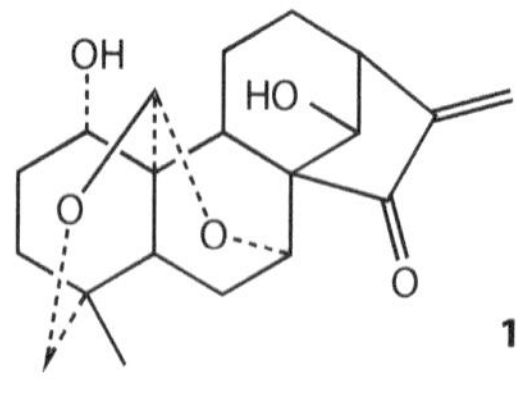

Herb Origination

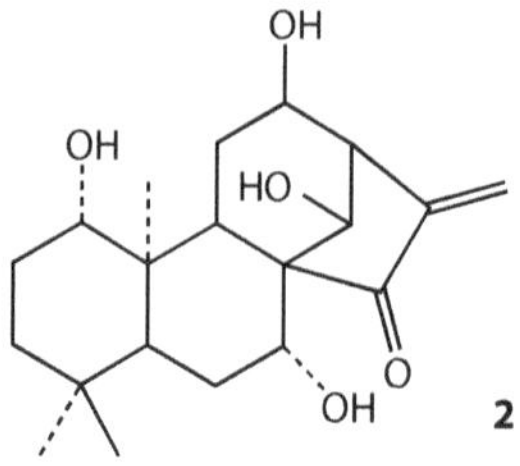

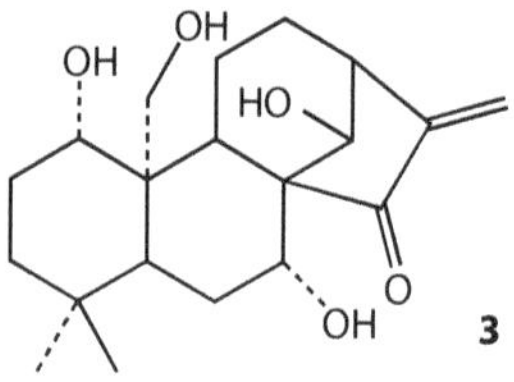

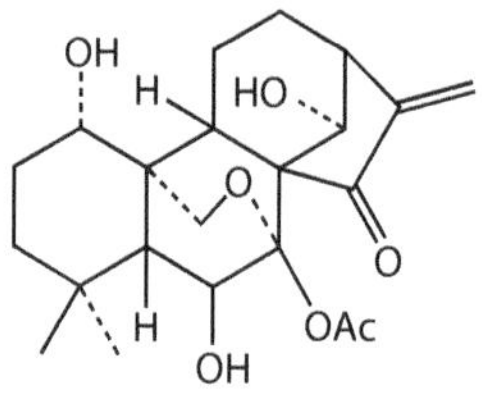

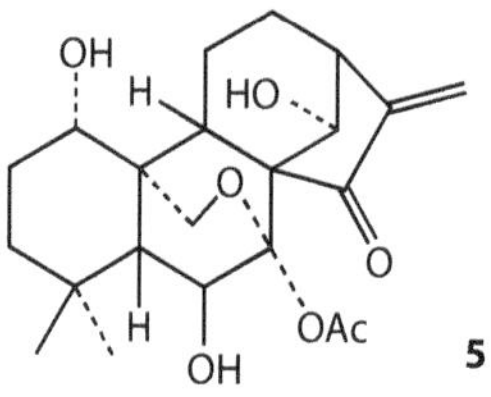

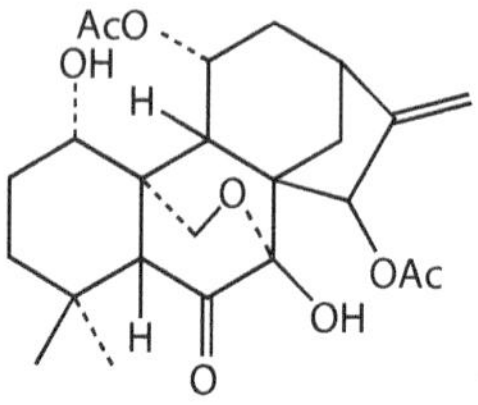

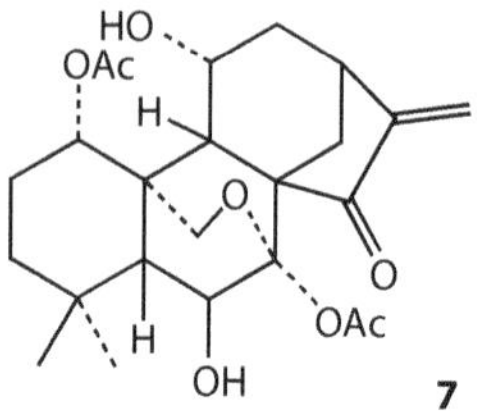

The herb Xi Huang Cao is the whole plants of *Rabdosia serra* and *R. lophanthoides* (Labiatae). The former species is broadly distributed in many Chinese provinces, and the latter one is wildly growing in the southern regions of Asia. In China, the whole plant can be collected annuall two to three times for folk medicinal purpose. A larger source of Xi Huang Cao was found in southwestern China.

Antitumor Constituents and Activity

ent-Kaurane-Type Diterpenoids

According to scientific reports, Xi Huang Cao (*R. serra*) was shown to have an antitumor-related property in the assay. A benzene fraction from the ethanolic extract of *R. serra* displayed a marked antitumor effect against the proliferation of human HepG2 hepatoma and HL-60 leukemia cell lines, and its inhibitory rates were up to 80% and 100% at a concentration of 100 μg/mL, respectively. From the low polarity fraction, a cytotoxic diterpenoid elucidated as II-5-3 (*ent*-1α,7α,12α,14β,20α-pentahydroxyhaur-16-en-15-one) was separated. Its antiproliferative rates on the HepG2 and HL-60 cells reached to 51.2% and 65.3% at the concentration of 12.5 μg/mL, respectively.[1] Rabdoserrin-A (**1**), excisanin-A (**2**), and kamebakaurin (**3**), the three diterpenoids isolated from herb *R. serra*, demonstrated a significant cytotoxic effect on human HeLa cervical cancer cells *in vitro*.[2]

In the continuing investigation, four more active *ent*-kaurane-type diterpenoids designated as 6β,14α-dihydroxy-1α,7β-diacetoxy-7α,20-epoxy-*ent*-kaur-16-en-15-one (**4**), lasiodin (**5**), effusanin-E (**6**), and nodosin, as well as three phenolics, pedalitin, rosmarinic acid, and methyl rosmarinate, were discovered from the leaves of *R. serra*. All these molecules were effective in the inhibition of human HepG3 hepatoma, MCF-7 breast cancer, and HL-60 leukemia cell lines *in vitro*. But only 6β,14α-dihydroxy-1α,7β-diacetoxy-7α,20-epoxy-*ent*-kaur-16-en-15-one (**4**) and lasiodin (**5**) displayed a marked cytotoxicity on the tested tumor cells (IC_{50}: <4.6 μM), whose antigrowth potencies were comparable to cisplatin.[3] Effusanin-E (**6**) also significantly inhibited the proliferation and induced the apoptosis of nasopharyngeal carcinoma cells *in vitro* and *in vivo* by blocking the NF-κB and COX-2 signaling, eliciting the cleavage of PARP and caspases-3/9, and inhibiting the nuclear translocation of p65 NF-κB proteins.[4] Similarly, by simultaneously activating Apaf-1/caspase-dependent apoptotic pathways and obstructing AKT/MAPK and COX-2/NF-κB signaling pathways, lasiodon (**5**) inhibited the proliferation of human nasopharyngeal carcinoma cells.[5] The results suggested that effusanin-E (**6**) and lasiodin (**5**) may be promising agents for the prevention and the treatment of neoplasm.

The cytotoxic effect of nodosin and serrin-B was shown on SGC7901 gastric carcinoma, HL-60 leukemia, LOVO colon cancer, U87 glioma cell lines, and serrin-B was also effective in the inhibition of human AGZY lung adenocarcinoma cell line.[6] Comparing the relationship between the structure and the activities with inactive parvifolin-G (**7**) revealed that the hydroxyl groups at C-7 and C-14β are important for the cytotoxicity, and the α-methylenecyclopentanone moiety is an active center for the tumor suppression. The substitution of a carbonyl group by acetoxy group at C-15 (like parvifolin-G) would diminish the inhibitory activity due to the loss of the hydrogen bond between the 6-OH and C-15 carbonyl groups.[3] Therefore, these findings may provide valuable clues for the development and design of new anticancer drug candidates.

Flavonoids

The flavonoid components derived from *R. lophanthoides* were found having an ability to induce the differentiation of malignant phenotypical reversion in human GHC-3 hepatocellular cancer cells *in vitro*. After 10 weeks treatment with the flavonoids, the synthesis of fetoprotein (AFP) and *ras* p21 were gradually decreased and the antigen of GHC-3 became weaker to bind on the cell membrane, leading the tumor cells to differentiation.[7]

References

1. Hu, S. Q. et al. 2009. Purification and identification of compounds with in vitro antitumor activity from *Rabdosia serra* (Maxim) Hara. *Bioinformatics and Biomedical Engineering, Third International Conference on Beijing, China, Issue Date*: 2009, Beijing, China, 11–3 June, IEEE, pp. 1–4.
2. Jin, R. L. et al. 1985. The structure of rabdoserrin A, isolated from *Rabdosia serra* (Maxim) Hara. *Yaoxue Xuebao* 20: 366–71.
3. Lin, L. Z. et al. 2012. Isolation and identification of *ent*-kaurane-type diterpenoids from *Rabdosia serra* (Maxim.) Hara leaf and their inhibitory activities against HepG2, MCF-7, and HL-60 cell lines. *Food Chem.* 131: 1009–14.
4. Zhuang, M. Z. et al. 2014. Effusanin E suppresses nasopharyngeal carcinoma cell growth by inhibiting NF-κB and COX-2 signaling. *PLoS One* 9: e109951.
5. Lin, L. Z. et al. 2014. Lasiodin inhibits proliferation of human nasopharyngeal carcinoma cells by simultaneous modulation of the Apaf-1/caspase, AKT/MAPK and COX-2/NF-κB signaling pathways. *PLoS One* 9: e97799.
6. Hai, G. F. et al. 2013. Toxic effects of serrin B and nodosin on HL60, SGC7901, LOVO, U87 and AGZY cells. *Xinxiang Yixueyuan Xuebao* 30: 345–6, 352.
7. Ge, Y. P. et al. 1995. Induction on the differentiation of malignant phenotypical reversion of human hepatocellular cancer cell line (GH-3) by *Rabdosia lophanthoides* flavones in vitro. *Xibao Shengwuxue Zazhi* 17: 83–6.

46 Hong Gen Cao 紅根草

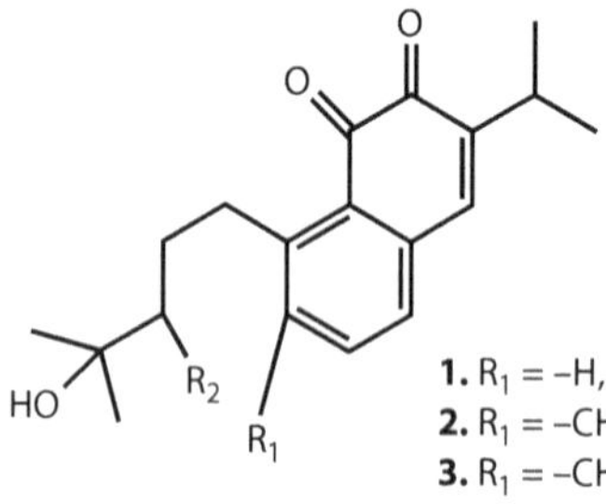

1. R_1 = -H, R_2 = -OH
2. R_1 = $-CH_3$, R_2 == O
3. R_1 = $-CH_3$, R_2 = -H

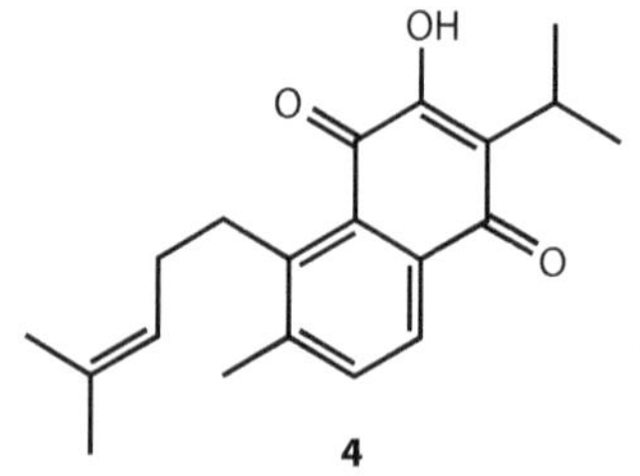

4 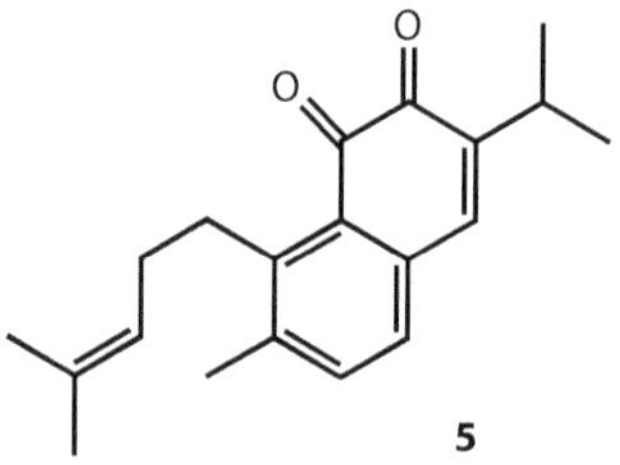 **5** 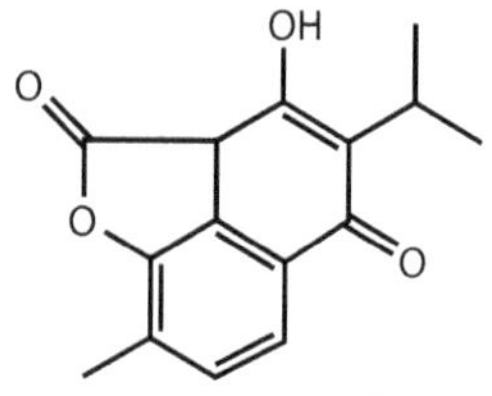 **6**

Herb Origination

The herb Hong Gen Cao originated from the dried whole plant of *Salvia prionitis* (Labiatae), whose plant is primarily distributed in the southern provinces of China. The herb is usually collected in spring and autumn and dried in the sun for Chinese medicinal application.

Antitumor Constituents and Activities

The principal bioactive components are diterpenoids in the root of Hong Gen Cao. Salvicine (**1**) is a diterpenoid quinone modified from a molecule isolated from the herb. As a nonintercalative Topo-II poison, salvicine (**1**) displayed potent *in vitro* and *in vivo* anticancer activities against various hematologic and solid tumor cells. In comparison with anticancer drugs, the cytotoxicity of salvicine (**1**) was as potent as that of etoposide but weaker than that of VCR in three leukemia cells but was over 5.41- and 4.15-fold stronger than those of VCR and etoposide, respectively, in 12 solid tumor cells. Especially, salvicine (**1**) exerted superior effects in the inhibition of human gastric and lung carcinoma cell lines.[1] The cotreatment with salvicine (6.25 μmol/L) and actinomycin-D (0.04–4 μmol/L) potentiated the cytotoxic effect against human K562 erythroleukemia cells, and the inhibitory rates were significantly raised from 8% to up to 69–71%.[2]

Importantly, salvicine (**1**) effectively obstructed the proliferation of both drug-sensitive and multidrug-resistant sublines, such as K562 and K562/A02, KB and KB/VCR, and MCF-7 and MCF-7/Adm, with an equivalent degree, and it induced similar levels of apoptosis in both the MDR and its parental cells. The drug-resistant reversal effect of salvicine (**1**) was much more potent than those of VCR, DOX, and etoposide, whose effect was mainly attributed to the diminishment of MDR-1 and P-gp expressions.[3,4] Moreover, salvicine (**1**) exerted a moderate antiproliferative effect on human A549 lung adenocarcinoma cells and human microvascular endothelial cells (HMECs) with IC_{50} values of 18.66 μM and 7.91 μM, respectively.[1–3] In the concentrations of 1.25–5.0 μM, salvicine (**1**) significantly restrained the endothelial cell migration by 56%, 73%, and 82%, respectively, and decreased the capillary-like tube formation of HMECs with high potency. When the concentration was increased to 30 μM, it markedly reduced the expression of bFGF-mRNA in the A549 cells.[5] Based upon the evidences, salvicine (**1**) was known to be a potent inhibitor of angiogenesis, which is capable of suppressing the angiogenic cascades, the proliferation, the migration, and the tube formation, in association with the decline of the bFGF expression. Due to the marked *in vitro* and *in vivo* antitumor properties and the obvious anti-MDR and anti-angiogenic activities, salvicine (**1**) is considered as a promising drug candidate currently in anticancer phases I and II clinical trials in China.[6]

Other diterpenoids isolated from the roots also demonstrated the inhibitory effects toward the cancer cell proliferation *in vitro*. 3-Keto-4-hydroxysaprorthoquinone (**2**) exerted the cytotoxic effect on human HL-60 leukemia cells and two human SGC-7901 and MKN-28 gastric carcinoma cells with IC_{50} values of 4.6, 0.2 and 0.3 μM, respectively.[7] 4-Hydroxysaprorthoquinone (**3**) was a marked inhibitor of Topo-I with an IC_{50} value of 0.8 μM.[7] The cytotoxicity of sapriparaquinone (**4**), saprorthoquinone (**5**), and sapriolactone (**6**) were established against murine P388 leukemia and human KB nasopharyngeal carcinoma cell lines,[8,9] whereas two dicycliditerpenoids, prionoid-D (**7**) and prionoid-E (**8**), significantly suppressed the proliferation of P388 leukemia cells (IC_{50}: 0.41 μM) and human lung carcinoma A549 cells (IC_{50}: 0.72 μM) *in vitro*.[10]

Mechanism Exploration

As a promising cancer therapeutic agent, salvicine (**1**) has attracted numerous scientists to subject the exploration of antineoplastic mechanism as their research projects. The approaches confirmed that salvicine provided a similar level of cytotoxic activity and mechanisms in both MDR and parental K562 cells, whose inhibitory mechanism was found to be related to the significant abilities of salvicine in (1) stabilizing DNA strand breaks, either through interactions with the enzyme alone or the DNA-enzyme complex; (2) stimulating intracellular H_2O_2 generation and GSH depletion in the early stage; (3) eliciting notable DNA double-strand breaks (DSBs) and downregulating DSBs repair proteins (Ku70, Ku86, and Rad51) through the apoptotic pathway; (4) activating ROS-related proteins p38 MAPK and JNK; and (5) diminishing Bcl-2 expression and activating caspase-1 and caspase-3, leading to the antigrowth-related mitochondrial-dependent apoptosis. The studies revealed a novel mechanism that H_2O_2 generation and GSH depletion play critical roles in salvicine-mediated DSBs and apoptosis in K562 cells. But, in MDR K562/A02 cells, the expressions of MDR-1 gene and PP-gp were additively downregulated by salvicine with no effect on the multidrug resistance associated protein (MRP) and lung resistance-related protein (LRP) gene expressions, suggesting that the decrease of MDR-1 and Bcl-2 expressions possibly contributed to the cytotoxic and apoptosis-inducing effects of salvicine in this MDR system. The potent cytotoxic activity of salvicine (**1**) on K562 cells was also reported to be accompanied by the blocking of the cell cycle at G1 phase.[1–4]

Moreover, in human HL-60 promyelocytic leukemia cells, the c-Myc P2 promoter-specific DNA damage was induced by salvicine (**1**) as an early event leading to the cell apoptotic death.[4] Salvicine could also induce evident DNA damage and double-strand breaks, which was highly correlated with the growth inhibition of human MCF-7 breast cancer cells. However, the MCF-7 cell apoptosis subsequent to DNA damage initiated by salvicine (**1**) was probably mediated through the p53-independent pathway concomitant with a dose-dependent decrease of c-Myc gene transcription and an increase of c-Jun expression.[11]

Other Bioactivities

The pharmacological study evidences suggested that the herb Hong Gen Cao possesses antianoxemia, coronary blood flow-increasing, anticoagulant, and antibacterial properties besides antitumor effect.

References

1. Qing, C. et al. 1999. In vitro cytotoxicity of salvicine, a novel diterpenoid quinine. *Zhongguo Yaoli Xuebao* 20: 297–302.
2. Qing, C. et al. 2003. Actinomycin D inhibiting K562 cell apoptosis elicited by salvicine but not decreasing its cytotoxicity. *Acta Pharmacol. Sinica* 24: 415–21.
3. Meng, L. H. et al. 2001. Salvicine, a novel topoisomerase II inhibitor, exerting its effect by trapping the enzyme-DNA cleavage complex. *Biochem. Pharmacol.* 62: 733–41.
4. Miao, Z. H. et al. 2003. Cytotoxicity, apoptosis induction and downregulation of MDR-1 expression by the anti-topoisomerase II agent, salvicine, in multidrug-resistant tumor cells. *Intl. J. Cancer* 106: 108–15.
5. Zhang, Y. L. et al. 2013. Anti-angiogenic activity of salvicine. *Pharm. Biol.* (London) 51: 1061–5.
6. Hu, C. X. et al. 2006. Salvicine functions as novel topoisomerase II poison by binding to ATP pocket. *Mol. Pharmacol.* 70: 1593–601.
7. Chen, X. et al. 2002. Bioactive abietane and seco-abietane diterpenoids from *Salvia prionitis*. *J. Nat. Prods.* 65: 1016–20.
8. Lin, L. Z. et al. 1990. A new diterpenoid quinine sapriparaquinone. *Yaoxue Xuebao* 25: 154–6.
9. Lin, L. Z. et al. 1989. Sapriolactone, a cytotoxic norditerpene from *Salvia prionitis*. *Phytochem.* 28: 3542–3.
10. Chang, J. et al. 2005. Novel Cytotoxic seco-abietane rearranged diterpenoids from *Salvia prionitis*. *Planta Med.* 71: 861–6.
11. Lu, H. R. et al. 2005. DNA damage, c-myc suppression and apoptosis induced by the novel topoisomerase II inhibitor, salvicine, in human breast cancer MCF-7 cells. *Cancer Chemother. Pharmacol.* 55: 286–94.

47 Shi Shang Bai 石上柏

Spikemoss or Great Selaginella

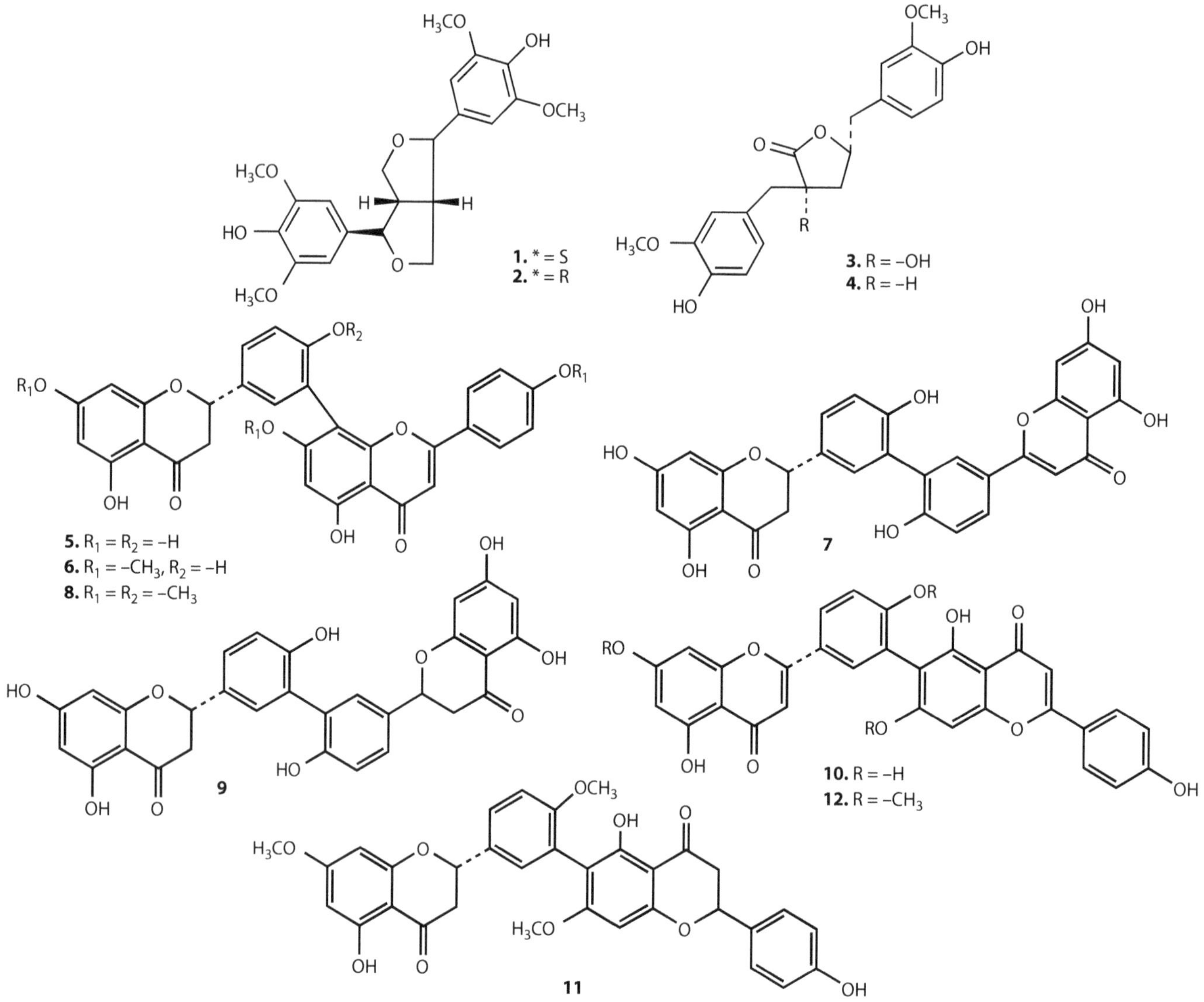

1. * = S
2. * = R

3. R = -OH
4. R = -H

5. $R_1 = R_2 = -H$
6. $R_1 = -CH_3, R_2 = -H$
8. $R_1 = R_2 = -CH_3$

7

9

10. R = -H
12. $R = -CH_3$

11

Herb Origination

The herb Shi Shang Bai (Spikemoss) originated from a Pteridophyte *Selaginella doederleinii* (Selaginellaceae). The perennial plant is generally distributed in southern China at a low altitude, as well as in India, Vietnam, Indonesia, and Japan. It normally grows wild on the edges of streams, wet rocks, cliffs, ravines, and shady places. The herb can be collected in all seasons and used fresh and in dried conditions for folk medical treatment.

Antitumor Activities and Constituents

Shi Shang Bai Extracts

Shi Shang Bai is a popular anticancer herb used in China. Its crude extract demonstrated a noticeable *in vitro* inhibitory effect against human HeLa cervix and TW03 nasopharyngy cancer cells.[1,2] The growth inhibition in the TW03 cells was accompanied by directing cell cycle arrest at S phase, as well as reducing Bcl-2 expression and upregulating Bax expression.[2] When orally given, its ethanolic extract to hepatoma-bearing mice for 12 continuous days significantly lengthened the living duration of the experimental mice, but the tumor tissue was not smaller.[3] Along with the increase of ROS generation, the loss of mitochondrial membrane potential, and the caspase activations, the ethanolic extract significantly triggered the cell apoptosis and inhibited the growth of human CNE nasopharyngeal carcinoma cells. When posttreatment with the ethanolic extract for two or three weeks is done, the tumor volume could be reduced by 68.4% and 72.5%, respectively, in a nude mice model.[4] The ethanolic extract also strongly restrained the activity of protein kinase-C (IC_{50}: 2.2 μg/mL), and the anti-PKC effect was more active than a well-known PKC inhibitor polymyxin-B (IC_{50}: 17.7 μg/mL).[5] In addition, its water extract showed a moderate inhibitory effect on mouse reverse transcriptase and human cellular DNA polymerase-α with IC_{50} values of 10 and 9.0 μg/mL, respectively, whose effects might be partly related to its tumor suppressive property.[6] Crude alkaloids isolated from the herb exhibited a marked inhibitory activity against the growth of murine sarcoma 180 cells *in vivo*.[3]

Lignans

From the ethanolic extract, four anticancer active lignans assigned as lirioresinol-A (**1**), lirioresinol-B (**2**), wikstromol (**3**), and matairesinol (**4**) were isolated. Their cytotoxicity against mouse L929 fibrosarcoma cells was verified to be moderate with IC_{50} values in the range of 9–20 μg/mL. The growth of P388 leukemia cells in mice was repressed by wikstromol (**3**) treatment.[7] Matairesinol (**4**) exerted a modest antigrowth effect against human HL-60 promyelocytic leukemia cells with IC_{50} value of 41 μg/mL, whose activity was almost equivalent to the effects of some current anticancer agents. During the treatment, the incorporations of thymidine, uridine, and leucine were strongly obstructed into HL-60 cells, indicating that the antileukemia effect in HL-60 cells was mediated by the cessation of DNA, RNA, and/or protein synthesis. On the contrary, matairesinol (**4**) was less effective against the growth of human Molt-4 T-lymphocytic leukemia cells, and it was not sensitive to mitogen-induced blastogenesis of normal human peripheral-blood lymphocytes.[8]

Biflavonoids

Six bioflavonoids were separated from the dichloromethane and acetic ether extracts and evaluated in a small panel of human neoplastic cell lines. All the biflavonoids were effective in the suppression of PC-9 human lung cancer cell line. The IC_{50} values were 6.41 μg/mL for amentoflavone (**5**), 6.74 μg/mL for heveaflavone (**6**), 8.12 μg/mL for 2″,3″-dihydro-3′,3‴-biapigenin (**7**), and 9.46 μg/mL for 7,4′,7″,4‴-tetra-*O*-methylamentoflavone (**8**). 3′,3‴-Binaringenin (**9**), amentoflavone (**1**), and 2″,3″-dihydro-3′,3‴-biapigenin (**7**) exhibited the moderate suppressive effect (IC_{50}: 19.3–42.0 μg/mL) on A549 lung cancer cells, whereas amentoflavone (**1**), heveaflavone (**6**), and robustaflavone (**10**) had the similar degree of antiproliferative activity on CNE2 nasopharyngeal carcinoma cells (IC_{50}s 15.8–42.8 μg/mL). The highest inhibitory effect was observed in K562 erythroleukemia cells by amentoflavone (**1**) (IC_{50}: 5.25 μg/mL), but heveaflavone (**6**), 7,4′,7″,4‴-tetra-*O*-methylamentoflavone (**8**), 3′,3‴-binaringenin (**9**), and robustaflavone (**10**) were not active in the K562 cells. Compared to the four cell lines mentioned earlier, HL-60 acute promyelocytic leukemia cells were resistant to the bioflavonoids; thus, the biflavonoids amentoflavone (**1**), heveaflavone (**6**), 7,4′,7″,4‴-tetra-*O*-methylamentoflavone (**8**), and robustaflavone (**10**) exerted a relatively lower antileukemia effect (IC_{50}: 46.0–49.2 μg/mL) in the HL-60 cells.[9]

Two biflavanones, 2,2″,3,3″-tetrahydrorobustaflavone 7,4′,7″-trimethyl ether (**11**) and robustaflavone 7,4′,7″-trimethyl ether (**12**), were isolated as cytotoxic constituents from Shi Shang Bai. Both were effective in the inhibition of human HCT8 (colon), NCI-H358 (lung), and K562 (leukemia) carcinoma cell lines with EC_{50} values of 15.6–28.8 μM *in vitro*.[10]

Clinical Practice

Shi Shang Bai tablet was manufactured in China by a method of water decoction and then ethanolic extraction. The tablet contains about 0.3 g of crude extracts and has been successfully used for the clinical treatment of lung carcinoma, throat carcinoma, gastrointestinal cancer, and chorioepithelioma with an oral dose of seven tablets per time and three times per day.[3] Eighty patients with terminal nasopharyngeal carcinoma were treated by radiotherapy in combination with taking 30 g of the herb extract daily in the whole course. The cure rate of nasopharyngeal primary lesion and neck lymph of the patients was 37.50% (30/80) and 56.25% (45/80), respectively, showing an obvious improvement, compared to another 80 patients in the same disease condition with radiotherapy alone. Also, the acute irradiation-caused side effects were markedly minimized in the patients taking the herb.[11] Up to now, only one case was reported about its side effect. A 52 year-old female patient with cholangiocarcinoma developed severe bone marrow inhibition when taking Shi Shang Bai daily. It was accompanied by severe pancytopenia with initial presentations of skin ecchymosis, itching, and gum bleeding. However, approximately one week after stopping the treatment, the hemogram returned to previous levels.[12] Now, Shi Shang Bai has been clinically combined with radiotherapy for the treatment of human nasopharyngeal carcinoma in China.

Other Bioactivities

The herb Shi Shang Bai (Spikemoss) displayed a significant effect in various infectious inflammations, and it can be partially used instead of antibiotics for the cure of acute tonsillitis, pneumonia, cholecystitis, urinary tract infections, and upper respiratory infections. The herb is often used in the treatment of cardiovascular diseases, acute and chronic hepatitis, and cirrhosis because it accelerates the restoration of liver functions in China.

References

1. Chao, L. R. et al. 1987. New alkaloid glycosides from Selaginella doederleinii. *J. Nat. Prod.* 50: 422–6.
2. Jing, Y. et al. 2009. Effects of *Selaginella doederleinii* on human nasopharyngeal carcinoma TW03 cells *in vitro* and its mechanism. *J. Chin. Med. Mater.* 32: 1864–7
3. *Quanguo Zhongcaoyao Huibian* (Compilation of Chinese Materia Medica), First Edition, (A), (1976), 2400, People's Health Publisher, Beijing, China.
4. Liu, H. H. et al. 2011. Reactive oxygen species-mediated mitochondrial dysfunction is involved in apoptosis in human nasopharyngeal carcinoma CNE cells induced *by Selaginella doederleinii* extract. *J. Ethnopharmacol.* 138: 184–91.
5. Huang, C. et al. 1995. Effects of *Selaginella doedealeinii* and *Livistona chinensis* on the activity of PKC. *Zhongcaoyao* 26: 414–8.
6. Lee, N. Y. et al. 2008. Identification of a new cytotoxic biflavanone from *Selaginella doederleinii. Chem. Pharm. Bull.* 56: 1360–1.
7. Lin, R. C. et al. 1994. Phenolic constituents of *Selaginella doederleinii. Planta Med.* 60: 168–70.

8. Hirano, T. et al. 1994. Natural flavonoids and lignans are potent cytostatic agents against human leukemic HL-60 cells. *Life Sci.* 55: 1061–9.
9. Li, S. G. et al. 2014. Preparative isolation of six antitumour biflavonoids from *Selaginella doederleinii* hieron by high-speed counter-current chromatography. *Phytochem. Analysis* 25: 127–33.
10. Oho, K. et al. 1989. Differential inhibitory effects of various herb extract on the activities of reverse transcriptase and various deoxyribonucleic acid (DNA) polymerases. *Chem. Pharm. Bull.* 37: 1810–2.
11. Zhou, T. C. et al. 2006. Clinical observation of selaginella combined with radiotherapy for terminal nasopharyngeal carcinoma. *Chin. J. Cancer Prevent. Treat.* 13: 772–3.
12. Pan, K. Y. et al. 2001. Severe reversible bone marrow suppression induced by *Selaginella doederleinii*. *J. Toxicol. Clin. Toxicol.* 39: 637–9.

48 Shui Fei Ji 水飛薊

Milk thistle

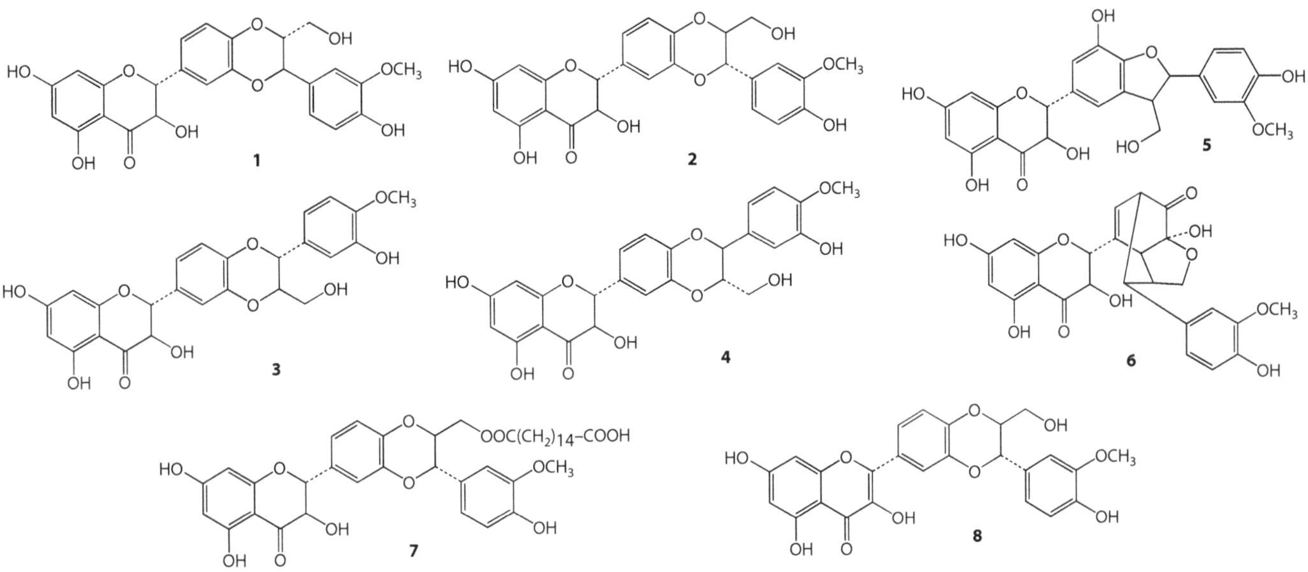

Herb Origination

The herb Shui Fei Ji is the ripe seeds of an Asteraceae plant *Silybum marianum* (= *Carduus marianus*). This annual or biannual plant is native to southern Europe, the Mediterranean, and Northern Africa, and it now spreads to the most temperate areas of the world as an invasive weed growing in wastelands and irrigation banks. The seeds have been used for 2000 years as an herbal remedy for a variety of ailments. Currently, the plant is cultivated in Austria, Germany, Hungary, Poland, China, and Argentina in a larger scale for the production of raw material affording to the pharmaceuticals.

Antitumor Activities and Constituents

Silymarin is a standardized extract prepared from the seeds of *S. marianum*, which contains 70–80% flavonolignans in the herb. The flavonolignan complex consists of six constituents, such as silibinin (= silybins)-A (**1**) and silibinin-B (**2**), isosilibinin-A (**3**), isosilibinin-B (**4**), silicristin (**5**), and silidianin (**6**). Silibinin-A (**1**) and silibinin-B (**2**), which are distereomers with approximately equimolar ratio, were the major bioactive constituents to exert bioactivities related to anticancer and anticarcinogenesis. The *in vitro* and *in vivo* investigations demonstrated that the silibinins as well as silymarin were effective in the growth suppression of a variety of cancer cells, especially, the solid tumors in the prostate, the breast, the lung, the bladder, the colon, the cervix, and the skin, with multiple and characteristic mechanisms.

Inhibition of Prostate Carcinoma Cells

Silymarin and silybins (**1** and **2**) demonstrated a marked suppressive effect against the growth of both types of human prostate cancer cells (androgen-dependent LNCaP cells and androgen-independent Du-145 and PC3 cells) *in vitro* and *in vivo* concomitantly causing cell cycle arrest and apoptosis, whose mechanism was revealed to be involved in multiple pathways, i.e., (1) blocked cell cycle progression by marked decrease of CDKs, elevation of the levels of CDK inhibitors (such as Cipl/p21 and Kipl/p27), and increase of their binding to CDK2 and/or CDK4; (2) inhibited the ligand binding to erbB1 receptor, ligand internalization, and erbB1 activation and inactivated the cytoplasmic mitogenic target ERK1/2 to block EGFR-MAPK/ERK1/2 signaling (such as in LNCaP and DU145 cells); (3) augmented IGFBP-3 accumulation and suppressed insulin receptor substrate-1 tyrosine phosphorylation (such as in PC3 cells); (4) inhibited the STAT3 constitutive activation and the STAT3-DNA binding and activated caspase-9 and caspase-3, leading to apoptotic death (such as in DU-145 cells); (5) diminished the basal- and hypoxia-induced HIF-1α protein expression level in association with the suppression of global protein translation (such as in LNCaP and PC3 cells); (6) suppressed the constitutive activation of NF-κB and the nuclear translocation of its p65 and p50 subunits and blocked IκBα phosphorylation (such as in DU-145 cells); (6) downregulated the telomerase activity and the CD44 expression (such as in osseous metastatic PC3M cells); (7) declined the secreted VEGF level and blocked the vessel tube formation to exert an antiangiogenic effect; and (9) raised the absolute amount of unphosphorylated Rb protein and Rb-E2F interaction that are leading to cellular growth inhibition and induction of differentiation (such as in LNCap cells).[1–9]

In the androgen-dependent LNCaP cells, the antigrowth effect was also followed by decreasing the intracellular and secreted levels of PSA under both serum- and androgen-stimulated conditions and reducing the androgen-stimulated secretion of both PSA and human glandular kallikrein-2. Isosilybin-A (**3**) and isosilybin-B

(**4**) at a concentration of 90 μM more effectively diminished the PSA secretion to nearly undetectable levels in LNCaP cells compared to silybin-A, silybin-B, and silybins mixture. At a concentration of 30 μmol/L, silybin-B (**2**) and isosilybin-B (**4**) exerted the strongest growth inhibition in androgen-independent PC3 cells and the significant growth suppression in androgen-independent DU-145 cells. The *in vitro* and *in vivo* potencies in the DU-145 cells were isosilybin-B > isosilybin-A > silybin-A > silybin-B.[1,2] Therefore, isosilybin-B (**4**) was recognized to rank as the most attractive flavonolignan in Milk thistle.

The *in vivo* treatment with silybins achieved obvious antiproliferative, proapoptotic, and antiangiogenic efficacies against advanced human prostate tumor xenograft growth in athymic nude mice, whose results correspond to the evidences from *in vitro* assays.[5–9] In the combination with chemotherapeutic agents to treat prostate cancer cells, silybins notably synergized the growth inhibitory effect of DOX and mitoxantrone in the Du-145 and/or PC3 cell lines and enhanced the induction of apoptosis and cell cycle arrest. The inhibitory effect of carboplatin (20 μg/mL) and cisplatin (2 μg/mL) were augmented from 68% to 80–90% and from 48% to 63–80%, respectively, in silybin (50100 μM) sensitized DU145 cells. In addition, silymarin displays a significant anticarcinogenic property. The dietary feeding of silymarin (500 ppm) could largely attenuate the incidence of DMAB-induced prostatic adenocarcinoma in male F344 rats.[1–9]

Inhibition of Breast Carcinoma Cells

The *in vitro* treatment with silymarin resulted in a significantly high to complete inhibition of estrogen-negative human MDA-MB-468 breast cancer cell growth in dose- and time-dependent manners and in both anchorage-dependent and anchorage-independent conditions. Simultaneously, silymarin elicited the MDA-MB-468 cells to a G1 cell arrest via the stimulation of a CDK inhibitor Cip1/p21 activity by 19-fold.[10] Through p53-involved and caspase-8-activated mitochondrial pathway, silibinins/silybins exerted the chemotherapeutic potential in two estrogen-positive human breast cancer cell lines (MCF-7 and T-47D), where the T-47D cells were more sensitive to silibinins than the MCF-7 cells.[11] More evidences revealed that silibinins also upregulated the expressions of Fas ligand (FasL) and Fas-associated death domain protein (FADD) and Bax and induced a conspicuous translocation of Bax to the mitochondria and the release of cytochrome c to cytosol in the MCF-7 cells, implying that both extrinsic Fas death receptor and intrinsic mitochondrial death pathways are involved in the silibinin-induced apoptosis of MCF-7 cells. Also, the blockage of IGF-1R markedly reinforced the silibinin-induced apoptosis[12] and the silibinin-elicited protective superoxide generation clearly enhanced the apoptosis of MCF-7 cells.[13] Likewise, through the suppression of NF-κB activation, silibinin elicited the apoptosis and obstructed the proliferation of ER-negative SKBR3 breast cancer cells with ErbB2-overexpression.[14]

Synergistic anticancer effects of silibinins with anticancer agents (DOX, cisplatin, and carboplatin) were demonstrated in both estrogen-dependent and estrogen-independent human breast cancer cell lines (MDA-MB468 and MCF-7), where the strongest synergistic growth inhibition and apoptosis induction were evident at a silibinin dose of 100 μM plus DOX (25 nM) in both cell lines, but silibinins combined with carboplatin showed the apoptotic effect only in the MCF-7 cells.[15] Moreover, silibinins also played an important role in the suppression of invasion and metastasis of MCF-7 cells. The inhibitory effect on phorbol-12-myristate-13-acetate (PMA)- or TPA-induced breast cancer cell invasion was found to correlate with (1) a specific inhibition of AP-1-dependent MMP-9 gene expression mediated by the blockage of MAPK signaling pathways and (2) a suppression of VEGF expression by the blockage of Raf/MEK/ERK pathway.[16,17] Also, silibinins acted as marked inhibitors on the COX-2 expression to obstruct the MMP-9 expression in the both MCF-7 cells and MDA-MB-231 breast neoplastic cells.[18] By restraining the P-gp activity, silymarin amplified the accumulation of daunomycin and decremented the efflux of daunomycin for reversing the MDR of MCF-7/Adm human breast cancer cell subline.[19]

Additionally, IdB 1016 is a complex of silybins with phosphatidylcholine. The treatment of IdB 1016 delayed the development of spontaneous mammary tumors, reduced the number and size of breast tumor masses, and diminished the lung metastasis in HER-2/neu transgenic mice. The treatment also enlarged the p53 mRNA activity in human SKBR3 breast cancer cells *in vitro*. Accordingly, the anticancer effects were revealed to be associated with the downregulation of HER-2/neu expression and the induction of senescent-like growth arrest and apoptosis through a p53-mediated pathway in the mammary tumor cells.[20]

Inhibition of Cervical Cancer Cells and Ovarian Cancer Cells

Silymarin and silibinins were reported to have a capability to cause the death of human HeLa cervical cancer cells via both apoptotic and necrotic pathways, i.e., silymarin induced the cell apoptosis at low concentrations (<80 μM) and caused the necrosis at a high concentration (160 μM). The silymarin- and silibinins-induced cell deaths were provoked by increases in ROS and in reactive nitrogen species (RNS) and was regulated by the activation of p38 and JNK-MAPKs in the HeLa cells, where the mitochondria-respiring function was interrupted and the ROS production and oxidative damage were elicited.[21,22] By the multiple pathways, i.e., mitogenic signaling, mitochondrial, and death receptor-mediated pathways, silibinin promoted G2 cell cycle arrest and apotosis of the HeLa cells. Moreover, silibinins effectively restrained HIF-1 transcriptional activity and HIF-1α accumulation and against hypoxia-induced VEGF, indicating the antigrowth effect of silibinins in the HeLa cells also involved in the blockage of HIF-1α and mTOR/p70S6K/4E-BP1 signaling pathway.[23,24]

Besides exerting the suppression against human A2780 ovarian cancer cells, silibinins also restored paclitaxel sensitivity to drug-resistant A2780/taxol cells and boosted paclitaxel-induced apoptosis and G2/M arrest.[25] The co-treatment with silybins (0.1–1 μM) could potentiate the cytotoxicity of cisplatin (0.1–1 μg/mL) on OVCA 433 and A2780 ovarian carcinoma cells and their corresponding cisplatin-resistant cells.[26] The MDR-reversing activity was consistent with its ability in the downregulation of survivin and P-gp.[26] When a silybin–phospholipid complex termed IdB 1016 was combined with cisplatin, a significant increase of the cisplatin activity was dose dependently achieved *in vitro* and *in vivo*. Importantly, the tested mice received the combinational treatment that could recover earlier in terms of body weight loss, and antiangiogenic effect also displayed in the *in vivo* model.[27]

Inhibition of Bladder Cancer Cells

Milk thistle is often used for treating a wide array of gallbladder diseases and symptoms. The tests in the treatment with silibinins *in vitro* and *in vivo* found the effective suppression on four types of human bladder cancers (5637 bladder cancer, T-24 high-grade bladder cancer, RT-4 bladder transitional cell papilloma, and TCC-SUP high-grade invasive bladder transitional cell cancer).[28–31] The oral gavage of silibinins (100 and 200 mg/kg doses, five days per week for 12 weeks) to nude mice xenografted with RT-4 cells obviously diminished the tumor volume by 51–58% and reduced the tumor weight by 44–49% in association with the moderate inhibition on the proliferation and the microvessel density and the strong induction of the cell apoptosis without any gross signs of toxicity, whose mechanism was revealed to correlate with (1) reduction of survivin levels and increase of AIF translocation, (2) activation of PARP cleavage and caspase-3 or caspase-9, (3) disruption of mitochondrial membrane potential and selective release of cytochrome c and Omi/HtrA2 from the mitochondria (such as in 5637 cell line), and (4) activation of p53/caspase-2 pathway and augment of caspase-mediated Cip1/p21 cleavage (such as in RT-4 cell line).[28–32]

The treatment with silibinins resulted in obvious dose- and time-dependent growth inhibitions in the highly invasive TCC-SUP cells together with a G1 arrest at lower doses and a G2/M arrest at higher doses. The strong induction of the expression of Cip1/p21 and Kip1/p27 and the reductions of CDKs and cyclins were found to be involved in the blockage of G1 progression, and the decreases in the levels of pCdc25c (Ser216), Cdc25c, pCdc2 (Tyr15), Cdc2, and cyclin-B1 in the TCC-SUP cells led the cells to G2/M arrest. Moreover, silibinins promoted the apoptosis of TCC-SUP cells via the activation of caspase-3 and PARP.[33] The evidences confirmed that the regulation of CDKI-CDK-cyclin cascade and caspase-3/PARP cleavages predominantly is involved in the mechanism of silibinins for the growth inhibition, the cell cycle interruption, and the apoptosis induction toward the bladder transitional cell carcinoma.[32] In addition, silymarin and silibinins were effective in preventing a bladder carcinogenesis provoked by tobacco smoke carcinogen N-butyl-N-(4-hydroxybutyl) nitrosamine in mice.[34] N-methyl-N-nitrosourea-initiated carcinogenesis and cancer progression in bladder were efficiently inhibited by silibinins in a rat model evidenced by declining the incidence of superficial and invasive bladder lesions without side effects.[28]

Inhibition of Colon Cancer Cells

The preventive effect of silymarin and silibinins was demonstrated *in vivo* against colon carcinogenesis caused by chemicals. The daily oral administration of silibinins to rats effectively inhibited colonic aberrant crypt foci and multicrypt AC/foci induced by carcinogens and improved enzymic antioxidant levels. By the treatment, azoxymethane or 1,2-dimethylhydrazine-elicited colon carcinogenesis was obstructed.[35–38] The antiproliferative and apoptotic effects of silybins/silibinins has been shown in four human colon cancer cell lines, HT-29, LoVo, SW480, and SW620 (a TRAIL-resistant metastatic cells) *in vitro*.[37–41] Silybins at 50–100 μg/mL doses elicited G0/G1 cell arrest and at its higher dose, and the longer treatment caused G2/M-cell cycle arrest, thereby dose and time dependently obstructing the proliferation of HT-29 cells.[39] The proliferation of HCT116 and SW480 cell lines was suppressed by silymarin concomitant with the decrease of cellular accumulation of exogenously induced cyclin D1 protein but did not change the level of cyclin D1 mRNA, whose cyclin D1 downregulation was resulted from proteasomal degradation through its threonine-286 phosphorylation via NF-κB activation.[42]

Recent advanced investigations in xenograft model corroborated that silibinins also obstructed the maintenance ability (self-renewal and sphere-formation) of human colorectal cancer stem-like cells by blocking the PP2Ac/AKT Ser473/mTOR pathway.[40] In addition, the antiangiogenesis effect can also be achieved by silymarin and silibinins in LoVo colon cancer cells.[41] Due to silymarin-inhibited P-gp-mediated efflux, the accumulation of digoxin and vinblastine in Caco-2 colon carcinoma cells was significantly enhanced by silymarin (50 μM) in a dose-dependent manner, and the MDR in colon carcinoma cells was reversed by the flavonolignan.[43] The remarkable results might provide a treatment option for the chemotherapy of colon cancer with silymarin and silibinins.

TRAIL is a promising anticancer agent, which selectively induces the apoptosis of cancer cells. Silibinins was able to synergistically enhance the TRAIL-elicited mitochondrial apoptosis in SW480 and SW621 colon cancer cell lines in association with the upregulation of DR4 and DR5, the downregulation of antiapoptotic proteins Mcl-1 and XIAP, the activation of caspase-3, caspase-8, and caspase-10, and the promotion of both intrinsic and extrinsic apoptotic pathways.[37] Therefore, the results evidenced that the combination of silibinins and TRAIL is a promising strategy for the improvement of colon cancer chemotherapy.[36]

Inhibition of Hepatoma Cells

Silymarin and silibinins are capable of protecting the liver cells from toxins by suppressing the oxidative stress and the ROS generation and restraining cytochrome P4502E1 and ethanol metabolism.[44] More data showed that the treatment with silimarin at doses of 50 and 75 μg/mL for 24 h obviously augmented the apoptosis of human HepG2 hepatoma.[45] The apoptosis of human HepG2 (HBV negative/p53 intact) and Hep3B (HBV positive/p53 mutated) hepatoma cells was markedly promoted by silybins. Simultaneously, silybins caused G1 arrest in HepG2 cells and both G1 and G2/M arrests in Hep3B cells via the increases of Kip1/p27 and the decreases of cyclins and CDKs levels and CDC2 kinase activity in both cell lines, where silybins displayed a stronger cytotoxicity in the Hep3B cells than in the HepG2 cells.[46] By activating the TRAIL death receptor apoptotic signaling pathway, i.e., the upregulation of apoptotic mediators (TRAIL, DR5) and the activation of caspase-3 and caspase-8 along with the downregulation of MMP-7 and MMP-9, silibinins enhanced the extrinsic apoptotic pathway to significantly repress the growth of murine orthotopic hepatocarcinoma Hep-55.1C cells *in vitro* and *in vivo*.[47]

Moreover, the silymarin treatment was able to attenuate the recruitment of the mast cell density and the MMP-2 and MMP-9 expressions in hepatoma induced N-nitrosodiethylamine in Wistar albino male rats.[48] By silibinins treatment, the proliferation of ethanol-dependent hepatoma cells was restrained and the ethanol metabolism in the hepatic cells were inhibited.[49] Therefore, these evidences suggested that silymarin and silybins/silibinins may be useful as adjunct agents in the prevention or the treatment of liver dysfunction in patients undergoing anticancer therapy.

Inhibition of Lung Cancer Cells

Besides the apoptosis induction by a mitochondria-dependent caspase cascade pathway, silymarin significantly exerted the inhibitory effect against the proliferation of highly metastatic human Anip973 lung adenocarcinoma cells within 48 h in a dose-dependent and a time-response manner.[50] In addition of the antiproliferative effect, silybins also showed dose- and time-dependent inhibitory effects on the motility and the invasion of human A549 non-small-cell lung carcinoma cells, whose mechanism was associated with (1) down-expressing MMP-2 and u-PA transcriptional levels, (2) up-expressing TIMP-2 translational and posttranslational level, (3) inhibiting ERK1/2 phosphorylation, and (4) restraining NF-κB and AP-1 nuclear translocation and these factors' binding activity on DNA.[51,52] The antigrowth and antiinvasive activities of silybins were also shown in athymic mice implanted with A549 cell xenograft. The oral feeding silybins (60 μM) to tumor-bearing nude mice suppressed the proliferation and the angiogenesis of A549 cells and elicited the apoptosis.[53] In an *in vivo* experiment silybins markedly lessened the DOX-induced systemic toxicity and the NF-κB signaling-involved chemoresistance, leading to the enhancement of the therapeutic response of DOX.[53]

More evidences revealed that the lung tumorigenesis and the migration of mouse lung epithelial LM2 cells could be obstructed by the silibinin treatment, whose inhibition was partly mediated by targeting the tumor microenvironment, such as (1) modulating TNFα and IFNγ-involved signaling; (2) repressing the phosphorylation of STAT3, STAT1, and Erk1/2 and blocking NF-κB-DNA binding; and (3) retarding the expressions of COX2, iNOS, MMPs-2/-9.[54] An advanced investigation found that combinations with silibinins synergistically augmented the cytotoxicity of histone deacetylase inhibitors (HDACi) (such as trichostatin-A and suberoylanilide hydroxamic acid) against NSCLC cells *in vitro* and *in vivo*, associated with the dramatic increases in p21 (CDKn1a) and global histone acetylation states of histones H3 and H4 and the potentiation of transcription, the degradation of cyclin-B1, and then the induction of G2/M arrest and apoptotic death.[55] These findings evidently established a safe and effective treatment for NSCLC cells and suggested that the HDACi/silibinins combination is ready for further evaluations in preclinical models.

In addition, the radical-scavenging and cell membrane-stabilizing potencies of silybins made it to be effective in the protection of cardiomyocytes from antitumor drugs such as DOX-induced oxidative stress and damages in heart microsomes and mitochondrion. The combinational treatment is beneficial for carcinoma patients, especially children and old people.[56,57]

Inhibition of Skin Cancer Cells

The topical application and the dietary feeding of silymarin achieved highly significant protection of skin carcinogenesis induced by chemicals in several mouse models. The anticarcinogenetic property was correlated with its capabilities in the inhibition of myeloperoxidase activity and IL-1α protein level, the decline of lipoxygenase and COX-2 activities, as well as a significant protection against tumor promoters (such as superoxide dismutase, GSH peroxidase, and catalase-induced lipid peroxidation and depletion of antioxidant enzymes). Some of the chemopreventive effects of silymarin were mediated by the suppression of receptor tyrosine kinases, CDK, and tumor necrosis factor mRNA expression. By the mechanism-related events, silymarin manifested the marked effects to (1) reduce tumor incidence, multiplicity, and volume; (2) inhibit papilloma growth; and (3) regress the established melanoma cells.[58] Moreover, the treatment with silymarin also concentration dependently restrained the migration of metastasis-specific human melanoma cell lines (A375 and Hs294t) and β-catenin-activated melanoma cells (Mel 1241) but there was no such effect on β-catenin-inactivated melanoma cells (Mel 1011). The mechanistic exploration displayed that the suppression of melanoma cell migration by silymarin was targeting the β-catenin signaling pathway, i.e., degradation or inactivation of β-catenin, elevation of casein kinase-1α and glycogen synthase kinase-3β levels, and inhibition of MMPs-2/-9, which were the downstream targets of β-catenin.[59] In anti-Fas agonistic Ab CH11-treated human A375-S2 malignant melanoma cells, the pretreatment with silymarin (3×10^{-4} mol/L) markedly amplified the apoptosis in association with the increase of the expression of FADD, the diminution of mitochondrial transmembrane potential, and the cleavage of procaspase-8.[60] Also, silymarin significantly potentiated the cisplatin-induced apoptosis of human G361 malignant melanoma cells *in vitro*.[1,61,62]

Both silymarin and silybins displayed the preventive effects against photocarcinogenesis in various animal models. The topical application or the dietary feeding of silymarin/silybins to SKH-1 nude mice reduced the ultraviolet-B (UVB) (290–320 nm)-caused skin cell oxidative stress, inflammation, DNA damage, apoptosis, and immune suppression, and then declined the incidence, the multiplicity, and the size of the melanoma caused by UVB in association with suppressing the intracellular production of hydrogen peroxide and NO and reducing the catalase depletion.[1,2] The mechanisms in cutaneous photoprotection triggered by the silymarin and silybins were demonstrated to be mainly correlated with (1) the inhibition of MAPK (i.e., ERK1/2, JNK1/2, SAPK2) activation; (2) the blockage of survival signaling by the inhibition of Akt phosphorylation to decrease survivin level; (3) the enhancement of Cip1/p21 and Kip1/p27 activities and decreases of CDK-2, CDK-4, cyclin-A, cyclin-E, and cyclin-D levels and the reduction of CDK-cyclin kinase activity; (4) the increase of p53-positive cells and the activation of suppressor p53 protein, which plays a crucial role in response to DNA damage; (5) the suppression of the form of cyclobutane pyrimidine dimers and the expression of COX-2 and its prostaglandin metabolites (PGE2, PGF2, PGD2); and (6) the downexpression of inflammatory cytokines TNFα and IL-1α.[1] *In vitro* studies using A431 human epidermoid carcinoma cells and JB6 mouse epithelial cells evidently also identified that the modulation of apoptosis, mitogenic signaling, and cell cycle progression is involved in silymarin and silybins efficacies against skin damage and carcinogenesis induced by UVB irradiation or endogenous tumor promoters.[1,62]

All these evidences observed from the experiments substantiated that silymarin and silybins may be beneficial in skin photoprotection against carcinogenesis, suggesting its development as a preventive agent for skin cancer.

Inhibition of Tongue Carcinoma Cells

The anticancer and anticarcinogenetic potentials of silymarin and silibinins were demonstrated in tongue malignant cells *in vitro* and/or *in vivo*. The treatment with 100 μM of silibinins markedly suppressed the invasion and the motility of human SCC-4 tongue squamous cancer cells by 89% and 66.4%, respectively. The metastasis-reducing effect was associated with the down-expression of MMP-2 and u-PA, the up-expression of TIMP-2 and PAI-1, and the attenuation of ERK1/2 phosphorylation. When combined with 20 μM U0126 (a specific mitogen-activated protein kinase (MEK) inhibitor) in the treatment, the expressions of MMP-2 and u-PA were restrained by 48.9–51.4% and the cell invasion was retarded by 45.7%.[63] In addition, the feeding of silymarin (500 ppm) during the promotion phase of 4-NQO-induced rat tumorigenesis exerted a chemopreventive effect against tongue squamous cell carcinoma in male F344 rats, whose effect was probably mediated by the modification of phase II enzyme activity and the decreases of PGE2 content.[64]

Inhibition of Renal Carcinoma Cells

At a ≥2 μmol/L concentration of silibinins, the DNA synthesis in metastatic SN12K1 renal cancer cells was inhibited, whereas at >80 μmol/L concentration, the growth of SN12K1 cells was obstructed in the presence of necrotic and apoptotic promotions, whose effect was independent of IGFBP-3.[65] Moreover, the dietary supplementation of silymarin was able to markedly protect against chemically induced nephrotoxicity and renal tumor promotion response by its antioxidant, antiinflammatory, and antiproliferative activities. For instance, the pretreatment with 25–200 μM of silymarin significantly protected against cisplatin-induced nephrotoxicity (cell death, apoptosis, and necrosis) of human renal proximal tubular HK-2 cells in a dose-dependent manner.[65–67]

Inhibition of Glioma Cells

By the treatment with silibinins, TRAIL-resistant glioma cells could be sensitized to the TRAIL by modulating multiple components in the death receptor-mediated apoptotic pathway, i.e., the upregulation of DR5 (a death receptor of TRAIL) in a transcription factor CHOP-dependent manner and the downregulation of the levels of pro-survival FLICE-like inhibitory protein (c-FLIP) and survivin by proteasome-mediated degradation. Therefore, the combinational treatment with subtoxic doses of silibinins and TRAIL was able to provoke a rapid apoptosis to exert a strong cytotoxic activity to various glioma cell lines (U251MG, U87MG, A172, and U251N) but not affect the normal astrocyte viability, implying that the co-treatment may offer a helpful strategy for safely treating TRAIL-resistant gliomas.[68] When silibinins is combined with arsenic trioxide (a newly introduced treatment for glioma), the synergical antitumor effect would be achieved in U87MG glioblastoma multiforme cells, evidenced as the suppressions of metabolic activity, cell proliferation, and gelatinase-A and gelatinase-B activities and the promotion of apoptosis. Simultaneously, silibinins diminished the mRNA level of cathepsin-B, u-PA, BCL2, CA9, MMPs-2/-9, membrane type 1-MMP, and survivin.[69] Therefore, the results suggested that the cotherapy may be efficient for the highly invasive human glioma treatment and pointed out that silymarin and silybins are useful in the treatment and the prevention of some neurodegenerative and neurotoxic processes, whose activity is partly attributed to their marked antioxidative activity.

Inhibition of Leukemia Cells

Only a few reports mentioned the antileukemia activity of silymarin. In association with lessening the telomerase activity, the *in vitro* treatment with silymarin significantly inhibited the growth of human K562 erythroleukemia cells.[70] Silymarin was effective in the moderate inhibition of a DOX-sensitive acute T lymphoblastic leukemia cell line (CCRF-CEM) but was inactive for its multidrug-resistant subline (CEM/ADR5000).[71]

Antineoplastic Silybin Derivatives

For the discovery of more efficient antitumor agents, the structure modification of silybins has been attempted on the C-23 hydroxyl group by acylation with three dicarboxylic acids. The monoester of silybins with hexadecanedioic acid displayed a greater antiproliferative effect against K562 human lymphoblastoma cells in concentration- and time-dependent manners, compared to the other derivatives and silybins. The treatment of K562 cells with 100 μM of silybins, silybin-23-*O*-dodecanedioate, and silybin-23-*O*-hexadecanedioate (**7**) also reduced the secretion of VEGF by 16.2%, 40.6%, and 49.3% after 48 h, and by 38.1%, 59.3%, and 76.6% after 72 h, respectively.[72] The findings highlighted that the acylated silybin derivatives with dicarboxylic acids improved the antitumor and antiangiogenic effects.

2,3-Dehydrosilybin (DHS) (**8**) is another derivative of silybin. After a 24 h treatment, DHS at 30–50 μM markedly promoted the apoptosis of transformed HepG2 and transformed cells with spindle fibroblastic-shape morphology (FIB) cancer cells, and DHS only induced necrosis markedly in HT-29 colon cancer cells but marginally in less transformed nontransformed cells with epithelium-like morphology (EPI) cells.[71] For killing human HepG2 hepatoma cells, the LD_{50} data of DHS (8 μM) were much lower than those of silybins (40 μM).[71] When DHS is combined with TNFα in a 6 h treatment, TNFα obviously accelerated the DHS-induced apoptotic death in the HepG2, HT29, and FIB cells, but not in EPI cells.[73] DHS is also a potent inhibitor DNA Topo-I, whose property rendered to sensitize TNFα for enhancing the cytotoxicity.[73] Also, the antioxidant activity of DHS (IC_{50}: 0.74 μM) was three to four times better than that of silybins (IC_{50}: 2.57 μM), and the inhibitory ability of DHS was sixfold stronger than that of silybins on MMP-2 and MMP-9 as well as invasiveness.[74]

Moreover, both silybins and DHS (**8**) are capable of suppressing the cellular glucose uptake by directly obstructing

GLUT4-mediated glucose transport in Chinese hamster ovary cells. The restriction of glucose transport and supply was confirmed in human HuH7 hepatoma cells and human Caco2 colon cancer cells, whose effect should partially contribute to the cancer cell death-inducing activities of DHS and silybin.[75] Overall, the superior activities of DHS suggest that DHS (**8**) may be more useful therapeutically than silybins in the treatment of cancer and other related diseases. In addition, some *O*-alkyl derivatives of DHS were reported to exert the improved an inhibitory effect against P-gp-mediated efflux activity and the enhanced cytotoxicity against CCRF-CEM T lymphoblastic leukemia, K562 myeloid leukemia, MCF-7 breast cancer, A549 lung adenocarcinoma, and murine L1210 leukemia cells, as well as multidrug-resistant leukemia cell sublines.[76]

Clinical Studies

1. Silipide, which is formulated with silibinins and phosphatidylcholine, was subjected to patients with colorectal adenocarcinoma at corresponding dosages of 360, 720, or 1440 mg silibinins daily for seven days. The repeated administration of silipide was safe, by which the levels of silibinins were 0.3 to 4 μmol/L in the plasma, 0.3–2.5 nmol/g in the liver tissue, and 20–141 nmol/g in colorectal tissue. The high levels of silibinins were detected in the human colorectal mucosa after the consumption of safe silibinins doses, and the intervention with silipide did not affect the circulating levels of IGFBP-3, IGF-I, or M1dG. The clinical data support the further exploration of silibinins as a potential agent for human colorectal cancer chemoprevention.[77]
2. A silybin phytosome was orally given to 13 patients with prostate cancer in daily doses of 2.5–20 g (divided to three doses, per day) for four weeks. No objective PSA responses were observed but also no obvious toxicity was seen. The results appeared to be well tolerated in patients with advanced prostate cancer and recommended a phase II dose.[78] Patients with prostate cancer in the treatment received silybins phytosome daily for 14–31 days (mean was 20 days) prior to surgery. Although silybin phytosome in a high oral dose achieved high blood concentrations transiently, low levels of silibinins were detected in the prostate tissue. The short half-life of silibinins should be attributed to its lack of tissue penetration.[79]

Microspheric Formulation

A microspheric form of silymarin was formulated by using various polymers like chitosan, pectin, carbopol 934P, ethyl cellulose, and eudragit RS100. The prepared ethyl cellulose and eudragit RS100 microspheres exhibited extended drug release for 12 h and, therefore, potentially improving the bioavailability of the silymarin. An *in vitro* cytotoxic test showed that 75% deaths occurred in DU145 cells after a 12 h treatment, implying the enhanced anticancer activity of silymarin microspheres against human DU145 prostate adenocarcinoma cells.[80]

Other Bioactivities

Silymarin and silybins have been proven to possess multiple pharmacological functions including hepatoprotective, neuroprotective, skin-protecting, antioxidative, antilipoperoxidative, nephropathy-preventing, anticardiotoxic, antiatherogenic, and antihypercholesterolemic activities. However, due to poor water solubility and low bioavailability, silymarin has been developed as enhanced formulations for clinical uses. Silipide, a complex of silymarin and phosphatidylcholine (lecithin), is about 10 times more bioavailable than silymarin.

References

1. Radek, G. 2007. Silybin and silymarin—New and emerging applications in medicine. *Current Med. Chem.* 14: 315–38.
2. Ajit, K. K. 2011. Milk thistle (*Silybum marianum*): A review. *Intl. J. Pharma Res. Develop.* 3: 1–10.
3. Raina, K. et al. 2007. Combinatorial strategies for cancer eradication by silibinin and cytotoxic agents: Efficacy and mechanisms. *Acta Pharmacol. Sinica*, 28: 1466–75.
4. Agarwal, C. et al. 2007. Silibinin inhibits constitutive activation of Stat3, and causes caspase activation and apoptotic death of human prostate carcinoma DU145 cells. *Carcinogen.* 28: 1463–70.
5. Jung, H. J. et al. 2009. Silibinin inhibits expression of HIF-1α through suppression of protein translation in prostate cancer cells. *Biochem. Biophys. Res. Commun.* 390: 71–6.
6. Handorean, A. M. et al. 2009. Silibinin suppresses CD44 expression in prostate cancer cells. *Am. J. Translat. Res.* 1: 80–6.
7. Deep, G. et al. 2012. Angiopreventive efficacy of pure flavonolignans from milk thistle extract against prostate cancer: Targeting VEGF-VEGFR signaling. *PloS One* 7: e34630.
8. Flaig, T. W. et al. 2007. Silibinin synergizes with mitoxantrone to inhibit cell growth and induce apoptosis in human prostate cancer cells. *Intl. J. Cancer* 120: 2028–33.
9. Deep, G. et al. 2007. Chemopreventive efficacy of silymarin in skin and prostate cancer. *Integr. Cancer Therapies* 6: 130–45.
10. Zi, X. et al. 1998. Anticarcinogenic effect of a flavonoid antioxidant, silymarin, in human breast cancer cells MDA-MB 468: Induction of G1 arrest through an increase in Cipl/p21 concomitant with a decrease in kinase activity of cyclin-dependent kinases and associated cyclins. *Clin Cancer Res.* 4: 1055–64.
11. Prabha, T. A. et al. 2011. Silibinin-induced apoptosis in MCF7 and T47D human breast carcinoma cells involves caspase-8 activation and mitochondrial pathway. *Cancer Invest.* 29: 12–20.
12. Wang, H. J. et al. 2008. Inhibition of insulin-like growth factor 1 receptor signaling enhanced silibinin-induced activation of death receptor and mitochondrial apoptotic pathways in human breast cancer MCF-7 cells. *J. Pharmacol. Sci.* 107: 260–9.
13. Wang, H. J. et al. 2010. Silibinin induces protective superoxide generation in human breast cancer MCF-7 cells. *Free Radical Res.* 44: 90–100.
14. Yousefi, M. et al. 2014. Silibinin induces apoptosis and inhibits proliferation of estrogen receptor (ER)-negative breast carcinoma cells through suppression of NF-κB activation. *Archiv. Iranian Med.* 17: 366–71.

15. Tyagi, A. K. et al. 2004. Synergistic anti-cancer effects of silibinin with conventional cytotoxic agents doxorubicin, cisplatin and carboplatin against human breast carcinoma MCF-7 and MDA-MB468 cells. *Oncol. Rep.* 11: 493–9.
16. Lee, S. O. et al. 2007. Silibinin suppresses PMA-induced MMP-9 expression by blocking the AP-1 activation via MAPK signaling pathways in MCF-7 human breast carcinoma cells. *Bioche. Biophys. Res. Commun.* 354: 165–71.
17. Kim, S. et al. 2009. Silibinin prevents TPA-induced MMP-9 expression and VEGF secretion by inactivation of the Raf/MEK/ERK pathway in MCF-7 human breast cancer cells. *Phytomed.* 16: 573–80.
18. Kim, S. et al. 2009. Silibinin prevents TPA-induced MMP-9 expression by down-regulation of COX-2 in human breast cancer cells. *J. Ethnopharmacol.* 126: 252–7
19. Chung, S. Y. et al. 2005. Inhibition of P-glycoprotein by natural products in human breast cancer cells. *Arch. Pharm. Res.* 28: 823–8.
20. Provinciali, M. et al. 2007. Effect of the silybin-phosphatidylcholine complex (IdB 1016) on the development of mammary tumors in HER-2/neu transgenic mice. *Cancer Res.* 67: 2022–9.
21. Huang, Q. et al. 2005. Silymarin augments human cervical cancer HeLa cell apoptosis via P38/JNK MAPK pathways in serum-free medium. *J. Asian Nat. Prod. Res.* 7: 701–9.
22. Fan, S. M. et al. 2011. Silibinin induced-autophagic and apoptotic death is associated with an increase in reactive oxygen and nitrogen species in HeLa cells. *Free Radical Res.* 45: 1307–24.
23. Zhang, Y. et al. 2012. Cellular and molecular mechanisms of silibinin induces cell-cycle arrest and apoptosis on HeLa cells. *Cell Biochem. Function* 30: 243–8.
24. Garcia-Maceira, P. et al. 2009. Silibinin inhibits hypoxia-inducible factor-1α and mTOR/p70S6K/4E-BP1 signalling pathway in human cervical and hepatoma cancer cells: Implications for anticancer therapy. *Oncogene* 28: 313–24.
25. Zhou, L. G. et al. 2008. Silibinin restores paclitaxel sensitivity to paclitaxel-resistant human ovarian carcinoma cells. *Anticancer Res.* 28: 1119–27.
26. Scambia, G. et al. 1996. Antiproliferative effect of silybin on gynecological malignancies: Synergism with cisplatin and doxorubicin. *Eur. J. Cancer,* Part A 32A: 877–82.
27. Giacomelli, S. et al. 2002. Silybin and its bioavailable phospholipid complex (IdB 1016) potentiate in vitro and in vivo the activity of cisplatin. *Life Sci.* 70: 1447–59.
28. Zeng, J. et al. 2011. Chemopreventive and chemotherapeutic effects of intravesical silibinin against bladder cancer by acting on mitochondria. *Mol. Cancer Therap.* 10: 104–16.
29. Sun, Y. et al. 2007. Effect of silibinin on proliferation of human bladder cancer cell 5637 in vitro and related mechanism. *J. Xi'an Jiaotong Univ.* (*Med. edit.*) 28: 559–62.
30. Tyagi, A. K. et al. 2003. Silibinin down-regulates survivin protein and mRNA expression and causes caspases activation and apoptosis in human bladder transitional-cell papilloma RT4 cells. *Bioche. Biophys. Res. Commun.* 312: 1178–84.
31. Singh, R. P. et al. 2008. Oral silibinin inhibits in vivo human bladder tumor xenograft growth involving down-regulation of surviving. *Clin. Cancer Res.* 14: 300–8.
32. Tyagi, A. et al. 2006. Silibinin activates p53-caspase 2 pathway and causes caspase-mediated cleavage of Cip1/p21 in apoptosis induction in bladder transitional-cell papilloma RT4 cells: Evidence for a regulatory loop between p53 and caspase 2. *Carcinogen.* 27: 2269–80.
33. Tyagi, A. et al. 2004. Silibinin causes cell cycle arrest and apoptosis in human bladder transitional cell carcinoma cells by regulating CDKI-CDK-cyclin cascade, and caspase 3 and PARP cleavages. *Carcinogen.* 25: 1711–20.
34. Tyagi, A. et al. 2007. Chemopreventive effects of silymarin and silibinin on N-butyl-N-(4-hydroxybutyl) nitrosamine-induced urinary bladder carcinogenesis in male ICR mice. *Mol. Cancer Therap.* 6(12, Pt.1): 3248–55.
35. Kauntz, H. et al. 2012. Silibinin, a natural flavonoid, modulates the early expression of chemo-prevention biomarkers in a preclinical model of colon carcinogenesis. *Intl. J. Oncol.* 41: 849–54.
36. Kauntz, H. et al. 2012. The flavonolignan silibinin potentiates TRAIL-induced apoptosis in human colon adenocarcinoma and in derived TRAIL-resistant metastatic cells. *Apoptosis* 17: 797–809.
37. Kauntz, H. et al. 2011. Silibinin triggers apoptotic signaling pathways and autophagic survival response in human colon adenocarcinoma cells and their derived metastatic cells. *Apoptosis* 16: 1042–53.
38. Sangeetha, N. et al. 2010. Silibinin ameliorates oxidative stress induced aberrant crypt foci and lipid peroxidation in 1,2 dimethylhydrazine induced rat colon cancer. *Investig. New Drugs* 28: 225–33.
39. Agarwal, C. et al. 2003. Silibinin upregulates the expression of cyclin-dependent kinase inhibitors and causes cell cycle arrest and apoptosis in human colon carcinoma HT-29 cells. *Oncogene* 22: 8271.
40. Wang, J. Y. et al. 2012. Silibinin suppresses the maintenance of colorectal cancer stem-like cells by inhibiting PP2A/AKT/mTOR pathways. *J. Cell. Biochem.* 113: 1733–43.
41. Yang, S. H. et al. 2003. Anti-angiogenic effect of silymarin on colon cancer Lovo cell line. *J. Surg. Res.* 113: 133–8.
42. Eo, H. J. et al. 2015. Silymarin induces cyclin D1 proteasomal degradation via its phosphorylation of threonine-286 in human colorectal cancer cells. *International Immunopharmacol.* 24: 1–6.
43. Zhang, S. Z. et al. 2003. Effect of the flavonoids biochanin A and silymarin on the P-glycoprotein-mediated transport of digoxin and vinblastine in human intestinal Caco-2 cells. *Pharm. Res.* 20: 1184–91.
44. Brandon-Warner, E. et al. 2010. Silibinin inhibits ethanol metabolism and ethanol-dependent cell proliferation in an in vitro model of hepatocellular carcinoma. *Cancer Lett.* 291: 120–9.
45. Ramakrishnan, G. et al. 2009. Silymarin inhibited proliferation and induced apoptosis in hepatic cancer cells. *Cell Prolifer.* 42: 229–40.
46. Varghese, L. et al. 2005. Silibinin efficacy against human hepatocellular carcinoma. *Clin. Cancer Res.* 11: 8441–8.
47. Bousserouel, S. et al. 2012. Silibinin inhibits tumor growth in a murine orthotopic hepatocarcinoma model and activates the TRAIL apoptotic signaling pathway. *Anticancer Res.* 32: 2455–62.
48. Ramakrishnan, G. et al. 2009. Silymarin attenuated mast cell recruitment thereby decreased the expressions of matrix metalloproteinases-2 and 9 in rat liver carcinogenesis. *Investig. New Drugs* 27: 233–40.
49. Brandon-Warner, E. et al. 2012. Silibinin (Milk Thistle) potentiates ethanol-dependent hepatocellular carcinoma progression in male mice. *Cancer Lett.* 326: 88–95.

50. Li, W. H. et al. 2011. Molecular mechanism of silymarin-induced apoptosis in a highly metastatic lung cancer cell line Anip97. *Cancer Biother. Radiopharma.* 26: 317–324.
51. Chu, S. C. et al. 2004. Silibinin inhibits the invasion of human lung cancer cells via decreased productions of urokinase-plasminogen activator and matrix metalloproteinase-2. *Mol. Carcinog.* 40: 143–9.
52. Chen, P. N. et al. 2005. Silibinin inhibits cell invasion through inactivation of both PI3K-Akt and MAPK signaling pathways. *Chem.-Biol. Interact.* 156: 141–50.
53. Singh, R. P. et al. 2004. Oral silibinin inhibits lung tumor growth in athymic nude mice and forms a novel chemocombination with doxorubicin targeting nuclear factor κB–mediated inducible chemoresistance. *Clin. Cancer Res.* 10: 8641–7.
54. Tyagi, A. et al. 2012. Silibinin modulates TNFα and IFNγ mediated signaling to regulate COX2 and iNOS expression in tumorigenic mouse lung epithelial LM2 cells. *Mol. Carcinogenesis* 51: 832–42.
55. Mateen, S. et al. 2012. Epigenetic modifications and p21-cyclin B1 nexus in anticancer effect of histone deacetylase inhibitors in combination with silibinin on non-small cell lung cancer cells. *Epigenetics* 7: 1161–72.
56. Chlopcíková, S. et al. 2004. Chemoprotective effect of plant phenolics against anthracycline-induced toxicity on rat cardiomyocytes. Part I. Silymarin and its flavonolignans. *Phytother. Res.* 18: 107–10.
57. Psotová, J. et al. 2002. Influence of silymarin and its flavonolignans on doxorubicin-iron induced lipid peroxidation in rat heart microsomes and mitochondria in comparison with quercetin. *J. Phytother. Res.* 16(Suppl. 1): S63–67.
58. Vaid, M. et al. 2010. Molecular mechanisms of inhibition of photocarcinogenesis by silymarin, a phytochemical from milk thistle (*Silybum marianum* L. Gaertn.) (review). *Intl. J. Oncol.* 36: 1053–60.
59. Vaid, M. et al. 2011. Silymarin targets β-catenin signaling in blocking migration/invasion of human melanoma cells. *PLoS One* 6: e23000.
60. Li, L. H. et al. 2007. Silymarin enhanced cytotoxic effect of anti-Fas agonistic antibody CH11 on A375-S2 cells. *J. Asian Nat. Prod. Res.* 9: 593–602.
61. Chen, X. W. et al. 2011. Pharmacokinetic profiles of anticancer herbal medicines in humans and the clinical implications. *Current Med. Chem.* 18: 3190–210.
62. Fan, S. M. et al. 2012. P53 activation plays a crucial role in silibinin induced ROS generation via PUMA and JNK. *Free Radical Res.*, 46: 310–9.
63. Chen, P. N. et al. 2006. Silibinin inhibits invasion of oral cancer cells by suppressing the MAPK pathway. *J. Dental Res.* 85: 220–5.
64. Yanaida, Y. et al. 2002. Dietary silymarin [Silybum Marianum] suppresses 4-nitroquinoline 1-oxide-induced tongue carcinogenesis in male F344 rats. *Carcinogen.* 23: 787–94.
65. Cheung, C. W. et al. 2007. Silibinin inhibits renal cell carcinoma via mechanisms that are independent of insulin-like growth factor-binding protein-3. *BJU Intl.* 99: 454–60.
66. Kaur, G. et al. 2010. Dietary supplementation of silymarin protects against chemically induced nephrotoxicity, inflammation and renal tumor promotion response. *Investigational New Drugs* 28: 703–13.
67. Ninsontia, C. et al. 2011. Silymarin selectively protects human renal cells from cisplatin-induced cell death. *Pharm. Biol.* 49: 1082–90.
68. Son, Y. Y. et al. 2007. Silibinin sensitizes human glioma cells to TRAIL-mediated apoptosis via DR5 up-regulation and down-regulation of c-FLIP and survivin. *Cancer Res.* 67: 8274–84.
69. Dizaji, M. Z. et al. 2012. Synergistic effects of arsenic trioxide and silibinin on apoptosis and invasion in human glioblastoma U87MG cell line. *Neurochemical Res.* 37: 370–80.
70. Faezizadeh, Z. et al. 2012. The effect of silymarin on telomerase activity in the human leukemia cell line K562. *Planta Med.* 78: 899–902.
71. Righeschi, C. et al. 2012. Microarray-based mRNA expression profiling of Leukemia cells treated with the flavonoid, casticin. *Cancer Genomics Proteomics* 9: 143–52.
72. Theodosiou, E. et al. 2011. Biocatalytic synthesis and antitumor activities of novel silybin acylated derivatives with dicarboxylic acids. *New Biotechnol.* 28: 342–8.
73. Thongphasuk, P. et al. 2008. Potent direct or TNF-α-promoted anti-cancer effects of 2,3-dehydrosilybin: Comparison study with silybin. *Chemother.* 54: 23–30; 2009. 2,3-Dehydrosilybin is a better DNA topoisomerase I inhibitor than its parental Silybin. *Chemother.* 55: 42–8.
74. Huber, A. et al. 2008. Significantly greater antioxidant anticancer activities of 2,3-dehydrosilybin than silybin. *Biochimica et Biophysica Acta* 1780: 837–47.
75. Zhan, T. Z. et al. 2011. Silybin and dehydrosilybin decrease glucose uptake by inhibiting GLUT proteins. *J. Cell. Biochem.* 112: 849–59.
76. Dzubak, P. et al. 2006. New derivatives of silybin and 2,3-dehydrosilybin and their cytotoxic and P-glycoprotein modulatory activity. *Bioorg. Med. Chem.* 14: 3793–810.
77. Hoh, C. et al. 2006. Pilot study of oral silibinin, a putative chemopreventive agent, in colorectal cancer patients: Silibinin levels in plasma, colorectum, and liver and their pharmacodynamic consequences. *Clin. Cancer Res.* 12: 2944–50.
78. Flaig, T. W. et al. 2007. A phase I and pharmacokinetic study of silybin-phytosome in prostate cancer patients. *Investigational New Drugs* 25: 139–46.
79. Flaig, T. W. et al. 2010. A study of high-dose oral silybin-phytosome followed by prostatectomy in patients with localized prostate cancer. *The Prostate* 70: 848–55.
80. Krishna, P. M. et al. 2014. Silymarin microspheres and its antiproliferative action on human prostate adenomatous cancer DU145 cells. World *J. Pharm. Pharmaceut. Sci.* 3: 1447–57.

49 Bai Ying 白英

Bittersweet herb

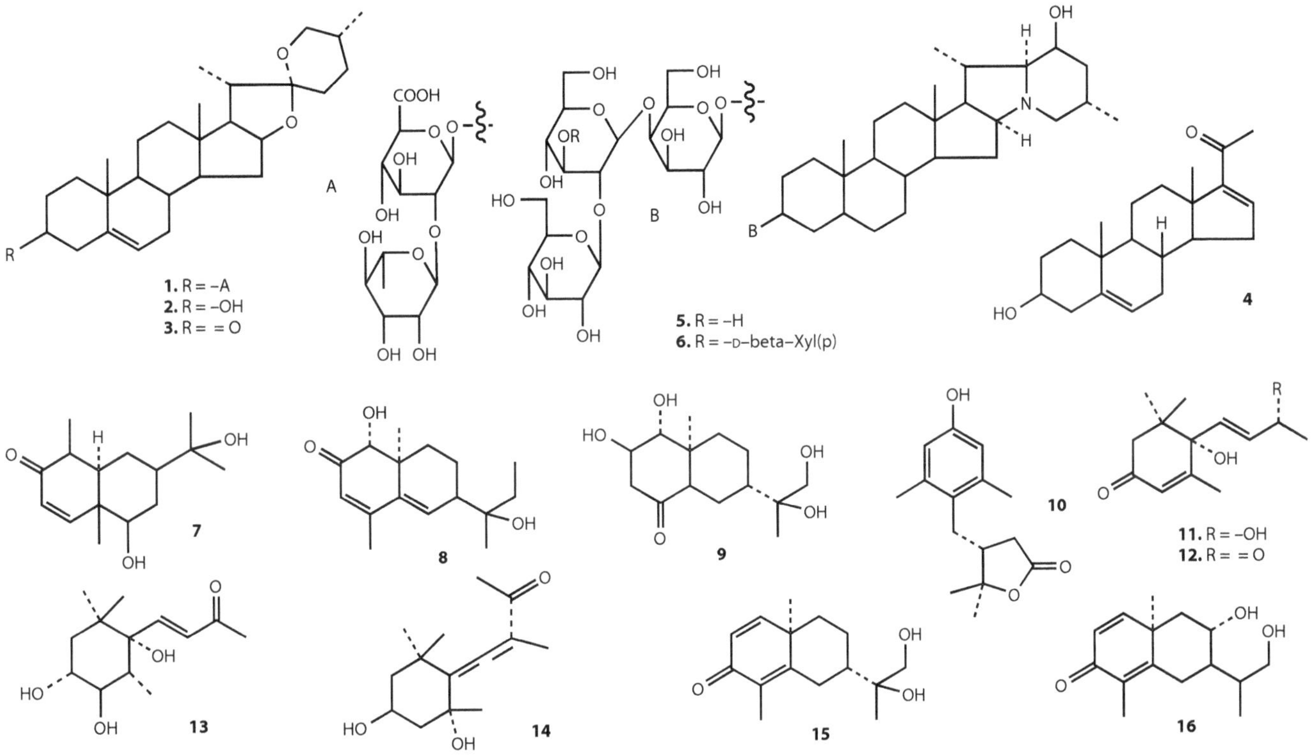

1. R = -A
2. R = -OH
3. R = =O

5. R = -H
6. R = -D-beta-Xyl(p)

11. R = -OH
12. R = =O

Herb Origination

The herb Bai Ying (Bittersweet herb) originated from a Solanaceae plant of *Solanum lyratum*. This perennial climbing plant is widely distributed in eastern and southeastern Asia. The whole plants are traditionally collected in summer and autumn and dried in the sun for the folk remedy in traditional Chinese medicine. The herb also can be used fresh.

Antitumor Activities

Bai Ying has been usually used as a folk anticancer drug in China to treat various solid tumors in the liver, the lung, the esophagus, and so on. Modern studies provided many scientific evidences to support the treatment and the development of the herb. Its aqueous extract exhibited an obvious inhibitory effect against the proliferation of a variety of human cancer cell lines, such as SGC-7901 and SGC-823 (stomach), A549 (lung), Colo205 and SW1116 (colon), SMMC-7721 and Bel-7402 (liver), HL-60 and U937 (leukemic), MCF-7 (breast), A2780 (ovary), HeLa, (cervix), and A375 (skin) cells, *in vitro*,[1–13] and against the growth of murine WEHI-3 leukemia, H22 hepatoma, and sarcoma 180 *in vivo*.[14] The inhibitory effect of its ethanolic extract primarily showed in SGC-7901 (stomach), Bel-7402 and Bel-7404 (liver), SPC-A-1 (lung), H08910 (ovary), HeLa (cervix), MCF-7 (breast), A375 (skin), and U937 (leukemic) human tumor cell lines, whose antiproliferative effect was reported to be closely concomitant with the stimulation of apoptosis and cell cycle arrest.[15–22] The ethanolic extract at high dosages exerted the antigrowth effect against sarcoma 180 and H22 hepatoma in mice for approximately 41.15% and 45.00%, respectively, leading to the diminishment of the tumor size and to the prolongation of the life duration without acute toxic effect.[23]

Usually, the alcoholic and aqueous extracts were relatively sensitive to these cancer cell lines such as SGC-7901, A375, Bel-7402, HeLa, and L929 cells but lower on MCF-7 and U937 cells.[22] The sensitivity of its alcoholic extract often appeared greater than that of its aqueous extract on the same cancer cells.[22] An ethyl acetate partition layer derived from the aqueous extract moderately obstructed human A375 amelanotic melanoma cells and human HeLa cervical cancer cells *in vitro* (respective IC_{50}: 9.69 and 20.90 μg/mL), and its n-butanolic layer showed a lower suppressive effect on the A375 cells and HeLa cells (respective IC_{50}: 31.72 and 64.42 μg/mL).[23] A hexane partition fraction derived from its methanolic extract exhibited the strongest cytotoxicity toward mouse LLC cells among the solvent partition fractions, and the marked growth inhibitory and apoptosis-increasing effects were further demonstrated in the *in vivo* treatment of LLC with this hexane fraction at a dose 50 mg/kg.[24] Besides notably inhibiting the viability of sarcoma 180 in mice, the n-butanolic extract was also able to remarkably improve the immune responses, i.e., potentiating splenocyte proliferation, enhancing IL-2 and interferon-γ productions and NK cell activities, augmenting the CTL, and elevating the levels of serum antigen-specific

Ab in the tumor-bearing mice.[25–28] In addition, the ethanolic extract could also improve the sensitivity of the HeLa cells to cisplatin, a chemotherapeutic drug.[18]

Antitumor Constituents and Activities

Through a bioassay-related phytochemical investigation, three types of major constituents, i.e., steroidal saponins, steroidal alkaloids, and sesquiterpenoids, were isolated from Bai Ying and discovered possessing marked an antiproliferative property against a variety of neoplastic cells *in vitro* or *in vivo.*

Steroids

The major anticancer ingredients in Bai Ying are a group of sperosteroidal saponins as well as their sapogenins. The total saponins inhibited the proliferation of Bel-7402 (liver), SGC-7901 (stomach), and MCF-7 (breast) human cancer cell lines *in vitro* and induced cell apoptosis.[29–30] After the total saponin treatment, HeLa cervical cancer cells and Ec-9706 esophagus cancer cells were accelerated to apoptotic death.[31,32] More study results suggested that apoptosis induction is involved in multiple routes such as death receptor and mitochondrial pathways.[30,31] The apoptosis of MCF-7 cells elicited by the total saponins was correlated with the upregulation of Bax and the downregulation of survivin expression.[33] The mechanism in the Ec-9706 cells was found to be associated with the upregulation of Fas expression in the Bel-7402 cells and the stimulation of p53 function.[32,34] *In vivo* assays evidenced the dose-dependent suppressive effect of total saponins against mouse sarcoma 180, and the inhibitory rate was 33.7% in a high dose with no acute toxic effect; however, it showed no influence on the growth of H22 hepatoma in mice.[30]

A group of steroid-related compounds were isolated from the herb, showing a dose-dependent tumor growth suppressive effect in *in vitro* assays. Two steroidal saponins designated as diosgenin 3-*O*-α-L-rhamnosyl-(1–2)-β-D-glucuroniduronic acid (**1**) and its methyl ester, three steroids assigned as diosgenin tigogenin (**2**) and tigogenone (**3**), as well as a pregnane-type steroid identified as 16-dehydropregnenolone (**4**), demonstrated moderate cytotoxicity on A375-S2, HeLa, SGC-7901, Bel-7402, or HepG2 human neoplastic cell lines *in vitro.*[35,36] The IC_{50} values of 16-dehydropregnenolone (**4**) were 13.1–49.8 μg/mL in the first four tumor cell lines.[35] Additionally, the antileukemia property of diosgenin was demonstrated in mouse WEHI-3 cells *in vitro* and *in vivo.*[27]

Steroidal Alkaloids

SLT-A is a total alkaloid extract prepared from Bai Ying, which moderately restrained the growth of HeLa cells (IC_{50}: ~82 μg/mL). In a concentration of 80 μg/mL, SLT-A was able to induce G2/M cell arrest and apoptosis of the HeLa cells via the up-expression of p53 and Bax and the activation of caspase-3.[37] The treatment with the total alkaloid could enhance the proliferation of human A549 lung adenocarcinoma cells in a dose-dependent manner. The apoptotic death of A549 cells was elicited by the activation of a Fas-mediated death receptor pathway and the inhibition of NF-κB signaling pathway, i.e., stimulation of Fas and FasL expressions, activation of caspase-8 and caspase-3, increase of IκBα expression, and inhibition of NF-κB/p65, survivin, and p-IκBα.[38,39] The *in vivo* treatment with the steroid alkaloids in a dose of 24 mg/kg repressed the growth of H22 hepatoma with a T/C value of 66.24% and the inhibitory rate of 50.14% in mice,[40] and in a dose of 48 mg/kg restrained the growth of A549 lung cancer with a T/C value of 45.24% and the inhibitory rate of 48.93% in nude mice.[41] Three steroidal alkaloid glycosides, tentatively named SL-b, SL-c (**5**), and SL-d (**6**), were isolated from the stems of *S. lyratum.* The SL-c (**5**) and SL-d (**6**) in a 8 μg/mL concentration as well as SL-b in a 15 μg/mL concentration completely obstructed the proliferation of human JTC-26 cervical cancer cells *in vitro* with 100% inhibitory rate.[42]

Sesquiterpenoids

Three antitumor sesquiterpenoids determined as lyratol-A (**7**), lyratol-B (**8**), lyratol-C (**9**), lyratol-D (**10**), dehydrovomifoliol (**11**), and blumenol-A (**12**) were separated from the whole plant of Bai Ying. Lyratol-A (**7**) and lyratol-B (**8**) were found to elicit a noticeable antitumor effect against murine P388 leukemia cells and human HT-29 colorectal adenocarcinoma cells. Lyratol-C (**9**), lyratol-D (**10**), dehydrovomifoliol (**11**), and blumenol-A (**12**) moderately obstructed the proliferation of KB (oral), HONE-1 (nasopharynx), and HT-29 (colon) human cancer cell lines *in vitro* (IC_{50}: 3.7–8.1 μM).[43,44] Two C13-norisoprenoids named lyratol-E (**13**) and lyratol-F (**14**) exhibited a selective and noticeable cytotoxic effect against the P388 and HT-29 cell lines in *in vitro* models.[44] The ED_{50} values were 3.1 and 2.7 μg/mL in P388 cells and 2.5 and 1.9 μg/mL in HT-29 cells, respectively, whose activities were comparable to those of etoposide (ED_{50}: 2.1 and 1.9 μg/mL).[45] Other eudesmane-type sesquiterpenoids assigned as solajiangxin-F (**15**), solajiangxin-G (**16**), solajiangxin-D, lyratol-G and 1β-hydroxy-1,2-dihydro-α-santonin, and vetispirane-type sesquiterpenoids identified as 2-hydroxysolajiangxin-E and solajiangxin-E were markedly cytotoxic to three cancer cell lines (P388, HONE-1, HT-29) with ED_{50} values of 3–7 μg/mL.[46–48]

Polysaccharides

S. lyratum total polysaccharides (SLTPs) are polysaccharide components prepared from the plant of *S. lyratum*, which obviously displayed antigrowth and apoptosis-inducing effects against human MCF-7 breast cancer and Ec-9706 esophageal cancer cell lines *in vitro* at different concentrations. The effective inhibition was probably correlated with the decrease of Bcl-2 expression level and the improvement of caspase-3 gene activity.[49,50]

Mechanism Exploration

The marked antineoplastic activity of Bai Ying extracts has attracted researchers to investigate the anticancer mechanism. The approach suggested that the apoptosis-inducing mechanism caused by the Bai Ying extracts may be selectively related to following multiinteractions: (1) diminishment of Bcl-2 and Bcl-xL expression and increase of Bax and/or Bid expression levels; (2) loss of mitochondrial membrane potential and release of cytochrome c to cytosol; (3) upregulation of Fas expression and downregulation of fasL expression (such as in HeLa, A549, SW1116,

SPC-A-1, BGC-823 cells); (4) reduction of survivin expression (such as in HeLa, MCF-7, SGC-7901 cells); (5) stimulation of p53 and/or p27 activities (such as in A549, MCF-7, Colo 205 and WEHI-3 cells); (6) enhancement of ROS production (such as in Colo 205 and WEHI-3 cells); (7) decline of c-Myc mRNA level (such as in SMMC-7721 cells); (8) activation of phospho-JNK and decrease of phospho-p38 MAPK (such as in LLC cells); and (9) activation of caspase-3, caspase-8 and/or caspase-9, then finally leading to the increase of the apoptotic rate.[1–28] In addition, the WEHI-3 leukemia cell apoptosis provoked by the Bai Ying extracts was found to be modulated by both extrinsic and intrinsic signaling pathways via p53 activation.[27]

Other Bioactivities

The herb Bai Ying (Bittersweet herb) has been used as antiinflammatory, immunomodulatory, antianaphylactic, and antioxidant agents for the treatment of febrifuge, diarrhea, and eye disease besides cancer in Eastern countries for years. Research reports showed Bai Ying is able to stimulate TNFα secretion via the signal transduction pathway of PKC activation and to promote the production of NO from rIFNγ-primed peritoneal macrophages in mice.[51]

References

1. Wu, J. et al. 2009. Apoptosis of human stomach SGC-7901 cells induced by *Solanum lyratum* Thunb. extract. *Shizhen Guoyi Guoyao* 20: 2509–11.
2. Yu, L. H. et al. 2008. Influence of *Solanum lyratum* Thunb extract on apoptosis and the expression of bcl-xl/bid genes in human stomach cancer SGC-7901 cells. *Zhongchengyao* 30: 1744–8.
3. Zhao, L. W. et al. 2007. Apoptosis-induced effect of solanum lyratum thunb extract on human cervical cancer Hela cells. *Chin. J. Clin. Pharmacol. Therap.* 12: 883–7.
4. Wei, X. et al. 2006. The influence of *Solanum lyratum* Thunb extract on apoptosis and the expression of Fas/FasL genes in HeLa cells. *Zhongyaocai* 29: 1203–6.
5. Tu, S. et al. 2008. The influence of *Solanum lyratum* Thunb. Extract on apoptosis and the expression of Fas/FasL genes in human lung cancer A549 cells. *Shizhen Guoyi Guoyao* 19: 603.
6. Yang, X. D. et al. 2010. Study of *Solamum lyratum* Thunb on inducing apoptosis of human lung cancer cell A549 and its mechanism. *Traditional Chin. Med. J.* 9: 61–3.
7. Zhu, H. J. et al. 2009. Apoptosis-induced effect of solanum lyratum thunb extract on human cancer A2780 cells. *Xibei Guofang Yixue Zazhi* 30: 126–8.
8. Shi, W. L. et al. 2002. Effects of *Solanum lyratum* Thunb on multiplication in human acute promyelocytic HL-60 cells. *J. Fujian TCM Coll.* 12: 36–8.
9. Hsu, S. C. et al. 2008. Crude extracts of *Solanum lyratum* induced cytotoxicity and apoptosis in a human colon adenocarcinoma cell line (Colo 205). *Anticancer Res.* 28: 1045–54.
10. Lan, F. F. et al. 2006. Inhibitory effects of *Solanum lyratum* Thunb extracts on c-myc gene expression and proliferation of human hepatoma SMMC-7721 cells. *Guangdong Med. J.* 27(12 J): 1779–82.
11. Yang, X. D. et al. 2010. Study on Solanum vine's inducing human gastric cancer apoptosis and its mechanisms. *J. Changchun TCM Univ.* 26: 572–3.
12. Yang, X. D. et al. 2010. Effect of *Solanum lyratum* Thunb on the apoptosis of MCF-7 human breast cancer cells. *Modern Chin. Med.* 12: 34–6.
13. Yang, X. D. et al. 2010. Study on Solanum vine's inducing human colon cancer SW1116 apoptosis and its mechanisms. *Zhejiang Tradit. Chin. J.* 45: 919–20.
14. Zhu, H. J. et al. 2009. Experimental study of ampelopsis on anti-sarcoma A2780 effect. *Sci. Technol. Engineering* 9: 2304–6.
15. Shan, C. M. et al. 2002. Study of apoptosis in human liver cancers. *World J. Gastroenterol.* 8: 247–52.
16. Chan, C. M. et al. 2001. Apoptosis of hepotoma cell line BEL-7404 induced by extracts of solanum lyratum thumb. *Chin. J. Clin. Pharmacol. Therap.* 6: 200–3.
17. Wei, X. et al. 2007. Apoptosis-inducing effect of *Solanum lyratum* Thunb extract on human breast cancer MCF-7 cells and the expression of apoptosis associated genes. *Youjiang Med. J.* 35: 357–9.
18. Huang, H. S. et al. 2009. Effects of *Solanum lyratum* thunb extract only or combined with cisplatin on growth of HeLa cells of cervical cancer. *Maternal and Child Health Care of China* 20: 2850–2.
19. Wei, X. et al. 2008. Experimental study on apoptosis induced by ethanol extracts of *Solanum lyratum* Thunb in human lung cancer SPC-A-1 cells. *China Pharmacy* 19: 256–28.
20. Huang, H. S. et al. 2011. Effects of *Solanum lyratum* Thunb extracts on growth of HO8910 of ovarian cancer cells. *Xiandai Zhongliu Yixue* (7): 1279–81.
21. Pu, H. Q. et al. 2008. Apoptosis-inducing effect of *Solanum lyratum* thunb extract on human gastric carcinoma SGC-7901 cells and the expression of apoptosis associated proteins. *Xiandai Zhongliu Yixue* 137–8.
22. Ren, J. et al. 2006. Preliminary study on the antitumor effect of the extracts of *Solanum lyratum* Thunb. *Zhongguo Zhongyao Zazhi* 31: 497–500.
23. Sun, L. X. et al. 2005. Preliminary study on the antitumor effect of the extracts of *Solanum lyratum*. *Shenyang Yaoke Daxue Xuebao* 22: 210–2.
24. Lee, J. H. et al. 2009. Caspase and mitogen activated protein kinase pathways are involved in *Solanum lyratum* herba induced apoptosis. *J. Ethnopharmacol.* 123: 121–7.
25. Liu, S. H. et al. 2011. Immunomodulatory activity of butanol extract from *Solanum lyratum* in tumor-bearing mice. *Immunopharmacol. Immunotoxicol.* 33: 100–6.
26. Yang, J. S. et al. 2010. *Solannm lyratum* extract affected immune response in normal and leukemia murine animal in vivo. *Human Experim. Toxicol.* 29: 359–67.
27. Yang, J. S. et al. 2012. *Solanum lyratum* extracts induce extrinsic and intrinsic pathways of apoptosis in WEHI-3 murine leukemia cells and inhibit allograft tumor. *Evidence-based Complem. Altern. Med.* 2012: 254960.
28. Yang, X. D. et al. 2011. Effect of total glycosides of *Solanum lyratum* on expression of survivin and bax in MCF-7 human breast cancer cells. *Zhongguo Xinyao Zazhi* 20: 1123–6.
29. Yao, X. S. et al. 1999. Steroid saponin compounds for curing cancer and their preparation method. *Faming Zhuanli Shenqing Gongkai Shuomingshu* CN 1237583 A 19991208.

30. Ren, J. et al. 2006. The Primary study on the antitumor effect of total saponin of *Solanum lyratum* Thunb. *Cancer Res. Prevent. Treat.* 33: 262–4.
31. Liu, H. R. et al. 2008. Antiproliferative activity of the total saponin of *Solanum lyratum* Thunb in Hela cells by inducing apoptosis. *Pharmazie* 63: 836–42.
32. Yang, X. D. et al. 2011. Study of Solanum lyratum total saponin inducing apoptosis of human esophageal epithelia Ec-9706 cells and its mechanism. *J. Mudanjiang Med. Univ.* 32: 7–9.
33. Yang, X. D. et al. 2011. Effect of total glycosides of *Solanum lyratum* on expression of survivin and bax in MCF-7 human breast cancer cells. *Zhongguo Xinyao Zazhi* 20: 1123–6.
34. Zhang, J. et al. 2011. The hepatoma Bel-7402 cell apoptosis-inducing mechanism of total saponin from Bai-Ying. J. *Mudanjiang Med. Univ.* 32: 4–6.
35. Li, Y. et al. 2009. Chemical constituents from herb of *Solanum lyratum. Zhongguo Zhongyao Zazhi* 34: 1805–8.
36. Sun, L. X. et al. 2006. Cytotoxic constituents from *Solanum lyratum. Archiev. Pharm. Res.* 29: 135–9.
37. Lu, W. Z. et al. 2010. Total alkaloids from *Solanum lyratum* Thunb. inhibited HeLa cells proliferation through induction of apoptosis and cell cycle arrest. *Latin Am. J. Pharmacy* 29: 1396–402.
38. Tu, S. et al. 2013. *Solanum lyratum* Thunberg alkaloid induces human lung adenocarcinoma A549 cells apoptosis by activating Fas-pathway. *Shizhen Guoyi Guoyao* 24: 66–8.
39. Wei, X. et al. 2013. *Solanum lyratum* Thunberg alkaloid induces human lung adenoearcinoma A549 cells apoptosis by inhibiting NF-κB signaling pathway. *Zhongyaocai* 36: 787–90.
40. Po, J. et al. 2013. Pharmacodynamic studies on *Solanum lyratum* steroid alkaloids for the inhibition of liver cancer H22 cells in rats. *Shizhen Guoyi Guoyao* 24: 1593–5.
41. Wang, J. N. et al. 2013. In vivo inhibiting activity of total steroidal alkaloids from *Solanum lyratum* Thunb. on A549 lung cancer malignant cell lines in nude mice. *Zhongyao Xinyao Yu Linchuang Yaoli* 24: 469–472.
42. Murakami, K. et al. 1985. Studies on the constituents of *S. lyratum* Thunb. II. *Chem. Pharm. Bull.* 33: 67–73.
43. Dai, S. J. et al. 2009. Two new eudesmane-type sesquiterpenoids from *Solanum lyratum. Nat. Prods. Res.* 23: 1196–200.
44. Ren, Y. et al. 2009. Two new sesquiterpenoids from *Solanum lyratum* with cytotoxic activities. *Chem. Pharm. Bull.* 57: 408–410.
45. Li, G. S. et al. 2013. Two new cytotoxic sesquiterpenoids from *Solanum lyratum. Chin. Chem. Lett.* 24: 1030–2.
46. Yue, X. D. et al. 2012. Two new C13-norisoprenoids from *Solanum lyratum. J. Asian Nat. Prod. Res.* 14: 486–90.
47. Nie, X. P. et al. 2014. New eudesmane-type sesquiterpenoid from *Solanum lyratum* with cytotoxic activity. *Nat. Prod. Res.* 28: 641–5.
48. Yao, F. et al. 2013. Three new cytotoxic sesquiterpenoids from *Solanum lyratum. Phytochem. Lett.* 6: 453–6.
49. Yang, X. D. et al. 2011. Study of the *Solamum lyratum* Thunb polysaccharides inhibiting proliferation of human breast cancer cells. *Zhongguo Meirong Yixue* 20: 1245–7.
50. Yang, X. D. et al. 2011. Study of the *Solamum lyratum* Thunb polysaccharides inhibiting proliferation of human esophageal epithelia cells. *Sichuan J. Physiol. Sci.* 33: 53–5.
51. Kim, H. M. et al. 1999. The nitric oxide-producing properties of *Solanum lyratum. J. Ethnopharmacol.* 67: 163–9.

50 San Ke Zhen 三颗针

Chinese barberry

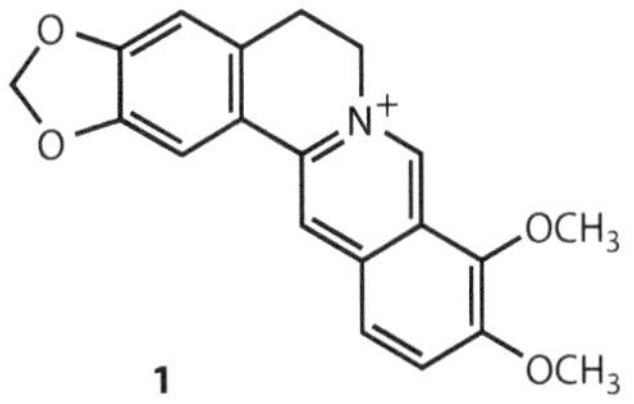

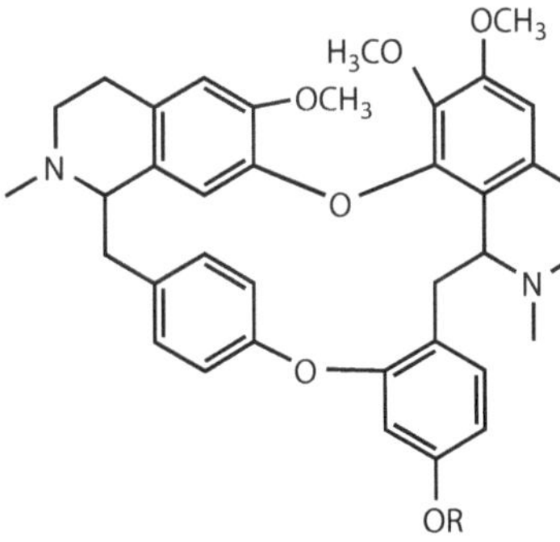

3. R = $-OCH_2CH_2CH_2CH_2-OCH_2CH_3$
4. R = -OOC-Ph-4-Cl
5. R = -OOC-Ph-2-Cl
6. R = -OOC-Ph-4-Br
7. R = -OOC-Ph-2-Br
8. R = $-OOC-Ph-4-OCH_3$
9. R = $-OOC-Ph-2-CH_3$
10. R = $-OOC-Ph-3-CH_2Cl$
11. R = $-O-CH_2-Ph-4-NO_2$
12. R = $-OOC-Ph-3,4,5-(OCH_3)_3$
13. R = -O
14. R = -OOC

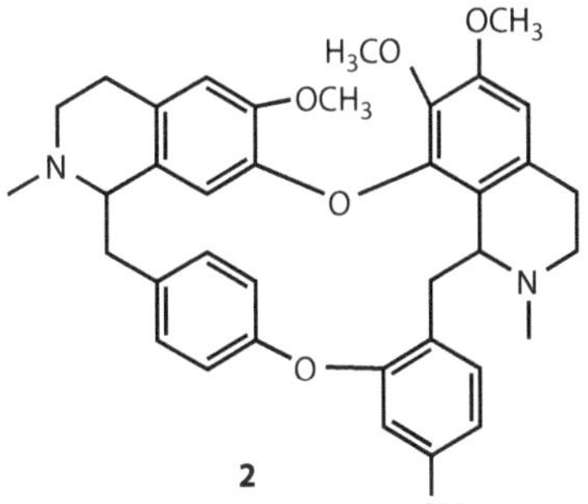

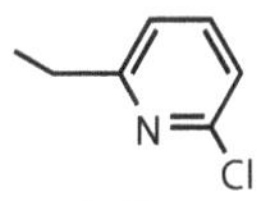

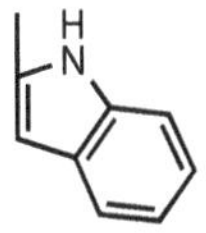

Herb Origination

The herb San Ke Zhen (Chinese barberry) originated from several *Berberis* genus plants such as *Berberis poiretii*, *B. sargentiana*, *B. veitchii*, *B. soulieana*, and *B. vernae* (Berberidaceae). The roots and the stems with the leaves are used as sources of the herb. The roots are generally collected in spring and autumn, whereas the stems with leaves are collected in any season. Also, San Ke Zhen is a large pharmaceutical source for the extraction of berberine.

Antitumor Constituents and Activities

The principal components in San Ke Zhen are two isoquinoline alkaloids assigned as berberine (**1**) and berbamine (**2**), which both are used for the treatment of many diseases. Many studies demonstrated two alkaloids as potentially useful agents for targeting a wide spectrum of neoplastic cells.

Berberine

Anticancer Effect

The investigation has established that berberine (**1**) broadly suppressed many types of human and murine carcinoma cell lines *in vitro* such as SMMC-7721 and HepG2 (liver), PG (lung), SW620 (colon), SNU-5 (gastric), PC3 and LNCaP (prostate), MCF-7 and MDA-MB-231 (breast), KB and 5-8F (nasopharynx), SCC-4 (tongue squamous), B16 and A431 (skin), T98G (glioblastoma), HSC-3 (oral squamous), SK-N-SH and SK-N-MC (neuroblastoma), U937 (lymphoma), HL-60, Molt-4 and WEHI-3 (leukemia), osteosarcoma, and Ehrlich ascites carcinoma cells.[1–7] The anticancer effect of berberine (**1**) was associated with the induction of cell cycle arrest and apoptosis but no such effects in noncancer human prostate epithelial (PWR-1E) cells and cortical neuronal cells.[7]

Induction of Cell Cycle Arrest and Apoptosis

The mechanism of cell cycle arrest in many cancer cell lines was found to correlate with (1) increase of CDC2 and p27 expressions; (2) decrease of CDC25c or CDC25A levels; (3) promotion of Weel and 14-3-3σ expressions; (4) inhibition of CDKs (CDK1, CDK2, and CDK4) and cyclin-B1, cyclin-D and cyclin-E; and (5) upregulation of p21 expressions p53-dependently.[7–14] The berberine-induced apoptosis was mediated by (1) up-expression of Bax and increase of Bax/Bcl-2 ratio, (2) disruption of mitochondrial membrane potential and release of cytochrome c and Smac/DIABLO, and (3) activation of PARP and caspase-3. However, in SNU-5 (stomach), HSC-3 (oral), PC3 (prostate), and SW620 (colon) tumor cell lines, berberine triggered the apoptosis by an ER stress response elicited by ROS generation and induction of mitochondria dysfunctions.[11,15–17] The cell cycle arrest and apoptotic activities of berberine (**1**) were revealed to be more effective in p53-expressing cancer cell lines (such as LNCaP prostate cancer, SK-N-SH neuroblastoma, and osteosarcoma) than in p53-deficient cancer cell lines (such as PC3 prostate cancer and SK-N-MC neuroblastoma).[7,14,18] While berberine (**1**) facilitated the apoptosis of human colorectal cancer cells, two proapoptotic genes (NAG-1 and ATF3) were up-expressed and then ATF3 was activated independent of p53-activation.[19] *In vivo* xenograft studies also confirmed that the reduction of tumor weights and volumes by berberine (**1**) was more marked in mice bearing p53-expressing LNCaP cells than that of p53-deficient PC3 cells.[18] The results indicated that berberine (**1**) prefer to serve as a p53-dependent agent in the growth inhibition of neoplastic cells. In addition, some specific effectors regulated by berberine

(**1**) were found to be partly involved in the antiproliferative and apoptotic activities; for instance, the decreases of side population cells and the ABCG2 expression were associated with the antigrowth effect of berberine in MCF-7 breast cancer cells,[20] and the acetylation of α-tubulin-induced by berberine (**1**) was linked to the apoptosis of leukemia HL-60 cells.[10]

Antiinvasive and Antimetastatic Activities

Berberine (**1**) was investigated in several highly invasive and metastatic cancer cells. Normally, three important factors, u-PA, ezrin, and MMPs, play critical roles in the invasion, the metastasis, and the angiogenesis of cancer cells. Thus, the inhibition of the ezrin, u-PA, and MMPs may lead to the inhibition of cancer cell migration and invasion. By repressing filopodia formation and retarding ezrin phosphorylation at threonine 567, berberine (**1**) at a concentration of 20 μM dose and time dependently restrained the invasion and the motility of 5-8F nasopharyngeal cancer cells by 73% and 67%, respectively, and obstructed tumor metastasis to lymph nodes, whose antimetastatic effect of berberine was further confirmed in a mouse model implanted with 5-8F cancer.[21] Berberine (**1**) inhibited the invasive capacity of SCC-4 tongue squamous malignant cells via the down-expression of u-PA, MMP-2, and MMP-9 and the inhibition of p-JNK, p-ERK, p-p38, IKK, and NF-κB signaling pathways.[22] The suppressive effect of berberine (**1**) on cell migration, adhesion invasion, and metastasis was also found in PG cells derived from a high metastatic human giant lung carcinoma cell line *in vitro*, whose mechanism was revealed to closely correlate with the significant inhibition of the cell adhesion and Martrigel-coated transwell, the down-expression of MMP-2, and the up-expression of TIMP2.[23,24] When berberine (**1**) was combined with As_2O_3 to treat glioma cells, the antimetastatic effect was significantly enhanced most likely by blocking the PKC-mediated signaling pathway involved in the cancer cell migration.[25]

Synergistic Activity

Berberine (**1**) might notably strengthen the radio- and chemosensitization by the increase of ROS and NO. When γ-irradiation is combined with berberine, the tumoricidal effect of radiotherapy was apparently augmented toward human HepG2 hepatoma cells.[26] The integration of berberine (**1**) with evodiamine significantly promoted the apoptosis of human SMMC-7721 hepatoma cells and amplified the level of TNFα, finally resulting in 50% inhibition on the cell growth.[27]

Anticarcinogenic Activity

Berberine (**1**) demonstrated an excellent antihepatocarcinogenetic potential. Berberine (**1**) in an oral dose of 50 mg/kg markedly obstructed the growth of hepatoma cells in the early phase of hepatocarcinogenesis induced by diethylnitrosamine plus phenobarbital in rats.[28] All these data evidenced that berberine (**1**) has more potential for the development of novel therapeutics in the treatment and the prevention of malignant tumor diseases.

Berbamine

Anticancer Effect

Berbamine (**2**), a *bis*-benzylisoquinoline alkaloid, has been used for the clinical treatment of patients with cancer for many years in China. In lab murine models, berbamine (**2**) effectively inhibited the growth of sarcoma 180 cells by 75–78% and prolonged the life span of mice bearing ascites hepatoma or Ehrlich cancer by 68–80%.[29] Berbamine (**2**) also exerted an obvious inhibitory effect against W256 sarcoma cells in rats.[30] The anticancer effect was revealed to be mediated by the significant acceleration of tumor cell necrosis and the blockage of nucleic acidic metabolism in the cancer cells.[29,30] In recent years, berbamine (**2**) was further proven to be effective in various human cancer cell lines, especially leukemia (K562, NB4, HL-60 and Jurkat), hepatoma (SMMC7721 and HepG2), highly metastatic breast cancer (MDA-MB-231 and MDA-MB-435S), prostate cancer (PC3), myeloma (KM3), and lymphoma cells, *in vitro*. The IC_{50} values were 3.86 μg/mL (at 48 h) in NB4 cells and 34.5 μM in HepG2 cells.[31–34]

Proapoptotic Mechanisms

The anticancer activity of berbamine (**2**) was revealed to be accompanied by the apoptosis-accelerating and cell cycle disturbing abilities. The mechanism was related to the concomitant events, (1) inhibition of telomerase activity and Bcl-2 expression,[35] (2) upregulation of Bax expression and p53 activity,[36,37] (3) blockage of NF-κB signaling pathway and decrease of survivin mRNA,[31,32] and (4) depolarization of mitochondrial membrane and loss of mitochondrial transmembrane potential and activation of caspases.[37,38] In highly metastatic breast cancer cell lines (MDA-MB-231 and MDA-MB-435S), the inhibitory effect of berbamine (**2**) was achieved by promoting apoptosis and suppressing cell migration and invasion, associated with the inhibition of Akt and NF-κB signaling pathways via the reduction of phosphorylation of Akt and c-Met and the inhibition of their downstream targets such as NF-κB, p65, Bcl-2/Bax, osteopontin, VEGF, MMP-9, and MMP-2.[31–37,39]

Synergistic and Anti-MDR Activities

Berbamine (**2**) also displayed significant synergistic effects with anticarcinoma agents such as trichostatin-A (a histone deacetylase inhibitor), celecoxib (an inhibitor of COX-2), and carmofur to inhibit the growth of the MDA-MB-231 cells.[38] When it combined with dexamethasone, DOX, or arsenic trioxide, the inhibitory effect on KM3 multiple myeloma cells was mediated by promoting G1 arrest and apoptosis and diminishing p65 nuclear translocation and NF-κB expression.[31,36] By inhibiting MDR-1 gene expression, activating caspase-3 and drug excretion capacity of cells, and downregulating p210 bcr/abl oncoprotein level, berbamine (**2**) effectively reversed the MDR of human K562/Adm cells and K562-R leukemia cells, to exert the inhibitory effect against the cell proliferation.[40–44] In the combination with a clinic anticancer drug imatinib/Gleevec, berbamine (**2**) was able to enhance the chemosensitivity of K562-R cells to imatinib. The results suggested that berbamine may be useful in the clinical treatment of drug-resistant CML patients.[44–46]

Immunoenhancing Effect

Berbamine (**2**) was capable of remarkably amplifying the number of leukocyte for the immunoenhancement. The combination with berbamine (**2**) in current cancer chemotherapies may play an additional role for the protection of leukocyte and marrow.[30]

Berbamine Derivatives

The research results provided strong evidences for the wide or the adjuvant therapeutic applications of berbamine (**2**) in cancer treatment. The significant property also suggested that berbamine (**2**) is a good starting point for the development of a novel drug candidate. The structural modification further found that etherification, esterification, or sulfonylation of the phenolic hydroxyl group in the berbamine markedly amplified the cytotoxicity against leukemia, lymphoma, hepatoma, breast cancer, and fibrosarcoma cell lines *in vitro* or *in vivo*. Eleven berbamine derivatives (**3–13**) were synthesized showing a great antileukemia activity 8–25 times more potent than its parental molecule. In particular, **3–13** displayed a consistent higher inhibitory effect against multidrug-resistant type of K562 leukemia cells.[47,48] 4-Chlorobenzoyl berbamine (**4**) demonstrated a significant suppressive effect on the proliferation of human lymphoma cell lines (Raji, L428, Namalwa, and Jurkat) *in vitro* as well in association with the induction of apoptosis and G2/M cell cycle arrest via PI3K/Akt and NF-κB signaling pathways in a caspase-dependent manner.[49]

O-(4-Ethoxybutyl) berbamine (**3**), an antagonist of calmodulin and trypsin-activated Ca^{2+}-Mg^{2+}-ATPase, exerted a significant inhibitory effect on human 7402 hepatoma, mouse H22 hepatom, and human HT1080 fibrosarcoma cell lines *in vitro* (IC_{50}: 1.2–8.2 μg/mL).[50,51] The antihepatoma effect was substantiated in mice implanted with H22 ascites hepatoma, and the life span of the tested mice was remarkably prolonged to more than three months. In the experiment, **3** markedly lessened the amount of calmodulin in the hepatoma cells and augmented the p53 translation to block the cell cycle at G2/M phase.[50] Through the decrease of MMP-2 and MMP-9 activities and the increase of TIMP-1 (a tissue inhibitor of metalloproteinase) mRNA levels, **3** was obviously effective in suppressing the invasion of HT1080 fibrosarcoma cells besides the proliferative inhibition.[51] Moreover, *O*-(4-ethoxybutyl) berbamine (**3**) was also shown to have a greater activity in reversing the MDR of human MCF-7/Adm breast neoplastic cells and significantly amplifying cytoplastic Ca^{2+} level in the cells.[52,53] Similar to berbamine (**2**), the synergistic effects of **3** was greatly demonstrated against H22 hepatoma in *in vivo* combinational treatments with DOX or PEGylated liposomal DOX and against sarcoma 180 with mitomycin-C or CTX, thereby improving the chemotherapeutic efficacy of these drugs. Concurrently, it augmented the host immune function to lessen the drug-caused toxicities and obviously prolonged the survival time of the experimented animals.[54,55] These evidences proved that the important anticancer derivative deserves further preclinical investigation and suggested that the structural modification of berbamine (**2**) should be continued for the discovery of more potentially useful drugs against malignant diseases.

Other Bioactivities

The herb San Ke Zhe (Chinese barberry) shows antibacterial and hypertensive effects in pharmacological studies. It is commonly used as an herbal medicine for patients with gastrointestinal disorders and diarrhea. Both berberine (**1**) and berbamine (**2**) exert multiple bioactivities such as antiarrhythmia and antimyocardial infarctions. Berberine (**1**) also displays antidiarrhetic, antiinflammatory, antilipid-peroxidative, antithrombocyte-agglutinative, antiulcer, and antimalarial activities.

References

1. Yu, F. S. et al. 2007. Berberine inhibits WEHI-3 leukemia cells in vivo. *In vivo* 21: 407–12.
2. Issat, T. et al. 2006. Berberine, a natural cholesterol reducing product, exerts antitumor cytostatic/cytotoxic effects independently from the mevalonate pathway. *Oncol. Reports* 16: 1273–6.
3. Jantova, S. et al. 2007. Berberine induces apoptosis through a mitochondrial/caspase pathway in human promonocytic U937 cells. *Toxicol. in vitro* 21: 25–31.
4. Letasiova, S. et al. 2006. Effect of berberine on proliferation, biosynthesis of macromolecules, cell cycle and induction of intercalation with DNA, dsDNA damage and apoptosis in Ehrlich ascites carcinoma cells. *J. Pharm. Pharmacol.* 58: 263–70.
5. Letasiova, S. et al. 2006. Berberine-antiproliferative activity in vitro and induction of apoptosis/necrosis of the U937 and B16 cells. *Cancer Lett.* 239: 254–62.
6. Jiang, Y. et al. 2005. Apoptosis of Molt-4 cells induced by berberine in vitro. *Yiyao Daobao* 24: 568–70.
7. Choi, M. S. et al. 2008. Berberine inhibits human neuroblastoma cell growth through induction of p53-dependent apoptosis. *Anticancer Res.* 28: 3777–84.
8. Zhang, W. D. et al. 2008. Berberine induces cell cycle arrest and apoptosis in human hepatocellular carcinoma Hep G2 cell line. *J. Wuhan Univ. (Med. edit.)* 29: 766–8, 786.
9. Lin, C. C. et al. 2006. Down-regulation of cyclin B1 and up-regulation of Weel by berberine promotes entry of leukemia cells into the G2/M-phase of the cell cycle. *Anticancer Res.* 26: 1097–104.
10. Khan, M. S. et al. 2010. Berberine and a *Berberis lycium* extract inactivate Cdc25A and induce α-tubulin acetylation that correlate with HL-60 cell cycle inhibition and apoptosis. *Mutation Res.* 683: 123–30.
11. Lin, C. C. et al. 2007. Berberine induces apoptosis in human HSC-3 oral cancer cells via simultaneous activation of the death receptor-mediated and mitochondrial pathway. *Anticancer Res.* 27: 3371–8.
12. Mantena, S. K. et al. 2006. Berberine inhibits growth, induces G1 arrest and apoptosis in human epidermoid carcinoma A431 cells by regulating Cdki-Cdk-cyclin cascade, disruption of mitochondrial membrane potential and cleavage of caspase 3 and PARP. *Carcinogen.* 27: 2018–27.
13. Eom, K. et al. 2008. Berberine induces G1 arrest and apoptosis in human glioblastoma T98G cells through mitochondrial/caspases pathway. *Biol. Pharm. Bull.* 31: 558–62.
14. Liu, Z. J. et al. Berberine induces p53-dependent cell cycle arrest and apoptosis of human osteosarcoma cells by inflicting DNA damage. *Mutation Res.* 662: 75–83.
15. Meeran, S. M. et al. 2008. Berberine-induced apoptosis in human prostate cancer cells is initiated by reactive oxygen species generation. *Toxicol. Applied Pharmacol.* 229: 33–43.
16. Lin, J. P. et al. 2008. Berberine induced down-regulation of matrix metalloproteinase-1, -2 and -9 in human gastric cancer cells (SNU-5) in vitro. *In vivo* 22: 223–30.
17. Hsu, W. H. et al. 2007. Berberine induces apoptosis in SW620 human colonic carcinoma cells through generation of reactive oxygen species and activation of JNK/p38 MAPK and FasL. *Archiv. Toxicol.* 81: 719–28.
18. Choi, M. S. et al. 2009. Berberine inhibits p53-dependent cell growth through induction of apoptosis of prostate cancer cells. *Intl. J. Oncol.* 34: 1221–30.

19. Piyanuch, R. et al. 2007. Berberine, a natural isoquinoline alkaloid, induces NAG-1 and ATF3 expression in human colorectal cancer cells. *Cancer Lett.* 258: 230–40.
20. Kim, J. B. et al. 2008. Berberine diminishes the side population and ABCG2 transporter expression in MCF-7 breast cancer cells. *Planta Med.* 74: 1693–700.
21. Tang, F. Q. et al. Berberine inhibits metastasis of nasopharyngeal carcinoma 5–8F cells by targeting Rho kinase-mediated Ezrin phosphorylation at threonine 567. *J. Biol. Chem.* 284: 27456–66.
22. Ho, Y. T. et al. 2009. Berberine suppresses in vitro migration and invasion of human SCC-4 tongue squamous cancer cells through the inhibitions of FAK, IKK, NF-κB, u-PA and MMP-2 and -9. *Cancer Lett.* 279: 155–62.
23. Hao, Y. et al. Effect of berberine on invasion and migration of PG cells from a high metastatic human giant lung carcinoma cell line. *Zhongguo Bingli Shengli Zazhi* 23: 474–8.
24. Kim, S. M. et al. 2008. Berberine suppresses TNFα-induced MMP-9 and cell invasion through inhibition of AP-1 activity in MDA-MB-231 human breast cancer cells. *Mol.* 13: 2975–85.
25. Lin, T. H. et al. 2008. Berberine enhances inhibition of glioma tumor cell migration and invasiveness mediated by arsenic trioxide. *BMC Cancer* 8: 58.
26. Hu, J. M. et al. 2009. The combination of berberine and irradiation enhances anticancer effects via activation of p38 MAPK pathway and ROS generation in human hepatoma cells. *J. Cell. Biochem.* 107: 955–64.
27. Wang, X. N. et al. 2008. Enhancement of apoptosis of human hepatocellular carcinoma SMMC-7721 cells through synergy of berberine and evodiamine. *Phytomed.* 15: 1062–8.
28. Zhao, X. et al. 2008. Effect of berberine on hepatocyte proliferation, inducible nitric oxide synthase expression, cytochrome P450 2E1 and 1A2 activities in diethylnitrosamine- and phenobarbital-treated rats. *Biomed. Pharmacother.* 62: 567–72.
29. Zhu, X. W. et al. 1986. Experimental study on the antitumor action of berbamine in mice. *Zhongxiyi Jiehe Zazhi* 10: 611–3, 582.
30. Liu, C. X. et al. (a) 1979. *Zhongcaoyao Tongxun* 8: 36; (b) 1999. *Chinese Materia Medica.* Vol. 3, 3–1897, 294. Shanghai Science and Technology Press, Shanghai, China.
31. Zhao, X. Y. et al. 2007. Berbamine selectively induces apoptosis of human acute promyelocytic leukemia cells via survivin-mediated pathway. *Chin. Med. J.* (Beijing, China, Eng. Edit.) 120: 802–6.
32. Wang, G. Y. et al. 2009. Berbamine induces Fas-mediated apoptosis in human hepatocellular carcinoma HepG2 cells and inhibits its tumor growth in nude mice. *J. Asian Nat. Prod. Res.* 11: 219–28.
33. Shen, Q. et al. 2008. Influences of berbamine on proliferation and apoptosis of leukemia K562 cells. *J. Zhengzhou Univ.* (Med. Edit.) 43: 1154–6.
34. Huang, Z. Y. et al. 2007. Experimental study of berbamine inducing apoptosis in human leukemia Jurkat cells. *Zhongguo Zhongliu* 16: 722–4.
35. Ji, Z. Y. et al. 2002. Inhibition of telomerase activity and bcl-2 expression in berbamine-induced apoptosis in HL-60 cells. *Planta Med.* 68: 596–600.
36. Liang, Y. et al. 2009. Berbamine, a novel nuclear factor κB inhibitor, inhibits growth and induces apoptosis in human myeloma cells. *Acta Pharmacol. Sinica* 30: 1659–65.
37. Sun, P. et al. 2007. Induction of apoptosis by berbamine in androgen-independent prostate cancer PC-3 in vitro. *Zhonghua Shiyan Waike Zazhi* 24: 957–9.
38. Wang, S. et al. 2009. Suppression of growth, migration and invasion of highly-metastatic human breast cancer cells by berbamine and its molecular mechanisms of action. *Mol. Cancer* 8: 81.
39. Wang, G. Y. et al. 2007. Berbamine induces apoptosis in human hepatoma cell line SMMC 7721 by loss in mitochondrial transmembrane potential and caspase activation. *J. Zhejiang Univ., Sci. B.* 8: 248–55.
40. Dong, Q. H. et al. 2004. Study on effect of berbamine on multidrug resistance leukemia K562/Adr cells. *Zhongguo Zhongxiyi Jiehe Zazhi* 24: 820–2.
41. Wei, Y. L. et al. 2009. Berbamine exhibits potent antitumor effects on imatinib-resistant CML cells in vitro and in vivo. *Acta Pharmacol. Sinica* 30: 451–7.
42. Zhao, X. Y. et al. 2003. Studies on effects of berbamine as a calmodulin antagonist on reversing multidrug resistance in human leukemia cells. *Yaowu Fenxi Zazhi* 23: 402–6.
43. Zhao, X. Y. et al. 2005. Studies on effects of berbamine on human leukemia cell line NB4. *Yaowu Fenxi Zazhi* 25: 1207–10.
44. Wu, D. et al. 2004. Apoptosis induced by berbamine in K562 cells correlates with the expression levels of bcr/abl gene and P210. *Zhongguo Bingli Shengli Zazhi* 20: 1396–401.
45. Xu, R. Z. et al. 2005. Berbamine: A novel inhibitor of bcr/abl fusion gene with potent anti-leukemia activity. *Leukemia Res.* 30: 17–23.
46. Wei, Y. L. et al. 2009. The antiproliferation effect of berbamine on K562 resistant cells by inhibiting NF-κB pathway. *Anatomical Record* 292: 945–50.
47. Xie, J. W. et al. 2009. Berbamine derivatives: A novel class of compounds for anti-leukemia activity. *Eur. J. Med. Chem.* 44: 3293–8.
48. Zou, L. L. et al. 2009. The Growth inhibiting effect of calmodulin antagonist *O*-(4-ethoxybutyl)-berbamine on leukemia cells K562 and K562/A02. *Zhongguo Yaolixue Tongbao* 25: 1313–7.
49. Du, H. P. et al. 2010. 4-Chlorobenzoyl berbamine induces apoptosis and G2/M cell cycle arrest through the PI3K/Akt and NF-κB signal pathway in lymphoma cells. *Oncol. Reports* 23: 709–16.
50. Liu, J. W. et al. 2002. The effect of calmodulin antagonist berbamine derivative-EBB on hepatoma in vitro and in vivo. *Chin. Med. J.* 115: 759–62.
51. Pan, B. et al. 2005. Effect of calmodulin antagonist EBB on invasion of human fibrosarcoma cell HT1080. *Zhongguo Yixue Kexueyuan Xuebao* 27: 311–4.
52. Cheng, Y. H. et al. 2006. Reversal of multidrug resistance in drug-resistant human breast cancer cell line MCF-7/Adr by calmodulin antagonist *O*-(4-ethoxyl-butyl)-berbamine. *Zhongguo Yixue Kexueyuan Xuebao* 28: 164–8.
53. Shi, X. et al. 2008. Influence of the calmodulin antagonist EBB on cyclin B1 and Cdc2-p34 in human drug-resistant breast cancer MCF-7/Adr cells. *Chin. J. Clin. Oncol.* 5: 108–12.
54. Fang, B. J. et al. 2004. Effect of *O*-4-ethoxylbutylberbamine in combination with pegylated liposomal doxorubicin on advanced hepatoma in mice. *World J. Gastroenterol.* 10: 950–3.
55. Zhang, J. H. et al. 1998. Effect of berbamine derivative (EBB) on anticancer and immune function of tumor-bearing mice. *Zhongcaoyao* 29: 243–6.

51 Zi Bai Pi 梓白皮

Chinese catalpa

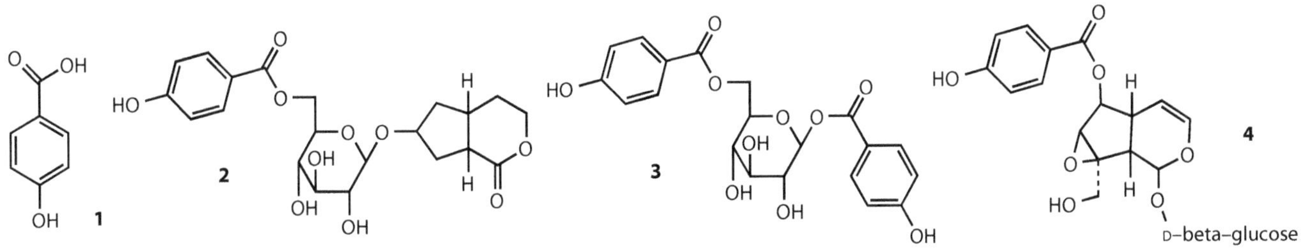

1 2 3 4

D-beta-glucose

Herb Origination

The herb Zi Bai Pi (Chinese catalpa) is the root barks and the stem barks of a deciduous tree *Catalpa ovata* (Bignoniaceae). This plant is broadly distributed in regions surrounding the Yangtze River and is also cultivated in North America and Europe. For Chinese medicinal uses, the barks in the tree roots and the stems can be annually collected and dried in the sun. The herb Zi Bai Pi was used as a traditional Chinese medicine for a thousand years, and it was documented in the first Chinese classic of materia medica entitled *Shennong Ben Cao Jing.*

Anticarcinogenic Constituents and Activities

In *in vitro* experiments, the barks and the seed oil of *C. ovata* exerted anticarcinogenic and anticancer effects. A methanolic extract of the barks displayed an obvious inhibitory effect against mutation, and its n-hexane partition layer strongly suppressed the carcinogenic rate of AFB-1.[1]

Naphthoquinones

The bioassay-directed investigation of the extract led to the isolation of eight antitumorigenic α-lapachone analogs. All the α-lapachones exerted a significant inhibitory activity against TPA-induced EBV-EA activation in Raji cells,[2] showing the antitumor-promoting activity.

Iridoids and Phenols

The isolation of *C. ovata* leaves led to the obtainment of four bioactive compounds identified as 4-hydroxybenzoic acid (**1**), ovatolactone-7-*O*-(6′-*p*-hydroxybenzoyl)-β-D-glucoside (**2**), 1,6-di-*O*-*p*-hydroxybenzoyl-β-D-glucoside (**3**), and catalposide (**4**). In a 100 μg/mL concentration, the compounds (4-hydroxybenzoic acid (**1**) and ovatolactone-7-*O*-(6′-*p*-hydroxybenzoyl)-β-D-glucoside (**2**)) were effective in the inhibition of leukemia cell lines (U937, HL-60, and Molt-4), and 1,6-di-*O*-*p*-hydroxybenzoyl-β-D-glucoside (**3**) showed only a mild cytotoxic effect in Molt-4 and HL-60 cell lines. The antileukemia property of 1,6-di-*O*-*p*-hydroxybenzoyl-β-D-glucoside (**3**) was found to closely correlate with the augmentation of p53 and IL-4 expressions and the decrease of IL-2 and IFNγ genes in Molt-4 cells. More test showed that the compound 1,6-di-*O*-*p*-hydroxybenzoyl-β-D-glucoside (**3**) was able to stimulate T cell-mediated immune responses.[3] Catalposide (**12**) displayed the effect in *in vivo* models with. The oral administration of catalposide (**4**) in a daily dose of 25 mg/kg exerted the suppressive effect for 60.68% and 50.80% against S180 and Heps carcinoma, respectively, with no influence on the immune function.[4]

Seed Oil

The seed oil of Chinese catalpa (CPO) is rich in 9-*trans*,11-*trans*,13-*cis*-conjugated linolenic acid (9*t*,11*t*,13*c*-CLN). The dietary administration of 1% CPO to rats for four weeks could suppress the development of colonic aberrant crypt foci induced by azoxymethane and inhibit the tumor cell proliferation in rats.[5,6] The CLNs were cytotoxic to U937 human monocytic leukemia cells at concentrations of >10 μM. The cytotoxic effect of 9*c*,11*t*,13*c*-CLN, 9*c*,11*t*,13*t*-CLN, and 9*t*,11*t*,13*c*-CLN were much stronger than that of 8*t*,10*t*,12*c*-CLN, whose mechanism of the CLNs might be attributed to lipid peroxidation.[5] These findings indicated the CPO may have a possible chemopreventive activity in the early phase of colon and lymphoblast of carcinogeneses.

Other Bioactivities

Catalposide, a major iridoid glycoside isolated from the herb, is a potent inducer of heme oxygenase-1 (HO-1), whose HO-1 as a stress response protein is known to play a protective role against oxidative injury. Therefore, catalposide was considered to have to ability to markedly protect Neuro 2A cells, a kind of neuronal cell lines, from oxidative damage.[7]

References

1. Kim, M. S. et al. 1992. Separation of antimutagenic substance from stem bark *of Catalpa ovata. Environ. Mutagens. Carcinog.* 12: 147–55.
2. Fujiwara, A. et al. 1998. Antitumor-promoting naphthoquinones from *Catalpa ovata. J. Nat. Prod.* 61: 629–62.
3. Oh, C. H. et al. 2010. Effects of isolated compounds from *Catalpa ovata* on the T cell-mediated immune responses and proliferation of leukemic cells. *Archiv. Pharm. Res.* 33: 545–50.
4. Wang, Q. Z. et al. 2012. Antitumor activity of catalposide. *Zhongchengyao* 34: 2381–4.
5. Suzuki, R. et al. 2001. Cytotoxic effect of conjugated trienoic fatty acids on mouse tumor and human monocytic leukemia cells. *Lipids* 36: 477–82.

6. Suzuki, R. et al. 2006. Catalpa seed oil rich in 9t,11t,13c-conjugated linolenic acid suppresses the development of colonic aberrant crypt foci induced by azoxymethane in rats. *Oncol. Reports* 16: 989–96.

7. Moon, M. K. et al. 2003. Catalposide protects neuro 2A cells from hydrogen peroxide-induced cytotoxicity via the expression of heme oxygenase-1. *Toxicology Lett.* 145: 46–54.

52 Bai Xian Pi 白鲜皮

Dittany root bark

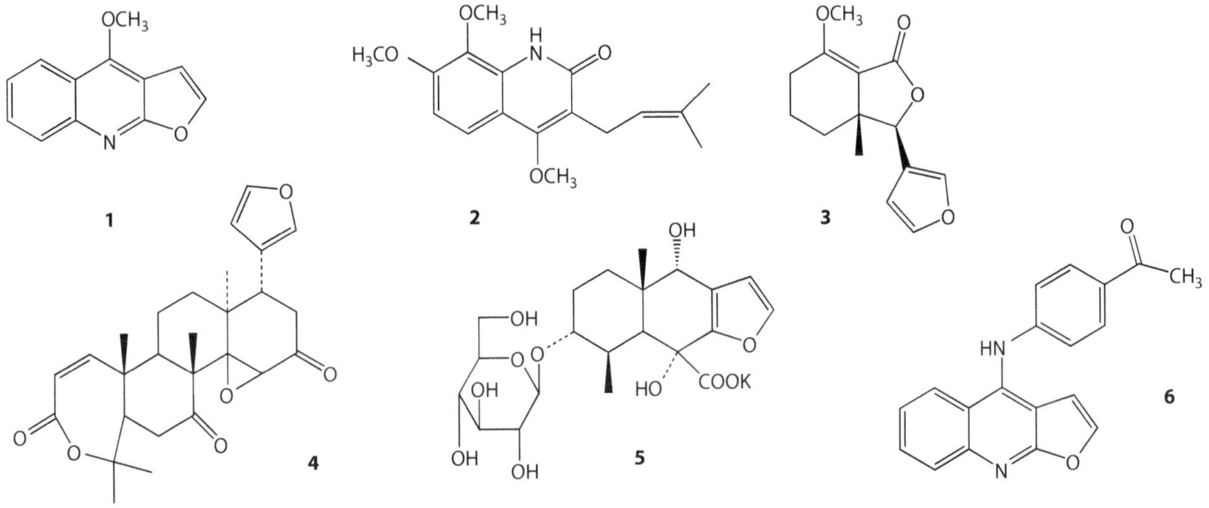

Herb Origination

The origin of the herb Bai Xian Pi is the root bark of a Rutaceae plant *Dictamnus dasycarpus*. The plant is distributed in the northeast, the north, and the southeast of China, as well as in Mongolia, Korea, and Russian Far East. The first Chinese classic of materia medica entitled *Shennong Ben Cao Jing* documented Bai Xian Pi (Dittany root bark). According to Chinese medicines, the root back is normally collected in spring and autumn for the medicinal use.

Antitumor Constituents and Activities

The lipophilic extract and its volatile oil derived from Bai Xian Pi exhibited *in vitro* antineoplastic effect. Three bioactive components, dictamnine (**1**), preskimmianine (**2**), and fraxinellone (**3**), isolated from the extract displayed cytotoxicity against L1210 lymphocytic leukemia cells and tumoricidal effect toward Ehrlich ascites tumor, sarcoma 180, and U14 cervical tumor cells *in vitro* in their 0.5% concentration. Among them, preskimmianine (**2**) exerted the most potent inhibition against L1210 cells (IC_{50}: 3.13 μg/mL); however, it was toxic to lymphocytes at a 50 μg/mL concentration.[1,2]

Obacunone (**4**), a limonoid triterpene in Bai Xian Pi, showed no direct cytotoxicity on cancer cells but could potentiate the cytotoxicity of VCR on murine L1210 leukemia cells by approximately tenfold and enhance the anticancer effect of vinblastine and taxol on both drug-sensitive KB-3-1 cells, and multidrug-resistant KB-V1 cells was greatly augmented in the presence of obacunone (**4**). However, it did not exert the similar additive action if combined with other drugs such as adriamycin, cisplatin, and 5-FU.[3]

A glycoside component designated as dasycarpuside-A (**5**) was isolated from the aqueous extract of Bai Xian Pi, which exhibited only weak cytotoxicity on lung carcinoma A549 cells.[4] In addition, an isofraxinellone derived from the lipophilic extract of Bai Xian Pi displayed an antimutagenic effect.[5]

Structural Modification

A group of 4-anilinofuro[2,3-b]quinoline derivatives were structurally modified from dictamnine (**1**) and evaluated by using the NCI's full panel of 60 human cancer cell lines. 1-[4-(Furo[2,3-b] quinolin-4-ylamino) phenyl] ethanone (FQPE) (**6**) (average GI_{50}: 0.025 μM for all tested cell lines) was found to be more potent than both clinical-used anticancer drugs, m-AMSA (average GI_{50}: 0.44 μM), and daunomycin (average GI_{50}: 0.044 μM). FQPE (**6**) was capable of obstructing all types of tested cancer cells with GI_{50} values of <0.04 μM except for NSCLC cells (average GI_{50}: 1.75 μM).[6,7] Although FQPE (**6**) was relatively resistant to HOP-92 cancer NSCLC cells (GI_{50}: 12.4 μM), it was sensitive to other NSCLC cell lines, HOP-62 (GI_{50}: <0.01 μM), NCl-H460 (GI_{50}: 0.01 μM), and NCI-H522 (GI_{50}: <0.01 μM). The sensitivity order of different cancer cell lines to FQPE (**6**) were colon cancer > CNS cancer > breast cancer > melanoma > prostate cancer > renal cancer > ovarian cancer > NSCLC.[6,7] According to the potent cytotoxicity, FQPE (**6**) can be considered to be a promising agent for further development of a new anticancer drug candidate.

Other Bioactivities

Bai Xian Pi (Dittany root bark) is one of the most commonly used Chinese herbs for the treatment of eczema. Biological studies showed that Bai Xian Pi has protective and therapeutic effects on the digestive system, where it prominently inhibits medicine-caused diarrhea, water-immersed stress ulcer, and gastric ulcer and markedly enlarges the choleresis amount. Bai Xian Pi also shows antibacterial and antiinflammatory effects. The major constituents, dictamnine (**1**) and fraxinellone (**3**), demonstrated a significant antiplatelet aggregation, antimutiagenic, and vascular relaxing activity, and dictamnine (**1**) can enhance heart and vascular constrictions as well.[8]

References

1. Kang, S. L. et al. 1983. Bioactive constituents in *Dictamnus dasycarpus. J.* Shenyang *Pharm. College* (18): 11–6.
2. Kim, S. W. et al. 1997. Isolation and characterization of antitumor agents from *Dictamnus albus. Saengyak Hakhoechi* 28: 209–14.
3. Jung, H. J. et al. 2000. Potentiating effect of obacunone from *Dictamnus dasycarpus* on cytotoxicity of microtubule inhibitors, vincristine, vinblastine, and taxol. *Planta Med.* 66: 74–6.
4. Chang, J. et al. 2002. Cytotoxic terpenoid and immunosuppressive phenolic glycosides from the root bark of *Dictamnus dasycarpus. Planta Med.* 68: 425–9.
5. Miyazawa, M. et al. 1995. Antimutagenic activity of isofraxinellone from *Dictamnus dasycarpus. J. Agricul. Food Chem.* 43: 1428–31.
6. Chen, I. L. et al. 2002. Synthesis and cytotoxic evaluation of some 4-anilinofuro[2,3-*b*] quinoline derivatives. *Helv. Chim. Acta* 85: 2214–21.
7. m-AMSA: N-[4-(acridin-9-yl-amino)-3-methoxyphenyl]methane sulfonamide.
8. Lv, M. Y. et al. 2015. Medicinal uses, phytochemistry and pharmacology of the genus *Dictamnus* (Rutaceae). *J. Ethnopharmacol.* 171, 247–63.

53 Ku Shen 苦參

Light yellow sophora

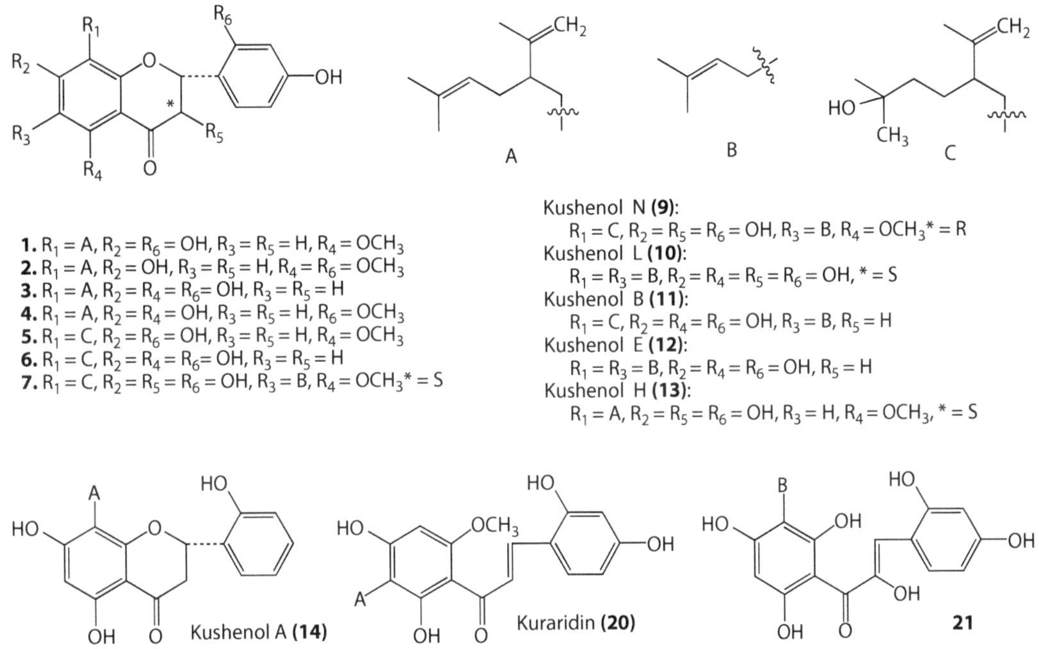

A 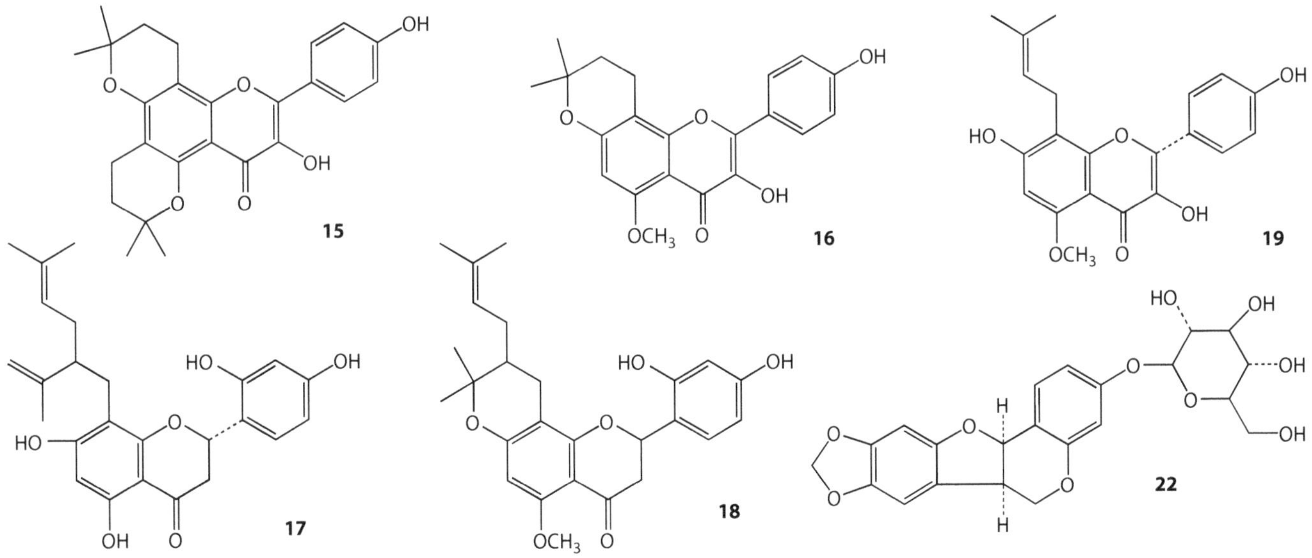 B 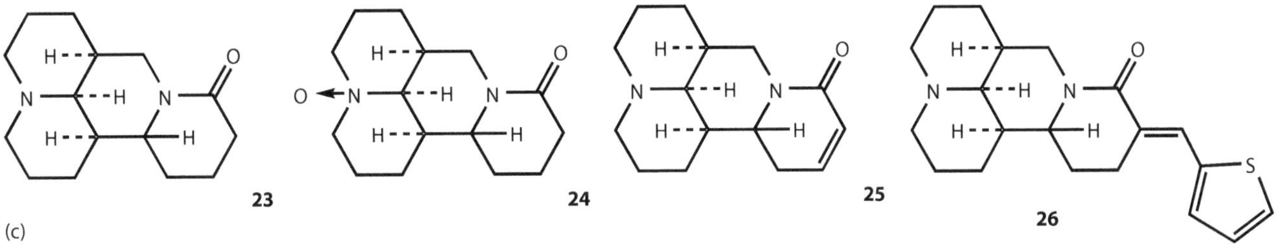 C

1. $R_1 = A, R_2 = R_6 = OH, R_3 = R_5 = H, R_4 = OCH_3$
2. $R_1 = A, R_2 = OH, R_3 = R_5 = H, R_4 = R_6 = OCH_3$
3. $R_1 = A, R_2 = R_4 = R_6 = OH, R_3 = R_5 = H$
4. $R_1 = A, R_2 = R_4 = OH, R_3 = R_5 = H, R_6 = OCH_3$
5. $R_1 = C, R_2 = R_6 = OH, R_3 = R_5 = H, R_4 = OCH_3$
6. $R_1 = C, R_2 = R_4 = R_6 = OH, R_3 = R_5 = H$
7. $R_1 = C, R_2 = R_5 = R_6 = OH, R_3 = B, R_4 = OCH_3{}^* = S$

Kushenol N **(9)**:
$R_1 = C, R_2 = R_5 = R_6 = OH, R_3 = B, R_4 = OCH_3{}^* = R$
Kushenol L **(10)**:
$R_1 = R_3 = B, R_2 = R_4 = R_5 = R_6 = OH, {}^* = S$
Kushenol B **(11)**:
$R_1 = C, R_2 = R_4 = R_6 = OH, R_3 = B, R_5 = H$
Kushenol E **(12)**:
$R_1 = R_3 = B, R_2 = R_4 = R_6 = OH, R_5 = H$
Kushenol H **(13)**:
$R_1 = A, R_2 = R_5 = R_6 = OH, R_3 = H, R_4 = OCH_3, {}^* = S$

Kushenol A **(14)** Kuraridin **(20)** **21**

(a)

15 **16** **19** **17** **18** **22**

(b)

23 **24** **25** **26**

(c)

Herb Origination

The herb Ku Shen is a frequently prescribed herb in traditional Chinese medicine, which was recorded as a top-grade drug in the first Chinese classic of materia medica *Shennong Ben Cao Jing*. The herb originated from a nationwide distributed evergreen shrub *Sophora flavescens* (Leguminosae). The best quality of root tube is traditionally collected between September and October and then dried in the sun for uses in folk medicinal practice.

Antitumor Activities

Ku Shen extract demonstrated a significant antineoplastic activity. Ku Shen (5–20 μg/mL) obviously inhibited the proliferation and induced the apoptosis of human HL-60 acute myelogenous leukemia cells in a dose-dependent fashion. Ku Shen (15 μg/mL) notably obstructed the proliferation of HL-60 cells and also augmented the differentiation of HL-60 cells to mononuclear macrophages but showed no apparent effect in human normal CFU-GM.[1–4] CRSFI (a compound radix *S. flavescens* injection) displayed a suppressive effect on the growth of lung adenocarcinoma cells *in vitro* and showed a depressant effect on the solid tumor cell lines such as Lewis lung cancer, H22 hepatoma, and ascetic hepatoma *in vivo*.[5] The *in vitro* treatment with CRSFI effectively inhibited the proliferation of human ACC-2 adenoid cystic carcinoma cells with the induction of cell cycle arrest and caspases-3 expression.[6] CRSFI could also augment the sensitivity of HepG2 hepatoma cells to chemotherapy through the down-expression of survivin mRNA.[7] After 48 h of being treated by 100 μL/mL CRSFI, the apoptosis of human gastric cancer SGC-7901 cells was promoted through the up-expressions of Bak and caspase-3 proteins.[8]

The combination of antitumor agents and Ku Shen greatly obstructed the proliferation of acute myelogenous leukemia cells and elicited the cell apoptosis with the down-expression of c-Myc.[9] In addition, an ethyl acetate fraction of Ku Shen at a concentration of 16.3 μg/mL markedly augmented the activity of QR and sequentially enhanced the antitumor effect of phase II enzyme in murine Hepa 1c1c7 hepatoma cells *in vitro*.[10]

Antitumor Constituents and Activities

The major cancer inhibitors in Ku Shen were well characterized to be flavonoids (KS-Fs) and alkaloids (KS-As). The KS-As is currently marketed in China as a drug for cancer treatment. KS-Fs and KS-As are valuable to be developed as adjuvants for the treatment of neoplastic disorders.

Flavonoids

Anticancer Activity

The anticancer efficacies of KS-Fs was demonstrated in a variety of carcinoma cell lines, such as three types of human lung cancer cell lines (A549, H460, and SPC-A-1) *in vitro*, two murine models (H22 hepatoma and sarcoma 180) *in vivo* with 60–80% suppressive rates, and two xenograft human Eca-109 esophageal cancer and H460 lung cancer in nude mice with 41–47% inhibitory rates. The KS-Fs also showed the ability to synergistically enhance the taxol in growth inhibition against the H460 and Eca-109 xenograft cancer cells *in vivo*.[11,12]

By cytotoxicity-guided separation, a group of cancer inhibitory flavonoids have been discovered from Ku Shen. Of them, the 12 flavornoids (**1**, **3**, **5–14**) whose unusual flavonoids with special side chains exhibited the antigrowth effect against five types of human tumor cell lines, i.e., A549 (lung), SKOV-3 (ovary), SK-MEL-2 (skin), XF498 (brain), and HCT-15 (colon), *in vitro*.[13] Kurarinone (**1**), 2′-methoxykurarinone (**2**), vexibinol (**3**), and vexibidin (**4**) showed moderate antiproliferative and apoptotic effects on human HL-60 leukemia cells (IC_{50}: 11.3–18.5 μM) and on human HepG2 hepatoma cells (IC_{50}: 13.3–36.2 μM).[14,15] The ED_{50} values of vexibinol (**3**) on A549 (lung), HeLa (cervix), and K562 (leukemic) cancer cell lines were 0.78, 1.57, and 2.14 μg/mL, respectively.[16] Also, kurarinone (**1**) exerted the cytotoxicity on MCF-7/6 (breast), H460, and SPC-A-1 (lung) human cancer cells,[11,12,17] and kurarinol (**5**) dose dependently provoked the apoptosis of HepG2, Huh-7, and H22 hepatoma cells by suppressing the STAT3 transcriptional effect.[18] Moreover, a mixture of norkurarinone and kuraridin (**20**) in a ratio of 10:9 exerted growth suppression on human SGC-7901 gastric adenocarcinoma cells with the induction of apoptosis and G2/M cell arrest.[19] However, the flavonoids (**1**, **3**, **5–7**) had no cytotoxic to human P-gp-expressing HCT15 colon carcinoma cells and its multidrug-resistant subline HCT15/CL02 cells *in vitro*, indicating that these flavonoids lack the ability to reverse the MDR through P-gp.[20]

Other isolated cytotoxic flavonoids assigned as flavenochromanes, sophoraflavanones, and sophoflavescenol hold two isoprenylpyran moieties on two sides of the molecules. Flavenochromane-C (**15**) displayed the cytotoxicity against A549 (lung), 1A9 (ovary), KB (oral), and KB-Vin (drug-resistant variant KB) human cancer cell lines (IC_{50}: <1.7 μM) and exhibited the inhibitory effect toward MCF-7 breast cancer cells (IC_{50}: 3.6 μM), while flavenochromane-B (**16**) demonstrated the inhibitory effects (IC_{50}: 3.2–6.9 μM) on these tumor cells.[21] The obvious in vitro antiproliferative effects were showed in KB cells for sophoraflavanone-G (**17**) and in HepG2 cells for sophoraflavanone-J (**18**). The apoptosis of HepG2 cells promoted by sophoraflavanone-J (**18**) was dose dependently triggered by nutrient depletion, ROS generation, mitochondrial dysfunction, and an intrinsic mitochondrial death pathway.[22–24] Despite the low effect on the MCF-7 breast cancer cells, sophoflavescenol (**19**) exerted the cytotoxicity against HL-60 leukemia, A549 lung cancer, and Lewis lung carcinoma cells. The antigrowth activity of sophoflavescenol (**19**) was demonstrated in a mouse model with the LLC without severe side effects.[25] According to the delightful anticarcinoma property, the Ku Shen flavonoids were strongly recommended for further development in the treatment of various carcinogenesis and neoplastic disorders.

Antiangiogenic Effect

Kushecarpin-D and (2S)-7,2′,4′-trihydroxy-5-methoxy-8-dimethylallyl flavanone exerted an antiangiogenic activity in HUVEC line (ECV304) *in vitro* concomitantly with the induction of G0/G1 cell arrest, the inhibitions of cell proliferation, migration, adhesion, and tube formation, and the decline of VEGF expression but without inducing apoptosis.[26,27]

Other Types of Flavones

Two isolated chalcone-type flavones were assigned as kuraridin (**20**) and 7,9,2′,4′-tetra-hydroxy-8-isopentenyl-5-methoxy-chalcone (**21**). The antiproliferative effects of flavenochromane-C (**15**) were showed in A549 (lung), SKOV-3 (ovary), HCT-15 (colon), SK-MEL-2 (skin), and XF498 (brain) human cancer cell lines *in vitro* (ED_{50}: 5.0–7.1 μg/mL)[13] and of matrine (**23**) were displayed in three leukemia cell lines such as human HL-60 promyelocytic leukemia, human U937 histiocytic leukemia, and mouse L1210 lymphocytic leukemia.[28] Trifolirhizin (**22**) was a pterocarpan, which belongs to a special group of isoflavonoid. The *in vitro* inhibitory effects were observed in human A2780 (ovary) and H23 (lung) cancer cell lines after being treated with trifolirhizin (**22**) with ED_{50} values of 15.0–37.8 μg/mL.[13]

Quinolizidine Alkaloids

The alkaloid components in Ku Shen have been prominently investigated for their chemical biology. Matrine (**23**), oxymatrine (**24**), sophocarpine (**25**), oxysophocarpine, sophoridine, and sophoramine were found being responsible for the biological activity of Ku Shen alkaloids. *In vivo* experiments showed that Ku Shen total alkaloids and its alkaloid compounds, such as matrine (**23**), oxymatrine (**24**), and sophocarpine (**25**), markedly suppressed the growth of murine solid and ascrites sarcoma 180, U14 cervical cancer, sarcoma 17, and Ehrlich ascites tumor.[29,30]

Marein

Both *in vitro* and *in vivo* models revealed that matrine (**23**) exerted a significant antiproliferative and proapoptotic activities against human BxPC-3 and PANC-1 pancreatic cancer, HL-60 leukemia, and mouse H22 hepatoma cells but had no such effects on normal human HL-7702 liver cells.[31,32] The broad *in vitro* antitumor spectrum of matrine (**23**) were observed in a variety types of human cancer cell lines such as MKN45 and SGC-7901 (stomach), K562 and U937 (leukemic), HepG2 (liver), LNCaP and PC3 (prostate), SW1116 and HT-29 (colon), MCF-7 (breast), A375 (skin), CNE1 and CNE2 (nasopharynx) cancer, HXO-Rb44 (Rb), MG-63, U-2OS, Saos-2, and N-methyl-N′-nitro-N-nitrosoguanidine (MNNG) (osteosarcoma), multiple myeloma, as well as mouse 4T-1 breast carcinoma and rat C6 glioma cells.[30–45] Matrine (**23**) was also effective in the inhibition of human MNNG/HOS osteosarcoma *in vivo* and rat UMR-108 osteosarcoma cells *in vitro* concomitantly with eliciting the cell apoptosis in a dose- and a time-dependent manner.[46,47] Matrine (**23**) was also able to notably obstruct the colonial formation of hematopoiesis progenitor cells in the peripheral blood of patients suffering from chronic granulocytic leukemia.[48] In the cotreatments, the apoptosis of K562 leukemia cells induced by etoposide or imatinib (two clinical drugs against leukemia) could be noticeably potentiated by matrine (**23**).[35,49] Similarly, matrine (**23**) significantly enhanced the apoptosis of human HepG2 hepatoma cells induced by resveratrol (a potential chemopreventive agent) and exhibited a synergistic antiproliferative effect.[50] Furthermore, the investigations found that matrine (**23**) also exerted antiangiogenesis-related antimetastatic effects. In a mice model with highly metastatic 4T1 breast cancer, the administration of matrine (**23**) dose dependently repressed the growth of primary tumors and inhibited the metastases to the lung and the liver in association with the downregulation of VEGF and VEGFR-2 expressions and the increase of caspase-3 and caspase-9 activation.[40]

14-Thienyl methylene matrine (YYJ18) (**26**) is derivative of matrine, which induced the apoptotic death of all three human nasopharyngeal cancer cell lines (CNEl, CNE2, and HONEl) through the modulation of MAPK and PI3K/Akt pathways and markedly inhibited the proliferation of all tested cell lines in a dose-dependent manner. In a concentration of 600 μM, the inhibition of YYJ18 (**26**) was most pronounced in the CNE2 cells, which was much lower than the reported dose of matrine (1.5 mg/mL),[51] implying that 14-thienyl methylene matrine (**26**) might provide better outcomes and less toxicity than matrine (**23**).

Oxymatrine

The antiproliferative effect of oxymatrine (**24**) was demonstrated in human SGC-7901 gastric cancer, human PANC-1 pancreas cancer, and rat H4IIE hepatoma cell lines *in vitro*.[52–54] Together with the inhibition of telomerase activity by means of its effects on hTERT and the upstream regulating genes, oxymatrine (**24**) dose dependently killed human SW1116 colon cancer cells and elicited G1/G0 cell arrest.[55] Oxymatrine (**24**) elicited the mitochondria-dependent apoptosis of human MNNG/HOS osteosarcoma cells and human MG-63 osteosarcoma cells via inhibition of PI3K/Akt pathway and the stimulation of caspase-triggered signaling pathway, respectively.[56,57] In the *in vitro* and *in vivo* experiments, oxymatrine (**24**) significantly suppressed the proliferation of prostate cancer cells in a time- and a dose-dependent manner concomitant with the induction of the cell apoptosis.[58] The proliferation and the invasion of human gastric cells was obstructed by oxymatrine (**24**) via the inhibition of EGFR/Cyclin Dl/CDK4/6, EGFR/Akt and MEK-1/ERK1/2/MMP2 pathway by suppressing EGFRp-Tyr845 phosphorylation and decreasing phospho-Cofilin (Ser3) and phospho-LIMK1 (Thr508) without changes in the total Cofilin and LIMK1 expressions.[50,59] Moreover, by cotreatment with oxymatrine (**24**), the cytotoxicity of CTX could be additively augmented in mice against Ehrlich tumor, and the toxic/side effects of CTX was also simultaneously diminished by oxymatrine (**24**).[60]

When the concentration exceeded to 1 mg/mL, oxymatrine (**24**) could retard the angiogenesis in SGC-7901 tumor by reducing VEGF expression besides significantly obstructing the growth of SGC-7901 cells and blocking the cell cycle.[53] The antiproliferative and antiangiogenic effects of oxymatrine (**24**) were also confirmed in nude mice with PANC-1 pancreatic cancer xenograft, whose effect was revealed to be correlated with the inhibition of NF-κB-mediated VEGF signaling pathway.[61] In addition, the treatments with oxymatrine (**24**) or Ku Shen total alkaloids demonstrated a positive effect on the leukopenia caused by either chemotherapy or radiotherapy (X-ray and ^{60}Co-γ) through the marked elevation of peripheral leukocyte level.[62]

Taken together, these remarkable results recommended that matrine (**23**) and oxymatrine (**24**) may be applied as promising adjunct agents in cancer clinics. The broad anticancer spectrum strongly advised that matrine (**23**) and oxymatrine (**24**) are potential drug leads for the development of cancer chemotherapies. The Ku Shen total alkaloids was also currently marketed in China being prepared through various types of medical preparation (such as injection, tablet, capsule, pill, oral solution, granule, etc.) for treating malignant solid tumors (e.g., sarcoma, gastric cancer, lung carcinoma, hepatoma, intestine tumor, and other cancers).[63]

Lectin

A lectin prepared from Ku Shen (SFL) displayed cytotoxicity against human HeLa cervical cancer cells *in vitro* and human MCF-7 breast cancer cells *in vitro* and *in vivo*. The apoptosis of HeLa cells and MCF-7 cells was elicited by a typical caspase-dependent proapoptotic mechanism in time- and dose-dependent manners after the treatment. The investigations also found that SFL was able to bind on a particular mannose-containing receptor on the HeLa cell surface, thereby initiating a downstream caspase cascade activity to trigger the apoptosis.[64,65] In the proapoptosis of MCF-7 cells, Bcl-2 and Bcl-xL were down-expressed, Bax and Bid were up-expressed, p53 and p21 levels were amplified, and NF-κB and ERK activities were reduced, leading to the release of cytochrome c from mitochondria into cytoplasm and the activation of s-3 and caspase-9. SFL also triggered the G2/M phase cell cycle arrest.[65]

Polysaccharide

Sophora flavescens polysaccharide (SFPW1) effectively inhibited the tumor growth in H22 hepatoma-bearing mice and promoted the splenocyte proliferation, resulting in a prolonged life survival. SFPW1, in an *in vivo* model, displayed no direct cytotoxic effect on the H22 cells, but it significantly strengthened peritoneal macrophages to devour H22 tumor cells and stimulated macrophages to produce NO via the upregulation of iNOS activity. These findings proved that the antitumor effect of SFPW1 should be associated with its potent immunostimulating effect and suggested that the polysaccharide may be a potential candidate for improving cancer chemotherapy as an immune regulator.[66]

Exploration of Mechanisms

Matrine (**23**) has been extensively investigated for its pro-apoptotic, antiviability, antiproliferative, and antiinvasive mechanisms. The mechanisms were revealed to be mediated by various characteristic events/pathways in different types of cancer cells, such as (1) inhibited telomerase activity by depressing hTERT expression (such as in SW1116 cells)[43]; (2) down-expressed PCNA and AFP (such as in BxPC-3, PANC-1, and HepG2 cells)[37]; (3) suppressed the activity of a translation factor eIF4E by dephosphorylating 4E-BP1 and inactivated Erk1/2 (such as in MKN45 cells)[34]; (4) collapsed mitochondrial membrane potential, released mitochondrial cytochrome c from to cytosol, and declined the levels of p-Akt and p-ERK1/2 (such as in AML cells)[36,48]; (5) up-expressed E2F-1 and Apaf-1 and down-expressed Rb (such as in K562 and U937 cells) and inhibited a bcr-abl-mediated MEK-ERK pathway and IL-6/JAK/STAT3 signaling cohort (such as in K562 cells)[35]; (6) increased ROS production and disrupted mitochondrial transmembrane potential and cleaved PARP and improved caspases-3/9 (such as in UMR-108 cells)[47]; (7) reduced Bcl-2/Bax ratio and c-Myc activity, upregulated Fas/FasL, and activated caspases (such as in BxPC-3 and PANC-1 cells)[31]; (8) reduced VEGF-A level, inactivated ERK1/2, and activated caspase-3 (such as in CNE1 and CNE2 cells)[67]; (9) elicited ROS-activated p38 pathway and activated caspase-3 (such as in NSCLC cells)[68]; and (10) augmented Bax/Bcl-2 ratio, released mitochondrial cytochrome c to cytosol, stimulated caspase-3 and caspase-9 as well as arrested G0/G1 cell cycle (such as in HT-29 cells).[69]

Furthermore, in androgen-dependent LNCaP prostate cancer cells, the anticancer mechanism of matrine (**23**) was also associated with the obvious diminishment of the AR level and the decline of PSA expression.[38] The mechanism linked to the inhibition of A375 cell invasion and metastasis by matrine (**23**) was associated with the down-expression of heparanase mRNA and protein for reducing the adhesion ability.[41]

Other Bioactivities

The herb Ku Shen is frequently used in China in different herbal formulations for the treatment of viral hepatitis, viral myocarditis, gastrointestinal hemorrhage, and skin diseases (such as psoriasis, colpitis, and eczema) besides cancer. Pharmacological studies have proven that the herb possesses a wide biologically active spectrum such as antiulcerative, antimyocardial ischemia, antioxidant, hypolipidemic, antiinflammatory, antiallergic, antiarrhythmic, coronary dilative, vasodilative, hypotensive, hypoglycemic, antipyretic, antiasthmatic, antispasmodic, antitussive, analgesic, expectorant, and antibacterial effects besides cancer suppression.

Extensive investigations in chemical biology exhibited that matrine (**23**) has antipyretic, anticonvulsant, antiliver injury, and antifibrosis activities and a stable effect on the CNS, whereas oxymatrine (**24**) displayed liver fibrosis- and cirrhosis-preventing, oxidative stress-reducing, antiarrhythmic, antiinflammatory, cardiotonic, antianaphylaxis, and smooth wheezing effects. In current clinics, oxymatrine (**24**) is used to treat chronic hepatitis B and chronic hepatitis C.[70]

Toxic and Side Effects

The toxic and side effects of Ku Shen were mainly ascribed to its alkaloid components. A large dose of the total alkaloids would cause agitation and even spasmodic convulsion in a mouse. The LD_{50} values of the Ku Shen extract in oral and intramuscular injection are 14.5 g/kg and 14.4 g/kg in mice. The oral administration of the total alkaloids showed the LD_{50} value to be 1.18 g/kg in mice.[48]

References

1. Tan, M. Q. et al. 2000. Antileukemic effect of *Sophora flavescens* and its mechanism. *J. Hunan Med. Univ.* 25: 443–5.
2. Xu, J. G. et al. 1990. Sophora decoction induces the differentiaon of human promyelocytic leukemia cells. *Zhongcaoyao* 15: 625–6.
3. Xiang, Q. et al. 2004. Effect of *Sophora flavescens* on acute myloid leukemia. *Acta Med. Sinica* 17: 10–1.
4. Qin, J. P. et al. 1994. Differentiation of K562 leukemia cells induced by *Sophora flavescens. J. Chongqin Med. Univ.* 19: 150–1.
5. Lin, L. Z. et al. 2009. Experimental study of antitumor effect of compound radix *Sophora flavescens* injection on lung cancer cells and hepatic carcinoma cells. *Zhongyao Xinyao Yu Linchuang Yaoli* 20: 21–3.

6. Wang, J. J. et al. 2011. Expression of survivin mRNA and protein induced by compound radix *Sophorae flavescentis* injection in human hepatoma cell line HepG2. *Zhongguo Yiyuan Yaoxue Zazhi* 31: 1770–3.
7. Shi, B. et al. 2012. Effects of compound radix *Sophorae flavescentis* injection on proliferation, apoptosis and caspase-3 expression in adenoid cystic carcinoma ACC-2 cells. *Huanqiu Zhongyiyao* 5: 721–4.
8. Zhang, W. L. et al. 2012. Inductive effect of compound *Sophora flavescens* injection on apoptosis of gastric cancer SGC-7901 cells and the mechanism. *Guangdong Yixue* 33: 2061–3.
9. Xiang, Q. et al. 2002. Anti-leukemia effect of *Sophora flavescens* combined with the low molecular weight natural tumor suppressor of the human fetal liver and its mechanism. *J. Hunan Med. Univ.* 27: 108–10.
10. Kim, Y. M. et al. 1997. Effects of natural products on the induction of NAD(P)H: Quinone reductase in Hepa 1clc7 cells for the development of cancer chemopreventive agents. *Nat. Prods. Sci.* 3: 81–3.
11. Sun, M. Y. et al. 2007. Novel antitumor activities of Kushen flavonoids in vitro and in vivo. *Phytother. Res.* 21: 269–77.
12. Sun, M. Y. et al. 2008. Antitumor activities of kushen flavonoids in vivo and in vitro. *Zhongxiyi Jiehe Xuebao* 6: 51–9.
13. Ryu, S. Y. et al. 1997. In vitro antitumor activity of flavonoids from *Sophora flavescens*. *Phytother. Res.* 11: 51–3.
14. Ko, W. G. et al. 2000. Lavandulylflavonoids: A new class of in vitro apoptogenic agents from *Sophora flavescens*. *Toxicol. in Vitro* 14: 429–33.
15. Kang, T. Y. et al. Cytotoxic lavandulyl flavanones from *Sophora flavescens*. *J. Nat. Prods.* 63: 680–1.
16. Kim, Y. K. et al. 1997. A cytotoxic constituent from *Sophora flavescents*. *Archiv. Pharm. Res.* 20: 342–5.
17. Naeyer, A. et al. 2004. Estrogenic and anticarcinogenic properties of kurarinone, a lavandulyl flavanone from the roots of *Sophora flavescens*. *J. Nat. Prod.* 67: 1829–32.
18. Shu, G. W. et al. 2014. Kurarinol induces hepatocellular carcinoma cell apoptosis through suppressing cellular signal transducer and activator of transcription 3 signaling. *Toxicol. Applied Pharmacol.* 281: 157–65.
19. Rasul, A. et al. 2011. Induction of mitochondria-mediated apoptosis in human gastric adenocarcinoma SGC-7901 cells by kuraridin and Nor-kurarinone isolated from *Sophorae flavescentis*. *Asian Pacific J. Cancer Prev.* 12: 2499–504.
20. Choi, S. U. et al. 1999. P-glycoprotein (P-gp) does not affect the cytotoxicity of flavonoids from *Sophora flavescens*, which also have no effects on Pgp action. *Anticancer Res.* 19: 2035–40.
21. Ding, P. L. et al. 2004. Cytotoxic isoprenylated flavonoids from the roots of *Sophora flavescens*. *Helv. Chim. Acta* 87: 2574–80.
22. Zhou, H. P. et al. 2009. Antiinflammatory and antiproliferative activities of trifolirhizin, a flavonoid from *Sophora flavescens* roots. *J. Agricul. Food Chem.* 57: 4580–5.
23. Cheung, C. S. et al. 2007. Proteomic characterization of sophoraflavone J-induced apoptosis in HepG2 cells. *Proteomics Clin. Appl.* 1: 1532–44.
24. Cha, J. D. et al. 2007. Induction of apoptosis in human oral epidermoid carcinoma cells by sophoraflavanone G from *Sophora flavescens*. *Food Sci. Biotechnol.* 16: 537–42.
25. Jung, H. A. et al. 2011. Antitumorigenic activity of sophoflavescenol against Lewis lung carcinoma in vitro and in vivo. *Archiv. Pharm. Res.* 34: 2087–99.
26. Zhang, X. L. et al. 2013. A novel flavonoid isolated from *Sophora flavescens* exhibited anti-angiogenesis activity, decreased VEGF expression and caused G0/G1 cell cycle arrest in vitro. *Pharmazie* 68: 369–75.
27. Pu, L. P. et al. 2013. The antiangiogenic activity of Kushecarpin D, a novel flavonoid isolated from *Sophora flavescens*. *Life Sci.* 93: 791–7.
28. Lee, J. H. et al. 2007. A new cytotoxic prenylated chalcone from *Sophora flavescens*. *Archiv. Pharm. Res.* 30: 408–11.
29. Liang, C. Z. et al. 2012. Matrine induces caspase-dependent apoptosis in human osteosarcoma cells in vitro and in vivo through the upregulation of Bax and Fas/FasL and downregulation of Bcl-2. *Cancer Chemother. Pharmacol.* 69: 317–331.
30. Li, X. R. et al. 1982. Sophora alkaloids inhibits mouse transplantable tumor. *Zhongxiyi Jiehe Zazhi* 2: 42–3.
31. Liu, T. Y. et al. 2010. Matrine inhibits proliferation and induces apoptosis of pancreatic cancer cells *in vitro* and *in vivo*. *Biol. Pharm. Bull.* 33: 1740–5.
32. Ma, L. D. et al. 2008. Antitumor effects of the Chinese medicine matrine on murine hepatocellular carcinoma cells. *Planta Med.* 74: 245–51.
33. Dai, Z. J. et al. 2009. Matrine induces apoptosis in gastric carcinoma cells via alteration of Fas/FasL and activation of caspase-3. *J. Ethnopharmacol.* 123: 91–6.
34. Jiang, T. J. et al. 2007. Matrine inhibited the activity of translation factor eIF4E through dephosphorylation of 4E-BP1 in gastric MKN45 cells. *Planta Med.* 73: 1176–81.
35. (a) Jiang, H. et al. 2007. Matrine upregulates the cell cycle protein E2F-1 and triggers apoptosis via the mitochondrial pathway in K562 cells. *Eur. J. Pharmacol.* 559: 98–108; (b) He, L. Y. et al. 2015. Matrine suppresses the growth of human chronic myeloid leukemia K562 cells via inhibiting bcr-abl-mediated MEK-ERK pathway. *Zhongliu Yanjiu and Linchuan* 27: 433–7; (c) Ma, L. et al. 2015. Matrine suppresses cell growth of human chronic myeloid leukemia cells via its inhibition of the interleukin-6/Janus activated kinase/signal transducer and activator of transcription 3 signaling cohort. *Leuk Lymphoma.* 56: 2923–30.
36. Liu, X. S. et al. 2006. Matrine-induced apoptosis in leukemia U937 cells: Involvement of caspases activation and MAPK-independent pathways. *Planta Med.* 72: 501–6.
37. Qin, X. G. et al. 2010. Effects of matrine on HepG2 cell proliferation and expression of tumor relevant proteins in vitro. *Pharm. Biol.* (London) 48: 275–81.
38. Chen, K. et al. 2008. Inhibitory effect of matrine on the expression of PSA and AR in prostate cancer cell line LNCaP. *J. Huazhong Univ. Sci. Technol., Med. Sci.* 28: 697–9.
39. Zhang, P. 2012. Matrine inhibits proliferation and induces apoptosis of the androgen-independent prostate cancer cell line PC-3. *Mol. Med. Reports* 5: 783–7.
40. Li, H. L. et al. 2010. Therapeutic effects of matrine on primary and metastatic breast cancer. *Am. J. Chin. Med.* 38: 1115–30.
41. Han, Y. X. et al. 2010. Matrine induces apoptosis of human multiple myeloma cells via activation of the mitochondrial pathway. *Leukemia Lymphoma* 51: 1337–46.
42. Zhou, L. H. et al. 2009. Effects of matrine on proliferation and telomerase activity of colon cancer SW1116 cells. *Zhongyaocai* 32: 923–5.
43. Liu, X. Y. et al. 2008. Matrine inhibits invasiveness and metastasis of human malignant melanoma cell line A375 in vitro. *Intl. J. Dermatol.* 47: 448–56.

44. Yu, W. et al. 2006. The effects of matrine on cell proliferation and telomerase activity in retinoblastoma cells in vitro. *Zhonghua Yanke Zazhi* 42: 594–599.
45. Zhang, S. J. et al. 2009. Matrine induces programmed cell death and regulates expression of relevant genes based on PCR array analysis in C6 glioma cells. *Mol. Biol. Reports* 36: 791–9.
46. Yan, F. et al. 2013. Matrine inhibited the growth of rat osteosarcoma UMR-108 cells by inducing apoptosis in a mitochondrial-caspase-dependent pathway. *Tumor Biol.* 34: 2135–40.
47. Zhang, S. H. et al. 2012. Matrine induces apoptosis in human acute myeloid leukemia cells via the mitochondrial pathway and Akt inactivation. *PLoS One* 7: e46853.
48. Xiao, S. Y. et al. (a) 1991. *Zhonghua Xueyexue Zazhi* 12: 89; (b) 1999. *Chinese Materia Medica*. Vol. 4, 4–3383, 637. Shanghai Science and Technology Press, Shanghai, China.
49. Liu, X. S. et al. 2006. Enhancement of imatinib-induced apoptosis by matrine in bcr/abl-positive leukemia K562 cells. *Pharm. Biol.*(Philadelphia) 44: 287–91.
50. Ou, X. Y. et al. 2014. Potentiation of resveratrol-induced apoptosis by matrine in human hepatoma HepG2 cells. *Oncol. Reports* 32: 2803–9.
51. Xie, M. et al. 2014. 14-Thienyl methylene matrine (YYJ18), the derivative from matrine, induces apoptosis of human nasopharyngeal carcinoma cells by targeting MAPK and PI3K/Akt pathways in vitro. *Cell. Physiol. Biochem.* 33: 1475–83.
52. Liu, Y. J. et al. 2010. Influence of oxymatrine on cell proliferation and VEGF expression in human gastric cancer cell line SGC-7901. *Zhongguo Aizheng Zazhi* 20: 22–6.
53. Ho, J. W. et al. 2009. Effects of oxymatrine from Ku Shen on cancer cells. *Anti-Cancer Agents in Med. Chem.* 9: 823–6.
54. Ling, Q. et al. 2011. Oxymatrine induces human pancreatic cancer PANC-1 cells apoptosis via regulating expression of Bcl-2 and IAP families, and releasing of cytochrome c. *J. Experim. Clin. Cancer Res.* 30: 66.
55. Zou, J. et al. 2005. Experimental study of the killing effects of oxymatrine on human colon cancer cell line SW1116. *Chin. J. Digestive Diseases* 6: 15–20.
56. Zhang, Y. et al. 2014. Oxymatrine induces mitochondria dependent apoptosis in human osteosarcoma MNNG/HOS cells through inhibition of PI3K/Akt pathway. *Tumor Biol.* 35: 1619–25.
57. Wei, J. H. et al. 2014. Oxymatrine extracted from Sophora flavescens inhibited cell growth and induced apoptosis in human osteosarcoma MG-63 cells in nitro. *Cell Biochem. Biophys.* 70: 1439–44.
58. Wu, C. Z. et al. 2015. Oxymatrine inhibits the proliferation of prostate cancer cells in vitro and in vivo. *Mol. Med. Reports* 11: 4129–34.
59. Guo, B. Y. et al. 2015. Oxymatrine targets EGFRp-Tyr845 and inhibits EGFR-related signaling pathways to suppress the proliferation and invasion of gastric cancer cells. *Cancer Chemother. Pharmacol.* 75; 353–63.
60. Yuan, C. et al. 1987. Effects of oxymatrine on the antitumor activity and toxicity of cyclophosphamide in mice. *Yaoxue Xuebao* 22: 245–9.
61. Chen, H. et al. 2013. Antiangiogenic effects of oxymatrine on pancreatic cancer by inhibition of the NF-κB-mediated VEGF signaling pathway. *Oncol. Reports* 30: 589–95.
62. Kojima, L. et al. (a) 1972. *Yigaku Shebutugaku* 84: 65; (b) 1999. *Chinese Materia Medica*. Vol. 4, 4–3383, 637. Shanghai Science and Technology Press, Shanghai, China.
63. Zhou, Y. W. et al. 2003. Alkaloid of *Sophora flavescens* for treating malignant solid tumor and its preparation. *Faming Zhuanli Shenqing Gongkai Shuomingshu* CN 2001–118472 A 20030108.
64. Liu, Z. et al. 2008. A mannose-binding lectin from *Sophora flavescens* induces apoptosis in HeLa cells. *Phytomed.* 15: 867–75.
65. Shi, Z. et al. 2014. Antitumor effects of concanavalin A and *Sophora flavescens* lectin in vitro and in vivo. *Acta Pharmacol. Sinica* 35: 248–56.
66. Bai, L. et al. 2012. Antitumor and immunomodulating activity of a polysaccharide from *Sophora flavescens* Ait. *Intl. J. Biol. Macromol.* 51: 705–9.
67. Xie, M. et al. 2014. Matrine-induced apoptosis of human nasopharyngeal carcinoma cells via in vitro vascular endothelial growth factor-a/extracellular signal-regulated kinase1/2 pathway inactivation. *Hormone Metabolic Res.* 46: 556–60.
68. Tan, C. H. et al. 2013. Matrine induction of reactive oxygen species activates p38 leading to caspase-dependent cell apoptosis in non-small cell lung cancer cells. *Oncol. Reports* 30: 2529–35.
69. Chang, C. et al. 2013. Effects of matrine on the proliferation of HT29 human colon cancer cells and its antitumor mechanism. *Oncol. Lett.* 6: 699–704.
70. Zhang, L. H. et al. 2009. The advanced studies on the pharmacological activities of matrine. *Zhongcaoyao* 40: 1000–3.

54 Da Ye Ma Wei Lian 大葉馬尾連

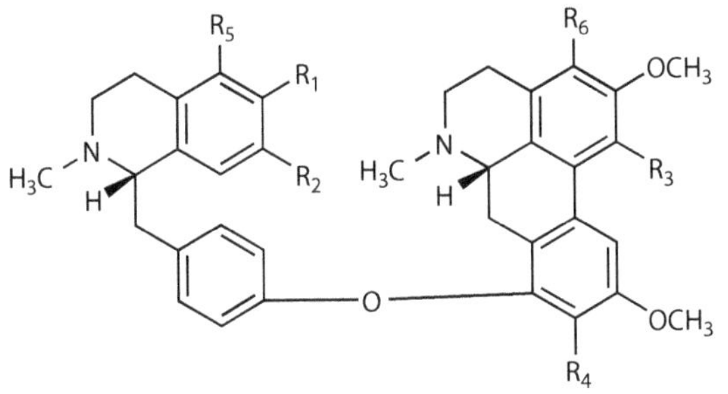

1. $R_1 = R_2 = R_3 = R_4 = R_6 = OCH_3, R_5 = H$
3. $R_1 = R_2 = R_4 = R_6 = OCH_3, R_3 = OH, R_5 = H$
4. $R_1 = R_6 = OH, R_2 = R_3 = R_4 = OCH_3, R_5 = H$
5. $R_1 = R_4 = R_6 = OH, R_2 = R_3 = OCH_3, R_5 = H$
6. $R_1 = R_4 = R_6 = OH, R_5 = R_6 = H$
7. $R_1 = R_2 = R_3 = OCH_3, R_5 = R_6 = OH$
8. $R_1 = R_4 = OH, R_2 = R_3 = R_6 = OCH_3, R_5 = H$
9. $R_1 = OH, R_2 = R_3 = R_4 = R_6 = OCH_3, R_5 = H$
10. $R_1 = R_2 = R_3 = OCH_3, R_4 = R_5 = OH, R_6 = H$

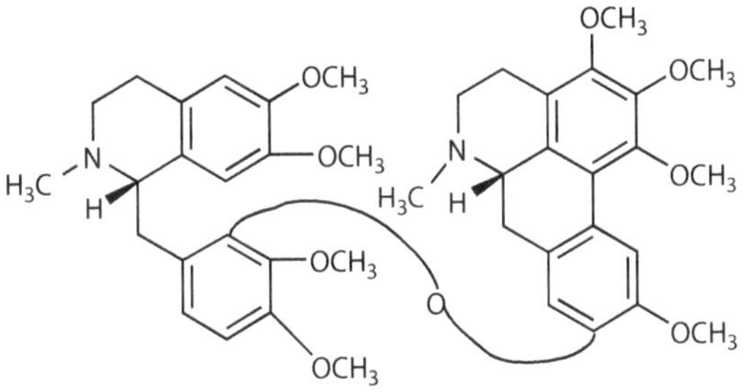

2

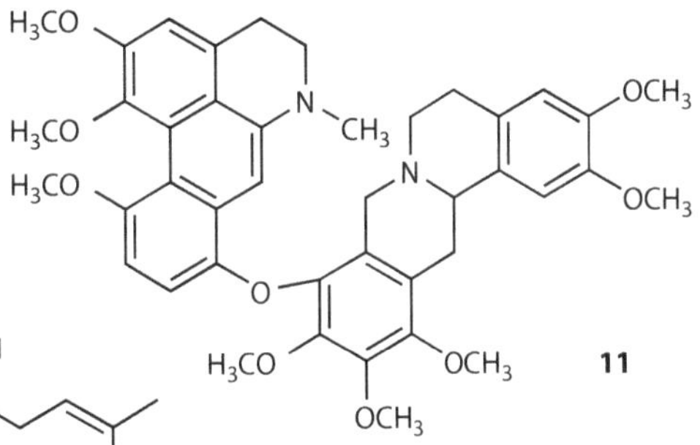

11

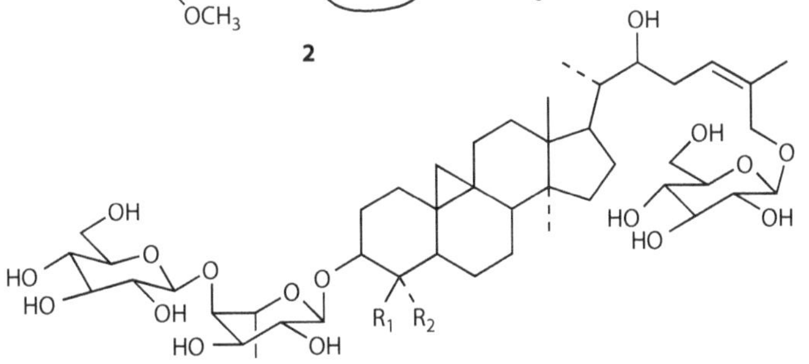

12. $R_1 = -CH_2OH, R_2 = -CH_3$
13. $R_1 = -CH_3, R_2 = -CH_2OH$
14. $R_1 = R_2 = -CH_3$

Herb Origination

The herb Da Ye Ma Wei Lian originated from three Raunculaceae plants, *Thalictrum faberi*, *T. acutifolium*, and *T. fortunei*. The distributions of these perennial plants mostly ranged in the southern and/or the southeastern regions of China. Their rhizomes are collected in spring and autumn and dried in the sun for Chinese folk medical practice. The herb also can be used fresh after collection.

Antitumor Constituents and Activities

Agents from T. faberi

Several anticancer dimeric aporphinebenzylisoquinoline alkaloids were discovered from the rhizomes of *T. faberi*. Of the isolated alkaloids, thalifaberine (**1**) and thalifabine (**2**) exhibited cytotoxicity on Walker 256 sarcoma cells.[1] 3-Hydroxy-6′-desmethylthalifaboramine (**3**), 3-hydroxythalifaboramine (**4**), 6′-desmethylthalifaboramine (**5**), 3,5′-dihydroxythalifaboramine (**6**), and 5′-hydroxythalifaboramine (**7**) showed moderate cytotoxicity on human Lu-1 (lung), ZR-75-1 (hormone-dependent breast), LNCaP (hormone-dependent prostate), KB (oral epidermoid), and KB-V (VLB-resistant oral) cancer cell lines *in vitro*.[2] Thalifaberine (**1**), thalifaberidine (**8**), and thalifasine (**9**) inhibited the growth of human BCA-1 breast cancer, Col-2 colon, HT-1080 fibrosarcoma, U373 glioblastoma, and A432 epidermoid tumor cancer cell lines as well as P388 murine leukemia cells.[3] The antiproliferative effect of thalifalandine (**10**) was present in mouse P388 and L1210 leukemia cell lines *in vitro* (IC_{50}: 0.7 and 1.8 μg/mL, respectively).[4]

The remarkable *in vivo* anticancer activity of thalidasine (= thalicarpine) was observed in animal models. The i.p. injection of thalidasine (70 mg/kg per day) to tumor-bearing mice for 10 days repressed Ehrlich ascites carcinoma and sarcoma 180 by 50% and 25%, respectively. In *in vivo* mouse models, it retarded the murine Lewis lung cancer by 50–58% in a dose of 100 mg/kg per day and markedly obstructed W256 sarcoma in a dose of 200 mg/kg/day. If it is changed to hypodermic injection, thalidasine in a dose of 42 mg/kg per day for 7 days restrained the growth of W256 sarcoma cells by 38.8% in rats.[5–7] The formulation of this bioactive alkaloid to a multiliposome was reported to be capable of enhancing its antitumor property.[8]

Agents from T. acutifolium

A dimeric aporphinebenzylisoquinoline alkaloid assigned as acutiaporberine (**11**) was separated from the rhizomes of *T. acutifolium*, which displayed a moderate cytotoxic activity in four cultured human carcinoma cell lines such as HeLa cervical epitheloid cancer, PLA-801 NSCLC, and MGC gastric cancer cells, and it was less active to HepG2 hepatoma cells and MCF-7 breast cancer cells *in vitro* (IC_{50}: 37–82 μg/mL) but was also cytotoxic to two normal cells (L-02 and NIH 3T3).[9–12] Furthermore, acutiaporberine (**11**) was able to dose and time dependently accelerate the apoptosis of PLA-801 lung cancer cells and highly metastatic human 95-Da lung cancer cells. The apoptosis-inducing mechanism was found to be closely associated with the down-expression of Bcl-2 and the up-expression of Bax and c-Myc.[13,14] The findings highlighted that the acutiaporberine (**11**) is has a potential to be developed as an agent to improve the treatment of highly metastatic lung cancer.

Agents from T. fortunei

Two bisbenzylisoquinoline alkaloids (thalifortine and aromoline) were isolated from the whole plant of *T. fortune*, but there were no antitumor activity reported.[13] Ten active triterpenoids, fortunei-saponins-A–J, were separated from the aerial part of *T. fortune*, showing a marked to weak suppressive effect against human Bel-7402 hepatoma, LoVo colon carcinoma, NCI-H460 NSCLC, and/or SGC-7901 gastric cancer cell lines *in vitro*.[14–16] Of the compounds, fortunei-saponin-I (**12**) and fortunei-saponin-J (**13**) demonstrated a marked antiproliferative effect against NCI-H460, Bel-7402, and Lovo cell lines (IC_{50}: 5.61, 6.83, 24.33 µg/mL and 3.08, 3.32, 7.79 µg/mL, respectively).[15] The inhibitory effects of fortunei-saponin-A (**14**) were weak on the four tumor cell lines (IC_{50}: 66.4, 84.8, 73.5, 89.6 µM, respectively), whose activities were much lower than those of fortunei-saponin-I and fortunei-saponin-J but greater than those of fortunei-saponins-B–H. The mechanism-related experiments revealed that fortunei-saponin-A (**14**) induced the apoptosis of Bel-7402 cells by (1) markedly provoking intracellular ROS and causing mitochondrial membrane potential loss and (2) significantly decreasing the expression level of Bcl-2 and increasing the expression levels of p53, Bax, and cleaved caspase-3.[16]

Other Medical Uses

The three origins of the herb Da Ye Ma Wei Lian, in most of the times, are used in local folk medical treatments. Many alkaloids isolated from the herb also displayed antibacterial, antimalarial, and hypertensive effects. The LD_{50} value of thalidasine in mice was 120 mg/kg by intravenous injection and 520 mg/kg by i.p. injection. The aerial part of *T. fortunei* is employed as an antibacterial, antiinflammatory, and immunoregulatory herb for the remedy of ophthalmia, dysentery, and jaundice.

References

1. Lin, L. Z. et al. 1983. Thalifaberine, thalifabine and huangshanine, three new dimeric aporphine-benzylisoquinoline alkaloids. *Planta Med.* 49: 55.
2. Lin, L. Z. et al. 1999. Phenolic aporphine-benzylisoquinoline alkaloids from *Thalictrum faberi*. *Phytochem.* 50: 829–34.
3. Lin, L. Z. et al. 1994. Thalifaberidine, a cytotoxic aporphine-benzylisoquinoline alkaloid from *Thalictrum faberi*. *J. Nat. Prod.* 57: 1430–6.
4. Lin, L. Z. et al. 1986. A new cytotoxic alkaloid, thalifalandine. *Heterocycles* 24: 2731–3.
5. Lin, L. C. et al. 1980. Studies on the chemical constituents of *Thalictrum faberi*. *Yaoxue Tongbao* 15: 46.
6. Lin, L. Z. et al. 1981. Chemical constituents of the anticancer plant *Thalictrum aberi* Ulber: I. Thalidasine and N-desmethylthalidasine. *Huaxue Xuebao* 39: 159–63.
7. Kupchan, S. M. et al. 1967. Isolation and structural elucidation of thalidasine, a novel bis(benzyl-isoquinoline) alkaloid tumor inhibitor from Thalictrum dasycarpum. *J. Am. Chem. Soc.* 89: 3075–6.
8. Gu, X. Q. et al. 1981. Studies on polyphase liposome—A new dosage form for antitumor agents. Part I. *Yaoxue Tongbao* 16: 501–2.
9. Lin, C. W. et al. 2000. Structure determination of a new ether-linkage bisalkaloid acutiaporberine. *Gaodeng Xuexiao Huaxue Xuebao* 21: 1820–3.
10. Chen, Q. et al. 2001. Cytotoxic activity of acutiaporberine, a novel bisalkaloid of plant origin, on several human carcinoma cell lines. *J. Zhongshan Univ.* (Sci. Edit.) 40: 9–12.
11. Chen, Q. et al. 2002. Apoptosis of a human non-small cell lung cancer (NSCLC) cell line, PLA-801, induced by acutiaporberine, a novel bisalkaloid derived from Thalictrum acutifolium (Hand.-Mazz.) Boivin. *Biochem. Pharmacol.* 63: 1389–96.
12. Chen, Q. et al. 2002. Apoptosis of human highly metastatic lung cancer cell line 95-D induced by acutiaporberine, a novel bisalkaloid derived from Thalictrum acutifolium. *Planta Med.* 68: 550–3.
13. Wu, Z. X. et al. 1990. Studies on the alkaloids from *Thalictrum fortunei*. *Acta Botanica Sinica* 32: 210–4.14.
14. Fortunei-saponin-A: 3-*O*-β-D-glucopyranosyl-(1-4)-β-D-fucopy ranosyl(22S,24Z)-cycloart-24-en-3β,22,26-triol 26-*O*-β-D-glucopyranoside; fortunei-saponin-B: 3-*O*-β-D-glucopyranosyl-(1-4)-β-D-fucopyranosyl(22S,24Z)-cycloart-24-en-3β,22,26-triol 26-*O*-α-L-arabinopyranosyl-(1-6)-β-D-glucopyranoside; fortunei-saponin-C: 3-*O*-β-D-glucopyranosyl-(1-4)-β-D-fucopy ranosyl(22S,24Z)-cycloart-24-en-3β,22,26-triol 26-*O*-β-D-xylopyranosyl-(1-6)-β-D-glucopyranoside; fortunei-saponin-D: 3-*O*-β-D-glucopyranosyl-(1-4)-β-D-fucopyranosyl(22S, 24Z)-cycloart-24-en-3β,22,26-triol 26-*O*-β-D-quinovopyranosyl-(1-6)-β-D-glucopyranoside; fortunei-saponin-I (1): 3-*O*-β-D-glucopyranosyl (1-4)-β-D-fucopyranosyl-(22S,24Z)-cycloart-24-en-3β,22,26,30-tetraol 26-*O*-β-D-glucopyranoside; and fortune-saponin-J: 3-*O*-β-D-glucopyranosyl (1-4)-β-D-fucopyranosyl-(22S,24Z)-cycloart-24-en-3β,22,26,29-tetraol 26-*O*-β-D-glucopyranoside.
15. Zhang, X. T. et al. 2012. Two new saponins from *Thalictrum fortune*. *J. Asian Nat. Prod. Res.* 14: 327–32.
16. Zhang, X. T. et al. 2011. A triterpenoid from *Thalictrum fortunei* induces apoptosis in BEL-7402 cells through the p53-induced apoptosis pathway. *Mol.* 16: 9505–19.

55 Zi Cao 紫草

Shikon or Arnebia root or Gromwell root

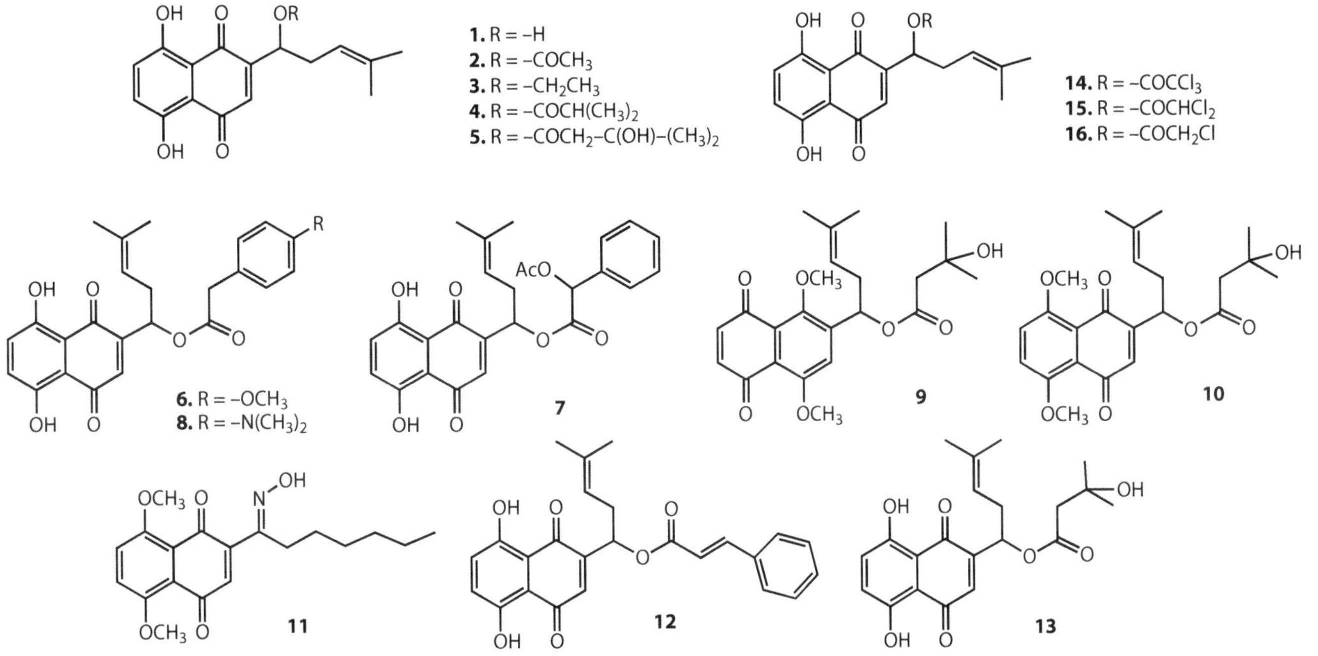

1. R = -H
2. R = $-COCH_3$
3. R = $-CH_2CH_3$
4. R = $-COCH(CH_3)_2$
5. R = $-COCH_2-C(OH)-(CH_3)_2$

14. R = $-COCCl_3$
15. R = $-COCHCl_2$
16. R = $-COCH_2Cl$

6. R = $-OCH_3$
8. R = $-N(CH_3)_2$

Herb Origination

The origin of Zi Cao is known from three plants of the Boraginaceae family, two *Arnebia* genus plants, *A. euchroma* and *A. guttata*, and one *Lithospermum* plant, *L. erythrorhizon*. Their roots are collected in the spring and the autumn and then dried in the sun for medical application. The first documentation of Zi Cao was in the first Chinese classic materia medica entitled *Shennong Ben Cao Jing*.

Antitumor Activities and Constituents

In vitro tests demonstrated that the Zi Cao extract terminated the proliferation of human Eca-109 esophageal carcinoma cells irreversibly and diminished the rate of spontaneous adenocarcinogenesis in rat breast.[1–3] Its anticarcinogenic and antitumor-promoting effects were clearly demonstrated by *in vivo* experiments with a two-stage carcinogenesis. By inhibiting the hyperproliferation and the oxidative damage, the extract obviously suppressed the two-stage skin carcinogenesis caused by DMBA and croton oil. The pretreatment with the Zi Cao extract at doses of 5–10 mg/kg could significantly restore the reduced levels of GSH and cellular protective enzymes with lessened oxidative stress and diminish the marker parameters of tumor promotion in two mice models initiated with benzoylperoxide followed by exposure to ultraviolet-B (UV-B) radiation or TPA. At the active dose range, the *in vivo* hydrogen peroxide content, MDA formation, ornithine decarboxylase activity, and DNA synthesis were significantly lessened.[4] The extensive investigations have revealed that the properties of Zi Cao (from all three origin plants) regarding the anticancer and anticarcinogenetic effects were attributed to a number of naphthoquinone derivatives of shikonin, especially the major constituent termed shikonin (**1**).

Shikonin

Shikonin (**1**) has been demonstrated in multiple pharmacological activities including the potent and broad spectrum of anticancer.[5] At doses of 5–10 mg/kg/day, shikonin (**1**) completely inhibited the cell growth of ascites sarcoma 180 in mice and prolonged the life span of the S180-bearing mice up to 92.5%.[6] The *in vivo* treatment with shikonin notably obstructed the cell growth of murine H22 hepatoma and human PC3 prostate carcinoma and lengthened the survival period of mice implanted with P388 leukemia.[7] The proliferation of stomach cancer cells and esophagus cancer cells was apparently obstructed by shikonin *in vitro* at the effective concentrations of 3–5 μg/mL, and the colony efficiency of cancer cells was significantly decreased by shikonin at concentrations of 5–10 μg/mL, without showing any damage to human normal cells, whose anticancer effect might be correlated to its role in obstructing the amount of RNA and the ultrastructure of cancer cells.[8] The moderate inhibitory effect of shikonin (**1**) was also demonstrated in a series of human cancer cell lines such as HL-60 (leukemic), HT-29 and Colo205 (colorectal), 143B (osteosarcoma), HepG2, Huh7 and Bel 7402 (liver), MCF-7 and T47D (ERα-positive breast), Tea8113 (tongue), U87MG, Hs683, and M059K (brain) cells, with respective IC_{50} values of 14.8, 5.5, 3.12, and 4.55 μM and 4.3 μg/mL in the first five cell lines.[7,9–15]

The anticancer activity of shikonin was closely associated with the promotion of apoptotic death. According to the continuous approaches, shikonin (**1**) was found to have a remarkable ability to stimulate the apoptosis of various types of human cancer cell lines such as melanoma (A375-S2), hepatoma (SK-Hep-1, HepG2, Bel7402, and Huh7), breast cancer (MFC-7), cervical cancer (HeLa), leukemia (K562 and HL-60), bladder cancer (T24), colon cancer (Colo205), glioma (U87MG, Hs683, and M059K), osteosarcoma (143B), and choriocarcinoma (JEG-3) cell lines.[7,9–28] Moreover, by inhibiting the expression of survivin and Bcl-2 and then enhancing the apoptosis, shikonin amplified the sensitivity of radiation against mouse hepatoma and Lewis lung cancer *in vivo* and also reversed the MDR of human JAR/MTX choriocarcinoma cells to methotrexate.[29,30] The results from a clinical approach using a shikonin-containing mixture demonstrated its safety and efficacy for the inhibition of late-stage lung cancer. Through the inhibition of MMP-9, shikonin (**1**) suppressed the migration and the invasion of MCF-7 and MDA-MB-231 human breast cancer cells.[31,32] In addition, an interesting approach showed that shikonin (**1**) elicited the breakage of the supercoiled plasmid pBR322 DNA in the presence of Cu(II) or Fe(II), increased intracellular ROS, finally resulting in DNA damage and apoptosis in the HeLa cells.[31,32] Consequently, shikonin (**1**) may be considered as a promising chemotherapeutic agent for advanced development in cancer clinics.

Shikonin Derivatives

Many shikonin derivatives, such as acetylshikonin, isobutyrolylshikonin, deoxyshikonin, isobutylshikonin, and β,β-dimethylacrylshikonin, were isolated from the herb Zi Cao, especially from the roots of *L. erythrorhizon*. Most of these naphthaquinone molecules displayed significant antiproliferative and apoptosis-inducing effects against the malignant cells. *In vitro* experiments in human MGC-803 gastric cancer cells and human Bel-7402 hepatoma cells revealed that the β,β-dimethylacrylshikonin, deoxyshikonin, 5,8-dihydroxy-2-(1-methoxy-4-methyl-3-pentenyl)-1,4-naphthalene-dione, as well as shikonin (**1**) showed more potent suppressive effects than cisplatin (DDP), an anticancer drug in clinics, showing respective IC_{50} values of 0.5–1.7 μg/mL and 1.3–1.5 μg/mL of the derivatives versus 4.4 and 7.6 μg/mL of DDP.[33] Acetylshikonin (**2**) dose dependently restrained the growth of A549, Bel-7402, MCF-7, and LLC (Lewis lung cancer) cells (IC_{50}: 2.72–6.82 μg/mL).[34] The treatment with β,β-dimethylacrylshikonin dose and time dependently reduced the cell viability of SGC-7901 gastric cancer and SMMC-7742 hepatoma and induced the cell apoptosis or blocked the cell cycle.[35–37] With the treatment with acetylshikonin in a dose of 2 mg/kg, a 42.85% growth inhibitory rate was resulted in mice bearing LLC,[34] whereas by β,β-dimethylacrylshikonin, the antigrowth effect was shown in mice against H22 hepatoma.[36] Meanwhile, the β-hydroxylnaphthoquinone derivatives, i.e., acetylshikonin (**2**), ethylshikonin (**3**), isobutylshikonin (**4**), 3′-hydroxyisovalerylshikonin, (**5**) as well as shikonin (**1**) were isolated from the roots of *L. erythrorhizon*. All the molecules exerted the potent growth inhibitory effect against HCT-116 (colon) and HepG2 (liver) human cancer cell lines, with IC_{50} values of 0.34–0.45 and 0.22–0.59 μM for the derivatives and IC_{50} values of 0.23 and 0.22 μM for shikonin (**1**), respectively.[38] These findings indicated that the shikonin derivatives exerted a potent antitumor activity similar to or a little lower than shikonin (**1**) and suggested that most of these shikonin derivatives may be the potential candidates for further development.

ShD, an extract mainly containing shikonin derivatives, exerted marked antitumor and immunomodulatory effects in murine models inoculated with sarcoma 180 or H22 hepatoma. Moreover, in daily doses of 2.5–5.0 mg/kg ShD, the survival time of the test animals was notably prolonged and the reduced $CD3^+$ and $CD19^+$ cells were recovered. The impairment of the immune function by ShD mostly is demonstrated in protecting the immune organs from damage and improving the life quality through enhancing the immune responses, as noted by the protected normal thymic structure, the enlarged splenic corpuscles, the augmented lymphocyte transformation and NK cell activity, and the amplified IL-2 production in the ShD-treated mice.[39]

Polysaccharide

A polysaccharide component (ARPS) was isolated from the roots of *Arnebia*, which exhibited significant dose-dependent antitumor and immunoregulating activities on human HepG2 hepatoma and SPC-A-1 lung cancer cells. When ARPS was treated to two tumor cell lines and mouse spleen lymphocyte, the proliferation of HepG2 cells and SPC-A-1 cells was markedly suppressed, whereas the proliferation of T lymphocytes was significantly promoted in the ARPS concentration of 121–364 μg/mL.[40] The *in vivo* antitumor effect of ARPS was further demonstrated obviously against mouse U14 uterine cervical carcinoma with prolonged life duration. At a medium dose, ARPS augmented the effect on the spleen index, but at high dose, it decreased the effect on the thymus index.[41]

Antitumor Mechanisms of Shikonin

The anticancer mechanism of shikonin (**1**) and its derivatives have been extensively explored, finding the effect to be concomitant with (1) inducing tumor cell apoptosis and cell cycle arrest, (2) activating MAPK, and (3) restraining the activities of tyrosine kinase and DNA Topo-I. These events affect the metabolite processes, the signal transduction, and the gene expression, proliferation and differentiation, leading to the growth inhibition against the cancer cells.[42] Shikonin (**1**) also provokes mammalian Topo-II-mediated DNA cleavage with no intercalation to the DNA.[43] The shikonin (**1**)-induced anticancer-related mechanisms were primarily summarized as follows, where shikonin was shown to normally have similar mediators but also have some unique characteristic roles and additional pathways in a variety of tumor cells.

Apoptosis Induction

The proapoptotic mechanism of shikonin in various cancer cell lines is preceded by multiple pathways including common morphological changes and characteristic regulations, such as (1) upregulating p27, p53, and Bad activities and down-expressing Bcl-2 and Bcl-xL; (2) triggering a series of events such as increase of ROS, loss of mitochondrial membrane potential, release of cytochrome c, cleavage of PARP, and activation of caspase-3 and caspase-9; (3) eliciting oxidative stress-mediated pathway and inducing ROS/Akt and RIP-1/NF-κB pathways (such as in

SK-Hep-1, Huh7, and Bel-7402 hepatoma cells)[7,21]; (4) attenuating catalase activity and upregulating SOD-1 expression (such as in U87MG glioma cells)[5,15]; (5) decreasing the phosphorylation levels of EGFR, ERK1/2, and Tyr kinases and augmenting apoptosis-related JNK1/2 protein intracellular phosphorylation levels (such as in HeLa cervical cancer, epidermoid carcinoma, 143B osteosarcoma, and JEG-3 chorio-carcinoma cells)[12,23,27]; (6) inducing caspase-activated DNase and/or digesting DNA fragmentation factor (DFF-45) to block cell cycle progression (such as in HeLa, Colo205 colon cancer, and A375-S2 melanoma cells)[6,17,18,20,28,44]; (7) amplifying the percentage lipid peroxidation and causing interactions between shikonin and cellular thiols such as GSH and protein thiols, then resulting in chromatin condensation and DNA fragmentation (such as in HL-60 leukemia cells)[8]; and (8) restraining 2-aminofluorene (AF) acetylation and AF-DNA adduct formation, suppressing NAT activity and expression, and blocking NAT Ag-Ab formation (such as in T24 bladder carcinoma cells).[19]

Moreover, upon treatment with 10 μM shikonin, ERα-positive human MCF-7 breast cancer cells underwent marked apoptotic morphological changes but not ERα-negative breast cancer cells, implying that the ERα level is important for MCF-7 cell apoptosis. Shikonin was capable of degrading ERα protein and decreasing ERα level through a proteasome-mediated pathway, leading the MCF-7 cells to apoptosis.[13,26,45] The β,β-dimethylacrylshikonin-promoted apoptosis of human SGC-7901 gastric cancer cells was found to be associated with multiple pathways, i.e., attenuation of Notch-1 activation, reduction of Jagged-1 and its downstream target Hes-1 expressions, and down-expression of XIAP and cIAP-2, besides induction of Bak and Bax expressions, ERK phosphorylation, loss of mitochondrial membrane potential, release of cytochrome c, cleavage of PARP, and activation of caspase-9, caspase-8, and caspase-3.[35,37]

Antiangiogenesis

Shikonin is also an inhibitor of tumor angiogenesis, whose effect was confirmed in mice implanted with B16 melanoma. The anti-angiogenesis mechanism of shikonin was revealed to be mediated by (1) blocking the expression of integrin-αvβ3, (2) inhibiting the proliferation and the migration of endothelial cells, (3) suppressing the proliferation of VEGF, and (4) reducing the network formation by endothelial cells on the Matrigel.[46] Through the down-expression of u-PA but not its receptor (u-PAR), shikonin (**1**) and acetylshikonin (**2**) significantly disrupted VEGF-induced tube formation in LLC-bearing mice.[47] The evidences suggested that the antiangiogenic property of shikonin should be correlated with its inhibitory effect against the carcinoma cell proliferation and migration/invasion.

Antioxidation

Shikonin (**1**) is an inhibitor of COX-2 retarded PMA-induced stimulation of ERK1/2 mitogen-activated protein kinases and restrained AP-1 in human mammary epithelial cells.[48] Shikonins (**1**) also showed the potent activity on superoxide anion radical (O^{2-}) scavenging and radical scavenging.[49,50] The results confirmed the potential of shikonins (**1**) in inhibiting oxidation-related carcinogenesis as well as inflammation.

Inhibition of HSP

HSPs is found at elevated levels in many human carcinomas, indicating that HSP might be highly involved in the response to stresses and survival. A further study demonstrated that HSP27 is related to the metastases of cancer cells and the resistance to radio- and chemotherapies. Shikonin (**1**) at a concentration of 1 μM strongly suppressed the expression of HSP27 in human KATO III gastric cancer cells.[51]

Reversal of Drug Resistance

In many clinical cases with drug resistance, P-gp was observed in overexpressed status in cancer cells. Shikonin (**1**) was able to exert the suppressive activity toward both drug-sensitive cancer cells (such as MCF-7 and HEK293) and their corresponding drug-resistant carcinoma cells. The drug resistance overturned by shikonin was not only due to the suppression of the overexpressed P-gp to reverse the drug resistance, but was also attributed to its ability in the induction of a necrotic death of neoplastic cells, such as MCF-7 cells and HEK293 cells.[52]

Structure Modification

For the optimization of the bioactivity, the structure modification of shikonin (**1**) has largely been conducted in the substitution of various acetic acid groups at its side chain. The created shikonin derivatives were claimed as tyrosine kinase inhibitors, displaying the improved anticancer effect against the carcinomas in the breast, the brain, the lung, the colon, the stomach, the ovary, the kidney, the skin, and the blood.[53]

Phenylacetylshikonin Analogs

The introduction of α-acetyl or of a 4-dimethyl amino group to the molecule of shikonin could improve the water solubility. Most of phenylacetylshikonin analogs expressed a potent cytotoxicity (ED_{50}: 0.1–1.80 μg/mL) against L1210 and K562 leukemia cells. Among them, 4-methoxyphenylacetylshikonin (**6**) (ED_{50}: 0.098 μg/mL) and α-acetoxyphenylacetylshik onin (**7**) (ED_{50}: 0.13 μg/mL) exerted the most potent antileukemia effect on the L1210 cells. 4-Methoxyphenylacetylshikonin (**6**) also exerted a more potent cytotoxicity on the K562 cells (ED_{50}: 0.033 μg/mL) than α-substituted phenylacetylshikonin (ED_{50}: 0.1 μg/mL).[53,54] However, the derivatives were much less sensitive to A549 lung cancer cells with ED_{50} values of 1.5–13.5 μg/mL, compared to shikonin. In *in vivo* assays with sarcoma 180, α-acetoxyphenylacetylshikonin (**7**) and 4-dimethylaminophenylacetylshikonin (**8**) resulted in a higher suppression (T/C value of 192–195%) and a significant prolongation of the life period of mice. Also, other analogs, such as 4-(N,N-dimethylamino)phenylacetylshikonin, 3,4-methylenedioxyphenylacetylshikonin, α-methoxyphenylacetylshikonin, and α-acetoxyphenylacetylshikonin displayed a higher antiadhesive activity in human A549 lung cancer cells.[54,55]

In addition, a series of the 6-isomers of 5,8-*O*-dimethylacylshikonin were synthesized from the starting shikonin. A derivative 5p (**9**) exerted more cytotoxicity than shikonin (**1**) against human MCF-7 and MDA-MB-231 breast carcinoma cells *in vitro*

(IC_{50}: 0.35 μM versus 1.9 μM and 0.2 μM versus 6.6 μM, respectively), with no toxicity in normal cells. The *in vivo* data from the mouse sarcoma 180 model suggested that the 6-isomers of 5,8-*O*-dimethylacylshikonin derivatives (such as 1-(1,4-dihydro-5,8-dimethoxy-1,4-dioxonaphthalen-6-yl)-4-methylpent-3-enyl-2-hydroxy-2-methylpropanoate (**9**)) were more active than the corresponding 2-isomers (such as 1-(1,4-dimethoxy-5,8-dihydro-5,8-dioxonaphthalen-6-yl)-4-methylpent-3-enyl-2-hydroxy-2-methylpropanoate (**10**)).[56]

2-Hyim-DMNQ-S33 and 93/637

A potent anticancer derivative of shikonin named 2-hyim-DMNQ-S33 (**11**) showed a suppressive effect against the proliferation of radiation-induced fibrosarcoma cells in a dose-dependent manner and significantly prolonged the survival time of mice bearing sarcoma 180 by 239%. After the treatment with 2-hyin-DMNQ-S33 for 4 h, the phosphorylation of ERK (pERK) was obviously restrained by the activation of c-jun-N-terminal kinase and PKCα. By moderating the expressions of pERK, c-jun-N-terminal kinase, and PKCα, 2-hyim-DMSQ-S33 (**11**) exerted the antitumor activity.[57] An acryloylshikonin analog called 93/637 (**12**) obstructed the growth of human PC3 prostate cancer cells dose dependently and inhibited the growth of other types of human prostate cancer cells (DU-145 and LNCaP) moderately in association with the down-regulation of IGF-II mRNA in DU-145 cells, of IGF-I and IGF-IR mRNAs in LNCaP, and of IGF-II mRNA and VEGF in PC3 cells, and the activation of IGF binding protein-3 in both DU-145 and PC3 cell lines. The results revealed that the antiprostate cancer property of 93/637 (**12**) is selectively correlated with the inhibitory effect on IGFs expression, especially in the PC3 cells.[58]

β-Hydroxyisovaleryl Shikonin

β-Hydroxyisovalerylshikonin (β-HIVS) (**13**) showed the growth inhibitory effect on various tumor cells. The most efficient cell death induced by β-HIVS was in two human lung cancer cell lines (NCI-H522 and DMS114). The IC_{50} values of β-HIVS (**13**) against the growth of human K562 and U937 leukemia cells were 0.12–0.14 μM. At a higher concentration, β-HIVS (**13**) retarded the growth of rat SR-3Y1, KDR/Flk-1-NIH3T3 cells, and human A431 epidermoid cells (IC_{50}: 1.2, 2.5, 11.0 μM, respectively). Due to the three cell lines expressing high levels of tyrosine kinases, the studies indicated that the anticancer property of β-HIVS is related to its capacity in the suppression of PTK activity.[59,60] When Bcr-Abl-positive K562 cells were treated with a combination of β-HIVS (**13**) and STI571 (Gleevec), a synergistic inhibitory effect was achieved in the induction of K562 cell apoptosis and the inhibition of PTK phosphorylation activity.[61] In addition, a derivative assigned as 5,8-dimethyl-2-β-hydroxyisovalerylshikonin (SK36) exerted the antiproliferative effect against human HL-60 leukemia cell line *in vitro*.[62]

Haloacetyl Shikonin Analogs

Haloacetylation of the secondary hydroxyl group at the side chain of shikonin could augment the antileukemia activity on the L1210 cells. 4-Halogenation tended to decrease the antileukemia effect on L1210 cells, but it enhanced the effect against K562 leukemia cells.[54] The cytotoxicity of monohaloacetylshikonin derivatives against the L1210 cells is shown in the following order (ED_{50} of μg/mL): monochloroacetylshikonin (0.142) > monobromoacetylshikonin (0.158) > monoiodoacetylshikonin (0.173), implying that the introduction of larger halogen atoms would lower the cytotoxicity. The ED_{50} (μg/mL) data of the chloroacetylshikonin derivatives would be influenced by the chlorine numbers, i.e., trichloroacetylshikonin (**14**) (0.032), dichloroacetylshikonin (**15**) (0.059), and monochloroacetylshikonin (**16**) (0.142). The results advocated that the electron-withdrawing effect of haloacetylation might be important for the cytotoxicity of chloroacetylshikonin derivatives. In a mouse model with L1210 cells, the T/C values of dichloroacetylshikonin (182%) and trifluoroacetylshikonin (195%) were greater than those of monoiodoacetylshikonin (117%), monochloroacetylshikonin (122%), and monobromoacetylshikonin (154%).[63]

A series of β-hydroxyisovalerylshikonin analogs were designed and synthesized by the connection of oxygen-containing substituents at the hydroxyl site of the shikonin side chain. Most of them exhibited a significant inhibitory activity on both multidrug-resistant DU-145 (prostate) and HeLa (cervical) cancer cell lines *in vitro*. The SAR showed that the analogs with ether substitution displayed the most potent antitumor activity and selective cytotoxicity toward the DU-145 cells. But the cytotoxicity would be declined if a steric hindrance in the carbon bearing β-hydroxyl is increased or a β-hydroxyl with acetoxy or methoxy in the shikonin derivatives having ether substituents is replaced.[64]

SYUNZ-7

SYUNZ-7 is a shikonin derivative (= 2 or 3,11-bis(phenylsulfanyl)-6-isohexenylnaphthazarin), displaying marked antiproliferation effects against a group of human cancer cell lines, including GLC-82 lung adenocarcinoma, CNE2 nasopharyngeal cancer, KB oral cavity cancer, MGC-803 gastric cancer, and HepG2 hepatoma (IC_{50}: 2.18–9.99 μg/mL). The anticancer activity was further demonstrated by using animal models implanted with EAC ascetic carcinoma or CNE2 nasopharyngeal cancer, and the inhibitory rates were 40.5–61.7% and 24.7–41.2%, respectively, in doses of 1–4 mg/kg. Simultaneously, SYUNZ-7 dose and time dependently induced the apoptosis of CNE2 cells and blocked the transition of CNE2 cells from the S phase to the G2/M phase. SYUNZ-7 was also able to obstruct the angiogenesis of CNE2 nasopharyngeal cancer xenografts in nude mice in a dose-dependent fashion.[65]

SYUNZ-4 and SYUNZ-16

SYUNZ-4 (= 3,11-bis(2-hydroxyethanesulfonyl)-6-isohexenylnaphthazarin) and SYUNZ-16 are the derivatives of alkannin, which is an optical isomer of shikonin at C-11. SYUNZ-4 presented a significant cytotoxicity on seven kinds of human cancer cells (IC_{50}: 0.30–7.8 μg/mL) *in vitro*. Its obvious suppression was also shown in MCF-7/Adm and KBV200 MDR carcinoma cells (IC_{50}: 1.96 and 7.78 μg/mL, respectively). The prominent growth inhibition of SYUNZ-4 was further confirmed in *in vivo* experiments. The i.p. administration of SYUNZ-4 in doses of 2.0–10 mg/kg for 10 days to tumor-bearing mice resulted in the antigrowth effect against sarcoma 180 for 31.5–69.7% and against HepS hepatoma for 45.9–67.5%. The inhibition rates were 48.4% and 61.7% on GLC-82 lung adenocarcinoma xenografts and 41.9% and 48.3% on CNE2 nasopharyngeal carcinoma xenografts, respectively, after the i.p. injection of SYUNZ-4 to nude mice in doses of 6.0 and 10 mg/kg for 18 days.[66]

SYUNZ-16 is a potent inhibitor of AKT signaling pathway in various neoplastic cell lines. The *in vitro* experiments demonstrated that SYUNZ-16 was effective in the growth inhibition of the GLC-82 cells and the Hep3B cells with the stimulation of apoptosis. The *in vivo* anticancer effect of SYUNZ-16 was proven in two animal models with xenograft GLC-82 and allograft S180.[67]

SH-7

SH-7, a shikonin derivative, 1-(1,4-dihydro-5,8-dihydroxy-1,4-dioxonaphthalen-2-yl)-4-methylpent-3-enylfuran-2-caroxylate, is a noticeable suppressor of Topo-I and Topo-II. SH-7 significantly elevated the expression of phosphorylated H2AX and stabilized the Topo-II-DNA cleavable complex, and the inhibitory potency on Topo-II was much stronger than that on Topo-I. The *in vitro* assay confirmed that SH-7 possesses a broad cytotoxicity on diversified neoplastic cell lines. SH-7 remarkably promoted the apoptosis of leukemia HL-60 cells in mitochondria dependence. The inhibitory activities of SH-7 were also demonstrated in mice bearing sarcoma 180 and in nude mice implanted with human PC3 prostate cancer, human SMMC-7721, or BEL-7402 hepatoma. Importantly, SH-7 displayed the marked inhibitory activity in three multidrug-resistant cancer cell lines as well with an average IC_{50} value nearly quivering to those of the corresponding parental cells. Hence, SH-7 was considered as a potential antitumor drug candidate for advanced investigation and development.[68]

Other Naphthoquinones

Two series of shikonin derivatives, 6- and 2-(1-acylsulfanylalkyl)-5,8-dimethoxy-1,4-naphthoquinones and 6- and 2-(1-substituted-thio-4-methylpent-3-enyl)-5,8-dimethoxynaphthalene-1,4-diones, were designed and synthesized. The *in vitro* assay results exhibited that most of the prepared compounds displayed the excellent selective suppressive effect toward human HT-29 colorectal cancer cells and the moderate activity against human BEL-7402 hepatoma and SPC-A1 lung cancer cell lines. Two derivatives assigned as 2-(1-acetylsulfanylpropyl)-5,8-dimethoxy-1,4-naphthoquinone, 6-(1-alkylthio-4-methylpent-3-enyl)-5,8-dimethoxynaphthalene-1,4-dione and 2-(1-alkylthio-4-methylpent-3-enyl)-5,8-dimethoxynaphthalene-1,4-dione displayed more potent inhibitory effects on the HT-29 cells among the naphthoquinones, whose activities were superior to shikonin (**1**).[69,70]

Nanoformulation

To limit its cytotoxic impact solely to tumor cells within the tumor microenvironment, shikonin-loaded Ab-armed PEGylated PLGA-nanoparticles have been formulated by using a single/double emulsion solvent evaporation/diffusion technique with sonication and then decoration of the surface of NPs with solubilizing agent PEG and tumor endothelial marker 1 (TEM1)/endosialin-targeting Ab through carbodiimide/N-hydroxysuccinimide chemistry. The engineered nanoparticles showed a smooth spherical shape with a size range of 120–250 nm and zeta potential value of −30 to −40 mV. The long-term exposure of the created nanoparticles was significantly toxic to TEM1-positive endothelial MS1 cells and OVCAR-5 ovarian epithelial cancer cells, while a 2 h exposure of the nanoparticles was not toxic to the lymphocytes. According to the findings, SHK-loaded Ab-armed PEGylated PLGA- nanoparticles may be a possible novel nanomedicine for targeted therapy of solid ovarian tumor, whose targeting moiety is specifically toward tumor microvasculature.[71] Likewise, to enhance antiproliferation properties, acetylshikonin (**2**) was successfully incorporated in solid lipid nanoparticles (SLN) by hot homogenization, whose regular nanoparticles is in the range of 70–120 nm with a polydispersity index of less than 0.10. The formulated shikonin-Act-SLN showed a higher antitumor/cytotoxic activity *in vitro* and *in vivo* than intact shikonin in terms of IC_{50} and DNA damage.[72] Consequently, the nanoformulation works provided sufficient information about improving the therapeutic efficacy and biodistribution of shikonin.

Other Bioactivities

The root extracts of Zi Cao have been used to treat macular eruption, measles, sore throat, carbuncles, and burns in east Asia areas for a thousand years. Pharmacological studies have proved shikonin (**1**) to possess pleiotropic, antigonadotropic, granuloma formation-enhancing, antiinflammatory, antiangiogenesis, platelet activation-inhibiting, DNA Topo-inhibiting, selective chemokine ligands-inhibiting, wound healing, anti-HIV-1, and antimicrobial activities. In addition, the aqueous water extract of Zi Cao showed anticomplement and antimutation effects.

References

1. Wang, L. et al. 1984. Effect of shikonin combined with high temperature heat on cultured Eta-109 cell proliferation and ^{3}H-TdR incorporation into DNA. *Jilin Yixue* 5: 30.
2. Zhu, M. Y. et al. 2012. Antitumor effect research progress of shikonin and its derivatives. *Acta Pharm. Sinica* 47: 588–93.
3. Tang, X. X. et al. 2015. Advances in tumor cell apoptosis induced by shikonin. *Zhejiang Yixue* 37: 265–8.
4. Sharma, S. et al. 2004. Effect of Onosma echioides on DMBA/croton oil mediated carcinogenic response, hyperproliferation and oxidative damage in murine skin. *Life Sci.* 75: 2391–410.
5. Chen, X. et al. 2002. Cellular pharmacology studies of shikonin derivatives. *Phytother. Res.* 16: 199–209.
6. Sankawa, U. et al. 1977. Antitumor activity of shikonin and its derivatives. *Chem. Pharm. Bull.* 25: 2392–5.
7. Gong, K. et al. 2011. Shikonin, a Chinese plant-derived naphthoquinone, induces apoptosis in hepatocellular carcinoma cells through reactive oxygen species: A potential new treatment for hepatocellular carcinoma. *Free Radical Biol. Med.* 51: 2259–71.
8. Lu, G. R. et al. 1990. Antitumor activity of naphthoquinone derivatives. *Zhongxiyi Jiehe Zazhi* 10: 422–5, 390.
9. Hsu, P. C. et al. 2004. Induction of apoptosis by shikonin through coordinative modulation of the Bcl-2 family, p27,

and p53, release of cytochrome c, and sequential activation of caspases in human colorectal carcinoma cells. *J. Agr. Food Chem.* 52: 6330–7.
10. Liu, R. T. et al. 2014. Studies on molecular mechanisms of shikonin induced programmed cell death in human hepatocellular carcinoma cells. *Chin. J. Biochem. Pharm.* 34: 1–7.
11. Nie, Y. K. et al. 2010. Shikonin inhibits the proliferation and induces the apoptosis of human HepG2 cells. *Can. J. Physiol. Pharmacol.* 88: 1138–46.
12. Chang, I.-C. et al. 2010. Shikonin induces apoptosis through reactive oxygen species/extracellular signal-regulated kinase pathway in osteosarcoma cells. *Biol. Pharm. Bull.* 33: 816–24.
13. Yao, Y. et al. 2010. A novel antiestrogen agent Shikonin inhibits estrogen-dependent gene transcription in human breast cancer cells. *Breast Cancer Res. Treatment* 121: 233–40.
14. Ruan, M. et al. 2010. Role of NF-κB pathway in shikonin induced apoptosis in oral squamous cell carcinoma tea-8,113 cells. *Shanghai Kouqiang Yixue* 19: 66–71.
15. Chen, C. H. et al. 2012. Novel multiple apoptotic mechanism of shikonin in human glioma cells. *Annals of Surgical Oncol.* 19: 3097–106.
16. Yang, H. J. et al. 2009. Shikonin exerts antitumor activity via proteasome inhibition and cell death induction *in vitro* and *in vivo*. *Intl. J. Cancer* 124: 2450–9.
17. Yoon, Y. et al. 1999. Shikonin, an ingredient of Lithospermum erythrorhizon induced apoptosis in HL60 human premyelocytic leukemia cell line. *Planta Med.* 65: 532–5.
18. Gao, D. Y. et al. 2002. Direct reaction between shikonin and thiols induces apoptosis in HL60 cells. *Biol. Pharm. Bull.* 25: 827–32.
19. Wu, Z. et al. 2004. Shikonin regulates HeLa cell death *via* caspase-3 activation and blockage of DNA synthesis. *J. Asian Nat. Prod. Res.* 6: 155–66.
20. Wu, Z. et al. 2004. p53-mediated cell cycle arrest and apoptosis induced by shikonin via a caspase-9-dependent mechanism in human malignant melanoma A375-S2 cells. *J. Pharmacol. Sci.* (Tokyo) 94: 166–76.
21. Yeh, C. C. et al. 2004. The inhibition of N-acetyltransferase activity and gene expression in human bladder cancer cells (T24) by shikonin. *In Vivo* 18: 21–32.
22. Wu, Z. et al. 2005. Phosphorylated extracellular signal-regulated kinase up-regulated p53 expression in shikonin-induced HeLa cell apoptosis. *Chin. Med. J.* (Eng. Edit.) 118: 671–7.
23. Chen, C. H. et al. 2003. Involvement of reactive oxygen species, but not mitochondrial permeability transition in the apoptotic induction of human SK-Hep-1 hepatoma cells by shikonin. *Planta Med.* 69: 1119–24.
24. Li, Y. M. et al. 2003. Shikonin inhibiting the catalytic activity of DNAtopoisomerase I and inducing the apoptosis of K562 leukemia cells. *Zhongguo Tianran Yaowu* 1: 165–8.
25. Singh, F. et al. 2003. Shikonin modulates cell proliferation by inhibiting epidermal growth factor receptor signaling in human epidermoid carcinoma cells. *Cancer Lett.* 200: 115–21.
26. Hou, Y. et al. 2006. Effect of shikonin on human breast cancer cells proliferation and apoptosis in vitro. *Yakugaku Zasshi* 126: 1383–6.
27. Huang, W. W. et al. 2009. Mechanisms of shikonin-induced apoptosis in JEG-3 cells. *Carcinog. Teratog. Mutag.* 21: 426–30.
28. Wu, Z. et al. 2004. Shikonin induce HeLa cell apoptosis via a caspase-dependent mechanism. *Chin. Pharmacol. Bull.* 20: 540–4.
29. Hu, Y. P. et al. 1991. Initial studies about radiosensitizing effect of shikonin for mice hepatoma 22 and Lewis lung carcinoma (LLC). *Zhongliu Fangzhi Yanjiu* 18: 71–3.
30. Yu, Y. X. et al. 2007. Relationship between the reverse effect of shikonin on methotrexate-resistant human choriocarcinoma cell line JAR/MTX and expressions of survivin and Bcl-2. *Acta Academiae Medicinae Militaris Tertiae* 29: 1880–2.
31. Jang, S. Y. et al. 2014. Shikonin blocks migration and invasion of human breast cancer cells through inhibition of matrix metalloproteinase-9 activation. *Oncol. Reports* 31: 2827–33.
32. Cheng, H. M. et al. 2011. DNA damage induced by shikonin in the presence of Cu(II) ions: Potential mechanism of its activity to apoptotic cell death. *J. Asian Nat. Prod. Res.* 13: 12–9.
33. Han, J. et al. 2007. Antitumor effects of constituents from *Lithospermum erythrorhizon* in vitro. *Jingxi Huagong* 24: 473–6.
34. Xiong, W. B. et al. 2009. In vitro and in vivo antitumor effects of acetylshikonin isolated from *Arnebia euchroma* (Royle) Johnst (Ruanzicao) cell suspension cultures. *Chin. Med.* 4: 14.
35. Shen, X. J. et al. 2012. β,β-Dimethylacrylshikonin induces mitochondria dependent apoptosis through ERK pathway in human gastric cancer SGC-7901 cells. *PLoS One* 7: e41773.
36. Wu, Y. Y. et al. 2012. Inhibitory effects of β,β-dimethylacrylshikonin on hepatocellular carcinoma in vitro and in vivo. *Phytother. Res.* 26: 764–71.
37. Shao, Z. J. et al. 2012. β,β-Dimethylacrylshikonin exerts antitumor activity via Notch-1 signaling pathway in vitro and in vivo. *Biochem. Pharmacol.* 84: 507–12.
38. Cui, X. R. et al. 2008. Comparison of the cytotoxic activities of naturally occurring hydroxylanthraquinones and hydroxynaphthoquinones. *Eur. J. Med. Chem.* 43: 1206–15.
39. Su, L. et al. 2012. Shikonin derivatives protect immune organs from damage and promote immune responses in vivo in tumor-bearing mice. *Phytotherapy Res.* 26: 26–33.
40. Chen, X. N. et al. 2008. Studies on the immunoregulation- and antitumor activity of polysaccharide from Arnebia root. *J. Zhejiang Univ.* (Sci. Edit.), 35: 674–7.
41. Chen, H. Y. et al. 2010. Effect of *Arnebia euchroma* (Royle) Johnst polysaccharide on mice bearing in U14 cervical cancer in vivo. *Zhongguo Xiandai Yingyong Yaoxue* 27: 1061–4.
42. Huang, H. et al. 2005. Anticancer effect of shikonin and derivatives. *Zhongliu Fangzhi Zazhi* 12: 75–8.
43. Fujii, N. et al. 1992. Induction of topoisomerase II-mediated DNA cleavage by the plant naphtha-quinones plumbagin and shikonin. *Antimicrobial Agents Chemother.* 36: 2589–94.
44. Yuan, Y. et al. 2010. A novel antiestrogen agent shikonin inhibits estrogen-dependent gene transcription in human breast cancer cells. *Breast Cancer Res. Treat.* 121: 233–40.
45. Wu, Z. et al. 2005. Studies on the mechanisms of shikonin-induced A375-S2 cell apoptosis. *Zhongguo Yaolixue Tongbao* 21: 202–5.
46. Yuki, H. et al. 1998. Shikonin, an ingredient of *Lithospermum erythrorhizon*, inhibits angiogenesis in vivo and in vitro. *Anticancer Res.* 18: 783–90.
47. Lee, H. J. et al. 2008. Shikonin, acetylshikonin, and isobutyroylshikonin inhibit VEGF-induced angiogenesis and suppress tumor growth in Lewis lung carcinoma-bearing mice. *Yakogaku Zasshi* 128: 1681–8.

48. Subbaramaiah, K. et al. 2001. Development and use of a gene promoter-based screen to identify novel inhibitors of cyclooxygenase-2 transcription. *J. Biomol. Screening* 6: 101–10.
49. Sekine, T. et al. 1998. Evaluation of superoxide anion radical scavenging activity of shikonin by electron spin resonance. *Intl. J. Pharma.* 174: 133–9.
50. Han, J. et al. 2008. Antioxidants from a Chinese medicinal herb *Lithospermum erythrorhizon*. *Food Chem.* 106: 2–10.
51. Morino, M. et al. 1998. Heat-shock protein 27 (HSP27) formation inhibitors containing shikonin. *Jpn. Kokai Tokkyo Koho* 7 pp. JP 96–216664 19960730.
52. Han, W. D. et al. 2007. Shikonin circumvents cancer drug resistance by induction of a necroptotic death. *Mol. Cancer Therapy* 6: 1641–9.
53. Nakaya, K. et al. 2002. Shikonin derivatives as tyrosine kinase inhibitors and antitumor agents *Jpn. Kokai Tokkyo Koho* JP 2002212065 A 20020731.
54. Kim, S. H. et al. 1996. Antitumor activity of arylacetylshikonin analogues. *Archiv. Pharm. Res.* 19: 416–22.
55. Kim, S. H. et al. 1997. Anti-cell adhesive effect of phenylacetylshikonin analogues related to their cytotoxicity in A549 cells. *Archiv. Pharm. Res.* 20: 155–7.
56. Zhou, W. et al. 2011. Semi-synthesis and antitumor activity of 6-isomers of 5, 8-O-dimethyl acylshikonin derivatives. *Eur. J. Med. Chem.* 46: 3420–7.
57. Kim, S. H. et al. 2001. Anticancer activities of a newly synthesized shikonin derivative, 2-hyim-DMNQ-S-33. *Cancer Lett.* 172: 171–175.
58. Gaddipali, J. P. et al. 2000. Inhibition of growth and regulation of IGFs and VEGF in human prostate cancer cell lines by shikonin analogue 93/637 (SA). *Anticancer Res.* 20: 2547–52.
59. Hashimoto, S. et al. 2002. β-hydroxyisovalerylshikonin is a novel and potent inhibitor of protein tyrosine kinases. *Jpn. J. Cancer Res.* 93: 944–51.
60. Xu, Y. et al. 2003. Growth inhibitory effects of β-hydroxyisovalerylshikonin on tumor cells expressing high levels of tyrosine kinases. *Shenyang Yaoke Daxue Xuebao* 20: 203–6.
61. Nakaya, K. et al. 2003. A shikonin derivative, [beta]-hydroxyisovalerylshikonin, is an ATP-non-competitive inhibitor of protein tyrosine kinases. *Anti-Cancer Drugs* 14: 683–93.
62. Cheng, L. J. et al. 2010. Effects of shikonin derivative SK36 on proliferation and apoptosis of HL-60 cells. *Zhongliu* 30: 581–5.
63. Zheng, X. G. et al. 1998. Haloacetylshikonin derivatives: Synthesis and evaluation of antitumor activity. *Yakhak Hoechi* 42: 159–64.
64. Rao, Z. et al. 2011. Synthesis and antitumor activity of β-hydroxyisovalerylshikonin analogues. *Eur. J. Med. Chem.* 46: 3934–41.
65. Huang, H. et al. 2005. Anticancer effect and mechanism of Shikonin derivative SYUNZ-7. *Aizheng* 24: 1453–8.
66. Xie, B. F. et al. 2007. Antitumor effect of alkannin derivative, SYUNZ-4. *Chin. Pharm. J.* 42: 1384–8.
67. Deng, R. et al. 2010. SYUNZ-16, a newly synthesized alkannin derivative, induces tumor cells apoptosis and suppresses tumor growth through inhibition of PKB/AKT kinase activity and blockade of AKT/FOXO signal pathway. *Intl. J. Cancer* 127: 220–9.
68. Yang, F. et al. 2006. SH-7, a new synthesized shikonin derivative, exerting its potent antitumor activities as a topoisomerase inhibitor. *Intl. J. Cancer* 119: 1184–1193.
69. Zhao, L. M. et al. 2008. Synthesis and antitumor activity of 6- and 2-(1-acylsulfanylalkyl)-5,8-dimethoxy-1,4-naphthoquinones. *Chin. Chem. Lett.* 19: 1206–8.
70. Zhao, L. M. et al. 2009. Synthesis and antitumor activity of 6- and 2-(1-substituted-thio-4-methylpent-3-enyl)-5,8-dimethoxynaphthalene-1,4-diones. *Eur. J. Med. Chem.* 44: 1410–4.
71. Matthaiou, E.-I. et al. 2014. Shikonin-loaded antibody-armed nanoparticles for targeted therapy of ovarian cancer. *Intl. J. Nanomed.* 9: 1855–70.
72. Eskandani, M. et al. 2014. Self-reporter shikonin-Act-loaded solid lipid nanoparticle: Formulation, physicochemical characterization and geno/cytotoxicity evaluation. *Europ. J. Pharm. Sci.* 59: 49–57.

56 Ku Di Dan 苦地膽

Elephant foot

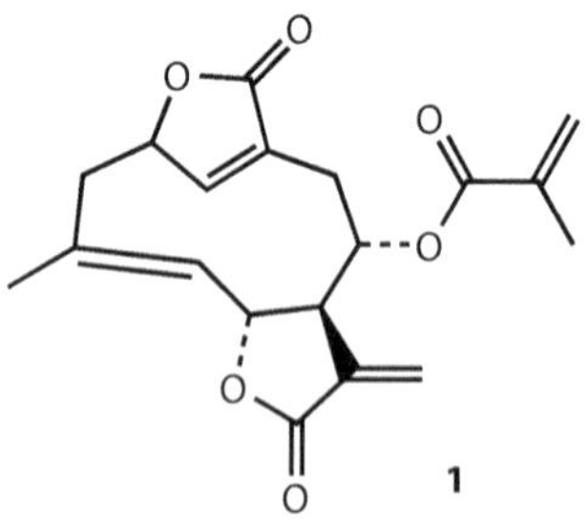

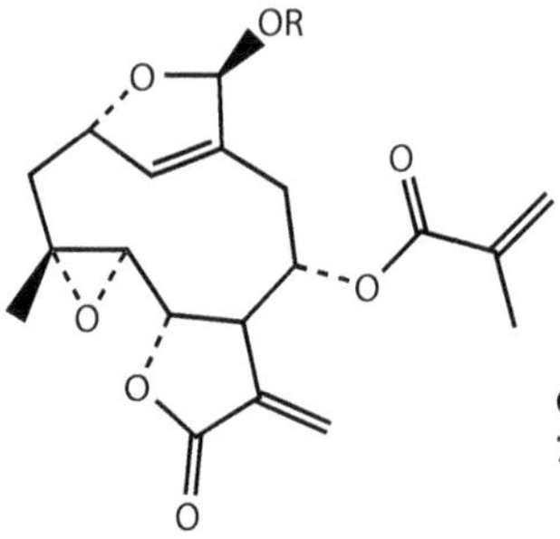

6. R = $-CH_3$
7. R = $-H$

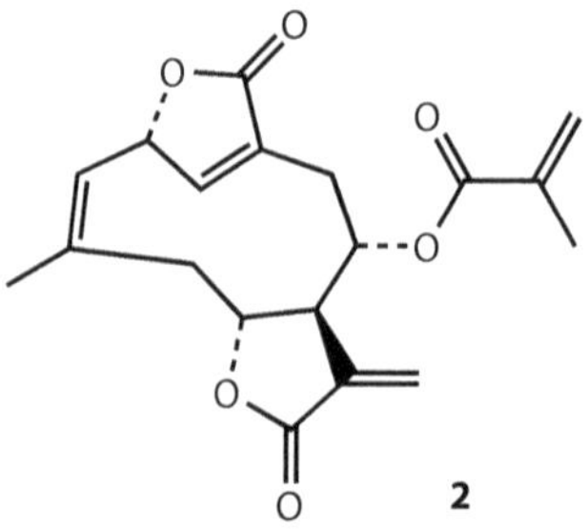

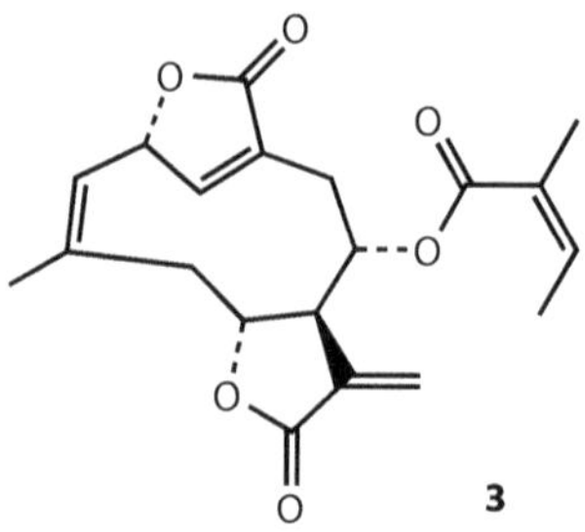

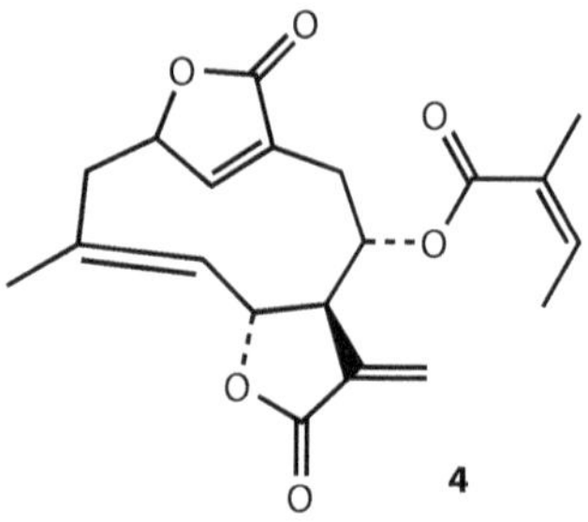

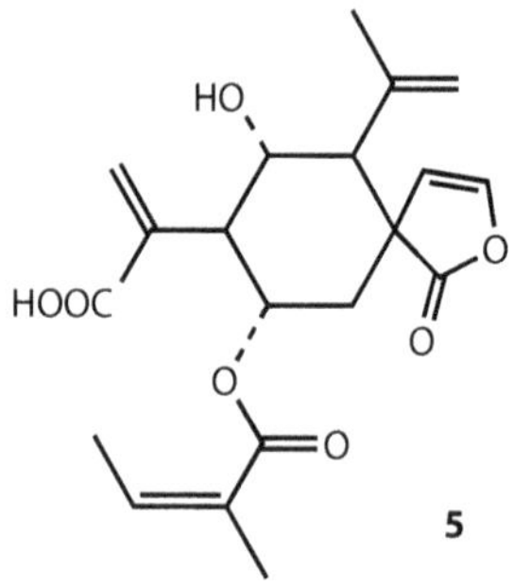

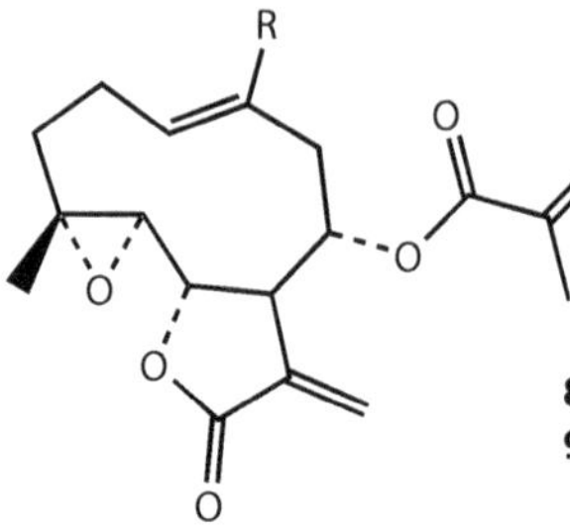

8. R = $-CH_2OH$
9. R = $-CHO$

Herb Origination

Two perennial herbaceous Compositae plants of *Elephantopus scaber* L. and *E. tomentosus* L. are the origins of Ku Di Dan. The former plant is widely found in the neotropical areas of the world, and the latter plant is distributed in both the southeastern regions of China and United States. The main producer of the herb is Chinese southeastern provinces, and the whole plant is collected in late summer and dried in the sun for medicinal application. The herb can also be used fresh after being collected.

Antitumor Constituents and Activities

Sesquiterpene lactones are the major tumor inhibitors discovered in Ku Di Dan. These anticancer sesquiterpenes found from both sources of the herb hold a similar germacrenolide-type structure but not quite same.

Agents from the Plant of E. scaber

An ethanolic extract of *E. scaber* exerted cytotoxicity on MCF-7 breast cancer cells (IC_{50}: 15 μg/mL) and triggered p53-dependent apoptosis.[1] An enriched dichloromethane fraction exerted a dose-dependent cytotoxicity in human epithelial cancer cells and showed hall mark property of apoptosis in human HeLa (cervix), A549 (lung), MCF-7 (breast), and Caco-2 (colon) cancer cell lines. Interestingly, the fraction inhibited multidrug-resistant transporters (ABC B1 and ABC G2) in human epithelial cancer cells.[2] The sesquiterpene lactones isolated from the herb as the major component exerted a marked inhibitory effect against various cancer cell lines. Deoxyelephantopin (DOE) (**1**), isodeoxyelephantopin (IDOE) (**2**), and scabertopin (**3**) displayed the antiproliferative activity on human HeLa (cervix), SMMC-7721 (liver), and Caco-2 (colon) cancer cell lines in a concentration-dependent manner *in vitro*.[3] The IC_{50} value of deoxyelephantopin (**1**) was 5.4 μM in the HeLa cells, whereas the respective IC_{50} of isodeoxyelephantopin (**2**) and scabertopin (**3**) were 25.39 and 22.19 μM in the HeLa cells after 48 h of treatment, 9.54 and 29.27 μM in the SMMC-7721 cells, and 25.76 and 35.99 μM in the Caco-2 cells.[4,5] The apoptosis and the G2/M phase cell arrest were elicited when the HeLa cells are exposed to deoxyelephantopin (**1**) and isodeoxyelephantopin (**2**) for 48 h.[3–5] Both deoxyelephantopin (**1**) and isodeoxyelephantopin (**2**) also caused a dose-dependent reduction in the viability of mouse L929 fibroblast cells *in vitro* (IC_{50}: 2.7–3.3 μg/mL).[6] Isoscabertopin (**4**) was also effective in the inhibition of the proliferation of HeLa and Caco-2 cells, while an elemanolide-type of sesquiterpene lactone assigned as elescaberin (**5**) diminished the viability of the SMMC-7721 cells.[3,7]

Among these major constituents, deoxyelephantopin (**1**) and isodeoxyelephantopin (**2**) have been paid more attention in anticancer investigations. More scientific data were disclosed as discussed separately as follows.

Deoxyelephantopin

DOE (**1**) and two analogs, 17,19-dihydrodeoxyelephantopin and 17,19-isodihydrodeoxyelephantopin, pronounced *in vitro* antiproliferative activities on MAXF 401NL (breast) RXF944L (renal), LXFL 529L (lung), and MEXF 394NL (skin) human cancer cell lines *in vitro*, whose respective IC_{70} values were 1.1, 4.0, and 4.3 μg/mL in MEXF 394NL cells.[8] When human CNE nasopharyngeal cancer cells are treated with DOE (**1**), both intrinsic and extrinsic apoptotic pathways plus Akt, ERK, and JNK interactions were found to be involved in the induction of apoptosis and S and G2/M phase cell arrests in both caspase-independent and caspase-dependent manners, leading to the suppression of the proliferation of CNE cells.[9] At a concentration of 3 μg/mL, DOE (**1**) provoked the maximum apoptosis of Daltons lymphoma ascites tumor cells and human HCT-116 colorectal cancer cells *in vitro*.[6] By targeting multiple signaling pathways, DOE (**1**) impaired the growth of SiHa cervical carcinoma cells and triggered G2/M phase arrest and apoptotic death, where PI3k/Akt/mTOR and MAPK pathways, STAT3/p53/p21 signaling, caspase cascades, and ROS generation played critical roles in the proapoptosis of SiHa cells.[10] The antiproliferative effect of DOE (**1**) was also shown in human A549 lung cancer cells and human HGC gastric cancer cells *in vitro* (IC_{50}: 4.2–4.7 μM), but there was no toxicity toward normal human lymphocytes.[4,11] During the inhibition on A549 cells, DOE (**1**) induced G2/M cell cycle arrest and cell apoptosis through both extrinsic and intrinsic pathways.[11] In association with the down-expression of MMP-2, MMP-9, u-PA, and u-PA receptor, the up-expression of TIMP-2, p-JNK, and p-p38, the decrease of p-ERK1/2 and p-Akt levels, and the inactivation of NF-κB and IκBα, DOE (**1**) exerted the antiinvasive and antimigratory effects in the A549 cells, showing a potential against the metastasis of NSCLC cells.[12]

The remarkable anticancer property of DOE (**1**) has also been demonstrated by several *in vivo* studies. In the animal models, DOE (**1**) was responsible for markedly inhibiting the growth of W256 ascites sarcoma in rats (T/C = 226% at a dose of 2.5 mg/kg) and for extending the life period of mice bearing Dalton's lymphoma ascites tumor (67.64–72.51% at i.p. doses of 50–100 mg/kg) with no toxicity.[5,13] The pretreatment with DOE (**1**) and paclitaxel (an antineoplastic drug), separately, to mice implanted with TS/A mammary adenocarcinoma cells resulted in a notable inhibitory effect against the colony formation, cell growth, migration and invasion of both orthotopic and metastatic TS/A tumor cells *in vivo*. The results showed that the decrease of tumor sizes was 99% versus 68%; the reduction of metastatic pulmonary foci in lung metastasis of TS/A cells was 82% versus 63%; and the prolonged life span (days) was 56 versus 37, indicating that DOE (**1**) was more effective than paclitaxel on the TS/A cells. During the treatment, c-JNK-mediated p21Waf1/Cip1 expression and caspase cascade activation were upregulated, TNFα-induced MMP-9 and NF-κB activities were abolished, and COX-2 and VEGF levels were diminished concurrently in mice bearing the metastatic TS/A lung tumor.[14] According to *in vitro* and *in vivo* evidences, deoxyelephantopin (**1**) can be considered as an effective inhibitor in tumor proliferation, growth, metastasis, and angiogenesis.

Isodeoxyelephantopin

The antiproliferative activity of IDOE (**2**) was demonstrated in *in vitro* models with four different human nasopharyngeal cancer cell lines, KB (epidermal), CNE1 (with high differentiation), CNE2 (with low differentiation), and SUNE1 (with poor differentiation and high metastasis). IDOE (**2**) obstructed the viability and the colony formation of KB cells (IC_{50}: 11.45 μM in 48 h), where G2/M phase cell cycle arrest and proapoptosis were accompanied to the treated KB cells.[15] In the SUNE1, CNE1, and CNE2 cell lines, IDOE (**2**) exerted its antitumor effects, associated with ROS-dependent DNA damage, G2/M arrest, mitochondrial-mediated apoptosis, and an antitumor inflammation factor pathway, such as the up-expression of IL-12α, IFNα, and IFNβ via both ROS-dependent and independent manners.[16] Similarly, IDOE (**2**) inhibited the growth of A549 lung carcinoma cells and T47D breast cancer cells in a dose- and a time-dependent manner (respective IC_{50}: 10.46 and 1.3 μg/mL) and induced caspase-3-mediated apoptosis and G2/M cell cycle arrest in the treated cells.[17] Likewise, in NF-κB ligand-induced osteoclastogenesis, IDOE (**2**) also has ability to lessen the expression of TNF-induced and NF-κB-regulated gene products regarding proliferation, apoptosis, and metastasis.[18]

All these investigations for the anticancer-related activities of DOE (**1**) and IDOE (**2**) not only provided insight of their multiple mechanisms, but also suggested that the two drug leads have a development potential for cancer chemotherapy and chemoprevention.

Agents from the Plant of E. tomoutosus

Some germacrenolide-type sesquiterpene lactones have been isolated from the plant of *E. tomentosus*. The isolated tomenphantopin-A (**6**), tomenphantopin-B (**7**), tomenphantin-A (**8**), tomenphantin-B (**9**), as well as dihydroelephantopin (**1**) demonstrated the obvious cytotoxic effects against the proliferation of human KB oral carcinoma cells, *in vitro*, with ED_{50} values of 5.0, 3.0, 2.7, and 2.5 μg/mL, respectively.[19,20]

Structure–Activity Relationship

Structurally, DOE (**1**), IDOE (**2**), tomenphantopins (tomenphantopin-A (**6**) and tomenphantopin-B (**7**)), and tomenphantins (tomenphantin-A (**8**) and tomenphantin-B (**9**)) possess C11-C13 exocyclic methylene conjugated to γ-lactone, exerting the inhibitory effect against the growth of cancer cells.[21,22] The hydrogenation of a double bond in the α-methylene-γ-lactone moiety or in the cyclodecane ring could markedly reduce the cytotoxicity. The evidences indicated that the presence of α-methylene-γ-lactone system in the skeleton of germacrenolide sesquiterpene lactones is essential for the cytotoxicity and the potent suppressive effects against the activities of DNA polymerase and thymidylate synthetase and against aerobic basal respiration and oxidative phosphorylation in the tumor cells.[21,22] When a double bond in the cyclodecane ring was epoxidized, the anticancer property could be enhanced. If the epoxidation occurred in double bonds both inside and outside the cyclodecane ring but not in the α-methylene-γ-lactone moiety, the antitumor potency would be augmented obviously.[23]

Other Medical Uses

The herb Ku Di Dan (Elephant foot) has been well known as a folk medicine in many countries in Southeast Asia, Latin America, and Africa for a long time. The herb is widely used for the treatment of nephritis, edema, dampness, chest pain, fever and cough of pneumonia, scabies, and arthralgia due to wounding. In Brazil, the infusion and the decoction of the whole plant (*E. scaber*) are used to stimulate diuresis, reduce fever, and eliminate bladder stones.

References

1. Ho, W. Y. et al. 2011. *Elephantopus scaber* induces cytotoxicity in MCF-7 human breast cancer cells via p53-induced apoptosis. *J. Med. Plants Res.* 5: 5741–9.
2. Beeran, A. A. et al. 2015. The enriched fraction of *Elephantopus scaber* triggers apoptosis and inhibits multidrug resistance transporters in human epithelial cancer cells. *Pharmacognosy Magazine* 11: 257–68.
3. Xu, G. et al. 2006. Antitumor activities of the four sesquiterpene lactones from *Elephantopus scaber* L. *Experim. Oncol.* 28: 106–9.
4. Liang, Q. L. et al. 2008. The antitumor effects in vitro of sesquiterpene lactones from *Elephantopus scaber. Tianran Chanwu Yanjiu Yu Kaifa* 20: 436–9.
5. Zou, G. et al. 2008. Deoxyelephantopin inhibits cancer cell proliferation and functions as a selective partial agonist against PPARγ. *Biochem Pharmacol.* 75: 1381–92.
6. Geetha, B. S. et al. 2012. Sesquiterpene lactones isolated from *Elephantopus scaber* L., inhibits human lymphocyte proliferation, growth of tumor cell lines and induces apoptosis in vitro. *J. Biomed. Biotech.* 2012: 721285, 8 pp.
7. Liang, Q. L. et al. 2008. A new elemanolide sesquiterpene lactone from *Elephantopus scaber. J. Asian Nat. Prods. Res.* 10: 403–7.
8. Than, N. N. et al. 2005. Sesquiterpene lactones from *Elephantopus scaber. Zeitschrift fuer Natur-forschung, B: Chem. Sci.* 60: 200–204.
9. Su, M. X. et al. 2011. Deoxyelephantopin from *Elephantopus scaber* L. induces cell-cycle arrest and apoptosis in the human nasopharyngeal cancer CNE cells. *Biochem. Biophys. Res. Commun.* 411: 342–7.
10. Farha, A. K. et al. 2014. Deoxyelephantopin impairs growth of cervical carcinoma SiHa cells and induces apoptosis by targeting multiple molecular signaling pathways. *Cell Biol. Toxicol.* 30: 331–43.
11. Farha, A. K. et al. 2013. Antineoplastic effects of deoxyelephantopin, a sesquiterpene lactone from *Elephantopus scaber*, on lung adenocarcinoma (A549) cells. *J. Integrative Med.* 11: 269–77.
12. Farha, A. K. et al. 2015. Anti-metastatic effect of deoxyelephantopin from *Elephantopus scaber* in A549 lung cancer cells in vitro. *Nat. Prod. Res.* Feb. 17: 1–5.
13. Lee, K. H. et al. 1975. Deoxyelephantopin, an antitumor principle from *Elephantopus carolinianus* Willd. *J. Pharm. Sci.* 64: 1572–3.
14. Huang, C. C. et al. 2010. Deoxyelephantopin, a novel multifunctional agent, suppresses mammary tumor growth and lung metastasis and doubles survival time in mice. *British J. Pharmacol.* 159: 856–71.
15. Farha, A. K. et al. 2013. Apoptosis mediated cytotoxicity induced by Isodeoxyelephantopin on nasopharyngeal carcinoma cells. *Asian J. Pharm. Clin. Res.* 6(Suppl. 2): 51–6.
16. Yan, G. R. et al. 2013. Quantitative proteomics characterization on the antitumor effects of isodeoxyelephantopin against nasopharyngeal carcinoma. *Proteomics* 13: 3222–32.
17. Kabeer, F. K. et al. 2014. Isodeoxyelephantopin from *Elephantopus scaber* (Didancao) induces cell cycle arrest and caspase-3-mediated apoptosis in breast carcinoma T47D cells and lung carcinoma A549 cells. *Chinese Med.* (London) 9: 14/1–14/9.
18. Ichikawa, H. et al. 2006. Isodeoxyelephantopin, a novel sesquiterpene lactone, potentiates apoptosis, inhibits invasion, and abolishes osteoclastogenesis through suppression of NF-κB activation and NF-κB-regulated gene expression. *Clin. Cancer Res.* 12: 5910–18.
19. Hayashi, T. et al. 1999. Antitumor agents. 190. Absolute stereochemistry of the cytotoxic germacranolides, tomenphantins A and B, from *Elephantopus tomentosus. J. Nat. Prods.* 62: 302–4.
20. Hayashi, T. et al. 1987. Structure and absolute stereochemistry of tomenphantopin-A and -B two cytotoxic sesquiterpene lactones from Elephantopus tomentosus. *Phytochem.* 26: 1065–8.
21. Hall, I. H. et al. 1978. Antitumor agents 190: Evaluation of α-methylene-γ-lactone-containing agents for inhibition of tumor growth, respiration, and nucleic acid synthesis. *J. Pharm. Sci.* 67: 1235–9.
22. Kupchan, S. M. et al. 1971. Tumor inhibitors: 69. Structure-cytotoxicity relationships among the sesquiterpene lactones. *J. Med. Chem.* 14: 1147–52.
23. Liang, Q. L. et al. 2007. Structure modification on sesquiterpene lactones from *Elephantopus scaber. Yaoxue Xuebao* 42: 1159–61.

57 Shao Yao 芍藥

Chinese peony root

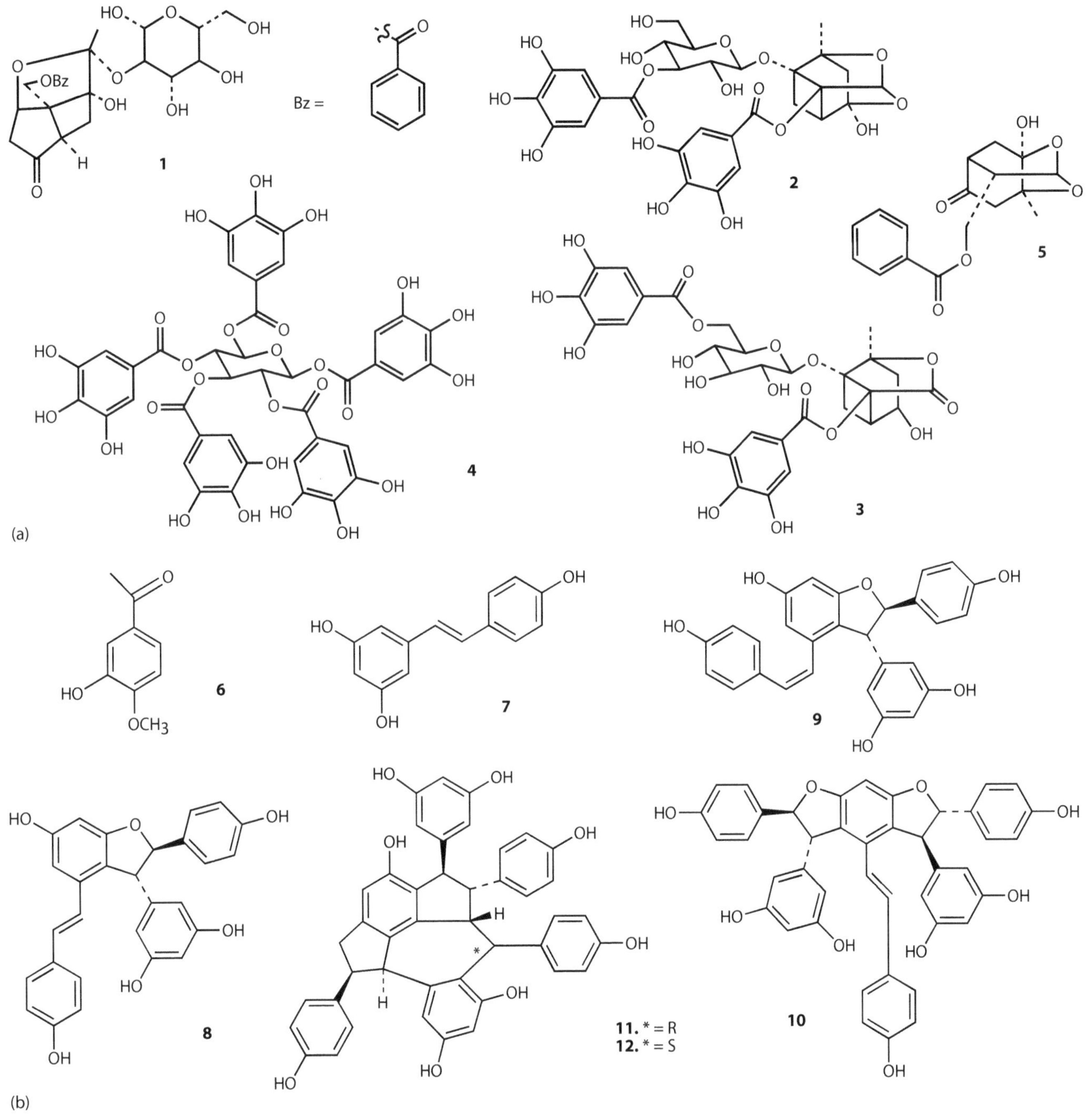

(a)

(b)

Herb Origination

The herb Shao Yao (Chinese peony root) is usually divided into two types from ancient China, namely Bai Shao (White peony) and Chi Shao (Red peony), and both peonies are important traditional Chinese medicines. Shao Yao was recorded in the first Chinese classic of materia medica titled as *Shennong Ben Cao Jing*. Customarily, Bai Shao is made from the dried roots of cultured *Paeonia lactiflora* and *P. lactiflora* var. *trichocarpa* (Paeoniaceae), and Chi Shao originated from the roots of wild *P. lactiflora* and six other *Paeonia* plants. Bai Shao is collected in summer and autumn, while Chi Shao is in spring and autumn.

Antitumor Activities

Peony roots are commonly used to treat liver diseases in China for centuries. Its water extract exhibited an inhibitory effect on the growth of both human HepG2 and Hep3B hepatoma cell lines *in vitro* with the promotion of apoptosis and cell cycle arrest. During its early apoptosis of the HepG2 cells, BNIP3 was up-expressed and RAD23B, HSPD1, and ZK1 were down-expressed by a p53-independent pathway.[1] The i.p. administration of Chi Shao n-butanolic extract (1–2 g/kg) to mice exerted the suppressive effect against the growth of entity sarcoma 180 cells and the obvious decrease of plasma fibrin contents in the tumor.[2,3] Also, its n-butanolic extract, water extract, and 70% ethanolic extract could raise the cAMP level in the tumor tissues of entity and ascites sarcoma 180 and Lewis lung carcinoma.[4]

The Bai Shao extract also could induce synergic interaction when combined with mitomycin (an anticancer drug) in the treatment of P388 leukemia-bearing mice. The extract not only strengthened the tumor inhibitory effect but also augmented the number of leukocyte, which was reduced by the mitomycin.[5] The combination of the n-butanolic extract with a small dose of anticancer drug cylcophosphamide markedly reduced the spontaneous metastasis of Lewis lung carcinoma *in vivo*.[6] The herbs also demonstrated an antimutagenic activity against BAP-induced mutation in *Sulmonella tyhimurium* TA98 and TA100 tests.[4–7]

Anticancer Constituents and Activities

Agents from Peony Roots

The total glucosides prepared from Red peony roots notably restrained the growth of HepA hepatoma cells and promoted cell apoptosis *in vitro*.[8] Seven monoterpene glycosides, albiflorin-R1 (**1**), 3′-*O*-galloylpaeoniflorin (**2**), 6′-*O*-galloylalbiflorin (**3**), 4′-*O*-galloylpaeoniflorin, 6′-*O*-galloylpaeoniflorin, 6′-*O*-benzoylpaeoniflorin, 4-*O*-galloylalbiflorin, and one polyphanol glycoside, pentagalloylglucose (PGG) (**4**), were isolated from the peony roots. All the glycosides demonstrated anticarcinogenic and antiproliferative activities on the tumor cells. When *in vitro* treatment with albiflorin-R1 (**1**) was done, the proliferation of HeLa cervical cancer and K562 leukemia cell lines were suppressed by 35% in a 50 μg/mL concentration, but the proliferation of J774 macrophages were also inhibited in a 32.5 μg/mL concentration,[9] implying albiflorin-R1 (**1**) has anticancer and immunosuppressive properties besides antiinflammation. Paeoniflorigenone (**5**) displayed a mild inhibitory activity against BT 483 (breast) and OVCA 429 (ovary) cancer cell lines (IC_{50}: 20.84 and 53.60 μM, respectively).[10]

Moreover, PGG (**4**) showed prominent anti-proliferative, antiinvasive, antioxidative, and antimutagenic effects on cancer cells and also showed the inhibitory effect on iNOS and COX-2.[11] PGG (**4**) and 6′-*O*-galloyl-albiflorin (**3**) as well as all seven monoterpene glycosides are antagonists for AR binding, wherein PGG (**4**) exerted a stronger inhibition on the AR-binding activity (IC_{50}: 4.1 μg/mL), compared to other paeoniflorin and albiflorin analogs. Therefore, PGG (**4**) showed better ability to restrain the proliferation of androgen-dependent human LNCa-PFGC prostate carcinoma cells *in vitro*.[12,13] Importantly, PGG (**4**) is also an antiangiogenic agent because it was capable of efficiently inhibiting the VEGF-induced proliferation of HUVECs and the growth of immortalized HMECs by obstructing VEGF binding to its receptor tyrosine kinase KDR/Flk-1 and blocking VEGF-induced capillary-like tube formation of endothelial cells on the Matrigel.[14] Based upon the evidences, PGG (**4**) may be a potential agent for development in cancer chemoprevention, antiangiogenesis, and antiinflammation. However, the anti-VEGF activity of PGG (**4**) did not affect the growth of human HT1080 fibrosarcoma cells and DU-145 human prostate cancer cells.[15]

Paeonol (**6**) is a major constituent in its essential oil from the root bark, which has been found to have antiproliferative and proapoptotic activities against hepatocelluar carcinoma and gastric cancer *in vitro* and *in vivo* and against Ece9706 esophageal carcinoma, LoVo colorectal cancer, and DLD-1 colon cancer cell lines *in vitro*. The regulative roles of paeonol (**6**) in apoptosis induction were found to be mediated by the blockage of multiple key signal pathways, including NF-κB, PI3K/PTEN/AKT, and ERK/JNK/P38/MAPKs.[16] Also, at a noncytotoxic concentration, paeonol (**6**) obstructed the migration and the invasion of human chondrosarcoma cells through the upregulation of miR-141 by modulating PKCδ and c-Src signaling pathways, indicating that paeonol (**6**) may be a potential anti-metastasis agent for the treatment of metastatic chondrosarcoma.[17] In addition, several polyphenol components isolated from the peony root were claimed as leukemia inhibitors and apoptosis promoters on leukemia cells.[11]

Agents from Peony Seeds

A methanolic extract from the seeds was found to exert different degrees of antiproliferative activities against HeLa (cervix), MCF-7 (breast), HepG2 (liver), and HT-29 (colon) human neoplastic cell lines.[8] Six cytotoxic stilbenes, assigned as *trans*-resveratrol (**7**), *trans*-ε-viniferin (**8**), *cis*-ε-viniferin (**9**), gnetin-H (**10**), suffruticosol-A (**11**) and suffruticosol-B (**12**), were isolated from the extract. The six stilbenes exhibited a significant cytotoxic effect against mouse C6 glioma cells (IC_{50}: 8.2–20.5 μg/mL). *Trans*-resveratrol (**7**) also modestly exerted the inhibitory effect against the HT-29 and HepG2 cells (respective IC_{50}: 25.2 and 11.8 μg/mL), whereas *trans*-ε-viniferin (**8**), *cis*-ε-viniferin (**9**), and gnetin-H (**10**) displayed a moderate cytotoxic effect on the HeLa and MCF-7 cell lines (IC_{50}: 12.9–21.5 μg/mL). However, suffruticosol-A (**11**) and suffruticosol-B (**12**) had less cytotoxicity on all these cancer cells *in vitro* except on the C6 glioma cells.[18] Likewise, resveratrol (**7**), *trans*-ε-viniferin (**8**), and gnetin-H (**10**) exerted the antiproliferative effect against human MCF-7 breast cancer cells in a similar manner as genistein (an isoflavone from soybean) at a concentration of >25 μM.[19] The stilbenes (**7–10** and **12**) were also reported to show moderate to weak antiproliferative and apoptosis-inducing effects in human HL-60 leukemia cells *in vitro* (IC_{50}: 20–90 μM). Concurrently, each 25 μM of resveratrol (**7**) and suffruticosol-B (**12**) lessened the mRNA level of cytochrome P450 (CYP1B1) and promoted the expression of caspase-3.[20,21]

In addition, the antimutagenic activity of the six stilbenes (**7~12**) was shown in *Salmonella typhimurium* TA100 in a dose-dependent fashion. Of them, resveratrol (**7**) displayed the strongest inhibitory effect against the mutation induced by MNNG, resulting in the IC_{50} value of 27 μg/plate.[22]

Other Bioactivities

Bai Shao (White Shao) and Chi Shao (Red Shao) are historically used as common herbs in traditional Chinese medicine.

Pharmacological approaches established that Bai Shao has antiinflammatory, antianoxemia, analgesic, antipyretic, hepatoprotective, immunoaugmentative, phagocytosis-enhancing, leukocyte-increasing, sedative, antiulcer, vasodilative, platelet aggregation-inhibiting activities, antispasmodic, and antimicrobial activities, whereas Chi Shao showed the biological activities in hepatoprotection, antithrombosis, antithrombocyte aggregation, blood lipid-reduction, cardiac promotion, antiarteriosclerosis, and lung vessel expansion.

References

1. Lee, S. M. Y. et al. 2002. Paeoniae radix, a Chinese herbal extract, inhibit hepatoma cells growth by inducing apoptosis in a p53 independent pathway. *Life Sci.* 71: 2267–77.
2. Huang, K. W. et al. 1985. Influences of red shao on anticancer and cAMP level. *Zhongliu Linchuang* 12: 179–83.
3. Huang, K. W. et al. (a) 1982. *Yaoxue Tongbao* 17: 303, 749; (b) 1999. *Chinese Materia Medica.* Vol. 3, 3–2105, 525. Shanghai Science and Technology Press, Shanghai, China.
4. Huang, K. W. et al. 1983/1984. Effect of Red shao on the growth and metastasis of experimental tumor cells and its pharmacological activities. *Zhonghua Zhongliu Zazhi* 5: 24–7; 6: 319.
5. Tsumura Juntendo Company. 1984. Isolation of biologically active natural products by chromatography. *Jpn. Kokai Tokkyo Koho* JP 59062312 A 19840409.
6. Sakai, Y. et al. 1990. Inhibitory action of peony root extract on the mutagenicity of benzo[a] pyrene. *Mutation Res.* 244: 129–34.
7. Sakai, Y. et al. 1989. Effects of constituents of Paeony root on the mutagenicity of benzo[α] pyrene. *Eisei Kagaku* 35: 433–43.
8. Xu, H. Y. et al. 2007. Effect of total glucosides from radix *Paeoniae rubra* on apoptosis of hepatoma cell in mice. *Zhongcaoyao* 38: 1364–6.
9. Wang, W. J. et al. 2005. Studies on in-vitro biological activity of albiflorin R1 in counteracting cell proliferation. *J. Guangzhou College TCM* 22: 53–5.
10. Li, P. et al. 2014. Monoterpene derivatives from the roots of *Paeonia lactiflora* and their anti-proliferative activity. *Fitoterapia* 98: 124–129.
11. Oba, H. et al. 2001. Plant polyphenols as leukemia inhibitors. *Jpn. Kokai Tokkyo Koho* 11 pp, JP 2000–38873.
12. Lee, S. J. et al. 2003. Inhibition of inducible nitric oxide synthase and cyclooxygenase-2 activity by 1,2,3,4,6-penta-*O*-galloyl-β-D-glucose in murine macrophage cells. *Archiv. Pharm. Res.* 26: 832–9.
13. Washida, K. et al. 2009. Androgen modulators from the roots of *Paeonia lactiflora* (Paeoniae radix) grown and processed in Nara prefecture, Japan. *Chem. Pharm. Bull.* 57: 971–4.
14. Washida, K. et al. 2009. Two new galloylated monoterpene glycosides, 4-*O*-galloylalbiflorin and 4′-*O*-galloylpaeoniflorin, from the roots of *Paeonia lactiflora* (Paeoniae radix) grown and processed in Nara prefecture, Japan. *Chem. Pharm. Bull.* 57: 1150–2.
15. Lee, S. J. et al. 2004. 1,2,3,4,6-Penta-*O*-galloyl-β-D-glucose blocks endothelial cell growth and tube formation through inhibition of VEGF binding to VEGF receptor. *Cancer Lett.* 208: 89–94.
16. Wu, J. et al. 2014. Antitumor effect of paeonol via regulating NF-κB, AKT and MAPKs activation: A quick review. *Biomed. Prevent. Nutr.* 4: 9–14.
17. Horng, C. T. et al. 2014. Paeonol suppresses chondrosarcoma metastasis through up-regulation of miR-141 by modulating PKCδ and c-Src signaling pathway. *Intl. J. Mol. Sci.* 15: 11760–72.
18. Billard, C. et al. 2002. Comparative antiproliferative and apoptotic effects of resveratrol, ε-viniferin and vine-shoots derived poly-phenols (vineatrols) on chronic B lymphocytic leukemia cells and normal human lymphocytes. *Leukemia Lymphoma* 43: 1991–2002.
19. Kim, H. J. et al. 2003. Differential effects of resveratrol and its oligomers isolated from seeds of *Paeonia lactiflora* (peony) on proliferation of MCF-7 and ROS 17/2.8 cells. *J. Food Sci. Nut.* 8: 356–64.
20. Nishida, S. et al. 2003. Induction of apoptosis in HL-60 cells treated with medicinal herbs. *Am. J. Chin. Med.* 31: 551–62.
21. Kang, J. et al. 2003. Resveratrol derivatives potently induce apoptosis in human promyelocytic leukemia cells. *Exper. Mol. Med.* 35: 467–74.
22. Kim, H. J. et al. 2002. Cytotoxic and antimutagenic stilbenes from seeds of *Paeonia lactiflora*. *Archiv. Pharm. Res.* 25: 293–9.

58 Di Huang 地黄

Chinese foxglove

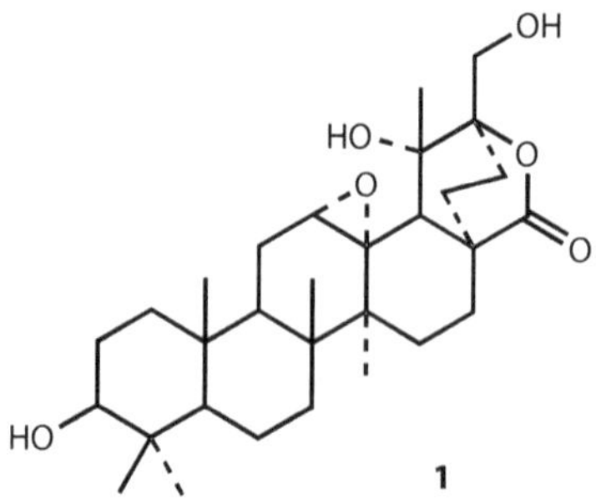

1 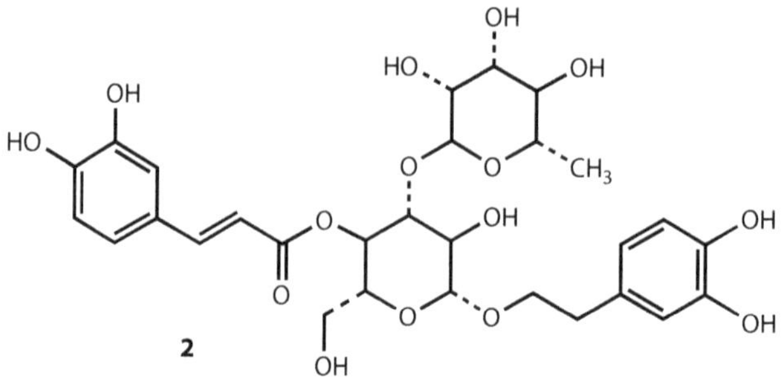 2 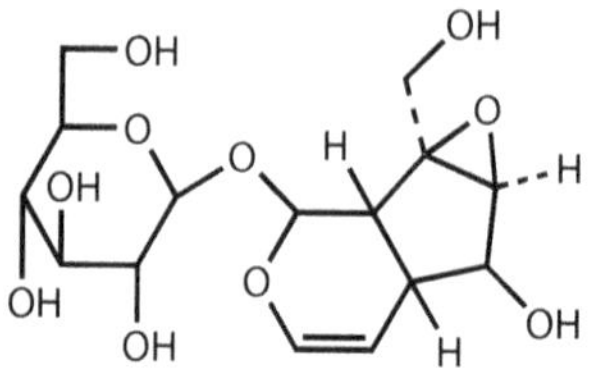 3

Herb Origination

The herb Di Huang (Chinese foxglove) is one of the 50 fundamental herbs used in traditional Chinese medicine, which was documented in the first Chinese materia medica entitled *Shennong Ben Cao Jing*. Di Huang is derived from the tuberous rhizomes of *Rehmannia glutinosa* (Scrophulariaceae). This perennial plant is distributed in many Chinese provinces, but, today, the herb is primarily produced by cultivation. The climatic and edaphic conditions in Jiaozuo of Henan province are conducive for the cultivation of a high-quality Di Huang product. Normally, there are three varieties of the herb, i.e., fresh Di Huang, dried Di Huang (Sheng Di), and cooked Di Huang (Shu Di) for current clinical use.

Antitumor Activity and Constituents

An ethyl acetate fraction derived from Di Huang showed chemopreventive effects on the carcinogenesis.[1] The Di Huang extract was effective in enhancing the cytotoxicity of mitomycin-C against murine P388 leukemic cells in mice and preventing the decrease of leukocyte counts caused by mitomycin-C.[2]

Polysaccharides

The major antitumor ingredients in Di Huang were demonstrated to be polysaccharides, whose antitumor effect was found to be attributed to its marked immunopotentiating property. The crude polysaccharides of Di Huang could significantly augment the proliferation and the tumoricidal effect of T-activated killer cells against Raji lymphoblastoid cells and leukemia L1210 cells in the presence of IL-2 and enhanced IL-2R expression.[3]

RGP-b is a polysaccharide (160 kDa) isolated from the herb, which is composed of five kinds of monosaccharides. RGP-b obviously enhanced the T lymphocyte proliferation of normal mice either *in vitro* or *in vivo* and increased IL-2 secretion simultaneously. The RGP-b suppressed the growth of murine solid tumors (sarcoma 180, Lewis lung, B16 melanoma, and H22 hepatoma) in mice by i.p. injection of 20–40 mg/kg daily for eight days. However, RGP-b was inactive in inhibiting the growth of S80 and HL-60 leukemia cells *in vivo*. To S180-bearing mice, the i.p. administration with RGP-b in doses of 10 or 20 mg/kg resulted in positive immunoregulatory activity, leading to the prolongation of splenic T lymphocyte proliferation. With the RGP-b treatment, the reduced CTL activity by the excessive tumor growth was obviously restored and the descent of IL-2 level and NK activity were also partly ameliorated. RGP-b also kept the ratio of $L3T4^+$ to lyt-2^+ subset lower, whose immune effect on lyt-2^+ T lymphocyte was parallel to that on CTL cytotoxicity, demonstrating the improvement of the lyt-2^+ CTL production, and the cytotoxicity was essential in the cellular immunoenhancing antitumor effect for RGP-b.[4–6]

Lower molecular Rehmannia polysaccharides (LRPS), another kind of Di Huang polysaccharide with a low molecular weight, is the main contents in Di Huang. It evidently inhibited the growth of LLC cells in mice, whose effect was correlated with the marked increase of p53 expression after administration of LRPS. Simultaneously, the expression of c-fos was amplified and the expression of c-Myc was lessened in the LLC cells, showing that these interactions should be involved in the antitumor mechanisms of LRPS.[7,8]

Triterpenoid

Three ursane-type triterpenes assigned as glutinosalactones-A–C were isolated from the 50% aqueous acetone extract of the leaves of *R. glutinosa* (collected in Jiaozuo, China). An *in vitro* assay showed that glutinosalactone-C (**1**) moderately suppressed the proliferation of the three tested human neoplastic cell lines. The IC_{50} values were 8.35 μM in MCF-7 breast cancer cells, 17.29 μM in HepG2 heptoma cells, and 39.25 μM in MG63 osteosarcoma cells.[9]

Phenylpropanoid Glycoside

From the leaves of the Di Huang plant, a phenylpropanoid glycoside elucidated as acteoside (**2**) was extracted, which displays various bioactivities. The antiproliferative effect of acteoside (**2**) was observed in B16-F10 melanoma cells (GI_{50}: 8 μM) and human HL-60 promyelocytic leukemia cells (IC_{50}: 26.7 μM).[10,11] The treatment of the HL-60 cells with acteoside (**2**) blocked the cell cycle progression at G1 phase prior to the induction of differentiation, associated with the increases of p21CIP1/WAF1 and p27KIP1 levels and the decreases in CDK2, CDK4, and CDK6 activities.[12] Moreover, by repressing Ca^{2+}-dependent CaMK/ERK and JNK/NF-κB signaling, acteoside (**2**) inhibited MMP-9 activity and exerted the suppressive effect against PMA-induced invasion and migration of human HT-1080 fibrosarcoma cells.[13] The anti-metastatic activity of acteoside (**2**) was also demonstrated in mice implanted with B16 melanoma cells. The i.p. administration of acteoside (**2**) in a dose of 50 mg/kg every other day obstructed the lung metastasis of B16 melanoma cells.[14] Additionally, acteoside (**2**) was found to have an antiestrogen activity in MCF-7 breast cancer cells and KS483 osteoblasts but no such effect on Ishikawa endometrial cells.[15] In the B16-F10 melanoma cells, acteoside (**2**) showed suppressive effects on the tyrosinase activity and melanin biosynthesis through the activation of a ERK signaling pathway.[16] The antiestrogen and antimelanogenic activities of acteoside (**2**) are considered to be conducive to the chemotherapies of breast cancer and melanoma, respectively.

Iridoid Glucoside

Catalpol (**3**), an effective iridoid glucoside isolated from the herb, demonstrated cardioprotective effects against DOX-induced toxicity without affecting its antitumor activity of the anthracycline. During this action, catalpol (**3**) reduced the level of intracellular ROS and the concentration of MDA and augmented the activities of antioxidant enzymes in DOX-treated H9c2 cells (rat heart cell line), thereby leading to the significant diminishment of DOX-caused damage. Catalpol (**3**) showed no negative interference with the antitumor activity of DOX in HeLa cervical cancer cells[17] but it could ameliorate sodium taurocholate-induced acute pancreatitis in rats by inhibiting the activation of NF-κB,[18] whose activity may be beneficial to the prevention of pancreas carcinogenesis.

Other Bioactivities

The herb Di Huang (Chinese foxglove) has hypoglycemic, hypotensive, immunoincremental, endocrine-regulating, antiinflammatory, hematopoietic stem cell-promoting, antithrombotic, antioxidant, and antifungi properties. Di Huang ethanolic extract displayed a strong scavenging activity against superoxide radical, hydroxyl radical, hydrogen peroxide, and DPPH radical. Through the scavenging activities of free radical and the inhibition of lipid peroxidation, the cooked Di Huang exerted the protective effect against cisplatin-induced HEI-OC1 auditory cell damage in a dose-dependent manner.[19] In addition; catalpol (**3**) also has a broad range of pharmacological activities including antiinflammation, analgesic, and aneuroprotection.

References

1. An, G. H. et al. 1997. Protein kinase-C receptor binding assay for the detection of chemopreventive agents from natural products. *Nat. Prod. Sci.* 3: 29–37.
2. Tsumura Juntendo Co., Ltd. 1984. Enhancement of the antitumor activity of mitomycin-C by plant extracts. *Jpn. Kokai Tokkyo Koho* 4 pp. JP 82–145431 19820824.
3. Wei, H. L. et al. 2002. Enhancement of proliferation and tumoricidal activities of T-AK cells by plant polysaccharides. *Zhongcaoyao* 33: 140–3.
4. Chen, L. Z. et al. 1995. Effects of *Rehmannia glutinosa* polysaccharide b on T-lymphocytes in mice bearing sarcoma 180. *Zhongguo Yaoli Xuebao* 16: 337–40.
5. Chen, L. Z. et al. 1994. Effects of *Rehmannia glutinosa* polysaccharide b on T-lymphocyte function in normal and S180 tumor bearing mice. *Zhongguo Yaolixue Yu Dulixue Zazhi* 8: 125–7.
6. Chen, L. Z. et al. 1993. Immuno-tumoricidal effect of *Rehmannia glutinosa* polysaccharide b and its mechanism. *Zhongguo Yaolixue Yu Dulixue Zazhi* 7: 153–6.
7. Wei, X. L. et al. 1998. Effect of low molecular weight *Rehmannia glutinosa* polysaccharides on the expression of oncogenes. *Zhongguo Yaolixue Yu Dulixue Zazhi* 12: 159–60.
8. Wei, X. L. et al. 1997. Effects of low-molecular-weight *Rehmannia glutinosa* polysaccharides on p53 gene expression. *Zhongguo Yaoli Xuebao* 18: 471–4.
9. Zhang, Y. L. et al. 2013. Three new ursane-type triterpenes from the leaves *of Rehmannia glutinosa. Fitoterapia* 89: 15–9.
10. Nagao, T. et al. 2001. Antiproliferative constituents in the plants: 7. Leaves of *Clerodendron bungei* and leaves and bark of C. trichotomum. *Biol. Pharm. Bull.* 24: 1338–41.
11. Inoue, M. et al. 1998. Induction of apoptotic cell death in HL-60 cells by acteoside, a phenylpropanoid glycoside. *Biol. Pharm. Bull.* 21: 81–3.
12. Lee, K. W. et al. 2007. Acteoside inhibits human promyelocytic HL-60 leukemia cell proliferation via inducing cell cycle arrest at G0/G1 phase and differentiation into monocyte. *Carcinogen.* 28: 1928–36.
13. Hwang, Y. P. et al. 2011. Acteoside inhibits PMA-induced matrix metalloproteinase-9 expression via CaMK/ERK- and JNK/NF-κB-dependent signaling. *Mol. Nutrit. Food Res.* 55(Suppl. 1): S103–S116.
14. Ohno, T. et al. 2002. Antimetastatic activity of acteoside, a phenylethanoid glycoside. *Biol. Pharm. Bull.* 25: 666–8.
15. Papoutsi, Z. et al. 2006. Acteoside and martynoside exhibit estrogenic/antiestrogenic properties. *J. Steroid Biochem. Mol. Biol.* 98: 63–71.
16. Son, Y. O. et al. 2011. Acteoside inhibits melanogenesis in B16F10 cells through ERK activation and tyrosinase down-regulation. *J. Pharmacy Pharmacol.* 63: 1309–19.
17. Wu, X. et al. 2012. Effect of catalpol on doxorubicin-induced cytotoxicity in H9c2 cells. *J. Med. Plants Res.* 6: 849–54.
18. Xiao, W. Q. et al. 2014. Catalpol ameliorates sodium taurocholate-induced acute pancreatitis in rats via inhibiting activation of NF-κB. *Intl. J. Mol. Sci.* 15: 11957–72.
19. Yu, H. H. et al. 2006. Protective effect of *Rehmannia glutinosa* on the cisplatin-induced damage of HEI-OC1 auditory cells through scavenging free radicals. *J. Ethnopharmacol.* 107: 383–8.

3

Anticancer Potentials of Antirheumatics Plant Herbs

CONTENTS

59 Liang Tou Jian 两頭尖

Radde anemone

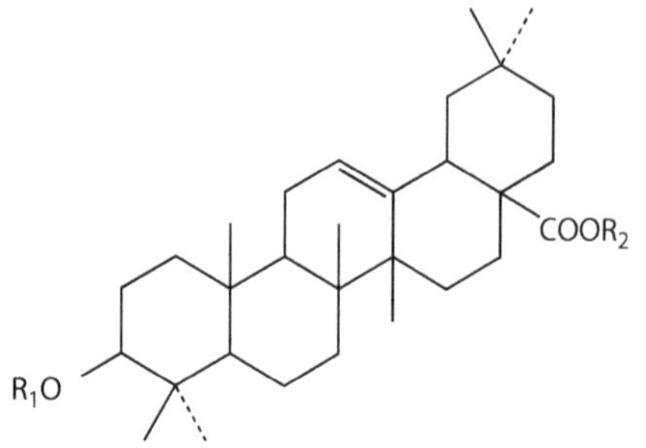

R_1O ... $COOR_2$

1. R_1 = –Ara–(2–1)–Glc–(2–1)–Rhm, R_2 = –H
2. R_1 = –Ara–(2–1)–Glc, R_2 = –H
3. R_1 = –Ara–(2–1)–Rhm, R_2 = –H
5. R_1 = R_2 = –Ara–(2–1)–Glc–(2–1)–Rhm
4. R_1 = –Ara–(2–1)–Rhm, R_2 = –H
(4–1)–Glc

Ara: Alpha-L-arabinopyranosyl
Glc: beta-D-glucopyranosyl
Rham: Alpha-L-rhamnopyranosyl

Herb Origination

The herb Liang Tou Jian (Radde anemone) is the dried rhizomes of a Ranunculaceae plant, *Anemone raddeana*. The herbaceous plant is distributed from the northeast and the east of China to the Far East of Russia, Korea, and Japan. The rhizomes are normally collected in summer and dried in the sun for use in Chinese folk medicine.

Antitumor Constituents and Activities

Saponins

Triterpene saponin components obtained from Liang Tou Jian demonstrated the inhibitory effect against the growth of carcinoma cells *in vitro*. The crude saponin of Liang Tou Jian markedly suppressed human neoplastic cell lines such as KB (nasopharynx), HCT8 (colon), MCF-7WT (breast), and MCF-7/adriamycin (Adm) (Adm-resistant) cells *in vitro* (IC_{50}: 7.68–19.43 μg/mL) and had no cross-resistance to epirubicin. The intragastric infusion of the crude saponin to mice at a dose of 1 g/kg notably restrained the growth of several types of carcinoma cells *in vivo*. The inhibitory rates were 68.1%, 62.5%, and 69.3%, respectively, on sarcoma 180, H22 hepatoma, and EAC.[1]

Raddeanin-A (**1**) is the major component that accounted for 20% of the crude saponin. The inhibitory effects of raddeanin-A (**1**) were demonstrated not only on the proliferation of human KB (nasopharynx), SKOV-3 (ovary), BGC823 (stomach), H460 (lung), and K562 (erythroleukemia) cancer cell lines, *in vitro*, but also on the growth of sarcoma 180, hepatoma 22, and U14 cervical carcinoma cells implanted in mice when injected with raddeanin-A at a dose of 4.5 mg/kg. The IC_{50} values were 4.64 μg/mL on the KB cells and 1.40 μg/mL on the SKOV-3 cells *in vitro*, and the growth inhibition rates were 60.5% on the S180, 36.2% on H22 cells, and 61.8% on U14 cells *in vivo*.[2,3] The dose- and time-dependent antiproliferative effects on H460 cells was accompanied with the induction of cell cycle G2/M arrest and apoptosis, associated with the decline of Bcl-2 protein expression, the inactivation of Akt, and the activation of PARP cleavages.[3] Besides the antiproliferative and apoptosis-promoting effects on BGC-823 cells, raddeanin-A (**1**) was also capable of inhibiting the invasion, the migration, and the adhesion of the gastric carcinoma cells. The apoptotic mechanism on the BGC-823 cells was found to be correlated with the downregulation of Bcl-2, Bcl-xL, and survivin expressions, the upregulation of Bax expression, and the significant activation of caspase-3, caspase-8, caspase-9 and PARP. Raddeanin-A (**1**) also enhanced the expressions of reversion-inducing cysteine-rich protein with Kazal motifs, E-cadherin (E-cad) and diminished the expressions of MMP-2, MMP-9, MMP-14, and Rhoc during the treatment of the BCG-823 cells. These interactions were probably responsible for the inhibitory abilities of raddeanin-A (**1**) on the invasion, migration, and adhesion of the BCG-823 cells.[4]

Other oleanolic acid-based saponins isolated from the herb exerted an obvious antiproliferative effect against the cancer cells *in vitro*. Raddeanin-R2 (**2**), eleutheroside-K (**3**), oleanolic acid 3-*O*-α-L-rhamnosyl (1-2)-[β-D-glucosyl(1-4)]-α-L-arabinoside (**4**) dose dependently suppressed the proliferation of human K562 erythroleukemia cells and human BGC823 gastric carcinoma cells with inhibitory rates of 89.0–97.6% and 88.1–90.0%, respectively.[5] The antigrowth effect of raddeanin-D (**5**) was demonstrated in various solid tumor models such as liver, gastric, lung, and breast carcinomas.[6,7]

By alkali hydrolysis, the total saponins were degraded at C-28 to give the hydrolyzate mixtures, which contains oleanolic acid and oligosaponins R0, RII, and RIII. The anticancer activity of RII and RIII was shown in three tumor cell lines such as SMMC-7721 human hepatoma, HeLa human cervical cancer, and L929 murine fibrosarcoma. The result implied that the hydrolyzation can enhance the cancer inhibitory effect by shortening the sugar chain in the saponins.[8]

Coumarins

Two coumarins identified as 4,7-dimethoxyl-5-methyl-6-hydroxycoumarin (**6**) and 4,7-dimethoxyl-5-formyl-6-hydroxycoumarin (**7**) were isolated from the dried rhizomes. *In vitro* assays showed that these coumarins could moderately inhibit the proliferation of human K562 (leukemia), A549 (NSCLC), and HCT-15 (colon cancer) cell lines with IC_{50} values of 1.37–15.4 μg/mL and 23.5–41.2 μg/mL, respectively.[9]

Polysaccharides

Neutral polysaccharides (ARP) were prepared from the roots of *Anemone raddeana*. The proliferation of human HepG2 hepatocellular carcinoma (HCC) and HCT-22 intestinal neoplastic cell lines could be significantly retarded by ARP treatment *in vitro*.[10] The oral administration of ARP not only significantly inhibited the growth of transplantable H22 hepatoma, but also remarkably promoted splenocytes proliferation, NK cell and CTL activities, serum IL-2 and TNFα productions in tumor-bearing mice, without toxicity to the body weight, the liver, and the kidney. The ARP could also improve the immune response to reverse the hematological parameters lessened by 5-FU to a near normal level.[11] The data evidenced that ARP acts as a immunostimulating agent for anticancer therapy, which may be potential drug leads for the development of a chemopreventive supplement.

Other Bioactivities

The saponin components from Liang Tou Jian (Radde anemone) displayed sedative, analgesic, anticonvulsive, and antiinflammatory effects in the pharmacological researches. The median lethal dose (LD_{50}) of raddeanin-A (**1**) by lavage was 1.1 g/kg and by injection was 16.1 mg/kg.[1]

References

1. Wang, M. K. et al. 2008. Antitumor activity of crude saponin from *Anemone raddeana* Regel. *Yingyong Yu Huanjing Shengwu Xuebao* 14: 378–82.
2. Wang, M. K. et al. 2008. Antitumor effects of raddeanin A on S180, H22 and U14 cell xenografts in mice. *Aizheng* 27: 910–3.
3. Gao, Y. R. et al. 2010. Inhibitory effect of raddeanin A in human non-small cell lung cancer H460 cells. *Yingyong Yu Huanjing Shengwu Xuebao* 16: 637–41.
4. Xue, G. et al. 2013. Raddeanin A induces human gastric cancer cells apoptosis and inhibits their invasion in vitro. *Biochem. Biophys. Res. Commun.* 439: 196–202.
5. Ren, F. Z. et al. 2005. Antitumor active components of rhizome of *Anemone raddeana* Regel. *Zhongcaoyao* 36: 1775–8.
6. Liu, D. Y. et al. 1984. Bioactive triterpane saponins from *Anemone raddeana*. *Zhongcaoyao* 15: 178.
7. Liu, D. Y. et al. 2001. Application of *Anemone raddeana* Regel extract and its preparation. *Faming Zhuanli Shenqing Gongkai Shuomingshu* CN 1312253 A 20010912.
8. Zhang, J. M. et al. 2003. Studies on anticancer activities of triterpenoid in *Anemone raddeana* Regel. *Zhongguo Xinyao Zazhi* 12: 191–3.
9. Ren, F. Z. et al. 2012. Coumarins of *Anemone raddeana* Regel and their biological activity. *Acta Pharm. Sinica* 47: 206–9.
10. Sun, Y. X. et al. 2009. Optimization of extraction technology of the *Anemone raddeana* polysaccharides (ARP) by orthogonal test design and evaluation of its antitumor activity. *Carbohydrate Polymers* 75: 575–9.
11. Liu, Y. et al. 2012. Anti-hepatoma activity in mice of a polysaccharide from the rhizome of *Anemone raddeana*. *Intl. J. Biol. Macromol.* 50: 632–6.

60 Du Huo 獨活

Biserrat Angelica root or Angelica root

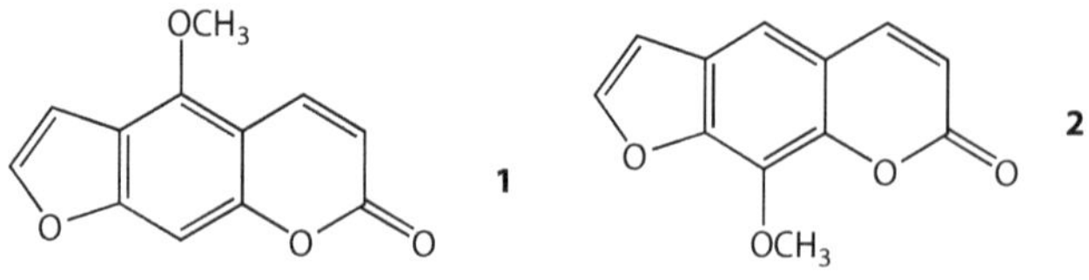

Herb Origination

The herb Du Huo (Angelica root) is one of the traditional Chinese medicines documented in the first Chinese classic of meteria medica titled as *Shennong Ben Cao Jing*. Du Huo is the dried roots of *Angelica biserrata* (Umbelliferae), whose plant distribution ranged in some southern provinces of the Yangtze River, and it is also cultured in the high elevation areas of Sichuan, Hubei, and Shaanxi provinces. Its roots are normally collected in autumn and dried at low temperature for application in Chinese medical practices.

Antitumor Activities and Constituents

Two furancoumarins assigned as bergapten (= 5-methoxypsoralen) (**1**) and xanthotoxin (= 8-methoxypsoralene) (**2**) were the major neoplastic inhibitors in Du Huo. Both coumarins demonstrated the suppressive effect against the growth of human HeLa (cervix) and MK-1 (stomach) cancer cell lines and blocked the incorporation of phosphorus to the tumor cells.[1–3] The coumarins also displayed the tumoricidal activity toward Ehrlich ascites cancer cells but the inhibitory potency of bergapten (**1**) was greater compated to that of xanthotoxin (**2**).[4,5] Bergapten (**1**) in a 100 μg/mL concentration obstructed the growth of human HepG2 hepatoma and SGC-7901 stomach cancer cell lines by 95.0% and 79.6%, respectively.[6] *In vitro* experimental results also showed that either bergapten (**1**) or bergapten plus ultraviolet radiation (PUVA) irritation were able to significantly restrain the proliferation of human neoplastic cell lines including breast cancer cells (MCF-7, ZR-75, SKBR-3, and BCAP), hepatoma cells (J5 and HepG2), gastric cancer cells (SGC-7901), and melanoma cells (B16-F10), together with enhancing cell cycle arrest and apoptosis.[6–10] The mechanism of inducing apoptotic responses in hormone-dependent MCF-7 breast neoplastic cells were investigated, showing that bergapten (**1**) amplified the mRNA and protein levels of p53 and p21waf through p38 MAPK activation and impaired the PI3Kinase/AKT survival signal. Besides PUVA upregulating the p53 expression and decreasing DNA replication, the UV photoactivated bergapten (**1**) also elicited membrane signaling pathways and counteracted the stimulatory effect of IGF-I/E2 mitogenic factors.[7,8]

Xanthotoxin (**2**) as a potent inhibitor of human cytochrome P4502A6 (CYP2A6) markedly exerted a short-term mitogenic effect (24 h) and a long-term antiproliferative effect (48–72 h) on two human melanoma cell lines (SK-Mel28 and C32TG)[11] and inhibited the growth of human A432 epidermal carcinoma cells and a highly metastatic human Mc3 mucoepidermoid cancer cells *in vitro*.[10–13] A synergistic activity could be achieved in the inhibition of Mc3 mucoepidermoid cell proliferation if xanthotoxin (**2**) was combined with homoharringtonine in the treatment.[12] However, xanthotoxin (**2**) was not effective in suppressing the growth of human EJ bladder cells *in vitro* and mouse lung carcinogenesis in the promotion or the progression stages *in vivo*, although it inhibited lung adenoma development elicited by 4-(methylnitrosamino)-1-(3-pyridyl)-1-butanone in mice.[14,15]

Moreover, xanthotoxin (**2**) plus long-wavelength UVA (320–400 nm) was used to clinically treat cutaneous T cell lymphoma as well as other various diseases such as systemic scleroderma, rheumatoid arthritis, and rejection of heart transplants. The xanthotoxin + UVA could modulate the immunogenicity of murine RL1 T cell leukemia cell lines, i.e., enhance both RL1-specific allogenic and syngeneic immune responses in association with the increase of intercellular adhesion molecule-1 expression.[16] In malignant Th2 neoplasms, the xanthotoxin + UVA treatment promoted the Th1-skewing biological action in the T cells and the phototreated T cells, and then stimulated the IL-8 production from monocytes. The xanthotoxin (**2**) combined with phototreated $CD4^+$ T cells could tolerate monocytes to be converted into effective tumor antigen-presenting cells for tumor-specific cytotoxic T cells.[17] In addition, the preexposure of the tumor cells to xanthotoxin (**2**) for 24 h could augment the photocytotoxicity of photofrin-II against EMT-6 murine mammary cancer cells by two to threefold.[18]

Therefore, based on the summary, furancoumarins, bergapten (**1**), and xanthotoxin (**2**) may be considered to be potential drug leads for the further development of photochemotherapeutic agents.

Other Bioactivities

The herb Du Huo (Angelica root) was identified to possess antiplatelet aggregation, antiinflammatory, sedative, antithrombotic, sedative, antiarrhythmic, hypnotic, antispasmodic, and light-sensitive effects by pharmacological studies. Also, bergapten (**1**) shows moderate protection on gastric ulcer.

References

1. Gawron, A. et al. 1987. Cytostatic activity of coumarins in vitro. *Planta Med.* 53: 526–9.
2. Okuyama, T. et al. 1990. Inhibition of tumor-promoter-enhanced phospholipid metabolism by Umbelliferous materials. *Chem. Pharm. Bull.* 38: 1084–6.
3. Fujioka, T. et al. 1999. Antiproliferative constituents from Umbelliferae plants: V. A new furano-coumarin and falcarindiol furanocoumarin ethers from the root of *Angelica japonica. Chem. Pharm. Bull.* 47: 96–100.
4. Meng, Z. M. et al. 1996. Studies of chemical constituents of *Ficus carica* L. *Zhongguo Yaoke Daxue Xuebao* 27: 202–4.
5. Wang, Y. S. et al. 1983. *The Pharmacology and Application of Chinese Medicines*, pp. 796, First Edition. People's Health Publisher, Beijing.
6. Dong, F. et al. 2010. Isolation and identification of bergapten in dry root of glehnia littoralis and preliminary determination of its antitumor activity in vitro. *Zhiwu Ziyuan yu Huanjing Xuebao* 19: 95–6.

7. Panno, M. L. et al. 2010. Breast cancer cell survival signal is affected by bergapten combined with an ultraviolet irradiation. *FEBS Lett.* 584: 2321–6.
8. Panno, M. L. et al. 2009. Evidence that bergapten, independently of its photoactivation, enhances p53 gene expression and induces apoptosis in human breast cancer cells. *Current Cancer Drug Targets* 9: 469–81.
9. Lee, Y. M. et al. 2003. Effect of 5-methoxypsoralen (5-MOP) on cell apoptosis and cell cycle in human hepatocellular carcinoma cell line. *Toxicol. in Vitro* 17: 279–87.
10. Yang, X. W. et al. 2006. Inhibitory effects of coumarins compounds against the growth of human epidermal carcinoma cell line S432 and human mammary cancer cell line BCAP in vitro. *Zhongguo Xiandai Zhongyao* 8: 9–10, 18.
11. Isoldi, M. C. et al. 2004. The role of calcium, calcium-activated K^+ channels, and tyrosine/kinase in psoralen-evoked responses in human melanoma cells. *Braz. J. Med. Biol. Res.* 37: 559–68.
12. Li, Y. et al. 2003. Inhibitory effects of homoharringtonine (HHT) and/or methoxsalen (8-OMP) on highly metastatic human mucoepidermoid carcinoma Mc3 cells. *Shiyong Kouqiang Yixue Zazhi* 19: 339–42.
13. Wu, J. Z. et al. 2000. Effects of psoralen and 8-methoxypsoralen on proliferation and metastatic potential of mucoepidermoid carcinoma Mc3 cells. *Disi Junyi Daxue Xuebao* 21: 911–4.
14. Kuno, T. et al. 2008. Lack of modifying potential of 8-methoxypsoralen in the promotion or progression stages of lung carcinogenesis in A/J female mice. *Oncol. Reports* 20: 767–72.
15. Takeuchi, H. et al. 2009. 8-methoxypsoralen, a potent human CYP2A6 inhibitor, inhibits lung adeno-carcinoma development induced by 4-(methylnitro-samino)-1-(3-pyridyl)-1-butanone in female A/J mice. *Mol. Med. Reports* 2: 585–8.
16. Cheng, T. Y. et al. 1996. The immunological effect of 8-methoxypsoralen and UVA treatment on murine T cell leukemia. *Photochem. Photobiol.* 64: 594–600.
17. Tokura, Y. et al. 2001. Photoactivational cytokine-modulatory action of 8-methoxy-psoralen plus ultraviolet A in lymphocytes, monocytes, and cutaneous T cell lymphoma cells. *Annals of the New York Academy of Sciences* 941 (Cutaneous T cell Lymphoma): 185–93.
18. Sousa, C. et al. 1998. 8-Methoxypsoralen potentiates the photocytotoxic effect of photofrin II towards EMT-6 murine mammary tumor cells. *Cancer Lett.* (Shannon, Ireland) 128: 177–82.

61 Wei Ling Xian 威靈僊

Chinese clematis

COOH
H_3CO
OH
A
R_2
R_1

1. R_1 = –CH_3, R_2 = –O–Ara–(2–1)–Rham–(3–1)–Rib–(4–1)–Glc–(4–1)–Glc–(6–1)–Rham
2. R_1 = –CH_3, R_2 = –O–Ara–(2–1)–Rham–(3–1)–Rib
3. R_1 = –CH_2OH, R_2 = –O–Ara–(2–1)–Rham–(3–1)–Rib–(4–1)–Glc–(6)–A
4. R_1 = –CH_3, R_2 = –O–Ara–(2–1)–Rham–(3–1)–Rib–(4–1)–Glc–(6)–A
8. R_1 = –CH_3, R_2 = –O–Ara–[(4–1)–Rham]–(2–1)–Rib
5. R_1 = –CH_2OH, R_2 = –O–Ara–(2–1)–Rham–(3–1)–Rib–(4–1)–Glc (4–1)–Glc
6. R_1 = –CH_2OH, R_2 = –O–Ara–(2–1)–Rham–(3–1)–Rib–(4–1)–Glc(4–1)–Glc–(4)–A
7. R_1 = –CH_2OH, R_2 = –O–Ara–(2–1)–Rham–(3–1)–Rib–(4–1)–Glc
9. R_1 = –CH_3, R_2 = OH

Ara: alpha–L–arabinopyranosyl; Glc: beta–D–glucopyranosyl; Rham: alpha–L–rhamnopyranosyl; Rib: beta–D–ribopyranosyl

Herb Origination

The herb Wei Ling Xian (Chinese clematis) is the dried rhizomatic roots of five Ranunculaceae plants such as *Clematis chinensis* and *C. mandshurica*. The first plant is the major source of the herb, and it is broadly distributed in the central, the eastern, and the southern regions of China as well as in the Ryukyu Islands and Vietnam. The herb was documented in *Kaibao Ben Cao*, the pharmacopeia of the Chinese Song dynasty, and the herb is predominantly produced in eastern China now.

Antitumor Constituents and Activities

Three kinds of constituents, protoanemonin, triterpend saponins, and polysaccharides, isolated from the herb have been reported to have the antineoplastic property.

Triterpene Saponins

The total triterpene saponins derived from the herb effectively suppressed the growth of two human promyelocytic leukemia cell lines (HL-60 and NB4) *in vitro* concomitantly with the promotion of apoptotic death and the disturbance of the cell cycle progression.[1,2] *In vitro* and *in vivo* investigations also demonstrated that the total saponins were effective in the growth inhibition of three murine tumor cells (HepA hepatoma, P388 leukemia, and sarcoma 180) and human HL-60 leukemia cells associated with the induction of apoptosis and cell cycle arrest. At doses of 0.3, 0.6, and 1.2 g/kg, the oral administration of the saponins to tumor transplanted to mice markedly inhibited the cell growth by 42.78–58.25% in S180 cells, 37.44–59.36% in HepA cells, and 34.50–54.39% in P388 cells.[3–5] From the total saponins, eight saponin compounds were isolated from *C. chinensis* and a group of saponin compounds from *C. mandshurica*. Two monodesmosidic saponins (3β-[(O-α-L-rhamnopyranosyl-(1-6)-O-β-D-glucopyranosyl-(1-4)-O-β-D-glucopyranosyl-(1-4)-O-β-D-ribopyranosyl-(1-3)-O-α-L-rhamnopyranosyl-(1-2)-α-L-arabinopyranosyl)oxy] olean-12-en-28-oic acid and 3β-[(O-β-D-ribopyranosyl-(1-3)-O-α-L-rhamnopyranosyl-(1-2)-α-L-arabinopyranosyl)oxy] olean-12-en-28-oic acid) from *C. chinensis* displayed an obvious cytotoxic effect against HL-60 leukemia cells (respective IC_{50}: 2.8 and 2.3 μM). Other types of BSY-1 (breast), PC3 (prostate), and SF-295 and U251 (CNS) human cancer cell lines were relatively sensitive to the saponin (**1**) (LC_{50}: 5.9–6.3 μM), but MKN28 (gastric), NCI-H460 (lung), and OVCAR-8 and OVCAR-3 (ovary) tumor cell lines were relatively resistant to the saponin (**1**) (LC_{50}: of 30–71 μM).[6] The antiproliferative effect of mandshunosides-A–E (**3–7**) derived from *C. mandshurica* were markedly present on two human colorectal cancer cell lines (HCT-116 and HT-29) *in vitro*. Their respective IC_{50} values were 0.6 and 0.9 μM for mandshunoside-D (**6**) and 2.1–3.0 and 2.8–4.2 μM for mandshunoside-A–C and mandshunoside-E.[7,8] The inhibition on the HCT-116 and HT-29 cells was moderately exerted by clematiganoside-A, clematichinenoside-C, clematochinenoside-A, and huzhongoside-B. In human PC3 prostate cancer cells, the isolated clematomandshurica saponin-J and clematomandshurica saponin-K exhibited the inhibitory effect (respective GI_{50}: 1.29 and 1.50 μM), and another monodesmosidic saponin (**8**) exerted a better antiproliferative effect (GI_{50}: 0.71 μM).[9] Based upon the scientific facts, the Wei Ling Xian saponins may be a potential candidate for further development to a clinic chemotherapeutic adjuvant against the carcinomas.

Saponin Aglycone

The saponin aglycone identified as oleanolic acid (**9**) was also found to have apoptosis-enhancing, antiproliferative, and anti-invasive effects against human HeLa cervical cancer cells *in vitro* in association with the activation of caspase-3 and the inhibition of MMP-3 and MMP-9 expressions.[10,11] An *in vivo* experiment showed that oleanoic acid (**9**) not only restrained the proliferation of hepatoma cells in mice but also protected the function of the liver that was injured by the tumor. Simultaneously, oleanoic acid (**9**) diminished the vascular endothelial growth factor (VEGF) and microvessel density (MVD) levels and suppressed aspartate aminotransferase (AST) and alanine aminotransferase (ALT) activities.[12] Therefore, the data demonstrated the therapeutic and preventive potentials of oleanoic acid in hepatoma and liver disease.

Protoanemonin Derivatives

Protoanemonin isolated from the herb only had some weak suppressive effects on the tumor cells, but three synthetic protoanemonin derivatives (Br-, I-, OAc) in concentrations of ~20 μg/mL displayed noticeable growth inhibition and S cell-arresting effects against human MCF-7 breast cancer cells *in vitro* in concentration- and time-dependent manners. 5-Bromo-methylfuran-2-one, one of the derivatives, exerted the relatively strongest antiproliferative activity on the MCF-7 cells.[13] The *in vitro* assays found that 5-bromomethylfuran-2-one was also effective in the suppression of HepG2 (liver) and A549 (lung) human neoplastic cell lines in association with the promotion of apoptosis and cell cycle arrest.[14,15] Its apoptotic mechanisms were revealed to be mediated by mitochondrial and extrinsic or death receptor pathways, i.e., (1) reduction of Bcl-2 expression and upregulation of Bax activity, (2) increase of Fas expression level and decrease of NF-κB signal transduction, and (3) activation of caspase-3 and caspase-8.[14,15]

Polysaccharides

The polysaccharide fraction prepared from *C. chinensis* displayed the growth inhibitory effect against human Tca-8113 tongue squamous cell cancer cells *in vitro*.[16] It was also capable of promoting the apoptotic death of SKOV-3 ovarian cancer, MCF-7 breast carcinoma, and Bel-7402 hepatoma cells. The apoptosis-inducing mechanism was associated with the activation of Fas expression and the inhibition of Bcl-2 expression.[17–19]

In conclusion, from the experimental findings, the antitumor activity of Wei Ling Xian (Chinese clematis roots) was revealed to be mostly attributed to some of its saponin constituents and polysaccharides. These results provide a scientific support for the application of Wei Ling Xian in Chinese medicine prescriptions for cancer treatment in clinics.

Other Medical Uses

The herb Wei Ling Xian (Chinese clematis) in traditional Chinese medicine is used in many herbal remedies exerting a variety of intriguing biological properties such as diuretic, antiperiodic, anodyne, choleretic, odinopoeia, antispasmodic, and anti-microorganism. The herb also has a history of folk practices in the treatment of arthritis and rheumatism, tetanus, and cold-type stomachache. But due to containing protoanemonin, the herb is a mild skin irritant. The protoanemonin can be polymerized to produce anemonin, which is toxic to the heart and the CNS, but the toxic principle can be dissipated by heat and by drying. Additionally, the whole plant extract has antirheumatic activity in the pharmacological test.

References

1. Zhou, Y. et al. 2011. Radix clematidis saponins inhibits NB4 cells and through inducement of apoptosis. *Zhongliu Fangzhi Yanjiu* 38: 881–5.
2. Chen, Y. R. et al. 2011. Study on clematis saponins inhibiting HL-60 cell growth. *J. Luzhou Med. College* 34: 231–4.
3. Qiu, G. Q. et al. 1999. The antitumour activity of total saponin of *Clematis chinensis*. *Zhongyaocai* 22: 351–3.
4. Zhao, Y. et al. 2010. Antitumor effects of *Clematis chinensis* saponins and its influences on proliferation and cell cycle of tumor cells. *Shizhen Guoyi Guoyao* 21: 1908–9.
5. Huang, L. et al. 2012. Effect of total saponin from radix Clematidis on acute promyelocytic leukemia HL60 cell line in vitro. *Zhongguo Shiyan Fangjixue Zazhi* 18: 311–5.
6. Mimaki, Y. et al. 2004. Triterpene saponins from the roots of *Clematis chinensis*. *J. Nat. Prod.* 67: 1511–6.
7. He, Y. X. et al. 2011. Cytotoxic triterpene saponins from *Clematis mandshurica*. *J. Asian Nat. Prod.* 13: 1104–9.
8. Li, L. et al. 2013. Mandshunosides C-E from the roots and rhizomes *of Clematis mandshurica*. *Phytochem. Lett.* 6: 570–4.
9. Gong, Y. X. et al. 2013. Triterpene saponins from *Clematis mandshurica* and their antiproliferative activity. *Planta Med.* 79: 987–94.
10. Huang, Z. Q. et al. 2011. Study on inhibitive effect of oleanolic acid on transplanted hepatocarcinoma in mice. *J. Anhui Agricul. Sci.* 39: 10807–8, 10851.
11. Wang, J. et al. 2011. Effect of oleanolic acid on the apoptosis of cervical cancer HeLa cells. *J. Heilongjiang Med. Pharmacy* 34: 31–2.
12. Ma, Y. et al. 2012. Effect of oleanolic acid on the apoptosis and invasion of cervical cancer HeLa cells. *Shandong Med. J.* 52: 47–9.
13. Jiang, F. Y. et al. 2012. Effects of protoanemonin derivatives on inducing apoptosis of human breast carcinoma MCF-7 cell line in vitro. *Tianjin Med. J.* 40: 876–878; *Shandong Med. J.* 49: 19–21.
14. Liu, B. X. Z. et al. 2012. Weilingxian antitumor research progress. *J. Changchun TCM Univer.* 28: 165–7.
15. Chan, G. H. et al. 2011. Effect of protoanemonin derivatives on inducing apoptosis of human hepatoma HepG2 cells. *J. Yanbian Univ.* 31–3.
16. Li, J. Y. et al. 2011. Polysaccharide from *Clematis chinensis* Osbeck inhibiting the growth of tongue squamous cell carcinoma. *Shengwu Jishu Tongxun* 22: 255–7.
17. Zhang, J. et al. 2011. Polysaccharides from *Clematis chinensis* induces the apoptosis of human hepatoma Bel-7402 cells. *J. Mudanjiang Med. Univ.* 32: 9–11.
18. Zhang, J. et al. 2011. Polysaccharides from *Clematis chinensis* induces the apoptosis of human breast cancer MCF-7 cells and influences the Bcl-2-Fas expression. *Chin. J. Birth Health and Heredity* 19: 17–8, 22.
19. Yang, X. D. 2011. Effects of radix Clematidis polysaccharide on the apoptosis of human ovary cancer SKOV3 cells. *Zhongyiyao Tongbao* 10: 61–2.

62 Chi Geng Teng 匙羹藤

Gurmar or Gymnema

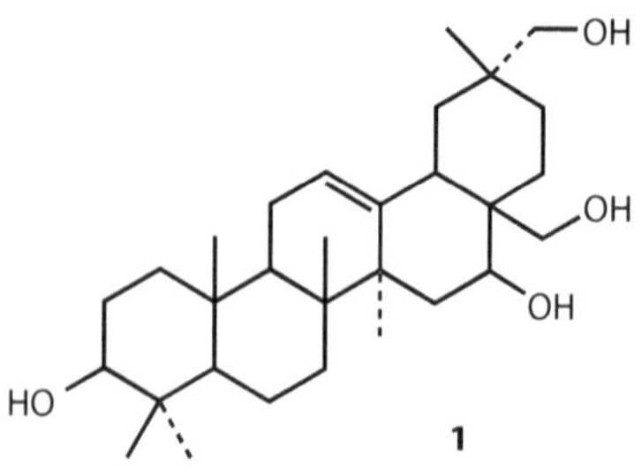

OH OH OH HO 1

Herb Origination

A woody slender plant *Gymnema sylvestre* (Asclepidaceae) is the origin of Chi Geng Teng (Gurmar). This annual climber is widespread in Asian tropical and subtropical regions from India to southern China and parts of Africa with a long history of traditional medicine. For local medicinal practice in China, its roots are collected any seasons and dried in the sun, and its leaves with twigs are commonly collected in spring. Also, the leaves and roots of *G. sylvestre* can be used fresh for the medical purpose.

Antitumor Activities

The extracts derived from Chi Geng Teng were investigated for antineoplastic activity on human MCF-7 (breast) and A549 (lung) epithelial carcinoma cell lines, *in vitro.* All three extracts (alcohol, chloroform, and ethyl acetate) were effective in the inhibition of MCF-7 cell proliferation with IC_{50} values of 9.0, 8.5, and 17 μg/mL, respectively, whereas etoposide (a current clinic anticancer drug) showed a similar IC_{50} value of 9.5 μg/mL in the same testing condition. But, the inhibitory effect of the extracts on A549 cells (IC_{50}: >88 μg/mL) was much lower than that of etoposide (IC_{50} 19.5 μg/mL).[1] An ethanolic extract of *G. sylvestre* leaves, which is used as an antihyperglycemic agent, showed anticancer and proapoptotic potentials in human A375 melanoma cells, whose effect was mediated by the stimulation of reactive oxygen species generation and mitochondria-dependent caspase pathway, including the decrease of the expressions of ICAD, EGFR, and Bcl-2 and the increases of mRNA expressions of apoptotic signal-related genes (cytochrome c, caspase-3, PARP, Bax).[2] The leave extract (containing 10.5% gymnemic acid) at a 1 mg/mL concentration almost completely obstructed the breast cancer resistance protein-mediated transport of methotrexate (MTX), to potentiate the antitumor activity of the chemotherapeutic drug.[3]

Antitumor Constituents and Activities

Triterpenoid

A triterpenoid assigned as gymnemagenol (**1**) isolated from the leave extracts demonstrated a moderate cytotoxicity on human HeLa cervical cancer cells *in vitro* (IC_{50}: 37 μg/mL, at 48 h). Gymnemagenol (**1**) at a concentration of 50 μg/mL displayed a 63% inhibitory effect against the HeLa cells, while a chemotherapeutic agent 5-FU had 57.5% suppression (IC_{50}: 36 μg/mL). After being treated with gymnemagenol (**1**) for 96 h, the induced percentage of HeLa cell death could reach to a maximum of 73%.[4] The antigrowth activity of gymnemagenol (**1**) was also observed on human HepG2 hepatoma cells (IC_{50}: 18.5 μg/mL at 24 h) *in vitro*, although the activity was less than that of 5-FU (IC_{50}: 1.34 μg/mL).[5]

Polysaccharides

From a crude polysaccharide component of *G. sylvestre* leaves, five water-soluble polysaccharides were purified and labeled as GSP11 (xylose: glucose, 1:2.47), GSP22 (rhamnose: galactose: glucose, 1.6:1.22:1), GSP33 (rhamnose: galactose: glucose, 1:1.1:1.5), GSP44 (xylose: glucose: galactose, 1:1.03:1.2), and GSP55 (xylose: glucose: rhamnose: galactose, 1.21:1.81:1:2.58). Their molecular weights were established as 5.3×10^4, 5.4×10^5, 9.5×10^5, 1.0×10^6, and 1.9×10^6 Da, respectively. These polysaccharides except for GSP22, in the *in vitro* assay, displayed antiproliferative effects in a dose-dependent manner in AGS gastric tumor cells. At the same concentration of 640 μg/mL, GSP11 and GSP33 showed great activities in U937 histiocytic lymphoma cells with respective inhibitory rates of 78.6% and 83.8%, while GSP22 exerted a similar degree of activity in SGC gastric cancer cells with an inhibitory rate of 78.2%. In addition, these polysaccharides, at a concentration of 300 mg/kg, also presented marked immunological properties, especially on blood serum hemolysin formation.[6] These results provided not only a scientific support for the herb application in folk prescription but also a suggestion of the potential polysaccharides used as natural supplements for cancer prevention and treatment.

Other Bioactivities

The extracts of Chi Geng Teng (Gurmar) are widely used as a folk drug in Australia, Japan, Vietnam, India, and southern China. It has been used as a natural treatment of diabetes for nearly two millennia in India, because it acted as a sugar destroyer to maintain the blood glucose of the body in healthy levels and to regulate sugar metabolism. The powdered Chi Geng Teng roots (Gymnema) are often used to treat snakebites, constipation, stomach complaints, water retention, and liver disease in southern Asian countries. Pharmacological studies characterized its multiple curative properties responsible for antimytotoxic, antioxidant, antihepatotoxic, antiperlipedemic, antihaemorrhagic, antihyperglycemic, analgesic, immunomodulatory, antiinflammatory, hair growth-promoting, and antibacterial activities.

References

1. Srikanth, A. V. et al. 2010. Anticancer activity of *Gymnema sylvestre* R. Br. *Intl. J. Pharm. Sci. Nanotechnol.* 3: 897–9.
2. Chakraborty, D. et al. 2013. Anti-hyperglycemic drug *Gymnema sylvestre* also shows anticancer potentials in human melanoma A375 cells via reactive oxygen species generation and mitochondria-dependent caspase pathway. *Integr. Cancer Therapies* 12: 433–41.

3. Tamaki, H. et al. 2010. Inhibitory effects of herbal extracts on breast cancer resistance protein (BCRP) and structure-inhibitory potency relationship of isoflavonoids. *Drug Metabol. Pharmacokinetics* 25: 170–9.
4. Khanna, V. G. et al. 2009. Anticancer-cytotoxic activity of saponins isolated from the leaves of *Gymnema sylvestre* and *Eclipta prostrata* on HeLa cells. *Intl. J. Green Pharmacy* 3: 227–9.
5. Khanna, V. G. et al. 2010. Non-proliferative activity of saponins isolated from the leaves of *Gymnema sylvestre* and *Eclipta prostrata* on HepG2 cells-in vitro study. *Intl. J. Pharm. Sci. Res.* 1: 38–42.
6. Wu, X. Y. et al. 2012. Isolation, purification, immunological and anti-tumor activities of polysaccharides from *Gymnema sylvestre. Food Res. Intl.* 48: 935–9.

63 Kun Ming Shan Hai Tang 昆明山海棠

Whiteback Thundergod Vine

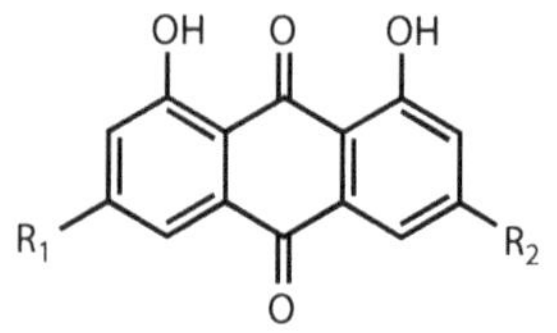

OH O OH

R_1 R_2

O

1. $R_1 = -CH_3$, $R_2 = -OCH_3$
2. $R_1 = -H$, $R_2 = -COOCH_2CH_3$

Herb Origination

The herb Kun Ming Shan Hai Tang (KMSHT) originated from a Celastraceae plant, *Tripterygium hypoglaucum*. This perennial plant is distributed in some Chinese provinces in the south of the Yangtze River. Normally, its roots are collected in late autumn and dried in the sun for folk medical practices. The herb was first documented as a toxicant in *Ben Cao Gangmu*, the most comprehensive medical book written in Chinese Ming dynasty.

Antitumor Activities and Constituents

The herb exerted significant cytotoxic and genotoxic effects on human HL-60 promyelocytic leukemia cells, and it concentration-dependently induced the mutagenesis of HL-60 cells. The mutation of HL-60 cells elicited by the extract was mainly mediated by the deletion of the hypoxanthine-guanine phosphoribosyl transferase gene.[1,2] The alcoholic extract of KMSHT exhibited the inhibitory activity against mouse U14 cervical carcinoma and S180 and S37 sarcomas for 40% and 33–52%, respectively.[3]

Alkaloids

Alkaloids in KMSHT were demonstrated to be potent antineoplastic components. Its total alkaloids (THHta) at a concentration of 100 μg/mL exerted the *in vitro* growth inhibitory effect on MOLT-4 and Jurkat leukemia, B16-F10 melanoma, and SW480 colon carcinoma cell lines with about 80% inhibitory rates.[4] In the Jurkat cells, the THHta promoted the cell cycle G1 arrest and the apoptosis in association with the augmentation of the activities of caspase-3, caspase-7, and PARP, enhancing the expressions of FasL and Bid, suppressing DNA synthesis and repairing DNA damage.[5,6] The apoptosis-inducing and growth inhibitory effects in the HL-60 cells by THHta was mediated by increasing the activities of c-Myc binding protein and caspase-3 and caspase-8 and upregulating the expressions of 16 genes related to the disturbance of the NF-κB signaling pathway.[7] However, the alkaloids also exerted toxic and mutagenic effects on TK gene in mouse lymphoma L5178Y cells *in vitro*.[8]

The growth inhibitory property of THHta on human HCT116 colon cancer was also demonstrated in both *in vitro* and *in vivo* models. In nude mice implanted with HCT116 cells, the tumor size and weight of the xenografts were significantly lessened by 80.2% in the treatment with THHta at a dose of 200 mg/kg. The antineoplastic effect may be closely correlated with the downregulation of proliferation cell nuclear antigen (PCNA) expression level and the increase of G0/G1 phase arrest and apoptotic death in the HCT116 cells.[9,10] The apoptosis induction of THHta was found to be mediated by the activation of caspase-3 and PARP and the inhibition of Bcl-2, Bcl-xL, and XIAP.[11] Also, THHta significantly inhibited the tumor-promoter TPA-induced cell neoplastic transformation in mouse JB6 Cl41 epidermal cells.[11] In these alkaloids, the most potent antiproliferative alkaloid in KMSHT was established to be triptolide (see Section Lei Gong Teng).[12]

Anthraquinones

Two anthraquinones determined as rhein ethyl ester (**1**) and physcion (**2**) were isolated from KMSHT, which were both responsible for the cytotoxicity against neoplasm. Rhein ethyl ester (**1**) and physcion (**2**) were moderately effective in the inhibition of human ovarian carcinoma cell lines (A2780 and OVCAR-3) with IC_{50} values in a range of 12.1–20.0 μg/mL, but physcion (**2**) also retarded the growth of IOSS144 cells, a normal cell line with the similar IC_{50} data.[13]

Other Bioactivities

The herb KMSHT is used in traditional Chinese medicine for the treatment of rheumatoid arthritis, autoimmune diseases, and various skin disorders, exhibiting many medicinal benefits such as antiarthritic, antiinflammation, immunosuppression, antifertility, and pregnancy-termination besides antineoplasm. The herb also causes no fertility on both man and woman in during KMSHT administration period. The alkaloid extract has been proven as a potent HSV-1 inhibitor in the *in vitro* experiments.

Toxicity

Because of its toxicity, the herb KMSHT should be used very carefully when treating children and fertile women, and it is better not to allow its use for the treatment of pregnant women. Use of the herb is not advisable in high doses and for long-term administration. Tea has been reported being able to release the toxicity of KMSHT when administration of the decoction with tea.

References

1. Liu, S. X. et al. 2000. Molecular analysis of *Tripterygium hypoglaucum* (Levl) Hutch-induced mutations at the HPRT locus in human promyelocytic leukemia cells by multiplex polymerase chain reaction. *Yichuan* (Chinese) 22: 305–8.
2. Liu, S. X. et al. 2002. Molecular analysis of THH-induced mutations at HPRT locus in human promyelocytic leukemia cells with multiplex polymerase chain reaction. *J. Med. Colleges of PLA* 17: 105–11.
3. Wang, Y. S. et al. 1983. *The Pharmacology and Application of Chinese Medicines* (*Zhongyao Yaoli yu Yingyong*), pp. 666, First Edition. People's Health Publisher, Beijing.

4. Huang, X. C. et al. 2006. In vitro experimental study of the anticancer effect of total alkaloids of *Tripterygium hypoglaucum. Zhongguo Yiyuan Yaoxue Zazhi* 26: 442–5.
5. Yang, L. J. et al. 2003. Tripterygium hypoglaucum (Levl) Hutch alkaloids induce PARP cleavage and caspase-3 activation in Jurkat T lymphoma cells. *Disan Junyi Daxue Xuebao* 25: 1505–20.
6. Zhao, Q. J. et al. 2003. *Tripterygium hypoglaucum* (Levl) Hutch alkaloids induce apoptosis of Jurkat lymphoma cells via the Fas receptor-mediated pathway. *Disan Junyi Daxue Xuebao* 25: 1521–3.
7. Zhuang, W. J. et al. 2004. Involvement of NF-κB and c-myc signaling pathways in the apoptosis of HL-60 cells induced by alkaloids of Tripterygium hypoglaucum (levl.) Hutch. *Phytomed.* 11: 295–302.
8. Lin, S. X. et al. 2003. Effects of total alkaloids of *Tripterygium hypoglaucum* Hutch on tk gene of mouse lymphoma cells. *Zhongguo Zhongyao Zazhi* 28: 954–7.
9. Huang, X. C. et al. 2009. Effects of total alkaloids of *Tripterygium hypoglaucum* Hutch on the growth of xenografts of human colon cancer cell line HCT116 in nude mice. *Mianyixue Zazhi* 25: 547–9, 553.
10. Huang, X. C. et al. 2009. Effects of total alkaloids of *Tripterygium hypoglaucum* Hutch on proliferation and apoptosis of human colon cancer cell line HCT116. *Di-San Junyi Daxue Xuebao* 31: 2246–8.
11. Jiang, X. et al. 2014. Total alkaloids of *Tripterygium hypoglaucum* (levl.) Hutch inhibits tumor growth both in vitro and in vivo. *J. Ethnopharmacol.* 151: 292–8.
12. Cao, J. et al. 2003. Molecular mechanisms of apoptosis in leukemia cells induced with *Tripterygium hypoglaucum* (Levl) Hutch alkaloids. *Disan Junyi Daxue Xuebao* 25: 1499–500.
13. Li, W. et al. 2011. A new natural compound with cytotoxic activity from *Tripterygium hypoglaucum. Chin. Herbal Med.* 3: 232–4.

64 Shan Hu Shu 珊瑚樹

Sweet Viburnum

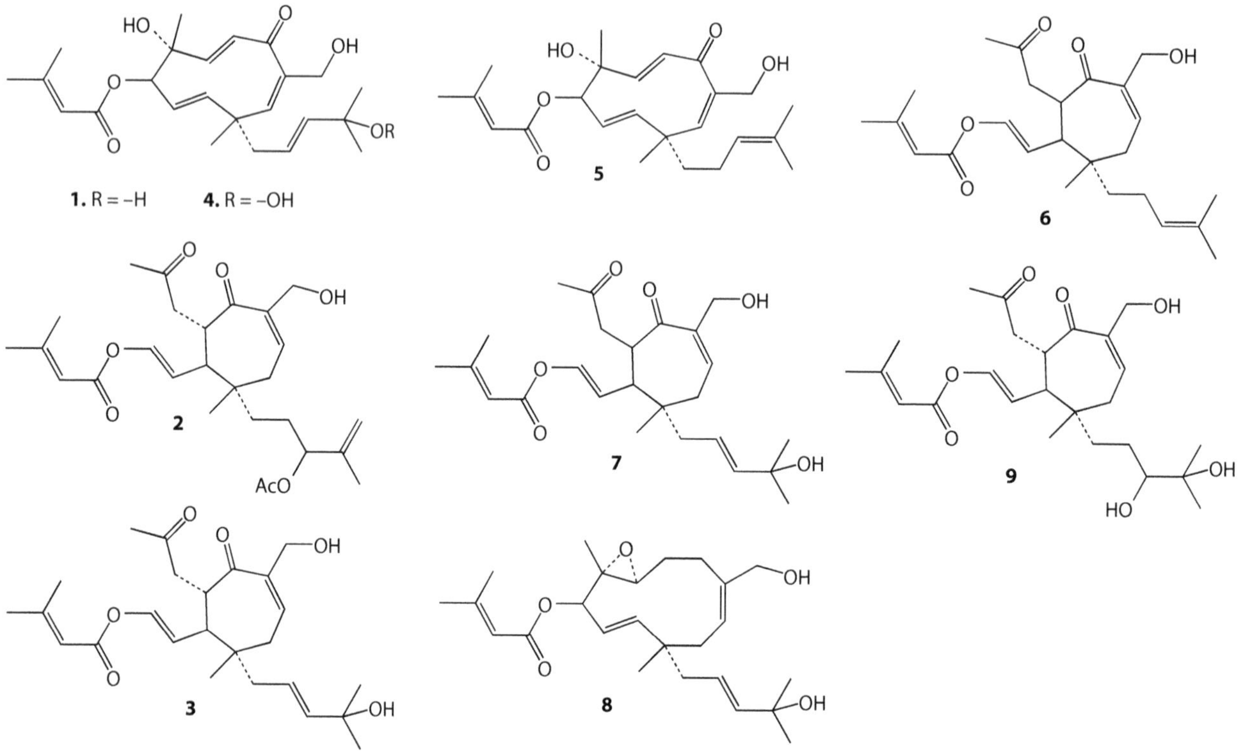

1. R = -H 4. R = -OH

5

6

2

7

9

3

8

(a)

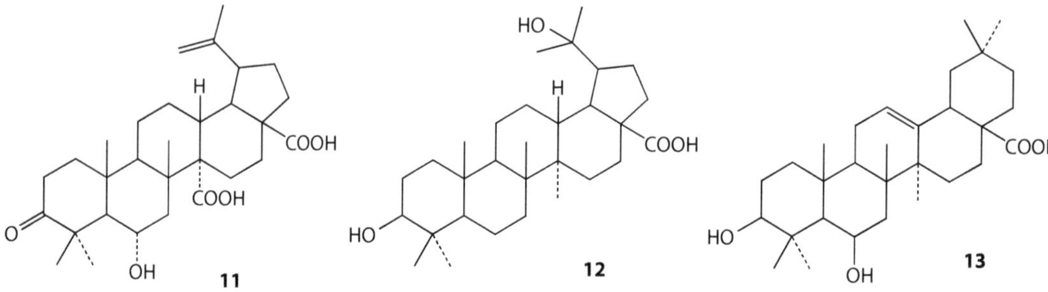

11

12

13

(b)

Herb Origination

The herb Shan Hu Shu (Sweet Viburnum) originates from a Caprifoliaceae tree, *Viburnum odoratissimum*. It is a large evergreen shrub native to Asia, which is generally distributed in the southern region of the Yangtze River and is widely cultivated in semitropical and tropical gardens in the world. Its leaves, barks and roots are collected for use in folk medical treatment. A same genus plant *V. awabuki* (Chindo Viburnum) was also found to have bioactivities in recent years.[1] Also, the two evergreen shrubs are now extensively planted in the southern United States and in other semitropical areas today.

Antitumor Constituents and Activities

Up to now, several types of molecules, such as triterpenes, diterpenes, sesquiterpenes, coumarines, flavonoids, and lignans, have been discovered from the two Viburnum plants. The two plants *V. awabuki* and *V. odoratissimum* are very rich in vibsane-type diterpenoids that are the characteristic components, and some of them are major anticancer constituents. However, under strong light irritation or high temperature, the rearrangement can be elicited in this type of diterpenes. The triterpenoid components were shown as another type of antitumor agents derived from the plants.

Diterpenes from V. odoratissimum

The bioassay-directed fractionation of the extracts of its leaves and/or flowers led to the isolation of a group of vibsane-type diterpenes. Vibsanol-A (**1**) at a concentration of 10 μM showed an obvious cytotoxicity against human NUGC gastric tumor cells,[2] and 5-epi-vibsanin-G at a concentration of 20 μg/mL had only a weak inhibition against the NUGC-3 cells (58% survival).[3] 18-*O*-methylvibsanin-G acetate (**2**) and a vibsane diacetate (**3**) at concentrations of 20 μg/mL moderately inhibited the survival of human NUGC-3 gastric and HONE-1 nasopharyngeal cancer cells.[3] From an acetone extract of its small twigs, the isolated vibsanin-K (**4**) was effective in the suppression of the NUGC cell proliferation at a concentration of 50 μg/mL.[4] In addition, another vibsane-type diterpenoid at concentrations of 5–10 μmol/L dose- and time-dependently inhibited the proliferation of HepG2 hepatoma cells concomitant with the induction of G0/G1 cell cycle arrest and apoptosis via a dose-dependent activation of caspase-3 and caspase-7.[5]

Diterpenoids from V. awabuki

More vibsane-type diterpenes with an antitumor activity have been isolated from the leaves and/or the twigs of *V. awabuki*. Vibsanin-B (**5**), vibsanin-C, and 5-epi-vibsanin-C (**6**) moderately suppressed the growth of human KB oral epidermal cancer cells *in vitro* (IC_{50}: 3.5, 11.3, and 10.7 μM, respectively), while 5-epi-vibsanin-H (**7**) only exhibited a weak effect on KB cells (IC_{50}: 45.5 μM).[6,7] However, vibsanin-K (**4**), which has a hydroperoxy function, showed no cytotoxicity on the KB cells, demonstrating that the hydroperoxy group is not related to the antitumor activity.[7] Vibsanin-P (**8**) and vibsanin-W (**9**) displayed a marked cytotoxic effect against mouse P388 leukemia cells (ED_{50}: 2.18–2.25 μg/mL), human A549 lung carcinoma cells (ED_{50}: 4.62–5.60 μg/mL), and human colon cancer HT-29 cells (ED_{50}: 9.97–8.15 μg/mL). Other isolated diterpenes designated as vibsanins-Q–V were moderately cytotoxic (ED_{50}: <10.0 μg/mL) to the P388 cell line.[8]

Triterpenes

Two triterpenoids, ursolic acid and 6β-hydroxylup-20(29)-en-3-oxo-27,28-dioic acid, were isolated from *V. odoratissimum*. At a concentration of 50 μg/mL, ursolic acid obviously restrained the two carcinoma cell lines (NUGC and HONE-1),[5] while 6β-hydroxylup-20(29)-en-3-oxo-27,28-dioic acid (**11**) at a concentration of 10 μM was notably cytotoxic to the NUGC cells *in vitro*.[2] From the separation of *V. awabuki* leaves and twigs, nine cytotoxic lupane-, secolupane-, and oleanane-type triterpenoids were obtained and demonstrated the inhibitory effect on the neoplastic cell lines *in vitro*.[9] For instance, 3β,20-dihydroxyl-lupane-28-oic acid (**12**) and 3β,6β-dihydroxyl-oleanene-12-en-28-oic acid (**13**) displayed a modest suppressive effect against the proliferation of mouse P388 leukemia cells (IC_{50}: 6.5 and 35 μg/mL, respectively) and human HT-29 colon cancer cells (IC_{50}: 9.0 and 19 μg/mL, respectively).[9]

References

1. Kim, T. H. 2002. Extracts derived from *Viburnum awabuki* containing physiological activity. *Repub. Korean Kongkae Taeho Kongbo* KR 2002067081 A 20020822.
2. Shen, Y. C. et al. 2002. New vibsane diterpenes and lupane triterpenes from *Viburnum odoratissimum*. *J. Nat. Prod.* 65: 1052–5.
3. Shen, Y. C. et al. 2004. Vibsane diterpenoids from the leaves and flowers of *Viburnum odoratissimum*. *J. Nat. Prod.* 67: 74–7.
4. Shen, Y. C. et al. 2003. New triterpenoid fatty acid esters from the small twigs of *Viburnum odoratissimum*. *J. Chinese Chem. Soc.* 50: 297–302.
5. Zhang, H. F. et al. 2014. Study on effect of vibsane-type diterpenoids of *Viburnum odoratissimum* on human HepG2 cell growth and its underlying mechanism. *Zhongguo Yingyong Shenglixue Zazhi* 30: 343–7.
6. Fukuyama, Y. et al. 2002. Seven-membered vibsane-type diterpenes with a 5,10-*cis* relationship from *Viburnum awabuki*. *Chem. Pharm. Bull.* 50: 368–71.
7. Minami, H. et al. 1998. Structures of new seven-membered ring vibsane-type diterpenes isolated from leaves of *Viburnum awabuki*. *Chem. Pharm. Bull.* 46: 1194–8.
8. El-Gamal, A. A. 2004. New diterpenoids from *Viburnum awabuki*. *J. Nat. Prod.* 67: 333–6.
9. El-Gamal, A. A. 2008. Cytotoxic lupane-, secolupane-, and oleanane-type triterpenes from *Viburnum awabuki*. *Nat. Prod. Res.* 22: 191–7.

65 Nong Ji Li 農吉利

Rattle pod

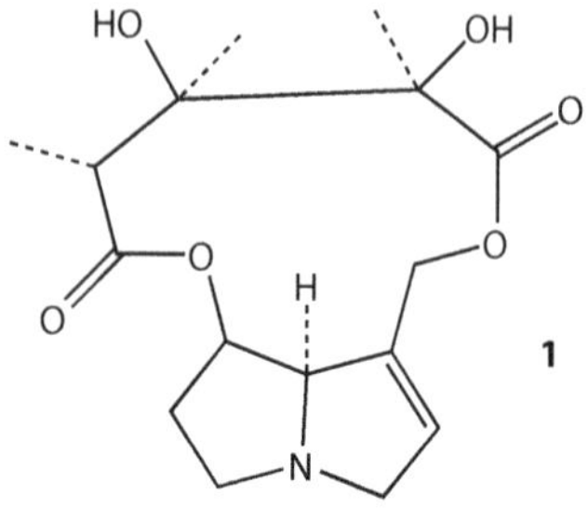

HO OH O O O H O N 1

Herb Origination

The herb Nong Ji Li (Rattle pod) is the dried whole plant of *Crotalaria sessiliflora* (Leguminosae). This annual plant has widely spread in central and east Asia from temperate to tropical regions. In China, the herb collection is generally done in summer and autumn and then dried in the sun for folk medicinal practice. The herb also can be used fresh.

Antitumor Activities and Constituents

Nong Ji Li has been used in Chinese folk medicine as an antitumor agent because it exerted a marked suppressive effect against several murine cancer cells in the experimental investigations. The cytotoxicity assay found that the extracts derived from its leaves, roots, and stems concentration-dependently inhibited the tumor cell survival. A cytotoxic pyrrolizidine alkaloid identified as monocrotaline (**1**) was separated from different portions of the plant, whose content was 9.18 mg/100 g in its leaves, 9.30 mg/100 g in its stems, 6.70 mg/100 g in its roots, and 8.86 mg/100 g in its seeds.[1–4] Monocrotaline (**1**) was effective in the inhibition of the cell growth of sarcoma 180, Walker sarcoma 256, and leukemia 615.[1–3] The treatment with monocrotaline (**1**) at a 0.5 mg/mL concentration restrained the DNA and RNA syntheses of cancer cells, thereby inhibiting mouse sarcoma 180 cells and human KB nasopharyngeal cancer cells, and at 0.3 and 0.5 mg/mL concentrations, it obstructed the growth of human Bel-7402 hepatoma cells and reduced the cell mitosis index.[5] The i.p. administration of monocrotaline (**1**) to tumor-bearing mice for 10 days resulted in 57.2% inhibition against sarcoma 180 in a dose of 150 mg/kg/day and 63–75% inhibition against sarcoma 37 in a dose of 100 mg/kg/day. The survival duration of the tested animals implanted with lymphoma-L1 (ascites type) could be prolonged by 62.5% after being injected with monocrotaline (**1**) in a dose of 155 mg/kg/day for 10 days.[1–3] The significant cytotoxicity of monocrotaline (**1**) was also proven in other types of cancer cell lines such as L1210 leukemia, metastatic Lewis lung cancer, adenocarcinoma 753, melanoma B16, Ehrlich tumor, and plasmacytoma, *in vitro*.[6] The antitumor effect of monocrotaline (**1**) on human BxPC-3 pancreatic cancer cells was mediated by blocking cell cycle, inducing apoptosis, and downregulating cyclin-B1 protein.[7]

Clinic Applications

During the early 1970s in China, Nong Ji Li and its major active constituent, monocrotaline (**1**), had been tested in several clinical trials for the treatment of patients suffering from malignant diseases.[6]

1. Twenty-five cases of leukemia were treated with monocrotaline (**1**) by intravenous injection or a drop in a daily dose of 100–200 mg, resulting in the total effectivity rate of 56%.
2. Three hundred sixty-five cases of digestive tract, lung, and cervical cancers were given a 30% ethanolic extract injection or a 100% water extract injection of Nong Ji Li together with Nong Ji Li decoction or tablets administered orally. The final effectivity rates were 60–62%.
3. By local external use of monocrotaline (**1**), a 72.3% effectivity rate resulted from 112 cases of melanoma, whereas a 50% effectivity rate from 60 cases of cervical cancer.
4. Forty-five cases of cancer patients (including squamous cell carcinoma, mouth/lip squamous cell carcinoma, testis carcinoma) were treated with Nong Ji Li, and the effectivity rate reached 75.6%.

Both Nong Ji Li extract and monocrotalin (**1**) have been proven to be chemotherapeutic agents in China for clinical application, which are generally used for the treatment of cervical cancer, esophagus carcinoma, hepatoma, gastric carcinoma, melanoma, and breast adenocarcinoma. However, because both cancer cells and hepatocytes are sensitive to monocrotalin (**1**) in clinical trials, a larger toxicity, which primarily injured the liver cells and secondly irritated the kidney and digestive tract, were found, and leucopenia and thrombocytopenia were also elicited.[6] Therefore, the treatment dose and schedule must be carefully managed, and a short-term schedule is suggested for using Nong Ji Li extract and monocrotalin (**1**) as the chemotherapeutic agents.

Other Medical Uses

The herb Nong Ji Li (Rattle pod) is mainly used in Chinese folk medicine to treat the diseases of dysentery and sore furuncle, besides cancers such as squamous cell skin cancer, esophageal cancer, and cervical cancer and so on.

References

1. Hsu, B. 1980. The use of herbs in anticancer agents. *Am. J. Chin. Med.* 8: 301.
2. Huang, L. et al. 1980. The isolation of antitumor active principle of *Crotalaria sessiliflora* and synthesis of its derivatives. *Yaoxue Xuebao*. 15: 278–83.
3. Roder, E. et al. 1992. Pyrrolizidine alkaloids from the seeds of *Crotalafia sessiliflora*. *Planta Med.* 58: 283.
4. Kim, T. et al. 2007. Growth-inhibitory effect on cancer cells of the extract from *Crotalaria sessiliflora* L. and identification of anticancer agents. *FASEB J.* 21: 842.9.
5. Ge, B. L. et al. 1985. The effects of monocrotaline on nucleic acids biosynthesis of human and animal cancer cells. *Chin. J. Pathophysiol.* 19: 30–4.
6. State Administration of Traditional Chinese Medicine of China. 1999. *Zhonghua Bencao* (Chinese Materia Medica). Vol. 4, 427–30, Shanghai Science and Technology Press, Shanghai, China.
7. Zeng, J. Y. et al. 2014. Effect of monocrotaline on induction of pancreatic cancer cell BxPC-3 into polyploid giant cells. *Zhongcaoyao* 45: 2042–6.

66 Zhu Sha Ren 竹砂仁

Stroma Hypocrellae

Herb Origination

The herb Zhu Sha Ren is the dried stroma of Hypocreaceae fungi, *Hypocrella bambusae*. The fungi, which are parasites on a kind of special bamboo *Sinarundinaria bamboos*, are distributed in the Chinese provinces of Yunnan, Sichuan, and Tibet. The herb is generally collected annually and dried in the sunlight for Chinese medical practices.

Antitumor Constituents and Activities

Hypocrellin-A (**1**) and hypocrellin-B (**2**) were two photodynamic perylenequinone pigments extracted from the Zhu Sha Ren, demonstrating a notable suppressive effect against the proliferation of several neoplastic cells *in vitro* and *in vivo*.[1–3] The treatment with hypocrellin-A (HA) (**1**) in a concentration of 25 μg/mL plus the illumination of a high-voltage Na-lamp (105 mW/cm^2) for 10 min intensively repressed the activities of mitochondrial ATPase and microsomal glucose-6-phosphatase in mouse hepatoma cells and reduced the sulphydryl (SH) contents of the mitochondrial and microsomal membrane proteins. Simultaneously, the lipid peroxidation of mitochondrial and microsomal membrane lipids were greatly enhanced in the hepatoma cells. The evidences implied that the mitochondria and microsomes are sensitive targets in the hepatoma cells with respect to the photosensitization of HA.[3] In human HeLa cervical cancer cells, HA (**1**) promoted the apoptosis and the oligonucleosomal fragmentation of the DNA by upregulating the expression of apoptosis-inducer Bax mRNA and downregulating the expression of apoptosis-suppressor, Bcl-2 mRNA, in the mitochondria.[4]

Human bladder carcinoma cells treated by hypocrellin-B (**2**) with light irritation displayed a significant neoplasm regression. The hypocrellin-B (**2**) that exerted a photodynamic therapeutic effect was characteristic of a predominantly vascular inhibition-mediated anticancer effect.[5] Hypocrellin (**3**) (EDSHB) was derived from hypocrellin-B (**2**) by structural modification with an ethyldiamino substitution. The EDAHB (**3**) could markedly improve the red light absorption and enhance the generation of active oxygen species, indicating that EDAHB (**3**) is a more potent photodynamic therapeutic anticancer agent than its parent hypocrellins.[6]

Nanoformulation

By controlling the charge properties of the drugs and the ion strength of the environment, a series of HA self-assembled nanostructures were formulated. The HA nanostructures significantly enhanced its water dispersion ability and $^1O_2$ generation efficiency, thereby improving the phototoxicity to human HeLa cervical cancer cells.[7] The photosensitive HA was also encapsulated with silica nanoparticle (SN) material. The HA–SN complex exhibited an improved performance in both stability and hydrophilicity than natural HA (**1**).[8]

References

1. Wang, Z. J. et al. 1999. Pharmacokinetics, tissue distribution and photodynamic therapy efficacy of liposomal-delivered hypocrellin A, a potential photosensitizer for tumor therapy. *Photochem. Photobiol.* 70: 773–80.
2. Diwu, Z. J. et al. 1995. Novel therapeutic and diagnostic applications of hypocrellins and hypericins. *Photochem. Photobiol.* 61: 529–39.
3. Fu, N. W. et al. 1989. Photodynamic action of hypocrellin A on hepatoma cell mitochondria and microsomes. *Zhongguo Yaoli Xuebao* 10: 371–3.
4. Fei, X. F. et al. 2006. Apoptotic effects of hypocrellin A on HeLa cells. *Chem. Res. in Chinese Univ.* 22: 772–5.
5. Chin, W. et al. 2004. Evaluation of hypocrellin B in a human bladder tumor model in experimental photodynamic therapy: Biodistribution, light dose and drug-light interval effects. *Int. J. Oncol.* 25: 623–9.
6. Xu, S. J. et al. 2014. Hypocrellin derivative with improvements of red absorption and active oxygen species generation. *Bioorg. Med. Chem. Lett.* 14: 1499–501.
7. Zhou, L. et al. 2015. Modulating the photo-exciting process of photosensitizer to improve in vitro phototoxicity by preparing its self-assembly nanostructures. *RSC Advances* 5: 2794–805.
8. Wang, F. et al. 2010. Characterization of anticancer hypocrellin A encapsulated with silica nanoparticles. *J. Thermal Analysis Calorim.* 102: 69–74.

67 Lao Guan Cao 老鸛草

Chinese cranesbill

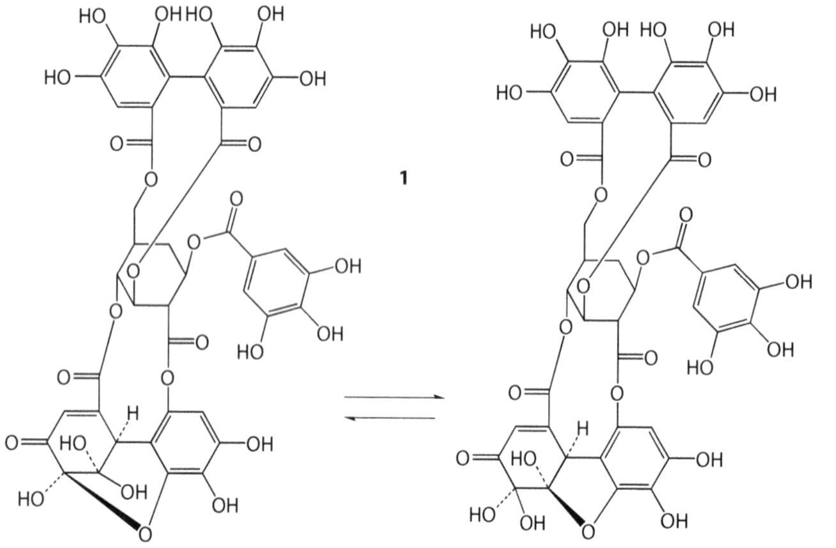

1

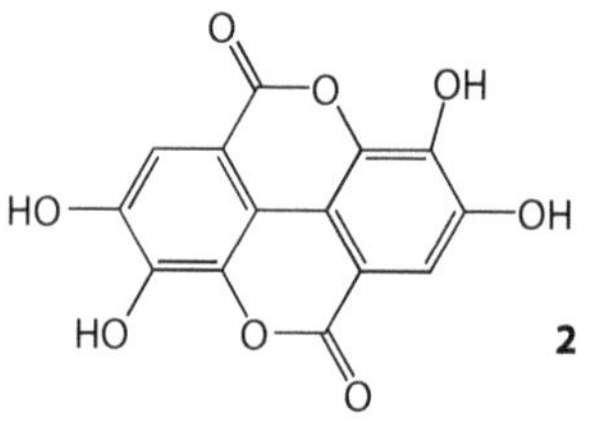

2

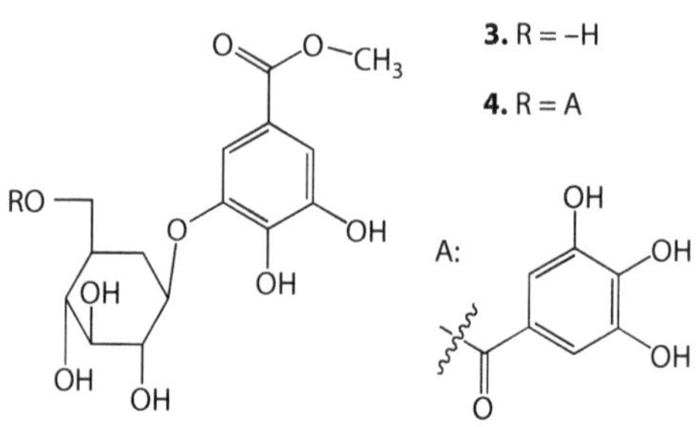

3. R = –H

4. R = A

Herb Origination

The herb Lao Guan Cao (Chinese cranesbill) is the dried whole plant *Geranium wilfordii* (Geraniaceae). The herbal plant is widely distributed in China. As a Chinese folk medicine, the whole plant is generally collected just before its fruit ripens in autumn and dried in the sun for folk medicinal application.

Antitumor Constituents and Activities

The EAF of Lao Guan Cao showed the significant inhibitory effect against human A549 (lung), SKOV-3 (ovarian), K562 (leukemic), HT-1080 (fibrosarcoma) cancer cell lines, and murine sarcoma cells.[1] Tannin-type components are the major antineoplastic substances in Lao Guan Cao, and the quantity of geraniin (**1**) is up to 2.2% in the herb. In the experiments, geraniin (**1**) prominently suppressed the carcinogenesis induced by a mutagen Trp-P-2. Ellagic acid (**2**), one of the hydrolyzates of geraniin, markedly obstructed the mutagenic action caused by benzopyrene-7,8-diol-9,10-epoxide.[2–4] The treatment with geraniin (**1**), prior to being given okadaic acid (a tumor promoter) on mouse skin carcinogenesis initiated with DMBA, could markedly diminish the percentage of tumor-bearing mice from 80% to 40% and reduce the average numbers of tumor per mouse from 3.8 to 1.1 within a 20-week treatment.[3] Geraniin (**1**) also exhibited a selective cytotoxicity against PRMI-7951 melanoma cells *in vitro* with ED_{50} values of 0.1–0.8 μg/mL, but it is inactive to human A549 lung cancer, HCT-8 intestinal adenocarcinoma, KB nasopharyngeal epidermoid carcinoma, and TE-671 medulloblastoma cell lines in its concentration of over 10 μg/mL.[4,5]

Three hydrolyzed tannins and a related compound, gallic acid, 1,2,3,4,6-penta-*O*-galloyl-β-glucopyranose, chebulagic acid, and chebulinic acid, were isolated from the active fractions, displaying a moderate cytotoxic activity toward the human tumor cell lines (A549, SKOV-3, HT-1080, K562, and S180) *in vitro*. Their ED_{50} values ranged from 2.9 to 16.9 μg/mL.[1] From the 70% acetone extract of the herb, two phenolic glycosides assigned as methylgallate-3-D-β-glucoside (**3**) and methylgallate-3-(6′-gallate)-D-β-glucoside (**4**) were isolated as anticancer agents.[6]

Other Bioactivities

The herb Lao Guan Cao (Chinese cranesbill) in traditional Chinese medicine is used to treat diarrhea, diarrhea dysentery, rheumatism, etc., as antirheumatic, antiseptic, and astringent. Pharmacological studies demonstrated that the herb possesses multiple biological properties including antiviral, antibacterial, antiinflammatory, antioxidative, antitussive, and hepatoprotective effects. Lao Guan Cao tannins and its hydrolyzate ellagic acids exhibited free radical-scavenging and antioxidant activities. Thus, the herb remarkably suppresses lipid peroxidation and liver cell damage.

References

1. Li, P. et al. 2013. Hydrolysable tannins and related compound having cytotoxic activity of *Geranium wilfordii* Maxim. *Advance J. Food Sci. Technol.* 5: 255–7.
2. Okuta, T. et al. 1979. Isolation of geraniin from plants of Geranium and Euphorbiaceae. *Yakugaku Zasshi* 99: 543–5.
3. Ahemed, K. M. et al. 1999. An anticancer tannin and other phenolics from *Limonium axaillare*. *Asian J. Chem.* 11: 261–3.
4. Okabe, S. et al. 2001. New TNF-α releasing inhibitors, geraniin and corilagin, in leaves of *Acer nikoense*, Megusurinoki. *Biol. Pharm. Bull.* 24: 1145–8.
5. Kashiwada, Y. et al. 1992. Antitumor agents: 129. Tannins and related compounds as selective cytotoxic agents. *J. Nat. Prod.* 55: 1033–43.
6. Wei, L. X. et al. 2000. Antitumor compounds extracted from heroubill herb and its medicinal preparation. *Faming Zhuanli Shenqing Gongkai Shuomingshu* CN 1249308 A 20000405.

68 Ci Tian Jia 刺天茄

Poison berry

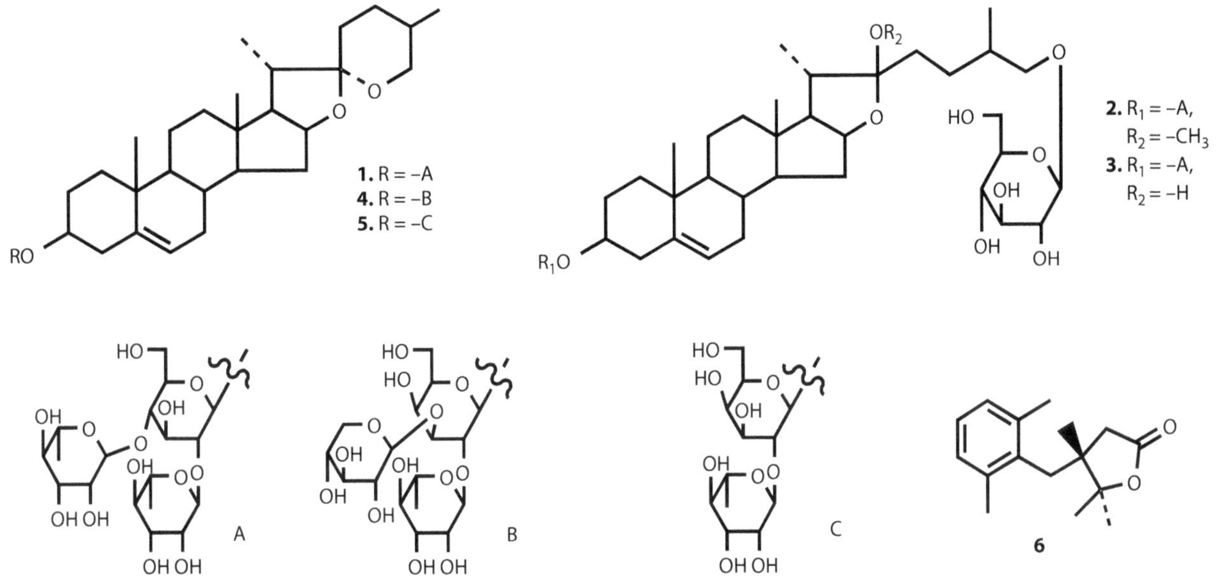

1. R = –A
4. R = –B
5. R = –C

2. R_1 = –A, R_2 = –CH_3
3. R_1 = –A, R_2 = –H

A B C **6**

Herb Origination

The herb Ci Tian Jia originated from a Solanaceae plant, *Solanum indicum* L. This herbal plant is distributed in the southern regions of China and Asia. Its whole plant, root, and fruit can be collected year-round and dried in the sun for the folk medicinal practice. The herb also can be used fresh.

Antitumor Activities and Constituent

The ethanolic extract prepared from whole plant of Ci Tian Jia demonstrated a significant cytotoxic activity against human Colo205 (colon), HeLa (cervix), KB (nasopharynx), HA22T (liver), HEp2 (larynges), GBM8401/TSGH (brain), and H147 (skin) cancer cell lines *in vitro*. A group of anticancer steroid saponins were discovered from the extract. Dioscin (**1**), methylprotodioscin (**2**), protodioscin (**3**), and methylprotoprosapogenin-A of dioscin showed cytotoxicity on rat C6 glioma cells *in vitro* and *in vivo*.[1] Dioscin (**1**) at a 10 μg/mL concentration obstructed the DNA synthesis of C6 glioma cells.[1] Indioside-E (**4**) inhibited the proliferation of human BEL-7402 hepatoma cells (IC_{50}: 4.2 μg/mL, in 72 h) and apparently augmented the BEL-7402 cell apoptosis via a mitochondria-dependent pathway, i.e., the reduction of Bcl-2 expression, the release of cytochrome c, the proteolysization of PARP, and the activation of caspase-3.[2–4] The *in vitro* assay also demonstrated that indioside-E (**4**) and its analog (5,6-dihydrogenated indioside-E) were effective in the inhibition of human MCF-7 breast cancer, KB nasopharynx cancer, K562 erythroleukemia, and U87 astrocytoma cell lines (IC_{50}: 1.32–3.77 μM) and also in the inhibition of human normal HL7702 hepatocytes and EVC304 umbilical vein endothelial *cells*. If the E-ring and F-ring formed spiro-link in indioside-E (**4**) were completely opened or were deoxidized to become a side chain, the cytotoxicity in the same cell lines would be attenuated for three to nine times.[5]

Three synthetic, indioside I-5 (= indioside-E) (**4**), indioside I-2 (**5**), and indioside I-1 were found to have an obvious inhibitory activity against the proliferation of BEL-7402 cells dose-dependently together with the promotion of the cell apoptosis. The IC_{50} values were 6.2–6.5 μg/mL (in 72 h) for the indioside I-5 and indiosides I-2.[6–8] Indioside I-5 (**4**) was also sensitive to human Bel-7404 (liver), HT-29 (colon), and CNE (brain) cancer cell lines *in vitro*, and exerted ~70% growth inhibition on the cancer cell lines *in vitro*. In NCI-H460 large-cell lung cancer cells, indioside I-5 (**4**) showed a lower antiproliferative effect.[9]

Additionally, solavetivone (**6**) is a different type of constituent discovered from this herb, which repressed the proliferation of human OVCAR-3 ovarian cancer cells with an IC_{50} value of 0.1 mM *in vitro*.[10]

Other Medicinal Uses

The herb Ci Tian Jia (Poison berry) has been used in folk medicine for the treatment of inflammation, bronchitis, toothache, ascites, edema, and wound infection. Its leaves are useful in cutaneous disorders. A decoction of the root is prescribed as a tonic, and it can also be used in difficult parturition.

References

1. Chiang, H. C. et al. 1991. Experimental antitumor agents from *Solanum indicum* L. *Anticancer Res.* 11: 1911–7.
2. Gu, G. F. et al. 2004. Facile synthesis of saponins containing 2,3-branched oligosaccharides by using partially protected glycosyl donors. *J. Org. Chem.* 69: 5497–500.
3. Ma, P. et al. 2005. Apoptosis-inducing activity of synthetic saponin in *Solanum indicum* on human hepatocarcinoma BEL-7402 cells. *Zhongguo Zhongliu Linchuang* 32: 481–5.

4. Ma, P. et al. 2006. Inducement effect of synthetic indiosides from *Solanum indicum* on apoptosis of human hepatocarcinoma cell line Bel-7402 and its mechanism. *Aizheng* 25: 438–42.
5. Gao, J. et al. 2011. Efficient synthesis of trisaccharide saponins and their tumor cell killing effects through oncotic necrosis. *Bioorg. Med. Chem. Lett.* 21: 622–7.
6. Ma, P. et al. 2008. Anti-proliferation effect of synthetic indioside from *Solanum indicum* L. on human hepatocarcinoma cells. *Jiepouxue Zazhi* (*Chin. J. Anatomy*) 31: 25–7.
7. Cao, T. T. et al. 2006. Cytotoxic effect of saponin I-2 in *Solanum indicum* L. on human hepatocarcinoma cells. *J. Binzhou Med. Univ.* 29: 255–6.
8. Ni, Y. H. et al. 2008. Study on antineoplastic activity and blood cell haemolysis test to saponin. *J. Binzhou Med. Univ.* 31: 85–6.
9. Cao, T. T. et al. 2008. Antitumor effects of saponin I-5 in *Solanum indicum* L. on different tumor cell lines. *J. Binzhou Med. Univ.* 31: 185–6.
10. Syu, W. Jr. et al. 2001. Cytotoxic and novel compounds from *Solanum indicum*. *J. Nat. Prod.* 64: 1232–3.

69 Fen Fang Ji 粉防己

Stephania root

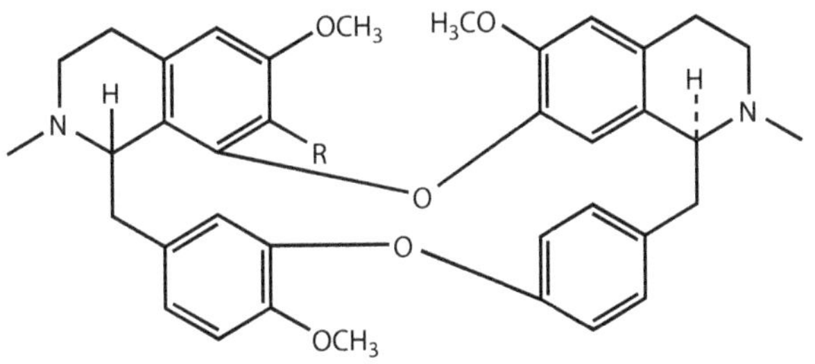

1. R = $-OCH_3$

2. R = $-OH$

Herb Origination

The herb Fen Fang Ji (Stephania root) is one of the fundamental herbs used in traditional Chinese medicine, which originated from the tuberous roots of *Stephania tetrandra* (Menispermaceae). This perennial vine plant is widely distributed in the southern and central regions of China. For obtaining a good quality of the herb, the roots are normally harvested in autumn and then dried in the sun for utilization in Chinese herbal remedy.

Antitumor Constituents and Activities

Tetrandrine

An aporphine–bisbenzylisoquinoline-type alkaloid termed tetrandrine (**1**) is a principal anticancer component in Fen Fang Ji. It suppressed the synthesis of DNA or RNA and the metabolism of protein in human HeLa (cervix) and Bel-7402 and Bel-7405 (liver) cancer cells, as well as in murine sarcoma 180 cells, and induced the cell apoptosis of human hepatoblastoma and other carcinomas.[1–3] The proliferative inhibition of tetrandrine (**1**) was also observed on four other different hepatoma cell lines (HepG2, PLC/PRF/5, Hep3B, and Huh-7). The IC_{50} values were 4.35, 9.44, and 10.41 μM in the first three hepatoma cell lines, respectively, but was 31.12 μM in mouse normal liver cells.[4] The antihepatoma activity and selectivity on HepG2 cells and PLC/PRF/5 cells were better than those of cisplatin.[4] After being treated with tetrandrine e (**1**), the cycle of PLC/PRF/5 hepatoma cells was arrested at G2/M phase in a dose-dependent manner but no such effect in the Hep3B cells, although the apoptotic effect of tetrandrine was induced in both hepatoma cells.[4] Its antihepatoma effect on the Huh-7 cells was concomitant with p53-independent and caspase-related pathways and G2/M-cell cycle arrest.[5] Tetrandrine (**1**) was also capable of provoking a mitochondrial dysfunction via the increase of ROS and the activation of ATG7 transcriptionally, leading to the promotion of autophagy in human hepatoma cells and other types of cancer cells *in vitro* and *in vivo*.[6,7] These data supported that tetrandrine (**1**) may have a wide range of applications in the fields of antitumor therapy and basic scientific research.

Moreover, the exposure of tetrandrine (**1**) moderately hindered the proliferation of SUM-149 (inflammatory) and SUM-159 (a noninflammatory metaplastic) breast cancer cell lines and blocked the mammosphere formation in the two breast cancer cell lines and restrained the aldehyde dehydrogenase positive population in SUM-159 cells, indicating that tetrandrine was able to kill the breast tumor-initiating cells preferentially, whose potency was similar to that of salinomycin, a known inhibitor targeting breast cancer initiation cells.[8] Through the initiation of ROS-induced JNK1/2 activation and JNK1/2-elicited proteasomal degradation of c-FLIPL/S and Bcl2, tetrandrine (**1**) promoted Fas- and mitochondria-mediated intrinsic and extrinsic apoptosis of PC3 and DU145 prostate cancer cell lines.[9] *In vitro* and *in vivo* experiments also demonstrated that tetrandrine (**1**) significantly inhibited the viability and induced the apoptosis of human BGC-823 gastric cancer cells in both dose- and time-dependent manners.[10] The antineoplastic activity of tetrandrine (**1**) also was confirmed in *in vivo* model with mouse ascites tumor.[1–3]

Importantly, tetrandrine (**1**) has a great potential for the improvement of current chemotherapy. A cotreatment with tetrandrine (**1**) and antitumor agents (Adm or VCR) synergistically restrained human cancer cell lines such as MCF-7, and its Adm-resistant MCF-7/Adm breast cancer cells, and KB, and its VCR-resistant KBv200 nasopharyngeal cancer cells *in vitro*, where tetrandrine (**1**) acted as a cancer sensitizer to potentiate the anticancer drugs via the induction of apoptosis and reversal of MDR.[11,12] Similarly, the synergistic cytotoxicity of tetrandrine (**1**) and anticancer agents was also observed in two gastric cancer cell lines (BGC-823 and MKN-28) but also associated with the down-expression of the mRNAs of ERCC1, TS, β-tubulin-III, and tau.[13]

Likewise, tetrandrine (**1**) is capable of sensitizing the radioactivity and blocking the metastatic ability of cancer cells.[1,14] The i.p. injection of tetrandrine (**1**) to mice in a dose of 10 mg/kg per day for five consecutive days notably declined the pulmonary metastatic rate by 40.3% and significantly prolonged the survival time of mice implanted with metastatic murine CT26 colorectal cancer. When combined with an antitumor agent 5-FU and tetrandrine, the antimetastatic effect was amplified with no acute toxicity and no obvious changes in the body weight of mice.[14] The suppression of ADAM17 and the downregulation of EGFR-PI3K-AKT signaling pathways might contribute to tetrandrine-induced decrease of proliferation, migration, and invasion in U87 glioma cells.[15] According to these evidences, tetrandrine (**1**) can be recommended as an adjunct agent for improving clinical chemotherapy and radiotherapy to fight cancer and to prevent cancer metastasis.

Fangchinoline

Fangchinoline (**2**) is another important bisbenzylisoquinoline in the herb with pain-relieving, blood pressure-depressing, and antibiotic activities, whose structure is only one methyl group less compared to that of tetrandrine (**1**). Fangchinoline (**2**) dose- and time-dependently restrained the cell proliferation of human PC3 prostate cancer cells *in vitro* and in nude mouse xenograft concomitantly with the promotion of apoptotic death and the arrest cell cycle progression at G1/S phase.[16] Both tetrandrine (**1**) and fangchinoline (**2**) at the same concentration of 3.0 μM could reduce the concentration of paclitaxel (a clinical drug) required to achieve a 50% inhibition in human HCT15 (P-gp positive) colon cancer cells by 3100- and 1900-fold, and also reduce the EC_{50} value of actinomycin-D by 36.0- and 45.9-fold in the HCT15 cells, respectively, but both had no additive effect on the drugs to SKOV-3 (P-gp negative) cells.[17] By repressing the P-gp activity in MDR1-MDCK II monolayer cells, fangchinoline (**2**) apparently diminished the efflux of paclitaxel and augmented the drug concentration in the tumor cells, thereby reversing the MDR and enhancing the cytotoxicity of paclitaxel.[18] Similarly, by the same pathway, fangchinoline (**2**) and tetrandrine (**1**) augmented the intracellular concentration of anticancer drugs and exerted the synergistic cytotoxicity in Caco-2 MDR and CEM/ADR5000 cancer cell lines in combination with Adm.[19] The anti-MDR activity of fangchinoline (**2**) and tetrandrine (**1**) were more significant than that of verapamil hydrochloride in the same molar concentration.[17] From these results, fangchinoline (**2**) and tetrandrine (**1**) could be considered as potential agents to reverse the MDR of chemotherapeutic drugs.

Exploration of Mechanisms

In recent years, the anticancer mechanism of tetrandrine (**1**) was indeed investigated. Its cytotoxicity toward human HepG2 hepatoma cells (IC_{50}: 9.0 μM) was closely accompanied with the blockage of cell cycle progression at G1 stage and the induction of apoptosis, whose proapoptotic effect was achieved by the downregulation of Bcl-xL, the upregulation of p53, the cleavage of Bid and Bax, the release of cytochrome c, the augmentation of p53 and p21/WAF1 expressions, the activation of caspase-3, caspase-9, and caspase-8, and the subsequent proteolytic cleavage of PARP. An up-expression of Fas/APO-1 and its two form ligands (membrane-bound Fas ligand and soluble Fas ligand) were also responsible for apoptosis promotion.[2,3,20] Similarly, the inhibitory effect of tetrandrine (**1**) against the growth of lymphoma U937 cells was associated to apoptotic acceleration as well. But early oxidative stress and chromatin fragmentation were found to be involved in the JNK-activated apoptosis of U937 lymphoma cells, and a catalytically active fragment of PKC-δ was generated to play a role in the activation of caspases.[21]

Upon treatment of human A549 lung carcinoma cells and murine epidermal JB6 Cl 41 cells with tetrandrine (**1**), many of the hallmark features of apoptosis and cell cycle arrest were elicited with a time-dependent inhibition of the cell growth. The signaling pathways of growth arrest and apoptosis in A549 cells and JB6 Cl41 cells were revealed to correlate with (1) augmenting CDK inhibitor p21 activity and inhibiting cyclin-D1, which further amplified the populations of both apoptotic sub-G1 and G1 phases; (2) downregulating ERK phosphorylation; (3) blocking Akt activation and activating caspase-3; and/or (4) suppressing AP-1 expression. Also, tetrandrine (**1**) concurrently influenced the expression patterns of cytoskeletons including distribution of F-actin and microtubule expression.[22–24]

The irreversible inhibition of tetrandrine (**1**) against the proliferation of human HT-29 colon carcinoma cells was accompanied by the G1 phase cell cycle arrest, whose effect was found to be at least mediated by different events, i.e., (1) inhibiting CDK2/cyclin-E and CDK4 without affecting CDK2/cyclin, CDK1/cyclin-B, and CDK6; and (2) triggering the proteasome-dependent degradation of CDK4, CDK6, cyclin-D1, and E2F1. The up-expression of p53 and p21Cip1 was also observed in wild-type p53 HCT116 colon cancer cells after the tetrandrine treatment.[25] The apoptosis promotion in BGC-823 gastric cancer cells was found to be associated with a mitochondrial pathway, i.e., (1) upregulation of Bax, Bak, and Bad and downregulation of Bcl-2 and Bcl-xL; (2) upregulation of apaf-1 and release of cytochrome c; and (3) activation of caspase-3 and caspase-9.[10]

The mechanism of fangchinoline (**2**) inhibiting human PC3 prostate cancer cells was explored as well. The G1/S phase cell cycle arrest in the PC3 cells was induced through the repression of a cyclin-regulated signaling pathway including the increase of p27 expression and the decrease of cyclin-D and PCNA expressions.[16] The apoptosis of PC3 prostate cancer cells and MDA-MB-231 breast cancer cells was provoked through a mitochondrial pathway, such as the up-expression of Bax, the decrease of Bcl-2 expression and Akt phosphorylation, the release of cytochrome c, the cleavage of PARP, and the activation of caspase-3, caspase-8, and caspase-9.[16,26]

Nanoformulation

Tetrandrine–phospholipid complex-loaded lipid nanocapsules (TPC-LNCs) were prepared, and the TPC-LNCs were spherical particles with a small size of 40 nm and a high encapsulation efficiency of 93.9%. The formulated lipid nanocapsules displayed greatly improved oral bioavailability of tetrandrine in rats.[27]

Other Bioactivities

In the Chinese pharmacopeia, Fen Fang Ji (Stephania root) is recommended for treating general symptoms such as fever, pain, and inflammation, and it has also been extensively used to promote diuresis, eliminate stagnant bronchial mucous, and detoxify diseases of rheumatism, rheumatoid arthritis, edema, and dysuria. Tetrandrine (**1**) is well known as a major constituent in Fen Fang Ji possessing antioxidant, hypertensive, antiarrhythmogenic, antithrombotic, anti-inflammatory, coronary vessel-dilative, antithrombocyte agglutinative, smooth muscle relaxant, antifibrotic and antiangina pectoris, antisilicosis, and neuroprotective activities.[28] However, an overdose of tetrandrine (**1**) may cause respiratory paralysis.

References

1. Yan, H. F. et al. (a) 1979. *Zhongyiyao Yanjiu Cankao* (2): 46; (b) 1999. *Chinese Materia Medica.* Vol. 3, 3–1986, 387. Shanghai Science and Technology Press, Shanghai, China.
2. Yoo, S. M. et al. 2002. Inhibition of proliferation and induction of apoptosis by tetrandrine in HepG2 cells. *J. Ethnopharmcol.* 81: 225–9.

3. Oh, S. H. et al. 2003. Induction of apoptosis in human hepatoblastoma cells by tetrandrine via caspase-dependent Bid cleavage and cytochrome c release. *Biochem. Pharmacol.* 66: 725–31.
4. Ng, L. T. et al. 2006. Antiproliferative and apoptotic effects of tetrandrine on different human hepatoma cell lines. *Am. J. Chin. Med.* 34: 125–35.
5. Yu, V. W. L. et al. 2013. Tetrandrine inhibits hepatocellular carcinoma cell growth through the caspase pathway and G2/M phase. *Oncol. Reports* 29: 2205–10.
6. Gong, K. et al. 2012. Autophagy-related gene 7 (ATG7) and reactive oxygen species/extracellular signal-regulated kinase regulate tetrandrine-induced autophagy in human hepatocellular carcinoma. *J. Biol. Chem.* 287: 35576–88.
7. Wang, H. Q. et al. 2015. Tetrandrine is a potent cell autophagy agonist via activated intracellular reactive oxygen species. *Cell. Biosci.* 5: 4/1–4/9.
8. Xu, W. et al. 2011. Tetrandrine, a compound common in Chinese traditional medicine, preferentially kills breast tumor initiating cells (TICs) in vitro. *Cancers* 3: 2274–85.
9. Chaudhary, P. et al. 2014. c-Jun NH2-terminal kinase-induced proteasomal degradation of c-FLIPL/S and Bcl2 sensitize prostate cancer cells to Fas- and mitochondria-mediated apoptosis by tetrandrine. *Biochem. Pharmacol.* (Amsterdam, Netherlands) 91: 457–73.
10. Qin, R. et al. 2013. Tetrandrine induces mitochondria-mediated apoptosis in human gastric cancer BGC-823 cells. *PLoS One* 8: e76486.
11. Ye, Z. G. et al. (a) 1999. Synergistic interaction between Ys-96, a bibenzylisoquinoline compound derived from *Stephania tetrandra*, and adriamycin or vincristine against human cancer cell lines in vitro. *Zhongguo Zhongyao Zazhi* 24: 556–9; (b) 2001. Potentiation of vincristine-induced apoptosis by tetrandrine, neferine and dauricine in the human mammary MCF-7 multidrug-resistant cells. *Yaoxue Xuebao* 36: 96–9.
12. Wang, J. H. et al. 2002. Reversal of anti-apoptotic action by tetrandrine in human breast carcinoma multidrug-resistant MCF-7 cells. *Zhongguo Zhongyao Zazhi* 27: 46–50.
13. Wei, J. et al. 2007. Synergistic interaction between tetrandrine and chemotherapeutic agents and influence of tetrandrine on chemotherapeutic agent-associated genes in human gastric cancer cell lines. *Cancer Chemother. Pharmacol.* 60: 703–11.
14. Chang, K. W. et al. 2004. Inhibitory effect of tetrandrine on pulmonary metastases in CT26 colorectal adenocarcinoma-bearing BALB/c mice. *Am. J. Chin. Med.* 32: 863–72.
15. Wu, Z. H. et al. 2014. Effects of tetrandrine on glioma cell malignant phenotype via inhibition of ADAM17. *Tumor Biol.* 35: 2205–10.
16. Wang, C. D. et al. 2010. Fangchinoline induced G1/S arrest by modulating expression of p27, PCNA, and cyclin D in human prostate carcinoma cancer PC3 cells and tumor xenograft. *Bioscience, Biotechnol. Biochem.* 74: 488–93.
17. Choi, S. et al. 1998. The bisbenzylisoquinoline alkaloids, tetrandrine and fangchinoline, enhance the cytotoxicity of multidrug resistance-related drugs via modulation of P-glycoprotein. *Anticancer Drugs* 9: 255–61.
18. He, L. et al. 2010. Transmembrane transport activity of paclitaxel regulated by fangchinoline in MDR1-mDCK II cells. *Zhongguo Zhongyao Zazhi.* 35: 1478–81.
19. Sun, Y. F. et al. 2014. Tetrandrine and fangchinoline, bisbenzylisoquinoline alkaloids from *Stephania tetrandra* can reverse multidrug resistance by inhibiting P-glycoprotein activity in multidrug resistant human cancer cells. *Phytomed.* 21: 1110–9.
20. Kuo, P. L. et al. 2003. Tetrandrine-induced cell cycle arrest and apoptosis in HepG2 cells. *Life Sci.* 73: 243–52.
21. Jang, B. et al. 2004. Tetrandrine-induced apoptosis is mediated by activation of caspases and PKC-δ in U937 cells. *Biochem. Pharmcol.* 67: 1819–29.
22. Lee, J. Y. et al. 2002. Tetrandrine-induced cell cycle arrest and apoptosis in A549 human lung carcinoma cells. *Intl. J. Oncol.* 21: 1239–44.
23. Cho, H. S. et al. 2009. Synergistic effect of ERK inhibition on tetrandrine-induced apoptosis in A549 human lung carcinoma cells. *J. Veterinary Sci.* 10: 23–8.
24. Nomura, M. et al. 2007. Inhibition of tetrandrine on epidermal growth factor-induced cell transformation and its signal transduction. *Anticancer Res.* 27: 3187–94.
25. Meng, L. H. et al. 2004. Tetrandrine induces early G1 arrest in human colon carcinoma cells by down-regulating the activity and inducing the degradation of G1-S-specific cyclin-dependent kinases and by inducing p53 and p21Cip1. *Cancer Res.* 64: 9086–92.
26. Xing, Z. B. et al. 2011. Fangchinoline inhibits breast adenocarcinoma proliferation by inducing apoptosis. *Chem. Pharm. Bull.* 59:1 476–80.
27. Zhao, Y. Q. et al. 2012. Preparation and characterization of tetrandrine-phospholipid complex loaded lipid nanocapsules as potential oral carriers. *Intl. J. Nanomed.* 8: 4169–81.
28. Xing, Z. B. et al. 2014. Advance on study of chemical components and pharmacological effect of *Stephania tetrandra*. *Zhongguo Shiyan Fangjixue Zazhi* 20: 241–6.

70 Hei Man 黑蔓

Regels three wingnut

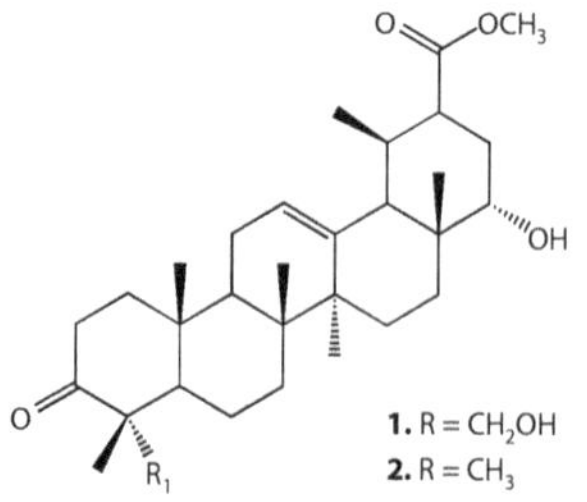

1. R = CH_2OH
2. R = CH_3

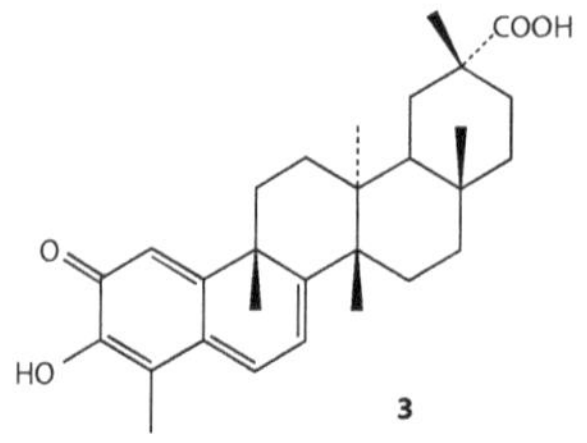

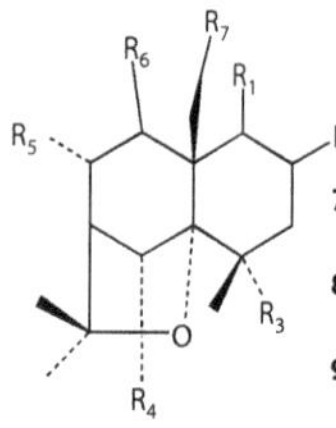

7. $R_1 = R_2 = R_7 = -OAc$, $R_3 = R_4 = -OH$, $R_5 = R_6 = -OOCC_6H_6$
8. $R_1 = R_2 = R_5 = R_6 = -OOCC_6H_6$, $R_4 = -OAc$ $R_3 = R_7 = -H$
9. $R_1 = R_2 = R_4 = R_5 = R_7 = -OAc$, $R_5 = -OH$ $R_6 = -OOCC_6H_6$

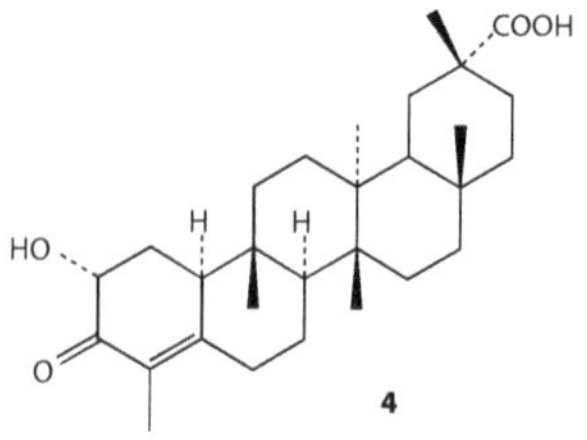

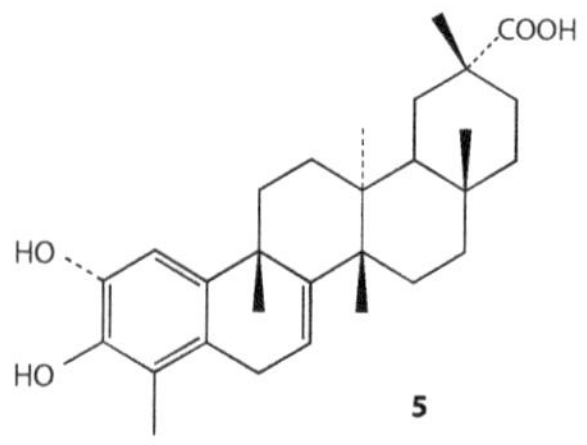

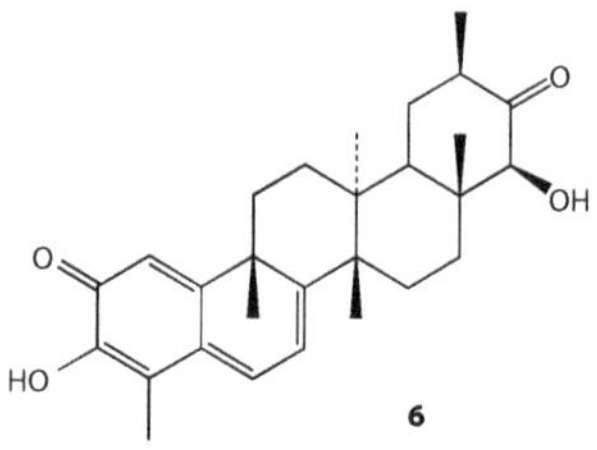

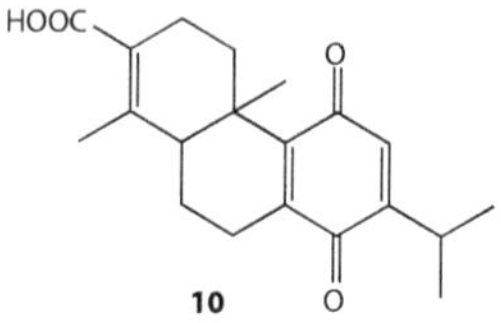

Herb Origination

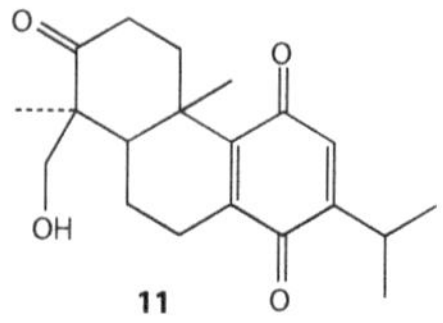

The herb Hei Man (Regels three wingnut) is the dried roots and vine stems of a Celastraceae plant, *Tripterygium regelii*. This vine has another common Chinese name, Dong Bei Lei Gong Teng (東北雷公藤). The shrubby perennial deciduous yellow vine plant is only distributed in northeast of China as well as in Korea and Japan. The root and vine can be collected annually for folk medical application.

Antitumor Activities and Constituents

Triterpenoids

Several anticancer triterpenoids were discovered from Hei Man. Of them, regelin (**1**) and regelinol (**2**) showed the suppressive effect against human KB nasopharyngeal carcinoma cells with ED_{50} values of 4.2 and 10.6 μg/mL, respectively.[1] Celastrol (**3**), whose structure holds a quinone methide moiety, is a major biological active triterpane of Hei Man. With the apoptosis induced by a mitochondrial-dependent caspase pathway, celastrol (**3**) restrained the proliferation of human MCF-7 breast adenocarcinoma cells and three glioma cell lines (U251, SHG44, and C6).[2,3] Also, celastrol (**3**) demonstrated a potent cytotoxic effect on human HL-60 promyelocytic leukemia cells *in vitro* with the apoptotic increase.[4] In both *in vitro* and *in vivo* models, celastrol (**3**) effectively induced the cell apoptotic death and inhibited the growth of B16 melanoma cells, via the activation of ROS-mediated caspase-dependent and -independent pathways and the inhibition of PI3K/AKT/mTOR signaling.[5]

Moreover, celastrol (**3**) is a radiosensitizer, exerting the greatest additive effect on ionizing radiation-induced human lung cancer cell death *in vitro*, wherein the quinone methide moiety is essential for radiosensitization. *In vivo* nude mouse xenografting data also validated that the treatment with I-radiation plus celastrol (**4**) synergistically delayed the lung cancer growth in mice. During the treatment, ROS production was simultaneously enhanced and the activities of antioxidant molecules (such as GSH and thioredoxin reductase) were obstructed, resulting in the potentiation of the I-radiation therapy.[6] Celastrol (**3**), rheol-B (**4**), triptohypol-C (**5**), and their acetates obviously obstructed EBV-EA activation promoted by TPA,[7] indicating that they have anticarcinogenic- and antitumor-promoting potentials. Celastrol (**3**), triptohypol-C (**5**), tingenine-B (**6**), and their acetates also exhibited potent inhibitory activities against lipopolysaccharide (LPS)-elicited human peripheral mononuclear cells to release interleukin-1α and interleukin-1β,[7] displaying certain immunodepressive effect.[8]

Other Terpenes

Three dihydroagarofuran sesquiterpenes from Hei Man, i.e., triptofordin-F2 (**7**), triptogelin-A1 (**8**), and 1,2,6,8,15-pentaacetoxy-9-benzoyloxy-4-hydroxydihydroagarofuran (**9**), exerted the inhibitory effects against TPA-induced EBV-EA activation in Raji cells at low doses.[9] Triptogelin-A1 (**8**) remarkably suppressed mouse skin tumor promotion in an *in vivo* two-stage carcinogenesis model.[10] All the evidences suggested that the sesquiterpenes possess an anticarcinogenetic property. Additionally, two diterpenequinones, triptoquinonoic acid-A (**10**) and triptoquinone-B (**11**) isolated from Hei Man, demonstrated inhibitory activities toward mouse P388 leukemia cells *in vitro*.[11]

References

1. Hori, H. et al. 1987. Isolation and structure of regelin and regelinol, new antitumor ursene-type triterpenoids from *Tripterygium regelii*. *Chem. Pharm. Bull.* 35: 2125–8.
2. Yang, H. S. et al. 2011. Celastrol isolated from *Tripterygium regelii* induces apoptosis through both caspase-dependent and -independent pathways in human breast cancer cells. *Food and Chem. Toxicol.* 49: 527–32.

3. Zhou, Y. X. et al. 2002. Several monomes from *Tripterygium wilfordii* inhibit proliferation of glioma cells in vitro. *Aizheng* 21: 1106–8.
4. Oto, J. et al. 1998. Biological activity of the triterpene celastrol: Analysis from the viewpoint of the apoptosis induction. *Kagawa Daigaku Nogakubu Gakujutsu Hokoku* 50: 79–87.
5. Lee, J. H. et al. 2012. Celastrol inhibits growth and induces apoptotic cell death in melanoma cells via the activation ROS-dependent mitochondrial pathway and the suppression of PI3K/AKT signaling. *Apoptosis* 17: 1275–86.
6. Takaishi, Y. et al. 1997. Triterpenoid inhibitors of interleukin-1 secretion and tumor-promotion from *Tripterygium wilfordii* var. *regelii*. Phytochem. 45: 969–74.
7. Seo, H. G. et al. 2011. Radiosensitization by celastrol is mediated by modification of antioxidant thiol molecules. *Chemico-Biol. Interact.* 193: 34–42.
8. Zhou, B. N. et al. 1991. Some progress on the chemistry of natural bioactive terpenoids from Chinese medicinal plants. *Memorias do Instituto Oswaldo Cruz* 86 (Suppl. 2): 219–26.
9. Takaishi, Y. et al. 1992. Inhibitory effects of dihydroagarofuran sesquiterpenes on Epstein-Barr virus activation. *Cancer Lett.* 65: 19–26.
10. Ujita, K. et al. 1993. Inhibitory effects of triptogelin A-1 on 12-O-tetradecanoylphorbol-13-acetate-induced skin tumor promotion. *Cancer Lett.* 68: 129–33.
11. Shen, J. H. et al. 1992. Studies on diterpene-quinones of *Tripterygium regelii* Sprague. *Chin. Chem. Lett.* 3: 113–6.

71 Lei Gong Teng 雷公藤

Triptolide

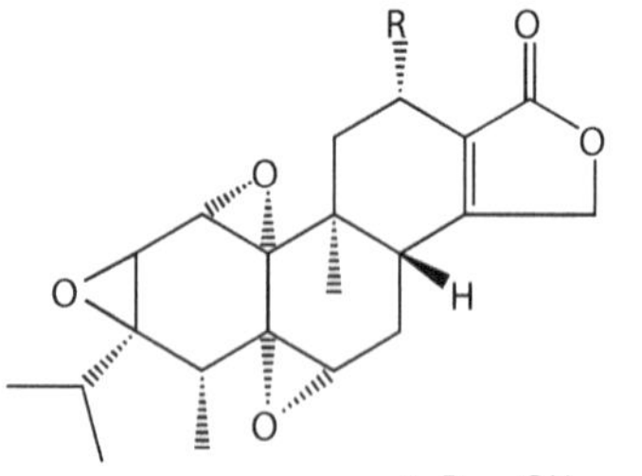

1. R = -OH
2. R = -H

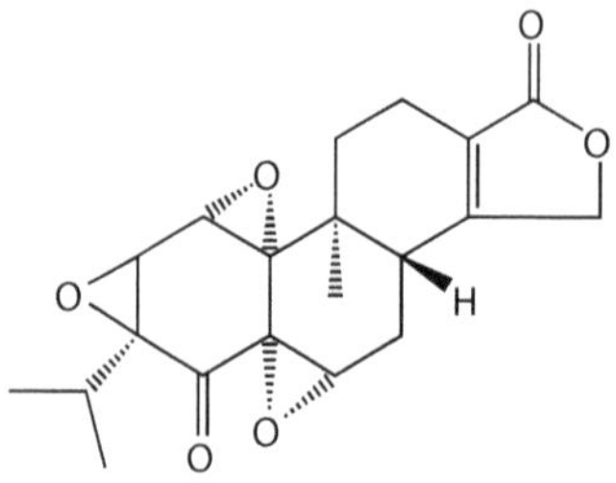

3

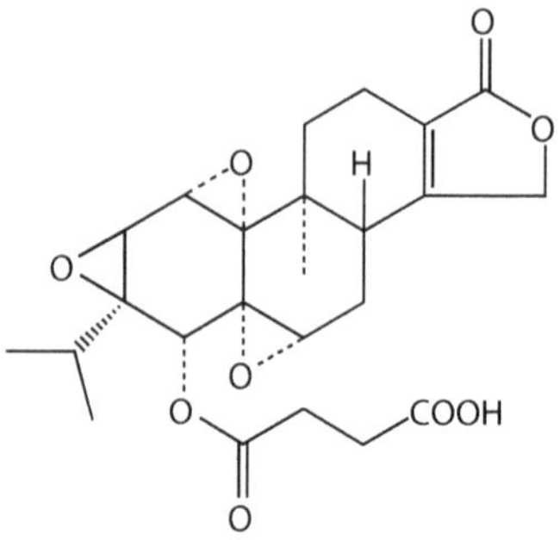

4

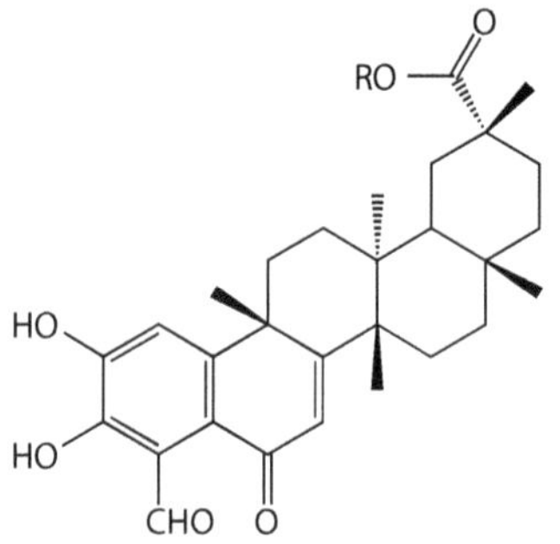

5. R = -H

6. R = -N(CH$_2$CH$_2$OH)$_2$ (CH$_3$)

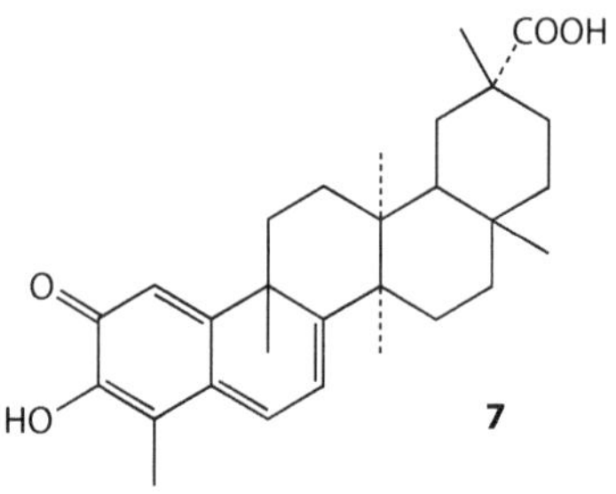

7

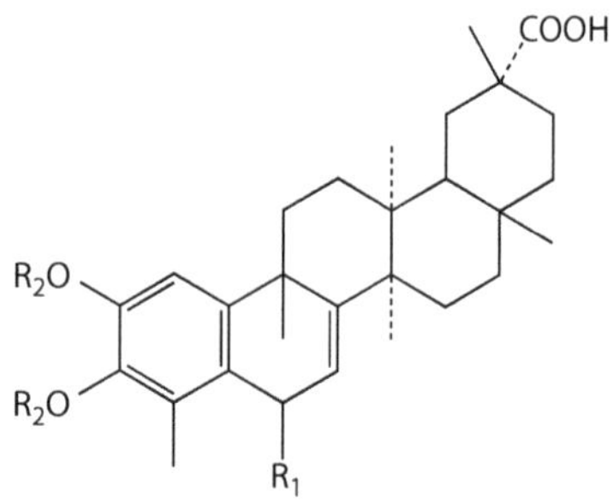

A = -S(p-C$_6$H$_4$)CH$_3$
B = -S(p-C$_6$H$_4$)NHCOCH$_3$
C = -SCH$_2$CH(COOH)NHCOCH$_3$

NST001 R$_1$ = -SO$_3$Na, R$_2$ = -H
NST001A R$_1$ = -SO$_3$Na, R$_2$ = -COCH$_3$
NST001B R$_1$ = -SO$_3$Na, R$_2$ = -COC$_2$H$_5$
NST6A-B R$_1$ = -A, R$_2$ = -COCH$_3$
NST6A-C R$_1$ = -B, R$_2$ = -COCH$_3$
NST6A-D R$_1$ = -C, R$_2$ = -COCH$_3$

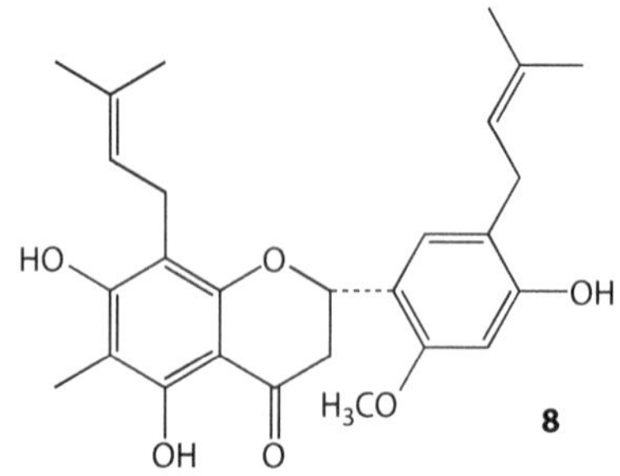

8

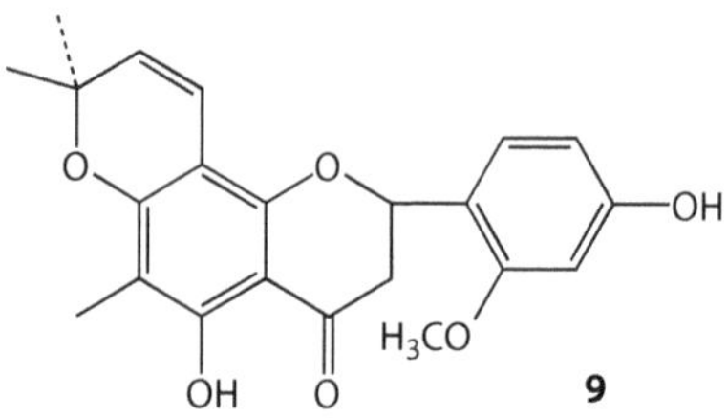

9

Herb Origination

The herb Lei Gong Teng (Triptolide) is the dried roots and stems of a Celastraceae plant, *Tripterygium wilfordii*. According to its Chinese name, the herb is sometimes translated as thunder god vine or thunder duke vine. This deciduous climbing vine is native to the southern part of China and to Burma. In China, it is generally distributed in the southern region of Yangtze River, Taiwan, and the southwest region. Its roots and vines can be annually collected for folk medicinal use, but the root bark is normally scraped off because its toxicity is too strong in this portion.

Antitumor Constituents and Activities

Over the past three decades of continuous investigation, over 46 diterpenoids, 20 new triterpenoids, 26 alkaloids, and other types of small molecules were identified from Lei Gong Teng. The antineoplastic components in the herb are primarily classified as two types of terpenoids: diterpenoids and triterpenoids. The diterpenoids such as triptolide (**1**), tripdiolide (**2**), triptonide (**3**), and wilforlides; and the triterpenoids, such as demethylzeylasteral, tripchlorolide, celastrol, and its N-methyldiethanolamine salt, were found to be truly responsible for the significant cytotoxic activity.

Triptolide and Tripdiolide

Triptolide (**1**) and tripdiolide (**2**) are characterized as abeoabietane-type diterpenoids with an α,β-unsaturated-5-membered lactone and triepoxides, exhibiting a broad cytotoxicity and an apoptosis-inducing property against various neoplastic cells with either wild-type p53 or mutant form of p53. *In vitro* and *in vivo* experiments have revealed the extensive spectrum of triptolide (**1**) in the anticancer activities,[1–3] for which reason it has indeed been paid attention for advanced investigations.

Anticarcinoma Effect in Female Sexual Organs

Four kinds of human breast cancer cell lines were evaluated in the presence of triptolide (**1**). At very low concentrations (2–10 ng/mL), triptolide (**1**) exhibited more suppressive activity than taxol toward the growth and the colony formation of MCF-7 and BT-20 breast cancer cell lines.[4] The treatment with 25 nM of triptolide for 48 h exhibited marked inhibitory effects on the cell viability of the three types of cells with greater effects observed in BT-474 EGFR2+ breast cancer cells compared with the other two cell types (MCF-7 and MDA-MB-231).[5] The MCF-7 (wild-type p53 and ERα-positive) cells were more sensitive to triptolide (**1**) than MDA-MB-231 (ERα-negative and mutant p53) breast cancer cells by almost 10 times. A 50 nM triptolide treatment resulted in the significant apoptosis of MDA-MB-231, BT-474 and MCF7 cells via a mechanism associated with the Wnt/β-catenin signaling pathway.[5] However, triptolide (**1**) induced only the slight S cell arrest of MCF-7 cells but elicited a significant S cell arrest of MDA-MB-231 cells, indicating that triptolide (**1**) mediated by particular pathways on different breast cancer cell lines. The decrease of ERα expression was one of the important events for the antigrowth potency on the breast cancer cell lines *in vitro* and *in vivo*.[4,6] The marked suppression of triptolide (**1**) on the anchorage-independent growth of the MCF-7 cells was found to be also mediated by inducing the cleavage of FAK and PARP, activating caspases, and decreasing cell adhesion potential concentration-dependently, but no cleaved FAK was observed in the triptolide-treated MDA-MB-231 cells.[7] The antiproliferative effect was also observed in other breast cancer cell lines (UISO-BCA-1, UISO-BCA-2, SK-BR-3, ZR-75-1, and HBL-100) with respective ED_{50} values of 6, 20, 10, 10, and 1 ng/mL.[6] The anti-breast-cancer activity of triptolide (**1**) was further proven in animal model implanted with MDA-435 or MCF-7 breast cancer cells. The i.p. injection of 25 μg triptolide (**1**) per time (three times weekly) to nude mice resulted in the significant inhibitory effect against human UISO-BCA-1 breast carcinoma.[6–9]

The remarkable anticancer activity of triptolide (**1**) was also observed in other types of human sexual organ-related cancer cell lines *in vitro*, such as endometrial tumor (Ishikawa, HEC-1B, and HHUA), ovarian cancer (SKOV-3, OVCAR-3, and A2780), and cervical cancer (SKG-II), concomitant with multiple regulations of cell cycle arrest, apoptotic death, and cell proliferative inhibition.[10,11] Triptolide (**1**) elicited a marked apoptosis promotion of the HEC-1B cells via a p53-independent mitochondrial pathway, including the downregulation of Bcl-2 level and the upregulation of Bax level and caspase-3 and caspase-9 activities.[12,13] At the same lower concentration (<5 μg/ml), the inhibition of triptolide (**1**) was greater than that of cisplatin (a chemotherapeutic agent) on A2780 cells. When a combined treatment was used with these two agents (triptolide and cisplatin), the growth inhibition on the A2780 cells was notably enhanced with the prolongation of the affected time.[12] In association with the repression of MMP-7 and MMP-19 expressions and the augmentation of E-cad expression in the tumor dose-dependently, the triptolide (**1**) treatment restrained the migration and the invasion of human SKOV-3 and A2780 ovarian cancer cells at a concentration of 15 nM *in vitro* and obstructed the tumor formation and metastasis in nude mice implant with SKOV-3 cells.[14]

Anticarcinoma Effect in Prostate

A water-soluble form of triptolide (**1**) is a promising drug candidate with the admission to phase I clinical trial for the treatment of prostate carcinoma. Triptolide (**1**) displayed dose-dependent suppressive effects on both normal and adenocarcinomas-derived primary cultures of human prostatic epithelial cells. Triptolide (**1**) in a lower dose retarded the cell proliferation and elicited a senescence-like phenotype in prostate cancer cells, and in a higher concentration, promoted tumor cell apoptosis, associated with the activation of p53 and the decrease of p21 WAF1/CIP1, hdm-2, and Bcl-2 expressions.[15,16] The exposure of two human prostate cancer cell lines (PC3 and LNCaP) to triptolide (**1**) markedly inhibited the cell growth and enhanced the cell death *in vitro* and gave an ED_{50} value of 10 ng/mL in the LNCaP cells.[6] The antigrowth activity was proven in nude mice-xenografted PC3 prostate cancer cells, whose inhibitory activity was mediated by the decline of SENP1 expression and the blockage of AR and c-Jun expressions and their mediated transcription in the prostate cancer cells.[17]

Antileukemia Effect

Both triptolide (**1**) and tripdiolide (**2**) were effective in the growth inhibition of murine L1210 and P388 lymphocytic leukemia cells at a dose of 0.1 mg/kg and of HL-60 human promyelocytic leukemia cells in a dose of 2–10 ng/kg *in vivo*.[3,18,19] Because HL-60 cells is a p53-deficient leukemia, the apoptosis-promoting effect by triptolide (**1**) was mediated by an activated p53-independent and mitochondria-dependent pathway.[20] In the concentration of 25 nM, triptolide (**1**) was able to promote the apoptosis of human U937 monocytic leukemia cells, associated with the downregulation of XIAP and the activation of caspase-3.[16] The treatment with triptolide (**1**) notably enhanced the apoptosis of human K562 erythroleukemia cells in dose- and time-dependent manners and obstructed the cell proliferation (IC_{50}: 40 ng/mL), whose apoptosis induction was associated with a strong inhibition on inflammatory factors COX-2 and iNOS and the down-expression of Bcl.[21,22] In MDM2-overexpressed ALL cells, the presence of triptolide (**1**) could elicit the cell apoptosis through the decrease of MDM2 expression and its transcriptional level, the increase of p53 levels, and the repression of XIAP, leading to the inhibition of the proliferation of ALL cells.[23] Furthermore, *in vivo* experiments disclosed that the treatment with triptolide (**1**) obviously prolonged the life duration of mice bearing L615 leukemia by 87.8% and 159.8%, respectively, at 0.20 and 0.25 mg/kg doses.[24] More *in vitro* and *in vivo* findings revealed that triptolide dramatically induced Rho-associated coiled-coil-containing protein kinase (ROCK1) cleavage/activation and myosin light chain (MLC) and myosin binding subunit of MLC phosphatase (MYPT) phosphorylation in human leukemia cell lines. The ROCK1 activation and the MLC phosphorylation were associated with the antileukemia effect of triptolide.[25] All these remarkable evidences strongly supported the further development of triptolide (**1**) as a new antileukemia drug lead.

Antimyeloma Effect

Triptolide (**1**) is capable of time- and dose-dependently inducing G2/M cell cycle arrest and caspase-dependent apoptosis and retarding the proliferation of U266 multiple myeloma cells, where the downregulation of histone H3K4, H3K27, and H3K36 trimethylation was involved in the antimyeloma mechanism of the triptolide.[26] The apoptosis of various myeloma cell lines could be rapidly induced by triptolide, associated with the loss of the mitochondrial transmembrane potential, the release of cytochrome c and Smac/DIABLO to cytosol, the activation of caspase-3 and caspase-9, and the rapid inhibition of Mcl-1 transcription.[27] More importantly, by replacing PI3k/Akt/NF-κB and MAPK pathways, triptolide (**1**) effectively restrained the proliferation of both dexamethasone-sensitive MM.1S myeloma cells and dexamethasone-resistant MM.1R multiple myeloma cells.[28] In a cotreatment, the cytotoxicities of dexamethasone and bortezomib/PS-341 could be potentiated by triptolide (**1**) against both multiple myeloma cell lines. These findings suggested a potential development of triptolide (**1**) to overcome the drug resistance for clinic patients with this universally fatal hematological malignancy.[28]

Anticarcinoma Effect in the Digestive System

Four gastric cancer cell lines with different p53 status such as AGS and MKN-45 (wild type p53), SGC-7901, and MKN-28 (mutant p53) were treated with triptolide (**1**). The growth of AGS cells with wild-type p53 was inhibited, and the apoptosis and G0/G1 cell cycle arrest was promoted in association with the up-expressions of p53, p21waf1/cip1 and Bax proteins, the activation of caspases, and the blockage of NK-κB and AP-1 transactivation. With the triptolide (**1**) treatment, the growth-restraining and apoptosis-increasing effects were observed in MKN-45 cells with wild-type p53 but no such effects in MKN-28 and SGC-7901 cells with mutant p53.[29] Moreover, the suppressive effect of triptolide was also demonstrated in various types of stomach cancer cell lines (KATO-III, MKN-7, and MKN-45) *in vitro*[1] and in MGC803 gastric carcinoma *in vivo*.[8] All these findings revealed that triptolide (**1**) exerted the differential inhibitory effects on the gastric cancer cells with different p53 status, and a functional p53 preferred for the proapoptotic and antitumor effects of triptolide (**1**).[29]

Triptolide (**1**) is a potent inhibitor of colon cancer proliferation and migration. The *in vivo* treatment with triptolide (**1**) could decline the incidence of tumor formation and elevate the survival rate of mice/nude mice inoculated with colon cancer cells dose-dependently. In the *in vitro* assays, the proliferation of human SW114 colon cancer cells was dose-dependently obstructed by triptolide (**1**) at 5–50 ng/mL concentrations, concomitant with the inhibition on two inflammatory factors COX-2 and iNOS activities.[22] Triptolide (**1**) potently obstructed the growth of HCT116 and HT-29 colon cancer cells and reduced the migration of HCT116 cells through the collagen by 65–80%. During the inhibitions, triptolide retarded the mRNA expression of the positive cell cycle regulators (c-Myc and A-, B-, C-, and D-types of cyclins), declined the expressions of VEGF and COX-2, and restrained the expressions of multiple cytokine receptors (CXCR4, TNF receptors, and TGF-β receptors). All these interactions subsequently led to the potent inhibition of the proliferation, migration, invasion, and metastasis of the multiple colon cancer cell lines.[30] Moreover, the *in vitro* experiments also demonstrated that triptolide (**1**) has marked capacities in diminishing the incidences of colon cell inflammation, inhibition of the proliferation, colony formation, and migration of colon cancer cells induced by colitis through the interruption of an IL6R-JAK/STAT pathway, i.e., reducing the secretion of IL-6 and the levels of JAK1, IL6R, and phosphorylated STAT3 and obstructing Rac1 activity and cyclin-D1 and CDK4 expressions, and then elongating the survival rate of mice/nude mice implanted with colon cancer cells dose-dependently.[31]

Moreover, the treatment with triptolide (**1**) in a dose of 0.5 μg/mL effectively promoted the apoptosis of highly fatal cholangiocarcinoma cells with the ED_{50} value of ≥0.05 μg/mL. The administration of triptolide (**1**) to hamster bearing carcinoma in a dose of 0.12 mg 10 times obviously inhibited the choledochus cancer cell growth and lessened the tumor size after one month of treatment.[32] When combined with TRAIL, the TRAIL-induced apoptotic killing ability was susceptibility enhanced by triptolide (**1**) even in TRAIL-resistant cholangiocarcinoma cells, offering synergistic suppression against cholangiocarcinoma.[33] Similarly, triptolide (**1**) could sensitize pancreatic cancer cells to the TRAIL-induced activation of death receptor pathway by increasing the levels of death receptor DR5 and decreasing the c-FLIP, which contribute to caspase-8 activation. Therefore, the cotreatment elicited both lysosomal and mitochondrial membrane permeabilizations, resulting in the cell death of pancreatic cancer cells.[34]

Anticarcinoma Effect in Lung

Triptolide (**1**) remarkably restrained the growth of squamous lung cancer caused by 3-methylcholanthrene by 65.13%.[17] Human UISO-LUC-1 lung carcinoma cell line treated by triptolide (**1**) exhibited the significant ED_{50} value of 10 ng/mL.[4] Through the suppression of NF-κB activation and regardless of the p53 phenotype, triptolide (**1**) sensitized both A549 (wild p53) and NCI-H1299 (null p53) human lung carcinoma cells to Apo2L/TRAIL-induced apoptosis, whose effect was mediated by the activations of ERK2 and caspases and the inhibition of p65 transactivation. The events elicited by triptolide (**1**) were also observed in the *ex vivo* culture of lung cancer tissue from four patients who underwent surgery.[35,36]

Anticancer Effect in Head Part

The prominent growth inhibitory and apoptosis-inducing activities of triptolide (**1**) was demonstrated at a nanomolar concentration in two human SCC25 and OEC-M1 oral cancer cells and in human KB nasopharynx cancer cells *in vitro* and *in vivo*.[37] The anticancer property of triptolide (**1**) was showed not only in the drug-sensitive parental KB and KB-3 cells but also in the multidrug-resistant KB-7D, KB-VI, and KB-tax cells. The MDR protein and MDR in both KB-7D and KB-tax cells were significantly lessened, and the apoptotic death was markedly augmented by triptolide (**1**) by activating caspase-3 and reducing Mcl-1 and XIAP expressions in both *in vitro* and xenograft mouse models. When the triptolide (**1**) was combined with 5-FU, the therapeutic value of triptolide (**1**) on multidrug-resistant cells could be obviously amplified.[8,38]

Moreover, triptolide (**1**) treatment remarkably obstructed the proliferation of SHG44, C6, and U251 glioma cell lines *in vitro* and accelerated the apoptotic death by promoting Bax expression and restraining Bcl-2 expression.[39] The *in vitro* assay also showed that triptolide (**1**) inhibited the cell growth, proliferation, and colony-forming ability of BE2-C neuroblastoma cells, together with the induction of cell apoptosis and cell cycle arrest in S phase. The tumorigenicity of neuroblastoma cells was confirmed by an *in vivo* tumorigenic assay.[40]

Antimelanoma Effect

The *in vivo* treatment of mice with triptolide (**1**) for two to three weeks restrained the growth of xenografts formed by B16 melanoma and obstructed the experimental metastasis of B16-F10 melanoma cells to the spleens and the lungs of mice.[8,9] The suppressive potency of triptolide (**1**) was comparable or superior to that of conventional antitumor drugs (cisplatin, Adm, and mitomycin). Importantly, the triptolide treatment could reverse the drug-resistance of tumor cells to taxol by inhibiting the overexpressed multidrug resistant gene-1.[9] Moreover, the *in vivo* treatment with triptolide (**1**) also notably decreased the proportion of regulatory T cells, lowered the Foxp3 level in spleen and auxiliary lymph nodes, reduced IL-10 production and transforming growth factor-β in peripheral blood and spleen, and remarkably inhibited VEGF production, which all interactions contributed to the antigrowth effect in mice implanted with B16-F10 melanoma.[41]

Anticancer Effect in Other Body Parts

Triptolide (**1**) showed a marked tumoricidal effect on Hodgkin's lymphocyte sarcoma Daudi cells *in vitro* in 10–42 μg/mL doses[22] and dose-dependently inhibited the proliferation of human HT-1080 fibrosarcoma and SAS squamous carcinoma and SKG-II uterine cervical cancer cell lines, whose effect was found to be initiated by a decrease in PI3K activity, in turn leading to the increase of JNK1 phosphorylation via Akt and/or PKC-independent pathway(s). The results indicated that JNK1 activation was a key required for the antitumor activity of triptolide (**1**) on HT-1080, SAS, and SKG-II carcinoma cells.[10] Also, by activating both death receptor and mitochondrial apoptotic pathways, triptolide (**1**) exerted antigrowth and proapoptotic effects in human osteosarcoma U2OS cells.[42] During the marked suppression on the proliferation, migration, and survivability of laryngocarcinoma HEp-2 cells, triptolide (**1**) promoted G1 cell cycle arrest and apoptosis through p53-dependent intrinsic and extrinsic pathways including the activation of p53 through the damage of DNA and the inhibition of E6-mediated p53 degradation.[43] Likewise, the growth of TSU bladder cancer cells could be restrained in mice by the *in vivo* treatment with triptolide (**1**) for two to three weeks.[8] The cotreatment with triptolide and cisplatin synergistically enhanced the antitumor effect on cisplatin-resistant human T24R2 bladder cancer cells, together with the induction of cell cycle arrest and apoptosis via cyclin-D1 and cyclin-E1 expression, release of cytochrome c, and activation of caspase-3, caspase-8, caspase-9, and PARP.[44]

Antiangiogenesis

Various angiogenesis assays established that triptolide (**1**) is an angiogenesis inhibitor with an IC_{50} value of 45 nM in HUVEC cells *in vitro*. When dosed at 0.75 mg/kg/day *in vivo*, triptolide (**1**) potently blocked the tumor angiogenesis and retarded the tumor progression in a murine tumorigenesis assay. The finding implied that the *in vivo* anticancer property of triptolide (**1**) was partly contributed by the inhibition of angiogenesis. The antiangiogenic mechanism was closely parallel with the attenuation of two endothelial receptor-mediated signaling pathways by lessening the expressions of proangiogenic Tie2 and VEGFR-2.[45]

Triptolide Derivatives

Due to its severe toxicity and water insolubility, triptolide (**1**) was often limited for clinical use. PG490-88 (**4**) and F60008, two new water-soluble triptolide derivatives, have been synthesized, presenting safe and potent antitumor benefits. F60008 is a prodrug that can be converted to triptolide (**1**) *in vivo*. In the *in vitro* and *in vivo* models, PG490-88 (**4**) obviously stimulated the cell apoptosis and sensitized the cancer cells to Topo inhibitors by blocking the p53-mediated induction of p21. A combined treatment with PG490-88 (**4**) and CPT-11 could force the regression of lung and colon cancer xenografts.[46] Now, PG490-88 (**4**) has been introduced to phase I clinical trial for the treatment of prostate neoplasm in the United States, whereas F60008 entered phase I dose escalation study in patients with advanced solid tumors.[47]

By the continuing investigations for design and synthesis of more valuable agents with the start molecule of triptolide, a series of triptolide derivatives have been reported, in which the C-14-hydroxyl were substituted by different amine esters. Many of the derivatives showed a potent inhibitory activity on KBM5 CML cells and KBM5-T315I (imatinib-resistant) leukemia cells concomitantly with the obvious downregulation of Bcr-AblmRNA *in vitro*.[48] The results clearly disclosed that the stereo-hindrance of C-14 group is largely responsible for the antitumor potentials.[49]

Other Diterpene Components

Five diterpenes assigned as 3-epi-triptobenzene-B, triptobenzene-B, wilforol-E, triptohairic acid, and hypoglic acid were isolated from the herb, displaying the inhibitory effects against the proliferation of human HeLa cervical cancer and murine L929 fibrosarcoma cell lines *in vitro*.[50] The transformed diterpenoid derivatives such as 17-hydroxytriptonide, 16-hydroxytriptonide, and 5-hydroxytriptonide were cytotoxic to most of the human cancer cell lines, but the degree of cytotoxicities were less than those of triptonide (**3**).[50]

Glycosides

The total glycosides (TGs) prepared from Lei Gong Teng exerted the suppressive effects on the DNA synthesis and the growth and the division of HeLa neoplastic cells *in vitro*.[51] Thirty patients with hysteromyoma had been treated by a combined oral administration of a steroid drug mifepristone (10 mg/day) and TGs (20 mg/day) for three months. The cochemotherapy reduced the uterine tumor volume from 16% to 37% and enlarged the effectivity rate from 73% to 93% in comparison with the treatment with mifepristone alone. Simultaneously, the clinical symptoms were markedly improved after the cotreatment, implying that TGs integrated with mifepristone is useful for treating hysteronmyoma to exert the definite and stable therapeutic effect with high effectivity rate.[52]

Nortriterpenoids

Demethylzeylasterals

Two nortriterpenoids, demethylzeylasteral (**5**) and its N-methyldiethanolamine salt (**6**) separated from Lei Gong Teng, were found to markedly suppress the growth of fibrosarcoma cells.[53] Also the nortriterpenoids are inhibitors of vascularization. Demethylzeylasteral (**5**) inhibited the proliferation of vascular endothelial cells about 30 times more effectively than it did with its antiproliferative effect on human cancer cells.[54] Demethylzeylasteral (**5**) at nontoxic doses repressed cell migration as well as reduced u-PA mRNA expression and activity. The daily oral administration of demethylzeylasteral (**5**) at a dose of 3 mg/kg for five days showed a partial inhibition, but at a daily dose of 30 mg/kg, it almost completely abrogated the development of human hepatoblastoma cells. Similarly, the growth of mouse B16-F10 melanoma cells was partially retarded by demethylzeylasteral (**5**) at a dose of 0.3 mg/kg per day and was almost completely blocked at doses of 3 or 30 mg/kg per day in the tumor implantation assay. According to the marked inhibition against the growth of well-vascularized tumor cells and the density of the microvessels in the tumors, demethylzeylasteral (**5**) may be considered as a promising drug lead in the treatment of highly vascularized and metastatic tumors as well as other angiogenic diseases.[55]

In addition, *in vitro* experiments also evaluated other isolated triterpenoids from the herb. Of them, triptotin-G and wilforol-A displayed the antiproliferative effect against several neoplastic cell lines. Both triterpenoids significantly obstructed the proliferation of P388 murine leukemia cells, and triptotin-D also selectively restrained the human A549 lung adenocarcinoma cells (see Sections Kun Ming Shan Hai Tang and Hei Man).[56]

Celastrol

A quinone methide triterpene termed celastrol (**7**) is one of the characteristic bioactive components in the herb, which is normally used as a remedy of chronic inflammatory and autoimmune diseases, e.g., rheumatoid arthritis.[55] An *in vitro* assay showed that celastrol (**7**) promoted the apoptosis of leukemia cells and repressed the proteasome activity in human 26S prostate cancer cells. Celastrol (**7**) could elicit the accumulation of three natural proteasome substrates (IκBα, Bax, and p27) in either of the two types of prostate cancer cell lines, PC3 (AR-neg.) and LNCaP (AR-pos.), and the suppression of AR protein expression in LNCaP cells, subsequently inducing cell apoptosis. An *in vivo* treatment of the PC3 tumor with celastrol (**7**) in daily doses of 1–3 mg/kg by i.p. injection for ~31 days resulted in a marked growth inhibition (65–93%) in nude mice.[57] Celastrol (**7**) markedly induced the apoptosis of LP-1 human multiple myeloma cells and inhibited the proliferation of LP-1 cells (IC_{50}: 0.88 μmol/L).[58] The *in vitro* assay exhibited that celastrol (**7**) obviously retarded proteasomal activity and potently elicited apoptosis and G0/G1 cell cycle arrest to inhibit the cell proliferation of the PC3 cells via the down-expression of IL-6 through a NF-κB-dependent pathway.[57–59] *In vitro* and *in vivo* experiments showed the down-regulating effect of celastrol (**7**) on HIF-1α expression, leading to antigrowth and antiproliferative effects on Hep3B hepatoma cells.[60] Through the down-expression of antiapoptotic proteins (cIAP1 and cIAP2, cellular FLIP, and Bcl-2) and the activation of caspase-8, caspase-3 and PARP cleavage, celastrol (**7**) potentiated TNF-α-induced apoptosis of MDA-MB-231 human breast cancer cells, and also through the down-expression of TNFα-induced MMP-9, celastrol prominently reduced the invasion of the MDA-MB-231 cells.[61] Moreover, the capability of celastrol (**7**) in inducing TNF-induced apoptosis and inhibiting the invasion of tumor cells was also found to be parallel with the inactivation of TAK1-mediated NF-κB pathway.[62]

Besides effectively enhancing the antiproliferative and apoptotic effects on NSCLC cells, celastrol (**7**) also potentiated the inhibitory effect of the cytotoxic agent cisplatin on NSCLC cells *in vitro* and *in vivo* via the inhibition of a CIP2A-Akt pathway.[63] The apoptosis of two gefitinib-resistant NSCLC cell lines (H1650 and H1975) could be promoted in dose- and time-dependent manners, whose effects were mediated by caspase-dependent mitochondria pathways and degradation of Hsp90 client proteins (EGFR and AKT).[64] By a cotreatment, celastrol (**7**) enhanced the ability of lapatinib to synergistically exert the antigrowth and apoptosis-inducing effects against HepG2 hepatoma cells concomitant with the downregulation of EGFR expression.[65] Celastrol (**7**) also showed its marked ability to play hypoxia-mediated antiangiogenic and antimetastatic effects via a HIF-1α pathway.[66] At a 0.2 μg/mL concentration, celastrol (**7**) significantly suppressed the proliferation of ECV-304 vascular endothelial cells with an IC_{50} value of 1.33 μg/mL, and it also obstructed the cell migration and the tube formation.[67] Further studies by using human glioma xenografts revealed that celastrol (**7**) retarded the expressions of VEGFR-1 and VEGFR-2, reduced the signal transduction between VEGF and VEGF receptors, and markedly attenuated the microvessel density in nude mice. Based on these great antiangiogenetic properties, the subcutaneous administration of celastrol (**7**) for four consecutive weeks achieved a significant suppression on the size of SHG-44 glioma in a xenograft model.[68] Moreover, the antimetastatic activity of celastrol (**7**) was proven in human 95-D lung carcinoma cells *in vitro* and in mouse B16-F10 melanoma cells *in vitro* and *in vivo*. Simultaneously, celastrol (**7**) inhibited the cell extracellular matrix adhesion by blocking the β1-integrin ligand affinity and retarding the formation of focal adhesion by activating the p38-MAPK pathway and reducing the focal adhesion kinase phosphorylation.[69] Consequently, the evidences highlighted that celastrol (**7**) is a potential agent for effectively fighting the proliferation, angiogenesis, and metastasis of malignant tumors and promoting the efficacy of anticancer drugs.

Celastrol Analogs

Based on semisynthetic derivatives of celastrol, the structure and activity analysis revealed that a quinone methide moiety is required for the antitumor activity.[70] Celastrol (**7**) and its analogs (Cel-1, Cel-3, Cel-6, Cel-13) exhibited the antiproliferative effect on rat PC12 pheochromocytoma cells and rat C6 glioma cells *in vitro*. The IC_{50} values of celastrol (**7**) and its analogs were 3.2 and 1.3–2.4 μmol/L in the PC12 cells, while IC_{50} values of celastrol (**7**) and Cel-6 were 1.5 and 0.6 μmol/L in the C6 cells, respectively, whose inhibitory activities were largely superior to those of cisplatin on the PC12 and C6 cell lines.[71] Likewise, six C6-celastrol derivatives were designed and synthesized, and their potent inhibitory activities were shown against BGC823 (stomach), H4 (liver), and Bel7402 (liver) human cancer cell lines *in vitro* (IC_{50}: 0.39–1.84 μM).

The C(6)-sulfided celastrol derivatives, NST6A-B, NST6A-C, and NST6A-D, showed a more potent anticancer effect on the three cancer cell lines (IC_{50}: 0.35–0.54 μM), and the potencies were about five to eight times higher than that of the parent molecule celastrol (**7**). The C(6)-sulfonted celastrol derivatives, NST001 and NST001A, also showed the potent inhibition against H522 (lung), Colo205 (colon), HepG2 (liver), and MDA-MB-468 (breast) human neoplastic cell lines (IC_{50}: 0.06–0.89 μM) and NST001A exerted the most potent effect toward Colo205 cells (IC_{50}: 0.06 μM) *in vitro* and *in vivo*.[72] But NST001 was more potent than NST001A in the antitumor profile on BGC823 gastric cancer cells (IC_{50}: 0.77 versus 1.53 μM). Subsequently, the C(6) derivatives of celastrol may be considered as potential drug candidates for further development in cancer treatment.[72]

Liposomes of Celastrol

Due to its low water solubility, the intestinal absorption and the anticancer effect of celastrol are poor when orally administrated. A liposome formulation composed of phospholipid, cholesterol, and Tween-80 resulted in a favorable encapsulation efficiency and exhibited an improved effective permeability.[73] PEGylated 1,2-distearoyl-sn-glycero-3-phosphocholine (DSPC) celastrol liposomes improved the efficient cellular uptake and anticancer efficacy in prostate cancer cells, comparable to that of free celastrol (**7**). By embedding celastrol in a liposomal bilayer, its release can be over an extended period, enhancing its bioavailability and reducing its frequency of dosing.[74]

Flavanones

Two unusual and antitumor active prenylated and C-methylated flavanones were isolated from the stems and the roots of *T. wilfordii* and were elucidated as (2S)-5,7,4′-trihydroxy-2′-methoxy-8,5′-di-(3-methyl-2-butenyl)-6-methyflavanone (**8**) and (±)-5,4′-dihydroxy-2′-methoxy-6′,6″-dimethypyrano-(2″,3″,7,8)-6-methyflavanone (**9**).[75] The two flavanones ((2S)-5,7,4′-trihydroxy-2′-methoxy-8,5′-di-(3-methyl-2-butenyl)-6-methyflavanone (**8**) and (±)-5,4′-dihydroxy-2′-methoxy-6′,6″-dimethypyrano-(2″,3″,7,8)-6-methyflavanone (**9**)) exerted a moderate antiproliferative effect against human HT-29 (colon) and ZR-75-1 (breast) carcinoma cell lines *in vitro*, with IC_{50} values of 22.9–35.1 and 10.3–13.2 μM, respectively. Additionally, the flavanone (±)-5,4′-dihydroxy-2′-methoxy-6′,6″-dimethypyrano-(2″,3″,7,8)-6-methylflavanone (**9**) exhibited an inhibitory effect on LPS-triggered NO production in RAW cells with IC_{50} value of 15.0 μM.[75]

Other Bioactivities

The herb Lei Gong Teng has similar bioactivities as KMSHT. Currently available data suggest that triptolide (**1**) is a promising immunosuppressive and antiinflammatory agent. For these activities, it could be used for the treatment of a variety of autoimmune diseases (rheumatoid arthritis) and transplantation. Triptolide (**1**) also displayed male antifertility effect. Moreover, tripterifordin exhibited an anti-HIV replication activity, and salaspermic acid was identified as an inhibitor of HIV reverse transcriptase. Celastrol (**7**) was proven to be a strong immunosuppressor and inhibited free radical damage in the models with experimental arthritis.

Toxic and Side Effects

The herb possesses a strong toxicity that causes marked side effects, especially in gastrointestinal tract. The toxicities of triptolide (**1**) are associated with hematopoietic, renal, cardiac, and reproductive systems. Thus, patients suffering from diseases of the heart, the liver, and the kidney as well as the lower level of leukocyte have to be very careful in the treatment with the herb and must follow doctor's instruction. It is prohibited for pregnant woman to use this herb.

References

1. Wang, C. Y. et al. 2014. Traditional Chinese medicine: A treasured natural resource of anticancer drug research and development. *Am. J. Chin. Med.* 42: 543–59.
2. Li, Q. Y. et al. 2011. Triptolide and its expanding multiple pharmacological functions. *Intl. Immunopharmacol.* 11: 377–83.
3. Wei, Y. S. et al. 1991. Inhibitory effect of triptolide on colony formation of breast and stomach cancer cell lines. *Zhongguo Yaoli Xuebao* 12: 406–10.
4. Liu, J. et al. 2009. Effects of triptolide from *Tripterygium wilfordii* on ERα and p53 expression in two human breast cancer cell lines. *Phytomed.* 16: 1006–13.
5. Shao, H. M. et al. 2014. Triptolide induces apoptosis of breast cancer cells via a mechanism associated with the Wnt/β-catenin signaling pathway. *Experim. Therap. Med.* 8: 505–8.
6. Li, H. et al. 2015. Triptolide inhibits human breast cancer MCF-7 cell growth via downregulation of the ERα-mediated signaling pathway. *Acta Pharmacol. Sinica* 36: 606–13.
7. Tan, B. J. et al. 2011. Effect of triptolide on focal adhesion kinase and survival in MCF-7 breast cancer cells. *Oncol. Reports* 26: 1315–21.
8. Shamon, L. A. et al. 1997. Evaluation of the mutagenic, cytotoxic, and antitumor potential of triptolide, a highly oxygenated diterpene isolated from Tripterygium wilfordii. *Cancer Lett.* 112: 113–7.
9. Yang, S. M. et al. 2003. Triptolide inhibit the growth and metastasis of solid tumors. *Mol. Cancer Therap.* 2: 65–72.
10. Miyata, Y. et al. 2005. Triptolide, a diterpenoid triepoxide, induces antitumor proliferation via activation of c-Jun NH2-terminal kinase 1 by decreasing phosphatidylinositol 3-kinase activity in human tumor cells. *Biochem. Biophys. Res. Communic.* 336: 1081–6.
11. Li, H. L. et al. 2010. Novel target genes responsive to the anti-growth activity of triptolide in endometrial and ovarian cancer cells. *Cancer Lett.* 297: 198–206.
12. Zhang, X. M. et al. 2008. Study of the effect of triptolide in ovarian cancer cell line A2780. *Huaxi Yixue* 23: 324–6.
13. Wang, X. F. et al. 2014. Triptolide induces apoptosis in endometrial cancer via a p53-independent mitochondrial pathway. *Mol. Med. Reports* 9: 39–44.
14. Zhao, H. X. et al. 2012. Triptolide inhibits ovarian cancer cell invasion by repression of matrix metalloproteinase 7 and 19 and upregulation of E-cadherin. *Exp. Mol. Med.* 44: 633–41.
15. Kiviharju, T. M. et al. 2002. Antiproliferative and proapoptotic activities of triptolide (PG490), a natural product entering clinical trials, on primary cultures of human prostatic epithelial cells. *Clin. Cancer Res.* 8: 2666–74.

16. Chang, W. et al. 2001. Triptolide and chemotherapy cooperate in tumor cell apoptosis: A role for the p53 pathway. *J. Biol. Chem.* 276: 2221–7.
17. Huang, W. W. et al. 2012. Triptolide inhibits the proliferation of prostate cancer cells and down regulates SUMO-specific protease 1 expression. *PLoS One* 7: e37693.
18. Choi, Y. J. et al. 2003. Immunosuppressant PG490 (triptolide) induces apoptosis through the activation of caspase-3 and downregulation of XIAP in U937 cells. *Biochem. Pharmacol.* 66: 273–80.
19. Xu, J. Y. et al. 1992. Antitumor effect of *Tripterygium wilfordii*. 1992. *Zhongguo Zhongxiyi Jiehe Zazhi* 12: 161–4.
20. Wan, C. K. et al. 2006. Triptolide induces Bcl-2 cleavage and mitochondria dependent apoptosis in p53-deficient HL-60 cells. *Cancer Lett.* 241: 31–41.
21. Lou, Y. J. et al. 2004. Triptolide downregulates Bcr-abl expression and induces apoptosis in chronic myelogenous leukemia cells. *Leukemia Lymphoma* 45: 373–6.
22. Tong, X. M. et al. 2007. Triptolide inhibits cyclooxygenase-2 and inducible nitric oxide synthase expression in human colon cancer and leukemia cells. *Acta Biochim. et Biophys. Sinica* 39: 89–95.
23. Huang, M. et al. 2013. Triptolide inhibits MDM2 and induces apoptosis in acute lymphoblastic leukemia cells through a p53-independent pathway. *Mol. Cancer Therap.* 12: 184–14.
24. Wang, Y. S. et al. 1983. *Pharmacology and Application of Chinese Materia Medica*, pp. 1186–97. People's Health Publisher, Beijing.
25. Liu, L. et al. 2013. Triptolide induces apoptosis in human leukemia cells through caspase-3-mediated ROCK1 activation and MLC phosphorylation. *Cell Death Disease* 4(Dec.): e941.
26. Zhao, F. et al. 2010. Role of triptolide in cell proliferation, cell cycle arrest, apoptosis and histone methylation in multiple myeloma U266 cells. *Eur. J. Pharmacol.* 646: 1–11.
27. Nakazato, T. et al. 2014. Triptolide induces apoptotic cell death of multiple myeloma cells via transcriptional repression of Mcl-1. *Intl. J. Oncol.* 44: 1131–8.
28. Yang, M. et al. 2008. Triptolide overcomes dexamethasone resistance and enhanced PS-341- induced apoptosis via PI3k/Akt/NF-κB pathways in human multiple myeloma cells. *Intl. J. Mol. Med.* 22: 489–96.
29. Jiang, X. H. et al. 2001. Functional p53 is required for triptolide-induced apoptosis and AP-1 and NF-κB activation in gastric cancer cells. *Oncogene* 20: 8009–18.
30. Johnson, S. M. et al. 2011. Triptolide inhibits proliferation and migration of colon cancer cells by inhibition of cell cycle regulators and cytokine receptors. *J. Surgical Res.* 168: 197–205.
31. Wang, Z. P. et al. 2009. Triptolide downregulates Rac1 and the JAK/STAT3 pathway and inhibits colitis-related colon cancer progression. *Exp. Mol. Med.* 41: 717–27.
32. Tengchaisri, T. et al. 1998. Antitumor activity of triptolide against cholangiocarcinoma growth in vitro and in hamsters. *Cancer Lett.* 133: 169–75.
33. Panichakul, T. et al. 2006. Triptolide sensitizes resistant cholangiocarcinoma cells to TRAIL-induced apoptosis. *Anticancer Res.* 26: 259–65.
34. Chen, Z. Y. et al. 2014. Triptolide sensitizes pancreatic cancer cells to TRAIL-induced activation of the death receptor pathway. *Cancer Lett.* 348: 156–66.
35. Frese, S. et al. 2003. PG490-mediated sensitization of lung cancer cells to Apo2L/TRAIL-induced apoptosis requires activation of ERK2. *Oncogene* 22: 5427–35.
36. Lee, K. Y. et al. 2002. Triptolide sensitizes lung cancer cells to TNF-related apoptosis-inducing ligand (TRAIL)-induced apoptosis by inhibitors of NF-κB activation. *Exp. Mol. Med.* 34: 462–8.
37. Chen, Y. W. et al. 2009. Triptolide exerts antitumor effect on oral cancer and KB cells in vitro and in vivo. *Oral Oncol.* 45: 562–8.
38. Chen, Y. W. et al. 2010. Triptolide circumvents drug-resistant effect and enhances 5-fluorouracil antitumor effect on KB cells. *Anti-Cancer Drugs* 21: 502–13.
39. Zhou, Y. X. et al. 2002. Several monomes from *Tripterygium wilfordii* inhibit proliferation of glioma cells in vitro. *Aizheng* 21: 1106–8.
40. Yan, X. M. et al. 2015. Triptolide inhibits cell proliferation and tumorigenicity of human neuroblastoma cells. *Mol. Med. Reports* 11: 791–6.
41. Liu, B. et al. 2013. Triptolide downregulates treg cells and the level of IL-10, TGF-β, and VEGF in melanoma-bearing mice. *Planta Med.* 79: 1401–7.
42. Kwon, H. Y. et al. 2013. Triptolide induces apoptosis through extrinsic and intrinsic pathways in human osteosarcoma U2OS cells. *Ind. J. Biochem. Biophys.* 50: 485–491.
43. Zhao, F. et al. 2013. Triptolide induces growth inhibition and apoptosis of human laryngocarcinoma cells by enhancing p53 activities and suppressing E6-mediated p53 degradation. *PLoS One* 8: e80784.
44. Ho, J. N. et al. 2015. Synergistic antitumor effect of triptolide and cisplatin in cisplatin resistant human bladder cancer cells. *J. Urol.* 193: 1016–22.
45. He, M. F. et al. 2010. Triptolide functions as a potent angiogenesis inhibitor. *Intl. J. Cancer* 126: 266–78.
46. Fidler, J. M. et al. 2003. PG490–88, a derivative of triptolide, causes tumor regression and sensitizes tumors to chemotherapy. *Mol. Cancer Therap.* 2: 855–62.
47. Kitzen, J. E. M. et al. 2009. Phase-I dose-escalation study of F60008, a novel apoptosis inducer, in patients with advanced solid tumors. *Eur. J. Cancer* 45: 1764–72.
48. Xu, F. et al. 2010. Design, synthesis, and biological evaluation of novel water-soluble triptolide derivatives: Antineoplastic activity against imatinib-resistant CML cells bearing T315I mutant Bcr-Abl. *Bioorg. Med. Chem.* 18: 1806–15.
49. Yao, Z. et al. 2007. Diterpenoid compounds from *Tripterygium wilfordii* and their anticancer activities. *Zhongcaoyao* 38: 1603–6.
50. Ning, L. L. et al. 2003. Cytotoxic biotransformed products from triptonide by *Aspergillus niger. Planta Med.* 59: 804–8.
51. Zhu, L. Q. et al. 1987. Effects of the total glycosides of *Tripterygium wilfordii* on HeLa cells and their possible mechanism. *Ziran Zazhi* 10: 877–8, 858.
52. Zhang, H. Y. et al. 2010. Observation on therapeutic effect of mifepristone combined with glycosides of *Tripterygium wilfordii* vine in patients with hysteromyoma. *Xiandai Zhongxiyi Jiehe Zazhi* 19: 168–9.
53. Ushiro, S. et al. 1997. New nortriterpenoid isolated from antirheumatoid arthritic plant, *Tripterygium wilfordii*, modulates tumor growth and neovascularization. *Intl. J. Cancer* 72: 657–63.
54. Ushiro, M. et al. 1997. Nortriterpenoids from *Tripterygium wilfordii* as vascularization inihibitors. *Jpn. Kokai Tokkyo Koho* JP 09100294 A 19970415.

55. Salminen, A. et al. 2010. Celastrol: Molecular targets of thunder god vine. *Biochem. Biophys. Res. Commun.* 394: 439–42.
56. Yang, G. Z. et al. 2006. Antitumor triterpenoids from *Tripterygium wilfordii* Hook F. *Chem. Indust. Forest Prods.* (China) 26: 19–22.
57. Yang, H. J. et al. 2006. Celastrol, a triterpene extracted from the Chinese "Thunder of God Vine," is a potent proteasome inhibitor and suppresses human prostate cancer growth in nude mice. *Cancer Res.* 66: 4758–65.
58. Ni, H. W. et al. 2012. Inductive effect of celastrol on apoptosis of human multiple myeloma cell line LP-1. *J. Anhui TCM College* 31: 59–63.
59. Chiang, K. C. et al. 2014. Celastrol blocks interleukin-6 gene expression via downregulation of NF-κB in prostate carcinoma cells. *PLoS One* 9: e93151.
60. Ma, J. et al. 2014. Celastrol inhibits the HIF-1α pathway by inhibition of mTOR/p70S6K/eIF4E and ERK1/2 phosphorylation in human hepatoma cells. *Oncol. Reports* 32: 235–42.
61. Mi, C. L. et al. 2014. Celastrol induces the apoptosis of breast cancer cells and inhibits their invasion via downregulation of MMP-9. *Oncol. Reports* 32: 2527–32.
62. Sethi, G. et al. 2007. Celastrol, a novel triterpene, potentiates TNF-induced apoptosis and suppresses invasion of tumor cells by inhibiting NF-κB-regulated gene products and TAK1-mediated NF-κB activation. *Blood* 109: 2727–35.
63. Liu, Z. et al. 2014. Cancerous inhibitor of CIP2A is targeted by natural compound celastrol for degradation in non-small-cell lung cancer. *Carcinog.* 35: 905–14.
64. Fan, X. X. et al. 2014. Celastrol induces apoptosis in gefitinib-resistant non-small cell lung cancer cells via caspases-dependent pathways and Hsp90 client protein degradation. *Mol.* 19: 3508–22.
65. Yan, Y. Y. et al. 2014. Celastrol enhanced the anticancer effect of lapatinib in human hepatocellular carcinoma cells in vitro. *J. Buon.* 19: 412–8.
66. Huang, L. L. et al. 2011. Inhibitory action of celastrol on hypoxia-mediated angiogenesis and metastasis via the HIF-1α pathway. *Intl. J. Mol. Med.* 27: 407–15.
67. Zhou, Y. X. et al. 2009. Antiangiogenic effect of celastrol on the growth of human glioma: An in vitro and in vivo study. *Chin. Med. J.* 122: 1666–73.
68. Huang, Y. L. et al. 2008. Celastrol inhibits the growth of human glioma xenografts in nude mice through suppressing VEGFR expression. *Cancer Lett.* 264: 101–6.
69. Zhu, H. et al. 2010. Celastrol acts as a potent antimetastatic agent targeting β1 integrin and inhibiting cell-extracellular matrix adhesion, in part via the p38 mitogen-activated protein kinase pathway. *J. Pharmacol. Exp Therap.* 334: 489–99.
70. Salvador, J. A. R. et al. 2014. Antitumor effects of celastrol and semi-synthetic derivatives. *Mini-Reviews in Org. Chem.* 11: 400–7.
71. Wang, L. et al. 2012. Antitumor effect of novel celastrol analogues in vitro. *Zhongguo Xinyao Yu Linchuang Zazhi* 31: 47–50.
72. Tang, K. Y. et al. 2014. Design, synthesis and biological evaluation of C(6)-modified celastrol derivatives as potential antitumor agents. *Mol.* 19: 10177–88.
73. Song, J. et al. 2011. Formulation and evaluation of celastrol-loaded liposomes. *Mol.*16: 7880–92.
74. Wolfram, J. et al. 2014. Evaluation of anticancer activity of celastrol liposomes in prostate cancer cells. *J. Microencapsul.* 31: 501–7.
75. Zeng, F. et al. 2010. Two prenylated and C-methylated flavonoids from *Tripterygium wilfordii*. *Planta Med.* 76: 1596–9.

72 Jiu Jie Long 九節龍

Small coralberry

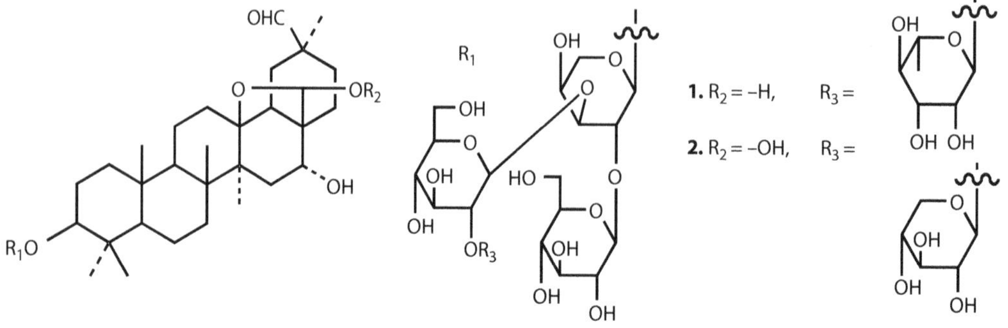

1. $R_2 = -H$, $R_3 =$

2. $R_2 = -OH$, $R_3 =$

Herb Origination

The herb Jiu Jie Long (Small coralberry) is the dried whole plant of *Ardisia pusilla* (Myrsinaceae). This evergreen shrub is native to eastern Asia, such as the southern region of the Yangtze River in China, south of Japan, Thailand, Malaysia, and the Philippines. The whole plant and its leaves can be collected annually and dried in the sun for folk medicinal practice.

Antitumor Activities and Constituents

The anticancer property of Jiu Jie Long was found to be primarily contributed by its triterpenoid saponins, which exerted a marked suppressive effect against the growth of sarcoma 180, U14 cervical cancer, H22 hepatoma, and LLC *in vitro* and *in vivo*.[1] Six triterpene saponins designated as ardipusilloside-I (**1**), ardipusilloside-III (**2**), ardipusilloside-IV, and ardipusilloside-V as well as ardipusilloside-A and ardipusilloside-B (see Zhu Sha Geng) were isolated from Jiu Jie Long. The saponins exerted both tumor inhibitory and immunoenhancing effects. *In vitro* investigations revealed a significant cytotoxicity of the six saponins on human U251MG glioblastoma cells without any effect on cultured human astrocytes.[2–5] Ardipusilloside-I (**1**) also markedly inhibited the viability and the proliferation of human cancer cell lines such as U87MG, U87, U373, and T98G glioblastoma, primary glioblastoma, NCI-H460 large cell lung cancer, and Mc3 mucoepidermoid cancer *in vitro* in time- and concentration-dependent manners, associated with the significant induction of apoptosis and cell cycle arrest.[5–8] The IC_{50} values of ardipusilloside-I (**1**) were 4.05 μM in U87MG cells, 8.2 μg/mL in U251MG cells, and 9.98 μg/mL in Mc3 cells.[3,6,7] The apoptotic mechanism of ardipusilloside-I (**1**) has been preliminarily explored in the U251MG cells, revealing a characteristic caspase-8-independent and FasL/Fas-signaling-mediated death receptor pathway involved in the apoptotic induction, i.e., augmentation of Fas and its ligand (FasL) expressions and activation of caspase-3 and caspase-8. The treatment of the U251MG cells with ardipusilloside-III (**2**) ran not only an intrinsic pathway mediated by BAD dephosphorylation and cleavage, but also an extrinisic pathway mediated by caspase-8 and caspase-3 activations.[3,5] Interestingly, a low dose of ardipusilloside-III (**2**) could provoke G2/M phase cell cycle arrest which is preceded by the apoptosis of the U251MG cells, but a higher dose of it induced the apoptosis only with no cell cycle arrest.[3] Besides the induction of G2/M phase cell cycle arrest and cell apoptosis, ardipusilloside-I (**1**) also activated the autophagy of both U373 and T98G glioma cells through the formation of autophagosomes and the up-expression of both autophagic protein Beclin 1 and LC3 in the glioma cells.[8] These mechanism characters may provide a valuable clue for the development of the ardipusilloside-I (**1**) and ardipusilloside-III (**2**) as candidates for chemotherapeutic treatment of human glioblastomas.

The antigrowth activity of ardipusilloside-I (**1**) was further established in nude mice xenografted human A549 NSCLC cells.[9] Both *in vitro* and *in vivo* assays demonstrated that ardipusilloside-I (**1**) lessened the survival of HepG2 and SMMC-7721 human hepatoma cells partially through the inhibition of Mek/Erk and Akt pathways, and it also effectively retarded the invasion and the metastasis of the hepatoma cells through the reduction of MMP-2 and MMP-9 activities. Concurrently, ardipusilloside-I (**1**) enhanced Rac1 activity that then enhanced E-cad activity, resulting in markedly less metastasis of the hepatoma cells.[10] The suppression of MMP-2 activity by ardipusilloside-I (**1**) was also observed in human U87 glioma cells, exerting antimigratory and antiinvasive effects.[11] In addition, its antiangiogenic activity was demonstrated in a chicken chorioallantoic membrane neovascularization model, where ardipusilloside-I (**1**) prominently suppressed an MVD protein and mRNA expressions of VEGF and VEGFR.[9]

In addition, the metabolism and pharmacokinetic investigations disclosed that the metabolites of ardipusilloside-I (**1**), not itself, were absorbed into the plasma after oral administration to tested rats. The produced M3 and M4 metabolites should be responsible for the antitumor activity *in vivo*.[12]

References

1. Bian, B. L. et al. 2000. Total triterpenoid saponin in coral ardisa root or other plants in same family and preparing process thereof. *Faming Zhuanli Shenqing Gongkai Shuomingshu* 5 pp. CN 99–105451, 19990408.
2. Tian, Y. et al. 2009. Triterpenoid saponins from *Ardisia pusilla* and their cytotoxic activity. *Planta Med.* 75: 70–5.
3. Lin, H. et al. 2008. Apoptosis induced by ardipusilloside III through BAD dephosphorylation and cleavage in human glioblastoma U251MG cells. *Apoptosis* 13: 247–57.

4. Tang, H. F. et al. 2009. Two new triterpenoid saponins cytotoxic to human glioblastoma U251MG cells from *Ardisia pusilla*. *Chem. Biodivers.* 6: 1443–52.
5. Zhang, Y. M. et al. 2010. Ardipusilloside I purified from *Ardisia pusilla* competitively binds VEGFR and induces apoptosis in NCI-H460 cells. *Phytomed.* 17: 519–26.
6. Xiong, J. et al. 2009. Ardipusilloside I induces apoptosis in human glioblastoma cells through a caspase-8-independent FasL/Fas-signaling pathway. *Environmental Toxicol. Pharmacol.* 27: 264–70.
7. Xu, X. F. et al. 2013. Ardipusilloside I induces apoptosis by regulating Bcl-2 family proteins in human mucoepidermoid carcinoma Mc3 cells. *BMC Complem. Altern. Med.* 13: 322/1–322/9.
8. Wang, R. et al. 2014. Stimulation of autophagic activity in human glioma cells by anti-proliferative ardipusilloside I isolated from *Ardisia pusilla*. *Life Sci.* 110: 15–22.
9. Wang, R. et al. 2012. Inhibition of tumor-induced angiogenesis and its mechanism by ardipusilloside I purified from *Ardisia pusilla*. *J. Asian Nat. Prods. Res.* 14: 55–63.
10. Lou, L. Q. et al. 2012. Ardipusilloside inhibits survival invasion and metastasis of human hepatocellular carcinoma cells. *Phytomed.* 19: 603–8.
11. Wang, L. et al. 2012. Effects of ardipusilloside-I on cell migration and invasion ability of glioma U87 cells. *Zhongchengyao* 34: 1861–5.
12. Wang, X. J. et al. 2012. Metabolism and pharmacokinetic study of ardipusilloside I in rats. *Planta Med.* 78: 565–74.

73 Zhu Ye Lan 竹葉蘭

Bamboo orchid

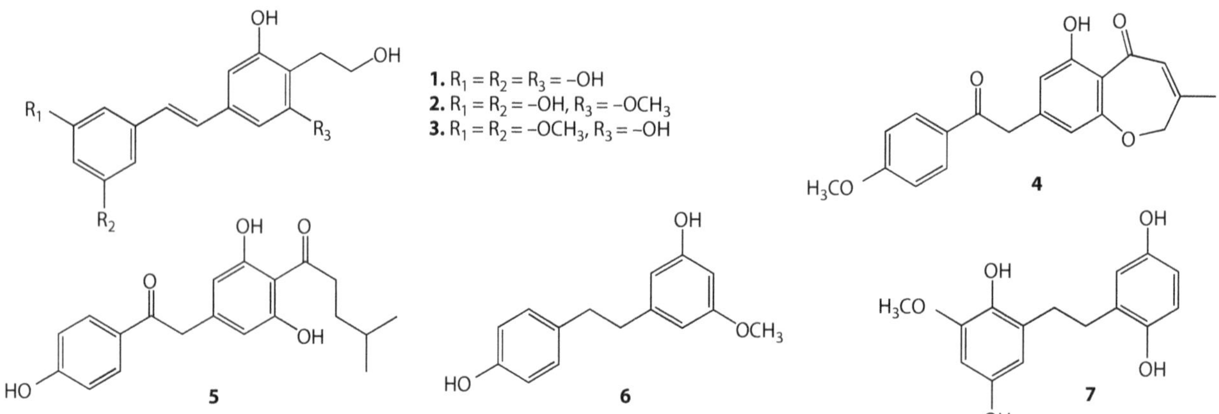

1. $R_1 = R_2 = R_3 =$ -OH
2. $R_1 = R_2 =$ -OH, $R_3 = -OCH_3$
3. $R_1 = R_2 = -OCH_3$, $R_3 =$ -OH

(a)

8. $R_1 =$ -beta-D-glucosyl, $R_2 = -CH_3$
11. $R_1 = -CH_3$, $R_2 =$ -beta-D-glucosyl

9. $R_1 = -CH_3$, $R_2 =$ -H
10. $R_1 =$ -H, $R_2 = -CH_3$

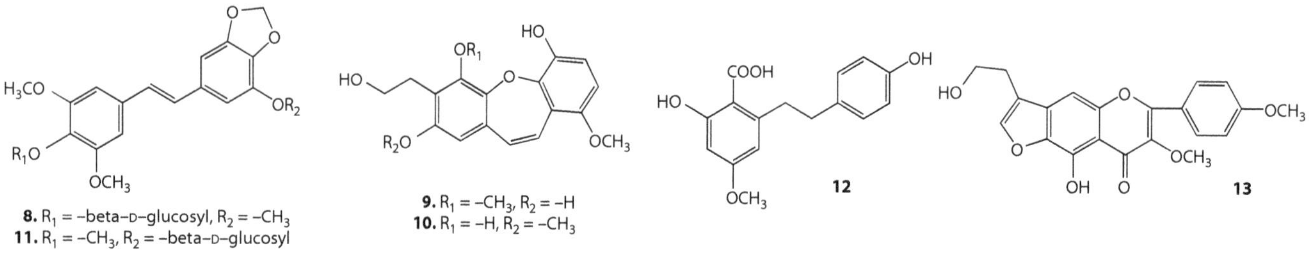

(b)

Herb Origination

The herb Zhu Ye Lan (Bamboo orchid) originates from the rhizomes of an Orchidaceae plant, *Arundina graminifolia* (= *Arundina chinensis* and *Bletia graminifolia*). This perennial and evergreen orchid is distributed in south Asian regions from tropical to south subtropical. The plant also extends to the Pacific Islands and Hawaii. The herb can be collected annually and dried in the sun after being sliced for Chinese folk medical practice. It also can be used fresh.

Antitumor Constituents and Activities

A phytochemical investigation of the bamboo orchid led to the separation of a series of diphenylethylenes and deoxybenzoins. A group of diphenylethylenes discovered from the herb displayed a moderate degree of antiproliferative effect against various human neoplastic cell lines selectively.

Diphenylethylenes

Five isolated diphenylethylenes elucidated as gramistilbenoids-A–C (**1**–**3**) and gramideoxybenzoin-D (**4**) and gramideoxybenzoin-E (**5**) exerted a moderate cytotoxicity against five human tumor cell lines (NB4, A549, SHSY5Y, PC3, and MCF-7) in an *in vitro* assay (IC_{50}: 1.8–8.7 μM). Gramistilbenoid-B (**2**) exhibited a relatively stronger cytotoxic effect against NB4 leukemia and PC3 prostate cancer cells (respective IC_{50}: 3.3 and 2.2 μM), and gramideoxybenzoin-D (**4**) was relatively sensitive to A549 lung adenocarcinoma, SHSY5Y neuroblastoma, and PC3 prostate cancer cells lines (respective IC_{50}: 2.2, 1.8, and 3.4 μM). Gramideoxybenzoin-E (**5**) was better cytotoxic to the NB4 and SHSY5Y cell lines (respective IC_{50}: 2.1 and 3.2 μM).[1] A bibenzyl derivative designated as 3,3′-dihydroxy-5-methoxybibenzyl (**6**) (batatasin-III), which was also isolated from 95% alcohol extract of the tuber of *A. graminifolia*, demonstrated the inhibitory effect against human BGC-823 gastric cancer cells and human Bel-7402 hepatoma cells. At a 10 mg/L concentration, the suppressive rates of batatasin-III (**6**) were 68.66% on Bel-7402 cells and 47.45% on BGC-823 cells *in vitro*.[2]

Continuing biology-related phytochemistry investigation discovered more bibenzyl derivatives and diphenylethylenes from the herb. Five of them exhibited different degrees of moderate cytotoxic effect on a small panel of human tumor cell lines (NB4, A549, SHSY5Y, PC3, and MCF-7). Only 2,5,2′,5′-tetrahydroxy-3-methoxybibenzyl (**7**) was effective in the moderate suppression of all tested cancer cell lines (IC_{50}: <10 μM). Graminibibenzyl-A (**8**), gramniphenol-H (**9**) and gramniphenol-I (**10**) showed the inhibitory activity against PC3 prostate cancer cells (IC_{50}: 3.5–3.8 μM), whereas gramniphenol-K was cytotoxic to MCF-7 (breast), A549 (lung), and SHSY5Y (brain) human cancer cell lines (respective IC_{50}: 6.2, 7.5, and 4.7 μM) and graminibibenzyl-B (**11**) to MCF-7 cells (IC_{50}: 2.1 μM). The higher antiproliferative effect was also presented by 5,12-dihydroxy-3-methoxybibenzyl-6-carboxylic acid

(**12**) in A549 cells (IC_{50}: 2.2 μM) and by gramniphenol-I (**10**) in NB4 leukemia cells (IC_{50}: 3.6 μM). Similar to the five compounds, 3-hydroxy-4,3,5-trimethoxy-*trans*-stilbene, 3,5-dihydroxystilbene-3-*O*-β-D-glucoside, 2,3-di-hydroxy-3,5-dimethoxystilbene, 3-hydroxy-5-methoxybibenzyl, rhapontigen, and bauhiniastatin-D exhibited cytotoxicity (IC_{50}: <10 μM) in some cancer cells lines (NB4, A549, SHSY5Y, PC3, or MCF-7).[3–5]

Flavone

An active flavone derivative was also derived from Zhu Ye Lan, whose structure was determined as 5-hydroxy-8-(2-hydroxyethyl)-3-methoxy-2-(4-methoxyphenyl)-4h-furo[2,3-h] chromen-4-one (**13**). According to a notable inhibitory effect shown in human Bel-7402 (hepatoma), MKN-28 (gastric cancer), and K562 (chronic granulocytic leukemia) cell lines, this flavone has been patented for use in the preparation of medical formulations as an antitumor agent.[6]

Other

The isolated 3S,4S-3′,4′-dihydroxyl-7,8-methylenedioxylptero carpan exerted a relatively higher cytotoxicity against HSY5Y human neuroblastoma cells (IC_{50}: 2.2 μM) and moderate cytotoxic effects against other four tested cancer cell lines (IC_{50}: 5–10 μM).[7]

References

1. Hu, Q. F. et al. 2013. Cytotoxic deoxy-benzoins and diphenyl-ethylenes from *Arundina graminifolia*. *J. Nat. Prod.* 76: 1854–9.
2. Liu, M. F. et al. 2012. Antitumoral bibenzyl derivatives from tuber of *Arundina graminifolia*. *Zhongguo Zhongyao Zazhi* 37: 66–70.
3. Du, G. et al. 2014. Bibenzyl derivatives of *Arundina graminifolia* and their cytotoxicity. *Chem. Nat. Compds.* 49: 1019–22.
4. Li, Y. K. et al. 2013. Two new diphenyl-ethylenes from *Arundina graminifolia* and their cytotoxicity. *Bull. Korean Chem. Soc.* 34: 3257–60.
5. Meng, C. Y. et al. 2014. A new cytotoxic stilbenoid from *Arundina graminifolia*. *Asian J. Chem.* 26: 2411–3.
6. Hu, Q. F. et al. 2012. Method for preparing 5-hydroxy-8-(2-hydroxyethyl)-3-methoxy-2-(4-methoxyphenyl)-4h-furo[2,3-h]chromen-4-one as flavones compound from *Arundina graminifolia* and its application in preparing the medical formulations as antitumor agent. *Faming Zhuanli Shenqing* CN 102675330 A 20120919.
7. Shu, L. D. et al. 2013. Flavonoids derivatives from *Arundina graminifolia* and their cytotoxicity. *Asian J. Chem.* 25: 8358–60.

74 Hong Sheng Ma 紅昇麻

Chinese astilbe

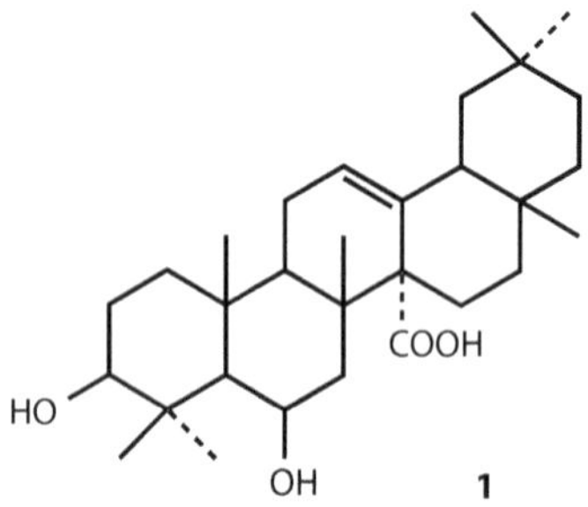

1

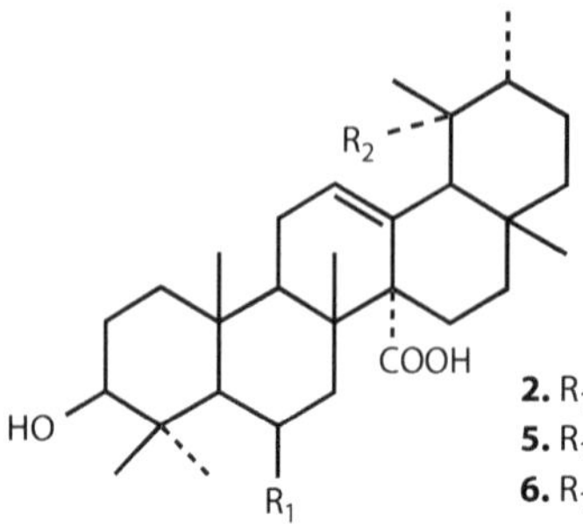

2. $R_1 = R_2 = -H$
5. $R_1 = -OH; R_2 = -H$
6. $R_1 = -OAc; R_2 = -OH$

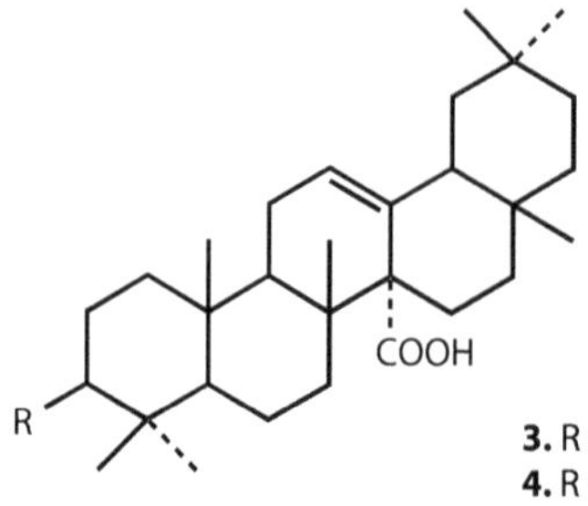

3. R = –OH
4. R = –OAc

Herb Origination

The herb Hong Sheng Ma (Chinese astilbe) is the rhizomes of two Saxifragaceae plants, *Astilbe chinensis* and *A. gradis*. The herb originated from the first plant is wildly produced in many places in China, and it also grows well in many areas of the United States as a very popular shade and woodland perennial. The herb from the secondary source is only produced in a small region of southern Yangtze River. Normally, their rhizomes are collected between summer and autumn and dried in the sun for Chinese folk medicine use. The herb also can be used fresh.

Antitumor Activities and Constituents

The oral administration of Hong Sheng Ma decoction (4 g/kg) for 10 days was able to retard the growth of sarcoma 180 by 51–54% in mice and prolong the vital stage of Ehrlich ascites carcinoma by 44% in mice. Hong Sheng Ma also raised the spleen lymphocyte transformation rate in its lower concentration *in vitro*.[1] The bioassay-guided separation of the rhizomes of *A. chinensis* discovered four cytotoxic pentacyclic triterpenoids assigned as astilbic acid (**1**), α-peltoboykinolic acid (**2**), β-peltoboykinolic acid (**3**), and its acetate (**4**). The triterpenoids (astilbic acid (**1**), α-peltoboykinolic acid (**2**), β-peltoboykinolic acid (**3**), and its acetate (**4**)) showed the growth inhibitory effect on human HL-60 promyelacytic leukemia, HO-8910 ovarian cancer, and HeLa cervical carcinoma cell lines *in vitro*. In concentrations of >2.5 μg/mL, β-peltoboykinolic acid (**3**) dose-dependently induced the HO-8910 cells to apoptotic death.[2–4]

Recently, more antineoplastic triterpenoids were discovered from *A. chinensis*. The isolated three olean-based triterpenoids (3β,6β-dihydroxyolean-12-en-27-oic acid, 3β,6β,24-trihydroxyolean-12-en-27-oic acid, and 3β-hydroxyolean-12-en-27-oic acid) and three ursane-based triterpenoids (astlibotriterpenic acid, 3β,19α-dihydroxy-6β-acetoxyursane, and 3β-acetoxy-6β-hydroxyurs-12-en-27-oic acid) displayed a modest inhibitory property against the growth of carcinoma cells.[6–13] 3β-Hydroxyolean-12-en-27-oic acid (**3**) (= β-peltoboykinolic acid) was effective in the suppression of human HL-60 (leukemia), HeLa (cervix), HepG2 (liver), Colo-205 (colorectal), and HO-8910 (ovary) cancer cell lines with IC_{50} values of 3.64, 3.94, 6.69, 7.31, and 8.01 μg/mL, respectively.[10,14] whose effect was found to closely relate to its ability of apoptosis-induction via downregulation of Bcl-2 expression, upregulation of Bax expression, lower of mitochondrial membrane potential, and activation of caspase-3.[10] The cytotoxic activity of astlibotriterpenic acid (**5**) was observed in seven human Bcap37 (breast), HeLa (cervix), HO-8910 (ovary), HepG2 (liver), SGC-7901 (stomach), PAA (lung), and K562 (leukemic) cancer cell lines and murine P388 leukemia cells,[6,7] which was found to be accompanied by dose-dependent inducing G0/G1 phase arrest and stimulating apoptosis by amplifying ROS generation and mitochondria-related mechanisms in the HeLa cells.[6,7] In the *in vitro* assay with the same cancer cell lines, α-peltoboykinolic acid (**2**), which lacks a hydroxyl at C-6, showed more potent antigrowth effect than astlibotriterpenic acid (**5**) (IC_{50}: 3.90–8.97 versus 7.73–19.28 μg/mL), implying that the hydroxylation at C-6 negatively influenced the antitumor potency.[6] The antiproliferative effect of 3β,19α-dihydroxy-6β-acetoxyursane (**6**) was present in human HeLa cervical cancer cells and murine fibrosarcoma L929 cells *in vitro*,[13] and the effect of 3β,6β-dihydroxyolean-12-en-27-oic acid (**1**) (= astilbic acid) was also demonstrated in the *in vivo* experiments. Oral treatment with 3β,6β-dihydroxyolean-12-en-27-oic acid (**1**) to mice in doses of 40–80 mg/kg for 10 days notably restrained the growth of mouse transplantable sarcoma 180 and H22 hepatoma cells.[8]

Moreover, the 3β,6β-dihydroxyolean-12-en-27-oic acid (**1**) was also capable of improving both cellular and humoral immune responses. It could augment the activities of cytotoxic T lymphocytes and NK cells and augment the splenocyte proliferation and the level of IL-2 secreted by splenocyte in tumor-bearing mice, whereas it remarkably promoted delayed-type hypersensitivity reaction and enhanced anti-sheep red blood cell antibody titers in naive mice. These evidences indicated that its antitumor effect was contributed by both antiproliferative and immunoregulatory activities.[8] Likewise, the levels of splenocyte proliferation and NK cells activity and the production of IL-2 from splenocytes are especially lower in mice bearing sarcoma 180 after the treatment with CTX, a common anticancer agent. The triterpenoid fractions derived from *A. chinensis* was able to markedly enlarge the peripheral white blood cell count and bone marrow cellularity in CTX-treated mice bearing sarcoma 180, providing a remarkable security against CTX-caused hematotoxicity, immunotoxicity, hepatotoxicity, and nephrontoxicity.[15] The findings highlighted that the triterpenoids from Chinese astilbe may also be beneficial in the abrogation of chemotherapy-induced toxicity besides the anticancer properties.

Other Medical Uses

The herb Hong Sheng Ma (Chinese astilbe) has been traditionally utilized in Chinese medicine for the treatment of enteritis, stomachache, snakebite, chronic arthritis, trauma, asthenia, and so on. The pharmacological investigations have substantiated that the herb possesses potent antielastase and antityrosinase activities.[5]

References

1. Chen, P. F. et al. 1996. A research on the antitumor effects of Heiji (radix *Astilbe chinensis*). *Zhongguo Zhongyao Zazhi* 21: 302–3.
2. Sun, H. X. et al. 2003. Cytotoxic pentacyclic triterpenoids from the rhizome of *Astilbe chinensis*. *Helv. Chim. Acta* 86: 2414–23.
3. Sun, H. X. et al. 2004. Cytotoxic oleanane triterpenoids from the rhizomes of *Astilbe chinensis* (Maxim.) Franch. et Savat. *J. Ethnopharmacol.* 90: 261–5.
4. Sun, H. X. et al. 2004. 3β,6β-dihydroxyolean-12-en-27-oic acid: A cytotoxic and apoptosis-inducing oleanane triterpenoid from the rhizome of *Astilbe chinensis*. *Acta crystallographica. Section-C*, 60(Pt 4): o300–2.
5. Lee, S. H. et al. 2009. Potent antielastase and antityrosinase activities of *Astilbe chinensis*. *Am. J. Pharmacol. Toxicol.* 4: 125–7.
6. Zhang, Y. B. et al. 2009. Astlibotriterpenic acid induces growth arrest and apoptosis in HeLa cells through mitochondria-related pathways and reactive oxygen species (ROS) production. *Chem. Biodivers.* 6: 218–30.
7. Zhang, Y. B. et al. 2008. A new cytotoxic, apoptosis-inducing triterpenoid from the rhizomes of *Astilbe chinensis*. *Chem. Biodivers.* 5: 189–96.
8. Deng, W. et al. 2009. Immunomodulatory activity of 3β,6β-dihydroxyolean-12-en-27-oic acid in tumor-bearing mice. *Chem. Biodivers.* 6: 1243–53.
9. Cai, X. F. et al. 2009. Cytotoxic triterpenoids from the rhizomes of *Astilbe chinensis*. *J. Nat. Prod.* 72: 1241–4.
10. Tu, J. et al. 2006. 3β-Hydroxyolean-12-en-27-oic acid: A cytotoxic, apoptosis-inducing natural drug against Colo-205 cancer cells. *Chem. Biodivers.* 3: 69–78.
11. Sun, H. X. et al. 2006. Induction of apoptosis in HeLa cells by 3β-hydroxy-12-oleanen-27-oic acid from the rhizomes of *Astilbe chinensis*. *Bioorg. Med. Chem.* 14: 1189–98.
12. Hu, J. Y. et al. 2006. Two new triterpenes from *Astilbe chinensis*. *Chin. Chem. Lett.* 17: 628–30.
13. Xu, Y. Q. et al. 2013. A new triterpene from *Astilbe chinensis*. *Chem. Nat. Compd.* 49: 268–70.
14. Ying, X. et al. 2011. Chemical constituents from *Astilbe chinensis*. *J. Asian Nat. Prod. Res.* 13: 188–91.
15. Sun, H. X. et al. 2008. Protective effect of triterpenoid fractions from the rhizomes of *Astilbe chinensis* on cyclophosphamide-induced toxicity in tumor-bearing mice. *J. Ethnopharmacol.* 119: 312–7.

75 Can Sha 蠶沙

Silkworm excreta or Silkworm feces

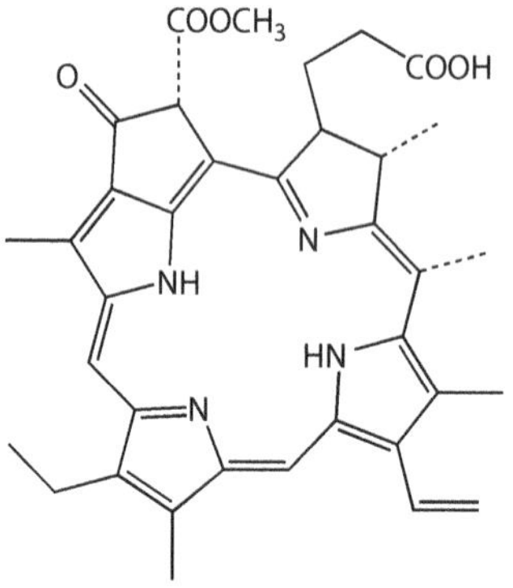

Herb Origination

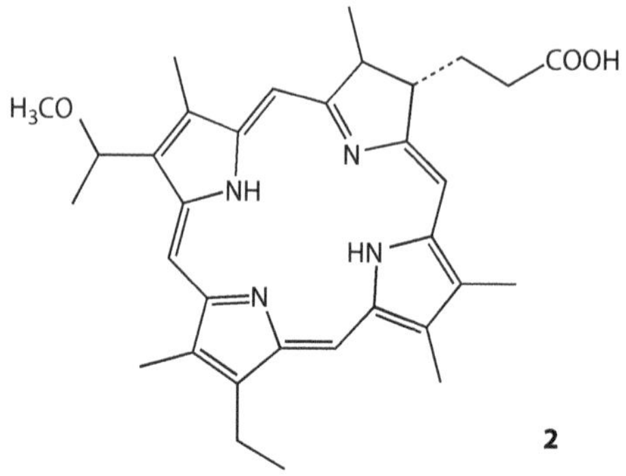

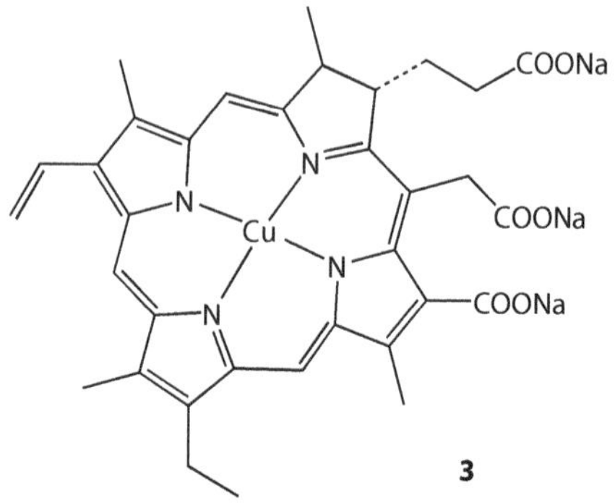

The herb Can Sha is the dried excreta of the larva of silkworm *Bombyx mori* L., which has long been used for its medicinal activities as a traditional Chinese medicine. The herb is majorly produced in the famous Chinese silk provinces, Zhejiang and south of Jiangsu.

Antitumor Constituents and Activities

The anticarcinoma ingredients in Can Sha are elucidated as chlorophyll metabolites which are photosensitizers, exhibiting a strong photodynamic inhibition on the human tumor cell lines *in vitro* and *in vivo*. The administration of the photosensitive extract in doses of 50–550 mg/kg intravenously or by intraduodenal injection to tumor-bearing mice, plus a light irradiation (near 650 nm) on the tumor site for 10 minutes, resulted in a potent growth inhibitory effect against cancer cells for 69–98% and 62–79%, respectively.[1–3] The anticancer activity could remarkably increase by an early light irradiation after the administration of chlorophyll derivatives.[4] More than 80% of the normal human and mouse control cells kept a safe condition for life after receiving the treatment.[3]

Several chlorophyll photosensitizers were separated from Can Sha, but the strongest photodynamic active derivative was CRD7 in the Can Sha.[5,6] Other photosensitizers, phorbin (chlorophyll without Mg) and purpurin derivatives, were obtained from the crude chlorophyll by selective hydrolysis and allomerization. Their structures were identified as chlorophyll-a, pheophytin-a, pheophorbide-a (**1**), pheophorbide-b, pyropheophorbide-a, 10-hydroxymethylpheophorbide-a methylpheophoribde-a, methylpyropheophorbide-a, and purpurin 7-lactone dimethyl ester.[2,7,8]

Pheophorbide-a

Pheophorbide-a (**1**) (PhA) was identified as a photosensitizer to exert cytotoxicity on a number of tumor cells in a PDT, whose molecule was also found in the herb Ban Zhi Lian (*Scutellaria barbata*). The *in vitro* and *in vivo* proliferations of mouse B16-F10 melanoma cells were significantly inhibited by the necrotic response after the pheophorbide-a (**1**) treatment with light illumination (1.2 J/cm^2, 665 nm).[9] The combined PDT with pheophorbide-a or pheophorbide-b demonstrated the antigrowth effect against hepatoma cell line *in vitro*.[10] A further investigation provided more evidences and mechanism-related clues for the PhA-PDT as a potentially promising treatment. The PhA-PDT could dose- and light dose-dependently increase significant cytotoxic photodamage and apoptosis or necrosis of many types of human neoplastic cell lines, including HepG2 and Hep3B (liver), HT-29 (colon), HeLa (cervix), LNCaP (prostate), MCF-7 and MDA-MB-231 (breast), HO-8910 (ovary), and Jurkat (leukemia),[9–17] but it was nontoxic to normal human WRL-68 liver cells.[13] The IC_{50} values at 14 J/cm^2 light irradiation were 0.07 μM on MCF7 cells, 0.095 μM on HepG2 cells, 0.15 μM on HeLa cells, 0.40 μM on HT-29 cells, and 0.70 μM on Jurkate cells, as well as 0.25 μM on B78-H1 (murine melanoma) cells.[15] At low doses ($<IC_{50}$), the photosensitizer induced a temporary growth arrest in HeLa cells and HepG2 cells, and it promoted the tumor cells to apoptotic death and/or necrosis when the doses were elevated to over its IC_{50} data. The response of HepG2 cells was more sensitive to the PhA-PDT treatment than that of HeLa cells.[15] Moreover, light-emitting diode (LED)-activated PhA could remarkably cause the apoptotic death of ovarian cancer cells and exert significant cytotoxicity and apoptosis of ovarian cancer cells.[18]

The *in vivo* exploration of the PhA-PDT afforded more support to the PhA-PDT treatment. Pheophorbide-a (**1**) with PDT in an intravenous dose of 9 mg/kg and light of 660 nm in a dose 100 J/cm^2 to treat azaserine-induced pancreatic carcinoma in a rat elicited the selective necrosis of the tumor and lengthened the rat lifetime markedly, but the curative therapy also injured the rat duodenum.[19] In xenografts of human HT-29 colon cancer cells, a combined treatment with pheophorbide-a liposome at an i.p. dose 30 mg/kg and the illumination of 665 nm in a dose of 100 J/cm^2 effectively delayed the growth of HT-29 cells.[12] When pheophorbide-a (**1**) in an intravenous dose of 0.3 mg/kg is combined with a light dose of 126 J/cm^2 for two weeks, the treated Hep3B tumor size could be significantly diminished by 57% in a nude mice model.[16]

Mechanistic studies demonstrated that the antigrowth and apoptosis-promoting activities of PDT-activated pheophorbide-a

is strictly related to (1) remarkable increase of intracellular ROS level and oxidative stress level, (2) induction of peroxidation, (3) depolarization of mitochondrial membrane potential and release of cytochrome c to the cytosol, and (4) activation of caspases cascade and cleavage of PARP. In estrogen receptor-negative human breast adenocarcinoma MDA-MB-231 cells, the antitumor effect of PhA-PDT was found to be not only dependent on the mitochondria-mediated apoptosis but also on the ERK-mediated autophagy.[20] Moreover, the PhA-PDT treatment could also trigger phagocytic capture by human macrophages and enhance the immunogenicity of HepG2 cells.[12] The evidences revealed that the PhA-PDT could be effectively potentiated on the cell lines of HepG2 hepatoma and HeLa cervical cancer if combined with siRNA specific for activating HO-1 and/or GSTA1, which are the responses to the lipid peroxidation.[15] Therefore, these positive results demonstrated that PhA-PDT may be a potentially promising treatment for some localized types of cancers, which can be a therapeutic option after the failures of radiotherapy and hormone therapy.

In addition, PhA (**1**) was conjugated with chemotherapeutic drugs such as DOX and paclitaxel. The conjugates in excitation at a lightwave 420 or 440 nm more potently displayed great inhibition against various carcinoma cell growth, suggesting that PhA conjugates with anticancer drugs have a development potential for selective cancer therapy as well as for the fluorescence detection of cancer.[21] A analog, pheophorbide-a methyl ester (MPPa), cooperated with LED activation, remarkably deactivated cisplatin-resistant ovarian COC1/DDP cells and enhanced the cell apoptotic death by localizing in the intracellular membrane system and increasing the collapse of mitochondrial membrane potential. The findings recommended that the LED-activated MPPa may be developed as a new modality for treating multidrug-resistant carcinomas, especially cisplatin-resistant ovarian neoplasm.[22]

CPD4

A phlorophyll-derivative 2-devinyl-2-(1-methoxylethyl) chlorine-f normally called CPD4 (**2**) is a photosensitizer. Associated with laser irritation at 630 or 670 nm, CDP4 (**2**) treatment could display a potent photodynamic effect against human neoplastic cell lines, such as MCF-7 (breast) and HR8384 (colon) *in vitro*, and against mouse colon cancer CT26 and sarcoma 180 *in vivo*.[23–27] The inhibitory rate of CPD4-PDT could reach to 97.9% and 55% toward the growth of sarcoma 180 and CT26 colon cancer, respectively, *in vivo*, and the mouse survival times were also significantly extended.[23,24] The studies further revealed that the laser-activated CPD4 (**2**) could enter into MCF-7 cells and bind the cells mainly in the cellular membrane and the mitochondria by electrostatic or hydrogen binding interaction strongly.[25] If combined with a chemotherapy drug Adm, the photodynamic effect of CPD4 could augment the G0/G1 cell arrest and the apoptosis, exerting an important synergistic effect against the MCF-7 cells.[26] The synergistic antineoplastic effect was also observed in the combination of CPD4-PDT with cinobufotalin on mice transplanted with H22 hepatoma with the suppressive rate of 51.69%. The PDT-combined treatment obviously strengthened the photosensitive killing effect of CPD4 and markedly improved the overall situation of mice bearing H22 hepatoma cells through the collapse of the tumor cell chromosome.[28] The results may provide scientific evidences for CPD4 (**2**) as a kind of promising photosensitizer for photodynamic therapy of malignant tumor cells.

Chlorophyllin

Chlorophyllin (**3**) (CHL) is a sodium–copper salt of chlorophyll derivative originated from Can Sha, which is a commonly used food dye for green coloration. At a 25–400 μg/mL concentration range, CHL could suppress the proliferation of human carcinoma cells such as HL-60 and K562 (leukemia), MCF-7 (breast), and murine sarcoma 180 cells *in vitro* by 8.2–95.7%. The antineoplastic effect in MCF-7 cells is mainly accompanied by the blockage of the cell cycle arrest at G2/M stage through cyclin level changes and promotion of apoptosis by deactivating ERKs.[29,30]

CHL (**3**) also demonstrated antimutagenic and anticarcinogenic activities together with its potent antioxidant property, which can form strong noncovalent complexes with several carcinogens to reduce DNA adduct and tumor formation. By the mechanistic actions, CHL (**3**) obstructed the carcinogenesis caused by AFB1, dibenzo(a,l)pyrene (DBP), or 2-amino-1-methyl-6-phenylimidazo-[4,5-b]pyridine.[31] In Caco-2 cell model, the intestinal epithelial transport of AFB1 and DBP was inhibited by CHL by directly binding CHL in the intestinal tract to the carcinogens, resulting in the blockage of the bioavailability of carcinogens.[31] A randomized, double-blind, placebo-controlled chemoprevention trial in Qidong, China, further proved that prophylactic interventions with CHL or supplementation of diets with foods rich in chlorophylls displayed practical means and resulted in chemical prevention against the development of HCC or other environmentally induced neoplastic diseases.[32] The efficient chemopreventive agent has also been used as a dietary supplement to reduce the intensity of the side effects of chemotherapy with CTX, indicating that CHL (**3**) may have beneficial effects when used in combination with anticancer drugs in clinical therapy.[33] However, the excess of chlorophyll in the diet may not only sequester the accessibility of aromatic mutagens to the cells but also disturb anticancer drugs with a heterocyclic structure (if taken orally) to affect the targeted cells, thereby reducing their bioavailability.[34]

Other Chlorophyll Derivatives

Several derivatives such as chlorin e6, 2-(1-hydroxyethyl) chlorin f, chlorin f methyl ether, chlorophyllin-manganese (III) selenite, polymeric chlorophylles, purpurin-18-N-butylimide, purpurin-18 methyl ester, and others were semisynthesized by utilizing pheophorbides and chlorophylls as starting materials.[35–39] Na chlorophyllin-manganese (III) selenite exhibited a marked inhibitory effect against the growth of H22 hepatoma cells in rats with 45–47% inhibitory rates.[36] The pyrazole and cyclopropane derivatives such as purpurin-18 methyl ester and purpurin-18-N-butylimide displayed similar photocytotoxic activity against the viability of human A549 lung carcinoma cells.[40] The recent approaches in the discovery of more potent and stable photodynamic chlorophyll derivatives have been continuously developed.

Other Biobenefits

The herb Can Sha (Silkworm feces) has been used as a traditional Chinese herb for a thousand years to treat hypertension, hyperlipidemia, and so on.

References

1. Zhong, J. X. et al. 1993. Photodynamic effects of Can-Sha photosensitizer (CPS) on transplanted tumors in mice. *Proceedings of SPIE-The International Society for Optical Engineering* 1616 (International Conference on Photodynamic Therapy and Laser Medicine, 1991), 283–5.
2. Dai, R. K. et al. 1992. Characterization of silkworm chlorophyll metabolites as an active photosensitizer for photodynamic therapy. *J. Nat. Prod.* 55: 1241–51.
3. Lee, W. Y. et al. 1990. Chlorophyll derivatives (CpD) extracted from silkworm excreta are specifically cytotoxic to tumor cells in vitro. *Yonsei Med. J.* 31: 225–33.
4. Park, W. J. et al. (a) 1990. *C. A* 112: 51380n; (b) 1999. *Chinese Materia Medica*. Vol. 9, 9–8097, 183, Shanghai Science and Technology Press, Shanghai, China.
5. Jin, X. L. et al. (a) 1992. Extraction and development of Chinese medicine photosensitizer from silkworm excrement. *Xiandai Yingyong Yaoxue* 9: 91; (b) 1999. *Chinese Materia Medica*. Vol. 9, 9–8097, 183, Shanghai Science and Technology Press, Shanghai, China.
6. Teng, L. S. et al. 1993. Photodynamic effect of chlorophyll derivative *with pulsed copper* vapor laser on human rectal carcinoma in vitro. *Proceedings of SPIE-The International Society for Optical Engineering* 1616 (International Conference on Photodynamic Therapy and Laser Medicine, 1991), 312–8.
7. Hu, L. Q. et al. 1988. Separation and identification of pheophorbides a from acid degradation products of silkworm excrement crude chlorophyll mixture. *Yiyao Gongye* 19: 157–61.
8. Zhu, Q. et al. 1992. Separation, preparation, and identification of phorbin derivatives. *Zhongguo Yiyao Gongye Zazhi* 23: 212–4.
9. Lim, D. S. et al. 2004. Silkworm-pheophorbide a mediated photodynamic therapy against B16F10 pigmented melanoma. *J. Photochem. Photobiol.* 74: 1–6.
10. Nakatani, Y. et al. 1981. Chemistry and biochemistry of Chinese drugs: VII. Cytostatic pheophytins from silkworm excreta, and derived photocytotoxic pheophorbides. *Chem. Pharm. Bull.* 29: 2261–9.
11. Xu, D. D. et al. 2011. Photo-activated pheophorbide a inhibits the growth of prostate cancer cells. *Laser Physics* 21: 1670–4.
12. Tang, P. M. K. et al. 2010. Pheophorbide a-mediated photodynamic therapy triggers HLA class I-restricted antigen presentation in human hepatocellular carcinoma. *Transl. Oncol.* 3: 114–22.
13. Chen, J. Y. et al. 2006. Pheophorbide a, a major antitumor component purified from *Scutellaria barbata*, induces apoptosis in human hepatocellular carcinoma cells. *Planta Med.* 72: 28–33.
14. Hajri, A. et al. 2002. In vitro and in vivo efficacy of photofrin and pheophorbide a, a bacterio-chlorin, in photodynamic therapy of colonic cancer cells. *Photochem Photobiol.* 75: 140–8.
15. Rapozzi, V. et al. 2009. Evidence that photoactivated pheophorbide a causes in human cancer cells a photodynamic effect involving lipid peroxidation. *Cancer Biol.Ther.* 8: 1318–27.
16. Tang, P. M. K. et al. 2006. Pheophorbide a, an active compound isolated from *Scutellaria barbata*, possesses photodynamic activities by inducing apoptosis in human hepatocellular carcinoma. *Cancer Biol. Therapy* 5: 1111–6.
17. Lee, W. Y. et al. 2004. Pheophorbidea induces a mitochondrial-mediated apoptosis in Jurkat leukaemia cells. *J. Photochem Photobiol B.* 75: 119–26.
18. Liu, L. et al. 2011. LED-activated pheophorbide a in ovarian cancer cells: Cytotoxicity and apoptosis induction. *Lase. Physics* 21: 423–6.
19. Evrard, S. P. K. et al. 1994. Experimental pancreatic cancer in the rat treated by photodynamic therapy. *Br. J. Surg.* 81: 1185–9.
20. Bui-Xuan, N. H. et al. 2010. Photo-activated pheophorbide-a, an active component of *Scutellaria barbata*, enhances apoptosis via the suppression of ERK-mediated autophagy in the estrogen receptor-negative human breast adenocarcinoma cells MDA-MB-231. *J. Ethnopharmacol.* 131: 95–103.
21. You, H. et al. 2011. Synthesis of pheophorbide-a conjugates with anticancer drugs as potential cancer diagnostic and therapeutic agents. *Bioorg. Med. Chem.* 19: 5383–91.
22. Tan, Y. et al. 2009. Photodynamic action of LED-activated pheophorbide a methyl ester in cisplatin-resistant human ovarian carcinoma cells. *Laser Phys.* 6: 321–7.
23. Zhang, J. L. et al. 2006. Photodynamic effect of two kinds of CPD photosensitizers on sarcoma S180 transplanted in mice. *Tianjin Yiyao* 34: 705–7.
24. Cui, J. H. et al. 1994. Photodynamic effect of chlorophyll derivative (CPD4) with pulsed copper-vapor laser on mouse transplanted tumor. *Zhonghua Zhongliu Zazhi* 16: 106–10.
25. Liu, Y. et al. 2009. Distribution and binding of novel photosensitizer 2-devinyl-2-(1-methoxylethyl) chlorin f in human breast cancer cells MCF-7. *Laser Physics Lett.* 6: 465–71.
26. Leng, L. et al. 2009. Effects of new photosensitizer combined with adriamycin on cell proliferation and cell cycle of breast cancer. *Zhongguo Zhongliu Linchuang* 36: 1416–9.
27. He, L. M. et al. 1995. Photodynamic effect of 2 photosensitizers on colon cancer line HR-8348 measured with MTT assay. *Zhongguo Jiguang* A22: 847–50.
28. He, D. Q. et al. 2009. The effect of photodynamic therapy combined cinobufotalin on mice transplanted H22 liver cancer. *Zhonghua Zhongyiyao Xuekan* 27: 2206–9.
29. Chiu, L. C. M. et al. 2003. Antiproliferative effect of chlorophyllin derived from a traditional Chinese medicine Bombyxmori excreta on human breast cancer MCF-7 cells. *Intl. J. Oncol.* 23: 729–35.
30. Chiu, L. C. M. et al. 2005. The chlorophyllin-induced cell cycle arrest and apoptosis in human breast cancer MCF-7 cells is associated with ERK deactivation and cyclin D1 depletion. *Intl. J. Mol. Med.* 16: 735–40.
31. Mata, J. E. et al. 2004. Effects of chlorophyllin on transport of dibenzo(a,l)pyrene, 2-amino-1-methyl-6-phenylimidazo-[4,5-b]pyridine, and aflatoxin B1 across Caco-2 cell monolayers. *Toxicol.* 196: 117–25.
32. Egner, P. A. et al. 2001. Chlorophyllin intervention reduces aflatoxin-DNA adducts in individuals at high risk for liver cancer. *Proceedings of the National Academy of Sciences of the United States of America* 98: 14601–6.
33. Te, C. et al. 1997. In vivo effects of chlorophyllin on the antitumor agent cyclophos-phamide. *Int. J. Cancer* 70: 84–9.
34. Ardelt, B. et al. 2001. Chlorophyllin protects cells from the cytostatic and cytotoxic effects of quinacrine mustard but not of nitrogen mustard. *Intl. J. Oncol.* 18: 848–53.

35. Yao, J. Z. et al. 2000. Synthesis, photosensitizing abilities and tumor-photobiological activities of chlorin f methyl ether. *Yaoxue Xuebao* 35: 63–6.
36. Han, M. J. et al. 1990. Biologically active polymer-targeting polymeric antitumor agents. *Makromolekulare Chemie, Macromolecular Symposia* 33 (Int. Symp. Mol. Des. Funct. Polym. 1989), 301–9.
37. Li, X. Y. et al. 2000. Synthesis of sodium chlorophyllin-manganese (III) selenite and its acute toxicity and preliminary test of inhibiting effect on hepatoma (H22) of rats. *Huaxi Yaoxue Zazhi* 15: 6–8.
38. Yao, J. Z. et al. 2000. Synthesis and photosensitizing abilities and tumor-photobiological activities of chlorin e6. *Zhongguo Yiyao Gongye Zazhi* 31: 215–7.
39. Yao, J. Z. et al. 2001. Synthesis and tumor-photobiological activities of 2-(1-hydroxyethyl) chlorin f and its ether derivatives. *Zhongguo Yaowu Huaxue Zazhi* 11: 1–4.
40. Yoon, I.-L. et al. 2011. Synthesis and photodynamic activities of pyrazolyl and cyclopropyl derivatives of purpurin-18 methyl ester and purpurin-18-N-butylimide. *Bull Kor Chem Soc* 32: 169–74.

76 Xu Chang Qing 徐長卿

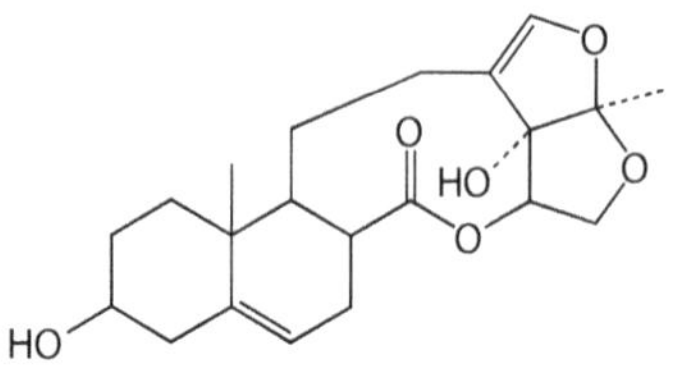

Herb Origination

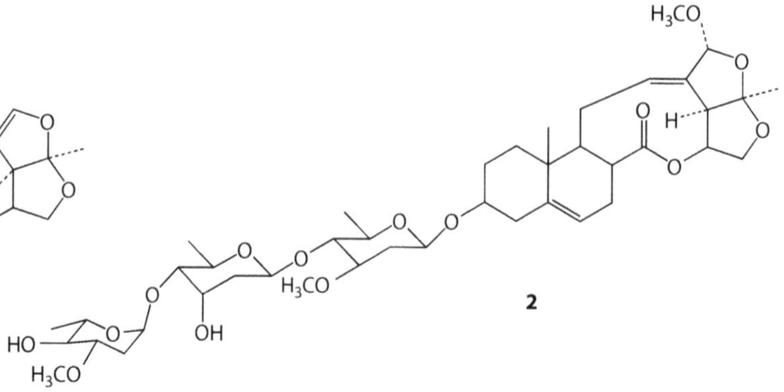

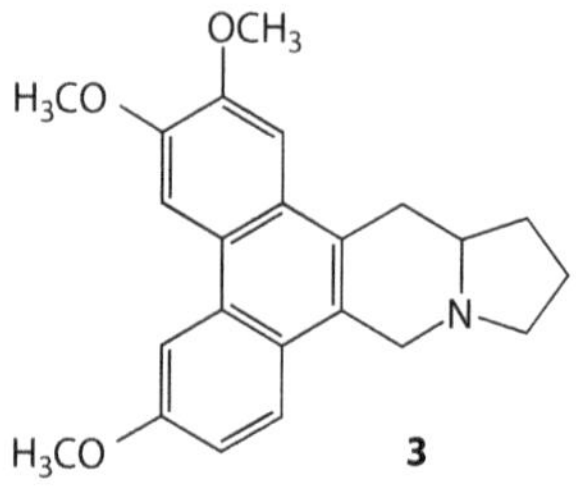

The herb Xu Chang Qing originates from the roots and the rhizomes of an Asclepiadaceae plant, *Cynanchum paniculatum.* This perennial climber plant is broadly distributed in eastern Asia, especially in China, Mongolia, Korea, and Japan. Its roots and rhizomes are normally collected in summer and autumn and dried in the shade for application in traditional Chinese medicine.

Antitumor Activities

C21 Steroidals

Three C21 steroidal glycosides assigned as cynanside-A (**1**) and cynanside-B, neocynapanogenin-F 3-*O*-β-D-thevetoside, and its aglycone neocynapanogenin-F (**2**), whose structures hold an aberrant 13,14:14,15-disecopregnane-type skeleton, exerted certain cytotoxic activities on human tumor cell lines *in vitro.* Cynanside-A (**1**) and cynanside-B showed a selective and moderate inhibitory effect against the proliferation of SK-MEL-2 melanoma cells with IC_{50} values of 26.55 and 17.36 μM, respectively, but their IC_{50} data on A549 (lung), SKOV-3 (ovary), and HCT-15 (colon) tumor cell lines were >30 μM.[1] Neocynapanogenin-F (**2**) demonstrated a marked cytotoxic activity on HL-60 leukemia cell line, and its maximum suppressive rate reached 98.14% at a concentration of 10 μg/mL *in vitro.* However, neocynapanogenin-F (**2**) and its 3-*O*-β-D-thevetoside only showed a weak antiproliferative effect on other tested human cancer cell lines such as A549 (lung), SMMC-7721 (liver), and BGC-823 (stomach) cells.[2]

Alkaloids

Antofine (**3**) is a phenanthroindolizidine alkaloid isolated from the herb as an important bioactive principle. In an *in vitro* assay, antofine (**3**) displayed potent antiproliferative effects in several human cancer cells with IC_{50} values in the nanomolar range. The treatment of two human colon carcinoma cell lines (HCT116 and SW480) with antofine (**3**) for 24 h did not result in the induction of apoptotic cell death but moderately elicited cell cycle arrest at G0/G1 phase and inhibited the expression of cyclin-D1, cyclin-E, and CDK4 and the transcriptional activity of β-catenin. The antigrowth activity of antofine (**3**) was also proven in a nude mouse model with HCT116 cells xenograft.[3] By arresting the cell cycle at G2/M phase after 48 h of incubation, antofine (**3**) significantly suppressed the proliferation of two tested human cancer cells *in vitro* and showed the IC_{50} values as 7.0 ng/mL in A549 lung cancer cells and 8.6 ng/mL in Col2 colon cancer cells.[4] Moreover, in a paclitaxel-resistant A549-PA lung cancer cell line, antofine (**3**) treatment notably reversed the MDR of A549-PA cells via a downregulation of P-gp mRNA and protein expression and an increase of intracellular rhodamine-123 accumulation, thereby effectively obstructing the growth of drug-resistant A549-PA cells.[5] These findings suggest that antofine (**3**) might be a potential drug lead for the development of cancer chemotherapeutic agents, particularly in overcoming cancer cell drug resistance.

Other Bioactivities

The herb Xu Chang Qing has been used in Chinese traditional medicine for a long history in the treatment of rheumatoid arthritis, lumbago, abdominal pain and vomiting, acute gastroenteritis, chronic bronchitis, hepatitis, liver cirrhosis, ascites, snakebites, and traumatic injuries. Pharmacological studies designated that the extracts of *C. paniculatum* possess analgesia, sedative, antibiosis, antiallergic, antiinflammatory activities, and so on. Also, its ethanolic extract shows a protective effect for treating herpes simplex encephalitis, and its steroidal glycoside and phenolic components have neuroprotective and analgesic activities.

References

1. Kim, C. S. 2013. Chemical constituents from the roots of *Cynanchum paniculatum* and their cytotoxic activity. *Carbohydrate Res.* 381: 1–5.
2. Dou, J. et al. 2007. New C21 steroidal glycoside from *Cynanchum paniculatum. Chin. Chem. Lett.* 18: 300–2.
3. Min, H. Y. et al. 2010. Inhibition of cell growth and potentiation of tumor necrosis factor-α-induced apoptosis by a phenanthroindolizidine alkaloid antofine in human colon cancer cells. *Biochem. Pharmacol.* 80: 1356–64.
4. Lee, S. K. et al. 2003. Cytotoxic activity and G2/M cell cycle arrest mediated by antofine, a phenanthroindolizidine alkaloid isolated from cynanchum paniculatum. *Planta Med.* 69: 21–5.
5. Kim, E. H. et al. 2012. Anti-proliferative activity and suppression of P-glycoprotein by (-)-antofine, a natural phenanthroindolizidine alkaloid, in paclitaxel-resistant human lung cancer cells. *Food Chem. Toxicol.* 50: 1060–5.

77 Da Ma Yao 大麻藥

Falcate dolichos

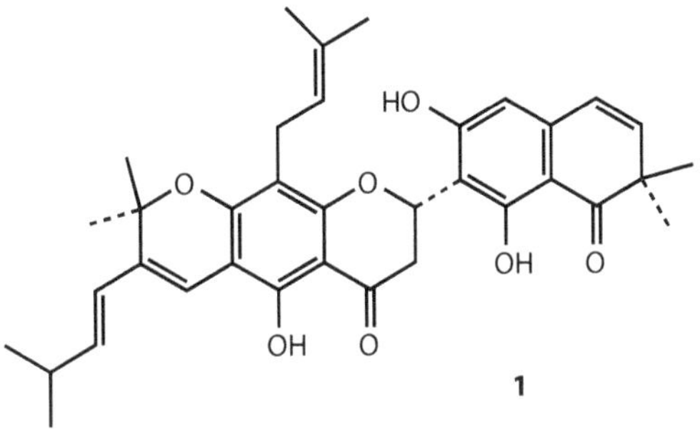

Herb Origination

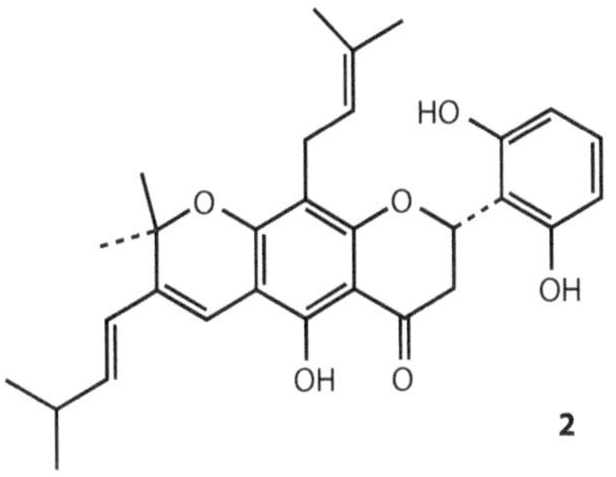

The herb Da Ma Yao (Falcate dolichos) originated from the dried roots and leaves of a Leguminosae plant, *Dolichos tenuicaulis*. Its distribution is broad in the regions of southern China and south and southeast Asia. In China, its leaves are generally collected in autumn, whereas its roots are collected in any season for traditional Chinese medical application.

Antitumor Activities and Constituents

The roots of Da Ma Yao showed an antineoplastic effect; especially, its aqueous extract at a concentration of 20 mg/kg markedly suppressed the cell respiration of mouse Ehrlich ascites carcinoma, sarcoma 180, sarcoma 37, and U14 cervical carcinoma, while its alcoholic extract in a 40 mg/kg concentration showed a marked inhibitory effect on the growth of Ehrlich ascites carcinoma and sarcoma 180 cells *in vitro*.[1] A direct inhibitory effect was achieved on sarcoma 37 cells *in vitro* by the total saponin component isolated from Da Ma Yao roots. The i.p. injection of the total saponin to tumor-bearing mice in a dose of 8 mg/kg for 10 days obstructed the growth of sarcoma 37 cells by 34.9–43.6%, but it showed no obvious antitumor effect on mouse models with U14 cervical carcinoma, sarcoma 180, or Ehrlich ascites cancer.[2]

Dolichnin-A (**1**) and dolichnin-B (**2**), two prenylated dihydroflavonoids, were isolated from the plant roots.[3] Both flavonoids demonstrated a marked *in vitro* inhibitory effect against the proliferation of human neoplastic cells *in vitro*. Three human cancer cell lines such as BEL-7402 (liver), SGC-7902 (stomach), A549 (lung), and K562 (leukemia) cells were relatively more sensitive to dolichnin-A (**1**), and the IC_{50} values ranged between 0.11 and 0.84 μg/mL in the three cell lines. Also, the IC_{50} values were 1.24–2.32 μg/mL for dolichnine-A (**1**) in human Hep3B and SMMC-7721 (liver), HT-29 (colon), MCF-7 (breast), A498 (renal), and PC3 (prostate) carcinoma cell lines, and 1.28–3.61 μg/mL for dolichnin-B (**2**) in K562, A549, Bel-2704, A498, HT-29, and MCF-7 cell lines.[4,5]

References

1. Guiyang Yixueyuan. 1975. *Dolichos tenuicaulis* extract influences the respiration of transplanted mouse tumor cells. *Kexue Tongbao* 20: 339–42.
2. Huang, H. P. et al. 1982. Antitumor activity of total saponins from *Dolichos falcatus* Klein. *Zhongguo Yaoli Xuebao* 3: 286–8.
3. Dolichnin-A: (2S)-5,2′,6′-trihydroxy-8-prenyl-6,7-(3-prenyl-2,2-dimethylpyrano)-3″4′-(2,2-dimethyl-1-ketone-cyclo hexadiene)-flavanone, and Dolichnin-B: (2S)-5,2′,6′-trihydroxy-8-prenyl-6,7-(3-prenyl-2,2-dimethyl-1-ketone-cyclohexadiene)-flavanone.
4. Peng, J. Y. et al. 2007. A new bioactive prenylated dihydroflavanoid from *Dolichos tenuicaulis* (Baker) Craib. *Chin. Chem. Lett.* 18: 293–6.
5. Peng, J. Y. et al. 2008. Two new bioactive prenylated dihydroflavanoids from the medicinal plant *Dolichos tenuicaulis* (Baker) Craib. *J. Asian Nat. Prod. Res.* 10: 169–175.

78 Tou Gu Cao 透骨草

Garden balsam

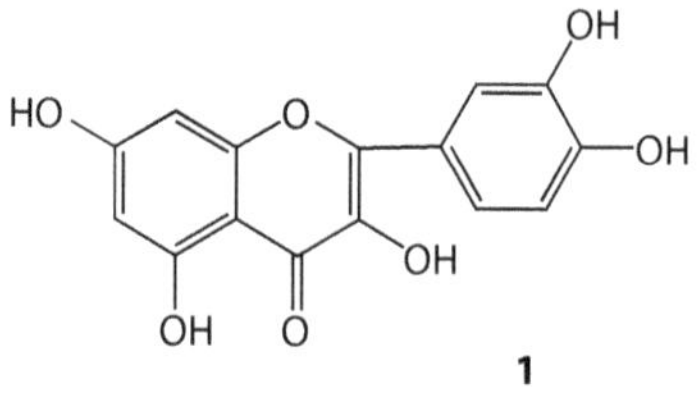

HO OH OH OH OH O 1 | O OCH3 O 2 | O O O H3CO OR 3. R = -H 4. R = -D-glucosyl | O O O HO O O 5

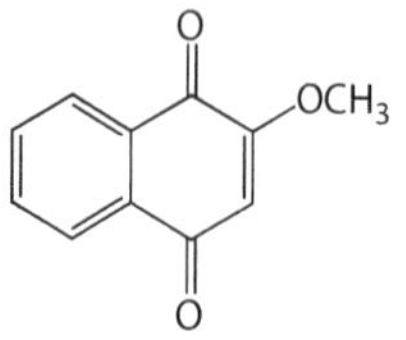

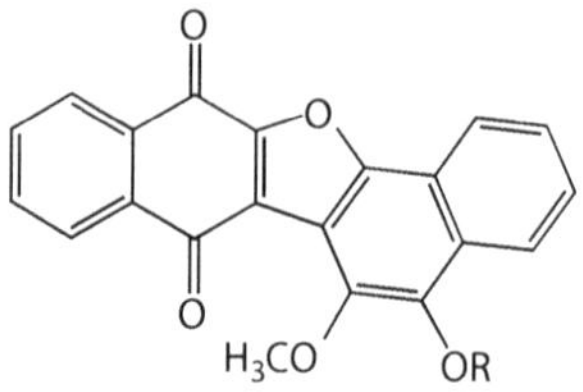

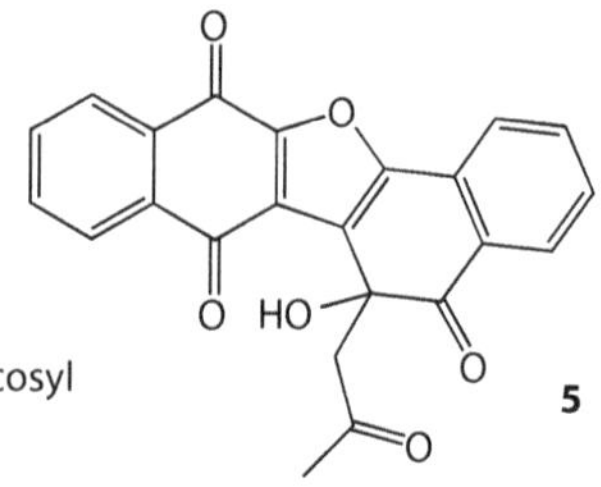

Herb Origination

The herb Tou Gu Cao (Garden balsam) is the dried whole plant *Impatiens balsamina* (Balsaminaceae), whose herbal plant is broadly cultivated in China. Its seed, stem, root, and flower have been independently used as Chinese medicines since the Ming dynasty. These herbs were firstly documented in *Jiuhuang Ben Cao*, a book regarding materia medica especially for the relief of famine. In Chinese herbal medicine, the plant seed was usually called Ji Xing Zi (急性子), while its flower was termed Feng Xian Hua (鳳僊花).

Antitumor Constituents and Activities

The plant has an extensive range of phytoconstituents like naphthoquinones, anthocyanidins, phenolic acids, flavonoids, coumarins, glycosides, and steroids, which have effective bioactivities. The two types of cancer inhibitors, flavonoids and naphthoquinones, were extracted from the different parts of the plant. The potent naphthoquinones like lawsone, lawsone methyl ether, and methylene-3,3′-bilawsone were present in the leaf of the plant that was proven to possess an intensive antitumor activity. One of the major constituents in Tou Gu Cao was found to be quercetin (**1**), which could inhibit the proliferation of human MDA-MB-435 breast cancer cells *in vitro* and *in vivo*, associated with the downregulation of signal transductions in the MDA-MB-435 cells.[1] 2-Methoxy-1,4-naphthoquinone (**2**) was isolated from the whole plant and the leaves, which demonstrated the intensive inhibition against human HepG2 hepatoma cells *in vitro*.[2] Naphthoquinone (**2**) was also capable of inducing human MKN45 gastric adenocarcinoma cells to necrotic and apoptotic deaths. When at low treatment doses (25–50 μM), the MKN45 cell apoptotic death was increased through a caspase-dependent pathway, but if the doses were higher than 50 μM, the cell necrosis was elicited via a superoxide anion catastrophe.[3] Moreover, three dinaphthofuran-7,12-dione derivatives identified as balsaminone-A (**3**), balsaminone-B (**4**), and balsaminone-C (**5**) were separated from the seeds (Ji Xing Zi), which all displayed a moderate cytotoxicity against A549 (lung), Bel-7402 (liver), and HeLa (cervix) human neoplastic cell lines.[4] The antigrowth effect might be related to the blockage of cell cycle arrest, but their mechanisms exhibited some differences.[5]

Additionally, a methanolic extract of Tou Gu Cao demonstrated the suppressive effect against the viability of HSC-2 human oral cancer cells and the proapoptotic activity by markedly amplifying AMP-activated protein kinase (AMPK) signaling and up-expressing mitochondria-related proteins (t-Bid, Bak, and Bad).[6]

Other Bioactivities

The herbs Tou Gu Cao and Ji Xing Zi have been widely used in traditional Chinese medicine to treat rheumatism, isthmus, and crural aches, fractures, superficial infections, fingernail inflammation, etc. Pharmacological approaches have identified some of flavonol and naphthoquinone derivatives from the herbs having marked antimicrobial, antianaphylaxis, antiinflammatory, itch-alleviating, and antidermatitis activities. 2-Methoxy-1,4-naphthoquinone (**2**) is a strong inhibitor against helicobacter pylori.[3]

References

1. Singhal, R. L. et al. 1995. Quercetin downregulates signal transduction in human breast carcinoma cells. *Biochem. Biophys. Res. Commun.* 208: 425–31.
2. Ding, Z. S. et al. 2008. Isolation and identification of an antitumor component from leaves of *Impatiens balsamina Mol.* 13: 220–9.
3. Wang, Y. C. et al. 2012. Anti-gastric adenocarcinoma activity of 2-methoxy-1,4-naphthoquinone, an anti-helicobacter pylori compound from *Impatiens balsamina* L. *Fitoterapia* 83: 1336–44.
4. Pei, H. et al. 2012. A new cytotoxic dinaphthofuran-7,12-dione derivatives from the seeds of *Impatiens balsamina. Zhongyaocai* 35: 407–10.
5. Pei, H. et al. 2012. Effects of balsaminone A and balsaminone B from Impatiens balsamina seed on growth and cycle of human lung cancer A549 cells. *Zhiwu Ziyuan Yu Huanjing Xuebao* 20: 15–8.
6. Shin, J.-A. et al. 2015. AMPK-activated protein kinase activation by *Impatiens balsamina* L. is related to apoptosis in HSC-2 human oral cancer cells. *Pharmacognosy Magazine* 11: 136–42.

79 Xiang Pai Cao 香排草

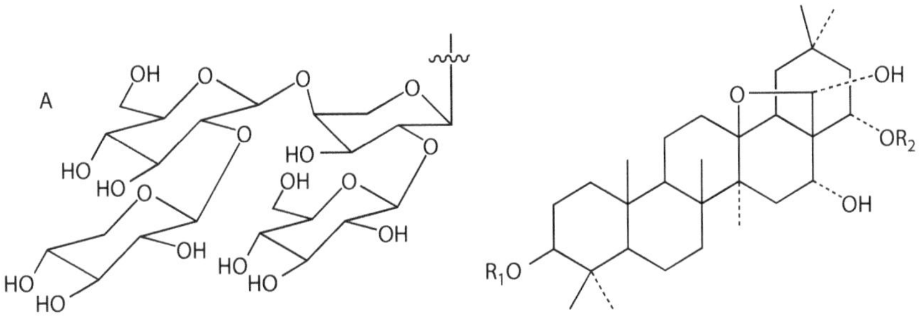

1. R_1 = –A, R_2 = –CO–$CH_2CH_2CH_2CH_2CH_3$
2. R_1 = –A, R_2 = –$COCH_2CH(CH_3)_2$
3. R_1 = –A, R_2 = –D-beta-glucopyranosyl

Herb Origination

The herb Xiang Pai Cao is a perennial Primulaceae plant, *Lysimachia capillipes*. The distribution of Xiang Pai Cao is in southern China from the eastern parts of Sichuan and Yunnan provinces to Zhejiang and Fujian provinces, as well as extended to Taiwan and the Philippines. The whole plant is collected in summer when its flowers are blooming and then dried in the sun for folk medicinal practices. The herb also can be used fresh.

Antitumor Constituents and Activities

Capilliposides that are triterpenoid glycosides extracted from the herb Xiang Pai Cao demonstrated a dose-dependent inhibitory effect on the proliferation of three types of human tumor cells in nude mice implanted with BGC-823 gastric cancer, PC3 prostate cancer, or SKOV-3 ovarian cancer without overt toxicity.[1] Both *in vitro* and *in vivo* assays confirmed that the capilliposides were capable of retarding the proliferation of NSCLC cells in a dose-dependent manner with the induction of apoptosis and cell cycle arrest at S phase. The NSCLC cell apoptotic death was promoted by capilliposides through a mitochondrial-mediated and ROS-activated apoptotic pathway.[2,3] Capilliposide-B (**1**) and capilliposide-D (**2**) exerted a significant cytotoxic activity against human A2780 ovarian cancer cells *in vitro*, and their IC_{50} values were 0.1 and 0.2 μg/mL, respectively, but capilliposide-A and capilliposide-C (**3**) were cytotoxic to the A2780 cells.[4,5] At concentrations within a range of 1.08–17.20 μmol/L, the treatment with capilliposide-D (**2**) for 48 h dose-dependently suppressed the proliferation of human BGC-823 (stomach), A549 (lung), Bel-7402 (liver), and PC3 and DU145 (prostate) carcinoma cell lines *in vitro* (respective IC_{50}: 3.74, 4.32, 5.35, 5.53, and 9.99 μmol/L). Through the downregulation of Bcl-2, JNK, and P38α/β, the upregulation of Bax, p-JNK, and p-P38, and the activation of caspases, the apoptotic death of PC3 and DU145 prostate cancer cells could be promoted by capilliposide-D (**2**).[6] Therefore, the capilliposides, especially, capilliposide-D (**2**), may have a developing potential in the prevention and the treatment of cancers.

Other Bioactivities

The herb Xiang Pai Cao (*Lysimachia capillipes*) is often used to treat colds and arthritis and is also used in cooking as a spice in southern China. Pharmacological studies proved that the herb possesses antiviral and antifebrile properties besides antitumor effect.

References

1. Xu, Y. et al. 2012. Studies on the antitumor activity of the total saponins from *Lysimachia capilllipes* Hemsl. *China Pharmacol. Bull.* 28: 545–9.
2. Fei, Z. H. et al. 2014. Capilliposide isolated from *Lysimachia capillipes* Hemsl. induces ROS generation, cell cycle arrest, and apoptosis in human nonsmall cell lung cancer cell lines. *Evidence-based Complem. Altern. Med.* 2014: 497456.
3. Fei, Z. H. et al. 2014. Capilliposides inhibits proliferation and induces apoptosis of human lung cancer H460 cells. *Zhejiang Yixue* 36: 742–6.
4. Tian, J. K. et al. 2006. Three novel triterpenoid saponins from *Lysimachia capillipes* and their cytotoxic activities. *Chem. Pharm. Bull.* 54: 567–9.
5. Tian, J. K. et al. 2006. New antitumor triterpene saponin from *Lysimachia capillipes. Chem. Nat. Compds.* 42: 328–31.
6. Li, R. Y. et al. 2014. Capilliposide C derived from *Lysimachia capillipes* Hemsl inhibits growth of human prostate cancer PC3 cells by targeting caspase and MAPK pathways. *Intl. Urol. Nephrol.* 46: 1335–44.

80 Bai Hua Dan 白花丹

White leadwort or Citraka or Chitrak

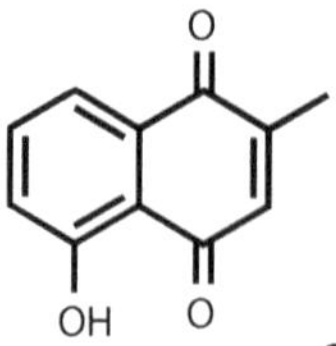

OH O 1

HO H H COOH COOH 2

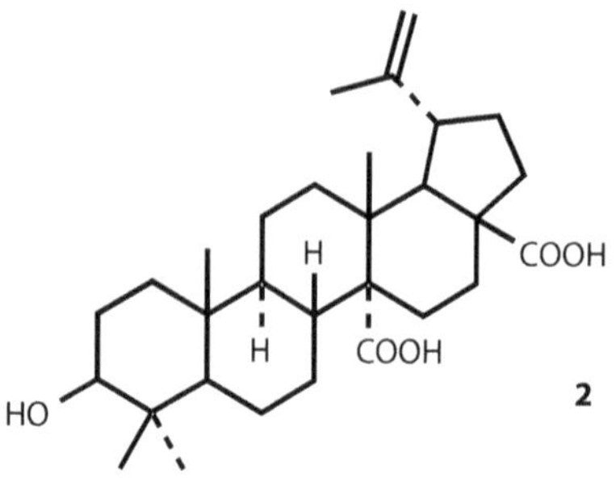

Herb Origination

The herb Bai Hua Dan (White leadwort) originates from a Plumbaginaceae plant, *Plumbago zeylanica*. This plant is native to the southeast regions of Asia. In China, the whole plant can be collected annually for use in Chinese folk medicine.

Antitumor Constituents and Activities

Naphthoquinones

In Vitro *Anticancer Effects*

A naphthoquinone assigned as plumbagin (**1**) was separated from Bai Hua Dan, which showed significant and broad antigrowth and apoptosis-inducing effects against many types of cancer cell lines, such as lung cancer (Calu-1, H460, A549), cervical cancer (HeLa, ME-180), breast cancer (MDA-MB-231SA, MCF-7), prostate cancer (PC3, LNCaP, C4-2, DU145), pancreatic cancer (PANC1, BxPC3, ASPC1), gastric cancer (AGS, SGC-7901, MKN-28), melanoma (Bowes), lymphoma (Raji), and leukemia (NB4, P388).[1–11] Plumbagin (**1**) was more effective in the growth inhibition of H460 cells compared to that of A549 cells, both of which are types of NSCLC cell lines.[3] The IC_{50} values in the MCF-7 cells and Bowes cells were 1.28 and 1.39 μM, respectively,[4] and the IC_{50} values in the AGS, MKN-28, and SGC-7901 cells was 10.12–19.12 μmol/L.[5] Plumbagin (**1**) at a 2.5–20 μmol/L concentration range dose-dependently inhibited the cell viability and induced the apoptosis of MDA-MB-231SA breast cancer cells (IC_{50}: 14.7 μmol/L).[6] At 5–20 μmol/L concentrations, plumbagin (**1**) was able to enhance the sensitivity of SGC-7901 gastric cancer cells to TNFα and cisplatin.[5] Also, the plumbagin (**1**) treatment showed an obvious inhibition on human U2OS osteosarcoma cells concomitantly with the promotion of apoptosis via the increase of p53 activity and the decrease of MDM2 expression.[7] Among several leukemia cell lines, U937 monocytic leukemia cells appeared to be more sensitive to plumbagin treatment in terms of cytotoxicity and level of apoptotic death compared to the more resistant Raji Burkitt lymphoma cells, whose effect might be related to plumbagin-generated tenfold higher ROS in U937 cells than in Raji cells.[8]

In Vivo *Anticancer Effects*

The *in vivo* anticancer effect of plumbagin (**1**) was confirmed in mouse models by using NB4 (leukemic), Panc-1 (pancreas), and DU145 (prostate) tumor xenografts.[9–11] The i.p. injection of plumbagin in a daily dose of 2 mg/kg for three weeks resulted in a 64.49% reduction of NB4 tumor volume.[9] Before the days of ectopic implantation of hormone-refractory DU145 tumor cells, the administration of plumbagin (**1**) by the same route could retard the growth of prostate cancer cells by three weeks and reduce both tumor weight and volume by 90%.[11] In a pancreatic tumor nude mice model, plumbagin (**1**) markedly inhibited the growth of the Panc-1 xenograft with no marked effect on the leukocyte counts and no overt toxic manifestation (such as body weight loss, tissue damage, and behavior change) in the treated animals.[9,10] Moreover, the tumor inhibitory and radio-modifying properties of plumbagin (**1**) were also demonstrated on mouse Ehrlich ascites carcinoma *in vivo* with the survival extension of the animal at 120 days.[12–14] The significant enhancement of the mean survival time and peritoneal cell counts were also present in mice bearing plumbagin-treated DAL as well.[12]

Anticarcinogenic Effects

Plumbagin (**1**) was proven as a promising anticarcinogenic agent. In experiments using rats, the oncogenesis in intestinal tumor provoked by azoxymethane and in hepatoma induced by 3-methyl-4-dimethylaminoazobenzene were obviously obstructed by the plumbagin treatment.[13–16] Intratumoral or oral administration of plumbagin (**1**) in a 2 mg/kg dose significantly diminished the growth of fibrosarcoma induced by methylcholanthrene in rats by 60–70%.[17–19] Also, plumbagin (**1**) restrained Nox-4 (a renal NAD(P)H oxidase) activity in human 293 embryonic kidney cells and LN229 brain tumor cells in time- and dose-dependent manners and repressed the superoxide production in Nox-4 transfected COS-7 cells (an African green monkey kidney fibroblast cells). During the *in vivo* tests, plumbagin (**1**) simultaneously reduced the activities of pathophysiological enzymes in the plasma, the liver, and the kidney. The results implied that the anticarcinogenic effect exerted by plumbagin (**1**) should be intimately correlated with its marked antioxidant activity.[17,20]

Antiinvasive and Antimetastatic Effects

Importantly, following the dose-dependent down-expressions of MMP-2 and u-PA and reduction of NF-κB and AP-1 binding abilities, plumbagin (**1**) showed an inhibitory effect on the abilities of adhesion, migration, and invasion of human hepatoma HepG2 cells *in vitro*.[21,22] The i.p. administration of plumbagin (2 mg/kg body weight, five days in a week) for eight weeks demonstrated a significant inhibitory effect against the growth and the metastasis of PC-3M-luciferase prostate cancer cells into liver in nude mice, but the blockage of metastasis into the lungs and the lymph nodes was not significant.[23] Similarly, in an *in vivo* model, the administration of plumbagin (2, 4, or 6 mg/kg, i.p. five times per week) for seven weeks to mice delayed the tumor growth by two to three weeks and reduced the tumor volume by 44–74% and also dose-dependently inhibited the MDA-MB-231SArfp breast tumor bone metastasis and osteolytic lesions.[6,24,25] Besides the suppression of the proliferation and the colony formation of SK-Hep-1 hepatoma cells and glioma cells associated with the induction of apoptosis and cell cycle arrest, plumbagin (**1**) was also capable of obstructing the migratory and invasive abilities of the cancer cell lines and exerting the antimetastatic effect.[26,27] Based upon these positive evidences, plumbagin (**1**) noticeably demonstrated the developing potential for the suppression of tumor growth and metastasis in cancer chemotherapy and chemoprevention.

Naphthoquinone Conjugators

Conjugated plumbagin (**1**) with cyclodextrin (a cyclic oligosaccharide) not only increased its solubility and stability but also enhanced its growth suppressive efficacy in mice implanted with B16F1 melanoma cells at a dose of 5 mg/kg (subcutaneous).[28] When plumbagin (**1**) was encapsulated in microspheres using poly(D,L-lactide)-coglycolide or niosomal, the toxicity could be attenuated and the antineoplastic effect was augmented in mice implanted with sarcoma 180 or Ehrlich ascites tumor.[29,30] In addition, two metal-linked plumbagins, $[Cu(PLN)_2]\text{-}2H_2O$ and $[Cu(PLN)(bipy)(H_2O)]_2\,(NO_3)_2\text{-}4H_2O$, were afforded by the reaction of plumbagin (**1**) with CuII salt or CuII and 2,2′-bipyridine (bipy), respectively. The Cu addition synergistically augmented the anticancer activity of plumbagin (**1**) and the inhibition activity to Topo-I and also augmented its capacity of generating DNA single-strand breaks through ROS production and noncovalent binding intercalation of DNA neighboring base pairs in neoplastic cells, leading to apoptosis promotion.[30,31] However, the complex $[Cu(PLN)_2]\text{-}H_2O$ exhibited lower antioxidant activities toward scavenging DPPH free radical and inhibiting lipid peroxidation, compared to plumbagin (**1**).[32] The findings provide a strong impact for designing anticancer drugs as conjugators and complexes with the cytotoxic and antioxidant activities.

Triterpenoids

An antiproliferative and antimetastatic triterpenoid identified as melaleucic acid (**2**) was discovered from the herb. Melaleucic acid (**2**) was capable of promoting the apoptosis of human MDA-MB-231 breast carcinoma cells by the induction of multiple events, such as loss of mitochondrial membrane potential with the downregulation of Bcl-2, the increase of Bad expression, the release of cytochrome c, the activation of caspase-3, and the cleavage of PARP leading to DNA fragmentation. The melaleucic acid (**2**) was also able to suppress the adhesion of MDA-MB-231 cell to fibronectin-coated substrate and to influence the extracellular matrix in correlation with the inhibition of the expressions of p-PI3K, p-Akt, p-JNK, MMP-2, MMP-9, p-ERK1/2, VEGF, and HIF-1α, leading to the antiadhesion, antiinvasive, and antimigratory effects in the MDA-MB-231 breast cancer cells.[33]

Exploration of Mechanisms

Antigrowth and Proapoptotic Mechanisms

The mechanism of plumbagin (**1**) in diminishing the viability of cancer cells has been explored to find the growth inhibition and the apoptosis induction correlated to the following events: (1) a mitochondrial pathway, i.e., upregulation of Bax, downregulation of phosphoinositide 3-kinase activity, loss of mitochondrial transmembrane potential, release of cytochrome c, activation of caspase-3 and caspases-9, and cleavage of PARP[9–11,33,34]; (2) reduction of EGFR/Neu expression and its downstream signaling (Akt, NF-κB, Bcl-2, and survivin), up-expression of p53 and p21CIP1/WAF1, and activation of JNK/p38 signaling, leading to caspase-3 activation (such in H460 lung cancer cells)[3]; (3) decrease of DNA-binding activity of transcription factors (AP-1, NF-κB, and Stat3)[11]; (4) induction of cell cycle arrest by downregulating regulatory proteins (cyclin-B1 and CDC25B)[3,35] and inhibition of NF-κB activation pathway that leads to the suppression of NF-κB-regulated gene products such as antiapoptotic (IAP1, IAP2, Bcl-2, Bcl-xL, cFLIP, Bfl-1/A1, and survivin), proliferative (cyclin-D1 and COX-2), and angiogenetic (MMP-9 and VEGF)[33]; and (5) alteration of gene expressions that are responsible for ROS metabolism and superoxide dismutase (SOD), where the generation of ROS plays a critical role in the plumbagin-induced apoptotic death (especially in NB4 [leukemic], ME-180 [cervical], and prostate cancer cells).[10,11,33,34] The established mechanisms of plumbagin (**1**) contributed to the antigrowth, apoptosis-inducing, anticarcinogenic, and radiosensitizing properties.

However, the characteristic mechanisms normally correspond to the anticancer effect of plumbagin (**1**) in the different neoplastic cells. For example, during the treatment of the pancreatic cancer cells (PANC1, BxPC3, and ASPC1), plumbagin (**1**) obstructed (1) the constitutive expressions of EGFR, pStat3Tyr705, and pStat3Ser727; (2) the DNA binding of Stat3; (3) the interaction of EGFR with Stat3; the (4) phosphorylation and DNA-binding activity of NF-κB; and (5) the activities of cyclin-D1, MMP-9, and survivin, whose events were responsible for the antigrowth mechanism.[36] In human prostate cancer cell lines (PC3, LNCaP, and C4-2), the antigrowth and antiviability effects of plumbagin (**1**) was largely associated with the modulation of cellular redox status and the generation of ROS but irrespective of their androgen responsiveness or p53 status.[33] The potentiated apoptosis and restrained growth of human gastric carcinoma cell lines (SGC-7901, MKN-28, and AGS) by plumbagin (**1**) was correlated with (1) a NF-κB pathway including the blockage of the expression of NF-κB-regulated gene products (Bcl-xL, Bcl-2, IAP1, XIAP, tumor factor, and VEGF), inhibition of NF-κB p65 nuclear translocation and degradation of IκBα and (2) reduction of TNFα-induced phosphorylation of p65 and IKK.[5] In the treatment of HT-29 colon cancer cells, AMPK might be a key mediator in the cancer inhibition and apoptotic induction of plumbagin, i.e., plumbagin induces AMPK/ASK1/TRAF2 association to activate proapoptotic JNK-p53 signal axis. Also, the AMPK activation of plumbagin might be enhanced by exogenously added short-chain ceramide to promote colon neoplastic cell apoptosis and growth inhibition.[37]

Antiinvasive and Antimetastatic Mechanism

The evidences showed that the antigrowth and antiinvasive activities of plumbagin (**1**) in hormone-refractory prostate cancer were mediated by the inhibition of multiple molecular targets, i.e., (1) inhibition of JAK-2, AKT, and Stat3 phosphorylation; (2) down-expression of PKCε (a predictive biomarker of PCa aggressiveness) and phosphatidylinositol 3-kinase; and (3) blockage of DNA-binding activity of transcription factors (AP-1, NF-κB, and Stat3) and lessening of Bcl-xL, CDC25A, and COX expressions.[11] The antigrowth and antimetastatic effects of plumbagin (**1**) in prostate cancer PC-3M-luciferase cells were found to be associated with the inhibition against multiple expressions of (1) pStat3Tyr705, pStat3Ser727, and PKCε; (2) Stat3 downstream target genes (survivin and BclxL); (3) proliferative markers Ki-67 and PCNA; (4) metastatic marker MMP9, MMP2, and u-PA; and (5) angiogenesis markers CD31 and VEGF.[22] The effects on MDA-MB-231SArfp breast tumor bone metastasis were mediated by (1) down-expressed IL-1β, TGF-β, MMP-2, and MMP-9; (2) restrained STAT3 signaling; (2) lessened secretion of osteoclast-activating factors through the decline of NF-κB activity; (3) altered neoplastic cell-induced RANKL/OPG ratio in osteoblasts; and (4) abrogated RANKL-induced NF-κB and MAPK pathways by blocking the connection of RANK to TRAF6, leading to the suppression of both cancer cell- and RANKL-stimulated osteoclastogenesis and improvement of the microenvironment in the bone,[6,24,25] whose mechanisms in SK-Hep-1 hepatoma cells and glioma cells were revealed to correlate with the upregulation of p21 and the down regulation of MMP-2 and MMP-9 in the hepatoma cells and the increase of p21CIP1 and p27KIP1 expressions and the decrease of FOXM1 expression and activity in the glioma cells.[26,27] The inhibitory effect of plumbagin (**1**) on the abilities of adhesion, migration, and invasion of human hepatoma HepG2 cells was mediated by the dose-dependent suppression of MMP-2 and u-PA expressions, reduction of NF-κB and AP-1 binding abilities, and enhancement of TIMP-2 and PAI-1 expressions.[21,22]

Anti-UVR Mechanism

The topical application of plumbagin (**1**) even in nontoxic doses (100–500 nmol) to mouse skin could elicit a dose-dependent inhibition against the ultraviolet radiation (UVR)-induced development of squamous cell carcinoma and augment the cell apoptosis induction and inhibition of the cell proliferation with no signs of toxicity during the entire period of the experiment. The mechanism in the plumbagin treatment was revealed to be associated with (1) restrained UVR-induced DNA binding of AP-1, NF-κB, Stat3 transcription factors, and Stat3-regulated molecules (CDC25A and survivin); (2) declined protein levels of Bcl-2, Bcl-xL, pERK1/2, PI3K85, pAKTSer473, and proliferating cell nuclear antigen; (3) augmented cell cycle inhibitory proteins p27 and p21; and (4) amplified UVR-induced Fas-associated death domain expression, Bax expression, and PARP cleavage.[38]

Other Bioactivities

The roots of *P. zeylanica* have been used in Indian medicine for >2500 years as an antiatherogenic, cardiotonic, hepatoprotective, and neuroprotective agent. Pharmacological studies have revealed that plumbagin (**1**) possesses pregnancy-terminating, microvasodilative, hypotensive, and antibacterial properties. The excitation of the CNS can be induced by a small dose of plumbagin, and the nervous excitation is turned to paralysis by a large dose. The acute LD_{50} of plumbagin were 9.4 mg/kg in normal mice by i.p. injection and 65 mg/kg in rat and 164 mg/kg in mouse by oral administration.[12] Also, plumbagin (**1**) is a GHS S-transferase inhibitor and a DNA cleaver, which was mediated by mammalian Topo-II.[39,40]

References

1. Lin, L. W. et al. 2003. Cytotoxic naphthoquinones and plumbagic acid glucosides from *Plumbago zeylanica*. *Phytochem.* 62: 619–22.
2. Nguyen, A. T. et al. 2004. Cytotoxic constituents from *Plumbago zeylanica*. *Fitoterapia* 75: 500–4.
3. Gomathinayagam, R. et al. 2008. Anticancer mechanism of plumbagin, a natural compound, on non-small cell lung cancer cells. *Anticancer Res.* 28: 785–92.
4. Nguyen, A. T. et al. 2006. Cytotoxicity of five plants used as anticancer remedies in Vietnamese traditional medicine. *Recent Progress in Med. Plants* 15: 137–47.
5. Li, J. et al. 2012. Plumbagin inhibits cell growth and potentiates apoptosis in human gastric cancer cells in vitro through the NF-κB signaling pathway. *Acta Pharmacol. Sinica* 33: 242–9.
6. Yan, W. et al. 2014. Plumbagin attenuates cancer cell growth and osteoclast formation in the bone microenvironment of mice. *Acta Pharmacol. Sinica* 35: 124–34.
7. Tian, L. Q. et al. 2012. Effect and mechanism of plumbagin in human osteosarcoma cell line U2OS. *Zhongliu Fangzhi Yanjiu* 39: 1285–8.
8. Gaascht, F. et al. 2014. Plumbagin modulates leukemia cell redox status. Mol. 19: 10011–32.
9. Chen, C. A. et al. 2009. Plumbagin, isolated from *Plumbago zeylanica*, induces cell death through apoptosis in human pancreatic cancer cells. *Pancreatol.* 9: 797–809.
10. Xu, K. H. et al. 2010. Plumbagin induces ROS-mediated apoptosis in human promyelocytic leukemia cells in vivo. *Leukemia Res.* 34: 658–65.
11. Aziz, M. H. et al. 2008. Plumbagin, a medicinal plant-derived naphthoquinone, is a novel inhibitor of the growth and invasion of hormone-refractory prostate cancer. *Cancer Res.* 68: 9024–32.
12. Kavimani, S. et al. 1996. Antitumor activity of plumbagin against Dalton's ascitic lymphoma. *Ind. J. Pharm. Sci.* 58: 194–6.
13. Prasad, V. S. et al. 1996. Radiosensitizing effect of plumbagin on mouse melanoma cells grown in vitro. *Ind. J. Experim. Biol.* 34: 857–8.
14. Devi, P. U. et al. 1999. Plumbagin, a plant naphthoquinone with antitumor and radiomodifying properties. *Pharm. Biol.* 37: 231–6.
15. Sugie, S. et al. 1998. Inhibitory effects of plumbagin and juglone on azoxymethane-induced intestinal carcinogenesis in rats. *Cancer Lett.* 127: 177–83.
16. Parimala, R. et al. 1993. Effect of Plumbagin on some glucose metabolising enzymes studied in rats in experimental hepatoma. *Mol.Cell. Biochem.* 125: 59–63.
17. Jayamathi, P. et al. 2010. Antioxidant property of plumbagin on fibrosarcoma induced rats. *Recent Research in Science and Technol.* 2: 1–3.
18. Chandrasekaran, B. et al. 1983. Growth inhibitory effect of echitamine and plumbagin on fibrosarcoma in rats. *Arogya* (Manipal, India) 9: 60–3.
19. Krishnaswamy, M. et al. 1980. Plumbagin: A study of its anticancer, antibacterial and antifungal properties. *Ind. J. Experim. Biol.* 18: 876–7.
20. Ding, Y. X. et al. 2005. Inhibition of Nox-4 activity by plumbagin, a plant-derived bioactive naphthoquinone. *J. Pharmacy Pharmacol.* 57: 111–6.
21. Sandur, S. K. et al. 2006. Plumbagin suppresses NF-κB activation and NF-κB-regulated gene products through modulation of p65 and IκBκ kinase activation, leading to potentiation of apoptosis induced by vytokine and chemotherapeutic agents. *J. Biol. Chem.* 281: 17023–33.

22. Shih, Y. W. et al. 2009. Plumbagin inhibits invasion and migration of liver cancer HepG2 cells by decreasing productions of matrix metalloproteinase-2 and urokinase-plasminogen activator. *Hepatology Res.* 39: 998–1009.
23. Hafeez, B. B. et al. 2013. Plumbagin, a medicinal plant (Plumbago zeylanica)-derived 1,4-naphthoquinone, inhibits growth and metastasis of human prostate cancer PC-3M-luciferase cells in an orthotopic xenograft mouse model. *Mol. Oncol.* 7: 428–39.
24. Li, Z. et al. 2012. Plumbagin inhibits breast tumor bone metastasis and osteolysis by modulating the tumor-bone microenvironment. *Current Mol. Med.* 12: 967–81.
25. Yan, W. et al. 2013. Suppressive effects of plumbagin on invasion and migration of breast cancer cells via the inhibition of STAT3 signaling and down-regulation of inflammatory cytokine expressions. *Bone Res.* 1: 362–70.
26. Cao, X. C. et al. 2013. The effects of plumbagin on proliferation and metastasis in human liver cancer SK-hep-1 cells. *Zhongguo Aizheng Zazhi* 23: 721–7.
27. Liu, X. J. et al. 2015. Plumbagin induces growth inhibition of human glioma cells by downregulating the expression and activity of FOXM1. *J. Neuro-Oncol.* 121: 469–77.
28. Naresh, R. A. R. et al. 1996. Niosomal plumbagin with reduced toxicity and improved anticancer activity in BALB/c mice. *J. Pharmacy Pharmacol.* 48: 1128–32.
29. Chen, Z. F. et al. 2009. Cytotoxicity of the traditional Chinese medicine (TCM) plumbagin in its copper chemistry. *Dalton Transactions* (48): 10824–33.
30. Nazeem, S. et al. 2009. Plumbagin induces cell death through a copper-redox cycle mechanism in human cancer cells. *Mutag.* 24: 413–8.
31. Tan, M. X. et al. 2011. Antioxidant activities of plumbagin and its Cu (II) complex. *Bioinorg. Chem. Applic.* 898726.
32. Sathya, S. et al. 2010. 3β-Hydroxylup-20(29)-ene-27,28-dioic acid dimethyl ester, a novel natural product from Plumbago zeylanica inhibits the proliferation and migration of MDA-MB-231 cells. *Chemico-Biol. Interactions* 188: 412–20.
33. Srinivas, P. et al. 2004. Plumbagin induces reactive oxygen species, which mediate apoptosis in human cervical cancer cells. *Mol. Carcinog.* 40: 201–11.
34. Powolny, A. A. et al. 2008. Plumbagin-induced apoptosis in human prostate cancer cells is associated with modulation of cellular redox status and generation of reactive oxygen species. *Pharm. Res.* 25: 2171–80.
35. Zhao, Y. L. et al. 2006. Effects of plumbagin on the human acute promyelocytic leukemia cells in vitro. *Zhongguo Bingli Shengli Xuehui* 14: 208–11.
36. Hafeez, B. B. et al. 2012. Plumbagin, a plant derived natural agent inhibits the growth of pancreatic cancer cells in in vitro and in vivo via targeting EGFR, Stat3 and NF-κB signaling pathways. *Intl. J. Cancer* 131: 2175–86.
37. Chen, M. B. et al. 2013. Activation of AMP-activated protein kinase (AMPK) mediates plumbagin-induced apoptosis and growth inhibition in cultured human colon cancer cells. *Cell. Signalling* 25: 1993–2002.
38. Sand, J. M. et al. 2012. Plumbagin (5-hydroxy-2-methyl-1,4-naphthoquinone), isolated from Plumbago zeylanica, inhibits ultraviolet radiation-induced development of squamous cell carcinomas. *Carcinogenesis* 33: 184–90.
39. SivaKumar, V. et al. 2005. In vivo micronucleus assay and GST activity in assessing genotoxicity of plumbagin in Swiss albino mice. *Drug Chemical Toxicol.* 28: 499–507.
40. Fujii, N. et al. 1992. *Antimicrobial Agents and Chemother.* 36: 2589.

81 Chou Bai 臭柏

Savin or Savin juniper

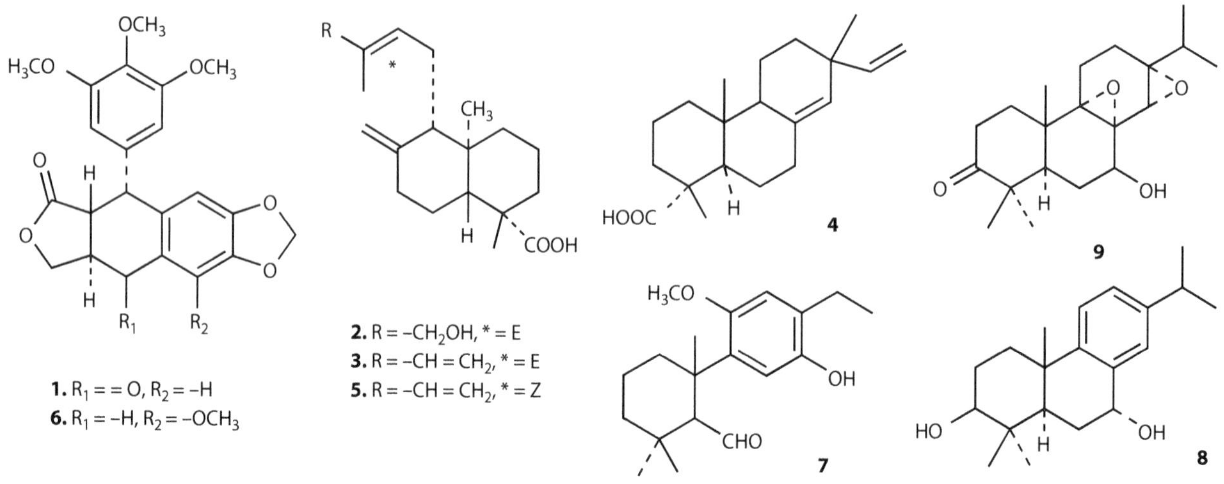

1. $R_1 = =O, R_2 = -H$
6. $R_1 = -H, R_2 = -OCH_3$

2. $R = -CH_2OH, * = E$
3. $R = -CH = CH_2, * = E$
5. $R = -CH = CH_2, * = Z$

Herb Origination

The herb Chou Bai (Savin juniper) is the twigs and the leaves of a Cupressaceae plant, *Sabina vulgaris* (= *Juniperus sabina*). The plant is distributed in the northwest of China and the inner Mongolian province as well as Europe. The herb is usually collected in spring and autumn and dried in the sun for folk medicinal application in China. It also can be used fresh.

Antitumor Activities and Constituents

The Chou Bai contains a toxic constituent podophyllotoxin (**1**), but the administration of 2% podophyllotoxin could cause sarcoma bleeding and necrosis in mice.[1] In the *in vitro* assays, podophyllotoxin (**1**) noticeably suppressed the growth of mouse P388 leukemia and two human A549 (lung) and HT-29 (colon) carcinoma cell lines with the same IC_{50} values of 0.25 μg/mL.[2]

Six other antitumor active compounds, i.e., *trans*-communic acid (**2**), *cis*-communic acid (**3**), sandaracopimaric acid (**4**), isocupressic acid (**5**), β-peltatin-A methyl ether (**6**), and 12-hydroxy-6,7-secoabieta-8,11,13-triene-6,7-dial (**7**), were isolated from Chou Bai. All the six compounds demonstrated cytotoxicity against murine P388 leukemia cells *in vitro*.[2] The most potent cytotoxicity among the six substances was achieved by β-peltatin-A methyl ether (**6**) with IC_{50} values in the range of 2.5–4 ng/mL against three neoplastic cell lines (P388, A549, and HT-29) *in vitro*.[3] Among the isolated diterpenoids from the herb, sabiperone-F (**9**) and 3β,7α-dihydroxyabieta-8,11,13-triene (**8**) demonstrated the moderate cell growth inhibitory activities against five human cancer cell lines, MCF-7 (breast), A549 (lung), HepG2 (liver), HCT-116 (colon), and HL-60 (leukemia) *in vitro*. The greater effect was shown in HL-60 cells and A549 cells by exposure to sabiperone-F (**9**), and the IC_{50} values were 6.37 and 5.59 μM, respectively. The treatment with 12.5 μM concentration of sabiperone-F (**9**) resulted in the growth arrest of both A549 and HepG2 cells by 21% and 51%, whereas 50 μM of 3β,7α-dihydroxyabieta-8,11,13-triene (**8**) exerted the growth inhibition against the MCF-7 and HCT116 cells by 37% and 39%, respectively.[4]

In addition, an extract derived from the berries of *S. vulgaris* also exerted the inhibitory activities against human HeLa (cervix) and KB (nasopharynx) carcinoma cell lines *in vitro*.[5] From the stems and the leaves of a close plant *Juniperus rigida*, which is distributed in northeast China, Korea, and Japan, two lignans (savinin and desoxypodophyllotoxin) and two labdane diterpenes (*trans*-communic acid and 13-epi-torulosal) were isolated and the considerable cytotoxic activity of these compounds were showed in four human cancer cell lines *in vitro*.[6]

Side Effects

While Chou Bai (Savin juniper) is orally administrated for a relatively long period, the containing volatile oil would induce severe dermatitis and mucositis. Overdoses can incur serious reactions of gastroenteritis with diarrhea, vomiting, abdominal pain, and death.

Other Bioactivities

As a traditional medicine in western countries, the Chou Bai (Savin juniper) foliage had been used as an abortifacient. For this reason, the cultivation of this species was long prohibited in France. In addition, β-peltatin-A methyl ether (**6**) also showed an antiviral activity against herpes simplex virus type-1 infecting the fibroblasts of monkey kidney (HSV-1/CV-1) and vesicular stomatitis virus infecting fibroblasts of hamster kidney (VSV/BHK) in the concentration of below 1 μg/mL.[3]

References

1. State of National Administration of Chinese Medicine. 1999. *Chinese Materia Medica*. Vol. 2, 2–0804: 330–1. Shanghai Science and Technology Press, Shanghai, China.
2. Fang, S. D. et al. 1989. The chemical nature of antitumor compounds *from Sabina vulgaris* Ant. *Zhiwu Xuebao* 31: 3882–8.
3. San, F. A. et al. 1993. Antineoplastic and antiviral activities of some cyclolignans. *Planta Med*. 59: 246–9.
4. Janar, J. et al. 2012. Sabiperones A-F, new diterpenoids from *Juniperus sabina*. *Chem. Pharm. Bull*. 60: 154–9.
5. Sadeghi-aliabadi, H. et al. 2009. Evaluation of *in vitro* cytotoxic effects of *Juniperus foetidissima* and *Juniperus sabina* extracts against a panel of cancer cells. *Iran. J. Pharm. Res*. 8: 281–6.
6. Woo, K. et al. 2011. A new lignan glycoside from *Juniperus rigida*. *Archiv. Pharm. Res*. 34: 2043–9.

82 Zhong Jie Feng 腫節風

Glabrous sarcandra

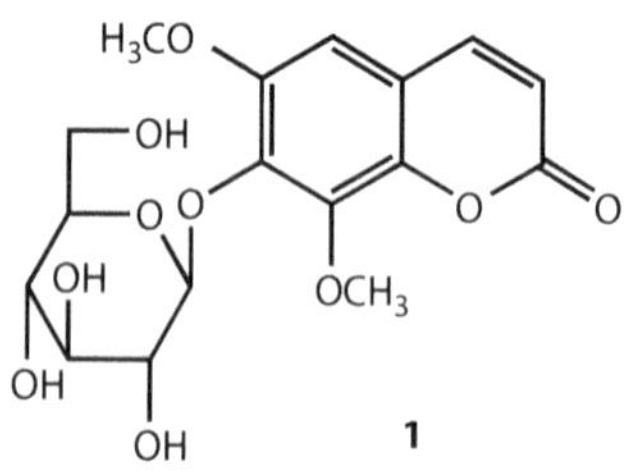

Herb Origination

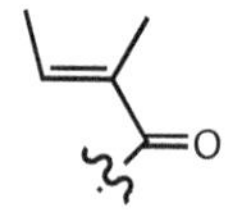

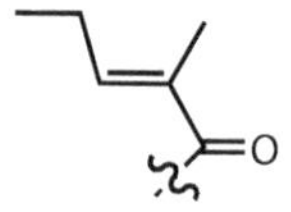

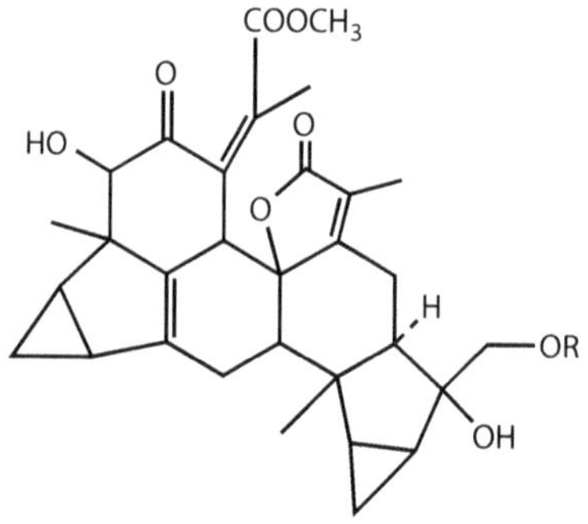

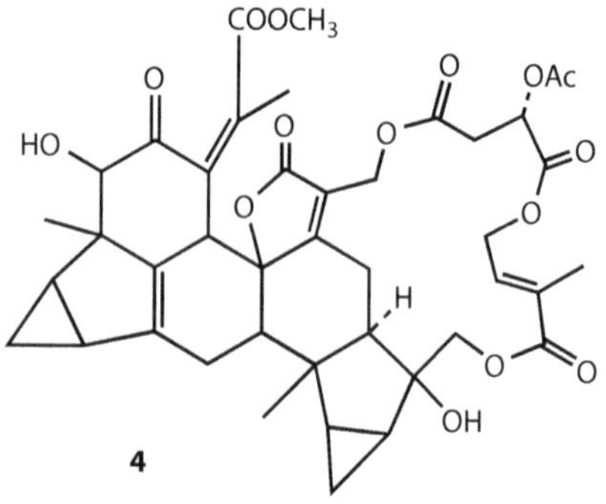

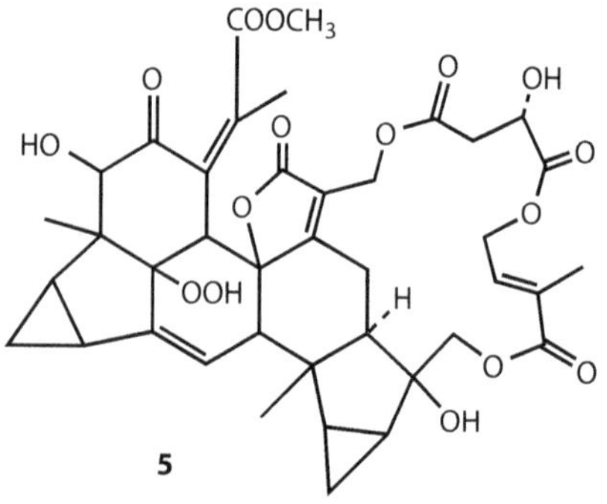

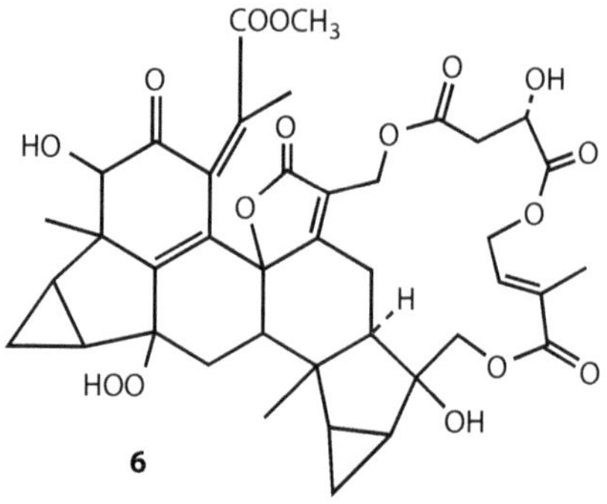

The herb Zhong Jie Feng (Glabrous sarcandra) is the dried root and the whole plant of *Sarcandra glabra* (Chloranthaceae). The herbaceous plant is native to southeast Asia as well as south of Japan and Korea, and it is widely distributed in the southern region of China. The herb can be collected and used in all seasons.

Antitumor Activities

The extract and volatile oil obtained from Zhong Jie Feng demonstrated a certain *in vitro* inhibitory property toward many murine carcinoma cells such as leukemia 615 and TM755 cells, spontaneous breast adenocarcinoma cells, lung adenocarcinoma 15 cells, sarcoma 180 and S37 cells, Ehrlich ascites cancer cells, AL771 spontaneity ascites cancer cells, L-415 ascites cells, and Walker 256 sarcoma cells.[1] An ethyl acetate extract derived from Zhong Jie Feng exerted the growth inhibition on human HL-60 leukemic cells *in vitro* together with the induction of S phase cell cycle arrest and the upregulation of proapoptotic Bax/Bcl-2 ratio.[2] The antitumor activity of Zhong Jie Feng extract was further confirmed in the animal models. The extract notably inhibited the growth of human nasopharyngeal cancer cells in xenograft nude mice, whose effect was associated with the decrease of Bcl-2 expression and the increase of Bax expression to accelerate the cell apoptosis.[3] The oral administration of the extract to tumor-bearing mice in a dose of 5 g/kg inhibited the Ehrlich entity carcinoma by 16%, but the growth inhibition on the Ehrlich cells could be augmented by 10% when combined with 5-FU or CTX.[4] An injection prepared from the herb demonstrated a marked suppressive effect against human A549 (lung), HCT-29 (colon), and BGC-823 (gastric) cancer cell lines *in vitro*. In a combinational treatment, the injection of Zhong Jie Feng could additively enhance the cytotoxicity of Adm on human HCT-8 colorectal cancer cells.[5]

Moreover, Zhong Jie Feng is an inhibitor of cellular respiration, whose effect could directly lessen the oxygen-consumptive ability of hepatoma H22 cells in mice.[6,7] Simultaneously, the lipoperoxide levels and the activities of GSH peroxidase and SOD were influenced by the Zhong Jie Feng extract in hepatoma H22 cells *in vitro* and *in vivo*.[8] It also affected the activities of other lysosomal enzymes (acid phosphatase, DNase, and RNase) as well as liver succinic dehydrogenase and catalase in tumor-bearing mice.[6] Preliminary clinical trials in patients also showed that the administration of the extract could obviously reduce the tumor size and improve the patients' appetite and body weight.[1]

Antitumor Constituents and Activities

Flavonoids

The flavonoid components isolated from Zhong Jie Feng possess a relatively strong ability to destroy cultured Ehrlich ascites cancer cells. The i.p. injection of the flavonoids to tumor-bearing mice for eight days suppressed the cell growth to up to 70.8%.[9] In the treatment, the incorporation of glycine into the synthesis of DNA and RNA was obstructed by the flavonoids in the Ehrlich tumor cells through the blockage of glycine assimilation.[10] A fraction containing flavone glycosides obtained from the 80% ethanolic extract exhibited the suppressive effect on the growth of ascitic sarcoma 150 cells *in vitro*,[11] and the total flavonoids prepared from Zhong Jie Feng displayed a marked inhibitory effect *in vivo* against solid and ascitic sarcoma 180 in mice.[12]

Polyphenols

An isolated coumarin glycoside elucidated as eleutheroside-B1 (**1**) exhibited an obvious cytotoxicity on human BGC-823 (stomach) and A2780 (ovary) cancer cell lines *in vivo* (respective IC_{50}: 2.53 and 1.85 μM).[13] Caffeic acid 3,4-dihydroxyphenethyl ester (CADPE) obtained from the separation of *S. glabra*, has a potent *in vitro* anticancer activity through multiple targets. The i.p. administration of CADPE at 2.5 mg/kg dose for eight days significantly inhibited the growth of H22 hepatoma and sarcoma 180 in mice, whose *in vivo* efficacies in these tumor models were equivalent to those of 5-FU (10 mg/kg, i.p.) and CTX (10 mg/kg, i.p.). The significant inhibition of CADPE was also shown in H22 hepatoma-induced acute ascites development with no toxicity.[14]

Sesquiterpenoids

Five dimeric sesquiterpenoids, sarcandrolides-A–E isolated from the whole plant of Zhong Jie Feng, have been evaluated in their cytotoxicity in three human cancer cell lines, HL-60 (leukemia), A549 (lung adenocarcinoma), and BEL-7402 (hepatoma) *in vitro*. The bioassay demonstrated that sarcandrolides-A–C (**2**–**4**) obviously restrained the growth of HL-60 cells (respective IC_{50}: 3.1, 8.4, and 8.5 μM), and sarcandrolide-A (**2**) and sarcandrolide-C (**4**) were effective to the A549 cells (IC_{50}: 7.2 and 4.7 μM, respectively) but no such effect in the BEL-7402 cells.[15] The IC_{50} values of sarcandrolide-F (**5**) and sarcandrolide-H (**6**) in the HL-60 cell line were 0.03 and 1.2 μM, respectively.[16]

Other Small Molecules

The isolated other constituents from Zhong Jie Feng, such as pinostrobin, isofraxidin, scoparone, 3,3′-biisofraxidin, istanbulin-A, atractylenolide-III, palmitic acid, chloranthalactone-E, pentadecanoic acid, vangoletin, showed only weak cell inhibitory activities in the *in vitro* experiments with neoplastic cell lines.[17]

Polysaccharides

SGP-2, an acidic polysaccharide (1880 kDa), was purified from *S. glabra*, which is mainly composed of glucose, galactose, mannose, arabinose, and galacturonic acid in a molar ratio of 12.19:8.68:6.03:1.00:15.24. In the viability assay and the colony formation assay, SGP-2 showed potent antiproliferation and apoptosis-inducing effects on human MG-63 osteosarcoma cells. Also, SGP-2 obstructed the migratory capacity of MG-63 cells accompanied with the inhibition of RAGE and NF-κB.[18]

Clinical Practices

The Zhong Jie Feng extract has been commercially marketed in China for the clinical treatment of neoplastic diseases. The extract is therapeutically effective on various types of cancers but has better responses to the treatment of colon carcinoma, pancreatic cancer, hepatoma, esophageal cancer, and leukemia. In the clinical practices, the Zhong Jie Feng extract could potentiate the antitumor efficacies of chemotherapy drugs (such as CTX, 5-FU, ADM) and ^{60}coradiotherapy by 11.17–39.80% when coadministered. The extract has been applied to treat 373 patients with various late-stage carcinomas. In the clinical trial, 53.9% of the patients showed improvement including 15.7% marked effectivity. Another small clinical trial in 14 patients with acute leukemia was treated with the Zhong Jie Feng extract, demonstrating 71.43% effective responses, wherein 4 patients had a complete remission and 6 had a partial remission without obvious side effects observed. However, the cancer recrudescence would happen if withdrawal of the administration.[19] A Zhong Jie Feng injection had been clinically employed with radiotherapy to treat 33 cases of late-stage gastrointestinal cancer. The clinical trial showed that 19 cases were improved and 6 cases were markedly effective.[5] According to these clinical trial results, using Zhong Jie Feng alone and in combination were much greater than using chemotherapy or radiotherapy alone.

Other Bioactivities

The herb Zhong Jie Feng (Glabrous sarcandra) has been used in traditional Chinese medicine for the treatment of bone fractures, bruises, arthritis, nausea, internal pain, joint swelling, cough, etc. Pharmacological studies have proven its nonspecific medical potentials such as antiinflammatory, detoxifying, immunoenhancing, antibacterial and antivirus activities. The herb has also been suggested for the clinical treatment of chemotherapy-induced thrombocytopenia and idiopathic thrombocytopenic purpura.

References

1. *Zhonghua Ben Cao*. 2000, Vol. 3, 456. Shanghai Science and Technology Press, Shanghai, China.
2. Li, W. Y. et al. 2007. Ethyl acetate extract of Chinese medicinal herb *Sarcandra glabra* induces growth inhibition on human leukemic HL-60 cells, associated with cell cycle arrest and up-regulation of pro-apoptotic Bax/Bcl-2 ratio. *Oncol. Reports* 17: 425–31.
3. Kang, M. et al. 2008. Study on the apoptosis of nasopharyngeal carcinoma cell line administrated with *Sarcandra glabra* extracts in vivo and its mechanism. *Zhongyaocai* 31: 1529–33.
4. Zhou, J. X. et al. 1988. Antitumor activity of *Sarcandra glaber. Zhongliu* 8: 261.
5. Zhou, B. et al. 2009. Advances on chemical constituents and pharmacological activity of *Sarcandra glaber. Chin. J. Modern Applied Pharmacy* 26: 982–6.
6. Cai, X. L. et al. 1981. The influence of total flavonoids from *Sarcandrae glaber* on the nucleic acid metabolism in Ehrlich ascites tumor cells. *Yiyao Gongye* 5: 26–8.
7. Zhang, Y. H. et al. 1985. The influence of cantharidin sodium and Sarcandrae on the hepatic energy metabolism and cyclic nucleotide metabolism in mice bearing ascites hepatoma H22 cells. *Zhongxiyi Jiehe Zazhi* 5: 686.
8. Liu, C. C. et al. 1981. Preliminary study on antitumor constituents in *Sarcandra glaber* (Thunb). *J. Beijing Univ. (Sci. Edit.)*. (2): 94–6.

9. Lin, J. et al. 1981. Effect of total flavanoids from *Sarcandra glaber* on immune function in tumor bearing mice. *J. Beijing Univ.* (*Sci Edit.*) (2): 80–4.
10. Wu, G. L. et al. 1985. Lipoperoxide levels, GSH-Px and SOD activity in regenerating liver hepatoma H22a cells and livers of control and tumor-bearing mice. *J. Beijing Normal Univ.* (*Sci. Edit.*). (3): 71–4.
11. Wu, G. L. et al. 1982. Biochemical actions of some anticancer agents. *J. Beijing Normal Univ.* (*Sci. Edit.*). (2): 57–66.
12. Su, M. et al. 2009. The tumor-suppressing effect of total flavonoids in *Sarcandra glabra* in mice bearing sarcoma 180. *Xibei Yaoxue Zazhi* 24: 272–4.
13. Wu, H. F. et al. 2012. Benzyl 2-β-gluco-pyranosyloxybenzoate, a new phenolic acid glycoside from *Sarcandra glabra*. *Mol.* 17: 5212–8.
14. Guo, X. et al. 2013. Antitumor activity of caffeic acid 3,4-dihydroxyphenethyl ester and its pharmacokinetic and metabolic properties. *Phytomed.* 20: 904–12.
15. He, X. F. et al. 2010. Sesquiterpenes and dimeric sesquiterpenoids from *Sarcandra glabra*. *J. Nat. Prod.* 73: 45–50.
16. Ni, G. et al. 2013. Cytotoxic sesquiterpenoids from *Sarcandra glabra*. *Tetrahedron* 69: 564–9.
17. Wang, F. et al. 2007. Active components of antitumor fraction from *Sarcandra glabra*. *Zhongguo Tianran Yaowu* 5: 174–8.
18. Zhang, Z. Z. et al. 2014. SGP-2, an acidic polysaccharide from *Sarcandra glabra*, inhibits proliferation and migration of human osteosarcoma cells. *Food Function* 5: 167–175.
19. Zhang, Y. et al. 2006. Studies on pharmacology of *Sarcandra glabra*. *Zhonghua Shiyong Zhongxiyi Zazhi* 19: 1839–41.

83 Tao Er Qi 桃兒七

Himalayan mayapple

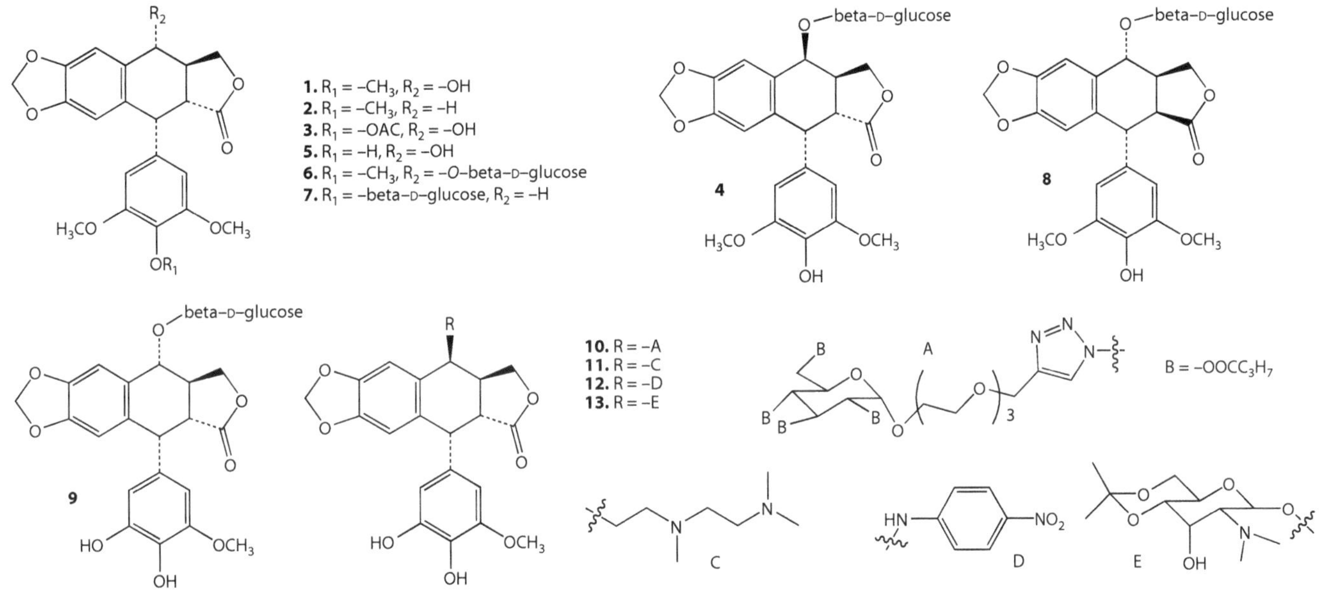

1. R_1 = $-CH_3$, R_2 = -OH
2. R_1 = $-CH_3$, R_2 = -H
3. R_1 = -OAC, R_2 = -OH
5. R_1 = -H, R_2 = -OH
6. R_1 = $-CH_3$, R_2 = -*O*-beta-D-glucose
7. R_1 = -beta-D-glucose, R_2 = -H

10. R = -A
11. R = -C
12. R = -D
13. R = -E

B = $-OOCC_3H_7$

(a)

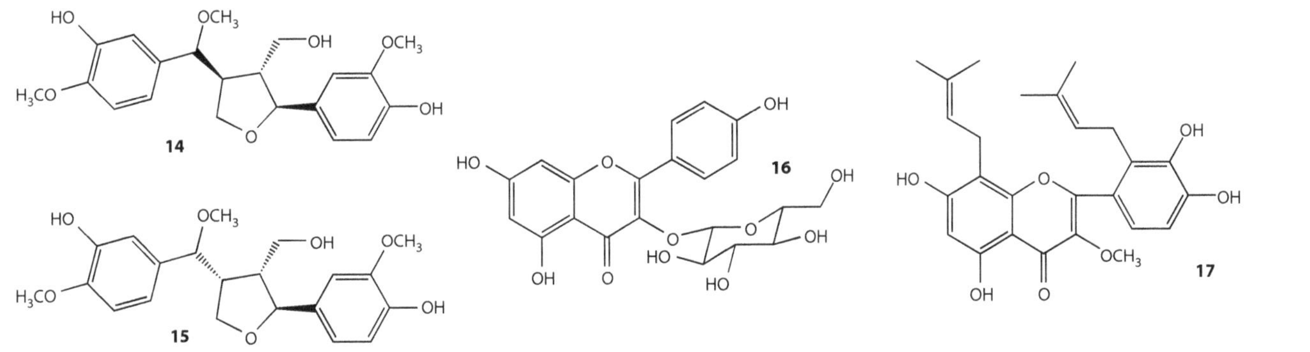

(b)

Herb Origination

The herb Tao Er Qi (Himalayan mayapple) is the dried roots and rhizomes of a Berberidaceae plant, *Sinopodophyllum hexandrum* (= *S. emodi* and *Podophyllum hexandrum*). This perennial herbage is native to the Himalayan region and its adjacent range from east Afghanistan, Bhutan, northern India, Kashmir, Nepal, and Pakistan to western China (i.e., Qinghai, Shaanxi, Gansu, Tibet, Sichuan, and Yunnan provinces). Its roots and rhizomes are generally collected in the spring and autumn and then dried in the sun. Also, its fruits are employed as another herb traditionally.

Antitumor Constituents and Activities

Tao Er Qi has a long history of folk herb usages in Chinese, Tibetan, and Indian traditional medicinal systems. Especially, in the three recent decades, Tao Er Qi has been paid more attention for its uses in the treatment of certain cancers due to the presence of bioactive aryltetralin lignans in the herb. The alcohol extract of *S. emodi* roots and rhizomes showed cytocidal effects on human K562 erythroleukemia cells, mouse L1210, and L7712 leukemia cell lines in an *in vitro* assay. After exposed the extract to cancer cell lines in a concentration of 10 μg/mL, the survival rates in K562 cells were reduced to 44.17%, and in L1210 and L7712 cells, the rates were reduced to 42.84% and 39.76%, respectively.[1] In the *in vivo* models, the administration of the extract at doses of 14 and 7 mg/kg inhibited the growth of transplanted mouse tumors (EAC, U14, and Hc) by 42.2% and 37.8%, 38.8% and 33.3%, and 41.5% and 35.6%, respectively.[1] The extract at 1, 2, and 3 mg/mL concentrations obviously restrained the proliferation of human MCF-7 breast cancer cells in time- and concentration-dependent manners with respective inhibitory rates of 43.0%, 54.9%, and 78.5%. Simultaneously, the extract elicited the G2/M cell cycle arrest and the cell apoptosis through the increase of the protein expressions of p21waf1/cip1 and c-Myc and the decrease of the protein expressions of Bcl-2 and PCNA.[2] Moreover, then 90%

ethanolic extract of *S. emodi* fruits also demonstrated the antiproliferative effect against human KB mouth epidermal carcinoma cells and its drug-resistant cancer cells and human LNCaP prostate cancer cells with IC_{50} values of 0.22, 4.1, and 2.1 μg/mL, respectively. The proliferation of rat ASK neuroglia tumor cells could be obstructed by 75% after being treated with the 90% ethanolic extract at a 4 μg/mL concentration.[3] Currently, the prepared Tao Er Qi extract has been used in the prescriptions for treating tumors including prostate cancer, liver cancer, cervical cancer, breast cancer, or glioma in China.

Aryltetralin Lignans

Chemical and pharmacological investigations have revealed that the aryltetralin lignans are the important bioactive components in Tao Er Qi (*S. emodi*). Especially, podophyllotoxin (**1**) is a major cytotoxic agent, showing a potent and broad antineoplastic spectrum. The mechanic approaches have proven that the cytotoxicity of podophyllotoxin (**1**) is attributed to its powerful interaction with β-tubulin, leading to disruptive microtubule organization and mitotic arrest, in a manner that is similar to the action of colchicines.[4,5] Due to its strong toxicity and its unacceptable levels of cytotoxicity, the herb (*S. emodi* rhizomes) is limited to be used in internal medicine, and podophyllotoxin (**1**) is precluded for use as an anticancer drug. However, podophyllotoxin (**1**) in persistent efforts served as a precursor for the chemical synthesis of anticancer drugs such as etoposide (VP-16), etopophose, and teniposide (VM-26). These podophyllotoxin-type drugs have been successfully utilized in clinics for curing lung cancer, testicular cancer, neuroblastoma, hepatoma, and other tumors.[4,5]

Meanwhile, several analogs of podophyllotoxin have been separated from the rhizomes of *S. emodi*, showing pronounced antineoplastic and antiviral effects. In the *in vitro* experiments, deoxypodophyllotoxin (**2**), 4′-acetyl-4′-demethylpodophyllotoxin (**3**) and 4′-demethylepipodophyllotoxin-7-*O*-β-D-glucopyranoside (4′DPG) (**4**) exerted the significant suppressive effect against the growth of HeLa cervical cancer cells and KB oral cancer cells (respective IC_{50}: 0.0069 and 0.0089 μM, 0.076 and 0.05 μM, and 0.048 and <0.01 μM).[6] 4′-Demethylpodophyllotoxin (**5**) and podophyllotoxin-7-D-β-glucopyranoside (**6**) demonstrated more potent cytotoxicity than podophyllotoxin (**1**) against PC3 (prostate), HCT116 (colon), HEK293 (kidney), MCF-7 (breast), HeLa (cervix), and KB (oral) human tumor cell lines *in vitro*. The IC_{50} values were 0.018–0.234 μM for 4′-demethylpodophyllotoxin (**5**) in all the cell lines and 0.022–0.054 μM for podophyllotoxin-7-D-β-glucopyranoside (**6**) in the first three cell lines. The glycosylation of the podophyllotoxin (**1**) with a β-D-glucose at 7-OH could enlarge the IC_{50} data from 0.056 to 9.25 μM in the KB cells but reduce its IC_{50} value from 40.5 to 3.15 μM in the HEK293 cells.[6,7] However, the same glycosylation of 4′-demethylpodophyllotoxin (**5**) at 7-OH remarkably lessened the cytotoxicity (IC_{50}: 3.95–46.3 μM).[6] 4′-Demethyl-7-deoxypodophyllotoxin (**7**) was another one showing similar and superior cytotoxic effect to podophyllotoxin (**1**) in PC3, HCT116, HEK936, and MCF-7 cell lines (IC_{50}: 0.208–0.291 μM), but its activities on the HeLa and KB cell lines were not comparable to those of podophyllotoxin (respective IC_{50}: 0.216 and 2.09 μM versus 0.075 and 0.056 μM).[6,7] Also, many of the derivatives mentioned earlier were more active than etoposide in the same condition.[6,7] Consequently, the podophyllotoxin derivatives (such as **2–7**) were the most interesting agents for further approach and development.

Furthermore, the *in vitro* experiments revealed that 4′DPG (**8**) induced a significant inhibition of the proliferation in the tested neoplastic cell lines (SH-SY5Y, CNE, HeLa, and K562), whereas 4′5′-didemethylpodophyllotoxin 7-O-β-D-glucopyranoside (4′5DPG) (**9**) at 10 μg/mL for 48 h was effective in the inhibition of CNE, HeLa, and K562 cells. Compared with etoposide, 4′DPG (**8**) had much more potent cytotoxic to CNE and K562 cells and 4′5DPG (**9**) was more cytotoxic to the CNE cells.[8,9] The IC_{50} values in the K562 cells were 7.79×10^{-9} mol/L for 4′DPG (**8**) but 2.23×10^{-5} mol/L for etoposide. The cytotoxicity of 4′DPG was found to be due to the blockage of the microtubule assembly of cancer cells at a low concentration and the promotion of the cell cycle arrest at mitotic phase and the apoptosis with caspase-3 activation.[8] Similar to 4′DPG (**8**) and etoposide, 4′DPG (**4**) treatment displayed a dose- and a time-dependent cytotoxic effect in HepG2 hepatoma cells together with the elicitation of the cell apoptotic death and DNA fragmentation, associated with the downregulation of Bcl-2 expression and the upregulation of Bax expression.[10]

Structural Modification of Podophyllotoxin

The success of etoposide and teniposide encouraged researchers to develop more efficient, pharmaceutically available, and safe antitumor drug candidates by semisynthetic techniques starting from podophyllotoxin (**1**). A series of 4β-triazole-linked glucose podophyllotoxin conjugates have been designed and synthesized. Most of these triazole derivatives have a good anticancer activity in a panel of five human cancer cell lines (HL-60, SMMC-7721, SW480, A549, and MCF-7). Among them, derivative-35 (**10**) showed the highest potency against all tested five cancer cell lines (IC_{50}: 0.59–2.90 μM), which is significantly more active than etoposide. The safe promotion of antitumor effect was found to be attributed to a perbutyrylated glucose residue, a suitable length of oligoethylene glycol linker and 4′-demethylation of podophyllotoxin.[11]

TOP-53 (**11**) is a derivative originated from podophyllotoxin, which showed extremely high selectivity against lung cancer and lung metastatic cancers. Its cytotoxicity was assessed to have IC_{50} values of 0.26–8.9 μg/mL against NSCLC cell lines (Lx-1, Lu-99, and PC-14) and was 0.016–0.37 μg/mL against murine Lewis lung cancer, Colon 16 colorectal cancer, P388 leukemia, and B16 melanoma. The *in vivo* investigations confirmed the marked inhibitory activity of TOP-53 against Lewis lung carcinoma, NSCLC, and four lung metastatic tumors (NL-22 and NL-17 colon carcinoma, UV2237M fibrosarcoma, and K1735M2 melanoma), where TOP-53 exerted potent antitumor activity superior to that of etoposide and showed twice the activity of etoposide in targeting Topo-II and inducting DNA strand breaks. Also, the high selectivity of TOP-53 was attributed to its high distribution into the lung and its persistence.[12] Therefore, TOP-53 has a promising potential in clinical field for the high effectivity against NSCLC and various lung metastatic tumors.

GL331 and NK611 are two promising antitumor active agents derived from podophyllotoxin, and both have been explored in clinical trials against various cancers. GL331 (**12**), a homolog of etoposide, has demonstrated more efficacious anticancer activity in both *in vitro* and *in vivo* lymphoma systems and more efficacy than etoposide in killing several other types of cancer cells, whose ID_{50} values were 2.5- to 17-fold lower than those of etoposide. Importantly, more cell-killing activities of GL331 were also observed even in MDR-1-overexpressing cell lines such as HCC36 NSCLC cells and SW620 colon cancer cells, whose cytotoxicity was attributed to the elevated abilities of inducing apoptosis, inhibiting Topo-II catalytic activity and microtubules assembly, and causing DNA strands breaking. Besides the greater inhibitory activity both *in vitro* and *in vivo*, NK611 (**13**), which can be easily semisynthesized in industrial scale, displayed more advantage in overcoming the MDR of many drug-resistant cancer cell lines (e.g., KB/VP-16, KB/Vcr, P388/Adm, L1210/Adm, MCF-7/Adm, HL-60/Adm, and HL-60/Vcr). Interestingly, phase I clinical trials of NK611 showed marked chemotherapeutic efficacy against four types of carcinomas, i.e., NSCLC, small cell lung cancer, head/neck cancer, and colon cancer, with minimal side effects.[13–15]

Tetrahydrofuranoid Lignans

Several tetrahydrofuranoid lignans were isolated from the roots and the rhizomes of *S. emodi.* Among these lignans, (−)-tanegool-7′-methyl ether (**14**) exerted the most potent cytotoxic effect against the tested human HeLa (cervix) and KB (oral) tumor cell lines, with moderate IC_{50} values of 9.7 and 4.7 μM, respectively, whose cytotoxicity on the KB cells was superior to that of etoposide (IC_{50}: 10.0 μM). (+)-7′-Methoxylariciresinol (**15**), which is a stereoisomer of (−)-tanegool-7′-methyl ether (**14**), only showed a weak inhibitory effect on the HeLa cells (IC_{50}: 32.2 μM), indicating a critical requirement of stereochemistry for the anticancer effect of the tetrahydrofuranoid lignans.[16]

Flavonoids

The fractionation of Sinopodophyllum hexandrum (= *S. emodi* and = *Podophyllum hexandrum*) root extract led to the obtainment of two flavones identified as kaempferol and quercetin and a flavone glycoside assigned as astragalin. In an *in vitro* assay, astragalin (**16**) markedly suppressed the proliferation of all the tested five lines, such as human PC3 (prostate), HeLa (cervix), HCT116 (colon), HEK293 (kidney), and MCF-7 (breast) neoplastic cells, with IC_{50} values ranging from 0.25 to 0.30 μM, whose antitumor potency was greater than that of etoposide (IC_{50}: 0.81–1.75 μM). Kaempferol and quercetin in the assay showed moderate to weak anti-proliferation (IC_{50}: 20.7–46.3 μM) except quercetin had obvious activity on the HEK293 cells (IC_{50}: 3.46 μM).[6] A group of flavonoid components were also isolated from the fruits of *S. hexandrum.* A prenyl flavonoid elucidated as 8,2′-diprenylquercetin 3-methyl ether (**17**) exerted a marked cytotoxicity effect against two human breast cancer cell lines (MDA-231 and T47D). The inhibitory rates could reach up to 67.84% and 98.56% in the MDA-231 cells and 82.19% and 92.08% in the T47D cells after being treated with 8,2′-diprenylquercetin 3-methyl ether (**17**) in 50 and 100 μmol/mL concentrations for 48 h. However, the isolated quercetin, kaempferol, and rutin were not effective in the experiment.[17]

Other Bioactivities

The herb Tao Er Qi (Himalayan mayapple) is used as a Chinese folk medicine for the treatment of various verrucoses, as a cathartic and anthelminthic agent, as well as rheumatoid ache and pyogenic infection of the skin tissue. In Tibet, the roots are used to treat patients who suffer from gynecological inflammation, and the fruits are employed to regulate menstruation, promote the circulation of blood in the treatment of amenorrhea, and help to treat difficult labor and retention of dead fetus or placenta.

References

1. Wang, D. W. et al. 1997. The antitumour activity of *Sinopodophyllum emodi. Zhongyaocai* 20: 571–4.
2. Li, G. Y. et al. 2006. Effect of ethanol extract from *Podophyllum emodi* var. Chinense on proliferation and apoptosis of breast carcinoma cell line MCF-7. *Chin. J. New Drug* 15: 1064–7.
3. Zong, Y. Y. et al. 2000. Antitumor screening research from 110 Tibetan medicines. *J. Pharm. Practices* 18: 290–1.
4. Bruschi, M. et al. 2010. Podophyllotoxin and antitumor synthetic aryltetralines: Toward a biomimetic preparation. *Biomimetics Learning from Nature*, Mukherjee, A. (ed.), pp. 305–24, InTech, Rijeka, Croatia.
5. Nagar, N. et al. 2011. Podophyllotoxin and their glycosidic derivatives. *Pharmacophore* 2: 124–34.
6. Zillaa, M. K. et al. 2014. 4′-Demethyl-deoxypodophyllotoxin glucoside isolated from *Podophyllum hexandrum* exhibits potential anticancer activities by altering Chk-2 signaling pathway in MCF-7 breast cancer cells. *Chemico-Biol. Interactions* 224: 100–7.
7. Sun, Y. J. et al. 2011. Three new cytotoxic aryltetralin lignans from *Sinopodophyllum emodi. Bioorg Med Chem Lett.* 21: 3794–7.
8. Qi, Y. L. et al. 2005. Antitumor pharmacology cytotoxicity, apoptosis induction, and mitotic arrest by a novel podophyllotoxin glucoside, 4DPG, in tumor cells. *Acta Pharmacol. Sinica* 26: 1000–8.
9. Zhao, C. Q. et al. 2011. Lignan glucoside from *Sinopodophyllum emodi* and its cytotoxic activity. *Chin. Chem. Lett.* 22: 181–4.
10. Liu, Y. F. et al. 2010. Cytotoxicity and apoptosis induced by a new podophyllotoxin glucoside in human hepatoma (HepG2) cells. *Can. J. Physiol. Pharmacol.* 88: 472–9.
11. Zi, C. T. 2013. Separation and purification of podophyllotoxin in *Sinopodophyllum emodi* Wall. *Mol.* 18: 13992–4012.
12. Utsugi, T. et al. 1996. Antitumor activity of a novel podophyllotoxin derivative (TOP-53) against lung cancer and lung metastatic cancer. *Cancer Res.* 56: 2809–14.
13. Liu, Y. Q. et al. 2015. Recent progress on C-4-modified podophyllotoxin analogs as potent antitumor agents. *Med. Res. Rev.* 35: 1–62.
14. Huang, T. S. et al. 1999. A novel podophyllotoxin-derived compound GL331 is more potent than its congener VP-16 in killing refractory cancer cells. *Pharm. Res.* 16: 997–1002.
15. Takigawa, N. et al. 1993. In vitro comparison of podophyllotoxin analogues; etoposide, teniposide and NK 611 using human lung cancer cell lines. *Gan To Kagaku Ryoho* 20: 473–7.
16. Sun, Y. J. et al. 2012. Four new cytotoxic tetrahydrofuranoid lignans from *Sinopodophyllum emodi. Planta Med.* 78: 480–4.
17. Kong, Y. et al. 2010. A new cytotoxic flavonoid from the fruit of *Sinopodophyllum hexandrum. Fitoterapia* 81: 367–70.

84 San Fen Dan 三分丹

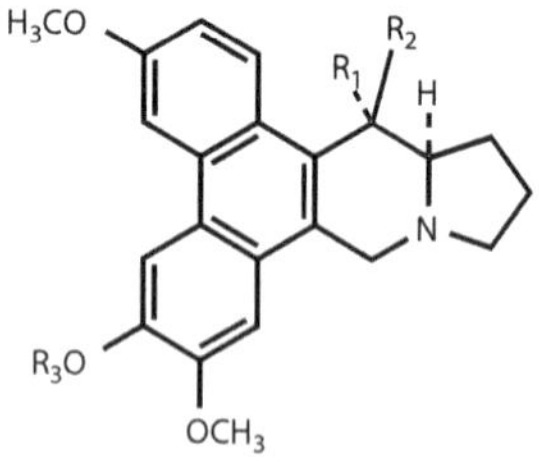

1. $R_1 = R_2 = R_3 = -H$
2. $R_1 = -OH, R_2 = -H, R_3 = -CH_3$
3. $R_1 = -OH, R_2 = R_3 = -H$
5. $R_1 = -H, R_2 = -OH, R_3 = -CH_3$
6. $R_1 = R_2 = -H, R_3 = -CH_3$

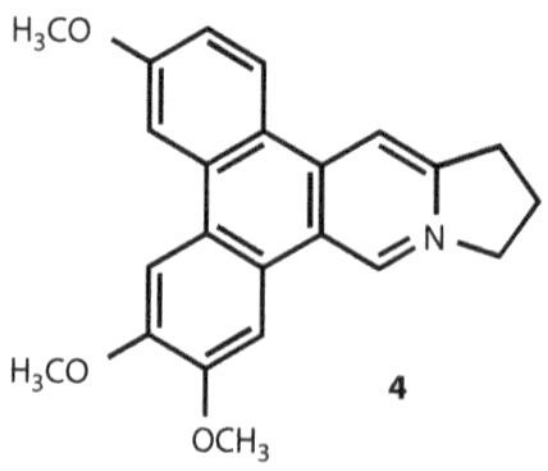

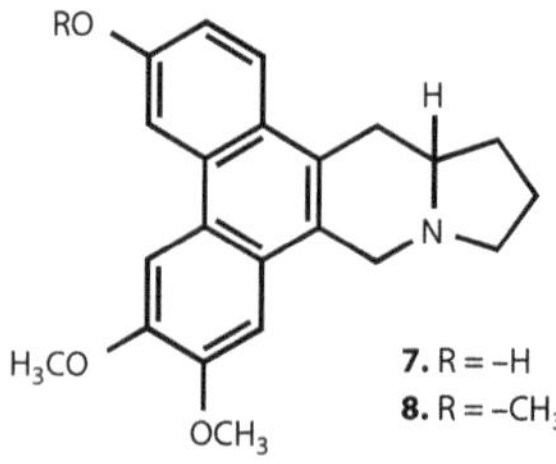

7. R = -H
8. $R = -CH_3$

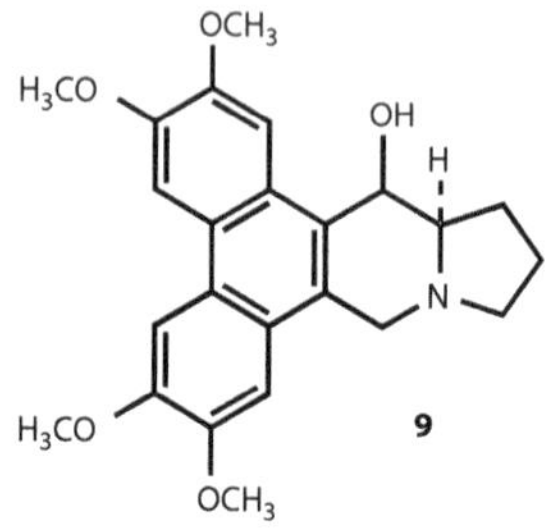

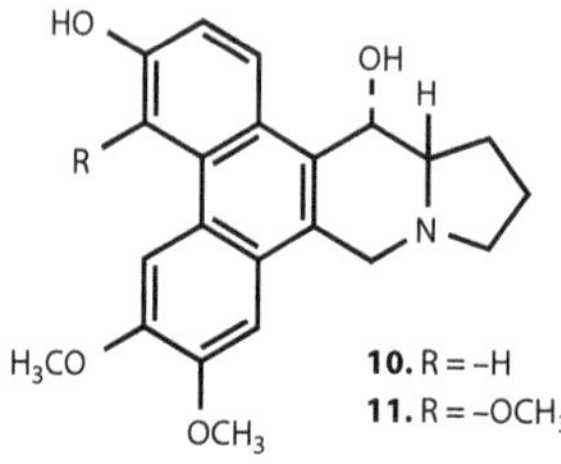

10. R = -H
11. $R = -OCH_3$

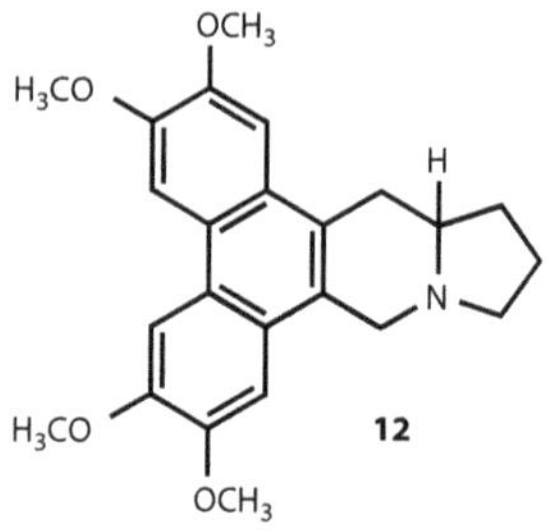

Herb Origination

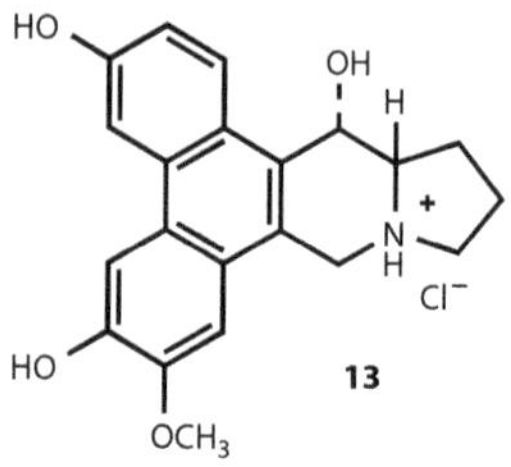

The herb San Fen Dan is the dried root of an Asclepiadaceae plant, *Tylophora atrofolliculata* (= *T. ovata*). The distribution of this scandent shrub ranged only in the southern provinces of China, as well as in India, Pakistan, Myanmar, Nepal, and Vietnam. Its roots are collected in winter and dried in the sun for Chinese folk medicinal application.

Antitumor Constituent and Activities

Alkaloids from the Roots

Phenanthroindolizidine alkaloids isolated from the herb were demonstrated to be responsible for the antitumor effect of San Fen Dan. The total alkaloids, in *in vitro* models, displayed an inhibitory effect against the proliferation of U14 cervical cancer, sarcoma 180, L615 leukemia, Walker 256 sarcoma, and HeLa cervical cancer cell lines.[1,2] The investigations of San Fen Dan alkaloids led to the separation of many bioactive phenanthroindolizidine alkaloids. Tylophoridicine-A (**1**), *O*-methyltylophorinidine (**2**), and tylophorinidine (**3**) exerted the antiproliferative effect against two tested human neoplastic cell lines, and the ED_{50} values were 0.029, 0.20, and <0.005 μg/mL in KB oral cancer cells and 6.36, 7.86, and 5.1 μg/mL in A549 lung tumor cells, respectively.[3] Tylophoridicine-D (**4**) showed a significant cytotoxic effect on human KB (oral) and HCT-8 (colon) carcinoma cell lines, giving the same IC_{50} values of <0.01 μM, while R-(+)-deoxytylophorinidine (= tylophoridicine-A) (**1**) displayed the similar degree of cytotoxic activity on the KB cells with an IC_{50} value of 0.083 μM, whose antiproliferative effects were more potent than Adm (IC_{50}: 0.40 and 0.20 μM) on the KB and HCT-8 cells. In the *in vitro* experiment, tylophorinidine (**3**) and tylophorinine (**5**) were moderately effective in the suppression of the KB and HCT-8 cells (IC_{50}: 3.56–6.60 μM), while tylophoridicine-C, tylophoridicine-E, and tylophoridicine-F showed a moderate to weak inhibitory effect on the HCT-8 and KB cell lines.[4] Tylophoridicine-C and tylophoridicine-F, which both have an N-oxide form, also exhibited the marked antiproliferative activity against HepG2 hepatoma cells and PANC1 pancreatic cancer cells. Their GI_{50} values were 98 and 71 nM in the HepG2 cells and 67 and 63 nM in the PANC1 cells, respectively. But tylophorinidine (**3**), tylophorinine (**5**), and R-(+)-deoxytylophorinidine (**1**), which have non-N-oxide form, displayed a more potent anticancer effect with GI_{50} values of 11, 20, and 13 nM in the HepG2 cells and 7, 11, and 11 nM in the PANC1 cells, respectively, in the same assay.[5] The results implied that the unshared pair of electrons on a nitrogen atom was at least partially responsible for the cytotoxic potency due to the oxidization to form an N-oxide corresponding to a lower antitumor activity.[4,5] More data revealed that the potent antigrowth activity correlated with their potent NF-κB-suppressive effects and cyclin-D1 downregulatory effects.[5] The growth-inhibitory activity of tylophorinidine (**3**) was further proven in nude mice implanted with HepG2 cells at a dose of 9 mg/kg given by i.p. injection (twice a day, every third day) for four cycles. However, in the same dose and administration scheme, R-(+)-deoxytylophorinidine (**1**) did not show activity against the HepG2 cell growth *in vivo*, whose lack of *in vivo* effect for R-(+)-deoxytylophorinidine (**1**) could be due to the different stereochemistry at C-13 from tylophorinidine (**3**), i.e., (R)-configuration at C-13 in R-(+)-deoxytylophorinidine (**1**) and (S)-configuration at C-13 in tylophorinidine (**3**). Also, tylophorinidine (**3**) has a (S)–OH group at C-14 position, whose (S)–OH group at C-14 may favor the pharmacokinetics and the antitumor activity *in vivo*.[5]

An important anticancer active phenanthroindolizidine alkaloid designated as (+)-(13aS)-deoxytylophorinine (**6**) (= S-(+)-desoxytylophorinine = S-(+)-deoxytylophorinidine) was separated from the roots of *T. atrofolliculata* and *T. ovata*. Both *in vitro* and *in vivo* models evidenced the potent anticancer activity of S-(+)-deoxytylophorinidine (**6**), which extremely obstructed the proliferation of a panel of human HCT-8 (colon cancer), HepG2 (hepatoma), U251 (glioma), SH-3Y-5Y (neuroblastoma), A549 (NSCLC), A375 (melanoma), A2780 (ovarian cancer), BGC-823 (gastric cancer), SW1990 (pancreatic cancer), and MCF-7 (breast cancer) cell lines, with IC_{50} values in the range of 1.16×10^{-7}–9.11×10^{-7} mol/L.[6,7] *In vivo* treatment with S-(+)-deoxytylophorinidine (**6**) in doses of 12.5 and 15 mg/kg markedly restrained the growth of H22 hepatoma in mice by 48.37% and 75.90%, respectively.[6,7] 3-*O*-Desmethyl-13α-(S)-deoxytylophorinine (**7**) was synthesized as a monodesmethyl metabolite of (+)-13α-(S)-deoxytylophorinine (**8**). The metabolite (**7**) demonstrated a significant cytotoxic effect on A375 malignant melanoma cells (IC_{50}: 0.011 nM), whose cytotoxicity was much greater than its parent molecule and anticancer drugs, DOX and paclitaxel.[8]

Alkaloids from the Stems and the Leaves

The cytotoxicity-related phytochemical investigations of the stems of *T. ovata* let to seven isolated phenanthroindolizidine alkaloids. Tylophovatine-C (**9**) was the major constituent in this part of *T. ovata*. All these alkaloids display growth suppression on HONE-1, NUGC-3, HepG2, SF-268, MCF-7, and NCI-H460 cancer cell lines, with GI_{50} values ranging from 0.004 to 0.78 μM. The most potent alkaloids were elucidated as 13α(S)-14(S)-(+)-3, 14-dihydroxy-6,7-dimethoxyphenanthroindolizidine (**10**) and 13α(S)-14(S)-(+)-3,14-dihydroxy-4,6,7-trimethoxyphenanthroindolizidine (**11**). The GI_{50} values ranged from 0.005 to 0.013 μM for 13α(S)-14(S)-(+)-3, 14-dihydroxy-6,7-dimethoxyphenanthroindolizidine (**10**) and from 0.004 to 0.008 μM for 13α(S)-14(S)-(+)-3,14-dihydroxy-4,6,7-trimethoxyphenanthroindolizidine (**11**) in these tested human carcinoma cell lines. Other alkaloids, such as *O*-methyl-tylophorinidine (**2**), tylophovatine-C (**9**), 13a(S)-(+)-tylophorine (**12**), 13a(S)-(+)-6-desmethyltylophorine, and 13α(S)-(+)-3-desmethylisotylocrebrine, exhibited a marked antigrowth effect on these cancer cell lines with GI_{50} values in a range of 0.029–0.780 μM. In addition, these isolated alkaloids displayed *in vitro* antiinflammatory effects in RAW264.7 cells via the inhibition of nitric oxide production.[9]

From the leaves of *T. ovata*, four septicine alkaloids and two phenanthroindolizidine alkaloids were isolated. The septicines determined as tylophovatine-A, tylophovatine-B, and (S)-(+)-hispidine only exerted a marked to moderate inhibitory effect against the proliferation of HONE-1, NUGC-3, HepG2, SF-268, MCF-7, and NCI-H460 cancer cell lines, with GI_{50} values between 0.714 and 7.704 μM, whereas (S)-(+)-septicine showed a moderate to weak growth inhibition in the bioassay (GI_{50}: 14.513–24.221 μM). Tylophovatine-C (**9**) and 13a(S)-14(S)-(+)-3,14-dihydroxy-4,6,7-trimethoxy-phenanthroindolizidine (**11**) were the two isolated phenanthroindolizidine from the leaves.[9] In addition, a similar phenanthroindolizidine assigned as 3-*O*-demethyltylophorinidine (**13**) was found in a close plant *T. indica* leaves and stems, whose alkaloid (**13**) showed a marked antigrowth activity with an IC_{50} value in the range of 0.89–1.40 μM on a panel of human ACHN (renal), PANC1 (pancreas), Calu1 and H460 (lung), and HCT-116 (colon) tumor cell lines, but it was shown to be nontoxic on MCF-10A normal breast cell line.[10]

Taken together, the phenanthroindolizidine alkaloids may be considered as encouraging anticancer drug leads that indeed deserve development for cancer chemotherapy in clinics. Based upon the remarkable potential, S-(+)-desoxytylophorinine (**6**) has been patented in China as a promising new drug candidate for treating hepatoma, fibroblast tumor, NSCLC, nephrotic cancer, oral epithelium carcinoma, prostatic carcinoma, melanoma, oral epidermoid carcinoma, ovarian carcinoma, gastric cancer, colon carcinoma, breast cancer, and Adm drug-resistant breast cancer.[11]

Other Bioactivities

In the distribution regions of the plant, San Fen Dan has been employed as a traditional herb to treat leukemia, rheumatism, asthma and coughing, traumatic injury, rheumatoid backaches, pains in the stomach and abdomen, and poisonous snakebites, even though it possesses mildly toxic properties. Pharmacological studies have shown that the phenanthroindolizidine alkaloids possess antianaphylactic, antiasthma, and antiinflammatory activities besides antileukemia and antineoplastic potentials.

References

1. Guangxi Institute of Medicine. 1977. Experimental studies on antitumor agents of *Tylophora ovata* Hook. et Steud. (Asclepiadaceae): II. Antitumor activity and pharmacology. *Shengwu Huaxue Yu Shengwu Wuli Xuebao* 9: 139–45.
2. Wang, Y. X. et al. 2008. Effects of *Tylophora ovata* (Lindl) Hook. et Steud. alkaloids (TOHa) on proliferation and apoptosis of HeLa cells in vitro. *Shipin Kexue* 29: 609–11.
3. Zhen, Y. Y. et al. 2002. Antitumor alkalois from *Tylophora ovate*. *Acta Botanica Sinica* 44: 349–53.
4. Huang, X. S. et al. 2004. Cytotoxic alkaloids from the roots of *Tylophora atrofolliculata*. *Planta Med.* 70: 441–5.
5. Gao, W. L. et al. 2007. Structure-activity studies of phenanthroindoli-zidine alkaloids as potential antitumor agents. *Bioorg. Med. Chem. Lett.* 17: 4338–42.
6. Liu, Z. J. et al. 2011. Anticancer effect and neuro-toxicity of S-(+)-deoxy-tylophorinidine, a new phenanthroindolizidine alkaloid that interacts with nucleic acids. *J. Asian Nat. Prod. Res.* 13: 400–8.
7. Liu, Z. J. et al. 2011. Interaction studies of an anticancer alkaloid, (+)-(13aS)-deoxytylophorinine, with calf thymus DNA and four repeated double-helical DNAs. *Chemother.* (Basel, Switzerland) 57: 310–20.
8. Yu, P. F. et al. 2012. Stereospecific synthesis and biological evaluation of monodesmethyl metabolites of (+)-13a-(S)-deoxytylophorinine as potential antitumor agents. *Synthesis* 44: 3757–64.
9. Lee, Y. Z. et al. 2011. Isolation and biological activities of phenanthro-indolizidine and septicine alkaloids from the Formosan *Tylophora ovata*. *Planta Med.* 77: 1932–8.
10. Dhiman, M. et al. 2013. A new phenanthroindolizidine alkaloid from *Tylophora indica*. *Chem. Papers* 67: 245–8.
11. Yu, S. S. et al. 2007. S-(+)-desoxytylophorinine, its preparation method, medicinal composite and application in tumor therapy. *Faming Zhuanli Shenqing* CN 101058578 A 20071024.

85 Qi Ceng Lou 七層樓

Coast Tylophora

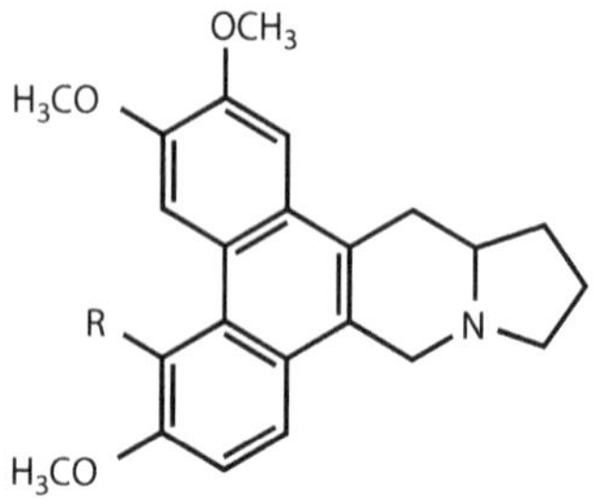

1. R = $-OCH_3$

2. R = $-H$

Herb Origination

The herb Qi Ceng Lou is the roots of an Asclepiadaceae plant, *Tylophora floribunda*. This perennial vine plant is mainly distributed in the southern and southeastern regions of China, as well as Korea and Japan. In China, the roots are collected in the seasons of autumn and winter and it can be used as fresh and sun-dried herbs for medical treatment.

Antitumor Activities and Constituents

From Qi Ceng Lou roots, several phenantoindolizidine alkaloids were separated as chemotherapeutic agents for the treatment of gastric cancer. The i.p. administration of the alkaloids elicited the growth inhibition against TMK gastric carcinoma cells transplanted in nude mice.[1] One of the alkaloids elucidated as tylocrebrine (**1**) demonstrated an obvious suppressive effect against the cell proliferation of lymphosarcoma, adenocarcinoma (755), leukemia (P388 and L1210), and nasopharyngeal carcinoma (KB), in association with the blockage of both protein and nucleic acid synthesis in the *in vitro* models.[2,3] In the treatment of HONE-1 (nasopharynx), NUGC-3 (stomach), and HepG2 (liver) cancer cell lines, tylophorine (**1**) dominantly arrests the cell cycle progression at G phase through the downregulation of cyclin-A2 expression.[4] Besides significantly reduced the volume of Ehrlich solid tumor in mice, tylophorine (**1**) notably restrained VEGF-induced angiogenesis processes including proliferation, migration, and tube formation of the endothelial cells. The antiangiogenic effect of tylophorine (**1**) was found to correlate with the direct inhibition of VEGFR2 tyrosine kinase activity and its downstream signaling pathways including Akt, Erk, and ROS in the endothelial cells. Tylophorine (**1**) could also obstruct the VEGF-stimulated inflammatory responses including IL-6, IL-8, TNFα, IFNγ, MMP-2, and NO secretion in HUVECs[5] Thus, tylophorine (**1**) may be a viable drug candidate for antiangiogenesis in the anticancer therapies. However, tylocrebrine (**1**) was reported to have less clinic value due to its irreversible toxicity on the CNS.[2,3]

A same type of alkaloid assigned as antofine (**2**), which was also derived from another Chinese herb Xu Chang Qing (*Cynanchum paniculatum*), displayed potent antiproliferative effects against several human carcinoma cells with IC_{50} values of ~10 nM.[6,7] The *in vitro* EC_{50} values of antofine (**2**) were 0.16 ng/mL in A549 lung carcinoma cells, 0.43 ng/mL in KB cells, 0.83 ng/mL in KB-VIN cells (a multidrug-resistant cells), and 4.5 ng/mL in MCF-7 breast neoplastic cells, and the IC_{50} value was 6 nM in HCT-116 colon cancer cells.[7,8] In the *in vivo* cancer xenograft model transplanted with HCT-116 cells, the treatment with antofine (**2**) in a dose of 8 mg/kg exerted the noticeable inhibitory effect against the growth of colon cancer cells.[7] However, further investigation found that the anticancer activity of antofine (**2**) in HCT-116 cells was neither attributed to the promotion of apoptosis nor related to the induction of cell cycle arrest. But, it has marked ability to moderately inhibit the expression of cyclin-A, cyclin-B1, and c-Myc and to decline the basal expression of p53 and p21 in time- and dose-dependent manners. The regulation of these biomarkers might partially participate in the anticancer mechanism.[7] All these discoveries recommend that antofine (**2**) has a potential to be a novel cancer chemotherapeutic agent.

Other Bioactivities

The roots of Qi Ceng Lou have been used as a local medicine for the treatment of infantile convulsions, diphtheria, traumatic injury, toothache, and snakebites. The total alkaloids derived from the Qi Ceng Lou displayed a significant antiinflammatory effect, whose mechanism was probably related to the inhibition of prostaglandin synthesis.

References

1. Koyama, K. et al. 1999. *Jpn. Kokai Tokkyo Koho* JP 98–97859, 19980409.
2. Peng, J. P. et al. 1989. Review of tylophora alkaloids. *Xibei Yaoxue Zazhi* 4: 424.
3. Duan, J. Y. et al. 1991. Antiinflammatory effect of total alkaloids of manyflower tylophora (*Tylophora floribunda*). *Zhongcaoyao* 22: 316–8.
4. Wu, C. M. et al. 2009. Tylophorine arrests cancer cells at G1 phase by downregulating cyclin A2 expression. *Biochem. Biophys. Res. Commun.* 386: 140–5.
5. Saraswati, S. et al. 2013. Tylophorine, a phenanthraindolizidine alkaloid isolated from *Tylophora indica* exerts antiangiogenic and antitumor activity by targeting vascular endothelial growth factor receptor 2-mediated angiogenesis. *Mol. Cancer* 12: 82.
6. Wang, H. G. et al. 2006. Antitumor constituents from root of *Tylophora floribunda*. *Zhongguo Tianran Yaowu* 4: 352–4.
7. Min, H. T. et al. 2005. Suppressive effects of antofine, a phenanthroindolizidine alkaloid isolated from *Cynanchum paniculatum*, on the *in vitro* cancer cell proliferation and in vivo tumor growth. *96th Annual Meeting of the American Association for Cancer Research*. Anaheim, CA, USA, April 16–20, 2005.
8. Su, C. R. et al. 2008. Total synthesis of phenanthroindolizidine alkaloids (±)-antofine, (±)-deoxy-pergularinine, and their dehydro congeners and evaluation of their cytotoxic activity. *Bioorg. Med. Chem.* 16: 6233–41.

86 Zi Yu Pan 紫玉盘

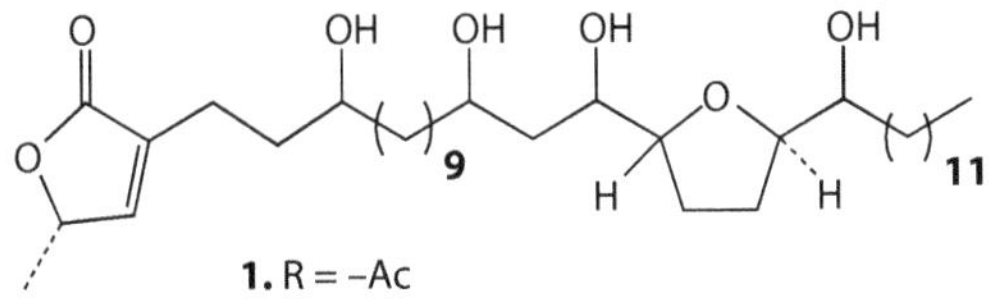

1. R = -Ac
2. R = -H

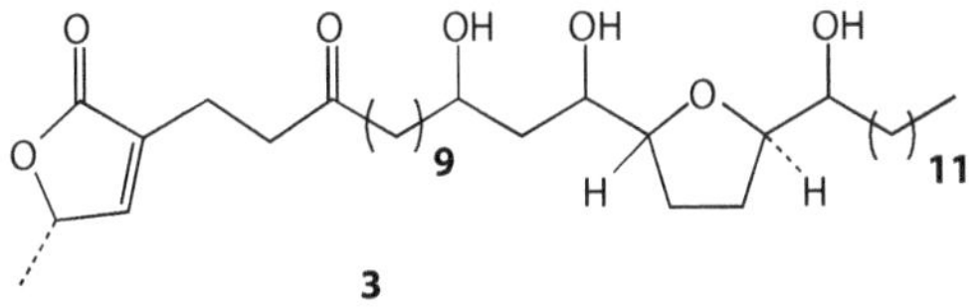

3

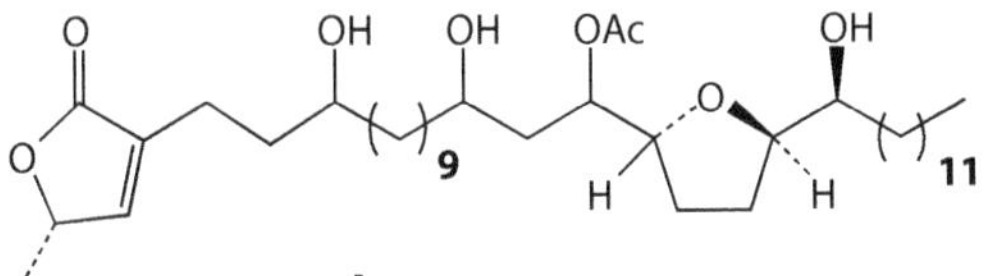

4

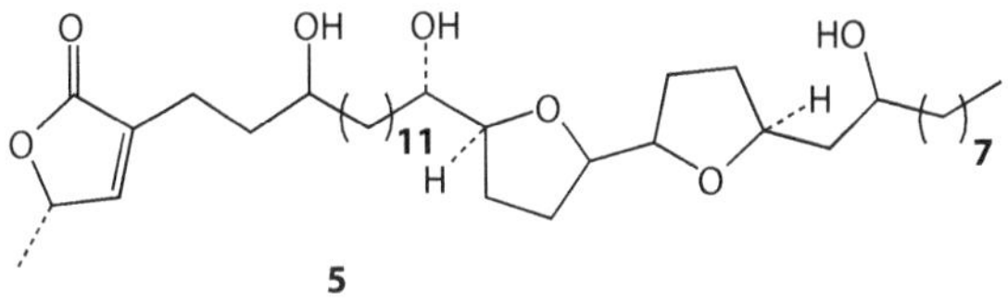

5

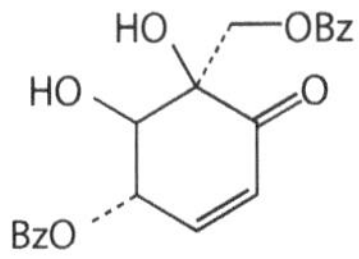

6

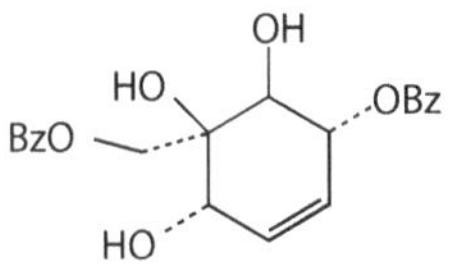

7

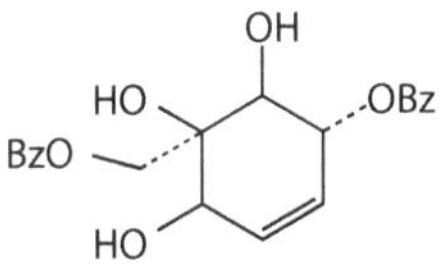

8

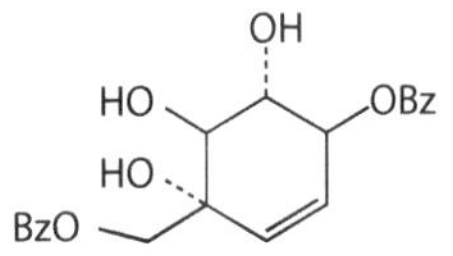

9

10

Bz = -OC-C_6H_5

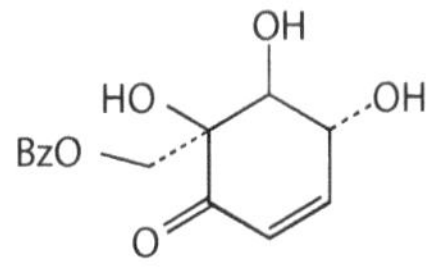

Herb Origination

The herb Zi Yu Pan originates from an Annonaceae bush, *Uvaria microcarpa*. Its roots and leaves are collected for use in local folk medicine. Several close plants belonging to the same genus, such as *U. boniana*, *U.calamistrata*, *U. kweichowensis*, *U. tonkinensis*, and *U. grandiflora* (Shan Jiao Zi), have been investigated due to their interesting bioactivities. All the plants of the *Uvaria* genus are distributed in parts of the southern and/or southwestern regions of China and southeast Asia countries.

Antitumor Activities

The ethanolic extract of Zi Yu Pan stems demonstrated an antiproliferative effect against three human carcinoma cell lines *in vitro*, and its inhibitory rates in 40 μg/mL concentration were 57.94% in HeLa cervical cancer cells, 73.82% in SGC-7901 gastric cancer cells, and 68.28% in Bel-7404 hepatoma cells. Four fractions obtained from partition of the extract with organic solvents showed some different degrees of the inhibitory effect on the three tumor cell lines. Its petroleum ether fraction at a 40 μg/mL concentration suppressed >50% of the SGC-7901 and Bel-7404 cells and <50% of the HeLa cells, while its chloroform fraction (CF) at 40 μg/mL and 10 μg/mL concentrations exerted >60% and >41% inhibitions on the tested cell lines, respectively. Its EAF and n-butanol fraction only showed a moderate or weak inhibitory effect on Bel-7404 cells but exerted comparable activity in the inhibition of HeLa and SGC-7901 cells *in vitro*, and the inhibitory rates of its EAF at a 10 μg/mL concentration could reach to >50%.[1] A petroleum ether fraction derived from 95% ethanolic extract of the stems and the leaves of *U. microcarpa* also displayed the obvious antiproliferative effect against three cell lines such as human KB (oral), SGC-7901 (stomach), and SMMC-7721 (liver) cancer cells at a 20 μg/mL concentration.[2] The treatment with this active fraction in a 600 mg/kg dose obstructed the tumor weight by 51.04% in a mice model implanted with entity sarcoma 180.[2]

Antitumor Constituents and Activities

A number of acetogenins, polyoxygenated cyclohexenes, benzylated flavanones, chalcones, lactams, and terpenes, have been discovered from the Uvaria plants by phytochemical studies. They were reported to possess diverse biological activities such as cytotoxic, antimalarial, antimicrobial, and/or antibacterial effects. Some of the acetogenins and polyoxygenated cyclohexenes are obviously responsible for the cytotoxic and antineoplastic activities.

Acetogenins

From U. microcarpa and U. boniana

The antitumor active acetogenins have not been reported from the isolation of *U. microcarpa*. But uvaribonin, uvaribonone, and uvaribonianin were isolated from the CF of *U. boniana*. The three acetogenins exhibited different degrees of antigrowth activity in *in vitro* models with human neoplastic cell lines.[3] Uvaribonin (**1**) was found to have an obvious inhibitory effect against KM20L2 colon tumor cells (IC_{50}: 0.0013 μg/mL) and MCF-7 breast cancer cells (IC_{50}: 0.011 μg/mL). The inhibitory effects of the acetogenins were also observed in other types of human cancer cell lines, such as H460 (lung), DU-145 (prostate), BXPC3 (pancreas), and SF-268 (brain) cells (IC_{50}: 1.0–1.4 μg/mL).[4]

From U. tonkinesis

Six monotetrahydrofuran acetogenins, tonkinesin-A (**2**), tonkinesin-B, tonkinesin-C (**3**), tonkinin-A, tonkinin-B, and tonkinin-C (**4**), were separated from the root of *U. tonkinesis*. Tonkinins-A and tonkinin-B and tonkinesin-A and tonkinesin-B are two isomeric pairs. Tonkinin-C and tonkinesin-C are the acetogenins with an unusual flanking acetoxy group adjacent on one side of the THF ring. Tonkinesin-A (**2**), tonkinesin-B, and tonkinesin-C (**3**) were selectively cytotoxic to human HCT-8 colon cancer cells (IC_{50}: 0.59, 2.44, 0.86 μM, respectively) and human leukemia HL-60 cells (IC_{50}: 0.016, 0.060, 0.00042 μM, respectively), but the three were inactive to human A2780 (breast) and KB (oral) cancer cell lines. The results indicated that the tonkinesins, especially tonkinesin-C (**3**), were potent to the HL-60 cells.[5] Moreover, tonkinesin-C (**3**) and tonkinin-C (**4**) were superactive to suppressing mouse L1210 leukemia cells with the same ED_{50} value of 0.0004 μg/mL.[6] Other active acetogenins named tonkinelin and tonkinecin (**5**) were isolated from the root bark of *U. tonkinensis*, exhibiting an obvious inhibitory effect against the HL-60 and HCT-8 cells with IC_{50} values of 1.0 and 0.52 μM and 6.7 and 0.8 μM, respectively.[7,8] Tonkinecin (**5**) also displayed a moderate inhibitory effect against the proliferation of Bel-7402 hepatoma cells (IC_{50}: 1.5 μM) and BGC gastric cancer cells (IC_{50}: 5.1 μM), *in vitro*.[8]

From U. calamistrata

Ten acetogenins were separated and their cytotoxicities were evaluated. Five mono-THF acetogenins designated as calamistrins-A–E and two bis-THF acetogenins assigned as calamistrin-F, and calamistrin-G (**5**) demonstrated a marked cytotoxic effect against the tested human A2780 (breast), KB (nasopharynx), and HCT-8 (colon) neoplastic cell lines but showed no cytotoxicity to MCF-7 breast cancer cells *in vitro*. The HCT-8 cells were sensitive to calamistrins-A–G, and the three cancer cell lines were resistant to calamistrin-H and calamistrin-I, two non-THF acetogenins, even at *in vitro* at a 100 μg/mL concentration.[9–11] Calamistrin-J exerted a moderate to weak suppressive effect on five kinds of human neoplastic cell lines (NCI-H460, HepG2, HeLa, Lovo, S180) but also on normal human embryonic lung fibroblast (HELF) cells. According to the IC_{50} values, its antiproliferative intensities were on LoVo (colon cancer) > S180 (sarcoma) > HELF > HeLa (cervix cancer) > HepG2 (hepatoma) > H460 (lung cancer). After being exposed to calamistrin-J (100 μg/mL) for 12 h, the cellular ROS level in LoVo cells significantly increased and the mitochondrial membrane potential began to decrease, thereby triggering the LoVo colon tumor cells to apoptosis.[12,13] The *in vivo* experiment also confirmed the anticarcinoma activity of calamistrin-J in mice implanted with sarcoma 180, and the inhibitory rates in its doses of 90, 30, and 10 mg/kg were 51%, 30%, and 17%, respectively.[12,13]

Polyoxygenated Cyclohexenes

Seven polyoxygenated cyclohexenes elucidated as uvaribonols-A–G were isolated from the stem of *U. boniana*. An *in vitro* cytotoxicity tests showed uvaribonols-A–G being inactive on several tumor cells, but the oxidized derivative (**6**) of uvaribonol-B could markedly restrain the proliferation of KB, Bel-7402, and A2780 tumor cells with the IC_{50} value of <1 μg/mL, implying that the α,β-unsaturated ketone was probably the effective center for the anticancer effect.[14] Kweichowenols-A–D, zeylenol (**7**), and uvarigranol-G (**8**) were from the leaves of *U. kweichowensis*. The six polyoxygenated cyclohexenes displayed a moderate suppressive effect against three human bronchogenic cancer cell lines (A549, SK-MES-1, and NCI-H446).[15,16] Among these compounds, kweichowenol-B (**9**) exerted a relatively higher antiproliferative activity on the three neoplastic cells (IC_{50}: 18–23 μg/mL), whereas kweichowenol-A was less active to these tumor cell lines (IC_{50}: 50–65 μg/mL).[15,16] Zeylenol (**7**) and (–)-3-*O*-debenzoylzeylenone (**10**) were also isolated from the stems/aerial parts of *U. grandiflora*. (–)-3-*O*-Debenzoyl-zeylenone (**10**) exhibited cytotoxicity obviously against LU-1 (lung) and SK-Mel-2 (skin) cancer cell lines (respective IC_{50}: 4.68 and 3.63 μM), modestly against HL-60 (leukemic), MKN-7 (stomach), HepG2 (liver), SW-480 (colon), and KB (epidermal) cancer cell lines (IC_{50}: 6.22–13.35 μM), and weakly against LNCaP (prostate) and MDA-BA-231 (breast) cancer cell lines (IC_{50}: 45–64 μM).[17,18] Zeylenol (**7**) also exerted moderate to weak inhibition against MDA-MB231 (breast) and HepG2 (liver) cancer cells in a dose-response manner.[17]

Saponins

Ardisiacrispin-B was a cytotoxic triterpene saponin isolated from *U. grandiflora*, which displayed a potent inhibitory activity against the proliferation of LU-1, KB, HepG2, MKN-7, and SW-480 cell lines (IC_{50}: 1.24–1.60 μM) and moderate cytotoxicities against the MDA-BA-231, LNCaP, and HL-60 cell lines (IC_{50}: 9.70–22.58 μM). However, it was also cytotoxic to normal 3T3 cell line (IC_{50}: 7.65 μM), which was significantly lower than that of the positive control, ellipticine.[18]

References

1. Mei, L. R. et al. 2010. Experimental study on antitumor activity of *Uvaria microcarpa* extracts. *Lishizhen Med. Mat. Med. Res.* 21: 2530–1.
2. Dai, Z. K. et al. 2008. Study on anticancer effects of petroleum ether fraction from stem and leaves extract of *Uvaria microcarpa*. *China J. Modern Med.* 18: 47–50.
3. Yang, X. N. and Chen, H. S. 2009. Advances in studies on chemical constituents and pharmacology of Uvaria. *J. Pharm. Practice* 27: 81–3.
4. Pettit, G. R. et al. 2008. Antineoplastic agents: 558. Ampelocissus sp. cancer cell growth inhibitory constituents. *J. Nat. Prod.* 71: 130–3.
5. Chen, Y. et al. 1996. Six acetogenins from *Uvaria tonkinesis*. *Phytochem.* 43: 793–801.
6. Sinz, A. et al. 1998. Novel acetogenins from the leaves of *Dasymaschalon sootepense*. *Helv. Chim. Acta* 81: 1608–15.
7. Chen, Y. et al. 1996. Tonkinelin: A novel annonaceous acetogenin from *Uvaria tonkinensis*. *Planta Med.* 63: 512–4.
8. Chen, Y. et al. 1996. Tonkinecin, a novel bioactive Annonaceous acetogenin from *Uvaria tonkinesis*. *J. Nat. Prod.* 59: 507–9.
9. Zhou, G. X. et al. 1999. Calamistrins A and B, two new cytotoxic monotetrahydrofuran annonaceous acetogenins from *Uvaria calamistrata*. *J. Nat. Prod.* 62: 261–4.
10. Zhou, G. X. et al. New annonaceous acetogenins from the roots of *Uvaria calamistrata*. *J. Nat. Prod.* 63: 1201–4.

11. Zhou, G. X. et al. 2008. Calamistrins H and I, two linear annonaceous acetogenins from the roots of *Uvaria calamistrata* Hance. *Heterocycles* 75: 933–8.
12. Ren, X. D. et al. 2007. Antitumor activity of calamistrin J in vivo and in vitro. *Zhongcaoyao* 38: 1527–30.
13. Ren, X. D. et al. 2007. The effect of calamistrin J on inducing Lovo cells apoptosis. *Jinan Daxue Xuebao, Ziran Kexue yu Yixueban* 28: 142–6.
14. Pan, X. P. et al. 1998. Study on the polyoxygenated cyclohexenes from *Uvaria boniana*. *Yaoxue Xuebao* 33: 275–81.
15. Xu, Q. M. et al. 2005. New polyoxygenated cyclohexenes from *Uvaria kweichowensis* and their antitumour activities. *Chem. Pharm. Bull.* 53: 826–8.
16. Xu, Q. M. et al. 2009. Two new polyoxygenated cyclohexenes from *Uvaria kweichowensis*. *J. Asian Nat. Prod. Res.* 11: 24–8.
17. Seangphakdee, P. et al. 2013. Antiinflammatory and anticancer activities of (–)zeylenol from stems of *Uvaria grandiflora*. *Sci. Asia* 39: 610–4.
18. Ho, D. V. et al. 2015. A new polyoxygenated cyclohexene and a new megastigmane glycoside from *Uvaria grandiflora*. *Bioorg. Med. Chem. Lett.* 25: 3246–50.

87 Cang Er 蒼耳

Siberian cocklebur

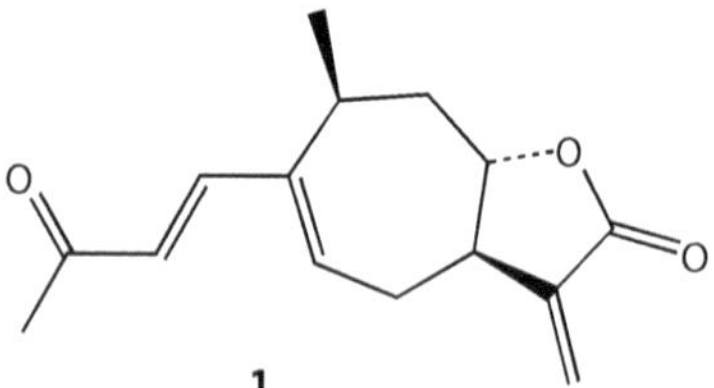

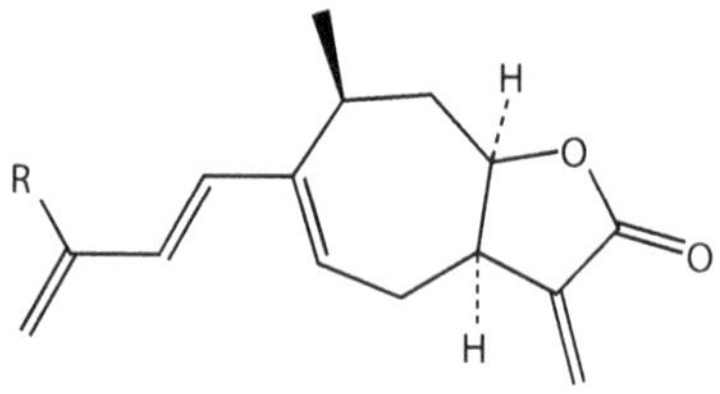

7. R = –CN
8. R = –COOH
9. R = –CONHC(CH$_3$)$_3$

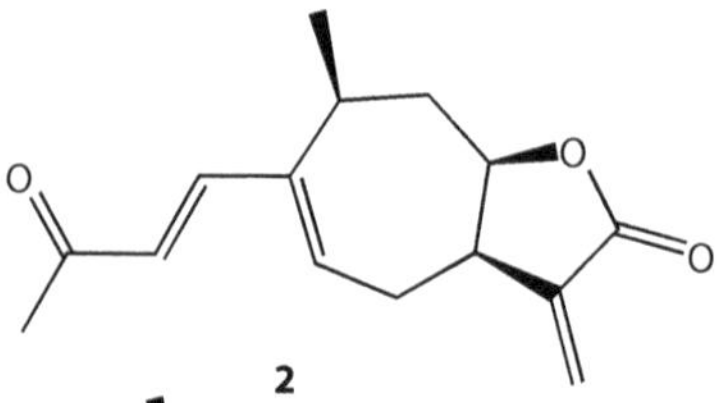

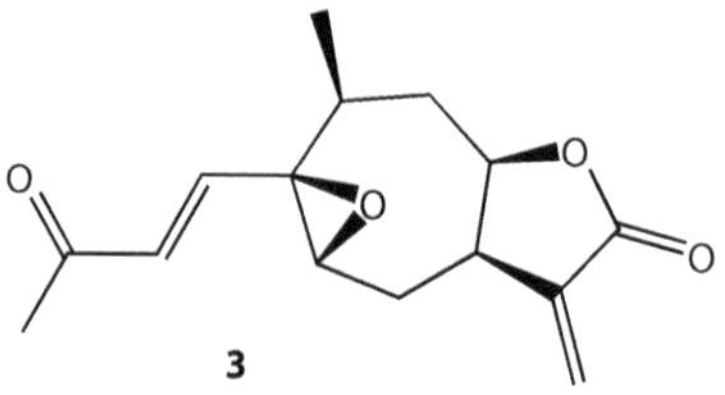

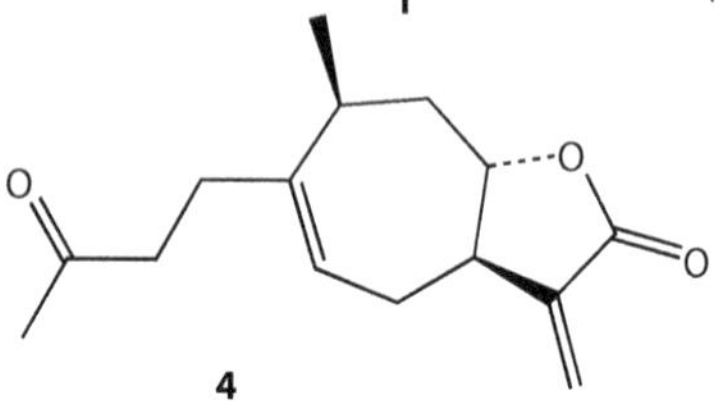

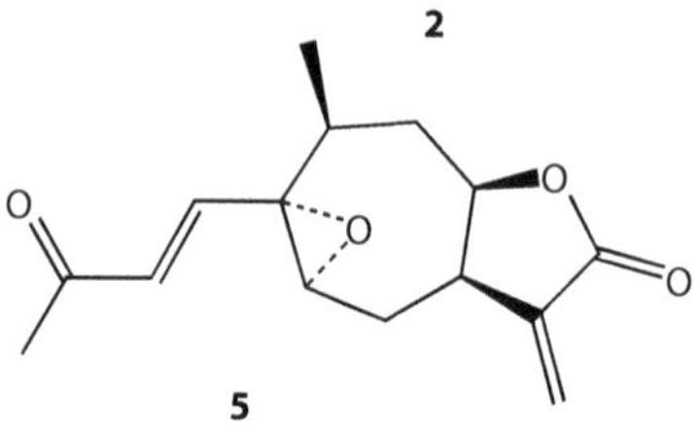

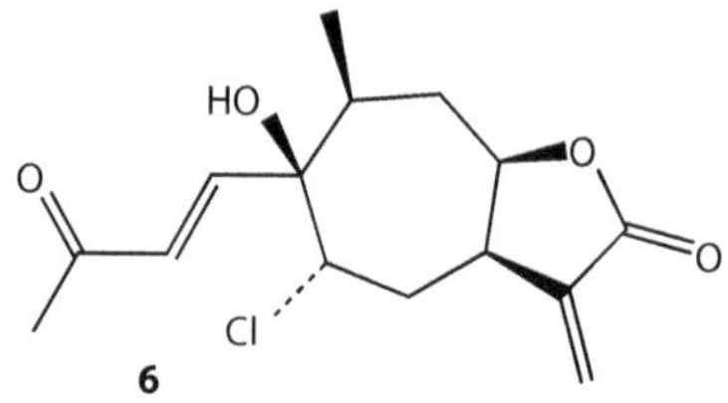

10. R = –CONH–X
11. R = –CON(CH$_2$CH$_3$)$_3$
12. R = –CONH–Y

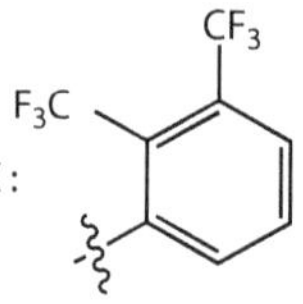

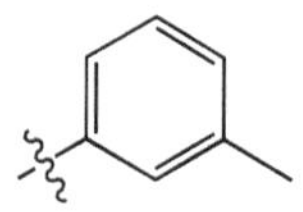

Herb Origination

The herb Cang Er (Siberian cocklebur) originated from an Asteraceae plant, *Xanthium sibiricum* (= *X. strumarim*). This annual herbaceous plant is extensively distributed in the world, but it mainly grows in northern Iran, China, and parts of Asia. In Chinese folk medicine, its whole plant, roots, flowers, and fruits can be individually employed and also prescribed in combination with other herbal products. Normally, the whole plant of Cang Er is collected in summer and dried in the sun for medicinal application. The herb also can be used fresh.

Antitumor Activities and Constituents

An *in vitro* screening research demonstrated that the 90% ethanolic extract of the Cang Er plant obviously suppressed the proliferation of human tumor cell lines, and the IC_{50} values were 5.4, 6.6, 13.2, and 15.5 μg/mL on Col2 (colon), BC1 (breast), KB (oral), and LNCaP (prostate) neoplastic cells, respectively.[1] Similarly, a methanolic extract of Cang Er leaves were found to have cytotoxic activities against human A549 (lung), SK-MEL-2 (skin), SK-OV-3 (ovary), XF-298 (brain), and HCT-115 (colon) cancer cell lines[2] and against A431 (epidermoid), HepG2 (liver), and MCF-7 (breast) cancer cell lines with IC_{50} values of 2.2, 1.5, and 3.0 μg/mL, respectively.[3] A dichloromethane extract from the Cang Er leaves was effective in the inhibition of mouse P388 and L1210 leukemia cell lines, and the IC_{50} values were 1.64 μg/mL in P388 cells and 1.1 μg/mL in L1210 cells.[4]

Likewise, a water extract of the Cang Er plant exerted a >30% growth inhibition in HeLa cervical cancer cells and a 54% growth inhibition in A549 lung cancer cells at a concentration of 2.5 mg/mL. The water extract (2.5 mg/mL) also restrained the BAP-DNA adduct formation and free radical formation by 41% and 32%, respectively, showing the cancer chemopreventive potential.[5] A chloroform extract of *X. strumarium* burs at a concentration of 100 μg/mL exhibited a potent cytotoxicity for all cell lines tested, such as WiDr (colon), MDA-MB-231 (breast), and NCI-417 (lung) cancer cells, with IC_{50} values ranging from 0.1 to 6.2 μg/mL.[6] The antitumor activity of the Cang Er fruit extract was demonstrated in an *in vivo* model with sarcoma 180, and the antigrowth rates reached to 26.22% and 44.51%, respectively, in doses of 10 and 20 g/kg. The fruit extract also showed an immunostimulating effect by dose-dependently enlarging the weights of the thymus and the spleen in mice bearing sarcoma 180.[7]

Essential Oil

An essential oil prepared from the leaves of Cang Er by water-steam distillation displayed a marked inhibitory activity against the proliferation of SGC-7901 gastric cancer and Bel-7402 hepatoma cell lines with the IC_{50} values of 14.56 and 17.99 μg/mL, respectively. A GC-MS analysis further revealed that the major components of the essential oil were caryophyllene (5.24%), phytol (12.25%), and (1E, 6E, 8S)-1-methyl-5-methylene-8-(1-methylethyl)-1,6-cyclodecadiene (28.49%).[8] 3,4-Dihydroxybenzaldehyde, which was separated from *X. strumarium* fruit, could cause cell apoptosis and 50% growth inhibition of human U937 histiocytic lymphoma cells at its concentration of 300 μM.[9]

Sesquiterpene Lactones

A group of xanthanolide-type sesquiterpene lactones was isolated from the aerial parts and/or leaves of *X. sibiricum*, and some of them were demonstrated to have antitumor properties.

Xanthatin (**1**) was the most reported bioactive of xanthanolide, which showed a wide antiproliferative spectrum on various neoplastic cell lines. Its IC_{50} values were 0.018 and 0.009 µg/mL in P388 and L1210 (leukemic), 3 µg/mL in NSCLC-N6 (bronchial epidermoid), 6.15 µg/mL in WiDr (colon), 13.9 µg/mL in MDA-MB-231 (breast), 3.9 µM (48 h) in MKN-45 (stomach), 7.36 µM (24 h) in B16-F10 (skin), and <20 µM (48 h) in A549, H1975, H1650, and HCC827 (lung) carcinoma cells.[3–12] The treatment of B16-F10 murine melanoma cells with xanthatin (**1**) at 10 µM *in vitro* for 24 h induced about 69.35% inhibition of cell proliferation and elicited cell apoptosis in a dose-dependent manner. Daily i.p. injection of xanthatin in doses of 0.2 and 0.4 mg/10 g to mice resulted in 30.81% and 42.57% inhibitions against the growth of B16-F10 melanoma, respectively, *in vivo*, whose antimelanoma activity of xanthatin (**1**) was found to correlate with the activation of Wnt/β-catenin pathway and the inhibition of angiogenesis markedly.[13] Moreover, the cytotoxicity of xanthatin (**1**) was also observed in HepG2 human hepatoma cell line, and its strong antiangiogenesis capacity was confirmed again by other research groups.[14]

The antiproliferative effect of xanthatin (**1**) on A549 NSCLC and KN-45 gastric cancer cells was executed via the induction of G2/M cell cycle arrest and intrinsic apoptosis, whose mechanism was elucidated to be associated with (1) the down-expression of Chk1 and Chk2 and the phosphorylation of CDC2; (2) the activation of p53, the reduction of Bcl-2/Bax ratio and downstream procaspase-9 and procaspase-3 levels; (3) the blockage of NF-κB (p65) and IκBα phosphorylation and the decrease of TNFα induced NF-κB (p65) translocation.[10,11] The disruption of GSK3β activity was also essential for xanthatin (**1**) to exert its anticancer properties in human NSCLC cells, concurrent with the preferable suppression of constitutive activation of STAT3.[12] In human breast cancer MDA-MB-231 cells, a unique mechanism was involved in the antiproliferative effect of xanthatin (**1**), where it triggered a caspase-independent cell death, associated with repression of Topo-IIα activity and concomitant increase of ROS production, stimulation of DNA damage-inducible GADD45γ expression and extension of c-Fos expression, and GADD45γ-primed JNK and p38 signaling pathways. Due to the marked induction of c-fos/GADD45γ and ROS production, xanthatin (**1**) in particular showed a stronger antiproliferative potential than etoposide on breast cancer.[15–17]

In a similar fashion, some xanthatin analogs that were isolated from *X. sibiricum* plant and/or its related Xanthium plants demonstrated a similar or a less degree of cytotoxic effect against the human carcinoma cell lines. 8-epi-Xanthatin (**2**) and 8-epi-xanthatin epoxide (**3**) were effective in the suppression of five tested human neoplastic cell lines *in vitro*, where the ED_{50} values were 4.5 µM versus 3.0 µM in A549 lung cancer cells, 6.1 µM versus 4.6 µM in SKOV-3 ovarian cancer cells, 0.8 µM versus 0.8 µM in SK-MEL-2 melanoma cells, 4.9 µM versus 3.8 µM in XF298 glioma cells, and 2.0 µM versus 1.5 µM in HCT115 colon cancer cells.[18] The inhibitory effect of xanthinosin (**4**) was greater than that of xanthatin (**1**) in WiBr (colon) and MDA-MB-231 (breast) human cancer cells (IC_{50}: 2.65 and 4.8 µg/mL, respectively).[6] 8-epi-Xanthatin-1α,5α-epoxide (**5**) and 1β-hydroxyl-5α-chloro-8-epi-xanthatin (**6**) exhibited the suppressive activity with IC_{50} values of 9.5 and 5.1 µM on SNU387 human HCC cells and of 9.5 and 20.7 µM on A549 human NSCLC cells, respectively. Two isolated xanthanolide dimers, pungiolide-D and pungiolide-E only showed a moderate cell growth inhibitory activity against the SNU387 cells (IC_{50}: 14.6 and 11.7 µM, respectively) but no cytotoxicity against the A549 cells.[19] In addition, the xanthanolides isolated from *X. italicum* were assigned as 4-epi-xanthanol, 4-epi-isoxanthanol, 2-hydroxyxanthinosin, as well as xanthatin (**1**), whose sesquiterpene lactones were demonstrated to exert an obvious antiproliferative activity against human HeLa cervix adenocarcinoma, A431 skin carcinoma, and MCF-7 breast adenocarcinoma cell lines.[20]

In conclusion, the summarized scientific data confirmed that the many xanthanolides, especially xanthatin, play important roles in the antitumor and antiangiogenic effects, which are potential agents and/or drug leads for tumor treatment and anticancer drug discovery, but further *in vivo* and preclinical studies are required for a detailed evaluation of this class of compounds.

Structural Modification

For improvement of the bioavailability and the pharmacodynamic profile, the molecule of xanthatin has been modified in its unsaturated side chain. The created 15 derivatives were created and evaluated in the *in vitro* model with A549 NSCLC and HepG2-B16 hepatoma cell lines. These derivatives displayed improved physical and chemical properties and enhanced cell permeability, thereby markedly increasing the bioavailability. Especially, derivative-I2 (**7**), derivative-I5 (**8**), derivative-I12 (**9**), and I15 (**10**) at a concentration of 2.5 mg/mL could kill both tested A549 and HepG2-B16 cells completely (100%). Their IC_{50} values were 8.6, 4.5, 12, and 6.5 µmol/L in the A549 cells and 2.5, 3.2, 2.9, and 1.1 µmol/L in the HepG2-B16 cells, whose cytotoxic activities were much superior to those of xanthatin (**1**). Derivative-I9 (**11**) and derivative-I14 (**12**) at the same concentration exerted the complete inhibitory effect on the A549 cells but lower suppression on the hepatoma cells (42% and 85%, respectively).[21] The findings have afforded several valuable xanthatin derivatives that may have a developing potential for cancer chemotherapy and prevention and also provide essentials for further design and development of more effective drug candidates.

Other Bioactivities

The herb Cang Er (Siberian cocklebur) and its fruit have been traditionally used to relieve aches, pains, and headaches associated with nasal congestion and sinusitis in combination with other herbs and are also often used for the treatment of sinus congestion, chronic nasal obstructions and discharges, and respiratory allergies. In pharmacological studies, the xanthanolide sesquiterpenes exhibited a broad spectrum of biological effects, including antimicrobial, fungicidal, antiviral, antibacterial, antimalarial, antitrypanosomal, antiulcerogen, and antiinflammatory activities beside antitumor.[22] However, the herbs contain toxic chemicals, which may cause severe hepatitis with fatal liver failure or interactions with the liver's detoxification systems. Overdosing of Cang Er and its fruit cause severe side effects including coma and death.

References

1. Zong, Y. Y. et al. 2000. Antitumor screening research from 110 Tibetan medicines. *Yaoxue Shijian Zazhi* 18: 290–1.
2. Ahn, J. W. et al. 1995. Isolation of cytotoxic compounds from the leaves of *Xanthium strumarium* L. *Nat. Prod. Sci.* 1: 1–4.
3. Sato, Y. et al. 1997. A xanthalonide with potent antibacterial activity against methicillin-resistant *Staphylococcus aureus. J. Pharm. Pharmacol.* 49: 1042–4.
4. Roussakis, C. et al. 1994. Cytotoxic activity of xanthatin and the crude extracts of *Xanthium strumarium. Planta Med.* 60: 473–4.
5. So, M. S. et al. 2010. Effect of *Xanthium sibiricum* Patr. on carcinogenesis in human cell lines. *J. Kor. Biol. Nurs. Sci.* 12: 127–32.
6. Ramirez-Erosa, I. et al. 2007. Xanthatin and xanthinosin from the burs of *Xanthium strumarium* L. as potential anticancer agents. *Can. J. Physiol. Pharmacol.* 85: 1160–72.
7. Pan, J. H. et al. 2013. Inhibitory effect of xanthium extract on S180 cells growth and the impact on immune functions in tumor-bearing mice. *Chin. J. Clin. Res.* 26: 317–9.
8. Liu, W. J. et al. 2013. Composition and antitumor activities of essential oil of leaves of xanthium sibiricum. *Tianran Chanwu Yanjiu Yu Kaifa* 25: 1680–4.
9. Lee, B. H. et al. 2008. Apoptotic cell death through inhibition of protein kinase CKII activity by 3,4-dihydroxybenzaldehyde purified from Xanthium strumarium. *Nat. Prod. Res.* 22: 1441–50.
10. Zhang, L. et al. 2012. Xanthatin induces G2/M cell cycle arrest and apoptosis in human gastric carcinoma MKN-45 cells. *Planta Med.* 78: 890–5.
11. Zhang, L. et al. 2012. Xanthatin induces cell cycle arrest at G2/M checkpoint and apoptosis via disrupting NF-κB pathway in A549 non-small-cell lung cancer cells. *Mol.* 17: 3736–50.
12. Tao, L. et al. 2013. Concerted suppression of STAT3 and GSK3β is involved in growth inhibition of non-small cell lung cancer by xanthatin. *PLoS One* 8: e81945.
13. Li, W. D. et al. 2013. Characterization of xanthatin: Anticancer properties and mechanisms of inhibited murine melanoma in vitro and in vivo. *Phytomed.* 20: 865–73.
14. Romero, M. et al. 2015. Optimization of xanthatin extraction from *Xanthium spinosum* L. and its cytotoxic, anti-angiogenesis and antiviral properties. *Eur. J. Med. Chem.* 90: 491–6.
15. Takeda, S. et al. 2011. (-)-Xanthatin selectively induces GADD45γ and stimulates caspase-independent cell death in human breast cancer MDA-MB-231 cells. *Chem. Res. Toxicol.* 24: 855–65.
16. Takeda, S. et al. 2013. (-)-Xanthatin induces the prolonged expression of c-Fos through an N-acetyl-L-cysteine (NAC)-sensitive mechanism in human breast cancer MDA-MB-231 cells. *J. Toxicol. Sci.* 38: 547–57.
17. Takeda, S. et al. 2013. (-)-Xanthatin up-regulation of the GADD45γ tumor suppressor gene in MDA-MB-231 breast cancer cells: Role of topoisomerase IIα inhibition and reactive oxygen species. *Toxicol.* 305: 1–9.
18. Kim, Y. S. et al. 2003. Two cytotoxic sesquiterpene lactones from the leaves of *Xanthium strumarium* and their in vitro inhibitory activity on farnesyltrans-ferase. *Planta Med.* 69: 375–7.
19. Wang, L. et al. 2013. Cytotoxic sesquiterpene lactones from aerial parts of *Xanthium sibiricum. Planta Med.* 79: 661–5.
20. Kovacs, A. et al. 2009. Xanthanolides with antitumour activity from *Xanthium italicum. Zeitschrift fuer Naturforschung, C* 64: 343–9.
21. Li, W. D. et al. 2013. Xanthatin derivative useful in treatment of various diseases and its preparation. *Faming Zhuanli Shenqing* CN 103193742 A 20130710.
22. Vasas, A. H. J. et al. 2011. Xanthane sesquiterpenoids: Structure, synthesis and biological activity. *Nat. Prod. Rep.* 28: 824–42.

88 Gui Zhen Cao 鬼針草

Beggarticks or Spanish needle

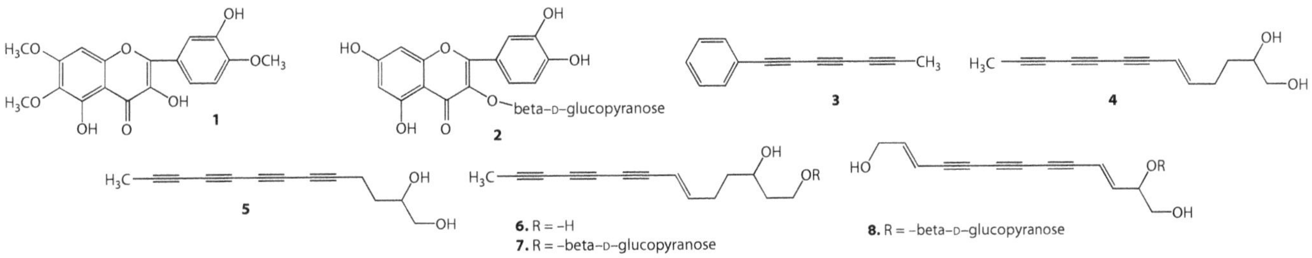

6. R = -H
7. R = -beta-D-glucopyranose
8. R = -beta-D-glucopyranose

Herb Origination

Two Asteraceae weeds, *Bidens pilosa* and *Bidens bipinnata*, are termed with the same Chinese name as Gui Zhen Cao used in traditional Chinese medicines. *B. alba* was originally grown in tropical America and spread to the tropics and the subtropics everywhere in the world. All the three plants were considered as herb by Chinese tradition and/or some South American cultures. The collection of the whole plants is in spring and autumn as a Chinese herb.

Antitumor Activities and Constituents

Agents from B. pilosa

In an *in vitro* assay, a crude hydroalcoholic extract (HAE) and a CF showed a certain cytotoxic effect on Ehrlich ascites cancer cells (IC_{50}: 83–97 μg/mL). The i.p. administration with HAE or CF to tumor-bearing mice in a respective dose of 150 or 300 mg/kg per day for nine days significantly diminished the tumor volume and markedly augmented nonviable tumor cell count, resulting in a notable increase of life span (41.7% and 54.2%) as well as decreases of LDH activity (30.6% and 39.5%) in serum and GSH concentration (50.7% and 94.6%) in the ascitic fluid, respectively.[1] Its methanolic extract and n-hexane extract showed a prominent cytotoxic effect against human HeLa cervical cancer cells *in vitro*.[2] Its water extract was demonstrated to have growth suppressive effects on human T cell leukemia virus type-1-infected T cells and adult T cell leukemia cells *in vitro* and *in vivo* in association with the induction of G1 cell arrest and apoptotic death. During the treatment, the activity of NF-κB and the expression of JunB and JunD were inhibited, thereby blocking NF-κB-DNA binding and AP-1-DNA binding.[3] A hot water extract derived from *B. pilosa* var. *minor* weakly inhibited four leukemic cell lines (L1210, P3MR1, Raji, and K562) with IC_{50} values below 200 μg/mL.[4] An EAF, which was prepared from extract of *B. pilosa* var. *radiate*, displayed the most remarkable antiproliferative effect against MGC-803 (stomach), MCF-7 (breast), HepG2 (liver), and RKO (colon) human tumor cell lines, particularly RKO cells.[5]

Almost 200 constituents including alkaloids, steroids, saponins, flavonoids, tannins, carotene, ascorbic acid, essential oils, polyacetylenes, and many others have been isolated from *B. pilosa*. The polyacetylenes might be the constituents responsible for its antitumor activity, while the flavonoid contents and total phenolic were highly correlated with its antioxidant activity. An active ingredient BP-6 elucidated as 5,7,4′-trihydroxy-3,3′-dimethylflavonol was separated from the EtOAc fraction. BP-6 could induce the cell apoptosis and inhibit the proliferation of RKO cells (IC_{50}: 6.66 μmol/L).[5] Centaureidin (**1**) is a cytotoxic flavone separated from *B. pilosa*, which acted as an inhibitor of tubulin polymerization.[6] It exerted an obvious antiproliferative effect on human cancer cell lines *in vitro* with IC_{50} values of 0.18 μM in HeLa cervical cancer, 0.43 μM in HepG2 hepatoma, 0.67 μM in A549 lung cancer, 0.85 μM in MCF-7 breast cancer, and 1.52 μM in U2-OS osteosarcoma.[7] Isoquercitrin (**2**), which was isolated from both origins of the herb (*B. pilosa* and *B. bipinnata*), was capable of obstructing the progression of human liver cancer cells and human pancreatic cancer cells *in vivo* and *in vitro*, whose molecular mechanisms were found to be closely associated with the activation of MAPK signaling pathway and the inhibition of PKC in the hepatoma cells and with the regulation of opioid receptors and MAPK signaling pathway in the pancreatic cancer cells.[8,9]

The isolated phenyl-1,3,5-heptatriyne (**3**) exerted a noticeable suppressive activity in terms of IC_{50} values of 8.0 μg/mL in KB oral cancer, 0.49 μg/mL in HepG2 hepatoma, 0.70 μg/mL in Caco2 colon tumor, and 10 μg/mL in MCF-7 breast cancer and an ED_{50} value of >4 μg/mL in mouse P388 leukemia. However, more data revealed the toxicity profiles of phenyl-1,3,5-heptatriyne (**3**) on normal blood cells.[10,11] Moreover, an EAF of *B. pilosa* was found to have antiproliferative and antitube formation activities against HUVECs. The bioassay-guided isolation of the fraction led to the separation of three polyacetylenes, 1,2-dihydroxy-5(E)-tridecene-7,9,11-triyne (**4**), 1,2-dihydroxytrideca-5,7,9,11-tetrayne (**5**), and 1,3-dihydroxy-6(E)-tetradecene-8,10,12-triyne (**6**), which manifested highly specific and significant activities on HUVEC proliferation (respective IC_{50}: 5.7, 2.5 and 0.375 μg/mL). At a concentration of 2.5 μg/mL, 1,2-dihydroxy-5(E)-tridecene-7,9,11-triyne (**4**) completely blocked the formation of tube-like structures and markedly reduced the ability of HUVECs to migrate toward bFGF or VEGF-A, and 1,3-dihydroxy-6(E)-tetradecene-8,10,12-triyne (**6**) exhibited a more potent effect on preventing the tube formation of HUVEC, whose significant antiangiogenesis activities correlated with the regulation of the expression of cell cycle mediators such as p27(Kip1), p21(Cip1), or cyclin-E.[12,13] Also, 1,2-dihydroxy-5(E)-tridecene-7,9,11-triyne (**4**) was also found to be able to promote the apoptosis of human endothelial cells prominently via the activation of CDK inhibitors and caspase-7.[13] However, an isolated polyacetylenic glucoside, identified as β-D-glucopyranosyloxy-3-hydroxy-6(E)-tetradecen-8,10,12-triyne (**7**), showed an overgrowing action on normal and transformed human cell lines in culture and exhibited an inhibitory activity on papilloma inducer in rat esophagus.[11]

Agents from B. bipinnata

The extract of *B. bipinnata* showed a moderate inhibitory effect *in vitro* against HepG2 (liver) and HeLa (cervix) human cancer cell lines (respective IC_{50}: 14.80 and 13.50 μg/mL, 48 h).[14] Its CF was able to retard the proliferation of K562 (leukemic) and HepG2 (liver) human cancer cell lines (respective IC_{50}: 12.74 and 9.17 μg/mL).[15] Mixed polyacetylene glycosides and a bipannat polyacetyloside (**8**) were isolated from the 70% ethanolic extract, which both exhibited a modest antileukemia effect against two types of human leukemia cell lines (HL-60 and U937) *in vitro* (IC_{50}: ≥60 μg/mL).[16] The *in vivo* anticancer activity of *B. bipinnata* was demonstrated in three mouse models with U14 cervix cancer, H22 primary hepatoma, or Ehrlich ascites carcinoma. Oral administration of its 90% ethanolic extract to tumor-bearing mice in two doses of 43.34 and 21.67 g/kg for 15 days inhibited the growth of U14 cells by 45.52% and 19.93%, respectively, and extended the survival duration of mice. The inhibitory effect was less active compared to CTX and cisplatin, but the 90% ethanolic extract significantly augmented the indexes of the spleen and the thymus and enhanced the nonspecific immune function in the tumor-bearing mice.[17–19]

Agents from B. alba

A crude extract was prepared from the fresh leaves of *Bidens alba*, whose major components are sesquiterpenes, and its minor ones are oxygenated sesquiterpenes and flavonoids. The extract and its fractions showed a concentration-dependent antiproliferative activity *in vitro* against three types of leukemia cell lines (K562, HL-60, and Nalm6), concomitant with the decline of the content of thymidine in the cells.[20] Also, a protein extract was prepared from the whole plant of *B. alba*. The treatment with the protein extract could induce the apoptosis of human SW480 colorectal cancer cells in association with the increase of ROS production and the decrease of GSH depletion, indicating that the protein extract of *B. alba* might have a therapeutic value against the human colorectal cancer.[21]

Other Bioactivities

Gui Zhen Cao (*B. pilosa*) is a popular nutraceutical herbal tea and folk medicine in the world. The herb has been reported to possess potent pharmacological properties like antiinflammatory, antihypertensive, antihyperglycemic, antiulcerogenic, hepatoprotective, antipyretic, antivirus, antiangiogenic, antibiotic, antirheumatic, and antidiabetes. Biological investigations proved that Gui Zhen Cao (*B. bipinnata*) have marked antiinflammatory, antihyperglycemic, antigastroelcosis, anti-thrombotic, hypnogenesis, and analgesic activities.

References

1. Kviecinski, M. R. et al. 2008. Study of the antitumor potential of *Bidens pilosa* (Asteraceae) used in Brazilian folk medicine. *J. Ethnopharmacol.* 117: 69–75.
2. Sundararajan, P. et al. 2006. Studies of anticancer and antipyretic activity of *Bidens pilosa* whole plant. *Afri. Health Sci.* 6: 27–30.
3. Nakama, S. et al. 2011. Anti-adult T cell leukemia effects of *Bidens pilosa*. *Intl. J. Oncol.* 38: 1163–73.
4. Chang, J. S. et al. 2001. Antileukemic activity of *Bidens pilosa* L. var. *minor* (Blume) Sherff and Houttuynia cordata Thunb. *Am. J. Chin. Med.* 29: 303 -12.
5. Wu, J. G. et al. 2013. Investigation of the extracts from *Bidens pilosa* Linn. var. *radiata* Sch. Bip. for antioxidant activities and cytotoxicity against human tumor cells. *J. Nat. Med.* 67: 17–26.
6. Beutler, J. A. et al. 1993. Centaureidin, a cytotoxic flavone from *Polymnia fruticosa*, inhibits tubulin polymerization. *BioMed. Chem. Lett.* 3: 581–4.
7. Fu, D. H. et al. 2013. Extraction and isolation of centaureidin from *Bidens pilosa* L. and evaluation of its inhibitory activity on human tumor cells in vitro. *Strait Pharm. J.* 25: 27–9.
8. Chen, Q. et al. 2015. Isoquercitrin inhibits the progression of pancreatic cancer in vivo and in vitro by regulating opioid receptors and the mitogen-activated protein kinase signaling pathway. *Oncol. Reports* 33: 840–8.
9. Huang, G. H. et al. 2014. Isoquercitrin inhibits the progression of liver cancer in vivo and in vitro via the MAPK signalling pathway. *Oncol. Reports* 31: 2377–84.
10. Kumari, P. et al. 2009. A promising anticancer and antimalarial component from the leaves of *Bidens pilosa*. *Planta Med.* 75: 59–61.
11. Alvarez, L. et al. 1996. Bioactive polyacetylenes from *Bidens pilosa*. *Planta Med.* 62: 355–7.
12. Wu, L. W. et al. 2004. Polyacetylenes function as antiangiogenic agents. *Pharm. Res.* 21: 2112–9.
13. Wu, L. W. et al. 2007. A novel polyacetylene significantly inhibits angiogenesis and promotes apoptosis in human endothelial cells through activation of the CDK inhibitors and caspase-7. *Planta Med.* 73: 655–61.
14. Yang, Q. H. et al. 2013. Study on in vitro antitumor activity of *Bidens bipinnata* L. extract. *Afri. J. Tradit. Complem. Alternat. Med.* 10: 543–9.
15. Lin, L. Q. et al. 2010. Antitumor activity of extracts of *Bidens bipinnata* L. in vitro. *J. Fujian Med. Univ.* 44: 83–5.
16. Wang, J. P. et al. 1997. Inhibition of 5 compounds from *Bidens bipinnata* on leukemia cells in vitro. *Zhongyaocai* 20: 247–9.
17. Feng, T. et al. 2007. Antitumor effect of 90% ethanol extract of *Bidens bipinnata* on tumor bearing U14 mice. *J. Anhui Agri. Sci.* 35: 1037–8.
18. Teng, R. et al. 2013. The investigations on antitumor activity of Bidens plants. *Strait Pharm. J.* 25: 63–5.
19. Zhu, L. H. et al. 2013. The inhibitory effect of *Binens bipinnata* L. extract on U14 tumour in mice. *Afr. J. Tradit. Complemen. Altern. Med.* 10: 66–9.
20. Nowill, A. E. et al. 2007. Process for obtaining an antineoplastic phytotherapeutic compound from an extract of *Bidens alba*. *PCT Intl. Appl.* WO 2007068071 A2 20070621.
21. Ong, P. L. et al. 2008. The anticancer effect of protein-extract from *Bidens alba* in human colorectal carcinoma SW480 cells via the reactive oxidative species- and glutathione depletion-dependent apoptosis. *Food Chem. Toxicol.* 46: 1535–47.

89 Ba Qie 菝葜

China root

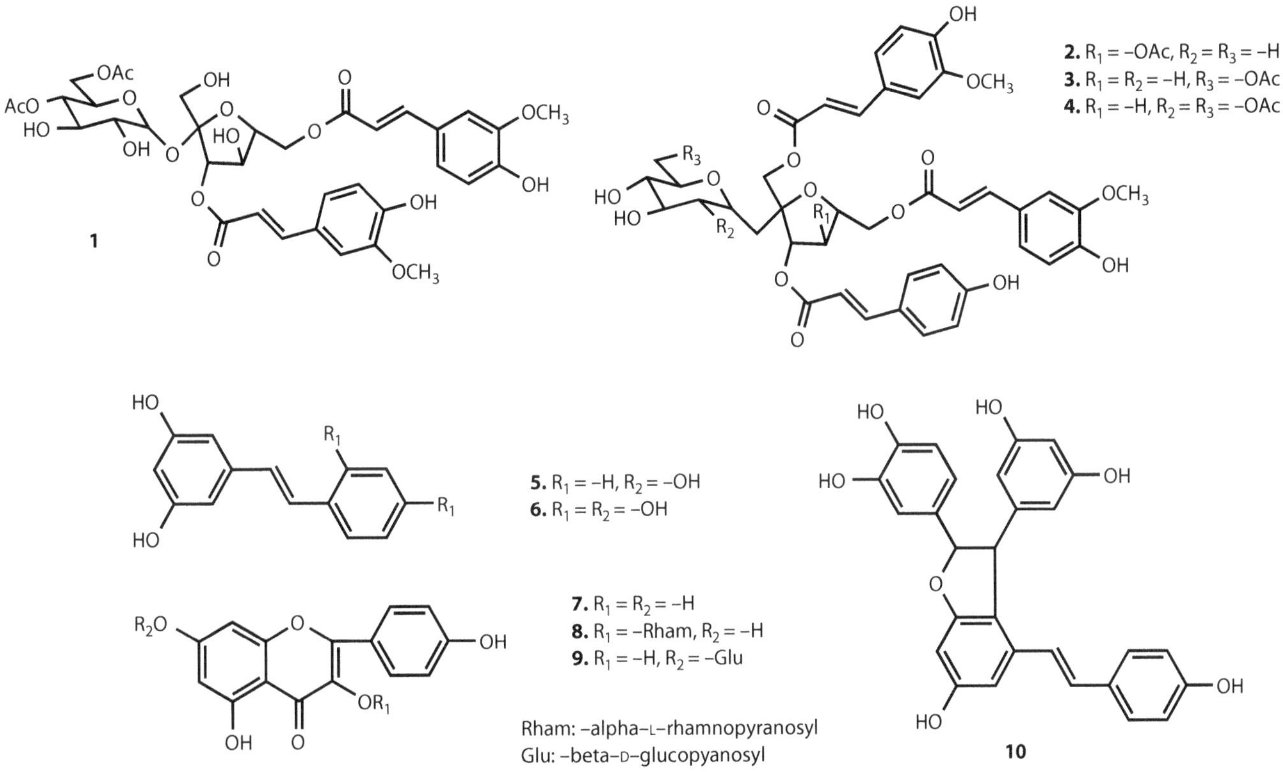

2. R_1 = -OAc, R_2 = R_3 = -H
3. R_1 = R_2 = -H, R_3 = -OAc
4. R_1 = -H, R_2 = R_3 = -OAc

5. R_1 = -H, R_2 = -OH
6. R_1 = R_2 = -OH

7. R_1 = R_2 = -H
8. R_1 = -Rham, R_2 = -H
9. R_1 = -H, R_2 = -Glu

Rham: -alpha-L-rhamnopyranosyl
Glu: -beta-D-glucopyranosyl

Herb Origination

The herb Ba Qie is the dried rhizome of a small vine *Smilax china* L. (Liliaceae). The plant is native to China and Japan. Its distribution is from southern China and Japan to Southeast Asian areas and islands. The rhizome of Ba Qie is normally collected in February or August and dried in the sun to be a functional folk medicine.

Antitumor Activities and Constituents

The crude extracts of Ba Qie could completely inhibit the mutagenicity of BAP.[1] Daily feeding of the alcoholic extract to tumor-bearing mice in a dose of 90 g/kg obviously inhibited the growth of sarcoma 180 cells and U14 cervical cancer cells but no such action on EACs.[2] The methanolic extract and an EAF of Ba Qie demonstrated a moderate antiproliferative effect against human HepG2 hepatoma cells and promoted the effect for the induction of G2/M cell cycle arrest and a late apoptosis and also showed radical-scavenging capacity.[3] The apoptosis of human MC-3 oral mucoepidermoid cancer cells enhanced by the methanolic extract was mediated by an ERK pathway, i.e., damaged mitochondrial membrane potential, activated caspase-8, and elevated death receptor-5 protein level, then leading to growth inhibition.[4] In association with the reduction of the mRNA levels of u-PA and u-PAR (molecules related to extracellular matrix (ECM) degradation) and the amplification of the mRNA levels of TIMP1 and TIMP2, the ethanolic extract of Ba Qie markedly inhibited the proliferation and the migration of MDA-MB-231 cells, showing antimetastatic potential.[5] Oral administration of the EAF to tumor-bearing mice in a high dose (0.6 g) for 14 days notably restrained the growth of mouse H22 hepatoma cells by 43.3%. Simultaneously, the immune system was stimulated through augmenting indexes of spleen and thymus and enhancing phagocytic rate.[6] In addition, the EAF also significantly augmented the quinone reductase activity in a murine Hepa 1c1c7 hepatoma cell culture system. Because the quinone reductase is a protective phase-II enzyme, the herb was considered to have a cancer chemopreventive property.[7]

Polyphenols

The bioassay-guided separation of Ba Qie ethanolic extract led to the discovery of nine phenylpropanoids including smilasides-A–F. Smilaside-A (**1**), smilaside-D (**2**), smilaside-E (**3**), and smilaside-F (**4**) were found to exert the antiproliferative effect against DLD-1 (colon), KB (oral epithelium), HeLa (cervix), MCF-7 (breast), A549 (lung), and Med (medulloblastoma) human tumor cell lines (IC_{50}: 2.7–13 μg/mL).[8] Other polyphenols were separated from the EAF and were characterized as resveratrol (**5**), oxyresveratrol (**6**), dihydrokaempferol (**7**), dihydrokaempferol-3-*O*-α-L-rharmnoside (**8**), kaempferol-7-*O*-β-D-glucoside (**9**), and scirpusin-A (**10**). The antitumor and apoptosis-inducing activities of these polyphenols (**5–10**) were demonstrated in the *in vitro* assay with human MCF-7 and MDA-MB-231 breast cancer cell lines, showing IC_{50} values ranging from 2.1 to 38.9 μg/mL.[9]

Kaempferol-7-*O*-β-glucoside (**9**) was also sensitive to human HeLa cervical cancer cells, A375 melanoma cells and HL-60 leukemia cells, displaying a remarkable antitumor effect concomitantly with the induction of cell cycle arrest and apoptosis via the decrease of the levels of certain cyclins and CDK in a p53-independent manner and the diminishment of Bcl-2 expression and NF-κB nuclear translocation.[10,11]

Steroidal Glycosides

Two steroids assigned as dioscin and diosgenin-3-*O*-[α-L-rhamnosyl-(1-3)-α-L-rhamnosyl-(1-4)-α-L-rhamnosyl(1-4)]-β-D-glucoside were isolated from Ba Qie, exerting a marked cytotoxic effect on human K562 leukemia cells *in vitro* at a 5 mg/L concentration and resulting in 89.1% and 90.1% inhibitory rates, respectively.[12]

Other Bioactivities

Pharmacological studies proved that Ba Qie possesses various biological properties including promotion of blood circulation, suppression of blood glucose, antiinflammatory, radical scavengers, antitrypanosomal, and antibacterial properties besides antineoplastic and antimutagenesis effects.

References

1. Lee, H. et al. 1988. Antimutagenic activity of extracts from anticancer drugs in Chinese medicine. *Mutation Res.* 204: 229–34.
2. Du, D. J. et al. 1989. The studies on the inflammation, antitumor and toxicity of a prescription with Ba-Qie as a major component. *Zhongchengyao* 11: 29–31.
3. Zhang, Q. F. et al. 2012. Antioxidant and anti-proliferative activity of Rhizoma Smilacis Chinae extracts and main constituents. *Food Chem.* 133: 140–5.
4. Yu, H. J. et al. 2014. Extracellular signal-regulated kinase inhibition is required for methanol extract of *Smilax china* L.-induced apoptosis through death receptor 5 in human oral mucoepidermoid carcinoma cells. *Mol. Med. Reports* 9: 663–8.
5. Nho, K. J. et al. 2015. Anti-metastatic effect of *Smilax china* L. extract on MDA-MB-231 cells. *Mol. Med. Reports* 11: 499–502.
6. Wang, H. Y. et al. 2012. Study on antitumor effect of ethyl acetate extract of *Smilax china* L. *Straint Pharm. J.* 24: 23–5.
7. Kim, Y. M. et al. 1997. Effects of natural products on the induction of NAD(P)H: Quinone reductase in Hepa 1c1c7 cells for the development of cancer chemopreventive agents. *Nat. Prod. Sci.* 3: 81–8.
8. Kuo, Y. H. et al. 2005. Cytotoxic phenylpropanoid glycosides from the stems of *Smilax china*. *J. Nat. Prods* 68 1475–8.
9. Wu, L. S. et al. 2010. Cytotoxic polyphenols against breast tumor cell in *Smilax china* L. *J. Ethnopharmacol.* 130: 460–4.
10. Xu, W. et al. 2008. Kaempferol-7-O-β-D-glucoside (KG) isolated from *Smilax china* L. rhizome induces G2/M phase arrest and apoptosis on HeLa cells in a p53-independent manner. *Cancer Lett.* 264: 229–40.
11. Li, Y. L. et al. 2007. A flavonoid glycoside isolated from *Smilax china* L. rhizome in vitro anticancer effects on human cancer cell lines. *J. Ethnopharmacol.* 113: 115–24.
12. Xu, Y. et al. 2011. Studies on steroidal saponins from *Smilax china* and their cytotoxic activities. *Zhongguo Shiyan Fangjixue Zazhi* 17: 92–6.

90 Niu Wei Cao 牛尾草

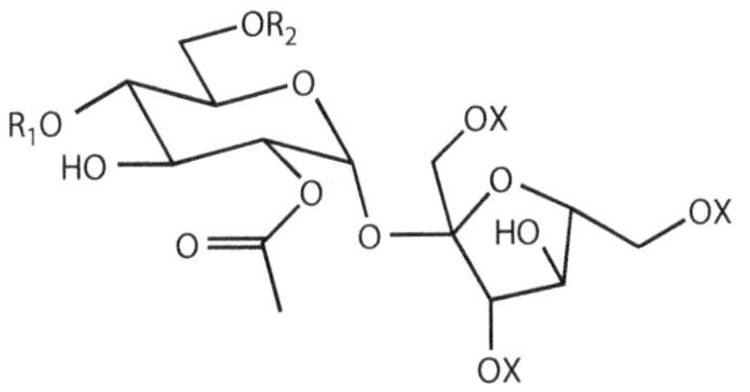

1. $R_1 = -R_2 = -Ac$
2. $R_1 = -H, R_2 = -Ac$
3. $R_1 = R_2 = -H$

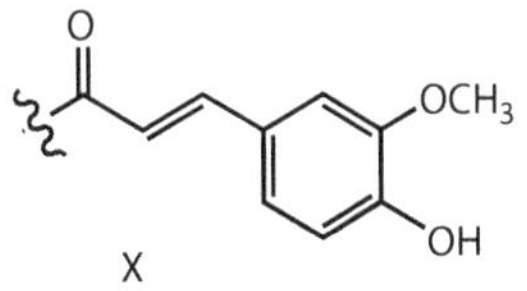

Herb Origination

The herb Niu Wei Cao is the dried roots and rhizomes of a small climbing plant *Smilax riparia* (Liliaceae). This edible plant is native to east Asia such as the southern regions of China, Japan, Korea, as well as the Philippines. As a functional Chinese folk medicine, its roots and rhizomes are normally collected in summer and autumn and then desiccated in the sun.

Antitumor Constituents and Activities

Phenylpropanoid glycosides such as smilasides and smiglasides are the major constituents in Niu Wei Cao. In an *in vitro* model, smiglaside-A (**1**), smiglaside-B (**2**) and smilaside-P (**3**) displayed moderate effects in the suppression of HL-60 (leukemic), SMMC-7721 (liver), MCF-7 (breast), SW480 (colon), and A549 (lung) human tumor cell lines and also showed moderate scavenging activities against DPPH radical. The greatest cytotoxic activity was achieved by smiglaside-A (**1**), which has three feruloyl groups and three acetyl groups, toward the five tumor cell lines (IC_{50}: 2.70, 3.79, 3.80, 3.93, and 11.91 μM, respectively).[1,2]

Other Medical Uses

The herb Niu Wei Cao has been utilized in the treatment of bronchitis, lumbago of renal asthenia, traumatic injury, and asthenia edema in China.

References

1. Wang, W. X. et al. 2013. Tumoral cytotoxic and antioxidative phenylpropanoid glycosides in *Smilax riparia* A. DC. *J. Ethnopharmacol.* 149: 527–32.
2. Sun, T. T. et al. 2012. Smilasides M and N, two new phenylpropanoid glycosides from *Smilax riparia. J. Asian Nat. Prod. Res.* 14: 165–70.

91 Nan She Teng 南蛇藤

Oriental bittersweet

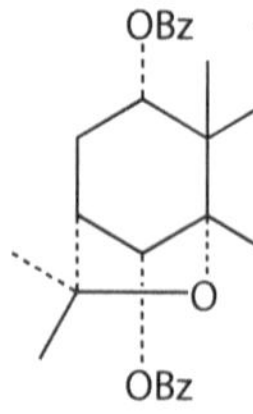

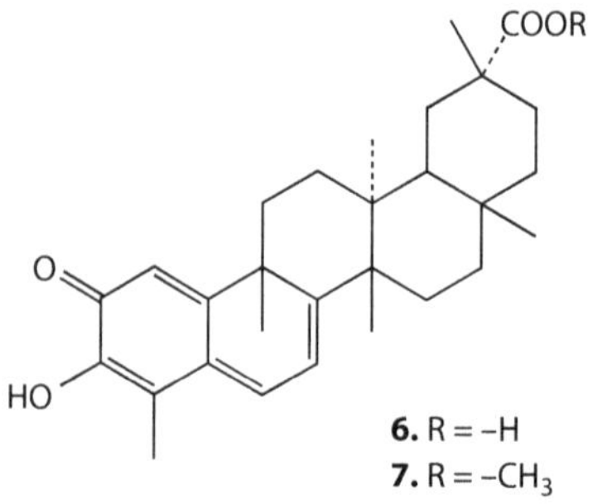

6. R = –H
7. R = $-CH_3$

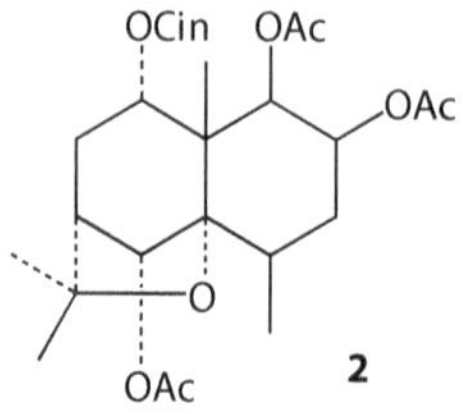

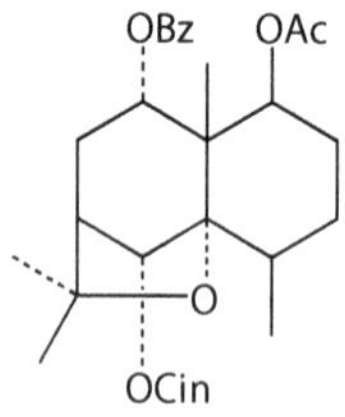

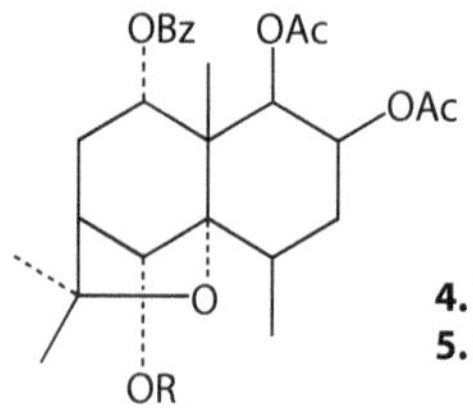

4. R = –Bz
5. R = –P

Bz = $-COC_6H_5$

Cin = $-COCH = CHC_6H_5$

P =

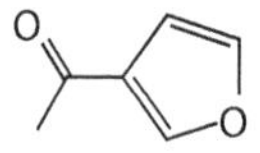

Herb Origination

The herb Nan She Teng (Oriental bittersweet) originates from a woody vine plant *Celastrus orbiculatus* (Celastraceae). The distribution of this deciduous vine is broadly in eastern Asia including China, Korea, and Japan. In 1879, the plant was introduced to North America, probably for ornamental uses, and was naturalized in eastern North America. Its stem is usually collected in spring and autumn, and its leaves, roots, and fruits are also used for folk medical application in China. The herb can be utilized fresh as well.

Antitumor Activities

Celastrus orbiculatus extract (COE), which is an EAF derived from the 95% ethanolic extract of Nan She Teng stalks, demonstrated the moderate inhibitory effect against HeLa (cervix), SGC-7901 and MGC-803 (stomach), HepG2 and Hepa1-6 (liver), and B16BL6 (skin) cancer cell lines, and it promoted the apoptosis of tumor cells in time- and/or concentration-dependent fashions.[1–7] After being treated COE at a 100 μg/mL concentration for 24 h, the inhibitory rates in HeLa (cervix), SMMC-7721 (liver), SGC-7901 (gastric), K562 (leukemic), and its K562/Adm human tumor cell lines were over 50%. COE treatment at a 40 mg/L concentration for 24–48 h notably enhanced the apoptosis of these cancer cells and arrested the cell cycle of HepG2 cells at G0/G1 stage.[8] The antihepatoma activity of COE was further proven in nude mice models xenografted with hepatoma HepA1-6 cells or HepG2 cells, and the growth of red fluorescent protein-xenografted human HCC was effectively inhibited by the extract in a nude mouse model. Early treatment with the extract could exert a marked inhibitory efficacy against the HCC cells, whose activity was very similar to that achieved by oxaliplatin (an anticancer drug) treatment.[4–7] Besides notably reducting the solid tumor volume and weight, COE also markedly restrained VEGF expression at both mRNA and protein levels and down-expressed bFGF and microvessel density (MVD), indicating that the antitumor activity of COE may be partially attributed to its effects against tumor angiogenesis by targeting the VEGF signaling pathway.[4–7] Also, the serum obtained from COE-treated animals was able to exert the similar anticancer effect against the proliferation of hepatoma cell lines (SMMC 7721 and Hepa1-6) and to exert the inhibition of the invasion and the migration of cancer cells and the decline of VEGF expression.[9,10] Also, a butanolic fraction of Nan She Teng showed the antiproliferative effect against the tumor cells as well, but it was less active than the EAF COE.[11]

By combinational treatments, both fractions of ethyl acetate and butanol in their IC_{50} concentrations could additively enhance the cytotoxicity of chemotherapeutic agents such as CTX, paclitaxel, carboplatin, cisplatin, Adm, and 5-FU, implying that the fractions have a potential as chemosensitizers in cancer treatment.[1,2] Moreover, in the treatment of MGC-803 cells and B16-F10 cells, COE and a methanolic extract of the herb significantly restrained the invasion and the migration activity of the tumor cells in a concentration-dependent manner through the dramatical inhibition of MMP-2 and MMP-9 activities via the down-regulation of NF-κB translocation to the nucleus.[12] In an *in vivo* model implanted with B16-F10 melanoma, the methanolic extract obviously suppressed lung metastasis.[12,13] Moreover, *in vitro* and *in vivo* treatments with different dosages of COE found that COE was capable of stimulating IL-2 and IFNγ secretions of dendritic cells (DCs), reducing IL-10 and IL-4 production of DCs, and enhancing the maturation of DCs in association with strongly augmented $CD8^+$ CTL responses. Through these COE-elicited events, the immune system in mice implanted with Hepa 1-6 hepatoma was markedly potentiated, leading to the growth inhibition against HCC.[14] During the significant growth inhibition of sarcoma 180 and Heps carcinoma in mice, the extracts amplified the SOD content and diminished malondialdehyde content in the serum obviously, signifying the antioxidative capacity along with the antitumor effect.[11]

Taken together, the findings demonstrated that Nan She Teng (Oriental bittersweet) can serve as a potential candidate for cancer chemotherapy. The antineoplastic property of Nan She Teng was mostly manifested in (1) the inhibition of the cancer cell proliferation, (2) the enhancement of the cell apoptotic death, (3) the repression of the cancer cell invasion and migration, (4) the suppression of angiogenesis in tumor, (5) the enhancement of chemotherapeutic agents synergistically, as well as (6) the regulation of immune functions and antioxidation.

Antitumor Constituents and Activity

The EAFs of Nan She Teng (COE), which were prepared from its stalks, roots, fruits, and leave, are rich in terpenoids. The major cancer growth-inhibitory activity of Nan She Teng has been found to be contributed by the terpenoid constituents, especially triterpenoids and sesquiterpenes. The total terpenoid extract of Nan She Teng was used for the exploration of its possible mechanisms in the inhibition of invasion and adhesion in hepatoma SMMC-7721 cells. The downregulations of VEGF secretion and MMP-2 protein expression were confirmed to play a critical role in the suppression of invasive, adhesive, and metastatic capacities of the SMMC-7721 cells after the terpenoid treatment, associated with the diminishment of the expression levels of GSH and P-gp in the SMMC-7721 cells dose-dependently.[15] The presence of the total terpenoid extract at noncytotoxic concentrations (5 and 10 μg/mL) could reverse the drug resistance of MCF-7/Adm breast cancer cells, where the terpenoids attenuated the drug resistance and augmented the Adm accumulation in the MCF-7/Adm cells, leading to the induction of the apoptotic MCF-7/Adm cells and its parent MCF-7 cells.[16]

Sesquiterpenoids

Many β-dihydroagarofuran-type sesquiterpenoids have been separated from the roots and the fruits of Nan She Teng. Most of them displayed a moderate to weak cytotoxicity on neoplastic cells, but only a few of the sesquiterpenoids showed marked anticancer effect. 1β-Acetoxy-6α,9α-dibenzoyloxy-β-dihydroagarofuran (**1**) and 1β,2β,6α-triacetoxy-9α-benzloxy-β-dihydroagarofuran (**2**), which were isolated from the plant fruits, exerted the most inhibitory effect against the proliferation of human A375-S2 melanoma and Hela cervical carcinoma cell lines *in vitro*. The IC_{50} values were 2.9 and 3.89 μM in the HeLa cells and 7.3 and 3.64 μM in A375-S2 cells, respectively.[17,18] From the seeds of *C. orbiculatus*, 22 β-dihydroagarofuran sesquiterpenoids were isolated and 8 of them were observed to exhibit cytotoxic effect on human HL-60 promyelocytic leukemia cells with IC_{50} values ranging from 1.9 to 8.3 μM. The three most active sesquiterpenoids were identified as celafolin A-1 (**3**) (IC_{50}: 1.9 μM), 9α-acetoxy-1β,6α-dibenzoyloxydihydro-β-agarofuran (IC_{50}: 2.8 μM), and 2α,9β-diacetoxy-1α-cinnamyloxydihydro-β-agarofuran (IC_{50}: 3.3 μM). The other sesquiterpenoids demonstrated less than 50% of cell growth inhibition at a concentration of up to 10 μM.[19]

Twelve β-dihydroagarofuran sesquiterpenoids were separated from the roots of *C. orbiculatus*, and three of them, which were identified as celafolin A-1 (**3**), celorbicol ester (**1**), and orbiculin-A (**4**), showed a moderate to weak cytotoxicity against various human cancer cell lines including SKOV-3 ovarian cancer, SNB-19 glioblastoma, NCI-H23 lung cancer, UACC-62 melanoma, KM-12 colon cancer, KB oral cancer, and MCF-7 breast cancer. The IC_{50} values of the sesquiterpenoids (celorbicol ester (**1**), celafolin A-1 (**3**), and orbiculin-A (**4**)) were in the ranges of 8.64–17.56 μM, 9.26–19.29 μM, and 38.56–64.90 μM, respectively. Their strongest inhibitory effect was found on MOLT leukemia cell line with respective IC_{50} values of 1.51, 3.05, and 7.33 μM.[20] Furthermore, these sesquiterpenoids were examined *in vitro* using drug-sensitive KB-3-1 and multidrug-resistant KB-V1 cells. The sesquiterpenoids with triesters (except orbiculin-B) demonstrated modest cytotoxicity in both drug-sensitive KB-3-1 cells and drug-resistant KB-V1 cells with IC_{50} values of 8.6–17.8 μM, whereas their tetra- and pentaesters exhibited weak toxicity with IC_{50} values of 26.4–85.3 μM. Orbiculin-A (**4**) and orbiculin-E (**5**), in particular, were capable of restoring the sensitivities of KB-V1 cells to anticancer drugs (Adm, taxol, and vinblastine) besides inhibiting drug-sensitive KB-3-1 cells. Celorbicol ester (**1**), celafolin A-1 (**3**), and orbiculin-A (**4**) were able to partially or completely reverse the resistance of Adm, vinblastine, and paclitaxel in the multidrug-resistant MCF7/Adm and KB-V1 cells. Also, some other sesquiterpenoids derived from the herb were shown to be more active than verapamil in the reversal of vinblastine resistance in the KB-V1 cells.[20,21]

Triterpenoids

The isolated major anticancer triterpenoids in Nan She Teng were acknowledged as celastrol (**6**) and pristimerin (**7**), which both demonstrated obvious cytotoxic effect against various human neoplastic cell lines such as A549 (lung), MCF-7 (breast), HCT-8 (colon), U87-MG (brain), PC3 (prostate), 1A9 and PTX10 (ovarian), KB (oral) tumor cells, and its drug-resistant KB-VIN cells, as well as P388 mouse leukemia cells, *in vitro*, with ED_{50} values ranging from 0.076 to 0.34 μg/mL.[22] The IC_{50} values of pristimerin (**7**) were 0.018 μg/mL in LAX cells and 0.267 μg/mL in P388 cells.[23] In the *in vitro* assays, celastrol (**6**) was also effective in enhancing the cell apoptosis and suppressing the proliferation of human cancer cell lines (including SHG44 glioma cells, Y79 retinoblastoma cells, HL-60 leukemia cells, KU7 and 253JB-V bladder cancer cells, and hepatoma cells).[24–27] The apoptotic mechanisms were found to be characteristic in the different types of cancer cells, e.g., being correlated with (1) the upregulation of the expressions of Fas and FasL and the downregulation of NF-κB expression and Topo-II activity (such as in HL-60 cells), (2) the increase of ROS and ROS-mediated specificity protein repressors (ZBTB4 and ZBTB10) through the downregulation of miR-27a and miR-20a/17-5p (such as in 253JB-V cells), (3) the inhibition of STAT3/JAK2 signaling cascade (such as in hepatocellular cancer cells), and (4) the decline of thymidine incorporation and the inhibition of NF-κB expression (such as in Y79 cells).[25–27] The antihepatoma activity of celastrol (**6**) was also demonstrated by an *in vivo* experiment in athymic nu/nu mice.[27]

The i.p. administration with celastrol (**6**) in a dose of 3 mg/kg (every two days) to mice inoculated with sarcoma 180 for five times markedly retarded the tumor growth by 46.86%. The inhibitory rate could be raised to 60.2% when combined with 5-FU. During the treatment, celastrol (**6**) also significantly obstructed the vessel formation and attenuated the microvessel density in the S180 tissue through the downregulation of VEGF and bFGF expressions.[28] Similarly, *in vivo* treatment with celastrol (**6**) by i.p. or subcutaneous administration in doses of 4 and 2 mg/kg inhibited the growth of human SHG-44 glioma xenografts in mice, which concurred with the suppression of angiogenesis through its roles in repressing VEGF receptors expression (VEGFR-1 and VEGFR-2) and their mRNA levels and inhibiting the expression of bFGF, cyclin-D1, and PCNA.[29–33] The antiangiogenic effect of celastrol (**6**) was also evidenced by the investigations using human endothelial ECV-344 cells, where celastrol (**6**) markedly obstructed the proliferation of ECV-344 cells with an IC_{50} value of 1.33 μg/mL. After the treatment, the cell cycle of ECV cells was arrested in S phase at its lower concentrations (5, 10, and 15 μg/mL) and the necrosis of ECV cells was elicited at its higher concentration (20 μg/mL). Moreover, the treated concentration of celastrol (**6**) even lowered to 0.2 μg/mL still significantly restrained the migration and the tube formation in the ECV cells.[29–33]

The described *in vitro* and *in vivo* studies substantiated that celastrol (**6**) plays an interesting inhibitory role in the proliferation, the survival, the metastasis, and the angiogenesis against a variety of carcinomas with low toxicity and side effects. The encouraging results supported celastrol (**6**) as a potential drug lead for further development in the treatment of malignant cancers. Currently, several drug candidates containing celastrol have been carried on clinical trials in China.

Celastrol Formulation

However, the poor water solubility of celastrol (**6**) restricts therapeutic applications. In order to improve the hydrophilicity, celastrol nanoparticles (CNPs), i.e., celastrol-loaded PEG-block-poly (ε-caprolactone) nanopolymeric micelles, were developed and evaluated on an Rb SO-Rb 50 cells. Both *in vitro* and *in vivo* experiments demonstrated that CNPs suppressed the growth of Rb by promoting the apoptosis in SO-Rb 50 cells in dose- and time-dependent manners, and the IC_{50} value of CNPs (celastrol-loading content: 7.36%) was 17.733 μg/mL. Its apoptosis-inducing mechanism might be correlated to the increased Bax/Bcl-2 ratio and the decreased NF-κB p65 and phospo-NF-κB p65 expressions.[34] Thus, the nanopolymerization can be considered as a helpful technique for the enhancement of celastrol (**6**), and the CNPs may be used as a potential alternative agent for the improvement of cancer chemotherapy.

Other Bioactivities

The herb Nan She Teng (Oriental bittersweet) has been widely used as a traditional Chinese medicine for the treatment of many diseases including rheumatoid arthritis and odontalgia. Pharmacological studies have established the herb to possess notable properties such as antiinflammatory, analgesia, antifertility, antivirus, and antibacterial effects besides antitumor. Celastrol (**6**) and flavonoid components in the herb showed a significant antiperoxidative activity, and the potency of celastrol (**6**) is fifteen times greater than that of vitamin E. Celastrol (**6**) showed a potent apoptogenic action in human HaCaT keratinocytes, suggesting that it may be a promising candidate for further development into an antipsoriatic agent.[35]

References

1. Wang, W. M. et al. 2012. Proliferation effects of *Celastrus orbiculatus* effective constituents combined with chemotherapeutic agents on SGC-7901 and HeLa cell in vitro. *Chin. J. Clinic.* 6: 5149–52.
2. Xiong, X. et al. 2011. Empirical study of acetoacetate extractive of *Celastrus orbiculatus* Thunb. Cytostasis and inducing apoptosis to human hepatocellular liver carcinoma cell line (HepG2). *Chin. J. Clinic Hepatol.* 14: 249–52.
3. Wang, M. R. et al. 2012. Acetoacetate extract from *Celastrus orbiculatus* Thunb inhibits growth of RFP-xenografted human liver carcinoma. *Chin. J. Hepatol.* 20: 377–80.
4. Wang, M. R. et al. 2012. Efficacy of the Chinese traditional medicinal herb *Celastrus orbiculatus* Thunb on human hepatocellular carcinoma in an orthothopic fluorescent nude mouse model. *Anticancer Res.* 32: 1213–20.
5. Hou, Y. et al. 2011. Celastrus orbiculatus extract inhibits the xenograft tumor growth of HepA1–6 hepatoma in mice. *Zhongliu* 31: 999–1003.
6. Yang, Q. W. et al. 2008. Anti-proliferation and apoptosis-induction of *Celastrus orbiculatus* extract on mouse melanoma B16BL6 cells. *Pharmacol. Clin. Chin. Materia Med.* 24: 61–3.
7. Qian, Y. Y. et al. 2012. *Celastrus orbiculatus* extract inhibits tumor angiogenesis by targeting vascular endothelial growth factor signaling pathway and shows potent antitumor activity in hepatocarcinomas in vitro and in vivo. *Chin. J. Integr. Med.* 18: 752–60.
8. Zhang, J. et al. 2006. In vitro study on the antitumor activity of *Celastrus orbiculatus* extract. *Pharmacol. Clin. Chin. Materia Med.* 22: 99–101.
9. Yuan, L. et al. 2011. Effect of serum containing *Celastrus orbiculatus* extract on proliferation and VEGF-c expression in hepatoma cells in mice. *Zhongguo Shiyan Fangjixue Zazhi* 11: 157–60.
10. Zhang, H. et al. 2011. Proliferation, migration and adhesion effects of extracted *Clastrus orbiculatus* containing serum on hepatoma cells line SMMC 7721. *J. Nanjing TCM Univ.* 17: 44–8.
11. Zhang, J. et al. 2006. Experimental study on antitumor effect of extractive from *Celastrus orbiculatus* in vivo. *China J. Chinese Materia Med.* 31: 1514–6.
12. Zhu, Y. D. et al. 2012. Effect of *Celastrus orbiculatus* extract on the invasion and migration in human gastric carcinoma MGC-803 cells. *Zhongguo Shiyan Fangjixue Zazhi* 18: 180–3.
13. Jeon, H. et al. 2011. Anti-metastatic effects of Celastrus orbiculatus extract in B16F10 melanoma cells. *Nat. Prod. Sci.* 17: 135–41.
14. Qian, Y. Y. et al. 2010. Enhancement of extracts from *Celastrus orbiculatus* on maturation and function of dendritic cells in vitro and in vivo. *Chin. Herbal Med.* 2: 195–203.
15. Yang, Q. W. et al. 2009. Influences of total terpenoid extract from *Celastrus orbiculatus* Thunb. on invasion and metastasis of liver carcinoma 7721 cell line. *Zhongcaoyao* 40: 434–7.

16. Wang, M. R. 2010. Research progress of a Chinese herbs Celastrus on anti-tumor effect. *J. Chin. Med.* (6): 1055–7.
17. Xu, J. et al. 2008. Cytotoxic β-dihydroagarofuran sesquiterpenoids from the fruits of *Celastrus orbiculatus. Z. Naturforsch.* 63C: 515–8.
18. Xu, J. et al. 2008. Cytotoxic sesquiterpenoids from the ethanol extract of fruits of *Celastrus orbiculatus. J. Ethnopharmacol.* 117: 175–7.
19. Zhu, Y. D. et al. 2008. Cytotoxic dihydroagarofuranoid sesquiterpenes from the seeds of *Celastrus orbiculatus. J. Nat. Prod.* 71: 1005–10.
20. Kim, S. E. et al. 1998. A new sesquiterpene ester from *Celastrus orbiculatus* reversing multidrug resistance in cancer cells. *J. Nat. Prod.* 61: 108–11.
21. Kim, S. E. et al. 1999. Sesquiterpene esters from *Celastrus orbiculatus* and their structure-activity relationship on the modulation of multidrug resistance. *J. Nat. Prod.* 62: 697–700.
22. Chang, F. G. et al. 2003. Antitumor agents: 228. Five new agarofurans, reissantins A-E, and cytotoxic principles from *Reissantia buchananii. J. Nat. Prod.* 66: 1416–20.
23. Zhou, Y. X. et al. 2002. Several monomes from *Tripterygium wilfordii* inhibit proliferation of glioma cells in vitro. *Chin. J. Cancer* 21: 1106–8.
24. Xu, Y. L. et al. 2008. Effect and possible mechanism of tripterine on inducing apoptosis of human acute myelocytic leukemia HL-60 cells. *J. Zhejiang Univ.* (Med. Edition) 35: 311–4.
25. Zuo, H. B. et al. 2004. Tripterine induces apoptosis and effect on NF-κB in human retinoblastoma Y79 cells. *Chin. J. Chin. Ophthalmol.* 14: 146–8.
26. Chadalapaka, G. et al. 2012. Celastrol decreases specificity proteins (Sp) and fibroblast growth factor receptor-3 (FGFR3) in bladder cancer cells. *Carcinogenesis* 33: 886–94.
27. Rajendran, P. et al. 2012. Celastrol suppresses growth and induces apoptosis of human hepatocellular carcinoma through the modulation of STAT3/JAK2 signaling cascade in vitro and in vivo. *Cancer Prev. Res.* (Phila.) 5: 631–43.
28. Wang, M. R. 2010. Research progress of a Chinese herbs Celastrus on antitumor effect. *China J. Chinese Med.* 151: 29–31.
29. Huang, Y. L. et al. 2007. The inhibition effect of tripterine on human glioma xenograft. *Jiangsu Yiyao* 33: 37–9.
30. Huang, Y. L. et al. 2008. Celastrol inhibits the growth of human glioma xenografts in nude mice through suppressing VEGFR expression. *Cancer Lett.* 264: 101–106.
31. Zhou, Y. X. et al. 2009. Antiangiogenic effect of celastrol on the growth of human glioma: An in vitro and in vivo study. *Chin. Med. J.* 122: 1666–73.
32. Zhang, L. J. et al. 2005. Experimental study on inhibiting angiogenesis in tumor by celastrol. *Cancer Res. Prevent. Treat.* 32: 719–20.
33. Huang, Y. L. et al. 2003. Celastroin the inhibition of neovascularization. *Chin. J. Oncol.* 25: 429–32.
34. Li, Z. et al. 2012. Antitumor activity of celastrol nanoparticles in a xenograft retinoblastoma tumor model. *Intl. J. Nanomed.* 7: 2389–98.
35. Zhou, L. L. et al. 2011. Celastrol-induced apoptosis in human HaCaT keratino-cytes involves the inhibition of NF-κB activity. *Eur. J. Pharmacol.* 670: 399–408.

92 Shui Gui Jiao 水鬼蕉

Spider lily

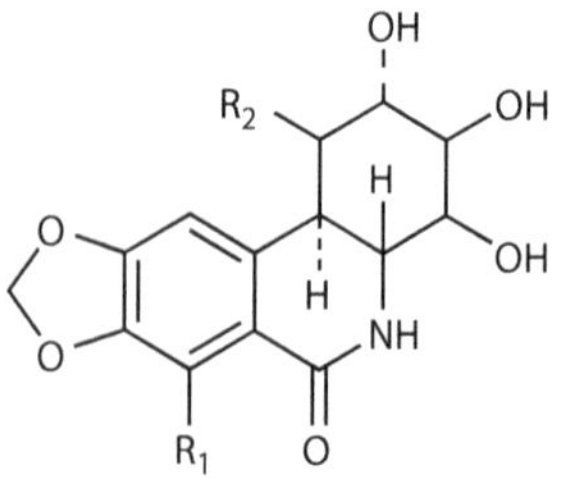

1. $R_1 = R_2 = -OH$
2. $R_1 = R_2 = -H$

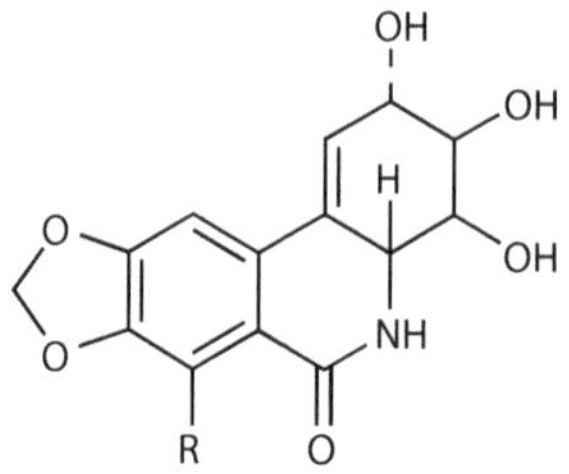

3. R = -H
4. R = -OH

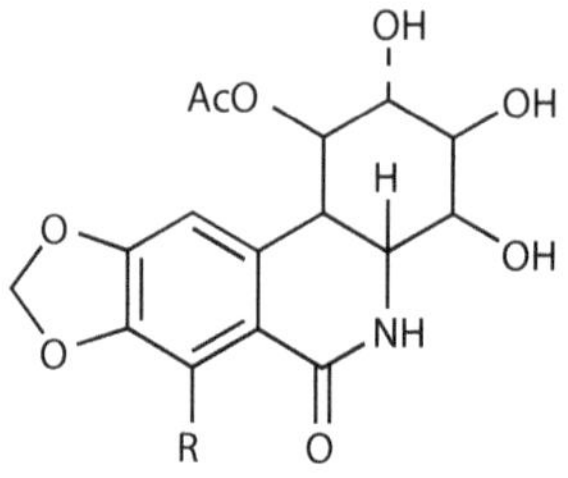

7

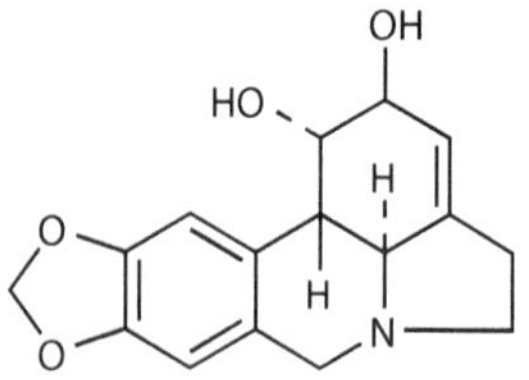

5

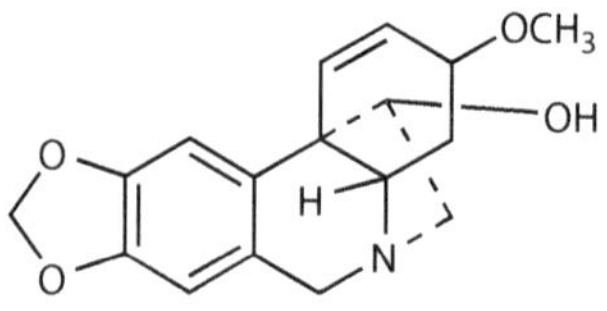

6

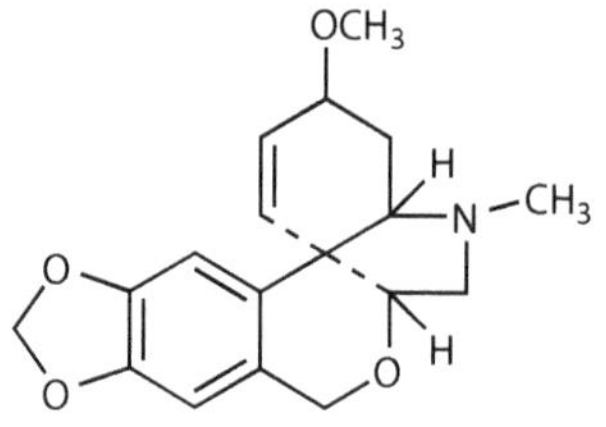

8

Herb Origination

The herb Shui Gui Jiao is the fresh leave of a bulbous perennial plant, *Hymenocallis littoralis* (Amaryllidaceae). This vigorous evergreen species is native to the coastal regions of southern Mexico and Central America. It is cultivated in the southern provinces of China and the rainforest of Southeast Asia, whose leaves are collected in summer and autumn in China and cut into small pieces for fresh use in the medical practice.

Antitumor Constituents and Activities

Although there is no report regarding the cancer inhibitory effect of the herb leaves, the alkaloid components (HLA) is isolated from the bulbs of Shui Gui Jiao displaying pronounced cytotoxic and apoptosis-inducing effects against human HepG2 hepatoma cell line *in vitro*, whose alkaloids are major ingredients of Shui Gui Jiao, holding an isocarbostyril skeleton. The antigrowth activity of HLA were also approved by *in vivo* experiments in mice transplanted with P388 leukemia cells or human M-5076 ovarian carcinoma cells, providing solid evidences for further investigation and development.[1]

Alkaloids

From the separation of HLA, a group of cytotoxic alkaloids named pancratistatin (**1**), narciclasine (**2**), 7-deoxy-*trans*-dihydronarciclasine (**3**), and 7-deoxynarciclasine (**4**) have been discovered. Pancratistatin (**1**) has shown to effectively induce cytotoxicity selectively in numerous cancer cell types. The four alkaloids were found to have cancer cell growth inhibitory effect (GI_{50}: 0.1–<0.01 μg/mL) against murine P388 lymphocytic leukemia and five human cancer cells *in vitro*.[2] The ED_{50} values of pancratistatin (**1**) and narciclasine (**3**) were in the range of 0.029–0.048 μg/mL and 0.012–0.024 μg/mL, respectively, on BXPC-3 (pancreas), MCF-7 (breast), NCI-H460 (lung), SF268 (brain), DU-145 (prostate), and KM20L2 (skin) human cancer cell lines.[3] Importantly, pancratistatin (**1**) is a highly selective inducer for cancer cell apoptosis via the activation of membrane-Fas-receptor-associated caspase-3. Thus, by the same pathway, pancratistatin (**1**) promoted the apoptosis of Jurkat acute human T cell leukemia cells.[4] Through the increase of ROS production and the collapse of mitochondrial membrane potential, pancratistatin treatment reduced the cell viability and induced the apoptosis in androgen-responsive (LNCaP) and androgen-refractory (DU145) prostate cancer cell lines in dose- and time-dependent manners. Pancratistatin also inhibited the migration capacity and induced the autophagy levels in androgen-independent, p53-mutant metastatic DU145 prostate cancer cells.[4] By selectively diminishing the cancer cell mitochondrial membrane potential, pancratistatin (**1**) triggered the apoptotic nuclear morphology in p53 wild-type HCT116 and p53-mutant HT-29 colorectal cancer cell lines in a manner independent of Bax and caspase activation.[5] In addition, tamoxifen, an estrogen receptor antagonist, could sensitize pancratistatin (**1**)-elicited apoptosis of human melanoma cells in a cotreatment, whose effect was found to be related to the depolarization of mitochondrial membrane potential initiated by ROS overgeneration.[5,6] But pancratistantin (**1**) displayed no effect on the viability of normal noncancerous human fibroblasts and only minimal effect on the noncancerous peripheral blood mononuclear cells.[6–8]

In vivo experiments further confirmed its antineoplastic property. The administration of pancratistatin (**1**) in doses of 0.38–3.0 mg/kg significantly extended the life span of mice bearing M5076 ovary sarcoma by 53–84%. A dose of 1.25 mg/kg of pancratistantin (**1**) markedly prolonged the life duration of mice bearing P388 leukemia by 106%.[9,10] The intratumor administration of pancratistatin in a dose of 3 mg/kg (twice a week for five weeks for HT-29 and four times over three weeks for DU145) significantly reduced the growth of human HT-29 colon carcinoma cells and androgen-refractory/p53-mutant DU145 prostate cancer cells in nude mice, with no apparent toxicity to the liver or the kidneys.[4,5] All the results evidenced that pancratistatin (**1**) may be an effective and selective anticancer agent with a potential for the advancement of clinical trials.

Moreover, these four alkaloids (**1**–**4**) showed a highly characteristic differential cytotoxicity profile against 60 diverse human tumor cell lines comprising the NCI panel. The most sensitive to the isocarbostyril alkaloids was a group of melanoma subpanel lines, and certain tumor cell lines were next (e.g., NSC lung, colon, brain, renal).[11] However, the reduction of the lactam carbonyl group in the structures of narciclasine (**2**) and 7-deoxy-*trans*-dihydronarciclasine (**3**) with lithium aluminum hydride lessened the anticancer activity ≤10 times.[9–11] Two isolated other types of alkaloids, haemanthamine (**6**) and lycorine (**5**), exerted remarkable cytotoxic effect on COL-2 (colon), BCA-1 (breast), A431 (skin epidermoid), KB (oral epithelium) and KB-V (vinblastine-resistant), ZR-75–1 (hormone-dependent breast), LNCaP (hormone-dependent prostate), and HT-1080 (fibrosarcoma) cancer cell lines (ED_{50}: 0.2–1.3 μg/mL). The two alkaloids (lycorine (5) and haemanthamine (**6**)) also showed the inhibitory effect against human Luc-1 lung cancer cells *in vitro* (respective ED_{50}: 1.6 and 3.6 μg/mL).[12]

Synthetic Analogs

The pancratistatin (**1**) is limited for preclinical and clinical investigations due to its low availability in its natural source and the difficulty in its chemical synthesis. In order to overcome the bottleneck, several synthetic analogs of 7-deoxypancratistatin with different modifications at C-1 were synthesized and found that a C-1 acetoxymethyl analog entitled JC-TH-acetate-4 (JCTH-4) (**7**) possessed similar degrees of cytotoxicity compared to pancratistatin (**1**). By increasing the ROS level, dissipating the mitochondrial membrane potential, and releasing the endonuclease-G and AIF, JCTH-4 (**7**) was effective in inducing apoptosis and autophagy in both p53-positive (HCT 116) and p53-negative (HT-29) human colorectal cancer cell lines and BxPC-3 and PANC-1 human pancreatic cancer cell lines, whose efficacy was similar to that of pancratistatin (**1**).[13,14] By the similar mitochondrial mechanism, JCTH-4 enhanced the apoptosis and autophagy of Saos-2 and U-2 OS chemoresistant osteosarcoma cells, thereby resulting in a cytotoxic effect.[15] In combination with tamoxifen, JCTH-4 (**7**) exerted an addictive effect in the promotion of apoptosis and autophagy of colorectal cancer cell lines.[13,14] But such cytotoxic effect of JCTH-4 was not found in normal human osteoblasts and normal human fetal fibroblasts cell lines,[15] and the minimal toxicity of JCTH-4 was shown in normal human fetal fibroblast cells and normal colon fibroblast (CCD-18Co) cell lines. Therefore, JCTH-4 (**7**) may potentially serve as a safer and more effective chemotherapeutic agent in several cancer chemotherapies.

Other Bioactivities

Pancratistatin (**1**) is a potent inhibitor of RNA viruses. Littoraline (**8**), an alkaloid in Shui Gui Jiao, demonstrated a suppressive effect on HIV reverse transcriptase.[16]

References

1. Zhang, W. C. et al. 2013. Apoptosis effect of *Hymenocallis littoralis* alkaloid on human hepatoma cell HepG-2. *Harbin Shangye Daxue Xuebao, Ziran Kexueban* 29: 18–21.
2. Pettit, G. R. et al. 2006. Isolation and structural modification of 7-deoxynarciclasine and 7-deoxy-trans-dihydronarciclasine. *J. Nat. Prods.* 69: 7–13.
3. Pettit, G. R. et al. 2005. Antineoplastic agents. 553. The Texas grasshopper *Brachystola magna*. *J. Nat. Prod.* 68: 1256–8.
4. Griffin, C. et al. 2011. Pancratistatin induces apoptosis and autophagy in metastatic prostate cancer cells. *Intl. J. Oncol.* 38: 1549–56.
5. Griffin, C. et al. 2011. Pancratistatin selectively targets cancer cell mitochondria and reduces growth of human colon tumor xenografts. *Mol. Cancer Therap.* 10: 57–68.
6. Griffin, C. et al. 2007. Pancratistatin a novel highly selective anticancer agent that induces apoptosis by the activation of membrane-Fas-receptor associated caspase-3. *Cell Apoptosis Res. Trends.* Edited by Zhang, Charles V. p. 93–109.
7. Griffin, C. et al. 2010. Pancratistatin induces apoptosis in clinical leukemia samples with minimal effect on non-cancerous peripheral blood mononuclear cells. *Cancer Cell Intl.* 10: 6.
8. Chatterjee, S. J. et al. 2011. Sensitization of human melanoma cells by tamoxifen to apoptosis induction by pancratistatin, a nongeno-toxic natural compound. *Melanoma Res.* 21: 1–11.
9. Pettit, G. R. et al. 2005. Antineoplastic agents. 527. Synthesis of 7-deoxynarcistatin, 7-deoxy-trans-dihydronarcistatin, and trans-dihydronarcistatin-1. *J. Nat. Prod.* 68: 207–11.
10. Pettit, G. R. et al. 1995. Antineoplastic agents, 294. Variations in the formation of pancratistatin and related isocarbostyrils in Hymenocallis littoralis. *J. Nat. Prods.* 58: 37–43.
11. Pettit, G. R. et al. 1993. Antineoplastic agents, 256. Cell growth inhibitory isocarbostyrils from Hymenocallis. *J. Nat. Prod.* 56: 1682–7.
12. Lin, L. Z. et al. 1995. Lycorine alkaloids from *Hymenocallis littoralis*. *Phytochem.* 40: 1295–8.
13. Ma, D. et al. 2012. A novel synthetic C-1 analogue of 7-deoxypancratistatin induces apoptosis in p53 positive and negative human colorectal cancer cells by targeting the mitochondria: Enhancement of activity by tamoxifen. *Investigat. New Drugs* 30: 1012–27.
14. Ma, D. et al. 2011. Induction of apoptosis and autophagy in human pancreatic cancer cells by a novel synthetic C-1 analogue of 7-deoxypancratistatin. *Am. J. Biomed. Sci.* 3: 278–91.
15. Ma, D. et al. 2011. Selective cytotoxicity against human osteosarcoma cells by a novel synthetic C-1 analogue of 7-deoxypancratistatin is potentiated by curcumin. *PLoS One* 6: e28780.
16. Gabrielsen, B. et al. 1992. Antiviral (RNA) activity of selected Amaryllidaceae isoquinoline constituents and synthesis of related substances. *J. Nat. Prods.* 55: 1569–81.

93 Ji Li 蒺藜

Caltrop or Puncture vine

1. R_1 = -H, R_2 = -beta-D-glucopyranosyl
3. R_1 = -alpha-L-rhamnopyranosyl
R_2 = -beta-D-xylopyranosyl

2

4. R_1 = -H, R_2 = -alpha-L-rhamnopyranosyl
5. R_1 = R_2 = -H
6. R_1 = -beta-D-glucopyranosyl, R_2 = -H

7. R = -H
8. R = $-CH_3$

Herb Origination

The herb Ji Li (Caltrop) is the fruit of an annual creeping plant, *Tribulus terrestris* (Zygophyllaceae), which is native to warm temperate and tropical regions of southern Europe, southern Asia, throughout Africa, and Australia. The fruits and the leaves are used as folk herbs in its many distribution areas.

Antitumor Activities

The chemopreventive property of the aqueous extracts of *T. terrestris* roots and fruits was demonstrated on *in vivo* papillomagenesis caused by DMBA and croton oil, whose tumorigenetic incidence was markedly diminished after continuous oral administration with the extracts at 800 mg/kg doses to mice. At the same doses, the root extract displayed greater inhibitory effect than the fruit extract on the skin papillomagenesis.[1] The aqueous extract of the Ji Li fruits could restrain the clonogenesis and the proliferation of human HepG2 hepatoma cells *in vitro* and promoted the HepG2 cell apoptosis through the decrease of NF-κB signaling and the blockage of NF-κB-dependent reporter gene expression and NF-κB subunit p50 expression.[2] The 70% ethanol extract from the plant leaves (collected in Bulgaria) exerted a marked dose-dependent inhibitory effect on the viability of human MCF-7 breast cancer cells (IC_{50}: 15 μg/mL) but a modest reduction on normal MCF10A breast epithelial cells.[3] The methanol extract from the plant fruits exhibited a weak antiproliferative effect against Dalton's lymphoma ascites and EAC cell lines *in vitro* (IC_{50}: 380–420 μg/mL). The oral administration of the extract in a dose of 100 and 250 mg/kg considerably attenuated the tumor volume and extended the life span of the tested mice by 31% and 45%, respectively, in a mouse model implanted with EAC.[4] When the extract prior to γ-radiation for seven days is orally given, the root extract at a daily dose of 800 mg/kg achieved a significant radioprotective effect by suppressing radiation-induced GSH depletion and diminishing lipoperoxidation level in the liver of mice.[5]

Antitumor Constituents and Activities

The major antitumor active compounds found in *T. terrestris* are believed to be steroidal saponins, which include protodioscin, prototribestin, pseudoprotodioscin, dioscin, tribestin, and tribulosin. However, from different parts (leaf, stem, and fruit) of *T. terrestris* collected from different regions (such as China, India, and Bulgaria), the isolated steroidal glycosides and the antitumor activity of the saponins are not the same.[6] The total saponins from this Chinese herb were cytotoxic to 786-0 (renal), Bel-7402 (liver), SKOV-3 (ovary), MCF-7, and Bcap-37 (breast) human cancer cell lines, associated with the stimulation of the cell apoptosis and the stoppage of the cell cycle progression.[7–10] The photoprotective effect of the saponins was present in normal human keratinocytes, where the saponins attenuated the UVB-induced skin damages and apoptotic death via the inhibition of an intrinsic apoptotic pathway, the enhancement of NER gene expression, and the blockage of UVB-mediated NF-κB activation.[11] These findings provided the evidences for the great developing potential of saponins from *T. terrestris* for cancer prevention and therapy.

Spirostanol Saponins

Three isolated spirostanol-based steroidal saponins from Ji Li exhibited a broad range of anticancer activity against a small panel of human cancer cell lines such as SK-MEL (skin), BT-549 (breast ductal), SKOV-3 (ovary), and KB (oral epidermoid) cells. The maximum inhibitory effect on SK-MEL, KB, BT-549, and SKOV-3 cell lines was achieved by a hecogenin glycoside (**1**) (TTS14) with IC_{50} values of 6.0–8.2 μg/mL, whereas isoterrestrosin-B (**2**) and another hecogenin glycoside (**3**) showed mild and selective cytotoxic effects against the SK-MEL cells at 6.7 and 9.1 μg/mL, respectively.[12,13] TTS14 (**1**) was also effective in growth suppression against NCI-H460 (lung), MCF-7 (breast), and SF-268 (brain) human cancer cell lines (respective IC_{50}: 5.3, 11.9, and 4.0 μM).[14] *In vitro* and *in vivo* experiments demonstrated that terrestrosin-D obstructed the growth of human PC3 prostate cancer cells and induced cell cycle arrest and apoptosis of PC3 cells through a caspase-independent mitochondrial pathway. Terrestrosin-D also demonstrated the antiangiogenic activity evidenced by the anti-growth and proapoptotic effects against HUVECs.[15]

Remarkably, dioscin (**4**) showed a broad spectrum of inhibitory activity against the proliferation of a variety of human tumor cell lines. The IC_{50} values were 0.8, 2.6, 4.5, and 7.5 μM, respectively, on H14 (lung), MDA-MB-435 (breast), HeLa (cervix), and HL-60 (leukemic) human tumor cell lines,[16] and the IC_{50} values were 1.1, 1.5, 1.6, 1.6, 2.5, and 5.2 μg/mL, respectively, on H1477 (skin), HEp-2 (larynx), Colo-205 (colon), 8401/TSGH (brain), HA22T (liver), and KB (nasopharynx) neoplastic cell lines.[17] Dioscin (**4**) at a 10 μg/mL concentration had an inhibitory effect on the DNA synthesis of C6 glioma cells.[17] Dioscin (**4**), prosapogenin-A of dioscin (**5**), and gracillin (**6**) displayed the inhibitory effect on K562 erythroleukemia cells (respective IC_{50}s 1.0, 1.2 and 7.0 μM).[18] The antiproliferative activity of dioscin (**4**) was importantly accompanied by the promotion of the tumor cell apoptosis. The apoptosis-inducing mechanisms were showed to be mediated by characteristic pathways in different types of cancer cells, such as (1) AIF-facilitating caspase-independent pathway and downregulating antiapoptotic proteins (Bcl-2, cIAP-1, and Mcl-1) in breast neoplastic cell lines (MDA-MB-231, MDA-MB-453, and T47D),[19] (2) caspase-3-dependent pathway in LNCaP prostate cancer cells,[20] (3) ROS-accumulated and mitochondrial signal-activated pathway in C6 glioma cells,[21] and (4) caspase-9-activated and caspase-8-reduced mitochondrial pathway in HeLa cervical cancer cells.[22] Also, dioscin (**4**) could elicit both autophagy and apoptosis in hepatoma cells and NSCLC cells (A549 and H1299).[23] After dioscin (**4**) treatment, the autophagy of A549 and H1299 cells occurred earlier than the apoptosis, whose apoptosis of A549 cells induced by dioscin was associated with dose-dependent augmentation of ERK1/2 and JNK1/2 activity and diminishment of PI3K expression and Akt and mTOR phosphorylation.[22] In addition, the induction of both differentiation and apoptosis by dioscin (**4**) was also found to be involved in the marked inhibition on the growth of human HL-60 leukemia cells.[24]

Moreover, dioscin (**4**) is capable of reversing the resistance degree of carcinoma cells and augmenting the concentration levels of chemotherapeutic agents in the tumor cells. By the dioscin (**4**) treatment, the MDR1 mRNA and protein expressions and the NF-κB signaling pathway were significantly obstructed, and/or P-gp expression was notably restrained in the multidrug-resistant neoplastic cell lines (such as K562/Adm cells, HepG2/Adm cells, and Caco-2/MTX cells), thereby effectively enhancing the transepithelial flux and the chemosensitivity of anticancer drugs in the absorptive direction.[25–27] The MDR-reversal potential of dioscin (**4**) was also proved in a rat model implanted with Caco-2 colon cancer cells.[27] According these evidences, dioscin (**4**) may have a developing value as a potential adjunctive agent for improving neoplastic chemotherapy. In addition, prosapogenin-A of dioscin (**5**) and tribestin also displayed a moderate MDR reversal activity.

Furostanol Saponins

Although the three isolated furostanol-based saponins assigned as terrestroside-B, tribulosaponin-A, and tribulosaponins-B showed no antitumor activity on the SK-MEL, BT-549, KB, and SKOV-3 cell lines,[11] terrestrinin-B, terrestrosides-A, chloromaloside-E, and terrestroneoside-A that were isolated from the same herb were reported to have potential antitumor activity *in vitro*.[28] Especially, protodioscin (**7**), a main steroidal saponin isolated from *T. terrestris*, was tested for cytotoxicity *in vitro* against 60 human cancer cell lines in NCI's (United States) anticancer drug screen. The result revealed that protodioscin (**7**) was selectively cytotoxic to MOLT-4 leukemia, A549 NSCLC, SW-620 and HCT-116 colon cancer, SNB-75 glioblastoma, LOX IMVI melanoma, and 786-0 renal cancer cell lines, with a GI_{50} value of ≤2.0 μM, and moderately cytotoxic to EKVX NSCLC, SK-MEL-2 melanoma, OVCAR-3 and OVCAR-5 ovarian cancer, ACHN and TK-10 renal cancer, and MDA-MB-231 and HS 578T breast cancer cell lines with GI_{50} values of 10–35 μM.[28] Protodioscin (**7**) also displayed marked antigrowth effect against HL-60 leukemia cells and only weak effect on KATO-III gastric cancer cells but no activity on A498 renal cancer cells.[29,30]

The NCI *in vitro* screening system similarly revealed that methyl protodioscin (**8**) exerted strong cytotoxic activity against most solid tumor cell lines with GI_{50} values of ≤10.0 μM, including against HCT-15 colon cancer cells and MDA-MB-435 breast cancer cells (GI_{50}: 2.0 μM), and moderate cytotoxicity against leukemia cell lines with GI_{50} values of 10–30 μM.[31] Moreover, methyl protodioscin (**8**) showed the antiproliferative effect on Colo205 (colon), KB (nasopharynx), HeLa (cervix), HA22T and HepG2 (liver), HEp-2 (larynx), H1477 (skin) cancer cell lines, and GBM8401/TSGH glioma cells (IC_{50}: 3.0–16.1 μg/mL), but the potencies were less than those of dioscin (**4**) in the same assay.[17,32] The IC_{50} values (1.6 μM) of K562 leukemia cells were the same with protodioscin (**7**) and methyl protodioscin (**8**).[33] Both saponins were also effective in the inhibition of rat C6 glioma cells *in vitro* and *in vivo*.[17] Additionally, a moderate MDR reversal activity was also observed on MDR-1 gene-transfected mouse lymphoma cells after the treatment with methyl protodioscin (**8**).[34]

All the summarized evidences highlighted that protodioscin (**7**) and methyl protodioscin (**8**) are the most important furostanol saponins in the herb Ji Li (Caltrop) for the antitumor property, although they were less active compared to dioscin (**4**). However, methyl protodioscin (**8**) could be biologically transformed to dioscin (**4**) as a main urinary metabolite in rats after oral administration.[35]

Other Bioactivities

The herb Ji Li (Caltrop) is an indigenous herb that has been used for centuries in China and India as a folk medicine with tonic, analgesic, astringent, stomachic, antihypertensive, diuretic, and urinary antiinfective properties. Pharmacological investigations evidenced the multiple bioactivities of Ji Li extract such as antiurolithic, aphrodisiac, diuretic, immunomodulatory, antidiabetic, antiinflammatory, hepatoprotective, cholesterin-reducing, hypolipidemic, analgesic, antispasmodic, antidepressant, heart muscle-strengthening, anthelmintic, and larvicidal activities. Also, the *Tribulus terrestris* extract has been heavily marketed by many supplement companies as a potential natural testosterone booster.

References

1. Kumar, M. et al. 2006. Chemopreventive potential of *Tribulus terrestris* against 7,12-dimethylbenz(a) anthracene induced skin papillomagenesis in mice. *Asian Pac. J. Cancer Prev.* 7: 289–94.
2. Kim, H. J. et al. 2011. Aqueous extract of *Tribulus terrestris* Linn induces cell growth arrest and apoptosis by down-regulating NF-κB signaling in liver cancer cells. *J. Ethnopharmacol.* 136: 197–203.
3. Angelova, S. et al. 2013. Antitumor activity of Bulgarian herb *Tribulus terrestris* L. on human breast cancer cells. *J. BioSci. Biotech.* 2: 25–32.
4. Divya, M. K. et al. 2014. Cytotoxic and antitumor effects of *Tribulus terrestris* fruit methanolic extract. *J. Pharmacogn. & Phytochem.* 3: 1–4.
5. Kumar, M. et al. 2009. Evaluation of radiomodulatory influence of *Tribulus terrestris* root extract against gamma radiation: Hematological, biochemical and cytological alterations in Swiss albino mice. *Pharmacol. Online.* (1): 214–28.
6. Dinchev, D. et al. 2007. Distribution of steroidal saponins in *Tribulus terrestris* from different geographical regions. *Phytochem.* 69: 176–86.
7. Sun, B. et al. 2004. Investigation of inhibitory and apoptosis-inducing effects of saponins from *Tribulus terrestris* on hepatoma cell line BEL-7402. *Zhongguo Zhongyao Zazhi* 29: 681–4.
8. Yang, H. J. et al. 2005. Experimental study of saponins from *Tribulus terrestris* on renal carcinoma cell line. *Zhongguo Zhongyao Zazhi* 30: 1271–4.
9. Sun, B. et al. 2003. The inhibitory effect of saponins from *Tribulus terrestris* on Bcap-37 breast cancer cell line in vitro. *Zhongyaocai* 26: 104–6.
10. Chen, Z. W. et al. 2013. Effect of saponins from *Tribulus terrestris* on proliferation of human ovarian cancer cell SKOV3. *Zhongguo Laonianxue Zazhi* 33: 4485–7.
11. Sisto, M. et al. 2012. Saponins from *Tribulus terrestris* L. protect human keratinocytes from UVB-induced damage. *J. Photochem. Photobiol. B: Biol.* 117: 193–201.
12. Bedir, E. et al. 2002. Biologically active steroidal glycosides from *Tribulus terrestris. Pharmazie* 57: 491–3.
13. Bedir, E. et al. 2000. New steroidal glycosides from the fruits of *Tribulus terrestris. J. Nat. Prod.* 63: 1699–1701.
14. Chen, P. Y. et al. 2011. Cytotoxic steroidal saponins from *Agave sisalana. Planta Med.* 77: 929–33.
15. Wei, S. H. et al. 2014. Terrestrosin D, a steroidal saponin from *Tribulus terrestris* L., inhibits growth and angiogenesis of human prostate cancer in vitro and in vivo. *Pathobiol.* 81: 123–32.
16. Wang, Z. et al. 2001. Effects of dioscin extracted from *Polygonatum zanlanscianense* Pamp on several human tumor cell lines. *Tsinghua Sci. Technol.* 6: 239–42.
17. Chiang, H. C. et al. 1991. Experimental antitumor agents from *Solanum indicum* L. *Anticancer Res.* 11: 1911–7.
18. Hu, K. et al. 1996. Antineoplastic agents: I. Three spirostanol glycosides from rhizomes of *Dioscorea collettii* var. *hypoglauca. Planta Med.* 62: 573–5.
19. Kim, E. A. et al. 2014. Dioscin induces caspase-independent apoptosis through activation of apoptosis-inducing factor in breast cancer cells. *Apoptosis* 19: 1165–5.
20. Chen, J. et al. 2014. Dioscin-induced apoptosis of human LNCaP prostate carcinoma cells through activation of caspase-3 and modulation of Bcl-2 protein family. *J. Huazhong Univ. of Sci. Techn., Med. Sci.* 34: 125–30.
21. Lv, L. L. et al. 2013. Dioscin, a natural steroid saponin, induces apoptosis and DNA damage through reactive oxygen species: A potential new drug for treatment of glioblastoma multiforme. *Food Chem. Toxicol.* 59: 657–69.
22. Cai, J. et al. 2002. Apoptosis induced by dioscin in HeLa cells. *Biol. Pharm. Bull.* 25: 193–6.
23. Hsieh, M. J. et al. 2013. Dioscin-induced autophagy mitigates cell apoptosis through modulation of PI3K/Akt and ERK and JNK signaling pathways in human lung cancer cell lines. *Archiv. Toxicol.* 87: 1927–37.
24. Wang, Z. et al. 2001. Effects of two saponins extracted from the *Polygonatum zanlanscianense* Pamp on the human leukemia (HL-60) cells. *Biol. Pharm. Bull.* 24: 159–62.
25. Sun, B. T. et al. 2011. Reversal effect of Dioscin on multidrug resistance in human hepatoma HepG2/adriamycin cells. *Eur. J. Pharmacol.* 654: 129–34.
26. Wang, L. J. et al. 2013. Dioscin restores the activity of the anticancer agent adriamycin in multidrug-resistant human leukemia K562/adriamycin cells by down-regulating MDR1 via a mechanism involving NF-κB signaling inhibition. *J. Nat. Prod.* 76: 909–14.
27. Wang, L. J. et al. 2014. Dioscin enhances methotrexate absorption by down-regulating MDR1 in vitro and in vivo. *Toxicol. Applied Pharmacol.* 277: 146–54.
28. Wang, J. et al. 2009. Five furostanol saponins from fruits of *Tribulus terrestris* and their cytotoxic activities. *Nat. Prod. Res.* 23: 1436–44.
29. Hu, K. et al. 2002. Protodioscin (NSC-698 796): Its spectrum of cytotoxicity against sixty human cancer cell lines in an anticancer drug screen panel. *Planta Med.* 68: 297–301.
30. Hibasami, H. et al. 2003. Protodioscin isolated from fenugreek (*Trigonella foenumgraecum* L.) induces cell death and morphological change indicative of apoptosis in leukemic cell line HL-60, but not in gastric cancer cell line KATO III. *Intl. J. Mol.Med.* 11: 23–26.
31. Hu, K et al. 2003. The cytotoxicity of methyl protodioscin against human cancer cell lines in vitro. *Cancer Investig.* 21: 389–93.
32. Wang, G. H. et al. 2006. Methyl protodioscin induces G2/M cell cycle arrest and apoptosis in HepG2 liver cancer cells. *Cancer Lett.* 241: 102–9.
33. Hu, K. et al. 1997. Antineoplastic agents. Part 2. Four furostanol glycosides from rhizomes of *Dioscorea collettii* var. *hypoglauca. Planta Med.* 63: 161–5.
34. Ivanova, A. et al. 2009. Screening of some saponins and phenolic components of *Tribulus terrestris* and *Smilax excelsa* as MDR modulators. *In vivo* (Athens, Greece) 23: 545–50.
35. He, X. J. et al. 2006. Structural identification of methyl protodioscin metabolites in rats' urine and their antiproliferative activities against human tumor cell lines. *Steroids* 71: 828–33.

94 Hu Ji Sheng 槲寄生

Chinese mistletoe

Herb Origination

The herb Hu Ji Sheng (Chinese mistletoe) is the dried twigs with leaves of a Loranthaceae plant, *Viscum coloratum*. The plant is native to the wide region of China as well as Korea and Japan, which grows attached to and within the branches of trees or shrubs. The herb is normally collected in the winter in China and dried for traditional medical uses.

Antitumor Activity and Constituents

EAF and butanol fraction derived from the mistletoe extract demonstrated a significant inhibition on the proliferation of human neoplastic cells such as A549 (lung), SKOV-3 (ovary), SK-MEL-2 (skin), HCT-15 (colon), and XF498 (brain) lines *in vitro*.[1] Some mixtures of triterpenoid and a large quantity of free fatty acid in the two fractions were identified as active components responsible for the anticancer property.[1] A chloroform extract from the mistletoe collected in Korea exhibited cytotoxicity toward various human and murine tumor cells *in vitro*.[2,3] The mistletoe has been coated with a biodegradable polymer wall in its formulation. Oral administration of 4% (430 mg/kg/day) enteric-coated mistletoe significantly lessened the tumor volume and extended the survival time of mice inoculated with B16-F10 melanoma.[4] Several types of ingredients isolated from the mistletoe were demonstrated to possess the antiproliferative activity against neoplastic cells, but the major antitumor substances in the mistletoe were found to be lectins.

Lectins

Anticancer and Antimetastatic Activities

The water extract of mistletoe abounds with lectins, which are used as a supplementary medicine in European carcinoma therapies.[5,6] Mistletoe lectins could accelerate the apoptosis of a variety of cancer cell lines including U937 lymphoma, HL-60 promyelocytic leukemic, DLD-1 and Colo colon carcinoma, Jurkat T-lymphoma, B16-BL6 melanoma, A253 squamous cancer, and SK-Hep-1 and Hep3B hepatoma.[5–11] A water extract (KM-110) and a lectin KLM-C derived from mistletoe in Korea were effective in suppressing the metastasis of three highly metastatic cancer cell lines (such as 26-M3.1 colon cancer, L5178Y-ML25 lymphoma, and B16-BL6 melanoma). The intravenous administration of KM-110 (100 μg/mouse) or KLM-C (50 ng/mouse) to tumor-bearing mice by various routes for two days significantly suppressed the lung metastasis of the B16-BL6 cells and 26-M3.1 cells and the liver/spleen metastasis of the L5178Y-ML25 cells in a dose-dependent behavior, and the treatment markedly prolonged the survival rates *in vivo*.[7–13] Giving KM-110 or KLM-C in the same doses to each mouse for one to three days obviously augmented the cytotoxicity of NK cells to Yac-1 lymphoma cells *in vivo*. The KLM-C (50 ng/mouse) treatment also induced the tumoricidal activity of peritoneal macrophages against the B16-BL6 cells. Moreover, *in vivo* assay for tumor-induced angiogenesis showed that the intravenous administration of KM-110 retarded the number of blood vessels oriented toward the tumor mass and restrained the growth of tumor cells. Even the KM-110-treated culture medium was also found to markedly suppress the growth of rat lung endothelial cells *in vitro*.[12–14]

Likewise, the mistletoe lectin could elicit a significant G0/G1 arrest of both B16BL6 and B16-F10 melanoma cells and promote both early and late apoptosis of the cells concomitant with the activation of multiple caspases.[4] When the lectin was combined with DOX, a strong synergistic anticancer effect was shown in the suppression of MCF-7 (estrogen receptor$^+$) and MDA-MB231 (estrogen receptor$^-$) human breast cancer cell lines. The cotreatment simultaneously induced S cell cycle arrest and stimulated apoptosis in both cell lines.[15] Accordingly, the results substantiated that the chemotherapeutic potency of mistletoe lectins including KLM-C in the inhibition of tumor growth and metastasis should be correlated with their abilities in promoting apoptotic death, potentiating immune functions and repressing angiogenesis. The prophylactic effect of mistletoe lectins was mainly mediated by the immunosimulation such as the activation of NK cells and macrophages and the modulation of lymphocytes, and then the host defense system was principally enhanced to fight cancers.

Immunotoxin of Lectin A Chain

Because toxin moiety in immunotoxin plays a distinct role in cytotoxicity of target tumor cells, a recombinant immunotoxin has been created, which was composed of a recombinant lectin A chain from Korean mistletoe and a single chain Fv of an anti-carcinoembryonic antigen (CEA) monoclonal antibody, and then this single-chain immunotoxin was expressed in *E. coli*. The resulting recombinant protein was strongly cytotoxic to CEA-expressing cancer cells but only minimally cytotoxic to non-CEA-expressing cells.[16]

Proteins

Heparin-binding protein (HBP) fractions were isolated from the Korean mistletoe extract, displaying strong cytotoxicity and anti-angiogenic effect against human and murine tumor cell lines in the *in vitro* assay. The HBP fractions were also able to elicit the production of several cytokines such as TNFα, IL-1β, and IL-6 in mouse peritoneal cells. The findings suggested that the isolated HBP fractions may be potential agents for cancer inhibition and immunomodulation.[17]

Polypeptide and Polysaccharide

A polypeptide viscotoxin-B2 isolated from the mistletoe (*V. coloratum*), which has high similarity with viscotoxins from *V. album*, showed distinct cytotoxic activity against tumor cells.[18] The IC_{50} value of viscotoxin-B2 was 1.6 μg/mL on the rat osteoblast-like sarcoma 17/2.8 cells *in vitro*. Moreover, mistletoe polysaccharides could restrain the proliferation of human SMMC-7721 hepatoma cells *in vitro* time- and dose-dependently.[19]

Alkaloids

The total alkaloids demonstrated the survival prolongation of mice bearing tumors and the prominent growth inhibitory effect on the carcinoma cells *in vitro* and *in vivo*.[20] The administration of the total alkaloids to tumor-bearing mice in abdominal injection with doses of 50–75 mg/kg/day for 7–10 days continuous significantly repressed the growth of various of murine tumor cells (entity sarcoma 37, sarcoma 180, L1210 leukemia, Ehrlich ascites cancer, and Lewis lung cancer) as well as human SMMC-7721 hepatoma cells *in vivo*.[21,22] The alkaloids at doses <40 μmol/L notably obstructed the growth of gastric cancer cells in a dose-dependent manner, and the highest inhibitory rate reached to 79.2%.[23] The alkaloids also obviously restrained the proliferation and induced the apoptosis of human SK-MES-1 lung squamous carcinoma cells (IC_{50}: 6.43 μg/mL) and human SPC-A1 lung adenocarcinoma cells (IC_{50}: 12.11 μg/mL) *in vitro*.[24] In the *in vitro* assays, the mistletoe alkali also played an important role in the suppression of salivary adenoid cystic carcinoma (SACC) cell proliferation, apoptosis, and invasion in association with markedly down-expression of PCNA and activation of caspases in the SACC cells.[25] The alkaloids also notably suppressed the metastasis of Lewis lung cancer cells and restrained the tumorigenesis of murine sarcoma virus.[21,22] These evidences provide an experimental information for the application and the development of mistletoe alkaloids for the treatment of human carcinomas.

Triterpenoids

Four triterpenoids elucidated as oleanolic acid, epi-oleanolic acid, 3-epi-betulinic acid, and betulonic acid were isolated as the cytotoxic principles from the CH_2Cl_2 extract. Oleanolic acid demonstrated the moderate to weak antineoplastic activity on five human tumor cell lines such as HO-8910 (ovary), SMMC7721 and HepG2 (hepatomas), T24 (bladder), and SHG (glioma), while 3-epi-betulinic acid and betulonic acid only showed weak activity against some tested tumor cell lines *in vitro*.[26,27] Several tumor cell lines treated with epi-oleanolic acid elicited a typical pattern of apoptotic death with apparent morphological changes and DNA fragmentation.[2,3,27]

Lignans

Two isolated lignans from the dried stems of *V. coloratum* were identified as (+)-epipinoresinol and (+)-syringa-resinol. The *in vitro* inhibitory effects of (+)-epipinoresinol was weak in the human carcinoma cell lines such as HO-8910 (ovary), T24 (bladder), and SMMC7721 and HepG2 (hepatomas), and (+)-syringaresinol was only active on HepG2 cells with low suppressive degree.[27]

Phenolic Compounds

7,3′,4′-Trimethylquercetin showed no antiproliferative effect on the HO-8910, T24, and SHG cells but only weak inhibition against the HepG2 cells.[9] 5-Hydroxy-3,7,3′-trimethoxyflavone-4′-*O*-β-D-glucoside and 1,7-bis(4-hydroxyphenyl)-1,4-heptadien-3-one exerted some degree of antitumor activities against four tested human tumor cell lines, HeLa (cervix), SGC-7901 (liver), MCF-7 (breast), and U251 (brain), in an *in vitro* assay.[28]

Mechanism Exploration

Apoptosis-Inducing Mechanisms

The apoptosis mechanism of the mistletoe lectins in both SK-Hep-1 (p53-pos.) and Hep3B (p53-neg.) hepatoma cell lines were revealed to be provoked by a mitochondrial controlled pathway in p53- and p21-independent manners, associated with the downregulation of Bcl-2 and telomerase expressions and the upregulation of Bax and caspase-3 activities.[26] The destructive apoptotic mechanism by mistletoe lectins in Hep3B hepatoma cells and U937 lymphoma cells was initiated by strongly induced prooxidant generation such as H_2O_2 and ROS, subsequently augmenting the phosphotransferase activities of JNK and SAPK, advancing DNA fragmentation, losing mitochondrial membrane potential, translocating Bax, releasing cytochrome c, and activating caspase-3, caspase-8, and caspase-9 in time- and dose-dependent manners. Concurrently, both PARP and PKCδ were also cleaved. If U937 cells were treated by lectin-II after being differentiated by IFNγ, the proteolytic effect of caspase-3 and caspase-9 was markedly elevated and that of caspase-8 was also prolonged for 18 h. The evidences indicated that the IFNγ-elicited U937 cell differentiation could augment the susceptibility to lectin-II-induced apoptosis.[26–32]

The apoptosis of human A253 squamous cell carcinoma cells induced by mistletoe lectins was followed by an Akt signaling pathway in correlation with the inhibition of telomerase activity and the activation of caspase-3.[28] A series of expressions were found to be involved in the apoptosis-inducing mechanism in human colon carcinoma Colo cells treated with the lectins, including the downregulation of receptor interacting protein, NF-κB, X-linked inhibitor of apoptosis protein, and Akt/protein kinase-B besides the activation of caspase-2, caspase-3, caspase-8, and caspase-9.[29] Furthermore, some research reports also proved that the cytotoxic activity of a lectin KML-C against both human cancer (U937, HL60, THP-1, and Jurkat) and murine tumor (L5178Y and 3T3) cells was correlated to apoptotic death mediated by Ca^{2+}/Mg^{2+}-dependent endonucleases in a dose-dependent manner,[33] but the apoptotic effect of lectins in HL-60 cells was not related with the blockage of cell cycle progression.[34] The findings confirmed the characteristic mechanisms of mistletoe lectins in a variety of cancers, whose specific targets might be used in cancer treatment.

Immunostimulating Mechanisms

The investigations also revealed that two specific routes of mistletoe lectins are involved in the regulation of macrophage responses. The lectins were able to manage various macrophage-mediated innate and adaptive responses, and the immunoregulation of mistletoe lectins was mediated by an important step, i.e., the lectins bind to surface proteins with D-galactose.[28] The upregulation of macrophage functions by mistletoe lectins were found to be also primarily organized by an ERK signaling and strongly augmented by the ERK phosphorylation in a time-dependent manner.[35–37] These positive results further evidenced the mistletoe lectins also having the immunopotentiating anti-tumor activity besides the notable therapeutic potential in cancer growth inhibition and apoptosis promotion.

Other Bioactivities

Pharmacological approaches confirmed that the Hu Ji Sheng (Chinese mistletoe) possesses multiple therapeutic benefits in lessening blood pressure, improving microcirculation, resisting arrhythmia, expanding coronary artery, relieving rheumatic symptoms, suppressing thrombocyte agglutination and lipid peroxidation, replenishing the liver and the kidney, strengthening the tendons and the bones, as well as preventing abortion.

References

1. Seo, J. H. et al. 2004. Active principles of the methanol extract of Korean mistletoe responsible for the inhibitory effect on the proliferation of human tumor cell lines. *Saengyak Hakhoechi* 35: 134–8.
2. Jung, M. J. et al. 2004. Isolation of epi-oleanolic acid from Korean mistletoe and its apoptosis-inducing activity in tumor cells. *Arch. Pharm. Res.* 27: 840–4.
3. Jung, M. J. et al. 2003. Anticancer compound from *Viscum album coloratum*, process for isolation thereof, and pharmaceutical and nutritional composition comprising the same. *Repub. Korean Kongkae Taeho Kongbo* KR 2003092170 A 20031206.
4. Han, S. Y. et al. 2015. Anticancer effects of enteric-coated polymers containing mistletoe lectin in murine melanoma cells in vitro and in vivo. *Mol. Cell. Biochem.* 408: 73–87.
5. Park, R. et al. 2000. Activation of c-Jun N-terminal kinase 1 (JNK1) in mistletoe lectin II-induced apoptosis of human myeloleukemic U937 cells. *Biochem. Pharm.* 60: 1685–91.
6. Lyu, S. Y. et al. 2004. Preparation of alginate/chitosan microcapsules and enteric coated granules of mistletoe lectin. *Arch. Pharm. Res.* 27: 118–26.
7. Park, W. B. et al. 2001. Inhibition of tumor growth and metastasis by Korean mistletoe lectin is associated with apoptosis and antiangiogenesis. *Cancer Biother. Radiopharm.* 16: 439–47.
8. Lyu, S. Y. et al. 2002. Korean mistletoe lectin-induced apoptosis in hepatocarcinoma cells is associated with inhibition of telomerase via mitochondrial controlled pathway independent of p53. *Archiv. Pharmacal Res.* 25: 93–101.
9. Kim, M. S. et al. 2001. Gamma-interferon (IFNγ) augments apoptotic response to mistletoe lectin-II via upregulation of Fas/Fas L expression and caspase activation in human myeloid U937 cells. *Immunopharm. Immunotoxicol.* 23: 55–66.
10. Lyu, S. Y. et al. 2002. Intitumor activities of extract of *Viscum album* var. *coloratum* modified with *Viscum album* var. *coloratum* agglutinin. *Nat. Prod. Sci.* 8: 155–61.
11. Choi, S. H. et al. 2004. Mistletoe lectin induces apoptosis and telomerase inhibition in human A253 cancer cells through dephosphorylation of Akt. *Archiv. Pharm. Res.* 27: 68–76.
12. Yoon, T. J. et al. 1998. Prophylactic effect of Korean mistletoe (*Viscum album coloratum*) extract on tumor metastasis is mediated by enhancement of NK cell activity. *Intl. J. Immunopharmacol.* 20: 163–72.
13. Yoon, T. J. et al. 1995. Inhibitory effect of Korean mistletoe (*Viscum album coloratum*) extract on tumor angiogenesis and metastasis of hematogenous and non-hematogenous tumor cells in mice. *Cancer Lett.* 97: 83–91.
14. Yoon, T. J. et al. 2003. Antitumor activity of the Korean mistletoe lectin is attributed to activation of macrophages and NK cells. *Archiv. Pharm Res.* 26: 86–7.
15. Hong, C. E. et al. 2014. Synergistic anticancer effects of lectin and doxorubicin in breast cancer cells. *Mol. Cell. Biochem.* 394: 225–35.
16. Cho, J. et al. 2013. Cytotoxicity of recombinant immunotoxin containing lectin A chain from Korean mistletoe. *Mol. Cell. Toxicol.* 9: 29–36.
17. Yoo, J. Y. et al. 2013. Isolation and partial characterization of heparin-binding protein from Korean mistletoe (*Viscum album coloratum*). *J. Med. Plants Res.* 7: 234–42.
18. Kong, J. L. et al. 2004. Purification and primary structure determination of a novel polypeptide isolated from mistletoe *Viscum coloratum*. *Chin. Chem. Lett.* 15: 1311–4.
19. Li, X. et al. 2006. Growth inhibition of human hepatocarcinoma cells induced by Chinese herbs Huqi San and its principal drug mistletoe extracts. *Shijie Huaren Xiaohua Zazhi* 14: 1963–9.
20. Peng, H. Y. et al. 2005. Studies on the anticancer effects of total alkaloid from *Viscum coloratum*. *Zhongguo Zhongyao Zazhi* 30: 381–2, 387.
21. Wang, Q. R. et al. 1994. The antitumor activity of total alkaloid from *Viscum coloratum*. *Zhongguo Zhongyao Zhazhi* 14: 45–7.
22. Park, J. H. et al. 1998. Cytotoxicity of heat-treated Korean mistletoe. *Cancer Lett.* 126: 43–8.
23. Qu, Y. K. et al. 2013. Antitumor effect of *Viscum coloratum* alkaloid on gastric cancer cells. *Zhongguo Laonianxue Zazhi* 33: 103–4.
24. Sun, L. et al. 2013. Inhibitory effects of mistletoe alkali on human lung adenocarcinoma SPC-A1 and squamous SK-MES-1 cells. *Zhonghua Zhongliu Fangzhi Zazhi* 20: 1653–6.
25. Li, M. H. et al. 2013. Inhibitory effects of mistletoe alkali on salivary adenoid cystic carcinoma cells. *Chem. Res. Chin. Univ.* 29: 275–9.
26. Chen, B. N. et al. 2009. Chemical constituents from *Viscum coloratum* (Kom.) *nakai* and their antitumor activities. *Tianran Chanwu Yanjiu Yu Kaifa* 21: 441–444, 452.
27. Chen, B. N. et al. 2009. Cytotoxic constituents from *Viscum coloratum*. *Chem. Nat. Compds.* 45: 547–9.
28. Zhao, Y. L. et al. 2012. Cytotoxic constituents of *Viscum coloraetum*. *Zeitschrift fuer Naturforschung, C: J. Biosci.* 67: 129–34.
29. Khil, L. Y. et al. 2007. Mechanisms involved in Korean mistletoe lectin-induced apoptosis of cancer cells. *World J. Gastroenterol.* 13: 2811–8.
30. Kim, M. S. et al. 2000. Activation of caspase cascades in Korean mistletoe (*Viscum album* var. *coloratum*) lectin-II-induced apoptosis of human myeloleukemic U937 cells. *General Pharmacol.* 34: 349–55.

31. Kim, W. H. et al. 2003. Involvement of hydrogen peroxide in mistletoe lectin-II-induced apoptosis of myeloleukemic U937 cells. *Life Sci.* 73: 1231–43.
32. Kim, W. H. et al. 2004. Critical role of reactive oxygen species and mitochondrial membrane potential in Korean mistletoe lectin-induced apoptosis in human hepatocarcinoma cells. *Mol. Pharmcol.* 66: 1383–96.
33. Yoon, T. J. et al. 1999. Lectins isolated from Korean mistletoe (*Viscum album coloratum*) induce apoptosis in tumor cells. *Cancer Lett.* 136: 33–40.
34. Lyu, S. Y. et al. 2001. Involvement of caspase-3 in apoptosis induced by *Viscum album* var. *coloratum* agglutinin in HL-60 cells. *Biosci. Biotech. Biochem.* 65: 534–41.
35. Lee, J. Y. et al. 2007. In vitro immunoregulatory effects of Korean mistletoe lectin on functional activation of monocytic and macrophage-like cells. *Biol. Pharm. Bull.* 30: 2043–51.
36. Byeon, S. E. et al. 2009. Extracellular signal-regulated kinase is a major enzyme in Korean mistletoe lectin-mediated regulation of macrophage functions. *Biomol. Therap.* 17: 293–8.
37. Lee, C. H. et al. 2009. Immunomodulating effects of Korean mistletoe lectin in vitro and in vivo. *Intl. Immunopharmacol.* 9: 1555–61.

4

Anticancer Potentials of Internal Cold-Dispelling Herbs

CONTENTS

95 Hong Dou Kou 紅豆蔻

Galana fruit

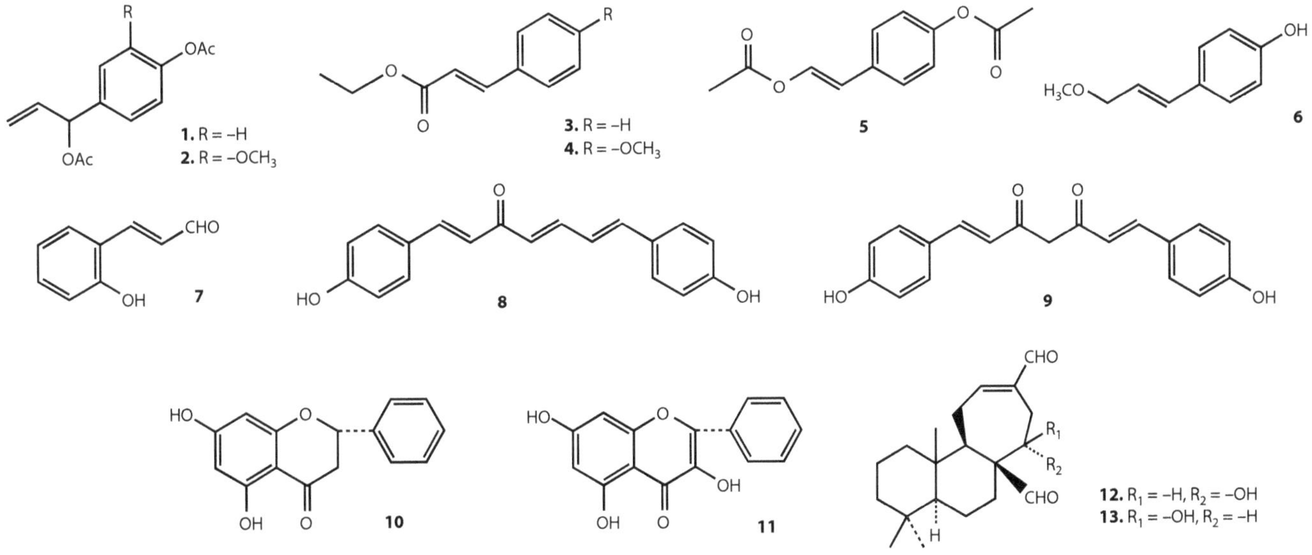

1. R = –H
2. R = –OCH$_3$
3. R = –H
4. R = –OCH$_3$
5
6
7
8
9
10
11
12. R$_1$ = –H, R$_2$ = –OH
13. R$_1$ = –OH, R$_2$ = –H

Herb Origination

The herb Hong Dou Kou (Galana fruit) is the dried fruit of a Zingiberaceae plant, *Alpinia galangal*. The plant is native to south Asia and cultivated in the south of China and other south Asian countries. Its red fruits and the galana rhizomes are used as two herbs in China. The rhizomes are normally collected in February and March, which are termed as Da-Gao-Liang-Jiang (大高良姜) as another Chinese herb.

Antitumor Constituents and Activities

The aqueous extract of the galangal rhizomes displayed a broad range of cytotoxic activities on four human cancer cell lines, A549 (p53$^+$ lung cancer), CRL2321 (p53$^+$ breast cancer), CRL2335 (p53$^-$ breast cancer), and 2800T (p53$^-$ skin fibroblast) but a considerably weaker response in the CRL2335 and 2800T cell lines, implying that the extract is more sensitive to p53 active cells than to p53 inactive cells.[1] Two nonpolar solvent extracts of the rhizomes were found to exert cytotoxic activity against a human HL-60 promyelocytic leukemia cells *in vitro* (IC$_{50}$: <6 μg/mL).[2]

Phenolics

Two major ingredients, 1′-acetoxychavicol acetate (ACA) (**1**) and 1′-acetoxyeugenol acetate (**2**), in the Galena fruit possess antitumor activity against mouse ascites sarcoma 180 *in vivo* and human HeLa cervical cancer cells *in vitro*.[3] ACA (**1**) also exerted cytotoxic effect on human COR L23 lung carcinoma, MCF-7 breast cancer, multiple myeloma, and various myeloid leukemia cell lines *in vitro*.[4–6] The IC$_{50}$ values (48 h) were 7.8 μM in the COR L23 cells and 23.9 μM in the MCF-7 cells.[4] ACA (**1**) showed a promising inhibitory effect against skin tumorigenesis in K5.STAT3C mice concomitantly with the suppression of phospho-p65 NF-κB activation[7] and against breast cancer metastasis *in vivo* by regulating the SHP-1/STAT3/MMPs signaling pathway, inhibiting MMP-2 and MMP-9 activities, as well as potently restraining the human breast cancer cell-induced osteolysis.[8] The cotreatment with ACA (**1**) and sodium butyrate (a short chain fatty acid) synergistically induced apoptosis of hepatoma cells via an increase in intracellular ROS and phosphorylation of AMPK.[9]

ACA (**1**) is also an inhibitor of xanthine oxidase, showing marked inhibition on TPA-induced superoxide (O^{2-}) generation in dimethyl sulfoxide-differentiated HL-60 leukemia cells and on DMBA-induced and TPA-promoted hydrogen peroxide production in mouse skin. It also markedly retarded rat tongue carcinogenesis induced by 4-nitroquinoline-1-oxide (4-NQO) in the initiation or postinitiation phases and inhibited tumor promoter-induced EVB-EA activation in Raji cells. The investigations revealed that the anticarcinogenic activity of ACA (**1**) was associated with blocking the generation of anions and superoxide from xanthine oxidase and NADPH oxidase, and both phenolic and benzylic acyloxy groups in the ACA (**1**) are essential for the anticarcinogenic activity.[10–12]

Feed diet containing 100 or 500 ppm of ACA (**1**) could restrain azoxymethane-induced colonic aberrant crypt foci and colonic mucosal cell proliferation by 54–77%. At the same time, ACA (**1**) not only diminished ornithine decarboxylase activity in the colonic mucosa, number of silver-stained nucleolar organizer regions' protein in the colonic mucosal cell nuclei, and blood/colonic mucosal polyamine contents, but also elevated the activities of phase II enzymes, QR, and glutathione S-transferase (GST) in the liver and the colon.[13,14] The observations designated that ACA (**1**) is a potential chemopreventive agent for restraining colon and skin tumourigenesis.

Two isolated ingredients from the root oil were identified as ethyl *trans*-cinnamate (**3**) and ethyl 4-methoxy-*trans*-cinnamate (**4**). Both could notably elevate GST activity in the mouse intestines and liver.[15] Ethyl 4-methoxy-*trans*-cinnamate (**4**) also exerted cytotoxicity against the growth of HeLa cervical cancer cells *in vitro*.[16] Because the escalation of GST activity is one of the characteristic action in anticarcinogenesis, the two cinnamates (ethyl *trans*-cinnamate (**3**) and ethyl 4-methoxy-*trans*-cinnamate (**4**)) was considered to be promising potential chemopreventive agents.[15] The significant antiproliferative effect of *trans*-p-coumaryl diacetate (**5**), which was derived from the herb rhizome, was present in MCF-7 breast neoplastic cells in an *in vitro* model.[17] Two other phenylpropanoids, *trans*-p-coumaryl alcohol (**6**) and *trans*-o-hydroxycinnamaldehyde (**7**) exhibited obvious anticancer activities against A549 (lung), Colo-205 and HT-29 (colon), A431 (skin), and NCI H460 (lung) human cancer cell lines (respective IC_{50}: 1.3–4.4 and 5.2–19.7 μg/mL), and both were moderately cytotoxic to PC3 prostate cancer cells (respective IC_{50}: 13.5 and 17.7 μg/mL), while ACA (**1**) and 1′-acetoxyeugenol acetate (**2**) only showed moderate to weak inhibition on these tested cancer cell lines.[18]

Diarylheptanoids

From the rhizomes of *A. galangal*, 1,7-bis(4-hydroxyphenyl)-1,4,6-heptatrien-3-one (**8**) and bisdemethoxycurcumin (**9**) were isolated, and their bioeffectivenesses were evaluated in human A2058 melanoma cells, showing significant inhibition against the proliferation of A2058 cells *in vitro*. In B16-F10 melanoma cells, both agents also exerted minor inhibitory effect on cellular tyrosinase activity and melanin content besides the antiproliferative effect.[19]

Flavonoids

Pinocembrin (**10**) and galangin (**11**) are two bioactive flavonoids separated from the rhizomes. The cytotoxicity of pinocembrin (**10**) was shown in HeLa (cervix), HCT-116, SW480 (colon) human cancer cell line, and human LF-1 lung fibroblasts cells at a concentration of 50 μM but nontoxic to HUVEC *in vitro*. The pinocembrin (**10**) treatment could trigger the apoptosis of human HCT-116 colon cancer cells via a Bax-dependent mitochondrial pathway,[16] whereas galangin (**11**) moderately inhibited the proliferation of MCF-7 breast cancer cells and EAC cells (IC_{50}: 34.11 and 22.29 μg/mL, respectively). In an animal model system, galangin (**11**) suppressed the EAC tumor growth by 73.51%. During the antigrowth action, galangin (**11**) inferenced the expressions of 19 different proteins involved in tumorigenesis and tumor cell apoptosis.[20] (See Section Gao-Liang-Jiang.)

Diterpenes

From the seeds of *A. galangal*, two cytotoxic diterpenes elucidated as galanal-A (**12**) and -B (**13**) were discovered. Both displayed marked cytotoxicity on human KB nasopharyngeal carcinoma cells *in vivo* (IC_{50}: 3.25 and 15 μg/mL, respectively).[21]

Exploration of Mechanisms

The mechanism studies revealed that the antineoplactic activity of ACA (**1**) is largely parallel to the acceleration of tumor cell apoptosis. ACA (**1**) dramatically inhibited the cell growth of multiple myeloma cells *in vivo* and *in vitro* accompanied by the induction of apoptosis and cell cycle arrest at G0/G1 phase. Its apoptosis-inducing and invasion-inhibiting mechanisms were correlated with (1) the downregulation of antiapoptotic proteins (survivin, IAP1, IAP2, X-chromosome-linked IAP, Bcl-2, Bcl-xL, Bfl-1/A1, and FLIP), (2) the activation of caspase-8, and (3) the inactivation of NF-κB and metastatic gene products (COX-2, ICAM-1, VEGF, and MMP-9). More evidences also suggested that ACA-induced apoptosis of myeloma cells was mediated by both mitochondrial- and Fas-dependent pathways and TRAIL death signaling pathway by enhancing the expressions of TRAIL/Apo2L and TRAIL receptor death receptor-5.[5,22,23] The stimulated apoptotic death of human NB4 promyelocytic leukemic cells by a low dose of ACA (**1**) was parallel to the loss of mitochondrial transmembrane potential and the activation of caspase-9. The ACA-induced death signaling in the NB4 cells was triggered by two pathways independently, i.e., mitochondrial oxygen stress pathway and casapse-8 elicited Fas-activating pathway.[6]

The initial induction of the mitochondrial apoptosis by pinocembrin (**8**) in HCT-116 colon cancer cells was accompanied with the translocation of cytosolic Bax protein to mitochondria, wherein the upregulation of proapoptotic Bax elicited the loss of mitochondrial membrane potential with subsequent release of cytochrome c and activation of caspase-9 and caspase-3.

The overexpression of Bax sensitized the HCT-116 cells to pinocembrin (**8**)-induced apoptosis.[16]

Other Bioactivities

The herb Hong Dou Kou (Galena fruit) has been proven to possess various therapeutic activities, i.e., antiallergic, anti-inflammatory, analgesic, antidiabetic, antiulcer, antioxidant, anti-amoebic, immunostimulating, antidermatophytic, antifungal, antibacterial, and so on. The rhizomes showed expectorant, antiulcerative, and antibacterial effects. The extract of galena fruit is also a potent inhibitor of fatty acid synthetase.

References

1. Zheng, G. Q. et al. 1993. Potential anticarcinogenic natural products isolated from lemongrass oil and galanga root oil. *J. Agricul. Food Chem.* 41: 153–6.
2. Muangnoi, P. et al. 2007. Cytotoxicity, apoptosis and DNA damage induced by *Alpinia galanga* rhizome extract. *Planta Med.* 73: 748–54.
3. Itokawa, H. et al. 1987. Antitumour principles from *Alpinia galanga. Planta Med.* 53: 32–3.
4. Lee, C. C. et al. 2005. Cytotoxicity of plants from Malaysia and Thailand used traditionally to treat cancer. *J. Ethnopharmacol.* 100: 237–43.
5. Ito, K. et al. 2005. 1′-Acetoxychavicol acetate induces apoptosis of myeloma cells via induction of TRAIL. *Biochem. Biophys. Res. Commun.* 338: 1702–10.
6. Morita, H. et al. 1988. Cytotoxic and antifungal diterpenes from the seeds of *Alpinia galangal. Planta Med.* 54: 117–20.
7. Batra, V. et al. 2012. Effects of the tropical ginger compound, 1′-acetoxychavicol acetate, against tumor promotion in K5.Stat3C transgenic mice. *J. Experim. Clin. Cancer Res.* 31: 57.
8. Wang, J. Q. et al. 2014. Small molecule 1′-acetoxychavicol acetate suppresses breast tumor metastasis by regulating the SHP-1/STAT3/MMPs signaling pathway. *Breast Cancer Res. Treatment* 148: 279–89.
9. Kato, R. et al. 2014. The synergistic effect of 1′-acetoxychavicol acetate and sodium butyrate on the death of human hepatocellular carcinoma cells. *Chemico-Biol. Interactions* 212: 1–10.
10. Kondo, A. et al. 1993. 1′-Acetoxychavicol acetate as a potent inhibitor of tumor promoter-induced Epstein-Barr virus activation from *Languas galanga*, a traditional Thai condiment. *Biosci. Biotechnol. Biochem.* 57: 1344–5.
11. Murakami, A. et al. 1999. Cancer preventive phytochemicals from tropical zingiberaceae. *Food for Health in the Pacific Rim, International Conference of Food Science and Technology*, Davis, Calif., Oct. 19–23, 1997, pp. 125–33.
12. Ohigashi, H. et al. 1997. Antitumor promoters from edible Thai plants: Isolation, cancer preventive potential, and action mechanisms. *Food Factors for Cancer Prevention*, (Int. Conference on Food Factors: Chemistry and Cancer Prevention), Hamamatsu, Japan, Dec., 1995 Meeting Date, pp. 188–93.
13. Tanaka, T. et al. 1997. Chemoprevention of azoxymethane-induced rat colon carcinogenesis by a xanthine oxidase inhibitor, 1′-acetoxychavicol acetate. *Jpn. J. Cancer Res.* 88: 821–30.
14. Tanaka, T. et al. 1997. A xanthine oxidase inhibitor 1′-acetoxychavicol acetate inhibits azoxy-methane-induced colonic aberrant crypt foci in rats. *Carcinogenesis* 18: 1113–8.
15. Sukari, M. A. et al. 2010. Antileukemic activity and chemical constituents of some Zingiberaceae species. *Asian J. Chem.* 22: 7891–6.
16. Kumar, M. A. S. et al. 2007. Pinocembrin triggers Bax-dependent mitochondrial apoptosis in colon cancer cells. *Mol. Carcinogenesis* 46: 231–41.
17. Wang, W. J. et al. 2012. Chemical constituents of *Alpinia galanga* rhizomes and their cytotoxicity in MCF-7 cells. *Shipin Yu Yaopin* 14: 88–91.
18. Chourasiya, S. S. et al. 2013. Isolation, synthesis and biological evaluation of phenylpropanoids from the rhizomes of *Alpinia galangal. Nat. Prod. Commun.* 8: 1741–6.
19. Lo, C. Y. et al. 2013. Antimelanoma and antityrosinase from *Alpinia galangal* constituents. *Scientific World J.* 186505.
20. Jaiswal, J. V. et al. 2012. The bioflavonoid galangin suppresses the growth of Ehrlich ascites carcinoma in Swiss albino mice: A molecular insight. *Applied Biochem. Biotechnol.* 167: 1325–39.
21. Ito, K. et al. 2004. Induction of apoptosis in human myeloid leukemia cells by 1′-acetoxychavicol acetate through a mitochondrial- and Fas-mediated dual mechanism. *Clin. Cancer Res.* 10: 2120–30.
22. Ito, K. et al. 2005. 1′-Acetoxychavicol acetate is a novel nuclear factor κB inhibitor with significant activity against multiple myeloma in vitro and in vivo. *Cancer Res.* 65: 4417–24.
23. Ichikawa, H. et al. 2005. Identification of a novel blocker of IκB kinase that enhances cellular apoptosis and inhibits cellular invasion through suppression of NF-κB-regulated gene products. *J. Immunol.* 174: 7383–92.

96 Gao Liang Jiang 高良姜

Eugenia or Galangal

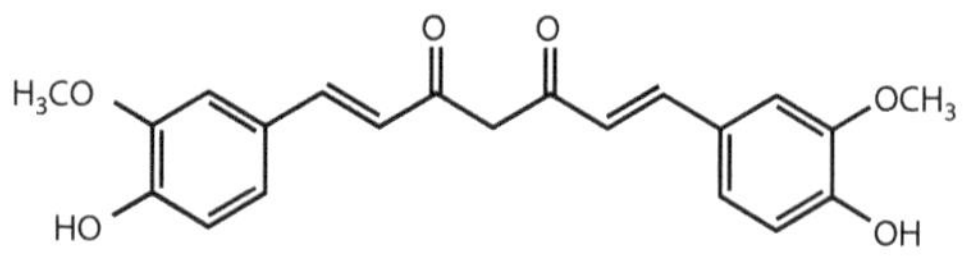

1

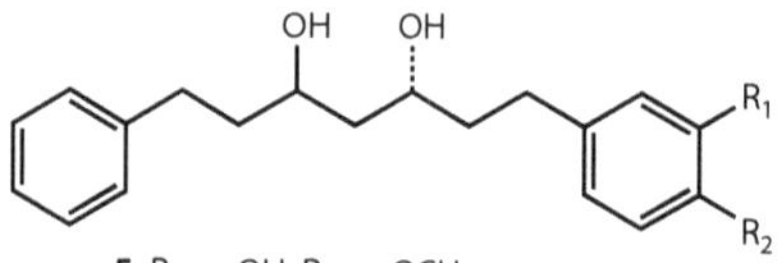

5. R_1 = –OH, R_2 = –OCH_3
8. R_1 = R_2 = –H

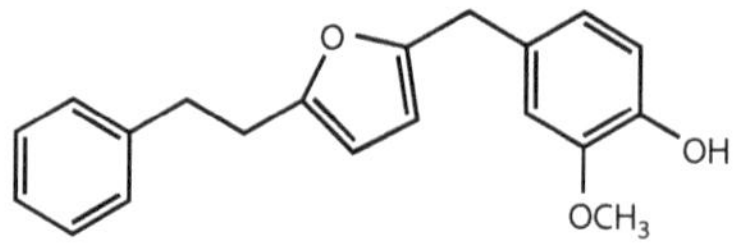

10

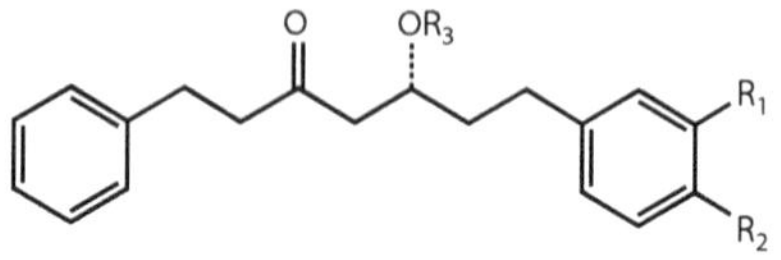

3. R_1 = R_3 = –OCH_3, R_2 = –OH
4. R_1 = –OCH_3, R_2 = –OH, R_3 = –H
6. R_1 = –H, R_2 = –OH, R_3 = –OCH_3
9. R_1 = R_2 = R_3 = –H

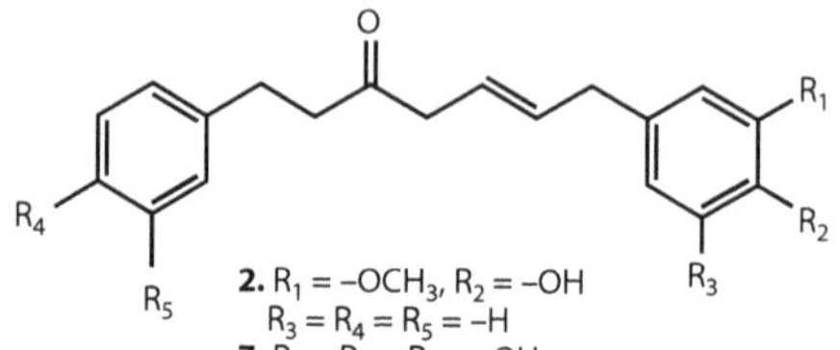

2. R_1 = –OCH_3, R_2 = –OH
R_3 = R_4 = R_5 = –H
7. R_2 = R_3 = R_4 = –OH
R_1 = –H, R_5 = –OCH_3

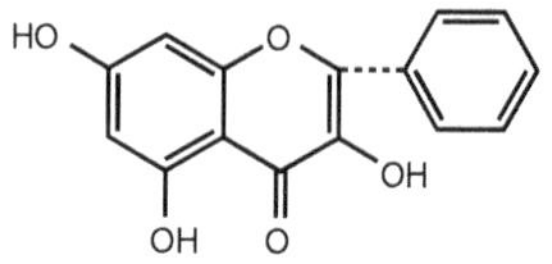

11

Herb Origination

The herb Gao Liang Jiang (Eugenia) is the dried rhizomes of a Zingiberaceae plant, *Alpinia officinarum*. The perennial plant is native to southern China, in particular, to the coast of southeast China, and now it is widely cultivated in southern Asia. In China, the rhizomes are collected between the end of summer and early autumn and dried in the sun for traditional medical use.

Antitumor Constituents and Activity

The methanolic extract of the herb exerted remarkable antitumor-promoting activity against *in vivo* two-stage carcinogenesis in mouse skin using 7,12-dimethylbenz[a]anthracene as an initiator and TPA as a promoter.[1] Up to now, the major constituents isolated from the herb were diarylheptanoids, flavonoids, phenylpropanoids, and its volatile oil. The diarylheptanoids and the flavonoids in Gao Liang Jiang have been paid more attention in the investigations related to anticancer and anticarcinogenetic effects.

Diarylheptanoids

As promising antitumorigenetic agents, a group of diarylheptanoids assigned as curcumin (**1**) and its analogs was isolated from the rhizomes of Eugenia. Curcumin (**1**) is a well-recognized bioactive molecule, whose anticancer property was discussed in detail in Jiang-Huang section. Other antitumor diarylheptanoids are majorly discussed in this section. 7-(4″-hydroxy-3″-methoxyphenyl)-1-phenyl-4*E*-hepten-3-one (**2**) and (5R)-5-methoxy-7-(4″-hydroxy-3″-methoxy-phenyl)-1-phenyl-3-heptanone (**3**) clearly showed cytotoxic effect against three neuroblastoma cell lines (IMR-32, SK-N-SH, and NB-39) *in vitro*, whose effect was correlated with their ability to induce cell cycle arrest and apoptotic death.[2] (5*R*)-5-Hydroxy-7-(4″-hydroxy-3″-methoxyphenyl)-1-phenyl-3-heptanone (**4**), 7-(4″-hydroxy-3″-methoxyphenyl)-1-phenyl-3,5-heptanediol (**5**), (5*S*)-7-(4″-hydroxyphenyl)-1-phenyl-5-methoxy-3-heptanone (**6**), and (5*R*)-7-(4″-hydroxy-3″-methoxyphenyl)-5-methoxy-1-phenyl-3-heptanone exerted significant antigrowth activities on the IMR-32 cells (IC_{50}: 0.23–1.26 μM). The most potent cytotoxicity on the IMR-32 cells was 7-(4″-hydroxy-3″-methoxyphenyl)-1-phenyl-4*E*-hepten-3-one (**2**) (IC_{50}: 0.11 μM).[3] The proliferation of SH-SY5Y neuroblastoma cells could be restrained by 1-(4-hydroxy-3-methoxyphenyl)-7-(3,4-dihydroxyphenyl)-4*E*-en-3-heptanone (**7**) in parallel with the elicitation of S phase cell arrest and apoptosis via the upregulation of ATF3 and the stabilization of p53.[4] Others such as 7-(4″-hydroxy-3″-methoxyphenyl)-1-phenyl-4*E*-hepten-3-one (**2**), 3,5-dihydroxy-1,7-diphenylheptane (**8**), 5-hydroxy-7-(4″-hydroxy-3″-methoxy-phenyl)-1-phenyl-3-heptanone, and 5-hydroxy-1,7-diphenyl-3-heptanone (**9**) were effective in the inhibition of murine B16 melanoma promoted by theophylline.[5] The cytotoxicity of 7-(3,4-dihydroxyphenyl)-1-(4-hydroxy-3-methoxyphenyl)-4-en-3-heptanone (**10**) was demonstrated in three human neoplastic cell lines such as HepG2 (liver), MCF-7 (breast), and SF-268 (brain), with a moderate degree, *in vitro*.[6]

Galangin

Anticancer Activities

Galangin (**11**) is a flavonol present in the herb with high concentrations, which is a potent inhibitor of the aryl hydrocarbon receptor (AhR) and a strong inhibitor on the proliferation of human breast cancer Hs578T (AhR-high) cells. During the inhibition against the Hs578T cells, galangin (**11**) blocked the cell cycle transition from G0/G1 to S phase, via nearly total elimination of cyclin-D_3 cyclin-A, and cyclin-E but not related to the AhR.[7] By binding to estrogen receptor ER, blocking the formation of mutagen-DNA adducts, and inhibiting CYP1A1 activity, galangin (**11**) apparently exerted the antiproliferative activity on an ER^+-human MCF-7 breast cancer cells (IC_{50}: 4.2 μg/mL) *in vitro*.[8–10] The anticancer effect of galangin (**11**) on two types of human colon cancer cells (HCT-15 and HT-29) was mediated by the promotion of apoptotic death via mitochondrial dysfunction and caspase-dependent pathway,[11] and human head and neck squamous cell carcinoma cells was associated with the induction of significant G0/G1 cell cycle arrest and apoptosis.[12] The treatment of human hepatoma cell lines (HepG2, Hep3B, and PLC/PRF/5) with galangin (**11**) obviously prolonged the ER stress and increased the free cytosolic Ca^{2+} concentration, resulting in the apoptosis induction and the growth suppression of hepatoma cells. The research revealed that the activation of MAPKs is involved in the ER stress stimulated by galangin.[13] Galangin (**11**), during the effect in HepG2 cells, also induced the autophagy of hepatoma cells by enhancing AMPK and LKB1 phosphorylation and reducing AKT and mTOR phosphorylation.[14]

Antiinvasive and Antimetastatic Activities

The TPA-induced invasion and migration of HepG2 cells could be effectively obstructed by galangin through a PKC/ERK pathway, i.e., strong down-expressions of PKCα, PKCδ, c-Fos, c-Jun, phospho-IκBα and NF-κB, phosphorylated ERK1/2 and suppression of MMP-2/-9 activity.[15] Similarly, besides markedly inhibiting the viability and proliferation of B16F10 melanoma cells and inducting the cell apoptosis through the disruption of mitochondrial membrane potential and the activation of phosphor-p38 MAPK and caspases, galangin (**11**) was also capable of exerting antiadhesion and antimetastatic functions via the blockage of focal adhesion kinase (FAK) expression and the reduction of FAK (Tyr397) phosphorylation. The inhibitory effect of galangin (**11**) on tumor growth and metastasis was proven in C57BL/6J mouse lung metastatic model using B16-F10 melanoma cells by the fact that it could retard the tumor colony formation in the lung tissue.[16,17]

Anticarcinogenic and Immunotoxicity-Reducing Activities

Galangin (**11**) exerted a marked suppressive effect against mutagenesis and carcinogenesis caused by 7,12-dimethyl benzo[a] anthracene, AFB1, or BAP. An *in vivo* study further confirmed that galangin (**11**) could lessen the micronuclei induced by N-Nitroso-N-methylurea = N-methyl-N-nitrosourea (NMU), N-methyl-N′-nitrosoguanidine or ethyl methane sulfonate in polychromatic erythrocytes, and bone marrow of mice.[18–21] But high doses galangin (**11**) increased the frequency of micronuclei in bone marrow cells and blood erythrocytes of mice.[22–24] The BAP-elicited cytochrome P450-dependent hydroxylation in human liver microsome was restrained by galangin (**11**), which also displayed a potent inhibition on CYP1A1 and CYP1A2 activities in a dose-dependent manner and a strong induction of the phase II enzyme QR, as well as a noticeable suppression of P-form phenolsulfotransferase (PST)-mediated sulfation.[23–26] Additionally, the suppressive effect of galangin (**11**) was also demonstrated on mitomycin c (MMC)-induced micronucleated reticulocytes of mice, implying that galangin (**11**) is capable of lessening MMC-caused immunotoxicity.[27] Galangin (**11**) acted as a potent inhibitor of the environmental chemical-mediated immunotoxicity in B-lymphopoesis to rescue normal pre-B-cells from DMBA-induced apoptosis.[28]

Antioxidant Activities

In the galangin treatment, antioxidative/antiperoxidative and free radical-scavenging effects were also observed characteristically.[29,30] Galangin (**11**) could prevent the superoxide anion radical formation by scavenging alkyl radical and/or blocking the reaction between genotoxic ion and DNA.[22,31] Galangin (**11**) acted as a potent COX-2 inhibitor to block the formation of colorectal polyps in colorectal cancer and hepatoma cells where it showed high levels of COX-2 expression.[32–35] These results established that the flavonoid has favorable characteristics for protecting from oxidative stress to lessen the incidents of carcinogenesis.

Consequently, the *in vitro* and *in vivo* evidences clearly demonstrated that galangin (**11**) may be useful as an adjuvant agent for carcinoma chemotherapeutics and chemoprevention.

SAR of Galangin

Galangin (**11**) has a higher lipophilic property among its similar flavonols such as quercetin, morin, kaempferol, and myricetin, etc. The 2,3-double bond and 3,5,7-hydroxyl groups in the flavonoid molecules might be essential for the inhibition of CYP450 enzymes, activation of QR, free radical-scavenging, and antioxidative activities to exert the cancer chemopreventive effect.[36]

Other Bioactivities

The herb Gao Liang Jiang (Eugenia) has extensive pharmacological effects, like antiulcer, antidiarrhea, antianoxemia, analgesia sedative, antiinflammation, antiplatelet aggregation, antithrombosis, antioxidative, antibacterial besides antitumor. Galangal (**11**) can potently suppress the fatty acid synthase, whose effect included both biphasic slow-binding inactivation and reversible inhibition.[37]

References

1. Yasukawa, K. et al. 2008. Inhibitory effect of the rhizomes of *Alpinia officinarum* on TPA-induced inflammation and tumor promotion in two-stage carcinogenesis in mouse skin. *J. Nat. Med.* 62: 374–8.
2. Tabata, K. et al. 2009. Diarylheptanoids derived from *Alpinia officinarum* induce apoptosis, S-phase arrest and differentiation in human neuroblastoma cells. *Anticancer Res.* 29: 4981–8.
3. Sun, Y. et al. 2008. New cytotoxic diarylheptanoids from the rhizomes of *Alpinia officinarum. Planta Med.* 74: 427–31.
4. Tian, Z. et al. 2009. Cytotoxic diarylheptanoid induces cell cycle arrest and apoptosis via increasing ATF3 and stabilizing p53 in SH-SY5Y cells. *Cancer Chemother. Pharmacol.* 63: 1131–9.
5. Matsuda, H. et al. 2009. Melanogenesis inhibitors from the rhizomes of *Alpinia officinarum* in B16 melanoma cells. *Bioorg. Med. Chem.* 17: 6048–53.
6. An, N. et al. 2008. Diarylheptanoids from the rhizomes of *Alpinia officinarum* and their anticancer activity. *Fitoterapia* 79: 27–31.
7. Murray, T. J. et al. 2006. Growth of a human mammary tumor cell line is blocked by galangin, a naturally occurring bioflavonoid, and is accompanied by down-regulation of cyclins D3, E, and A. *Breast Cancer Res.* 8: R17.
8. So, F. V. et al. 1997. Inhibition of proliferation of estrogen receptor-positive MCF-7 human breast cancer cells by flavonoids in the presence and absence of excess estrogen. *Cancer Lett.* 112: 127–33.

9. Ciolino, H. P. et al. 1999. The flavonoid galangin is an inhibitor of CYP1A1 activity and an agonist/antagonist of the aryl hydrocarbon receptor. *British J. Cancer* 79: 1340–6.
10. Heo, M. Y. et al. 2001. Anti-genotoxicity of galangin as a cancer chemopreventive agent candidate. *Mutation Res.* 488: 135–50.
11. Ha, T. W. et al. 2013. Galangin induces human colon cancer cell death via the mitochondrial dysfunction and caspase-dependent pathway. *Experim. Biol. Med.* (London, UK) 238: 1047–54.
12. Zhu, L. P. 2014. Galangin inhibits growth of human head and neck squamous carcinoma cells in vitro and in vivo. *Chemico-Biol. Interactions* 224: 149–56.
13. Su, L. J. et al. 2013. Galangin inhibits proliferation of hepatocellular carcinoma cells by inducing endoplasmic reticulum stress. *Food Chem. Toxicol.* 62: 810–6.
14. Zhang, H. T. et al. 2013. Galangin inhibits proliferation of HepG2 cells by activating AMPK via increasing the AMP/TAN ratio in a LKB1-independent manner. *Eur. J. Pharmacol.* 718. 235–44.
15. Chien, S. T. et al. 2015. Galangin, a novel dietary flavonoid, attenuates metastatic feature via PKC/ERK signaling pathway in TPA-treated liver cancer HepG2 cells. *Cancer Cell International* 15: 1–21.
16. Zhang, W. J. et al. 2013. Galangin induces B16F10 melanoma cell apoptosis via mitochondrial pathway and sustained activation of p38 MAPK. *Cytotechnol.* 65: 447–55.
17. Zhang, W. J. et al. 2013. Galangin inhibits tumor growth and metastasis of B16F10 melanoma. *J. Cell. Biochem.* 114: 152–61.
18. Heo, M. Y. et al. 1992. Anticlastogenic effects of galangin against mitomycin C-induced micro-nuclei in reticulocytes of mice. *Mutat. Res.* 360: 37–41.
19. Quadri, S. A. et al. 2000. The bioflavonoid galangin blocks aryl hydrocarbon receptor activation and polycyclic aromatic hydrocarbon-induced pre-B-cell apoptosis. *Mol. Pharmacol.* 58: 515–25.
20. Francis, A. R. et al. 1989. Modulating effect of plant flavonoids on the mutagenicity of *N*-methyl-*N*-nitro-*N*-nitrosoguanidine. *Carcinogen.* 10: 1953–5.
21. Sohn, S. J. et al. 1995. Inhibition of *N*-methyl-*N*-nitrosourea-induced sister-chromatid exchange and DNA methylation by galangin. *Yakhak Hoeji* 39: 94–101.
22. Sohn, S. J. et al. 1998. Antigenotoxicity of galangin against *N*-methyl-*N*-nitrosourea. *Mutat. Res.* 402: 231–6.
23. Varanda, E. A. et al. 1999. Tavares, Inhibitory effect of propolis and bee venom on the mutagenicity of some direct- and indirect-acting mutagens. *Teratog. Carcinog. Mutagen* 19: 403–3.
24. MacGregor, J. T. et al. 1983. In vivo exposure to plant flavonols: Influence on frequencies of micro-nuclei in mouse erythrocytes and sister-chromatid exchange in rabbit lymphocytes. *Mutat. Res.* 124: 255–20.
25. Zhai, S. et al. 1998. Comparative inhibition of human cytochromes P450 1A1 and 1A2 by flavonoids. *Drug Metabol. Dispos.* 26: 989–92.
26. Buening, M. K. et al. 1981. Activation and inhibition of benzo[*a*]pyrene and aflatoxin B_1 metabolism in human liver microsomes by naturally occurring flavonoids. *Cancer Res.* 41: 67–72.
27. Uda, Y. et al. 1997. Induction of the anticarcinogenic marker enzyme, quinone reductase, in murine hepatoma cells in vitro by flavonoids. *Cancer Lett.* 120: 213–6.
28. Eaton, E. A. et al. 1996. Flavonoids, potent inhibitors of the human P-form phenolsulfotransferase: Potential role in drug metabolism and chemoprevention. *Drug Metabol. Dispos.* 24: 232–7.
29. Silva, I. D. et al. 2000. Chemical features of flavonols affecting their genotoxicity: Potential implications in their use as therapeutical agents. *Chem. Biol. Interact.* 124: 29–51.
30. MacGregor, I. T. et al. 1983. In vivo exposure to plant flavonols: Influence on frequencies of micronuclei in mouse erythrocytes and sister-chromatid exchange in rabbit lymphocytes. *Mutat. Res.* 124: 255–70.
31. Imamura, Y. et al. 2000. Inhibitory effects of flavonoids on rabbit heart carbonyl reductase. *J. Biochem. Tokyo* 127: 653–8.
32. Kang, S. S. et al. 2000. Isolation of COX-2 inhibitors from *Alpinia officinarum. Korean J. Pharmacogn.* 31: 57–62.
33. Kune, G. A. et al. 1988. Colorectal cancer risk, chronic illnesses, operations, and medications: Case control results from the melbourne colorectal cancer study. *Cancer Res.* 48: 4399–404.
34. Oshima, M. et al. 1996. Suppression of intestinal polyposis in Apc delta-716 knockout mice by inhibition of cyclooxygenase 2 (COX-2). *Cell* 48: 803–9.
35. Reddy, B. S. et al. 1996. Evaluation of cyclooxygenase-2 inhibitor for potential chemopreventive properties in colon carcinogenesis. *Cancer Res.* 56: 4566–9.
36. Hatch, F. T. et al. 2000. Quantitative structure-activity relationship of flavonoids for inhibition of heterocyclic amine mutagenicity. *Environ. Mol. Mutagen* 35: 279–99.
37. Li, B. H. et al. 2003. Presence of fatty acid synthase inhibitors in the rhizome of *Alpinia officinarum* hance. *J. Enzyme Inhibit. Med. Chem.* 18: 349–56.

97 Rou Gui 肉桂

Chinese cinnamon

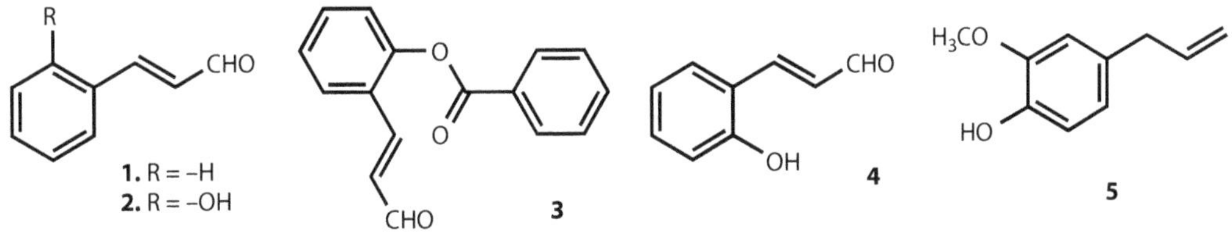

1. R = –H
2. R = –OH

Herb Origination

The herb Rou Gui (Chinese cinnamon) is the dried stem bark of a Lauraceae plant, *Cinnamomum cassia* and *C. cassia* var. *macrophyllum*. The aromatic-rich tree is native to southern China, Burma, Bangladesh, India, and Vietnam. It is one of the 50 fundamental herbs, and it was recorded in the earliest Chinese herbal book, *Shennong Bencao Jing*. The herb was introduced to Europe by Arabian and Phoenician traders, in classical times. The herb is mainly produced in the southern provinces of China and Vietnam. The better quality of Rou Gui should be collected in the autumn.

Antitumor Activities

Rou Gui demonstrated the cytotoxic effect toward human HeLa (cervix), A549 (lung), SK-OV-3 (ovary), SK-MEL-2 (skin), HCT-15 (colon), and XF-498 (central nervous system) cancer cell lines *in vitro* and showed the inhibitory effect against Ehrlich ascites carcinoma in mice.[1–3] The apoptosis-inducing and antiproliferative effects in mouse melanoma cells were elucidated to directly link with the abilities to repress NF-κB and AP-1 activities and their target gene (Bcl-2, BcL-xL, and survivin) expressions. The antigrowth effect of the extract on neoplasm was further shown in melanoma transplantation model *in vivo* by oral administration.[4]

Moreover, ACE-c, an aqueous extract prepared from the herb, markedly exhibited two interesting effects in human SiHa cervical cancer cells, i.e., (1) apoptosis-inducing effect through loss of mitochondrial membrane potential and increase in intracellular calcium signaling and (2) migration-reducing effect by diminishing the expressions of MMP-2 and Her-2 (an oncoprotein).[4] In addition, the butanolic fractions of Rou Gui displayed a remarkable inhibitory effect against the activity of tumor metastasis-related MMP-9 at a concentration of 100 μg/mL with its suppressive rate of >90%.[5] These findings suggested that the aqueous extract is valuable for further development as a chemopreventive remedy in cervical cancer.

Antitumor Constituents and Activities

The principal and active constituent in the herb was characterized as *trans*-cinnamaldehyde (Cin) (**1**), whose cytotoxic effect on HeLa, SK-MEL-2, and HCT-15 carcinoma cells was comparable to that of cisplatin and mitomycin-C with ED_{50} values of 0.63–8.1 μg/L but not sensitive to A549, SKOV-3, and XF-498 tumor cells *in vitro*.[3] The injection of Cin (**1**) to mice completely obstructed the carcinogenesis caused by SV40 viruses.[2] Cin (**1**) potently promoted the apoptosis of human HL-60 promyelocytic leukemia cells.[6] Cin (**1**), cinnamic acid (Ca), and cinnamyl alcohol (Cal) also exerted the antiproliferative and apoptosis-inducing activities in human HepG2 hepatoma cells. At the same of 30 μM, the order of antiproliferative potency on the HepG2 cells was Cin > Ca > Cal, where Cin (**1**) displayed almost the same anticancer potency level as 5-FU (IC_{50}: 9.76 versus 9.57 μM).[7]

Two cinnamaldehyde derivatives were found exerting a significant anticarcinoma effect. 2′-Hydroxycinnamaldehyde (HCA) (**2**) was isolated from Rou Gui and 2′-benzoyloxycinnamaldehyde (BCA) (**3**) was prepared by the reaction of HCA and PhCOCl. Both HCA (**2**) and BCA (**3**) significantly inhibited the proliferation of human tumor cells *in vitro* and restrained the growth of human SW-620 colon tumor xenograft in nude mice without losing body weight.[8] The treatment with HCA (**2**) and BCA (**3**) for 10 weeks, respectively, delayed the development of H-ras12V-induced hepatocellular carcinoma, associated with an inhibition of farnesyl transferase and an immunostimulation on T cells.[6] HCA (**4**) exhibited antiproliferative and antigrowth effects in HCT116 human colorectal cancer cells *in vitro* and *in vivo* (IC_{50}: 6.17 μM, 72 h), accompanied by the suppression of a Wnt/β-catenin cell signaling pathway.[9] Eugenol (**5**) demonstrated the moderate suppressive effects on the SKOV-3 (ovary), HCT-15 (colon), and XF-498 (CNS) human neoplastic cell lines *in vitro*.[3]

In addition, the bark and the roots of another plant of the same genus *C. osmophloeum* are widely used in Taiwan as spice substitutes for *C. cassia*. From its heartwood and roots, several lignan components were isolated. Cytotoxicity assays of these lignans revealed that a cyclolignan ester assigned as (7′S,8′R,8R)-lyoniresinol-9,9′-di-*O*-(E)-feruloyl ester was effective in the inhibition of human HepG2 and Hep3B hepatoma cells and oral carcinoma Ca9-22 cells *in vitro*, with IC_{50} values of 7.87, 4.31, and 2.51 μg/mL, respectively.[10]

Mechanism Exploration

The anticancer and apoptosis-inducing mechanisms of the cinnamaldehydes was found to mainly to be associated with (1) increase of ROS; (2) transduction of apoptotic signals including the downregulation of Bcl-2 and the activation of caspase-3; (3) inhibition of DNA-binding activity of AP-1 accompanied by the decrease of c-Jun and c-Fos expressions; (4) decline of proteasome activity that leads to increase of ER stress and mitochondrial perturbation; (5) induction of mitochondrial permeability transition and release of cytochrome c to cytosol; as well as (6) orientation of a T cell differentiation through the suppression of farnesyl-protein transferase.[5–14] The apoptosis-induction in HepG2 cells was mediated by the p53- and CD95 (APO-1)-signaling pathways, i.e., the downregulation of Bcl-xL expression, the upregulation of CD95 (APO-1), p53, and Bax proteins, and the cleave of the PARP.[8] The hepatoma development delayed by BCA (**3**) was also correlated to a long-term immunostimulating effect on T cells, including the augmentation of the splenocyte proliferation and the lymphocyte infiltration into the liver.[11]

In general, the activation of p38-mitogen-activated protein kinase, an increase of ROS generation, and the downregulation of Bcl-2 occurred in both nondrug-resistant and drug-resistant cancer cell lines. Most likely through the pathways, BCA (**3**) treatment was able to exert similar growth inhibitory effects and apoptotic death on the drug-resistant cancer cells and their parental cancer cells, implying that BCA (**3**) may be developed as a useful drug candidate for treating drug-resistant tumor cells.[5,15]

Other Bioactivities

The herb Rou Gui (Chinese cinnamon) demonstrated multiple biological activities such as antiulcerative, hypotensive, antiinflammatory, leukogenic, radiation protective, antithrombocyte-agglutinative effects. Rou Gui also notably augments coronary flow and cerebral flow, improves acute myocardial ischemia, promotes secretion of gastric juice and salivary gland, and enhances digestive function.

An investigation reported a significant additional benefit of the herb for the treatment of patients with type II diabetes, where Rou Gui (cinnamon) markedly decreased fasting blood sugar, but it does not have an effect on hemoglobin A1C (a biological marker of long-term diabetes). The effects on enhancing insulin sensitivity might be mediated by the polyphenols of Rou Gui.[16,17] In addition, Rou Gui is commonly used as a flavoring agent for desserts, pastries, confectionary, and meat. But some cinnamon oil-entrained agents (such as styrene, cinnamaldehyde, and coumarin) were proven to be toxic in their high concentrations.

References

1. Haranaka, K. et al. 1985. Antitumor activities and tumor necrosis factor producibility of traditional Chinese medicines and crude drugs. *Cancer Immunol. Immunother* 20: 1–5.
2. Kwon, B. M. et al. 1998. Synthesis and *in vitro* cytotoxicity of cinnamaldehydes to human solid tumor cells. *Archiv. Pharm. Res.* 21: 147–52.
3. Lee, H. et al. 2004. Cytotoxic and mutagenic effects of *Cinnamomum cassia* bark-derived materials. *J. Microbiol. Biotechnol.* 14: 1176–81.
4. Koppikar, S. J. et al. 2010. Aqueous cinnamon extract (ACE-c) from the bark of *Cinnamomum cassia* causes apoptosis in human cervical cancer cell line (SiHa) through loss of mitochondrial membrane potential. *BMC Cancer* 10: 210.
5. Seo, U. K. et al. 2005. Large-scale and effective screening of Korean medicinal plants for inhibitory activity on matrix metalloproteinase-9. *J. Ethnopharmacol.* 97: 101–6.
6. Ka, H. et al. 2003. Cinnamaldehyde induces apoptosis by ROS-mediated mitochondrial permeability transition in human promyelocytic leukemia HL-60 cells. *Cancer Lett.* (Oxford, U.K.) 196: 143–52.
7. Ng, L. T. et al. 2011. Antiproliferative activity of Cinnamomum cassia constituents and effects of pifithrin-alpha on their apoptotic signaling pathways in HepG2 cells. *Evidence-Based Complem. Alternat. Med.* 2011: 492148.
8. Lee, C. W. et al. 1999. Inhibition of human tumor growth by 2′-hydroxy- and 2′-benzoyloxycinnam-aldehydes. *Planta Med.* 65: 263–6.
9. Lee, M.-A. et al. 2013. Antitumor activity of 2-hydroxycinnamaldehyde for human colon cancer cells through suppression of β-catenin signaling. *J. Nat. Prod.* 76: 1278–84.
10. Moon, E. Y. et al. 2006. Delayed occurrence of H-ras12V-induced hepatocellular carcinoma with long-term treatment with cinnamaldehydes. *Eur. J. Pharmacol.* 53: 270–5.
11. Hong, S. H. et al. 2007. Apoptosis induction of 2′-hydroxycinnamaldehyde as a proteasome inhibitor is associated with ER stress and mitochondrial perturbation in cancer cells. 2007. *Biochem. Pharmacol.* 74: 557–65.
12. Lee, C. W. et al. 2007. 2-Hydroxycinnamaldehyde inhibits SW620 colon cancer cell growth through AP-1 inactivation. *J. Pharmacol. Sci.* (Tokyo, Jpn) 104: 19–28.
13. Koh, W. S. et al. 1998. Cinnamaldehyde inhibits proliferation and modulates T-cell differentiation. *Intl. J. Immunopharmacol.* 20: 643–60.
14. Chung, Y. M. et al. 2007. The activity of 2′-benzoyloxycinnamaldehyde against drug- resistant cancer cell lines. *J. Chemother.* 19: 428–37.
15. Lu, T. et al. 2012. Cinnamon extract improves fasting blood glucose and glycosylated hemoglobin level in Chinese patients with type 2 diabetes. *Nutri. Res.* 2002. 32: 408–22.
16. Howard, M. E. et al. 2013. Potential benefits of cinnamon in Type 2 diabetes. *Am. J. Lifestyle Med.* 7: 23–6.

98 Wu Zhu Yu 吴茱萸

Evodia fruit

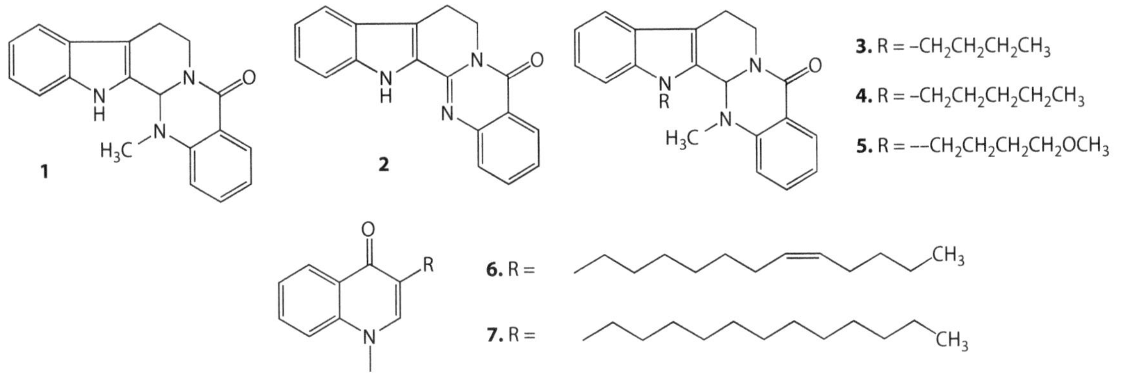

3. R = $-CH_2CH_2CH_2CH_3$

4. R = $-CH_2CH_2CH_2CH_2CH_3$

5. R = $-CH_2CH_2CH_2CH_2OCH_3$

6. R =

7. R =

Herb Origination

The major source of Wu Zhu Yu (Evodia fruit) is the dried immature fruits of a Rutaceae plant, *Evodia rutaecarpa*, as well as its two varieties var. *officinalis* and var. *bodinieri*. The immature fruits are generally collected in July and August and dried in the sun or at a low temperature for Chinese folk medicinal uses. Wu Zhu Yu was documented as a middle class medicine in *Shennong Bencao Jing*, the first Chinese classic of materia medica.

Antitumor Constituents and Activity

Indoloquinazoline Alkaloids

Two indoloquinazoline alkaloids, evodiamine (**1**) and rutaecarpine (**2**), are the major components in Wu Zhu Yu. Both displayed a cytotoxic effect against CCRF-CEM leukemia cells *in vitro* with IC_{50} values of 2.64–4.53 μM.[1] Compared to rutaecarpine (**2**), evodiamine (**1**) exhibited a broader spectrum of antineoplastic property, whose cytotoxic effect was observed in various human carcinoma cell lines, such as KB (nasopharyngeal), HeLa (cervix), A375-S2 (skin), Colo205 (colorectal), SPC-A-1 and NCI-H446 (lung), MCF-7 (breast), PC3 and DU-145 (prostate), SGC-7901 (stomach), THP-1 (monocytic leukemia), U937 (lymphoma), ARO (thyroid), and K562 and CCRF-CEM/C1 (leukemia) cells, and a variety of murine carcinoma cell lines: Lewis (lung), B16-F10 (skin), 26-L5 (colon), P388 (leukemia), and L929 (fibrosarcoma) cells.[2–8] The IC_{50} values were 0.43 μg/mL on P388 cells, 0.98 μg/mL on KB cells, and 1.25 μg/mL on 26-L5 cells.[2–5] At a 1 μM concentration, evodiamine (**1**) strongly repressed the expression of HSP27 gene in HeLa cervical cancer, Colo205 colon carcinoma, and SK-N-Mc neuroblastoma cell lines.[4] The antigrowth effect of evodiamine (**1**) was further verified in mouse models against MFC forestomach carcinoma, sarcoma 180, and HepA hepatoma,[2–5] whose antitumor activity were similar to those of cisplatin (a chemotherapeutic drug), but cisplatin did seriously lessen the body weight of mice, whereas evodiamine (**1**) did not. Rutaecarpine (**2**) was *in vitro* effective in the inhibition of neoplastic cell lines such as U251 (CNS), HT-29 (colon), A549/ATCC (lung), OVCAR-4 (ovary), and HS-578T (breast). Its most active was in U251 cells with GI_{50} value of 0.02 μM, and its moderate suppression was shown on other four carcinoma cell lines with GI_{50} values in a range of 14.5–31.6 μM.[9] At a dose of 5 mg/kg, rutaecarpine (**2**) significantly restrained the growth of both sarcoma 180 and H22 hepatoma *in vivo* but showed little toxicity to the spleen and the thymus.[10]

Moreover, evodiamine (**1**) also dose-dependently obstructed the invasion of B16-F10 melanoma cells, Lewis lung cancer cells, and 26-L5 colon cancer cells with IC_{50} values of 2.4, 4.8, and 3.7 μM, respectively. Its inhibitory rate on 26-L5 cell invasion and migration reached to about 70% at 10 μg/mL of evodiamine (**1**).[5] The preadministration of evodiamine (**1**) at a dose of 10 μg/mL to mice before the inoculation of the Lewis cells or B16-F10 cells elicited a significant suppressive effect on the lung metastasis and the liver metastasis. When evodiamine (**1**) was administered to mice in a dose of 10 μg/mL from the sixth day after tumor inoculation, the numbers of tumor nodules in the lungs was attenuated by 48%.[11,12] Evodiamine (**1**) is also a dual catalytic inhibitor of human Topo-I and Topo-II (important targets for anticancer drugs) with IC_{50} values of 60.74 and 78.81 μM, respectively. Due to the property, it could enhance the antigrowth effect against camptothecin-resistant carcinoma cells.[13] Both *in vitro* and *in vivo* experiments demonstrated that evodiamine (**1**) exerts the anti-proliferative effect against Adm-resistant human breast cancer NCI/ADRRES cells in a concentration-dependent manner, concomitant with the induction of a substantial apoptosis and G2/M cell arrest and the enhancement of tubulin polymerization.[14] The results evidenced that evodiamine (**1**) may be useful for reversing MDR and blocking cancer invasion and metastasis. Additionally, a bioactivity–structure relationship analysis revealed that the presence of a methyl group at N14 and a proton of β-configuration at C-13b may be largely responsible for the anticancer potency of evodiamine (**1**).[11]

N13-Evodiamine Derivatives

For improving the anticancer activity and the bioavailability of evodiamine, 38 N13-substituted evodiamine derivatives were designed, synthesized, and assessed in six kinds of human cancer cell lines, i.e., prostate cancer (PC3 and DU-145), lung cancer (H460), breast cancer (MCF-7), colon cancer (HCT-5), and glioblastoma (SF-268). Of them, N13-butylevodiamine (**3**), N13-pentylevodiamine (**4**), N13-(4-methoxybutyl)evodiamine (**5**), and N1,6-bis-(evodiamin-N13-yl)hexane displayed obviously improved solubility and antiproliferative effects on the cancer cell lines, and N13-(4-methoxybutyl)evodiamine (**5**) showed the most potent inhibitory activity and a broader spectrum of activity against the tested cancer cell lines (IC_{50}: 1–2 μM).[15] The appropriate substitution on N13-position of evodiamine could augment the cytotoxicity and broaden the antitumor spectra, but the derivatives are still unsuitable for clinical application because of its poor solubilities.

Quinolone Alkaloids

Seventeen quinolone alkaloids isolated from the dried and nearly ripe fruits of *E. rutaecarpa* were evaluated in four human neoplastic cell lines, HL-60 (leukemia), HepG2 (hepatoma), H460 (lung tumor), and N87 (gastric cancer), *in vitro*. These alkaloids such as evocarpine (**6**), dihydroevocarpine (**7**), 1-methyl-2-[7-hydroxy-(E)-9-tridecenyl]-4(1H)-quinolone, 1-methyl-2-[(Z)-4-nonenyl]-4(1H)-quinolone, 1-methyl-2-[(1E,5Z)-1,5-undecadienyl]-4(1H)-quinolone, and 1-methyl-2-[(E)-1-undecenyl]-4(1H)-quinolone showed a moderate inhibitory activity against the proliferation of the tested cancer cell lines with IC_{50} values of 14–22 μM.[16,17] The major structural differences in the 17 alkaloids are the length of the aliphatic side chain and the number of double bonds. The bioassay results indicated that the longer aliphatic side chain at C-2 of the quinolone alkaloids conferred a relatively stronger antiproliferative effect, and the presence of double bonds could slightly improve the inhibitory effect on the tested carcinoma cell lines.[16] Also, evocarpine (**6**) was able to activate protein kinase-A and promote the apoptosis of HL-60 promyeocytic leukemia cells in a concentration-dependent manner.[18] Two quinolones, dihydroevocarpine (**7**) and 1-methyl-2-undecyl-4-quinolone were shown to be modest inhibitors of P-gp activity, implying that they might have an antidrug-resistant potential.[1]

Exploration of Mechanism

The remarkable anticancer property of evodiamine (**1**) attracted researchers to explore its mechanisms. The studies revealed four distinct pathways involved in the anticancer mechanisms of evodiamine (**1**) in human A375-S2 melanoma cells, i.e., (1) induction of the cell apoptotic death at an early stage, accompanied by the down-expression of Bcl-2, the up-expression of Bax, and the activation of caspase-3; (2) initiation of MAPK-dependent necrosis at a later stage via the increase of p38 phosphorylation and the decrease of ERK expression and phosphorylation; (3) repression of PI3-K/PKC survival pathway and subsequent inhibition of ERK cascade; and (4) reduction of an antiapoptotic protein SIRT1 expression and augmentation of p53 activity and its phosphorylation, whose p53 activation was found to correlate with the activation of a proapoptotic pathway and the inhibition of a PI3-K/PKC survival pathway.[19,20]

Moreover, the synchronized role of autophagy and apoptosis was activated in the evodiamine-treated human SGC-7901 gastric adenocarcinoma cells besides the cell cycle arrest at G2/M phase, leading to growth suppression.[21] The mitotic arrest and the subsequent mitotic slippage were also participated in the evodiamine-promoted SGC-7901 cell apoptosis.[22] Similarly, the treatment of human glioblastoma cells with evodiamine not only elicited intracellular calcium/JNK signaling-mediated autophagy but also enlarged calcium/mitochondria-mediated apoptosis in dose- and time-dependent manners.[23] The antiproliferative effect of evodiamine (**1**) on Colo205 colon cancer cells was primarily accompanied by the promotion of apoptosis and G2/M cell arrest by upregulating p53 activity and Bax expression, declining Bcl-2 expression, and provoking loss of mitochondrial transmembrane potential and caspase-3 activation.[24] In addition, a typical apoptotic death of L929 cells initiated by evodiamine (**1**) was closely accompanied by the induction of cell cycle arrest at G0/G1 phase.[25]

Hepatocyte growth factor (HGF) is one of the factors that significantly stimulate the invasion and migration of cancer cells. The suppressive effect of evodiamine (**1**) on HGF-induced invasion and migration was confirmed in colon 26-L5 cancer, B16-F10 melanoma, and LLC cell lines in a concentration-dependent manner. At a 30 μM concentration, it displayed complete inhibition against the metastasis of three cancer cell lines *in vitro*, whose mechanism was partly correlated with the inhibition of cell spreading.[26] Furthermore, evodiamine (**1**) is a highly potent inhibitor of NF-κB activation, and it can abrogate both inducible and constitutive NF-κB activation and sequentially obstruct the NF-κB-dependent reporter gene expression such as IκBα phosphorylation, IκBα kinase activity, IκBα degradation, p65 phosphorylation, p65 acetylation, and p65 nuclear translocation. Evodiamine (**1**) also markedly suppressed TNF-induced Akt activation and all NF-κB-regulated gene products (such as cyclin-D1, c-Myc, COX-2, MMP-9, ICAM-1, MDR1, survivin, XIAP, IAP1, IAP2, FLIP, Bcl-2, Bcl-xL, and Bfl-1/A1). All the interactions might provide the multiple mechanism characteristics for evodiamine (**1**) in obstructing the tumor cell proliferation, promoting the apoptosis and cell cycle arrest, and repressing the invasion and metastasis.[27]

Nanoformulation

EVO-NPs is a nanoparticle of evodiamine (**1**), which was established by the use of a gelatinase cleavage peptide with PEG and poly(ε-caprolactone). EVO-NPs were found to be transformed by gelatinases to significantly promote drug delivery and to enhance the cellular uptake of evodiamine. Both *in vitro* and *in vivo* data showed that the EVO-NPs exerted higher growth suppression than the free evodiamine on mouse H22 hepatoma model via intravenous administration. The finding suggested that the EVO-NPs may be promising for the improvement of antitumor efficacy in various overexpressed gelatinase cancers.[28]

Other Bioactivities

The herb Wu Zhu Yu (Evodia fruit) is often used in traditional Chinese medicine to treat inflammatory diseases (such as hemorrhage, dysentery, postpartum, and amenorrhea), painful conditions (such as headaches and abdominal pain), and cardiovascular and endocrine systems. Researches afforded more evidences for the herb possessing antigastric ulcer, digestive tonic, antidiarrheal, hepatoprotective, antiinflammatory, antithrombotic, antiemetic, antiobesity, anthelminthic, antiplatelet aggregation, analgesic, thermoregulatory, vasorelaxing, choleretic, immunomoderating, and antibacterial activities. The herb can obviously stimulate the secretion of IL-1β, IL-6, TNFα, and GM-CSF from mononuclear cells at a low dose.[29] However, the herb requires professional guidance for safe usage, and it is proscribed to be used by pregnant women in the Chinese herb tradition.

The two major constituents in Wu Zhu Yu have been studied to show that evodiamine (**1**) possesses antioxidant and anti-inflammatory activities, and trutaecarpine (**2**) has cardiovascular, antithrombosis, and antiplatelet aggregation, activities, etc.[3]

References

1. Adams, M. et al. 2007. Cytotoxicity and p-glycoprotein modulating effects of quinolones and indolo-quinazolines from the Chinese herb Evodia rutaecarpa. *Planta Med.* 73: 1554–7.
2. Li, G. Z. et al. 2005. Studies on the antitumor activities of alkaloid from Evodia rutaecarpa. *Zhongyao Yanjiu yu Xinxi* 7: 11–14.
3. Itokawa, H. et al. 1990. *Shioyaku Gaku Zashi* 444: 135.
4. Seiho, Y. et al. 1996. *Jpn. Kokai Tokkyo Koho* (1996), 7 pp., JP1996-214315.
5. Ogasawara, M. et al. 2001. Screening of natural compounds for inhibitory activity on colon cancer cell migration. *Biol. Pharm. Bull.* 24: 720–3.
6. Lee, T. J. et al. 2006. Caspase-dependent and caspase-independent apoptosis induced by evodiamine in human leukemic U937 cells. *Mol. Cancer Therapeutics* 5: 2398–2407.
7. Chen, M. C. et al. 2010. Anti-proliferative effects of evodiamine on human thyroid cancer cell line ARO. *J. Cell. Biochem.* 110: 1495–503.
8. Kan, S. F. et al. 2007. Anti-proliferative effects of evodiamine on human prostate cancer cells DU145 and PC3. *J. Cell. Biochem.* 101: 44–56.
9. Lee, S. H. et al. 2008. Progress in the studies on rutaecarpine. *Mol.* 13: 272–80.
10. Guo, H. et al. 2010. Synthesis, structure characterization of rutaecarpine and its antitumor activity in vivo. *Chem. Bioeng.* 27: 37–40.
11. Ogasawara, M. et al. 2002. Anti-invasive and metastatic activities of evodiamine. *Biol. Pharm. Bull.* 25: 1491–3.
12. Ogasawara, M. et al. 2001. Inhibitory effects of evodiamine on *in vitro* invasion and experimental lung metastasis of murine colon cancer cells. *Biol. Pharm. Bull.* 24: 917–20.
13. Pan, X. B. et al. 2012. Evodiamine, a dual catalytic inhibitor of type I and II topoisomerases, exhibits enhanced inhibition against camptothecin resistant cells. *Phytomed.* 19: 618–24.
14. Liao, C. W. et al. 2005. Antitumor mechanism of evodiamine, a constituent from Chinese herb *Evodiae fructus*, in human multiple-drug resistant breast cancer NCI/ADR-RES cells in vitro and in vivo. *Carcinogenesis* 26: 968–75.
15. Song, S. C. et al. 2013. Design, synthesis and evaluation of N13-substituted evodiamine derivatives against human cancer cell lines. *Mol.* 18: 15750–68.
16. Huang, X. et al. 2012. New cytotoxic quinolone alkaloids from fruits of *Evodia rutaecarpa. Fitoterapia* 83: 709–14.
17. Ishii, E. et al. 2000. Quinolone alkaloids for the inhibition of *Helicobacter pylori. Jpn. Kokai Tokkyo Koho* JP 2000302682 A 20001031.
18. Kim, N. Y. et al. 2000. Cyclic adenosine monophosphate inhibits quinolone alkaloid evocarpine-induced apoptosis via activation of protein kinase A in human leukaemic HL-60 cells. *Pharmacol. Toxicol.* (Copenhagen) 87: 1–5.
19. Wang, C. et al. 2005. Roles of SIRT1 and phosphoinositide 3-OH kinase/protein kinase C pathways in evodiamine-induced human melanoma A375-S2 cell death. *J. Pharmacol. Sci.* (Jpn) 97: 494–500.
20. Zhang, Y. et al. 2003. Intracellular regulation of evodiamine-induced A375-S2 cell death. *Biol. Pharm. Bull.* 26: 1543–7.
21. Rasul, A. et al. 2012. Cytotoxic effect of evodiamine in SGC-7901 human gastric adenocarcinoma cells via simultaneous induction of apoptosis and autophagy. *Oncol. Reports* 27: 1481–7.
22. Zhu, L. H. et al. 2011. Induction of apoptosis by evodiamine, involves both activation of mitotic arrest and mitotic slippage. *Oncol. Reports* 26: 1447–55.
23. Liu, A. J. et al. 2013. Evodiamine, a plant alkaloid, induces calcium/JNK-mediated autophagy and calcium/mitochondria-mediated apoptosis in human glioblastoma cells. *Chemico-Biol. Interactions* 205: 20–8.
24. Yang, Z. G. et al. 2009. Antiproliferation and apoptosis induced by evodiamine in human colorectal carcinoma cells (Colo-205). *Chem. Biodiv.* 6: 924–33.
25. Zhang, Y. et al. 2004. Atypical apoptosis in L929 cells induced by evodiamine isolated from *Evodia rutaecarpa. J. Asian Nat. Prod. Res.* 6: 19–27.
26. Ogasawara, M. et al. 2004. Inhibition by evodiamine of hepatocyte growth factor-induced invasion and migration of tumor cells. *Biol. Pharm. Bull.* 27: 578–82.
27. Takada, Y. et al. 2005. Evodiamine abolishes constitutive and inducible NF-κB activation by inhibiting IκBα kinase activation, thereby suppressing NF-κB regulated antiapoptotic and metastatic gene expression, upregulating apoptosis, and inhibiting invasion. *J. Biol. Chem.* 280: 17203–12.
28. Zhang, Q. N. et al. 2013. Tumor delivery efficiency and apoptosis enhancement by EVO nanoparticles on Murie hepatic carcinoma cell line H22. *J. Biomed. Nanotechnol.* 9: 1354–61.
29. Chang, C. P. et al. 1995. The effect of *Evodia rutaecarpa* extract on cytokine secretion by human mononuclear cells in vitro. *Am. J. Chin. Med.* 23: 173–80.

99 Rou Dou Kou 肉豆蔻

Nutmeg

1

9

14

2. $R_1 = -CH_2- = R_2$, $R_3 = -CH_2- = R_4$, $R_5 = -H$
6. $R_1 = -CH_3$, $R_2 = R_5 = -H$, $R_3 = -CH_2- = R_4$
7. $R_1 = -CH_2- = R_2$, $R_3 = -CH_3$, $R_4 = -H$, $R_5 = -OH$
8. $R_1 = R_3 = -CH_3$, $R_2 = R_4 = R_5 = -H$

3. $R_1 = -CH_2- = R_2$
10. $R_1 = R_3 = -CH_3$, $R_2 = R_4 = -H$

4. $R_1 = -CH_3$, $R_2 = -H$
5. $R_1 = -CH_2- = R_2$
13. $R_1 = R_2 = -H$

12

18. $R = -CH_3$
19. $R = -H$

15. $R = -H$
16. $R = -OH$

20

Herb Origination

The herb Rou Dou Kou (Nutmeg) is the dried seed kernel of a tropical Myristicaceae tree, *Myristica fragrans*. The plants are principally produced in Asian tropical regions such as Indonesia, Malaysia, and West Indian Islands. Thus, the herb used in traditional Chinese medicine is imported overseas. Mace is the aril covering the seed, which is commonly used as spice in cuisines.

Antitumor Activities

Mace (aril covering the seed) demonstrated a chemopreventive effect against cervical carcinogenesis induced by 3-methylcholanthrene in mice. If mace was preadministered orally at a dose of 10 mg/mouse per day for 7 days before and 90 days following the carcinogen thread insertion, the incidence of cervical carcinogenesis could be significantly declined from 73.9% of the control group to 21.4%.[1] DMBA-induced papillomagenesis in the skin of mice was obviously reduced 50% by giving a diet containing 1% mace during the tumorigenesis.[2] Besides the anticarcinogenetic activity, the methanol extract of mace at the concentrations of 50 and 100 μg/mL markedly inhibited the proliferation of Jurkat human leukemia T-cells and induced the cell apoptosis in a mechanism involving SIRTI mRNA downregulation.[3] The methanolic extract also demonstrated a potent suppressive effect on the proliferation of human A549 (lung), SKOV-3 (ovary), SK-MEL-2 (skin), XF498 (CNS), and HCT-15 (colon) tumor cell lines *in vitro*.[4] The essential oil of nutmeg, in an *in vitro* model, displayed the moderate antiproliferative effect against human HCT-116 (colorectal), and MCF-7 (breast) carcinoma cell lines with IC_{50} values of 78.61 and 66.45 μg/mL, respectively, implying that the nutmeg oil has a potential to be developed as an anticarcinogenic and antioxidant drug. According to a gas chromatography mass spectrometry analysis, 8 compounds were identified in nutmeg oil.[5]

Antitumor Constituents and Activities

In the continuous effort, many lignans and phenolic components were discovered as neoplastic inhibitors from the herb, i.e., safrole (**1**), machilin-A (**2**) and machilin-F (**3**), licarin-A (**4**) and licarin-B (**5**), macelignan (**6**), myristargenol-A (**7**), meso-dihydroguaiaretic acid (**8**), methoxyeugenol (**9**), nectandrin-B (**10**), 2-(4-allyl-2,6-dimethoxyphenoxy)-1-(4-hydroxy-3-methoxyphenyl) propan-1-ol (**11**), *erythro*-(7*S*,8*R*)-$\Delta^{8'}$-4,7-dihydroxy-3,3′,5′-trimethoxy-8-O-4′-neolignan-8′-ene (**12**), (7R,8R)-7,8-dihydro-7-(3,4-dihydroxyphenyl)-3′-methoxy-8-methyl-1′-(E-propenyl)-benzofuran (**13**), (7S,8S,7′R,8′S)-4,5′-dihydroxy-3,3′-dimethoxy-7,7′-epoxylignan (**14**), 1-(2,6-dihydroxyphenyl)-9-(4-hydroxyphenyl)-1-nonanone (**15**), 1-(2,6-dihydroxyphenyl)-9-(3,4-di-hydroxyphenyl)-1-nonanone (**16**), as well as (E)-3-(3-methyl-5-pentylfuran-2-yl) acrylic acid (**17**). *In vitro* assays showed that the lignans **1–11** and the fatty acid (**17**) repressed the proliferation of cultured human A549 (lung), SKOV-3 (ovary), SK-MEL-2 (skin), and HCT-15 (colon) tumor cell lines,[4–6] whereas the three other lignans **12–14** and two phenolics **15–16** displayed moderate cytotoxicity with IC_{50} values in a range of 2.11–4.92 μM in human K562 leukemia cells *in vitro*.[7] The i.p. injection of the phenolic inhibitor (1-(2,6-dihydroxyphenyl)-9-(3,4-di-hydroxyphenyl)-1-nonanone (16)) prolonged the life span of mice implanted with sarcoma 180.[8] The cytotoxicity of meso-dihydroguaiaretic acid (**8**) was present in human H358 lung carcinoma cells in allogeneic tumor-bearing mice model with an IC_{50} value of 10.1 μM.[9] Other isolated lignans were evaluated in human neoplastic cell lines (HL-60, MCF-7, and A549) *in vitro*, and some of them showed cytotoxicity.[10]

Three other antitumor agents, assigned as nordihydroguaiaretic acid (NDGA) (**18**), dihydroguaiaretic acid (DGA) (**19**), and curcumin (**20**), were also isolated from Mace. The anticancer property of NDGA (**18**), DGA (**19**), and curcumin (**20**) was also demonstrated *in vivo* and *in vitro* toward leukemia, lung carcinoma, and colon cancer cells.[11] Moreover, the ethanolic extract of Rou Dou Kou was also able to effectively improve the T cell percentage and increase the indexes of the spleen and the thymus.[12] Freeze-dried water extract from the leaves of *M. fragrans* demonstrated antimutagenic and free radicals-scavenging activities.[13]

In addition, the investigations further found that macelignan (**6**) showed the protective effect against cisplatin-induced hepatotoxicity in mice, whose mechanism was revealed to correlate to the activation of a MAPK signaling pathway. The finding recommended that the cotreatment of macelignan (**6**) with cisplatin may provide more advantage in the treatment and the prevention of hepatoma.

Other Bioactivities

In traditional Chinese medicine, Rou Dou Kou (Nutmeg) and its oil are usually employed for the treatment of disorders related to the nervous and digestive systems. Modern studies showed the herb possesses sedative, antiinflammatory, and smooth muscle-effective activities besides anticancer and anticarcinogenesis. Mace and nutmeg exhibited no noticeable side effects or neurological response at low doses, but their large overdoses may cause toxic symptoms and harm. Additionally, ground nutmeg is often used for flavoring many cuisines and foods in the world. The essential oil derived from the nutmeg is also widely used in perfumery, cosmetic, and pharmaceutical industries.

References

1. Husain, S. P. et al. 1991. Chemopreventive action of mace (*Myristica fragrans*, Houtt) on methylcholanthrene-induced carcinogenesis in the uterine cervix in mice. *Cancer Lett.* 56: 231–4.
2. Jannu, L. N. et al. 1991. Chemopreventive action of mace (*Myristica fragrans*, Houtt) on DMBA-induced papillomagenesis in the skin of mice. *Cancer Lett.* 56: 59–63.
3. Chirathaworn, C. et al. 2007. *Myristica fragrans* Houtt. methanolic extract induces apoptosis in a human leukemia cell line through SIRT1 mRNA down-regulation. *J. Med. Assoc. Thailand* 90: 2422–8.
4. Lee, J. W. et al. 2006. Inhibitory effects of the seed extract of Myristicae semen on the proliferation of human tumor cell lines. (II). *Saengyak Hakhoechi* 37: 206–11.
5. Piaru, S. P. et al. 2012. Chemical composition, antioxidant and cytotoxicity activities of the essential oils of Myristica fragrans and *Morinda citrifolia*. *J. Sci. Food Agricul.* 92: 593–7.
6. Lee, J. W. et al. 2005. Inhibitory effects of the seed extract of *Myristica fragrans* on the proliferation of human tumor cell lines. *Saengyak Hakhoechi* 36: 240–4.
7. Duan, L. et al. 2009. Cytotoxic and antioxidative phenolic compounds from the traditional Chinese medicinal plant, *Myristica fragrans*. *Planta Med.* 75: 1241–5.
8. Nakajima, I. et al. 1989. Myristica fragrans extract as neoplasm inhibitor. *Jpn. Kokai Tokkyo Koho* 5 pp. Application: JP 87-200400 19870811.
9. Thuong, P. T. et al. 2014. Cytotoxic and antitumor activities of lignans from the seeds of Vietnamese nutmeg *Myristica fragrans*. *Archiv. Pharm. Res.* 37: 399–403.
10. Cuong, T. D. et al. 2012. Compounds from the seeds of *Myristica fragrans* and their cytotoxic activity. *Nat. Prod. Sci.* 18: 97–101.
11. Park, S. Y. et al. 1998. Inhibition of fos-jun-DNA complex formation by dihydroguaiaretic acid and in vitro cytotoxic effects on cancer cells. *Cancer Lett.* 127: 23–8.
12. Pei, L. P. et al. 2009. Effect of *Myristica fragrans* Houtt on antitumor and immune regulate on in entrails. *Chin. J. Ethnomed. Ethnopharm* 18: 23–4.
13. Akinboro, A. et al. 2011. Antioxidants in aqueous extract of *Myristica fragrans* (Houtt.) suppress mitosis and cyclophosphamide-induced chromosomal aberrations in Allium cepa L. cells. *J. Zhejiang Univ. Sci. B.* 12: 915–22.

5

Anticancer Potentials of Vital Energy-Regulating Herbs

CONTENTS

100 Shan You Gan 山油柑

Acronychia

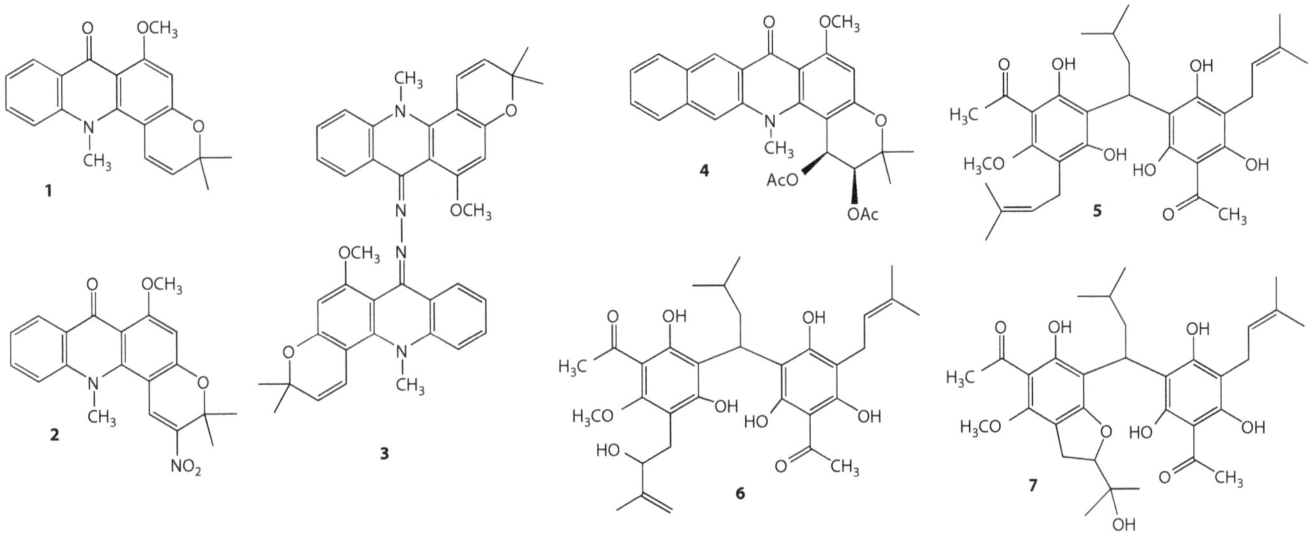

Herb Origination

The herb Shan You Gan (Acronychia) is the dried root or the marrow wood of a Rutaceae plant, *Acronychia pedunculata*. This plant is distributed in south and southeast Asia from India and Sri Lanka to South China, Indonesia, and Papua New Guinea. Generally, its roots and woods are collected in any season in China for folk medical application.

Antitumor Constituents and Activities

Alkaloids

From the marrow wood of Shan You Gan, an alkaloid elucidated as acronycine (**1**) was isolated that showed a broad spectrum of antineoplastic property. The oral administration of acronycine (**1**) in a dose of 40 mg/kg extremely extended the lifetime of mice implanted with L615 leukemia over 60 days and also prolonged the life span of mice inoculated with reticulum cell ascites tumor. A significant growth inhibitory activity of acronycine (**1**) was observed in mice bearing hepatoma or U14 cervical carcinoma in oral doses of 20 or 40 mg/kg.[1] Acronycine (**1**) also effectively obstructed the proliferation of X5563 plasmocyte myeloma cells, C1498 myeloid leukemia cells, and adenocarcinoma-755 cells *in vitro*.[2]

Acronycine (**1**) and its two modified analogs, i.e., 2-nitroacronycine (**2**) and acronycineazine (**3**), exhibited obvious cytotoxicity against several human breast, colon, lung, skin neoplastic cell lines as well as KB-3 and drug-resistant KB-V1. The cytotoxicity of the two derivatives was more potent than that of acronycine (**1**) on UISO-BCA-1 breast cancer cells *in vitro*. A single intraperitoneal (i.p.) administration of acronycine (**1**) at a dose of 25 mg/kg was effective at prolonging the life duration in mice implanted with MOPC-315 plasmacytoma.[3] Prominently, the sensitivity of these derivatives on drug-resistant KB-VI cells was greater than on its parent (drug-sensitive) KB cells.[4] The anticancer mechanism of acronycine azine (**3**) was revealed to be partly mediated by the arrest of cell cycle at G0/G1 phase and the inhibition of catalytic activities of DNA polymerase and RNA polymerase in the UISO-BCA-1 cells.[4]

Despite the marked antitumor properties against a small panel of solid tumor models, the moderate potency and the low water solubility of acronycine (**1**) sternly limited its usage in the succeeding clinical trials. When the lipophilic acronycine was solubilized in the cosolvent system used for etoposide, the solubility improved the acronycine showing a broad cytotoxic effect in fresh human tumor cells from patients with renal cell cancer, ovarian cancer, uterine cancer, or metastatic tumors of unknown primary. In P-gp-positive multidrug-resistant tumor cell lines, acronycine (**1**) in the etoposide diluent was active in the suppression of multidrug-resistant Chinese hamster ovary cells but not against MDR-L1210 murine leukemia cells, 8226 human myeloma cells, and human CCRF-CEM lymphoblasts. The i.p. injection of the acronycine containing 10% etoposide (v/v%) showed significant tumor growth delays in nude mice transplanted with human MCF-7 breast cancer xenografts and in mice implanted with colon 38 tumor.[3]

The investigations on SARs revealed the crucial role of the 1,2-double bond in the structure of acronycine (**1**). By the transformation of the 1,2-double bond into the corresponding oxirane or 1,2-epoxide, a group of acronycine derivatives with a broadened spectrum of antitumor were developed. Of these derivatives, 1,2-dihydroxy-1,2-dihydrobenzo-[b]acronycine esters, and its diesters demonstrated the suppressive effect on a human orthotopic model of cancers xenografted in nude mice.[5] S23906-1 (**4**) which is a benzo[b]acronycine derivative also exerted the impressive broad anticancer efficacy. By intravenous or oral administration, S23906-1 (**4**) showed comparable or better suppressive activity than the clinically used chemotherapeutic drugs in nude mice implanted with aggressive human neoplasm of the lung, the ovary, or the colon. In the *in vivo* experiments, S23906-1 (**4**) demonstrated selectivity to human solid carcinomas as compared to murine-transplantable tumors. The treatment with S23906-1 (**4**) could notably promote the apoptosis of human HL-60 promyelocytic leukemia cells and murine B16 melanoma cells, but the apoptosis-inducing effect was poorer in the B16 cells than in the HL-60 cells, whose antineoplastic mechanism was found to correlate with the cell cycle perturbations (G2/M arrest), covalent adducts with DNA, DNA alkylation, inhibition of DNA synthesis, and apoptosis promotion through the induction of chromatin condensation, cyclin-E protein modulation, ROS production, and activation of caspase-3.[6,7]

Acetophenones

An acetophenone dimer, assigned as acrovestone (**5**), was isolated from the stems and the root bark of *A. pedunculata*, which showed potent cytotoxicity toward human KB epidermoid cancer cells and against human A549 lung cancer cells, murine P388, and L1210 lymphocytic leukemia cells with ED_{50} of 0.98, 3.28, and 2.95 μg/mL, respectively. At its 0.5 μg/mL concentration, acrovestone (**5**) was able to exert 100% inhibition against the growth of KB cells.[8] From the trunk bark of *A. pedunculata*, three acetophenone dimers elucidated as acrovestone (**5**), acrovestenol (**6**), and acrofolione-A (**7**) were separated together with several acronychia-type acetophenones and furoquinoline alkaloids. In *in vitro* models, acrovestone (**5**) and acrovestenol (**6**) exhibited substantial cytotoxicity with IC_{50} values of 0.38 and 2.8 μM on human A2058 melanoma cells and 0.93 and 2.7 μM on human DU145 prostate cancer cells, respectively, whose inhibitory potencies were greater than the anticancer drug sorafenib. The antiproliferative effect of acrofolione A (**7**) was present only in the A2058 melanoma cell line (IC_{50}: 4.2 μM).[9] In addition, six acetophenone monomers were separated from the leaves and the twigs of *A. pedunculata*, which showed a lower effect on human HCT-116 colon carcinoma cells *in vitro*. Among them, acronyculatin-F was the most potent molecule on the HCT-116 cells. At a concentration of 100 μM, the cell viability was 8% after being treated with acronyculatin-F. Compared to the relatively weak effects of the acetophenone monomers, the acetophenone dimeric skeleton contributed more marked cytotoxic activity.[10]

Other Medical Uses

The decoction of Shan You Gan roots, barks, and leaves is traditionally used to treat scabies, sores, ulcers, intestinal infections, and a variety of stomach diseases based on their antifungal and antimicrobial properties. In addition, the roots are used as a fish poison in southern Vietnam, and the tender leaves are used in salads as a condiment. Fragrant oil prepared from its stem and leaves can be used in cosmetic perfumery.

References

1. Liu, C. X. et al. 1999. *Chinese Materia Medica*, Vol. 4, 4-3686, 868. Shanghai Science and Technology Press, Shanghai, China.
2. Jiangsu Xin Yixueyuan. 1977. *Zhongyao Dacidian (Encyclopedia on Chinese Medicinal. Substances)*, First Edition, 1: 66. Shanghai Science and Technology Press, Shanghai, China.
3. Dorr, R. T. et al. 1989. Antitumor activity and murine pharmacokinetics of parenteral acronycine. *Cancer Res.* 49: 340–4.
4. Shieh, H. L. et al. 1992. Evaluation of the cytotoxic mechanisms mediated by the broad-spectrum antitumor alkaloid acronycine and selected semisynthetic derivatives. *Chemicobiol. Interactions* 81: 35–55.
5. Nguyen, Q. C. et al. 2009. Acronycine derivatives: A promising series of anticancer agents. *Anti-Cancer Agents in Med. Chem.* 9: 804–15.
6. Guilbaud, N. et al. 2002. Acronycine derivatives as promising antitumor agents. *Anti-Cancer Drugs* 13: 445–9.
7. Kluza, J. et al. 2002. Induction of apoptosis in HL-60 leukemia and B16 melanoma cells by the acronycine derivative S23906–1. *Biochem. Pharmacol.* 63: 1443–52.
8. Wu, T. S. et al. 1989. X-ray crystal structure of acrovestone, a cytotoxic principle from *Acronychia pedunculata*. *J. Nat. Prod.* 52: 1284–9.
9. Kouloura, E. et al. 2012: Cytotoxic prenylated acetophenone dimers from *Acronychia pedunculata*. *J. Nat. Prod.* 75: 1270–6.
10. Kozaki, S. et al. 2014. Three acetophenones from *Acronychia pedunculata*. *J. Nat. Med.* 68: 421–6.

101 Zhi Shi 枳實

Immature bitter orange

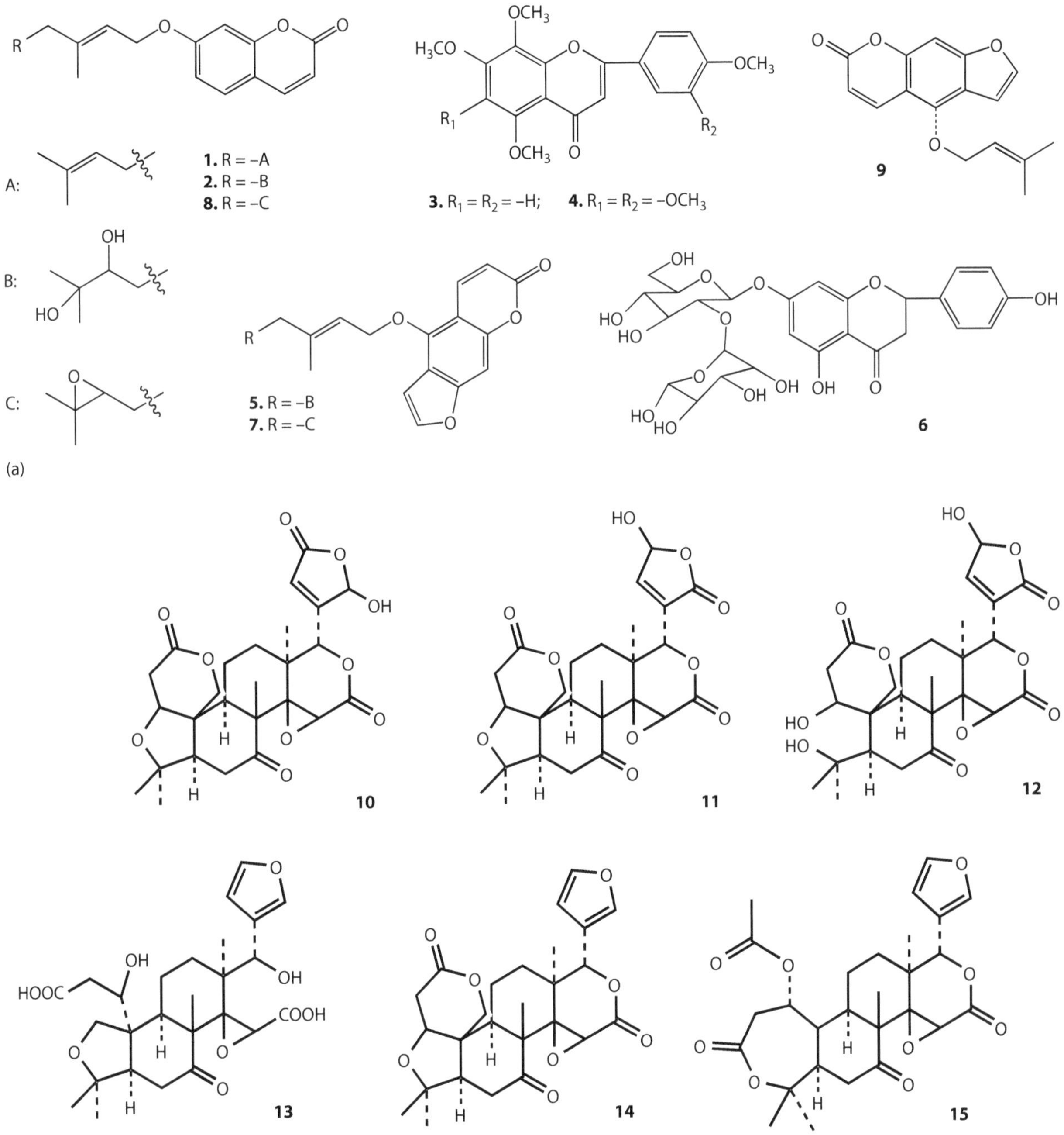

1. R = –A
2. R = –B
8. R = –C

3. $R_1 = R_2 = –H$; 4. $R_1 = R_2 = –OCH_3$

9

5. R = –B
7. R = –C

6

(a)

10 11 12

13 14 15

(b)

Herb Origination

The herb Zhi Shi (Immature bitter orange) is one of the popular Chinese folk medicines used for thousands of years. The documentation of Zhi Shi could be found in the first Chinese classic of materia medica entitled *Shennong Ben Cao Jing*. The immature fruits originated from *Citrus aurantium* and *C. sinensis* (Rutaceae) are the herb sources of Zhi Shi. The two kinds of bitter orange trees are broadly cultured along the Yangtze River and southern China. The fallen immature fruits are collected in May and June and dried in the sun or by gentle heat for traditional Chinese medicine use.

Antitumor Constituents and Activities

Coumarins and Flavonoids from the Immature Fruits

An ethanol extract of Zhi Shi was confirmed to possess the antitumor activity *in vivo* and *in vitro*; for instance, it effectively obstructed the proliferation of murine P388 leukemia cells.

The flavonoid component isolated from Zhi Shi (Korean *Citrus aurantium*) displayed obvious inhibitory effect against the proliferation of human A549 lung cancer cells in a dose-dependent manner but only a weak inhibition on WI-38 cells (a lung-derived human embryonic fibroblast cell line). The anti-A549 cell activity was found to be parallel with multiple cellular pathways, i.e., (1) the promotion of apoptosis through upregulation of caspase expression and augmentation of cleaved PARP and Bax/Bcl-xL ratio and (2) the induction of G2/M cell arrest moderated by downregulation of the expression levels of cyclin-B1, CDC2, CDC25c, and p21WAF1/CIP1.[1,2]

Five anticancer phenolic compounds identified as auraptene (**1**), marmin (**2**), tangeretin (**3**), nobiretin (**4**), and 5-[(6′,7′-dihydroxy-3′,7′-dimethyl-2-octenyl)-oxy]-psoralen (DDOP) (**5**) were isolated from Zhi Shi. All compounds showed a growth suppressive effect against L1210 and K562 leukemia cell lines *in vitro*.[1] Auraptene (**1**) also inhibited the proliferation of 320 colon carcinoma cells and amplified the apoptosis,[3] while tangeretin (**3**) effectively repressed the growth and the invasion of human MCF 7/6 breast cancer cells *in vitro*.[4] Along with disturbing the tumor cell cycle and promoting the apoptotic death, tangeretin (**3**) markedly obstructed the proliferation of human HL-60 promyelocytic leukemia cells. Tangeretin (**3**) and nobiletin (**4**) at concentrations of 2–8 μg/mL significantly retarded the growth of HTB43 squamous cell carcinoma cells and 9L colloidal sarcinoma cells *in vitro*.[5,6] A flavonoid glucoside identified as naringin (**6**) could markedly hinder the DNA formation in human (breast, colon, liver) cancer tissue but had no such action in human normal bone marrow and spleen tissues. Both naringin (**6**) and its aglycon naringenin were able to selectively restrain the growth of cancer cells and the mutagenesis induced by some chemicals.[7,8] Hesperidin isolated from orange peel was moderately active as an antioxidant agent, but it also exerted pronounced anticancer activity against the selected larynx, cervix, breast, and liver carcinoma cell lines with IC_{50} values ranging from 1.67 to 4.58 μg/mL.[9]

Moreover, a 20 μg/mL dose of auraptene (**1**) has a potential to overcome drug resistance and to enhance the tumoricidal effect in association with the inhibition on P-gp activity.[10] Nobiletin (**4**) exhibited the antiproliferative and antiinvasive effects in TMK-1 gastric carcinoma cells concomitantly with decrease of the production of MMPs, and it suppressed the formation of peritoneal dissemination nodules from the TMK-1 cells in a mouse model.[11] By interfering phosphatidylinositol-3 activation and diminishing MMP production, nobiletin (**4**) restrained the invasion of HT-1080 fibrosarcoma cells,[12] indicating that nobiletin (**4**) has a potential for the prevention of the solid tumor cell invasion and metastasis. In addition, the polymethoxyflavonoids such as tangeretin (**3**) and nobiletin (**4**) showed inhibitory effects on melanogenesis in a human melanoma.[13]

The noticeable anticarcinogenetic activity of Zhi Shi was also demonstrated by other experimental studies. The i.p. injection of auraptene (**1**) in a dose of 100 mg/kg to mice for five successive days obstructed the Diethylnitrosamine (DEN)-induced hepatomagenesis and repressed the tumor cell proliferation, but it was not active in the cell apoptosis and cytochrome P450 (CYP) expression,[14] whose anticarcinogenic mechanism was found to partially correlate with the suppression of antiproliferation-relating gene expression, activation of tumoricidal phase II enzymes (such as quinonereductase and GST) in the intestine and the liver, and inhibition of the micronuclear mutation.[14,15] Naringenin was able to restrain the activity of AFB1 for protecting the liver from carcinogenesis.[16] A diet of either naringenin or apigenin to mice could lessen the multiplicity aberrant crypt foci (ACF) caused by the injection of azoxymethane through the promotion of the tumor cell apoptosis, showing the two flavonoids were effective in the inhibition of colon carcinogenesis at the ACF stage.[17] In addition, the treatment with individual components such as auraptene (**1**), DDOP (**5**), 5-[3′,7′-dimethyl-6′-epoxy-2-octenyl] psoralen (**7**), epoxyauraptene (**8**), and isoimperatonin (**9**) obviously reduced TPA-promoting activation of EBV-EA and markedly inhibited the DMBA and TPA two-stage-induced mouse skin carcinogenesis.[18] Hence, the coumarins and the flavonoids prepared from the immature fruits of bitter oranges were proven to exert antitumor, anticarcinogenic, and antimutagenic effects, which may be beneficial to cancer prevention and therapy as a supplement.

Flavonoids and Triterpenoids from the Flowers

A methanolic extract prepared from *C. aurantium* bloom mainly contains phenolics and flavonoids, which exerted moderate to appreciable activities against human HT-29 colon adenocarcinoma cells and human MCF-7 and MDA-MB-231 breast carcinoma cells *in vitro*.[19] 5-Hydroxy-6,7,3′,4′-tetra-methoxyflavone and limonexic acid (**10**) were isolated from the flowers of *C. aurantium* var. *amara* as major constituents. Both compounds exhibited marked antioxidant and inhibitory effects on mouse B16 melanoma cells at concentrations from 6.25 to 50 μg/mL and on human SMCC-7721 hepatoma cells at concentrations from 12.5 to 200 μg/mL.[20]

Triterpanoids from the Seeds

Several limonin-type oxygenated triterpenoids such as limonexic acid (**11**), ichanexic acid (**12**), isolimonic acid (**13**), limonin (**14**), and nomilin (**15**) were discovered from the seeds of the bitter orange, showing antiproliferative effect on human colon cancer cells and/or human pancreas cancer cells *in vitro*.[21–24] A significant antigrowth effect was noticed by isolimonoic acid (**13**) within 24 h of treatment on HT-29 colon cancer cells at a concentration of as low as 5.0 μM and also by ichanexic acid (**12**) at a concentration of 10.0 μM, but no apparent cytostatic effect happened on the noncancerous COS-1 fibroblast cells *in vitro*.[22] The treatment with limonin (**14**) or its glucoside at concentrations of 25 and 6.25 μM for 24 h have shown a marked inhibitory activity against human SW480 colon adenocarcinoma cells for 42% and 61%, respectively.[23] Limonexic acid (**11**), limonin (**14**), and nomilin (**15**) at a concentration of 40 μM diminished the growth of human Panc-28 pancreatic carcinoma cells by 71%, 80%, and 86%, respectively, after an *in vitro* treatment for 48 h.[24] According to these results, the bioactive limonoids may be the possible drug leads for the development of cancer chemopreventive and chemotherapeutic agents.

Volatile Oil from the Peels

The volatile oil prepared from the fruit peels interestingly displayed anti-proliferative effect on human SW480 colon neoplastic cells at different concentrations, but no cytotoxicity on normal NIH 3T3 cells, at the similar doses. At a dose of 100 ppm, the oil showed 67.4% and 91.5% inhibition against the proliferation of SW480 cells *in vitro* after 24 h and 48 h treatment, respectively.[25]

Other Bioactivities

Pharmacological studies have proven that the herb Zhi Shi (Immature bitter orange) also has antiinflammatory, antiulcerative, antioxidant, antiviral, and antibacterial properties. It can augment heart contraction, increase heart export and coronary flow amounts, and promote gastrointestinal function. The pigment in Zhi Shi is a valuable antioxidant that is able to neutralize free radicals and improve vitamin C absorption.

References

1. Satoh, Y. et al. 1996. Bioactive constituents of *Aurantii fructus immaturus*. *Yakugaku Zasshi*. 116: 244–50.
2. Park, K. I. et al. 2012. Induction of the cell cycle arrest and apoptosis by flavonoids isolated from Korean *Citrus aurantium* L. in non-small-cell lung cancer cells. *Food Chem*. 135: 2728–35.
3. Mori, H. et al. 2001. Cell proliferation in cancer prevention; effects of preventive agents on estrogen-related endometrial carcinogenesis model and on an in vitro model in human colorectal cells. *Mutation Res*. 480: 201–7.
4. Depypere, H. T. et al. 2000. Inhibition of tamoxifen's therapeutic benefit by tangeretin in mammary cancer. *Eur. J. Cancer* 36(suppl.4): S73.
5. Kandaswami, C. et al. 1992. Differential inhibition of proliferation of human squamous cell carcinoma, gliosarcoma and embryonic fibroblast-like lung cells in culture by plant flavonoids. *Anti-Cancer Drugs* 3: 525–30.
6. Kandaswami, C. et al. 1991. Antitproliferative effects of citrus flavonoids on a human squamous cell carcinoma in vitro. *Cancer Lett*. 56: 147–52.
7. Beljanski, M. et al. 1990. Separation of naringin and naringenin from plant material as neoplasm inhibitors. *Eur. Pat. Appl*. EP 352147 A2 19900124.
8. Francis, A. R. et al. 1989. Modulating effect of plant flavonoids on the mutagenicity of N-methyl-N′-nitro-N-nitrosoguanidine. *Carcinogen*. 10: 1953–5.
9. Al-Ashaal, H. A. et al. 2011. Antioxidant capacity of hesperidin from citrus peel using electron spin resonance and cytotoxic activity against human carcinoma cell lines. *Pharm. Biol*. (London, U.K.) 49: 276–82.
10. Simon, P. N. et al. 2003. A two-complementary method assay for screening new reversal agents of cancer cell multidrug resistance. *Pharm. Biol*. 41: 72–7.
11. Minagawa, A. et al. 2001. The citrus flavonoid, nobiletin, inhibits peritoneal dissemination of human gastric carcinoma in SCID mice. *Jpn J. Cancer Res*. 92: 1322–8.
12. Sato, T. et al. 2002. Inhibition of activator protein-1 binding activity and phosphatidylinositol 3-kinase pathway by nobiletin, a polymethoxy flavonoid, results in augmentation of tissue inhibitor of metalloproteinases-1 production and suppression of production of matrix metalloproteinases-1 and -9 in human fibrosarcoma HT-1080 cells. *Cancer Res*. 62: 1025–9.
13. Tsukayama, M. et al. 2003. Improved, rapid and efficient synthesis of polymethoxyflavones under microwave irradiation and their inhibitory effects on melanogenesis. *Heterocycles* 60: 2725–84.
14. Kitano, M. et al. 2000. Chemopreventive effects of coumaperine from pepper on the initiation stage of chemical hepatocarcinogenesis in the rat. *Jpn. J. Cancer Res*. 91: 674–80.
15. Tanaka, T. et al. 1997. Citrus auraptene inhibits chemically induced colonic aberrant crypt foci in male F344 rats. *Carcinogen*. 18: 2155–61.
16. Guengerich, F. P. et al. 1990. In vitro inhibition of dihydropyridine oxidation and aflatoxin B1 activation in human liver microsomes by naringenin and other flavonoids. *Carcinogenesis* 11: 2275–9.
17. Leonardi, T. et al. 2010. Apigenin and naringenin suppress colon carcinogenesis through the aberrant crypt stage in azoxymethane-treated rats. *Experim. Biol. Med*. 235: 710–7.
18. Takashi, Y. et al. 1997. Inhibitory effects of coumarin derivatives from citrus fruits on Epstein-Barr virus early antigen activation. *Jpn. Kokai Tokkyo Koho* JP 09157166 A 19970617.
19. Karimi, E. et al. 2012. Phenolic compounds characterization and biological activities of *Citrus aurantium* bloom. *Mol*. 17: 1203–18.
20. Zhao, H. Y. et al. 2012. Bioactivity evaluations of ingredients extracted from the flowers of *Citrus aurantium* L. var. *amara* Engl. *Food Chem*. 135: 2175–81.
21. Jayaprakasha, G. K. et al. 2010. Bioactive compounds from sour orange inhibit colon cancer cell proliferation and induce cell cycle arrest. *J. Agricul. Food Chem*. 58: 180–6.
22. Jayaprakasha, G. K. et al. 2008. Novel triterpenoid from *Citrus aurantium* L. possesses chemo-preventive properties against human colon cancer cells. *Bioorg. Med. Chem*. 16: 5939–51.
23. Murthy, K. N. et al. 2007. Potential of citrus limonoids in pancreatic cancer prevention. *Abstracts of Papers, 234th ACS National Meeting*, Boston MA, U.S., August 19–23, 2007, AGFD-243.
24. Murthy, K. N. et al. 2009. Limonin and its glucoside from citrus can inhibit colon cancer: Evidence from in vitro studies. *Acta Horticulturae*, 841(Proceedings of the 2nd International Symposium on Human Health Effects of Fruits and Vegetables, 2007), 145–50.
25. Jayaprakasha, G. K. et al. 2007. Volatile oil from sour oranges (*Citrus aurantium* L.) has potential benefit in colon cancer prevention. *Abstracts of Papers, 234th ACS National Meeting*, Boston, MA, U.S., August 19–23, 2007, AGFD-244.

102 Tu Mu Xiang 土木香

Elecampane or Horse-heal

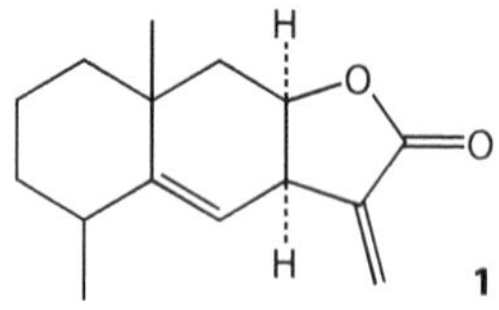

Herb Origination

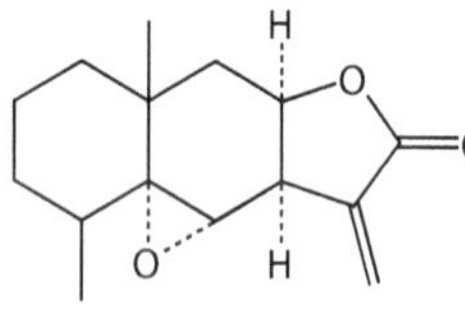

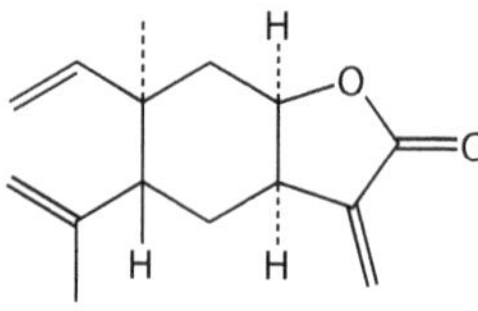

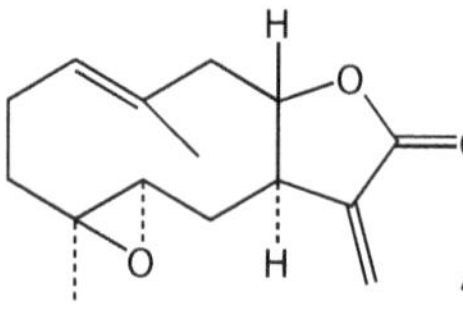

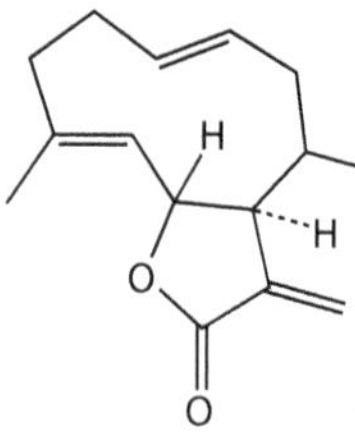

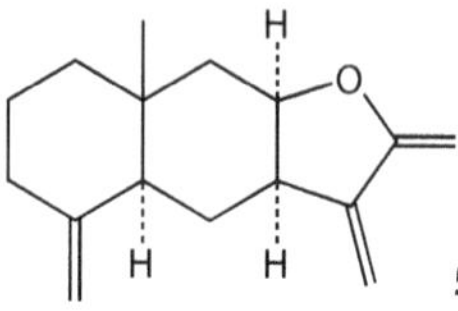

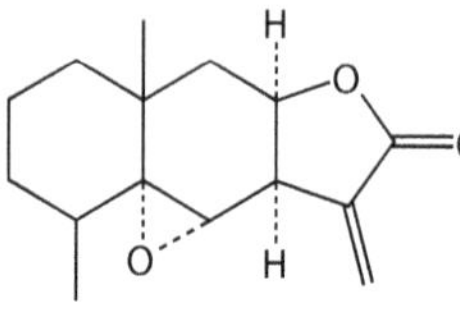

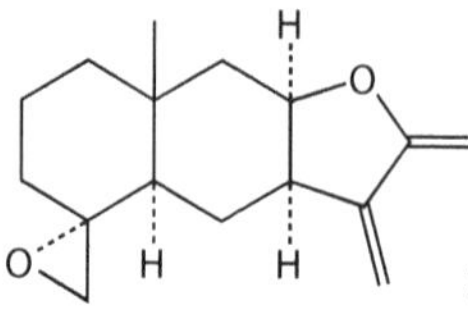

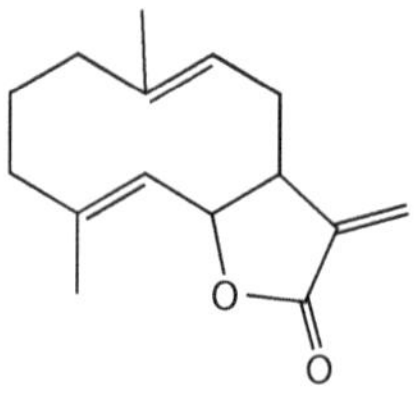

The herb Tu Mu Xiang (Elecampane) is the dried rhizomes and roots of a Composite plant, *Inula helenium*, whose perennial plant is wildly distributed throughout continental Europe and the temperate region of Asian as far as southern Siberia and northwest India. As a plant of naturalization, it has spread to North America, where it grows abundantly from northern Carolina to Missouri.

Antitumor Activities

The crude ethanolic extract of Tu Mu Xiang demonstrated marked inhibitory effect against the proliferation of Raji lymphoblastoid cells *in vitro* at a 10–50 μg/mL concentration.[1] Its methanolic extract notably suppressed the growth of human MK-1-expressing tumor, human HeLa cervical carcinoma, and mouse B16F10 melanoma cell lines.[2] Its significant necrotic-like toxicity was demonstrated in four human neoplastic cells, HT-29 (colon), MCF-7 (breast), Capan-2 (pancreas), and G1 (astrocytoma), *in vitro*, but it has over 120 times lower toxicity on healthy peripheral blood lymphocytes from two separated human donors. The LD_{50} values on the four cancer cells were in a range of 0.015–0.020 μL/mL.[3] After the treatment, the antigrowth and proapoptotic effects were observed in human KB oral cancer cells, associated with DNA fragmentation and increase of caspase-3, caspase-7, and caspase-9 proteolytic processing.[4]

Antitumor Constituents and Activities

Sesquiterpene lactones are the major antineoplastic constituents in *Inula helenium*. The five isolated sesquiterpene lactones with a 11,13-dehydrolactone moiety from n-hexane partitioned fraction of the methanolic extract presented an antiproliferative property against the three cancer cell lines (MK-1, HeLa, and B16F10) *in vitro*. Alantolactone (**1**) and 5α-epoxyalantolactone (**2**) displayed a similar level of inhibition against the proliferation of the cancer cell lines (GI_{50}: 3.6–6.9 μM). 1,3,11(13)-Elematrien-8β,12-olide (**3**) exhibited the same level of inhibitory effect against the MK-1 and B16F10 cancer cell lines but had about half less activity on the HeLa cells. 4β,5α-Epoxy-1(10),11(13)-germacradiene-8,12-oilde (**4**) and isoalantolactone (**5**) exerted only moderate inhibition on MK-1 and B16F10 (GI_{50}: 12–33 μM and 29–44 μM).[2] Alantolactone (**1**) was also effective in the growth inhibition and the cell cycle retardation of human A549 lung cancer cells.[5] The cell viability of human RKO colon cancer cells was retarded, and the ROS-mediated mitochondria-dependent apoptotic death was elicited after the treatment of alantolactone (**1**).[6] Two other isolated sesquiterpenes that have non-11,13-dehydrolactone moiety were inactive, implying that the 11,13-dehydrolactone moiety in the sesquiterpenes must closely contribute to the neoplasm-inhibitory activity.[2] These findings revealed that Tu Mu Xiang may be advantageous for promoting clinic treatment.

The marked antigrowth activities of isoalantolactone (**5**) were extensively substantiated in multiple types of human cancer cell lines such as U251SP (brain), HLE (liver), MM1-CB (skin), HeLa (cervix), KT (breast), SHIN3, HOC-21 and HAC-2 (ovary), and UM-SCC-10A (head/neck), *in vitro*.[7–12] The exposure of isoalantolactone (**5**) elicited the UM-SCC-10A cells to apoptosis via a mitochondrial pathway, whose proapoptosis was also found to associate with G1 cell cycle arrest via the downregulation of cyclin-D and the upregulation of p53 and p21.[13] In other *in vitro* assays, isoalantolactone (**5**), santamarine, and/or dehydrocostuslactone exhibited the antiproliferative activities to human breast cancer cell lines (MCF-7 and KT) and human gynecologic carcinoma cell lines (HeLa, SHIN3, HOC-21, and HAC-2). The IC_{50} values were 4.40–4.57 μmol/L in the MCF-7 and KT cell lines.[13–15] The anticancer activity of isoalantolactone (**5**) was also confirmed in mice implanted with murine H22 hepatoma or sarcoma 180 but no toxicity was shown on human embryonic lung cells.[7–12] Through ROS-mediated caspase-dependent apoptotic pathways, S phase arrest, and down-expression of Bcr/Abl, isoalantolactone (**5**) markedly inhibited the growth of drug-resistant K562/A02 human erythroleukemia cells.[16] By analysis of the correlations between antitumor potencies and the structures of eudesmane sesquiterpene lactones, the SAR (structure and activity relationship) was designated as (1) β-unsaturated five-membered lactone ring is necessary for the antitumor activities; (2) 1,10-seco, i.e., the ring-A opening led to decrease of antigrowth activity; and (3) the bond between C-5 and C-10 of ring-A and ring-B broken to form a 10-membered macroring can reduce or lose the inhibitory property.[7–11] Furthermore, the structural modification of alantolactone (**1**) and isoalantolactone (**5**) gave two derivatives 5α,6α-epoxyalantolactone (**6**) and epoxyisoalantolactone (**7**), which both performed higher antiproliferative activity against HepG2 hepatoma cells than the starting molecules (alantolactone (**1**) and isoalantolactone (**5**)), also indicating that the formation of an epoxy group on the skeleton of this type of sesquiterpenes could further augment the anticancer activity.[17]

Moreover, another type of isolated sesquiterpene termed isocostunolide (**8**) efficiently induced cytotoxicity in A2058 (skin), HT-29 (colon), and HepG2 (liver) cancer cell lines (respective IC_{50}: 3.2, 5.0, and 2.0 μg/mL).[18] The apoptosis-inducing mechanism in the A2058 cells was revealed to activate a mitochondria pathway, i.e., down-expression of Bcl-2 family proteins, marked increase of Fas level and mitochondrial membrane depolarization to facilitate cytochrome c, and decline of Bid, pro-caspase-8, pro-caspase-3, PARP levels.[18] Among the three separated germacrene-type sesquiterpene lactones from the herb, only eupatolide (**9**) exerted a significant suppressive effect against the growth of four human lung cancer cell lines *in vitro*, whereas other two analogs had no such activity due to no 6-hydroxy group in the ring-A,[16] whose inhibitory effect of eupatolide (**9**) and isoalantolactone (**5**) was known to be stronger than that of cisplatin and similar to cisplatin in small cell lung tumor cell lines (PG-6 and QG-90).[11,19]

In addition, isoalantolactone (**5**) and alantolactone (**1**) as well as the methanolic extract of Tu Mu Xiang showed a marked potential to induce detoxifying enzymes such as NAD(P)H: (quinone acceptor) oxidoreductase-1 (NQO1, QR). The isoalantolactone (**5**) could also dose-dependently activate other phase II detoxifying enzymes such as γ-glutamyl-cysteine synthetase, GST, GSH reductase, and heme oxygenase-1 in the cultured cells by accumulating Nrf2 in the nucleus, suggesting that isoalantolactone (**5**) is also a potent phase II enzyme inducer, having profitable potentials in carcinogenetic chemoprevention besides the cancer chemotherapy.[20]

Other Medicinal Uses

The herb Tu Mu Xiang (Elecampane) has been used broadly as a herbal medicine throughout the world for a long history, for instance, as therapeutic agents to treat tuber culoticenterorrhea, chronic enterogastritis, and bronchitis in China, and as diaphoresis, diuretic, and expectorant agents in Europe. The Native Americans used the infusion and the decoctions of this herb to take care of lung disorders and against tuberculosis. Recently, modern studies have shown that Tu Mu Xiang is able to play medicinal functions with antioxidant, antihelminthic antiulcer, antiinflammatory, and antibacterial effects.[21]

References

1. Spiridonov, N. A. et al. 2005. Cytotoxicity of some Russian ethnomedicinal plants and plant compounds. *Phytother. Res.* 19: 428–32.
2. Konishi, T. et al. 2002. Antiproliferative sesquiterpene lactones from the roots of *Inula helenium. Biol. Pharma. Bull.* 25: 1370–2.
3. Dorn, D. C. et al. 2006. Tumor cell specific toxicity of *Inula helenium* extracts. *Phytother. Res.* 20. 970–80.
4. Lee, M. J. et al. 2011. Growth inhibition of human oral cancer cells by *Inula helenium. Pharmacol. Therap. Toxicol. IIADR/AADR/CADR 89th General Session and Exhibition* (March 16–19, 2011) San Diego.
5. Zong, M. R. et al. 2011. Inhibitory effects of natural compound alantolactone on human non-small cell lung cancer A549 cells. *Chem. Res. Chin. Univ.* 27: 241–4.
6. Zhang, Y. et al. 2013. Alantolactone induces apoptosis in RKO cells through the generation of reactive oxygen species and the mitochondrial pathway. *Mol. Med. Reports* 8: 967–72.
7. Li, Y. et al. 2010. In vivo and in vitro antitumor activity studies of five sesquiterpenoids from *Inula helenium. Chin. Pharmacol. Bull.* 26: 112–5.
8. Yu, F. et al. 2010. Studies on the anti-growth activity of three sesquiterpene compounds to human tumor cell lines. *Tianran Chanwu Yanjiu Yu Kaifa* 22: 506–9.
9. Si, Y. R. et al. 2010. Study of the anti-proliferative activity and mechanism of three sesquiterpene compounds on gynecologic tumor cell lines. *Aibian, Jibian, Tubian* 22: 28–31.
10. Chen, J. J. et al. 2010. Anti-human hepatoma activity of five sesquiterpenoids from *Inula helenium. Aibian, Jibian, Tubian* 22: 440–3.
11. Li, Y. et al. 2010. Antitumor effects of three sesquiterpene lactones of *Inula helenium* and their structure-activity relationship. *Zhongcaoyao* 41: 1336–8.
12. Wu, M. J. et al. 2013. Isoalantolactone inhibits UM-SCC-10A cell growth via cell cycle arrest and apoptosis induction. *PLoS One* 8: e76000.
13. Li, Y. et al. 2012. Antitumour activities of sesquiterpene lactones from *Inula helenium* and *Inula japonica. Zeitschrift fuer Naturforschung, C: J. Biosci.* 67: 375–80.
14. Li, M. et al. 2013. In vitro anti-human breast tumor activity of sesquiterpenoid lactones from *Inula helenium. Hebei Yike Daxue Xuebao* 34: 869–72.
15. Li, M. et al. 2013. Anti-proliferative activity of sesquiterpenoids from *Inula helenium* and *Artemisia frigida* on human breast tumor cell lines and their structure-activity relationship investigation. *Tianran Chanwu Yanjiu Yu Kaifa* 25: 555–7, 529.
16. Cai, H. et al. 2014. Growth inhibition effects of isoalantolactone on K562/A02 cells: Caspase-dependent apoptotic pathways, S phase arrest, and downregulation of Bcr/Abl. *Phytother. Res.* 28: 1679–86.
17. Du, H. J. et al. 2013. Structural modification of isoalantolactone and alantolactone isolated from *Inula helenium. Tianran Chanwu Yanjiu Yu Kaifa* 25: 156–60.
18. Chen, C. N. et al. 2007. Isocostunolide, a sesquiterpene lactone, induces mitochondrial membrane depolarization and caspase-dependent apoptosis in human melanoma cells. *Cancer Lett.* 246: 237–52.
19. Li, Y. et al. 2010. In vitro anti-human lung tumor activity studies of three sesquiterpenoids from *Inula helenium. Hebei Yike Daxue Xuebao* 31: 621–4.
20. Seo, J. Y. et al. 2009. Isoalantolactone from *Inula helenium* caused Nrf2-mediated induction of detoxifying enzymes. *J. Med. Food* 12: 1038–45.
21. Iuliana, S. et al. 2013. Antioxidant and chemical properties of *Inula helenium* root extracts. *Cent. Eur. J. Chem.* 11: 1699–709

103 He Tao Qiu 核桃楸

Manchurian walnut

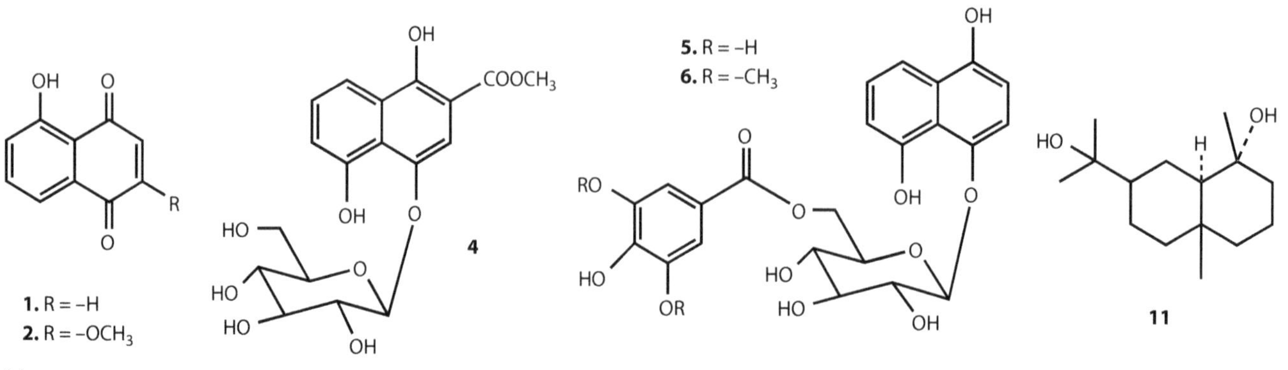

1. R = -H
2. R = -OCH₃

(a)

7. R_1 = -H, R_2 = -H, R_3 = =O
8. R1 = -CH_3, R_2 = R_3 = -OH

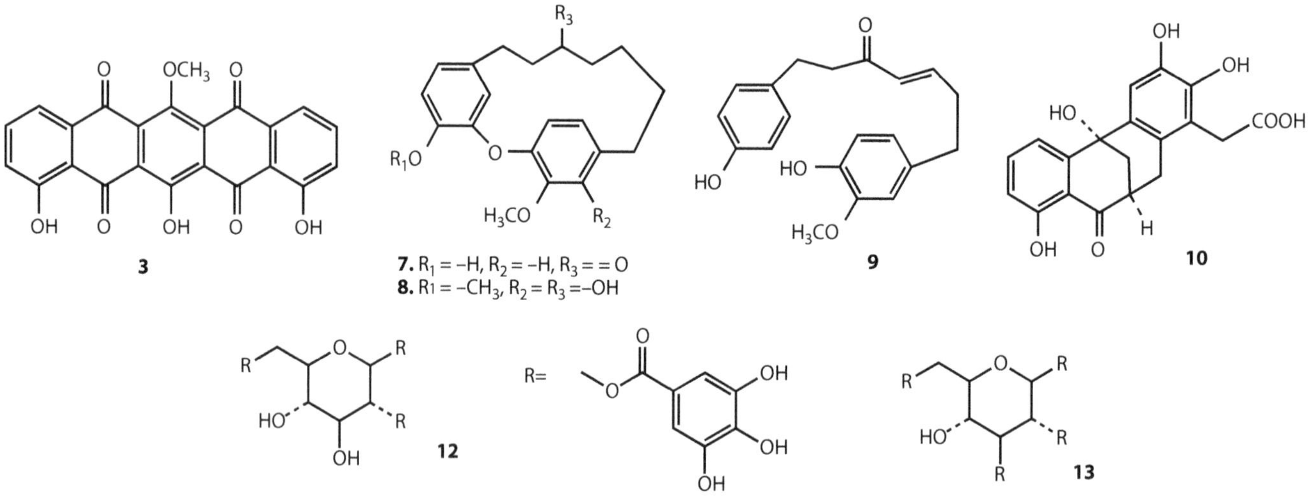

(b)

Herb Origination

The herb He Tao Qiu (Manchurian walnut) originated from a Juglandaceae plant, *Juglans mandshurica*, whose unripe or ripe fruit peels are used as a traditional Chinese medicine. The plant is native to the eastern Asiatic region (China, Russian Far East, and Korea). The herb is normally collected in spring and autumn, which can be applied as fresh and dried herb in folk medical practice. Its dried root is another herb used in Korea.

Antitumor Activity

Extract from He Tao Qiu Fruits

The decoction of He Tao Qiu green husk by gavage to mice showed obvious suppressive effect on the transgenic entity hepatoma and sarcoma 180.[1,2] Besides a prominent performance of tumor inhibition *in vivo*, the extract at a high dose also enhanced immune functions, such as augmentation of the phagocytic function of macrophage and the proliferation of T lymphocyte and leukocyte and the promotion of the production levels of IL-2 and TNFα in mice.[2]

Extract from He Tao Qiu Leaves

The leaf extract of He Tao Qui was capable of markedly protecting HS68 human skin fibroblasts from H_2O_2-induced damage by regulating oxidative defense system and ROS production, activating NF-E2-related factor-2, and increasing levels of GSH and heme oxygenase-1. The leaf extract also restrained H_2O_2-induced phosphorylation of ERK, p38, and JNK and restrained H_2O_2-induced MMP-1 and COL1A1, leading to the anticarcinogenic and apoptosis-inducing effects.[3]

Extract from He Tao Qiu Stems

A chloroform extract from the stem bark of the plant was effective in the antiproliferation against human HeLa cervical cancer cells and mouse Hca-F ascites hepatoma cells in concentrations of 25–100 μg/mL *in vitro* and against sarcoma 180 cells in doses of 9 and 18 mg/kg *in vivo*.[4] An extract derived from He Tao Qiu bark could also restrain the growth/proliferation of sarcoma 180 and H22 hepatoma in dosages 50–200 mg/kg *in vivo* and in concentrations of 25–100 mg/kg *in vitro*, resulting in the inhibition ratios of 61.76–69.85% and 65.92–73.18%, respectively.[5] The bark extracts exhibited the cytotoxic effects on HT-29 (colon) and A599 (lung) human carcinoma cell lines.[6]

Antitumor Constituents and Activities

The research in anticarcinoma and anticarcinogenic constituents have been indeed approached in different portions of the He Tao Qiu plant such as fruit, fruit peel, root, leave, and stem bark. A variety of natural agents with cancer inhibitory property has been isolated, but naphthoquinones and naphthalene glycosides were considered to be largely in charge of the tumor suppression of He Tao Qiu.

Naphthoquinones

Juglone (**1**) isolated from He Tao Qin fruits was capable of obviously prolonging the life duration of mice bearing HepA ascites hepatoma by 95% when juglone (**1**) is abdominally injected in doses of 5–8 mg/kg/day for seven days *in vivo*. The DNA inhibition reached the highest degree in the HepA cells after the treatment of juglone (**1**) for 5 h in doses of 0.1–0.25 mg/kg. Juglone (**1**) could promote mitochondrial-dependent apoptosis in human HL-60 leukemia cells and mouse HepA hepatoma cells, accompanied by the elevation of Bax/Bcl-2 ratio, loss of mitochondrial membrane potential, release of Smac, cytochrome c and apoptosis-inducing factor (AIF) to cell cytoplasm, cleavage of PARP, and activation of caspase-9 and caspase-3.[7,8] ROS generation played a significant role in triggering the juglone-induced apoptosis of HL-60 cells, and its IC_{50} value was ~8 μM.[9] By down-expressing the levels of AR and PSA, juglone (**1**) promoted capase-activated apoptosis of AR-sensitive LNCaP prostate cancer cells.[10] However, the apoptosis-inducing and antiproliferative effects on human PC3 prostate cancer cells were in a higher concentration of juglone (**1**).[10,11] Juglone (**1**) also exhibited moderate cytotoxicities against MGC-803 (gastric), A549 (lung), K562 (leukemia), and HeLa (cervical) tumor cell lines (IC_{50}: 25.9, 28.6, 39.1, 44.9 μM, respectively).[12–14] Moreover, juglone (**1**) synergistically potentiated the cytotoxicity of cisplatin (an anticancer drug) against the HeLa cells in the cotreatment.[12,13]

Four other antitumor compounds were obtained from the isolation of *J. mandshurica* exocarp. 2,5-Dihydroxy-1,4-naphthoquinone and 2,5-dihydroxy-1,4-naphthoquinone presented moderate suppressive effects against human HepG2 hepatoma cells with IC_{50} values of 5.0 and 7.0 μmol/L, whereas 5-hydroxy-1,4-naphthoquinone and 2,5-dihydroxy-1,4-naphthoquinone showed the similar degree of inhibitory effect against human HL-60 leukemia cells with IC_{50} value of 9.3 and 2.3 μmol/L, respectively.[14] A marked tumor inhibitor named 5-hydroxy-2-methoxy-1,4-naphthoquinone (**2**) was isolated from the roots of He Tao Qiu. Its IC_{50} values were 0.08, 1.2, and 2.63 μg/mL in A549 (lung), MCF-7 (breast), and HT-29 (colon) human cancer cell lines[15,16]; 2.0–2.7 μM in MGC-803 (gastric), K562 (leukemic), and SiHa (cervical) cancer cell lines; 4.0–6.9 μM in HeLa and CaSKi cervical cancer and JAR choriocarcinoma cell lines.[17] Juglanthraquinone-C (isolated from the plant stem bark) exerted the suppressive effect on the viability and the proliferation of various human neoplastic cells *in vitro*. Its IC_{50} values were 9 μg/mL in the HepG2 cells but 36 μg/mL in human L02 normal liver cells. The antihepatoma activity of juglanthraquinone-C was associated with the induction of S phase cell cycle arrest and apoptosis of HepG2 cells.[18]

In addition, p-hydroxymethoxybenzobijuglone (HMBBJ) (**3**) was discovered from the plant leaves. HMBBJ (**3**) displayed moderate cytotoxic effects against three human neoplastic cell lines, MCF-7 (breast), HeLa (cervix), and BGC823 (stomach), with IC_{50} values ranging from 7.5 to 26.8 μmol/L *in vitro*.[19,20] The proliferative inhibition on HeLa cells and BGC823 cells by HMBBJ (**3**) were found to be closely accompanied by cell cycle arrest at G2/M phase and efficient promotion of apoptosis through a mitochondria-dependent pathway.[21,22]

Naphthalene Glycosides

A group of naphthalene glycosides was separated from He Tao Qiu fruits. Almost all of them exhibited cytotoxic activity against human HL-60 leukemia cells, but only α-tetralonyl glucosides were inactive.[22] 1,4,8-Trihydroxy-3-naphthalenecarboxylic acid 1-*O*-β-D-glucoside methyl ester (**4**) exerted the growth inhibitory effect against HT-29 colon cancer and A549 lung cancer cell lines *in vitro* with IC_{50} values of 8.06 μg/mL and 7.79 μg/mL, respectively.[15] Three other analogs, 1,4,8-trihydroxynaphthalene-1-*O*-β-D-glucoside, 4-hydroxynaphthalene-1-*O*-β-D-glucoside, and 1,4,8-trihydroxynaphthalene-1-*O*-β-D-[6′-*O*-(3″,4″,5″-trihydroxybenzoyl)]-glucoside (**5**) displayed cytotoxicity against human SMMC-7721 hepatoma cells, and the third naphthalenyl glucoside (**5**) was also cytotoxic to human MCF-7 breast carcinoma cells.[23] However, the effect of 1,4,8-trihydroxynaphthalene-1-*O*-β-*D*-[6′-*O*-(3″,4″,5″-trihydroxybenzoyl)]-glucoside (**5**) and 1,4,8-trihydroxynaphthalene-1-*O*-β-*D*-[6′-*O*-(3″,5″-dimethoxy-4″-hydroxybenzoyl)]-glucoside (**6**) were weak on human U937 histiocytic lymphoma cells (IC_{50}: 30 and 50 μg/mL, respectively).[24] The results indicated that the naphthalenyl glucosides are important components in response to the antitumor effect of this herb.

In addition, the compounds 1,4,8-Trihydroxy-3-naphthalene-carboxylic acid 1-*O*-β-d-glucoside methyl ester (**4**), 1,4,8-trihydroxynaphthalene-1-*O*-β-D-[6′-*O*-(3″,4″,5″-trihydroxybenzoyl)]-glucoside (**5**) and 1,4,8-trihydroxynaphthalene-1-*O*-β-D-[6′-*O*-(3″,5″-dimethoxy-4″-hydroxybenzoyl)]-glucoside (**6**) are mostly inhibitors of DNA Topo-I and Topo –II, and some of them showed greater anti-Topo activity than chemotherapeutic agents, etoposide and camptothecin.[15,16] The fractionation of the extract derived from the fresh rejuvenated fruits afforded four cytotoxic fractions, which were effective in the inhibition of human stomach cancer BGC803 cells. From the active fractions, four naphthalenyl glucosides were isolated and their structures were elucidated as 1,4,8-trihydroxy-naphthalene-1-*O*-β-D-[6′-*O*-(3″,4″,5″-trihydroxybenzoyl)]-β-D-glucoside (**5**), 1,4,5-trihydroxynaphthalene-1,5-di-*O*-β-D-glucoside, 1,4,8-trihydroxynaphthalene-1-*O*-β-D-glucoside, and 1,4,5-trihydroxynaphthalene-1,4-di-*O*-β-D-glucoside.[25]

Diarylheptanoids

From the roots of He Tao Qiu, three antitumor active diarylheptanoids elucidated as galleon (**7**), galleol (**8**), and cleavaged galleon (**9**) were isolated. They demonstrated moderate cytotoxic activity against human HT-29 colon cancer and A549 lung cancer cell lines *in vitro*. The IC_{50} values of galleon (**7**) and cleavaged galleon (**9**) were 5.3 and 8.2 μg/mL in HT-29 cells and 2.2 and 5.4 μg/mL in A549 cells, respectively.[26]

α-Tetralonyl Derivative

Juglanone (**10**), α-tetralonyl derivative, was isolated from the fresh unripe fruits, which is a marked antioxidant agent with radical-scavenging and superoxide dismutase-like activities. The cytotoxic activity of juglanone (**10**) was demonstrated *in vitro* against HL-60 human myeloid leukemia with an IC_{50} value of 19.7 μM.[27]

Terpenoids

Only one sesquiterpenoid designated as eudesmane-4α,11-diol (**11**) was isolated from the root of He Tao Qiu, which displayed obvious antiproliferative effect against the HT-29 cells *in vitro* with an IC_{50} value of 12.9 μg/mL.[15,16] A triterpenoid identified as ursolic acid-3-caffeate derived from the roots exerted its moderate cytotoxicity in human HT-29 (colon) and MCF-7 (breast) cancer cell lines *in vitro*, and it was also an inhibitor of DNA Topos.[15,16]

Flavones

The effects of a flavone extract originated from the stem barks of He Tao Qiu plant were present in the proliferative inhibition on Bel-7402 hepatocarcinoma cells and the apoptosis promotion, whose apoptotic effect was implemented by obstructing the over-expression of the p73 gene.[28]

Tannins

Two galloyl monosaccharides were isolated from a water extract of He Tai Qiu's stem-bark and were identified as 1,2,6-trigalloylglucose (TEgG) (**12**) and 1,2,3,6-tetragalloylglucose (TRgG) (**13**). Both galloylglucoses at 100 or 150 μM concentration showed cytotoxic activity in leukemia HL-60 cells and concurrently enhanced caspase-3 activity and caused internucleosomal DNA fragmentation. TEgG (**12**) displayed greater apoptosis-inducing activity in HL-60 cell lines as compared to TRgG (**13**).[29]

Polysaccharide

A water-soluble polysaccharide, named JRP1 (molecular weight: 38,400), was extracted from the epicarp of immature fruits of *J. mandshurica*, which was composed of 51.8% neutral sugar, 1.39% protein, and 37.5% uronic acid, and its sugar components were galactose (43.1%), glucose (23.6%), arabinose (16.2%), rhamnose (9.8%), and fructose (7.3%). JRP1 not only significantly inhibited the growth of mouse sarcoma 180 cells *in vivo* but also markedly enhanced the proliferative ability of lymphocytes, the phagocytic activity of macrophages, and the serum immune cytokine levels such as IL-2, TNFα, and IFNγ,[30] indicating the effective antitumor and immunoregulative functions of JRP1.

Clinical Practice

One hundred twenty patients suffering esophagus-cardia carcinoma had been treated with the ethanolic extract of He Tao Qiu fruits via oral administration (10–20 mL × three times, per day) for one year. The final total effective rate reached to 53%. But the effective rate could be 76% for patients in early stage. After a two-month treatment, most of the patients had obvious improvement in symptoms, appetite, and pain without any side effects.[24]

References

1. Li, X. F. et al. 2007. Progress of research on the chemical components and pharmaceutical action of walnut green husk. *Shipin Keji* (4): 241–2.
2. Guo, J. H. et al. 2007. Inhibitory effects and immunoregulation of *Juglans mandshurica* maxim extract on S180 mouse sarcoma. *J. Jilin Univ.* (*Med. Edit.*) 33: 286–9.
3. Park, G. H. et al. 2012. *Juglans mandshurica* leaf extract protects skin fibroblasts from damage by regulating the oxidative defense system. *Biochem. Biophys. Res. Commun.* 421: 343–8.
4. Liu, C. et al 2013. Investigation into the antitumor activity of *Juglans mandshurica* Maxim. extracts. *Shenyang Yaoke Daxue Xuebao* 30: 799–802.
5. Zou, P. W. et al. 2010. Antitumor effect of *Juglans mandshurica* maxim bark extraction. *Zhongguo Yiyuan Yaoxue Zazhi* 30: 308–10.
6. Kim, S. H. et al. 1998. Cytotoxic compounds from the roots of *Juglans mandshurica. J Nat Prod.* 61: 643–5.
7. Zhang, Y. P. et al. 1987. Antitumor effect of Juglone. *J. Shenyang Pharm. College* 4: 166–9.
8. Xu, H. L. et al. 2010. Anti-proliferative effect of Juglone from *Juglans mandshurica* Maxim on human leukemia cell HL-60 by inducing apoptosis through the mitochondria-dependent pathway. *Eur. J. Pharmacol.* 645: 14–22.
9. Xu, H. L. et al. 2012. Juglone, from *Juglans mandshurica* Maxim, inhibits growth and induces apoptosis in human leukemia cell HL-60 through a reactive oxygen species-dependent mechanism. *Food Chem. Toxicol.* 50: 590–6.
10. Xu, H. L. et al. 2013. Juglone, isolated from *Juglans mandshurica* Maxim, induces apoptosis via down-regulation of AR expression in human prostate cancer LNCaP cells. *Bioorg. Med. Chem. Lett.* 23: 3631–4.
11. Fang, F. et al. 2013. Inhibitory effect of juglone on human prostate cancer PC3 cells. *Lishizhen Med. Materia Medica Res.* 24: 1120–1.
12. Zhang, W. et al. 2013. Effect of juglone alone or combined with cisplatin on survival and apoptosis of human cervical cancer HeLa cells. *Chin. J. Pharmacol. Toxicol.* 27: 663–7.
13. Zhang, W. et al. 2012. Anticancer activity and mechanism of juglone on human cervical carcinoma HeLa cells. *Can. J. Physiol. Pharmacol.* 90: 1553–8.
14. Dong, M. et al. 2011. Study on cytotoxic active constituents of *Juglans mandshurica* exocarp. *Tianran Chanwu Yanjiu Yu Kaifa* 23: 805–8.
15. Kim, S. H. et al. 1998. Cytotoxic compounds from the roots of *Juglans mandshurica. J. Nat. Prod.* 61: 643–5.
16. Li, G. et al. 2003. DNA topoisomerases I and II inhibitory activity of constituents isolated from *Juglans mandshurica. Arch. Pharm. Res.* 26: 466–70.
17. Yao, D. L. et al. 2014. A new phenolic glycoside from *Juglans mandshurica. Nat. Prod. Res.* 28: 998–1002.

18. Yao, Y. et al. 2012. Juglanthraquinone C, a novel natural compound derived from *Juglans mandshurica* Maxim, induces S phase arrest and apoptosis in HepG2 cells. *Apoptosis* 17: 832–41.
19. Li, Z. B. et al. 2007. A cytotoxic compound from the leaves of *Juglans mandshurica. Chin. Chem. Lett.* 18: 846–8.
20. Li, Z. B. et al. 2007. Benzobijuglone, a novel cytotoxic compound from *Juglans mandshurica*, induced apoptosis in HeLa cervical cancer cells. *Phytomed.* 14: 846–52.
21. Li, Z. B. et al. 2009. Apoptosis of BGC823 cell line induced by p-hydroxymethoxybenzobijuglone, a novel compound from *Juglans mandshurica. Phytotherapy Res.* 23: 551–7.
22. Liu, L. J. et al. 2004. Studies on the cytotoxicity of compounds from fruits of *Juglans mandshurica. Nat. Med.* 58: 226–9.
23. Liu, L. J. et al. 2010. Studies on the cytotoxicity of naphthoquinone derivatives from the fresh rejuvenated fruits of *Juglans mandshurica. Zhongguo Xiandai Yingyong Yaoxue* 27: 574–577.
24. Joe, Y. K. et al. 1996. New naphthalenyl glucosides from the roots of *Juglans mandshurica. J. Nat. Prod.* 59: 159–60.
25. Liu, L. J. et al. 2010. Naphthalenyl glucosides from the cytotoxic portion of the fresh rejuvenated fruits of *Juglans mandshurica. Zhongguo Xiandai Yingyong Yaoxue* 27: 704–8.
26. Lee, K. et al. 2002. Cytotoxic diarylheptanoids from the roots of *Juglans mandshurica. J. Nat. Prods.* 65: 1707–8.
27. Liu, L. J. et al. 2010. Juglanone, a novel α-tetralonyl derivative with potent antioxidant activity from *Juglans mandshurica. J. Nat. Med.* 64: 496–9.
28. Min, B. S. et al. 2004. Apoptosis-inducing activity of galloylglucoses from *Juglans mandshurica* in human promyeloid leukemic HL-60 cells. *Nat. Prod. Sci.* 10: 48–53.
29. Lin, G. F. et al. 2010. Effect of flavones extract from *Juglans mandshurica* maxim stem-barks on p73-gene expression in hepatocarcinoma cell Bel-7402. *Shandong Yiyao* 50: 10–2.
30. Wang, R. J. et al. 2015. Antitumor effects and immune regulation activities of a purified polysaccharide extracted from *Juglan regia. Intl. J. Biol, Macromol.* 72: 771–5.

104 Hou Po 厚樸

Magnolia bark or Honokiol bark

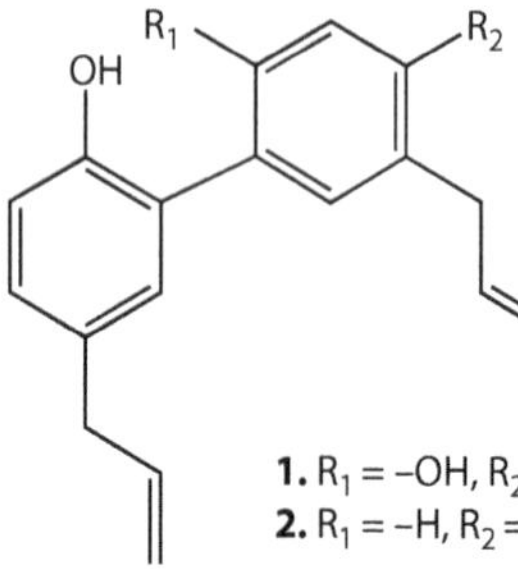

1. R_1 = -OH, R_2 = -H
2. R_1 = -H, R_2 = -OH

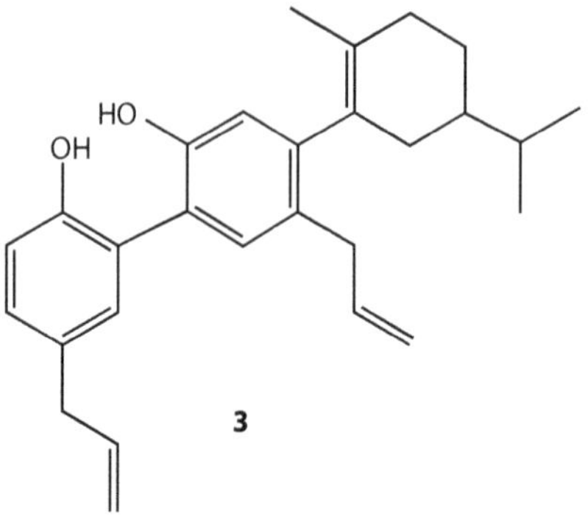

3

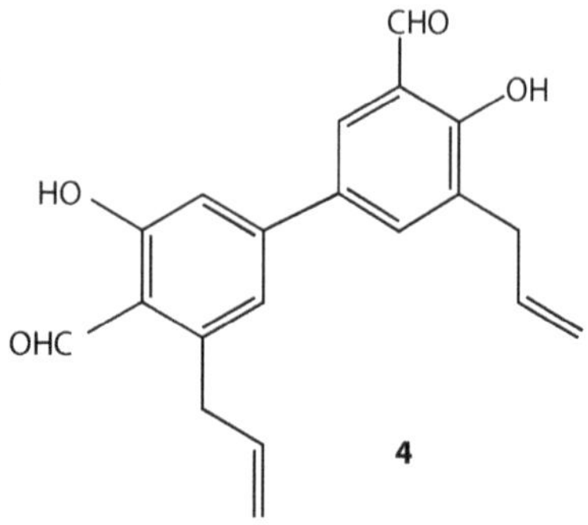

4

Herb Origination

The herb Hou Po is the dried barks of stem, root, and branch of two Magnoliaceae plants, *Magnolia officinalis* and *M. officinalis* var. *biloba*. The herb is a common traditional Chinese medicine recorded in *Shennong Ben Cao Jing*, the first Chinese classic of materia medica. These trees are native to the mountains and the valleys of China at 300–1500 m altitudes. Traditionally, the great quality of Hou Po is produced in Sichuan, Hubei, and Zhejiang provinces in China. Today, the bulk of bark for commercial and domestic uses is supplied by the plants in cultivation.

Antitumor Activities

The methanolic extract of Hou Po showed a potent cytotoxic potential on A549 (lung) and Col-2 (colon) human cancer cell lines *in vitro* but weak on human SK-Hep hepatoma cells,[1,2] whereas its n-butanol and chloroform partitioned fractions presented cytotoxicity on the SK-Hep cells (IC_{50}: 80–90 μg/mL).[2] The aqueous extract of Hou Po demonstrated the inhibitory effect against the cell viability of human c5637 urinary bladder cancer cells, associated with the upregulation of proapoptotic molecules (Bax, cytochrome c, and caspase-3), the down-expression of MMP-2 and MMP-9, and the blockage of DNA synthesis.[3] The methanolic extract and the derived n-butanol and ethyl acetate fractions also exerted marked inhibition on the activity of MMP-2, a key enzyme closely related to cancer metastasis.[2,4] An *in vivo* investigation confirmed that the suppression of the aqueous extract was achieved against carcinogen N-butyl-N-(4-hydroxybutyl) nitrosamine-induced urinary bladder tumors and the tumor cell invasion.[3]

Antitumor Constituents and Activities

Many types of constituents such as lignans (including neolignans, dilignans, monoterpene lignans), polyphenols, alkaloids, monoterpenes, and polysaccharides have been discovered from phytochemistry studies of Hou Po. Its neolignans are the most important components in response to the biological benefits of the herb. Magnolol (**1**) and honokiol (**2**) are the principal neolignans that contribute to the antitumor-related activities. According to the following summarized chemotherapeutic potential, magnolol (**1**) and honokiol (**2**) may be considered as promising agents for improving the poor response of both chemo- and radiotherapies against cancer.

Magnolol and Honokiol

Anticarcinogenic- and Antitumor-Promoting Effects

Three neolignans, magnolol (**1**), honokiol (**2**), and monoterpenyl-magnolol, were separated from the methanolic extract and exerted obvious suppression against TPA-induced EBV-EA activation. In an *in vivo* test of two-stage carcinogenesis, magnolol (**1**) showed the inhibitory effect against mouse skin tumor promotion.[5,6] Magnolol (**1**) and honokiol (**2**) also displayed chemopreventive effects against melanoma development induced by chemicals and UVB in mice. The pretreatment of combinations of α-santalol with magnolol or honokiol additively diminished the skin tumor multiplicity up to 75% in mice implanted with human A431 epidemoid carcinoma cells, whose α-santalol is an active agent from sandalwood oil having skin permeation-enhancing effect. The cotreatment restrained the cell proliferation and elicited the apoptosis of A431 cells, whose chemopreventive and anticarcinogenic effects were greater than those of α-santalol, honokiol and magnolol alone.[7]

Antiproliferative and Apoptosis-Inducing Effects

Magnolol (**1**) and honokiol (**2**) were able to enhance the cell apoptosis, thereby obstructing the cancer cell proliferation.[8] At 10–40 μM concentrations, magnolol (**1**) restrained the proliferation of human Colo-205 (colon) and HepG2 (liver) cancer cell lines with the blockage of DNA synthesis, and it also displayed the antiproliferative effect on human CH27 lung carcinoma and U373 astrocytoma cells *in vitro*.[9–11] Daily i.p. injections of magnolol (**1**) to nude mice bearing Colo-205 colon cancer led to the decrease of the tumor regression up to 85%.[9] The treatment with magnolol (**1**) in 40–80 μM concentration exhibited the cytotoxic effect and G2/M cell cycle arrest in two human androgen-independent PC3 and DU-145 prostate cancer cell lines, associated with the inhibition of cell cycle regulatory proteins including cyclin-A, cyclin-B1, cyclin-D1, and cyclin-E, CDK-2, and CDK-4.[12] Magnolol (**1**) also notably promoted the apoptosis of PC3 cells via EGFR-mediated signaling transduction pathway and alteration of the expressions of IGF-1 and its associated proteins, but magnolol (**1**) did not influence the viability of normal human prostate epithelial cells and human normal bronchial epithelial cells at the same concentration.[13–15] Similarly, magnolol (**1**) elicited the apoptosis of human T98G glioblastoma, A549, H441, and H520 NSCLC, MCF-7b breast cancer, and HCT116 colon cancer cell lines by diverse and characteristic pathways.[16–19] Through G2/M phase arrest pathway and ROS-involved/caspase-independent intrinsic pathway with release of AIF from mitochondrial, magnolol (**1**) effectively induced the apoptosis and inhibited the proliferation of MCF-7 cells.[17] Also, magnolol (**1**) and honokiol (**2**) demonstrated moderate cytotoxicity against OVCAR-3 (ovary), HepG2 (liver), and HeLa (cervix) human tumor cell lines.[20]

Honokiol (**2**) was a little toxic to normal cells but exerted potent anticancer activity *in vitro* and *in vivo*. By causing G1 cell cycle arrest and inducing apoptosis, honokiol (**2**) exerted antigrowth effects on both MiaPaCa and Panc1 pancreatic cancer cell lines in association with the marked down-expression of cyclin-D1, cyclin-E, CDK-2, and CDK-4, and activation of p21 and p27.[21] In nude mice incubated with human RKO colon cancer, honokiol (**2**) inhibited the cell growth and prolonged the life duration of tumor-bearing mice. The treatment of the RKO cells with honokiol (**2**) in doses of 5–10 μg/mL for 48 h significantly accelerated the cell apoptosis by activating caspase cascades.[22] In human SMMC-7721 hepatoma, JJ012 and SW1353 chondrosarcoma, and U87 glioblastoma cell lines, honokiol (**2**) markedly promoted the apoptotic death of all the four cell lines and dose-dependently suppressed the proliferation of SMMC-7721 cells *in vitro*.[23,24] The *in vivo* treatment with honokiol (**2**) for 21 days dramatically diminished the volume of chondrosarcoma by 53%.[24] Similarly, honokiol (**2**) exerted the suppressive effect against AML cells *in vitro* and *in vivo* concomitantly with the elicitation of apoptosis by inhibiting the activity of histone deacetylases and also prominently restraining the clonogenic activity of hematopoietic progenitors in bone marrow mononuclear cells from patients with AML.[25] In addition, by the cotreatment with honokiol (**2**), the cytotoxic effect of gemcitabine could be potentiated against the pancreatic cancer cells, whose effect was in part mediated by restricting the gemcitabine-induced nuclear accumulation of NF-κB.[21]

Autophagy-Inducing Effects

In addition to the stimulation of tumor cell apoptosis, honokiol (**2**) induced ROS-mediated cytoprotective autophagy in the PC3 prostate cancer cells *in vitro* and *in vivo* through the increase of LC3BII protein activity.[26] Honokiol (**2**) at a concentration of 50 μM significantly augmented Beclin-1 and LC3-II activities and markedly decreased Rb protein expression, then leading DBTRG-05MG glioblastoma multiforme (GBM) cells to type II-programmed cell death (autophagy).[27] The results may provide a potential strategy for improving the clinical outcome of GBM treatment.

Antiinvasive and Antimetastatic Effects

In vitro treatment with magnolol (**1**) at a 20 μM concentration could exert 98% inhibition on the invasion of PC3 prostate cancer cells by downregulating both protein and mRNA levels of MMP-2 and MMP-9.[13,14] In association with the dose-dependent inhibition of the expressions of ICAM-1 and VCAM-1, honokiol (**2**) markedly reduced the adhesion and the invasion of human T98G glioblastoma cells, indicating antimetastatic potential.[15] The antiinvasive and antimetastatic effects of honokiol (**2**) on U87MG human glioblastoma cells were mediated by obstructing the adhesion of U87MG to brain microvascular endothelial cells (BMECs) by inhibiting the VCAM-1 expression and blocking the invasion of U87MG through BMECs by reducing membrane permeability and epithelial-mesenchymal transition (EMT) processes.[28] Also, magnolol (**1**) and honokiol (**2**) were capable of suppressing the proliferation, migration, and invasion of human HONE1 nasopharyngeal carcinoma cells.[29]

Antiangiogenic Effect

Magnolol (**1**) was demonstrated to be an inhibitor of VEGF-induced angiogenesis. The treatment of HUVECs with magnolol (**1**) resulted in the inhibition of the proliferation, migration, and vessel sprouting through the decline of VEGF-induced Ras activation, inhibition of Ras-dependent MAPK and ERK, and blockage of PI3K/Akt and p38 signaling pathways.[30] Honokiol (**2**) was able to restrain the cell viability and the DNA synthesis in vascular smooth muscle cells and to increase G1 cell cycle arrest through the reduction of cyclin and CDK expressions and marked activation of p38/MAPK and JNK.[31] In hypoxic human T24 bladder carcinoma cells, the magnolol treatment restrained VEGF secretion and hypoxia-stimulated H_2O_2 formation and diminished HIF-1α expression and transcriptional levels. Magnolol (**1**) also acted as a VEGFR2 antagonist to attenuate the activation of downstream AKT/mTOR/p70S6K/4E-BP-1 kinase in both the T24 cells and the tissues. The antigrowth and antiangiogenic activities of magnolol (**1**) were also demonstrated in a T24 xenograft mouse model. The data evidenced that the antiangiogenic activity of magnolol (**1**) is largely mediated by suppressing HIF-1α/VEGF-dependent pathways and suggested that magnolol (**1**) and honokiol (**2**) may be potential antiangiogenic agents to be developed for chemotherapy in patients with cancer.[32]

Differentiation-Inducing Effect

By increasing the cell-expressing membrane differentiation markers CD11b and CD14, both magnolol (**1**) and honokiol (**2**) at doses of 10–30 μM were able to enhance the differentiation of human HL-60 acute promyelocytic leukemia cells initiated by low doses of all-*trans*-retinoic acid (ATRA) or 25-dihydroxyvitamin-D3 (VD3). Combining magnolol or honokiol to the treatment of HL-60 cells with ATRA or VD3 also enlarged the G0/G1 cell population and the expression of p27 Kip1 (a CDK inhibitor). These findings highlighted that the potential strategy of magnolol and honokiol in combination with the low doses of VD3 and ATRA can improve the clinical treatment for acute promyelocytic leukemia.[33]

Drug-Resistant Reversal Effect

The investigation confirmed that magnolol (**1**), honokiol (**2**), as well as 4-*O*-methylhonokiol also have an ability to dose- and time-dependently restrain P-gp expression and to enhance intracellular accumulation of calcein (a P-gp substrate), leading to the reversal of the drug-resistance in NCI/ADR-RES cells and the potentiation of daunorubicin-induced cytotoxic activity. These positive data evidenced that the neolignans (honokiol, magnolol, and 4-*O*-methylhonokiol) may be promising agents for reducing the MDR of cancer cells to anticancer drugs via the downregulation of P-gp expression.[34]

Antioxidant Activity

Honokiol (**2**) is also an effective scavenger of both superoxide and peroxyl radicals, whose reactivity was 20 times higher than a vitamin E analog trolox. The antioxidative property might be important for the antitumor and antiangiogenetic activities of honokiol.[35]

Other Neolignans

Several other neolignans were isolated from Hou Po, showing antitumor-related potentials in *in vitro* and *in vivo* experiments. 4′-Methoxymagndialdehyde and magnaldehyde-B could promote the apoptotic death of human HeLa cervical epitheloid carcinoma cells concomitantly with cleavage of procaspase-8 and procaspase-3 and PARP into active forms. *In vivo*, the administration of magnaldehyde-B in a dose 20 mg/kg to mice inoculated with Lewis lung carcinoma resulted in a 28.7% reduction of tumor volume.[36] 4-*O*-Methylhonokiol in concentrations of ~30 μM could cause G0/G1 phase cell cycle arrest followed by the induction of apoptotic death in human colon cancer cell lines (SW620 and HCT116), thereby retarding the tumor cell growth, whose effects were validated *in vivo* using a nude mice xenograft model implanted with SW620 colon cancer cells. The antitumor activity was revealed to correlate with the decrease of constitutive activated NF-κB-DNA-binding activity and antiapoptotic protein expressions and the increase of the expression of p21 and apoptotic proteins.[37] Similarly, accompanied by the decreased NF-κB activity, the increased expression of apoptotic proteins and p21, and the enhanced PPARγ transcriptional activity, 4-*O*-methylhonokiol inhibited the growth of human prostate cancer cell lines (PC3 and LNCaP) and elicited G0/G1 cell cycle arrest and cell apoptosis. The growth inhibitory effect of 4-*O*-methylhonokiol was further proven in an animal model with xenograft prostate cancer cells.[38] 4-*O*-Methylhonokiol was also able to induce the apoptosis of SiHa cervical carcinoma cells through the inhibition of PI3K/Akt pathway, the induction of intrinsic pathway, and the activation of PPARγ.[39]

Piperitylmagnolol (**3**) was effective in the growth inhibition of K562 (leukemic), HeLa (cervix), A549 (lung), and HCT116 (colon) cancer cells *in vitro* (IC_{50}: 7.7–9.5 μg/mL), whereas magnolol monoacetate and magnolol diacetate were much less active.[40] Also, piperitylmagnolol (**3**) demonstrated moderate cytotoxicity against HepG2 (liver), OVCAR-3 (ovary), and HeLa (cervix) human tumor cell lines.[20]

Synthetic Honokiol Derivatives

In order to find more stable and less susceptible agent to bypass the drug resistance and to prevent angiogenesis-dependent tumor growth and metastasis, 47 honokiol analogs and derivatives have been synthesized and evaluated. The analogs hold an allylated biphenolic scaffold that displayed a unique mode of action in antiangiogenic and antitumor activities. Among them, a bisaldehyde derivative (**4**) exhibited the strongest inhibitory effects against the proliferation, migration, and tube formation of HUVECs, featuring its antiangiogenic effect by targeting VEGF or fibroblast growth factor to moderately block the newly grown segmental vessels. The bisaldehyde derivative (**4**) also exerted medium cytotoxicity against three selected tumor cell lines, A549 (lung cancer), HepG2 (hepatoma), and LL/2 (Lewis lung tumor), *in vitro*.[41]

Polysaccharides

Three polysaccharide fractions were prepared from the herb, and these polysaccharides were composed of fucose, xylose, mannose, glucose, galactose, and arabinose. The polysaccharides also displayed antioxidant effect, including scavenging activity of superoxide anion and hydrogen peroxide. Among them, a polysaccharide fraction with 3.9–4.2 kDa moleculular weight exhibited the highest antioxidant activities and the stronger cytotoxic activity on human MCF-7 breast carcinoma cell line *in vitro*.[42]

Exploration of Apoptotic Mechanisms

Magnolol (**1**) and honokiol (**2**) have been proposed to play a similar role in the tumor cell growth inhibition through cytotoxicity, apoptosis-inducing, antiangiogenic, differentiation, and antioxidant actions in several *in vivo* models but their mechanisms were not the same. Honokiol (**2**)-induced apoptotic mechanism in human CH27 squamous lung cancer cells was mediated by the upregulation of Bad and the downregulation of Bcl-xL, the release of cytochrome c to cytosol, and the sequential activation of caspases, without effects on the levels of Bcl-2, Bcl-xS, Bag-1, Bax, and Bak proteins,[7] but magnolol (**1**) significantly augmented the expressions of Bad and Bcl-xS and decreased the expression of Bcl-xL.[10] Concomitantly, magnolol (**1**) not only caused cytosolic cytochrome c and activated caspases but also induced a modest and persistent JNK activation and ERK inactivation in the apoptosis of CH27 cells.[10] Magnolol (**1**) showed the growth inhibitory activity toward human HepG2 hepatoma, Colo205 colon cancer, and U373 glioblastoma cell lines, whose antigrowth effect essentially depended on the abilities of magnolol in the induction of cell cycle arrest at G0/G1 phase via the decrease of cyclin-A and cyclin-D1 protein levels, the reduction of CDK2 activity, the increase of p21 activity and CDK2-p21/Cip1 complex, and the blockage of DNA synthesis.[9,11] The apoptosis induced by honokiol (**2**) in SMMC-7721 hepatoma cells was triggered by the increases of ROS production and Bax/Bcl-2 ratios, and chondrosarcoma cells was closely correlated to the increase of ER stress and changes of cytosol calcium levels.[22] A caspase-independent pathway involved in the magnolol (**1**) elicited the apoptosis of A549 NSCLC cells, which was mainly associated with the up-expression of Bax and Bid; the activation of p38, JNK, and endonuclease-G; the inhibition of PI3K/AKT and ERK1/2 activities; the release of cytochrome c from mitochondria; and the cleave of PARP.[17]

Besides the down-expression of Bcl-2, augmentation p53 and Bax expressions, and release of mitochondrial cytochrome c, magnolol (**1**) also displayed several other characteristic apoptotic features, including phosphorylation of AMPK, propidium iodide labeling, cleavage of PARP, and activation of caspase-3 in human HCT-116 colon carcinoma cells, which induced AMPK activation that also correlates to its antimigratory and anti-invasive effects of magnolol (**1**) in HCT-116 cells.[19] By reducing the DCLK1 level and inhibiting γ-secretase complex and Notch signaling pathway, honokiol (**2**) stimulated the sensitivity of colon cancer stem cells to ionizing radiation (IR). Therefore, the combination of honokiol and IR prominently elicited the apoptosis and suppressed the proliferation and colony formation of the colon cancer stem cells *in vitro* and *in vivo*.[43] The apoptosis of glioblastoma cells could be triggered by honokiol (**2**) through both caspase-independent and caspase-dependent pathways, the latter including both extrinsic pathway and intrinsic pathway. The suppression of ERK1/2 and STAT3 signaling and activation of p38 MAPK signaling pathway were found to be involved in human U87 glioblastoma cell apoptosis elicited by honokiol (**2**), whereas the apoptotic induction in T98G glioblastoma cells by honokiol (**2**) was associated with the downregulation of Bcl-2 (an anti apoptotic protein) and the upregulation of Bax (a proapoptotic protein).[15,44]

Collectively, the explorations concerning the mechanisms provided the theory basis for clinical approaches to the use of Hou Po or its major constituents, magnolol (**1**) and honokiol (**2**), in the promotion of chemotherapy on neoplastic diseases.

Other Bioactivities

Pharmacological studies have proven that Hou Po (Magnolia bark) has multiple therapeutic benefits such as muscle relaxant, antioxidant, antiinflammatory, antiseptic, astringent, antispasmodic, carminative, hypotensive, analgesic, stimulant, antiemetic, antiulcerative, central depressant, blood pressure reductive, antifungal, and antimicrobial properties. Its antioxidant activity was found to be more potent than vitamin E for up to a thousand times. The herb has also been used to break addiction to cigarettes and to treat amoebic dysentery. In Japan, the herb is used to help control stress and anxiety as well. Magnolol (**1**) and honokiol (**2**) have been demonstrated to have antianxiety activity, and they were shown to reduce allergic and asthmatic reactions.

References

1. Nam, K. A. et al. 2000. Evaluation of cytotoxic potential of natural products in cultured human cancer cells. *Nat. Prod. Sci.* 6: 183–8.
2. Lee, D. Y. et al. 2006. Inhibitory effect of methanol extract of *Magnolia officinalis* on matrix metalloproteinase-2. *J. Food Sci. Nutr.* 11: 191–7.
3. Lee, S. J. et al. 2009. Inhibitory effects of the aqueous extract of *Magnolia officinalis* on the responses of human urinary bladder cancer 5637 cells in vitro and mouse urinary bladder tumors induced by N-butyl-N-(4-hydroxybutyl) nitrosamine in vivo. *Phytother. Res.* 23: 20–7.
4. Seo, U. K. et al. 2005. Large-scale and effective screening of Korean medicinal plants for inhibitory activity on matrix metalloproteinase-9. *J. Ethnopharmacol.* 97: 101–6.
5. Konoshima, T. et al. 1991. Studies on inhibitors of skin tumor promotion: Neolignans from *Magnolia officinalis. J. Nat. Prods.* 54: 816–22.
6. Tokuta, T. et al. 1990. Inhibitory effects on Epstein-Barr virus activation and antitumor promoting activities of Coix seed. *Planta Med.* 56: 653.
7. Chilampalli, C. et al. 2013. Chemopreventive effects of combination of honokiol and magnolol with α-santalol on skin cancer developments. *Drug Discov. Therapeutics* 7: 109–15.
8. Yang, S. Y. et al. 2002. Down-modulation of Bcl-XL, release of cytochrome c and sequential activation of caspases during honokiol-induced apoptosis in human squamous lung cancer CH27 cells. *Biochem. Pharmacol.* 63: 1641–51.
9. Lin, S. Y. et al. 2001. Magnolol suppresses proliferation of cultured human colon and liver cancer cells by inhibiting DNA synthesis and activating apoptosis. *J. Cell. Biochem.* 84: 532–44.
10. Yang, S. E. et al. 2003. Effector mechanism of magnolol-induced apoptosis in human lung squamous carcinoma CH27 cells. *British J. Pharmacol.* 138: 193–201.
11. Chen, L. C. et al. 2009. Magnolol inhibits human glioblastoma cell proliferation through upregulation of p21/Cip1. *J. Agricult. Food Chem.* 57: 7331–7.
12. McKeown, B. T. et al. 2014. Magnolol causes alterations in the cell cycle in androgen insensitive human prostate cancer cells in vitro by affecting expression of key cell cycle regulatory proteins. *Nutr. Cancer* 66: 1154–64.
13. Lee, D. H. et al. 2009. Magnolol induces apoptosis via inhibiting the EGFR/PI3K/Akt signaling pathway in human prostate cancer cells. *J. Cell. Biochem.* 106: 1113–22.
14. Hwang, E. S. et al. 2010. Magnolol suppresses metastasis via inhibition of invasion, migration, and matrix metalloproteinase-2/-9 activities in PC-3 human prostate carcinoma cells. *Biosci. Biotech. Biochem.* 74: 961–7.
15. Jeong, J. J. et al. 2012. Honokiol exerts an anticancer effect in T98G human glioblastoma cells through the induction of apoptosis and the regulation of adhesion molecules. *Intl. J. Oncol.* 41: 1358–64.
16. Zhou, Y. F. et al. 2013. Magnolol induces apoptosis in MCF-7 human breast cancer cells through G2/M phase arrest and caspase-independent pathway. *Pharmazie* 68: 755–62.
17. Tsai, J. R. et al. 2014. Magnolol induces apoptosis via caspase-independent pathways in non-small cell lung cancer cells. *Archiv. Pharm. Res.* 37: 548–57.
18. McKeown, B. T. et al. 2014. Magnolol affects expression of IGF-1 and associated binding proteins in human prostate cancer cells in vitro. *Anticancer Res.* 34: 6333–8.
19. Park, J. B. et al. 2012. Magnolol-induced apoptosis in HCT-116 colon cancer cells is associated with the AMP-activated protein kinase signaling pathway. *Biol. Pharm. Bull.* 35: 1614–20.
20. Syu, W. Jr et al. 2004. Antimicrobial and cytotoxic activities of neolignans from *Magnolia officinalis. Chem. Biodiv.* 1: 530–7.
21. Arora, S. et al. 2011. Honokiol arrests cell cycle, induces apoptosis, and potentiates the cytotoxic effect of gemcitabine in human pancreatic cancer cells. *PLoS One* 6: e21573.
22. Chen, F. et al. 2004. Honokiol: A potent chemotherapy candidate for human colorectal carcinoma. *World J. Gastroenterol.* 10: 3459–63.
23. Han, L. L. et al. 2009. Reactive oxygen species production and Bax/Bcl-2 regulation in honokiol-induced apoptosis in human hepatocellular carcinoma SMMC-7721 cells. *Envir. Toxicol. Pharmacol.* 28: 97–103.

24. Chen, Y. J. et al. 2010. Honokiol induces cell apoptosis in human chondrosarcoma cells through mitochondrial dysfunction and endoplasmic reticulum stress. *Cancer Lett.* 291: 20–30.
25. Li, H. Y. et al. 2015. Honokiol induces cell cycle arrest and apoptosis via inhibiting class I histone deacetylases in acute myeloid leukemia. *J. Cell. Biochem.* 116: 287–98.
26. Hahm, E. R. et al. 2014. Honokiol activates reactive oxygen species-mediated cytoprotective autophagy in human prostate cancer cells. *Prostate* (Hoboken, NJ, US). 74: 1209–21.
27. Chang, K. H. et al. 2013. Honokiol-induced apoptosis and autophagy in glioblastoma multiforme cells. *Oncol. Lett.* 6: 1435–8.
28. Joo, Y. N. et al. 2014. Honokiol inhibits U87MG human glioblastoma cell invasion through endothelial cells by regulating membrane permeability and the epithelial-mesenchymal transition. *Intl. J. Oncol.* 44: 187–94.
29. Qin, J. et al. 2015. Mechanism of anti-nasopharyngeal carcinoma effect of magnolol and honokiol. *Zhongcaoyao* 46: 226–30.
30. Kim, K. M. et al. 2013. Magnolol suppresses vascular endothelial growth factor-induced angiogenesis by inhibiting Ras-dependent mitogen-activated protein kinase and phosphatidylinositol 3-kinase/Akt signaling pathways. *Nutr. Cancer* 65: 1245–53.
31. Lee, B. B. et al. 2006. Honokiol causes the p21WAF1-mediated G1-phase arrest of the cell cycle through inducing p38 mitogen activated protein kinase in vascular smooth muscle cells. *FEBS Lett.* 580: 5177–84.
32. Chen, M. C. et al. 2013. Magnolol suppresses hypoxia-induced angiogenesis via inhibition of HIF-1α/VEGF signaling pathway in human bladder cancer cells. *Biochem. Pharmacol.* 85: 1278–87.
33. Fong, W. F. et al. 2005. Magnolol and honokiol enhance HL-60 human leukemia cell differentiation induced by 1,25-dihydroxyvitamin D_3 and retinoic acid. *Intl. J. Biochem. Cell Biol.* 37: 427–41.
34. Han, H. K. et al. 2012. Modulation of P-glycoprotein expression by honokiol, magnolol and 4-O-methylhonokiol, the bioactive components of *Magnolia officinalis. Anticancer Res.* 32: 4445–52.
35. Dikalov, S. et al. 2008. Honokiol is a potent scavenger of superoxide and peroxyl radicals. *Biochem. Pharmacol.* 76: 589–96.
36. Youn, U. J. et al. 2013. Apoptosis-inducing and antitumor activity of neolignans isolated from *Magnolia officinalis* in HeLa cancer cells. *Phytotherapy Res.* 27: 1419–22.
37. Oh, J. H. et al. 2012. 4-*O*-methylhonokiol inhibits colon tumor growth via p21-mediated suppression of NF-κB activity. *J. Nutr. Biochem.* 23: 706–15.
38. Lee, N. J. et al. 2013. 4-O-methylhonokiol, a PPARγ agonist, inhibits prostate tumour growth: P21-mediated suppression of NF-κB activity. *British J. Pharmacol.* 168: 1133–45.
39. Hyun, S. Y. et al. 2015. Peroxisome proliferator-activated receptor-gamma agonist 4-Q-methylhonokiol induces apoptosis by triggering the intrinsic apoptosis pathway and inhibiting the PI3K/Akt survival pathway in SiHa human cervical cancer cells. *J. Microbiol. Biotechnol.* 25: 334–42.
40. Youn, U. J. et al. 2011. A cytotoxic monoterpene-neolignan from the stem bark of *Magnolia officinalis. Nat. Prod. Sci.* 17: 95–9.
41. Ma, L. et al. 2011. Structural modification of honokiol, a biphenyl occurring in *Magnolia officinalis*: The evaluation of honokiol analogues as inhibitors of angiogenesis and for their cytotoxicity and structure activity relationship. *J. Med. Chem.* 54: 6469–81.
42. Lan, M. B. et al. 2012. Antioxidant and antitumor activities of purified polysaccharides with low molecular weights from *Magnolia officinalis. J. Med. Plants Res.* 6: 1025–34.
43. Ponnurangam, S. et al. 2012. Honokiol in combination with radiation targets notch signaling to inhibit colon cancer stem cells. *Mol. Cancer Therap.* 11: 963–72.
44. Zhang, Y. B. 2014. Downregulation of STAT3 and activation of MAPK are involved in the induction of apoptosis by HNK in glioblastoma cell line U87. *Oncol. Reports* 32: 2038–46.

105 Gan Song 甘松

Chinese spikenard

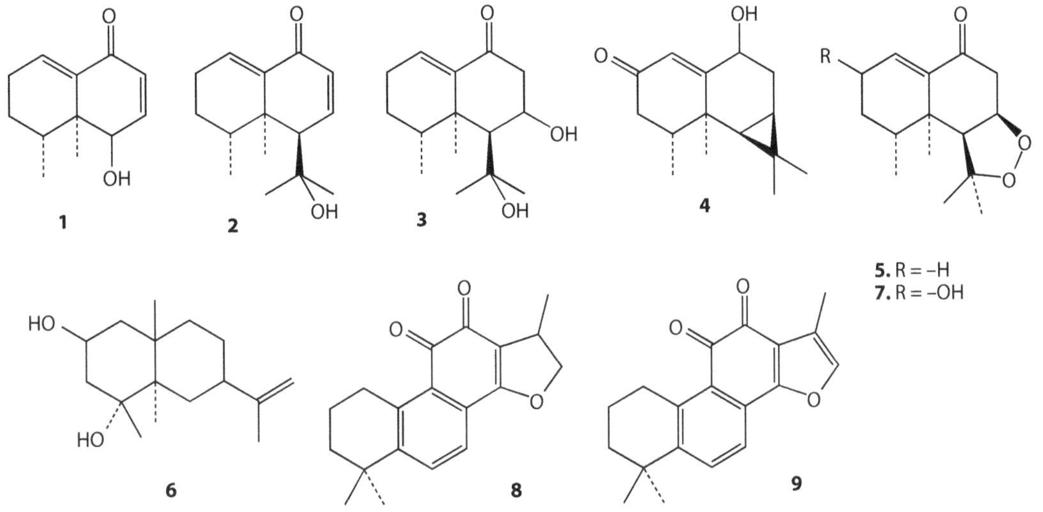

1 2 3 4 5. R = -H 7. R = -OH 6 8 9

Herb Origination

The herb Gan Song (Chinese spikenard) is the dried roots and rhizomes of two plants, *Nardostachys chinensis* and *N. jatamansi* (Valerianaceae). The distributions of these two perennial plants are in western China for the former origin of the herb and in the Himalayas of Nepal, China, and India for the latter one. The general collection season for the herb is in summer and autumn, but the autumn collection is considered to have better quality of the herb.

Antitumor Constituents and Activities

In recent years, Nardostachys rhizoma extracts have been patented as a promising drug candidate for the prevention and the treatment of several carcinoma diseases in the lung, the prostate, the pancreas, the kidney, and the brain. The extracts were reported to be capable of suppressing the growth of neoplastic cells and inducing the cell apoptosis.[1] Different classes of constituents such as alkaloids, sterols, neolignans, and lignans have been isolated from the herb, but sesquiterpenoids are particularly rich in the plants. The phytochemical experiments revealed that the two origins of Gan Song contain similar sesquiterpene type of inhibitors; however, their anticancer sesquiterpenes were not quite the same.

Agents from N. chinensis

An ethyl acetate partitioned fraction demonstrated cytotoxic effect on mouse P388 leukemia cells *in vitro* (IC_{50}: 12.5 μg/mL). A systemic investigation of the active fraction led to the isolation of six cytostatic sesquiterpenoids identified as desoxonarchinol-A (**1**), kanshone-A (**2**), nardosinonediol (**3**), debilon (**4**), nardosinone (**5**), and eudesm-11-en-2,4α-diol (**6**). They displayed moderate inhibitory effect (IC_{50}: 2.2–18.5 μg/mL) in the *in vitro* assay with P388 cell line. Of these terpenes, desoxonarchinol-A (**1**) and kanshone-A (**2**) exerted greater cytotoxicity on the P388 cells, and their IC_{50} values were 2.2 and 7.0 μg/mL, respectively.[2] When converted to esters of desoxonarchinol-A (**1**), the anti-P388 activity could be augmented by 3.67–15.7-fold. The IC_{50} value of desoxonarchinol-A benzoate was 0.14 μg/mL, which was the most potent one in the four types of esters. If desoxonarchinol-A was transformed to a quinone-type derivative, the IC_{50} value reached to 0.11 μg/mL and the antileukemia activity was enhanced by 20-fold.[2] An *in vitro* experiment with a small panel of human neoplastic cell lines showed that kanshone-A (**2**) restrained the proliferation of BGC-823 (gastric), Bel-7402 (liver), A2780 (ovary), HCT-8 (colon), and A549 (lung) human cancer cell lines (IC_{50}: 1.90–2.46 μg/mL), whereas kanshone-B (**7**) only showed modest suppressive effect on Bel-7402 hepatoma cells (IC_{50} 7.54 μg/mL).[3] Analyzing the relationship between the structure and the biology of these active sesquiterpenes suggested that the α,β-unsaturated ketone conjugated system in the rings is probably the key center for the cytotoxicity.

In addition, an aqueous extract from *N. chinensis* and an active 20% methanol chromatographic fraction derived from the ethyl acetate layer exerted melanogenesis inhibitory activity in B16-F10 melanoma cells via PI3K/Akt signaling and stimulation of MEK/ERK phosphorylation and obstruction of tyrosinase activity and tyrosinase-related proteins expression. The findings may be helpful for the design of melanoma-preventing and skin-whitening agents.[4,5]

Agents from N. jatamansi

Both aqueous and hydroalcohol extracts of *N. jatamansi* were genotoxic to the DNA of human HepG2 hepatoma cells *in vitro* in concentrations of 5 and 10 mg/mL, respectively.[6] The isolation of its chloroform–methanol (1:1) fraction led to obtainment of three triterpenoids and five sesquiterpenes. Of these compounds, only the two triterpenoids, i.e., ursolic acid and its 3-*O*-arabinoside, demonstrated moderate inhibitory effect against the proliferation of DU-145 (prostate), MCF-7 (breast), SK-N-SH (brain), and A549 (lung) human tumor cell lines *in vitro* (IC_{50}s 18–32 μM).[7] Compared to ER^+-MCF-7 breast cancer cells, its methanol extract (NJM) and subsequent diethyl ether fraction (NJDE) displayed relatively higher inhibition against ER^--MDA-MB-231 breast cancer cells (IC_{50}: 23.83 and 25.04 μg/mL, respectively). Both induced obvious cell apoptotic death, but NJM caused G2/M arrest, while NJDE caused G0/G1 phase arrest in the MDA-MB-231 cells.[8]

The herb (*N. jatamansi*) possesses marked protective activities on carcinogenesis-related oxidative injury and genotoxicity. The pretreatment with *N. jatamansi* extract by oral administration in a daily dose of 500 mg/kg for seven days could notably reverse the myocardial damage caused by a chemotherapeutic agent doxorubicin (15 mg/kg, i.p.) in rat by restoring the activity of antioxidant enzymes (such as superoxide dismutase, catalase, glutathione peroxidase, and GST), adjusting the lipid peroxides to near normal levels and elevating the serum marker enzymes (such as lactate dehydrogenase, creatine phosphokinase, aspartate aminotransaminase, and alanine aminotransaminase).[9]

Other Bioactivities

Pharmacological studies have demonstrated that the herb Gan Song possesses multiple biological functions including cognition and memory improvement, hypolipidemic, hepatoprotective, anticonvulsant, antidepressant, antiparkinson, neuroprotective, cardio-protective, and antifungal activities. Acaciin and ursolie acid are the active components for antihiotics and antiinflammatory. In addition, Nardostachys rhizomes, especially from *N. jatamansi* plant, is used in the manufacture of an intensely aromatic amber-colored essential oil. The oil has been utilized as a perfume and a medicine as well as in religious contexts since ancient times.

References

1. Hwang, S. Y. et al. 2012. (a) Nardostachys rhizoma extracts for preventing and treating lung cancer. *Repub. Korean Kongkae Taeho Kongbo* KR 2012109136 A 20121008; (b) Spikenard extracts for the treatment of prostate cancer. *PCT Int. Appl.* WO 2012030142 A2 20120308; (c) Nardostachys rhizoma extracts for the treatment of pancreatic cancer. *PCT Intl. Appl.* WO 2012134251 A2 20121004; (d) Nardostachys rhizoma extracts for the treatment of renal cancer. *PCT Intl. Appl.* WO 2012134250 A2 20121004; (e) Nardostachys rhizoma extracts for the treatment of brain cancer. *Repub. Korean Kongkae Taeho Kongbo* KR 2012092265 A 20120821.
2. Itokawa, H. et al. 1993. Cytotoxic sesquiterpenes from *Nardostachys chinensis. Chem. Pharm. Bull.* 41: 1183–4.
3. Masuyama, K. et al. 1993. Eudesm-11-en-2,4α-diol from *Nardostachys chinensis. Phytochem.* 34: 567–8.
4. Lee, S. J. et al. 2006. Inhibitory effects of aqueous extracts from *Nardostachys chinensis* on α-melanocyte stimulating hormone-induced melanogenesis in B16F10 cells. *Integrative Biosci.* 10: 233–6.
5. Jang, J. Y. et al. 2011. Partially purified components of *Nardostachys chinensis* suppress melanin synthesis through ERK and Akt signaling pathway with cAMP down-regulation in B16F10 cells. *J. Ethnopharmacol.* 137: 1207–8.
6. Etebari, M. et al. 2012. Evaluation of DNA damage of hydroalcoholic and aqueous extract of *Echium amoenum* and *Nardostachys jatamansi. J. Res. in Med. Sci.* 17: 782–6.
7. Rekha, K. et al. 2013. Two new sesquiterpenoids from the rhizomes of *Nardostachys jatamansi. J. Asian Nat. Prod. Res.* 15: 111–6.
8. Chaudhary, S. et al. 2015. Evaluation of antioxidant and anticancer activity of extract and fractions of *Nardostachys jatamansi* DC in breast carcinoma. *BMC Complem. Altern. Med.* 15: 1–13.
9. Subashini, R. et al. 2006. Protective effect of *Nardostachys jatamansi* on oxidative injury and cellular abnormalities during doxorubicin-induced cardiac damage in rats. *J. Pharm. Pharmacol.* 58: 257–62.

6

Anticancer Potentials of Blood-Activating and Stasis-Resolving Herbs

CONTENTS

106 He Huan Pi 合歡皮

Mimosa tree bark or Silk tree bark

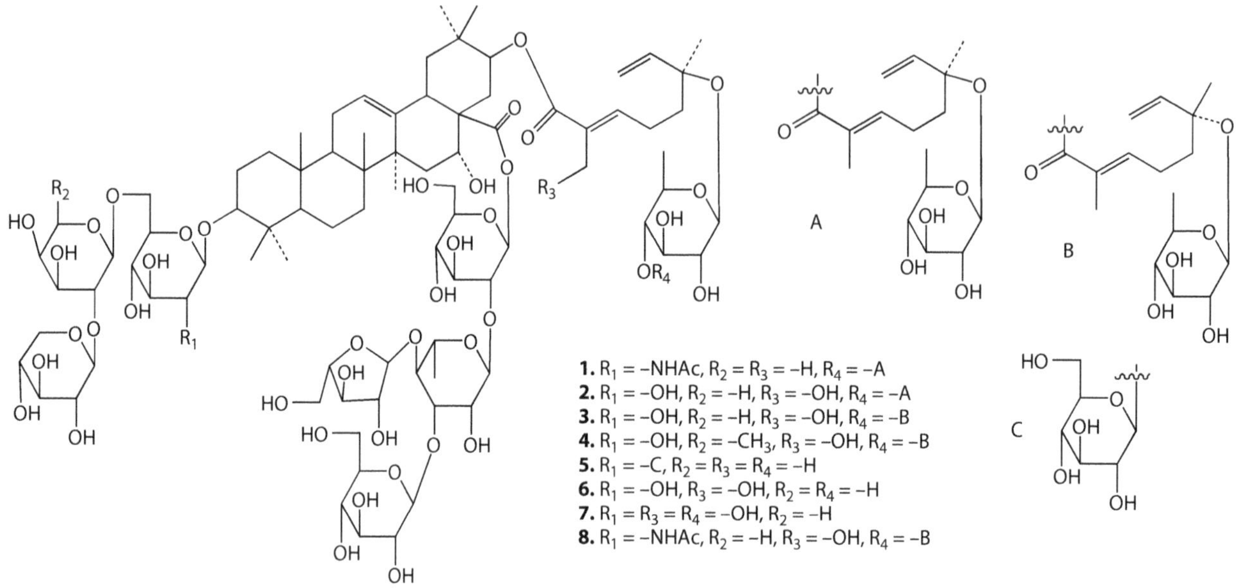

1. R_1 = –NHAc, R_2 = R_3 = –H, R_4 = –A
2. R_1 = –OH, R_2 = –H, R_3 = –OH, R_4 = –A
3. R_1 = –OH, R_2 = –H, R_3 = –OH, R_4 = –B
4. R_1 = –OH, R_2 = –CH_3, R_3 = –OH, R_4 = –B
5. R_1 = –C, R_2 = R_3 = R_4 = –H
6. R_1 = –OH, R_3 = –OH, R_2 = R_4 = –H
7. R_1 = R_3 = R_4 = –OH, R_2 = –H
8. R_1 = –NHAc, R_2 = –H, R_3 = –OH, R_4 = –B

Herb Origination

The herb He Huan Pi (Mimosa tree bark) is the dried stem barks of a Leguminosae tree, *Albizia julibrissin*. This small deciduous tree is native to southern and eastern Asia, from east Iran to China and Korea. The plant was introduced to Europe in the mid-eighteenth century and is now broadly cultivated throughout the southeastern United States along the roadsides. As an herb, the barks are stripped off from the tree stem between summer and autumn and dried in the sun for medical application.

Antitumor Activities

The water extract of Cortex albiziae has been claimed as a patent for treating glioma, hepatoma, and esophageal cancer because the extracts exerted the inhibitory effect against the proliferation of three human carcinoma cell lines (HepG2, Eca9706, and C6) and induced C6 glioma cells to apoptosis and cell cycle arrest.[1] A fraction prepared from the herb by partition and chromatography showed significant inhibitory effect on human U251 glioma cells.[2] More researches revealed that the herb contains antitumor angiogenesis components that could retard the proliferation of human vessel endothelial cells (HMEC-I), whose active components were identified as saponins.[3,4]

Antitumor Constituents and Activities

A saponin fraction prepared from the crude extract of He Huan Pi exhibited moderate cytotoxicity against human KB nasopharyngeal cancer cells *in vitro* (IC_{50}: 12.8 μg/mL). Many antitumor triterpenoidal saponins were separated from the fraction. Julibroside-III (**1**) obviously restrained the growth of KB cells (IC_{50}: 1.9 μg/mL or 0.9 μM)[5] and both julibroside-J1 (**2**) and julibroside-J9 (**3**) demonstrated prominent suppressive effect on KB cells by 94% in doses of 4 and 10 μM, respectively, *in vitro*.[6] Julibroside-J21 and julibroside -J28 exerted more potent inhibition on human Bel-7402 liver adenocarcinoma cells compared to julibroside-J8 and julibroside-J13.[7,8] At a 10 μM concentration, julibroside-J28, julibroside-J29, julibroside-J30, and julibroside-J31 significantly restrained the proliferation of PC3MIE8 (prostate), HeLa (cervix), and/or MDA-MB-435 (breast) human cancer cell lines *in vitro*.[9,10] The antiproliferative effect of julibroside-J8 (**4**) was shown in human BGC-823 (stomach), Bel-7402 (liver), and HeLa (cervix) cancer cell lines at a concentration of 100 μg/mL.[11] The *in vitro* assays also substantiated four other julibroside-J18, julibroside-J19, julibroside-J22, and julibroside-J25 possessing the antitumor property.[12,13]

The effect of julibroside-J8 (**4**) in the induction of apoptosis and DNA fragmentation of HeLa cells was shown to be associated with the initiation of morphologic changes such as an increase in Bax expression, a significant decrease in Bcl-2 expression in the mitochondria, downregulation of inhibitor of caspase-activated DNase (ICAD) expression, and activation of caspase-3.[11] Three artificial secondary saponins (**5–7**) obtained from the hydrolysis of the saponin fraction with $NaHCO_3$ displayed the inhibitory activity on the KB cells (IC_{50}: 9.1, 2.9, and 3.7 μg/mL, respectively).[5] Because julibroside-III (**1**) showed the stronger cytotoxic effect (IC_{50}: 1.9 μg/mL), the evidences revealed that a hydroxyl group at C-16 of the aglycon may play an important role in mediating the inhibition, and an N-acetyl-glucosamine moiety at C-3′ seems to enhance the anticancer effect.[5] In addition, HaBC18, a purified substance, was extracted from a n-butanolic fraction of the herb and displayed a noticeable inhibitory effect toward human acute leukemia Jurkat T cells *in vitro* (IC_{50}: 1.25 μg/mL) and less sensitive to a human normal PBMC cells. The effect against Jurkat T cells was revealed to be accompanied with apoptosis induction through Bcl-xL-regulated and mitochondria-dependent death-signaling pathways.[14]

The antiangiogenic activity of He Huan Pi has been paid more attention recently for further investigation. The saponin-rich extracts/fractions such as n-butanolic extract, 50% ethanolic, and 70% ethanolic fractions demonstrated significant *in vitro* inhibitory effect against the angiogenesis of HMEC-1 and 3B11 mouse vessel endothelial cells.[15] The total saponin extract was subjected to *in vivo* investigation in mice implanted with mouse H22 hepatoma. The oral administration of the saponin at a dose of 5 mg/kg per day for 7–14 days resulted in an obvious antiangiogenic effect by the repression of phosphorylated FAK, Akt, and ERK in a VEGF/VEGFR2 signaling pathway and the blockage of vascularization in basic fibroblast growth factor (bFGF)-induced Matrigel plugs and microvasculature formation.[16,17] By blocking the endothelial cell proliferation and the vascular formation, the saponin-rich extract significantly inhibited the growth of LLC cells and reduced the metastatic lesions in a mouse model.[18] The antiangiogenic activity was also observed in Ea.hy926 endothelial cells *in vitro* with significant inhibition of the VEGF-mediated endothelial cell proliferation, migration, and tube formation.[17] Furthermore, julibroside-J8 (**4**) and julibroside-J12 (**8**) were demonstrated as prominent antiangiogenic saponins, which blocked the formations of Matrigel tube and microvessel *in vitro*. When treated with 0.5–4 μg/mL julibroside-J8 or 0.1–0.5 μg/mL julibroside-J12, respectively, the growth, migration, and tube formation of HMEC-1 cells were dose-dependently obstructed, wherein the antiangiogenic activity of julibroside-J12 (**8**) was more potent than that of julibroside-J8.[19,20] The *in vivo* experiment proved the antiangiogenic activity of julibroside-J8 (**4**) in nude mice model implanted with colon cancer cells.[19] These findings strongly supported the further development of He Huan Pi saponins as effective angiogenesis inhibitors in clinics.

Additionally, a polysaccharide component prepared from the herb He Huan Pi was reported to have obvious anticancer activity in mice implanted with sarcoma 180 cells with the inhibitory rate of 73.0%.[21]

Other Bioactivities

The herb He Huan Pi (Mimosa tree bark) has been investigated in pharmacological studies, displaying abortifacient and antiallergic effects.

References

1. Chen, T. G. et al. 2013. Application of *Cortex albiziae* water extract in producing anticancer drugs. *Faming Zhuanli Shenqing* CN 103263461 A 20130828.
2. Yu, J. N. et al. 2013. *Albizia julibrissin* bark extract containing antitumor bioactive component, and preparation method and application thereof. *Faming Zhuanli Shenqing* CN 103006752 A 20130403.
3. Jin, J. et al. 2012. The effect of Chinese herb on tumor angiogenesis by inhibiting vessel endothelial cells. Ran, S. (ed.). *Tumor Angiogenesis* pp. 67–84.
4. Li, Q. et al. 2012. Screening antitumor angiogenesis components from *Cortex albiziae. Zhongchengyao* 34: 744–7.
5. Iketa, T. et al. 1997. Cytotoxic glycosides from *Albizia julibrissin. J. Nat. Prod.* 60: 102–7.
6. Zou, K. et al. 2000. Two diastereomeric saponins with cytotoxic activity from *Albizia julibrissin. Carbohydrate Res.* 324: 182–8.
7. Zou, K. et al. 2005. Diastereoisomeric saponins from *Albizia julibrissin. Carbohydrate Res.* 340: 1329–34.
8. Zou, K. et al. 2006. A cytotoxic saponin from *Albizia julibrissin. Chem. Pharm. Bull.* 54: 1211–2.
9. Liang, H. et al. 2005. An antitumor compound julibroside J28 from *Albizia julibrissin. Bioorg. Med. Chem. Lett.* 15: 4493–5.
10. Zheng, L. et al. 2006. Three antitumor saponins from *Albizia julibrissin. Bioor. Med. Chem. Lett.* 16: 2765–8.
11. Zheng, L. et al. 2006. Julibroside J8-induced HeLa cell apoptosis through caspase pathway. *J. Asian Nat. Prods. Res.* 8: 457–65.
12. Zou, K. et al. 2005. Structures and activity of two novel saponins from *Albizia julibrissin. Youji Huaxue* 25: 654–9.
13. Zou, K. et al. 2005. A pair of isomeric saponins with cytotoxicity from *Albizia julibrissin. J. Asian Nat. Prods. Res.* 7: 783–9.
14. Won, H. J. et al. 2006. Induction of apoptosis in human acute leukemia Jurkat T cells by extract *Albizia julibrissin* is mediated via mitochondria-dependent caspase-3 activation. *J. Ethnopharmacol.* 106: 383–9.
15. Liu, L. Y. et al. 2011. Effects of different extracts of *Albizia julibrissin* on HMEC cells and 3B11 cells. *Shizhen Guoyi Guoyao* 22: 762–4.
16. Wu, P. X. et al. 2012. The study on the antiangiogenesis effect of *Albizia julibrissin* saponins on the model of hepatocellular carcinoma in mice. *J. Xuzhou Med. College* 32: 36–40.
17. Cai, W. W. et al. 2015. Total saponins from *Albizia julibrissin* inhibit vascular endothelial growth factor-mediated angiogenesis in vitro and in vivo. *Mol. Med. Reports* 11: 3405–13.
18. Feng, L. et al. 2011. In vivo studies on the antiangiogenesis effect of *Albizia julibrissin* extract. *Nat. Prods. Res. Develop.* 23: 328–31.
19. Hua, H. et al. 2009. Anti-angiogenic activity of julibroside J8, a natural product isolated from *Albizia julibrissin. Phytomed.* 16: 703–11.
20. Hua, H. et al. 2011. Pharmacodynamics of julibroside J8 and J12 in inhibiting angiogenesis. *Asian Biomed.* 5: 755–63.
21. Moon, C. K. et al. 1985. Antitumor activities of several phytopolysaccharides. *Archiv. Pharm. Res.* 8: 42–4.

107 Ru Xiang 乳香

Frankincense or Olibanum

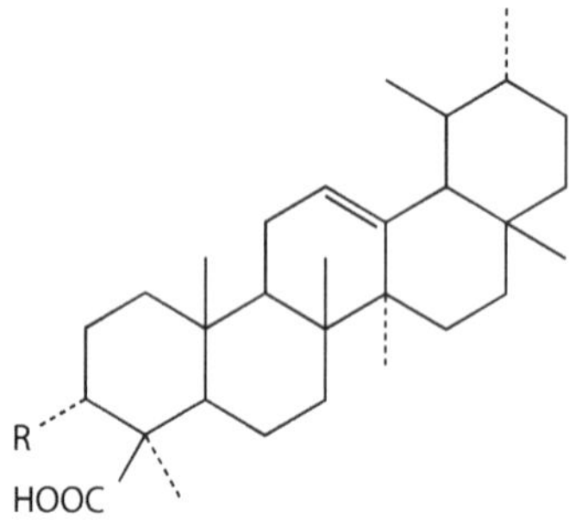

1. R = -OH
2. R = -OOCCH$_3$

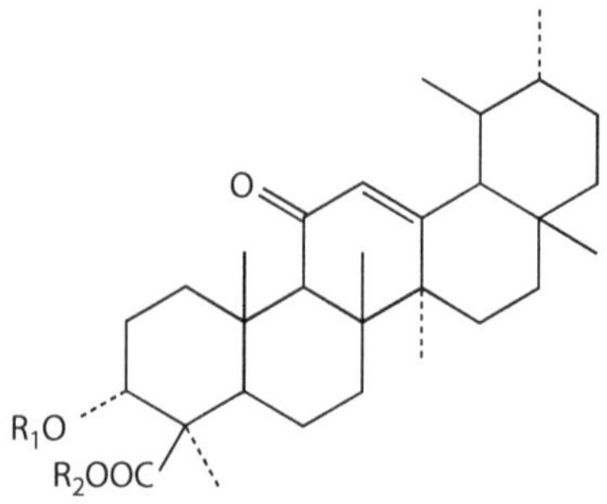

3. R$_1$ = R$_2$ = -H
4. R$_1$ = -OOCCH$_3$, R$_2$ = -H
5. R$_1$ = -H, R$_2$ = -CH$_3$
6. R$_1$ = -H, R$_2$ = -CH(CH$_3$)$_2$

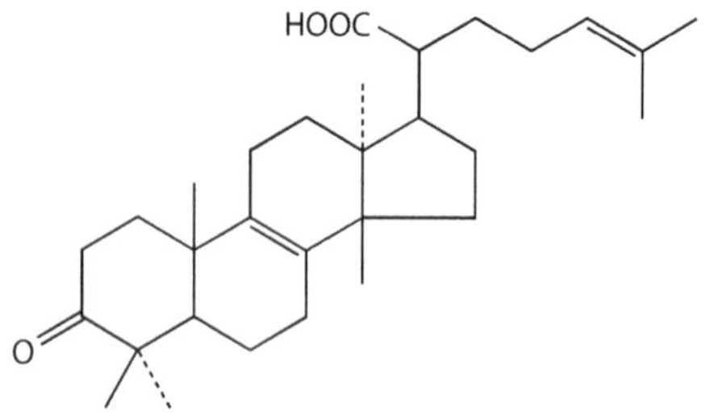

7

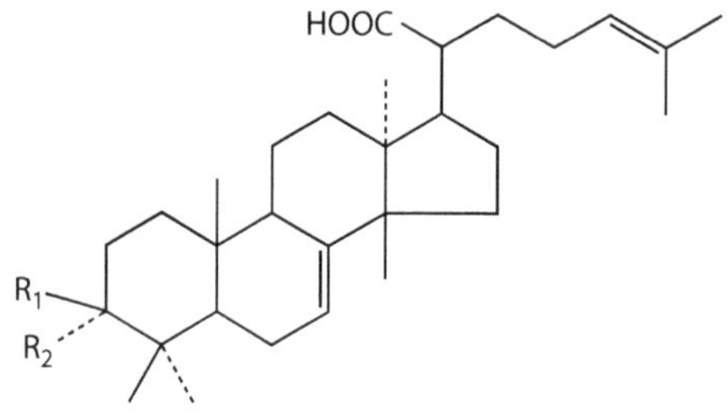

8. R$_1$ = -H, R$_2$ = -OOCCH$_3$
9. R$_1$ = -OOCCH$_3$, R$_1$ = -H

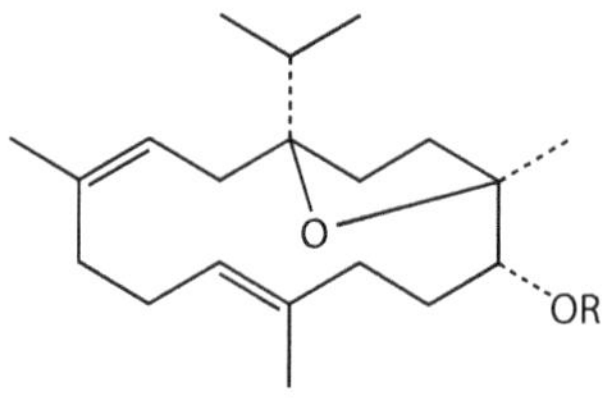

10. R = -CH$_3$
11. R = -H

Herb Origination

The herb Ru Xiang (Frankincense or Olibanum) is an aromatic resin obtained from the trees of *Boswellia carterii*, *B. neglecta*, and *B. bhaw-dajiana* and other trees of the same genus, particularly *B. sacra*, *B. thurifera*, and *B. frereana* (Burseraceae). Most of the Ru Xiang herb was produced in northeastern Africa and southern Arabia. The resin has been used in North Africa for more than 5000 years for perfumery and aromatherapy. Southern Arabia was a major exporter of frankincense in ancient times with some of it being traded to as far as China, being a traditional medicine in Asia.

Antitumor Activities

The extracts from the *Boswellia* genus gum resins might possess anticancer activities, based on their antiproliferative and proapoptotic properties *in vitro* and *in vivo*. The treatment with the extract to female rats inoculated with C6 glioma cells for 14 days (3 × 240 mg/kg) markedly lessened the tumor volume and enhanced the cell apoptosis, resulting in more than doubled survival time of rats compared with nontreated animals.[1] In a clinical study, the extract obviously diminished perifocal edema and urinary LTE4 excretion as a metabolite of leukotriene synthesis, leading to an improvement in patients with malignant glioma.[1] An extract from the resin of *B. serrata* in an *in vitro* model induced moderate antiproliferative effects in five leukemia (HL-60, K562, U937, Molt-4, THP-1) cell lines and two brain tumor (LN-18, LN-229) cell lines (GI_{50}: >57 μg/mL).[2] The herb extract also acted as a lipoxygenase inhibitor to successfully reverse multiple brain metastases in a breast cancer patient who had not shown improvement after the standard therapy.[3] The findings suggested that Ru Xiang may be useful as an adjuvant to the standard therapy in the treatment of brain cancer patients and breast cancer patients with brain metastases. Additionally, the methanolic extract of the gum resin, in mice models, notably restrained skin carcinogenesis initiated and promoted by chemicals.[4]

Antitumor Constituents and Activities

The varieties of frankincense trees produce slightly different types of resin due to the differences in soil and climate. These gum resins predominantly consist of triterpenes, diterpenes, sesquiterpenes, and monoterpenes. The major antineoplastic constituents in the resins were a group of tetracyclo- and pentacyclo-triterpenes, such as boswellic acid and its derivatives. From the methanolic extract of resins derived from *B. carterii*, 15 triterpene acids, viz., two α-boswellic acids (oleanane-type), seven β-boswellic acids (ursane-type), and two lupeolic acids (lupane-type), as well as four tirucallane-type and two cembrane-type diterpenes were isolated. *In vitro* and *in vivo* investigations proved that the triterpenoids exert profound cytotoxicity on cancer cells with a multiplicity of mechanisms. The boswellic acids were the major active components that obstructed leukotriene biosynthesis and 5-lipoxygenase and exerted antiproliferative activity toward a variety of tumor cells.

Boswellic Acids

The boswellic acids such as β-boswellic acid (**1**), keto-β-boswellic acid (K-BA), and acetyl-keto-β-boswellic acid (AK-BA) exhibited effective growth inhibition against human HepG2 hepatoma cells by inducing the cancer cell G2/M-phase arrest and apoptosis in association with increases of p21 and p53 expression levels and caspase-8 and caspase-3 activation levels.[5,6] When treated with β-boswellic acid (**1**), K-BA, or AK-BA, respectively, the boswellic acids (particularly AK-BA and K-BA) exerted antiproliferative and apoptosis-eliciting effects in human HT-29 colon cancer cells via a pathway-dependent caspase-8 activation but independent of Fas/FasL interaction.[7] The synthesis of DNA, RNA, and protein in human HL-60 leukemia cells could be dose-dependently retarded by the treatment with β-boswellic acid (**1**), 3-*O*-acetyl-β-boswellic acid (**2**), 11-keto-β-boswellic acid (**3**), and 3-*O*-acetyl-11-keto-β-boswellic acid (**4**), respectively, and their IC_{50} values ranged from 0.6 to 7.1 μM. Among them, 3-*O*-acetyl-11-keto-β-boswellic acid (**4**) acted as an inhibitor of Topo-I and 5-lipoxygenase to trigger the most pronounced inhibitory effects on the DNA, RNA, and protein syntheses with IC_{50} values of 0.6, 0.5, and 4.1 μM, respectively, leading to a significant inhibition on the growth of HL-60 cells, but it does not affect the cell viability.[8] *In vitro* assays also showed the inhibitory activity of 3-*O*-acetyl-11-keto-β-boswellic acid (**4**) on five other human neoplastic cell lines, such as MCF-7 (breast), HeLa (cervix), Bel-7402 and SMMC-7721 (liver), and K562 (leukemia) cells.[9] The treatment of primary human meningioma cells by 3-*O*-acetyl-11-keto-β-boswellic acid (**4**) resulted in a remarkable and rapid inhibition against the cell proliferation and the motility with IC_{50} values of 2–8 μM, whose effect was largely mediated by the blockage of ERK signal transduction pathway and direct repression of 5-lipoxygenase.[10] Acetyl-11-keto-β-boswellic acid (**4**) obstructed the proliferation of human prostate cancer cells and caused G1 phase cell cycle arrest parallel with the decrease of AR expression through the interruption of Sp1 binding activity on the AR promoter, the induction of p21WAF1/CIP1, and the reduction of cyclin-D1.[11] Moreover, its isomer 3α-acetyl-11-keto-α-boswellic acid also demonstrated the antigrowth and apoptosis-promoting effects against chemotherapy-resistant human PC3 prostate cancer cells *in vitro* and *in vivo*.[12] From the structural modification of 3-acetyl-11-oxo-β-boswellic acid (**4**), methyl and isopropyl esters of 11-oxo-β-boswellic acid (**5** and **6**) were derived. Both derivatives displayed more potent apoptotic activity and toxicity superior to its original molecule (of 3-acetyl-11-oxo-β-boswellic acid (**4**)) on human NB4 acute promyelocytic leukemia cells *in vitro*.[13]

Moreover, 16 triterpenoids derived from the herb were subjected to *in vitro* assays with three human neuroblastoma cell lines (IMR-32, NB-29, and SK-N-SH). Fourteen of them exhibited cytotoxic activities with IC_{50} values of 4.1–82.4 μM against all the three cell lines. The most potent inhibitory effect was presented by acetyl lupeoic acid on the IMR-32 and SK-N-SH cell lines, and the IC_{50} values were lower as 4.1 and 4.7 μM, respectively. 11-Keto-β-boswellic acid (**3**), acetyl-11α-methoxy-β-boswellic acid, and acetyl β-boswellic acid (**2**) were shown to be almost comparable with or has a higher activity (IC_{50}: 13.4–28.2 μM) than cisplatin (26.0 μM) against the NB-39 cells, whereas the IC_{50} data of acetyl lupeolic acid (4.7 μM) and acetyl β-boswellic acid (**2**, 24.0 μM) were comparable with or lower than that of cisplatin (23.0 μM) against the SK-N-SH cells, respectively.[14]

Boswellic Acid Acetates

The earlier investigations reported that α- and β-boswellic acid acetates without the 11-keto group also exert marked antineoplastic effect, especially on leukemia cells. BC-4 contains two isomers, i.e., β-boswellic acid acetate (BC-4-I) and α-boswellic acid acetate (BC-4-II). In *in vitro* tests with six human myeloid leukemia cell lines (NB4, SKNO-1, K562, U937, ML-1, and HL-60 cells), BC-4 strongly inhibited growth of the tested cancer cell lines dose- and time-dependently and induced these cell apoptosis through the activation of caspase-8 pathway. The caspase-8 pathway was activated in the leukemia cells by the increase of DR4 and DR5 expressions and the activated caspase-8, then stimulated caspase-3 either directly or indirectly by cleaving Bid, thereby in turn reducing the mitochondria membrane potential and eliciting the apoptotic death.[15,16] Also, BC-4 was able to trigger monocytic differentiation of HL-60, U937, and ML-1 myeloid leukemia cells at a dose <12.5 μg/mL (24.2μM), but BC-4 failed to induce the differentiation of erythroid leukemia K562 and DS-19 cells.[16] The dual apoptotic and differentiation effects of BC-4 resulted in the notable growth suppression in the treated myeloid leukemia cells. At a concentration of 38.8 μM, BC-4 reduced the viability of HL-60 cells by 60% at 24 h, but there were virtually no viable HL-60 cells when the exposure lasted for 3 days.[16] An *in vivo* treatment of the HL-60 cells with BC-4 at a dose of 50 mg/kg in mouse subrenal capsules or in diffusion chambers inoculated into mice further confirmed the antileukemia activity. The HL-60 cells treated by BC-4 in diffusion chambers also presented characteristics of mature granulocytic cells.[17] When BC-4 is combined with daidzein (S86019) in the treatment, 80% of HL-60 cells exhibited NBT reduction and 82% of the cells showed phagocytosis after four days of exposure, resulting in a better cellular differentiation of HL-60 cells than its single treatment.[18] Moreover, the BC-4 could induce the differentiation of B16-F10 mouse melanoma cells and inhibit the migration activity of B16-F10 cells, accompanied by the blockage of its G1 cell population and decrease of Topo-II activity. BC-4 was also effective in eliciting the apoptosis of human HT-1080 fibrosarcoma cells and lessening MMP secretion from the tumor cells.[19] Based upon the positive evidences, BC-4 may be considered as a potential candidate with no obvious side effects for the prevention of primary tumor growth, invasion, and metastasis.[19]

Tirucallic Acids and Lupeolic Acids

Three tetracyclic triterpenoids identified as 3-oxo-tirucallic acid (**7**), 3α-acetoxytirucallic acid (**8**), and 3-β-acetoxytirucallic acid (**9**) were separated from the oleogum resin of *B. carterii*. The tirucallic acids present a new class of Akt inhibitors with antitumor properties. When they were used to treat human prostate cancer cell lines (LNCaP and PC3), the antiproliferative activity was found to be correlated with predominantly expressed Akt1 and Akt2. In association with the inhibition of cellular Akt phosphorylation and Akt signaling pathways (including p65 nuclear accumulation and decrease of AR, β-catenin, and c-Myc), the tirucallic acids obstructed the growth of prostate cancer cells and promoted the apoptosis of the PC3 cells *in vitro* and in nude mice xenograft without overt systemic toxicity.[20] But the effects would not be observed in nontumorigenic cells treated by the tirucallic acids. Moreover, 3-oxo-tirucallic acid (= elemonic acid) (**7**) showed the antiproliferative activity against a mini panel of human MCF-7 (breast), Bel-7402 and SMMC-7721 (liver), HeLa (cervix), and K562 (leukemia) cancer cell lines *in vitro*.[9] Other triterpenic acids assigned as 3α-hydroxytirucalla-7,24-dien-21-oic acid (**8**), 3β-acetoxytirucalla-7,24-dien-21-oic acid, lupeolic acid, and acetyl lupeolic acid exhibited moderate to weak inhibitory effect against the proliferation of human neuroblastoma cell lines (IMR-32, SK-N-SH, and NB-39) *in vitro*, and 3β-acetoxytirucalla-8,24-dien-21-oic acid (**9**) only showed the same degree of inhibition on the SK-N-SH and NB-39 cells and inactive on the IMR-32 cells.[14]

Incensoles

Several cambrane diterpenes were isolated from the chloroform extract of Ru Xiang and tested by *in vitro* assay with a human leukemia HL-60 cell line. Among them, acetyl incensole (**10**) showed growth inhibitory effect against the HL-60 cells, and its IC_{50} value was measured to be around 16.3 μmol/L.[21] However, acetyl incensole (**10**) and incensole (**11**) only displayed weak antibrain carcinoma effect on the IMR-32, NB-29, and SK-N-SH cells *in vitro*.[14]

Essential Oil

By steam distillation of the tree resin, frankincense oil is produced in ≈3% yields. The oil was found to contain monoterpenes (13.1%), sesquiterpenes (1%), and diterpenes (42.5%).[22] The oil derived from *B. carterii* suppressed the viability of J82 bladder transitional carcinoma cells by multiple pathways without apoptosis promotion, and the oil was had inference to normal UROtsa bladder urothelial cells.[23] When assessed by a lymphocyte proliferation assay, the oil was able to strongly stimulate immune functions with 90% lymphocyte transformation.[22] The essential oil was also evaluated *in vitro* with a small panel of human neoplastic cell lines, showing moderate antiproliferative effect against MCF-7 breast cancer cells, HepG2 hepatoma cells, HeLa cervical cancer cells, A549 lung cancer cells, and HS-1 melanoma cells, and their IC_{50} values were between 39.7 and 60.3 μg/mL. The gas chromatography mass spectrometry (GC-MS) examination revealed that the major constituents in frankincense essential oil were n-octylacetate 34.66%, followed by nerolidol-isobutyrate, 3,7,11-trimethyl-1,6,10-dodecatrien-3-ylester-formic acid, δ-elemene, and n-octanol (18.29%, 9.61%, 5.61%, and 3.24%, respectively).[24]

Other Bioactivities

The herb Ru Xiang (Frankincense) is an edible resin that is used in traditional medicines in Asia for digestion and healthy skin and treating arthritis and healing wounds. Pharmacological studies evidenced that Ru Xiang has a great variety of biological properties such as analgesia, antiinflammatory, antileucopenia, gastric mucosa-protecting, antigastrohelcoma, antidepressant, antiviral, antibacterial, antifungal, and antiseptic activities. However, the herb can induce notable irritation on gastrointestinal tract. It is prohibited for pregnant woman to use the herb orally and must be careful of oral administration for people who have weak gastric ability.

References

1. Winking, M. et al. 2000. Boswellic acids inhibit glioma growth: A new treatment option? *J. Neuro-oncol.* 46: 97–103.
2. Hostanska, K. et al. 2002. Cytostatic and apoptosis-inducing activity of boswellic acids toward malignant cell lines in vitro. *Anticancer Res.* 22: 2853–62.
3. Flavin, D. F. et al. 2007. A lipoxygenase inhibitor in breast cancer brain metastases. *J. Neurooncol.* 82: 91–3.
4. Huang, M. T. et al. 2000. Antitumor and anticarcinogenic activities of triterpenoid, β-boswellic acid. *BioFactors* 13: 225–30.
5. Noaman, E. et al. 2009. Boswellic acid fractions induces apoptosis and cell cycle arrest in hepatocellular carcinoma cell line (HepG2) through p53 accumulation. *Egyp. J. Biochem. Mol. Biol.* 27: 101–21.
6. Liu, J. J. et al. 2002. Keto- and acetyl-keto-boswellic acids inhibit proliferation and induce apoptosis in HepG2 cells via a caspase-8 dependent pathway. *Intl. J. Mol. Med.* 10: 501–5.
7. Liu, J. J. et al. 2002. Boswellic acids trigger apoptosis via a pathway dependent on caspase-8 activation but independent on Fas/Fas ligand interaction in colon cancer HT-29 cells. *Carcinogenesis* 23: 2087–93.
8. Shao, Y. et al. 1998. Inhibitory activity of boswellic acids from *Boswellia serrata* against human leukemia HL-60 cells in culture. *Planta Med.* 64: 328–31.
9. Li, F. S. et al. 2002. Chemical constituents of *Boswellia carterii* (Frankincense). *Zhongguo Tianran Yaowu* 8: 25–7.
10. Park, Y. S. et al. 2002. Cytotoxic action of acetyl-11-keto-β-boswellic acid (AKBA) on meningioma cells. *Planta Med.* 68: 397–401.
11. Yuan, H. Q. et al. 2008. Inhibitory effect of acetyl-11-keto-β-boswellic acid on androgen receptor by interference of Sp1 binding activity in prostate cancer cells. *Biochem. Pharmacol.* 75: 2112–21.
12. Buechele, B. et al. 2006. Characterization of 3α-acetyl-11-keto-α-boswellic acid, a pentacyclic triterpenoid inducing apoptosis in vitro and in vivo. *Planta Med.* 72: 1285–9.
13. Meng, Y. Q. et al. 2005. Studies on the synthesis and antitumor activities of boswellic acid analogues. *Zhongguo Yaowu Huaxue Zazhi* 15: 16–21.
14. Akihisa, T. et al. 2006. Cancer chemopreventive effects and cytotoxic activities of the triterpene acids from the resin of *Boswellia carteri. Biol. Pharm. Bull.* 29: 1976–9.
15. Xia, L. J. et al. 2005. Boswellic acid acetate induces apoptosis through caspase-mediated pathways in myeloid leukemia cells. *Mol. Cancer Ther. March.* 4: 381–8.
16. Jing, Y. K. et al. 1999. Boswellic acid acetate induces differentiation and apoptosis in leukemia cell lines. *Leukemia Res.* 23: 43–50.
17. Jing, Y. K. et al. 1992. Growth inhibition and differentiation of promyelocytic cells (HL-60) induced by BC-4, an active principle from *Boswellia carterii* Birdw. *J. Chin. Acad. Med. Sci.* 7: 12–5.
18. Jing, Y. K. et al. 1993. Combination induction of cell differentiation of HL-60 cells by daidzein (S86019) and BC-4 or ARA-c. *Yaoxue Xuebao* 28: 11–6.
19. Zhao, W. et al. 2003. Boswellic acid acetate induces differentiation and apoptosis in highly metastatic melanoma and fibrosarcoma cells. *Cancer Detect. Prev.* 27: 67–75.

20. Estrada, A. C. et al. 2010. Tirucallic acids are novel pleckstrin homology domain-dependent Akt inhibitors inducing apoptosis in prostate cancer cells. *Mol. Pharmacol.* 77: 378–87.
21. Wang, F. et al. 2009. Cembrane diterpenes in olibanum. *Zhongguo Zhongyao Zazhi* 34: 2477–80.
22. Mikhaeil, B. R. et al. 2003. Chemistry and immunomodulatory activity of frankincense oil. Z. Naturforsch C. 58: 230–8.
23. Barton, F. M. et al. 2009. Frankincense oil derived from *Boswellia carteri* induces tumor cell specific cytotoxicity. BMC Complem. Altern. Med. 9: 6.
24. Chen, Y. L. et al. 2013. Composition and potential anticancer activities of essential oils obtained from myrrh and frankincense. *Oncology Lett.* 6: 1140–6.

108 Su Mu 蘇木

Sappanwood

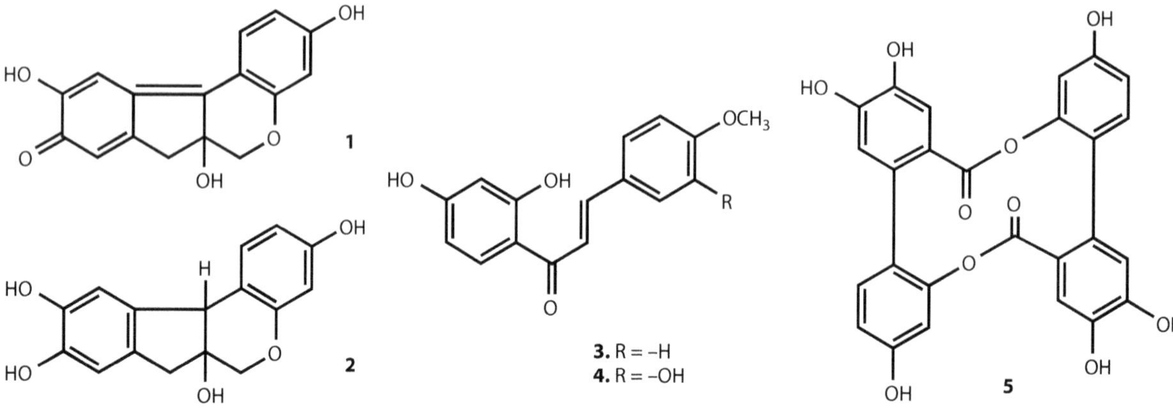

1

2

3. R = -H
4. R = -OH

5

Herb Origination

The herb Su Mu (Sappanwood) originated from the marrow wood of a Leguminosae plant, *Caesalpinia sappan*, whose tree is native to southeastern Asia, but the distribution is only in the valleys of the Jinsha River and the Red River in China. Now the tree is cultivated in the south and southwest regions of China.

Antitumor Activities

The extracts made from Su Mu with methanol, methanol–water, or water exhibited the growth inhibitory activity against various human neoplastic cell lines such as HeLa (cervix), A549 (lung), HT-1080 (fibrosarcoma), HL-60 and K562 (leukemia), and murine tumor cell lines such as 26-L5 (colon), B16-BL6 (skin), L929 (fibroblast), and LLC (Lewis lung) in a dose-dependent fashion. The ED_{50} values ranged from 8.2 to 27.8 µg/mL in the HT-1080, HeLa and LLC cells.[1] the water extract (0.5 mg/mL) showed cytotoxicity to human HL-60 leukemia cells and suppressive effect toward mouse Yac-1 lymphoma cells, L929 cells, and human K562 erythroleukemia cells.[2–4] By increasing the expression of caspase-3 and caspase-9 and decreasing the expression of survivin, its aqueous extracts obviously promoted the apoptosis of human SKOV-3 ovarian cancer cells *in vitro*.[5] Its chloroform extract noticeably inhibited the viability of two head and neck cancer cell lines (HNSCC4 and HNSCC31) *in vitro*. Concurrently, the expressions of p53 and p21WAF1/CIP1 were upregulated, leading to cell cycle arrest and apoptotic death, but no such effects were observed in normal epithelial cell lines.[6]

Furthermore, the antitumor activity of Su Mu was also proven by *in vivo* experiments. The i.p. injection of the Su Mu decoction obviously prolonged the life span of mice bearing Ehrlich ascites carcinoma. The daily injection of the decoction (1:1) 0.1 or 0.2 mL to tumor-bearing mice for seven continuous days extended the life span of the mice by 97.8% and 107.8% for P388 leukemia and 102.6% and 117.5% for L1210 leukemia, respectively.[7,8] In a mice model with ascetic H22 hepatoma, the Su Mu extract significantly lengthened the life duration of mice for 150.9% by intravenous injection and 193.4% by intraabdominal administration.[9] The Su Mu extract was also able to restrain the metastasis of Lewis lung cancer cells by reducing CD44 expression in the tumor and decreasing P-selectin level in serum.[10]

Antitumor Constituents and Activities

Pigments

From the dried heartwood of Su Mu, two natural red pigments, brazilein (**1**) and brazilin (**2**), were discovered to possess the anticarcinoma-related properties. The treatment of human HepG2 hepatoma cells with brazilein (**1**) in the concentrations of 5 and 10 µg/mL markedly demonstrated the apoptosis promotion and the growth inhibition on the HepG2 cells concomitant with the decrease of survivin mRNA expression and increases of caspase-9 and caspase-3 activities as well as PARP cleavage.[11] Also, brazilein (**1**) demonstrated similar cytotoxic effect against human K562 leukemia and ABCB1-overexpressed K562/AO2 cells (IC_{50}: 5.45–5.62 µmol/L), whose effect on the overexpressed ABCB1-mediated MDR was found to be attributed to escaping the excretion of ABCB1 transporter but not to modulating the ABCB1 expression and to have an ability to accumulate the intracellular DOX.[12] Similarly, brazilein (**1**) showed induced growth inhibition on human breast cancer MCF-7 cells (IC_{50}: 7.23 µmol/L) and MCF-7/DOX cells, where brazilein caused G1 cell cycle arrest in the MCF-7 cells via the downregulation of cyclin-D1 and GSK-3β/β-catenin pathway[13] and augmented the sensitivity ofDOX on the MCF-7/DOX cells via the inhibition of HER-2 activation.[14] Also, brazilein (**1**) inhibited human breast cancer MDA-MB-231 cell proliferation, migration, and invasion in association with the inactivation of both PI3K/Akt and p38 MAPK signaling pathways and the suppression of MMP-2 expression, leading to the inactivation of NF-κB.[15] Moreover, brazilein (**1**) and brazilin (**2**) have also been confirmed to have the inhibitory activity against angiogenesis in tumors.[16] These evidences suggested that brazilein (**1**) and/or brazilin (**2**) have a potential for circumventing MDR and restraining angiogenesis in tumors, which deserve further investigations as anticancer drug leads.

The exposure of brazilin (**2**) to human U87 glioma cells dose-dependently suppressed the proliferation and induced the cell apoptosis in association with the increased proportion of sub-G1 cells, activated caspase-3 expression, and subsequent cleavage of PARP.[17] The anticancer effect of brazilin (**2**) in human U266 multiple myeloma cells was found to be accompanied by the elicitation of cell cycle arrest and apoptosis. The induction of G2/M phase arrest in the U266 cells by brazilin (**2**) was mediated by enhancing the activities of p21 and p27 and attenuating the expression of CDKs such as cyclin-D1, cyclin-B1, and cyclin-E, whereas the apoptosis elicited by brazilin (**2**) was mediated by a mitochondria-dependent and caspase-3-activated pathway, as well as inhibiting transcription factors and histone deacetylases and activating histone acetyl-transferase.[18] In addition, the cytotoxicity of chemotherapeutic drugs (such as bortezomib or DOX) could be potentiated by brazilin (**2**) in the treated U266 cells.[18] Based upon these findings, brazilin (**2**) was recognized to be potential as a chemotherapeutic agent alone or in combination with an anticancer agent for the treatment of glioma and multiple myeloma.

Flavonoids

Isoliquiritigenin 2′-methyl ether (**3**) isolated from the heartwood was found to have the ability to inhibit the growth of both primary and metastatic oral cancer cells and to induce the cell apoptosis *in vitro* in time- and dose-dependent manners. Its antioral cancer mechanism was revealed to be parallel with (1) the upregulation of the expression of cell cycle regulatory proteins (p21 and p53); (2) the activation of HO-1 (heme oxygenase-1) via a pathway relating to the phosphorylation of MAPKs; and (3) the activation of NF-κB and Nrf2.[19] Sappanchalcone (**4**), a flavonoid separated from the herb, exerted protective activity on the oral carcinoma cells, where it activated the signaling of p53-dependent mitochondrial and moderating p38, ERK, JNK, and NF-κB in the tumor cells by the phosphorylation of each MAPKs, the increase of nuclear p65 expression, the degradation of IκB-α, and the NF-κB-DNA binding. Its antigrowth and apoptosis-inducing mechanisms in the oral cancer cells also are associated with the increase of cytosolic level of cytochrome c, the downregulation of Bcl-2 expression, the upregulation of Bax and p53 expressions, the activation of caspase-3 and caspase-9, and the cleavage of PARP.[20]

Phenolic Compounds

A biphenyl dimer designated as caesappanin-A (**5**) was isolated from the heartwood ethanolic extract, displaying cytotoxicity against four human neoplastic cell lines including HCT-8 (colon), BGC-823 (stomach), A549 (lung), and A2780 (ovary) cells (IC_{50}: 1.67–4.88 μM).[21] In addition, a phenol component derived from the herb Su Mu was reported to be effective in the inhibition of human HeLa cervical cancer cell proliferation *in vitro*.[22]

Other Bioactivities

The herb Su Mu (Sappanwood) has long been used in traditional medicine in China and India, demonstrating multiple medicinal abilities such as antiinflammatory, antioxidant, immunosuppressive, anticoagulant, and antibacterial properties. The herb also promotes circulation, increases coronary flow, and reduces blood viscosity. In addition, the plant normally produces a natural reddish dye called brazilin, used for dyeing fabric as well as making red paints and inks.

References

1. Ueda, J. Y. et al. 2002. Antiproliferative activity of Vietnamese medicinal plants. *Biol. Pharm. Bull.* 25: 753–60.
2. Xu, J. G. et al. (a) 1989. *Zhongliu Yanjiu yu Linchuang* (3): 15; (b) 1999. *Chinese Materia Medica* Vol. 4, 4-3014, 377-8. Shanghai Science and Technology Press, Shanghai, China.
3. Ma, J. Y. et al. 1990. Cytotoxicity of 15 herbs on HL-60, Yac-1, K562 and L929 cells in vitro. *Tianjin Yiyao* 18: 41.
4. Ren, L. S. et al. 2000. Studies of anticancer mechanism of aqueous extract of lignum sappan. *Shanxi Medical J.* 29: 201–3.
5. Zhang, X. M. et al. 2010. Study of *Caesalpinia sappan* aqueous extract's apoptosis-inducing effects on human ovarian cancer cell SKOV3. *Zhongliu Yanjiu yu Linchuang* 22: 388–90, 395.
6. Kim, E. et al. 2005. *Caesalpinia sappan* induces cell death by increasing the expression of p53 and p21WAF1/CIP1 in head and neck cancer cells. *Am. J. Chinese Med.* 33: 405–14.
7. Ren, L. S. et al. 1990. Antitumor action of lignum sappan. *Zhongguo Zhongyao Zazhi* 15: 306–7.
8. Xu, J. G. et al. 1991. The effect of *Caesalpinia sappan* L. extract on the tumor. *Zhongguo Zhongyao Zazhi* 16: 306.
9. Xu, J. G. et al. 2006. The effect of *Caesalpinia sappan* L extract on tumor. *Zhongliu Yanjiu yu Linchuang* 18: 726–7.
10. Tian, T. et al. 2010. Effects of lignum sappan on growth and metastases of Lewis lung carcinoma at different phases in C57BL/6 mice. *Zhongguo Zhongxiyi Jiehe Zazhi* 30: 733–7.
11. Zhong, X. et al. 2009. Brazilein inhibits survivin protein and mRNA expression and induces apoptosis in hepatocellular carcinoma HepG2 cells. *Neoplasma* 56: 387–92.
12. Yang, H.-O. et al. 2007. Use of the extract of *Caesalpinia sappan* and compounds therefrom. *PCT Intl. Appl.* WO 2007066928 A1 20070614.
13. Tao, L. Y. et al. 2013. Brazilein, a compound isolated from *Caesalpinia sappan* Linn., induced growth inhibition in breast cancer cells via involvement of GSK-3β/β-catenin/cyclin D1 pathway. *Chemico-Biol. Interactions* 206: 1–5.
14. Laksmiani, N. P. L. et al. 2015. Brazilein increases the sensitivity of doxorubicin on MCF-7 resistant doxorubicin (MCF-7/DOX) cells through inhibition of HER-2 activation. *Intl. J. Pharmacy Pharm. Sci.* 7: 525–8.
15. Hsieh, C. Y. et al. 2013. Brazilein suppresses migration and invasion of MDA-MB-231 breast cancer cells. *Chemico-Biol. Interactions* 204: 105–15.
16. Tao, L. Y. et al. 2011. Brazilein overcame ABCB1-mediated multidrug resistance in human leukemia K562/AO2 cells. *Afri. J. Pharmacy Pharmacol.* 5: 1937–44.
17. Lee, D. Y. et al. 2013. Brazilin inhibits growth and induces apoptosis in human glioblastoma cells. *Mol.* 18: 2449–57.
18. Kim, B. L. et al. 2012. Brazilin induces apoptosis and G2/M arrest via inactivation of histone deacetylase in multiple myeloma U266 cells. *J. Agricul. Food Chem.* 60: 9882–9.
19. Lee, Y. M. et al. 2010. Isoliquiritigenin 2′-methyl ether induces growth inhibition and apoptosis in oral cancer cells via heme oxygenase-1. *Toxicol. in Vitro* 24: 776–82.
20. Lee, Y. M. et al. 2011. Mechanism of sappanchalcone-induced growth inhibition and apoptosis in human oral cancer cells. *Toxicol. in Vitro* 25: 1782–8.
21. Shu, S. H. et al. 2011. Two novel biphenyl dimers from the heartwood of *Caesalpinia sappan*. *Fitoterapia* 82: 762–6.
22. Zou, S. S. et al. 2010. Effect of *Caesalpinia sappan* L phenol of cervical cancer cells. *J. Chongqing Univ.* (*Tech., Sci. Edit.*) 24: 33–5.

109 Cao Hong Hua 草紅花

Safflower or Carthami flos

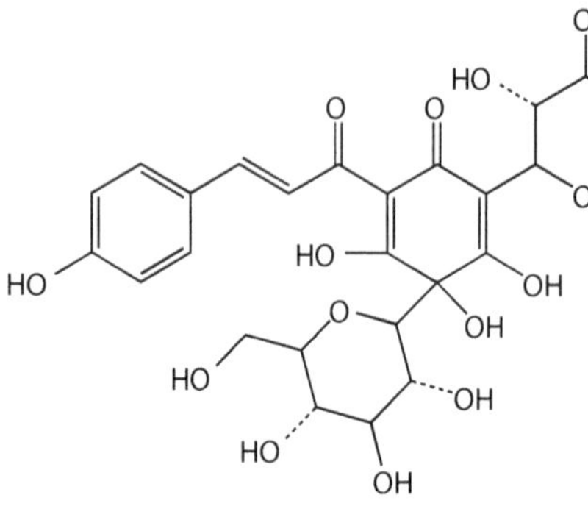

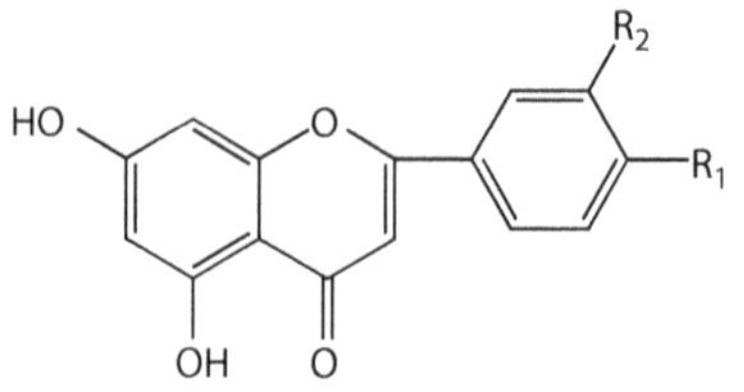

2. $R_1 = R_2 = -OH$
3. $R_1 = -OCH_3$, $R_2 = -H$

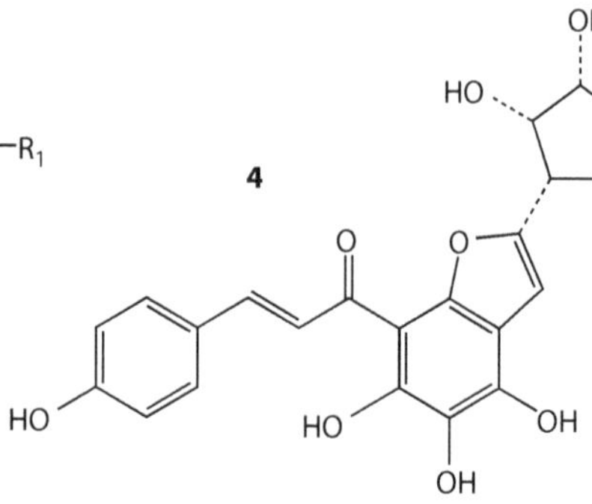

Herb Origination

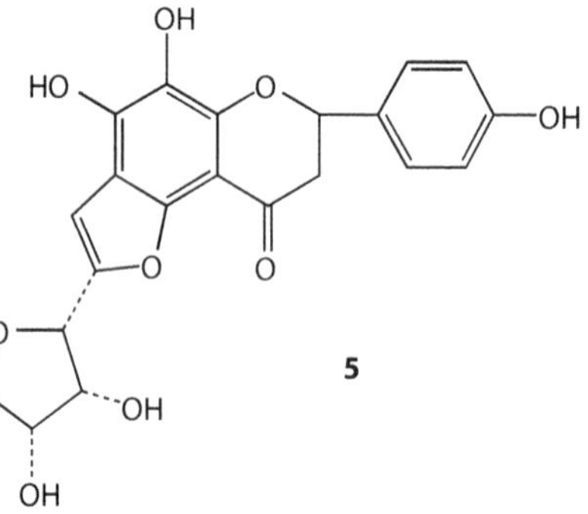

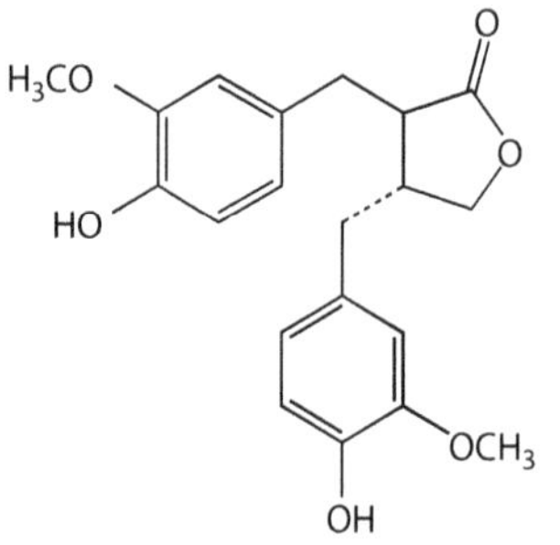

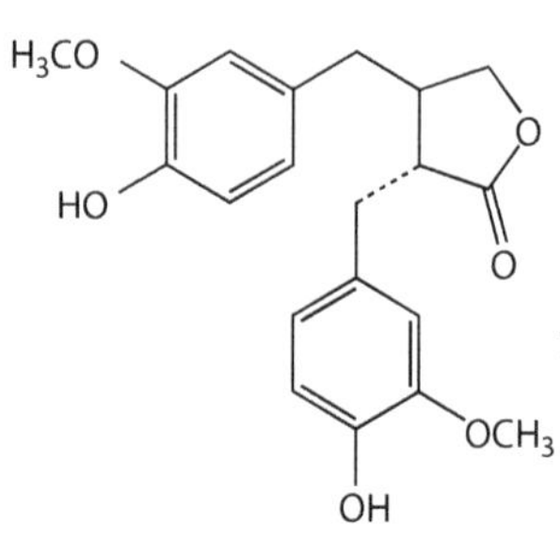

The herb Cao Hong Hua (Safflower) is the dried tubular flower of *Carthamus tinctorius* L. (Compositae). This annual plant is broadly distributed in China and mainly cultivated in the provinces of Henan, Xinjiang, Zhejiang, and Sichuan. The flowers are collected in its blooming season and then dried in the shade. Cao Hong Hua is extensively used in traditional Chinese medicine since the Han dynasty. In addition, this plant is primarily cultivated for its seeds, which are used as edible oil and medicine and also used in manufactures.

Antitumor Activities

The methanolic extract of the flower displayed moderate anticancer activity against human colorectal adenocarcinoma DLD-1 cell line (IC_{50}: 72 μg/mL), whereas the flower dichloromethane extract showed the weak inhibitory effect on the growth of human SW620 colon carcinoma cells (IC_{50}: 0.15 mg/mL), and it induced the cell apoptosis through the downregulation of Bcl-2 transcripts and the upregulation of caspase-3, caspase-7, and caspase-9.[1,2] A 95% alcohol elution fraction of the extract exhibited moderate cytotoxicity against five kinds of human tumor cell lines such as K562 (leukemic), SMMC7721 (liver), HeLa (cervix), H1299, and A549 (lung), especially human lung cancer cell lines (IC_{50}: 16.24–66.51 μg/mL).[3] Also, the dichloromethane extract showed stimulatory effect on lymphocyte proliferation with an increase of 8-fold, while the flower methanol and the hexane extracts augmented the stimulation by 12- and 14-fold, respectively.[2] The findings suggested that both apoptosis-enhancing and lymphocyte growth-promoting effects by the extracts might contribute to the anticolon cancer activity.[4] In addition, the flower was confirmed to have an ability to enhance the antitumor activity of dendritic cell (DC) vaccines via polarization toward Th1 cytokines and increase of cytotoxic T lymphocytes. A combinational treatment with the extract and the DC vaccine could attenuate 15.3% more of the weight of JC tumor in mice compared to the treatment with only DC vaccine.[5]

Moreover, a methanolic extract prepared from roasted safflower seeds exhibited moderate cytotoxicity against three human cancer cell lines, HepG2 (liver), MCF-7 (breast), and HeLa (cervix), in a dose-dependent manner. An EAF derived from the methanolic extract demonstrated greater cytotoxicity against these cancer cell lines *in vitro*.[6]

Antitumor Constituents and Activities

A variety of constituents has been isolated from the safflower extracts as well as the plant seeds. But some of them were demonstrated to have moderate to weak inhibitory effect against the proliferation of certain cancer cells and tumor promotion. Few of them also showed antiangiogenesis and immunoenhancing potentials. These scientific evidences reinforced the safflower being used in Chinese herbal prescriptions and preparations for cancer chemotherapy and prevention.

Polysaccharides

In vitro assays showed that safflower polysaccharide (SPS) restrained the proliferation of human SCG-7901 gastric cancer and SMMC-7721 hepatoma cell lines in time- and concentration-dependent manners and enhanced the two tumor cell lines to apoptosis and cell cycle arrest by the downregulation of Bcl-2, cyclin-B1, and Cdc25B; the upregulation of Bax; and the decline of mitochondrial membrane potential in a time-dependent manner.[7–10] The antiproliferative effect on SCG-7901 cells was found to also be associated with the reduced expression levels of Akt and p-Akt and the inhibited PI3K/Akt signaling pathway, and its IC_{50} values were 0.226 (48 h) and 0.048 mg/mL (72 h).[11] SPS inhibited the proliferation and metastasis of MCF-7 human breast cancer cells in dose- and time-dependent manners (IC_{50}: 0.12 mg/mL), associated with the down-expression of Bcl-2 and MMP-9 and the up-expression of BAX and TIPM-1.[12] However, SPS exhibited no such inhibitory effect on human HeLa cervical cancer cells, mouse sarcoma 180, and mouse LA795 lung neoplastic cells *in vitro*.

The *in vivo* anticancer activity of SPS was further proven in tumor-bearing mouse models. The i.p. administration of SPS to tumor-bearing mice in a 40 mg/kg dose for 10 days significantly inhibited the growth of sarcoma 180 by 51.33% and diminished the tumor volume and the growth of LA795 lung cancer cells in mice. The *in vivo* anticancer activity was closely concomitant with the increase of serum IL-12 and TNFα and the decrease of IL-10 content to modulate the cellular immune function in S180-bearing mice and the enhancement of cytotoxicity of splenic CTL cells and NK cells in LA795-bearing mice.[13,14] The evidences demonstrated that the antitumor mechanism of SPS in S180 and LA795 tumors might be tightly related to the enhancement of the host cellular immune function.

A Japanese research group had applied a patent for the isolation of a large molecular polysaccharide from a hot water extract of safflower, which comprised of rhamnose, mannose, arabinose, galactose, glucose, and xylose, wherein the weight ratio of mannose to rhamnose is 1.0:2.9. According to the immunological (such as promotion of IL-1 and IL-6 production and TNFα production), antiproliferative, antimetastatic, and prophylactic activities, the polysaccharide-contained substance was suggested to utilize in cancer prevention and therapy and as an additive to cosmetics and foods in addition to drugs.[15]

Hydroxysafflor Yellow A

Hydroxysafflor yellow A (HSYA) (**1**) is a chalcone glycoside separated from *C. tinctorius*. In a nude mice model, HSYA (**1**) treatment could inhibit the growth of transplanted human gastric adenocarcinoma BGC-823 cells together with the diminished microvessel count and microvessel density (MVD) and the obstructed MMP-9 and bFGF expressions in the tumor tissue.[16,17] Similarly, HSYA (**1**) considerably suppressed tumor growth in H22 hepatoma-bearing mice by (1) inhibiting the secretion of angiogenesis factors (VEGF A, bFGF) and VEGF receptor-1; (2) blocking ERK1/2 phosphorylation and NF-κB activity by down-expressing of p65 in nucleus, enhancing p65 level in cytoplasm, and inhibiting IκB phosphorylation and cytoplasmic degradation of IκB-α; (3) lessening mRNA expression levels of cell proliferation-related genes (cyclin-D1, c-Myc, c-Fos); as well as (4) improving spleen and thymus indexes to exert marked protective effect on the immune system.[18] Therefore, the antiproliferative and antigrowth activities of HSYA (**1**) on the hepatoma and the gastric carcinoma are dependent on the antiangiogenesis, which also strongly links with several signal transduction pathways associated with the cell proliferation and apoptosis.

Polyphenols

The isolation of the EAF from safflower seeds led to obtaining six phenolic compounds, which exerted comparable cytotoxic activity against three cancer cell lines. The moderate to weak potencies were flavones (luteolin and acacetin) > lignans (matairesinol and 8′-hydroxyarctigenin) > serotonins (p-coumaroyl serotonin and N-feruloyl serotonin).[6] The IC_{50} values of luteolin (**2**) and acacetin (**3**) were 33.6 and 37.7 μg/mL in MCF-7 breast cancer cells, 47.3 and 56.6 μg/mL in HepG2 hepatoma cells, and 51.8 and 62.1 μg/mL in HeLa cervical cancer cells, respectively.[6] Through the activation of MAPK-mediated signaling pathways with subsequent induction of a mitochondria- and caspase-dependent mechanisms, acacetin (**3**) elicited the apoptosis of HSC-3 oral squamous cell cancer (SCC) cells, leading to restrain the proliferation of HSC-3 cells (IC_{50}: 25 μg/mL, 24 h).[19] Two rearranged derivatives of flavonoid C-glycosides assigned as saffloflavoneside-A (**4**) and saffloflavoneside-B (**5**) were isolated from the florets of *C. tinctorius*. Both flavonoid C-glycosides at 10 μM showed strong inhibitory activity against PC12 pheochromocytoma cell damage induced by rotenone.[20]

The lignans such as matairesinol (**6**) and 2-hydroxyarctigenin (**7**) displayed the cytotoxicity on human HL-60 promyleocytic leukemia cells together with induced DNA damage and apoptosis *in vitro* (IC_{50}: 60 μM).[21] In addition, the lignans and the serotonins derived from the safflower seed oil exhibited the anti-tumor-promoting activity because both had an inhibitory activity on PMA-induced EBV-EA activation.[22]

Phytosterols

The methanolic extract of *Carthami flos* demonstrated an antitumor-promoting activity in a two-stage carcinogenesis experiment. Two active Δ5- and Δ7-sterol fractions were separated from the methanolic extract. Stigmasterol (71% in the mixture) was the most abundant of 14 sterols identified in the Δ5-sterol fraction, which markedly inhibited the tumor promotion in mouse skin the two-stage carcinogenesis in a murine animal model.[23]

Fatty Acids and Fatty Alcohols

Conjugated fatty acid (CFA-S), which is rich in conjugated linoleic acid, was derived from safflower oil. Giving a diet containing 1% dose of CFA-S to female Sprague–Dawley rats could suppress mammary and colon carcinogeneses caused by 1,2-dimethylhydrazine and DMBA. The result recommended that a diet containing the appropriate levels of CFA-S may be helpful for blocking mammary and colon carcinogeneses.[24] In a skin carcinogenic model, a mixture of erythroalkane-6,8-diols, which was prepared from the flowers of *C. tinctorius*, markedly suppressed the two-stage skin tumor formation initiated by DMBA and promoted by TPA in mice.[25]

Nanoformulation

The flower extract of *Carthamus tinctorius* has been formulated to its silver nanoparticles (AgNPs) at 50°C or room temperature;

the green synthesized silver nanocomplex (AgNPs) displayed significant cytotoxic effect on salivary gland tumors (SGT) oral cancer cell line *in vitro* in a concentration range from 0.2 to 1.0 mM.[4]

Other Bioactivities

The herb Cao Hong Hua (Safflower) is commonly used to treat many kinds of health problems such as cerebrovascular and cardiovascular diseases for its significant properties in promoting blood circulation and removing blood stasis. Based upon the current information, it is evident that safflower has multipharmacological functions including antiischemic injury, antimyocardial injury, antithrombus function, antiinflammation, analgesic, antioxidant, antidiabetic, hepatoprotective and antiherlipidemic activities.

Moreover, safflower oil contains rich n-6 polyunsaturated fatty acids. Animal studies showed that a high fat diet rich in n-6 polyunsaturated fatty acids may promote the initiation of colon tumor growth but no growth-promoting effect on the established colon tumor. Also, the high level of the n-6 polyunsaturated fatty acids were reported to have the ability to become precursors of intermediates involved in mammary tumor development.[26,27]

References

1. Bouraoui, N. K. et al. 2011. Antioxidant, antimicrobial, anti-inflammatory and anticancer activities of *Carthamus tinctorius* flowers. *Planta Med.* 77: PM136.
2. Arpornsuwan, T. et al. 2012. Effects of *Carthamus tinctorius* L. solvent extracts on anti-proliferation of human colon cancer (SW620 cell line) via apoptosis and the growth promotion of lymphocytes. *Songklanakarin J. Sci. Technol.* 34: 45–51.
3. Fan, L. et al. 2013. Antitumor activity of different effective fractions of safflower extract in vitro. *Aibian, Jibian, Tubian* 25: 348–51.
4. Sreekanth, T. V. M. et al. 2011. Green synthesis of silver nanoparticles from *Carthamus tinctorius* flower extract and evaluation of their antimicrobial and cytotoxic activities. *Current Nanosci.* 7: 1046–53.
5. Chang, J. M. et al. 2011. *Carthamus tinctorius* enhances the antitumor activity of dendritic cell vaccines via polarization toward Th1 cytokines and increase of cytotoxic T lymphocytes. *Evidence-based Complem. Altern. Med.* 2011: 2748–58.
6. Bae, S. J. et al. 2002. Cytotoxicity of phenolic compounds isolated from seeds of safflower (*Carthamus tinctorius* L.) on cancer cell lines. *Food Sci. Biotechnol.* 11: 140–6.
7. Liang Y et al. 2011. The inhibitory effect of safflower polysaccharide on the cell proliferation of SMMC-7721 of human liver cancer. *Zhongyiyao Xuebao* 39: 32–5.
8. Sun, Y. et al. 2014. Mechanism investigation of cell cycle arrest in hepatic cancer cell induced by safflower polysaccharide. *Zhongguo Shiyan Fangjixue Zazhi* 20: 156–9.
9. Zhang, X. L. et al. 2012. Effects of safflower polysaccharide on gene transcription and protein express on of Bcl-2 and Bax in human hepatocarcinoma cell line SMMC-7721. *Zhongguo Shiyan Fangjixue Zazhi* 18: 239–44.
10. Ma, X. B. et al. (a) 2012. The effects of safflower polysaccharide on the gene expression of Bcl-2 and Bax in gastric carcinoma cell line. *Guangdong Yixue* 33: 3698–700; (b) 2013. The effects of safflower polysaccharide on the mitochondrial membrane potential and proliferation of human gastric cancer SGC-7901 cells. *Guangdong Yixue* 34: 1002–5.
11. Tao, J. et al. 2012. Safflower polysaccharides inhibit PI3K/Akt signaling pathway induces apoptosis of human gastric cancer cells. *Practice Oncol. J.* 26: 119–24.
12. Luo, Z. B. et al. 2015. Safflower polysaccharide inhibits the proliferation and metastasis of MCF-7 breast cancer cells. *Mol. Med. Reports* 11: 4611–6.
13. Shi, X. K. et al. 2010. Antitumor activity of safflower polysaccharide (SPS) and effect on cytotoxicity of CTL cells, NK cells of T739 lung cancer in mice. *Zhongguo Zhongyao Zazhi* 35: 215–8.
14. Ma, X. B. et al. 2013. The effects of safflower polysaccharide on serum interleukin-10, interleukin-12 and tumor necrosis factor-α in S180 tumor-bearing mice. *Guangdong Yixue* 34: 1984–6.
15. Nagai, K. et al. 1998. Pharmacologically active substances from safflower extracts. *PCT Intl. Appl.* WO 9844005 A1 19981008.
16. Xi, S. Y. et al. 2012. Effects of hydroxy safflower yellow-A on tumor capillary angiogenesis in transplanted human gastric adenocarcinoma BGC-823 tumors in nude mice. *J. Tradit. Chin. Med.* 32: 243–8.
17. Xi, S. Y. et al. 2010. Effects of HSYA on expression of bFGF protein and MMP-9 in BGC-823 transplantation tumor of nude mice. *Zhongguo Zhongyao Zazhi* 35: 2877–81.
18. Yang, F. F. et al. 2015. Hydroxysafflor yellow A inhibits angiogenesis of hepatocellular carcinoma via blocking ERK/MAPK and NF-κB signaling pathway in H22 tumor-bearing mice. *Eur. J. Pharmacol.* 754: 105–14.
19. Kim, C. D. et al. 2015. The mechanism of acacetin-induced apoptosis on oral squamous cell carcinoma. *Archiv. Oral Biol.* 60: 1283–98.
20. He, J. et al. 2014. Saffloflavonesides A and B, two rearranged derivatives of flavonoid C-glycosides with a furan-tetrahydrofuran ring from *Carthamus tinctorius*. *Organic Lett.* 16: 5714–7.
21. Kim, J. H. et al. 2003. Lignan from safflower seeds induces apoptosis in human promyelocytic leukemia cells. *Nutraceuticals Food* 8: 113–8.
22. Nagatsu, A. et al. 2000. Tyrosinase inhibitory and antitumor promoting activities of compounds isolated from safflower (*Carthamus tinctorius* L.) and cotton (*Gossypium hirsutum* L.) oil cakes. *Nat. Prod. Lett.* 14: 153–8.
23. Kasahara, Y. et al. 1994. *Carthami flos* extract and its component, stigmasterol, inhibit tumor promotion in mouse skin two-stage carcinogenesis. *Phytother. Res.* 8: 327–31.
24. Cheng, J. L. et al. 2003. Dose response study of conjugated fatty acid derived from safflower oil on mammary and colon carcinogenesis pretreated with 7,12-dimethylbenz[a]anthracene (DMBA) and 1,2-dimethylhydrazine (DMH) in female Sprague-Dawley rats. *Cancer Lett.* (Oxford, UK) 196: 161–8.
25. Yasukawa, K. et al. 1996. Inhibitory effect of alkane-6,8-diols, the components of safflower, on tumor promotion by 12-O-tetradecanoyl-phorbol-13-acetate in two-stage carcinogenesis in mouse skin. *Oncol.* 53: 133–6.
26. Calder, P. C. et al. 1998. Dietary fish oil suppre human colon tumor growth in athymic mice. *Clin. Sci.* (Lond) 94: 303–11.
27. Bagga, D. et al. 2002. Long Chain n-3 to n-6 polyunsaturated fatty acid ratios in breast adipose tissue from women with and without breast cancer. *Nutr. Cancer* 42: 180–5.

110 Mian Teng 绵藤

Pale bittersweet

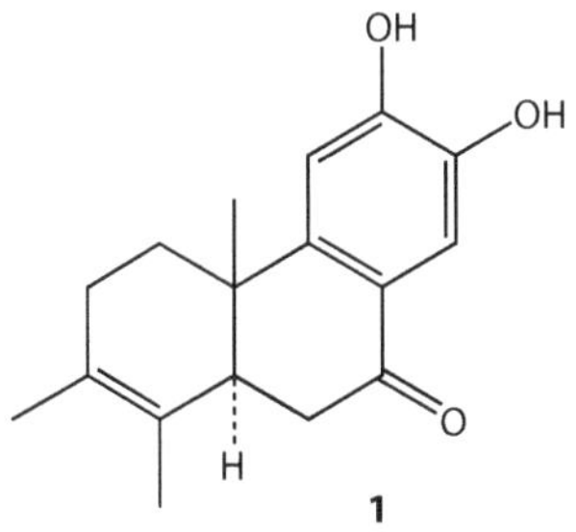

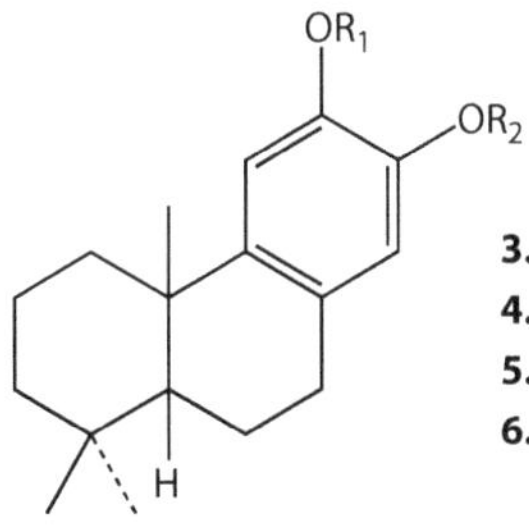

3. $R_1 = R_2 = -H$
4. $R_1 = R_2 = -CH_3$
5. R_1 = –p-fluorobenzyl, R_2 = –H
6. R_1 = –H, R_2 = –p-fluorobenzyl

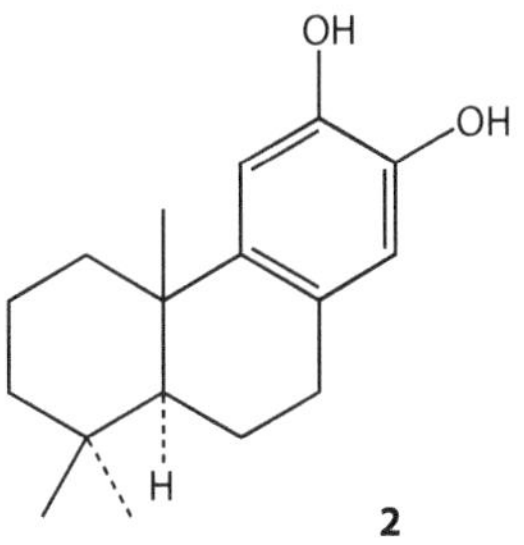

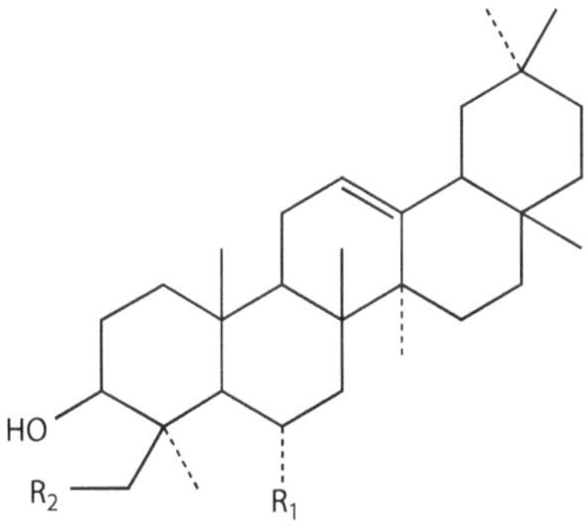

7. R_1 = –OH, R_2 = –H
8. R_1 = –H, R_2 = –OH

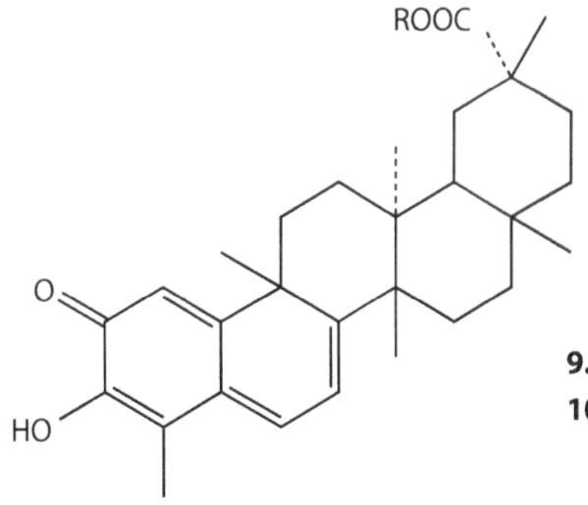

9. R = –H
10. R = $-CH_3$

Herb Origination

The herb Mian Teng (Pale bittersweet) originates from a woody twining shrub *Celastrus hypoleucus* (Celastraceae), whose vine plant is a native of forests elevated between 400–2700 m in China (e.g., in Shaanxi, Gansu, Sichuan, and Yunnan provinces). Generally, its roots and stalks are collected after autumn, and its leaves are collected in spring and summer and then dried in the sun, respectively, for Chinese traditional medicinal practices.

Antitumor Constituents and Activities

Several biological active diterpenoids and triterpenoids were discovered from the isolation of Mian Teng roots and stalks. The *in vitro* evaluation by using neoplastic cell lines found some of the terpenoids and their derivatives to possess the antiproliferative property.

Diterpenoids

Two unusual 17-carbon diterpenoids assigned as celahypodiol (**1**) and (+)-7-deoxynimbidiol (**2**) demonstrated to be moderate inhibitors against the proliferation of human cancer cells *in vitro*.[1,2] The IC_{50} values of celahypodiol (**1**) ranged between 16.21 and 38.03 μg/mL against K562 erythroleukemia, Bcap37 breast cancer, RKO colon cancer, and SMMC-7721 hepatoma cell lines, whereas the IC_{50} values of (+)-7-deoxynimbidiol (**2**) were 19.6–41.2 μg/mL on A549 lung cancer, HeLa cervical cancer, CNE nasopharyngeal tumor, and MCF-7 breast cancer cell lines.[1,2] By total synthesis, *cis*-(±)-7-deoxynimbidiol (**3**), a diastereoisomer of (+)-7-deoxynimbidiol, was produced along with a group of derivatives. This diastereoisomer (**3**) and its dimethoxide (**4**) demonstrated much improved suppressive effect toward the carcinoma cell lines (such as CNE, A549, MCF-7, and HeLa) with the IC_{50} values of 3.6 and 4.5 μg/mL, 5.7 and 9.6 μg/mL, 10.9 and 13.2 μg/mL, and 9.6 and 10.9 μg/mL, respectively. The experiments also revealed that the methoxylation of the molecules would attenuate the inhibitory activity.[2] Monofluorobenzylation of the *cis*-(±)-7-deoxynimbidiol (**3**) could slightly enhance the cytotoxic activity against the MCF-7 cell line. The IC_{50} values of two monofluorobenzylated derivatives *cis*-3-O-(p-fluorobenzyl)-7-deoxynimbidiol (**5**) and *cis*-2-O-(p-fluorobenzyl)-7-deoxynimbidiol (**6**) were 7.49 and 11.26 μg/mL on the MCF-7 cells, respectively.[3]

Triterpenoids

The isolated triterpenoids were responsible for the modest antiproliferative effect on a variety of human carcinoma cell lines. 12-Oleanene-3β,6α-diol (**7**) was effective in the inhibition of four cancer cell lines (K562, RKO, Bcap37, and SMMC-7721) with IC_{50} values between 11.21 and 22.68 μg/mL,[1] while 12-oleanene-3β,23-diol (**8**) showed moderate cytotoxic effect against human HeLa cervical squamous carcinoma cells with an IC_{50} value of 28.9 μg/mL.[4] At concentrations of 2.5–20 μg/mL for 48 h, 12-oleanene-3β,6α-diol (**7**) enhanced the apoptosis and disturbed the cell cycle progression, thereby restraining the proliferation of RKO colorectal cancer cells.[5] Three nortriterpenes elucidated as celastorol (**9**), pristimerine (**10**), and 2-hydroxy-3-methyl-21-oxo-12,24-dinor-D:B-friedooleana-1,3,5(10),7-tetraen-29-oic acid were also separated from the roots of *C. hypoleucus*. In the presence of pristimerine (**10**), the most marked anticancer effect was observed against HL-60 leukemia cells, A549 lung carcinoma cells, Bel-7402 hepatoma cells, and mouse P388 leukemia cells (IC_{50}: 4–13 μg/mL). Celastorol (**9**) was secondary effective in the antiproliferative action against P388, A549, and Bel-7402 cancer cell lines with IC_{50} values ranging from 3 to 10 μg/mL.[6]

Other Medical Uses

The herb Mian Teng (Pale bittersweet) has been traditionally used for antiinflammation and detumescence. Celastrol (**9**) and pristimerin (**10**) isolated from *C. hypoleucus* exhibit significant antifungal activity against plant pathogenic fungi *in vitro* and *in vivo*.[7]

References

1. Wang, K. W. et al. 2006. Novel skeleton terpenes from *Celastrus hypoleucus* with antitumor activities. *Bioorg. Med. Chem. Lett.* 16: 2274–7.
2. Xiong, Y. et al. 2006. Isolation, synthesis, and antitumor activities of a novel class of podocarpic diterpenes. *Bioorg. Med. Chem. Lett.* 16: 786–9.
3. Xiong, Y. et al. 2006. Synthesis and antitumor activities of a series of novel tricycle diterpenes. *Gaodeng Xuexiao Huaxue Xuebao* 27: 2101–5.
4. Wang, K. W. et al. 2005. Two novel olean triterpenoids from *Celastrus hypoleucus*. *Helv. Chim. Acta* 88: 990–5.
5. Mao, J. S. et al. 2006. Antitumor effects of novel triterpene from *Celastrus hypoleucus* on human colorectal cancer cell line RKO in vitro. Zhongguo Zhongyao Zazhi 31: 1450–3.
6. Wang, H. et al. 2010. A New nortriterpene from the root of *Celastrus hypoleucus*. *Helv. Chim. Acta* 93: 1628–33.
7. Luo, D. Q. et al. 2005. Antifungal properties of pristimerin and celastrol isolated from *Celastrus hypoleucus*. *Pest Manag. Sci.* 61: 85–90.

111 Mo Yao 沒藥

Myrrh

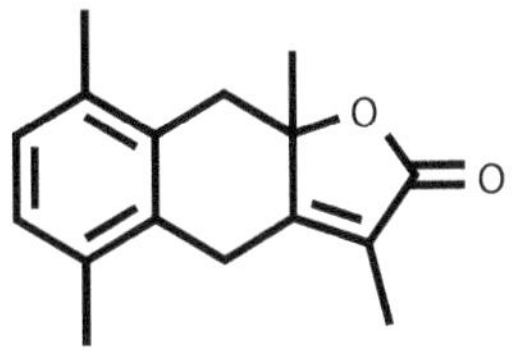

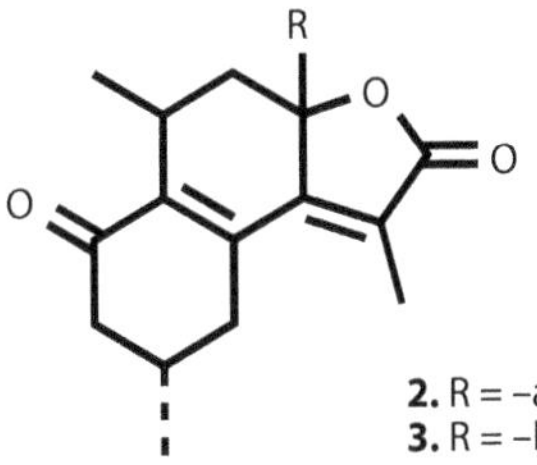

2. R = –alpha–OH
3. R = –beta–OH
5. R = –H
6. R = $–OOCH_3$

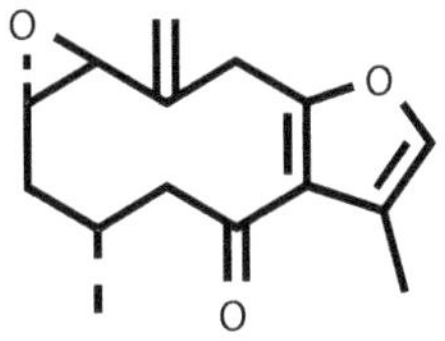

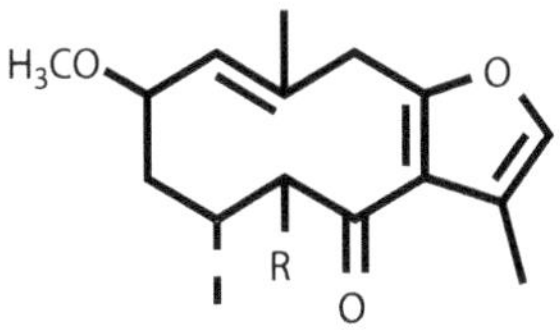

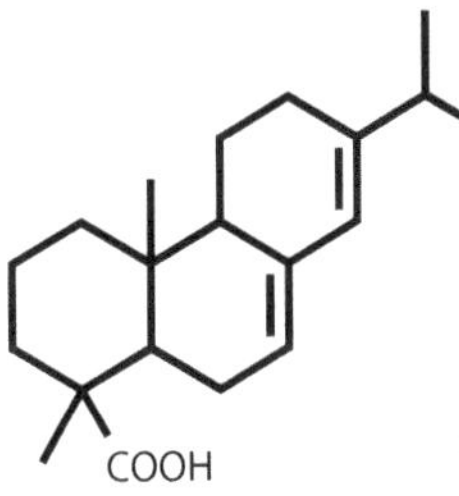

Herb Origination

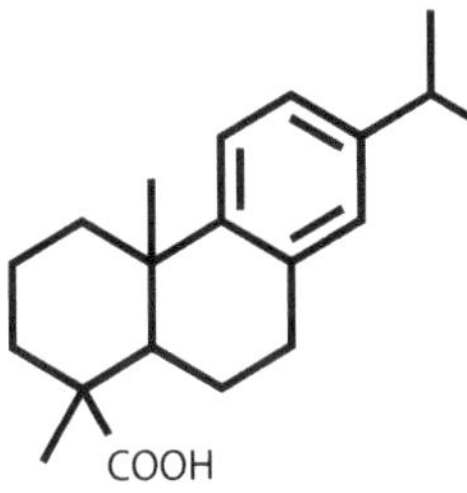

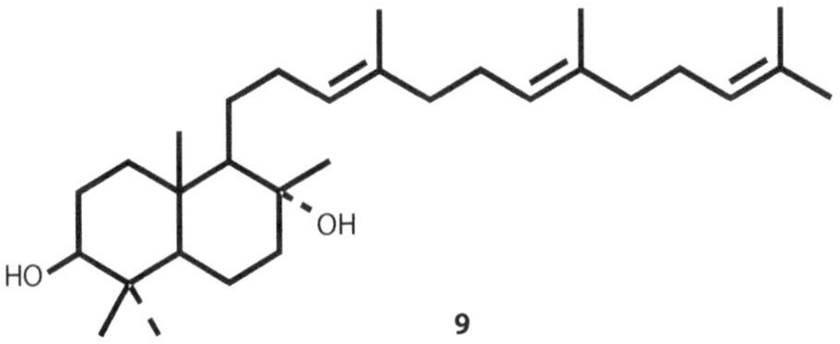

The herb Mo Yao (Myrrh) is the air-dried gum of oleoresin, which is primarily derived from a Burseraceae shrub tree, *Commiphora myrrha* and *C. molmol*. The shrubs grow in sandy and rocky areas in Somalia, Ethiopia, and South Arabia (Saudi Arabia, Yemen). Still other *Commiphora* species yield some types of myrrh. Myrrh was used by the ancient Egyptians for the embalming of mummies and used throughout history as a perfume, incense, and medicine.

Antitumor Activity and Constituents

The water extract of *C. myrrha* resin significantly inhibited the cell growth of six human cancer cell lines such as A549 (lung), Panc-1 and Panc02 (pancreas), MCF-7 (breast), PC3 and LNCaP (prostate), and two mouse tumor cell lines, LLC (lung) and MCNeuA (breast) cells, without such inhibition on normal cells. The suppressive ratios in the tumor cell lines (except of LNCaP cells) could reach >75%.[1] In other *in vitro* assay, the 85% ethanolic extract (AE) and the petroleum ether extract (PE) of the resin moderately restrained the proliferation of three human gynecologic neoplastic cell lines, A2780 and SKOV-3 (ovary) and Shikawa (endometrial), in a dose-dependent relation. The IC_{50} values of AE and PE were 15.8–20.73 μg/mL in the A2708 cells and 26.63–26.91 μg/mL in the Shikawa cells.[2]

Antitumor Constituents and Activities

A phytochemistry investigation led to the isolation of a series of metabolites such as flavonoids, terpenoids, steroids, lignans, carbohydrates, and long-chain aliphatic alcoholic derivatives from the *Commiphora* plants.

Terpenoids

The major anticancer constituents in the Myrrh resin were terpenoids, especially sesquiterpenoids. Although they showed only moderate anticancer property, the positive evidences provided a scientific base for using the herb in cancer chemoprevention and treatment. A 14(10→1)*abeo*-eudesmane sesquiterpenoid called myrrhanolide-A (**1**) and a mixture of two cadinane-type sesquiterpenoids named myrrhanolide-B (**2**) and myrrhanolide-C (**3**) were isolated from the resinous exudates, exhibiting cytotoxic effect against human PC3 prostate carcinoma cell line with IC_{50} values of 38.3–46.0 μM and displaying no inhibition against human DU-145 prostate cancer cells.[3] A germacrene-type sesquiterpenoid elucidated as *rel*-1S,2S-epoxy-4R-furanogermacra-10(15)-en-6-one (**4**) modestly suppressed the proliferation of human MCF-7 breast cancer cells with an IC_{50} value of 40 μM.[4] Two similar types of sesquiterpenoids assigned as [1(10)*E*,2R,4R]-2-methoxy-8,12-epoxygermacra-1(10),7,11-trien-6-one (**5**) and 2-methoxy-5-acetoxyfuranogermacra-1(10)-en-6-one (**6**) were effective in the suppression of hormone-independent prostate cancer cell lines (PC3, PC3M, and Du-145), but both had weak action on HT-29 colon cancer cells.[5] The antigrowth effect on the prostate cancer cell lines was accompanied by the induction of G0/G1 cell arrest via the increase of p21 expression and the decrease of cyclin-D.[6] Two abietane diterpenes assigned as abietic acid (**7**) and dehydroabietic acid (**8**) were also separated from Mo Yao, which displayed dose-dependent cytotoxicity on SKOV3, A2780, and Shikawa gynecologic cancer cell lines *in vitro*. The antiproliferative activity of dehydroabietic acid (**8**) was relatively higher in the SKOV-3 cells with an IC_{50} value of 26.93 μM, whereas abietic acid (**7**) in A2780 cells with an IC_{50} value of 46.89 μM. But both diterpenoids had no such suppressive effect on SiHa cervical cancer cells.[2]

In addition, a cytotoxic fraction-D was isolated from a similar gum resin of *C. wightii* and elucidated as a mixture of (Z)-5-tricosene-1,2,3,4-tetraol and (Z)-5-tetracosene-1,2,3,4-tetraol, which could diminish the viability of MCF-7 breast cancer cells and PC3 prostate tumor cells, showing the same IC_{50} values of 25 μM in the two tumor cell lines. Importantly, the fraction-D was able to overcome P-gp-mediated drug resistance to retard the cell viability of both transfected P388/MDR and its parental cell lines (IC_{50}: <25 μM).[7] A polypodane-type bicyclic triterpenoid elucidated as myrrhanol-C (**9**) was separated from the gum resin of *C. mukul*, which was found to play an inhibitory role against chemoresistant and androgen-dependent (AD) PC3 prostate cancer cells *in vitro* and *in vivo* (IC_{50}: 10 μM). During the inhibition, myrrhanol-C (**9**) potently attenuated the expression of cyclin-D1 and cyclin-E, thereby arresting the cell cycle arrest in G0/G1 stage and triggering the cell apoptosis. Myrrhanol-C (**9**) also obstructed the formation of prostate carcinoma colonies in soft agar and inhibited the proliferation and the angiogenesis of the prostate tumors xenografted onto chick chorioallantoic membranes (CAMs), without overt systemic toxicity.[8,9]

Essential Oil

The essential oil was obtained through hydrodistillation of the Myrrh resin for 3 h and evaluated *in vitro* with a small panel of human neoplastic cell lines, showing moderate antiproliferative effect against MCF-7 breast cancer, HepG2 hepatoma, HeLa cervical cancer, A549 lung cancer and HS-1 melanoma cell lines, and their IC_{50} values were between 19.8 and 41.4 μg/mL. Relatively, MCF-7 and HS-1 cell lines were sensitive to the myrrh essential oils, and the apoptosis of MCF-7 cells was elicited after the treatment. Based upon its GC-MS analysis, the major constituents in Myrrh essential oil were identified as 4-ethynyl-4-hydroxy-3,5,5-trimethyl-2-cyclohexen-1-one (12.01%), copaene (5.50%), β-elemene (6.18%), and dehydroaromaden-drene (4.62%).[10]

Other Bioactivities

The herb Mo Yao (Myrrh) has been traditionally utilized in China, India, Rome, Egypt, Greece, and Babylon for the treatment of various diseases, such as dysmenorhhea, amenorrhea, ache, fever, stomach complaints for stimulating the appetite, and flow of digestive juices, diseases of gall bladder, chest ailments, skin infections, and snake and scorpion bites. Pharmacological data demonstrated the myrrh resin to possess diverse biological properties such as antiinflammatory, antihyperlycemic, antidysmenorrheic, antifungal, anesthetic, and antibacterial activities besides the cytotoxicity.

References

1. Shoemaker, M. et al. 2005. In vitro anticancer activity of twelve Chinese medicinal herbs. *Phytother. Res.* 19: 649–51.
2. Su, S. L. et al. 2011. Cytotoxicity activity of extracts and compounds from *Commiphora myrrha* resin against human gynecologic cancer cells. *J. Med. Plants Res.* 5: 1382–9.
3. Shen, T. et al. 2009. A triterpenoid and sesquiterpenoids from the resinous exudates of *Commiphora myrrha. Helv. Chim. Acta* 92: 645–52.
4. Zhu, N. Q. et al. 2001. Furanosesquiterpenoids of *Commiphora myrrha. J. Nat. Prod.* 64: 1460–2.
5. Ji, K. et al. 2008. Separation and identification of myrrh sesquiterpenoids and their anti-proliferation effect on tumor cells. *J. Shandong Univ.* 46: 344–8.
6. Wang, X. L. et al. 2008. Overexpression of p21WAF/CIP1 involved in sesquiterpenoid-mediated inhibitory effect on proliferation of prostate cancer cells. *Dulixue Zazhi* 22: 10–3.
7. Zhu, N. Q. et al. 2001. Bioactive constituents from gum guggul (*Commiphora wightii*). *Phytochem.* 56: 723–7.
8. Samy, A. F. M. et al. 2011. (8R)-3β,8-Dihydroxypolypoda-13E,17E,21-triene induces cell cycle arrest and apoptosis in treatment-resistant prostate cancer cells. *J. Nat. Prod.* 74: 1731–6.
9. Domingo, V. et al. 2013. First synthesis of (+)-myrrhanol C, an anti-prostate cancer lead. *Org. Biomol. Chem.* 11: 559–62.
10. Chen, Y. L. et al. 2013. Composition and potential anticancer activities of essential oils obtained from myrrh and frankincense. *Oncol. Lett.* 6: 1140–6.

112 Fan Hong Hua 番紅花

Saffron

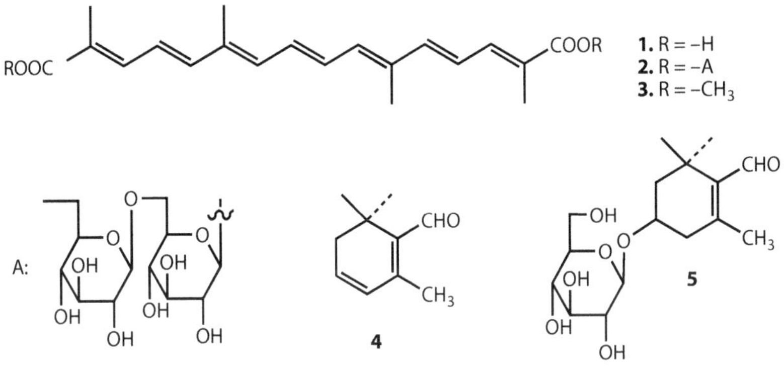

ROOC COOR **1.** R = –H **2.** R = –A **3.** R = $-CH_3$

A: O O OH OH OH OH OH OH CHO CH_3 **4** CHO CH_3 OH O O OH OH OH **5**

Herb Origination

The herb Fan Hong Hua (Saffron) is the dried stigmas of the flowers of an Iridaceae plant, *Crocus sativus* L., which is one of the famous and important Chinese traditional herbs and one of the food spices widely used in Middle Eastern cuisine. The herb is originally imported from Spain and south Europe and is now cultivated in some places in China.

Antitumor Activities

Saffron Stigmas

In Vivo *Anticancer Activity*

The dried red dark stigmas of Saffron displayed a wide spectrum of cytotoxicity against different types of murine and human cancer, sarcoma, and leukemia cells. In a mouse model, the Saffron extract decreased the incidence of squamous cell carcinoma and soft tissue sarcoma, delayed the growth of Ehrlich and Dalton's lymphoma ascites (DLA) tumors, and extended the life span of tumor-bearing mice.[1] The oral administration of the Saffron extract (100 mg/kg) remarkably delayed the onset of papilloma formation, reduced the mean number of papillomas per mouse,[2] and significantly suppressed the growth of S180 solid sarcoma and DLA by 41% and 87%, respectively.[3] When the dose was raised to 150 mg/kg, it delayed the onset of tumor formation and inhibited the growth of a delayed DLA and solid tumors by 80%.[4] The Saffron extract simultaneously elevated the levels of serum vitamin A and β-carotene.[4] The Saffron aqueous extract dose-dependently elicited the cell apoptosis and obstructed the progression of gastric cancer cells in rats, together with significantly increasing serum lactate dehydrogenase (LDH) and decreased plasma antioxidant activity.[5] The oral administration of 80% ethanolic extract of Saffron in doses of 75–300 mg/kg/day to mice significantly reduced the diethylnitrosamine (DEN)-induced increase in the number and the incidence of hepatic dyschromatic nodules in association with the decrease of placental GST-positive foci in livers; the counteraction of DEN-induced oxidative stress such as restoration of superoxide dismutase, catalase, GST levels; the diminishment of myeloperoxidase activity, malondialdehyde, and protein carbonyl formation in liver; and the inhibition of COX-2, iNOS, NF-κB p65, and phosphorylated TNF-receptor.[6] Similarly, Saffron also restored the levels of GSH, GSH reductase, and GST in mice implanted with sarcoma 180.[3] The *in vivo* evidences demonstrated that the proapoptotic and antioxidant activities of Saffron contributed to the antitumor and chemopreventive effects.

In Vitro *Anticancer Activity*

In the *in vitro* assays, five human tumor cell lines, i.e., HeLa cervical epitheloid carcinoma, A549 lung cancer, HepG2 hepatoma, A-204 rhabdomyosarcoma, WI-38 normal lung fibroblast, and VA-13 (WI-38 cells *in vitro* transformed by SV40 tumor virus), were found to be more sensitive than the normal cells to the suppressive effects of Saffron extract on colony formation and both DNA and RNA synthesis but not on the protein synthesis.[7–9] The Saffron extract concentration- and time-dependently decreased the cell viability of human HeLa, HepG2, A549, MCF-7, and HCT116 malignant cell lines, wherein apoptotic death was significantly promoted.[10–14] Compared to p53-/- HCT116 cells, Saffron was more sensitive to p53 wild-type HCT116 colon carcinoma cells in the induction of DNA damage, apoptosis, and cell cycle distribution.[13] The antigrowth effect on MCF-7 and MDA-MB-231 breast cancer cells after a 48 h treatment was demonstrated to be partially attributed to the Saffron-declined glycosylation degree.[15] Likewise, Saffron was markedly effective in anticarcinogenesis besides its antitumor property. Saffron also exerted the inhibition of NF-κB activity and the modulation of oxidative damage to suppress inflammatory response and to protect rat liver from carcinogenesis.[12] At a 100 μg/mL concentration, a 50% ethanolic extract of Saffron exerted marked inhibitory effects against EBV-EA activation and Raji tumor cells. The administration of the extract resulted in a suppression against the two-stage carcinogenesis of mouse skin papillomas induced by DMBA and TPA or DMBA and cotton oil.[2,16]

Synergistic Anticancer and Antitoxic Activities

Saffron extract could provide an addictive inhibitory effect on the colony formation and the nucleic acid synthesis in different human malignant cells *in vitro* when it is combined with low concentrations of antitumor agents such as sodium selenite and sodium arsenite.[9,17,18] The oral administration with Saffron extract in 20–80 mg/kg dose significantly repressed the cellular DNA damage (strand breaks) caused by well-known antitumor drugs (cisplatin, mitomycin-C, and cyclophosphamide) in mice.[19] More studies found that the Saffron has the abilities to disrupt protein–DNA interactions and to restrain Topo-II, which is an important enzyme for cellular DNA synthesis.[1] The treatment with Saffron could partially lessen cisplatin-induced toxic side effects including nephron toxicity and prolong the survival times of tumor-bearing mice by clearly reversing many of the kidney enzymes such as increase of the active glucose-6-phosphate dehydrogenase, decrease of phosphorylation to oxidation ratio in the mitochondria, and attenuation of the activities of phosphatase, alanine aminotransferase, aspartate aminotransferase, isocitrate dehydrogenase, malate dehydrogenase, sorbitol dehydrogenase, and γ-glutamyl transferase.[20] The Saffron methanolic extract also exerted high antioxidant and radical-scavenging activities.[21] These studies clearly confirmed the potential roles of Saffron stigmas extract as an antigenotoxic, antioxidant, and chemopreventive agent, which may be an adjuvant in chemotherapeutic applications.

Saffron Corm

The extracts of Saffron corm, which were prepared with *tris*-(hydroxymethyl) aminomethane buffer, polar solvent, or water, display a broad antitumor spectrum. In the *in vitro* experiments, the extract exerted significant inhibitory effect against six types of solid tumors and leukemia, with 50% lethal concentration (LC_{50}) ranging from 25 to 50 μg/mL and also exhibited toxicity on normal human cells with an LC_{50} value of about 250 μg/mL, which was 5–10 times lower than that of tumor cells.[22] The extract of Saffron corms have been demonstrated to contain a proteoglycan that consists of approximately 10% protein and 90% carbohydrate. This proteoglycan showed cytotoxicity on human cancer cells in culture, and the IC_{50} values were 7, 9, and 22 μg/mL, respectively, in the cells derived from fibrosarcoma, cervical epithelioid carcinoma, and breast cancer. The proteoglycan presented to be about eight times more cytotoxic for malignant cells than for their normal counterparts.[23,24] In the treatment of cervical neoplastic cells, the glycoconjugate caused plasma membrane damage and allowed movements of both calcium and macromolecules, leading to cell lysis, but the cell death induction was not mediated by apoptosis.[25] In addition, the glycoconjugate can be biosynthesized by the callus cultures of Saffron corms as well.[26]

Antitumor Constituents and Activities

More than 150 volatile and nonvolatile constituents and 40–50 of their structures have already been identified from Saffron. Carotenoids are the major active components in Saffron. The total carotenoid was found to have anticancer, anticarcinogenic, antimutagenic, antitoxic, antioxidant, and immunomodulating effects. A group of individual pigments such as crocetin (**1**), crocin (**2**), dimethylcrocetin (**3**), safranal (**4**), picrocrocin (**5**), diglucosyl crocetins, and triglucosyl crocetins were separated from the Saffron extract.

Carotenoids

Anticancer Activities

The Saffron carotenoids demonstrated antiproliferative effect on human K562 and HL-60 leukemia cells *in vitro*, and the IC_{50} value was 0.12 μM in HL-60 cells, which has the same potency as all-*trans*-retinoic acid (an anti-leukemia agent).[27] The IC_{50} values were 0.8, 2, and 2 μM, respectively, for dimethylcrocetin (**3**), crocetin (**1**), and crocin (**2**) in the HL-60 cells.[28] Crocin (**2**) exhibited mild cytotoxic effects on human Molt-4 T-cell leukemia cell line, and it increased DNA fragmentation and necrosis of Molt-4 cells at higher doses of crocin.[29] Considering that the carotenoids are not the precursors of provitamin A, Saffron carotenoids can be more suitable to cancer clinics compared to the retinoids, because the toxicity of retinoids is an important limiting factor for its use in medical treatment.[28] In other *in vitro* assays, crocin (**2**) showed weak cytotoxic effect on human and animal tumor cell lines such as HeLa (cervix), HT-29 (colon), AGS (stomach), and DHD/K12-PROb (colon) cells (respective LD_{50}: 3.0, 0.4, and 1.0 mM), together with the induced prominent apoptosis.[30,31] The long-term treatment with the crocin (**2**) selectively enhanced the survival of female rats with colon cancer without major toxic effects.[31] The incubation of HeLa, A549 (lung cancer), and VA13 (SV-40-transformed fetal lung fibroblast) cells with crocetin (**1**) for 3 h resulted in the inhibitory activities against the cell growth and the synthesis of nucleic acid and protein dose-dependently, and it also showed a dose-dependent inhibition on the synthesis of DNA and RNA in isolated nuclei and on RNA polymerase-II.[32,33] The treatment of HeLa, A549, and SKOV3 (ovary) cancer cells with crocetin (**1**) at concentrations of ~240 μmol/L time-dependently enhanced the apoptosis and the cell cycle arrest through both p53-independent and p53-dependent mechanisms accompanied by p21WAF1/Cip1 activation.[34] In the small panel of human cancer cell lines (HCT116, SKOV3, HeLa, A549, and HepG2,), crocetin (**1**) displayed approximately 5- to 18-fold higher cytotoxicity than crocin (**2**), whose IC_{50} values were 0.16–0.61 mmol/L for crocetin versus 2.0–5.5 mmol/L for crocin. A significant activation of Nrf2 was elicited in both HeLa cells treated with crocin and crocetin; however, the ROS level was markedly elevated by crocetin (**1**) only in the HeLa cells, indicating that both carotenoids followed different mechanisms for their anticancer activity.[35]

Likewise, crocin (**2**) at 1 mM significantly lessened the proliferation of three colorectal cancer cell lines (HCT-116, SW480, and HT-29) to 2.8%, 52%, and 16.8%, respectively,[36] and at 2 mM, it obviously reduced the proliferation of prostate cancer cell lines (LAPC-4, 22rv1, DU-145, and PC3) to 18%, 34.2%, 22%, 12%, and 30%, respectively.[37] The IC_{50} values were 0.26–0.95 mM in the seven prostate cancer cell lines, including hormone-sensitive LAPC-4, CWR22, and LNCaP cells and hormone-insensitive 22rv1, C4-2B, DU-145, and PC3 cells.[37] The oral gavage of crocetin (**1**) and crocin (**2**) exerted the antigrowth effect on two aggressive prostate cancer cells (PC3 and 22rv1) xenografted in male nude mice, where the inhibition of crocetin (**1**) was higher when compared to crocin (**2**).[38] Both carotenoids also promoted cell cycle arrest in prostate cancer cells and restrained prostate cancer cell invasion and migration by diminishing MMP and urokinase expression/activities.[38] With the treatment with crocetin (**1**), the proliferation of three pancreatic cancer cells (BxPC-3,

Capan-1, and ASPC-1) could be markedly suppressed via marked reductions of the expressions of CDC2, CDC25C, Cyclin-B1, and EGFR and H3-thymidine incorporation.[39] After 24 h of incubation, crocetin (**1**) at ~10 μM concentrations presented the remarkable suppressive effects not only on the proliferation but also on the invasion of a highly invasive MDA-MB-231 breast carcinoma cells, associated with the downregulation of MMP expression.[40] Furthermore, a liposomal encapsulation of crocin (**2**) could notably improve the cytotoxic effects in HeLa cells and MCF-7 cells compared to the crocin alone.[41]

The *in vivo* research displayed the marked antineoplastic effect in accordance with the results from *in vitro* assays. The oral administration of crocetin (**1**) to nude mice bearing highly aggressive MIA-PaCa-2 pancreatic cancer cells resulted in significant regression on cell growth and proliferation.[39] The *in vivo* treatment with crocin (**2**) markedly decreased the cell viability of Dalton's lymphoma and increased the life span of the tested animals by 37–44%. If the animals are given the treatment of crocin (**2**) before the induction of the lymphoma cells, the solid tumor showed a 95.6% reduction and the life duration of the tested animals had a 58% prolongation in the 31st day. Simultaneously, crocin (**2**) also showed significant impact on hematological parameters such as the hemoglobin count and the lymphocyte numbers.[42]

Anticarcinogenetic Activity

Most of the Saffron carotenoids exerted the inhibitory effect toward mutagen-induced carcinogenesis. The treatment with 20 mg/kg dose of crocetin (**1**) to mice bearing lung cancer induced by BAP (50 mg/kg) clearly diminished the marked increased levels of lipid peroxidetion and marker enzymes and returned these levels to near normal. At the same time, the decreased activities of the enzymic antioxidants and GSH-metabolizing enzymes in the BAP-induced animals were augmented.[43,44] The hepatotoxic lesions, the cytotoxicity, and the DNA adduct formation caused by AFB1 in C3H10/T1/2 fibroblast cells were remarkably inhibited by crocetin (**1**) treatment. It also exerted the inhibitory effects against skin tumor promotion induced by BAP in mice and against gastric carcinogenesis induced by MNNG in rats and conferred a protective effect on the bladder toxicity induced by CTX in mice.[45,46] Also, more data proved that crocetin (**1**) acted as a potent chemopreventive agent to scavenge free radical and to play an important role in cellular function. In addition, diglucosylcrocetin and crocin (**2**) inhibited the early tumor antigen expression of adenovirus-infected cells, but crocetin esters were less potent than crocin in the inhibition of EBV-EA expression,[19,47] indicating the anticarcinogenic potential.

Differentiational Activity

Carotenoids of 5 μM concentration could provoke the differentiation of HL-60 leukemia cells, whose differentiation-inducing rates were 70% for dimethylcrocetin (**3**), 50% for crocetin (**1**), and 48% for crocin (**2**). However, their differentiational effects were lower than that of all-*trans* retinoic acid (85%).[28]

Synergistic Activity

A significant synergistic effect was achieved by a combinational treatment with crocetin (60 μmol/L) and VCR (1 μmol/L), where crocetin (**1**) notably enhanced the cytotoxicity of VCR against human HeLa (cervix), A549 (lung), and SKOV-3 (ovary) cancer cell lines and against VCR-resistant MCF-7/VCR breast cancer cells.[34] The combination of crocin (**2**) and cisplatin exerted a strong killing effect and an antiinvasive effect on MG63 and OS732 osteosarcoma cell lines, associated with the up-expression of caspase-3 and caspase-8.[48] Moreover, the nephrotoxicity of cisplatin could be diminished by crocin (**2**) via the attenuation of ROS and oxidative damage. During the treatment, it also exerted the protective effect by reducing the levels of urea, creatinine, urinary glucose, and protein in the blood.[49] These evidences afforded the positive scientific support for using the synergistic effect of Saffron to improve the efficacy of current chemotherapies.

Antioxidant Activity

By inhibiting free radical-induced lipid peroxidation and stabilizing antioxidant enzyme system, 2 mg/kg of crocetin (**1**) markedly inhibited antitumor drug cisplatin-induced nephrotoxicity in fibrosarcoma bearing rats.[50,51] These antioxidant and radical-scavenging properties proved that carotenoids have noticeable potentials in antigenotoxin and diminution of the toxicity caused by chemotherapeutic drugs.

Cyclohexenes

Safranal (**4**), in the *in vitro* assays, showed the cytotoxic response to K562 human CML cells and HeLa human cervical cancer cells. The IC_{50} values were 0.8 mM for safranal (**4**) and 3.0 mM for picrocrocin (**5**) in the HeLa cells.[52,53] The inhibitory effect of safranal (**4**) on the K562 cells was accompanied by the down-expression of the Bcr-Abl gene.[52] Also, safranal (**4**) was found to be a useful agent for scavenging free radicals and attenuating renal ischemia/reperfusion injury through the decrease of lipid peroxidation level in rats.[20,54]

Nanoformulation

Crocin (**2**) (25 mg/mL) were formulated with hydrogenated soy phosphatidylcholine, cholesterol, and methoxypolyethylene glycol-distearoylphosphatidylcholine (m.w. 2000) at different molar ratios to yield four polyethylene glycolated nanoliposomes. The PEGylated nanoliposomes established the cytotoxicity and the antitumor activity against C26 colon carcinoma cells *in vitro* and *in vivo*. The crocin nanoliposome at doses of 50 and 100 mg/kg significantly decreased the tumor size and increased the survival rate in mice implanted with C26 colon carcinoma.[55] Similarly, the liposome encapsulation of safranal (**4**) was fabricated by a mixture of distearoylphosphatidylcholine, cholesterol, distearoylglycerophosphoglycerol, and safranal at a molar ratio of 1:1:0.4:0.1. The prepared safranal nanoliposome showed the enhanced dose-dependent cytotoxic and proapoptotic effects on HeLa and MCF-7 cell lines with IC_{50} values of 0.04 and 0.13 mM, respectively, compared to 0.06 and 0.5 mM of the safranal.[56]

Other Bioactivities

The herb Fan Hong Hua (Saffron) exhibited anticoagulant, antiplatelet aggregation, neuroprotectant, cardiovascular obstacle-modifying, memory function-promoting, and uterus-stimulating effects, but it also showed nontoxic, nonmutagenic, and noncomutagenic activities in pharmacological approaches. Saffron is used for the treatment of injuries from falls, typhoid, hemoptysis, and hematemesis in China for a long time. However, the administration of Saffron in a large dose can cause toxicity and side effects. The LD_{50} value of oral administrarion was 20.7 g/kg in mice, while the LD_{50} value of i.p. administration was 1.2–2.2 g/kg.

Crocetin (**1**) and crocin (**2**) were shown to be effective in the prevention and the treatment of several diseases such as atherosclerosis, myocardial ischemia, hemorrhagic shock, and cerebral injury. Their biological effects are largely attributed to their strong antioxidant activity. Clinical trials on the anti-Alzheimer effect of Saffron demonstrated that it was effective as donepezil. The skin care effects of Saffron such as antipruritis and complexion promoter were proved by two clinical trials.[57]

References

1. Nair, S. C. et al. 1995. Saffron chemoprevention in biology and medicine: A review. *Cancer Biotherapy* 10: 257–64.
2. Salomi, M. J. et al. 1991. Inhibitory effects of *Nigella sativa* and Saffron (*Crocus sativus*) on chemical carcinogenesis in mice. *Nutr. Cancer* 16: 67–72.
3. Nair, S. C. et al. 1992. Effect of Saffron on thymocyte proliferation, intracellular glutathione levels and its antitumor activity. *BioFactors* 4: 51–4.
4. Nair, S. C. et al. 1994. Effects of Saffron on vitamin A levels and its antitumor activity on the growth of solid tumors in mice. *Intl. J. Pharmacogn.* 32: 105–14.
5. Bathaie, S. Z. et al. 2013. Saffron aqueous extract inhibits the chemically-induced gastric cancer progression in the Wistar albino rat. *Iranian J. Basic Med. Sci.*16: 27–38
6. Amin, A. et al. 2011. Saffron: A potential candidate for a novel anticancer drug against hepatocellular carcinoma. *Hepatol.* 54: 857–867.
7. Abdullaev, F. I. et al. 1992. The effect of Saffron on intracellular DNA, RNA and protein synthesis in malignant and nonmalignant human cells. *BioFactors* 4: 43–5.
8. Abdullaev, F. I. et al. 2003. Use of in vitro assays to assess the potential anti-genotoxic and cytotoxic effects of Saffron (*Crocus sativus* L.). *Toxicol. in Vitro* 17: 731–6.
9. Abdullaev, F. I. et al. 1996. Inhibition of colony formation of HeLa cells by naturally occurring and synthetic agents. *BioFactors* 5: 133–8.
10. Mousavi, S. H. et al. 2009. Role of caspases and Bax protein in Saffron-induced apoptosis in MCF-7 cells. *Food Chem. Toxicol.* 47: 1909–13.
11. Tavakkol-Afshari, J. et al. 2008. Study of cytotoxic and apoptogenic properties of Saffron extract in human cancer cell lines. *Food Chem. Toxicol.* 46: 3443–7.
12. Amin, A. et al. 2011. Saffron: A potential candidate for a novel anticancer drug against hepatocellular carcinoma. *Hepatol.* 54: 857–67.
13. Bajbouj, K. et al. 2012. The anticancer effect of Saffron in two p53 isogenic colorectal cancer cell lines. *BMC Complem. Altern. Med.* 12: 69.
14. Samarghandian, S. et al. 2011. Suppression of pulmonary tumor promotion and induction of apoptosis by *Crocus sativus* L. extraction. *Applied Biochem. Biotech.* 164: 238–47.
15. Chryssanthi, D. G. et al. 2007. Inhibition of breast cancer cell proliferation by style constituents of different Crocus species. *Anticancer Res.* 27: 357–62.
16. Konoshima, T. et al. 1998. Crocin and crocetin derivatives inhibit skin tumor promotion in mice. *Phytother. Res.* 12: 400–4.
17. Riveron-Negrete, L. et al. (a) 2004. Additive inhibitory effect of Saffron in combination with sodium selenite on tumor cells. *Acta Horticulturae*, 650; (b) 2003. *Proc. First Int. Symp. Saffron Biol Biotechnol.* 477–84.
18. Riveron-Negrete, L. et al. 2002. The combination of natural and synthetic agents-a new pharmacological approach in cancer chemoprevention. *Proc. Western Pharmacol. Soc.* 45: 74–5.
19. Premkumar, K. et al. 2006. Protective effect of Saffron (*Crocus sativus* L.) aqueous extract against genetic damage induced by antitumor agents in mice. *Human Experim. Toxicol.* 25: 79–84.
20. Escribano, J. et al. 2000. The cytolytic effect of a glycoconjugate extracted from corms of Saffron plant (*Crocus sativus*) on human cell lines in culture. *Planta Med.* 66: 157–62.
21. Assimopoulou, A. N. et al. 2005. Radical scavenging activity of *Crocus sativus* L. extract and its bioactive constituents. *Phytother. Res.* 19: 997–1000.
22. Wu, P. et al. 2005. Saffron corm extract, and its preparation method and uses. *Faming Zhuanli Shenqing Gongkai Shuomingshu* CN 1009-3559 20041224.
23. Escribano, J. et al. 1999. Production of a cytotoxic proteoglycan using a callus culture of Saffron corms (*Crocus sativus* L.). *J. Biotechnol.* 73: 53–9.
24. Rubio, A. et al. (a) 2004. Presence of bioactive glycoconjugates on different stages of Saffron corm. *Acta Horticulturae* 650; (b) 2003. *Proc. First Int. Symp. Saffron Biol Biotechnol.* 485–9.
25. Escribano, J. et al. 2000. The cytolytic effect of a glycoconjugate extracted from corms of Saffron plant (*Crocus sativus*) on human cell lines in culture. *Planta Med.* 66: 157–62.
26. El Daly, E. S. et al. 1998. Protective effect of cysteine and vitamin E, *Crocus sativus* and *Nigella sativa* extracts on cisplatin-induced toxicity in rats. *J. de Pharmacie de Belgique* 53: 87–95.
27. Tarantilis, P. A. et al. (a) 2004. Chemical analysis and antitumor activity of natural and semi-natural carotenoids of Saffron. *Acta Horticulturae.* 650; (b) 2003. *Proc. First Int. Symp. Saffron Biol Biotechnol.* 447–61.
28. Tarantilis, P. A. et al. 1994. Inhibition of growth and induction of differentiation of promyelocytic leukemia (HL-60) by carotenoids from *Crocus sativus* L. *Anticancer Res.* 14: 1913–8.
29. Rezaee, R. et al. 2013. Cytotoxic effects of crocin on MOLT-4 human leukemia cells. *J. Complem. Integr. Med.* 10: 105–112, 8.
30. Hoshyar, R. et al. 2013. crocin triggers the apoptosis through increasing the Bax/Bcl-2 ratio and caspase activation in human gastric adenocarcinoma, AGS, cells. *DNA Cell Biol.* 32: 50–7.
31. Garciaolmo, D. C. et al. 1999. Effects of long-term treatment of colon adenocarcinoma with crocin, a carotenoid from Saffron (*Crocus sativus*): An experimental study in the rat. *Nutr. Cancer* 35: 120–6.
32. Abdullaev, F.-I. et al. 1994. Inhibitory effect of crocetin on intracellular nucleic acid and protein synthesis in malignant cells. *Toxicol. Lett.* 70: 243–51.
33. Ashrafi, M. et al. 2005. The effect of carotenoids obtained from Saffron on histone H1 structure and H1-DNA interaction. *Intl. J. Biol. Macromol.* 36: 246–52.

by diminishing the Bcl-2 expression and promoting the p53 expression.[16]

Clinical Trials

The E Zhu oil has been subjected to clinical trials in China for the investigation of cancer chemotherapies. One hundred sixty-one patients with cervical carcinoma had been treated with E Zhu oil by the methods as follows: (1) one of the injections (1% E Zhu oil, 2% E Zhu oil emulsion, and 0.5% E Zhu alcohol solution) was administrated into the cervical cancer area in patients, 5–10 mL per day, and was smeared on the cancer area at the same time. (2) 0.25% E Zhu oil (20 mL) was intravenously injected to patients. (3) 0.25% E Zhu oil injection (100 mL) was added to a 5% glucose solution (100 mL) and then was administered by venoclysis. After one month of treatment by local injection and using 1200 mL through intravenous injection, the results showed 52 healed, 25 curative, 41 effective, and 47 ineffective effects and also showed that the effect is much improved in early stages than in late stages.[1,3] The 4% E Zhu oil ointment and the 3% E Zhu oil emulsion had been also used locally for the treatment of 116 patients with cervicitis. The total curative rate reached to 98.2%, including 66 cured, 48 effective, and 2 ineffective (serious erosion).[1]

Other Bioactivities

Pharmacological researches have proven that E Zhu has antihepatotoxic, antiinflammatory, leucopenia-preventing, blood flow-increasing, antiplatelet aggregation, antiearly pregnancy, antithrombotic, and antibacterial activities. In addition, germacrone showed antiandrogenic effect on *in vitro* and *in vivo* assays.[17]

References

1. Li, Y. K. et al. 1992. *The Pharmacology of Chinese Traditional Medicines*, First Edition, p. 145. China Traditional Chinese Medicine Publishing House, Beijing, China.
2. Xu, H. X. et al. 1978. Antitumor activity of Curcuma aromatic part, V. *J. Shenyang Pharm. College* (10): 20.
3. Wang, Y. S. 1983. *Pharmacology and Application of Chinese Materia Medica*. 870–6. People's Health Publishing House, Beijing, China.
4. Zhu, J. C. et al. 1979. Pathological charges of cervical cancer cells after treated with E-Zhu oil. *J. Wenzhou Med. College* (1): 30–5.
5. Mi, F. S. et al. 1992. The radio-potentiating effects of E-Zhu oil on lung adenocarcinoma LA-795. *Zhonghua Fangshe Yixue yu Fanghu Zazhi* 12: 405–7.
6. Deng, R. et al. 2000. The usage of a gelatin microsome of E-Zhu oil in block of the liver artery. *Yaoxue Xuebao* 35: 539–43.
7. Kim, H. R. et al. 2004. P-glycoprotein inhibitory activity of Indonesian medicinal plants in human breast cancer cells. *Nat. Prod. Sci.* 10: 268–71.
8. Zeng, J. H. et al. 2012. (a) Spectrum-effect relationship between fingerprint of essential oil and of antitumor effect from *Curcuma kwangsiensis*. *Zhongguo Shiyan Fangjixue Zazhi* 18: 91–94; (b) Study on spectrum-effect relationship between fingerprint of essential oil and of antitumor effect from Curcuma kwangsiensis. *Afri. J. Pharmacy Pharmacol.* 6: 1348–51.
9. Lai, E. Y. C. et al. 2004. Antimicrobial activity and cytotoxicity of the essential oil of *Curcuma zedoaria*. *Am. J. Chin. Med.* 32: 281–90.
10. Tian, S. J. et al. 1985. Separation and identification of the essential oil from *Curcuma kwangsiensis* and comparison with the essential oil from *C. wenyujin* by gas chromatography and TLC. *J. Pharm. Analysis* 5: 325–8.
11. Tang, M. Y. et al. 2000. Studies on the chemical constituents of E-Zhu essential oil. *Linchang Huaxue yu Gongye* 20: 65–9.
12. Wang, Y. et al. 2001. Study on the quality of *Rhizoma curcumae*. *Yaoxue Xuebao* 36: 849–53.
13. Sun, H. J. et al. 1983. Study on antitumor effect of Curcuma aromatica salisb-synthesis of monosodium curcumol phosphate. *Yiyao Gongye* (8): 12–3.
14. Yuan, W. X. et al. 1984. Antitumor activity of curcumol monosodium phosphate. *Shenyang Yaoxueyuan Xuebao* 1: 210.
15. Sukari, M. A. et al. 2010. Bioactive sesquiterpenes from *Curcuma ochrorhiza* and *Curcuma heyneana*. *Nat. Prod. Res.* 24: 838–45.
16. Zeng, J. H. et al. 2012. Apoptosis-induced antitumor effect of *Curcuma kwangsiensis* polysaccharides against human nasopharyngeal carcinoma cells. *Carbohydrate Polymers* 89: 1067–72.
17. Suphrom, N. et al. 2012. Anti-androgenic effect of sesquiterpenes isolated from the rhizomes of *Curcuma aeruginosa* Roxb. *Fitoterapia* 83: 864–71.

114 Jiang Huang 姜黄

Turmeric

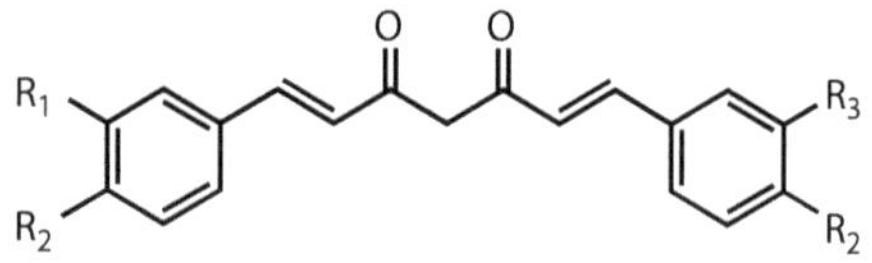

1. $R_1 = R_3 = -OCH_3$, $R_2 = -OH$
2. $R_1 = -OCH_3$, $R_2 = -OH$, $R_3 = -H$
3. $R_1 = R_3 = -H$, $R_2 = -OH$

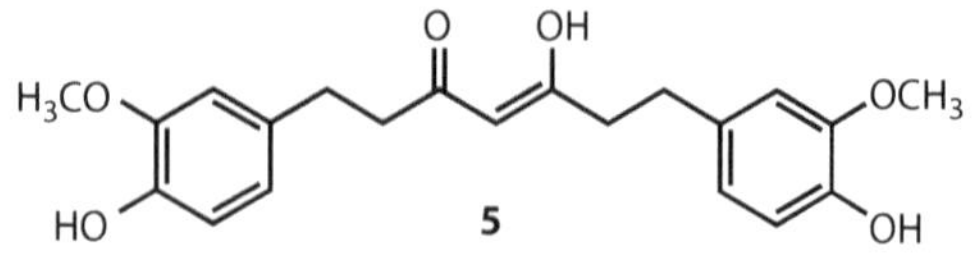

(a)

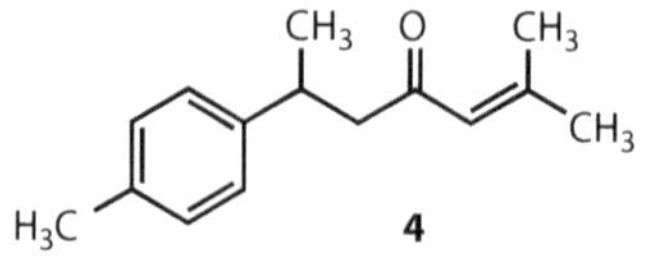

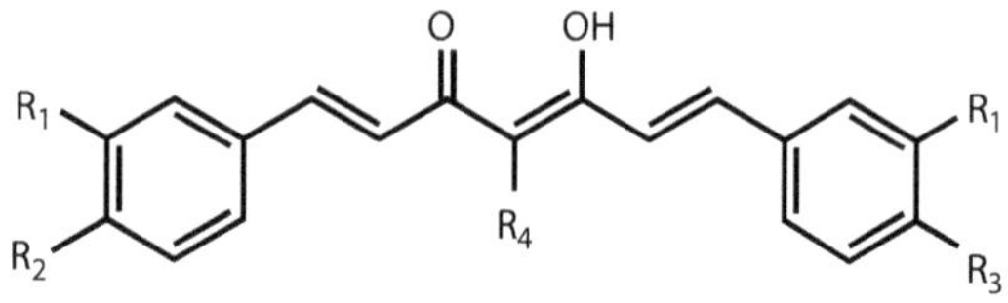

6. $R_1 = R_2 = R_3 = -OCH_3$, $R_4 = -H$
7. $R_1 = -OCH_3$, $R_2 = R_3 = -OCH_2COCH_3$, $R_4 = -H$
8. $R_1 = R_2 = -OCH_3$, $R_3 = -OH$, $R_4 = -H$
9. $R_1 = -OCH_3$, $R_2 = -OCH_2COCH_3$, $R_3 = -OH$, $R_4 = -H$

10. $R_1 = -OH$, $R_2 = R_3 = -OH$, $R_4 = -H$
11. $R_1 = R_2 = R_3 = -OCH_3$, $R_4 = -CH_3$
12. $R_1 = -H$, $R_2 = R_3 = -OGlc$, $R_4 = -H$
13. $R_1 = -OCH_3$, $R_2 = R_3 = -OSO_2NH_2$, $R_4 = -H$
14. $R_1 = -OCH_3$, $R_2 = R_3 = -OH$, $R_4 = -COOCH_3$
15. $R_1 = -OCH_3$, $R_2 = R_3 = -OH$, $R_4 = -COOH$
16. $R_1 = -OCH_3$, $R_2 = R_3 = -OH$, $R_4 = -CH = CH_2-$

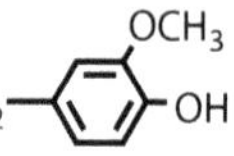

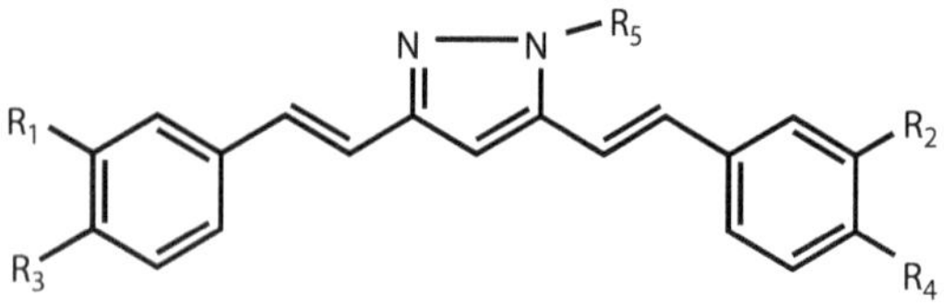

17. $R_1 = R_2 = -OCH_3$, $R_3 = R_4 = -OH$, $R_5 = -H$
18. $R_1 = -OCH_3$, $R_3 = R_4 = -OH$, $R_2 = R_5 = -H$
19. $R_1 = R_2 = R_5 = -H$, $R_3 = R_4 = -OH$
20. $R_1 = R_2 = -OCH_3$, $R_3 = R_4 = -OH$, $R_5 = -CH_3$

(b)

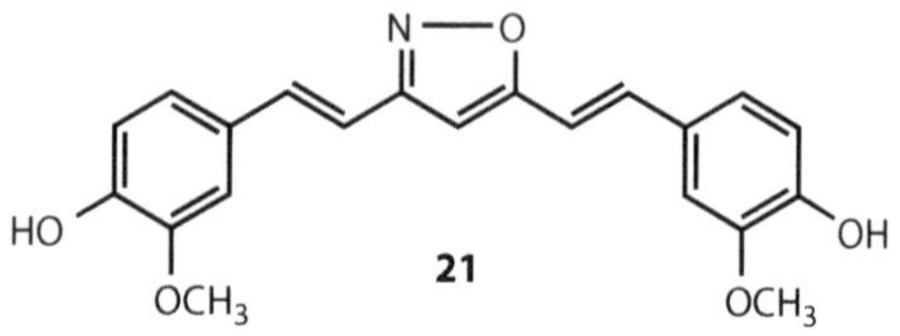

21

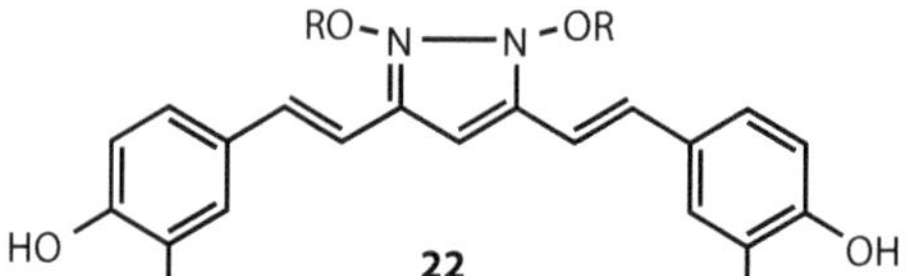

22 $R = -CH_2Ph$

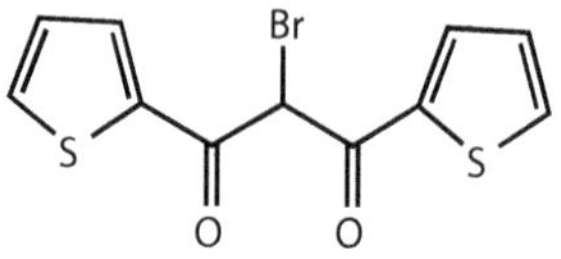

29

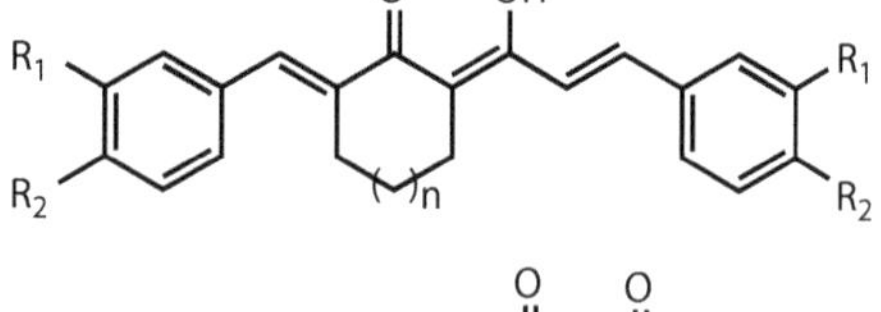

23. n = 0, $R_1 = R_2 = -OCH_3$
24. n = 1, $R_1 = -H$, $R_2 = -OH$
25. n = 1, $R_1 = -OCH_3$, $R_2 = -OH$

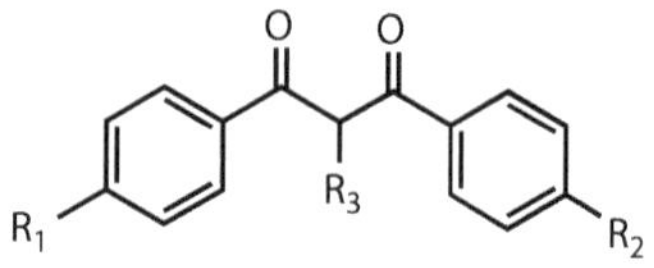

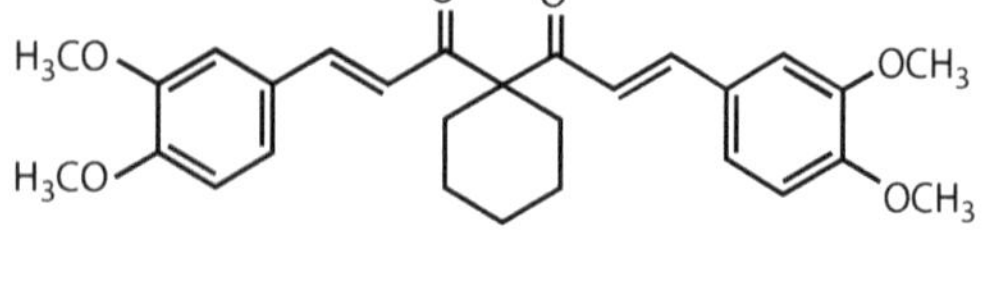

28

26. $R_1 = R_2 = -F$, $R_3 = -H$
27. $R_1 = -NO_2$, $R_2 = -OCH_3$, $R_3 = -Br$

(c)

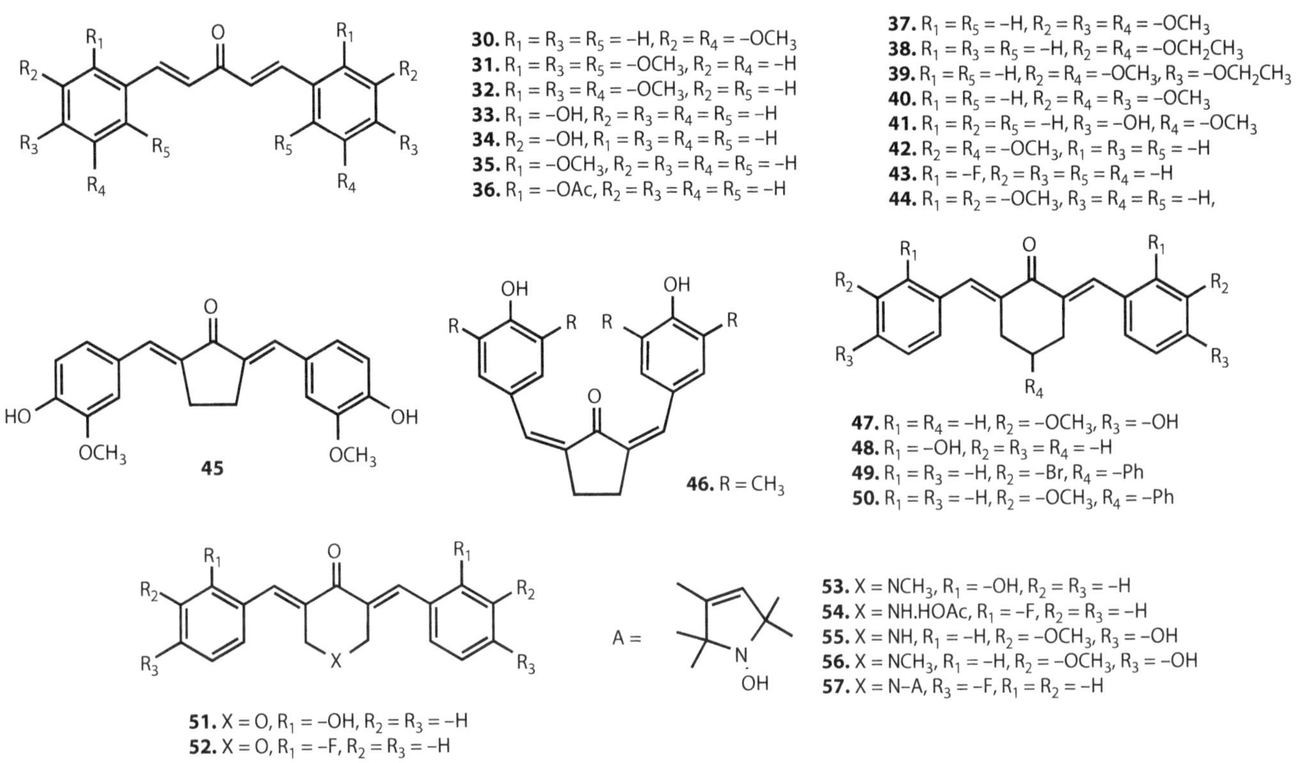

30. $R_1 = R_3 = R_5 = \text{-H}, R_2 = R_4 = \text{-OCH}_3$
31. $R_1 = R_3 = R_5 = \text{-OCH}_3, R_2 = R_4 = \text{-H}$
32. $R_1 = R_3 = R_4 = \text{-OCH}_3, R_2 = R_5 = \text{-H}$
33. $R_1 = \text{-OH}, R_2 = R_3 = R_4 = R_5 = \text{-H}$
34. $R_2 = \text{-OH}, R_1 = R_3 = R_4 = R_5 = \text{-H}$
35. $R_1 = \text{-OCH}_3, R_2 = R_3 = R_4 = R_5 = \text{-H}$
36. $R_1 = \text{-OAc}, R_2 = R_3 = R_4 = R_5 = \text{-H}$

37. $R_1 = R_5 = \text{-H}, R_2 = R_3 = R_4 = \text{-OCH}_3$
38. $R_1 = R_3 = R_5 = \text{-H}, R_2 = R_4 = \text{-OCH}_2\text{CH}_3$
39. $R_1 = R_5 = \text{-H}, R_2 = R_4 = \text{-OCH}_3, R_3 = \text{-OCH}_2\text{CH}_3$
40. $R_1 = R_5 = \text{-H}, R_2 = R_4 = R_3 = \text{-OCH}_3$
41. $R_1 = R_2 = R_5 = \text{-H}, R_3 = \text{-OH}, R_4 = \text{-OCH}_3$
42. $R_2 = R_4 = \text{-OCH}_3, R_1 = R_3 = R_5 = \text{-H}$
43. $R_1 = \text{-F}, R_2 = R_3 = R_5 = R_4 = \text{-H}$
44. $R_1 = R_2 = \text{-OCH}_3, R_3 = R_4 = R_5 = \text{-H},$

45

46. $R = CH_3$

47. $R_1 = R_4 = \text{-H}, R_2 = \text{-OCH}_3, R_3 = \text{-OH}$
48. $R_1 = \text{-OH}, R_2 = R_3 = R_4 = \text{-H}$
49. $R_1 = R_3 = \text{-H}, R_2 = \text{-Br}, R_4 = \text{-Ph}$
50. $R_1 = R_3 = \text{-H}, R_2 = \text{-OCH}_3, R_4 = \text{-Ph}$

51. $X = O, R_1 = \text{-OH}, R_2 = R_3 = \text{-H}$
52. $X = O, R_1 = \text{-F}, R_2 = R_3 = \text{-H}$

A =

53. $X = NCH_3, R_1 = \text{-OH}, R_2 = R_3 = \text{-H}$
54. $X = \text{NH.HOAc}, R_1 = \text{-F}, R_2 = R_3 = \text{-H}$
55. $X = NH, R_1 = \text{-H}, R_2 = \text{-OCH}_3, R_3 = \text{-OH}$
56. $X = NCH_3, R_1 = \text{-H}, R_2 = \text{-OCH}_3, R_3 = \text{-OH}$
57. $X = \text{N-A}, R_3 = \text{-F}, R_1 = R_2 = \text{-H}$

(d)

Herb Origination

The herb Jiang Huang (Turmeric) is the dried rhizomes of a Zingiberaceae family plant, *Curcuma longa*. This perennial plant is distributed in southern Asia and is also produced by cultivation in China and India today. Turmeric has been used as an herb with multiple health-restoring properties in southeast Asian countries and as a common spice, preservative, and coloring matter in south Asian and Middle Eastern culinary art. The first record of Jiang Huang (Turmeric) as an herb in China was found in Xinxiu Ben Cao (AD 659) of the Tang dynasty, which is the world first pharmacopoeia promulgated by the government.

Antitumor Constituents and Activities

Tremendous investigations of the *Curcuma* genus have revealed that curcuminoids are the major therapeutically valuable constituents, and curcumin (**1**) is the most important curcuminoid. The antitumor property of curcumin (**1**) is mainly presented in six aspects such as cancer cell growth inhibition, apoptotic induction, antimetastasis, antioxidation, anticarcinogenesis, and synergistic action with clinical chemotherapeutic drugs. For the summarization of the information comprehensively, each aspect as well as the major mechanisms of molecular and biological actions in a variety of cancers were individually discussed.

Antigrowth and Apoptosis-Inducing Activities

Effect on Carcinomas in the Blood and the Lymphocytes

Various types of leukemia cells and lymphoma cells seem sensitive to the curcuminoids. Curcumin (**1**) prominently demonstrated the suppressive effect against HL-60 and NB4 promyelocytic leukemia, K562 eythroleukemia, HTLV-1-infected T cell leukemia, Molt4 T-lymphoblast/acute lymphoblastic leukemia, primary newly diagnosed CML, B-chronic lymphocytic leukemia, CA46 Burkitt's lymphoma, TK6 B-lymphoblastoid, U937 leukemic monocyte lymphoma, Jurkat (T cell lymphoblast-like cells) cell lines, as well as against several multidrug-resistant leukemia cell lines (HL-60/Vinc, HL-60/Adr, K562/A02, and K562/Adm).[1–14] Curcumin (**1**) was also effective in the suppression of mouse leukemia L1210 cells, L1210/Adr cells, and rat RBL-2H3 basophilic leukemia mast cell lines.[15,16]

Extensive investigations on its mechanism revealed that these significant inhibitions on the growth of leukemia and lymphoma cells closely related to the induction of apoptosis and DNA damage. Curcumin (**1**) at a concentration of as low as 3.5 μg/mL accelerated the apoptotic death of HL-60 cells in dose- and time-dependent manners,[17] and at a concentration from 6.25 to 50 μM, it repressed the DNA synthesis in HL-60 cells.[18] During the apoptotic induction, curcumin significantly downregulated Bcl-2 and Wilms' tumor gene-1 (WT1) expressions in K562, HL-60, U937, and Molt4 cells[19–21] and suppressed NF-κB and activator protein-1 (AP-1) activities through direct interruption of the binding of NF-κB and AP-1 to their consensus DNA sequences in HL-60 cells.[22–24] The antigrowth effect of HL-60 cells by curcumin (**1**) was further confirmed in xenograft nude mice *in vivo* with a 54.35% inhibitory rate.[19] The cytotoxicity of curcumin against HL-60 cells could be enhanced by being combined with trichostatin-A or valproic acid due to promoting p38-dependent Bax expression, increasing histone acetylation, and/or hindering histone deacetylase.[20,25] According to the evidences, curcumin (**1**) was known to have a therapeutic potential in the chemotherapy of promyelocytic leukemia and sensitization of these cells to current antineoplastic drugs.

The mechanisms of curcumin (**1**) in other types of leukemia and lymphoma cell lines were characteristically observed. The antiproliferation on NB4 cells by curcumin was mediated by the increase of acetylated histone H3 level and tumor suppressor p53 expression.[2] In the curcumin-treated primary CML cells, the growth inhibition was attributed to the marked suppression of STAT5 pathway.[3] The CA46 cell apoptosis induced by curcumin was found to be associated with the downregulation of the expressions of c-Myc, Bcl-2, and mutant-type p53 and the upregulation of the expression of Fas.[7] The obstruction of telomerase activity and GST P1-1 expression was involved in K562 cell apoptotic induction by curcumin (**1**) besides the downregulation of Bcl-2 and upregulation of Bax and caspases.[5,26] The curcumin-induced apoptosis of multidrug-resistant leukemia K562/A02 cells was triggered by Cu^{2+}-increased ROS generation.[17] At the same time of the marked proteolytic activation of caspase-3 and caspase-8 and the cleavage of PARP, the Fas/FasL pathway was elevated in the curcumin-initiated apoptosis of U937 cells.[11] The treatment of WT1 isoform-transfected U937 cells with a noncytotoxic dose (15 μM) of curcumin dose-dependently declined the WT1 protein levels via protein kinase C (PKC) degradation during the posttranslational processing.[27] In HTLV-1-infected T cell leukemia cells, the antiproliferative effect of curcumin (**1**) was accompanied by the induction of cell cycle arrest and apoptosis by reducing the constitutive activation of AP-1 by decreasing the JunD protein expression.[12]

Human AML is an immunophenotypically heterogenous malignant disease, which holds CD34 positivity with poor prognosis. The $CD34^+$ AML cells are usually 10- to 15-fold more resistant to an anticancer drug daunorubicin (DNR) than $CD34^-$ AML cells. Curcumin (**1**) could synergistically enhance the cytotoxic effect of DNR in the treatment of two DNR-insensitive $CD34^+$ AML cell lines (KG1a and Kasumi-1) and primary $CD34^+$ AML cells. The apoptosis- and G1/S cell arrest-inducing effects of curcumin were observed in the DNR-insensitive and DNR-sensitive $CD34^+$ AML cells.[28] In addition, dimethoxycurcumin (**2**) and bisdemethoxycurcumin (**3**) isolated from the herb displayed the same degree of antigrowth effect as curcumin did against four leukemia cells (HL-60, K562, U937, and Molt4).[21] In addition, ar-turmerone (**4**), which is a noncurcuminoid compounds isolated from Turmeric, also exhibited moderate cytotoxic and apoptotic effects on the leukemia cell lines (Molt4B, HL-60, K562, U937, and RBL-2H3) with IC_{50} values of 20–50 μg/mL.[17,29,30] The inhibitory rate of ar-turmerone (**4**) reached 84% in the U937 cells. The upregulation of Bax and p53 expressions and caspase-3 activation is involved in the ar-turmerone-promoted U937 cell apoptosis.[14]

Effect on Carcinoma in the Stomach

Curcumin (**1**) demonstrated marked *in vitro* suppressive effect on the growth of four human gastric carcinoma cell lines (SGC-7901, NUGC-3, MGC803, and AGS) in dose- and time-dependent manners.[6,26–40] The IC_{50} values on MGC803 cells were 13 μM in 48 h and 8 μM in 96 h, and the LD_{50} value on NUGC-3 cells was 13 μM.[6,31,32] After the curcumin treatment at concentrations of 5–25 μmol/L for four days, the AGS cell proliferation was diminished by 34–92%. The significant inhibition on telomerase and DNA polymerase-λ by curcumin (**1**) was correlated with the promotion of a G2/M cell cycle arrest and an apoptotic response to gastric cancer cells.[30,32] The anticancer activity of curcumin (**1**) was also further approved in a nude mice model implanted with SGC7901 cancer cells.[33,34]

Prominently, in association with the activation of caspase-3 and the decline of overexpressed *P-gp, curcumin* (**1**) at noncytotoxic concentrations (5–20 μmol/L) reversed the drug resistance of SGC7901/Vcr gastric carcinoma cells.[35] When the concentration was up to 10–40 μmol/L, curcumin (**1**) could notably retard the invasion, adhesion, and migration of SGC-7901 cells.[31] When curcumin is combined with 5-FU, a significant synergistic effect could be dose-dependently achieved against the growth of AGS cells.[30] These results proved that curcumin (**1**) has multiple therapeutic potentials in the inhibition of both proliferation and metastasis of gastric carcinoma.

Effect on Carcinoma in the Colon

Various human colon/colorectal cancer cells emerged to be sensitive to curcumin (**1**). The antigrowth and apoptotic effects of curcumin were shown significantly in colon cancer cell lines (HT-29, HCT116, HCT15, SW480, SW48, Lovo, Caco-2, and Colo205). But curcumin (**1**) acted its characteristic mechanisms on different types of colon carcinoma cells.[36–38] HT-29 cells were relatively more sensitive to curcumin exposing than Caco-2 cells. Curcumin (**1**) induced G2/M-cell arrest and apoptosis of HT-29 cells by p53 activation, regulation of apoptosis-related proteins, as well as inhibition of COX-2 expression,[39–41] whereas curcumin (10–30 μM) dose-dependently hindered SW480 cell proliferation with apoptotic induction via a Akt signal pathway, i.e., decline of phosphorylated Akt and total Akt levels, and activation of caspase-3.[42] Curcumin (~20 μM) elicited DNA damage and mitosis arrest in HCT116 cells and blocked the cell cycle at S and G2/M stages, associated with the increase of GADD153 mRNA expression, leading the HCT116 cells to apoptotic death.[43–45]

In vitro experiments further revealed that curcumin significantly repressed the invasion of Colo 205 cells via the inhibition on MMP-2 and MMP-9, COX-2, and NF-κB.[46] Curcumin (**1**) also inhibited the EGFR expression in human Caco-2 and HT-29 colon cancer cell lines. The antigrowth effect of curcumin on Moser cells was found to be correlated with the stimulation of PPAR-γ and the inhibition of cyclin-D1 and EGFR.[47,48] Moreover, curcumin (**1**) was able to remarkably potentiate the anticancer effect of γ-radiotherapy against HCT116 colorectal cancer xenografts in nude mice. During the cotreatment, NF-κB activity and NF-κB-regulated gene products (such as c-Myc, Bcl-2, Bcl-xL, cyclin-D1, cellular inhibitor of AP-1, COX-2, VEGF, and MMP-9) were markedly restrained by curcumin, leading to the antiproliferative and angiogenic effects on HCT-116 cells.[49]

Effect on Carcinoma in the Liver

The studies have demonstrated marked therapeutic and preventive effects of curcumin (**1**) against cancer cell growth and carcinogenesis in the liver, as well as prominent hepatoprotective property. *In vitro* assays showed that curcumin dose-dependently restrained a panel of human hepatoma cell lines (HepG2, Hep3B, Bel7402, SMMC7721, and SK-hep-1) with the induction of apoptosis and cell cycle arrest and the reduction of telomerase activity. The IC_{50} values were 3.83 μM (in 24 h) in Bel7402 cells and 5.4 μg/mL in

SMMC7721 cells.[6,34,50–52] When 50–200 mg/kg doses of curcumin were orally administered to nude mice implanted with Bel7402 cells, the significant effect on the xenografts was exerted as inhibiting the hepatoma growth and prolonging the life duration of mice with no toxicity and weight loss during the treatment.[50] The expression and the distribution of subcellular PKC isoforms were obviously reduced in the curcumin-treated hepatoma Hep3B cells.[53] The antigrowth and the apoptosis- and cell cycle arrest-inducing effects in Sk-hep-1 cells by curcumin (**1**) were found to be associated with the blockage of MDR1 mRNA expression.[54] In Bel7402 cells and HepG2 cells, curcumin also exerted significant suppressive effect against the expressions of VEGF and hypoxia-inducible factor-1α (HIF-1α) through the blockage of signal transduction pathway of PI3K/AKT/FRAP, indicating that the antiangiogenetic activity of curcumin (**1**) also contributed to the antihepatoma effect.[55–57] Moreover, curcumin (**1**) could obstruct the migratory and invasive abilities of mouse hepatoma Hca-F cells via a mechanism involving the inactivation of caveolin-1 and EGFR.[58] By reducing the P-*gp*-mediated drug efflux, curcumin (**1**) was also active in reversing the drug resistance of Adm in HepG2/Adm cells and subsequently augmenting the concentration of Adm in the liver.[59]

In addition, the anticarcinogenic and hepatoprotecting properties of curcumin (**1**) was markedly demonstrated *in vivo* against N-bis-(2-hydroxypropyl) nitrosamine-induced liver adenoma formation and dimethylnitrosamine-induced hepatic injury, whose actions were associated with decrease of HO-1 (an important antioxidant enzyme) expression and activity.[60,61] Curcumin (**1**) was also effective in exerting the antiproliferative and apoptotic effects in KKU-M214 cholangiocarcinoma cells (a rare adenocarcinoma) dose- and time-dependently.[62] The promotion of apoptotic death in KKU-M214 cells was associated with (1) the obvious production of superoxide anion; (2) the repression of NF-κB and Bcl-xL levels; (3) the upregulation of p53 and Bax; and (4) the inhibition of cellular redox and collapse of mitochondrial transmembrane potential.[62]

Effect on Carcinoma in the Pancreas

A group of human pancreatic cancer cell lines (BxPC-3, MiaPaCa-2, Panc-1, and SUIT-2) and murine pancreatic cancer cells (Pan02) were significantly inhibited by curcumin (**1**) *in vitro*.[63–66] The antigrowth rates were 45.9% and 78.1% in Panc-1 cells in 30 and 60 μM concentrations of curcumin (**1**), respectively, whose effect was accompanied by S and G2/M cell arrest.[66] The treatment of the BxPC-3 cells with a low and single exposure of curcumin (2.5 μM) for 24 h triggered a significant apoptosis and G2/M cell cycle arrest with the induction of ATM/Chk1 expression.[67] The same apoptosis and G2/M cell cycle arrest were also promoted by curcumin (**1**) in Pan02 cells in correlation with the downregulation Bcl-2 and Bak expressions, the upregulation of Bax activity, as well as the reduction IL-8 expression and enhancement of IL-8 receptor on the cell surface.[65]

NF-κB and its gene products were known to relate to the proliferation, survival, angiogenesis, and chemoresistance of pancreatic cancer. Curcumin (**1**) acted as a significant NF-κB inhibitor, consistently repressing the NF-κB binding and diminishing the expressions of NF-κB-regulated gene products (including COX-2, PSG-E_2, and IL-8).[68] In association with the marked reduction of the activities of NF-κB and NF-κB-regulated gene products (such as cyclin-D1, c-Myc, Bcl-2, Bcl-xL, cellular IAP-1, COX-2, VEGF, and MMPs), the extensive *in vitro* and *in vivo* (nude mice) treatments with curcumin (**1**) or Turmeric Force (a product of Jiang Huang) could potentiate the growth inhibition and the apoptosis caused by gemcitabine on pancreatic carcinoma cells (BxPC-3, MiaPaCa-2, and Panc-1) and lessen the tumor cell resistance to gemcitabine and amplify the chemotherapeutic rate.[63,69] The cotreatment also diminished the $CD31^+$ microvessel, showing highly effective antiangiogenesis against the pancreatic cancer.[63] Curcumin (**1**) in the cotreatment also markedly enhanced the inhibitory effect of gemcitabine to limit the cell viability of p34 pancreatic carcinoma cells (high COX-2 expression) but not so potent in Panc-1 cells (low COX-2 expression), indicating that the inhibition on the p34 cells is strongly related to the decline of COX-2 and p-ERK1/2 levels.[70] When the BxPC-3 cells were cotreated by curcumin (**1**) plus docosahexaenoic acid, omega-3 fatty acids or genistin *in vivo* (nude mice) or *in vitro*, the significant synergistic effects were concomitantly achieved with the apoptotic and inhibitory effects (approximately 72%).[71] At the same time, the expressions of iNOS, COX-2, and 5-LOX were downregulated and the p21 activity was upregulated in the tumor xenograft.[72] When cotreatment with curcumin and WT1-targeting small inhibitory RNA (siRNA), the growth inhibition on the Panc-1 cells could be enhanced by notably decreasing WT1 expression.[73]

In order to improve the oral bioavailability and the drug delivery, the liposomal formulation of curcumin (**1**) had been developed, demonstrating greater activity against multiple cancers. The best dosing schedule for the liposomal curcumin was 20 mg/kg given once daily three times per week in a nude mice model xenografted with human MiaPaCa-2 pancreatic cancer, displaying optimal tumor growth inhibition without toxicity.[74] The evidences showed that curcumin might be used to the development of an effective treatment of pancreatic adenocarcinoma.

Effect on Carcinoma in the Lung

The growth of A549 and H1299 human lung cancer cell lines could be dose-dependently repressed by curcumin (**1**) with its IC_{50} values of 50 and 40 μM (in 24 h), respectively, whose effects were p53-independently mediated by inhibiting the antiapoptotic genes (Bcl-2, Bcl-xL, and c-Myc) and activating Bax, p53, and caspase-1 and caspase-3.[75] In the treated A549 cells, curcumin (**1**) simultaneously (1) prevented β-catenin from cytoplasm into the nucleus; (2) elicited oxidative DNA damage, (3) blocked Wnt signal transduction pathway and protein synthesis by modulating eukaryotic initiation factors (eIF2α and eIF4E); and (4) finally effectively resulted to cell cycle arrest and growth suppression.[75–78] In human A2 lung adenocarcinoma cells, curcumin (**1**) prompted the apoptosis by suppressing survivin expression to exert the antiproliferative effect (IC_{50} 40 μM).[79] The similar suppressive effect of curcumin against PC-9 human lung cancer cells was found to be associated with (1) the induction of growth arrest and DNA damage-inducible genes GADD45 and GADD153, (2) the activation of CDK inhibitor genes p21 and p27, and (3) the downregulation of numerous gene expressions (such as Bcl-2, cyclin-D1, CDK2, CDK4, and CDK6).[80]

Similar to the anticancer drugs vinorelbine and cisplatin, curcumin (**1**) could induce apoptosis of human H520 squamous cell lung carcinoma cells and human H460 NSCLC cells by declining Bcl-2 and Bcl-xL expressions, increasing Bax and Bcl-xS activities, releasing cytochrome c, and activating caspase-9 and caspase-3. Also, the expressions of COX-2, NF-κB, and AP-1 were lessened in the H520 cells, and the generation of superoxide anion was increased in the H460 cells after the curcumin treatment, leading to synergistically enhancing the cytotoxic activity of cisplatin and vinorelbine on the cancer cells.[81,82] The decline of ERK1/2 and ERCC1 expressions and thymidine phosphorylase (IP) activity were also observed to be involved in the synergistic effect exerted by the curcumin plus cisplatin against the NSCLC cells.[83]

Interestingly, the antiinvasive and antimetastatic effects of curcumin (**1**) were observed in a highly invasive CL1-5 lung adenocarcinoma cells. At a concentration range far below its cytotoxic level (20 μM), curcumin notably reduced the invasive capacity of the CL1-5 cells in a dose-dependent manner, whose effect was found to be correlated with the activation of a tumor suppressor DnaJ-like HSP 40 (HLJ1) through the activation of JNK/JunD pathway and the upregulation of E-cad expression.[84] During the interactions, several other invasion-related genes (such as integrins α6 and β4, MMP-14, and neuronal cell adhesion molecule) were also repressed, and several HSPs (Hsp27, Hsp70, and Hsp40-like protein) were concurrently activated.[85] Moreover, curcumin (**1**) showed a remarkable reversal capacity against Bcl-2-mediated cisplatin resistance in multidrug-resistant A549/DDP cells and H460/DDP cells, displaying the antiproliferative effect on the A549/DDP cells with promoted apoptosis and G2-phase cell cycle arrest.[86,87] In addition, the pulmonary adenoma formation and growth caused by N-bis-(2-hydroxypropyl) nitrosamine (a oncogenic agent) was significantly obstructed by curcumin (**1**) in a mouse model.[88]

All the evidences clearly demonstrated that curcumin (**1**) is a promising chemotherapeutic and chemopreventive agent for the improvement of lung neoplastic treatment and prevention.

Effect on Carcinoma in the Prostate

Epidemiological studies evaluated the effects of curcumin in prostate cancer cells *in vitro* and *in vivo*, revealing that curcumin (**1**) was able to interfere with growth factor signaling pathways, to restrain the transforming activities and to enhance apoptosis in both AD and androgen-independent (AI) human prostate cancer cells, but it is inactive in normal human prostate epithelial cells.[89,90] During the actions, curcumin (**1**) also potently inhibited EGFR signaling in both types of cells through three routes, i.e., (1) downregulating the EGFR protein, (2) diminishing tyrosine kinase activity in the intrinsic EGFR, and (3) repressing ligand-induced activation of the EGFR.[89] In both AD type of LNCaP cells and AI type of PC3 cells, curcumin (**1**) completely restrained the expression of a cell survival factor Akt but not in the AI type of DU-145 cells, suggesting that the inhibition of Akt activity is one of the antiprostate carcinoma mechanisms of curcumin.[91]

The extensive approaches discovered that the mechanisms of curcumin were much different in the AD and AI prostate tumor cells. For the induction of LNCaP (AD) cell apoptosis, curcumin influenced multiple interactions, i.e., (1) reducing the expressions of Bcl-2 and Bcl-xL; (2) translocating Bax and p53 to mitochondria; (3) increasing the generation of ROS, diminishing the mitochondrial membrane potential, and releasing the mitochondrial proteins (such as cytochrome c, Smac/DIABLO, and Omi/HtrA2); (4) activating the expressions of Bak, Bim, Noxa, PUMA, and caspase-3; (5) downregulating the transactivation and the expressions of AR; (6) restraining the expression of PI3K and phosphorylation of Ser473 AKT/PKB, NF-κB, AP-1, and CREB-binding protein; (7) repressing PSA protein function and blocking the expression of AR by decreasing luciferase activity; and (8) decreasing the microvessel-d in the LNCaP cells.[90,92–96] In the PC3 cells (AI), curcumin (**1**) followed p53-independent multimechanic routes to effectively elicit the apoptosis and the G2/M cell arrest, thereby suppressing the growth of PC3 cells *in vitro* and *in vivo*, whose multimechanisms in the AI cells were established to correlate with with (1) activating c-jun N-terminal kinase (and p38 MAPK; (2) augmenting expressions of Hesl, Notch1 and nuclear translocation; (3) inhibiting transcription factor (NF-κB and AP-1) signaling pathways; (4) reducing Jagged1 expression and an oncogene MDM2 level; (5) activating p21 Waf1/CIP1; (6) enhancing the activities of caspases and AIF; and (7) reducing VEGF expressions. These events might serve to explain the proliferative and angiogenetic effects of curcumin (**1**) on the AI prostate cancer cells.[97–104]

Moreover, curcumin (**1**) was able to potentiate the activities of chemotherapy and radiotherapy against prostate cancer. *In vitro* and *in vivo* treatments with curcumin and β-phenylethyl isothiocyanate (PEITC) in low doses displayed additive effects to suppress the growth of PC3 cells by interfering with EGFR, Akt, and NF-κB signaling pathways.[105,106] When combined with resveratrol, the liposomal forms of curcumin (**1**) notably obstructed the growth of prostatic adenocarcinoma cells and elicited the apoptosis in association with the reduced tumor suppressor gene phosphatase and tensin homolog (PTEN) and the downregulated cyclin-D1, p-Akt, m-TOR, and AR.[107] Further studies revealed that the prostate carcinoma cells have the osseomimetic properties as well, by which activities the propensity of osseous metastases would be developed, while the prostate cancer cells acquire these bone-like activities for surviving in the bony microenvironment. Experiments confirmed that curcumin was able to interfere with the development of osteoblast and osteoblast-like properties of C4-2B cells (a highly metastatic subline of the LNCaP cells) by significantly repressing the ligand-stimulated autophosphorylation of EGFR and CSF1-R and decreasing the expressions of NF-κB and core-binding factor a-1 in the C4-2B cells. When the C4-2B cells were grown under promineralization conditions, curcumin (**1**) prevented the mineralized nodule formation mainly through the blockage of the growth factor receptor pathways and the NF-κB activation.[108] Moreover, by obviously blocking CCL2 (a chemotactic factor of prostate cancer, playing important roles in the development of bone metastasis)-mediated actions in the invasion, the adhesion, and the motility, and also in part through the differential regulation of PKC and MMP-9 signalings, curcumin (**1**) exerted potential antimetastatic effect in bone derived by prostate cancer PC3 cells.[109] The curcumin treatment also affected the inhibition of invasive ability and the reduction of tumor volume of AI prostate carcinoma DU-145 cells *in vitro* and *in vivo*, associated with the significant decrease of MMP-2 and MMP-9 expressions.[110] Consequently, curcumin (**1**) may effectively restrain the growth factor collaboration between prostate cancer cells and osteoblast cells, showing a chemotherapeutic advantage in interfering with the metastatic potential of prostate cancer cells.

Effect on Carcinomas in the Bladder

Curcumin (**1**) was shown to be a potential agent to suppress oncogenesis (including cell survival, proliferation, and angiogenesis) and to promote apoptosis in various human bladder cancer cell lines such as T24, 253JB-V, UMUC, EJ, RT4V6 (IFNα-sensitive), KU-7 (IFNα-resistant), and murine MBT-2 bladder carcinoma cells *in vitro* or *in vivo*. An *in vivo* clonal growth assay exhibited that curcumin in a large dose (100 μM) and in a short term was completely lethal to three bladder cancer cell lines (T24, UMUC, and MBT-2).[111–114] The daily oral administration of curcumin (**1**) could notably decline the incidence of bladder tumorigenesis caused by aristolochic acid in rats.[115] In an orthotopic mouse model, a maximum reduction of the volume 253JB-V bladder tumor was achieved when curcumin (**1**) was given in combination with anticancer agents (such as gemcitabine and paclitaxel).[111] In addition, curcumin (**1**) significantly repressed the NF-κB activation and then reduced the COX-2 production and the VEGF activity, leading to the diminishment of the risk factors of bladder carcinogenesis caused by cigarette smoking.[116,117]

Furthermore, curcumin was capable of enhancing the chemotherapeutic effect of Bacillus Calmette–Guerin intravesical therapy (which is a standard treatment for bladder cancer in clinics), associated with inhibiting NF-κB activity and inducing TRAIL receptors in the bladder cancer cells.[118] N-Maleoyl-L-valine-curcumin (NVC) and N-maleoylglycine-curcumin (NGC) are two esterase-sensitive curcumin prodrugs. The treatment of a human EJ bladder cancer cells with NVC or NGC in a 40 μmol/L concentration significantly retarded the cell growth by 66.23% and 68.21%, respectively, in dose- and time-dependent manners. The IC_{50} values of curcumin (**1**) and its derivatives NVC and NGC were 16.5, 20.1, and 18.7 μmol/L on the EJ cells, respectively.[119,120] These evidences proposed that curcumin (**1**) is an effective nontoxic intravesical agent and drug lead, which can be used for the improvement of the current standard of care in chemoprevention and chemotherapy of bladder cancer.

Briefly, the antineoplastic mechanism of curcumin (**1**) in the bladder cancer cells was revealed to correlate with (1) the inhibition of NF-κB activation and NF-κB-dependent genes (such as Bcl-2, surviving, and cyclin-D1)[112–117,121,122]; (2) the decline of specificity protein transcription factor expression[121]; (3) the decrease of p300, c-fos and c-jun expressions, and acetyl histone H3 and H4 protein expressions[122,123]; (4) the abolishment of COX-2, c-Myc, and VEGF expressions[116,117,121]; (5) the upregulation of p21WAF1/CIP1 (a CDK inhibitor)[124]; (6) the augmentation of Bax and p53 expressions[112]; (7) the reduction of proliferation marker Ki-67 and microvessel-d (CD31)[112]; and (8) the diminution of prostaglandin E2 synthesis,[119] thereby finally eliciting cell cycle arrest and apoptotic death.[112]

Effect on Carcinoma in the Kidney

An *in vitro* assay demonstrated the marked antineoplastic activity of curcumin (**1**) on two human renal carcinoma cell lines (TK-10 and Caki). Curcumin (50 μM) effectively suppressed the TK-10 cells in a similar fashion to etoposide (an anticancer agent) with an IC_{50} value of 12.16 μM, whose effect was mediated by the inhibition of Topo-II activity and the induction of DNA damage and apoptosis.[125] The cytotoxicity induced by curcumin in the Caki cells was mainly followed by inactivating the Akt-related cell survival pathway and activating an apoptotic pathway, including downregulation of the expressions of Bcl-2, Bcl-xL, and IAP proteins; sequential dephosphorylation of Akt; cleavage of phospholipase C-γ1; release of cytochrome c; activation of caspase-3; and DNA fragmentation.[126] Moreover, *in vivo* experiments revealed that curcumin (**1**) could also enhance the activities of antioxidant and phase II-metabolizing enzymes to afford a substantial protection against oxidative damage and omithine decarboxylase (ODC) activity caused by ferric nitriletriacetate (a kidney-specific carcinogen).[127,128] The potent antioxidant and apoptotic effects evidenced that curcumin (**1**) is a potential chemopreventive agent for the treatment of renal carcinogenesis.

Effect on Carcinoma in the Cervix

Cervical cancer development and carcinogenesis have been revealed to be largely caused by the infection with high-risk human papillomaviruses (HPVs) predominantly through the action of viral oncoproteins E6 and E7.[129] *In vitro* and *in vivo* experiments confirmed that the curcumin (**1**) was capable of exerting dose-dependent suppressive effects against the proliferation of three types of HPV-positive human cervical cancer cell linrs (HeLa, SiHa, and Caski).[130] The injection of curcumin (0.2 mL, in a 250 μmol/L concentration, once per day for 10 days) into the abdominal cavity of mice bearing HeLa cancer could achieve the inhibition rate of 74.33%.[131]

Its anticervical cancer mechanism has been gradually found out to be mediated by multipathways. Importantly, the cytotoxicity of curcumin is more selective in HPV16- and HPV18-infected cervical cells compared to non-HPV infected cells due to the suppression of E6 and E7 expressions, the inhibition of NF-κB and AP-1, and the restoration of p53 function.[132,133] Curcumin (**1**) was also effective in the induction of cell cycle arrest at S stage and apoptosis of cervical cancer cells, wherein a series of alteractions successively occurred, such as (1) decline of Bcl-2 and Bcl-xL expressions and increase of Bax and AIF expressions and p53 and p21 activities; (2) disruption of microtubule assembly dynamics; (3) release of cytochrome c and activation of caspase-3 and caspase-9, (4) decrease of COX-2, iNOS, NF-κB, and cyclin-D1 levels; and (5) distinct inhibition of hTERT and XIAP protein.[134–138] The inhibitory effect of curcumin against the Caski cells was additionally associated with the dose-dependent downregulation of pleiotrophin.[139] Likewise, the treatment with 50 μmol/L curcumin markedly reduced the migration of Caski cells via significant blockage of MMP-2, MT1-MMP, and NF-κB expressions, suggesting that curcumin may be used as a potential antiinvasive and antimetastatic agent on the cervical cancer cells.[139,140]

Furthermore, in the presence of SOD, ascorbic acid, or N-acetylcysteine, the cellular levels of curcumin could be amplified by 31–66%, and the anticancer activity of curcumin was noticeably enhanced.[141] In combination with taxol (an anticancer drug in clinics), curcumin was able to potentiate the cytotoxic activity of taxol together with promoting the taxol-induced apoptosis and lessening the taxol-induced NF-κB activation and serine/threonine kinase Akt phosphorylation without affecting the taxol-induced tubulin polymerization and the CDK2 activation.[142] The pretreatment with curcumin (**1**) significantly and dose-dependently sensitized the activity of ionizing radiation against the two HeLa and SiHa cancer cells, indicating that the curcumin application is an effective radiation-modifying modality for cervical cancer therapeutic improvement. The radiosensitization of curcumin (**1**) was found to be parallel with the increase of ROS and the activation of ERK1/2.[143]

Prominently, curcuminoids such as curcumin (**1**), demethoxycurcumin (**2**) and bisdemethoxycurcumin (**3**) and their major metabolite form assigned as tetrahydrocurcumin (**5**), were found to possess potential ability to reduce MDR-1 gene expression and P-gp function in multidrug-resistant human KB-V1 cervical carcinoma cells. Treating the cells with nontoxic doses of curcuminoids, especially curcumin (**1**) and tetrahydrocurcumin (**5**), could enhance the cell sensitivity to vinblastine, mitoxantrone, and etoposide in the P-gp-expressing drug-resistant KB-V1 cells in association with retarding verapamil-stimulated ATPase activity and drug-binding site of transporter.[144–147] Curcumin (**1**) was able to amplify the concentration of vinblastine in the KB-V1 cells more effectively than other curcuminoids, whereas bisdemethoxycurcumin (**3**) displayed to be the most active in the MDR-1 gene inhibition.[145,146] These findings highlighted that the curcuminoids are effective MDR modulators, which may be employed to improve the conventional chemotherapy for cervical carcinoma in combination with anticancer drugs.

Effect on Carcinoma in the Ovary

Many studies demonstrated that curcumin (**1**) was able to effectively exert the antiproliferatory and apoptotic effects on a variety of human ovarian cancer cell lines (such as A2780, CAOV3, SKOV, OVCAR-3, HO-8910, 3AO, OC3, HeyA8, and HeyA8/MDR) *in vitro*. Curcumin (**1**), demethoxycurcumin (**2**), and bisdemethoxycurcumin (**3**) displayed the cytotoxicity on OC3 and OVCAR-3 cells with CD_{50} values ranging from 3.1 to 4.4 μg/mL.[148] *In vivo* models implanted with SKOV3i.p.1 cells or HeyA8 cells confirmed that curcumin (**1**) resulted in 49% and 55% reductions in mean tumor cell growth.[149]

The antigrowth mechanisms of curcumin (**1**) seems to be their respective feature in different types of ovarian cancer cells. For instance, in the inhibition of CAOV3 cells by curcumin (**1**), p53 phosphorylation was induced and AMPK was activated in a p38-dependent manner.[150] Curcumin also repressed EGFR and AKT/ERK activations and reduced aquaporin expression in the CAOV3 cells, resulting in the diminution of the cell migration.[151] The time- and dose-dependent cytotoxicities of curcumin (**1**) were present in other ovarian cancer cell lines with differing p53 statuses such as HEY and OVCA429 (wild-type p53), OCC1 (mutant p53), and SKOV-3 (null p53). The p53-independent cytotoxic and apoptotic effects of curcumin were found to correlate with the activation of p38-MAPK, the ablation of prosurvival Akt signaling, and the reduction of survivin expressions in the ovarian cancer cells.[152] The antiproliferative effect of curcumin (10–50 μmol/L) on A2780 cells was accompanied by the blockage of the cell cycle at G0/G1 stage and the promotion of apoptosis in association with the retardation of NF-κB and Bcl-2 expressions and activation of caspase-3,[153] whereas the effect of curcumin (40 μM) in HO-8910 and 3AO cell lines is closely related to the promotion of cell cycle arrest at S and/or G2/M stages and apoptosis through the increase of the levels of p53 and Bax and the decrease of the expressions of Bcl-2, Bcl-xL, and procaspase-3.[154–156] Besides the similar effects, curcumin (**1**) in an oral dose of 500 mg/kg also restrained the expression of angiogenic cytokine in athymic mice implanted with HeyA8/MDR, SKOV3i.p.1, or HeyA8 types of ovarian cancer cells.[149]

In the approaches for improving the treatment of ovarian cancer, curcumin (**1**) demonstrated more interesting features in the sensitization of anticancer drugs and the reversal of MDR. The cytotoxicity of cisplatin could be effectively augmented by the combination with curcumin in the treatment of CAOV3, 3AO, and SKOV-3 ovarian cancer cell lines, while the effect of carboplatin and topotecan were enhanced by curcumin (**1**) in 3AO cells.[157,158] Curcumin at a concentration of 5 mg/L improved the sensitization of OCC1 ovarian neoplastic cells to cisplatin (2.5–10 mg/L) by 2.66 times, via the blockage of Fanconi anemia/BRCA pathway.[159,160] Similarly, curcumin (**1**) combined with paclitaxel or docetaxel was capable of inhibiting the growth of OC3, HeyA8, and/or SKOV cell lines and together reducing the toxicity caused by the two anticancer drugs.[149,161] But the synergistic effect of curcumin on cisplatin was not found in human HO-8910PM ovarian cancer cells.[162] In addition, the cotreatment of paclitaxel and curcumin (**1**) in nanoemulsion formulation could improve the oral bioavailability and the therapeutic efficacy in mice bearing SKOV-3 tumor.[163]

Importantly, the cytotoxicity of therapeutic drugs in several multidrug-resistant ovarian cancer cells could also be synergistically augmented by curcumin. The oral administration of the mice with curcumin (**1**) at 50 mg/kg for three consecutive days markedly lessened the levels of intestinal P-gp and cytochrome P450 3A2 protein, indicating a potential for reversal of MDR.[163] In mice with drug-resistant HeyA8/MDR tumors, curcumin helped the docetaxel to obviously restrain the tumor cell growth by 58%.[149] When cisplatin is combined (2.5 μg/mL) with curcumin (20 μmol/L), the cisplatin sensitivity was enhanced and the proliferation of cisplatin-resistant ovarian cancer COCI/CDDP cells was markedly hindered, associated with activation of Smac and caspase-3 and inhibition of survivin and Bcl-2.[154,155,164–166] The drug-resistant SKOV-3TR ovarian adenocarcinoma cells were effectively restrained by the cotreatment of paclitaxel and curcumin by inhibiting NF-κB activity and P-gp expression. According to the significant efficacy in the preclinical models, the cochemotherapy with curcumin (**1**) may be attractive in clinics for patients with ovarian cancer, especially multidrug-resistant ovarian cancer.

Effect on Carcinoma in the Breast

Various studies provided solid evidences to substantiate that curcumin (**1**) obviously displayed antiproliferative and apoptosis-promoting effects on both types of breast cancer cell lines, estrogen receptor-positive MCF-7 cells and estrogen receptor-negative MDA-MB-231 cells, *in vitro* and *in vivo*. The IC_{50} values of curcumin (**1**) were 12–35 μM in MCF-7 cells and 30 μM in MDA-MB-231 cells,[138,167–169] where the cell cycle arrest and the apoptosis of the two types of breast cancer cells were promoted by curcumin in a low cytostatic dose of 20 μM.[168] When the dose was raised to 54 μM, curcumin (**1**) damaged the DNA and caused marked depolymerization of the interphase microtubules and the mitotic spindle microtubules in the MCF-7 cells, thereby destroying the breast cancer cells.[138,170]

The mechanism of curcumin on the breast cancer has been extensively explored, revealing that the antiproliferative effect was achieved by quite different multipathways in the estrogen receptor-dependent and estrogen receptor-independent breast neoplastic cells. In MCF-7 cells (estrogen receptor$^+$), the suppressive effect of curcumin was estrogen-dependent, followed by inhibiting the expression of estrogen receptor downstream genes including pS2 and transforming the growth factor-α.[171] The curcumin-induced MCF-7 cell apoptosis and growth suppression were also found to occur through (1) the increase of p53 and p21 levels, p53-DNA binding activity, and p53-dependent Bax expression; (2) the downregulation of IGF-1 axis, CD44V6, and PCNA expressions; and (3) the activation of AMPK and the blockage of AMPK downstream targets (PPAR-γ, MAP kinases, and COX-2).[169,172–175] The inhibitory effect in MDA-MB-231 cells (estrogen receptor$^-$) by curcumin was associated with (1) the downregulation of Notch1 gene expression and NF-κB activity and (2) the suppression of two major angiogenesis factors VEGF and bFGF in the transcript levels. Besides the different mechanisms, the anticancer activity of curcumin on both ER$^+$-MCF-7 cells and estrogen receptor$^-$ MDA-MB-231 cells also partially shared one same mechanism, i.e., curcumin-regulated Wnt/β-catenin signaling by markedly diminishing the nuclear expression of disheveled, β-catenin, cyclin-D1, and slug.[169] Curcumin (**1**), in addition, was effective in a specific triple negative breast carcinoma, whose cells lack the expressions of estrogen and progesterone receptors but have HER2 overexpression. In the triple negative breast cancer cells, curcumin (**1**) triggered the DNA damage and apoptosis and restrained the cell growth and migration in anchorage-independent manner in association with the increased expression and cytoplasmic retention of BRCA1 protein. These data recommended the use of curcumin to improve the survival of patients with the triple negative breast cancer.[176]

Furthermore, curcumin exerted strong antiinvasive effects in the MDA-MB-231 cells via (1) the downregulation of MMP-2 and MMP-9, (2) the reduction of NF-κB and AP-1 activities, (3) the decrease of TIMP-1, and (4) the blockage of RON tyrosine kinase expression.[171,177–179] These interactions lead to the significant attenuation of the cell invasions and the number of lung metastases in nude mice implanted with MDA-MB-231 cells through the obstruction of the cell adhesion/motility and a reconstituted basement membrane.[178–182] Also, by a Ca^{2+}-mitochondrial pathway including the increase of ROS and the decrease of Bcl-2 oncoprotein, curcumin (**1**) lessened the cell viability and the metastasis in mice implanted with highly metastatic murine ENU 1564 mammary gland cells.[183]

Curcumin (**1**) and tetrahydrocurcumin (**5**) are the marked inhibitors of mitoxantrone resistance protein (MXR), multidrug-resistant protein-1 (MRP1), and P-gp. Through the suppression of the efflux functions of P-gp, MXR, and MRP1, both curcumin and tetrahydrocurcumin could reverse the MDR and markedly augment the sensitivity of vinblastine, mitoxantrone, and etoposide in MCF-7/MDR and MCF7AdmVp3000 cells.[184,185] Many curcumin analogs (such as benzyloxime, isoxazole, and pyrazole heterocycles in a diketone system), especially the isoxazole analogue, demonstrated remarkable increases of the antitumor potency in both drug-sensitive MCF-7 cells and drug-resistant MCF-7 cells.[186] Moreover, a synergistical effect could be achieved by the cotreatment of curcumin and epigallocatechin gallate against MDA-MB-231 breast cancer cells with a 49% volume reduction in nude mice, wherein the protein levels of VEGFR-1, EGFR, and Akt were notably declined, and VEGFR-1 might play a key role in the inhibition against the growth of breast cancer cells.[187] Also, the cotreatment with curcumin and Adm or docetaxel showed the synergistic efficacy against the MCF-7 cells, and the xanthorrhizol–curcumin combination exerted the similar synergistic growth inhibition against the MDA-MB-231 cells.[188–190] Interestingly, a conjugation of curcumin to gold nanoparticles (10 nm) potentiated the bioavailability, the cellular uptake, and the antitumor efficacy in the cisplatin-resistant MDA-MB-231 cells.[191] Curcumin-PEG divinyl ether polymer conjugate showed similar but more potent cytotoxic effect on the MCF-7 cells than the free curcumin.[192] When combined with copper (II) sulfate, curcumin (**1**) could promote the apoptosis of ZR-75-1 human oxidation-resistant breast cancer cells, but it was effective only in the copper-oxidized cells.[193]

Based upon the results, curcumin (**1**) may be considered as a potential drug lead for the development of more effective agents against estrogen receptor-dependent or estrogen receptor-independent breast cancer and MDR breast cancer.

Effect on Carcinoma in the Brain

Curcumin (**1**) was found to effectively block many types of brain tumor formation and to promote cell apoptosis *in vitro*. In human glioma cell lines (SHG44, U87, and U251), curcumin demonstrated the antigrowth effect with enhanced cell cycle arrest and caspase-8-activated apoptosis.[194–196] G6P translocase (G6PT) plays a crucial role in transducing intracellular signalings in brain carcinoma cells. Curcumin (**1**) was capable of limiting the G6PT expression by >90% and triggering the U87 cells to death,[197] and demethoxycurcumin (**2**) more effectively induced the G2/M cell arrest and Bcl-2 mediated apoptosis in U87 cells than curcumin.[194] The inhibitory effect of curcumin (**1**) on human U87MG malignant glioblastoma cells was closely accompanied by a series of signal interactions, i.e., cleavage of Bid to tBid, increase of Bax/Bcl-2 ratio, elevation of Smac/DIABLO cytosolic level, release of cytochrome c from the mitochondria, activation of caspase-9, caspase-8, and caspase-3, and inhibition of NF-κB, then favoring the apoptosis.[198] In another type of DBTRG glioblastoma cells, curcumin exerted dose- and time-dependent cytotoxicities by either influencing p53 pathway (via the increase of p53 and p21 activities and the decrease of CDC2 expression) or inhibiting RB pathway (via the diminution of phosphorylated RB and the augmentation of CDKN2A/p16), leading the cells to apoptotic death and cell cycle arrest.[199]

The overexpression of transcription factors NF-κB and AP-1 generally is involved in the glioma cell survival, radioresistance, and chemoresistance. In the *in vitro* treatment of human (T98G, T67, and U87MG) and rat (C6) glioma cell lines, curcumin (**1**) significantly lessened the survival of glioma cells in a p53- and caspase-independent manner, associated with (1) restraining the AP-1 and NF-κB signaling pathways via the prevention of constitutive JNK and activation of Akt and (2) reducing the expressions of Bcl-2 and IAP family members as well as DNA repair enzymes (MGMT, DNA-PK, Ku70, Ku80, and ERCC-1). Through these interactions, curcumin (**1**) was capable of sensitizing the glioma cells to clinical radiotherapy and chemotherapeutic agents (such as camptothecin, cisplatin, etoposide, and doxorubicin), indicating the potential of curcumin (**1**) as an adjunct to current chemo- and radiotherapies in the treatment of brain cancer.[200]

Also, by the inhibition against the expressions of MMP and VEGF, curcumin (**1**) was able to significantly restrain the invasion of human astroglioma cells into the surrounding normal brain tissue.[201,202] If formulated to a water-soluble mode, curcumin (**1**) would easily cross the blood–brain barrier to demonstrate more effectivity in blocking the proliferation, survival, and invasion of human oligodendroglioma and mouse GL261 glioma and N18 neuroblastoma and also inhibiting the metastasis of mouse B16-F10 melanoma cells to the brain, without influencing the viability of normal brain cells. The further mechanic studies revealed that the antiglioma effect of solubilized curcumin was attributed to the effective suppression of cyclin-D1, P-NF-κB, Bcl-xL, P-Akt, and VEGF and the activation of caspase-3 and caspase-7.[203] In addition, *in vitro* and *in vivo* studies testified that curcumin (**1**) is also effective in the treatment of CNS disorders such as hypoxia-induced vascular leakage in brain, subarachnoid hemorrhage, and cerebral vasospasm, concomitant with attenuating oxidative brain injury and lipid peroxidation and reducing inflammatory gene expression and histone acetyl-transferase activity.[204,205]

Effect on Carcinoma in the Head and the Neck

In the *in vitro* assays, curcumin (**1**) demonstrated the inhibitory effect against the viability of many types of head and neck squamous cell carcinoma (HNSCC) cell lines such as SCC-1, SCC-9, CCL23, CAL27, NPC-TW076, UM-SCC1, UM-SCC14A, MDA686LN, and KB cells, giving the IC_{50} values of 15–22 μM for the first four HNSCC cell lines.[205–209] The growth suppression of HNSCC cells by curcumin (**1**) was also confirmed in nude mice xenografted with CAL27 cells or CNE-2Z-H5 cells,[208,210] where curcumin (**1**) in a 50 mg/kg dose restrained the proliferation of CNE-2Z-H5 cells by 59.75%.[211] The mechanism of curcumin was found to correlate with (1) disturbing the cell cycle by marked decrease of the expressions of cyclin-A, cyclin-B, cyclin-D1, and CDK1; (2) inducing apoptosis by the upregulation of Bax, the downregulation of Bcl-2, and the sequential activation of caspase-9 and caspase-3; (3) blocking EGFR phosphorylation; (4) inhibiting the NF-κB transcription; (5) inhibiting the expressions of COX-2 and MMP-9; and (6) markedly declining the IL-6 and IL-8 levels.[205–209,212] The IL-6 was reported to participate in the promotion of neoplastic cell proliferation and survival through the phosphorylation of STAT3, a cell-signaling protein, but curcumin (**1**) is an effective inhibitor of STAT3 in the HNSCC cells. Curcumin (**1**) showed more rapid and more potent suppressive effect on the STAT3 phosphorylation and HNSCC cell proliferation compared to AG490 (a well-characterized JAK2 inhibitor).[213] The mitochondria-, AIF- and caspase-3-dependent pathways were found to play an essential role in curcumin-induced apoptosis and G2/M phase arrest in NPC-TW 076 cells.[212] Additionally, the treatment of HEp-2 laryngeal cancer cells with curcumin could augment the cisplatin-induced apoptosis by 7.1% via the downregulation of Bcl-xL and the upregulation of Bax and nuclear AIF.[211]

When curcumin (**1**) was prepared as a liposomal formulation, its anti-HNSCC activity in CAL27 cells and UM-SCC1 cells would be potentiated *in vitro* and *in vivo* without demonstrable toxicity. The administration of the liposomal curcumin combined with a suboptimal dose of cisplatin to nude mice resulted in a marked antitumor effect against the xenografted HNSCC tumors, whose mechanism was found to be mediated by two different signaling pathways, i.e., AKT-independent pathway and NF-κB pathway.[214,215] All these remarkable results strongly recommended further investigation into the potential use of curcumin as an adjuvant in the treatment of nasopharyngeal carcinoma.

Effect on Carcinoma in the Skin

Curcumin (**1**) demonstrated potent growth inhibition against human melanoma cell lines (C32, G-361, WM 266-4, UACC-62, and A375) and murine melanoma cell lines (B16 and B16-F10) together with obvious apoptotic induction but no effect on normal melanocytes. The IC_{50} values of curcumin (**1**) were 4.28 μM in UACC-62 cells and 6.1–7.7 μM in three melanoma cell lines with B-raf mutation (C32, G-361, and WM266-4).[125,216] At a concentration of >20 μmol/L, curcumin markedly promoted the apoptosis and proliferatory inhibition of A375 melanoma cells *in vitro*. Eight melanoma cell lines (four with wild-type and four with mutant p53) were used for an *in vitro* investigation, where curcumin (**1**) dose- and time-dependently elicited the apoptosis of all tested melanoma cell lines through a p53-independent membrane-mediated mechanism including the advancement of Fas receptor/caspase-8 pathway and the blockage of NF-κB cell survival pathway.[217] In the *in vivo* experiment, the i.p. administration of curcumin (**1**) in a dose of 50 mg/kg to mice notably diminished the size and the weight of B16 melanoma by 55.61% and 55.56%, respectively, and reduced the level of MMP-2 activity by 50.94%,[218,219] whose antimelanoma mechanism was revealed to correlate with (1) the upregulation of p53, p21, p27, and checkpoint kinase-2; (2) the diminution of cyclin-D1 expressions to block the cell cycle progression and decrease of c-Myc and Bcl-2 expressions; (3) the activation of caspase-3 and caspase-8 and cleavage of PARP to elicit the cell apoptosis; (4) the suppression of STAT1 phosphorylation and COX-2, NF-κB, and IKK activities; (5) the reduction of iNOS expression; (6) the decline of MMP-2 activity by lessening MT1-MMP mRNA expression; and (7) the reduction of skin GSH quantity.[200–224]

Since the melanoma cells with mutant p53 normally showed a strong resistance to conventional chemotherapy, curcumin (**1**) was capable of providing potential avenues to overcome the chemoresistance for improving the type of melanoma treatment.[217] Importantly, curcumin (**1**) displayed remarkable inhibitory effects on the invasion and the lung metastasis caused by highly metastatic B16-F10 melanoma cells in mice. By the curcumin treatment, the lung metastatic tumor formation was repressed by 89.3% and the life span of mice bearing B16-F10 melanoma was prolonged by 143.9%,[225,226] whose antimetastatic property was found to be closely correlated with its abilities of (1) downregulation of focal adhesion kinase (FAK and MMP-2 activities, (2) reduction of α5β1 and αvβ3 integrin receptor expressions, (3) blockage of binding to extracellular matrix (ECM) proteins (such as fibronectin, vitronectin, and collagen-IV), (4) advancement of three antimetastatic protein expressions (included E-cad, nonmetastatic gene 23, and tissue inhibitor metalloproteinase-2), and (5) inhibition of PRL-3 oncogene.[226–229]

In addition, the *in vivo* tests also substantiated that curcumin, its derivatives (bisdemethoxycurcumin, tetra-hydrocurcumin, and salicyl curcumin), and C–HP-β-CD (a complex of curcumin and hydroxylpropyl-β-cyclodextrin) accomplished antiangiogenetic and antimetastatic effects via marked reduction of melanoma-directed capillaries and inhibition of serum NO and TNFα production.[229–231] When joined with DOX (an anticancer drug), the curcumin treatment showed the enhanced cytotoxic effect and the immune response in B16-R melanoma cells *in vitro* and *in vivo*, resulting in a significant increase of survival time.[225] The evidences demonstrated that curcumin (**1**) may have a potential to overcome the chemoresistance of melanoma cells and to promote the efficacy of clinical therapy against the melanoma.

Effect on Other Types of Carcinomas

Adenoid cystic cancer (ACC) is a highly malignant and aggressive neoplasm with weak response to currently available anticarcinoma drugs. Curcumin (**1**) was demonstrated to be a potent inhibitor of the ACC progression and a promoter of ACC cell apoptosis *in vitro* and *in vivo*, whose dose-dependent inhibition on ACC cell growth by curcumin was associated with dual inhibition by both NF-κB and mTOR pathways. Also, through the downregulation of VEGF and MMP-2 and MMP-9, curcumin (**1**) markedly attenuated the abilities of ACC cells to invade/migrate and angiogenesis. The findings provided promising evidences to support further clinical studies of curcumin (**1**) as a novel chemotherapeutic agent for ACC.[231]

Uterine leiomyosarcoma has an unfavorable response to chemotherapy, although rapamycin obviously restrained human SKN uterine leiomyosarcoma cells *in vitro*. The lack of PTEN protein, which generally causes AKT-mTOR activation, augments the leiomyosarcoma formation. By hindering the AKT-mTOR pathway, curcumin (**1**) at a high concentration obstructed the SKN cell growth and significantly promoted cell apoptosis, but no such effects were exerted by rapamycin.[232] The treatment with curcumin also effectively restrained the proliferation of osteosarcoma cells via the blockage of the Wnt/β-catenin pathway, i.e., reduction of both intrinsic and activated β-catenin/Tcf transcriptional activities. Moreover, curcumin (**1**) dose-dependently diminished the cell migration and the invasion of osteosarcoma and decreased the MMP-9 activity and its protein level.[233] With the treatment with 5 μmol/L curcumin (**1**) combined with Adm, a synergistic antineoplastic effect was achieved markedly against human HT1080 fibrosarcoma cells *in vitro*.[190]

Anticancer Immunity Activities

Besides the broad spectrum of inhibition against various cancer cells, curcumin (**1**) is also capable of activating the responses of immunotherapeutic cytokines that possess antitumor property. The administration of a low dose of curcumin (**1**) to mice bearing 3LL LLC once a day for 10 consecutive days obviously delayed the tumor growth and prolonged the survival period, whose effect was found to be partially contributed by T lymphocyte-mediated adaptive immune responses. Curcumin at a low dose augmented the T cells derived from the 3LL tumor-bearing mice, especially the amplified $CD8^+$ T cells could subsequently stimulate IFNγ secretion and cytotoxicity against the 3LL cells specifically.[233] With its conjunction with IL-2 therapy, the oral administration of curcumin to mouse model implanted with Meth-A ascites tumor markedly attenuated the IL-2 therapy-induced iNOS expression and NO production and enhanced the proliferation and the cytotoxicity of macrophages and lymphocytes, finally leading to the augmentation of the IL-2 therapy-induced survival prolongation of the tested mice. During the treatment, curcumin (**1**) also lessened the apoptosis of cocultured lymphocytes and macrophages.[234] Based upon the research results, the importance of the immunotherapeutic potential of curcumin (**1**) was evidenced in the treatment for anticancer and anticarcinogenesis.

Structure Alteration and Structural Biology

Due to the remarkable biological features in various aggressive and recurrent cancer models and negligible toxicity in normal cells, curcumin (**1**) has attracted great attentions in drug discovery and clinic oncology. The tremendous therapeutic potential made the agent a promising anticancer drug lead, but its clinic efficacy is poor due to its poor bioabsorption. Therefore, many scientists have targeted to develop more effective curcumin analogs with more bioavailability. The strategies of curcumin structural modification largely focused on altering the aryl substitution at the aromatic rings and amending the system of α,β-unsaturated 1,3-diketone for the improvement of its pharmacodynamic profile. The findings from the structural modifications and the biological evaluation have afforded several valuable curcumin derivatives that may have a translational potential for cancer chemotherapy and prevention and also promoted deeper understandings on the SAR of curcumin, which may be essential for further design and development of more effective drug candidates.

Modification in Aromatic Rings

According to SAR studies, a series of curcumin analogs was synthesized by the modification of aromatic rings in the curcumin. The results revealed that the dimethylation (such as **6**) of curcumin potentiated the antiandrogen activity and reduced dihydrotestosterone (DHT)-induced AR activity in wild-type AR^+ human PC3 prostate cancer cells and mutant-type AR^+ human DU-145 prostate cancer cells by 70% and 45%, respectively. Introducing two methoxycarbonylmethyl groups into the phenolic hydroxyls at C-4 of curcumin (such as **7**) markedly enhanced the anti-AR activity in a wild type of AR^+ DU-145 cells. But the monomethylation (such as **8**) and the monomethoxycarbonylmethylation (such as **9**) of curcumin at one benzene ring did not appear with such positive effect.[235] The studies further revealed that bis-(3,4-dimethoxyphenyl) moieties, conjugated β-diketone moiety, and intramolecular symmetry are the important factors related to the enlargement of antitumor and antiandrogenic activities of curcumin (**1**).[235]

A demethylated product (**10**) or a trimethylated product (**11**) of curcumin showed notably enhanced inhibitory effects against 1A9, KB, and HCT-8 cancer cell lines. Fluorination at the ortho position of both benzene rings without any other substitution showed a broad and amplified cytotoxic effect on many human neoplastic cell lines. When the introduction of a methoxy group into its meta position or the additional fluorination at the para position is done, the cytotoxic effect would be declined or abolished.[236] Glycosylation at its aromatic ring could elevate its water solubility, but the cytotoxicity toward cisplatin-sensitive human ovarian carcinoma 2008 cells and its cisplatin-resistant C13* cells would be reduced. But these curcumin derivatives showed greater kinetic stability and good selectivity since they are much less toxic. The combination with the most bioactive glycosylcurcuminoid (**12**) could improve the efficacy and the selectivity of cisplatin toward both ovarian carcinoma cells (2008 and C13*).[237] An analog (**13**) produced by the connection of sulfanate to 4-hydroxyl group in curcumin could augment the drug absorption, leading to improvement of the antiproliferative activity on four tumor cell lines (two prostate cancer cells, AI PC3 cells and AD LNCaP cells, and two breast carcinoma cells, estrogen-dependent MCF-7 cells and estrogen-independent MDA-MB-231 cells).[238] CDF, a diflourinated curcumin, which possesses antioxidant property, exerted obvious suppression on pancreatic cancer cell survival, clonogenicity, formation of pancreatospheres, and cell invasion and migration and also obstructed the pancreatic cancer stem cells (CSCs) function, in both *in vitro* and in an orthotopic xenograft models, whose effects were mainly associated with suppression of EZH2 expression and activation of a panel of tumor-suppressive micro-RNA expressions in the pancreatic cancer cells.[239]

Modification of β-Diketone (Keto-enol) System

The SAR analysis indicated that the diketone system is critical for the anticancer potency of curcumin. In an attempt to improve the pharmacodynamic profile of curcumin, its E,E-1,7-diarylhepta-1,6-diene-3,5-dione backbone was armed for modification to create a series of derivatives. The saturation of the olefinic bonds and the introduction of a methyl group to the double bond of enol form in curcumin would abolish or decrease the activity. However, if a group is brought such as ethoxycarbonylethyl or carbonyl acid, which can enhance the conjugation system to this site, the anti-AR effect of the products (**14** and **15**) was greatly amplified in the prostate cancer cells.[235] If a (4-hydroxy-3-methoxyphenyl) methylene moiety was introduced into a position between the β-diketone structure, the resulted derivative (**16**) markedly obstructed the proliferation of a variety of neoplastic cell lines such as K562, B16, HepG2, SW480, and SH-SY5Y.[240]

When the keto-enol moiety in curcumin was converted to a corresponding pyrazole (**17–19**), the cytotoxicity was enhanced but the antiandrogen potency was obviously attenuated. The derivative **19** also presented antiangiogenic activity.[235–238] If linking an N-methyl at the pyrazole ring (such as **20**), the antiproliferative activity would be reduced by threefold.[239] However, MR39 (**21**) and a benzyl oxime derivative (**22**) were derived by converting the keto-enol moiety to the corresponding isoxazole analogs, which exhibited the enhanced antitumor activity on hepatoma HA22T/VGH cells. Compared with curcumin (**1**), MR39 (**21**) exerted more potent antiproliferative effect on MCF-7 breast cancer cells and similar activity on multidrug-resistant MCF-7R cells and MDR HL-60 leukemia cells.[241,242]

For improving the absorption and the penetration through the cell membrane, a five-membered ring or a six-membered ring was introduced to the β-keto-enole system of curcumin to improve the lipophilicity and the rigidity. Among the two created series of analogs, three derivatives (**23–25**) displayed greater cytotoxicity to leukemic cell lines (L1210, Molt 4C/8, and CEM) and more cytotoxicity to eight other types of cancer cell lines (such as cancers of the skin, the non-small cell lung, the colon, the ovary, the kidney, the CNS, the prostate, and the breast). Exclusively, the derivative **23** demonstrated the best antitumor profile, whose potency was higher than curcumin (**1**) against all the neoplastic cell lines assayed.[243]

Simplification of β-Diketone System

Although the β-diketone system in curcumin is necessary for its antitumor and anticarcinogenetic properties, some investigations explored the simplification of E,E-1,7-diarylhepta-1,6-diene-3,5-dione in curcumin to 1,3-diaryl-1,3-diketo-propane-type derivatives. Two compounds **26** and **27** were demonstrated to have the significant cytotoxic effects against human 1A9 ovarian cancer cells with ED_{50} values of <0.25 and <0.63 μg/mL, respectively. FLLL-32 (**28**) was a curcumin analog made by the introduction of a cycle hexane located between the β-diketone. It specifically targeted the STAT3 signaling pathway to promote the apoptotic death of melanoma cells at a micromolar concentration with no adverse effect on the function or the viability of immune cells.[244] When the phenyl group was replaced with thiophenyl group, the afforded compound **29** still showed remarkable cytotoxicity against human osteogenic sarcoma (HOS) (bone) and 1A9 (ovary) cancer cell lines with ED_{50} values of <2.5 and 2.1 μg/mL, respectively. The compounds **27** and **29** were reported to have a broad spectrum of inhibitory effect on a variety of human tumor cell lines, including A549 (lung), MCF-7 (breast), HCT-8 (ileocecal), HOS (bone), PC3 (prostate), SK-MEL-2 (skin), U-87-MG (brain), KB (nasopharynx), and KB-VIN cells.[235,236]

The β-diketone structure in curcumin has been simplified to a group of monoketones to afford a series of 1,5-diaryl-3-oxo-1,4-pentadiene analogs. Some of these derivatives displayed potent antiproliferative activity against four human sexual organ cancer cell lines (PC3 and LNCaP prostate cancer cells and MCF-7 and MDA-MB-231 breast cancer cells) *in vitro* with IC_{50} values between 0.4 and 9.5 μM, whose potencies were 2–50 times superior than those of curcumin.[238] Derivatives **30–32** exhibited higher selectivity ratio on the mammary epithelial cancer cells than curcumin. Among them, **31** was the most potent derivative with the highest level of selectivity.[238] The derivatives **33–36**, especially compound **33**, displayed a higher degree of cytotoxicity in the NCI *in vitro* anticancer cell line screen and better effect in the antiangiogenesis assays.[245] Derivatives GO-Y016 (**37**), GO-Y030 (**38**), and GO-Y031 (**39**) inhibited the growth of cancer cells with a higher potency than 5-FU in the MDA-MB-231 breast cancer cell line and PANC-1, HPAC, and BXPC-3 pancreatic cancer cell lines and exerted the better effects than CPT-11 and cisplatin in some of the tumor cell lines.[246] By inhibiting STAT3 phosphorylation and its downstream target gene expression and inducing apoptosis, GO-Y030 (**37**) displayed an ability to lessen the viability and the tumorsphere formation in colon CSCs. The antigrowth activity of GO-Y030 (**37**) was also substantiated in the CSCs from both SW480 and HCT-116 colon cancer cell lines in mouse models.[247] GO-Y078 (**40**) showed the improved bioavailability and the most enhanced growth inhibition against the colorectal carcinoma cells *in vitro,* being superior to curcumin (**1**). In a mouse model with the colorectal cancer, GO-Y078 (**40**) demonstrated 1.4-fold more survival elongation that was not shown by GO-Y030 (**37**) and curcumin (**1**).[248]

Two derivatives, FLLL-11 (**41**) and FLLL-12 (**42**), exhibited more potent effect than curcumin in the inhibition of STAT3, AKT, and HER-2/neu pathways and the suppression of the cancer cell growth and migration in eight different prostate and breast neoplastic cell lines with IC_{50} values between 0.3 and 5.7 μmol/L.[249] GO-Y030 (**38**), FLLL-11 (**41**), and FLLL-12 (**42**) also exerted stronger antigrowth effect at a concentration much lower than curcumin in three human colorectal cancer cell lines (SW480, HT-29, and HCT116), and the IC_{50} values ranged between 0.51 and 4.48 μM.[250] The treatment with GL63 (**43**) dose-dependently retarded the proliferation of HepG2 hepatoma cells and promoted the apoptosis at a 20 μM concentration, showing more potential than curcumin (**1**) because GL63 was able to induce the ER stress response and to upregulate CHOP, XBP-1, ATF-4, and GRP78 expressions, but curcumin had no effect on the ER stress.[251] Another ER stress-inducer assigned as (1E,4E)-1,5-bis(2,3-dimethoxy-phenyl)penta-1,4-dien-3-one (**44**) could dose-responsively augment the apoptosis of H460 lung carcinoma cells in association with the ER stress-mediated apoptosis pathway and caspase activation. *In vivo*, (1E,4E)-1,5-bis(2,3-dimethoxy-phenyl)penta-1,4-dien-3-one (**44**) displayed a dramatic 53.5% reduction in H460 xenograft tumor size after 22 days of treatment.[252] These results corroborated that the structural modification at the symmetrical α,β-unsaturated ketone of curcumin is one of the resourceful routes for the augmentation of the anticancer and antiangiogenesis potencies.

Creation of Center Cycloketones

When the pentadienone moiety in curcumin was modified to have a cyclohexanone or a cyclopentanone in the center, another group of analogs was produced. PGV-0 (**45**) and its geometric isomer PGV-1 (**46**) could perform better cytotoxic effect against T47D breast cancer cells with IC_{50} values of ≤3.16 and 9.39 μM, respectively, whose potency was more effective than that of curcumin (IC_{50}: 19.05 μM). The treatment of the breast cancer cells with 5 μM of PGV-1 (**46**) exerted the antiangiogenic effect through the reduction of VEGF and COX-2 expressions.[253,254] A tetrahydropyran analog (**47**) has a marked ability for binding to nuclear type II sites on breast cancer cells with high affinity to obstruct cell proliferation, and it was also effective against leukemia and prostate cancer cells (GI_{50}: <1.0 μM).[245] Compound **48** has a broad spectrum of inhibitory activity against the viability of cancer cells and angiogenesis. In RPMI-8226 leukemia cells and RXF-393 renal cancer cells, **48** exhibited remarkable suppressive effects with GI_{50} values of 0.6 and 0.5 μM, respectively.[245] When a phenyl group was linked to 4-position of the cyclohexanone, the two created analogs **49** and **50** displayed significant cytotoxicity toward B16 and L1210 murine cancer cell lines, and the IC_{50} values were 1.6 and 0.51 μM in B16 melanoma cells and 0.35 and 1.2 μM in L1210 leukemia cells, respectively.[255]

Synthesis of Center Heterocycloketons

The derivatives (**51–54**) with tetrahydropyran or piperidine were obtained by introducing a heteroatom into the cyclohexanone. Their antitumor and antiangiogenesis effects were improved compared to the derivatives without cyclohexanone. The ortho-fluoro-substituted piperidone analog (**54**) was the most active one among them in the NCI anticancer cell line screen and NCI antiangiogenesis assays. The GI_{50} values for **54** was 0.7 μM, which was 13.6- and 10.4-fold better than cisplatin (GI_{50}: 9.5) and curcumin (GI_{50}: 7.3), respectively, against cancer types such as leukemia, colon, CNS, prostate, and breast cancers. The suppressive effect of **54** on the angiogenesis was almost as potent as an antiangiogenic drug TNP-470, which is undergoing in clinical trials. Furthermore, **54** showed no *in vivo* toxicity on the liver, the kidney, and the spleen, being much safer than cisplatin. Due to its greater activity plus lower toxicity, **54** can be considered as a promising chemotherapeutic agent leading to clinical development. Bioassays also revealed that derivatives **51**, **54**, as well as **48** were potent inhibitors against cord formation and tumor cell migration.[245]

Another well-studied curcumin derivative with piperidine in the pentadienone moiety was EF24 (**55**), which significantly promoted cell cycle arrest and apoptosis of human MDA-MB-231 (breast), DU-145 (prostate), SKOV-3, and IGROV1 (ovary) neoplastic cell lines. By inhibiting NF-κB signaling pathway and HIF-1α posttranscription, EF24 (**55**) disturbed the microtubule cytoskeleton of PC3 prostate cancer cells and MDA-MB-231 breast cancer cells. The anticarcinoma activity was further confirmed in a mouse xenograft model with human breast carcinoma at a dose much less than curcumin.[256–259] When EF24 (**55**) was conjugated to fVIIa (a transmembrane receptor) through a tripeptide-chloromethyl ketone, the formed complex displayed greater activities in arresting the MDA-MB-231 cells and RPMI-7951 melanoma cells than EF24 alone and in reducing tumor size and toxic side effects in athymic nude mice bearing human cancer xenografts. Also, the remarkable efficacy also proved EF24 (**55**) to be useful for treating drug-resistant tumors and micrometastases in addition to inhibiting the primary tumors.[260,261] PAC (**56**), a derivative with N-methyl substitution at the piperidine, was five times more efficient than curcumin in the breast cancer cell apoptosis induction via an internal mitochondrial route, whose effect was 10-fold higher against estrogen receptor$^-$ breast cancer cells (MDA-MB231 and BEC114) than against estrogen receptor$^+$ breast cancer cells (MCF-7 and T-47D), but the ectopic expression of ERα-rendered estrogen receptor$^-$ breast cancer cells was more resistant to PAC (**56**). Besides markedly reducing the tumor size and triggering the apoptosis *in vivo*, PAC (**56**) also demonstrated higher stability in the blood and greater biodistribution and bioavailability in nude mice.[262] A fluorinated analog labeled as HO-3867 (**57**) exhibited substantial cytotoxicity to all the tumor cells tested *in vitro* and exerted dose-dependent inhibition of tumor growth in nude mice bearing xenografts with human A2780 ovarian carcinoma cells, where HO-3867 (**57**) demonstrated 100-fold higher cellular uptake and bioabsorption compared to curcumin (**1**).[263]

Formulation Studies

Despite curcumin (**1**) having the broad spectrum of chemopreventive, anticarcinoma, radio- and chemosensibilizing activities, the poor systemic bioavailability such as low solubility and high metabolic instability in both plasma and tissues limited the therapeutic efficacy of curcumin in the clinical treatment of oncology. In order to improve the great therapeutic interest, the clinical potential of curcumin (**1**) has been extensively approached by using adjuvant and delivery vehicles in the formulation studies.

Microparticles

Some effective vehicles were selected for the localized delivery of curcumin over sustained periods of time to elevate the bioavailabilty. Poly(D-,L-lactide-co-glycolide), a biodegradable and biocompatible polymer, was used to formulate the curcumin microparticles, which could accumulate the curcumin levels in the lungs, the brain, and the frequent sites of breast cancer metastases by 10- to 30-fold in the blood and some tissues, showing marked anticancer efficacy in nude mice with MDA-MB-231 xenografts. The curcumin microparticles were also able to noticeably suppress the tumor angiogenesis via the decrease of VEGF expression.[264] Likewise, an encapsulation of curcumin was developed as injectable agents by using the self-assembling β-hairpin hydrogels as the drug delivery vehicle, whose formulation can effectively localize curcumin delivery over sustained periods.[265]

In addition, a liposomal formulation of turmeric oil was prepared by covalently conjugating insulin to the terminal of the PEG chain of sterically stabilized liposomes. The fabricated liposomes (ISSLs) of turmeric oil specially targeted the insulin receptor, demonstrating its potential for the treatment of insulin receptor-positive human SMMC-7721 hepatoma with overexpressing insulin receptors.[266]

Nanocapsules

In recent years, the techniques for formulating biodegradable nanoparticulates have been employed to encapsulate curcumin. The constructed nanoparticles can release active curcumin (**1**) in an effective intracellular environment, exhibiting greatly improved bioavailability with very rapid and more efficient cellular uptake. Curc–OEG nanoparticles, which were formed by the conjugation of curcumin with two short oligo (ethylene glycol) chains through β-thioester bonds, are an intracellular labile amphiphilic surfactant-like curcumin prodrug. Besides displaying high suppressive ability to several cancer cells *in vitro*, the Curc–OEG nanoparticles by intravenous injection significantly lessened the growth of MDA-MB-468 breast tumor and SKOV-3 ovarian tumor in nude mice xenograft without acute and subchronic toxicities to the mouse's visceral organs even at high doses.[267] Curcumin-loaded transferrin-mediated solid lipid nanoparticles (SLNs) were prepared, which could enhance the cytotoxicity, the ROS level, and the cell uptake in the MCF-7 breast cancer cells *in vitro*.[268] By using poly(lactide-co-glycolide) and a stabilizer PEG-5000, curcumin was encapsulated in a nanoparticulate formulation. The formed curcumin-loaded poly(lactic-co-glycolic acid) (PLGA) nanoparticles showed to be as potent as or more potent than curcumin in suppressing the proliferation of various neoplastic cells and eliciting the apoptosis of leukemic cells *in vitro* and more bioavailability *in vivo*. Also, it was more active than curcumin in inhibiting TNF-induced NF-κB activation and in suppressing NF-κB-regulated proteins involved in cell proliferation (cyclin-D1), invasion, (MMP-9) and angiogenesis (VEGF).[269]

Following the extensive utilization of nanotechnology, more and more curcumin nanoformulations have been reported. The curcumin-loaded chitosan/poly(butyl cyanoacrylate) nanoparticles and curcumin-loaded human serum albumin nanoparticles exhibited greater therapeutic effects in the growth inhibition of HCT116 colon cancer cells *in vitro* and the angiogenesis suppression in hepatocellular carcinoma *in vivo*. The potent antitumor activity was clearly attributed to the enhanced water solubility, the increased accumulation in tumors, and an ability to traverse vascular endothelial cells.[270,271] Moreover, a group of curcumin—PVP nanoparticles was fabricated by using a simple technique of nanoprecipitation with polyvinyl-pyrrolidone (PVP) as the hydrophilic carrier, which significantly enhanced the antigrowth and antioxidant effects of curcumin (**1**) against human hepatoma cells (HepG2, Hep3B, and PLC/PRF/5).[272] The cytotoxicity and the antioxidant activity of curcumin to K562 human leukemia cells were amplified in the treatment with the created β-casein–curcumin micelles.[273] The marked suppressive efficacy on human carcinoma of the colon, the breast, and the pancreas was notably achieved by the administration of curcumin–rubusoside nanoparticle.[274] The evidences established that the curcumin nanoformulation is one of the promising techniques to promote the potential of curcumin in clinics that merits further investigation. In recent years, nanotechnology has been extensively used for the development of new types of nanocurcumines, such as curcumin-loaded lipopolysaccharide nanocarriers, curcumin-entrapped folic acid-conjugated PLGA-PEG nanoparticles, curcumin-loaded PEGylated PLGA nanocapsules, PLGA curcumin nanoparticles, chitosan-coated curcumin nanoparticles, curcumin-loaded pH-sensitive O-carboxymethyl chitosan/fucoidan nanoparticles, dendrosomal curcumin nanoformulation, and PEG-cyclodextrin-coated curcumin-loaded zinc ferrite core nanocomposites.[275–283] All these achievements show a potential delivery strategy to improve the oral bioavailability and the anticancer efficacy of curcumin in the cancer treatment.

Conjugated Complexes

A group of backbone-type of polymer–curcumin conjugates (polycurcumins) was formulated by the condensation and the polymerization of curcumin. These polycurcumins display advantages of the tailored water solubility, high drug-loading efficiency, and fixed drug-loading contents. In the *in vitro* assays, the polycurcumins demonstrated many potential applications for their cytotoxicity to various cancer cells. A polyacetal-based polycurcumin (PCurc-8) was highly cytotoxic to human SKOV-3 and OVCAR-3 ovarian cancer cells and human MCF-7 breast cancer cells, associated with the promotion of cell cycle arrest and apoptosis. *In vivo* by intravenous injection, PCurc-8 exerted a remarkable antitumor activity against the SKOV-3 xenograft in nude mice model.[284] Also, three conjugates were synthesized by inserting succinic acid, glutaric acid, and methylcarboxylic acid as the respective spacers between curcumin and monomethoxy polyethylene glycol (m.w. 2000), to fabricate mPEG2000–succinyl–curcumin, mPEG 2000–glutaryl–curcumin, and mPEG2000–methylcarboxyl–curcumin, respectively. The cytotoxic effects of these conjugates were proven in human NCI-H187 (lung), Caco-2 (colon), MCF-7 (breast), and KB (oral cavity) cancer cell lines. The IC_{50} values were in the range of 1–6 μM, similar to the free curcumin, but these mono-PEGylated conjugates of curcumin were stable at physiological pH and curcumin release readily in human plasma.[285] Curcumin conjugated with a biodegradable polymer poly(lactic-co-glycolic acid) efficiently obstructed the proliferation and the survival of human HCT 116 colon carcinoma cells as compared to native curcumin.[286] Similar to nanoformulation, the approaches could be a promising strategy to improve the therapeutic index of cancer therapy.

Metal Complexes

A Zn(II)–curcumin complex was reported to be more potent in the antisarcoma activity as compared to their parent curcumin.[287] 1,7-Dianthryl-1,6-heptadiene-3,5-dione (A), 1,7-bis(2-hydroxylnaphthyl)-1,6-heptadiene-3,5-dione (B), 1,7-bis(4-me thoxyphenyl)-1,6-heptadiene-3,5-dione, and 1,7-bis(4-hydroxy-3-methoxyphenyl)-1,6-heptadiene-3,5-dione, four curcuminoid analogs, were used to link with aluminum (III) to form their corresponding aluminum chelates. All the produced complexes were remarkably cytotoxic to murine EACs and mouse L929 fibroblast cells compared to the free curcuminoid analogs. The concentrations needed for 50% cell death were ~4 μg/mL for the aluminum (III)–curcumin complexes but 10 μg/mL for the earlier curcuminoid analogs, implying that the aluminum chelates more potently reduce the tumor volume in mice. The aluminum complex B with hydroxyl group in the naphthyl ring was the most active toward the L929 cells (1 μg/mL produced 62.5% cell death), while the chelate A, which is the unsubstituted molecule, was the least active toward the life span extension in tumor-bearing mice for 29.5%.[288]

Other Bioactivities

From ancient China, Jiang Huang (Turmeric) has been used in the treatment of indigestion, hepatitis, atherosclerosis, diabetes, jaundice, and bacterial infections. Jiang Huang and its major ingredient curcuminoids have been proven to possess a myriad of therapeutic potencies ranging from antioxidant, antiinflammatory, antihepatotoxic, neuroprotective, hypolipidemic, anticoagulant, antidepressant, antispasmodic, antiparasitic, nematocidal, carminative, antifertility, antimicrobial activities, and many more. Curcumin (**1**) is also HIV-1 and HIV-2 protease inhibitors. The daily oral administration of 10 g of curcumin showed no evidence of toxicity in patients.

References

1. Kuo, M. L. et al. 1996. Curcumin, an antioxidant and antitumor promoter, induces apoptosis in human leukemia cells. *Biochim. et Biophys. Acta, Molecular Basis of Disease* 1317: 95–100.
2. Chen, Y. et al. 2004. Effects of curcumin on proliferation of NB4 cells and acetylation of histone H3 and p53. *Chin. J. Cancer Res.* 16: 256–9.
3. Chen, W. H. et al. 2004. Effect of curcumin on STAT5 signaling pathway in primary CML cells. *Zhongguo Shiyan Xueyexue Zazhi* 12: 572–6.
4. Duvoix, A. et al. 2003. Curcumin-induced cell death in two leukemia cell lines: K562 and Jurkat. *Annals New York Academy Sci.* 1010(Apoptosis), pp. 389–92.
5. Chakraborty, S. et al. 2006. Inhibition of telomerase activity and induction of apoptosis by curcumin in K562 cells. *Mutation Res.* 596: 81–90.
6. Xu, J. H. et al. 1998. Antitumor effects of curcumin on human tumor cell lines in vitro and stability of curcumin in water solution. *Zhongguo Yaolixue Tongbao* 14: 415–7.
7. Wu, Y. et al. 2002. Anticancer activities of curcumin on human Burkitt's lymphoma. *Zhonghua Zhongliu Zazhi* 24: 348–51.
8. Zhang, J. Q. et al. 2003. Effect of curcumin on proliferation and apoptosis of TK6 cells. *Acta Nutr. Sinica* 25: 268–71
9. Bielak-Zmijewska, A. et al. 2004. P-glycoprotein expression does not change the apoptotic pathway induced by curcumin in HL-60 cells. *Cancer Chemother. Pharmacol.* 53: 179–85.
10. Indap, M. A. et al. 2006. Inhibitory effect of cinnamoyl compounds against human malignant cell line. *Ind. J. Experim. Biol.* 44: 216–20.
11. Park, C. et al. 2007. Induction of apoptosis by curcumin in human leukemic U937 cells through activation of caspases and upregulation of Fas/FasL expression. *Kor. J. Genetics* 29: 177–84.
12. Tomita, M. et al. 2006. Curcumin suppresses constitutive activation of AP-1 by downregulation of JunD protein in HTLV-1-infected T-cell lines. *Leukemia Res.* 30: 313–21.
13. Angelo, L. S. et al. 2009. Turmeric and green tea: A recipe for the treatment of B-chronic lymphocytic leukemia. *Clin. Cancer Res.* 15: 1123–5.
14. Lee, Y. K. et al. 2009. Activation of apoptotic protein in U937 cells by a component of turmeric oil. *BMB Reports* 42: 96–100.
15. Choi, B. H. et al. 2008. Curcumin down-regulates the multidrug-resistance mdrlb gene by inhibiting the PI3K/Akt/NF-κB pathway. *Cancer Lett.* 259: 111–8.
16. Ji, M. J. et al. 2004. Induction of apoptosis by ar-turmerone on various cell lines. *Intl. J. Mol. Med.* 14: 253–6.
17. Lu, J. J. et al. 2012. The short-time treatment with curcumin sufficiently decreases cell viability, induces apoptosis and copper enhances these effects in multidrug-resistant K562/A02 cells. *Mol. Cell. Biochem.* 360: 253–60.
18. Gaurtam, S. C. et al. 1998. Nonselective inhibition of proliferation of transformed and nontransformed cells by the anticancer agent curcumin (Diferuloylmethane). *Biochem. Pharmacol.* 55: 1333–7.
19. Zhang, P. et al. 2005. Study on anticancer activities of curcumin in HL-60 cells in vitro and in vivo. *Zhongguo Yaoxue Zazhi* 40: 347–9.
20. Chen, J. et al. 2006. Trichostatin A improves the anticancer activity of low concentrations of curcumin in human leukemia cells. *Pharmazie* 61: 710–6.
21. Anuchapreeda, S. et al. 2008. Effect of pure curcumin, demethoxycurcumin, and bisde-methoxycurcumin on WT1 gene expression in leukemic cell lines. *Cancer Chemother. Pharmacol.* 62: 585–94.
22. Han, S. S. et al. 2002. Curcumin suppresses activation of NF-κB and AP-1 induced by phorbol ester in cultured human promyelocytic leukemia cells. *J. Biochem. Mol. Biol.* 35: 337–42.
23. Chuang, S. E. et al. 2002. Basal levels and patterns of anticancer drug-induced activation of nuclear factor-κB (NF-κB), and its attenuation by tamoxifen, dexamethasone, and curcumin in carcinoma cells. *Biochem. Pharmacol.* 63: 1709–16.
24. Surh, Y. J. et al. 2000. Inhibitory effects of curcumin and capsaicin on phorbol ester-induced activation of eukaryotic transcription factors, NF-κB and AP-1. *BioFactors* 12: 107–12.

25. Chen, J. et al. 2010. Curcumin p38-dependently enhances the anticancer activity of valproic acid in human leukemia cells. *Eur. J. Pharm. Sci.* 41: 210–18.
26. Duvoix, A. et al. 2003. Induction of apoptosis by curcumin: Mediation by glutathione S-transferase P1–1 inhibition. *Biochem. Pharmacol.* 66: 1475–83.
27. Semsri, S. et al. 2011. Pure curcumin inhibits exogenous Wilms' tumor (WT1) (+/+) isoform protein via degradation pathway and protein kinase C in transfected U937 cells. *African J. Pharmacy and Pharmacol.* 5: 1846–56.
28. Rao, J. et al. 2011. Curcumin reduces expression of Bcl-2, leading to apoptosis in daunorubicin-insensitive $CD34^+$ acute myeloid leukemia cell lines and primary sorted $CD34^+$ acute myeloid leukemia cells. *J. Translat. Med.* 9: 71.
29. Paek, S. Y. et al. 1996. Ar-turmerone and β-atlantone induce internucleosomal DNA fragmentation associated with programmed cell death in human myeloid leukemia HL-60 cells. *Archev. Pharm. Res.* 19: 91–4.
30. Aratanechemuge, Y. et al. 2002. Selective induction of apoptosis by ar-turmerone isolated from turmeric (*Curcuma longa* L) in two human leukemia cell lines, but not in human stomach cancer cell line. *Intl. J. Mol. Med.* 9: 481–4.
31. Koo, J. Y. et al. 2004. Curcumin inhibits the growth of AGS human gastric carcinoma cells in vitro and shows synergism with 5-fluorouracil. *J. Med. Food* 7: 117–21.
32. Zheng, X. Z. et al. 2008. Anti-invasion and anti-metastasis effect of curcumin on human gastric carcinoma SGC-7901 cells. *Zhongguo Yaoshi* 11: 1183–4.
33. Mizushina, Y. et al. 2003. Some anti-chronic inflammatory compounds are DNA polymerase lambda-specific inhibitors. *Biochem. Pharmacol.* 66: 1935–44.
34. Cui, S. X. et al. 2002. Study on antitumor effect of curcumin. *Zhongliu Fangzhi Zazhi* 9: 50–2.
35. Tang, X. Q. et al. 2005. Effect of curcumin on multidrug resistance in resistant human gastric carcinoma cell line SGC7901/VCR. *Acta Pharmacol Sin.* 26: 1009–16.
36. Wei, S. C. et al. 2004. Comparison of the anti-proliferation and apoptosis-induction activities of sulindac, celecoxib, curcumin, and nifedipine in mismatch repair-deficient cell lines. *J. Formosan Med. Assoc.* 103: 599–606.
37. Rashmi, R. et al. 2005. Human colon cancer cells lacking Bax resist curcumin-induced apoptosis and Bax requirement is dispensable with ectopic expression of Smac or downregulation of Bcl-XL. *Carcinogenesis* 26: 713–23.
38. Chen, H. et al. Study on anticancer role of curcumin in human colon carcinoma cell line. *Zhongliu Yanjiu Yu Linchuang* 18: 4–7.
39. Van Erk, M. J. et al. 2004. Time- and dose-dependent effects of curcumin on gene expression in human colon cancer cells. *J. Carcinogenesis* 3: 8.
40. Goel, A. et al. 2001. Specific inhibition of cyclooxygenase-2 (COX-2) expression by dietary curcumin in HT-29 human colon cancer cells. *Cancer Lett.* 172: 111–118.
41. Song, G. et al. 2005. Curcumin induces human HT-29 colon adenocarcinoma cell apoptosis by activating p53 and regulating apoptosis-related protein expression. *Braz. J. Med. Biol. Res.* 38: 1791–8.
42. Choi, O. S. et al. 2004. Effects of curcumin of apoptosis in SW480 human colon cancer cell line. *Hanguk Yongyang Hakhoechi* 37: 31–7.
43. Scott, D. W. et al. 2004. Curcumin-induced GADD153 gene up-regulation in human colon cancer cells. *Carcinogenesis* 25: 2155–64.
44. Watson, J. L. et al. 2008. Curcumin induces apoptosis in HCT-116 human colon cancer cells in a p21-independent manner. *Experim. Mol. Pathol.* 84: 230–3.
45. Lu, J. J. et al. 2011. Curcumin induces DNA damage and caffeine-insensitive cell cycle arrest in colorectal carcinoma HCT116 cells. *Mol. Cell. Biochem.* 354: 247–52.
46. Su, C. C. et al. 2006. Curcumin inhibits cell migration of human colon cancer colo 205 cells through the inhibition of NF-κB/p65 and down-regulates cyclooxygenase-2 and matrix metalloproteinase-2 expressions. *Anticancer Res.* 26: 1281–8.
47. Chen, A. P. et al. 2006. Curcumin inhibits human colon cancer cell growth by suppressing gene expression of epidermal growth factor receptor through reducing the activity of the transcription factor Egr-1. *Oncogene* 25: 278–87.
48. Chen, A. P. et al. 2005. Activation of PPAR-γ by curcumin inhibits Moser cell growth and mediates suppression of gene expression of cyclin D1 and EGFR. *Am. J. Physiol.* 288(3, Pt. 1): G447-G456.
49. Kunnumakkara, A. B. et al. 2008. Curcumin sensitizes human colorectal cancer xenografts in nude mice to γ-radiation by targeting NF-κB-regulated gene products. *Clin. Cancer Res.* 14: 2128–36.
50. Cui, S. X. et al. 2006. Curcumin inhibits telomerase activity in human cancer cell lines. *Intl. J. Mol. Med.* 18: 227–31.
51. Zhou, H. K. et al. 2006. Effects of curcumin on telomerase activity and on proliferation of human hepG2 cells. *Zhongguo Xiandai Yixue Zazhi* 16: 3525–8, 3533.
52. Shan, L. J. et al. 2009. Apoptosis of liver cancer SMMC7721 cell line induced by curcumin. *J. Dalian Med. Univ.* 31: 142–4.
53. Kao, H. H. et al. 2011. Kinase gene expression and subcellular protein expression pattern of protein kinase C isoforms in curcumin-treated human hepatocellular carcinoma Hep 3B cells. *Plant Foods for Human Nutr.* 66: 136–42.
54. Wang, W. Z. et al. 2010. Anticancer activities of curcumin on human hepatocarcinoma cell line sk-hep-1. *Zhongguo Zhongyao Zazhi* 35: 485–8.
55. Sun, J. et al. 2008. The expression of VEGF and HIF-1α protein by curcumin in human hepatocellular carcinoma BEL-7402 cells through PI3K/AKT/FRAP signal transduction pathway. *Zhongguo Yishi Zazhi* 10: 41–4.
56. Hou, W. et al. 2008. Effect of curcumin on vascular endothelial growth factor expression in HepG2 hepatocellular carcinoma cells under hypoxic conditions. *Shijie Huaren Xiaohua Zazhi* 16: 2234–8.
57. Hou, W. et al. 2008. Effect of curcumin on hypoxia-inducible factor-1α expression in hepatocellular carcinoma cells HepG2 under hypoxia and its possible mechanism. *Shijie Huaren Xiaohua Zazhi* 16: 2354–8.
58. Wang, S. J. et al. 2011. Curcumin inhibits the migration and invasion of mouse hepatoma Hca-F cells through down-regulating caveolin-1 expression and epidermal growth factor receptor signaling. *IUBMB Life* 63: 775–82.
59. Wei, M. et al. 2008. Reversion of drug resistance in a hepatocellular carcinoma by curcumin in vitro. *Zhongguo Xiandai Yixue Zazhi* 18: 2441–3, 2448.

60. Huang, A. C. et al. 2008. Effects of curcumin on N-bis(2-Hydroxypropyl) nitrosamine (DHPN)-induced lung and liver tumorigenesis in BALB/c mice in vivo. *In Vivo* 22: 781–6.
61. Farombi, E. et al. 2008. Curcumin attenuates dimethylnitrosamine-induced liver injury in rats through Nrf2-mediated induction of heme oxygenase-1. *Food Chem. Toxicol.* 46: 1279–87.
62. Suphim, B. L. et al. 2010. Redox modulation and human bile duct cancer inhibition by curcumin. *Food Chem. Toxicol.* 48: 2265–72.
63. Kunnumakkara, A. B. et al. 2007. Curcumin potentiates antitumor activity of gemcitabine in an orthotopic model of pancreatic cancer through suppression of proliferation, angiogenesis, and inhibition of nuclear factor-κB-regulated gene products. *Cancer Res.* 67: 3853–61.
64. Gong, A. et al. 2004. Inhibitory effect of curcumin on pancreatic carcinoma cell line and possible mechanisms. *Yi Xian Bing Xue* 4: 218–22.
65. Hidaka, H. et al. 2002. Curcumin inhibits interleukin 8 production and enhances interleukin 8 receptor expression on the cell surface impact on human pancreatic carcinoma cell growth by autocrine regulation. *Cancer* 95: 1206–14.
66. Xu, W. M. et al. 2008. Effects of curcumin on cell cycle of pancreatic carcinoma cells in vitro. *Zhongguo Redai Yixue* 8: 2115–6.
67. Sahu, R. P. et al. 2009. Activation of ATM/Chk1 by curcumin causes cell cycle arrest and apoptosis in human pancreatic cancer cells. *British J. Cancer* 100. 1425–33.
68. Li, L. et al. 2004. Nuclear factor-κB and IκB kinase are constitutively active in human pancreatic cells, and their down-regulation by curcumin (diferuloylmethane) is associated with the suppression of proliferation and the induction of apoptosis. *Cancer* 19: 127.
69. Ramachandran, C. et al. 2010. Potentiation of gemcitabine by Turmeric Force in pancreatic cancer cell lines. *Oncol. Reports* 23: 1529–35.
70. Shahar, L. A. et al. 2007. Curcumin augments gemcitabine cytotoxic effect on pancreatic adeno-carcinoma cell lines. *Cancer Investigation* 25: 411–8.
71. Duan, H. et al. 2004. Interaction between curcumin and genistein on human pancreatic carcinoma cell line BXPC-3. *Shiyong Zhongliu Zazhi* 19: 127–9.
72. Swamy, M. V. et al. 2008. Prevention and treatment of pancreatic cancer by curcumin in combination with omega-3 fatty acids. *Nutr. Cancer* 60(Suppl. 1): 81–9.
73. Glienke, W. et al. 2009. Wilms' tumour gene 1 (WT1) as a target in curcumin treatment of pancreatic cancer cells. *Eur. J. Cancer* 45: 874–80.
74. Mach, C. M. et al. 2009. Determination of minimum effective dose and optimal dosing schedule for liposomal curcumin in a xenograft human pancreatic cancer model. *Anticancer Res.* 29: 1895–900.
75. Radhakrishna, P. G. et al. 2004. Induction of apoptosis in human lung cancer cells by curcumin. *Cancer Lett.* 208: 163–70.
76. Li, H. et al. 2008. Curcumin protects against cytotoxic and inflammatory effects of quartz particles but causes oxidative DNA damage in a rat lung epithelial cell line. *Toxicol. & Applied Pharmacol.* 227: 115–24.
77. Yue, X. et al. 2008. Curcumin inhibits proliferation of lung cancer cell A549 through Wnt signaling pathway. *J. Chongqing Med. Univ.* 33: 1454–7.
78. Chen, L. X. et al. 2010. Curcumin modulates eukaryotic initiation factors in human lung adenocarcinoma epithelial cells. *Mol. Biol. Reports* 37: 3105–10.
79. Zheng, W. et al. 2008. Effects of curcumin in inhibiting proliferation and inducing apoptosis in human lung cancer cells. *Zhongguo Yike Daxue Xuebao* 37: 607–10.
80. Saha, A. et al. 2010. Apoptosis of human lung cancer cells by curcumin mediated through up-regulation of growth arrest and DNA damage inducible genes 45 and 153. *Biol. Pharm. Bull.* 33: 1291–9.
81. Sen, S. et al. 2005. Curcumin enhances vinorelbine mediated apoptosis in NSCLC cells by the mitochondrial pathway. *Biochem. Biophys. Res. Commun.* 331: 1245–52.
82. Chanvorachote, P. et al. 2009. Curcumin sensitizes lung cancer cells to cisplatin-induced apoptosis through superoxide anion-mediated Bcl-2 degradation. *Cancer Investigation* 27: 624–35.
83. Tsai, M. S. et al. 2011. Synergistic effect of curcumin and cisplatin via down-regulation of thymidine phosphorylase and excision repair cross-complementary 1 (ERCC1). *Mol. Pharmacol.* 80: 136–46.
84. Chen, H. W. et al. Curcumin inhibits lung cancer cell invasion and metastasis through the tumor suppressor HLJ1. *Cancer Res.* 68: 7428–38.
85. Chen, H. W. et al. 2004. Anti-invasive gene expression profile of curcumin in lung adenocarcinoma based on a high throughput microarray analysis. *Mol. Pharmacol.* 65: 99–10.
86. Cao, H. et al. 2008. Effects of curcumin combined with cisplatin on the proliferation and apoptosis of human lung cancer cell line A549 in vitro. *J. Wuhan Univ.* (*Sci. Edition*), 29: 213–7.
87. Chen, X. X. et al. 2007. Effect of curcumin on proliferation of human lung adenocarcinoma cell line A549/DDP. *Disi Junyi Daxue Xuebao* 28: 2287–90.
88. Huang, A. C. et al. 2008. Effects of curcumin on N-bis(2-Hydroxypropyl) nitrosamine (DHPN)-induced lung and liver tumorigenesis in BALB/c mice in vivo. *In Vivo* 22: 781–6.
89. Dorie, T. et al. 2000. Therapeutic potential of curcumin in human prostate cancer. II. Curcumin inhibits tyrosine kinase activity of epidermal growth factor receptor and depletes the protein. *Mol. Urol.* 4: 1–6.
90. Nakamura, K. et al. 2002. Curcumin down-regulates AR gene expression and activation in prostate cancer cell lines. *Intl. J. Oncol.* 21: 825–30.
91. Chaudhary, L. R. et al. 2003. Inhibition of cell survival signal protein kinase B/Akt by curcumin in human prostate cancer cells. *J. Cell. Biochem.* 89: 1–5.
92. Yang, L. et al. 2006. The effect of curcumin on proliferation and apoptosis in LNCaP prostate cancer cells. *Chin. J. Clin. Oncol.* 3: 55–60.
93. Guo, H. et al. 2006. Curcumin-induced apoptosis in androgen-dependent prostate cancer cell line LNCaP in vitro. *Zhonghua Nankexue Zazhi* 12: 141–4.
94. Shankar, S. et al. 2007. Involvement of Bcl-2 family members, phosphatidylinositol 3′-kinase/AKT and mitochondrial p53 in curcumin (diferulolylmethane)-induced apoptosis in prostate cancer. *Intl. J. Oncol.* 30: 905–18.

95. Deeb, D. et al. 2004. Curcumin sensitizes prostate cancer cells to tumor necrosis factor-related apoptosis-inducing ligand/Apo2L by inhibiting nuclear factor-κB through suppression of IκBα phosphorylation. *Mol. Cancer Therap.* 3: 803–12.
96. Dorai, T. et al. 2001. Therapeutic potential of curcumin in human prostate cancer: III. Curcumin inhibits proliferation, induces apoptosis, and inhibits angiogenesis of LNCaP prostate cancer cells in vivo. *Prostate* 7: 293–303.
97. Deng, G. et al. 2008. Curcumin inhibits the expression of vascular endothelial growth factor and androgen-independent prostate cancer cell line PC3 in vitro. *Zhonghua Nankexue Zazhi* 14: 116–21.
98. Li, M. et al. 2007. Curcumin, a dietary component, has anticancer, chemosensitization, and radio-sensitization effects by down-regulating the MDM2 oncogene through the PI3K/mTOR/ETS2 pathway. *Cancer Res.* 67: 1988–96.
99. Chen, Q. H. 2015. Curcumin-based anti-prostate cancer agents. *Anti-Cancer Agents in Med. Chem.* 15: 138–56.
100. Deng, G. et al. 2007. Effect of curcumin on the expression and distribution of Notch1 in androgen independent prostate cancer cell line PC3 in vitro. *Huazhong Keji Daxue Xuebao, Yixueban* 36: 740–3, 847.
101. Deng, G. et al. 2008. Effects of curcumin on Notch signaling pathway in androgen-independent prostate cancer cell line PC3 in vitro. *Zhonghua Shiyan Waike Zazhi* 25: 929–31.
102. Chendil, D. et al. 2004. Curcumin confers radiosensitizing effect in prostate cancer cell line PC3. *Oncogene* 23: 1599–607.
103. Liu, S. L. et al. 2011. Antitumor activity of curcumin against androgen-independent prostate cancer cells via inhibition of NF-κB and AP-1 pathway in vitro. *J. Huazhong Univ., Sci. Tech. (Med. Sci.)*, 31: 530–4.
104. Hilchie, A. L. et al. 2010. Curcumin-induced apoptosis in PC3 prostate carcinoma cells is caspase-independent and involves cellular ceramide accumulation and damage to mitochondria. *Nutr. Cancer* 62: 379–89.
105. Kim, J. W. et al. 2006. Inhibition of EGFR signaling in human prostate cancer PC3 cells by combination treatment with β-phenylethyl isothiocyanate and curcumin. *Carcinogenesis* 27: 475–82.
106. Barve, A. et al. 2008. Murine prostate cancer inhibition by dietary phytochemicals-curcumin and phenyethylisothiocyanate. *Pharm. Res.* 25: 2181–9.
107. Narayanan, N. K. et al. 2009. Liposome encapsulation of curcumin and resveratrol in combination reduces prostate cancer incidence in PTEN knockout mice. *Intl. J. Cancer* 125: 1–8.
108. Dorai, T. et al. 2004. Therapeutic potential of curcumin in prostate cancer: IV. Interference with the osteomimetic properties of hormone refractory C4–2B prostate cancer cells. *The prostate* 60: 1–17.
109. Herman, J. G. et al. 2009. Curcumin blocks CCL2-induced adhesion, motility and invasion, in part, through downregulation of CCL2 expression and proteolytic activity. *Intl. J. Oncol.* 34: 1319–27.
110. Hong, J. H. et al. 2006. The effects of curcumin on the invasiveness of prostate cancer *in vitro* and in vivo. *Prostate Cancer and Prostatic Diseases* 9: 147–52.
111. Tharakan, S. T. et al. 2010. Curcumin potentiates the antitumor effects of gemcitabine in an orthotopic model of human bladder cancer through suppression of proliferative and angiogenic biomarkers. *Biochem. Pharmacol.* 79: 218–28.
112. Tian, B. Q. et al. 2008. Effects of curcumin on bladder cancer cells and development of urothelial tumors in a rat bladder carcinogenesis model. *Cancer Lett.* 264: 299–308.
113. Sindhwani, P. et al. 2001. Curcumin prevents intravesical tumor implantation of the MBT-2 tumor cell line in C3H mice. *J. Urol.* 166: 1498–501.
114. Sindhwani, P. et al. 2000. Curcumin: A food spice with cytotoxic activity against urinary bladder cancer. *Surgical Forum* 51: 625–6.
115. Li, C. Z. et al. 2008. Preventive effects of curcumin in rat bladder tumor induced by aristolochic acid. *Zhongliu Fangzhi Yanjiu* 35: 483–6.
116. Kamat, A. M. et al. 2007: Curcumin potentiates the apoptotic effects of chemotherapeutic agents and cytokines through downregulation of NF-κB and NF-κB-regulated gene products in IFN-α-sensitive and IFN-α-resistant human bladder cancer cells. *Mol. Cancer Therapeutics* 6: 1022–30.
117. Tharakan, S. T. et al. 2010. Curcumin potentiates the antitumor effects of gemcitabine in an orthotopic model of human bladder cancer through suppression of proliferative and angiogenic biomarkers. *Biochem. Pharmacol.* 79: 218–28.
118. Kamat, A. M. et al. 2009. Curcumin potentiates the antitumor effects of Bacillus calmette-guerin against bladder cancer through the down-regulation of NF-κB and upregulation of TRAIL receptors. *Cancer Res.* 69: 8958–66.
119. Lu, P. et al. 2006. Targeted apoptosis-inducing effects of curcumin prodrug on bladder cancer cells. *Zhongguo Yaolixue Tongbao* 22: 1218–22.
120. Tong, Q. S. et al. 2006. Apoptosis-inducing effects of curcumin derivatives in human bladder cancer cells. *Anti-Cancer Drugs* 17: 279–87.
121. Chadalapaka, G. et al. 2008. Curcumin decreases specificity protein expression in bladder cancer cells. *Cancer Res.* 68: 5345–54.
122. Yang, J. R. et al. (a) 2008. Effects of curcumin on survivin expression in T24 cells. *Xinan Guofang Yiyao* 18: 352–4; (b) 2007. Curcumin inhibits proliferation of cell strain of bladder carcinoma and induces its apoptosis. *Di-San Junyi Daxue Xuebao* 29: 2350–3; (c) 2008. Effect of curcumin on cathepsin D expression of T24 cells. *Chongqing Yixue* 37: 1540–2.
123. Fang, W. et al. 2007. Effect of curcumin on expression of p300 in bladder cancer T24 cell. *Zhongliu Fangzhi Yanjiu* 34: 132–4.
124. Park, C. et al. 2006. Induction of G2/M arrest and inhibition of cyclooxygenase-2 activity by curcumin in human bladder cancer T24 cells. *Oncol. Reports* 15: 1225–31.
125. Martin-Cordero, C. et al. 2003. Curcumin as a DNA topoisomerase II poison. *J. Enzyme Inhibit. Med. Chem.* 18: 505–9.
126. Woo, J. Y. et al. 2003. Molecular mechanisms of curcumin-induced cytotoxicity: Induction of apoptosis through generation of reactive oxygen species, downregulation of Bcl-xL and IAP, the release of cytochrome c and inhibition of Akt. *Carcinogenesis* 24: 1199–208.
127. Iqbal, M. et al. 2009. Curcumin attenuates oxidative damage in animals treated with a renal carcinogen, ferric nitrilotriacetate (Fe-NTA): Implications for cancer prevention. *Mol. Cell. Biochem.* 324: 157–64.
128. Okazaki, Y. et al. 2005. Suppressive effects of dietary curcumin on the increased activity of renal ornithine decarboxylase in mice treated with a renal carcinogen, ferric nitrilotriacetate. *Biochimica et Biophysica Acta, Molecular Basis of Disease* 1740: 357–66.

129. Singh, M. et al. 2009. Molecular mechanism of curcumin induced cytotoxicity in human cervical carcinoma cells. *Mol. Cell. Biochem.* 325: 107–19.
130. Prusty, B. K. et al. 2005. Constitutive activation of transcription factor AP-1 in cervical cancer and suppression of human papillo-mavirus (HPV) transcription and AP-1 activity in HeLa cells by curcumin. *Intl. J. Cancer* 113: 951–60.
131. Zhao, J. et al. 2007. Antitumor effect of curcumin on human cervical carcinoma HeLa cells in vitro and in vivo. *Chin. J. Cancer Res.* 19: 32–6.
132. Wang, J. P. et al. 2006. Apoptosis of HeLa cells induced by curcumin and its mechanism of action. *Huaxia Yixue* 19: 623–5.
133. Divya, C. S. et al. Antitumor action of curcumin in human papilloma-virus associated cells involves downregulation of viral oncogenes, prevention of NF-κB and AP-1 translocation, and modulation of apoptosis. *Mol. Carcinogenesis* 45: 320–32.
134. Huang, M. M. et al. 2008. Effect of curcumin on proliferation and apoptosis of HeLa cells. *Zhongguo Shengwu Zhipinxue Zazhi* 21: 1094–7.
135. Zhao, J. et al. Effects of curcumin on proliferation and apoptosis of human cervical carcinoma HeLa cells in vitro. *Chin. J. Cancer Res.* 16: 225–8.
136. Wang, J. P. et al. 2006. Effect of anti-proliferation of curcumin on cervical carcinoma HeLa cells and its mechanism. *Xiandai Zhongliu Yixue* 14: 1001–3.
137. Li, J. et al. 2006. Effects of curcuma on different phases of Hela cell cycle. *Jilin Daxue Xuebao, Yixueban* 32: 675–7.
138. Gupta, K. K. et al. 2006. Dietary antioxidant curcumin inhibits microtubule assembly through tubulin binding. *FEBS J.* 273: 5320–32.
139. Fan, T. T. et al. 2008. Effect of curcumin on the protein expression of pleiotrophin in cervical cancer Caski cells. *Chongqing Yike Daxue Xuebao* 33: 825–7.
140. Xu, F. et al. 2009. Effects of curcumin on invasion and metastasis in the human cervical cancer cells Caski. *Chin. J. Cancer Res.* 21: 159–62.
141. Hong, J. et al. 2007. Curcumin-induced growth inhibitory effects on HeLa cells altered by antioxidant modulators. *Food Sci. Biotechnol.* 16: 1029–34.
142. Bava, S. V. et al. 2005. Sensitization of taxol-induced apoptosis by curcumin involves down-regulation of NF-κB and the serine/threonine kinase Akt and is independent of tubulin polymerization. *J. Biol. Chem.* 280: 6301–8.
143. Javvadi, P. et al. 2008. The chemopreventive agent curcumin is a potent radiosensitizer of human cervical tumor cells via increased reactive oxygen species production and overactivetion of the mitogen-activated protein kinase pathway. *Mol. Pharmacol.* 73: 1491–501.
144. Limtrakul, P. et al. 2007. Modulation of function of three ABC drug transporters, P-glycoprotein (ABCB1), mitoxantrone resistance protein (ABCG2) and multidrug resistance protein 1 (ABCC1) by tetrahydrocurcumin, a major metabolite of curcumin. *Mol. Cell. Biochem.* 296: 85–95.
145. Limtrakul, P. et al. (a) 2005. Modulation of human multidrug-resistance MDR-1 gene by natural curcuminoids. *Acta Horticulturae* 678. (b) 2003. *Proc. WOCMAP III: Third World Cong. Med. Aromat Plants.* 75–83.
146. Chearwae, W. et al. 2004. Biochemical mechanism of modulation of human P-glycoprotein (ABCB1) by curcumin I, II, and III purified from Turmeric powder. *Biochem. Pharmacol.* 68: 2043–52.
147. Anuchapreeda, S. et al. 2002. Modulation of P-glycoprotein expression and function by curcumin in multidrug-resistant human KB cells. *Biochem. Pharmacol.* 64: 573–82.
148. Syu, W. Jr. et al. 1998. Cytotoxicity of curcuminoids and some novel compounds from *Curcuma zedoaria*. *J. Nat. Prods.* 61: 1531–4.
149. Lin, Y. G. et al. 2007. Curcumin inhibits tumor growth and angiogenesis in ovarian carcinoma by targeting the NF-κB pathway. *Clin. Cancer Res.* 13: 3423–30.
150. Pan, W. et al. 2008. AMPK mediates curcumin-induced cell death in CaOV3 ovarian cancer cells. *Oncol. Reports* 20: 1553–9.
151. Ji, C. et al. 2008. Curcumin attenuates EGF-induced AQP3 up-regulation and cell migration in human ovarian cancer cells. *Cancer Chemother. & Pharmacol.* 62: 857–65.
152. Watson, J. L. et al. 2010. Curcumin-induced apoptosis in ovarian carcinoma cells is p53-independent and involves p38 mitogen-activated protein kinase activation and downregulation of Bcl-2 and survivin expression and Akt signaling. *Mol. Carcinogenesis* 49: 13–24.
153. Zheng, L. D. et al. (a) 2006. Growth inhibition and apoptosis inducing mechanisms of curcumin on human ovarian cancer cell line A2780. *Chin. J. Integrat. Med.* 12: 126–31; (b) 2004. Growth-inhibitory effects of curcumin on ovary cancer cells and its mechanisms. *J. Huazhong Univ. Sci. Technol.* (*Med. Sci.*) 24: 55–8; (c) 2003. Cell cycle arrest and apoptosis of human ovary cancer cell line A2780 induced by curcumin in vitro. *J. Huazhong Univ. Tech.* (*Med. Edition*), 32: 209–11, 215.
154. Wang, Q. et al. 2005. Effects of curcumin on proliferation and apoptosis of human ovarian cancer cell line HO-8910 in vitro. *J. Nanjing Med. Univ.* 25: 262–5, 277.
155. Shi, M. X. et al. 2006. Antiproliferation and apoptosis induced by curcumin in human ovarian cancer cells. *Cell Biol. Intl.* 30: 221–6.
156. Liang, H. M. et al. 2002. Effects of IFN-γ on curcumin's antiproliferative capacity of human ovarian cancer cell line 3AO. *J. Shandong Univ.* (*Med. Edit.*) 40: 307–9.
157. Li, Q. et al. 2004. Inhibition of curcumin and curcumin-based combination chemotherapy on human ovarian epithelial carcinoma cell line 3AO in vitro. *J. Shandong Univ.* (*Med. Edit.*), 42: 671–3.
158. Chan, M. M. et al. 2003. Inhibition of growth and sensitization to cisplatin-mediated killing of ovarian cancer cells by polyphenolic chemopreventive agents. *J. Cell. Physiol.* 194: 63–70.
159. Guan, S. L. et al. 2011. Antitumor effect of curcumin combining with cis-platin on human ovarian cancer cell line COC1 in vitro. *Yingyong Huaxue* 28: 1022–7.
160. Chirnomas, D. et al. 2006. Chemosensitization to cisplatin by inhibitors of the Fanconi anemia/BRCA pathway. *Mol. Cancer Therap.* 5: 952–61.
161. Liu, G. Y. et al. 2004. Anti-proliferation effect of paclitaxel with the combination of curcumin on human ovarian carcinoma cell line OC3. *J. Shandong Univ.* (*Med. Edit.*), 42: 325–7, 331.
162. Li, Y. C. et al. 2006. Preventive effects of curcumin on cisplatin-induced nephrotoxicity in rats. *Dulixue Zazhi* 20: 91–3.
163. Ganta, S. et al. 2010. Curcumin enhances oral bioavailability and antitumor therapeutic efficacy of paclitaxel upon administration in nanoemulsion formulation. *J. Pharm. Sci.* 99: 4630–41.

164. Ying, H. C. et al. 2007. Drug-resistant reversing effect of curcumin on COC1/DDP and its mechanism. *Xiandai Zhongliu Yixue* 15: 604–7.
165. Lu, J. et al. 2009. The enhancing effect of curcumin on the sensitivity of cisplatin-resistant human ovarian cancer cell line COCI/DDP. *Shiyong Yixue Zazhi* 25: 1183–6.
166. Ganta, S. et al. 2009. Coadministration of paclitaxel and curcumin in nanoemulsion formulations to overcome multidrug resistance in tumor cells. *Mol. Pharms.* 6: 928–39.
167. Wu, X. J. et al. 2005. Study of apoptotic effect of curcumin on human breast cancer cell of MCF-7. *Chongqing Yixue* 34: 1768–9, 1773; 2006. Anti-proliferative effect of curcumin on human breast cancer of MCF-7 cells. *Di-San Junyi Daxue Xuebao* 28: 1870–2.
168. Zhang, H. G. et al. 2007. Curcumin reverses breast tumor exosomes mediated immune suppression of NK cell tumor cytotoxicity. *Biochimica et Biophysica Acta, Mol. Cell Res.* 1773: 1116–23.
169. Prasad, C. P. et al. 2009. Potent growth suppressive activity of curcumin in human breast cancer cells: Modulation of Wnt/β-catenin signaling. *Chemico-Biol. Interactions* 181: 263–71.
170. Peng, J. H. et al. 2008. Effects of phytoestrogens on DNA damage of MCF-7 breast cancer cells. *Shipin Kexue* (Beijing, China) 29: 549–52.
171. Li, H. C. et al. 2003. Analysis of anti-proliferation of curcumin on human breast cancer cells and its mechanism. *Zhonghua Yixue Zazhi* 83: 1764–8.
172. Choudhuri, T. et al. 2002. Curcumin induces apoptosis in human breast cancer cells through p53-dependent Bax induction. *FEBS Lett.* 512: 334–40.
173. Wang, X. L. et al. 2007. Effect of curcumin on expressions of p21 and CD44V6 in human breast cancer xenografts. *Zhongguo Bingli Shengli Zazhi* 23: 1524–6.
174. Lee, Y. K. et al. 2009. Curcumin exerts antidifferentiation effect through AMPKα-PPAR-γ in 3T3-L1 adipocytes and antiproliferatory effect through AMPKα-COX-2 in cancer cells. *J. Agricul. Food Chem.* 57: 305–10.
175. Xia, Y. Q. et al. 2007. The potentiation of curcumin on insulin-like growth factor-1 action in MCF-7 human breast carcinoma cells. *Life Sci.* 80: 2161–9.
176. Rowe, D. L. et al. 2009. Modulation of the BRCA1 protein and induction of apoptosis in triple negative breast cancer cell lines by the polyphenolic compound curcumin. *Breast Cancer* 3: 61–75.
177. Long, L. et al. 2008. Down-regulation of Notch1 and NF-κB by curcumin in breast cancer cells MDA-MB-231. *Chin. J. Cancer Res.* 20: 294–300.
178. Narasimhan, M. et al. 2008. Curcumin blocks RON tyrosine kinase-mediated invasion of breast carcinoma cells. *Cancer Res.* 68: 5185–92.
179. Bang, M. H. et al. 2006. Effect of curcumin on cancer invasion and matrix metalloproteinase-9 activity in MDA-MB-231 human breast cancer cell. *Hanguk Yongyang Hakhoechi* 39: 756–61.
180. Bachmeier, B. et al. 2007. The chemopreventive polyphenol curcumin prevents hematogenous breast cancer metastases in immune-deficient mice. *Cell. Physiol. Biochem.* 19: 137–52.
181. Bachmeier, B. E. et al. 2008. Curcumin downregulates the inflammatory cytokines CXCL1 and -2 in breast cancer cells via NF-κB. *Carcinogen.* 29: 779–89.
182. Moulik, S. et al. 2008. Phosphatidylinositol 3-kinase and NF-κB involved in epidermal growth factor-induced matrix metallo-proteinase-9 expression. *J. Cancer Mol.* 4: 55–60.
183. Ibrahim, A. et al. 2011. Curcumin induces apoptosis in a murine mammary gland adenocarcinoma cell line through the mitochondrial pathway. *Eur. J. Pharmacol.* 668: 127–32.
184. Limtrakul, P. et al. 2007. Modulation of function of three ABC drug transporters, P-glycoprotein (ABCB1), mitoxantrone resistance protein (ABCG2) and multidrug resistance protein 1 (ABCC1) by tetrahydrocurcumin, a major metabolite of curcumin. *Mol. Cell. Biochem.* 296: 85–95.
185. Shukla, S. et al. 2009. Curcumin inhibits the activity of ABCG2/BCRP1, a multidrug resistance-linked ABC drug transporter in mice. *Pharm. Res.* 26: 480–7.
186. Labbozzetta, M. et al. 2009. Curcumin as a possible lead compound against hormone-independent, multidrug-resistant breast cancer. *Annals of the New York Academy of Sciences* 1155: 278–83.
187. Somers-Edgar, T. J. 2008. The combination of epigallocatechin gallate and curcumin suppresses ERα-breast cancer cell growth in vitro and in vivo. *Intl. J. Cancer* 122: 1966–71.
188. Cheah, Y. et al. 2009. Combined xanthorrhizol-curcumin exhibits synergistic growth inhibitory activity via apoptosis induction in human breast cancer cells MDA-MB-231. *Cancer Cell Intl.* 9: 1.
189. Fang, H. Y. et al. 2011. Proteomic identification of differentially expressed proteins in curcumin-treated MCF-7 cells. *Phytomed.* 18: 697–703.
190. Tian, J. et al. 2010. Synergistic antitumor efficacy of curcumin combination with adriamycin. *J. Yantai Univ. (Sci. Tech. Edit.)* 23: 297–303.
191. Criss, C. et al. 2008. Gold mediated cellular delivery of anticancer drugs. Abstracts of Papers, *235th ACS National Meeting, New Orleans, LA, April 6–10, 2008*, CHED-1298.
192. Tang, H. D. et al. 2009. Curcumin-containing polymers as anticancer prodrugs. Abstracts of Papers. *237th ACS National Meeting, Salt Lake City, UT,* March 22–26, 2009, POLY-373.
193. Quiroga, A. et al. 2010. Anti-breast cancer activity of curcumin on the human oxidation-resistant cells ZR-75-1 with γ-glutamyltrans-peptidase inhibition. *J. Experim. Therap. Oncol.* 8: 261–6.
194. Luthra, P. M. et al. 2009. Demethoxycurcumin induces Bcl-2 mediated G2/M arrest and apoptosis in human glioma U87 cells. *Biochem. Biophys. Res. Commun.* 384: 420–5.
195. Liu, T. et al. 2009. The regulatory effect of curcumin on the differential expression of Bcl-2 and caspase 8 and its promotional effect of apoptosis mechanism in human glioma cells. *Zhongguo Aizheng Zazhi* 19: 247–51.
196. Liu, E. Y. et al. 2007. Curcumin induces G2/M cell cycle arrest in a p53-dependent manner and upregulates ING4 expression in human glioma. *J. Neurooncol.* 85: 263–70.
197. Belkaid, A. et al. 2006. Silencing of the human microsomal glucose-6-phosphate translocase induces glioma cell death: Potential new anticancer target for curcumin. *FEBS Lett.* 580: 3746–52.
198. Karmakar, S. et al. 2007. Curcumin suppressed anti-apoptotic signals and activated cysteine proteases for apoptosis in human malignant glioblastoma U87MG cells. *Neurochem. Res.* 32: 2103–13.

199. Su, C. C. et al. 2010. The anti-cancer efficacy of curcumin scrutinized through core signaling pathways in glioblastoma. *Intl. J. Mol. Med.* 26: 217–24.
200. Dhandapani, K. M. et al. 2007. Curcumin suppresses growth and chemoresistance of human glioblastoma cells via AP-1 and NF-κB transcription factors. *J. Neurochem.* 102: 522–38.
201. Kim, S. Y. et al. 2005. Curcumin is a potent broad spectrum inhibitor of matrix metallo-proteinase gene expression in human astroglioma cells. *Biochem. Biophys. Res. Commun.* 337: 510–6.
202. Woo, M. et al. 2005. Curcumin suppresses phorbol ester-induced matrix metalloproteinase-9 expression by inhibiting the PKC to MAPK signaling pathways in human astroglioma cells. *Biochem. Biophys. Res. Commun.* 335: 1017–25.
203. Purkayastha, S. et al. 2009. Curcumin blocks brain tumor formation. *Brain Res.* 1266: 130–8.
204. Wakade, C. et al. 2009. Curcumin attenuates vascular inflammation and cerebral vasospasm after subarachnoid hemorrhage in mice. *Antioxidants Redox Signaling* 11: 35–46.
205. Kang, S. Y. et al. 2006. Curcumin-induced histone hypoacetylation enhances caspase-3-dependent glioma cell death and neurogenesis of neural progenitor cells. *Stem Cells Develop.* 15: 165–74.
206. Khafif, A. et al. 2009. Curcumin: A potential radio-enhancer in head and neck cancer. *Laryngoscope* 119: 2019–26.
207. Cohen, A. N. et al. 2009. Suppression of interleukin 6 and 8 production in head and neck cancer cells with curcumin via inhibition of ikappa beta kinase. *Arch. Otolaryngol. Head Neck Surgery* 135: 190–7.
208. LoTempio, M. M. et al. 2005. Curcumin suppresses growth of head and neck squamous cell carcinoma. *Clin. Cancer Res.* 11: 6994–7002.
209. Aggarwal, S. et al. 2004. Inhibition of growth and survival of human head and neck squamous cell carcinoma cells by curcumin via modulation of NF-κB signaling. *Intl. J. Cancer* 111: 679–92.
210. Yao, Y. H. et al. 2006. Anticancer activities of curcumin on nasopharyngeal carcinoma. *Zhongliu Fangzhi Yanjiu* 33: 487–9.
211. Kuhar, M. et al. 2007. Curcumin and quercetin combined with cisplatin to induce apoptosis in human laryngeal carcinoma Hep-2 cells through the mitochondrial pathway. *J. Cancer Mol.* 3: 121–8.
212. Kuo, C. L. et al. 2011. Apoptotic death in curcumin-treated NPC-TW 076 human naso-pharyngeal carcinoma cells is mediated through the ROS, mitochondrial depolarization and caspase-3-dependent signaling responses. *Intl. J. Oncol.* 39: 319–28.
213. Chakravarti, N. et al. 2006. Targeting constitutive and interleukin-6-inducible signal transducers and activators of transcription 3 pathway in head and neck squamous cell carcinoma cells by curcumin (diferuloylmethane). *Intl. J. Cancer* 119: 1268–75.
214. Wang, D. et al. 2008. Liposome-encapsulated curcumin suppresses growth of head and neck squamous cell carcinoma in vitro and in xenografts through the inhibition of NF-κB by an AKT-independent pathway. *Clin. Cancer Res.* 14: 6228–36.
215. Duarte, V. M. et al. 2010. Curcumin enhances the effect of cisplatin in suppression of head and neck squamous cell carcinoma via inhibition of IKKβ protein of the NF-κB pathway. *Mol. Cancer Therap.* 9: 2665–75.
216. Siwak, D. R. et al. 2005. Curcumin-induced antiproliferative and proapoptotic effects in melanoma cells are associated with suppression of IκB kinase and nuclear factor κB activity and are independent of the B-raf/mitogen-activated/extracellular signal-regulated protein kinase pathway and the Akt pathway. *Cancer* 104: 879–90.
217. Menon, L. G. et al. 1999. Anti-metastatic activity of curcumin and catechin. *Cancer Lett.* 141: 159–65.
218. Zhou, L. et al. 2007. Effect of curcumin on MT1-MMP-mediated promatrix metalloproteinase-2 activation of tumor-bearing mice. *Linchuang Pifuke Zazhi* 36: 54952.
219. Liu, Y. Q. et al. 2007. Curcumin inhibits mouse melanoma growth and influences nuclear factor κB activation and survivin expression. *Zhonghua Pifuke Zazhi* 40: 684–7.
220. Qiu, S. et al. 2005. Apoptosis induced by curcumin and its effect on c-myc and caspase-3 expressions in human melanoma A375 cell line. *Diyi Junyi Daxue Xuebao* 25: 1517–21.
221. Zheng, M. Z. et al. 2004. Inhibition of NF-κB and nitric oxide by curcumin induces G2/M cell cycle arrest and apoptosis in human melanoma cells. *Melanoma Res.* 14: 165–71.
222. Marin, Y. E. et al. 2007. Curcumin downregulates the constitutive activity of NF-κB and induces apoptosis in novel mouse melanoma cells. *Melanoma Res.* 17: 274–83.
223. Gui, F. et al. 2008. Preliminary study on molecular mechanism of curcumin anti-mouse melanoma. *Zhongyaocai* 31: 1685–9.
224. Bush, J. A. et al. 2001. Curcumin induces apoptosis in human melanoma cells through a Fas Receptor/Caspase-8 Pathway Independent of p53. *Exper. Cell Res.* 271: 305–14.
225. Odot, J. et al. 2004. In vitro and in vivo antitumoral effect of curcumin against melanoma cells. *Intl. J. Cancer* 111: 381–7.
226. Wang, L. et al. 2009. An anticancer effect of curcumin mediated by down-regulating phosphatase of regenerating liver-3 expression on highly metastatic melanoma cells. *Mol. Pharmacol.* 76: 1238–45.
227. Banerji, A. et al. 2004. Effect of curcumin on gelatinase A (MMP-2) activity in B16F10 melanoma cells. *Cancer Lett.* 211: 235–42.
228. Ray, S. et al. 2003. Curcumin exhibits antimetastatic properties by modulating integrin receptors, collagenase activity, and expression of Nm23 and E-cadherin. *J. Envir. Pathol. Toxicol. & Oncol.* 22: 49–58.
229. Varghese, L. et al. 2002. Inhibition of tumour specific angiogenesis by some synthetic curcuminoid derivatives. *Amala Res. Bull.* 22: 65–71.
230. Li, J. M. et al. 2008. Inhibitory effect of water-soluble preparation of curcumin on spontaneous metastasis of B16F10 melanoma in mice. *Zhongguo Zhongliu Shengwu Zhiliao Zazhi* 15: 286–8.
231. Sun, Z. J. et al. 2011. Curcumin dually inhibits both mammalian target of rapamycin and nuclear factor-κB pathways through a crossed phosphatidylinositol 3-kinase/Akt/IκB kinase complex signaling axis in adenoid cystic carcinoma. *Mol. Pharmacol.* 79: 106–18.
232. Leow, P. C. et al. 2010. Antitumor activity of natural compounds, curcumin and PKF118–310, as Wnt/β-catenin antagonists against human osteosarcoma cells. *Investigational New Drugs* 28: 766–82.
233. Luo, F. F. et al. 2011. Low-dose curcumin leads to the inhibition of tumor growth via enhancing CTL-mediated antitumor immunity. *Intl. Immunopharmacol.* 11: 1234–40.

234. Song, M. Y. et al. 2011. Use of curcumin to decrease nitric oxide production during the induction of antitumor responses by IL-2. *J. Immunother.* 34: 149–64.
235. Ohtsu, H. et al. 2002. Antitumor agents: 217. Curcumin analogues as novel androgen receptor antagonists with potential as anti-prostate cancer agents *J. Med. Chem.* 45: 5037–42.
236. Ishida, J. et al. 2002. Antitumor agents: Part 214: Synthesis and evaluation of curcumin analogues as cytotoxic agents. *Bioorg. Med. Chem.* 10: 3481–7.
237. Ferrari, E. et al. 2009. Synthesis, cytotoxic, and combined cDDP activity of new stable curcumin derivatives. *Bioorg. Med. Chem.* 17: 3043–52.
238. Fuchs, J. R. et al. 2009. Structure-activity relationship studies of curcumin analogues. *Bioorg. Med. Chem. Lett.* 19: 2065–9.
239. Bao, B. et al. 2012. Curcumin analogue CDF inhibits pancreatic tumor growth by switching on suppressor microRNAs and attenuating EZH2 expression. *Cancer Res.* 72:335–45.
240. Xu, J. H. et al. 2009. Preparation of curcumin derivative as antitumor agent. *Faming Zhuanli Shenqing Gongkai Shuomingshu* 9pp. Application: CN 2008-10071178 20080605.
241. Poma, P. et al. 2007. The antitumor activities of curcumin and of its isoxazole analogue are not affected by multiple gene expression changes in an MDR model of the MCF-7 breast cancer cell line: Analysis of the possible molecular basis. *Intl. J. Mol. Med.* 20: 329–35.
242. Simoni, D. et al. 2008. Antitumor effects of curcumin and structurally β-diketone modified analogs on multidrug resistant cancer cells. *Bioorg. Med. Chem. Lett.* 18: 845–9.
243. Youssef, D. et al. 2007. Design, synthesis, and cytostatic activity of novel cyclic curcumin analogues. *Bioorg. Med. Chem. Lett.* 17: 5624–9.
244. Bill, M. A. et al. 2010. The small molecule curcumin analog FLLL32 induces apoptosis in melanoma cells via STAT3 inhibition and retains the cellular response to cytokines with antitumor activity. *Mol. Cancer* 9: 165.
245. Brian, K. A. et al. 2004. Synthesis and biological evaluation of novel curcumin analogs as anticancer and antiangiogenesis agents. *Bioorg. Med. Chem.* 12: 3871–83.
246. Hutzen, B. et al. 2009. Curcumin analogue GO-Y030 inhibits STAT3 activity and cell growth in breast and pancreatic carcinomas. *Intl. J. Oncol.* 35: 867–72.
247. Lin, L. et al. 2011. Targeting colon cancer stem cells using a new curcumin analogue, GO-Y030. British J. Cancer 105: 212–20.
248. Kudo, C. et al. 2011. Synthesis of 86 species of 1,5-diaryl-3-oxo-1,4-pentadienes analogs of curcumin can yield a good lead in vivo. *BMC Pharmacol.* 11: 4.
249. Lin, L. et al. 2009. New curcumin analogues exhibit enhanced growth-suppressive activity and inhibit AKT and signal transducer and activator of transcription 3 phosphorylation in breast and prostate cancer cells. *Cancer Sci.* 100: 1719–27.
250. Cen, L. et al. 2009. New structural analogues of curcumin exhibit potent growth suppressive activity in human colorectal carcinoma cells. *BMC Cancer* 9: 99.
251. Xiao, J. et al. 2010. Synthesis and biological analysis of a new curcumin analogue for enhanced antitumor activity in HepG2 cells. *Oncol. Reports* 23: 1435–41.
252. Wang, Y. et al. 2011. A novel monocarbonyl analogue of curcumin, (1E,4E)-1,5-Bis(2,3-dimethoxyphenyl) penta-1,4-dien-3-one, induced cancer cell H460 apoptosis via activation of endoplasmic reticulum stress signaling pathway. *J. Med. Chem.* 54: 3768–78.
253. Muhammad, D. et al. 2007. Geometric isomers and cytotoxic effect on T47D cells of curcumin analogs PGV-0 and PGV-1. *Majalah Farmasi Indonesia* 18: 40–7.
254. Melyanto, E. et al. 2006. PGV-1 decreases angiogenic factor (VEGF and COX-2) expression non T47D cell inducted by estrogen. *Majalah Farmasi Indonesia* 17: 1–6.
255. Davis, R. et al. 2008. Syntheses and cytotoxic properties of the curcumin analogs 2,6-bis (benzylidene)-4-phenylcyclohexanones. *Archiv der Pharmazie* (Weinheim, Germany) 341: 440–5.
256. Kasinski, A. L. et al. 2008. Inhibition of IκB kinase-nuclear factor-κB signaling pathway by 3,5-bis(2-fluro-benzylidene) piperidin-4-one (EF24), a novel monoketone analog of curcumin. *Mol. Pharmacol.* 74: 654–61.
257. Brian, K. A. et al. 2005. EF24, a novel synthetic curcumin analog, induces apoptosis in cancer cells via a redox-dependent mechanism. *Anticancer Drugs* 16: 263–75.
258. Thomas, S. L. et al. 2008. EF24, a novel curcumin analog, disrupts the microtubule cytoskeleton and inhibits HIF-1α. *Cell Cycle* 7: 2409–17.
259. Tan, X. et al. 2010. Multiple anticancer activities of EF24, a novel curcumin analog on human ovarian carcinoma cells. *Reproductive Sci.* 17: 931–40.
260. Sun, A. M. et al. 2006. Synthesis of EF24-tripeptide chloromethyl ketone: A novel curcumin-related anticancer drug delivery system. *J. Med. Chem.* 49: 3153–8.
261. Shoji, M. et al. 2008. Targeting tissue factor-expressing tumor angiogenesis and tumors with EF24 conjugated to factor VIIa. *J. Drug Targeting* 16: 185–97.
262. Al-Hujaily, E. M. et al. 2011. PAC, a novel curcumin analogue, has anti-breast cancer properties with higher efficiency on ER-negative cells. *Breast Cancer Res. & Treatment* 128: 97–107.
263. Dayton, A. et al. 2010. Cellular uptake, retention and bioabsorption of HO-3867, a fluorinated curcumin analog with potential antitumor properties. *Cancer Biol. Therapy* 10: 1027–32.
264. Shahani, K. et al. 2010. Injectable sustained release microparticles of curcumin: A new concept for cancer chemoprevention. *Cancer Res.* 70: 4443–52.
265. Altunbas, A. et al. 2011. Encapsulation of curcumin in self-assembling peptide hydrogels as injectable drug delivery vehicles. *Biomaterials* 32: 5906–14.
266. Yang, Z. W. et al. 2010. Preparation and characterization of zedoary turmeric oil-loaded insulin-modified sterically stabilized liposomes. *J. Liposome Res.* 20: 9–15.
267. Tang, H. D. et al. 2010. Amphiphilic curcumin conjugate-forming nanoparticles as anticancer prodrug and drug carriers: In vitro and in vivo effects. *Nanomedicine* 5: 855–65.
268. Mulik, R. S. et al. 2010. Transferrin mediated solid lipid nanoparticles containing curcumin: Enhanced in vitro anticancer activity by induction of apoptosis. *Intl. J. Pharm.* 398: 190–203.
269. Anand, P. et al. 2010. Design of curcumin-loaded PLGA nanoparticles formulation with enhanced cellular uptake, and increased bioactivity in vitro and superior bioavailability in vivo. *Biochem. Pharmacol.* 79: 330–8.
270. Kim, T. H. et al. 2011. Preparation and characterization of water-soluble albumin-bound curcumin nanoparticles with improved antitumor activity. *Intl. J. Pharms.* 403: 285–91.

271. Duan, J. H. et al. 2010. Synthesis and in vitro/in vivo anticancer evaluation of curcumin-loaded chitosan/poly(butyl cyanoacrylate) nanoparticles. *Intl. J. Pharmaceutics* 400: 211–20.
272. Yen, F. L. et al. 2010. Curcumin nanoparticles improve the physicochemical properties of curcumin and effectively enhance its antioxidant and antihepatoma activities. *J. Agricul. Food Chem.* 28: 7376–82.
273. Esmaili, M. et al. 2011. Beta casein-micelle as a nano vehicle for solubility enhancement of curcumin; food industry application. *LWT-Food Sci. Technol.* 44: 2166–72.
274. Zhang, F. et al. 2011. A novel solubility-enhanced curcumin formulation showing stability and maintenance of anticancer activity. *J. Pharm. Sci.* 100: 2778–89.
275. Sawant, V. J. et al. 2014. PEG-cyclodextrin coated curcumin loaded zinc ferrite core nanocomposites as pH-responsive drug delivery system for anti-inflammation and anticancer application. *Archiv. Applied Sci. Res.* 6: 44–54.
276. Chaurasia, S. et al. 2015. Lipopolysaccharide based oral nanocarriers for the improvement of bioavailability and anticancer efficacy of curcumin. *Carbohydrate Polymers* 130: 9–17.
277. Pillai, J. J. et al. 2015. Curcumin entrapped folic acid conjugated PLGA-PEG nanoparticles exhibit enhanced anticancer activity by site specific delivery. *RSC Advances* 5: 25518–24.
278. Huang, Y. C. et al. 2015. O-carboxymethyl chitosan/fucoidan nanoparticles increase cellular curcumin uptake. *Food Hydrocolloids* 53: 261–9.
279. Loch-Neckel, G. et al. 2015. Orally administered chitosan-coated polycaprolactone nanoparticles containing curcumin attenuate metastatic melanoma in the lungs. *J. Pharm. Sci.* 104: 3524–34.
280. Hu, X. Y. et al. 2015. Curcumin attenuates opioid tolerance and dependence by inhibiting Ca^{2+}/calmodulin-dependent protein kinase II α activity. *J. Pharmacol. Experim. Therap.* 352: 420–8.
281. Mirgani, M. T. et al. 2014. Dendrosomal curcumin nanoformulation downregulates pluripotency genes via miR-145 activation in U87MG glioblastoma cells. *Intl. J. Nanomed.* 9: 403–17.
282. Zhang, J. F. et al. 2015. Self-carried curcumin nanoparticles for in vitro and in vivo cancer therapy with real-time monitoring of drug release. *Nanoscale* 7: 13503–10.
283. Klippstein, R. et al. 2015. Passively targeted curcumin-loaded PEGylated PLGA nanocapsules for colon cancer therapy in vivo. *Small* 11: 4704–22.
284. Tang, H. D. et al. 2010. Curcumin polymers as anticancer conjugates. *Biomaterials* 31: 7139–49.
285. Wichitnithad, W. et al. 2011. Effects of different carboxylic ester spacers on chemical stability, release characteristics, and anticancer activity of mono-PEGylated curcumin conjugates. *J. Pharm. Sci.* 100: 5206–18.
286. Waghela, B. N. et al. 2015. Curcumin conjugated with PLGA potentiates sustainability, anti-proliferative activity and apoptosis in human colon carcinoma cells. *PLoS One* 10: e0117526/1–e0117526/24.
287. Modi, G. et al. 2011. Increased anticancer activity of curcumin-Zn (II) complex by species sensitive method. *Chem. Sinica* 2: 91–9.
288. John, V. D. et al. 2010. Antitumour studies of aluminum complexes of synthetic curcuminoids. *Main Group Metal Chem.* 33: 157–66.

115 Yu Jin 鬱金

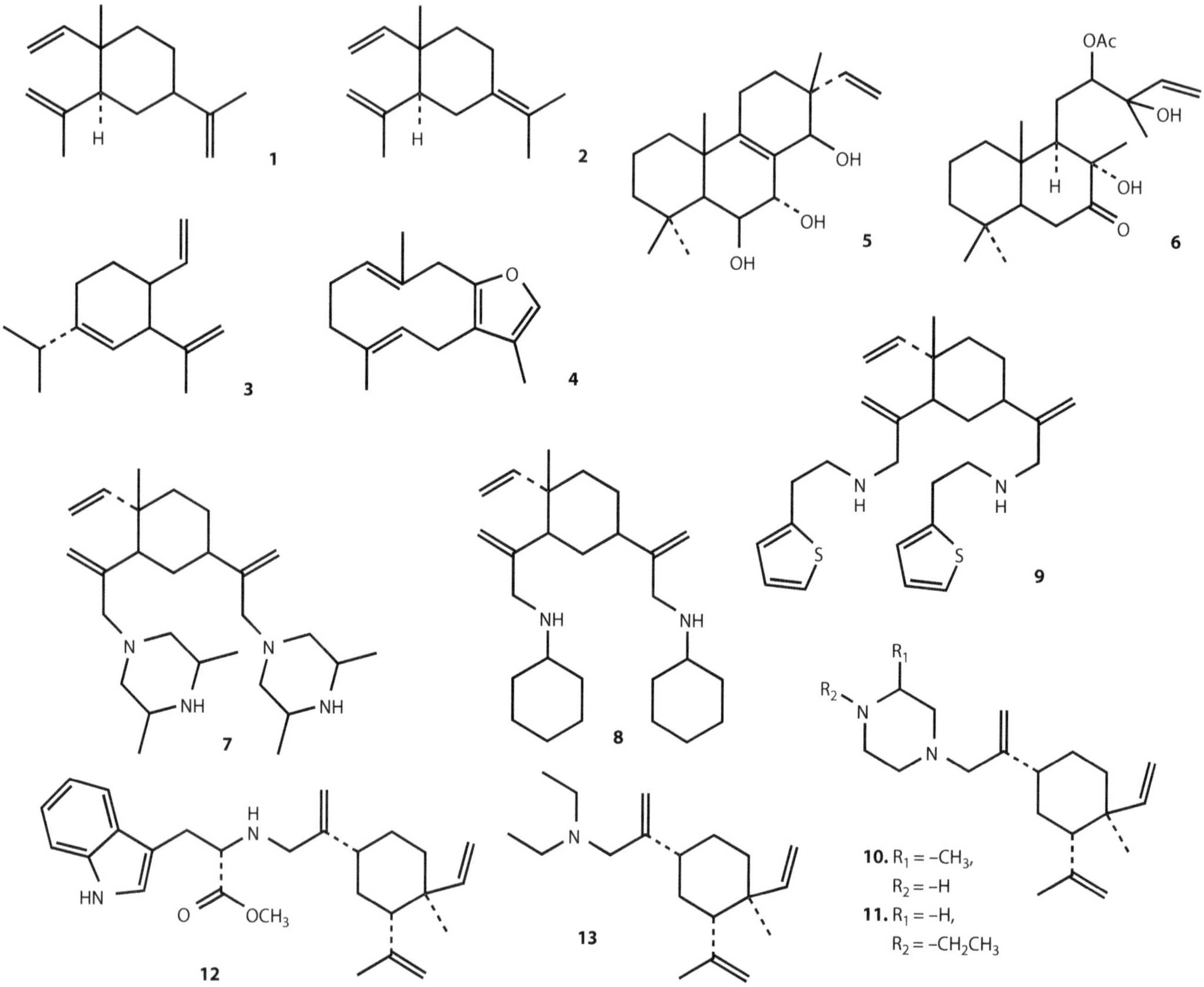

Herb Origination

The herb Yu Jin is normally prepared from the dried rhizomes of *Curcuma wenyujin*, which is mainly produced in the Zhejiang province. Traditionally, its major rhizomes are called Wen E Zhu (温莪術), and the small root tuber is the source of Wen Yu Jin (温鬱金). Moreover, the small rhizomes of other Zingiberaceae plants, *C. aeruginosa*, *C. longa* L., *C. kwangsiensis*, and *C. chuanyujin* are also sources of the herb Yu Jin. (See Sections E Zhu and Jiang Huang).

Antitumor Activities and Constituents

The essential oil of *C. wenyujin* demonstrated obvious antiproliferative effect against various neoplastic cells. The treatment with the oil inhibited the growth of human HepG2 hepatoma cells and promoted cell apoptosis and S/G2 cell cycle arrest.[1] The *C. wenyujin* oil extracted by CO_2 liquid restrained the proliferation of human SPC-A-1 lung adenocarcinoma cells for 62.57% in a 62.5 μg/mL concentration, whose activity was stronger than that of the oil isolated by normal methods.[2] The Yu Jin oil primarily contains three types of anticancer principals, (1) curcumanoids such as curcumin (see Section Jiang Huang); (2) sesquiterpenes such as curcumol, curcumenol, and curdion (see Section E Zhu), which can be extracted from the oil made by CO_2 liquid extraction in higher percentages; and (3) elemene and furanodiene, two important bioactive sesquiterpenes isolated from the essential oil derived from the rhizomes of *C. wenyujin* and *C. kwangsiensis*. In addition, an ethanolic extract derived from the stems and the leaves of *C. wenyujin* also showed the anticarcinoma effect against the proliferation of human HEp-2 larynx carcinoma cells obviously.[3]

Elemenes

The elemene normally showed three isomers, i.e., β-(**1**), γ-(**2**), and δ-(**3**) elemene, in Yu Jin essential oil wherein the content of β-elemene (**1**) is dominant.[4] From *in vitro* and *in vivo* experiments, the elemenes were found to possess significant antitumor activity. β-Elemene (**1**) demonstrated a broad spectrum of *in vitro* inhibitory effect against the proliferation of various human tumor cell lines, i.e., LoVo (colon); SMMC-7721, 7402, and HepG2 (liver); HEp-2 (laryngeal); HeLa (cervix); A549 (lung); SGC-7901 (stomach); HL-60 and K562 (leukemia); T24 (bladder); NSCLC (lung); RPMI-8226 (multiple myeloma); SHG-44 and U251 (glioma); U87 (glioblastoma); lung fibroblast and bronchial epithelial and breast cells; and many murine tumor cell lines, i.e., C6 (glioma), B16, (melanoma), Hca-F25/cL-16A3 (ascite hepatoma), and gastric cancer. The anticarcinoma effects of β-elemene were closely correlated with its abilities in disturbing cell cycles and inducing apoptotic death.[5–14] Animal pharmacodynamic studies of β-elemene (**1**) resulted in the life prolongation rates of 103–224% for hepatic ascites carcinoma and 47–286% for L1210 leukemia and the growth inhibition of 10–30% for a solid hepatoma, and they showed 50–70% inhibition of a murine subrenal capsule model with cerebral neuroglioma.[15] The i.p. injection of β-elemene (**1**) in a dose of 50 mg/kg markedly inhibited the growth of hepatoma H22 cells by 48% in mice.[5,6] Both oral administration and gastric serosal injection of β-elemene (**1**) could stimulate the cell apoptosis in mice implanted with gastric cancer with lymphatic metastasis, indicating that it is a useful agent for the prevention and the treatment of the lymph node metastasis of gastric cancer.[7] The life span extension in mice bearing Ehrlich ascites cancer or ascites reticulum cell sarcoma was found to be accompanied with the blockage of DNA and RNA syntheses after the β-elemene treatment.[15]

Another isomer δ-elemene (**3**) was reported to have the significant ability to promote the apoptosis of human cancer cell lines such as NCI-H292 lung cancer mucoepidermoid cells, DLD-1 colorectal adenocarcinoma cells, HL-60 leukemia cells, and HeLa cervical cancer cells.[16,17] An *in vivo* test further confirmed the *in vitro* inhibitory activity of elemenes on the hepatoma proliferation.[18] Moreover, the elemenes also could potentiate the antitumor immune system in H22 hepatome and HepG2 hepatoma cells. The immunoenhancing effect partially correlated with the activation of HSP70 in the H22 cells and the upregulation of 13 genetic protein expressions and the downregulation of 11 genetic protein expressions in the HepG2 cells.[19] The anticancer immunotherapeutic effect of the elemene emulsion was clinically proven in six patients with malignant tumor, where the rDNA transcription of lymphocytes was significantly enhanced.[20]

Furanodiene

Furanodiene (**4**) is another primary sesquiterpene component in the herb essential oil wherein it is more than 20% in content, which demonstrated a remarkable *in vitro* growth inhibition on a panel of human HeLa (cervix), HEp-2 (larynx), SGC-7901 (stomach), HL-60 (leukemia), PC3 (prostate), HT-1080 (sarcoma), and U251 (glioma) neoplastic cell lines, with IC_{50} values of 0.6–7.0 μg/mL. It also moderately repressed the proliferation of a group of human cancer cell lines, HepG2 and SMMC-7721 (liver), A549 (lung), K562 (leukemia), and MDA-MB-435s (breast), with IC_{50} values in a range of 9–20 μg/mL, but it showed moderate cytotoxic effect to normal embryonic fibroblast cells as well.[21,22] Furanodiene (**4**) obviously inhibited the proliferation in both human breast cancer cell lines (MCF-7 and MDA-MB-231) in a dose-dependent manner in association with increase of LDH release and induction of G0/G1 cycle arrest.[23] By downregulating the expressions of integrin αV and β-catenin, blocking the phosphorylations of FAK, Akt and, PI3 kinase p85, and inhibiting MMP-9, furanodiene (**4**) exerted antimetastatic effect in an *in vitro* model with the MDA-MB-231 cells.[24] The antitumor property of furanodiene (**4**) was further demonstrated by *in vivo* experiments with mouse models implanted with U14 uterine cervical tumor, sarcoma 180 or MCF-7 breast cancer.[21,22] The i.p. injection of 15 and 30 mg/kg furanodiene (**4**) dose-dependently suppressed the growth of MCF-7 cancer xenograft in nude mice, achieving 32% and 54% inhibition rates, respectively.[23]

The HL-60 cell apoptosis stimulated by furanodiene (**4**) was revealed to be mediated by TNFR1-mediated extrinsic apoptotic pathways, where the upregulation of TNFR1, the formation of TNFR1 complex, and the production of TNFα were provoked in the HL-60 cells.[25] The MARK signaling and mitochondria caspase apoptotic pathways played an important role in the furanodiene (**4**)-promoted cell cycle arrest and apoptosis of human hepatoma cells, associated with the blockage of ERK/MAPK signaling, the depolarization of mitochondrial transmembrane, the release of mitochondrial cytochrome c, the activation of p38 and caspases-3, and the cleavage of PARP. Furanodiene (**4**) displayed an obvious protective effect on the immune function as well.[26]

Curcumrinols

Curcumrinols-A–C are three cytotoxic diterpenoids isolated from the rhizomes of Yu Jin. Their cytotoxic activity were mainly present in two different types of neoplasm. Curcumrinol-A (**5**) displayed medium cytotoxicity against human HL-60 promyelocytic leukemia and K562 CML cell lines with IC_{50} values of 3.2 and 11.2 μg/mL, respectively, but curcumrinol-B (a 14S epimer of curcumrinol-A (**5**)) exhibited only weak activity on the leukemia cells.[27] Curcumrinol-C (**6**) was effective in the growth suppression of human SW620 colon cancer and SGC-7901 gastric cancer cell lines concomitant with stimulated apoptosis and cell cycle arrest.[28,29] The IC_{50} value was 24.16 μg/mL in SW620 cells, whose effect was moderate, but it was more potent than cisplatin (IC_{50}: 45.80 μg/mL). The SW620 cell apoptosis caused by curcumrinol-C (**6**) were associated with inhibiting MAPK signaling pathway and enhancing apoptotic activity of caspase-3.[30,31]

Other Bioactive Components

More cytotoxic components were found from a methylene chloride extract of the root tubers of Yu Jin under bioassay-directed phytochemistry approaches. Three isolated curcuminoids elucidated as curcumin, demethoxy-curcumin, and bis-demethoxy-curcumin, as well as a sesquiterpene assigned as gweicurculactone, exerted the antineoplastic effect when tested on five human cancer cell lines, HL-60, HepG2, K562, KB, and MCF-7, *in vitro*.[32]

Exploration of Mechanism of Elemene

The mechanism of elemenes for the induction of apoptosis and cell cycle arrest has been extensively investigated, revealing the characteristics of signaling pathways in the different types of cancer cells. In NSCLC cells, the β-elemene (**1**)-triggered apoptosis was mediated by a mitochondrial apoptotic pathway including decrease of Bcl-2 expression, release of cytochrome c, increase of cleaved PARP level, and activation of caspase-3, caspase-7, and caspase-9, whereas its G2/M phase cell cycle arrest was followed by the decreases in the levels of cyclin-B1 and phospho-CDC2 (Thr-161) and the increases in the levels of p27kip1 and phospho-CDC2 (Tyr-15), as well as the downregulation of CDC25C expression and the upregulation of Chk2 expression.[12] The stimulation of Ca^{2+} ion and the suppression of telomerase activity were also observed in human LoVo colon cancer cells after being treated with β-elemene (**1**), where Ca^{2+} ion plays an important role in the apoptotic process and G0/G1 phase blockage.[13,33] Human BIU-87 bladder cancer cell apoptosis provoked by β-elemene (**1**) was correlated with the changes of the transformation rate of the phospholipid metabolism. By a special signal transduction pathway, i.e., significantly diminishing the inositol incorporation into phosphatidylinositol and reducing the cell membrane fluidity, β-elemene (**1**) could accelerated the BIU-87 cell apoptosis.[34] The antiproliferation and the promotion of cell cycle arrest and apoptosis caused by β-elemene in human U87 glioblastoma cells were found to be mediated by p38 MAPK activation, GMFβ signaling activation, inactivation of ERK1/2-Bcl-2/survivin pathway, and regulation of p-MKK3 and p-MKK6 levels.[35–38] The proapoptotic mechanism in U87MG and C6 glioblastoma cell lines by β-elemene (**1**) was found to be also associated with the disruption of the Hsp90/Raf-1 complex formation, which was a key step in maintaining Raf-1 conformation stability and causing Raf-1 deactivation and ERK pathway inhibition, thereby leading to the apoptosis of glioblastoma cells.[39] The downregulation of c-Myc expression or Bcl-2/Bcl-xL expressions is also involved in the cell apoptosis and the cell cycle arrest induced by elemene in human U251 glioma cells and rat C6 glioma cells, respectively.[23,40]

Moreover, the remarkable growth inhibition of HEp-2 laryngeal cancer cells by elemenes was also revealed to be closely related to the apoptotic promotion, where elemenes repressed the expressions of eukaryotic initiation factors (eIF4E and eIF4G) and bFGF besides marked caspase-3 activation. In addition to the apoptosis promotion, elemenes also exerted antiangiogenetic and antivascular effects via the decrease of the MVD and VEGF expression in the HEp-2 cells.[41,42] In a mouse Lewis lung neoplastic model, elemenes were able to obstruct the metastasis of Lewis cells, whose antimetastatic mechanism was partially correlated with the reduction of matrix component expression and the protection of basement membrane and ECM barrier.[43]

The cell cycle arrest and the apoptosis in HL-60 cells and HeLa cells were triggered by δ-elemene (**3**) primarily through a caspase-3-dependent pathway,[17,44] whereas the apoptosis elicited by δ-elemene in human NCI-H292 lung cancer mucoepidermoid and DLD-1 colorectal adenocarcinoma cell lines was mediated by both MAPK-involved pathway and mitochondrial-involved pathway. Also, the rapid increase in the intracellular levels of ROS was found to be a key in the induction of the carcinoma cell apoptosis (HeLa, DLD-1, and NCI-H292).[17,45–47] During the apoptosis induction on the NCI-H292 cells, the expression of Bcl family proteins was downregulated, ERK and p38 were activated, p38 MAPK and iNOS levels were augmented, and release of cytochrome c and AIF from the mitochondria into the cytosol occurred.[3,25]

Antichemoresistant Activities

Besides the remarkable antineoplastic activity, elemenes as well as the EtOAc and CH_2Cl_2 extracts of Yu Jin also displayed a prominent chemoresistance reversal property to restore the sensitivity of multidrug-resistant cancer cells to antitumor agents.[48,49] β-Elemene (**1**) in a noncytotoxic dose (4 or 6 μg/mL) partly reversed the drug resistance and amplified the sensitivity of the cancer cells to DOX via the obvious downregulation of Bcl-2 and P-gp expressions. By the resistance-reversing effect, β-elemene (**1**) markedly enlarged the DOX-promoted apoptotic death in drug-resistant K562/ADM leukemia cells and MCF-7/ADM breast carcinoma cells.[50,51] The anti-MDR effect of β-elemene (**1**) was also substantiated in cisplatin-resistant human ovarian cancer cells, whose synergistic effect was partly parallel with the enhancement of cell cycle G2/M arrest by downregulating the expressions of cyclin-B1 and CDC2 and elevating the levels of p53, p21waf1/cip1, p27kip1, and Gadd45 in the multidrug-resistant ovarian cancer cells.[52] When β-elemene (1) is combined with tetramethylpyrazine in noncytotoxic doses, the drug resistance reversal effect could be improved by 4.65-fold as well as the intracellular ADM concentration, and the cell apoptosis were amplified in the K562/Adr cells.[53] Also, β-elemene treatment markedly increased the intracellular accumulation of DOX and rhodamine 123 to enhance the efficacy of DOX in both drug-resistant K562/DNR leukemia cells and SGC7901/Adr gastric cancer cells and significantly inhibited P-gp expression via the downregulation of Akt phosphorylation and the significant upregulation of E3 ubiquitin ligases, c-Cbl and Cbl-b. Likewise, β-elemene (**1**) significantly enhanced the antitumor activity of DOX in nude mice xenografted with SGC7901/Adm.[54]

Chemosensitive Activity

β-Elemene (**1**) was able to augment the sensitivity of U87 glioblastoma cells to a chemotherapeutic temozolomide, whose anticancer and chemosensitizing effects could be synergistically enhanced by PD98059.[38] Through the downregulation of mTOR to lessen survivin and HIP-1α expressions, β-elemene (**1**) potentiated the radiosensitivity of A549 anoxic lung adenocarcinoma xenograft *in vivo*.[55,56] Therefore, β-elemene may be considered as a promising chemosensitizer and drug resistance reverser for adjuvant uses in cancer therapies.

Clinical Trials

Elemene injections have been extensively used in clinical practices in China for the treatment of malignant tumors. No serious side effects such as myelosuppression occurred during and after the elemene treatment.[57]

Treatments for Malignant Brain Tumors

Elemenes were intravenously infused (via subclavical vein or intermedian cubital vein or via carotid artery by a pump) to treat 23 patients with malignant brain tumors (13 primary tumors and 10 metastatic tumors). A total dose of 400–800 mg per day, 6–12 g for a therapeutic course, and two to three courses with an interval of 1–1.5 month were scheduled. After the treatment, the tumor size was decreased by 62.0% and the survival time was prolonged to 25.8 months, showing the overall effective rate of up to 74%.[58,59] In another trial, 19 (aged from 12–74 years old) patients with malignant brain cancer, including 16 cases of recurrent tumors, were administrated with elemenes by intraarterial perfusion, intravenous infusion, and/or local use. The results showed that the overall response rate was 68.42% (four cases of complete response and nine cases of partial response).[60] Eleven patients with multiple brain metastatic tumors were treated with elemenes, resulting in a satisfactory efficacy. Four had complete response and two had partial response with 12 months of a median survival time.[61] Consequently, the clinical trials proved that the continuously infused elemenes resulted in a significant effect in the treatment of malignant brain tumor, whose chemotherapy has the benefit of prolonged life and high-quality survival time for patients.[53]

Treatment for Rectal Carcinoma

A retention enema of an elemene emulsion in combination with 5-FU had been utilized in clinical treatments of 31 patients with rectal carcinoma in the late stage. The clinical trial resulted in obvious symptomatic improvement and marked tumor regression concomitant with the elimination of the 5-FU-caused side effects such as nausea, vomiting, leucopenia, and anorexia by elemene.[62]

Treatment for Malignant Ascites Tumor

A total of 55 patients with malignant ascites tumor initiated from different carcinomas (8 ovarian, 21 gastric, 16 rectal, 5 hepatocellular, and 2 pancreatic carcinomas and 3 unknown cancer origins) were treated by the i.p. administration of the elemene emulsion in an effective dose of 400 mg/m^2 body surface. The therapeutic effects to the carcinomas in ovarian, colorectal, and gastric ascites exhibited to be better than in the liver and pancreatic ascites. The average effective rates reached to 95.5%.[63]

Treatment for Malignant Pleurisy

Twenty-four patients with malignant pleurisy initiated from breast cancer pleural metastasis were in this clinical trial. After the aspiration in combination with systemic chemotherapy regimen, 300 mg elemene, which was diluted into 40 mL saline, was administrated by pleural infusion, resulting in a satisfactory effect.[64] Four hundred eighty-four patients with malignant effusions (including 171 peritoneal and 313 pleural effusions) were received in a prospective multicenter phase III clinical trial in China during 1994–1995. A 0.5% emulsion of elemene was administered in a dose of 200 mg/m^2 by intrapleural injection once per week for one to two weeks and a dose of 300–400 mg/m^2 by i.p. injection once or twice per week for two weeks. The response rate in patients with malignant pleural effusion was 77.6%, and in patients with peritoneal effusion, it was 66.1%, showing no toxicities in the bone marrow, the liver, the heart, and the kidney.[65] From 34 patients with massive malignant pleurisy in remedy with closed drainage and cisplatin injection, 17 patients had been randomly selected to receive additional elemene. The total effective rate increased to 94.1% in the patients who received additional elemene, compared to 88.2% of the patients received the cisplatin alone, implying that the elemene displayed positive synergistic action with cisplatin in the treatment of malignant pleurisy.[66]

Treatment for Bladder Cancer

For low toxicity and high effectiveness, β-elemene (**1**) has been used for the prevention and the remedy of the recurrence of superficial bladder cancer in clinics. The trial proved that β-elemene (**1**) was capable of restraining the growth of the bladder cancer cells and inducing the cell apoptosis by various mechanisms. The side effect such as urinary stimulus symptoms in superficial bladder cancer perfusion was much lower than that of other chemotherapeutic drugs.[67]

Structural Modification

The structural modification of β-elemene (**1**) has been extensively approached, giving several promising derivatives with intensively enhanced antitumor activity. A mixture of derivatives with 13-monoethyl amide or 13,14-diethyl amide were obtained from the modification of β-elemene (**1**), which at a dose of 100 μg/mL exerted 100% inhibition against the growth of HeLa cervical cancer cells.[68] If it is transferred to organometallic molecules, the produced β-elemene metal oxides demonstrated the augmented suppressive effect against the carcinoma cells such as HeLa, Raji, K562, and J6-2 lines.[69] If β-elemene is connected to amino acid, carboxylic acid, or pharmaceutically acceptable salts, the inhibitory effect of these derivatives were markedly improved against human HL-60 leukemia cells.[70]

Three more derivatives of β-elemene (**1**), assigned as 13,14-bis(*cis*-3,5-dimethyl-1-piperazinyl)-β-elemene (**7**), 13,14-bis[2-(2-thiophenyl)ethylamino]-β-elemene (**8**), and 13,14-bis (cyclohexamino)-β-elemene (**9**), exerted potent antiproliferative activity against human K562 (leukemia), HeLa (cervix), and SGC-7901 (stomach) tumor cell lines *in vitro* with the IG_{50} values of <5 μM. 13,14-Bis(*cis*-3,5-dimethyl-1-piperazinyl)-β-elemene (**7**) was one of the most potent derivatives in the antigrowth of leukemia cells.[71] Four piperazine derivatives of β-elemene, i.e., 13-(3-methyl-1-piperazinyl)-β-elemene (DX1) (**10**), 13-(*cis*-3,5-dimethyl-1-piperazinyl)-β-elemene (DX2), 13-(4-ethyl-1-piperazinyl)-β-elemene (DX3) (**11**), 13-(4-isopropyl-1-piperazinyl)-β-elemene (DX4), and 13-piperazinyl-β-elemene (DX5), exhibited the enhanced inhibitory effect against the growth of four types of human leukemia cell lines (HL-60, NB4, K562, and HP100-1) with IG_{50} values of <10 μM. The molecules with a secondary amino moiety, such as DX1, DX2, and DX5, showed to be more potent in inhibiting the growth and in augmenting the apoptosis of leukemia cells than DX3 and DX4. The apoptosis elicited by these β-elemene piperazine derivatives were associated with the decrease of c-FLIP levels and the generation of H_2O_2, then provoking the activation of both death receptor- and mitochondrial-mediated apoptotic pathways. The HL-60 leukemia cells were more sensitive to DX1 (**10**)-induced apoptosis than its H_2O_2-resistant HP100-1 cells.[72]

Two other antileukemia derivatives designed as N-(β-elemene-13-yl) tryptophan (ET) and N-(β-elemene-13-yl) tryptophan methyl ester (ETME) were created. The apoptotic mechanism of ET and ETME (**12**) was similarly associated with H_2O_2

generation, decrease of mitochondrial membrane potential, and activation of caspase-3 in the NB4 leukemia cells. Importantly, ETME (**12**) could synergistically enhance the therapeutic effect of arsenic trioxide (As_2O_3) in the treatment of acute promyelocytic leukemia.[73,74] Two groups of β-elemene monosubstituted amine derivatives and aromatic heterocyclic derivatives were created by the nucleophilic substitution. The antineoplastic activity of these derivatives were extensively improved to be superior to the parent molecule, β-elemene (**1**).[75,76] Especially, β-elemene-13-N-diethyl amine (**13**) showed the most potent cytotoxic activity against K562 and HeLa cells *in vitro* with IC_{50} values around 0.29 and 0.04 μM, respectively.[76] Accordingly, β-elemene (**1**) is a valuable drug lead for the development of more pharmaceutically effective agents with low toxicity and side effect. The approaches using structural modification techniques have been continued in China especially in recent years.

Nanoformulation

Two types of superparamagnetic nanoparticles were prepared with elemene showing the improvement of antitumor activity. In the *in vitro* experiments, the superparamagnetic nanoelemene at a concentration range from 2.5 to 25 mg/L significantly reduced the proliferation and the invasion of human HCT116 colorectal cancer cells in a dose-dependent manner via the down-expression of miR-155,[77] whereas the elemene superparamagnetic stealth nanoliposome at a concentraions of 2.5–10 mg/L diminished the proliferation and the invasion of human HEp-2 laryngeal cancer cells.[78] For the optimization of intravenous delivery, β-elemene-loaded nanostructured lipid carriers (NLCs) were designed and prepared by high-pressure homogenization method using glycerol monostearate as the solid lipid and a mixture of Maisine 35-1 and Labrafil M1944 CS as the liquid lipid. Compared to elemene injection, β-elemene-loaded NLCs showed markedly higher bioavailability and antitumor efficacy with less irritation and less toxic effects.[79] β-elemene-contained SLNs were formulated, whose optimized formulation was composed of monostearin and precirol ATO 5 at a mass ratio of 3:7, which was quite stable for 8 months at room temperature. After the intravenous administration of the SLN for 5 minutes, the levels of β-elemene were 1.5, 2.9, and 1.4 times higher than those of β-elemene emulsion in the liver, the spleen, and the kidney, respectively, and were 30% lower in the heart and the lung.[80] Therefore, the nanoformulations presented a promising advantage for using elemene in the cancer clinic treatment.

References

1. Yu, X. et al. 2008. Essential oil of *Curcuma wenyujin* induces apoptosis in human hepatoma cells. *World J. Gastroenterol.* 14: 4309–18.
2. Nie, X. H. et al. 2003. Effect of extraction techniques on the components and antitumor activity in vitro of volatile oil from *Curcuma wenyujin*. *Yaowu Shengwu Jishu* 10: 152–4.
3. Tang, C. C. et al. 2007. Chemical constituents of stems and leaves of *Curcuma wenyujin* and its anticancer activities. *Wenzhou Yixueyuan Xuebao* 37: 110–3.
4. Guo, Y. T. et al. 1983. Separation and identification of elemenes from the volatile oil of *Curcuma wenyujin*. *Zhongyao Tongbao* 8: 31.
5. Wang, X. W. et al. 1998. Elemene: Antineoplastic. *Drugs of the Future* 23: 266–70.
6. Wang, Z. M. et al. 2004. The role for lymphatic absorption path of elemene emulsion in lymphatic metastasis of the gastric cancer in progression. *Zhongguo Zhongliu Linchuang* 31: 1396–400.
7. Zhou, H. G. et al. 2000. Antitumor effects of elemene. *Zhongguo Zhongliu Linchang* 27: 392–4.
8. Hua, W. F. et al. 2006. Foundation and clinical research on antitumor effects of β-elemene. *Zhongyaocai* 29: 93–7.
9. Li, W. X. et al. 2002. Experimental observation on apoptosis induced by elemene in laryngeal neoplasm cells. *Shanghai Dier Yike Daxue Xuebao* 22: 306–8.
10. Sun, D. J. et al. 2001. Elemene induces apoptosis and regulates expression of bcl-2 protein in human hepatic cancer 7402 cells and cervix cancer Hela cells. *Fudan Xuebao, Yixue Kexueban* 28: 403–5.
11. Wang, G. et al. 2005. Antitumor effect of β-elemene in non-small-cell lung cancer cells is mediated via induction of cell cycle arrest and apoptotic cell death. *Cell. Mol. Life Sci.* 62: 881–93.
12. Huang, FC et al. 2003. Effects of apoptosis induced by β-elemene in colon cancer lovo cell line. *Fudan Xuebao, Yixueban* 30: 49–51.
13. Yang, H. et al. 1996. The antitumor activity of elemene is associated with apoptosis. *Zhongguo Zhongliu Zazhi* 18: 169–72.
14. Chen, H. et al. 2010. Effect of β-elemene on proliferation of human multiple myeloma cells. *Zhongchengyao* 32: 730–2.
15. Chen, Y. R. et al. 1998. Method for preparing β-elemene and its use in the treatment of cancer. *PCT Int. Appl.* WO 9846553 A1 19981022.
16. Xu, Y. H. et al. 2005. Influences of elemene on expression of Bcl-2 family genes in rat C6 glioma cells. *Zhonghua Yixue Zazhi* 85: 1700–3.
17. Wang, X. S. et al. 2006. The effect of δ-elemene on Hela cell lines by apoptosis induction. *Yakugaku Zasshi* 126: 979–90.
18. Gao, Z. H. et al. 2002. Influence of elemene or heat shock treatment upon the expression of membrane HSP70 and HSPs genes in HepG2 cells. *Chin. J. Immunol.* 18: 790–4.
19. Wu, W. Z. et al. 1999. The studies on the immuno-protective mechanism of β-elemene in the antitumor activity. *Zhonghua Zhongliu Zazhi* 21: 405–7.
20. Zhang, X. J. et al. 1999. The inference of elemene on the activity of r-DNA transcription. *Zhongguo Zhongliu Linchuang* 26: 443–4.
21. Sun, X. Y. et al. 2009. Potential anticancer activities of furanodiene, a sesquiterpene from *Curcuma wenyujin*. *Am. J. Chin. Med.* 37: 589–96.
22. Ba, Z. Z. et al. 2009. Potential anticancer activity of furanodiene. *Chin. J. Cancer Res.* 21: 154–8.
23. Zhong, Z. F. et al. 2012. Furanodiene, a natural product, inhibits breast cancer growth both in vitro and in vivo. *Cell. Physiol. Biochem.* 30: 778–90.
24. Zhong, Z. F. et al. 2014. Furanodiene, a natural small molecule suppresses metastatic breast cancer cell migration and invasion in vitro. *Eur. J. Pharmacol.* 737: 1–10.

25. Ma, E. L. et al. 2008. Induction of apoptosis by furanodiene in HL60 leukemia cells through activation of TNFR1 signaling pathway. *Cancer Lett.* 271: 158–66.
26. Xiao, Y. et al. 2007. Furanodiene induces G2/M cell cycle arrest and apoptosis through MAPK signaling and mitochondria-caspase pathway in human hepatocellular carcinoma cells. *Cancer Biol. Therap.* 6: 104450.
27. Huang, W. et al. 2008. Cytotoxic diterpenes from the root tuber of *Curcuma wenyujin*. *Helv. Chim. Acta* 91: 944–50.
28. Jin, H. F. et al. 2011. Influence of diterpenoid curcumrinol C from ether extract of radix Curcumae on human gastric cancer cell SGC-7901 in expression of caspase-9, 3, 7, and PARP (89KD). *Zhonghua Zhongyiyao Zazhi* 26: 395–8.
29. Jin, H. F. et al. 2010. Effect of diterpenoid C from radix Curcumae on proliferation of human gastric cancer cells SGC-7901. *Zhonghua Zhongyiyao Zazhi* 25: 783–6.
30. Jin, H. F. et al. 2011. Effect of diterpenoid curcumrinol C from ether extract of *Curcuma wenyujin* on proliferation of human colon cancer cells SW620. *Yiyao Daobao* 30: 160–3.
31. Shen, Y. et al. 2011. Apoptosis of human colon adenocarcinoma cell line SW620 induced by diterpenoid C from radix Curcumae and its related pathways. *Zhongguo Yaolixue Tongbao* 27: 396–401.
32. Wang, D. et al. 2008. Isolation and cytotoxic activity of compounds from the root tuber of *Curcuma wenyujin*. *Nat. Prod. Communicat.* 3: 861–4.
33. Huang, F. C. et al. 2004. Effect of elemene on the telomerase activity, apoptosis and cell cycles of the colon cancer LoVo cell line. *Yiyao Daobao* 23: 712–4.
34. Li, C. G. et al. 2004. Effects of β-elemene on transformation rate of phospholipid metabolism and cell membrane fluidity in human bladder carcinoma BIU-87 cells. *Zhonghua Yixue Zazhi* 84: 416–7.
35. Zhu, T. Z. et al. 2011. β-elemene inhibits proliferation of human glioblastoma cells through the activation of glia maturation factor β and induces sensitization to cisplatin. *Oncol. Reports* 26: 405–13.
36. Zhu, T. Z. et al. 2011. β-elemene inhibits proliferation of human glioblastoma cells and causes cell-cycle G0/G1 arrest via mutually compensatory activation of MKK3 and MKK6. *Intl. J. Oncol.* 38: 419–26.
37. Yao, Y. Q. et al. 2008. Antitumor effect of β-elemene in glioblastoma cells depends on p38 MAPK activation. *Cancer Lett.* 264: 127–34.
38. Zhu, T. Z. et al. 2014. β-Elemene inhibits proliferation through crosstalk between glia maturation factor β and extracellular signal-regulated kinase 1/2 and impairs drug resistance to temozolomide in glioblastoma cells. *Mol. Med. Reports* 10: 1122–1128.
39. Zhao, Y. S. et al. 2012. β-Elemene inhibits Hsp90/Raf-1 molecular complex inducing apoptosis of glioblastoma cells. *J. Neuro-Oncol.* 107: 307–14.
40. Yang, W. Z. et al. 2005. Study on inhibition of c-myc gene expression in human glioma U251 cell line by elemene and its mechanism on apoptosis. *Zhongguo Zhongliu Linchuang* 32: 763–6.
41. Tao, L. et al. 2006. Elemene displays anticancer ability on laryngeal cancer cells in vitro and in vivo. *Cancer Chemother. Pharmacol.* 58: 24–34.
42. Tao, L. et al. 2005. Inhibiting and proapoptotic effects of elemene on laryngeal carcinoma cells. *Zhongguo Linchuang Yaoxue Zazhi* 14: 148–52.
43. Feng, L. et al. 2005. Experimental study of elemene on BM and ECM in mice with Lewis lung cancer. *Zhongguo Zhongliu Linchuang* 32: 891–4.
44. Ying, J. et al. 2011. Induction of caspase-3-dependent apoptosis in human leukemia HL-60 cells by δ-elemene. *Yakugaku Zasshi* 131: 1383–94.
45. Ying, J. et al. 2011. Cell apoptosis induced by δ-elemene in lung carcinoma mucoepidermoid cells takes place via activation of the MAPKs pathway. *Asian J. Tradit. Med.* 6: 89–103.
46. Xie, C. Y. et al. 2011. B-cell lymphoma-2 over-expression protects δ-elemene-induced apoptosis in human lung carcinoma mucoepidermoid cells via a nuclear factor κB-related pathway. *Biol. Pharm. Bull.* 34: 1279–86.
47. Xie, C. Y. et al. 2009. Cell apoptosis induced by δ-elemene in colorectal adenocarcinoma cells via a mitochondrial-mediated pathway. *Yakugaku Zasshi* 129: 1403–13.
48. Yang, L. et al. 2011. Reversal of multidrug resistance in human breast cancer cells by *Curcuma wenyujin* and *Chrysanthemum indicum*. *Phytomed.* 18: 710–8.
49. Yang, L. et al. 2011. Reversal effects of traditional Chinese herbs on multidrug resistance in cancer cells. *Nat. Prod. Res.* 25: 1885–9.
50. Hao, L. H. et al. 2005. Study on mechanism of reversal effects of β-elemene on K562/ADM cells. *Zhongguo Zhongliu Linchuang* 32: 548–50.
51. Hu, J. et al. 2004. Reversal of resistance to adriamycin in human breast cancer cell line MCF-7/ADM by β-elemene. *Zhonghua Zhongliu Zazhi* 26: 268–70.
52. Li, X. et al. 2005. Antiproliferative effect of β-elemene in chemoresistant ovarian carcinoma cells is mediated through arrest of the cell cycle at the G2/M phase. *Cell. Mol. Life Sci.* 62: 894–904.
53. Hao, L. H. et al. 2005. Studies of tetramethylpyrazine in combination with β-elemene on apoptosis and reversal of multidrug resistance in K562/ADM cell line. *Zhongguo Zhongliu Linchuang* 32: 25–8, 33.
54. Zhang, Y. et al. 2013. The role of E3 ubiquitin ligase Cbl proteins in β-elemene reversing multi-drug resistance of human gastric adeno-carcinoma cells. *Intl. J. Mol. Sci.* 14: 10075–10089.
55. Li, G. Q. et al. 2012. Down-regulation of survivin and hypoxia-inducible factor-1α by β-elemene enhances the radiosensitivity of lung adenocarcinoma xenograft. *Cancer Biother. Radiopharm.* 27: 56–64.
56. Zou, K. et al. 2014. Down-regulation of mammalian target of rapamycin decreases HIF-1α and survivin expression in anoxic lung adenocarcinoma A549 cell to elemene and/or irradiation. *Tumor Biol.* 35: 9735–41.
57. Dou, P. G. et al. 2005. Antitumour activity of concentrated elemene injection in vitro. *J. Dalian Med. Univ.* 27: 421–3.
58. Tan, P. G. et al. 2001. Continuously infused elemene chemotherapy in treatment of malignant brain tumors. *Zhongguo Zhongliu Linchang* 28: 682–4.
59. Xu, Y. H. et al. 2005. Research status of elemene in the treatment of malignant brain tumors. *Zhonghua Shenjing Waike Jibing Yanjiu Zazhi* 4: 284–5.

60. Jusheng, H. et al. 1994. Elemene in the treatment of primary brain tumors. *Proc. 16th Int. Cancer Congress, Free Papers and Posters. New Delhi*, October 30–November 5, 1994, 2: 877–9.
61. Yinghui, X. et al. 1994. Intra-arterial perfusion of elemene in the treatment of multiple metastatic brain tumors. Rao, R. S. (ed.), *Proc. 16th Int. Cancer Congress, Free Papers and Posters. New Delhi*, October 30–November 5, 1994, 2: 881–3.
62. Pan, Q. X. et al. 1996. Short-term efficacy of elemene emulsion retention enema in treatment of late-stage rectal carcinoma. *Hunan Yixue* 13: 306.
63. Huang, L. M. et al. 1996. Effect of elemene to different malignant ascites. *Hunan Yixue* 13: 241.
64. Dong, Z. L. et al. 1996. Combined elemene chemotherapy in treatment of malignant pleurisy. *Hunan Yixue* 13: 307.
65. Wang, J. et al. 1996. Phase III clinical trial of elemenum emulsion in the management of malignant pleural and peritoneal effusions. *Zhonghua Zhongliu Zazhi* 18: 464–7.
66. Jiang, Y. J. et al. 1997. Closed drainage and elemene plus cisplatin intrapleural injection in treatment of malignant pleurisy. *Jiangsu Yiyao* 23: 218–9.
67. Shang, Y. H. et al. 2009. Progress of β-elemene in preventing recurrence of superficial bladder cancer. *J. Dalian Med. Univ.* 31: 215–8.
68. Cheng, G. B. et al. 1997. Preparation of nitrogen-functionalized β-elemene analogs as anticancer drugs. *Faming Zhuanli Shenqing Gongkai Shuomingshu* CN 1153167 A 19970702.
69. Cheng, B. G. et al. 1997. Elemene-metal complexes and as anticancer drugs. *Faming Zhuanli Shenqing Gongkai Shuomingshu* CN 1153158 A 19970702.
70. Huang, J. H. et al. 2006. Preparation of β-elemene amino or carboxylic acid derivatives as antitumor agents. *Faming Zhuanli Shenqing Gongkai Shuomingshu* CN 1008–1623 20060510.
71. Xu, L. Y. et al. 2006. The synthesis and anti-proliferative effects of β-elemene derivatives with mTOR inhibition activity. *Bioorg. Med. Chem.* 14: 5351–6.
72. Yu, Z. Y. et al. 2011. β-Elemene piperazine derivatives induce apoptosis in human leukemia cells through downregulation of c-FLIP and generation of ROS. *Plos One* 6: e15843.
73. Yu, Z. Y. et al. 2010. Study on mechanism of β-elemene derivative (ET) inducing NB4 cell apoptosis. *Zhongguo Zhongyao Zazhi* 35: 1324–7.
74. Yu, Z. Y. et al. 2008. N-(β-Elemene-13-yl)tryptophan methyl ester induces apoptosis in human leukemia cells and synergizes with arsenic trioxide through a hydrogen peroxide dependent pathway. *Cancer Lett.* 269: 165–73.
75. Xu, L. Y. et al. 2006. Synthesis of substituted β-elemene derivatives and determination of their activity as antitumor agents. *Zhongguo Yaowu Huaxue Zazhi* 16: 277–80.
76. Liu, G. F. et al. 2007. Synthesis and in vitro antitumor activity of β-elemene monosubstituted amine derivatives. *Zhongguo Yaoke Daxue Xuebao* 38: 396–9.
77. Fan, Y. et al. 2013. Effects of superparamagnetic nano elemene on proliferation and invasion and microRNA-155 expression of human colorectal cancer cells. *Zhonghua Shiyan Waike Zazhi* 30: 2593–5.
78. Fan, Y. et al. 2014. Effects of elemene superparamagnetic stealth liposomes on clone formation and invasion of cancer Hep-2 cells. *Zhonghua Shiyan Waike Zazhi* 31: 619–620.
79. Shi, F. et al. 2012. Formulation design, preparation, and in vitro and in vivo characterizations of β-elemene-loaded nanostructured lipid carriers. *Intl. J. Nanomed.* 8: 2533–41.
80. Wang, Y. Z. et al. 2005. Characterization and body distribution of β-elemene solid lipid nanoparticles (SLN). *Drug develop. Indust. pharmacy* 31: 769–78.

116 Chuan Xiong 川芎

Szechuan lovage

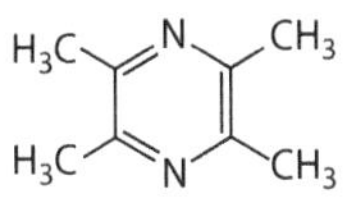

Herb Origination

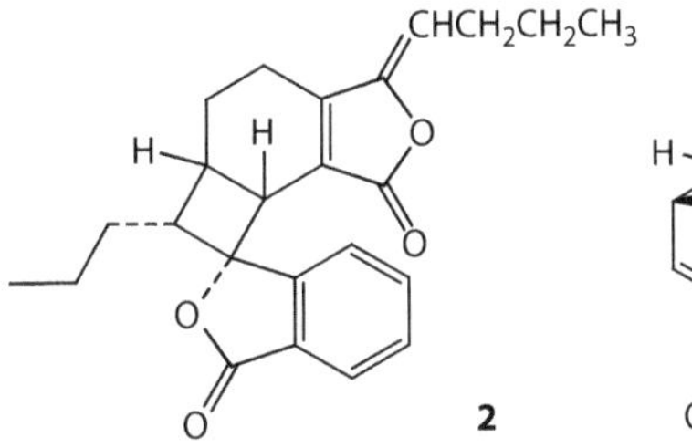

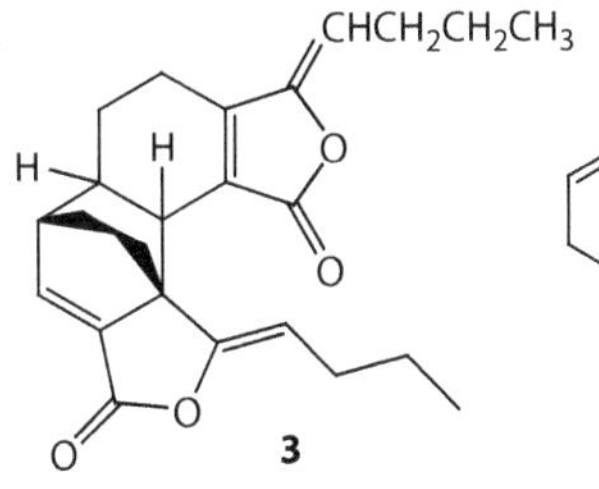

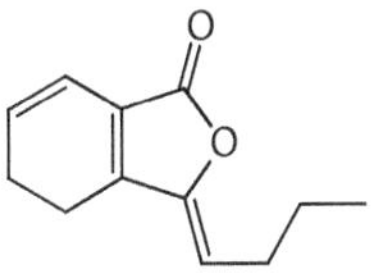

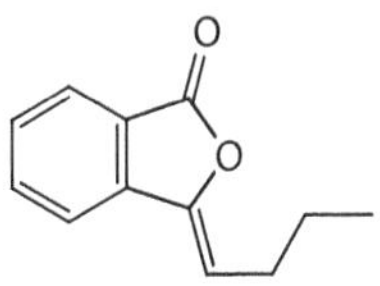

The herb Chuan Xiong (Szechuan lovage) is the dried rhizomes of an Umberlliferae plant, *Ligusticum chuanxiong* (= *L. wallichii*). Its rhizomes and roots are generally collected in early summer and dried in mild heat. Today, this perennial plant is cultivated in many places, and the Sichuan province in China is the major producing place of the herb.

Antitumor Activities and Constituents

Tetramethylpyrazine

The herb Chuan Xiong contains an important bioactive principle tetramethylpyrazine (TTMP) (**1**) which is a calcium channel blocker. In both *in vitro* and *in vivo* models, TTMP (**1**) dose-dependently suppressed the proliferation and the growth of human HepG2 hepatoma cells associated with the induction of apoptosis and autophagy in the HepG2 cells.[1] The TTMP treatment restrained the proliferation of osteosarcoma cell lines (MG-63, SAOS-2, and U2OS) in a dose-dependent manner and markedly induced the apoptosis and the G0/G1 arrest in the MG-63 cells via the down-expression of nuclear NF-κB p65, BCL-2 and cyclin-D1 and the up-expression of cytosolic NF-κB. The antiosteosarcoma activity was also demonstrated in nude mice with a low toxicity after the i.p. injection of TTMP at a dose of 100 mg/kg every other day for 28 days.[2] Besides the suppressive effect against the growth of human HL-60 myelocyte leukemia cells and K562 erythroleukemia cells, TTMP (**1**) importantly displayed marked ability in the reversal of MDR in some multidrug-resistant carcinoma cells and blockage of cancer metastasis. Through the increase of the intracellular concentration of DNR (an antitumor agent), TTMP (**1**) enhanced the sensitivity of multidrug-resistant HL-60/HT leukemia cells to DNR. In the combination with verapamil (a calcium channel blocker), the synergic treatment of TTMP (**1**) markedly reversed the MDR of the HL-60/HT cells.[3,4] Also, TTMP (**1**) could effectively reverse the MDR of hepatoma Bel-7402/Adr cells and ADR-resistant Ehrlich ascites cancer (EAC) cells, and augmented the cytotoxicity and the chemosensitivity of Adm in these multidrug-resistant cancer cells. Its anti-MDR mechanism was found to be related to the decrease of both mRNA and protein levels of multidrug-resistant genes, MDR1, MRP2, MRP3, and MRP5.[5–8] In addition, GST activity of Adm-resistant EAC was reduced by 26.05% after the administration of TTMP, whose action might partly contribute to the inhibition of drug resistance.[6,7] However, TTMP (**1**) had no reversal effect on cisplatin-induced drug resistance in human 3Ao/Cddp epithelial ovarian cancer cell line.[8] Moreover, the treatment of TTMP combined with As_2O_3 could exert significant effects on the proliferative inhibition of the HL-60 cells. During the inhibition, TTMP (300 μg/mL) synergistically potentiated the As_2O_3 (0.5 μM)-induced differentiation of HL-60 cells, associated with regulating the expressions and the activities of the factors related to G0/G1 phase arrest.[9]

In vivo experiments truly demonstrated that TTMP (**1**) was effective in the antimetastatic effect, where TTMP (**1**) elicited the suppressive effect on the pulmonary metastasis of mouse hepatoma cells.[10] The oral administration of TTMP (**1**) at a dose of 20 mg/kg per day to a mouse model for 18 days obviously diminished the pulmonary metastasis of B16-F10 melanoma, and the pulmonary metastasis nodules were significantly lessened from 134 to 72. A large dose of TTMP also exerted the inhibitory effect on biosynthesis of DNA, RNA, and protein in the B16-F10 cells in a dose-dependent manner.[9] The antimetastatic and multidrug-resistant reversal activities of TTMP (**1**) were found to be probably attributed to its abilities in diminishing the surface activity and the adhesion of carcinoma cells.[11,12] Also, the TTMP (**1**) treatment stimulated the lymphocyte proliferation response and potentiated NK cell activity in both normal mice and B16 melanoma-bearing mice.[12,13]

In addition, another inhibitory property of TTMP (**1**) was found against the growth of fibrocyte, suggesting that TTMP (**1**) can be used to retard the fibrocyte proliferation caused by radiotherapeutic treatment.[14] Two phthalides, levistolide-A (**3**) and Z,Z′-6,8′,7,3′-diligustilide (**2**), isolated from the Chuan Xiong, significantly abrogated platelet-derived growth factor (PDGF-BB)-activated proliferation in both rat and human hepatic satellites cell lines possibly through induction of cell cycle arrest and apoptosis, indicating that the phthalides may be potential antifibrotic drugs for the treatment and the prevention of hepatic fibrosis and liver carcinogenesis.[15]

Essential Oil

The essential oil from the rhizomes of *L. chuanxiong* and its two major components identified as Z-ligustilide (**4**) and butylidene phthalide (**5**) displayed significant cytotoxic and apoptosis-inducing activities for all three tested MCF-7 (breast), HeLa (cervix), and SK-Hep-1 (liver) cell lines, in a concentration-dependent manner.[16]

Polysaccharide

The Chuan Xiong polysaccharide obviously showed the anti-proliferative and antiviability effects on human hepatoma HepG2 cells *in vitro* and also induced the cell apoptosis by arresting the tumor cells in the G1 phase. At a concentration of 1 mg/mL, the inhibitory rate could reach 54.7% in the HepG2 cells.[17]

Other Bioactivities

The herb Chuan Xiong (Szechuan lovage) and its major component, tetramethylpyrazine (**1**), demonstrated multiple biological responses in pharmacological experiments, such as coronary, cardiotonic, hypotensive, brain, and kidney blood flow-increasing, lung and brain vasodilative, microcirculation-promoting, anti-myocardial ischemia, antianoxemia, antiplatelet aggregation, and immunopotentiating effects.

References

1. Cao, J. et al. 2015. Tetramethylpyrazine (TMP) exerts antitumor effects by inducing apoptosis and autophagy in hepatocellular carcinoma. *Intl. Immuno-pharmacol.* 26: 212–20.
2. Wang, Y. et al. 2013. Tetramethylpyrazine inhibits osteosarcoma cell proliferation via downregulation of NF-κB in vitro and in vivo. *Mol. Med. Reports* 8: 984–8.
3. Liang, R. et al. 1998. Inhibition of tetramethylpyrazine on HL-60 K562 leukemia cell lines. *Disi Junyi Daxue Xuebao* 19: 108–9.
4. Liang, R. et al. 1998. The expression of Bcl-xL in drug resistant leukemia K562/VCR cells. *Disi Junyi Daxue Xuebao* 19: 385.
5. Wang, X. B. et al. 2010. Inhibition of tetramethylpyrazine on P-gp, MRP2, MRP3 and MRP5 in multidrug resistant human hepatocellular carcinoma cells. *Oncol. Reports* 23: 211–5.
6. Hu, Y. P. et al. 1993. Tetramethylpyrazine and verapamil reverse the multidrug resistance of driamycin in mouse Ehrlich ascites tumor. *Yaoxue Xuebao* 28: 75–8.
7. Xie, Z. F. et al. 1993. Effect of tetramethylpyrazine and hydroxyurea on the inhibition of DNA synthesis by doxorubicin in K562 cell line. *Zhonghua Yixue Zazhi* 73: 559–60.
8. Chen, J. L. et al. 2000. Mechanism of drug resistance and reversal with ligustrazine and cyclo-sporin A in cisplatin-induced human epithelial ovarian cancer resistant cell line 3Ao/cDDP. *Chin. J. Cancer Res.* 12: 197–203.
9. Wu, Y. N. et al. 2012. Tetramethylpyrazine potentiates arsenic trioxide activity against HL-60 cell lines. *Braz. J. Med. Biol. Res.* 45: 187–96.
10. Li, X. T. et al. 1980. Several blood circulation promoting herbs inhibit the lung metastases of mouse hepatoma cells. *Zhongyi Zazhi* 21: 75.
11. Liu, J. R. et al. 1993. Anti-matastatic activity and mechanism of tetramethylpyrazine. *Zhongguo Yaolixue yu Dulixue Zazhi* 7: 149–52.
12. Liu, J. R. et al. 1995. The response of mouse spleen lymphocyte proliferation by tetramethylpyrazine. *J. Huaxi Med. Univ.* 26: 177–9.
13. Zhang, S. W. et al. 1990. The radiosensitization and radioprotection of Chuanxiong. *Zhongxiyi Jiehe Zazhi* 10: 697–8.
14. Chen, X. Z. et al. 1987. The inhibitory effect of *Salvia miltorrhiza* and tetramethylpyrazine on the growth of fibroblasts in vitro. *Zhongxiyi Jiehe Zazhi* 7: 547–8, 518.
15. Lee, T. F. et al. 2007. Studies on antiproliferative effects of phthalides from *Ligusticum chuanxiong* in hepatic stellate cells. *Planta Med.* 73: 527–34.
16. Shin, S. Y. 2011. Study on cytotoxic activities of the essential oil compounds from *Ligusticum chuanxiong* against some human cancer strains. *Yakhak Hoechi* 55: 398–403.
17. Wang, J. C. et al. 2014. Influence of Chuanxiong polysaccharide on proliferation and apoptosis of human hepatoma cell HepG2. *Nanjing Zhongyiyao Daxue Xuebao* 30: 461–4.

117 Zhen Zhu Cai 珍珠菜

Gooseneck loosestrife

1. $R_1 = -S_1$, $R_2 = -OH$, $R_3 = R_4 = -H$
2. $R_1 = -S_3$, $R_2 = -OH$, $R_3 = R_4 = -H$
3. $R_1 = -S_2$, $R_2 = =O$, $R_3 = R_4 = -H$
4. $R_1 = -S_3$, $R_2 = =O$, $R_3 = R_4 = -H$
5. $R_1 = -S_3$, $R_2 = -OH$, $R_3 = R_4 = -OAc$
6. $R_1 = -S_4$, $R_2 = -OH$, $R_3 = R_4 = -H$

S_1 = -Ara-[(2-1)-Glu]-(4-1)-Glu
S_2 = -Ara-[(2-1)-Glu]-(4-1)-Glu-(2-1)-Rham
S_3 = -Ara-[(2-1)-Glu]-(4-1)-Glu-(2-1)-Xyl
S_4 = -Ara-[(2-1)-Glu-6-Ac]-(4-1)-Glu-(2-1)-Rham
Ara: arabinopyanosyl, Glu: glucopyranosyl, Rham: rhamnopyranosyl, Xyl: xylopyranosyl

7

Herb Origination

The herb Zhen Zhu Cai (Gooseneck loosestrife) originated from a Primulaceae plant of *Lysimachia clethroides*. This perennial herbaceous plant is native of China, Korea, and Japan. The whole plant and its roots are normally collected in autumn and dried in the sun for Chinese medical utilization. The herb also can be used fresh annually.

Antitumor Activities

Zhen Zhu Cai extract was evidenced to possess obvious antineoplastic potentials by both *in vitro* and *in vivo* investigations. Its antileukemia effect was proven in human K562 erythroleukemia cells (IC_{50}: 39.87 μg/mL, 48 h) *in vitro* and in mouse L1210 leukemia cells *in vivo* with a 45% inhibitory rate.[1] Different organic solvent partitioned fractions from the extract showed the suppressive effect against sarcoma 180 in a mouse model. Its EAF and n-butanol fraction exerted relatively greater antiproliferative effect on mouse sarcoma 180 and human K562 and HL-60 leukemia cell lines.[2] Also, Zhen Zhu Cao extract was capable of reversing the DNA-inhibitory effect of CTX in the bone marrow, indicating that the herb may protect the bone marrow from CTX toxicity.[3]

Antitumor Constituents and Activities

Biological assay-combined phytochemistry investigations revealed that the flavonoids and triterpene saponins are the major antitumor active components in Zhen Zhu Cao. These components play important roles in suppressing the growth of multiple types of cancer cells. Their anticarcinoma potency cannot compare to the current chemotherapeutic drugs but show no obvious side effect. The evidences described in the following provided the scientific support for using the herb in the alternative treatment of cancer patients.

Flavonoids

In vitro morphological studies demonstrated that the total flavonoids significantly restrained the proliferation of SMMC-7721 hepatoma, HeLa cervical cancer, and leukemia (L615, K562 and HL-60) cell lines by the stimulation of apoptosis.[4–7] The antileukemia effect of the total flavonoids were associated with causing G2/M cell cycle arrest, directly damaging DNA, and interfering some related proteins synthesis in the HL-60 cells.[7] When the apoptosis occurred in K562 cells and SMMC-7721 cells by the flavonoids, Bcl-2 expression was markedly downregulated while the expressions of Fas, TRAIL, and DR5 were upregulated.[6,8] The results suggested that the apoptosis promotion should be an important anticancer mechanism for the flavonoids.

Daily i.p. administration of the flavonoid principles in a dose of 273 mg/kg for 7 continuous days inhibited the growth of W256 Walker sarcoma by 45.2% in rats. When the i.p. injection dose was 62.5 mg/kg per day for 10 days, the growth of carcinoma cells were obviously obstructed in mice, whose inhibitory rates were in a range of 46.7–58.3% against mouse L1 hypodermic tumor, sarcoma 180, U14 cervical cancer, hepatoma 22, and Ehrlich tumor cells. The flavonoids were also notably effective in the suppression of mouse ascetic primary reticulum cell sarcoma and the life span prolongation in mice by 63.6%.[3–6] The inhibitory rates were 57.8% against rat H22 hepatoma cells at a dose of 200 mg/kg and 49.9% against mouse U14 cervical cancer cells at a dose of 400 mg/kg.[5,7] After the i.p. administration of the total flavonoids in a daily dose of 500 mg/kg for 6 days into mice preinoculated with L615 leukemia, the mean survival time of the tested mice was outstandingly extended to 260.7%.[4]

The antineoplastic effects of the total flavonoids labeled as ZE4 were also evidenced by *in vivo* experiments with nude mouse models. Intragastric (i.g.)-adminstered ZE4 (200 mg/kg, per day) for 21 days notably restrained human Bel-7402 hepatoma cells by 52.1% and obviously attenuated the MVD in nude mice,[9,10] while i.p.-injected ZE4 (200 mg/kg, every other day) to the tested nude mice for 21 days significantly suppressed human HL-60 leukemia xenografts by 51.32% and lessened the expressions of Ki-67 and CD34 (a vascular endothelial cell membrane antigen).[11] Similarly, ZE4 was administered in doses of 100 and 200 mg/kg/day, resulting in the inhibitory rates of 44.57% and 48.32%, respectively, in nude mice implanted with human HeLa cervical cancer, together with the upregulation of p53, p21, and Bax expressions and the reduction of CD34 expression level.[12] The *in vivo* tests established that the antigrowth effect the total flavonoids (ZE4) was also correlated with the antiangiogenetic activity against the carcinoma cells.

Recently, 15 flavonoids have been isolated and identified from the total flavonoids, such as prunin, rutin, kaempferol, quercetin, isoquercitrin, dihydrokaempferol, naringenin, eriodictyol, quercetin-3-*O*-(2,6-dirhamnoosylglucoside), isorhamnetin-3-*O*-β-D-rutinoside, kaempferol-7-*O*-β-D-glucoside, kaempferol-3-*O*-β-D-rutinoside, kaempferol-3-*O*-(2,6-dirhamnosylglucoside), and (–)-epicatechin.[6,13] Some of them have been reported to exert moderate to weak anticarcinogenic effects in the experiments, showing potential for further development to be used as supplements in the cancer prevention.

Triterpenoid Saponins

The total saponins of Zhen Zhu Cai has been patented as a medicinal product for cancer treatment, especially for hepatoma.[14] *In vitro* experiments showed that the exposure of the total saponins in concentrations of ~100 μg/mL could reach the maximum inhibition rates to 91.92% in SMMC-7721 hepaoma cells, 81.98% in MCF-7 breast cancer cells, 73.94% in HeLa cervical cancer cells, and 34.16% in Caco-2 colon cancer cells. The oral administration of the total saponins to tumor-bearing mice in three doses of 100, 200, and 400 mg/kg for 10 days resulted in a marked effect with >30% inhibitory rate against the proliferation of cancer cells and exhibited 57.8% antihepatoma effect in a dose of 200 mg/mL. Also, the saponins were capable of blocking the metastasis of neoplastic cells to lung.[14,15]

Several oleanane-type triterpenoid saponins with 13β,28-epoxy were isolated from Zhen Zhu Cai, and seven of them showed antineoplastic property. Ardisianoside-E (**1**), lysikokianoside-1 (**2**), and clethroidoside-C (**3**), clethroidoside-D (**4**), clethroidoside-F (**5**) displayed moderate cytotoxic activity on human A549 (lung), HepG2 (liver), HT-29 (colon), BGC-823 (gastric), and A375 (skin) carcinoma cell lines, *in vitro* (IC_{50}: of 0.75–2.62 μM). Clethroidoside-E (**6**) selectively exerted the cytotoxic effect against the BGC-823, HepG2, and HT-29 cell lines (IC_{50}s: of 8.05, 6.26, and 1.4 μM, respectively).[16] At low concentrations between 0.05 and 0.1 μg/mL, Lclet 4 (another oleanane-type 13β,28-epoxy triterpene saponoside) and mitoxantrone showed no cytotoxic and/or proapoptotic effect on human DU-145 prostate cancer cells.[17,18] But the cocktails of the two agents could exert synergistic proapoptotic and antiinvasive effects on DU-145 cells, accompanied by the activation of caspase-3 and caspase-7 and the inhibition of MMP expression.[17]

Ecdysteroid Analog

An ecdysteroid compound (**7**) was extracted from *L. clethroides*, demonstrating the inhibitory effect against ovarian cancer cell proliferation with low toxicity *in vitro*.[19]

Other Medical Uses

The herb Zhen Zhu Cao (Gooseneck loosestrife) has been employed in China as a folk medicine to treat edema, jaundice diseases, hepatitis, and inflammations besides tumors.

References

1. Zhang, W. et al. 2007. Studies on the antileucemiaeffects of the extract from *Lysmachia clethroides* duby. *Antiinfect Pharm.* 4: 62–5.
2. Xu, X. Y. et al. 2003. Primary studies on the antitumor effect of *Lysimachia clethroides* extracts. *Chin. Wild Plant Resources* (2): 31–4.
3. Chinese Hankou Hospital of Hupei Air Force. (a) 1977. *Xinyixue* 8: 112; (b) 1999. *Chinese Materia Medica.* Vol. 6, 6–5359, 97. Shanghai Science and Technology Press, Shanghai, China.
4. Chinese Hankou Hospital of Hupei Air Force. 1981. Experimental study on the effect of a flavonoid preparation from *Lysimachia clethroides* on L615 leukemia. *Xinyixue* 12: 293–4.
5. Tang, L. H. et al. 2009. Effect of *Lysimachia clethroides* Duby extract to liver cancer. *Zhongcaoyao* 40: 108–11.
6. Liu, Y. L. et al. 2010. Growth inhibitory and apoptosis inducing by effects of total flavonoids from *Lysimachia clethroides* Duby in human chronic myeloid leukemia K562 cells. *J. Ethnopharmacol.* 131: 1–9.
7. Tang, L. H. et al. 2007. Study on apoptosis of HL-60 cell line induced by total flavones *Lysimachia clethroides* Duby. *J. Shanghai Univ. TCM* 21: 54–7.
8. Tang, L. H. et al. 2010. Induction of apoptosis of SMMC-7721 by ZE4 extracted from *Lysimachia clethroides. Shanghai J. TCM* 44: 58–62.
9. Wang, Y. Q. et al. 2007. Primary studies on the anti-uterine cervix cancer effects of the extract ZE4 from *Lysmachia clethroides* Duby. *Chin. Pharmacol. Bull.* 23: 925–7.
10. Wang, L. et al. 2012. Inhibition of antitumor effective part ZE4 from *Lysimachia clethroides* Duby on Bel-7402 cell xenografted hepatoma in nude mice. *Chin. J. Pharmacol. Toxicol.* 26: 635–40.
11. Yang, N. et al. 2013. Effect of total flavonoids from *Lysimachia clethroides* Duby on human leukemia HL-60 cell xenograft in nude mice. *Jiangsu Yiyao* 39: 1120–3.
12. Zhang, Q. Q. et al. 2012. Inhibitory effect of total flavonoids from *Lysimachia clethroides* Duby (ZE4) on xenograft human cervical cancer in nude mice. *Chin. Pharmacol. Bull.* 28: 204–8.
13. Wu, W. et al. 2011. Chemical constituents of antitumor active fraction of *Lysimachia clethroides. Zhongcaoyao* 42: 38–41.
14. Tang, L. H. et al. 2008. Application of total saponins of *Lysimachia clethroides* in preparation of medicine for treating tumor. *Faming Zhuanli Shenqing* CN 2007–10191737 20071214.
15. Tang, L. H. et al. 2008. Application of total saponins of *Lysimachia clethroides* in preparation of medicine for treating tumor. *Faming Zhuanli Shenqing* CN 101199563 A 20080618.
16. Liang, D. et al. 2011. Cytotoxic triterpenoid saponins from *Lysimachia clethroides. J. Nat. Prods.* 74: 2128–36.
17. Lclet4: 3-*O*-β-D-glucopyranosyl-(1–2)-[α-L-rhamnopyranosyl-(1–2)-β-D-glucopyranosyl-(1–4)-]-α-L-arabinopyranosylproto primulagenin-A.
18. Koczurkiewicz, P. et al. 2013. Lclet 4 enhances pro-apoptotic and anti-invasive effects of mitoxantrone on human prostate cancer cells—In vitro study. *Acta Biochimica Polonica* 60: 331–8.
19. Xuan, H. C. et al. 2015. Ecdysteroid compound capable of inhibiting ovarian cancer cell proliferation, pharmaceutical composition, preparation method and application. *Faming Zhuanli Shenqing* CN 104693261 A 20150610.

118 Hu Zhang 虎杖

Giant knotweed

1. $R_1 = -CH_3, R_2 = -OH$
5. $R_1 = -CH_2OH, R_2 = -H$
6. $R_1 = -COOCH, R_2 = -H$

2. $R_1 = R_2 = -H$
3. $R_1 = -H$, R_2 = –beta-D-glucoside
4. $R_1 = R_2 = -OCH_3$

7

Herb Origination

The herb Hu Zhang (Giant knotweed) is the dried roots and rhizomes of a Polygonaceae plant, *Polygonum cuspidatum*. The herbaceous plant is native to eastern Asia (in China, Japan, and Korea), and it is also distributed in Europe and North America. As a Chinese herb, the rhizomes are collected in spring and autumn and dried in the sun for folk medicinal treatment. It also can be used fresh.

Antitumor Constituents and Activities

The decoction of Hu Zhang showed 35.3–37.2% suppressive effect against mouse ascites carcinoma.[1] The ethyl acetate extract of the roots of *P. cuspidatum* exhibited a significant inhibition of STAT3 activity (100% of inhibition at its 40 μg/mL concentration). The inhibition of STAT3 transcription activity has been demonstrated to increase the apoptotic rate and to retard the proliferation of tumor cells. In Hu Zhang, anthraquinones, stilbenes, and quinones are the major components responsible for various biological activities, including anticarcinogenesis and antitumor. The contents of emodin, resveratrol, and resveratrol glucoside are 3.38%, 1.75%, and 4.8%, respectively, in Hu Zhang.

Emodin

Emodin (**1**), a major principle in the herb, is a strong inhibitor of protein tyrosine kinse (p561ck), whose potency is greater than those of emodin-8-*O*-D-β-glucoside and emodin methyl ester.[2] When the administration of emodin (**1**) is done by oral or subcutaneous/i.p. injection to tumor-implanted mice, the growth inhibitory effects were notably shown against sarcoma 180, hepatoma, lymphoma, breast adenocarcinoma, melanoma, and Ehrlich ascites tumor with the suppressive rates of 30–52%.[3] By blocking DNA and RNA syntheses, emodin (**1**) exerted the cytotoxicity in human HL-60 promyelocytic leukemic cells *in vitro*.[4] Moreover, further experiments demonstrated that emodin (**1**) has a marked ability to restrain tyrosine kinase-mediated phosphorylation of VEGFRs in human HCT-116 colon cancer cells. The treatment with 40 μM of emodin (**1**) could reduce the relative activities of VEGFR-1, VEGFR-2, and VEGFR-3 by 22.4%, 58.5%, and 31.6%, respectively. Concurrently, emodin (**1**) blocked the HCT116 cell cycle at G2/M phase and dose-dependently promoted cell apoptosis.[5] But it displayed weak cytotoxic effect in human A549 (lung), SKOV-3 (ovary), HepG2 (liver), and HT-29 (colon) carcinoma cell lines.[6] These results designated that emodin (**1**) may be used as an adjuvant inhibitor for certain types of tumor growth and angiogenesis. In addition, emodins (**1**) as well as the water extract of Hu Zhang could markedly obstruct the mutagenicity of 1-nitropyrene DNA adducts in *Salmonella typhimurium* TA98.[7]

Resveratrol

Resveratrol (**2**) is also highly enriched in grapes, peanuts, red wine, and other food sources, but it is also contained within the roots and the fruits of Hu Zhang as a natural phytoalexin. Up to now, numerous studies revealed that resveratrol has a remarkable ability to suppress the proliferation of a wide variety of tumor cell lines, including lymphoid and myeloid cancers, multiple myeloma, head and neck SCC, and other solid carcinomas in the breast, the ovary, the prostate, the cervix, the thyroid, the stomach, the colon, the pancreas, and the skin.[8–10] Including 1.2% or 3.6% crude resveratrol extract in a diet for 27 weeks significantly lowered the azoxymethane (AOM)-induced formation of aberrant crypt foci by 40–42%. The dietary intake of 1.2% resveratrol extract daily of mice for 37 weeks lessened the number of AOM-induced tumors per colon by 61% and diminished the percentage of mice with colon tumor by 49%. Similarly, the percentage of mammary carcinogenesis caused by DMBA in rats was attenuated by 44% when 1% resveratrol extract is added to the diet to female rats for 23 weeks.[11]

In *in vitro* experiments, resveratrol (**2**) retarded the proliferation of human MCF-7 breast cancer cells at S/G2/M phase[12] and also showed abilities to reverse MDR, exerting obvious inhibition on Adm-resistant MCF-7 cells.[10] The proliferation of human SGC7901 gastric cancer cells could be suppressed by resveratrol (**2**) concomitantly with the dose-dependent induction of the cell apoptosis through a PI3K/Akt signal pathway including downregulated Bcl-2 and p-Akt protein expressions and upregulated Bax and caspase-3.[13] The antitumor effects of resveratrol on human colorectal cancer cell lines (HCT116 and LoVo) were associated with the attenuation of Wnt/β-catenin signaling and MALAT1 expression and the inhibition of its target genes such as c-Myc and MMP-7. These elicited events also led to the suppression of colorectal cancer cell invasion and metastasis.[14] Through the strong blockage of DNA synthesis and the promotion of apoptosis, resveratrol (**2**) at doses of 2.5 and 10 mg/kg notably obstructed the tumor volume and size and the metastasis to the lung by 42–56% in mice bearing highly metastatic LLC. Besides the antineoplastic and anticarcinogenic activities, resveratrol (**2**) also has the abilities to suppress the angiogenesis of HUVEC *in vitro*, associated with the blockage of VEGF binding to HUVEC at 10–100 μmol/L concentrations, and it obstructed the tumor-induced neovascularization at doses of 2.5 and 10 mg/kg in an animal model.[15–17] Moreover, a combined treatment with resveratrol (**2**) and curcumin was found to exert a synergistic antiproliferative effect in colon carcinoma cells and hepatoma cells. The apoptosis of Hepal-6 hepatoma cells promoted by resveratrol plus curcumin was accompanied by the upregulation of intracellular ROS level, the downregulation of XIAP and survivin expressions, and the activation of caspase-3, caspase-8, and caspase-9.[18] Accordingly, the findings provided important preclinical evidences supporting the future development of resveratrol (**2**) in chemoprevention, chemotherapy, antiangiogenesis, and antimetastasis toward the malignant tumor disease. In addition, a technique of magnetic orcinol-imprinted poly(ethylene-co-vinyl alcohol) composite particles could not only improve the extraction of resveratrol (**2**) from the herb but also enhance the delivery of resveratrol to the tested HOS cells, resulting in an efficient suppressive effect.[19]

Other Stilbenes

Resveratrol-3-*O*-β-D-glucoside (**3**), a bioactive agent in Hu Zhang, was significantly effective in terms of adhesion and invasion on four colorectal neoplastic cell lines (HR8348, Hce8693, HT29, and LoVo) *in vitro* at a concentration of 3.2 mmol/L. The adhesion inhibition rate was 67.6–78.8%, and the invasion inhibition rate was 82.7–92.7%. Also, the PKC activity was diminished by resveratrol-3-*O*-β-D-glucoside (**3**) at the same concentration with an inhibition rate of 35.1–49.6%. The results implied that the antiadhesion and antiinvasive functions of resveratrol-3-*O*-β-D-glucoside is probably mediated through the inhibition of PKC in the colorectal carcinoma cells.[20]

3,4′-Dimethoxy-5-hydroxystilbene (**4**) was derived from the structural modification of resveratrol-3-*O*-β-glucoside (**3**) by methylation and acid hydrolysis. 3,4′-Dimethoxy-5-hydroxystilbene (**4**) could activate the expression of Bax and caspases and then promote human HL-60 promyelocytic leukemic cells to apoptotic death.[21]

Other Quinones

Other quinone analogs assigned as 2-methoxystypandrone (**5**), aloe emodin (**6**), and rhein (**7**) were effective in the inhibition of three human breast cancer cell lines (MDA-MB-453, MDA-MB-468, and MDA-MB-231), where 2-methoxystypandrone (**5**) showed the stronger inhibitory activity against the proliferation of human breast cells (IC_{50}: 2.7–7.8 μM) and induced the cell death more potently in the MDA-MB-231 and MDA-MB-468 cell lines (which contain constitutively activated STAT3) as compared to MDA-MB-453 cells (which lack aberrant STAT3 activation). Thus, the findings revealed that the anti-breast-cancer effect of 2-methoxystypandrone (**5**) was largely dependent to its significant inhibition on the IL-6-induced constitutive activation of STAT3 in the tumor cells. Aloe emodin (**6**) and rhein (**7**) exhibited modest activity in the suppression of the three breast cancer cell lines.[22]

Exploration of Mechanisms

The mechanism regarding the antitumor and anticarcinogenic effects of resveratrol (**2**) has been deeply explored, finding the following events primarily involved in the activities, such as (1) upregulation of p21Cip/WAF1, p53, Bax, and caspase activities; (2) downregulation of cyclin-D1 and cyclin-E, survivin, Bcl-2, Bcl-xL, and cIAPs expressions; (3) inhibition of transcription factors including NF-κB, AP-1, and Egr-1; (4) inhibition of protein kinases including IκBα kinase, JNK, MAPK, Akt, PKC, PKD, and casein kinase-II; and (5) reduction of gene products such as COX-2, 5-LOX, VEGF, IL-1, IL-6, IL-8, AR, and PSA.[8] Various cancer cells could be provoked by resveratrol (**2**) to apoptotic death by some characteristic multiple regulations. For instance, the apoptotic mechanism of resveratrol in human U251 giloma cells and primary gastric cancer cells was associated with the decrease of Bcl-2 activity, the increase of Bax expression, the cleavage of PARP, the release of cytochrome c from the mitochondria to the cytoplasm, and the activation of caspase-3 and caspase-9.[23] However, in human HL-60 leukemia cells, the FasL-related apoptosis elicited by resveratrol (**2**) was mainly mediated by CDC42 activation in ASK1/JNK-dependent signaling cascade.[24] The apoptotic induction of resveratrol (**2**) in nude mice transplanted with primary gastric carcinoma cells was mediated by downregulating the antiapoptotic Bcl-2 expression and upregulating the apoptotic Bax expression.[25] The inhibitory effect of resveratrol (**2**) on human MCF-10A breast epithelial cells was characteristically accompanied by the decrease of aryl hydrocarbon receptor–DNA binding activity, the decline of 2-hydroxyestradiol and 4-hydroxyestradiol formation, and the induction of cytochrome P450 1A1 and 1B1 expressions.[26] Also, resveratrol (**2**) obviously attenuated the intracellular ROS formation and oxidative DNA damage as well as the cytotoxicity induced by catechol estrogens, thereby obstructing the neoplastic transformation in human breast epithelial cells.[26] Moreover, the metastasis of breast cancer cells was obstructed by resveratrol (**2**) by rapidly inducing a global array of filopodia, retarding focal adhesions and FAK activity, and altering the cytoskeleton.[26,27]

Likewise, resveratrol (**2**) was capable of blocking NF-κB activation induced by an inflammatory agent TNF via the diminution of NF-κB-dependent reporter gene transcription and the repression of phosphorylation and nuclear translocation of p65 subunit in NF-κB, whose events were coincided with the inhibition of AP-1. Resveratrol (**2**) also restrained the TNF-induced activations of MAPK, JNK, and downregulated HER-2/neu gene expression and obstructed reactive oxygen intermediate generation and TNF-induced lipid peroxidation by the inhibition of COX-2 and MMP-9 activities.[28–30] These resveratrol-provoked multiinteractions were reported to also be complicatedly involved in the growth inhibition and the apoptosis-induction in many cell lines, such as MCF-7 (breast cancer), U937 (lymphoma), Jurkat (lymphoid leukemia), H4 (hepatoma), HeLa (cervical cancer), and melanoma.[31,32]

Other Bioactivities

In pharmacological studies, Hu Zhang (Giant knotweed) exerts antioxidative, laxative, sedative, antitussive, hemostasis, antiinflammatory, antiviral, and antibacterial effects. Hu Zhang is able to reduce blood pressure and blood lipid level, to promote microcirculation, to inhibit agglutination of thrombocyte, to raise leukocyte, and to enhance the contraction of the intestine tube. However, the herb might cause side effects such as nausea, vomiting, diarrhea, and indigestion in some cases. Also, Hu Zhang rarely causes peritonitis, hepatic cell damage, respiratory depression, and lipid increase in the marrow, but it does not influence the functions of the liver and the kidney as well as the hemogram indexes significantly.

References

1. Zhou, L. D. et al. 1989. Inhibitory effect of Hu-Zhang decoction on Ehrlich ascites tumor. *Zhongxiyi Jiehe Zazhi* 9: 111.
2. Jayasuriya, H. et al. 1992. Emodin, a protein tyrosine kinase inhibitor from *Polygonum cuspidatum*. *J. Nat. Prod.* 55: 696–8.
3. Liao, X. Y. et al. 1988. Antitumor pharmacology study of emdin in *Polygonum cuspidatum*. *Zhongguo Yiyuan Yaoxue Zazhi* 8: 214.
4. Yeh, S. F. et al. 1988. Effects of anthraquinones of *Polygonum cuspidatum* on HL-60 cells. *Planta Med.* 54: 413–4.
5. Lu, Y. Y. et al. 2008. The effect of emodin on VEGF receptors in human colon cancer cells. *Cancer Biother. Radiopharm.* 23: 222–8.
6. Hwangbo, K. et al. 2012. Inhibition of DNA topoisomerases I and II of compounds from *Reynoutria japonica*. *Archiv. Pharm. Res.* 35: 1583–9.
7. Su, H. Y. et al. 1995. Emodin inhibits the mutagenicity and DNA adducts induced by 1-nitropyrene. *Mutation Res.* 129: 205–12.
8. Aggarwal, B. B. et al. Role of resveratrol in prevention and therapy of cancer: Preclinical and clinical studies. *Anticancer Res.* 24: 2783–840.
9. Li, T. et al. 2008. Anti-leukemia effect of resveratrol of *Polygonum cuspidatum* exerts and possible molecular mechanism. *J. Xi'an Jiaotong Univ.* (*Med. Edit.*), 29: 340–5.
10. Feng, L. et al. Active substance of anticancer effect in *Polygonum cuspidatum*. *Zhongyaocai* 29: 689–91.
11. Huang, M. T. et al. 2001. Inhibitory effect of an extract of the root of the Chinese plant *Polygonum cuspidatum* on chemically induced several biomarker changes and tumorigenesis in mice. *Abst. Pap. 221st ACS National Meeting,* San Diego, CA, U.S. April 1–5, AGFD-023.
12. Banerjee, S. et al. 2002. Suppression of 7,12-dimethylbenz(a) anthracene-induced mammary carcinogenesis in rats by resveratrol: role of nuclear factor-κB, cyclooxygenase 2, and matrix metalloprotease 9. *Cancer Res.* 62: 4945–54.
13. Liu, J. et al. 2013. Effect of *Polygonum cuspidatum* extract resveratrol on human gastric cancer 7901 cell proliferation and apoptosis. *Shizhen Guoyi Guoyao* 24: 1627–9.
14. Ji, Q. et al. 2013. Resveratrol inhibits invasion and metastasis of colorectal cancer cells via MALAT1 mediated Wnt/β-catenin signal pathway. *Plos One* 8: e78700.
15. Kimura, Y. et al. 2001. Resveratrol isolated from *Polygonum cuspidatum* root prevents tumor growth and metastasis to lung and tumor-induced neovascularization in Lewis lung carcinoma-bearing mice. *J. Nat. Prod.* 131: 1844–9.
16. Wang, S. S. et al. 2004. Angiogenesis and anti-angiogenesis activity of Chinese medicinal herbal extracts. *Life Sci.* 74: 2467–78.
17. Cao, Y. et al. 2005. Anti-angiogenic activity of resveratrol, a natural compound from medicinal plants. *J. Asian Nat. Prods. Res.* 7: 205–13.
18. Du, Q. et al. 2013. Synergistic anticancer effects of curcumin and resveratrol in Hepa1-6 hepatocellular carcinoma cells. *Oncol. Reports* 29: 1851–8.
19. Lee, M. W. et al. 2012. Extraction of resveratrol from *Polygonum cuspidatum* with magnetic orcinol-imprinted poly(ethylene-co-vinyl alcohol) composite particles and their in vitro suppression of human osteogenic sarcoma (HOS) cell line. *J. Mat. Chem.* 22: 24644–51.
20. Li, X. N. et al. 2001. Inhibition of protein kinase C by 3,4′,5-trihydroxystibene-3-β-mono-D-glucoside in human colorectal carcinoma cell lines. *Shijie Huaren Xiaohua Zazhi* 9: 198–201.
21. Lee, S. H. et al. 2002. Induction of apoptosis by 3,4′-dimethoxy-5-hydroxystilbene in human promyeloid leukemic HL-60 cells. *Planta Med.* 68: 123–7.
22. Liu, J. W. et al. 2012. Small-molecule STAT3 signaling pathway modulators from *Polygonum cuspidatum*. *Planta Med.* 78: 1568–70.
23. Jiang, H. et al. 2005. Resveratrol-induced apoptotic death in human U251 glioma cells. *Mol. Cancer Therap.* 4: 554–61.
24. Su, J. L. et al. 2005. Resveratrol induces FasL-related apoptosis through Cdc42 activation of ASK1/JNK-dependent signaling pathway in human leukemia HL-60 cells. *Carcinogenesis* 26: 1–10.
25. Zhou, H. B. et al. 2005. Anticancer activity of resveratrol on implanted human primary gastric carcinoma cells in nude mice. *World J. Gastroenterol.* 11: 280–4.
26. Chen, Z. H. et al. 2004. Resveratrol inhibits TCDD-induced expression of CYP1A1 and CYP1B1 and catechol estrogen-mediated oxidative DNA damage in cultured human mammary epithelial cells. *Carcinogen.* 25: 2005–13.
27. Azios, N. G. et al. 2005. Resveratrol and estradiol exert disparate effects on cell migration, cell surface actin structures, and focal adhesion assembly in MDA-MB-231 human breast cancer cells. *Neoplasia* 7: 128–40.
28. Provinciali, M. et al. 2005. Effect of resveratrol on the development of spontaneous mammary tumors in HER-2/neu transgenic mice. *Intl. J. Cancer* 115: 36–45.
29. Woo, J. H. et al. 2004. Resveratrol inhibits phorbol myristate acetate-induced matrix metalloproteinase-9 expression by inhibiting JNK and PKC signal transduction. *Oncogene* 23: 1845–53.
30. Manna, S. K. et al. 2000. Resveratrol suppresses TNF-induced activation of nuclear transcription factors NF-κB, activator protein-1, and apoptosis: Potential role of reactive oxygen intermediates and lipid peroxidation. *J. Immunol.* 164: 6509–19.
31. Kundu, J. B. et al. 2004. Resveratrol inhibits phorbol ester-induced cyclooxygenase-2 expression in mouse skin: MAPKs and AP-1 as potential molecular targets. *BioFactors* 21: 33–9.
32. Pozo-Guisado, E. et al. 2005. Resveratrol-induced apoptosis in MCF-7 human breast cancer cells involves a caspase-independent mechanism with downregulation of Bcl-2 and NF-κB. *Intl. J. Cancer* 115: 74–84.

119 Xiang Cha Cai 香茶菜

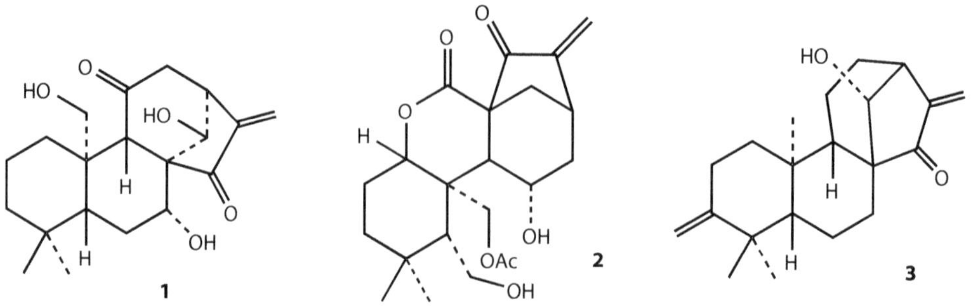

Herb Origination

The herb Xiang Cha Cai is the whole plant and root of *Rabdosia amethystoides* (Labiatae). The perennial and herbal plant is primarily distributed in southern and southeastern China. The herb can be utilized fresh any time, or its terrestrial parts can be collected at blooming season and dried in the sun for medicinal application.

Antitumor Constituents and Activity

Amethystoidine-A (**1**) is one of the anticancer constituents isolated from Xian Cha Cai, whose diterpenoid exhibited moderate cytotoxicity to repress the proliferation human QGY-7703 (liver), HeLa (cervix), and CaEs-17 (esophagus) cancer cell lines *in vitro* (IC_{50}: 1.33–2.74 μg/mL).[1] The antiproliferative effect was also demonstrated by the *in vivo* experiments. Daily i.p. administration of amethystoidin-A (**1**) for seven continuous days remarkably prolonged the life duration of mice bearing Ehrlich ascites tumor over 112%.[2] The acetylation of amethystoidine-A (**1**) could augment the growth suppression against the tested cancer cell lines.[2] A different type of diterpenoid, assigned as rabdophyllin-G (**2**) isolated from the herb, also exerted the significant inhibitory action against Ehrlich ascites carcinoma in mice.[3,4]

Glaucocalyxins were extracted from *R. amethystoides* and *R. japonica* var. *glaucocalyx* with 96% ethanol. An *in vitro* assay showed that glaucocalyxin-A (**3**) and glaucocalyxin-B dose-dependently restrained the growth of human HL-60 leukemia cells (respective IC_{50}: 6.15 and 5.86 μM at 24 h), together with the elicitation of apoptosis, G2/M phase cycle arrest, DNA damage and the accumulation of ROS in the HL-60 cells. Both also caused rapid decrease of the intracellular GSH content and reduction of GSH-related enzyme activity (such as GSH reductase and GSH peroxidase). The evidences revealed that the promotion of apoptosis was processed through a ROS-dependent mitochondrial dysfunction pathway, and the perturbation of intracellular GSH redox system was also important in regulating the glaucocalyxin-induced cytotoxic activity in the HL-60 leukemia cells.[5,6] Moreover, glaucocalyxin-A (**3**) was also a marked growth inhibitor of K562 (leukemic), PC3 (prostate), KB (oral), and MCF-7 and Hs578T (breast) human neoplastic call lines (IC_{50}: 3.0–8.4 μM).[7,8] The cytotoxic and proapoptotic activities of glaucocalyxin-A (**3**) in the KB cells were found to be mediated by a lysosomal–mitochondrial death pathway, i.e., induction of an early lysosomal rupture, increase of ROS, mitochondrial membrane permeabilization, release of cytochrome c, and activation of caspase-9 and caspase-3.[7] Glaucocalyxin-A (**3**)-induced MCF-7 and Hst578T cell death was due to the induction cell cycle arrest at G2/M transition and apoptosis in association with the activation of a JNK pathway.[8] In the treated human U87MG glioma cells, glaucocalyxin-A (**3**) dose-dependently promoted the cell apoptosis and retarded the cell proliferation in correlation with the blockage of Akt phosphorylation and BAD phosphorylation, lowered X-linked inhibitor of apoptosis protein, and activation of caspase-3.[9] Therefore, these results highlighted that glaucocalyxin-A (**3**) may be a promising candidate for cancer chemotherapy. Moreover, glaucocalyxin-A ferulic acid derivatives that were produced by esterification to form the monoester products demonstrated antitumor and anticarcinogenic potentials for the treatment of solid carcinomas in the stomach, the liver, the lung, the cervix, the colon, and the kidney.[10]

Other Bioactivities

Xiang Cha Cai has been found to possess antiinflammatory, hepatoprotective, and antibacterial properties besides anticancer activity in pharmacological investigations. Amethystoidine-A (**1**) is capable of enhancing nonspecific immune function.

References

1. Yao, Q. S. et al. 1984. Antitumor and antibiotic activities of amethystoidine A. *Jiangsu Med. J.* 10: 22–4.
2. Yao, Q. S. et al. 1984 Study on the antitumor constiteunts of *Rabdosia maerophlla. Jiangsu Med. J.* 10: 575.
3. Cheng, P. Y. et al. 1982. The antitumor constituents of *Rabdosia amethystoides. Acta Pharm. Sinica* 17: 33–7.
4. Cheng, P. Y. et al. 1982. The structure of rabdophyllin G, an antitumor constituent of *Rabdosia macrophylla. Yaoxue Xuebao* 17: 917–21.
5. Yang, W. H. et al. 2013. Glaucocalyxin A and B-induced cell death is related to GSH perturbation in human leukemia HL-60 cells. *Anticancer Agents Med. Chem.* 13: 1280–90.
6. Gao, L. W. et al. 2011. Glaucocalyxin A induces apoptosis in human leukemia HL-60 cells through mitochondria-mediated death pathway. *Toxicol In vitro* 25: 51–63.

7. Sun, L. M. et al. 2014. Glaucocalyxin A induces apoptosis in human squamous cell carcinoma KB cells through lysosomal-mitochondrial death pathway. www.paper.edu.cn/en_releasepaper/content/4581415
8. Gao, L. W. et al. 2013. Glaucocalyxin A activates FasL and induces apoptosis induction through the JNK pathway in human breast cancer cells. *Asian Pac J Cancer Prev.* 14: 5805–10.
9. Xiao, X. et al. 2013. Glaucocalyxin A, a negative Akt regulator, specifically induces apoptosis in human brain glioblastoma U87MG cells. *Acta Biochem. Sinica* 45: 946–52.
10. Li, Y. S. et al. 2011. Glaucocalyxin A ferulic acid derivatives, preparation and medical application. *Faming Zhuanli Shenqing* CN 102260173 A 20111130.

120 Si Leng Gan 四棱杆

Japanese Rabdisia

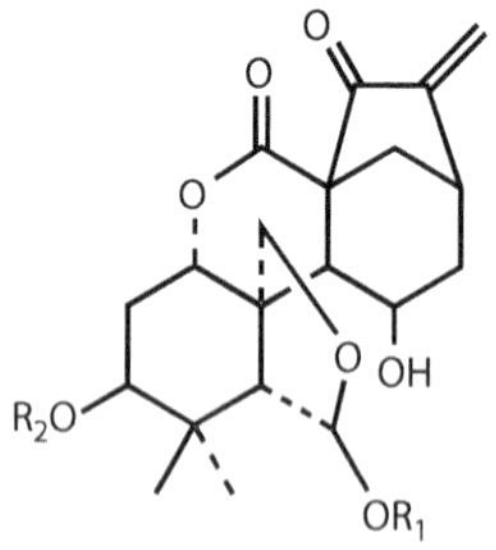

1. R_1 = –CH_3, R_2 = –H
6. R_1 = –H, R_2 = –OH
8. R_1 = –H, R_2 = –H

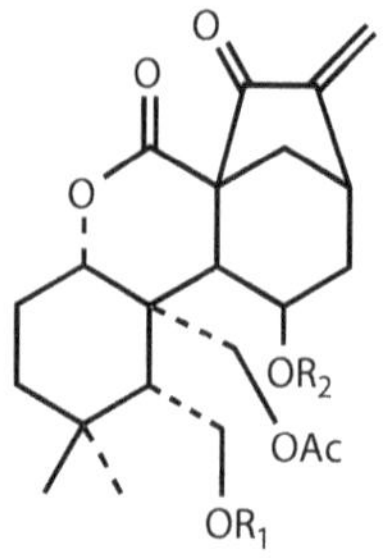

2. R_1 = R_2 = –Ac
3. R_1 = R_2 = –H

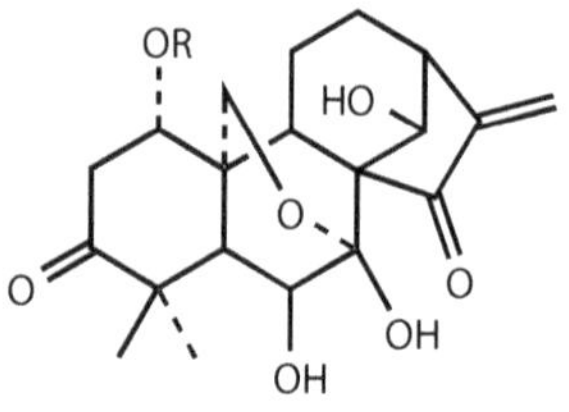

4. R = –H
5. R = –Ac

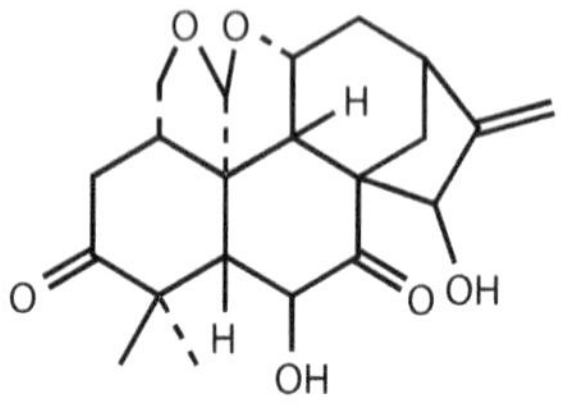

7

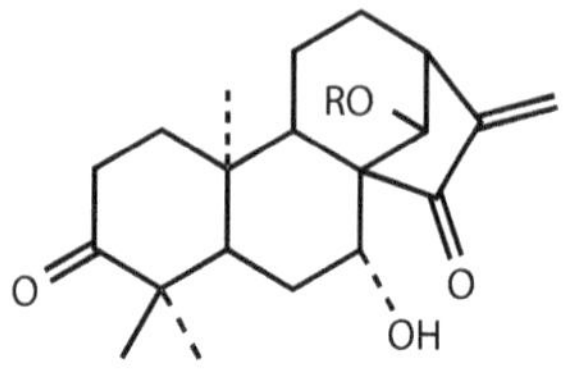

9. R = –H 10. R = –Ac

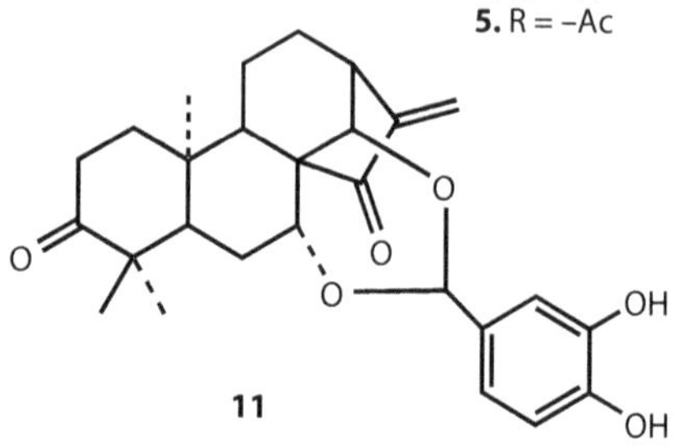

11

Herb Origination

The herb Si Leng Gan is the dried leaves of a Labiatae plant, *Rabdosia japonica* (= *Isodon japonica*). This plant is distributed in the Chinese provinces of Shanxi, Shaanxi, Gansu, Jiangsu, Henan, and Sichuan. Its varietal plant *I. japonica* var. *glaucocalyx* is widely distributed in northern China. The leaves are collected in autumn and dried in the sun for medical treatments.

Antitumor Activities and Constituents

The aqueous extract and the alcoholic extract isolated from the leaves of Si Leng Gan demonstrated remarkable suppressive effect against the growth of Ehrlich ascites cancer cells *in vitro* and *in vivo*. The daily i.p. administration of the alcoholic extracts in doses of ≥2.5 g/kg to mice bearing tumor for 7 continuous days significantly prolonged the life span to 80% and inhibited 46.6% of entity sarcoma 180 cells and 39% of reticulum cell sarcoma cells. However, its suppressive effect was lower toward ascites hepatoma cells.[1] Its ethanolic extract presented the cytotoxicity in five human cancer cell lines, and the IC_{50} values ranged from 2.70 to 6.94 μg/mL against the growth of K562 (leukemic), MKN-45 (gastric), HT-29 (colon), A549 (lung), and MCF-7 (breast) cancer cells. The most effective action was observed in K562 leukemia cells, whose inhibitory rate was 74.1% at a 4 μg/mL concentration (IC_{50}: 2.70 μg/mL).[2] Moreover, the ethanolic extract also exerted prominent antitumor-immunostimulating activity, i.e., markedly enhanced the proliferation of splenocyte, induced the significant enhancement of NK cell activity, and increased the production of IFNγ and TNFα against Yac-1 T-lymphoma cells.[2]

Diterpenoids

A group of *ent*-kaurane diterpenoids with anticarcinoma property was separated from the leaves of *R. japonica*. Rabdosin-A (**1**), rabdosin-B (**2**), rabdosin-C (**3**), and lasiokaurin (**4**) noticeably obstructed the growth of Ehrlich ascites cancer cells.[3] Rabdosin-B (**2**) evidently inhibited the proliferation of human HepG2 hepatoma cells *in vitro* at low concentrations (3.125–12.50 μmol/L) and prolonged the living periods of mice bearing L1210 leukemia by 122% *in vivo*.[4] When the concentrations of rabdosin-B was enlarged to 25–50 μmol/L, the HepG2 cell growth was completely obstructed and the cell apoptosis and necrosis were elicited.[5] The cytotoxic effects of lasiokaurin (**4**), oridonin (**5**), and shikokianin were demonstrated in human HL-60 leukemia and A549 lung neoplastic cell lines *in vitro*, and the IC_{50} values were 11.4–18.8 and 2.0–4.6 μM for lasiokaurin (**4**) and oridonin (**5**), respectively. Lasiokaurin (**4**) exerted moderate cytotoxicity against cervical cancer, reticulum cell sarcoma, and HO-8910 ovarian cancer as well.[6,7] The *in vivo* experiments by daily i.p. injection of rabdosin-C (**3**) or lasiokaurin (**4**) in doses of 10–20 mg/kg significantly restrained the cell growth of murine L1210 leukemia, Ehrlich ascites carcinoma, and ascites hepatoma.[6,7] Maoyecrystal-I (**7**) separated from the herb was comparably effective in the growth inhibition of human K562 erythroleukemia cells (IC_{50}: 7.30 μg/mL), in which the structure of the oxetane group might be the active center related to the antileukemia effect.[8] Moreover, oridonin (**5**), enmein (**6**), and nodosin (**8**) are also shown with potent antimutagenic effects.[9] The investigations clearly revealed that these diterpenoids are the major components responsible for the antineoplastic property of Si Leng Gan.

Furthermore, more cytotoxic diterpenoids such as glaucocalyxins-A–F, epinodosin, lasiokaourin, oridonin (**5**), epinodosinol, and rabdosinate were discovered from a varietal plant *R. japonica* var. *glaucocalyx*. The last five diterpenoids displayed significant cytotoxicity against human Bel-7402 and HepG2 hepatoma cells and human HO-8910 ovarian tumor cells.[10–12] Glaucocalyxins-A (**9**), glaucocalyxin-B (**10**), and glaucocalyxin-D showed an apparent activity against four human tumor cell lines (HL-60, 6T-CEM, LoVo, and A549) with IC_{50} values ranging from 0.049

to 2.65 μg/mL. The strongest effect was achieved by glaucocalyxin-A against T cell leukemia 6T-CEM cells (IC_{50}: 0.049 μg/mL), being more potent than DOX (IC_{50}: 0.081 μg/mL).[13] Glaucocalyxin-A (**9**) and glaucocalyxin-B (**10**) could induce apoptosis, cell cycle arrest at G2/M-phase, and DNA damage in the HL-60 cells, whose apoptosis promoted by glaucocalyxin-A and glaucocalyxin-B was confirmed to be through a ROS-dependent mitochondrial dysfunction pathway.[14] The two glaucocalyxins also decreased the activities of GSH-related enzymes and the intracellular GSH content to regulate the cytotoxicity in the treatment of HL-60 cells.[15] In human U87MG glioma cells, glaucocalyxin-A (**9**) restrained the proliferation and promoted the apoptosis in a dose-dependent manner associated with the decrease of Akt phosphorylation and BAD phosphorylation, the reduction of X-linked inhibitor of apoptotic protein expression, and the activation of caspase-3.[16] Glaucocalyxins-A (**9**) and glaucocalyxin-B (**10**) also showed marked to moderate cytotoxicity on U87, HepG2, HeLa, K562, EC-1, and A549 tumor cell lines, wherein the most potent cytotoxicity of glaucocalyxin-A (**9**) was observed in EC-1 esophageal cancer cells (IC_{50}: 0.29 μM).[17] In addition, glaucocalyxin-H (**11**) exhibited higher inhibitory activities than its parent glaucocalyxin-A (**9**) and 5-FU (an antitumor agent). Its IC_{50} values were 1.86, 1.97, 3.17, 3.64, 3.65, and 10.95 μM in K562, HepG2, EC-1, HeLa, U87, and MCF-7 cancer cell lines, respectively.[17] The antihepatoma activity of glaucocalyxin-H (**11**) was also proven *in vitro* together with the induction of HepG2 cells to apoptosis due to the decreased Bcl2 and increased Bax proteins.[18] By comparing these data, the SAR of the diterpenoids can be concluded that the α,β-unsaturated ketone moiety in the D-ring is the leading antitumor active sites, and the hydroxyl groups (OH-7 and OH-14) play an important role in the cytotoxic activity.[13] Collectively, the results signified that the glaucocalyxins, especially glaucocalyxin-A (**9**) and glaucocalyxin-H (**11**), may become a promising candidate in the treatment of several types of malignant tumor for chemotherapy and prevention.

Oridonin Nanoliposomes

Liposomal encapsulation can remarkably improve the potency and the specificity of antitumor agents. An oridonin (**5**)–nanoliposomes injection (O-NL) has been prepared for comparing the cytotoxic effect with its free oridonin solution (O-F) *in vitro* and *in vivo*. O-NL (1.84×10^{-7} μmol/L) dose- and time-dependently suppressed the proliferation of human cancer cells *in vitro*, and its inhibitory rates on HepG2 hepatoma cells and MGC-803 gastric cancer cells were 75.6% and 80.0% at a 96 h treatment with O-NL, whereas the maximum inhibitory rates of O-F were 42.1% and 22.1%, respectively. The *in vivo* antitumor effect was also proven in mice implanted with H22 hepatoma cells, and the inhibition ratio based on the weights for O-NL (in a dose of 1.68×10^{-2} g/kg/day) was 78.4%, being much greater than 25.4% obtained from O-F (in the same dose of 1.68×10^{-2} g/kg/day)-treated group.[19]

Polyphenols

The extract of *R. japonica* has been reported to have a high content of polyphenols. From the dried leaves of Si Leng Gan, a group of antioxidative phenolic compounds (such as pedalitin, quercetin, rutin, isoquercitrin, and rosmarinic acid) were isolated and then subjected to *in vitro* assay. These polyphenols and phenolics displayed superoxide-scavenging activity and an inhibitory effect on xanthine oxidase (EC 1.1.3.22). Among these molecules, the most potent antioxidative agent was pedalitin (**12**), which was capable of restraining the generation of superoxide radicals in part by competitively inhibiting xanthine oxidase.[20] Moreover, pedalitin (**12**) also demonstrated an *in vitro* cytotoxicity against the murine B16-F10 melanoma cells with an IC_{50} value of 30 μM (9.5 μg/mL).[21]

Other Medical Uses

The herb Si Leng Gan has been employed as a folk medicine in China for the treatment of hepatitis, gastritis, mastitis, cough, and snakebite.

References

1. Chen, Z. Y. et al. (a) 1982. *J. Henan Med. College* 17: 82; (b) 1999. *Chinese Materia Medica*. Vol. 7, 7–6165, 146. Shanghai Science and Technology Press, Shanghai, China.
2. Hwang, Y. J. et al. 2012. Study on the immunomodulation effect of *Isodon japonicus* extract via splenocyte function and NK antitumor activity. *Intl. J. Mol. Sci.* 13: 4880–8.
3. Li, J. C. et al. 1982. Studies on the antitumor diterpenoid constituents of *Rabdosia japonica* (Burm. F) Hara I. *Yaoxue Xuebao* 17: 682–7.
4. Liu, C. J. et al. 1982. Studies on the antitumor diterpenoid constituents of *Rabdosia japonica* (Burm. F) Hara II. *Yaoxue Xuebao* 17: 750–4.
5. Ding, L. et al. 2008. The effect of Rabdosin B, an *ent*-kaurane-diterpene on the proliferation of human liver cancer HepG2 cells. *J. NW. Normal Univ. (Nat. Sci. Edit.)* 44: 91–5.
6. Chen, Z. Y. et al. 1985. Antitumor effects of rabddosins C and lasiokaurin. *Zhongyao Tongbao* 10: 374–6.
7. Bai, S. P. et al. 2005. Two novel *ent*-kauranoid diterpenoids from *Isodon japonica* leaves. *Planta Med.* 71: 764–9.
8. Han, Q. B. et al. 2004. A novel cytotoxic oxetane *ent*-kauranoid from *Isodon japonicus*. *Planta Med.* 70: 581–4.
9. Kakinuma, K. et al. 1984. Antimutagenic diterpenoids from a crude drug Isodonis herba (Enmei-So). *Agricult. Biol. Chem.* 48: 1647–8.
10. Ding, L. et al. 2008. Chemical components of diterpenoids from *Isodon japonica* var. *galaucocalyx* from Gansu Province, China. *Guihaia* 28: 265–8.
11. Liu, J. G. et al. 2009. Use of diterpenoids from *Isodon japonica* var. *galaucocalyx* in preparing anticancer medicine. *China Patent* 200910044882.
12. Ding, L. et al. 2011. Comparison of cytotoxicity and DNA damage potential induced by *ent*-kaurene diterpenoids from Isodon plant. *Nat. Prod. Res.* 25: 1402–11.
13. Xiang, Z. B. et al. 2011. Cytotoxic activity of diterpenoids from *Rabdosia japonica* var. *glaucocalyx*. *Asian J. Chem.* 23: 3761–2.
14. Gao, L. W. et al. 2011. Glaucocalyxin A induces apoptosis in human leukemia HL-60 cells through mitochondria-mediated death pathway. *Toxicol. in vitro* 25: 51–63.

15. Yang, W. H. et al. 2013. Glaucocalyxin A and B-induced cell death is related to GSH perturbation in human leukemia HL-60 cells. *Anti-Cancer Agents in Med. Chem.* 13: 1280–90.
16. Xiao, X. et al. 2013. Glaucocalyxin A, a negative Akt regulator, specifically induces apoptosis in human brain glioblastoma U87MG cells. *Acta Biochim. et Biophys. Sinica* 45: 946–52.
17. Liang, H. J. et al. 2012. Isolation, structural elucidation, and cytotoxicity of three new *ent*-kaurane diterpenoids from Isodon japonica var. glaucocalyx. *Planta Med.* 78: 589–96.
18. Hai, G. F. et al. 2015. Anti-hepatoma activity of a novel compound glaucocalyxin H in vivo and in vitro. *AAPS PharmSciTech* 16: 496–504.
19. Wang, C. J. et al. 2008. Study on in vitro cytotoxicity and in vivo antitumor effect of nanoliposomes containing oridonin. *Asian J. Pharmacodyn. Pharmacokin.* 8: 324–8.
20. Nitoda, T. et al. 2008. Effects of phenolic compounds isolated from *Rabdosia japonica* on B16-F10 melanoma cells. *Phytother Res.* 22: 867–72.
21. Masuoka, N. et al. 2006. Antioxidants from *Rabdosia japonica. Phytother. Res.* 20: 206–13.

121 Ba Li Ma 八厘麻

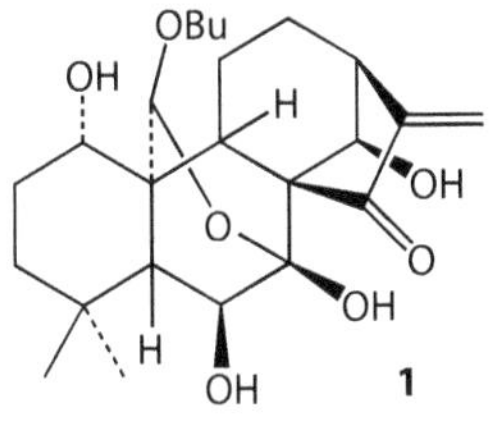

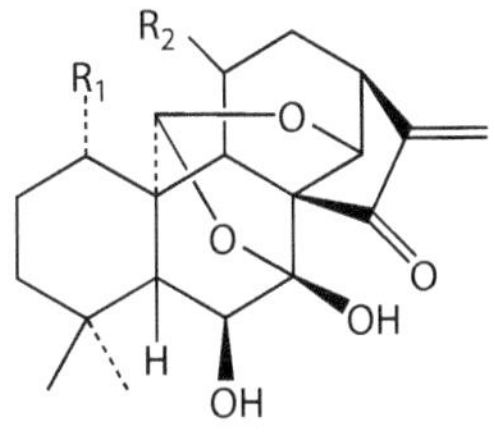

2. $R_1 = R_2 = -H$
8. $R_1 = -OH, R_2 = -H$
9. $R_1 = -H, R_2 = -OH$

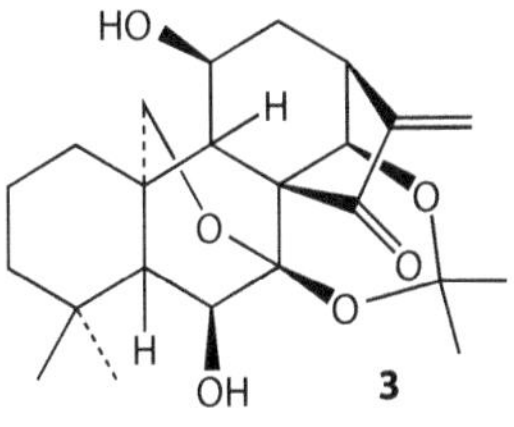

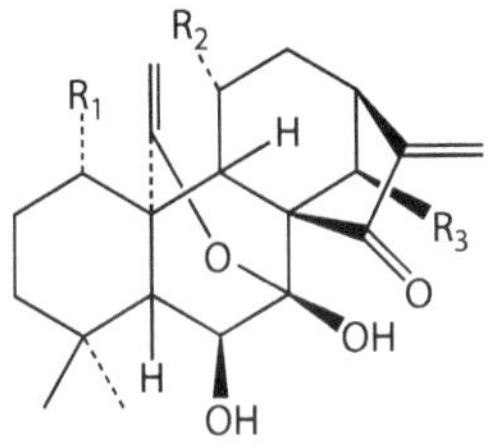

4. $R_1 = -OAc, R_2 = -H, R_3 = -OH$
5. $R_1 = -H, R_2 = R_3 = -OH$
6. $R_1 = -OH, R_2 = R_3 = -H$

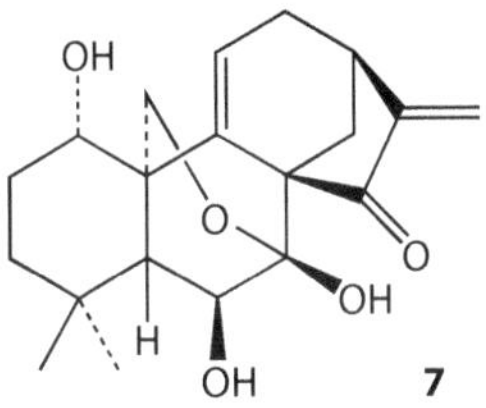

Herb Origination

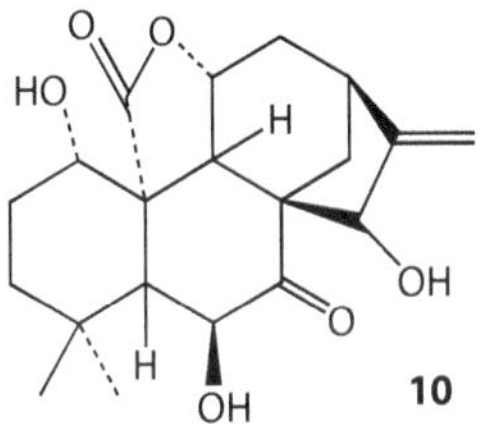

The herb Ba Li Ma originates from a whole plant, *Rabdosia rosthornii* (= *Isodon rosthornii*) (Lamiaceae). This perennial herb is distributed only in a small area between southern Sichuan province and northern Guizhou province in China. The herb is generally collected in summer and autumn and then dried in the sun for folk medicinal application. It also can be used fresh all the year round.

Antitumor Constituents and Activities

The plant *R. rosthornii* is a rich source of *ent*-kaurane type diterpenoids that are responsible for most of the cytotoxic effect of the herb against a variety of tumor cell lines. *In vitro* models demonstrated seven *ent*-kaurane diterpenoids that were separated from the aerial parts of Ba Li Ma exerted prominent suppressive effect against the tested small panel of human carcinoma cell lines (IC_{50}: 1.2–8.6 μM).[1–3] The activities of **1–7** were superior to those of cisplatin but much inferior to those of paclitaxel. Three other same type of diterpenoids (**8–10**) showed relatively lower activity on all five cell lines (IC_{50}: 7.3 to >40 μM), and the other eight (**11–16**) were selectively active in the some tumor cell lines.[1–3]

Compared to other cancer cell lines, the HL-60 leukemia cells were sensitive to the *ent*-kaurane diterpenoids and 20-norenmein diterpenoids. The most effective diterpenoids on the HL-60 cells were assigned to be isorosthin-O (**1**), xerophilurin-B (**2**), EDEKEO (**3**), and longikaurin-G (**4**) (IC_{50}: <2 μM), whereas xerophilurin-B (**2**), EDEKEO (**3**), and longikaurin-G (**4**) showed the highest cytotoxicity on the SMMC-7721 hepatoma cells (IC_{50}: <2.8 μM). EDEKEO (**3**) also exerted the most potent antiproliferative effect on A549 lung cancer, SW480 colon cancer, and MCF-7 breast cancer cell lines (respective IC_{50}: 3.4, 2.0, and 1.8 μM).[1–3] Furthermore, the analysis of the relationship between the *ent*-kaurane structures and the cytotoxicity suggested that (1) a carbonyl conjugated with the exocyclic double bond is a structural requirement and (2) the improvement of liposolubility may enhance the inhibitory potency. The *ent*-kaurane diterpenoids (**1–14**) characteristically displayed marked cytotoxic effect against the SW480 and HL-60 cell lines. When the carbonyl group was reduced to the hydroxyl group, the activity would be lessened or lost such as **10** and **16**, but they still showed the antileukemia potency in HL-60 cells.[3]

References

1. Zhan, R. et al. 2011. Isorosthornins A-C, new *ent*-kaurane diterpenoids from *Isodon rosthornii*. *Nat. Prod. Bioprospect.* 1: 116–20.
2. Zhan, R. et al. 2013. *ent*-Atisane and *ent*-kaurane diterpenoids from *Isodon rosthornii*. *Fitoterapia* 88: 76–81.
3. Zhan, R. et al. 2013. Bioactive *ent*-kaurane diterpenoids from *Isodon rosthornii*. *J. Nat. Prod.* 76: 1267–77.

122 Xiao Hong Shen 小红参

1. R_1 = -OCH_3, R_2 = -H

2. R_1 = -NH_2, R_2 = -Glucose

6. R_1 = R_3 = R_4 = -OH, R_2 = -CH_3
7. R_1 = R_4 = -H, R_2 = -CH_2OH, R_3 = -OH
8. R_1 = R_4 = -OH, R_2 = -CH_3
R_3 = -Glu-(2-1)-Rham (6'-OAc)

Herb Origination

The herb Xiao Hong Shen originated from a Rubiaceae plant, *Rubia yunnanensis*, and is native to the Yunnan province of China, and the roots of this perennial climbing plant have been used as an herbal medicine for a hundred years. The roots are normally collected between late autumn and winter and dried for folk medical treatment. Xiao Hong Shen is also used as an alternative herb for *R. cordifolia* (see Section Qian Cao 茜草), a well-known traditional Chinese medicine listed in the Chinese pharmacopoeia.

Antitumor Activity and Constituents

By phytochemical investigations, three different types of constituents were discovered from the roots of Xiao Hong Shen to have anticarcinoma-related activities. The most attractive principals are a group of cyclic hexapeptides, and others such as the arborinane-type triterpenoids and anthraquinones also showed obvious cytotoxic activities in the *in vitro* bioassays.

Cyclic Hexapeptides

An ethyl acetate extract derived from Xiao Hong Shen displayed the growth inhibitory effect *in vitro* against four human neoplastic cells such as BEL-7402 (liver), A549 (lung), BGC-823 (stomach), and U251 (brain) and a murine B16 melanoma cells with IC_{50} values of 2.18–14.32 μM, whereas its n-butanolic fraction was only moderately effective on the A549 and BGC-823 cells. Many valuable cyclic hexapeptides (RVs and rubiyunnanins) were obtained from the separation of the EtOAc extract. These cyclopeptides were evaluated in a panel of carcinoma cell lines including HepG2, Bel-7402, and SMMC-7721 (liver); MDA-M-231 (breast); DU-145 and PC3 (prostate); A549 (lung); BGC-823 (stomach); HeLa (cervix); U251 (brain); and B16 (skin) tumor cells *in vitro*. The most potent cytotoxic cyclic hexapeptides in the herb were identified as RA-V and RA-I, which were reported as anticancer drug candidates isolated from Qian Cao by Dr. Itokawa's group in the 1980s to the 1990s. The IC_{50} data were in the ranges of 0.001–0.14 μM for RA-V and 0.16–2.02 μM for RA-I against various carcinoma cell lines.[1–3] RA-V, for instance, significantly obstructed the growth of human MCF-7 and MDA-MB-231 breast cancer cells and murine 4T1 breast carcinoma cells *in vitro*, and the anticancer mechanism in the MCF-7 cells was found to be related to the initiation of mitochondrial apoptotic pathway through the blockage of the interaction between PDK1 and AKT.[1–4] The isolated rubiyunnanins were demonstrated to have moderate cytotoxicities on the 11 neoplastic cell lines. Among them, the most active agent was rubiyunnanin-C (**1**), and its IC_{50} values ranged from 0.67 to 10.69 μM. Almost all of the cyclic hexapeptides exhibited obvious inhibitory effects on NO production and NF-κB signaling pathway in LPS and IFNγ-induced RAW 264.7 murine macrophages and in TNFα-induced HEK-293-NF-κB luciferase stable cells, whereas

RA-V showed the best activity in the assay. The findings implied that the suppression of NF-κB signaling pathway may be partially related to the anticancer and anticarcinogenic mechanisms of these hexapeptides.[1–3]

Furthermore, RA-V also exerted marked antiproliferative effect against HUVECs and HMECs through the induction of cell cycle G2/M arrest and cell apoptosis in association with the blockage of ERK1/2 phosphorylation pathway and the downregulation of cell cycle regulatory proteins. RA-V could also restrain the migration and the tube formation of HUVECs and HMECs by the inhibition of MMP-2 expression. The evidences proved that RA-V may also play a role in antiangiogenesis.[5]

From the n-butanolic fraction, several antitumor glycocyclohexapeptides assigned as RY-I, RY-II, and RY-III were separated, which were elucidated to be the glycosides of RAs such as RA-V. Comparedto RY-I and RY-III, RY-II (**2**) exerted relatively greater antigrowth effect against the 11 tested carcinoma cell lines with IC_{50} values in the range of 2.89–14.4 μM. The potency of RYs were obviously less than the corresponding aglycones of RAs, indicating that the glycosidation of RAs would diminish the cytotoxic level.[6–8]

Arborinane-Type Triterpenoids

Twelve isolated arborinane-type triterpenoids designated as rubiyunnanols were assayed *in vitro* for the evaluation of their antineoplastic activity. Rubiyunnanol-B (**3**) and rubiabonol-G (**4**) demonstrated the suppressive effect on the proliferation of two human carcinoma cell lines with IC_{50} values of 8.2 and 7.0 μM in human A549 lung cancer cells and 5.3 and 2.2 μM in human HeLa cervical neoplastic cells, respectively. Rubiarbonone-E 19-acetate and rubiarboside-G 28-acetate exerted similar moderate level of inhibition against the HeLa cells (IC_{50}: 7.9 and 2.2 μM, respectively), whereas rubiyunnanol-A (**5**) had the antiproliferative effect on the A549 cells (IC_{50}: 9.8 μM).[3]

Anthraquinones

From Xiao Hong Shen, several anthraquinones were isolated in the antitumor-related phytochemical investigation. 1,3,6-Trihydroxy-2-methyl-9,10-anthraquinone (**6**) exerted cytotoxic effect in human HeLa cervical cancer cells together with the induction of apoptosis and G2/M cell cycle arrest. The apoptosis of HeLa cells was induced through a mitochondria-mediated pathway, i.e., translocation of Bax to the mitochondria, release of cytochrome c into cytosol, and cleavage of caspase and PARP, thereby triggering the apoptotic death. The block of cell cycle progression in the HeLa cells by 1,3,6-trihydroxy-2-methyl-9,10-anthraquinone (**6**) was correlated with the activation of p21 and cyclin-B1 and the inactivation of CDC2–cyclin-B1 complex of G2/M checkpoint.[9] The antiproliferative effect on the HeLa cells was also observed in the treatment with 3-hydroxy-2-hydroxymethyl-9,10-anthraquinone (**7**) and 1,3,6-trihydroxy-2-methyl-9,10-anthra quinone-3-*O*-(6′-*O*-acetyl)-α-L-rhamnosyl-(1–2)-β-D-glucoside (**8**), with IC_{50} values of 3.0 and 4.2 μM, respectively. In addition, 2-methoxy-1,4-naphthoquinone (**9**) was effective in the suppression of human SMMC-7742 hepatoma cells (IC_{50}: 4.3 μM).[3]

Nanoformulation

For the improvement of solubility and bioavalibility, a micelle-like nanoparticle of RA-V was prepared in a pH 7.4 aqueous solution with poly(β-amino ester)s copolymers. The RA-V-loaded micelles exhibited high antitumor efficiency toward MCF-7 cells and HeLa cancer cells and showed endocytic pathway and mitochondria-regulated apoptosis. The *in vivo* growth inhibition of RA-V micelles were further demonstrated in MCF-7 cell-xenografted nude mice with no toxicity, resulting in much improved anti-breast-cancer effect. Therefore, the RA-V micelles may be used as a potential nanoscaled cancer therapeutic agent.[10]

Other Medical Uses

The herb Xiao Hong Shen roots have a long history of use in Chinese folk medicine for the treatment of rheumatism, vertigo, insomnia, tuberculosis, menstrual disorders, and contusions besides malignant tumor disease.

References

1. Fan, J. T. et al. 2010. Rubiyunnanins A and B, two novel cyclic hexapeptides from *Rubia yunnanensis*. *Tetrahedron Lett.* 51: 6810–3.
2. Fan, J. T. et al. 2010. Rubiyunnanins C-H, cytotoxic cyclic hexapeptides from *Rubia yunnanensis* inhibiting nitric oxide production and NF-κB activation. *Bioorg. Med. Chem.* 18: 8226–34.
3. Fan, J. T. et al. 2011. Biologically active arborinane-type triterpenoids and anthraquinones from *Rubia yunnanensis*. *J. Nat. Prod.* 74: 2069–80.
4. Fang, X. Y. et al. 2013. Plant cyclopeptide RA-V kills human breast cancer cells by inducing mitochondria-mediated apoptosis through blocking PDK1-AKT interaction. *Toxicol. Applied Pharmacol.* 267: 95–103.
5. Yue, G. L. et al. 2011. Cyclopeptide RA-V inhibits angiogenesis by down-regulating ERK1/2 phosphorylation in HUVEC and HMEC-1 endothelial cells. *British J. Pharmacol.* 164: 1883–98.
6. Zou, C. et al. 1992. A new antitumor glycocyclohexapeptide and arborane type new triterpenoids from *Rubia yunnanensis*. *Yunnan Zhiwu Yanjiu* 14: 114.
7. Zou, C. et al. 1993. Antitumor glycocyclohexapeptide from *Rubiay yunnanensis*. *Acta Bot. Yunnanica* 15: 399–402.
8. He, M. et al. 1993. New antitumor glycocyclohexapeptide from *Rubia yunnanensis*. *Chin. Chem. Lett.* 4: 1065–6.
9. Zeng, G. Z. et al. 2013. Apoptosis induction and G2/M arrest of 2-methyl-1,3,6-trihydroxy-9,10-anthraquinone from *Rubia yunnanensis* in human cervical cancer HeLa cells. *Pharmazie* 68: 293–9.
10. Qiao, Z. Y. et al. 2015. A pH-responsive natural cyclopeptide RA-V drug formulation for improved breast cancer therapy. *J. Mater. Chem. B: Materials for Biol. Med.* 3: 4514–23.

123 Chou Cao 臭草

Common rue

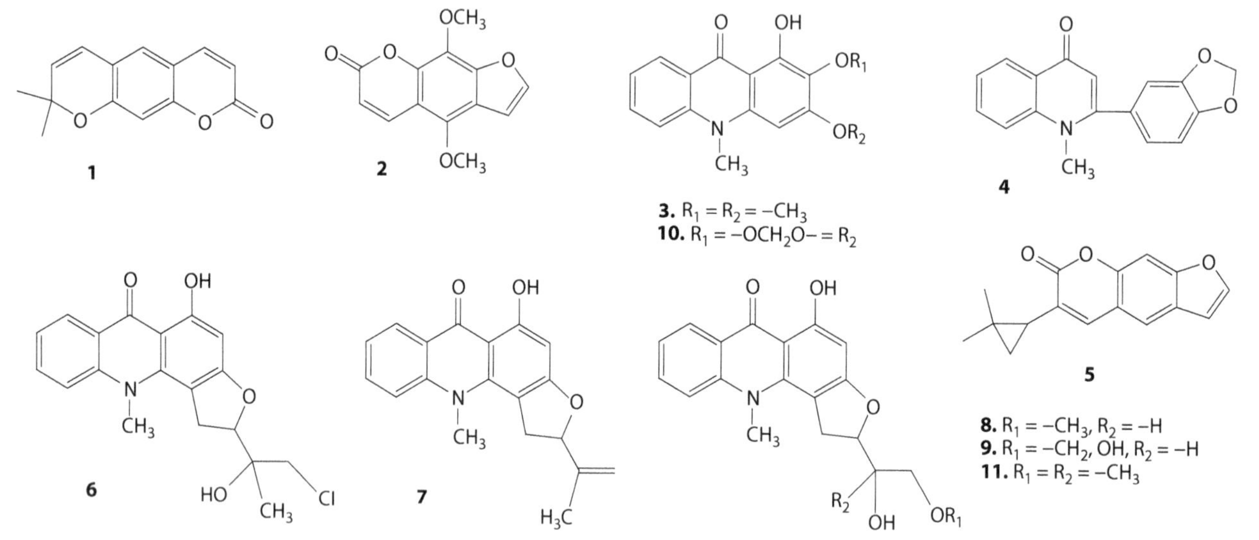

3. $R_1 = R_2 = -CH_3$
10. $R_1 = -OCH_2O- = R_2$

8. $R_1 = -CH_3, R_2 = -H$
9. $R_1 = -CH_2, OH, R_2 = -H$
11. $R_1 = R_2 = -CH_3$

Herb Origination

The herb Chou Cao (Common rue) originated from an evergreen shrub, *Ruta graveolens* L. (Rutaceae), which is native to southern Europe and northern Africa. The plant is widely distributed in southern China and is also naturalized along roadsides and waste areas in North America. In China, the whole plant is collected in July and August and used fresh or dried in the shade for folk medical application.

Antitumor Activities

The petroleum ether extract of Chou Cao showed significant cytotoxicity against Yoshita sarcoma *in vitro.*[1] A 70% ethanolic extract of Chou Cao aerial parts was found to be moderately cytotoxic to DLA, EAC, L929 aneuploid fibrosarcoma, two Burkitt's lymphoma (Raji and Ramos), LNCaP-FGC-10 prostate adenocarcinoma, and Mehr-80 large cell lung carcinoma *in vitro.*[2,3] The administration of the extract could diminish the possible development of the solid DLA and EAC tumor cells with the elongation of the life span of the animals bearing the tumors, but it is not effective in decreasing already developed DLA and EAC carcinomas.[2] A 80% methanolic extract of Chao Cao leaves was effective in the antiproliferation and anticolony formation of HCT116 (colorectal), MCF-7 (breast), and PC3 and DU-145 (prostate) human cancer cell lines *in vitro.* The suppression of the proliferation and the survival of the colon, the breast, and the prostate cancer cell lines were revealed to be complemented by the induction of the G2/M cell arrest and aberrant mitoses and the decrease of the clonogenicity through the activation of a p53-regulated pathway, the reduction of phospho-Akt and cyclin-B1 levels, and the activation of caspase-3.[4]

Ruta-6 is a Chou Cao alcohol extract. If combined with $Ca_3(PO_4)_2$, a different dose of Ruta-6 was effective in the inhibition of human brain carcinoma cells and normal B-lymphoid cells *in vitro.* Fifteen patients diagnosed with intracranial tumors had been treated with Ruta-6 plus $Ca_3(PO_4)_2$. Of these 15 patients, 6 of the glioma patients showed complete regression of the tumors. Both *in vivo* and *in vitro* research revealed that Ruta-6 plus $Ca_3(PO_4)_2$ caused telomere erosion in the brain cancer cells and elicited mitotic catastrophe events, then destroyed the brain cancer cells. The results suggested that the combination of Ruta-6 and $Ca_3(PO_4)_2$ may be a promising chemotherapy for brain cancers, particularly glioma.[5]

Antitumor Constituents and Activities

Coumarins and Alkaloids

Three antineoplastic constituents, which were isolated from Chou Cao and its cultured tissues, were identified as psoralen, isoimperatorin, and dictamnine. Besides the compounds, xanthotoxin (**1**) and isopimpinellin (**2**) exhibited the tumoricidal effect on the cancer cells, and xanthotoxin (**1**) also showed antimitotic effect.[6–8] Other growth inhibitory components found from the herb, such as isopimpinellin (**2**), arborinine (**3**), graveoline (**4**), clausindin (**5**), and dictamine, displayed the growth inhibitory effect against a series of NCI carcinoma cell lines including HeLa (cervix), KB (nasopharyngus), Hepa 1c1c7 (liver), and DLD (colon) tumor cells.[9] The proliferation of human MCF-7 (breast) and A431 (epidermoid) cancer cell lines were obviously inhibited by arborinine (**3**).[10] However, xanthotoxin (**1**) was reported to have a risk to initiate skin cancer after the i.p. injection to mice with UV light irradiation.[8] The treatment with graveoline (**4**) induced both apoptotic and autophagic cell death in A375 melanoma cells.[11]

A group of furanoacridone alkaloids isolated from the Chou Cao, was demonstrated to have the ability to reverse the MDR in human P-gp-transfected L5178 mouse lymphoma cells. At the same 40 μM concentration, arborinine (**2**), isogravacridone chlorine (**6**), rutacridone (**7**), gravacridonediol (**8**), and gravacridonetriol (**9**) inhibited the pump function of P-gp more efficiently in the L5178 cells than a positive control verapamil (40.6 μM). Gravacridonediol (**8**) was proven to have the most efficient MDR reversal effect, exerting over 100-fold increase in Rh-123 accumulation even at the lower concentration. The sequence of antiproliferative potency against the L5178 cell line *in vitro* was isogravacridone chlorine (**6**) > rutacridone (**7**) > evoxanthine (**10**) ≥ gravacridonediol (**8**) > gravacridonediol monomethyl ether (**11**) > gravacridonetriol (**9**) ≥ arborinine (**3**). Moreover, gravacridonetriol (**9**) and gravacridonediol monomethyl ether (**11**) markedly augmented the cytotoxic activity of DOX against the L5178 cells with the decline of the P-gp mRNA levels. Arborinine (**2**), evoxanthine (**3**), and gravacridonediol (**5**) also additively enhanced the anticancer effect of chemotherapeutic agents, but rutacridone (**7**) and isogravacridone chlorine (**6**) exerted antagonism with DOX to reduce its cytostatic activity. The results evidenced that the acridone skeleton in the alkaloids may be useful in the design of novel anticancer agents.[12]

Essential Oil

The essential oil extracted from Chou Cao exerted moderate antitumor activity against HepG2 (liver) and NCI-H460 (lung) human neoplastic cell lines (IC_{50}: 23.21 and 21.87 μg/mL, respectively). By GC-MS technique, 21 components were identified from the oil, where the major components in the oil were identified as 2-undecanone (46.15%), 2-nonanone (27.01%), and 2-acetoxytridecane (12.73%).[13]

Mutagenicity

Chou Cao extract, additionally, showed a strong mutagenicity toward *Salmonella typhimurium* strain TA98 without a liver cytosol S9 mix and presented moderate mutagenic effects in its strain TA100 with and without S9 mix. By GC-MS, the furoquinoline alkaloids such as dictamnine, skimmianine, γ-fagarine, kokusaginine, and pteleine were detected from the extract.[14] Likewise, the mutagenicity of rutacridone (**7**) and rutacridone epoxide were shown in the *S. typhimurium* strains TA98, TA100, and TA1538. In contrast to rutacridone epoxide as a direct-acting mutagen, the mutagenicity of rutacridone required a metabolic conversion.[15] Also, isogravacridon chlorine (**6**), another furanoacridone alkaloid from the roots, displayed the mutagenic activity on the same strains.[15]

Other Bioactivities

Pharmacological studies in China already confirmed that Chou Cao (Common rue) possesses antispasmodic, antibacterial, and pregnancy-terminating properties besides antitumor. The herb was noted in European folk medicine to relieve gas pains and colic, to improve appetite and digestion, and to promote the onset of menstruation and uterine contractions. The refined rue oil and pilocarpine (a constituent in the herb) were traditionally used as abortifacient among Hispanic people in New Mexico in the United States.

When the herb is made into an ointment for external use, it is effective against gout, arthritis, rheumatism, and neuralgia. However, the coumarin constituents in Chou Cao can cause photosensitive action on the skin. In addition, the rue is a traditional flavoring in Greece and other Mediterranean countries.

Toxic and Side Effects

The volatile oil of Chou Cao (Common rue) causes irritation on the skin. The oral administration of the oil can cause strong stomachache, emetic, twitch, and even prostration; thus, the dosing should be very careful.

References

1. Trovato, A. et al. 1996. In vitro cytotoxic effect of some medicinal plants containing flavonoids. *Bollettino Chim. Farmaceutico* 135: 263–6.
2. Preethi, K. C. et al. 2006. Antitumor activity of *Ruta graveolens* extract. *Asian Pacific J. Cancer Prev.* 7: 439–43.
3. Varamini, P. et al. 2009. Cell cycle analysis and cytotoxic potential of *Ruta graveolens* against human tumor cell lines. *Neoplasma* 56: 490–3.
4. Fadlalla, K. et al. 2011. Ruta graveolens extract induces DNA damage pathways and blocks Akt activation to inhibit cancer cell proliferation and survival. *Anticancer Res.* 31: 233–41.
5. Pathak, S. et al. 2003. Ruta 6 selectively induces cell death in brain cancer cells but proliferation in normal peripheral blood lymphocytes: A novel treatment for human brain cancer. *Intl. J. Oncol.* 23: 975–82.
6. Zobel, A. M. et al. 1997. Differences in antimitotic activity of natural products removed from plant surface and interior of *Ruta graveolens* and *Brassica oleracea. Can. Herba Polonica* 43: 334–7.
7. Gawron, A. et al. 1987. Cytostatic activity of coumarins in vitro. *Planta Med.* 53: 526–9.
8. Nieschulz, O. et al. 1999. *Chinese Materia Medica.* Vol. 4, 4–3783, 962. Shanghai Science and Technology Press, Shanghai, China.
9. Wu, T. S. et al. 2003. Cytotoxic and antiplatelet aggregation principles of *Ruta graveolens. J. Chin. Chem. Soc.* (Taiwan) 50: 171–8.
10. Rethy, B. et al. 2007. Investigation of cytotoxic activity on human cancer cell lines of arborinine and furanoacridones isolated from Ruta graveolens. *Planta Med.* 73: 41–8.
11. Ghosh, S. et al. 2014. Graveoline isolated from ethanolic extract of *Ruta graveolens* triggers apoptosis and autophagy in skin melanoma cells: A novel apoptosis-independent autophagic signaling pathway. *Phytother. Res.* 28: 1153–62.
12. Rethy, B. et al. 2008. Inhibition properties of acridone alkaloids on a murine lymphoma cell line. *Anticancer Res.* 28: 2737–43.
13. Tang, Z. N. et al. 2011. Chemical composition and biological activity of the essential oil of *Ruta graveolens. Zhongguo Xiandai Yingyong Yaoxue* 28: 834–8.
14. Paulini, H. et al. 1987. Mutagenic compounds in an extract from Rutae herba (*Ruta graveolens* L.). I. mutagenicity is partially caused by furoquinoline alkaloids. *Mutagenesis* 2: 271.
15. Paulini, H. et al. 1989. Mutagenicity testing of rutacridone epoxide and rutacridone, alkaloids in *Ruta graveolens* L., using the Salmonella/microsome assay. *Mutagenesis* 4: 45–50.

124 Shi Jian Chuan 石見穿

Chinese sage

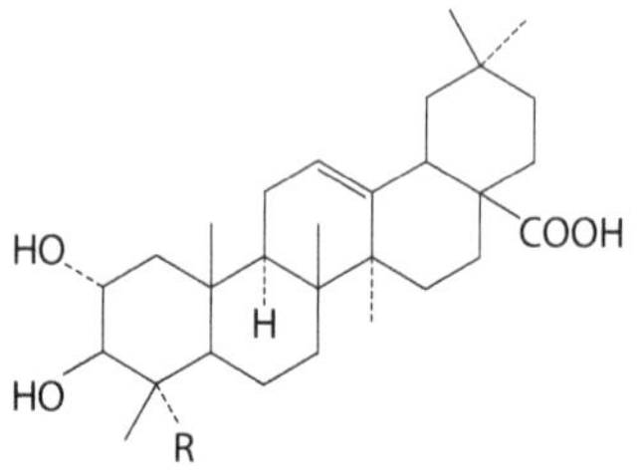

3. R = $-CH_3$
5. R = $-CH_2OH$

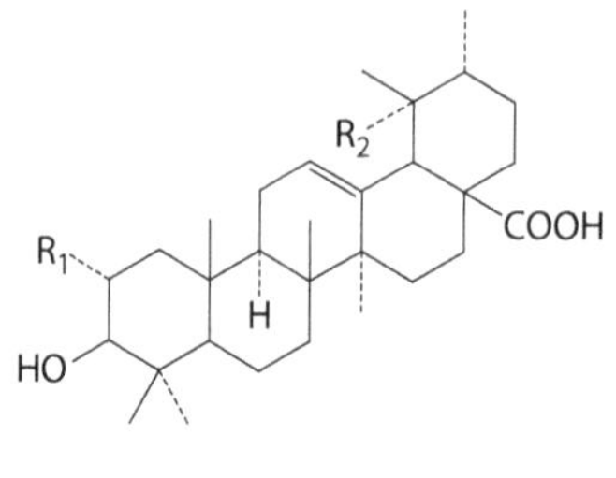

1. $R_1 = -H, R_2 = -OH$
2. $R_1 = -OH, R_2 = -H$
6. $R_1 = R_2 = -OH$

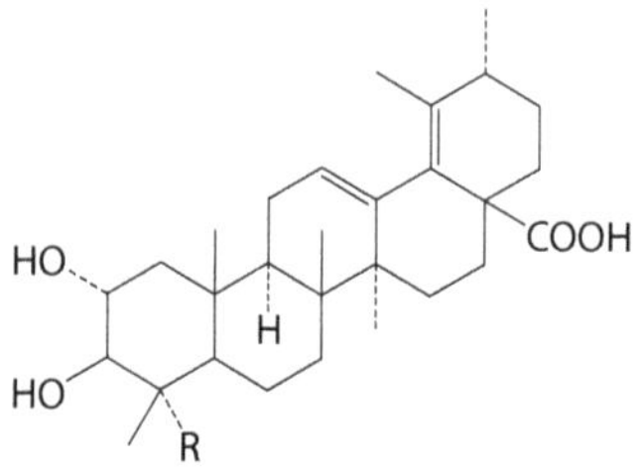

4. R = $-CH_2OH$
7. R = $-CH_3$

Herb Origination

The herb Shi Jian Chuan (Chinese sage) originates from an entire plant, *Salvia chinensis* (Lamiaceae), whose annual herbaceous plant is distributed in the southern region of the Yangtze River in China. The herb collection is usually done in the plant blooming season. The herb can be used fresh and sun-dried for folk medical practice.

Antitumor Activities and Constituents

An alcoholic extract of Shi Jian Chuan displayed certain antiproliferative effect against five human carcinoma cell lines, LoVo (colon), BGC823 and MKN-28 (stomach), A549 (lung) and HepG2 (liver), and mouse LLC cells *in vitro*, whose inhibitory rates were around 10%–70% in its concentrations of 50–400 μg/mL. The *in vitro* assay also revealed that the extract was able to suppress the proliferation of HUVEC cells and to markedly restrain the HUVEC tube formation in association with the increase of HUVEC cell apoptosis and G1 cell cycle arrest, whose inhibitory rates could reach to 18–59% in the concentrations of 12.5–200 μg/mL, and the effect on human umbilical vein endothelial cells (HUVEC) was notably greater than those on the six tumor cell lines mentioned earlier. The administration of the extract to tumor-bearing mice markedly inhibited the growth of Lewis lung cancer cells by 45.9% in a daily dose of 140 mg/kg and suppressed the growth of H22 hepatoma by 48.93% in a dose of 10 g/kg per day. After the treatment, the *in vivo* VEGF expression level and the MVD were also obviously diminished, indicating that the antitumor activity might correlate with its capacity of antiangiogenesis.[1–6] Biology-related phytochemical studies further revealed that Shi Jian Chuan constituents, such as triterpenoids, polyphenolics, polysaccharides, etc., were responsible for the biological activities of the *Salvia* genus.

Triterpenoids

Several triterpenoids separated from the aerial parts of Shi Jian Chuan displayed the moderate inhibitory effect against the proliferation of human HL-60 promyelocytic leukemia cells *in vitro*. Of these inhibitors, pomolic acid (**1**) and 2α-hydroxyursolic acid (**2**) were the most potent with GI_{50} values of 7.77 and 18.36 μM, respectively. The treatment of the triterpenoids such as pomolic acid (**1**), maslinic acid (**3**), pinfaenoic acid (**4**), arjunolic acid (**5**), tormentic acid (**6**), and goreishic acid-I (**7**) alone did not induce NBT (a marker of differentiated cells) reduction, but they notably enhanced the NBT reduction of all *trans*-retinoic acid (an agent used for the treatment of acute promyelocytic leukemia patients) to elicit the HL-60 cells to differentiation, suggesting that the triterpenoids as well as the herb extract can improve leukemia chemotherapy when combined with all *trans*-retinoic acid.[7] Moreover, another isolated triterpenoid assigned as ursolic acid was effective in the inhibition of five human solid tumor lines such as MCF-7 (breast), LoVo (colon), BGC-823 and MKN-28 (stomach), and A549 (lung) cells, *in vitro*.[8]

Flavonoids

The total flavonoids prepared from the *Salvia* dose-dependently induced the apoptosis of human HepG2 and Huh-7 hepatocellular carcinoma cells *in vitro* and significantly repressed the growth of transplanted murine H22 ascitic hepatoma cells *in vivo*. During the antihepatoma effects, the flavonoids substantially suppressed NF-κB activity in the hepatic cancer cells.[9]

Polysaccharides

A polysaccharide component was prepared from *S. chinensis* by a hot water–ethanol method. The polysaccharides could inhibit the growth of human SGC-7901 gastric cancer cell line in dose- and time-dependent manners.[10] The polysaccharide at 50 and 100 g/L concentrations inhibited the metastatic ability of human MGC-803 gastric cancer cells in correlation with the decline of IL-8 level in the MGC-803 cells.[11] More experiments clearly showed the antitumor immunostimulatory effect of the polysaccharide against the transplanted H22 hepatoma cells *in vivo*, whose effect was mediated by amplified cytotoxic activities of the natural killer and the $CD8^+$ T cells, alleviated tumor transplantation-induced $CD4^+$ T cell apoptosis, dysregulated serum cytokine profiles, reduced serum level of PGE2, and restrained transcription and translation of COX-2 in tumor-associated macrophages.[12] These findings noticeably supported the polysaccharide as an adjuvant reagent in the clinical treatment of cancers in the stomach and the liver.

Other Medical Uses

The herb Shi Jian Chuan (Chinese sage) is used as a Chinese folk medicine for the treatment of hepatitis, nephritis, and dysmenorrhea, besides neoplasm. The triterpenoids isolated from the *Salvia* genus exhibit various biological functions including antioxidant, antiinflammatory, and antiviral activities.

References

1. Liang, W. et al. 2014. Advances of chemical constituents and antitumor effects of *Salvia chinensis* Benth. *J. Modern Oncol.* 22: 2492–4.
2. Gao, J. F. et al. 2013. Advances on chemical constituents and pharmacological effects of *Salvia chinensis. Chin. J. Exper. Tradit. Med. Fomul.* 19: 348–51.
3. Zhang, S. et al. 2012. Effects of the extract of *Salvia chinensis* Benth on biological behavior of vascular endothelial cells. *Jiangsu Me. J.* 38: 1257–60, 1368.
4. Liu, F. et al. 2012. Inhibitory effect of extracts from *Salvia chinensis* against H22 tumor in mice. *Chin. J. Experim. Tradit. Med. Formul.* 18: 249–51.
5. Liu, F. et al. 2012. Effect of *Salvia chinensis* extraction on angiogenesis of tumor. *Zhongguo Zhongyao Zazhi* 37: 1285–8.
6. Xu, J. X. et al. 2011. Progress in research on chemical constituents and antitumor effect of *Salvia chinensis. Xiandai Zhongliu Yixue* 19: 587–90.
7. Wang, Y. L. et al. 2009. Triterpenoids isolated from the aerial parts of *Salvia chinensis. Phytochem. Lett.* 2: 81–4.
8. Qian, X. P. et al. 2012. In vitro anticancer activities of the ursolic acid isolated from *Salvia chinensis. Xiandai Zhongliu Yixue* 20: 2244–8.
9. Xiang, M. X. et al. 2013. Chemical composition of total flavonoids from *Salvia chinensia* Benth and their pro-apoptotic effect on hepatocellular carcinoma cells: Potential roles of suppressing cellular NF-κB signaling. *Food Chem. Toxicol.* 62: 420–6.
10. Liang, Q. C. et al. 2013. Extraction of polysaccharides from *Salvia chinensis* and its antitumor effect. *Guangpu Shiyanshi* 30: 1331–4.
11. Zhu, H. Y. et al. 2012. Effect of *Salvia chinensis* Benth polysaccharides on metastasis ability of human gastric cancer cells (MGC-803 cells). *Zhongguo Yiyao Daobao* 9: 5–7.
12. Shu, G. W. 2015. Antitumor immunostimulatory activity of polysaccharides from *Salvia chinensis* Benth. *J. Ethnopharmacol.* 168: 237–47.

125 Dan Shen 丹参

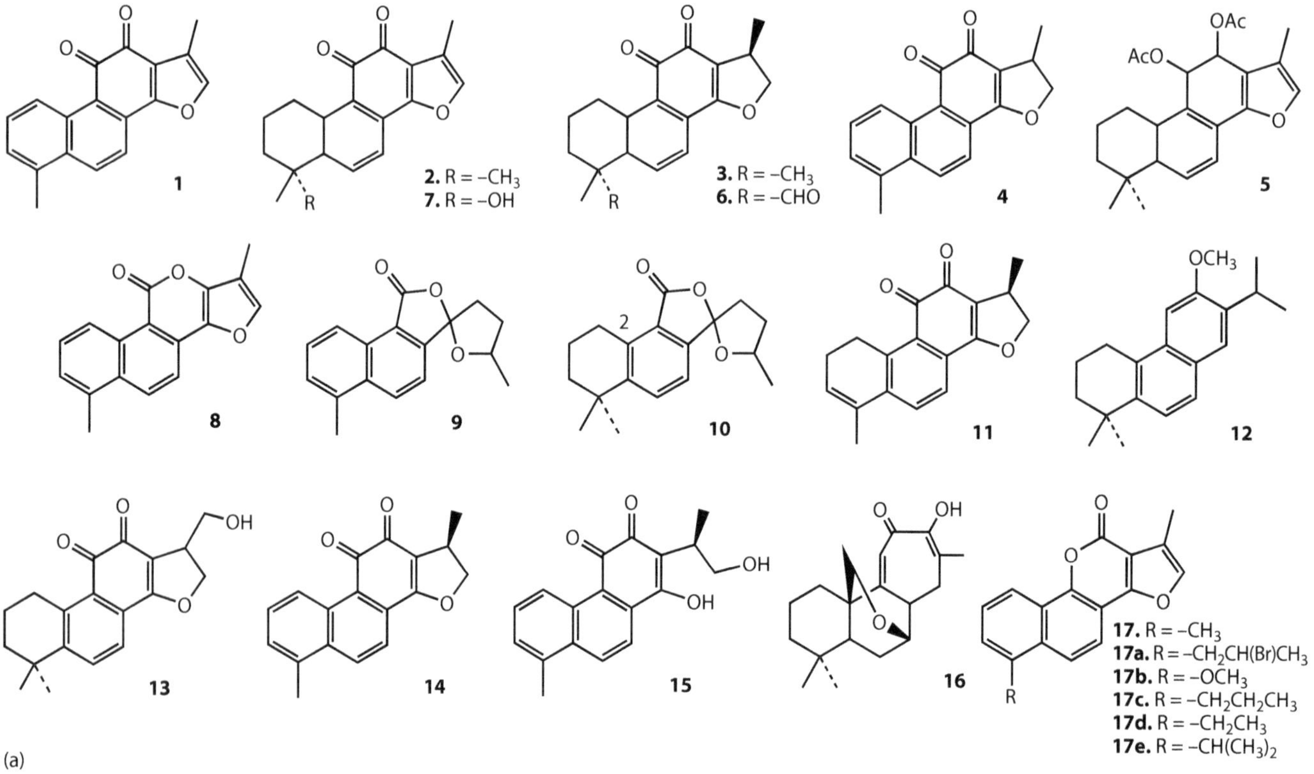

O O 1

O O 2. R = $-CH_3$ 7. R = $-OH$

3. R = $-CH_3$ 6. R = $-CHO$

4

OAc AcO 5

8 9 2 10 11 OCH_3 12

OH 13 14 OH OH 15 OH 16

17. R = $-CH_3$
17a. R = $-CH_2CH(Br)CH_3$
17b. R = $-OCH_3$
17c. R = $-CH_2CH_2CH_3$
17d. R = $-CH_2CH_3$
17e. R = $-CH(CH_3)_2$

(a)

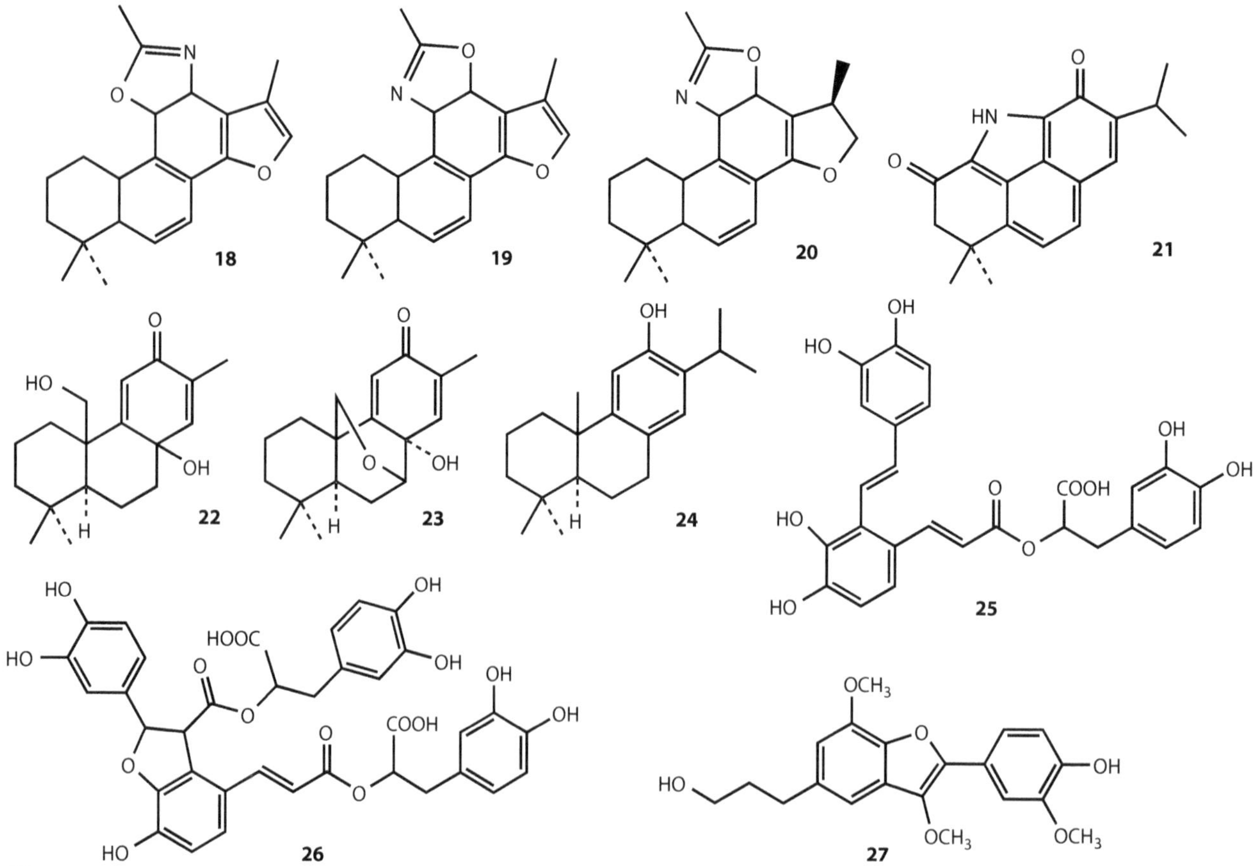

N O 18 N O 19 N O 20 HN O 21

HO OH 22 OH 23 OH 24

OH HO HO HO OH OH COOH 25

HO HO OH HOOC OH OH COOH OH HO 26

OCH_3 HO OH OCH_3 OCH_3 27

(b)

Herb Origination

The herb Dan Shen is one of the most valuable Chinese traditional medicines, which was recorded as a top-grade drug in the first Chinese classic of materia medica entitled *Shennong Ben Cao Jing*. The herb mainly originated from the dried roots of *Salvia miltiorrhiza* (Lamiaceae) and partially from the dried roots of *S. przewalskii*. The former plant is widely distributed in many Chinese provinces, and the latter plant is only found in some areas of western China.

Antitumor Activities

Because Dan Shen is widely used in China as an effective regimen, it has drawn attention from chemists and medicinal clinicians, especially in the two recent decades for the prevention and the treatment of cancers. Studies revealed that the Dan Shen extract was sensitive to inhibit multiple types of cancer cell lines. The significant cytotoxicity of Dan Shen was observed in human CAL-27 and FaDu head and neck epithelial tumor, HepG2 hepatoma, KB nasopharynx cancer cell lines, as well as murine sarcoma 180 and Ehrlich neoplastic cell lines. The antiproliferative activity was found to be related to the blockage of nucleoside transport (uridine and thymidine) and DNA synthesis in the carcinoma cells.[1–5] After the Dan Shen extract treatment, a rapid decline of intracellular GSH and protein thiol content was resulted in the HepG2 cells. Concurrently, the mitochondrial permeability transition and its membrane potential were disturbed, and the release of cytochrome c into the cytosol and the elevation of the intracellular ROS level subsequently occurred prior to the initiation of apoptosis.[5,6] Furthermore, Dan Shen also obstructed the invasion and the adhesion of human SMMC-7721 hepatoma cells by repressing the expression of cell membrane intercellular adhesive molecule (ICAM)-1. In nude mice implanted with human metastatic LCI-D20 hepatoma cells, the inhibitory activity of Dan Shen was demonstrated against the metastasis and the recurrence of human liver carcinoma after hepatectomy,[7] indicating that Dan Shen is able to exert antimetastasis and antiinvasion functions besides the antiproliferation.

Moreover, Dan Shen markedly potentiated the cytotoxicity of anticancer drugs such as 5-FU, mitomycin-C, and methotrexate (MTX) in KB nasopharyngeal cancer cells and BEL-7402 hepatoma cells *in vitro* and *in vivo*.[2] When Dan Shen extract and baicalin were applied together, a synergistic inhibitory effect was offered in human MCF-7 breast cancer cell proliferation to enhance the potential therapeutic benefits.[1] Eighty-two patients with breast cancer had been recruited to take Dan Shen (20 mg/kg) and Yun Zhi polysaccharopeptide (50 mg/kg) capsules every day for a total of six months. The absolute counts of T helper lymphocytes (CD4$^+$), the ratio of T helper (CD4$^+$)/T suppressor and cytotoxic lymphocytes (CD8$^+$), and the percentage of B-lymphocytes were significantly elevated, while the plasma sIL-2R concentration was obviously lessened in the patients. The findings indicated that the regular oral administration of Dan Shen can be beneficial for promoting immunological function and reducing the side effects caused by chemotherapeutic agents.[8] Additionally, Dan Shen with vitamin E could alleviate the damages of respiratory nasal and tracheal mucosa caused by pingyangmycin in Wistar rats, exerting the protective activity.[9]

Moreover, the Dan Shen extract exhibited significant antimutagenic action against AFB1-induced hepatocarcinogenesis in rats, whose inhibitory effect was accompanied by the activation of serum alanine aminotransferase and aspartate aminotransferase and the substantial reduction of GST-P mRNA expression and GST placenta form positive foci formation. The antihepatocarcinogenic effect was also found to be associated with the corresponding decrease of AFB1-DNA adduct formation as well as decline of AFB1-induced oxidative DNA damage in the rat liver.[10]

Antitumor Constituents and Activities

The discovered growth inhibitory components from Dan Shen have been demonstrated to be prominently conducive to clinical cancer chemotherapy and prevention. The bioactive ingredients, such as lipophilic constituents (tanshinone-IIA, tanshinone-I, dihydrotanshinon-I, ailantholide, cryptotanshinone, neotanshinlactone, miltirone, and nitrogen-containing compounds) and hydrophilic components (salvinal, salvianolic acid-A, and salvianolic acid-B), have been investigated in *in vitro* and *in vivo* experiments and approved the ingredients to play important roles in the suppression of different stages of tumor evolution, progression, and metastasis.

Abietane-Type Diterpene Quinones

The lipophilic constituents derived from Dan Shen are principally abietane-type diterpene quinones, which were demonstrated as the major anticancer agents in the herb extract.

Tanshinone-I and Its Analogs

Tanshinone-I (TSI) (**1**) and tanshinone-IIA (TSIIA) (**2**) were cytotoxic to P388 murine leukemia cells with 86.76% and 56.05% inhibitory rates, respectively, at a 25 μg/mL concentration.[11] Both *in vitro* and *in vivo* experiments provided the evidences in the suppression of human HepG2 hepatoma cells and the promotion of G0/G1 cell cycle arrest and apoptosis for TSI (**1**).[12] Through mitochondria-mediated intrinsic cell death pathway and p21-mediated G0/G1 cell cycle arrest, TSI (**1**) elicited the apoptotic death and obstructed the proliferation of human Colo205 colon neoplastic cells.[13] TSI (**1**) and its analog 15,16-dihydrotanshinone-I dose- and time-dependently restrained the growth of human MCF-7 breast cancer (estrogen receptor$^+$) and MDA-MB-231 breast cancer (estrogen receptor$^-$) cell lines and notably enhanced their apoptosis *in vitro*.[14,15] The onset of the apoptotic death of these cancer cells was mediated by the downregulation of the antiapoptotic protein Bcl-2, the upregulation of proapoptotic protein Bax, and the activation of caspase-3-dependent pathway.[12,14,15] The antigrowth effect of 15,16-dihydrotanshinone-I on the MDA-MB-231 cells was further confirmed in a nude mice xenograft experiment.[15] TSI (**1**) was effective in inhibiting the proliferation of three kinds of monocytic leukemia (U937, THP-1, and SHI-1) cell lines and inducing the apoptosis time- and dose-dependently. The apoptosis of three monocytic leukemia cell lines provoked TSI was highly correlated with the activation of caspase-3, the downregulation of survivin expression, and the decreases of telomerase activity and hTERT mRNA expression.[16] Compared TSIIA (**2**) and cryptotanshinone (CTS)

(**3**) (two other anticancer agents in Dan Shen), TSI (**1**) showed the most potent activity in the suppression of H1299 lung carcinoma cells and DU-145 prostate cancer cells. The treatment with TSI (**1**) at a dose of 200 mg/kg markedly reduced the tumor weight by 34% in a mouse model implanted with H1299 NSCLC cells and induced 54% antiproliferative, 193% apoptotic, and 72% antiangiogenic effects.[17] Similarly, the elicitation of apoptotic death, proliferative inhibition, and angiogenic repression by TSI (**1**) was demonstrated in human DU145 prostate tumor cells *in vitro* and *in vivo*.[18] The downregulation of Aurora-A function is also partially involved in the anticancer mechanism of TSI (**1**) against prostate and lung cancer cells.[17,18]

Moreover, in a highly invasive human CL1-5 lung adenocarcinoma cells, TSI (**1**) obviously obstructed the migration, invasion, and gelatinase activities in the macrophage-conditioned medium-stimulated CL1-5 cells *in vitro*, although no direct cytotoxicity to the CL1-5 cells. The antitumorigenic and antimetastatic effects were further proven in immunodeficient mice implanted with CL1-5 tumor. These effects were found to be mediated by multiple mechanisms such as reduction of interleukin-8 transcriptional activity and angiogenic factor, attenuation of DNA-binding activity of AP-1 and NF-κB, and suppression of ras-MAPK and Rac1 signaling pathways.[18] Importantly, TSI (**1**) dose-dependently suppressed ICAM-1 and VCAM-1 expressions in TNFα-stimulated HUVECs.[19] Therefore, the pretreatment with TSI (**1**) prominently reduced the adhesion of either MDA-MB-231 breast cancer cells or U937 monocyte lymphoma cells to HUVECs, efficiently reduced TNFα-induced VEGF production, and inhibited MDA-MB-231 migration. The diminution of the tumor mass volume and the metastatic incidents by TSI (**1**) was also demonstrated *in vivo*.[14,19] Taken together, these results evidenced the potential therapeutic values and mechanisms of TSI (**1**) on human cancer and suggested that TSI (**1**) may serve as an effective adjunctive drug for the cancer treatments.

Likewise, a naturally occurring analog, dihydrotanshinone-I (**4**), was reported to have cytotoxic activity on a variety of tumor cells; especially, it was effective in the growth arrest of a multidrug-resistant-type leukemia cells and the induction apoptosis of K562/ADR cells.[20] More interestingly, the studies showed that dihydrotanshinone-I (**4**) has the ability to block angiogenesis by suppressing endothelial cell proliferation, migration, invasion and tube formation, indicating that this analog has a potential to be developed as a novel antiangiogenic agent.[21]

Tanshinone-IIA and Its Analogs

TSIIA (**2**) established significant cytotoxicity on many types of human cancer cells, such as hepatoma (HepG2, Bel-7402 and SMMC-7721), breast cancer (MCF-7 and MDA-MB-231), colon cancer (Colo 205 and HCT-116), prostate cancer (PC3 and LNCaP), leukemia (HL-60, K562 and NB4), cervical and ovarian cancer (HeLa and SKOV3), gastric cancer (MKN-45), osteosarcoma (MG-63), and glioma cells.[22–41] The IC_{50} values were 0.1 μg/mL in giloma cells, 0.4 μM or 0.25 μg/mL in MCF-7 cells, 6.28 μg/mL in Bel-7402 cells, and 7.8 μM in PC3 cells. The inhibitory effect of TSIIA (**2**) was largely correlated with its ability in elicitating the cell apoptotic death and/or disturbing the cell cycle progression. But some characteristic pathways were found to be selectively involved in the inhibitory mechanisms for the specific carcinoma cells. The growth, proliferation, and colony-formation of human SMMC-7721 hepatoma cells were inhibited by TSIIA (**2**) by promoting the cell cycle arrest and apoptotic death, associated with the increase of intracellular calcium, the downregulation of Bcl-2 and c-Myc expressions, and the upregulation of p53, Fas, Bax, and MT-1A expressions.[22,42] Both mitochondria-mediated intrinsic death and Fas-mediated extrinsic death pathways participated in the TSIIA-promoted apoptotic death of Colo205 cells.[23] The suppressive effect against human MKN-45 gastric cancer cell proliferation closely correlated with the down-expression of integrin-β1 and MMP-7 mRNA,[24] whose inhibitory effect was further proven in a mouse xenograft model with gastric cancer.[43] By disrupting the mitotic spindle during the M-phase and subsequently triggering the tumor cells to apoptosis through the mitochondria-dependent apoptotic pathway, TSIIA (**2**) arrested the proliferation of HeLa cervical neoplastic cells in mitosis, whose apoptosis was advanced by TSIIA faster than by taxol and VCR.[25] The proapoptotic signaling pathway of TSIIA in HL-60 promyelocytic leukemia cells and K562 erythroleukemia cells was related to the increase of the cells hypodiploid DNA, the activation of caspase-3, and the cleavage of PARP.[26,27] Also, TSIIA (**2**) induced cytochrome c-mediated caspase cascade apoptosis and obstructed the proliferation of A549 human lung cancer cells (IC_{50}: 14.5–16.0 μM at 48 h) via the activation of JNK pathway,[44] whereas the anticancer mechanism in NCI-H460 lung cancer cells narrowly correlated with the decreases of Bcl-2 and c-Myc expressions and telomerase activity, the inhibition of DNA synthesis, and the changes of the cellular surface antigen expression.[2,29] The apoptosis-inducing effect of TSIIA (**2**) in rat C6 glioma cells was associated to the significant decrease of constitutive STAT3 activity parallel with the marked attenuation of expression of Bcl-xL and cyclin-D1.[30]

Similar to TSI (**1**), TSIIA (**2**) demonstrated a potential anticancer effect on both estrogen receptor$^+$-MCF-7 and estrogen receptor$^-$ MDA-MB-231 breast cancer cells *in vitro*. By subcutaneous injection of TSIIA to nude mice at a dose of 30 mg/kg (three times per week) for 10 weeks, the tumor mass volume was reduced by 44.91%, whose effect was stronger than tamoxifen in both the estrogen receptor$^+$ and estrogen receptor$^-$ breast carcinomas.[34,35] The activity was also correlated with the inhibition of multiple genes involved in the cell cycle regulation, the cell proliferation, the apoptosis, and the DNA synthesis.[35,36] Likewise, acetyltanshinone-IIA (**5**) preferentially inhibited the growth of estrogen receptor$^+$ breast cancer cell lines (MCF-7 and T-47D) by restraining GREB1 (estrogen receptor-responsive gene) transcription. Acetyltanshinone-IIA (**5**) was also effective in inhibiting estrogen receptor$^-$ breast cancer cells (MDA-MB-231), but it was more potent in the estrogen receptor$^+$ cells than in the estrogen receptor$^-$ cells.[45] The daily oral administration of TSIIA (25 mg/kg) retarded the growth of AD LNCaP prostate cancer xenograft in correlation with the downregulation of the tumor AR abundance and AR nuclear translocation in nude mice. Consequently, the inhibitory effect on the AI prostate carcinoma cells was less effective than on the AD cells, and the anti-LNCap potency of TSIIA (**2**) was superior to that of TSI (**1**) and 10–30 folds greater than that of Casodex (racemic).[46] The cotreatment of TSIIA (**2**) with cisplatin showed synergistic antitumor effects against human prostate cancer AI LNCaP cells and AD PC3 cells with the increase of the intracellular concentration of cisplatin and elicited cell cycle arrest and apoptosis via death receptor pathway and mitochondrial pathway.[47] Also, TIIA could enhance the TRAIL-induced apoptosis by upregulating DR5 receptors through ROS-JNK-CHOP signaling axis in human ovarian carcinoma cells.[48]

Moreover, TSIIA (**2**) not only enforces the tumor cell apoptosis but also induces the cell differentiation and inhibits the cell invasion and metastasis. The treatment of human glioma cells with TSIIA (0.025–0.10 μg/mL) could significantly provoke the cell differentiation through the enhancement of ADPRTL1 and CYP1A1 mRNA expression for one- to twofold and the suppression of BrdU incorporation besides the increase of apoptosis and the decrease of colony formation.[29] When TSIIA (**2**) caused the apoptosis of NB4 acute promyelocytic leukemia and MG-63 osteosarcoma cells, the tumor cell adhesion and invasion were concurrently restrained through the modulation of ECM and the secretion of MMP-2, MMP-9 and TIMP-2.[32,33,49–51]

The investigation further revealed that TSIIA (**2**) could repress HUVEC growth and tube formation with respective IC_{50} values of 0.5 and 1 μM.[35] TSIIA (**2**) elicited cytotoxicity and oxidative stress on human endothelial cells via the activation of quinone oxidoreductase (NQO1), followed by the induction of a Ca^{2+} imbalance and mitochondrial dysfunction and then the stimulation caspase activity.[38,50–52] The antiangiogenic function was shown in TSIIA (2)-treated carcinoma cells such as SKOV-3 ovarian cancer, SMMC-7721 hepatoma, HCT-116 colon cancer, and MG-63 osteosarcoma, whose marked effect on the vessel tube formation was partly attributed to its ability in the down-expression of VEGF.[40,50,51] The antiangiogenic effect was revealed to be involved in the downregulation of a VEGF/VEGFR2 pathway in vascular endothelial cells.[53] The results indicated that TSIIA (**2**) also has potent antiangiogenic property, whose effect contributed to its anticancer potency.

In addition, TSIIA (**2**) may potentially protect the heart from severe toxicity of DOX. The cardiomyocyte apoptosis caused by DOX was repressed by TSIIA (**2**) by stimulating Akt-signaling pathways.[49] The sodium sulfonate of TSIIA could protect the DOX-induced nephropathy by a notable effect against oxidative stress.[54,55] According to the remarkable evidences, TSIIA (**2**) deserves to be supported as a promising drug lead for further development in drug discovery and antineoplastic clinical trials.

Cryptotanshinone

The inhibition of CTS (**3**), 1,2-dihydrotanshinone-I, tanshindiol-A, tanshindiol-B, tanshindiol-C, and methylenetanshinquinone was similar or slightly stronger *in vitro*, compared to that of TSIIA (**2**) on the proliferation of XF-498 SKOV-3, SK-MEL-2, A549, and HCT-15 cancer cell lines.[56] Accompanied by the activation of p38/JNK and the inhibition of ERK1/2 by the induction of ROS, CTS (**3**) promoted caspase-independent cell death of the human Rh30 rhabdomyosarcoma, DU-145 prostate cancer, and MCF-7 breast cancer cell lines.[57] CTS (**3**) as a potent STAT3 inhibitor rapidly inhibited the phosphorylation of STAT3 Tyr705 and lessened the expression of STAT3 downstream target proteins such as cyclin-D1, Bcl-xL, and survivin in the DU-145 cells to exert the antiproliferative effect.[58] CTS (**3**), dihydrotanshinone-I (**4**), and dihydroisotanshinone-I were also effective in suppressing A549 lung cancer cells (IC_{50}: 2.4–2.7 μM), while CTS (**3**) inhibited HCT-8 (colon) and BGC-823 (stomach) cancer cell lines (respective IC_{50}: 3.9 and 8.3 μM), and dihydrotanshinone-I (**4**) obstructed BGC-823 cells (IC_{50}: 2.2 μM).[59] In a test with HUVECs, CTS (**3**) significantly reduced the cellular levels of VEGF and a downstream of HIF-1α, thereby blocking the tube formation. Similar to the reduction of VEGF expression and the blockage of HIF-1α binding to the VEGF promoter, CTS (**3**) at a dose of 10 mg/kg suppressed the growth of PC3 cells by 46.4% in nude mice. During the effect, CTS (**3**) lessened the expressions of Ki-67 (proliferation), carbonic anhydrase-IX (hypoxic marker) CD34 (blood vessel), VEGF (angiogenesis), and AEG-1.[60] Moreover, CTS (**3**) acted as a potent stimulator of ER stress to promote many types of cancer cells to apoptotic death. By eliciting ROS-generated ER stress, CTS (**3**) was able to sensitize a broad range of anticancer agents including etoposide, 5-FU, cisplatin, and TNFα in the treatment of human hepatoma and breast cancer.[61]

Importantly, CTS (**3**) has an ability to diminish the cell viability of some drug-resistant tumor cells (such as melanoma B16BL6 cells and leukemia K562/Adr cells) by eliciting cell cycle arrest and apoptosis by up-expressing p21 and down-expressing Cdk1/cdc2 and Bcl-2. The overactivated eIF4E was significantly reduced in K562/Adm leukemia cells after the treatment, whose interaction was responsible for the MDR-reversing action in human chronic myeloid leukemia cells.[62,63] By down-regulating P-gp mRNA and protein levels, and inhibiting P-gp ATPase activity, both CTS (**3**) and dihydrotanshinone amplified the cytotoxicity of DOX and irinotecan in P-gp-overexpressing SW620 Ad300 colon cancer cells.[64] Furthermore, CTS (**3**) was also able to suppress the lymphangiogenesis (which, like angiogenesis, plays an important role in promoting tumor growth and metastasis) in an *in vitro* model and inhibit the tube formation in lymphatic endothelial cells.[65] When CTS (3) is combined As_2O_3, the cytotoxicity on human U266 multiple myeloma cells was synergistically enhanced and the cell apoptosis was mainly promoted through the induction of a p38/JNK pathway.[66] Therefore, the findings suggest that cryptotanshinone could be further developed for sensitizing resistant cancer cells and used as an adjuvant therapy together with anticancer drugs.

Other Tanshinone Analogs

Many tanshinone analogs with dihydrofurano-1,2-naphthoquinone, furano-1,2-naphtho-quinone, or 2-hydroxy-1,4-naphthoquinone skeletons were isolated from the chloroform and ethanolic extracts of Dan Shen roots. These analogs were found to have cytotoxic activities against various human solid tumor cell lines, such as HeLa (cervix), SKOV-3 (ovary), KB (nasopharynx), A549 (lung), SK-MEL-2 (skin), HCT-15 and Colo-205 (colon), XF498 (brain), HEp-2 (larynx), and MCF-7 and MDA-MB-231 (breast) cells *in* vitro.[56,67] Several tanshinone analogs were effective at <1 μg/mL concentrations without selectivity.[66] Tanshinaldehyde (**6**), przewaquinone-C (**7**), tanshinlactone-A (**8**), danshenspiroketalactone-I (**9**) and danshenspiroketalactone-II (**10**), epi-danshenspiroketal-lactone, methyl dihydrotanshinonate, dihydronortanshinone, and dihydroiso-tanshinone showed significant cytotoxic effect against KB, Colo205, HeLa, and HEp-2 cell lines *in vitro*.[68] Tanshinlactone-A (**11**) also exerted moderate cytotoxicities against human OVCAR-3 ovary and HepG2 liver carcinoma cell lines.[69] Two analogs assigned as 1,2,15,16-tetrahydrotanshiquinone (**12**) and Ro-090680 (**13**) were the growth inhibitors of P388 leukemia cells.[70] The i.p. injection of przewaquinone-A (**14**) to tumor-bearing mice in doses of 120–150 mg/kg restrained the cell growth of Lewis lung cancer, B16 melanoma, and sarcoma 180 *in vivo* by 35.8–67.8% and obviously prolonged the life span of mice implanted with P388 lymphocytic leukemia.[71] The antitumor property of tanshinone-VI (**15**) was primarily shown in the suppression of cell adhesion, due to the blockage of the upregulation of cell adhesion molecules (ICAM-1 and VCAM-1), with the consequent inhibition of metastases formation and/or angiogenesis.[72]

In addition, dihydrotanshinone-I (**4**) suppressed the catalytic activity of Topo-I by the formation of a cleavable complex and partly intercalation into DNA.[73] A unique type of the diterpenoid in Dan Shen assigned as miltipolone (**16**) exerted potent antiproliferative effect against murine B16-F10 melanoma cells and human HCT-116 colon cancer cells *in vitro* (respective IC_{50}: 0.16 and 0.003 μg/mL,).[74] Danshenol-A, danshenol-B, and danshenol-C were the three other diterpenoids from Dan Shen, showing obvious antiproliferative effect against HCT-8, BGC-823, and A549 human cancer cell lines (IC_{50}: 1.0–3.9 μM), whose activities were comparable to those of TSIIA (**2**). Danshenol-B and danshenol-C were also moderately cytotoxic to A2780 ovarian cancer cells (IC_{50}: 4.6–5.2 μM).[59]

Neotanshinlactones

The extended studies exhibited that neotanshinlactone (**17**) was active in the inhibition of estrogen receptor $(ER)^+$ human MCF-7 and ZR-75-1 breast carcinoma cell lines *in vitro* with ED_{50} values of 0.6 and 0.3 μg/mL, respectively, but was inactive on estrogen receptor $(ER)^-$ breast cancer cells (MDA-MB-231 and HS-587-T). Interestingly, neotanshinlactone (**17**) also inhibited HER2-overexpressing SK-BR-3 breast cancer cells. The basis of these direct comparisons revealed that neotanshinlactone (**17**) was 10-fold more potent and 20-fold more selective than Nolvadex (an antagonist of the estrogen receptor in the breast tissue) against ER^+ and $HER2^+$ breast cancer cell lines *in vitro*, respectively.[75] The synthesized series of neotanshinlactone derivatives (**17a–17e**) were found to have potent and selective anti-breast-cancer activity with IC_{50} values of 0.1–0.3 μg/mL against human ZR-75-1 breast cancer cells *in vitro*. **17a** was two- to threefold more potent than the starting molecule **17** against HER2-overexpressed SK-BR-3 (ER^-) and ZR-75-1 (ER^+) breast cancer cell lines. Importantly, **17b** exerted high selectivity and was 23 times more active against estrogen receptor+ and HER2 overexpressed ZR-75-1 cells than against ER^+-MCF-7 cells, whereas **17c** displayed an approximately 12-fold ratio of ER^- SK-BR-3/ER^+ MCF-7 selectivity. In nude mice xenografts models, analog **17d** exerted potent inhibitory activity against the ZR-75-1 breast carcinoma, but no activity on MDA-MB-231 breast cancer and PC3 prostate carcinoma xenografts.[76] The extremely selective derivatives can be considered to have development potential for the treatment of breast cancer as clinical trial candidates.

N-Containing Tanshinones

Four N-containing tanshinone analogs, neosalvianen (**18**), salvianen (**19**), salvianan (**20**), and salviadione (**21**), were also isolated from Dan Shen roots. The most potent N-containing tanshinone was identified as salvianen (**19**), which showed dose-dependent and moderate cytotoxic effect against HeLa, HepG2, and OVCAR-3 neoplastic cell lines with a CD_{50} range of 30.4–39.5 μM.[77,78]

Structure–Activity Relationships

The investigations of the structure–bioactivity relationship disclosed that the tanshinone analogs with either olefinic feature or hydroxyl substitutions in the A-ring demonstrated higher antigrowth activities on the neoplastic cells. Meaningfully, the presence of a furanonaphthoquinone in the molecule, i.e., tanshinones, with an *o*-quinone in C-ring and an intact D-ring, exhibited significant cytotoxic effect, whereas the tanshinones with 2-hydroxy-p-quinone in C-ring and without D-ring or lack of an intact furan ring were found to be inactive.[79] These results suggested that the planar phenanthrene ring of the tanshinones is important for the interaction with DNA sequences, and the furano-o-quinone moiety is responsible for the production of reactive free radicals in the close vicinity of the bases to cause DNA damage in the tumor cells.[67]

Abietane-Type Norditerpenoids

From the roots of *S. miltiorrhiza* (collected in Tibet), three cancer growth inhibitory abietane-type norditerpenoids were elucidated as militibetin-A (**22**), yunnannin-A (**23**), and ferruginol (**24**). In an *in vitro* assay, the norditerpenoids exhibited marked cytotoxic effects against P388 (mouse lymphocytic leukemia), HONE-1 (human nasopharyngeal cancer), and HT-29 (human colon adeno-carcinoma) cell lines, and their ED_{50} values ranged from 2.9 to 5.4 μg/mL, whose potencies were less than those of chemotherapeutic agents, etoposide and cisplatin (ED_{50}: 1.4–1.9 μg/mL), on the same tumor cell lines.[80]

Caffeic Acid Derivatives

Salvianolic acid-A (SAA) (**25**) and salvianolic acid-B (SAB) (**26**), two caffeic acid derivatives isolated from the aqueous extract of Dan Shen, were found to possess anticancer activity and an ability to reduce the side effects of commonly used anticancer drugs. In the *in vitro* treatment, SAA (**25**) inhibited proliferation, caused cell cycle arrest at the S phase, and induced apoptosis dose-dependently to two kinds of cancer cells, MDR MCF-7 human breast cancer cells and their parental counterparts, where SAA downregulated the P-gplevel and increased the ROS level by 6.2-fold in MDR MCF-7 cells and by 1.6-fold in MCF-7 cells, indicating that SAA was capable of reversing the MDR of the resistant cells. SAA showed higher antitumor activity than DOX did in xenografts established from the resistant cells.[81] The present work raised a possibility that SAA might be considered a potential choice to overcome MDR for the selective susceptibility of the resistant breast cancer cells to SAA treatment. In the combinational treatments, SAA (**25**) synergistically augmented the antitumor activities of 5-FU, mitomycin-C, and MTX without increasing the toxicity in the *in vivo* test models.[82]

SAB (**26**) displayed marked suppression against the incidence of a SCC from 64.7% to 16.7%. Through the decreases of hypoxia-inducible factor-1 and VEGF protein, SAB (**26**) obstructed the malignant transformation of oral precancerous lesion, showing that the anticancer effect may be closely related to the antiangiogenic activity.[83] Similarly, the antiproliferative effect of SAB (**26**) on SCC4 and CAL27 oral SCC cells was partially contributed by the antiangiogenic potential by down-expressin the key regulator genes of angiogenesis.[84] The antigrowth effect of SAB (**26**) was also demonstrated in human JHU-022 and JHU-013 head and neck SCC cell lines (HNSCC) *in vitro* with IC_{50} values of 18 and 50 μM, respectively. The treatment of HNSCC xenografts in nude mice with SAB (**26**) in a dose of 80 mg/kg per day for 25 days markedly reduced the tumor volumes. The antineoplastic mechanism has been proposed to respect the inhibition of COX-2/PGE-2 pathway and lipid peroxidation, the promotion of apoptosis, and the blockage of angiogenesis.[85,86] Furthermore, the anticancer efficacy of low-dose celecoxib could be significantly enhanced by SAB (**26**) on the JHU-013 and JHU-022 cell lines in a cotreatment. The daily treatment with SAB (40 mg/kg/day) and celecoxib (2.5 mg/kg/day) together resulted in a more pronounced anti-HNSCC effect in nude mice implanted with JHU-013 xenograft compared to a full dose of SAB (80 mg/kg/day) or celecoxib (5 mg/kg/day) alone. The *in vitro* and *in vivo* combinational effect was fond to be associated with the profound inhibition of COX-2 activity and the promotion of apoptosis.[87]

In addition, SAB (**26**) was also capable of exerting a chemopreventive effect DMBA-induced oral carcinogenesis in a hamster model and alleviating the toxicity caused by cisplatin, a chemotherapeutic drug.[83] Consequently, SAB (**26**) may be considered as a promising drug candidate for the treatment of malignant tumors, especially HNSCC.

Phenolic Acid Analogs

Several phenolic and aromatic components separated from herb Dan Shen showed marked antiproliferative effect against the neoplastic cells as well. By arresting the cell cycle at mitosis, repressing the tubulin polymerization, and increasing the apoptotic death, salvinal (**27**) caused *in vitro* growth inhibition on a variety of human cancer cell lines (IC_{50}: 4–17 μM). Because salvinal (**27**) is a poor substrate for the transport by P-gp and MDR-associated protein, a similar inhibitory potency was achieved by salvinal (**27**) against both parental KB cells and multidrug-resistant KB cell sublines (such as P-gp-overexpressing KB/vin10 cells, KB/taxol-50 cells, and MRP-expressing etoposide-resistant KB/7D cells).[88] SAA had no inhibitory effects against the proliferation of B16-F10 melanoma cells and HUVEC cells, but it significantly obstructed the invasion and the migration of B16-F10 melanoma cells because it repressed VEGF-induced endothelial migration, tube formation, and new vessel formation dramatically in B16-F10 cells in association with the significant expressive decreases of MMP-2, MMP-9 and VEGF. The suppressive effect on lung metastasis in spontaneous and experimental B16-F10 melanoma models was approved *in vivo* in the treatment with SAA at doses of 20–40 mg/kg.[89]

Other isolated aromatic constituents, alvianonol, 2α-acetoxysugiol, and danshenxinkun-B, showed moderate cytotoxicity against three human cancer cell lines (HeLa, HepG2, and OVCAR-3). Arucadiol palmitate potently obstructed the proliferation of the HeLa and OVCAR-3 cells *in vitro*, and its respective CD_{50} values were 3.2 and 4.1 μg/mL, those CD_{50} values were comparable to those of cisplatin.[90] In a nude mice model, the injection of Dan Shen depside salts in a dose of 50 mg/kg every 3 days for 16 days inhibited the growth of human SMMC-7721 hepatoma cells and induced the cell apoptosis through a mitochondrial pathway and the down-expression of Ki–67 and VEGF.[91,92]

Polysaccharides

A polysaccharide (SMP-W1) was purified from the roots of *S. miltiorrhiza*, whose apparent molecular weight was estimated to be 6.9 × 10^5 Da. SMP-W1 contained 96.9% total sugar and a minor amount of uronic acid (0.12%) and consisted of mannose, rhamnose, arabinose, glucose, and galactose in a molar ratio of 2.14:2.35:1.27:0.99:1.11. The *in vitro* exposure to SMP-W1 at a concentration of 400 μg/mL resulted in aq 43% inhibition against the proliferation of H22 hepatoma cells. SMP-W1 that is orally fed to mice for 10 days at a high dose of 200 mg/kg exerted the antihepatoma effect with an inhibitory rate of 55.1%, which was near to the administration of 5-FU. During the inhibition, SMP-W1 also markedly improved the body weight, the spleen index, and the thymus index in the tumor-bearing mice. More investigations showed that SMP-W1 also augmented the activities of antioxidases such as serum SOD, CAT, and GSH-Px and enhanced TNFα secretion in mice bearing H22 hepatoma.[93] SMP-U1, a polysaccharide extracted from Dan Shen, displayed not only significant antioxidant activity but also antiproliferative effect on human Bcap-37 (breast) and Eca-109 (esophagus) cancer cell lines at a concentration of 0.30 mg/mL.[94] These results proved that the polysaccharides of Dan Shen may be developed as an antitumor adjuvant with antioxidant and immunoregulative functions.

Nano- and Microformulations

In order to amplify the tumor-targeting efficacy, TSIIA (**2**) was loaded into mPEG-PLGA-PLL-cRGD nanoparticles (methoxy polyethylene glycol, polylactic-co-glycolic acid, poly-L-lysine, cyclic arginine-glycine-aspartic acid). The TSIIA nanoparticles extended the TSIIA releasing time and improved tumor-targeting activity. In the *in vitro* and *in vivo* models, the nanoparticles significantly inhibited the development of hepatoma, proving a novel promising targeted treatment for hepatoma.[95] TSIIA (**2**) was also capsulated into a microemulsion, which was composed of phospholipid, ethyl oleate, glycerol, and pluronic F68. The created TSIIA microemulsion demonstrated the improved drug delivery system and the enhanced antihepatoma effect *in vitro* and *in vivo* with murine hepatoma H22 cells.[96]

Side Effects

Two earlier *in vivo* experiments exhibited that Dan Shen might promote the metastasis of cancer cells. The i.p. administration of the Dan Shen extract into murine animals could increase the metastasis percentage of Lewis lung cancer cells in mice and the spread rate of Walker sarcoma cells in rat.[97–100] However, in a metastatic LCI-D20 human liver cancer model, Dan Shen significantly suppressed the metastasis and the recurrence of liver cancer cells after the hepatectomy in nude mice.[7] In the two recent decades, the effect of Dan Shen regarding metastasis enhancement or metastasis inhibitiion is an important research topic in China.

Other Bioactivities

The herb Dan Shen is a commonly used traditional Chinese medicine, which is widely used as an effective remedy for angina pectoris, cerebrovascular disorders, myocardial infarction, and hypertension with minimal side effects. Pharmacological data implied that Dan Shen may bring remarkable medicinal benefits such as coronary flow-increasing, microcirculation-enhancing, vasodilative, antihepatotoxic, antiatheroscherosis, antiplatelet aggregation, anticoagulant, antianoxemia, antiinflammatory, immunoincremental, antiulcerative, antioxidative, etc. As the most abundant diterpene quinine in Dan Shen, TSIIA (**2**) has been extensively studied to have various biological activities including antioxidant, and prevention of angina pectoris and myocardial infarction besides antitumor.

References

1. Franek, K. J. et al. 2005. In vitro studies of baicalin alone or in combination with *Salvia miltiorrhiza* extract as a potential anticancer agent. *Intl. J. Oncol.* 26: 217–24.
2. Zhang, S. H. et al. 2004. Salvianolic acid A inhibits nucleoside transport and potentiates the antitumor activity of chemotherapeutic drugs. *Yaoxue Xuebao* 39: 496–9.
3. Zhang, Y. W. et al. 1989. An assessment of the clinical application of "Huo Xue Hua Yu" vegetable drug Danshen (*Salvia miltiorrhiza*) for malignant lymphoma—An analysis of 47 cases. *J. Xi-an Med. Univ.* 7: 403.
4. Zhang, W. W. et al. 2010. Advances in studies on antitumor activities of compounds in *Salvia miltiorrhiza*. Zhongguo Zhongyo Zazhi 35: 389–92.
5. Liu, J. et al. 2000. *Salvia miltiorrhiza* inhibits cell growth and induces apoptosis in human hepatoma HepG2 cells. *Cancer Lett.* 153: 85–93.
6. Liu, J. et al. 2001. Role of intracellular thiol depletion, mitochondrial dysfunction and reactive oxygen species in *Salvia miltiorrhiza*-induced apoptosis in human hepatoma HepG2 cells. *Life Sci.* 69: 1833–50.
7. Sun, J. et al. 1999. Studies on the inhibitory effect of Dan-Shen against hepatoma metastasis. *Zhongguo Zhongxiyi Jiehe Zazhi* 19: 292–5.
8. Wong, C. W. et al. 2005. Immunomodulatory activities of yunzhi and danshen in post-treatment breast cancer patients. *Am. J. Chin. Med.* 33: 381–95.
9. Chen, F. et al. 2003. Effect of pingyangmycin on mucous membrane of respiratory tract and its prevention. *Zhonghua Erbi Yanhouke Zazhi* 38: 285–8.
10. Liu, J. et al. 2001. Protection of *Salvia miltiorrhiza* against aflatoxin-B_1-induced hepatocarcino-genesis in Fischer 344 rats: Dual mechanisms involved. *Life Sci.* 69: 309–26.
11. Mosaddik, M. A. et al. 2003. In vitro cytotoxicity of tanshinones isolated from *Salvia miltiorrhiza* Bunge against P388 lymphocytic leukemia cells. *Phytomed.* 10: 682–5.
12. Zheng, G. C. et al. 2005. Study on the antitumor effect and mechanism of tanshinone I. *Shiyong Zhongliu Zazhi* (*J. Practical Oncol.*) 20: 33–5.
13. Su, C. C. et al. 2008. Growth inhibition and apoptosis induction by tanshinone I in human colon cancer Colo205 cells. *Intl. J. Mol. Med.* 22: 613–8.
14. Nizamutdinova, I. T. et al. 2008. Tanshinone I effectively induces apoptosis in estrogen receptor-positive (MCF-7) and estrogen receptor-negative (MDA-MB-231) breast cancer cells. *Intl. J. Oncol.* 3: 485–91.
15. Tsai, S. L. et al. 2007. Antitumor potential of 15,16-dihydrotanshinone I against breast adenocarcinoma through inducing G1 arrest and apoptosis. *Biochem. Pharmacol.* 74: 1575–86.
16. Liu, X. D. et al. 2010. Down-regulation of telomerase activity and activation of caspase-3 are responsible for tanshinone I-induced apoptosis in monocyte leukemia cells in vitro. *Intl. J. Mol. Sci.* 11: 2267–80.
17. Li, Y. L. et al. 2013. Bioactive tanshinone I inhibits the growth of lung cancer in part via downregulation of Aurora A function. *Mol. Carcinogen.* 52: 535–43.
18. Gong, Y. et al. 2011. Bioactive tanshinones in *Salvia miltiorrhiza* inhibit the growth of prostate cancer cells in vitro and in mice. *Intl. J. Cancer* 129: 1042–52.
19. Nizamutdinova, I. T. et al. 2008. Tanshinone I suppresses growth and invasion of human breast cancer cells, MDA-MB-231, through regulation of adhesion molecules. *Carcinogenesis* 29: 1885–92.
20. Lee, D. S. et al. 2000. Biological activity of dihydrotanshinone I: Effect on apoptosis. *J. Biosci. Bioeng.* 89: 292–3.
21. Bian, W. P. et al. 2008. Dihydrotanshinone I inhibits angiogenesis both *in vitro* and *in vivo. Acta Biochim. et Biophys. Sinica* 40: 1–6.
22. Yuan, S. L. et al. 2004. Growth inhibition and apoptosis induction of tanshinone IIA on human hepatocellular carcinoma cells. *World. J. Gastroenterol.* 10: 2024–8.
23. Su, C. C. et al. 2008. Growth inhibition and apoptosis induction by tanshinone IIA in human colon adenocarcinoma cells. *Planta Med.* 74: 1357–62.
24. Ye, Z. Y. et al. 2009. Inhibitory action of transhinone IIA on human gastric cancer cell line MKN-45. *Chin. J. Surg. Integr. Tradit. Western Med.* 15: 294–8.
25. Zhou, L. L. et al. 2008. Tanshinone IIA, an isolated compound from *Salvia miltiorrhiza* Bunge, induces apoptosis in HeLa cells through mitotic arrest. *Life Sci.* 83: 394–403.
26. Sung, H. J. et al. 1999. Tanshinone IIA an ingredient of *Salvia miltiorrhiza* BUNGE induces apoptosis in human leukemia cell lines through the activation of caspase-3. *Exp. Mol. Med.* 31: 174–8.
27. Yoon, Y. et al. 1999. Tanshinone IIA isolated from *Salvia miltiorrhiza* BUNGE induced apoptosis in HL-60 human premyelocytic leukemia cell line. *J. Ethnopharmacol.* 68: 121–7.
28. Yuan, S. L. et al. 2003. Anticancer effect of tanshinone and its mechanisms. *Aizheng* 22: 1363–6.
29. Hu, H. Y. et al. 2005. The proliferative inhibition and apoptosis-inducing effects of tanshinone IIA against NCI-H460 lung cancer cells. *Zhongyaocai* 28: 301–4.
30. Tanga, C. et al. 2010. Tanshinone IIA inhibits constitutive STAT3 activation, suppresses proliferation, and induces apoptosis in rat C6 glioma cells. *Neurosci. Lett.* 470: 126–9.
31. Wang, J. et al. Growth inhibition and induction of apoptosis and differentiation of tanshinone IIA in human glioma cells. *J. Neurooncol.* 82: 11–21.

32. Liu, J. J. et al. 2006. Induction of apoptosis and inhibition of cell adhesive and invasive effects by tanshinone IIA in acute promyelocytic leukemia cells in vitro. *J. Biomed. Sci.* 13: 813–23.
33. Meng, W. et al. 2002. Study on the relationship between NB4 cell apoptosis induced by tanshinone IIA and the cell mitochondrial transmembrane potential. *Zhonghua Xueyexue Zazhi.* 23: 297–300.
34. Su, C. C. et al. 2008. Tanshinone IIA inhibits human breast cancer cells through increased Bax to Bcl-xL ratios. *Intl. J. Mol. Med.* 22: 357–61.
35. Wang, X. J. et al. 2005. Potential anticancer activity of tanshinone IIA against human breast cancer. *Intl. J. Cancer.* 116: 799–807.
36. Lu, Q. et al. 2009. Experimental study of the anticancer mechanism of tanshinone IIA against human breast cancer. *Intl. J. Mol. Med.* 24: 773–780.
37. Lu, Y. et al. 2006. Tanshinone IIA, a major component of danshen possesses potent anticancer and antiangiogenic activities. *5th AACR Intl. Conference on Frontiers in Cancer Prev. Res.*, Nov 12–15, (2006), A118.
38. Yang, L. Y. et al. 2005. Tanshinone IIA isolated from *Salvia miltiorrhiza* elicits the cell death of human endothelial cells. *J. Biomed. Sci.* 12: 347–61.
39. Fu, H. et al. 2009. Effect of tanshinone IIA on vascular endothelial growth factor expression in hepatocellular carcinoma cell line SMMC-7721. *J. Xi'an Jiaotong Univ.* (*Med. Sci.*) 30: 115–8.
40. Tang, Z. et al. 2003. Growth inhibition and apoptosis induction in human hepatoma cells by tanshinone IIA. *J. Huazhong Univ. Sci Tech.* (*Med. Sci.*) 23: 166–8, 172.
41. Lee, W. Y. et al. 2008. Cytotoxicity of major tanshinones isolated from Danshen (*Salvia miltiorrhiza*) on HepG2 cells in relation to glutathione perturbation. *Food. Chem. Toxicol.* 46: 328–38.
42. Dai, Z. K. et al. 2012. Tanshinone IIA activates calcium-dependent apoptosis signaling pathway in human hepatoma cells. *J. Nat. Med.* 66: 192–201.
43. Chen, J. et al. 2012. Tanshinone-IIA induces growth inhibition and apoptosis in gastric cancer in vitro and in vivo. *Oncol. Reports* 27: 523–8.
44. Zhang, J. et al. 2014. Tanshinone IIA induces cytochrome c-mediated caspase cascade apoptosis in A549 human lung cancer cells via the JNK pathway. *Intl. J. Oncol.* 45: 683–90.
45. Yu, T. et al. 2014. A novel anticancer agent, acetyltanshinone IIA, inhibits oestrogen receptor positive breast cancer cell growth by down-regulating the oestrogen receptor. *Cancer Lett.* (NY, NY, US) 346: 94–103.
46. Zhang, Y. et al. 2012. Tanshinones from Chinese medicinal herb Danshen (*Salvia miltiorrhiza* Bunge) Suppress prostate cancer growth and androgen receptor signaling. *Pharm. Res.* 29: 1595–608.
47. Hou, L. L. et al. 2013. Synergistic antitumor effect of tanshinone IIA in combination with cisplatin on prostate cancer and its molecular mechanism. *Yaoxue Xuebao* 48: 675–9.
48. Chang, C. C. et al. 2015. Tanshinone IIA facilitates TRAIL sensitization by up-regulating DR5 through the ROS-JNK-CHOP signaling axis in human ovarian carcinoma cell lines. *Chem. Res. Toxicol.* 28:1574–83.
49. Tsai, M. Y. et al. 2011. Anti-angiogenic effect of tanshinone IIA involves inhibition of matrix invasion and modification of MMP-2/TIMP-2 secretion in vascular endothelial cells. *Cancer Lett.* 310: 198–206.
50. Zhang, Y. et al. 2012. Tanshinone IIA induces apoptosis and inhibits the proliferation, migration, and invasion of the osteosarcoma MG-63 cell line in vitro. *Anti-Cancer Drugs* 23: 212–9.
51. Zhuang, Y. Y. et al. 2011. The studies of apoptosis effect and its mechanisms of tanshinone IIA on human ovarian cancer cell SKOV3.*Guoji Fuchankexue Zazhi* 38: 328–31.
52. Zhou, L. H. et al. 2011. Tan II-A inhibits COX-2-regulated VEGF expression in human colon cancer HCT-116 cells. *Shijie Huaren Xiaohua Zazhi* 19: 1561–7.
53. Xing, Y. Y. et al. 2015. Anti-angiogenic effect of tanshinone IIA involves inhibition of the VEGF/VEGFR2 pathway in vascular endothelial cells. *Oncol. Reports* 33: 163–70.
54. Liu, X. et al. 2011. Proteomic assessment of tanshinone IIA sodium sulfonate on doxorubicin induced nephropathy. *Am. J. Chin. Med.* 39: 395–409.
55. Hong, H. J. et al. 2012. Tanshinone IIA prevents doxorubicin-induced cardiomyocyte apoptosis through Akt-dependent pathway. *Intl. J. Cardiol.* 157: 174–9.
56. Ryu, S. Y. et al. 1997. *In vitro* cytotoxicity of tanshinones from *Salvia miltiorrhiza. Planta Med.* 63: 339–42.
57. Chen, W. X. et al. 2012. Cryptotanshinone activates p38/JNK and inhibits Erk1/2 leading to caspase-independent cell death in tumor cells. *Cancer Prevention Res.* 5: 778–87.
58. Shin, D. et al. 2009. Cryptotanshinone inhibits constitutive signal transducer and activator of transcription 3 function through blocking the dimerization in DU145 prostate cancer cells. *Cancer Res.* 69: 193–202.
59. Zhang, D. W. et al. 2013. Two new diterpenoids from cell cultures of *Salvia miltiorrhiza. Chem. Pharm. Bull.* 61: 576–50.
60. Kim, S. H. et al. (a) 2012. Abstract A83: Inhibition of hypoxia inducible factor alpha and astrocyte elevated gene-1 mediates cryptotanshionone induced antitumor activity in hypoxic PC3 cells. *Cancer Prevent. Res.* 5(11-Suppl.): A83; (b) 2012. *Proc. 11th Annual AACR Int. Confer. Frontiers Cancer Prev. Res.*, October 16–19; Anaheim, CA. Philadelphia (PA).
61. Park, I. et al. 2012. Cryptotanshinone induces ER stress-mediated apoptosis in HepG2 and MCF7 cells. *Apoptosis* 17: 248–57.
62. Chen, L. et al. 2011. Cryptotanshinone has diverse effects on cell cycle events in melanoma cell lines with different metastatic capacity. *Cancer Chemother. Pharmacol.* 68: 17–27.
63. Ge, Y. Q. et al. 2012. Cryptotanshinone induces cell cycle arrest and apoptosis of multidrug resistant human chronic myeloid leukemia cells by inhibiting the activity of eukaryotic initiation factor 4E. *Mol. Cell. Biochem.* 368: 17–25.
64. Hu, T. et al. 2014. Reversal of P-glycoprotein (P-gp) mediated multidrug resistance in colon cancer cells by cryptotanshinone and dihydrotanshinone of Salvia miltiorrhiza. *Phytomed.* 21: 1264–72.
65. Luo, Y. et al. 2011. Cryptotanshinone inhibits lymphatic endothelial cell tube formation by suppressing VEGFR-3/ERK and small GTPase pathways. *Cancer Prev. Res.* 4: 2083–91.
66. Liu, P. et al. 2013. Anticancer activity in human multiple myeloma U266 cells: Synergy between cryptotanshinone and arsenic trioxide. *Metallomics* 5: 871–8.
67. Wu, W. L. et al. 1991. Cytotoxic activities of tanshinones against human carcinoma cell lines. *Am. J. Chinese Med.*19: 207–16.

68. Lin, H. C. et al. (a) 1993. Phytochemical and pharmacological study on *Salvia miltiorrhiza* (IV)-cytotoxic activity of tanshinones. *Zhonghua Yaoxue Zazhi* 45: 85–87; (b) 1995. Phytochemical and pharmacological study on *Salvia miltiorrhiza* (VI)-cytotoxic activity of tanshinones. *Zhonghua Yaoxue Zazhi* 47: 77–80.
69. Sun, C. M. et al. 2006. Isolation, structure elucidation, and syntheses of isoneocrypto-tanshinone II (I) and tanshinlactone A (II) from *Salvia miltiorrhiza*. *Heterocycles* 68: 247–55.
70. Li, Z. T. et al. 1991. Chemical constituents of *Salvia miltiorrhiza* f.alba. *Yaoxue Xuebao* 26: 209.
71. Yang, B. J. et al. 1981. Studies on the active principles of danshen V: Isolation and structures of przewaquinone A and przewaquinone B. *Yaoxue Xuebao* 16: 837.
72. Nicolin, V. et al. 2013. Tanshinone VI inhibits the expression of intercellular adhesion molecule-1 and vascular cell adhesion molecule-1. *Intl. J. Immunopathol. Pharmacol.* 26: 977–82.
73. Lee, D. S. et al. 1999. Inhibition of DNA topoisomerase I by dihydrotanshinone I, components of a medicinal herb *Salvia miltiorrhiza* Bunge. *Biosci. Biotechnol. Biochem.* 63: 1370–3.
74. Haro, G. D. et al. 1990. Miltipolone, a new diterpenoid tropolone possessing cytotoxic activities from *Salvia miltiorrhiza* Bunge. *Chem. Lett.* 19: 1599–602.
75. Wang, X. H. et al. 2004. Antitumor agents: 239. Isolation, structure elucidation, total synthesis, and anti-breast cancer activity of neo-tanshinlactone from *Salvia miltiorrhiza*. *J. Med. Chem.* 47: 5816–9.
76. Dong, Y. Z. et al. 2010. Antitumor agents. 272. Structure–activity relationships and in vivo selective anti-breast cancer activity of novel neo-tanshinlactone analogues. *J. Med. Chem.* 53: 2299–308.
77. Don, M. J. et al. 2005. Nitrogen-containing compounds from *Salvia miltiorrhiza*. *J. Nat. Prods.* 68: 1066–77.
78. Syu, W. J. et al. 2001. Cytotoxic and novel compounds from *Solanum indicum*. *J. Nat. Prod.* 64: 1232–3.
79. Lin, H. C. et al. 1991. Phytochemical and pharmacological study on *Salvia miltiorrhiza* (II)-cytotoxic activity of tanshinones. *Zhonghua Yaoxue Zazhi* 43. 501–4.
80. Yao, F. et al. 2012. New abietane norditerpenoid from *Salvia miltiorrhiza* with cytotoxic activities. *J. Asian Nat. Prod. Res.* 14: 913–7.
81. Wang, X. et al. 2015. Salvianolic acid A shows selective cytotoxicity against multidrug-resistant MCF-7 breast cancer cells. *Anti-Cancer Drugs* 26: 210–23.
82. Jiang, R. W. et al. 2005. Chemistry and biological activities of caffeic acid derivatives from *Salvia miltiorrhiza*. *Current Med. Chem.* 12: 237–46.
83. Zhou, Z. T. et al. 2006. The preventive effect of salvianolic acid B on malignant trans-formation of DMBA-induced oral premalignant lesion in hamsters. *Carcinogen.* 27: 826–32.
84. Yang, Y. et al. 2011. Modulation of growth and angiogenic potential of oral squamous carcinoma cells in vitro using salvianolic acid B. *BMC Complem. Alternative Med.* 11: 54.
85. Hao, Y. B. et al. 2009. Salvianolic acid B inhibits growth of head and neck squanous cell carcinoma in vitro and in vivo via cycloxygease-2 and apoptotic pathways. *Intl. J. Cancer* 124: 2200–9.
86. Zhao, Y. et al. 2011. Salvianolic acid B, a potential chemopreventive agent, for head and neck squamous cell cancer cells. *J. Oncol.* 534–48.
87. Zhao, Y. et al. 2010. Combination effects of salvianolic acid B with low-dose celecoxib on inhibition of head and neck squamous cell carcinoma growth *in vitro* and *in vivo*. *Cancer Prev. Res.* 3: 787–96.
88. Chang, J. Y. et al. 2004. Salvinal, a novel microtubule inhibitor isolated from *Salvia miltiorrhizae* Bunge (Danshen), with antimitotic activity in multidrug-sensitive and -resistant human tumor cells. *Mol. Pharmacol.* 65: 77–84.
89. Zhang, L. J. et al. 2010. Danshensu has antitumor activity in B16F10 melanoma by inhibiting angiogenesis and tumor cell invasion. *Eur. J. Pharmacol.* 643: 195–201.
90. Don, M. J. et al. 2006. Cytotoxic and aromatic constituents from *Salvia miltiorrhiza*. *Phytochem.* 67: 497–503.
91. Li, X. P. et al. 2015. Effect of depsides salts from *Salvia miltiorrhiza* on human hepatoma cell line SMMC-7721 subcutaneous xenografts in nude mice. *Zhongnan Daxue Xuebao, Yixueban* 40: 158–64.
92. Song, S. H. et al. 2010. Salvianolate induces apoptosis of human hepatoma SMMC-7721 cells through mitochondrial pathway. *Chinese J. Cancer Biother.* 17: 62–6.
93. Liu, L. et al. 2013. Studies on immuno-regulatory and antitumor activities of a polysaccharide from *Salvia miltiorrhiza* Bunge. *Carbohydrate Polymers* 92: 479–83.
94. Jiang, Y. Y. et al. 2014. Characterization, antioxidant and antitumor activities of polysaccharides from *Salvia miltiorrhiza* Bunge. *Intl. J. Biol. Macromol.* 70: 92–9.
95. Wang, Y. et al. 2014. Targeted delivery of tanshinone IIA-conjugated mPEG-PLGA-PLL-cRGD nanoparticles to hepatocellular carcinoma. *J. Biomed. Nanotechnol.* 10: 3244–52.
96. Ma, H. et al. 2013. Novel microemulsion of tanshinone IIA, isolated from *Salvia miltiorrhiza* Bunge, exerts anticancer activity through inducing apoptosis in hepatoma cells. *Am. J. Chin. Med.* 41: 197–210.
97. Chen, L. L. et al. 2006. Review on the research of the effect of Danshen and its extract on tumor metastasis. *J. Zhejiang Univ. TCM* 30: 449–52.
98. Li, C. Z. et al. 1983. Influence of *Salvia* on the blood dissemination of Walker256 cancer cells in rat. *Zhongliu* 3: 66.
99. Fu, N. W. et al. 1981. Primary studies on the inference of experimental hepatoma metastasis by Dan-Shen. *Zhonghua Zhongliu Zazhi* 3:165.
100. Ding, G. et al. 2001. The inferences of Dan-shen and Chi-shao on the live metastasis of rat Walker 256 sarcoma. *Chin. J. Cancer* 11: 264–6.

126 Tie Gu San 鐵箍散

Schisandra vine

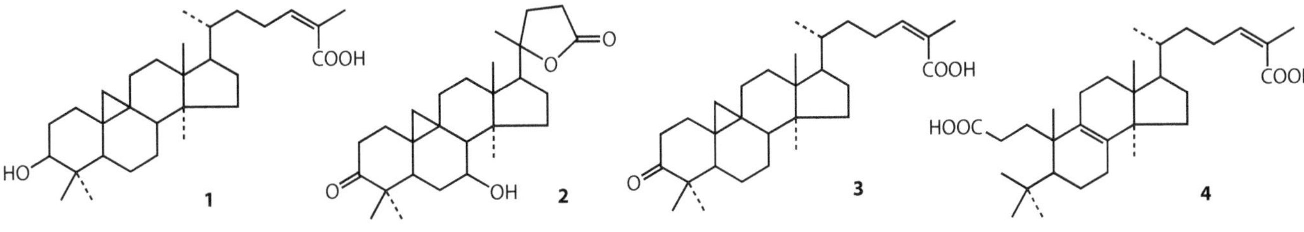

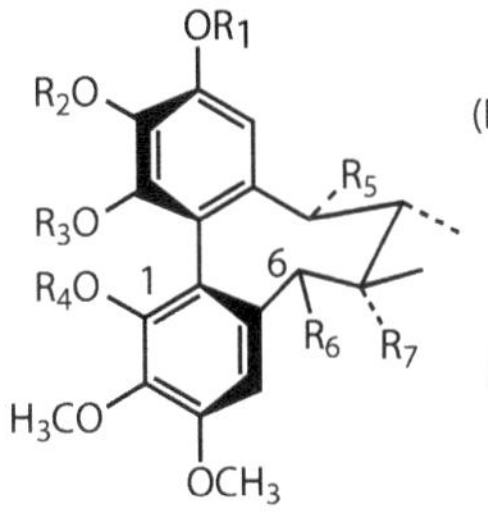

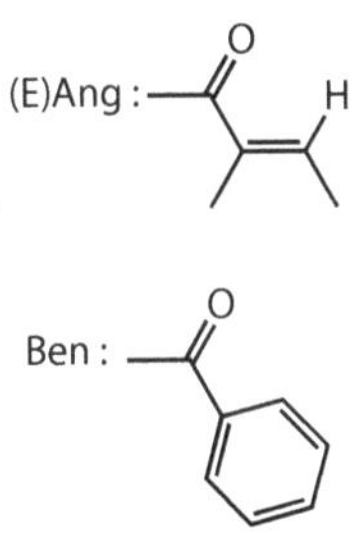

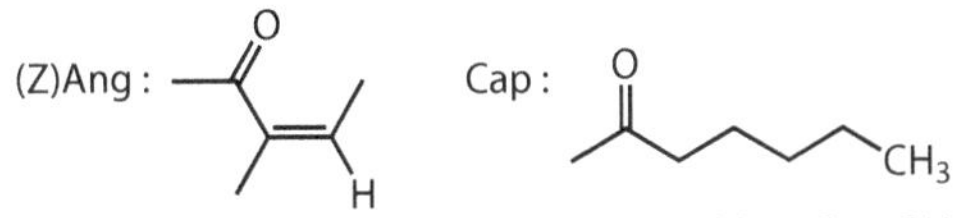

(E)Ang : Ben : (Z)Ang : Cap :

5. $R_1 = R_2 = CH_2$, $R_3 = R_4 = H$, $R_5 = R_6 = O$–(*Z*)Ang, $R_7 = OH$
6. $R_1 = R_2 = R_3 = CH_3$, $R_4 = O$–(*Z*) Ang, $R_5 = OH$, $R_6 = R_7 = H$
7. $R_1 = R_2 = CH_2$, $R_3 = H$, $R_4 = CH_3$, $R_5 = OAc$, $R_6 = O$–(*Z*)Ang, $R_7 = OH$
8. $R_1 = R_2 = CH_2$, $R_3 = R_4 = CH_3$, $R_5 = OAc$, $R_6 = O$–(*Z*)Ang, $R_7 = OH$
9. $R_1 = H$, $R_2 = R_3 = R_4 = CH_3$, $R_5 = O$–Cap, $R_6 = O$–(*E*)Ang, $R_7 = OH$
10. $R_1 = H$, $R_2 = R_3 = R_4 = CH_3$, $R_5 = O$–Cap, $R_6 = O$–Ben, $R_7 = OH$
11. $R_1 = H$, $R_2 = R_3 = CH_3$, $R_4 = O$–(*Z*)Ang, $R_5 = OH$, $R_6 = OAc$, $R_7 = H$
12. $R_1 = R_2 = CH_2$, $R_3 = R_4 = CH_3$, $R_5 = O$–Cap, $R_6 = O$–(*Z*)Ang, $R_7 = H$

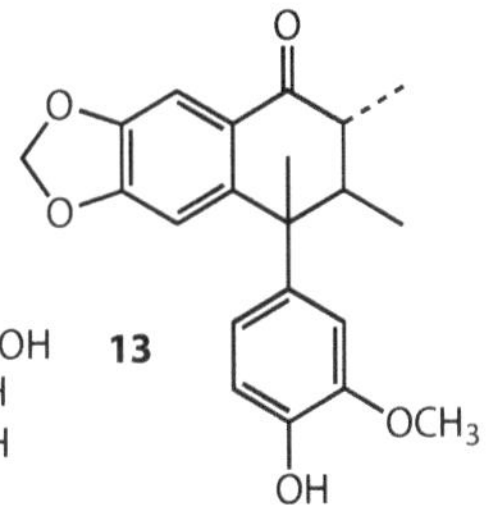

Herb Origination

The herb Tie Gu San (Schisandra vine) is the dried roots and stems of two Schisandraceae plants, *Schisandra propinqua* and *S. propinque* var. *sinensis*. The two plants are extensively distributed in southwestern region of China as well as in India and Nepal. The roots and the stems are usually collected in winter and dried in the sun for folk medicinal purpose in some areas of China.

Antitumor Constituents and Activities

Triterpenoids

Triterpenoids and lignans are the major constituents in the herb Tie Gu San, and several of them present marked antineoplastic potential. Three cycloartane triterpenoids designated as schisandrolic acid (**1**), isoschisandrolic acid, and schisanterpene-B (**2**) demonstrated moderate cytotoxic effect on human HepG2 hepatoma cells *in vitro* together with the induction of G0/G1 arrest and subsequent apoptosis.[1,2] Schisanterpene-B (**2**) and schisandronic acid (**3**) was effective in the inhibition of other human cancer cell lines such as HL-60 (leukemia), Bel-7402 (hepatoma), and KB (epidermoid) cells *in vitro*. The moderate cytotoxicity was also achieved by schisandrolic acid (**1**) on a drug-resistant R-HepG2 hepatoma cells with an IC_{50} value of 10.54 μM.[3] Interestingly, a secocycloartane triterpenoid, assigned as manwuweizic acid (**4**), notably suppressed the cell growth of Lewis lung carcinoma, brain tumor-22, and solid hepatoma only in the murine animal models but no cytotoxic action against these tumor cells *in vitro*.[4] Also, it showed significant cytotoxic effect against human decidual cells and rat luteal cells *in vitro*.[5]

Lignans

Tie Gu San also contains rich dibenzocyclooctadiene lignans, which generally possess a variety of pharmacological activities. The lignans such as propinquanin-E (**5**), propinquanin-F (**6**), propinquanin-G (**7**), and kadsurarin-II (**8**) as well as octadecanoic acid 2,3-dihydroxypropyl ester displayed moderate cytotoxicity on human cancer cell lines such as HepG2, KB, HL-60, and Bel-7402 cells with IC_{50} values in the range of 37–73 μM,[2] whereas propinquanin-B (**9**) and schisantherin-I (**10**) were significantly cytotoxic to these carcinoma cell lines and a drug-resistant R-HepG2 hepatoma cells *in vitro*.[3] The IC_{50} values for propinquanin-B (**9**) were less than 10 μM in HL-60 and HepG2 cells and were below 19 μM in R-HepG2, KB, and Bel-7402 cells. Moreover, two other lignans, propinquanin-D (**11**) and heteroclitin-A (**12**), showed the evidences of obvious cytotoxicity in R-HepG2 cells *in vitro* with IC_{50} values of 16.22–17.34 μM.[3] In comparison of the anticancer activities and structures, the analysis revealed that the C-6 and a hydroxyl group at C-1 in the dibenzocyclooctadiene lignans may play an important responsibility for the cytotoxic effect.[4,5] Additionally, a lignin elucidated as epienshicine (**13**) was isolated from another source of the herb *S. propinque* var. *sinensis*, and it displayed the growth suppressive activity *in vitro* against murine P388 leukemia cells with the inhibitory rate of 72.05% at a concentration of 10 μg/mL.[6] Additionally, several dibenzocyclooctadiene lignans derived from the herb exerted moderate to weak inhibitory effect against the proliferation of lymphocyte; especially, propinquanin-A, propinquanin-B (**9**), and schisantherin-I (**10**) showed the most obvious antiproliferative action on the lymphocytes (IC_{50}: 20–42 μmol/L) among these isolated lignans.[7]

Other Medical Uses

The herb Tie Gu San (Schisandra vine) has been used as a Chinese traditional medicine for the treatment of rheumatism, ulcer with pyogenic infections, stomachache, neurasthenia, and traumatic injury, etc.

References

1. Tian, Z. et al. 2007. Cytotoxic activity of schisandrolic and isoschisandrolic acids involves induction of apoptosis. *Chemother.* 53: 257–62.
2. Xu, L. J. et al. 2006. A new triterpene and dibenzocyclooctadiene lignans from *Schisandra propinqua* (Wall.) Baill. *Chem. Pharm. Bull.* 54: 542–5.
3. Xu, L. J. et al. 2006. New lignans and cytotoxic constituents from *Schisandra propinqua. Planta Med.* 72: 169–74.
4. Liu, J. S. et al. 1988. Anwuweizonic acid and manwuweizic acid, the putative anticancer active principle of *Schisandra propinqua. Can. J. Chem.* 66: 414–5.
5. Chen, Y. G. et al. 2001. Triterpenoid acids from *Schisandra propinqua* with cytotoxic effect on rat luteal cells and human decidual cells in vitro. *Fitoterapia* 72: 435 -7.
6. Liu, J. S. et al. 1988. Studies on the constituents of Schisandraceae plants in Shennongjia District: I. Constituents of *Schisandra propinqua* Hook F et al. Thoms. var. *sinensis* Oliv. *Huaxue Xuebao* 46: 345–8.
7. Jin, M. N. et al. 2012. Lignans from *Schisandra propinqua* with inhibitory effects on lymphocyte proliferation. *Planta Med.* 78: 807–13.

127 Zhu Huang 竹黄

Tabasheer or Stroma shiraiae

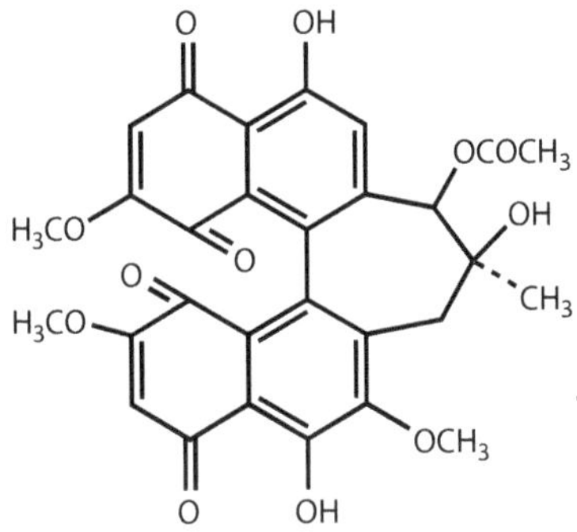

Herb Origination

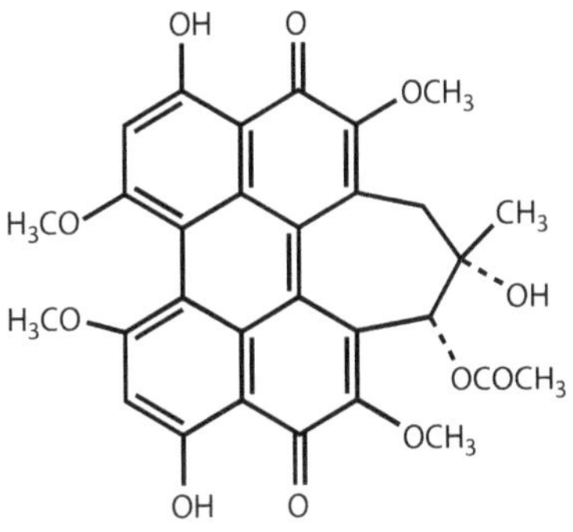

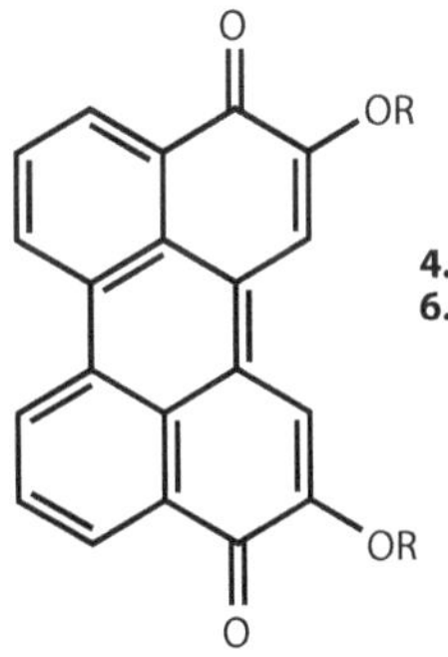

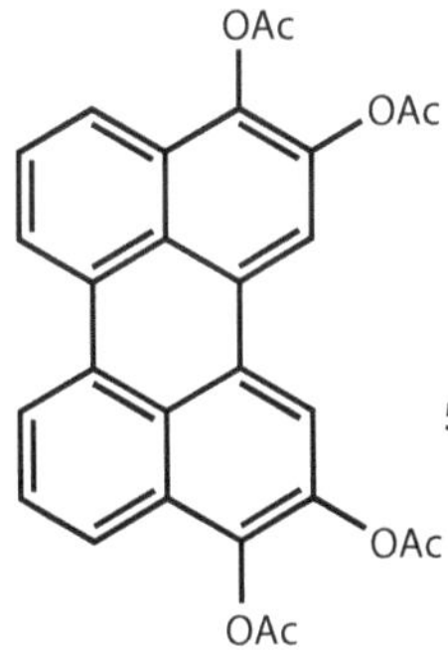

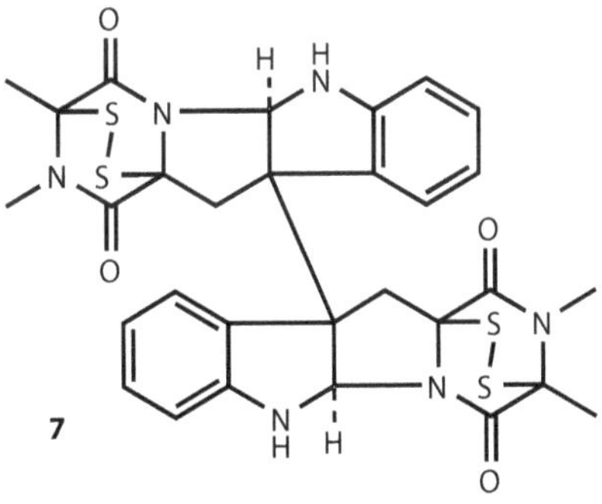

The herb Zhu Huang (Tabasheer) is the dried fruiting bodies of the fungi *Shiraia bambusicola* (Hypocreaceae). The fungi are parasite on the declining twigs of several genera of bamboos, whose fungi are broadly distributed in many southern provinces of China as well as in Japan. Its larger stromata is normally collected around April 5 and then dried in the sun for traditional Chinese medical application. The herb is mostly produced in the provinces of Jiangsu, Zhejiang, Anhui, and Sichuan in China.

Antitumor Constituents and Activities

Perylene Derivatives

Zhu Huang contains rich photosensitive pigments. Four cytotoxic perylenequinone derivatives, hypocrellin-A, hypocrellin-B, hypocrellin-C and hypocrellin-D (**1**), were isolated from the herb (see Section Zhu Sha Ren). Hypocrellin-D (**1**) significantly suppressed the growth of Bel-7721 (liver) and A549 and Anip-973 (lung) tumor cell lines *in vitro* (IC_{50}: 1.8, 8.8, and 38.4 μg/mL, respectively), whereas hypocrellin-A significantly inhibited the growth of CHO (ovary), HL-60 (leukemic), and A549 (lung) tumor cell lines in dose-dependent manner (IC_{50}: 0.47, 0.11, and 0.22 mg/mL, respectively).[1–3] Two other perylenequinone analogs assigned as shiraiachrome-A (**2**) and shiraiachrome-B (**3**) were also isolated from the mycelium of *S. bambusicola* as the cytotoxic principles. A bioassay confirmed that shiraiachrome-A (**2**) and shiraiachrome-B (**3**) were effective in the suppression of a group of human HCT-8 (intestinal), KB (nasopharynx), A549 (lung), and murine P388 leukemia carcinoma cell lines with ED_{50} values of 2.1 and 4.64, 5.5 and 0.55, 0.55 and 3.18, and 0.54 and 0.39 mg/mL, respectively. By structural modification of these two perylane derivatives, two more cytotoxic agents 2,11-Diacetoxy-3,10-perylenequinone (**4**) and 2,3,10,11-tetraacetoxyperylene (**5**) and a PKC inhibitor 2,11-Dihydroxy-3,10-perylenequinone (**6**) were created. The derivatives 2,11-Diacetoxy-3,10-perylene quinone (**4**) and 2,3,10,11-tetraacetoxyperylene (**5**) demonstrated greater antiproliferative effect on human tumor cell lines, such as HCT-8 (intestinal cancer), RPMI-7951 (melanoma), KB (nasopharynx cancer), and TE-671 (medulloblastoma), *in vitro*. The ED_{50} values of 2,11-Diacetoxy-3,10-perylenequinone (**4**) and 2,3,10,11-tetraacetoxyperylene (**5**) were the same as 0.05 mg/mL in the RPMI-7951 cells and 0.68 and 0.61 mg/mL in the TE-671 cells, respectively.[4]

Epidithiodioxopiprazine

11,11′-Dideoxyverticillin (**7**) isolated from Zhu Huang demonstrated potent anticancer and antiangiogenic effects *in vitro* and *in vivo*. An *in vitro* assay exhibited that 11,11′-dideoxyverticillin potently inhibited the proliferation of four human breast carcinoma cell lines with an average IC_{50} value of 0.2 μM and human HCT colon carcinoma cells with IC_{50} value of 0.03 μg/mL. After being treated with 11,11′-dideoxyverticillin (**7**) at concentrations of 0.5–2.0 μM for 36 h, the apoptotic morphological changes were remarkably promoted in MB-MB-468 breast cancer cells. Even at low concentrations (0.0625–0.5 μM) for 24 h, 11,11′-dideoxyverticillin (**7**) dose-dependently arrested the cell cycles of MB-MB-468 cells and HCT-116 cells at G2/M phase.[5,6] The G2/M cell arrest in HCT-8 cells was found to be associated with marked increases in the levels of p53, phosphor-p53, phospho-Chk2 (Thr 68), and p38-MAPK, suggesting that p53-mediated Chk2 phosphorylation may play a vital role in the induction of cell cycle arrest.[5] An *in vivo* test further substantiated the antineoplastic activity of 11,11′-dideoxyverticillin (**7**). The daily i.p. administration of 11,11′-dideoxyverticillin (0.5 or 0.75 mg/kg) could achieve remarkable efficacy against the cell growth of mouse sarcoma 180 and hepatoma 22 with inhibition rates ranging from 45% to 72.4%.[5,6]

11,11′-Dideoxyverticillin (**7**) is also a potent inhibitor of growth factor receptor tyrosine kinase. The *in vivo* anticancer effect was found to be closely correlated with its remarkable antiangiogenic property. The treatment with 11,11′-dideoxyverticillin (**7**) markedly inhibited the growth of HUVECs.[5,7] When EGFR-overexpressed MDA-MB-468 breast cancer cells and EGFR2-overexpressed SKOV-3 ovarian carcinoma cells are exposed, 11,11′-dideoxyverticillin (**7**) potently restrained the EGF-induced phosphorylation of EGFR and EGFR2 with IC_{50} values of 0.136 and 1.645 nM, respectively.[5,7] During the inhibition of angiogenesis progression, 11,11′-dideoxyverticillin (**7**) completely suppressed VEGF-induced microvessel sprouting and serum-induced HUVEC tube formation. The IC_{50} values were about 0.17 μM for VEGF-stimulated HUVEC cells and 0.39 μM for serum-stimulated HUVEC cells. In addition, 11,11′-dideoxyverticillin (**7**) could decrease the VEGF secretion in the MDA-MB-468 breast cancer cells, accompanied by the marked suppression of VEGF-induced tyrosine phosphorylation of Flt-1 and KDR/Flk-1.[5,7] These evidences clearly confirmed that 11,11′-dideoxyverticillin (**7**) is a potent angiogenesis inhibitor, having a potential for further development to be a new drug candidate for cancer chemotherapy.

Other Bioactivities

The herb Zhu Huang (Tabasheer) was demonstrated to have anticoagulant, antiinflammatory, and analgesic properties by pharmacological investigations.

References

1. Fang, L. Z. et al. 2006. Hypocrellin D, a cytotoxic fungal pigment from fruiting bodies of the ascomycete *Shiraia bambusicola*. *J. Antibiotics* 59: 351–4.
2. Ali, S. M. et al. 2002. Efficacy of hypocrellin pharmacokinetics in phototherapy. *Int. J. Oncol.* 21: 1229–37.
3. Shao, Y. et al. 2011. Stability and antitumor activity of hypocrellin from liquid-cultured mycelia of Shiraia bambusicola strain ZH-5-1. *Shipin Kexue* 32: 96–100.
4. Wang, H. K. et al. 1992. Antitumor agents. 134. New shiraiachrome-A- and calphostin-C-related perylene derivatives as cytotoxic and antiviral agents and inhibitors of protein kinase C. *J. Med. Chem.* 35: 2717–21.
5. Zhang, Y. X. et al. 2005. 11,11′-Dideoxyverticillin: A natural compound possessing growth factor receptor tyrosine kinase-inhibitory effect with anti-tumor activity. *Anti-Cancer Drugs* 16: 515–24.
6. Chen, Y. et al. 2005. The p53 pathway is synergized by p38 MAPK signaling to mediate 11,11′-dideoxyverticillin-induced G2/M arrest. *FEBS Lett.* 579: 3683–90.
7. Chen, Y. et al. 2005. Antiangiogenic activity of 11,11′-dideoxyverticillin, a natural product isolated from the fungus *Shiraia bambusicola*. *Biochem. Biophysic. Res. Commun.* 329: 1334–42.

128 Hei San Len 黑三棱

Sparganii

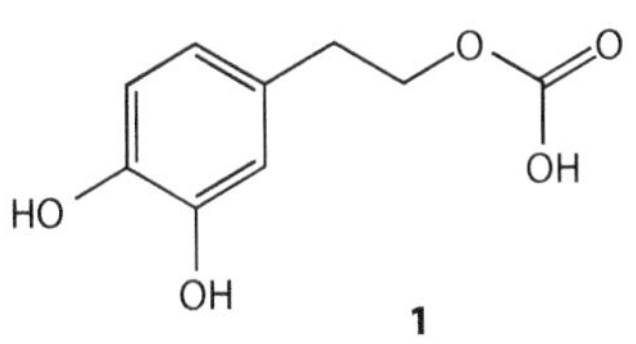

Herb Origination

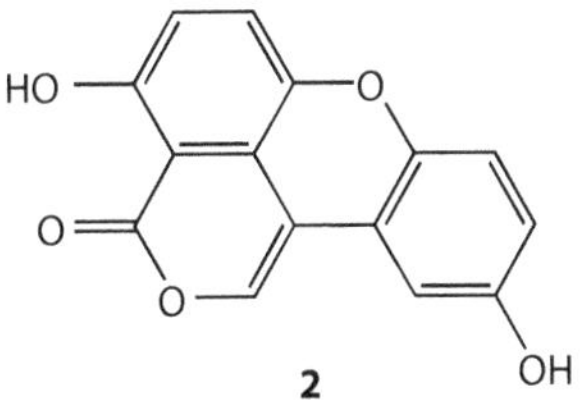

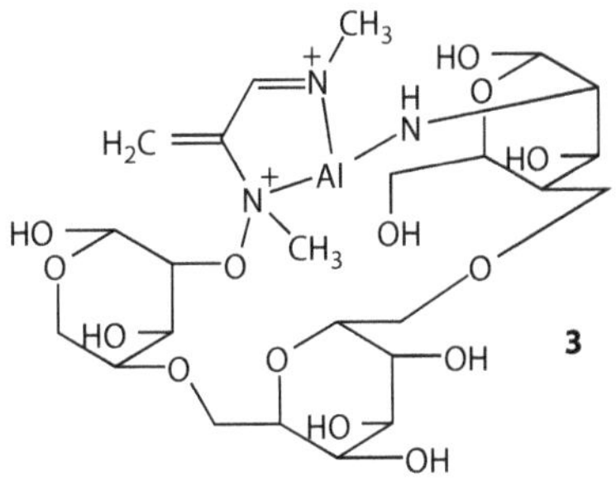

The herb Hei San Len is the dried tuber roots of a Sparganiaceae plant, *Sparganium stoloniferum*. This perennial and aquatic plant is broadly distributed in the wet valley areas of middle and east Asia (such as China, Mongolia, Pakistan, Afghanistan, Kazakhstan, Tajikistan, Uzbekistan, Russia, Korea, and Japan) as well as North America. Its tubers are generally collected in winter, and then the tuber skin is removed and dried in the sun for the traditional use in Chinese medicine.

Antitumor Activities and Constituents

In vitro experiments found that the extract of Hei San Len time- and dose-dependently inhibited the proliferation of human MCF-7 breast cancer cells in association with obvious caspase-3 activation and increase of PARP fragmentation.[1] The *in vivo* treatment with the aqueous extract of Hei San Len for 10 days given orally could reduce the tumor weight and restrain the tumor growth in mice bearing H22 hepatoma cells. At the same time, the aqueous extract also exerted immunomoderating function such as elevating the levels of IL-2 and TNFα in blood plasma and declining the indexes of the thymus and the spleen.[2] The cytotoxic strength on HeLa human cervical cancer cells was water extract > 75% methanol extract > 100% methanol extract.[3]

Flavonoids

Pharmacological studies have shown that flavonoids are one of the most important contributors to the biological effects of HeiSan Len, including anticancer, antiinflammatory, and antithrombotic activities. The flavonoids showed a notable cytotoxicity against estrogen receptor$^+$ MCF-7 breast cancer and A549 lung cancer cell lines *in vitro*. The antiproliferative effect was found to be accompanied by the induction of S/G2 cell arrest and apoptotic death.[4] The flavonoids have also been proven to have a cytotoxic effect on human HeLa cervical neoplastic cells *in vitro*, whereas the flavonoid aglycones were known to have less anti-HeLa activity.[3]

Phenolics

Hydroxytyrosol acetate (**1**) is an antineoplastic phenolic compound isolated from the methanolic extract of the Sparganii rhizome, which exhibited moderate to weak suppressive effect against SKOV-3 (ovary), SK-MEL-2 (skin), A549 (lung), and HCT-15 (colon) human cancer cell lines with respective IC_{50} values of 14.11, 23.67, 36.52, and 64.29 μM.[5] A phenylpropanoid glycerol designated as 1-*O*-*cis*-feruloyl-3-*O*-*trans*-*p*-coumaroylglycerol and a sucrose ester named β-D-(1-*O*-acetyl-3-*O*-*cis*-feruloyl)-fructofuranosyl-α-D-2′,3′,6′-*O*-triacetylglucopyranoside, which were both separated from the aqueous ethanolic extract of Hei San Len, showed only weak cytotoxic effect against mouse LA795 lung adenocarcinoma cell line.[6]

Isocoumarin Analog

A compound assigned as sparstolonin-B (**2**) isolated from the herb at a 10 μM concentration significantly inhibited the growth of both N-Myc-amplified (SK-N-BE2, NGP, and IMR-32) and N-Myc-nonamplified (SH-SY5Y and SKNF-1) neuroblastoma cell lines in association with the induction of G2-M cell cycle arrest and ROS generation-promoted apoptosis in the tested neuroblastoma cells of different genetic backgrounds.[7] Sparstolonin-B (**2**) also displayed antiangiogenenic property in microarray experiments with human coronary artery endothelial cells and HUVECs. The process of new capillary formation from existing blood vessels and the cell cycle progression of endothelial cells could be obstructed in the presence of sparstolonin-B (**2**), associated with the downregulation of cyclin-E2 and cell division cycle-6. The marked reduction in angiogenesis was also proven in a CAM assay in *ex vivo*.[8]

N-Heterocyclic Al Complex

From an aqueous extract of the Sparganii turber, a unique N-heterocyclic Al complex glycoside termed grailsine-Al-glycoside (**3**) was isolated, which obviously inhibited estrogen receptor$^+$ A549 (lung) and MCF-7 (breast) human cancer cell lines by inhibiting cell proliferation and inducing apoptosis and also obviously restrained estrogen receptor$^-$ Hela (cervix) and HepG2 (liver) human cancer cell lines. During the treatments, the cell cycles of A549 and MCF-7 cells were arrested at G2/S phase, whereas the HepG2 cell cycle was arrested at G1 phase by a high concentration of grailsine-Al-glycoside (**3**). The results implied that the anticancer mechanism was mediated by an estrogen receptor-independent pathway and showed a potential as chemotherapeutic agent for further investigation.[9]

Other Medical Uses

The herb Hei San Lin (Rhizoma Sparganii) has long been used as an emmenagogue and a galactagogue agent in Chinese folk medicine for the treatment of dysmenorrhea and lactogenesis. The biological activities including antispasmodic, antiinflammatory, antithrombosis, antiplatelet, analgesic, antioxidant, and aldose reductase inhibition have also been reported in the pharmacological investigations of Hei San Lin. However, Hei San Lin significantly depressed the levels of embryos' FGF-1 and the expressions of VEGF and estrogen receptor-α in pregnant ICR mice and its offspring, implicating anti-angiogenesis and anti-estrogen toxicity effects in pregnant rodents.[10]

References

1. Cho, S. I. et al. 2006. Anticancer activities of *Sparganium stoloniferum* on the proliferation of MCF-7 cells. *J. Biomed. Nanotechnol.* 2: 125–8.
2. Li, X. C. et al. 2010. Antitumor effect of Sparganii extract against mouse H22 hepatoma. *Heilongjiang Med. Pharm.* 33: 78.
3. Sun, J. et al. 2010. *Sparganium stoloniferum* flavonoids extraction and HPLC analysis of ingredients against HeLa cervical cancer. *Xibei Zhiwu Xuebao* 30: 2530–5.
4. Sun, J. et al. 2011. Flavonoids of Rhizoma Sparaganii induce S/G2 stage arrest in A549 and MCF-7 cells. *Tianran Chanwu Yanjiu Yu Kaifa* 23: 224–7, 282.
5. Lee, S. Y. et al. 2010. A new phenylpropane glycoside from the rhizome of *Sparganium stoloniferum*. *Archiv. Pharm. Res.* 33: 515–21.
6. Xiong, Y. et al. 2009. New chemical constituents from the rhizomes of *Sparganium stoloniferum*. *Archiv.Pharm. Res.* 32: 717–20.
7. Kumar, A. et al. 2014. Sparstolonin B, a novel plant derived compound, arrests cell cycle and induces apoptosis in N-Myc amplified and N-Myc nonamplified neuroblastoma cells. PLoS One 9: e96343/1-e96343/11.
8. Bateman, H. R. et al. 2013. Sparstolonin B inhibits pro-angiogenic functions and blocks cell cycle progression in endothelial cells. *PLoS One* 8: e70500.
9. Zhang, J. W. et al. 2014. Anticancer effects of grailsine-al-glycoside isolated from Rhizoma Sparganii. *BMC Complem. Altern. Med.* 14: 82/1–82/5.
10. Sun, J. et al. (a) 2011. Reproductive toxicity of Rhizoma Sparganii (*Sparganium stoloniferum* Buch.-Ham.) in mice: Mechanisms of anti-angiogenesis and anti-estrogen pharmacologic activities. *J. Ethno-pharmacol.* 137: 1498–503; (b) 2012. *J. Ethnopharmacol.* 139: 680.

129 Wang Bu Liu Xing 王不留行

Semen vaccariae

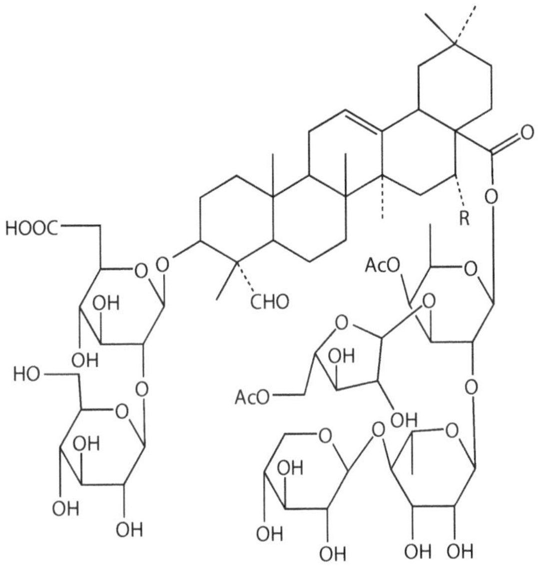

Segetoside-H (1) R = –H

Segetoside-I (2) R = –OH

Herb Origination

The herb Wang Bu Liu Xing (Semen vaccariae) is the dried seeds of a Caryophyllaceae plant, *Vaccaria segetalis* (= *V. pyramidata* and *Saponaria segetalis*). The distribution of Wang Bu Liu Xing is broad in Asia and Europe. Except in the southern region, it grows in most areas of China. Its seeds are harvested in May when the seeds turn yellow brown and then dried in shade for folk therapeutic use. The herb was documented in the first Chinese material medica entitled *Shennong Ben Cao Jing*.

Antitumor Activities

In vitro experiments demonstrated that a 70% methanolic extract derived from the powdered seeds of Wang Bu Liu Xing suppressed the proliferation of three human carcinoma cell lines, WiDr (colon), NCI-417 (lung), and MDA-MB-231 (breast), with IC_{50} values of 9.5, 18.7, and 19.4 μg/mL, respectively.[1] Interestingly, an aqueous extract of *V. segetalis* seeds could significantly suppress the proliferation and the migration of human mammary epithelial cells (HMECs) *in vitro* in a dose-dependent manner (IC_{50}: 50 μg/mL) and also obstruct the angiogenesis in the Matrigel plug mouse model.[2] The anticarcinoma and antineovascularizing effects of 70% ethanolic extract were demonstrated in mouse model inoculated with H22 hepatoma. The treatment with the extract in doses of 2.5 and 5 mg/kg for 10 days markedly improved the quality of life in mice and restrained the growth of hepatoma by 59.23% and 73.20%, respectively, whose antihepatoma mechanisms were found to be likely due to to the blockage of the angiogenesis and the induction of the apoptosis of tumor cells and vascular endothelial cells concomitant with the down-expression of CD31.[3] These results recommended that the marked antineovascularizing activity of Wang Bu Liu Xing is also useful for treating and preventing diseases related to angiogenesis, especially cancer development and metastasis. In addition, two extracts prepared from the dried whole plant of *V. segetalis* exerted the antiproliferative inhibition against human bladder carcinoma cell line. The IC_{50} values was 29.3 μg/mL for its methanolic extract and 19.5 μg/mL for its chloroform extract.[4]

Antitumor Constituents and Activities

The major antitumor constituents in Wang Bu Liu Xing were revealed to be several bisdesmosidic saponins, which showed cytotoxicity against human neoplastic cell lines, particularly on breast and prostate cancer cells with the IC_{50} values in the range of 1–4 μg/mL. Other constituents such as monodesmosidic saponins, phenolics, and cyclopeptides did not exert such inhibitory effect even at a 50 μg/mL concentration.[5] Six cytotoxic triterpenoid saponins assigned as vaccaroside-B, vaccaroside-E, vaccaroside-G, vaccaroside-I, segetoside-H (**1**), and segetoside-I (**2**) were isolated from Wang Bu Liu Xing. They displayed moderate cytotoxic activities against mouse P388 leukemia, human LNcaP prostate adenocarcinoma, and human A549 lung cancer cell lines with IC_{50} values in the range 0.1–12.9 μM.[6] The treatment of MDA-MB-231 breast and PC3 prostate neoplastic cell lines with segetalin-H (**1**) or segetalin-I (**2**) in small amounts (4–7 μM) stimulated the cell apoptosis and restrained the proliferation of tumor cells.[5] Both segetalins also exerted moderate inhibitory effect toward human WiDr (colon), MDA-MB-231 (breast), NCI-417 (lung), and PC3 (prostate) cancer cell lines but showed a similar degree of inhibition against human normal fibroblast JB cells. The IC_{50} values were 1.3 and 1.3 μg/mL in MDA-MB-231 cells, 11.8 and 4.0 μg/mL in PC3 cells, 14.1 and 4.0 μg/mL in JB cells, 15.9 and 16.7 μg/mL in WiDr cells, and 18.6 and 19.8 μg/mL in NCI-147 cells, respectively.[1]

Other Bioactivities

The herb Wang Bu Liu Xing (Semen vaccariae) has been traditionally used to activate blood circulation, to promote milk secretion and diuresis, to improve menstrual discharge, to treat amenorrhea and mastitis, and to heal wounds as an astringent in Chinese folk medicine. Pharmacological approaches corroborated that Wang Bu Liu Xing possesses antiearly pregnancy and antiimplantation functions; thus, the herb is also used for birth control locally.

References

1. Balsevich, J. J. et al. 2012. Antiproliferative activity of *Saponaria vaccaria* constituents and related compounds. *Fitoterapia* 83: 170–81.
2. Feng, L. et al. 2012. (a) Vaccaria segetalis extract can inhibit angiogenesis. *Asian Biomed.* 6: 683–92; (b) Study on antiangiogenesis effect of Vaccaria segetalis. *Zhong Yao Cai.* 32:1256–9.
3. Gao, Y. Y. et al. 2010. Antitumor effect and its mechanism of *Vaccaria segetalis* on mouse inoculated H22 solid carcinoma. *Intl. Conference on Bioinformatics and Biomedical Engineering—ICBBE*, pp. 1–4.
4. Sobirdjan, A. et al. 2012. In vitro screening of the cytotoxic, antibacterial and antioxidant activities of some Uzbek plants used in folk medicine. *Asian J. Tradit. Med.* 7: 73–80.
5. Hickie, R. et al. 2009. Saponin extract from Saponaria spp. for treating cancer. *PCT Int. Appl.* WO 2009117828 A1 20091001
6. Ma, C. H. et al. 2008. Cytotoxic triterpenoid saponins from *Vaccaria segetalis*. *J. Asian Nat. Prod. Res.* 10: 177–84.

130 Liang Mian Zhen 兩面針

Shiny leaf prickly ash

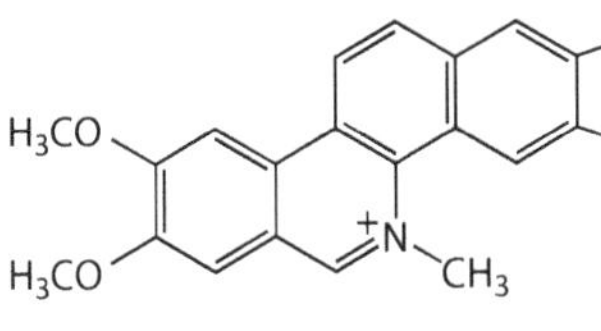

1. **2.** Cl^-

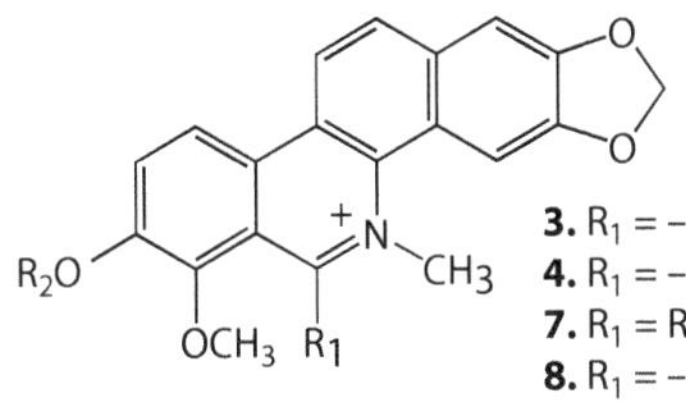

3. R_1 = -H, R_2 = $-CH_3$
4. R_1 = $-CH_2CH_3$, R_2 = $-CH_3$
7. R_1 = R_2 = -H
8. R_1 = -H, R_2 = $-CH_3$

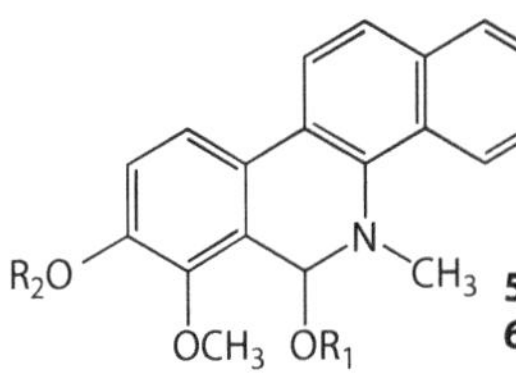

5. R_1 = R_2 = $-CH_3$
6. R_1 = R_2 = -H

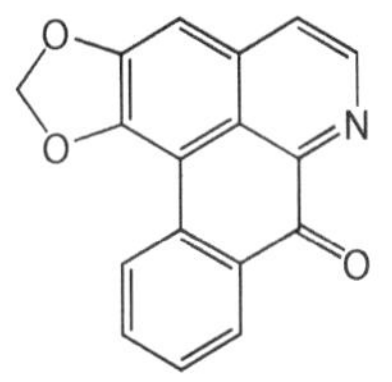

9

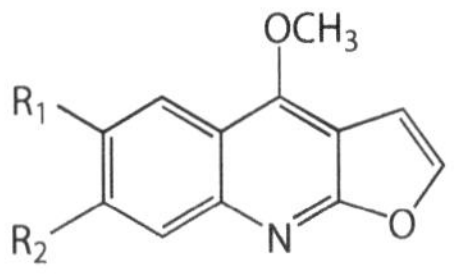

10. R_1 = R_2–OCH_3
11. R_1 = $-OCH_2O-$ = R_2

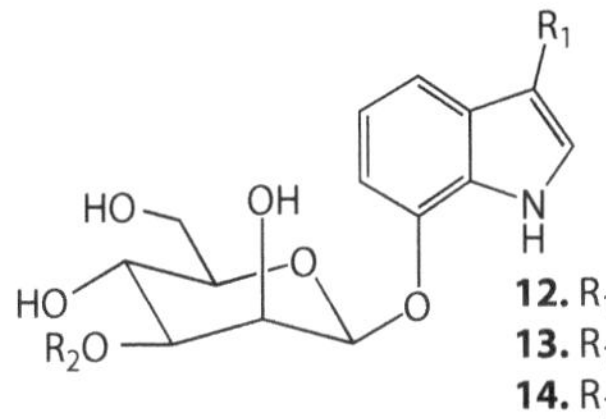

12. R_1 = $-COOCH_3$, R_2 = -H
13. R_1 = $-COOCH_3$, R_2 = -Ac
14. R_1 = $-CH_3$, R_2–H

Herb Origination

The earliest record of the herb Liang Mian Zhen (Shiny leaf prickly ash) was in the first Chinese classic of materia medica entitled *Shennong Ben Cao Jing*. The herb originated from the dried roots and twigs of a Rutaceae plant, *Zanthoxylum nitidum*. Its distribution is in southern China and south Asian areas and islands, Australia, and southwest Pacific islands.

Antitumor Constituents and Activity

Benzophenanthridine Alkaloids

The herb Liang Mian Zhen is rich in benzophenanthridine alkaloids, and many of them, discovered from Liang Mian Zhen, are responsible for the biological functions of the herb, including tumor-inhibiting effect in different potencies. The representative alkaloids were identified as nitidine (**1**) and its chloride (**2**) in the herb.

Nitidine and Nitidine Chloride

Both alkaloids effectively inhibited the growth and the proliferation of many murine and human carcinoma cells *in vitro*. The treatment with nitidine (**1**) in a 4 mg/kg dose prolonged the life duration of mice bearing P388 or L1210 leukemia by 109% and 36%, respectively.[1] Nitidine chloride (**2**) showed more potent inhibitory effect against the growth of nasopharyngeal cancer cell lines (7111 and Ecv2) *in vitro* and of Ehrlich ascites tumor, P388 leukemia, sarcoma 180, and HepG2 hepatoma *in vivo*.[2–4] By the *in vivo* treatment with nitidine chloride (**2**) in a dose of 10.0 mg/kg, the survival time of mice bearing H22 mouse ascitic hepatoma was significantly extended by 85.7%. The i.p. injection of nitidine chloride (**2**) in a dose of 20 mg/kg obviously declined the mitosis index of Ehrlich ascites cancer cells in mice and markedly restrained the proliferation and the cell cycle of the Ehrlich tumor. If the dose was increased to 40 mg/kg, nitidine chloride (**2**) killed the tumor cells at S phase and remarkably prolonged life span of the mice by 270%.[5–7] The significant antigrowth effect of nitidine chloride (**2**) on human HepG2 hepatoma in nude mice was probably correlated with the inhibitory effect against Topo-I and Topo-II.[4] Also, nitidine chloride (**2**) induced the cell apoptosis and obstructed the cell proliferation *in vitro* and/or *in vivo* by suppressing ERK signaling pathway in renal cancer cell lines (786-O and A498) and by restraining a RB/E2F pathway in hepatoms cell line (SMMC-7721).[8,9] Importantly, nitidine chloride (**2**) in a concentration of ~12 μg/mL was sensitive to multidrug-resistant KBV200 cells, eliciting the promotion of apoptosis, cell cycle arrest, and growth inhibition.[10]

Likewise, i.p. injection with nitidine chloride (**2**) to nude mice at a dosage of 7 mg/kg/day markedly inhibited the growth of xenografted human SGC-7901 gastric cancer cells and effectively suppressed the volume, weight, and MVD of the solid tumors. The potent anticancer and apoptosis-inducing activities exerted by nitidine chloride (**2**) were found to be closely related to STAT3 signaling cascade, i.e., (1) lessening the expressions of STAT3-dependent target genes, including cyclin-D1, CD31, Bcl-xL, and VEGF; (2) blocking Janus kinase-2/STAT3 signaling and STAT3/DNA-binding activity in endothelial cells; (3) restraining VEGF-induced endothelial cell migration, proliferation, and tubular formation; and (4) dramatically blocking VEGF triggered neovascularization in the cornea and the Matrigel plugs.[10] These evidences highlighted that nitidine chloride (**2**) as a potent inhibitor of STAT3 signaling and angiogenesis is a promising chemotherapeutic agent, which deserves to be in a proclinic investigation.

Furthermore, its methanolic extract and nitidine (**1**) were found to obstruct Topo-I-mediated DNA relaxation and stabilization of the covalent binary complex between the enzyme and the DNA. Both nitidine (**1**) and fagaronine markedly retarded the Topo-II function as well at a 10 μM concentration,[11,12] and nitidine (**1**) had been found to be inhibitors of viral RNA reverse transcriptase and mouse embryonic DNA polymerase.[13,14] These activities might be closely linked to the anticancer effect of the alkaloids. Taken together, the benzophenanthridines, especially nitidine chloride (**2**), may have a valid potential to develop new anticancer agents.

Other Nitidine Analogs

More benzophenanthridine alkaloids have been discovered from the Liang Mian Zhen with *in vitro* and *in vivo* biological evaluations. Chelerythrine (**3**) is a selective PKC inhibitor, capable of significantly displaying antitumor effects by inducing the tumor cell apoptosis, disturbing the cell cycle, and downregulating the expressions of multidrug-resistant genes. Thus, it markedly suppressed the growth of human cancer cell lines such as HL-60 (leukemic), LNCaP and DU-145 (prostate), KB (nasopharyngus), HeLa (cervix), gastric cancer, NSCLC, and SQ-20B (a radioresistant and chemoresistant SCC) *in vitro*.[15–21] In the chelerythrine (**3**) treatment, the expression profile of apoptosis-related genes p53, p21waf/cipl, c-Myc, and Bax was promoted in the gastric carcinoma cells, but Bcl-2 expression was kept unchanged.[18] In a cotreatment *in vitro* with cisplatin (a chemotherapeutic agent), chelerythrine (**3**) was able to additively augment the cytotoxic effect of cisplatin against six human head and neck SCC cell lines, such as UM-SCC-11B, 14A, 14C, 22B, 8029NA, and 8029DDP (a cisplatin-resistant subline).[22,23] The *in vivo* antigrowth effect of 6-methoxy-5,6-dihydronitidine (**5**) was demonstrated in a mouse model with P388 leukemia.[7] 6-Ethoxychelerythrine (**4**) and 6-methoxy-5,6-dihydronitidine (**5**) also exerted notable antigrowth effect against the EACs to prolong the life mduration of the tumor-bearing mice.[6,24]

Two other benzophenanthridines, 1-methoxy-12-methyl-12,13-dihydro-[1,3]dioxolo[4′,5′:4,5]benzo-[1,2-c]-phenanthridine-2,13-diol (**6**) and isofagaridine (**7**), showed moderate to weak inhibitory effect against human cancer cell lines such as HepG2 (liver), MDA-MB-231 (breast) and its MDR subline, U87MG (brain), and HCT-116 (colon) cells and exerted obvious suppressive effect against CCRF-CEM human lymphoblast cells (respective IC_{50}: 0.24 and 0.30 μM) and its MDR subline CEM/ADR5000 (respective IC_{50}: 31.58 and 20.37 μM).[25] Angoline (**8**) was a potent and selective inhibitor of STAT3 signaling pathway.[26] By the targeting, angoline (**8**) consequently exerted growth inhibition of human HepG2 (liver), MDA-MB-231 (breast), and H4 (brain) cancer cell lines (IC_{50}: 3.14–4.72 μM). Moreover, from *Z. nitidum* var. *fastuosum*, 13 benzophenanthridines were isolated and three compounds, 6-methoxydihydrochelerythrine, 6-methoxy-7-demethyldihydrochelerythrine, and 8-(1′-hydroxyethyl)-7,8-dihydrochelerythrine, exhibited moderate to weak cytotoxic effects on human A549 (lung), HeLa (cervix), SMMC-7721 (liver), and EJ (bladder) cancer cell lines *in vitro*.[27]

Other Types of Alkaloids

Other types of alkaloids were also separated from the herb *Z. nitidum* and showed anticancer potential. Among them, liriodenine (**9**) exerted the antigrowth activities against human MCF-7 breast cancer, NCI-H460 lung cancer, and SF-268 glioblastoma cell lines *in vitro* (IC_{50}: 2.19 and 3.19 μg/mL). The potent cytotoxicity of liriodenine (**9**) was also present on other types of human solid cancer cell lines: A549 (lung), HCT-8 (colon), HepG2 and SK-Hep-1 (live), and KB (nasopharyngus) cells and two murine leukemia cell lines (P388 and L1210), *in vitro*, but no obvious effect on normal human IMR-90 cells.[28,29] After being treated with liriodenine (**9**), the cell cycle was arrested at G1 stage and the DNA synthesis was obstructed in the HepG2 cells. Concurrently, both iNOS and p53 expressions were promoted and the NO level was elevated, implying that the NO production and the p53 activation are critical factors for the liriodenine-induced growth inhibition in the human p53 wild-type hepatoma cells.[29] Likewise, two isolated furoquinolines assigned as kokusaginine (**10**) and maculine (**11**) interestingly exerted better effect on the suppression of drug-resistant CEM/ADR5000 lymphoblast cells (respective IC_{50}: 44.56 and 63.09 μM) compared to the effects on the original CCRF-CEM lymphoblast cells (respective IC_{50}: 49.81 and 89.09 μM).[25]

Indole Alkaloid Glycosides

Three mannopyranosides of indole alkaloids were isolated from an ethanol extract of *Z. nitidum* roots and assigned as methyl 7-(β-D-mannopyranosyloxy)-1H-indole-2-carboxylate (**12**), methyl 7-[(3-O-acetyl-β-D-mannopyranosyl)oxy]-1H-indole-2-carboxylate (**13**), and 2-methyl-1H-indol-7-yl-β-D-mannopyranoside (**14**). An *in vitro* assay revealed that these alkaloid mannosides possess significant cytotoxicities against all the tested tumor cell lines (A549, BGC-823, HCT15, HeLa, HepG2, MCF-7, SGC-7901, and SK-MEL-2) with IC_{50} values of less than 30 μM. According to the IC_{50} values, the order of anticancer potencies were 2-methyl-1H-indol-7-yl-β-D-mannopyranoside (**14**) (IC_{50}: 9.21–12.75 μM) > methyl 7-(β-D-mannopyranosyloxy)-1H-indole-2-carboxylate (**12**) (IC_{50}: 18.11–21.04 μM) > methyl 7-[(3-O-acetyl-β-D-mannopyranosyl)oxy]-1H-indole-2-carboxy-late (**13**) (IC_{50}: 23.47–28.12 μM).[30]

Metal Complexes of Liriodenine

When liriodenine (**9**) was reacted with some specific metal salts such as MnII, FeII, CoII, ZnII, Pt(ii), and Ru(ii) to afford a group of metal complexes such as $[MnCl_2(\mathbf{9})_2]$, $[FeCl_2(\mathbf{9})_2]$, $[Zn_2(\mathbf{9})_2(\mu_2\text{-}Cl)_2Cl_2]$, *cis*-$[PtCl_2\ (\mathbf{9})]$, *cis*-$[PtCl_2(\mathbf{9})\ (DMSO)]$, $[Co(\mathbf{9})_2(H_2O)_2{\cdot}Co(\mathbf{9})_2\ (CH_3CH_2OH)_2](ClO_4)_4$, and *cis*-$[RuCl_2(\mathbf{9})(DMSO)_2]{\cdot}1.5H_2O$. All these metal-based complexes were found to effectively obstruct the activity of Topo-I even at a low concentration (≤10 μM) due to having an ability of intensively binding to the DNA helix.[31,32] Through G-quadruplex DNA stabilization, the *cis*-$[PtCl_2(\mathbf{9})\ (DMSO)]$ treatment resulted in obvious G2/M and S cell cycle arrest, apoptosis, and telomerase inhibition activity in Bel-7404 human hepatoma cells.[33] Compared to the liriodenine (**9**) alone, the metal complexes exhibited the enhanced synergic cytotoxicity to the selected human tumor cell lines.

Other Bioactivities

Pharmacological investigation demonstrated that Liang Miang Zhen (Shiny leaf prickly ash) possesses multiple biological properties such as analgesic, repercussive, antirheumatic, anti-inflammatory, blood circulation-promoting, antispasmodic, and antibacterial. The plant resin collected from the bark, especially from the roots, is a powerful stimulant and tonic. In addition, the plant is able to be used as an insecticide, and it is also toxic to fish.

References

1. Jiang, J. W. and Xiao, Q. Q. 1986. *Manual of Herbal Active Ingredients*. p. 956, People' Health Publishing House, Beijing, China.
2. Liu, L. M. et al. 2009. Antitumor effect of nitidine chloride in vitro and in vivo. *Chin. J. Pharmacol. Toxicol.* 23: 214–8.
3. Liu, H. G. et al. 2007. Effect of nitidine chloride-induced apoptosis in two nasopharyngeal carcinoma cell lines *in vitro*. *Yakugaku Zashi* 22: 514–6.
4. Liu, L. M. et al. 2010. Anti-hepatoma activity of nitidine chloride and its effect on topoisomerase. *Chin. Pharmacol. Bull.* 26: 497–500.
5. Fan, Y. J. et al. 1981. Effect of nitidine chloride on mouse Ehrlich ascites tumor cell cycle. *Zhongguo Yaoli Xuebao* 2: 46.
6. Huang, Z. X. et al. 1980. Studies on the antitumor constituents of *Zanthoxylum nitidum* (Roxb.) DC. *Acta Chimica Sinica* 38: 535–42.
7. Wall, M. E. et al. 1987. Plant antitumor agents: 27. Isolation, structure, and structure activity relationships of alkaloids from *Fagara macrophylla*. *J. Nat. Prods.* 50: 1095–9.
8. Fang, Z. Q. et al. 2014. Nitidine chloride induces apoptosis and inhibits tumor cell proliferation via suppressing ERK signaling pathway in renal cancer. *Food Chem. Toxicol.* 66: 210–6.
9. Huang, Y. et al. 2013. The mechanism of nitidine chloride for inhibiting proliferation of SMMC-7721 by RB/E2F pathway. *Yaowu Shengwu Jishu* 20: 17–20.
10. Chen, J. et al. 2012. Inhibition of STAT3 signaling pathway by nitidine chloride suppressed the angiogenesis and growth of human gastric cancer. *Mol. Cancer Therap.* 11: 277–87.
11. Fang, S. D. et al. 1993. Inhibitors of DNA topoisomerase I isolated from the roots of *Zanthoxylum nitidum*. *J. Org. Chem.* 58: 5025–7.
12. Wang, L. K. et al. 1993. Inhibition of topoisomerase I function by nitidine and fagaronine. *Chem. Res. Toxicol.* 6: 813–8.
13. Sethi, V. S. et al. 1976. Inhibition of mammalian and oncornavirus nucleic acid polymerase: Published activities by alkoxybenzophenanthridine alkaloids. *Cancer Res.* 36: 2390–5.
14. Sethi, V. S. et al. (a) 1977. *Ann. N.Y. Acad. Sci.* 284: 508; (b) 1999. *Chinese Materia Medica*. Vol. 4, 4–3821, 993 Shanghai Science and Technology Press, Shanghai, China.
15. Wang, B. L. et al. 2007. Anticancer activity of nitidine chloride from *Zanthoxylum nitidum* (Roxb.) DC. On multidrug resistant KBV200 cells in vitro. *Chin. J. Pharmacol. Toxicol.* 21: 512–5.
16. Vrba, J. R. et al. 2008. Chelerythrine and dihydrochelerythrine induce G1 phase arrest and bimodal cell death in human leukemia HL-60 cells. *Toxicol. in Vitro* 22: 1008–17.
17. Liu, F. et al. 2009. Inhibition effect of chelerythrine on Hela cells. *Progression in Modern Biomed.* (China) 9: 514–6.
18. Zhu, G. H. et al. 1999. Pharmacological inhibition of protein kinase C activity could induce apoptosis in gastric cancer cells by differential regulation of apoptosis-related genes. *Digestive Diseases Sci.* 44: 2020–6
19. Chmura, S. J. et al. 2000. In vitro and in vivo activity of protein kinase C inhibitor chelerythrine chloride induces tumor cell toxicity and growth delay in vivo. *Clin. Cancer Res.* 6: 737–42.
20. Gao, Z. Q. et al. 2007. Effects of PKC inhibitor, chelerythrine chloride, on drug-sensitivity of NSCLC cell lines. *Chin. J. Lung Cancer* 10: 455–60.
21. Malikova, J. et al. 2006. The effect of chelerythrine on cell growth, apoptosis, and cell cycle in human normal and cancer cells in comparison with sanguinarine. *Cell Biol. Toxicol.* 22: 439–53.
22. Weichselbaum, R. R. et al. 2002. Chelerythrine-based therapies for cancer. *PCT Intl. Appl.* WO 2002013803 A2 20020221.
23. Hoffmann, T. K. et al. 2002. Antitumor activity of protein kinase C inhibitors and cisplatin in human head and neck squamous cell carcinoma lines. *Anti-Cancer Drugs* 13: 93–100.
24. Wang, M. H. et al. 1981. Isolation of antitumor alkaloids from *Zanthoxylum nitidum* and structural study of its alkaloid C. *China J. Chin. Materia Medica* 16: 48.
25. Sandjo, L. P. et al. 2014. Cytotoxic benzophenanthridine and furoquinoline alkaloids from *Zanthoxylum buesgenii*. *Chem. Cen. J.* 8: 61.
26. Liu, J. W. et al. 2014. Angoline: A selective IL-6/STAT3 signaling pathway inhibitor isolated from *Zanthoxylum nitidum*. *Phytomed.* 21: 1088–91.
27. Wang, C. F. et al. 2015. Cytotoxicity of benzophenanthridine alkaloids from the roots *of Zanthoxylum nitidum* (Roxb.) DC. var. fastuosum How ex Huang. *Nat. Prod. Res.* 29: 1380–3.
28. Yang, C. H. et al. 2009. Secondary metabolites and cytotoxic activities from the stem bark of *Zanthoxylum nitidum*. *Chem. Biodiver.* 6: 846–57.
29. Hsieh, T. J. et al. 2005. Liriodenine inhibits the proliferation of human hepatoma cell lines by blocking cell cycle progression and nitric oxide-mediated activation of p53 expression. *Food Chem. Toxicol.* 43: 1117–26.
30. Hu, J. et al. 2014. Cytotoxic mannopyranosides of indole alkaloids from *Zanthoxylum nitidum*. *Chem. Biodiv.* 11: 970–4.
31. Liu, Y. C. et al. 2009. Divalent later transition metal complexes of the traditional Chinese medicine (TCM) liriodenine: coordination chemistry, cytotoxicity and DNA binding studies. *Dalton Trans.* (48): 10813–23.
32. Chen, Z. F. et al. 2009. Potential new inorganic antitumor agents from combining the anticancer traditional Chinese medicine (TCM) liriodenine with metal ions, and DNA binding studies. *Dalton Trans.* (2): 262–72.
33. Li, Y. L. et al. 2014. A platinum(II) complex of liriodenine from traditional Chinese medicine (TCM): Cell cycle arrest, cell apoptosis induction and telomerase inhibition activity via G-quadruplex DNA stabilization. *J. Inorg. Biochem.* 137: 12–21.

7

Anticancer Potentials of Hemostatic Herbs

CONTENTS

131 Xian He Cao 仙鶴草

Asian agrimony

Herb Origination

The herb Xian He Cao (Asian agrimony) is the dried aerial parts of a Rosaceae plant, *Agrimonia pilosa*. The plant is native to northern Asia and eastern Europe, and now it is widely distributed and cultured nationwide in China. The best collection season for the herb is normally in summer and autumn just before the flower season. Its roots are also used as another Chinese herb, which is collected in late autumn.

Antitumor Activities

The Xian He Cao decoction was effective in the growth inhibition and the apoptosis induction of cultured human HL-60 promyelacytic leukemia cells.[1] The Xian He Cao extract exerted the growth inhibitory activity against human JTC-26 cervical carcinoma for over 90% *in vitro* and against murine sarcoma 180 for 25–50% *in vivo*. The exposure of 500 μg Xian He Cao extract to the cancer cells for six days could kill all cells without any damage to the normal cells.[2] A nonsugar fraction of the roots with median polarity also showed antitumor property when the extract is given through i.p. injection to mice once for four days before the inoculation of the tumor cells such as MM2 breast carcinoma or solid sarcoma 180. This fraction significantly prolonged the life duration of mice implanted with sarcoma 180, MM-2 breast cancer, or Meth-A fibrosarcoma.[2,3] In an *in vitro* system, moderate anticarcinogenic and antimutagenic activities of Xian He Cao were also established against the environmental mutagens/carcinogens, for instance, BAP, 1,6-dinitro-pyrene, and 3,9-dinitro-fluoranthene.[4] Moreover, the Xian He Cao extract has potential inhibitory activity on CDC25 tyrosin phosphatase (an activator of the mitosis-inducing p34cdc2 kinase), which is used in a highly specific mechanism-based screen assay for antimitotic drug discovery.[5]

Antitumor Constituents and Activities

Tannins

From the active nonsugar fraction, agrimoniin (**1**) was isolated and elucidated as a dimer tannin. It demonstrated significant cytotoxic effect on MM2 breast carcinoma, E.L.4 lymphosarcoma, Meth-A fibrosarcoma, and L-929 fibrosarcoma cells *in vitro*.[3,6] When an i.p. injection of agrimoniin (**1**) at a dose over 10 mg/kg is done to mice inoculated with the MM2 tumor, the tumor growth was almost completely rejected and the life span of the mice was notably prolonged, where some tested mice were cured. Agrimoniin (**1**) also restrained the growth of murine ascites carcinomas such as MH134 hepatoma and Meth-A fibrosarcoma *in vivo*[3–8] and suppressed the growth of human solid carcinoma cells, such as MGC803 (stomach), SPC-A-1 (lung), and HeLa (cervix), obviously in nude mice xenograft.[9] The apoptosis of human SGC-7901 gastric neoplastic cells could be provoked by agrimoniin (**1**) through the increases of calcium concentration and intracellular ROS level and the decrease of mitochondrial transmembrane potential.[10] Gerannin, another unique tannin component isolated from the herb, was also reported exert antiproliferative effect against the SGC-7901 cells after being treated with ~15 μg/mL of gerannin for 72 h (IC_{50}: 11.5 μg/mL). The apoptosis-promoting effect occurred after the SGC-7901 cells were treated by gerannin for 24 h.[11] Gerannin also markedly restrained the growth of human HepG2 hepatoma cells *in vitro* in association with the promotion of the expression of a tumor suppressor gene p53.[12]

The i.p. injection of agrimoniin (**1**) to mice bearing tumor was also able to augment the number of peripheral WBCs and the ratio of monocytes and to enlarge the capacity of the spleen to take up thymidine.[7] The cytotoxicity of NK cells and peritoneal exudate cells was potentiated and the lytic activity of antibody-dependent cells was enhanced after the administration of agrimoniin (**1**) by i.p. injection to mice, leading to the growth inhibition of the MM2 cells.[13] IL-1β secretion in the culture supernatant of the human peripheral blood mononuclear cells was also notably stimulated by agrimoniin (**1**) in dose- and time-dependent manners, and IL-1 was secreted to the adherent peritoneal exudate cells in four days after i.p. administration with agrimoniin (10 mg/kg) to mice.[13] Consequently, the results indicate that the anticancer effect of agrimoniin (**1**) should be largely attributable to the potential of the host-mediated defense via the activation of macrophage, the secretion of IL-1, and the increase of cytotoxic immunocytes.[14,15]

Polysaccharides

Total polysaccharides were prepared from *A. pilosa* by optimum extraction technology, which could inhibit the hyperplasia of human U251 glioblastoma cells in a dose-dependent manner (IC_{50}: 1.35 mg/mL) *in vitro*. The treatment concurrently enhanced the apoptotic death of the U251 cells, whose apoptosis-induction should largely contribute to the growth suppressive effect of the polysaccharides on the tumor cells.[16]

Other Bioactivities

Pharmacological studies demonstrated that Xian He Cao (Asian agrimony) possesses multiple health functions, such as anticoagulant, antithrombosis, antiinflammatory, antiarrhythmic, anthelmintic, hypoglycemic, antipaludian, antihypertensive, antitoxic, analgetic, choleretic, hemostatic, teniacidal, and antibacterial activities. The herb extract also displayed a broad spectrum of antiviral effect on all three subtypes of human influenza viruses, including H1N1 and H3N2 influenza A subtypes and influenza B virus.[17] The flavonoid components derived from the separation of Xian He Cao are effective inhibitors of acetyl-cholinesterase.[18]

References

1. Gao, K. et al. 2000. Experimental study on decoctum *Agrimonia pilosa* Ledeb-induced apoptosis in HL-60 cells in vitro. *Zhongyaocai* 23: 561–2.
2. Wang, X. Q. et al. 1985. Review of clinical application and pharmacological activities of *Agrimonia pilosa*. *Xinzhongyi* (5): 55.
3. Miyamoto, K. et al. 1985. Isolation of agrimoniin, an antitumor constituent, from the roots of *Agrimonia pilosa* LEDEB. *Chem. Pharm. Bull.* 33: 3977–81.
4. Horikawa, K. et al. 1994. Moderate inhibition of mutagenicity and carcinogenicity of benzo[a]pyrene, 1,6-dinitropyrene and 3,9-dinitro-fluoranthene by Chinese medicinal herbs. *Mutagenesis* 9: 523–6.
5. Yang, H. et al. 2005. Screening the active constituents of Chinese medicinal herbs as potent inhibitors of Cdc25 tyrosine phosphatase, an activator of the mitosis-inducing p34cdc2 kinase. *J. Zhejiang Univ., Sci. B*, 6B: 656–63.
6. Xu, Q. et al. 1986. Antitumor activity of agrimoniin and its effect on immune responses. *Gifu Yakka Daigaku Kiyo* (35): 36–44.
7. Koshiura. R. et al. 1985. Antitumor activity of methanol extract from roots of *Agrimonia pilosa* LEDEB. *Jpn. J. Pharmacol.* 38: 9–16.
8. Miyamoto, K. et al. 1987. Antitumor effect of agrimoniin, a tannin of *Agrimonia pilosa*, on transplantable rodent tumors. *Jpn. J. Pharmacol.* 43: 187–95.
9. Wang, S. G. et al. 1998. Effect of *Agrimonia pilosa* Ledeb on nude mice bearing human cancerous xenograft. *Disi Junyi Daxue Xuebao* 19: 702–4.

10. Wang, B. Q. et al. 2011. Agrimoniin induced SGC7901 cell apoptosis associated mitochondrial transmembrane potential and intracellular calcium concentration. *J. Med. Plants Res.* 5: 3512–9.
11. Qing, W. B. et al. 2010. Induction of apoptosis in human gastric carcinoma cell by geraniin. *Intl. Conference on Biomed. Engineering of Informatics*, 3rd, Yantai, October 16–18, 5: 1951–4.
12. Xiong, J. Z. et al. 2010. Induction of P53 genes in human hepatoma cells by geraniin. *Intl. Conference on Biomed. Engineering & Informatics*, 3rd, Yantai, October 16–18, 5: 2071–4.
13. Miyamoto, K. et al. 1988. Induction of cytotoxicity of peritoneal exudate cells by agrimoniin, a novel immunomodulatory tannin of *Agrimonia pilosa* Ledeb. *Cancer Immunol. Immunother. CII,* 27: 59–62.
14. Miyamoto, K. et al. 1995. Anticarcinogenic activities of polyphenols in foods and herbs. *Book of Abstracts, 210th ACS National Meeting*, Chicago, IL, (Pt. 1), AGFD-231.
15. Miyamoto, K. et al. 1997. Anticarcinogenic activities of polyphenols in foods and herbs. *ACS Symposium Series* 662: 245–59.
16. Zhu, K. et al. 2012. Extraction of total polysaccharides from *Agrimonia pilosa* and evaluation of its inhibitory activity on human glioblastoma U251 cells in vitro. *Zhongguo Shiyan Fangjixue Zazhi* 18: 188–91.
17. Shin, W. J. et al. 2010. Broad-spectrum antiviral effect of *Agrimonia pilosa* extract on influenza viruses. *Microbiol. Immunol.* 54: 11–9.
18. Jung, M. et al. 2007. Acetylcholinesterase inhibition by flavonoids from *Agrimonia pilosa. Mol.* 12: 2130–9.

132 Bai Ji 白及

Chinese ground orchid

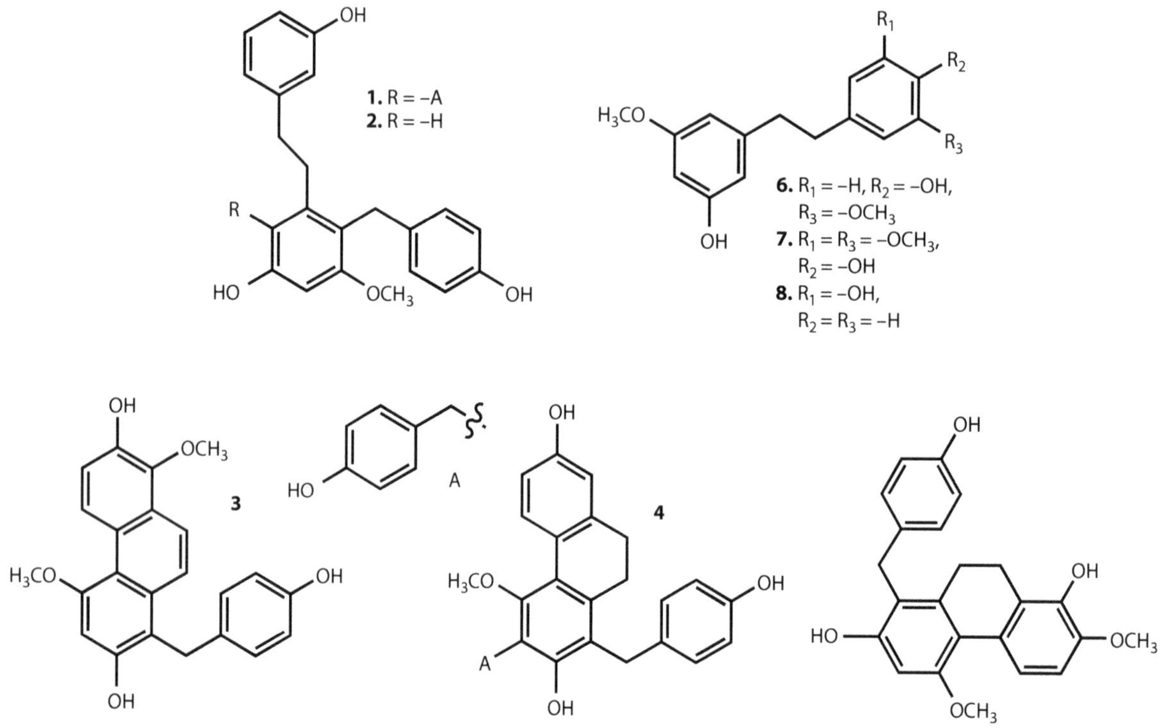

1. R = -A
2. R = -H

6. R_1 = -H, R_2 = -OH, R_3 = $-OCH_3$
7. R_1 = R_3 = $-OCH_3$, R_2 = -OH
8. R_1 = -OH, R_2 = R_3 = -H

Herb Origination

The herb Bai Ji (Chinese ground orchid) is the dried tuberous rhizomes of an Orchidaceae plant, *Bletilla striata*. This deciduous terrestrial orchid is native to the temperate areas of China and Japan. Usually, the tubers are collected in September and October and steamed and then dried in the sun for traditional Chinese medical practice.

Antitumor Activities

An injection prepared from the tubers of Bai Ji exhibited significant suppressive effect against the growth of hepatoma cells induced by DAB (an oncogenic agent) in rats.[1] The chloroform partition fraction elicited the apoptotic death of HL-60 human leukemia cells and B16 mouse melanoma cells.[2,3] The extracts prepared from the fibrous root part (FRP) and the pseudobulb part (PSP) of *B. striata*; especially, the FRP showed phenolic content, stronger DPPH-scavenging and tyrosinase-inhibiting activities and ferric-reducing antioxidant capacity. Both chloroform fractions of FRP and PSP dose-dependently induce the apoptosis of HepG2 human hepatoma cells.[4] Moreover, between 1990 and 1993, 56 patients with primary hepatoma were clinically treated by permanent hepatic arterial embolization with Bai Ji powders. The resulted vascular embolization, tumor necrosis, and long-term inhibitory effect were obviously enhanced, and the one, two, and three-year survival rates were amplified to 44.9%, 33.6%, and 33.6%, respectively.[5,6]

By emulsification–condensation–chemical cross-linking, cisplatin with Bai Ji microsphere and 5-FU with Bai Ji microsphere were prepared. The microspheres could clearly sustain and release their antitumor properties *in vitro*. The microsphere prepared with 5-FU and Bai Ji was infused into rabbits bearing VX2 transplanted with hepatoma through hepatic artery in a dose of 10 mg/kg, exerting intensive vessel embolization function, tumor growth inhibition, and higher grade of tumor necrosis. When the treatment was clinically used in 11 patients with primary hepatoma, the 5-FU/Bai Ji microsphere could improve the release of antitumor agent 5-FU to enhance the therapeutic effects and to reduce the toxicity, indicating that the microsphere of 5-FU/Bai Ji is a safe antihepatoma agent and an effective peripheral embolization agent.[7–9]

Antitumor Constituents and Activities

Stilbenoids

Many stilbenoids were isolated from Bai Ji by the guidance of suppressive effect on the tubulin polymerization. The two stilbenoids elucidated as 3′,5-dihydroxy-2-(p-hydroxybenzyl)-3-methoxybibenzyl (**1**) and 3,3′-dihydroxy-2′,6′-bis(p-hydroxybenzyl)-5-methoxybibenzyl (**2**) were able to restrain the polymerization of tubulin and mitosis with an IC_{50} value of 10 μM. Also, the bisbenzyl (**1**) and other two stilbenoids 1-(p-hydroxybenzyl)-4,8-dimethoxy-phenanthrene-2,7-diol (**3**) and 7 2,7-dihydroxy-1,3-bis(p-hydroxybenzyl)-4-methoxy-9,10-dihydro-phenanthrene

(**4**) at a 3 μM concentration strongly enhanced the cytotoxic activity of 7-ethyl-10-hydroxycamptothecin (SN-38, an active metabolite of CPT-11) in breast carcinoma resistance protein (BCRP)-transduced K562 (K562/BCRP) cells but not in human K562 leukemia cells. The results proved that the three stilbenoids (bisbenzyl (**1**), 1-(p-hydroxybenzyl)-4,8-dimethoxy-phenanthrene-2,7-diol (**3**), and 7 2,7-dihydroxy-1,3-bis(p-hydroxy-benzyl)-4-methoxy-9,10-dihydro-phenanthrene (**4**)) sensitized the multidrug-resistant leukemia K562/BCRP cells to SN-38 by inhibiting BCRP-mediated concurrent resistance to chemotherapeutic drugs.[10] Gigantol (**5**), batatasin-III (**6**), 3′,4″-dihydroxy-5′,3″,5″-trimethoxybibenzyl (**7**), and 9,10-dihydro-1-(4′-hydroxybenzyl)-4,7-dimethoxyphenanthrene-2,8-diol (**8**), in the *in vitro* assay, were cytotoxic to human SKOV-3 (ovary), A549 (lung), SK-MEL-2 (skin), and HCT-15 (colon) neoplastic cell lines, whose potencies were **5** (IC_{50}: 5.28–7.14 μM) > **8** (IC_{50}: 2.16–12.69 μM) > **6** (IC_{50}: 9.68–18.94 μM) > **7** (IC_{50}: 17.92–24.51 μM).[11]

Polysaccharide

A polysaccharide (BSPS) was extracted from the root tubers. When BSPS was sulfated, the solubility in the water and the biological activity were significantly improved. BSPS-sulfate demonstrated not only obvious inhibition against the growth of U937 lymphoma cells and H_2O_2-induced hemolysis but also increase of the proliferation of lymphocyte B and scavenging ability of O^{2-} and OH.[12]

Other Bioactivities

The herb Bai Ji (Chinese ground orchid) displays obvious pharmacological properties such as hemostatic, membrane-protecting, mucous antibacterial, and antifungal effects.

References

1. (a) Department of Pharmacy, Wuhan Medical University. 1978. *J. Wuhan Med. Univ.* (2): 116; (b) 1999. *Chinese Materia Medica*. Vol. 8, 8–7803, 674–9. Shanghai Science and Technology Press, Shanghai, China.
2. Wang, L. F. et al. 2013. Studies on active fraction in rhizoma *Bletillae striatae* for inducing apoptosis of HL60 cells and its related mechanisms. *Zhonghua Zhongyiyao Xuekan* 31: 2224–6.
3. Lu, X. F. et al. 2013. Study of rhizoma *Bietillae striatae* extracts in inducing apoptosis on mice melanoma B16 cells. *Zhonghua Zhongyiyao Xuekan* 31: 1619–21.
4. Jiang, F. S. et al. 2013. Antioxidant, antityrosinase and antitumor activity comparison: The potential utilization of fibrous root part of *Bletilla striata* (Thunb.) Reichb.f. *PLoS One* 8: e58004.
5. Feng, G. et al. 1996. Comparative study on the long-term effect of permanent embolization of hepatic artery with *Bletilla striata* in patients with primary liver cancer. *J. Tongji Med. Univ.* 16: 111–6.
6. Zheng, C. et al. 1998. *Bletilla striata* as a vascular embolizing agent in interventional treatment of primary hepatic carcinoma. *China Med. J.* (*Eng. Edit.*) 111: 1060–3.
7. Li, X. et al. 2003. Therapeutic efficacy of 5-FU *Bletilla striata* microspheres infused through hepatic artery against rabbit VX2 transplanted hepatoma. *Shijie Huaren Xiaohua Zazhi* 11: 1337–40.
8. Li, W. Y. et al. 2003. Preparation of cisplatin with *Bletilla striata* microspheres and their physicochemical properties. *Zhongguo Yaoxue Zazhi* 38: 517–20.
9. Li, W. Y. et al. 2001. Pharmacokinetics of Fu Bletilla microspheres after hepatic arterial embolization in patients with primary liver cancer. *Zhongguo Yiyuan Yaoxue Zazhi* 21: 643–4.
10. Morita, H. 2005. Antimitotic activity and reversal of breast cancer resistance protein-mediated drug resistance by stilbenoids from *Bletilla striata*. *Bioorg. Med. Chem. Lett.* 15: 1051–4.
11. Woo, K. Y. et al. 2014. Wan phytochemical constituents of *Bletilla striata* and their cytotoxic activity. *Nat. Prod. Sci.* 20: 91–4.
12. Chen, J. Y. et al. 2007. Comparison study on bioactivities of *Bletilla striata* (Thunb.) Reichb. f. polysaccharide and BSPSS. *Shipin Kexue* 28: 27–31.

133 Shan Cha 山茶

Camellia

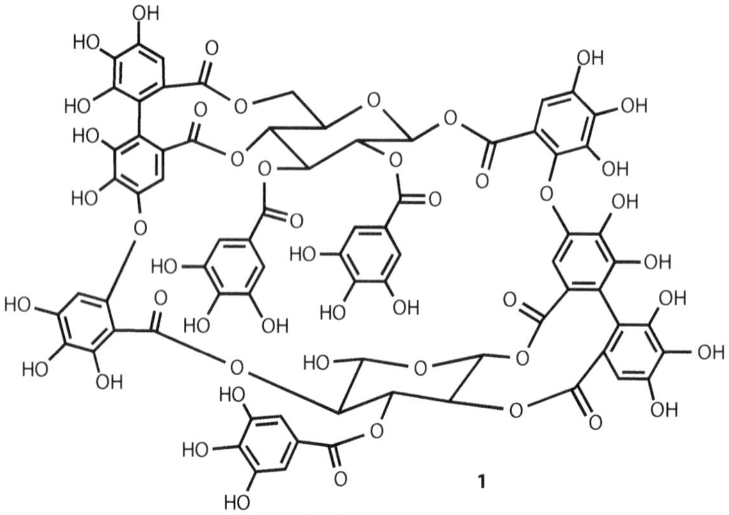

1

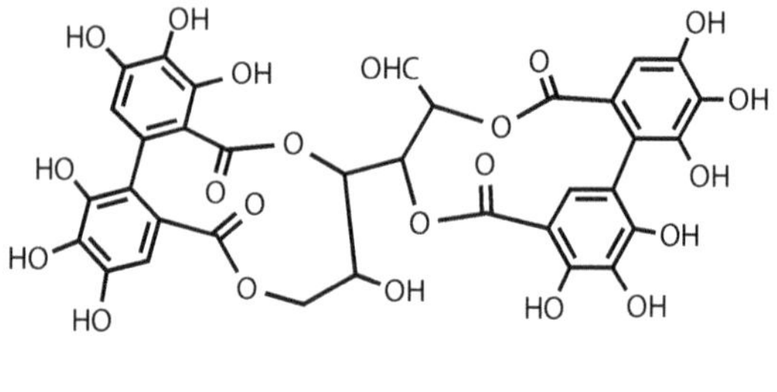

2

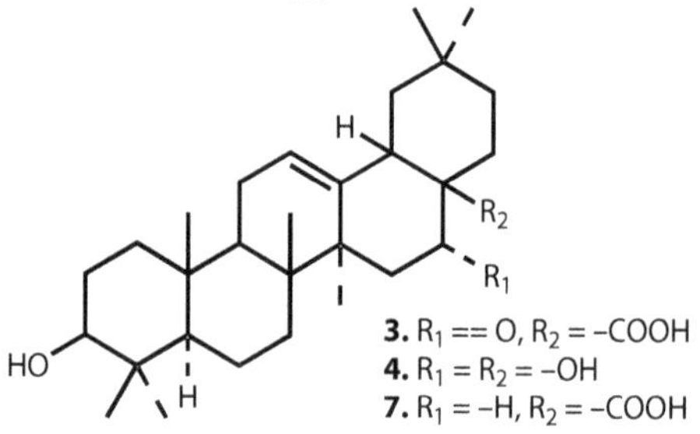

3. R_1 == O, R_2 = -COOH
4. R_1 = R_2 = -OH
7. R_1 = -H, R_2 = -COOH

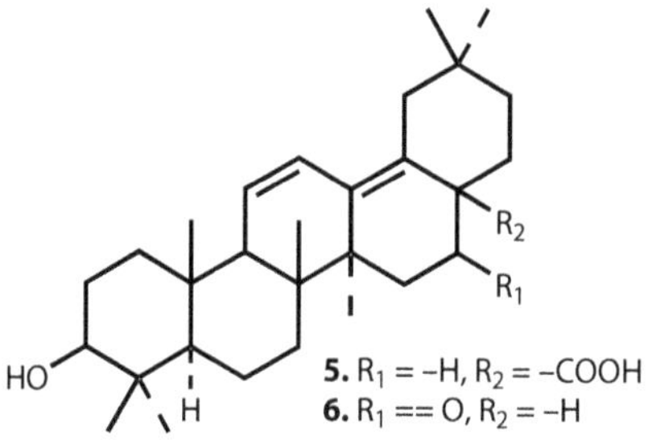

5. R_1 = -H, R_2 = -COOH
6. R_1 == O, R_2 = -H

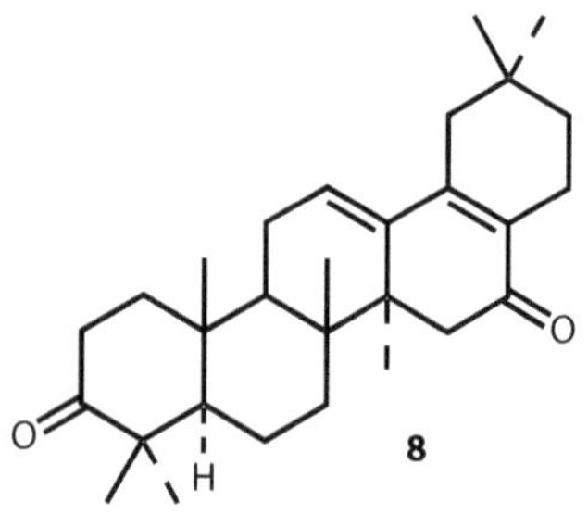

8

Herb Origination

The herb Shan Cha (Camellia) originated from an evergreen bush, *Camellia japonica* L. (Theaceae). The plant is native to China, Korea, and Japan, and it is widely cultured in eastern Asia as a common garden flower. It has been cultivated in China for thousands of years and was introduced to Europe during the eighteenth century. The flowers, the roots, the leaves, and the seeds of Camellia are used as folk medicines in China.

Anticarcinogenicity and Constituents

Camellia Oil

The antiproliferative and apoptosis-inducing effects of the water extract of Camellia flowers were shown in human MCF-7 breast cancer cells *in vitro*.[1] Camellia oil prepared from the flowers is rich in oleamide-like oleic acid. The Camellia oil and its distillate fractions were effective in suppressing the spontaneous lung metastasis of mouse melanoma B16 cells when administered orally or by i.p. injection to B16-bearing mice daily, and the i.p. injection was more potent.[2] Therefore, Camellia oil may be a potential supplement for people and patients to protect from carcinogenesis and metastasis, besides Camellia oil is quite safe to be used in foods.

Tannins

In the early studies, a tannin component derived from Camellia flowers showed the inhibitory effect toward striated muscle sarcoma induced by 9,10-dimethyl-1,2-benzoanthracene. The oral administration of the tannin component to rats or mice for one to three months suppressed the growth of implanted soft tissue tumor.[3] From the flower buds of the Camellia, a dimer of macrocyclic elladitannin assigned as camellin-B (**1**) was isolated and proven to possess marked host-mediated antineoplastic potential. Daily administration of camellin-B (**1**) to mice implanted with sarcoma 180 by intramuscular injection of 10 mg/kg per day for four days noticeably prolonged the life duration by 36%.[4] Another tannin named pedunculagin (**2**) separated from the acetone extract of Camellia leaves could significantly diminish the activity of Topo-I at a concentration of 0.03 μg/mL. Due to the most of Topoisomerase inhibitors are closely related to the cancer inhibition, pedunculagin (**2**) might be considered to have the anticancer potential.[5]

Triterpenoids

Three triterpenoids isolated from the nonsaponifiable lipid of the Camellia seed oil were elucidated as dammarenediol-II, (20R)-taraxastane-3β,20-diol, and lupane-3β,20-diol. The triterpenoids exerted potent inhibitory effects against the activation of EBV-EA in Raji cells, indicating the triterpenoids having anticarcinogenetic activity.[6] A cytotoxic triterpenoid assigned as 3β-*O*-acetyl-16β-hydroxyolean-12-ene was isolated from an EAF of the Camellia stem bark. It demonstrated moderate antileukemia effect on LLC cells and HL-60 cells *in vitro* with IC_{50} values (μM) of 25.2 and 21.7, respectively, but it was less active in human MCF-7 (breast) and A549 (lung) cancer cell lines.[7] A group of oleanane-type triterpenes were isolated from an ethyl acetate extract of Camellia fruit peels, and six of them demonstrated moderated cytotoxicity against human breast cancer cell lines (MDA-MB-231 and MCF-7) and MCF-7/ADR (ADR-resistant) cells with IC_{50} values ranging from 0.51 to 13.55 μM. The most potent triterpenoid in the *in vitro* assay was camellenodiol (**3**), and its IC_{50} values (μM) were 0.51, 1.19, and 0.82, respectively. Importantly, the suppressive effects of the triterpenoids were stronger on the MCF-7/Adm cells than on its original MCF-7 cells as evidenced by the IC_{50} data, i.e., the IC_{50} values were 1.52 versus 1.96 μM for 3β,16α,17-trihydroxyolean-12-ene (**4**), 2.37 versus 4.95 μM for 3β-hydroxyolean-11,13(18)-diene-28-oic acid (**5**), 2.51 versus 8.75 μM for 3β-hydroxy-16-oxo-olean-11,13(18)-diene (**6**), 8.06 versus 13.55 μM for oleanolic acid (**7**), and 17.37 versus >30 μM for 3,16-dioxo-olean-12(13),17(18)-diene (**8**), but the IC_{50} values were similar for 3β-acetoxyolean-12-ene-28-oic acid (5.17 versus 5.21 μM).[8] Accordingly, the results supported that the triterpenoids are new lead compounds for the development of potential agents in the treatment of breast cancer, and the camellia fruit peels are a good herb source for the prevention of breast cancer.

References

1. Eristavi, K. D. et al. (a) 1970. Effect of cameline on induced tumors. *Soobsh. Akad. Nauk Gruz. SSR* 59: 489–91; (b) 1999. *Chinese Materia Medica*. Vol. 3, 3–2146, 559. Shanghai Science and Technology Press, Shanghai, China.
2. Miura, D. al, 2007. Camellia oil and its distillate fractions effectively inhibit the spontaneous metastasis of mouse melanoma B16 cells. *FEBS Lett.* 581: 2541–8.
3. Way, T. D. et al. 2009. Beneficial effects of different tea flowers against human breast cancer MCF-7 cells. *Food Chem.* 114: 1231–6.
4. Yoshida, T. et al. 1989. Camelliin B and nobotanin I, macrocyclic ellagitannin dimers and related dimers, and their antitumor activity. *Chem. Pharm. Bull.* 37: 3174–6.
5. Oosishi, K. et al. 1994. Topoisomerase inhibitors containing tannins, especially pedunculagin, for treatment of cancer. *Jpn. Kokai Tokkyo Koho* JP92-247169.
6. Akihisa, T. et al. 2004. 3-epicabraleahydroxylactone and other triterpenoids from camellia oil and their inhibitory effects on Epstein-Barr virus activation. *Chem. Pharm. Bull.* 52: 153–6.
7. Thao, N. T. et al. 2010. Triterpenoids from *Camellia japonica* and their cytotoxic activity. *Chem. Pharm. Bull.* 58: 121–4.
8. Uddin, M. N. et al. 2014. Oleanane triterpenes as protein tyrosine phosphatase 1B (PTP1B) inhibitors from *Camellia japonica*. *Phytochem.* 103: 99–106.

134 Mai Jiao 麦角

Ergot

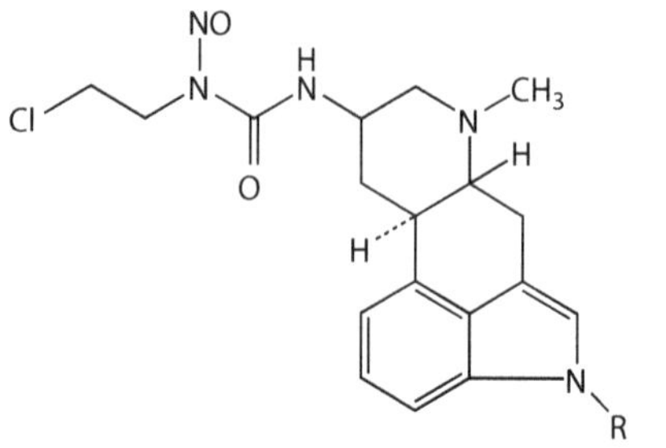

1. R = -NO
2. R = -H

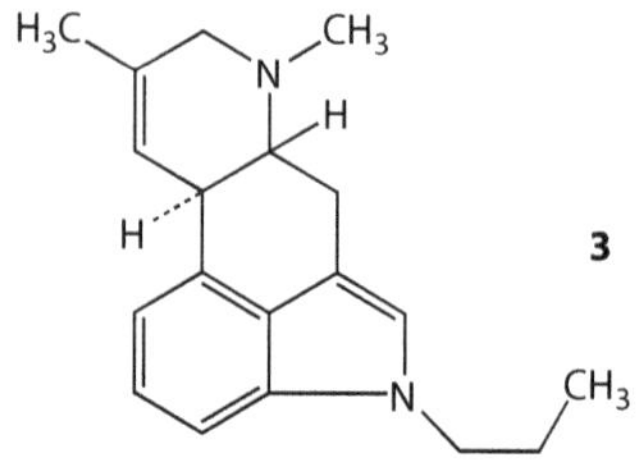

3

Herb Origination

The herb Mai Jiao (Ergot) is the black and dark purple sclerotia of lysergic fungi *Claviceps purpurea* and *C. aestivum* (Clavicipitaceae). When the parasite fungi are on grains such as wheat, barley, and others, it would cause a disease of rye. During wheat and barley harvest and ripening in the summer, the sclerotia of ergot are collected and dried in shade or by baking at a low temperature for folk medicine use in China.

Antitumor Constituents and Activities

Clavicepamines (molecular weight: 2–18 kDa), a mixture of stable and water-soluble basic proteins containing rich lysine (30–95%), were isolated from the fermentation of ergots (*C. purpurea*, *C. fusiformis*, and *C. paspali*). The fundamental structural units of clavicepamines were ε-lysine (poly)peptides. The proteins exhibited powerful antitumor activity, especially effectively against Yoshida rat sarcoma, NK/Ly ascites tumor, and Ehrlich ascites tumor *in vivo* without toxic/side effects. The daily administration of the protein fractions containing >40 mol% lysine in doses of 10–100 mg/kg for 5–10 days could receive 40–100% suppression of these tumors *in vivo*.[1–3]

The alkaloids isolated from ergot were not reported to have antitumor activity, but two derivatives assigned as 8-[3-(2-chloroethyl)-3-nitrosoureido]-1-nitroso-6-methylergoline (**1**) and 8-[3-(2-chloroethyl)-3-nitrosoureido]-6-methylergoline, which were derived from 8β-amino-6-methylergoline, displayed the suppressive effect on the growth of murine L1210 leukemia in mice.[4] An ergot alkaloid designated as ergotamine (**2**) had been applied in a dose of 5 mg/kg to treat mice implanted with solid sarcoma 180, whose agent could resensitize the antitumor activity of hydralazine to overcome the drug resistance in the tumor.[5] Ergotamine (**2**), 1-propyl agroclavine tartrate (**3**), dihydroergocristine, and ergocornin-E showed suppressive effect toward a panel of tumor cell lines of NCI, in the United States. 1-Propyl agroclavine tartrate (**3**) revealed the strongest cytotoxicity on leukemic, renal, colon, skin, lung, brain, and ovarian cancer cell lines. Especially, 1-propyl agroclavine tartrate (**3**) was the most active against leukemia cell lines and the least active against ovarian cancer cells.[6]

Other Bioactivities

The alkaloid components isolated from Mai Jiao (Ergot) displayed uterine muscle-exiting, peripheral vascular smooth muscle contraction-enhancing, and nerve system-influencing effects in the pharmacological experiments. But these alkaloids are toxic, so people must be careful in the dosage used for medical treatments.

References

1. Tyihak, E. et al. 1978. Clavicepamines. *Hung. Teljes* HU 72-GO1226 19721208.
2. Szokan, G. et al. 1997. Structure determination and synthesis of lysine isopeptides influencing on cell proliferation. *Biopolymers* 42: 305–18.
3. Szokan, G. et al. 1994. Chemical and biological investigations of natural and synthetic isopeptides. *Kemiai Kozlemenyek* 79: 139–57.
4. Crider, A. M. et al. 1979. Ergot alkaloids: Synthesis of nitrosourea derivatives of ergolines as potential anticancer agents. *J. Med. Chem.* 22: 32–5.
5. Jones, G. R. N. et al. 1982. Resensitization of drug-resistant S180 tumor cells with ergotamine. *Biochem. Soc. Transactions* 10: 502–3.
6. Mrusek, M. et al. 2015. Identification of cellular and molecular factors determining the response of cancer cells to six ergot alkaloids. *Investigational New Drugs* 33: 32–44.

135 Tuan Nang Cao 團囊草

Snake tongue truffle club

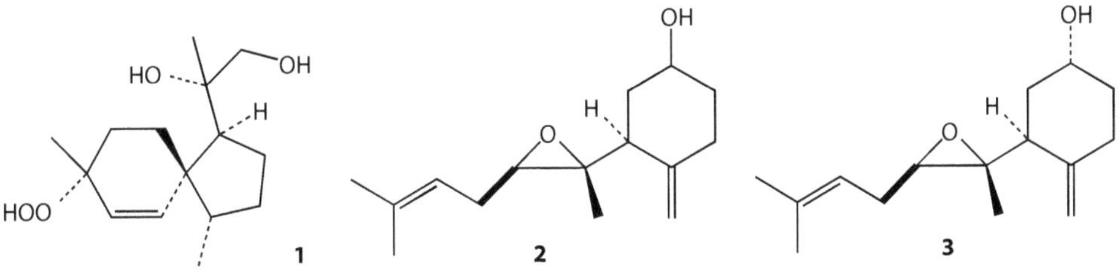

Herb Origination

The herb origin of Tuan Nang Cao (Snake tongue truffle club) is the stroma of a Clavicipitaceae fungi, *Cordyceps ophioglossoides*. Its mycelia grow on the bottom of bamboos and oak trees with distributions in southern China, as well as in North America and Europe. The herb is generally collected in summer and autumn and dried in the sunlight for traditional Chinese medicine use.

Antitumor Constituents and Activities

The bioactive constituents in Tuan Nang Cao have been known to be cordycepin and its derivatives, ergosterol, polysaccharides, glycoprotein, and β-aminoisobutyric acid-coupled peptides. The anticancer property of cordycepin was discussed in a section of the fungi *C. militaris* (see Section Yong Cao).

Protein-Bound Polysaccharide

Besides cordycepin, other types of components from the herb also displayed the suppressive effect against the tumor cell growth. A protein-bound polysaccharide (SN-C) obtained from the culture filtrate of Tuan Nang Cao is mainly composed of glucose and galactosamine in its saccharide potion. The proliferation on various murine tumor cells including P388 leukemia could be constricted by SN-C treatment *in vitro*. The i.p. administration of the SN-C into tumor-bearing mice markedly suppressed the growth of allogeneic and syngeneic tumor cells such as MM46 mammary carcinoma, sarcoma 180 and L5178Y leukemia, and markedly prolonged the life duration of mice inoculated with Ehrlich ascites tumor or X5563 plasmacyroma. SN-C also obviously blocked the incorporation of glucose into Meth-A fibrosarcoma cells and consequently retarded the DNA synthesis. Besides the direct cytocidal activity, SN-C could also stimulate host cell-mediated effects and restore the depressed capacity to raise delayed-type hypersensitivity in tumor-bearing mice.[1,2]

Polysaccharides

From the SN-C, a water-insoluble extracellular glucan (CO-1) and a water/alkali-insoluble galactosaminoglycan (CO-N) were derived by ultrasonication and heat treatment. CO-1 (molecular weight: from 2×10^6 to 6×10^4) is composed of a backbone of (1–3)-linked β-D-glucopyranosyl residues and branches of a glucosyl group at C-6 position of every second glucosyl units. CO-1 strongly obstructed the growth of sarcoma 180 cells *in vivo*, when given orally, and effectively inhibited the syngeneic MM46 mammary solid carcinoma in mice, but it had no effect on ascitic tumors. In addition, CO-1 was also able to amplify the number of peritoneal exudate cells and to markedly stimulate the chemiluminescence response of these exudate cells after the i.p. injection to normal mice, implying that the antitumor effect of CO-1 might be correlated with its immunoenhancing functions.[3–6] CO-N (average molecular weight: 50,000) was composed mainly of D-galactosamine (80.5%) and small proportions of glucose, galactose, mannose, protein, and acetyl groups. CO-N displayed direct cytotoxicity again cultured IMC and P388D1 cancer cell lines *in vitro*. When CO-N is given to tumor-bearing mice by i.p. injection, CO-N obstructed the growth of sarcoma 180 cells and significantly prolonged the survival duration of mice bearing ascitic tumors such as Ehrlich carcinoma and IMC carcinoma. By intra-tumoral administration, CO-N could inhibit the solid Ehrlich carcinoma in mice. The intravenous injection of CO-N even at a low dose exerted the suppressive effect against a syngeneic MM46 mammary carcinoma cells *in vivo*. The investigations also found that the higher molecular weight fraction of CO-N showed relatively greater antineoplastic effect, but the low molecular weight fraction (below 6600) of CO-N only had weak activity against the tumors.[6–8]

Sesquiterpenoids

Three antitumor active sesquiterpenoids designated as cordycepol-C (**1**), ophiocoridin-D (**2**), and cordycol (**3**) were isolated from the cultured mycelia of *C. ophioglossoides*. All these sesquiterpenoids were moderately effective in the growth suppression of human HeLa (cervix) and HepG2 (liver) cancer cell lines. Cordycepol-C (**1**) and cordycol (**3**) exhibited their IC_{50} values in a range of 12–33 μg/mL against the HeLa and HepG2 cell lines. In the *in vitro* models, cordycepol-C (**1**) and ophiocoridin-D (**2**) restrained the proliferation of human MCF-7 breast cancer cells and human A549 NSCLC cells, respectively. Among these tested tumor cell lines, HeLa cervical cancer cells were the most sensitive to the three sesquiterpenoids. No harmful effect was observed toward normal LO2 hepatic cell line for these sesquiterpenoids.[9,10] The apoptosis of HepG2 cells elicited by cordycepol-C (**1**) was associated with a p53-independent, caspase-independent, and Bax-mediated mitochondrial pathway, leading to the loss of mitochondrial membrane potential, cleavage of PARP-1, and nuclear translocation of AIF and Endo-G.[11]

Other Bioactivities

The herb Tuan Nang Cao (Snake tongue truffle club) has been demonstrated to possess diversified pharmacological actions including immunomodulatory, hypoglycemic, hypolipidemic, hypocholesterolemic, antiinflammatory, antiaging, antioxidant, neuroprotective, renoprotective, and antimicrobial effects.

References

1. Ohmori, T. et al. 1988. Component analysis of protein-bound polysaccharide (SN-C) from *Cordyceps ophioglossoides* and its effects on syngeneic murine tumors. *Chem. Pharm. Bull.* 36: 4505–11.
2. Ohmori, T. et al. 1986. Antitumor activity of protein-bound polysaccharide from *Cordyceps ophioglossoides* in mice. *Jpn. J. Cancer Res.* 77: 1256–63.
3. Ohmori, T. et al. 1988. Dissociation of a glucan fraction (CO-1) from protein-bound polysaccharide of *Cordyceps ophioglossoides* and analysis of its antitumor effect. *Chem. Pharm. Bull.* 36: 4512–8.
4. Kawaguchi, N. et al. 1987. Branching frequency of antitumor 6-*O*-branched (1–3)-β-D-glucan from *Cordyceps ophioglossoides. Agricul. Biol. Chem.* 51: 2805–6.
5. Yamada, H. et al. 1984. Structure and antitumor activity of an alkali-soluble polysaccharide from *Cordyceps ophioglossoides. Carbohydrate Res.* 125: 107–15.
6. Kawaguchi, N. et al. 1995. Structures and biological activities of polysaccharides produced by *Cordyceps ophioglossoides. Snow Brand R&D Reports* 103: 67–103.
7. Ohmori, T. et al. 1989. Isolation of galactosaminoglycan moiety (CO-N) from protein-bound polysaccharide of *Cordyceps ophioglossoides* and its effects against murine tumors. *Chem. Pharm. Bull.* 37: 1019–22.
8. Ohmori, T. et al. 1989. The correlation between molecular weight and antitumor activity of galactosamino-glycan (CO-N) from Cordyceps ophioglossoides. *Chem. Pharm. Bull.* 37: 1337–40.
9. Li, Y. Q. et al. 2011. Sesquiterpenoid compounds from *Cordyceps ophioglossoides* and their application in preparing antitumor drugs. *Faming Zhuanli Shenqing* CN 102229595 A 20111102.
10. Sun, Y. S. et al. 2013. Unusual spirodecane sesquiterpenes and a fumagillol analog from *Cordyceps ophioglossoides. Helv. Chim. Acta* 96: 76–84.
11. Sun, Y. S. et al. 2014. Cordycepol C induces caspase-independent apoptosis in human hepatocellular carcinoma HepG2 cells. *Biol. Pharm. Bull.* 37: 608–17.

136 Guan Ye Lian Qiao 貫葉連翹

St. John's wort

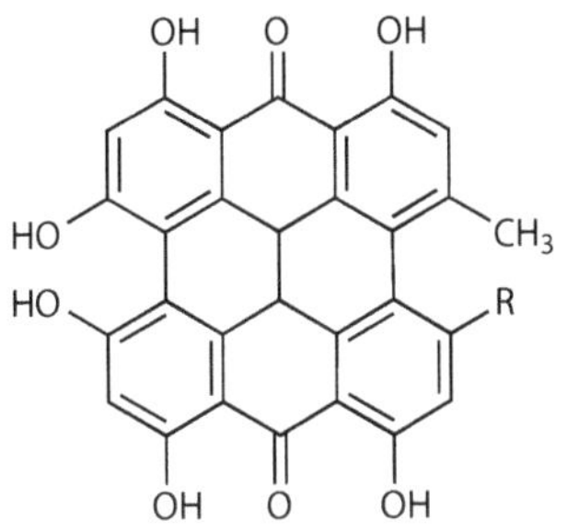

1. R = CH_3
2. R = CH_2OH

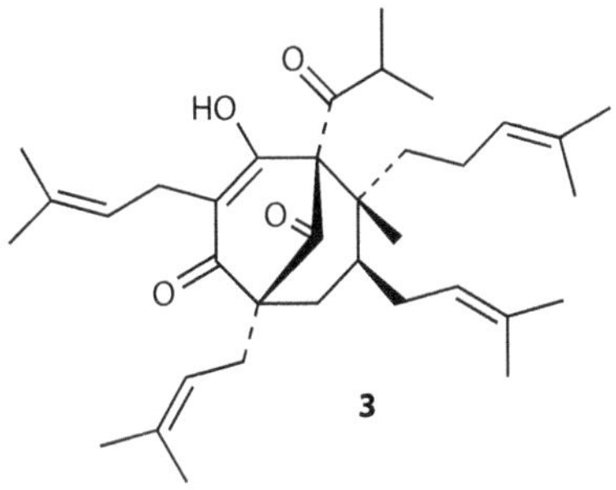

3

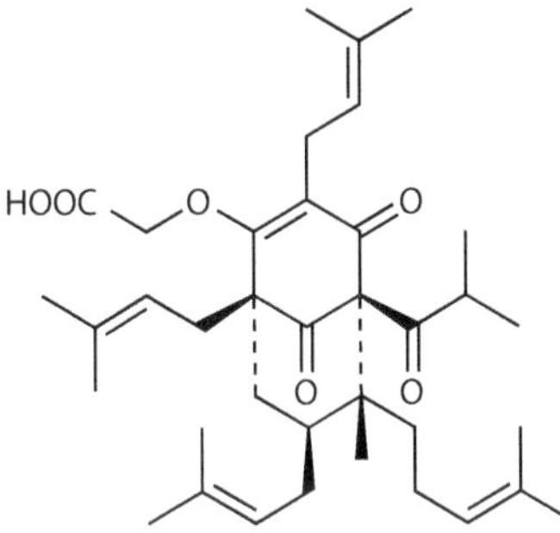

4

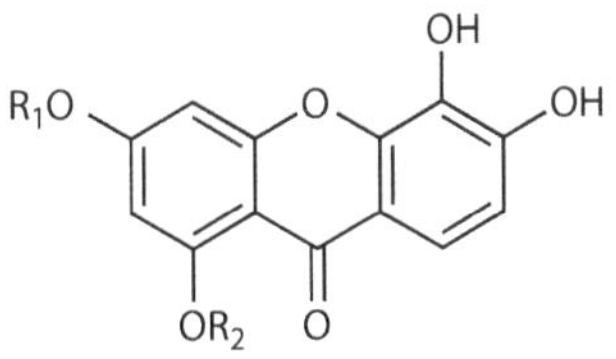

5. $R_1 = R_2 = -H$
6. $R_1 = -CH_3$, $R_2 = -H$
8. $R_1 = R_2 = -CH_3$

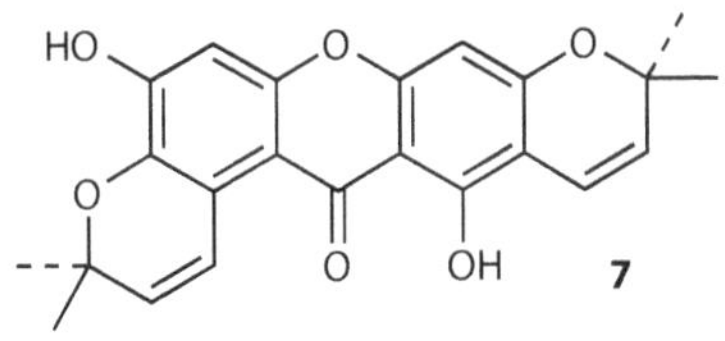

7

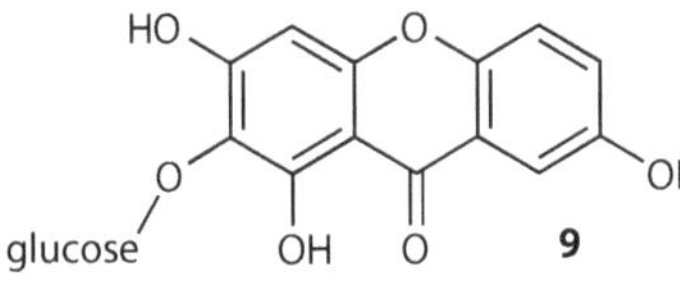

9

Herb Origination

The origin of Guan Ye Lian Qiao (St. John's wort) is a Hypericaceae plant, *Hypericum perforatum* L. The perennial plant is indigenous to Europe, western Asia, and north Africa, but it has been introduced to many temperate areas of the world. The broad distribution may also be ascribed to its cultivation as a medicinal and a garden plant. In China, the whole plant is usually collected between July and October and dried in the sun for use as a traditional Chinese medicine and a European herbal medicine.

Antitumor Activities and Constituents

The cytotoxic activity of the extracts prepared from fresh and dried St. John's wort were investigated in three human malignant tumor cell lines (K562 erythroleukemia, U937 histiocytic lymphoma, and LN229 glioblastoma) with white light illumination or exposure in the dark. Both extracts displayed light-dependent phototoxic properties to obstruct the tumor growth and to promote the apoptosis. The light activation extremely potentiated the cytotoxic activity of these extracts, but the fresh herb obviously showed to be more sensitive to the neoplastic cells than the dried herb.[1] HyTE-3 was a hydroalcoholic extract of St. John's wort, which was able to inhibit the proliferation of human A375 malignant melanoma cells and to augment antioxidant effect. In combination with UVA irradiation (1.8 J/cm^2), HyTE-3 showed remarkable phototoxicity in the A375 cells at a 78 μg/mL concentration to result in a 50% cell destruction.[2]

The major constituents isolated from the St. John's wort extracts such as hypericin (**1**), pseudohypericin (**2**), hyperforin (**3**), and quercetin demonstrated potent suppressive effects against the activity of cytochrome P4501A1 (CYP1A1, a human procarcinogen-activating enzyme) and against 7,8-diol-BAP (a mutagen)-caused diolepoxide-2 formation. The IC_{50} values against CYP1A1 were 0.5 μM for hypericin (**1**), 1.2 μM for hyperforin (**3**), 1.5 μM for quercetin, and 8 μM for pseudohypericin (**2**),[3] indicating that these molecules have anticarcinogenic potentials.

Naphthodianthrone-Type Components

Antileukemia Effect of Hypericins

Hypericin (**1**) and pseudohypericin (**2**) are photosensitive pigments and principal anticancer constituents in St. John's wort, where pseudohypericin (**2**) is two times more abundant than hypericin (**1**). Both agents demonstrated significant cytotoxic, phototoxic, and apoptosis-increasing effects on the neoplastic cells. The treatment with photoactivated hypericin (**1**) or pseudohypericin (**2**) inhibited the cell proliferation and amplified the DNA fragmentation of human Jurkat leukemic lymphoma cells dose-dependently *in vitro*. The IC_{50} values of hypericin (**1**) and pseudohypericin (**2**) were 0.1 and 0.2 μg/mL, respectively. But hypericin and pseudohypericin in nonphotoactivated conditions only showed lower activity at the same concentration.[4]

The methanolic extract of St. John's wort flower showed a marked concentration-dependent and long-lasting suppression on the K562 cell growth and acceleration of the apoptosis; however, hypericin (**1**) exerted only a weak inhibitory effect against the growth human K562 erythroleukemic cells *in vitro* with no effect in inducing apoptosis.[5] The phototoxicity of hypericin (**1**) on human HL-60 promyelocytic leukemic cells could be effectively potentiated by the cotreatment with 5′-(N,N-dimethyl)-amiloride (an inhibitor of Na^+/H^+ exchanger) or omeprazole (an inhibitor H^+-K^+-ATPase).[6] In addition, hypericin (**1**) could also scavenge superoxide anion radicals and inhibit PKC activity in human CMK-7 megakaryoblastic leukemia cells *in vitro*.[7] Therefore, hypericin (**1**) appears to have many potentials as a drug lead for further development to improve current leukemia chemotherapy.

Antisolid Tumor Effect of Hypericins

Hypericin (**1**) has been reported to have photodependent cytotoxicity in a variety of cancer cell lines. In recent years, the attention on hypericin (**1**) as a potential clinical anticancer agent has risen since photoactivated hypericin could cause irreversible cellular damage and tumor destruction *in vivo* and *in vitro*.[8] After the treatment of highly metastatic DA3Hi adenocarcinoma and SQ2 anaplastic squamous cell carcinoma with photosensitized hypericin (**1**), the primary tumor development was markedly obstructed and the tumor necrosis was extensively augmented by local, intratumoral, and systemic inflammatory reactions *in vivo*. Simultaneously, cytokine mRNA profiles were augmented and the survival of mice bearing tumor was significantly prolonged.[9]

In vitro experiments following the irradiation with red light (590 nm) for 30 min resulted in 50% lethality (LD_{50}) of hypericin (2.07–2.23 μM) in human LNCaP, PC3, and DU-145 prostate cancer cell lines. The treatment of the LNCaP prostate carcinoma in nude mice with photoactivated hypericin for over 28 days significantly diminished the tumor growth and the PSA levels, closely associated with serotonin reuptake inhibition and serotonin antagonist.[10,11] When treated with instillation into human bladders, hypericin (**1**) could selectively accumulate in the bladder and cause bladder carcinoma cell lesions. Based upon this specific property in bladder carcinoma lesions, hypericin (**1**) is now employed as a fluorescent diagnostic tool in the treatment of superficial bladder cancer.[12] Also, a polar methanolic fraction derived from the herb exerted significant photocytotoxicity on two urinary bladder carcinoma cell lines, such as T24 (high-grade metastatic cancer) and RT4 (primary low-grade papillary transitional cell cancer), at a concentration of 60 μg/mL with 4–8 J/cm^2 light dose, whose activity was comparable to a clinically proven photosensitizer photofrin under the same conditions.[13] Moreover, the photodynamic therapy of hypericin (**1**) was also significantly effective in other human carcinoma cells (HepG2 hepatoma and MDA-231 mammary cancer) and in basal cell carcinoma (BCC) (a nonmelanoma skin cancer cells) from patients. After being cotreated with 590 nm light irritation, the inhibitory rates were 51.5% for hypericin (**1**) and 81% for the herb extract in the same HepG2 cells *in vitro*.[14–17] When the photoactivated hypericin (**1**) is combined with manumycin-A (a selective farnesyltransferase inhibitor) to treat human HT-29 adenocarcinoma cells, the antiproliferation and apoptotic response were obviously enhanced via the inhibition of Ras processing and the elevation of caspase-3/caspase-7 activity.[18]

Interestingly, because cisplatin (CDDP) and mitoxantrone are potential substrates of ABC transporters and hypericin (**1**) is able to induce the expression of two ABC transporters, multidrug resistance-associated protein-1 and breast cancer resistance protein (BCRP), the cytotoxicity of CDDP could be attenuated by hypericin pretreatment in both A2780 and A2780cis ovarian cancer cell lines and the cytotoxicity of mitoxantrone in HL-60 leukemia cells. But hypericin (**1**) potentiated mitoxantrone-induced death in cBCRP cells due to hypericin being a potential substrate of BCRP transporter.[19]

Photodynamic Effect of Hypericin

Besides the growth inhibition in different tumor models, the photodynamic therapy (PDT) with hypericin (**1**) was also able to elicit tumor vascular damage. Intravenous hypericin administration at dose of 5 mg/kg and then exposure to laser light immediately markedly lessened the perfusion of RIF-1 fibrosarcoma and obviously injured the tumor vascular *in vivo*; simultaneously, the nucleosomal DNA fragmentation and the expressions of both Fas and Fas ligand were augmented.[20] The results evidenced that the antitumor effect was largely attributed to hypericin-mediated overall PDT-induced apoptotic response and vascular damage and strongly suggested that targeting the tumor vasculature by short drug light interval PDT with hypericin has a good prospect for further development to eradicate solid tumors. However, the PDT-shocked tumor cells and the arrested vascular perfusion would be interestingly restored if the first application of the laser irradiation was too long or the second application of the laser irradiation was performed within 24 h.[13,21] Hence, the approaches in reducing the lesions to normal tissues and enhancing the delivery of hypericin (**1**) using different types of light exposure procedures are still attractive research projects in the improvement of the clinical therapy.

Phloroglucinol-Type Components

Hyperforin (**3**), a prenylated phloroglucinol derivative, was found in St. John's wort as a bioactive component with prominent amounts, which exerted significant suppressive effect *in vitro* and *in vivo* against the growth of many human and murine lymphoma, leukemia, melanoma, breast cancer, and melanoma cell lines (IC_{50}: 3–15 μM). A431 squamous cell cancer and Jurkat lymphoma cell lines and three types of breast carcinoma cells (MT-450, MDA-MB-468, and MCF-7) were more sensitive to hyperforin (**3**) compared with malignant melanoma (HT-144, SB1, SB3, MV3, and IF6). Hyperforin (**3**) was also effective in the inhibition of rat prostate cancer cell lines (AT-2.1, AR42J, and ARIP) and human SKOV-3 ovarian cancer cell line (IC_{50}: 1.4–3.0 μM). But its inhibitory rates was lower in rat MAT-Lu prostate cancer cells (IC_{50}: 9.0 μM) and rat BDX2 fibrosarcoma cells (IC_{50}: 40 μM).[22] the daily subcutaneous administration of hyperforin by in a dose of 100 μL of 2 mM hyperforin solution to tumor-bearing rats for two successive weeks remarkably obstructed the growth of autologous MT450 breast carcinoma cells without signs of acute toxicity, whose inhibition was associated with the induction of apoptosis via the activation of a mitochondria-mediated apoptotic pathway and whose antigrowth potency was similar to that of paclitaxel.[22] In addition to the antiproliferative and proapoptotic activities, hyperforin (**3**) also exerted antiangiogenic effect by blocking the microvessel formation of human dermal microvascular endothelial cells in rats bearing MT-450 breast cancer.[23] In an *in vivo* treatment with hyperforin (**3**), the growth of Kaposi's sarcoma (a highly angiogenic tumor) was strongly restrained and the sarcoma was remarkably reduced in size and in vascularization through the blockage of NF-κB translocation.[24]

Likewise, the antigrowth and apoptosis-promoting effects of hyperforin (**3**) also displayed in K562 and U937 leukemia cells, LN229 brain glioblastoma cells, and human normal astrocytes *in vitro* (GI_{50}: 14.9–19.9 μM).[22,25] Hyperforin (**3**) induced the apoptosis of both CLL and AML cell lines. During the proapoptosis induction, hyperforin directly obstructed the activities of serine/threonine protein kinase B/AKT1, leading to activation of Bad through its nonphosphorylation by AKT1 in the AML cell lines and primary AML cells, and up-expressed Noxa (possibly through the inhibition of proteasome activity) in the primary CLL cells. Hyperforin (**3**) also inhibited MMP-2 activity in the AML cells and restrained VEGF and MMP-9 in the CLL cells, leading to the hindrance of the cell migration and angiogenesis.[26] *In vivo* experiments demonstrated that hyperforin (**3**) was effective in the suppression of B-cell CLL and also in the reversal of the CLL cell MDR through the down-regulation of overexpressed P-gp and the suppression of BCRP (which is normally expressed in most of CLL cells) activity.[27,28] Interestingly, the cotreatment with hyperforin (**3**) and hypericin (**1**) could act synergistically in the suppressive effect against the growth of K562 and U937 leukemic cell lines, whose finding gave the herb as an interesting option in the leukemia treatment.[22,25]

Dicyclohexylammonium salt of hyperforin (DCHA-HF) showed the anticancer and antiangiogenic activities in various neoplastic cells. DCHA-HF was more effective in dose- and time-dependent inhibitions of K562 chronic myeloid leukemia cells than hyperforin (**3**), with an IC_{50} value of 3.2 μM for 72 h of the treatment. The suppression of K562 cells by DCHA-HF was found to follow the induction of caspase-dependent apoptosis and G1 cell cycle arrest via a mitochondrial pathway, i.e., (1) activation of p53 and p27Kip1; (2) down-expression of antiapoptotic proteins and upexpression of proapoptotic proteins; (3) loss of mitochondrial transmembrane potential and release of cytochrome c; and (4) subsequent PARP cleavage and activation of caspase-3, caspase-8, and caspase-9 cascade.[29] In addition, aristoforin (**4**), a hyperforin derivative, is more soluble and stable in an aqueous solution than hyperforin (**3**) due to the improved pharmacological activity. The *in vivo* antitumor potential of aristoforn (**4**) were demonstrated in the treated animals without inducing toxicity.[30]

Xanthone-Type Components

Five xanthones were isolated from the adventitious roots of St. John's wort and elucidated as 1,3,5,6-tetrahydroxyxanthone (**5**), 1,5,6-trihydroxy-3-methoxyxanthone (**6**), brasilixanthone-B (**7**), ferrxanthone (**8**), and neolancerin (**9**). The first three xanthones (**5–7**) moderately diminished the viability of HL-60 leukemia cells with IC_{50} values (μM) of 31.5, 28.9, and 27.7, respectively. The five xanthones exhibited radical-scavenging activity with inhibition values of 27.4–33.2% at 10 μM concentrations.[31]

Protein-Type Component

A protein called CHP-10 (39 kDa) was isolated from the callus culture of St. John's wort, which is composed of a unique sequence with 20 amino acids. CHP-10 was found to have a repression effect against the growth of abnormally proliferating cells from cancerous and/or noncancerous proliferative disorders.[32]

Exploration of Mechanism

Hypericin (**1**) is one of the most powerful natural photosensitizer, showing high potency in the photodynamic treatment of neoplasms as described earlier. Extensive investigations further provided evidences to explore the mechanisms of anticancer and apoptosis-induction for hypericin (**1**). Photoactivated hypericin-induced apoptosis of cancer cells such as nasopharyngeal cancer and mucosa neoplasm should be mediated in part by the TRAIL/TRAIL-receptor system and subsequent activation of caspase-8 and caspase-3. It further induced the abbreviation of tumor cells and amplified the subdiploid DNA, finally resulting in the neoplastic cell death program.[33,34] The photoactivated hypericin (**1**) also upregulated the expressions of two NO-synthesizing enzymes NOS-I and NOS-II and augmented the production of gaseous free radical and NO, wherein NO plays an important role in the apoptosis induction. In addition, the NO is also an important modulator of immune, endocrine, and neuronal functions.[35]

Hypericin (**1**) was reported to have the ability to catalytically restrain the DNA relaxation activity of Topo-IIα and to block the cleavage complex stabilization in both wild-type and amsacrine-resistant HL-60 leukemia cells *in vitro*.[36] After the cotreatment with hypericin, the elicited apoptosis or necrosis was proceeded in both drug and light dose-dependent fashion before induction of G2/M phase cell cycle arrest, which PDT effect was mediated by a mitochondrial pathway including the activation of caspase and the inhibition of overexpressed Bcl-2.[37]

As known now, c-erB-2 oncoprotein is usually overexpressed in 20–30% of human ovary adenocarcinoma and breast cancer cells. Through the upregulation of p21WAF1 expression and the blockage of the c-erB-2 expression by hindering the autophosphorylation of c-erB-2 and the downstream kinases (MEK and ERK1/2), hypericin (**1**) promoted the apoptotic and growth inhibitory effects toward human SKOV-3 ovarian cancer cells with an IC_{50} value of 7.5 μM (in 72 h). Also, the SKOV-3 cell movement was obstructed by hypericin (**1**) by restraining MMP expression and acting in the Matrigel, implying that hypericin has antiinvasive activity in the SKOV-3 cells.[38] Furthermore, various pharmaceutically important enzymes such as telomerase, PKC, monoaminoxidase, reverse transcriptase, dopamine-β-hydroxylase, and cytochrome P450 were found to be involved in the suppression of hypericin (**1**).[37] According to these findings regarding medical photochemistry and photobiology, hypericin (**1**) was demonstrated to have potentials not only in cancer therapy but also in cancer diagnosis.[39]

Clinical Investigation

The photodynamic effect of the herb extract on nonmelanoma skin cancer cells had been investigated in a clinical trial. The study was carried out on a total 34 patients: 8 with actinic keratoses (AKs), 21 with BCC, and 5 with Bowen's disease (a carcinoma in situ). The herb extract was smeared over the skin lesions under occlusion where it was irradiated with 75 J/cm^{-2} of red light 2 h later, whose treatment was executed once a week. After an average of six weeks of treatment, the percentage of complete clinical response was 50% for patients with AKs, 28% for patients with superficial BCC, and 40% for patients with Bowen's disease. Only a partial remission was seen in patients with nodular BCCs, and a complete disappearance of tumor cells was found in 11% of patients with superficial BCCs and in 80% of patients with Bowen's disease. But all the patients complained of burning and pain sensations during the irradiation. The treatment protocol still has possibilities for the improvement of the drug delivery and other types of light exposure procedures.[16]

Nanoformulation

Hypericin-loaded lipid nanocapsules (LNCs) was formulated, which could suppress the aggregation of hypericin in aqueous media, amplify its apparent solubility, and enhance the generation of singlet oxygen as compared to its free molecule. The photodynamic activity of hypericin-loaded LNCs was tested in human HeLa cervical carcinoma cells. The cell viability radically decreased to 10–20% at a 1 μM concentration, implying that the hypericin-loaded LNC25 holds promise for the application in cancer treatment due to prolonged circulation time and accumulation in the tumor.[40]

Other Bioactivity

The herb Guan Ye Lian Qiao (St. John's wort) has been widely known as an herbal treatment for depression, especially in children and adolescents. Research evidences suggest that daily treatment with St. John's wort is able to relieve the most common physical and behavioral symptoms, as well as premenstrual syndrome. Hypericin (**1**) possesses antidepressive and antiviral (human immunodeficiency and hepatitis C virus) activities besides the antineoplastic potential. Hyperforin (**3**) may be useful for the treatment of alcoholism, and it has also been reported to have antidepressive, antioxidant, free radical-scavenging, photoprotective, antiinflammatory, and antibacterial (against gram-negative bacteria) properties.[41] A cream containing 1.5% w/w of a hyperforin-rich extract from *H. perforatum* can significantly reduce UVB-induced erythema without any skin irritation.[42]

References

1. Hostanska, K. et al. 2002. Aqueous ethanolic extract of St. John's wort (*Hyperricum perforatum* L.) induces growth inhibition and apoptosis in human malignant cells in vitro. *Pharmazie* 57: 323–31.
2. Menichini, G. et al. 2013. *Hypericum perforatum* L. subsp. perforatum induces inhibition of free radicals and enhanced phototoxicity in human melanoma cells under ultraviolet light. *Cell Proliferation* 46: 193–202.
3. Schwarz, D. et al. 2003. St. John's wort extracts and some of their constituents potently inhibit ultimate carcinoma formation from benzo[a]pyrene-7,8-dihydrodiol by human CYP1A1. *Cancer Res.* 63: 8062–8.
4. Schempp, C. M. et al. 2002. Phototoxic and apoptosis-inducing capacity of pseudohypericin. *Planta Med.* 68: 171.
5. Roscetti, G. et al. 2004. Cytotoxic activity of *Hypericum perforatum* L. on K562 erythroleukemic cells: Differential effects between methanolic extract and hypericin. *Phytotherapy Res.* 18: 66–72.
6. Mirossay, L. et al. 1999. Hypericin-induced phototoxicity of human leukemic cell line HL-60 is potentiated by omeprazole, an inhibitor of H^+K^+-ATPase and 5′-(N,N-dimethyl)-amiloride, an inhibitor of Na^+/H^+ exchanger. *Physiolog. Res.* 48: 135–41.
7. Shiono, Y. et al. 2002. Effects of polyphenolic anthrone derivatives, resistomycin and hypericin, on apoptosis in human megakaryoblastic leukemia CMK-7 cell line. *J. Biosci.* 57: 923–9.
8. Agostinis, P. et al. 2002. Hypericin in cancer treatment: More light on the way. *Intl. J. Biochem. Cell Biol.* 34: 221–41.
9. Blank, M. et al. 2001. Effects of photodynamic therapy with hypericin in mice bearing highly invasive solid tumors. *Oncol. Res.* 12: 409–18.
10. Xie, X. W. et al. 2001. Tumor-specific and photodependent cytotoxicity of hypericin in the human LNCaP prostate tumor model. *Photochem. Photobiol.* 74: 221–5.
11. Martarelli, D. et al. 2004. *Hypericum perforatum* methanolic extract inhibits growth of human prostatic carcinoma cell line orthotopically implanted in nude mice. *Cancer Lett.* 210: 27–33.
12. Kamuhabwa, A. et al. 2004. Hypericin as a potential phototherapeutic agent in superficial transitional cell carcinoma of the bladder. *Photochem. Photobiol. Sci.* 3: 772–80.
13. Stavropoulos, N. E. et al. 2006. *Hypericum perforatum* L. extract—Novel photosensitizer against human bladder cancer cells. *J. Photochem. Photobiol. B: Biol.* 84: 64–9.
14. Wang, X. et al. 2008. Effect of light wavelength on photodynamic therapy of hypericin and extract from *Hypericum perforatum* L. on HepG2 cancer cell line of human liver in vitro. *Huaxi Yaoxue Zazhi* 23: 47–9.
15. Wang, X. L. et al. 2008. Photocytotoxic effect of hypericin and extract in *Hypericum perforatum* L. on HepG2 cancer cell line of human liver in vitro. *Shizhen Guoyi Guoyao* 19: 69–71.
16. Kacerovska, D. et al. 2008. Photodynamic therapy of nonmelanoma skin cancer with topical *Hypericum perforatum* extract—A pilot study. *Photochem. Photobiol.* 84: 779–85.
17. Wang, X. L. et al. 2008. Photocytotoxic effect of hypericin extract from *Hypericum perforatum* L. on MDA231 human mammary carcinoma cell lines in vitro. *Zhongguo Xiandai Yingyong Yaoxue* 25: 1–4.
18. Sackova, V. et al. 2011. Enhanced antiproliferative and apoptotic response of HT-29 adenocarcinoma cells to combination of photoactivated hypericin and farnesyltransferase inhibitor manumycin A. *Intl. J. Mol. Sci.* 12: 8388–405.
19. Jendzelovska, Z. et al. 2014. Single pre-treatment with hypericin, a St. John's wort secondary metabolite, attenuates cisplatin- and mitoxantrone-induced cell death in A2780, A2780cis and HL-60 cells. *Toxicol. In Vitro* 28: 1259–73.
20. Chen, B. et al. 2002. Photodynamic therapy with hypericin induces vascular damage and apoptosis in the RIF-1 mouse tumor model. *Intl. J. Cancer* 98: 284–90.
21. Chen, B. et al. 2002. Antivascular tumor eradication by hypericin-mediated photodynamic therapy. *J. Photochem. Photobiol.* 76: 509–13.
22. Schempp, C. M. et al. 2002. Inhibition of tumor cell growth by hyperforin, a novel anticancer drug from St. John's wort that acts by induction of apoptosis. *Onogene* 21: 1242–50.
23. Schempp, C. M. et al. 2005. Hyperforin acts as an angiogenesis inhibitor in vitro and in vivo. *Planta Med.* 71: 999–1004.
24. Lorusso, G. et al. 2009. Mechanisms of hyperforin as an anti-angiogenic angioprevention agent. *Eur. J. Cancer.* 45: 1474–84.
25. Hostanska, K. et al. 2003. Hyperforin a constituent of St. John's wort (*Hyperricum perforatum*) extract induces apoptosis by triggering activation of caspases and with hypericin synergistically exerts cytotoxicity towards human malignant cell lines. *Eur. J. Pharm. Biopharm.* 56: 121–32.
26. Billard, C. et al. 2013. Mechanistic insights into the antileukemic activity of hyperforin. *Current Cancer Drug Targets* 13: 1–10.

27. Quiney, C. et al. 2007. Hyperforin inhibits P-gp and BCRP activities in chronic lymphocytic leukemia cells and myeloid cells. *Leukemia Lymphoma* 48: 1587–99.
28. Quiney, C. et al. 2006. Pro-apoptotic properties of hyperforin in leukemic cells from patients with B-cell chronic lymphocytic leukemia. *Leukemia* 20: 491–7.
29. Liu, J. Y. et al. 2011. Induction of apoptosis in K562 cells by dicyclohexylammonium salt of hyperforin through a mitochondrial-related pathway. *Chemico-Biol. Interactions* 190: 91–101.
30. Gartner, M. et al. 2005. Aristoforin, a novel stable derivative of hyperforin, is a potent anticancer agent. *ChemBioChem* 8: 171–7.
31. Li, W. et al. 2013. Isolation of xanthones from adventitious roots of St. John's wort (*Hypericum perforatum* L.) and their antioxidant and cytotoxic activities. *Food Sci. Biotechnol.* 22: 945–9.
32. Khalii, K. et al. 2003. Antiproliferative protein CHP-10 from *Hyperricum perforatum* and uses for cancer therapy. *PCT Int. Appl.* 40 pp. WO2003-US13154 A2 20031113.
33. Schempp, C. M. et al. 2001. Hypericin photo-induced apoptosis involves the tumor necrosis factor-related apoptosis-inducing ligand (TRAIL) and activation of caspase-8. *FEBS Lett.* 493: 26–30.
34. Ali, S. M. et al. 2001. Hypericin and hypocrellin induced apoptosis in human mucosal carcinoma cells. *J. Photochem. Photobiol. B.* 65: 59–73.
35. Ali, S. M. et al. 2003. Nitric oxide mediated photo-induced cell death in human malignant cells. *Intl. J. Oncol.* 22: 751–6.
36. Peebles, K. A. et al. 2001. Catalytic inhibition of human DNA topoisomerase IIα by hypericin, a naphthodianthrone from St. John's wort (*Hyperricum perforatum*). *Biochem. Pharm.* 62: 1059–70.
37. Vantieghem, A. et al. 2002. Signaling pathways involved in the regulation of apoptosis following photodynamic therapy. *Proc. Biennial Meet. Soc. Free Radical. Res. Int. 11th, Paris, France*, pp. 45–9.
38. Hwang, M. S. et al. 2001. Inhibition of c-erbB-2 expression and activity in human ovarian carcinoma cells by hypericin. *Anticancer Res.* 21: 2649–55.
39. Kubin, A. et al. 2005. Hypericin—The facts about a controversial agent. *Current Pharm. Design* 11: 233–53.
40. Barras, A. et al. 2013. Hypericin-loaded lipid nanocapsules for photodynamic cancer therapy in vitro. *Nanoscale* 5: 10562–72.
41. Woelfle, U. et al. 2014. Topical application of St. John's wort (*Hypericum perforatum*). *Planta Med.* 80: 109–20.
42. Meinke, M. C. et al. 2012: In vivo photoprotective and anti-inflammatory effect of hyperforin is associated with high antioxidant activity in vitro and ex vivo. *Eur. J. Pharma. Biopharm.* 81: 346–50.

137 Wu Se Mei 五色梅

Lantana or Sleeper weed

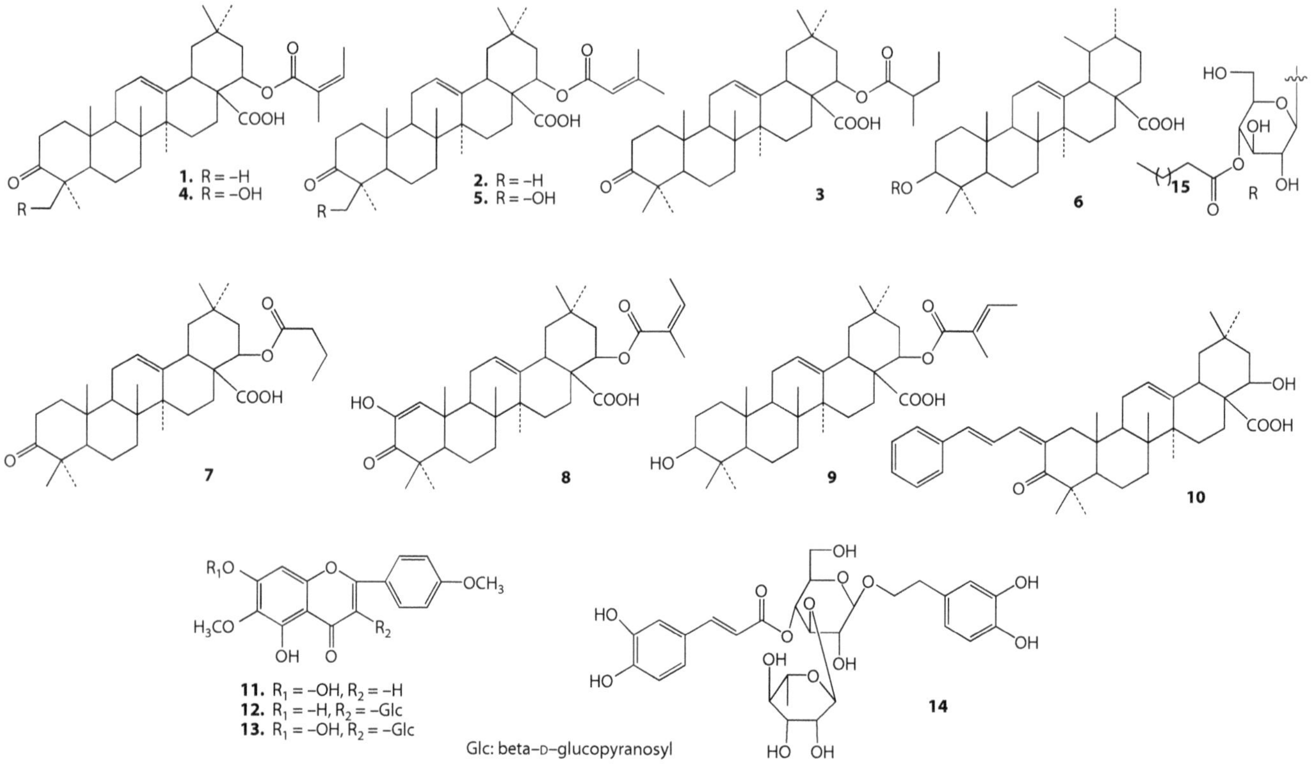

1. R = -H
4. R = -OH

2. R = -H
5. R = -OH

11. R_1 = -OH, R_2 = -H
12. R_1 = -H, R_2 = -Glc
13. R_1 = -OH, R_2 = -Glc

Glc: beta-D-glucopyranosyl

Herb Origination

The herb Wu Se Mei is the leaves of a Verbenaceae bush, *Lantana camara* L., which is one of the 10 most poisonous weeds in the world. The plant is indigenous to the tropical area of Middle America, especially Texas. Now, it has become naturalized in tropical and warm areas worldwide as an ornamental plant. The plant was introduced into China but was diffused in the Fujian, Taiwan, Guangxi, and Guangdong provinces. Its leaves are collected in spring and autumn and used as folk medicine both as fresh and dried herb in China.

Anticarcinogenetic Constituents and Activities

The extract of Wu Se Mei leaves demonstrated cytotoxicity against five tested carcinoma cell lines, HEp-2 (larynx), A549 (lung), B16F10 (skin), DLA, Jurkat (leukemia) cells, as well as NRK-49F normal rat kidney cells, *in vitro*.[1,2] The 95% ethanolic extract of the herb exhibited cell death properties in human MCF-7 breast cancer cell line in association with the regulation of Bcl family and the inhibition of caspases.[3] Several triterpenoids, napthaquinones, flavonoids, alkaloids, and glycosides isolated from this plant are known to exert diverse biological activities including cytotoxic and anticancer properties. The major poisonous constituents are two olean-12-ene triterpenoids identified as lantadene-A (**1**) and lantadene-B (**2**) in Wu Se Mei leaves. In addition, fraction LC-2 was derived from the fruits of *L. camara*, which showed anti-uterus-cancer potential against human endometrial carcinoma cells mediated through its anti-estrogenic activity.[4]

Pentacyclic Triterpenoids

Lantadene-A (**1**), lantadene-B (**2**), and the methyl ester of lantadene-A (**1**) displayed a significant decrease in the incidence of squamous cell carcinoma and the average number of papillomas initiated by DMBA followed by TPA promotion in mice. The result suggested that the three triterpenoids have potential chemopreventive property against the two-stage carcinogenesis of skin *in vivo*, where lantadene-A (**1**) showed stronger effect than lantadene-B. The anticarcinogenic activity was mediated by a significant decrease of transcription factor expressions such as the mRNA expressions of AP-1 (c-jun and c-fos), NF-κB (p65), and p53 in the lantadene-treated mouse melanoma.[5–7] In addition, lantadene-A (**1**) displayed the growth suppressive effect against mouse hepatoma cells induced by N-nitrosodiethylamine and phenobarbital.[6]

In the *in vitro* models, lantadene-A (**1**) induced marked concentration- and time-dependent inhibitions on HL-60 leukemia cell proliferation (IC_{50}: 19.8 μg/mL, 48 h). The antigrowth activities of lantadene-A (**1**) and its methyl ester were similar in the assays with HeLa (cervix), 502723 (colon), A549 (lung), and HL-60 (leukemic) human cancer cell lines (IC_{50}: 19.8–23.3 versus 19.2–21.5 μg/mL).[8–10] During the antileukemia action, lantadene-A (**1**) promoted G0/G1 cell cycle arrest and cell apoptosis via a caspase-3-dependent pathway including the down- and upregulations of Bcl-2 and Bax expressions, respectively.[8–10] Lantadene-A (**1**), lantadene-B (**2**), lantadene-C (**3**), icterogenin (**4**), and its region isomer (**5**) exerted moderate to weak suppressive effects on three human neoplastic cell lines, KB (oral), HCT-116 (colon), and MCF-7 (breast), and mouse L1210 leukemia cell line with an IC_{50} value ranging between 5.8 and 44.7 μM, where icterogenin (**4**) was the most active agent against the four tumor cell lines (IC_{50}: 5.8–15 μM) and was relatively sensitive to HCT-116 colon carcinoma and L1210 leukemia cell lines (IC_{50}: 5.8 and 6.8 μM, respectively).[11] Moreover, the isolated ursolic acid stearoyl glucoside (**6**) markedly restrained free radical formation by scavenging hydroxyl radicals, reduced diethylnitrosamine (DENA)-elevated level of lipid peroxidation (LPO), and reversed DENA-diminished activity of antioxidant enzymes (such as GSH transferase, GSH peroxidase, superoxide dismutase, and catalase), leading to the inhibitory effect against the DENA-induced hepatomagenesis.[12]

Lantadene Derivatives from Semisynthesis

For the optimization of the efficacy, the structure of lantadene-A (**1**) has been modified, especially, the groups attached to C-22 and C-17, which inferred the importance in relation to the antitumor effect. However, there were no derivatives with largely improved activity found in the investigation. Only a modified ester (**7**) showed a similar degree of anticancer and anticarcinogenic activities to its parent molecule.[10,13] 3-Oxo reduced lantadene-A and lantadene-B are the minor constituents of *L. camara* weed, but they could be prepared by a single step by reducing lantadene-A (**1**) and lantadene-B (**2**) under microwave irradiation with 98–99% yields. Both products demonstrated selective cytotoxic effect against HL-60, MCF-7, HSC-2, and HCT-116 cancer cell lines (IC_{50}: 1.2–6.4 μM) with no toxicity toward VERO normal cells. The 3-oxo-reduced lantadene-A and lantadene-B promoted the apoptosis of human HL-60 leukemia cells by marked decreasing NF-κB (p65) and Bcl-2 expressions and increasing Bax and caspase-3 activities. At a concentration of 15 μM, the reduced lantadene-A and lantadene-B also significantly lessened the production of nitrite and TNF-α and retarded iNOS gene expression in the HL-60 cells.[14] The results revealed that the 3-oxo-reduced lantadene-A and lantadene-B have the potential to be developed as anticancer agents, indicating that the augmentation of polarity in these triterpenoids obviously enhanced the antitumor activity.

Moreover, the introduction of a hydroxyl functionality in ring A of lantadene-A was designed for the enhancement of polarity and bioactivity. The newly synthesized derivative, 22β-angeloyloxymethyl-2-hydroxy-3-oxo-olean-1,12-dien-28-oate (**8**), showed better cytotoxicity on human cancer cell lines (HL-60, HeLa, 502713, and A549) *in vitro* and a greater tumor inhibition profile against DMBA/TPA-induced two-stage squamous cell carcinogenesis *in vivo*, compared to lantadene-A (**1**). The antitumor and anticarcinogenic effects were found to be correlated to the marked down-expressions of AP-1 (c-jun), NF-κB (p65), and p55.[15] 22β-Angeloyloxyoleanolic acid (**9**) and 2-(3-phenylprop-2-enylidene)-22β-hydroxy-3-oxoolean-12-en-28-oic acid (**10**) were the most active out of the synthesized congeners of lantadenes, and their GI_{50} values were <5 μM against more than 80% cancer cell lines of NCI, in the United States USA.[16] 2-(3-Phenylprop-2-enylidene)-22β-hydroxy-3-oxoolean-12-en-28-oic acid (**10**) displayed enhanced cytotoxicity against a panel of melanoma cell lines (M14, LOX IMVI, MALME-3M, MDA-MB-435, SK-MEL-2, SK-MEL-28, SK-MEL-5, UACC-257 UACC-62, and B16F10) and other types of cancer cell lines (Molt-4, HOP-92, Colo205, SF295, OVCR-3, A498, PC3, and MDA-MB-231) as compared to lantadene-A and cisplatin, but it was nontoxic to VERO normal cells. When treated in the B16-F10 cells, 2-(3-phenylprop-2-enylidene)-22β-hydroxy-3-oxoolean-12-en-28-oic acid (**10**) induced sub-G1 cell cycle arrest and cell apoptosis by inhibiting NF-κB, c-jun, and Bcl-2 and activating Bax and caspase-3. The derivative (**10**), in a B16-F10 allograft mice model, significantly suppressed the tumor growth and the tumor weight and obviously prolonged the survival rate *in vivo* and also showed a better profile than cisplatin in terms of hematological parameters and liver enzyme levels.[17] Hence, the semisynthesis results provided a great design idea for further optimization of the structure to create more valuable antitumor candidates.

Flavonoids

One flavonoid and two flavonol glycosides isolated from the leaves, i.e., 3,5,7-trihydroxy-4′,6-dimethoxyflavonol (**11**), pectrolinarigenin-7-*O*-β-glucoside (**12**), and camaraside (**13**), were found to be also responsible for the antitumor activity.[18]

Tannins

Verbascoside (**14**), another constituent isolated from *L. camara*, is an inhibitor of PKC with an IC_{50} value of 25 μM. An *in vitro* assay showed that verbascoside (**14**) markedly obstructed the proliferation of murine L1210 leukemia cells, whose antileukemia activity might be partially attributed to the inhibitory effect of PKC.[18,19]

Other Medical Uses

All the parts of Wu Se Mei (Sleeper weed) plant have been traditionally used for several ailments throughout the world. Pharmacological data revealed the methanolic extract of Wu Se Mei leaves has health benefits in healing gastric ulcers and preventing the development of duodenal ulcers in rats. The extract displayed antioxidant, antiinflammatory, antidiabetic, antiulcer, analgesic, antimotility, anticonvulsant, antifeedant, larval mortality/repellency, wound-healing, antifungal, and antibacterial properties. Lantadene-A (**1**) is responsible for the anti-pyretic effect, and verbascoside (**3**) has antimicroorganism and immunosuppressive activities.

References

1. Raghu, G. A. et al. 2009. In vitro cytotoxic activity of *Lantana camara* Linn. *Ind. J. Pharmacol.* 36: 94–5.
2. Badakhshan, M. P. et al. 2009. Anti-leukemia activity of methanolic extracts of *Lantana camara*. *Pharmacogn. Res.* 1: 274–9.
3. Han, E. B. et al. 2015. *Lantana camara* induces apoptosis by Bcl-2 family and caspases activation. *Pathol. Oncol. Res.* 21: 325–31.

4. Sarwar, S. et al. 2013. Novel anti-uterus cancer potential of fruit extract of *Lantana camara* as exhibited through the inhibition of alkaline phosphatase in human endometrial adenocarcinomatic cell line. *J. Med. Plants Res.* 7: 1216–21.
5. Kaur, J. et al. 2010. Antitumor activity of lantadenes in DMBA/TPA induced skin tumors in mice: Expression of transcription factors. *Am. J. Biomed. Sci.* 2: 79–90.
6. Inada, A. et al. 1997. Antitumor promoting activities of lantadenes on mouse skin tumors and mouse hepatic tumors. *Planta Med.* 63: 272–4
7. Kaur, J. et al. 2008. Chemopreventive activity of lantadenes on two-stage carcinogenesis model in Swiss albino mice: AP-1 (c-jun), NF-κB (p65) and P53 expression by ELISA and immunehistochemical localization. *Mol. Cell. Biochem.* 314: 1–8.
8. Inada, A. et al. 1995. Inhibitory effects of lantadenes and related triterpenoids on Epstein-Barr virus activation. *Planta Med.* 61: 558–9.
9. Litaudon, M. et al. 2009. Cytotoxic pentacyclic triterpenoids from *Combretum sundaicum* and *Lantana camara* as inhibitors of Bcl-xL/BakBH3 domain peptide interaction. *J. Nat. Prod.* 72: 1314–20.
10. Sharma, M. et al. 2008. Reduced lantadenes A and lantadenes and their esters as potential antitumor agents. *J. Nat. Prod.* 71: 1222–7.
11. Sharma, M. et al. 2007. Lantadene A-induced apoptosis in human leukemia HL-60 cells. *Ind. J. Pharmacol.* 39: 140–4.
12. Kazmi, I. et al. 2013. Anticancer effect of ursolic acid stearoyl glucoside in chemically induced hepatocellular carcinoma. *J. Physiol. Biochem.* 69: 687–95.
13. Sharma, M. et al. 2007. Synthesis, cytotoxicity, and antitumor activity of lantadene-A congeners. *Chem. Biodiver.* 4: 932–9.
14. Kumar, S. S. et al. 2013. Reduced lantadenes A and B: Semi-synthetic synthesis, selective cytotoxicity, apoptosis induction and inhibition of NO, TNFα production in HL-60 cells. *Med. Chem. Res.* 22: 3379–88.
15. Sharma, M. et al. 2011. Design, synthesis and evaluation of lantadene A congener with hydroxyl functionality in ring A as an antitumor agent. *Nat. Prod. Res.* 25: 387–96.
16. Tailor, N. K. et al. 2013. Synthesis and in vitro anticancer studies of novel C-2 arylidene congeners of lantadenes. *Eur. J. Med. Chem.* 64, 285–91.
17. Tailor, N. K. et al. 2013. Effective melanoma inhibition by synthetic pentacyclic triterpenoid 2-(3-phenylprop-2-en-1-ylidene)-22β-hydroxy-3-oxo-olean-12-en-28-oic acid: An in vitro and in vivo study. *J. Environm. Pathol. Toxicol. Oncol.* 32: 59–92.
18. Mahato, S. B. et al. 1994. Potential antitumor agents from *Lantana camara*: Structures of flavonoid-, and phenylpropanoid glycosides. *Tetrahedron* 50. 9439–46.
19. Herbert, J. M. et al. 1991. Verbascoside isolated from *Lantana camara*, an inhibitor of protein kinase C. *J. Nat. Prods.* 54: 1595–600.

138 Pu Kui 蒲葵

Chinese fan palm

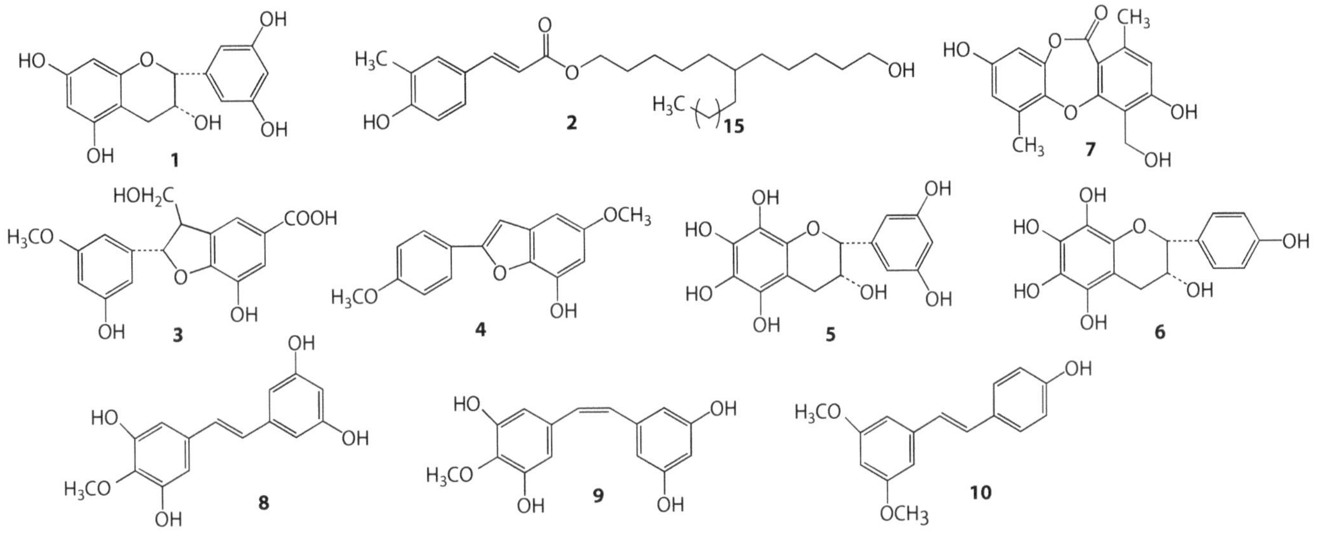

(a)

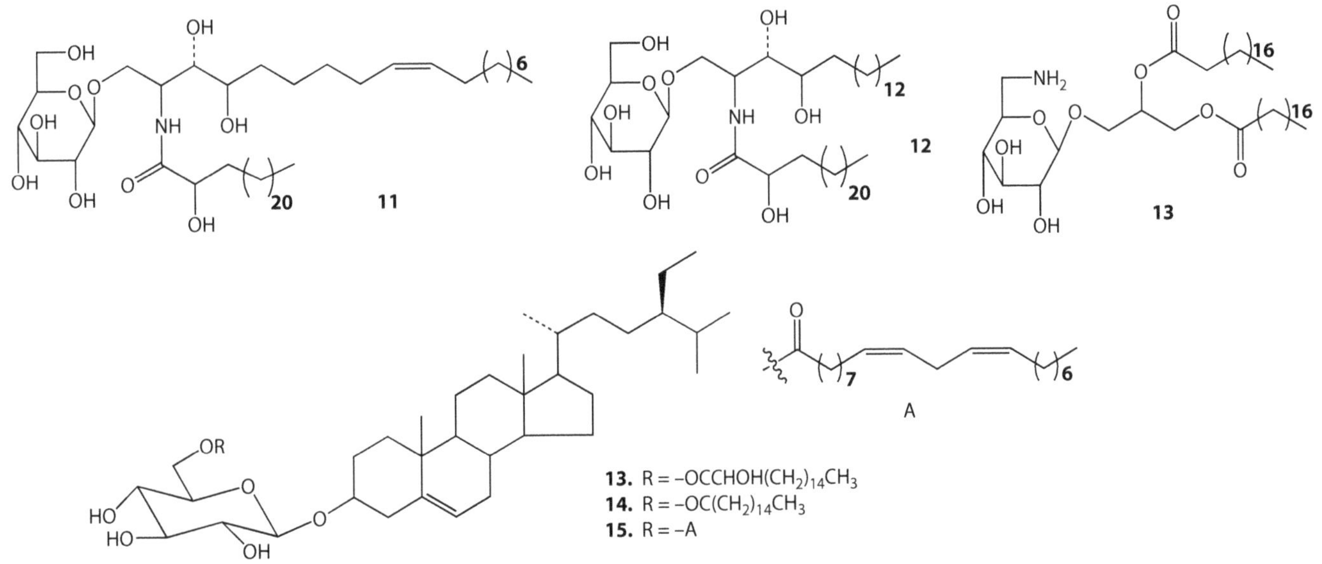

13. R = $-OCCHOH(CH_2)_{14}CH_3$
14. R = $-OC(CH_2)_{14}CH_3$
15. R = -A

(b)

Herb Origination

The herb Pu Kui (Chinese fan palm) originated from a species of subtropical palm tree, *Livistona chinensis* (Palmaceous). Its distribution mainly ranged in southern China, southern Japan, Taiwan, Ryukyu Islands, and Vietnam. This palm is increasingly popular for use in landscapes in Florida, California, Hawaii, South Africa, and other warm temperate climates. Its roots, leaves, and seeds are used as different folk medicines in China.

Antitumor Activities

In the *in vitro* assay, an aqueous extract of Pu Kui seed inhibited the proliferation of endothelial cells and multiple tumor cell lines including mouse fibrosarcoma, human breast, and colon carcinomas. The extract also suppressed the growth of the subcutaneous fibrosarcoma cells in a mouse model.[1] The oral administration of its decoction (0.2 mL) retarded the metastasis of B16-F10 melanoma cells in mice and also promoted spleen cell proliferation and increased mouse spleen weight, indicating that the antitumor activity was mediated by the activation of the host immune system.[2] The alcoholic extract of Pu Kui seed demonstrated significant inhibitory effect on PKC activity with the reduced rates of 56.2% and 66.6% in two concentrations of 40 and 100 μg/mL, respectively.[3] The ethanolic extract of Pu Kui seed showed considerable antineoplastic effect against three human tumor cell lines: HeLa (cervix), SGC-7901 (stomach), and Bel-7402 (liver) cells.[4] When the seed was separated into different components, the shell including the seed skin appeared to be more potent than the inner kernel in the suppression of tumor growth and angiogenesis. Based upon the potency, the extract derived from the Pu Kui shells may be a potential supplemental source for cancer treatment and prevention.[1] In addition, a EAF of the alcoholic extract of Pu Kui roots was found to have an antitumor effect against the proliferation of seven carcinoma cell lines such as L1210 and P388D1 leukemia, B16 melanoma, Hele7404 hepatoma, NG108-15 glioma, and HeLa cervical cancer at its concentration of 5.0 μg/mL *in vitro*.[5]

From the ethanolic extract of Pu Kui seeds, a highly purified fraction LC-X was separated, which is a marked inhibitor against the activities of various protein kinases *in vitro*, including PAK2, PKA, PKC, GSK-3α, CK2, MAPK, and JNK1, with IC_{50} values between 1 and 40 μg/mL. At doses of >50 μg/mL *in vitro*, the proliferation of two human nasopharyngeal carcinoma (NPC-TW02 and NPC-TW04) cells and human MCF-7 breast cancer cells were significantly blocked by the LC-X but no such effect on A431 epidermoid and HeLa cervical carcinoma cell lines. The antitumor activity of LC-X was found to be related to the induction of cell cycle arrest at G2/M phase and apoptotic death of the NPC-TW02 cells. Studies also revealed that EGFR and MAPK could be potently inhibited by LC-X in the NPC-TW02 and A431 cell lines in dose- and time-dependent manners, whose blockage of EGFR and MARK pathway might be involved in the antineoplastic mechanism.[6] An EAF of the alcoholic extract from Pu Kui seeds selectively inhibited the cell proliferation of human HT-29 colon neoplastic cells and human T24 bladder carcinoma cells in a dose-dependent manner, and the inhibitory rates were up to 74.66% and 86.52%, respectively, whose mechanism might be partially associated with the reduction of VEGF protein secretion and the inhibition of the expressions of Flk-1 mRNA and protein.[7]

Antitumor Constituents and Activities

From the Pu Kui seeds/fruits and roots, several different types of anticancer constituents were separated, which showed marked to weak inhibitory effects in the *in vitro* assay with human neoplastic cell lines.

Phenolic Compounds

A flavane designated as 2S,3S-3,5,7,3′,5′-pentahydroxyflavane (**1**) markedly inhibited the proliferation of human HL-60 promyelocytic leukemia and CNE-1 nasopharyngeal carcinoma cell lines with the IC_{50} values (μM) of 0.2 and 1.0, respectively, showing greater potency than cisplatin.[8] Most of the flavanes and flavanoids isolated from the herb exhibited potent antioxidant activity.[8] Among the five antioxidant phenolics isolated from Pu Kui fruits, E-[6′-(5″-hydroxypentyl)tricosyl]-4-hydroxy-3-methoxy-cinnamate (**2**), 1-{ω-isoferul[6-(4-hydroxybutyl)-pentadecanoic acid]}-glycerol, 2-(3′-hydroxy-5′-methoxyphenyl)-3-hydroxylmethyl-7-methoxy-2,3-dihydrobenzofuran-5-carboxylic acid (**3**), and 7-hydroxy-5,4′-dimethoxy-2-arylbenzofuran (**4**), exerted moderate antiproliferative activity on four tested human HL-60 and K562 (leukemic), HepG2 (liver), and CNE-1 (nasopharynx) cancer cell lines.[9] The treatment with 7-hydroxy-5,4′-dimethoxy-2-arylbenzofuran (**4**) elicited S cell cycle arrest and apoptosis of cervical cancer cells and exerted the anticancer function, together with the upregulation of cyclin-A2 and CDK2, the damage of DNA, and the inhibition of PARP activity.[10] A group of hydroxyflavans, such as (2S,3S)-3,5,7,3′,5′-pentahydroxyflavan (**1**), 3,5,6,7,8,3′,5′-heptahydroxyflavan (**5**), and 3,5,6,7,8,4′-hexahydroxyflavan (**6**), were isolated from its seeds, and these hydroxyl flavans were effective in the treatment of hepatoma, leukemia, nasopharyngeal cancer cell lines, etc.[11] In addition, one deposidone assigned as livistone-A (**7**) and three stilbenes (**8–10**) separated from the fruits also exerted remarkable cell protective activity against H_2O_2-induced cell damage of human SH-SY5Y neuroblastoma cells.[12]

Ceramides and Acylglycerols

Thirteen glycosyl ceramides and acylglycerols were isolated from the 70% ethanol extract of its roots. Of them, 1-*O*-β-D-gluco-pyranosyl-(2S,3S,4R,9Z)-2-[(2R)-2-hydroxydocosanoylamino]-9-octadecene-1,3,4-triol (**11**), 1-*O*-β-D-glucopyranosyl-(2S,3S,4R,9Z)-2-[(2R-2-hydroxytetracosan oylamino]-1,3,4-octadecanetriol (**12**), and 1-octadecanoyl-2-nonadecanoyl-3-*O*-(6-amino-6-deoxy)-β-D-glucopyranosyl-sn-glycerol (**13**) displayed moderate to weak inhibitory effects against the proliferation of tested human tumor cell lines (K562, HL-60, HepG2, and CNE-1). Their IC_{50} values (μM) were 14.2–20.6 in HL-60 cells, 12.38–18.70 in K562 cells, and 12.54–22.73 in CNE-1 cells, but their weak effects were observed in HepG2 cells (IC_{50}: 30.50–74.70 μM). 1-*O*-β-D-gluco-pyranosyl-(2S,3S,4R,9Z)-2-[(2R)-2-hydroxydocosanoylamino]-9-octadecene-1,3,4-triol (**11**) and 1-*O*-β-D-glucopyranosyl-(2S,3S,4R,9Z)-2-[(2R-2-hydroxytetracosanoylamino]-1,3,4-octadecanetriol (**12**) at a concentration of 100 μg/mL completely obstructed the viability of K562 cells, resulting in about 90.0% antiproliferative efficacy, whereas 1-octadecanoyl-2-nonadecanoyl-3-*O*-(6-amino-6-deoxy)-β-D-glucopyranosyl-sn-glycerol (**13**) exhibited 91.3% inhibitory efficacy on CNE-1 nasopharyngeal carcinoma at its highest concentration and showed the inhibitory efficacy of 67.3% and 71.5% at a 100 μg/mL concentration against HepG 2 and K562 cell lines.[13]

Steroid

Δ5-Isospirost-3β-ol, which was isolated from its seeds, displayed significant inhibitory effects against murine P388 leukemia, human HeLa cervical cancer, human Hele-7404 hepatoma, and human SGC-7901 gastric cancer cells *in vitro*.[14] Several 6′-*O*-acyl-β-D-glucosyl-β-sitosterols were isolated from the 70% ethanolic extract of *L. chinensis* roots. Four of them, 6′-*O*-(2″-hydroxy-heptadecanoyl)-β-D-glucosyl-β-sitosterol (**14**), 6′-*O*-hexadecanoyl-β-D-glucosyl-β-sitosterol (**15**), 6′-O-(icosa-9″Z,12″Z-dienoyl)-β-D-glucosyl-β-sitosterol (**16**), and 3-*O*-octadecanoyl-β-sitosterol, exhibited moderate to weak antiproliferative effects against human neoplastic cell lines (K562, HL-60, HepG2, and CNE-1) *in vitro*. The relatively better inhibitory effect was showed by 6′-*O*-(2″-hydroxy-heptadecanoyl)-β-D-glucosyl-β-sitosterol (**14**) (IC_{50}: 12.38–26.76 μM) and 6′-O-(icosa-9″Z,12″Z-dienoyl)-β-D-glucosyl-β-sitosterol (**16**) (IC_{50}: 12.77–24.76 μM).[15]

References

1. Sartippour, M. R. et al. 2001. Livistona extract inhibits angiogenesis and cancer growth. *Oncol. Reports* 8: 1355–7.
2. Liu, S. Y. et al. 1987. Antitumor metastatic components in *Trapa taiwanensis* Nakai and *Livistona chinensis* R.Br. *Bull. Institute Zool., Acad. Sinica* 26: 143–50.
3. Huang, C. et al. 1995. Effect of Selginella herb and Livistona seeds on the activity of PKC. *Zhongcaoyao* 26: 414–7.
4. Zhu, Y. L. et al. 2007. Chemical components and anticancer activity analysis of ethanol extract from seed of *Livistona chinensis. Huaxue Yu Shengwu Gongcheng* 24: 35–7.
5. Zhong, Z. G. et al. 2007. Study on the anticancer effects of extracts from roots of *Livistona chinensis* in vitro. *Zhongyaocai* 30: 60–3.
6. Huang, W. C. et al. 2007. Selective downregulation of EGF receptor and downstream MAPK pathway in human cancer cell lines by active components partially purified from the seeds of *Livistona chinensis* R. Brown. *Cancer Lett.* 248: 137–46.
7. Wang, H. et al. 2008. Screening of antitumor parts from the seeds of *Livistona chinensis* and its anti-angiogenesis effect. *Zhongyaocai* 31: 718–22.
8. Zeng, X. B. et al. 2011. Antioxidant flavanes from *Livistona chinensis. Fitoterapia* 82: 609–14.
9. Zeng, X. B. et al. 2012. Bioactive phenolics from the fruits of *Livistona chinensis. Fitoterapia* 83: 104–9.
10. Chen, H. B. et al. 2015. A new arylbenzofuran derivative functions as an antitumor agent by inducing DNA damage and inhibiting PARP activity. *Sci. Reports* 5: 10893.
11. He, X. J. et al. 2010. Hydroxy flavans from *Livistona chinensis* seeds and their application for antiaging and antitumor treatment. *Faming Zhuanli Shenqing* CN 101857584 A 20101013.
12. Yuan, T. et al. 2009. Phenolic compounds with cell protective activity from the fruits of *Livistona chinensis. J. Asian Nat. Prod. Res.* 11: 243–9.
13. Zeng, X. B. et al. 2012. Cytotoxic ceramides and glycerides from the roots of *Livistona chinensis. Fitoterapia* 83: 609–16.
14. Liu, Z. P. et al. 2007. Effective chemical components from seeds of *Livistona chinensis. Zhongcaoyao* 38: 178–80.
15. Zeng, X. B. et al. 2013. Unusual lipids and acylglucosylsterols from the roots of *Livistona chinensis. Phytochem. Lett.* 6: 36–40.

139 Zhe Shu 柘樹

Cudrang or Silkworm thorn

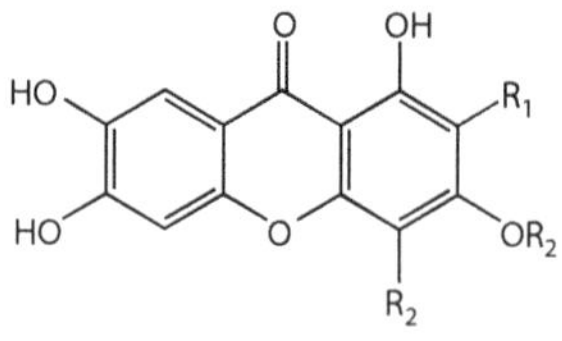

1. R_1 = –H; R_2 = $-CH_2-CH=C(CH_3)_2$
2. R_1 = $-CH_2-CH=C(CH_3)_2$; R_2 = –OH
5. R_1 = $-C(CH_3)_2-CH=CH_2$; R_2 = –OH

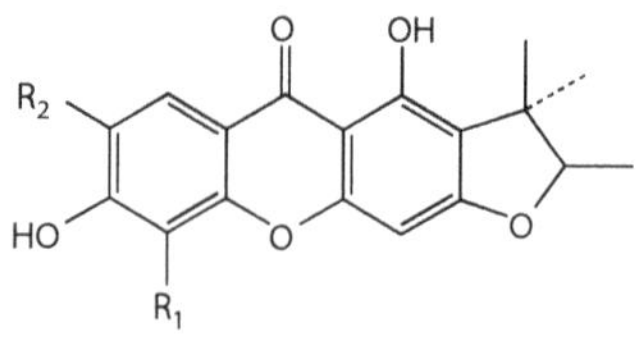

3. R_1 = $-CH_2-CH=C(CH_3)_2$; R_2 = –OH
4. R_1 = –H; R_2 = –OH

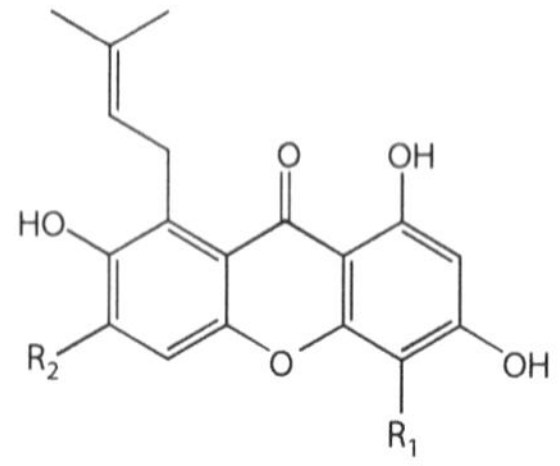

6. R_1 = $-CH_2-CH=C(CH_3)_2$; R_2 = –OH
8. R_1 = $-CH_2-CH=C(CH_3)_2$; R_2 = –H

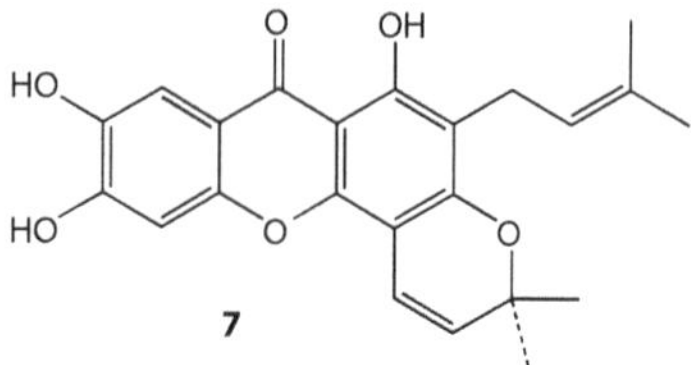

7

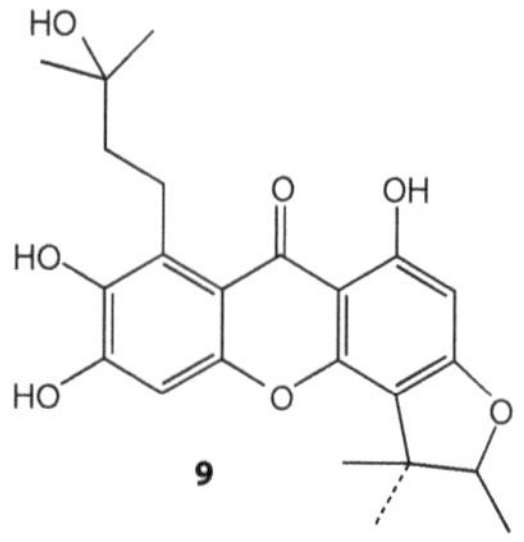

9

Herb Origination

The herb Zhe Shu (Cudrang) originated from a Moraceae plant, *Maclura tricuspidata* (= *Cudrania tricuspidata*). This deciduous shrub or tree is native to east Asia, especially in central, east, and south China and Korea, and it has been cultivated in Japan for a long time. Its roots, stems, leaves, barks, and fruits are used in Chinese herbal medicines independently.

Antitumor Constituents and Activities

The roots of Zhe Shu are applied in the clinics of China and Korea for the treatment of digestive apparatus carcinoma, especially gastric carcinoma. Its crude flavonoid components were reported to have inhibitory effect against human gastric neoplastic NKM cells *in vitro* together with the blockage of macromolecule synthesis in the tumor cells.[1] According to phytochemistry research, Zhe Shu was revealed to be a rich source of isoprenylated xanthones and isoprenylated flavonoids. Over 20 isoprenylated xanthones have been discovered from the roots and/or the root barks of *M. tricuspidata*, and the cytotoxicity of some of them mostly contributed to the antineoplastic effect of the herb. Cudratricusxanthone-G (**1**), cudratricusxanthone-E (**2**), cudraxanthone-M (**3**), and toxyloxanthone-C (**4**) were the first four strongest xanthones in the growth suppression of all four tested human carcinoma cells *in vitro* with IC_{50} values in a range of 1.6–11.8 μg/mL. Xanthone-V1a (**5**) and cudratricusxanthone-G (**1**) displayed greater cytotoxicity on human HCT-116 colorectal cancer cells (IC_{50}: 1.3–1.8 μg/mL), whereas cudratricusxanthone-G (**1**) and cudratricusxanthone-E (**2**) were mostly sensitive to human BGC-823 gastric cancer cells (IC_{50}: 1.6 and 1.6 μg/mL). Cudratricusxanthone-G (**1**) also exerted greater inhibitory effect against the growth of human hepatoma SMMC-7721 cells (IC_{50}: 2.7 μg/mL) *in vitro*, compared to other isolated xanthones.[2,3] Cudraxanthone-H (**8**) demonstrated higher cytotoxic effect against human SGC-7901 gastric cancer cells (IC_{50}: 1.8 μg/mL) than against BGC-823 (IC_{50}: 9.2 μg/mL) and SMMC-7721 cell lines (IC_{50}: 11.7 μg/mL) but no cytotoxicity against HCT-116 cells.[2] Macluraxanthone-B (**13**), cudraxanthone-L, and 2,3,6,8-tetrahydroxy-1-(3-methylbut-2-enyl)-5-(2-methylbut-3-en-2-yl)-9H-xanthen-9-one showed the moderate antigrowth activity against human A549 lung cancer cells and human SKOV3 ovarian carcinoma cells *in vitro* with IC_{50} values of 2.88 and 4.24 μM, 3.15 and 4.72 μM, and 5.93 and 7.09 μM, respectively.[4] Moreover, the isolated isoprenylated flavonoids were evaluated by the *in vitro* assays with the HCT-116, SMMC-7721, SGC-7901, and BGC-823 cell lines. However, only cudraflavanose-C (**17**) and cudraflavanose-A (**18**) displayed weak inhibitory effect and others were inactive.[3]

Taken together, these positive results suggested that the bioactive molecules of the isoprenylated xanthones are potential drug leads, which are worthy of further investigations in *in vivo* experiment and structural modification.

Other Medical Uses

The herb Zhe Shu has been used as a traditional medicine for curing neuritis and inflammation in Asia. The roots of Zhe Shu are also one of the sources of another Chinese folk medicine, Chuan Po Shi (穿破石) which is often employed in the treatment of gonorrhea, rheumatism, jaundice, dysmenorrhea, boils, bruising, and scabies. Also, its bark fibers are used for making paper; its leaves are used as food for silkworm; its fruit are edible; and its root and bark are largely used medicinally.

References

1. Xu, Y. T. et al. 1998. Effect of the flavonoids of Zheshu on the synthesis of macromolecules in human gastric cancer NKM cell line. *Zhongyiyao Xuebao* 26: 47–8.
2. Zou, Y. S. et al. 2004. Cytotoxic isoprenylated xanthones from *Cudrania tricuspidata*. *Bioorg. Med. Chem.* 12: 1947–53.
3. Zou, Y. S. et al. 2005. Isoprenylated xanthones and flavonoids from *Cudrania tricuspidata*. *Chem. Biodivers.* 2: 131–8.
4. Lee, B. W. et al. 2005. Cytotoxic xanthones from *Cudrania tricuspidata*. *J. Nat. Prod.* 68: 456–8.

140 Tian Qi 田七

Notoginseng

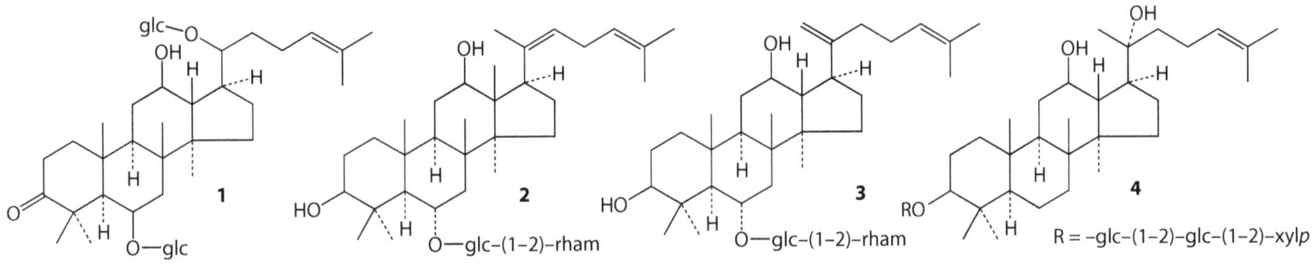

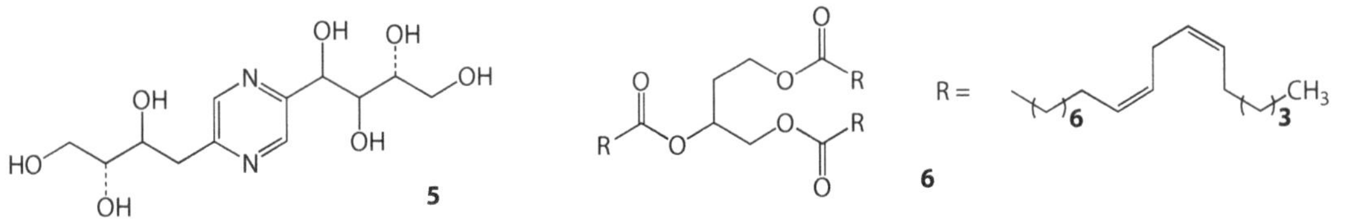

Herb Origination

The herb Tian Qi (Notoginseng) is the dried rhizomes of an Araliaceae plant, *Panax notoginseng* (= *P. pseudoginseng*). Tian Qi plant grows naturally in southern and southwestern China; its rhizomes and roots are normally harvested after being cultivated for three to seven years. As a famous Chinese herb, it was firstly documented in a Chinese compendium of material medica entitled *Ben Cao Gangmu* (AD 1596) and has been extensively used in China since the end of the nineteenth century. It has acquired a very favorable reputation for hemostatic proprietary herbal remedy.

Antitumor Activities

The water extract of Notoginseng dose-dependently exerted the growth inhibition on two human lung cancer cell lines (A549 and NIC-H460) and induced the cell apoptotic death in correlation with mitochondrial dysfunction and dephosphorylation of the Akt signaling pathway.[1] This antilung carcinoma effect was also proven in a nude mice model xenografted with NCI-H460 cells without any side effects.[2] The aqueous extracts derived from different plant parts (rhizome, root, flower, and berry) of *P. notoginseng* were evaluated in human SW480 colorectal carcinoma cells. The flower extract showed the most potent antiproliferative effect compared to the other three extracts. At a 1.0 mg/mL concentration, it obstructed the cell growth by 93.1%,[3] whereas the treatment with the root extract at the same concentration suppressed the growth of SW480 cells by 85.8%.[4] The anticarcinogenic property of the methanolic extract of the plant roots was presented in a noticeable inhibition of EBV-EA induced by a tumor promoter TPA.[5] The extract also demonstrated strong antitumor-promoting effects against three two-stage carcinogenesis such as in mouse skin initiated by DMBA and promoted by TPA, mycotoxin, or fumonisin-B1; in pulmonary induced by 4-nitroquinoline-N-oxide as an initiator and glycerol as a promoter; and in liver initiated by N-nitroso-diethylamine and promoted by phenobarbital in *in vivo* or *in vitro* tests.[5–7]

The raw and white Notoginseng was shown to be not strong, but its red Notoginseng (by steaming up to 24 h) exerted a significant increase in antiproliferative and proapoptotic effects, e.g., on hepatoma cell lines (SNU449, SNU182, and HepG2).[8] The heat treatment process may change the chemical profile and augment the efficacy of Notoginseng in the anticancer treatments.[8] Meaningfully, the red Notoginseng displayed the best inhibitory activity against the proliferation of cancer cells compared to two other kinds of red Ginsengs derived from Asian ginseng and American ginseng. Due to the high level of biological activity, the red Notoginseng is considered as a promising and useful botanical product in cancer chemoprevention.[9]

Antitumor Constituents and Activities

Similar to Asian ginseng and American ginseng, Notoginseng contains the same type of dammarane triterpenoid saponins as the major antitumor and anticarcinogenic constituents, but the white Notoginseng possesses the most abundant ginsenosides, i.e., two- and fivefold higher than white Asian ginseng and American ginseng. Moreover, some other constituents such as triterpenoids, polyacetylenes, and polysaccharides derived from the Notoginseng were also established to contribute to the antiproliferative effects against the neoplastic cells.

Total Saponins

The ginsenosides in *P. notoginseng* (PNS) includes two aglycone classifications: 20(S)-protopanaxadiol (PPD) and 20(S)-protopanaxatriol, which are the same types of aglycones involved in the saponins of *P. ginseng* and *P. quinquefolius*. The naturally occurring PNS at higher concentrations were found to be able to exert the cytotoxic, antiproliferative, apoptosis-inducing, and anticarcinogenic activities against various human tumor cell lines such as BGC-823 (stomach), SMMC-7721 and HepG2 (liver), Bel-7402 (liver), LoVo (colon), and RPMI8226 (multiple myeloma), in dose- and time-dependent behaviors, *in vitro*, where the cell cycle arrest was also induced in LoVo cells at S phase and in SMMC-7721 cells at G0/G1 phase.[10–14] After the treatment, the down-expression of Bcl-2 and the up-expression of Bax occurred in BGC823 and RPMI8226 cell lines, the increase of gap junction intercellular communication function was found in SMMC-7721 cells, and the contents of TNFα and IL-18 were markedly increased in HepG2 cells, whose characteristic events should be involved in the antitumor mechanisms in different types of cancer cells.[10–14] During the suppression on hepatoma cell lines (SMMC-7721 and Bel-7402), the PNS at a 400 μg/mL concentration significantly inhibited AFP-L3 and GP-73 activities. The antihepatoma activity of the PNS at the 400 μg/mL concentration was comparable to that of 5-FU at a 40 μg/mL concentration.[15,16] The PNS also has abilities to dose-and time-dependently diminish the survival rate of human lung adenocarcinoma A529 cells by stimulating apoptosis, whose effect can be synergistically enhanced when cotreated with LY294002 (a specific inhibitor of PI3K).[17] Moreover, the PNS exerted the antiproliferative effect against human promyelocytic leukemia NB4 cells and partially elicited the differentiation of NB4 cells.[18] The PNS also showed marked antioxidant capacities in 1,1-diphenyl-2-picrylhydrazyl free radical-scavenging assay and hydroxyl radical-scavenging assay *in vitro*.[10]

Besides the antiproliferative property, the PNS also act as a safe and effective agent for the reversal of MDR and the blockage of tumor cell metastasis. By attenuating the expressions of MDR-1 and P-gp, the PNS at a high concentration partially reversed the multidrug resistance of MCF-7/Adm (a human breast cancer MDR strain) *in vitro*.[19] After the treatment of human PC3 prostate cancer cells with the saponins (400 mg/L), the expressions of vascular cell adhesion molecule-1 and proliferating cell nuclear antigen (PCNA) were notably downregulated, the phosphorylation level of p38 MAPK pathway was dramatically augmented, and the expression of migration-related protein MMP-2 were markedly diminished, thereby leading to effectively restraining the proliferation and the migration of PC3 cells.[20] In a lung metastatic model of B16 melanoma, the PNS at a dose of 480 mg/kg not only obviously inhibited the growth and the colonies by 50.85% but also effectively repressed the lung metastasis of B16 cells, associated with the upregulation of connexin-32 expression.[21] Also, the treatment with a saponin-rich ethanolic extract also obviously obstructed the liver metastasis and improved the life quality of mice grafted the B16 melanoma.[22] By the treatment of 4T1 breast cancer cells with the PNS, the viability/growth was impaired and the lung metastasis was obviously inhibited in both spontaneous and experimental metastasis models *in vitro* and *in vivo*.[23]

The synergistic effect of PNS was investigated by the combination with chemotherapeutic agents. A saponin-rich Tian Qi root extract additively potentiated the chemotherapeutic effect of 5-FU or irinotecan against human SW480 colorectal cancer cells, whereas a saponin-rich Tian Qi flower extract at a 0.25 mg/mL concentration improved the antiproliferative effect of 5-FU and reduced the dosage of 5-FU needed for the treatment of human HCT-116 colorectal cancer.[4,24] In human T47D breast cancer cells, the PNS showed direct, time- and dose-dependent inhibitory effect, and it could also enhance the antitumor effect of tamoxifen at a high dose by impacting the cell cycle.[25] By the combinational treatment, the PNS significantly enhanced the cytotoxic effect of cisplatin and CTX and concurrently attenuated the toxicity of the two drugs.[26,27] By up-expressing Bcl-2 and down-expressing Bax, the integration with PNS and Adm synergistically retarded the proliferation of multiple myeloma RPMI8226 cells.[12]

Moreover, the cotreatment of the PNS (480 mg/kg/day) and CTX (20 mg/kg/day) promoted the cell transformation of T lymphocyte and amplified IL-2 and TNFα in a rat model with sarcoma 180, resulting in the enhancement of body immunity and the alleviation of toxicity reaction besides the enlarged cytotoxicity of CTX.[27] Probably due to the immunoenhancing function, the pretreatment of the PNS was capable of reducing DOX-caused myocardial damage and protecting the mice from DOX-induced cardiotoxicity *in vivo* and *in vitro* through significantly lowered levels of serum LDH, CK, and CK-MB and normalized activities of GSH peroxidase, catalase, and myocardial superoxide dismutase.[28,29] The PNS is also a prophylactic agent for cisplatin-induced nephrotoxicity, whose effect is closely associated with attenuating cisplatin-induced cytosolic free [Ca^{2+}] overload and blocking the formations of DNA–protein cross-link and DNA interstrand cross-link.[26]

These deepening research results evidenced that the PNS have multitarget antitumor activity and potential for clinical application. The PNS deserve to be further developed as a highly efficient, low toxicity, and tumor resistance-reversal agent.

Individual Saponins

To date, over 50 pure saponins including ginsenosides, notoginsenosides, and gypenosides have been isolated from Tian Qi, wherein ginsenoside-Rb1 (34.4%), ginsenoside-Rg1 (31.1%), ginsenoside-Rd, and notoginsenoside-R1 are considered to be the major constituents. The total content of the eight important saponins (ginsenoside-Rg1, ginsenoside-Re, ginsenoside-Rb1, ginsenoside-Rc, and ginsenoside-Rd; notoginsenoside-R1; and isomeric ginsenoside-Rb2 and ginsenoside-Rb3) was 81.7% in Tian Qi. During the steaming process, the original polar ginsenosides are degradable to less polar hydrolysates by shortening the carbohydrate chain, implying that the size of the sugar moiety within the ginsenosides highly impacted the anticancer activity, which enhances with the diminution of the sugar number. Therefore, the steaming significantly promoted the transformation of Rg3 and Rh2, which are recognized as the major inhibitors in the total saponins against cancer cell proliferation. By the steaming process, the contents of less active notoginsenoside-R1 and ginsenoside-Rg1, ginsenoside-Re, ginsenoside-Rc, ginsenoside-Rb1, ginsenoside-Rb2, ginsenoside-Rb3, and ginsenoside-Rd were diminished, and the contents of more antitumor active ginsenoside-Rk1, ginsenoside-Rk3, ginsenoside-Rh1, ginsenoside-Rh2, ginsenoside-Rg2, ginsenoside-Rg3, and 20R-Rg2 were correspondingly augmented.[10,30–32]

The two major inhibitors, ginsenoside-Rh2 and ginsenoside-Rg3, which have been also discussed in the sections of Ren Seng and Xi Yang Seng, displayed marked inhibitory effect against the formation of angiogenesis and vasculogenic mimicry in B16 melanoma and then obstructed the blood supply in the tumor tissue effectually.[33] Rg3 could hinder the invasion of mouse MM1 ascites hepatoma, B16-FE7 melanoma cells, human OC-10 small cell lung cancer, and PSN-1 pancreatic carcinoma cells. Rg3 restrained the metastasis of B16-FE7 melanoma and colon cancer cells to the lung as well in the *in vitro* assay. The antiproliferative and antimetastatic effects of Rg3 were proven in nude models implanted with human SKOV-3 ovarian cancer cells or SK-MES-1 lung squamous carcinoma cells, whose activities were mediated by the suppression of angiogenesis and MMP-9 expression and the down-expression of VEGF and bFGF. The antigrowth activity on the SK-MES-1 cells reached to 81.14% when Rg3 was given by intragastric (i.g.) for 28 days in a dose of 2 mg/kg/day.[33] According to the affirmative evidences, ginsenoside-Rh2 and ginsenoside-Rg3 were suggested to be deserving of a development as chemotherapeutic and chemopreventive agents for cancer patients.

Likewise, more ginsenosides were discovered from the Tian Qi plant to exert the antitumor effects in vitro as well. 6-*O*-β-D-Glucopyranosyl-20-*O*-β-D-glucopyranosyl-20(S)-protopanaxadiol-3-one (**1**) exhibited the inhibitory effect against the proliferation of HCT-8 (colon), Bel-7402 (liver), BGC-823 (stomach), A2780 (ovary), and A549 (lung) human cancer cell lines (IC_{50}: 5.4–8.6 μg/mL).[34] The antitumor effects of ginsenoside-Pn1 (isolated from the leaves of Tian Qi) was established in NCI-H460 (lung), HepG2 (liver), and SGC-7901 (stomach) human cancer cell lines, shown to be relatively greater than that of Rg3, an approved clinical agent for cancer therapy in China.[35] The antiproliferative effect of notoginsenoside-R1 on the HeLa cells was mediated by upregulating the gap junction function, and R1 could also markedly enhance the cytotoxicity of cisplatin.[35] When ginsenoside-Rg1, ginsenoside-Rb1, and notoginsenoside-R1 are used to treat human SW480 colon cancer cells in each concentration of 300 μM, respectively, for two days, the proapoptotic and antiproliferative effects were prominently elicited.[4] Through similar mechanisms, i.e., induction of mitochondrial dysfunction with Bax up-expression and Bcl-2 down-expression, ginsenoside-F4 (**2**) and ginsenoside-Rg6 (**3**) arrested the proliferation and elicited the apoptosis of human lymphocytoma Jurkat cells.[36,37] The induction of S and G2/M cell cycle arrest and apoptosis by notoginsenoside-Ft1 (**4**) in human neuroblastoma SH-SY5Y cells were associated with the enhancement of p38 MAPK and ERK1/2 pathways.[38] Accordingly, the investigations provided a remarkable scientific base for the application of Tian Qi and its saponins in cancer treatment and drug development.

Sapogenins

20(S)-25-Methoxyldammarane-3β,12β,20-triol (25-OCH_3-PPD) is the most safe and effective antitumor sapogenin that was isolated from the roots, the leaves, and the seeds of *P. notoginseng*. Their inhibitory effects were demonstrated in various human solid cancer cells such as in the liver, the colon, the lung, the pancreas, the breast, and the prostate organs.[39–44] 25-OCH_3-PPD decreased the survival, repressed the proliferation, and induced the apoptosis and G1 cell arrest in the lung cancer cells (A549, H358, and H838), prostate cancer cells (AD LNCaP and AI PC3), and breast cancer cells *in vitro* but showed almost no effect on the cell viability of Chang liver cells (a type of normal human liver cell line).[41–44] The growth inhibitory effect of 25-OCH_3-PPD was further demonstrated in nude mice xenografted with A549 lung carcinoma or LNCaP prostate tumor without any host toxicity.[43,44] In comparison with three structurally related molecules, ginsenoside-Rh2, ginsenoside-Rg3, and 20(S)-PPD, the potencies of cytotoxicity were in the order or 25-OCH_3-PPD $\gg$ 20(S)-PPD $\gg$ Rg3 and Ph2.[41]

The mechanisms of 25-OCH_3-PPD for antiproliferation and apoptosis and cell cycle arrest induction on the neoplastic cells were revealed to involve (1) decreasing the levels of proteins associated with the cell proliferation and the cell survival (such as MDM2, E2F1, cyclin-D1, and CDK-2 and CDK-4 in lung and prostate cancer cells),[43,44] (2) activating proapoptotic proteins (such as cleaved PARP, cleaved caspase-3, caspase-8, and caspase-9 in prostate cancer cells),[44] (3) downregulating the expression of β-catenin, a key mediator in the Wnt pathway and reducing the expressions of transcriptional targets of β-catenin (such as c-Myc, cyclin-D1, CDK-4 and T cell factor-4 in colon and lung cancer cells),[39] and (4) inhibiting MDM2 oncogene and related pathways (such as in pancreas cancer cells).[42] The growth inhibitory mechanism of 25-OCH_3-PPD in the LNCaP cells was mainly accompanied by retarding the expression of AR and PSA against the AD prostate cancer cells. Also, 25-OCH_3-PPD displayed therapeutic potential against AI prostate carcinoma, indicating that its antiprostate cancer effect was mediated by different mechanisms.[44] Particularly, the antihepatoma and apoptosis-promoting activities of 25-OCH_3-PPD were demonstrated to largely correlate with its marked abilities in (1) decreasing Bcl-2/Bax ratio and survinin expression via c-FLIP-mediated NF-κB activation; (2) activating caspase-3 level; and (3) diminishing fibrosis markers such as α-smooth muscle actin (α-SMA), TGF-β1, and TIMP-1.[40]

All the provided preclinical data obtained from *in vitro* and *in vivo* investigations suggested that 25-OCH_3-PPD may be used as a promising chemotherapeutic adjunct and a chemopreventive agent for anticancer clinical development.

Polyacetylenes

Panaxynol and panaxydol are naturally occurring polyacetylenes in the lipophilic fractions of *P. notoginseng* roots. Their antiproliferative properties against the malignant cells have been discussed in Sections Ren Seng and Xi Yang Seng. More investigation found that both panaxynol and panaxydol exerted marked antiproliferation and proapoptotic effects in human HL-60 promyelocytic leukemia cells time- and dose-dependently.[45] In rat C6 glioma cells, the panaxydol treatment dose-dependently inhibited the cell proliferation *in vitro* and elicited the G0/G1 cell arrest with the promotion of p27 expression and differentiation response, with an IC_{50} value around 39.5 μM.[46] Through cAMP- and MAPK-dependent mechanisms, i.e., increasing the albumin secretion and the alkaline phosphatase activity, elevating the p21 and p-ERK1/2 protein levels, and reducing the alpha-fetoprotein (AFP) secretion and the regulatory factors of Id1 expression, panaxydol dose-dependently restrained the proliferation of human SMMC-7721 hepatoma cells and stimulated apoptosis-related morphological and ultrastructure changes.[47] Panaxatrol, another polyacetylene derived from Tian Qi, had been investigated as a salt form of disucinate sodium in patients with advanced solid tumors and healthy volunteers, suggesting a 30-day continuous intravenous injection of panaxatrol in a dose of 100 mg/m^2 per day is a great scheme for further phase II trial.[48]

Other Small Molecules

A water-soluble alkaloid designated as 2-(1′,2′,3′,4′-tetrahydroxybutyl)-6-(2″,3″,4″-trihydroxybutyl)-pyrazine (**5**) was isolated from the aqueous extract of Tian Qi, displaying moderate or weak antiproliferative effect against human Bel-7404 hepatoma cells and human 803 gastric neoplastic cells *in vitro*.[49] Trilinolein (**6**), a bioactive component derived from Tian Qi, was effective in the suppression of human A549 NSCLC cells and the promotion of A549 cell apoptosis via the modulation of PI3K/Akt pathway.[50]

Polysaccharides

Four polysaccharides, designated PF3111, PF3112, PBGA11, and PBGA12, were prepared from Tian Qi, which are heteroglycans with molecular weights ranging from 37 to 760 kDa, composed of glucose, galactose, xylose, arabinose, and mannose in different molar ratios. The polysaccharides demonstrated anticarcinoma-related immunostimulating effects, i.e., inducing the production of significant amounts of TNFα and interferon-γ.[51] Likewise, an arabinogalactan termed RN1 was isolated from the flowers of *P. notoginseng*, whose structure has a backbone of 1,6-linked Gal with 1,3-linked Gal branches. The branches mainly contained 1,5-linked, 1,3,5-linked, terminal arabinose, and terminal galactose. RN1 was capable of reducing the migration of endothelial cells and obstructing the tube formation on the Matrigel to exert antiangiogenic effect via the inhibition of BMP2/Smad1/5/8/Id1 signaling. Thus, RN1 suppressed the microvessel formation in the BxPC-3 pancreatic cancer cell xenograft tumor in nude mice.[52]

Other Bioactivities

Tian Qi (Notoginseng) exerts significant beneficial effects in treating trauma and bleeding caused by internal and external injury, promoting blood circulation, and reducing blood clotting. Hence, Tian Qi is the important ingredient in Yunnan Baiyao, one of the most famous Chinese medicines. The Tian Qi saponins were demonstrated to possess multiple ranges of activities in cardiovascular and cerebrovascular system, CNS, hematopoietic system, immune system, as well as antifibrosis, antiaging hemostatic, antioxidant, hypolipidemic, hepatoprotective, and renoprotective activities.

References

1. Park, S. C. et al. 2009. Induction of apoptosis in human lung carcinoma cells by the water extract of *Panax notoginseng* is associated with the activation of caspase-3 through down-regulation of Akt. *Intl. J. Oncol.* 35: 121–7.
2. Park, S. C. et al. 2013. Antitumor effects of water extracts of *Panax notoginseng* on NCI-H460 tumor regression model. *J. Korean Oriental Med.* 31: 8–16.
3. Wang, C. Z. et al. 2009. Anti-proliferative effects of different plant parts of *Panax notoginseng* on SW480 human colorectal cancer cells. *Phytother. Res.* 23: 6–13.
4. Wang, C. Z. et al. 2007. Chemopreventive effects of *Panax notoginseng* and its major constituents on SW480 human colorectal cancer cells. *Intl. J. Oncol.* 31: 1149–56.
5. Konoshima, T. et al. 1996. Antitumor-promoting activities of the roots of *Panax notoginseng* I. *Nat. Med.* 50: 158–62.
6. Konoshima, T. et al. 1999. Anticarcinogenic activity of the roots of *Panax notoginseng*. II. *Biol. Pharm. Bull.* 22: 1150–2.
7. Konoshima, T. et al. 1997. Antitumor-promoting activities of ginsenoside Rg1 and *Panax notoginseng*. *Food Factors for Cancer Prevent., Int. Conf. Food Factors: Chem. Cancer Prev., Hamamatsu, Japan*, December 1995; pp. 235–9.
8. Toh, D. F. et al. 2011. Anti-proliferative effects of raw and steamed extracts of *Panax notoginseng* and its ginsenoside constituents on human liver cancer cells. *Chin. Med.* 6: 4.
9. Sun, S. et al. Red notoginseng: Higher ginsenoside content and stronger anticancer potential than Asian and American ginseng. *Food Chem.* 125: 1299–305.
10. He, N. W. et al. 2012. Antioxidant, antiproliferative, and pro-apoptotic activities of a saponin extract derived from the roots of *Panax notoginseng* (Burk.) F. H. Chen. *J. Med. Food* 15: 350–9.
11. Shang, X. L. et al. 2006. Inhibitory effects on human hepatocarcinoma cells with panax notoginseng saponins. *Zhongguo Linchuang Kangfu* 10: 121–3.
12. Wang, Q. X. et al. 2011. Antitumor effects and mechanisms of *Panax notoginseng* saponin on human multiple myeloma cell line RPMI8226. *Xiandai Zhongliu Yixue* 19: 1953–5.
13. Cheng, F. Y. et al. 2011. Effect of *Panax notoginseng* saponins on tumor proliferation of human HepG2 cells and its mechanis. *J. Hebei Med. Univ.* 32: 447–9.
14. Lu, X. R. et al. 2011. Expressions of Bcl2 and Bax in cell line BGC823 induced by *Panax notoginseng* saponins. *Yaowu Fenxi Zazhi* 31: 570–3.
15. Pei, X. D. et al. 2014. Influence of *Panax notoginsenosides* on AFP-L3 and GP-73 expressions in hepatoma cell lines. *Shijie Huaren Xiaohua Zazhi*, 22: 3619–24.
16. Wen, L. L. et al. 2013. Effects of *Panax notoginseng* saponins on the proliferation of three different kinds of human hepatoma cell line. *Zhongliu Yaoxue* 3: 100–3, 125.
17. Zhang, Z. L. et al. 2014. *Panax notoginseng* saponins induces the apoptosis of human lung adenocarcinoma A549 cells. *Xuzhou Yixueyuan Xuebao* 34: 515–9.
18. Li, X. H. et al. 2004. Effect of *Panax notoginseng* saponin on procoagulant activity and differentiation induction in NB4 cells. *Zhongguo Zhongyi Yanjiuyuan Zhuban* 24: 63–6.
19. Liu, L. L. et al. 2008. Reversal effect of *Panax notoginseng* saponins on multidrug resistance breast cancer cell MCF/ADM. *Shizhen Guoyi Guoyao* 19: 954–6.
20. Ni, X. C. et al. 2011. Inhibition of the proliferation and migration of human prostate cancer PC3 cells by total *Panax notoginseng* saponins. *Zhongguo Zhongliu Linchuang* 38: 638–41.
21. Zhang, B. et al. 2010. Effect of *Panax notoginseng* saponins on growth and metastasis of malignant melanoma. *Zhongguo Jiceng Yiyao* 17: 755–7.
22. Chen, P. F. et al. 2006. Effects of ethanol extracts of *Panax notoginseng* on liver metastasis of B16 melanoma grafted in mice. *J. Chin. Integr. Med.* 4: 500–3.
23. Wang, P. W. et al. 2014. *Panax notoginseng* saponins (PNS) inhibit breast cancer metastasis. *J. Ethnopharmacol.* 154: 663–71.
24. Wang, C. Z. et al. 2007. Notoginseng enhances anticancer effect of 5-fuorouracil on human colorectal cancer cells. *Cancer Chemother. Pharmacol.* 60: 69–79.

25. Huang, M. et al. 2011. Impact of Panax notoginsenoside and tamoxifen on breast cancer T47D cell. *Shijie Zhongyiyao* 6: 340–2.
26. Liu, S. J. et al. 2000. *Panax notoginseng* saponins attenuated cisplatin-induced nephrotoxicity. *Acta Pharmacol. Sinica* 21: 257–60.
27. Zhang, C. L. et al. 2008. Efficacy-enhancing and toxicity-attenuating effect of *Panax notoginseng* saponins on cyclophosphamide. *Nanjing Zhongyiyao Daxue Xuebao* 24: 254–6.
28. Liu, L. et al. 2008. Protective effect of saponins from *Panax notoginseng* against doxorubicin-induced cardiotoxicity in mice. *Planta Med.* 74: 203–9.
29. Shi, R. et al. 2007. Study on protective effects of *Panax notoginseng* saponins on doxorubicin-induced myocardial damage. *Zhongguo Zhongyao Zazhi* 32: 2632–5.
30. Sun, S. et al. 2009. Effect of steaming the root of *Panax notoginseng* on chemical composition and anticancer activities. *Food Chem.* 118: 307–14.
31. Qi, X. Y. et al. 2012. *Panax notoginseng* saponins R1 enhances the cytotoxicity of cisplatin via gap junction intercellular communication. *J. Bengbu Med. College* 37: 134–6, 141.
32. Mao, Q. et al. 2012. Target separation of a new antitumor saponin and metabolic profiling of leaves of *Panax notoginseng* by liquid chromatography with eletrospray ionization quadrupole time-of-flight mass spectrometry. *J. Pharm. Biomed. Anal.* 59: 67–77.
33. Gu, L. H. 2012. Research progress on the antitumor mechanisms of saponins. *Chin. J. Crit. Care Med.* (Elect. Edit.) 5: 344–50.
34. Fu, H. Z. et al. 2013. A new protopanaxadiol-type ginsenoside from the roots of *Panax notoginseng. J. Asian Nat. Prod. Res.* 15: 1139–43.
35. Yang, Z. G .et al. 2006. Ginsenoside Rd from *Panax notoginseng* is cytotoxic towards HeLa cancer cells and induces apoptosis. *Chem. Biodiver.* 3: 187–97.
36. Chen, B. et al. 2013. The apoptosis-inducing effect of ginsenoside F4 from steamed notoginseng on human lymphocytoma JK cells. *Nat. Prod. Res.* 27: 2351–4.
37. Chen, B. et al. 2013. Apoptosis-inducing effect of ginsenoside Rg6 on human lymphocytoma JK cells. *Mol.* 18: 8109–19.
38. Gao, B. et al. 2014. p38 MAPK and ERK1/2 pathways are involved in the pro-apoptotic effect of notoginsenoside Ft1 on human neuroblastoma SH-SY5Y cells. *Life Sci.* 108: 63–70.
39. Bi, X. L. et al. 2009. Anticancer activity of *Panax notoginseng* extract 20(S)-25-OCH_3-PPD: Targetting β-catenin signalling. *Clin. Exp. Pharmacol. Physiol.* 36: 1074–8.
40. Wu, Y. L. et al. 2011. 25-OCH_3-PPD induces the apoptosis of activated t-HSC/Cl-6 cells via c-FLIP-mediated NF-κB activation. *Chemico-Biol. Interactions* 194: 106–12.
41. Zhao, Y. et al. 2007. Isolation, structural determination, and evaluation of the biological activity of 20(S)-25-methoxyldammarane-3β,12β, 20-triol [20(S)-25-OCH_3-PPD], a novel natural product from *Panax notoginseng. Med. Chem.* 3: 51–60.
42. Wang, W. et al. 2009. Novel ginsenosides 25-OH-PPD and 25-OCH_3-PPD as experimental therapy for pancreatic cancer: Anticancer activity and mechanisms of action. *Cancer Lett.* 278: 241–8.
43. Wang, W. et al. 2009. Anti-lung cancer effects of novel ginsenoside 25-OCH_3-PPD. *Lung cancer* (Amsterdam, Netherlands) 65: 306–11.
44. Wang, W. et al. 2008. 20(S)-25-methoxyldammarane-3β,12β, 20-triol, a novel natural product for prostate cancer therapy: Activity in vitro and in vivo and mechanisms of action. *British J. Cancer* 98: 792–802.
45. Yan, Z. H. et al. 2011. Induction of apoptosis in human promyelocytic leukemia HL60 cells by panaxynol and panaxydol. *Mol.* 16: 5561–73.
46. Hai, J. et al. 2008. Growth inhibition and induction of differentiation by panaxydol in rat C6 glioma cells. *Neurological Res.* 30: 99–105.
47. Wang, Z. J. et al. 2011. Induction of differentiation by panaxydol in human hepatocarcinoma SMMC-7721 cells via cAMP and MAP kinase dependent mechanism. *Yakugakuzasshi* (*J. Pharm. Soc. Jpn.*) 131: 993–1000.
48. Zhao, Y. et al. 2010. Pharmacokinetics of panaxatrol disuccinate sodium, a novel anticancer drug from *Panax notoginseng*, in healthy volunteers and patients with advanced solid tumors. *Acta Pharmacol. Sinica* 31, 1515–22.
49. Li, Q. et al. 2001. Isolation, identification and physiological activities of 2-(1′,2′,3′,4′-tetrahydroxybutyl)-6-(2″,3′,4″-trihydroxybutyl) pyrazine from *Panax notoginseng. Chem. J. Chin. Univ.* 22: 1824–8.
50. Chou, P. Y. et al. 2011. Trilinolein inhibits proliferation of human non-small cell lung carcinoma A549 through the modulation of PI3K/Akt pathway. *Am. J. Chin. Med.* 39: 803–15.
51. Gao, H. et al. 1996. Immunostimulating polysaccharides from *Panax notoginseng. Pharm. Res.* 13: 1196–200.
52. Wang, P. P. et al. 2015. An arabinogalactan from flowers of *Panax notoginseng* inhibits angiogenesis by BMP2/Smad/Id1 signaling. *Carbohydr. Polym.* 121: 328–35.

141 Sang Huang 桑黄

False tinder polypore or Flecked flesh polypore

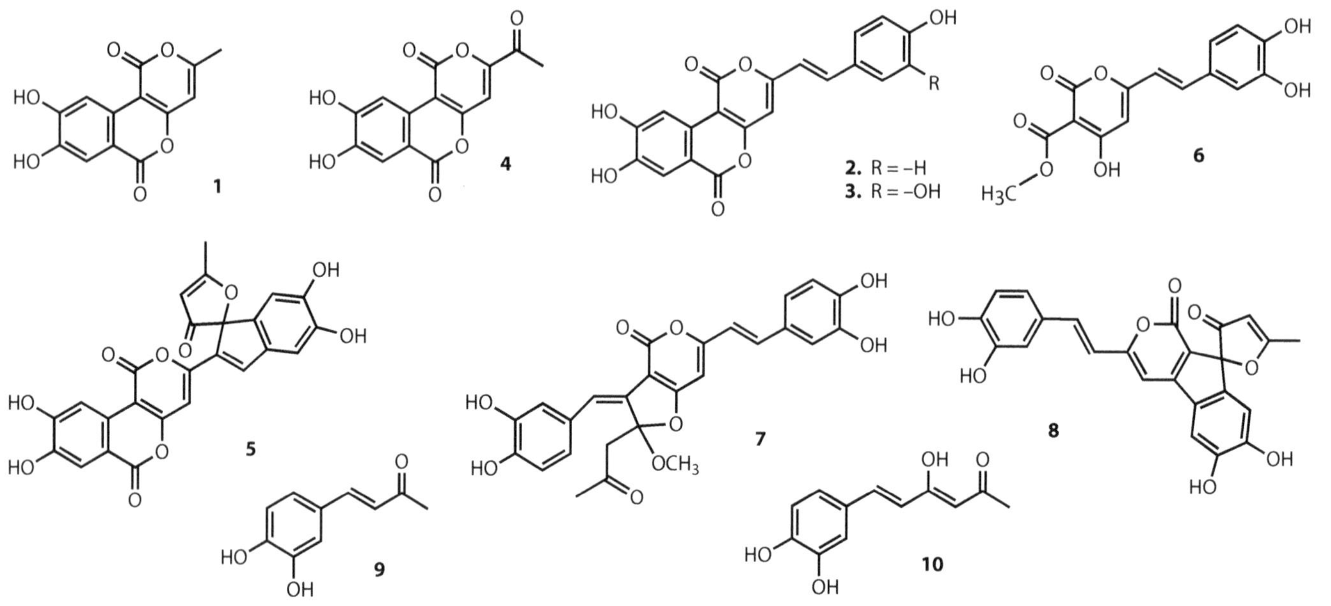

Herb Origination

The herb Sang Huang (Flecked flesh polypore) is the dried fruit body of fungi *Phellinus igniarius.* (Polyporaceae). It is a parasite on the stems of many hardwoods such as mulberry, birch, pine, poplar, and aspen, and the mulberry is the best host tree for the herb quality. The fungi are widely distributed in many places in Chinese forests. Two other fungi in the same genus, *P. linteus* and *P. baumii*, have similar biological activities and can be used as supplemental sources of the herb Sang Huang. The commercial cultivation of the fungi has been successful.

Antitumor Activities

Sang Huang extracts displayed obvious antineoplastic and immunoregulative effects. In sarcoma 180 and MFC gastric cancer models implanted in mice, its extract (*P. linteus*) given in an oral dose of 0.5 g/kg/day to the mice for 14 days markedly suppressed the cell growth with inhibitory rates of 46.07% and 43.09%, respectively.[1] When i.g. administration of its water extract in doses of 0.5–2.0 g/kg per day for 10 days is done to tumor-bearing mice, the inhibitory rates were 38.0–53.6% on sarcoma 180, 44.83–51.15% on MFC, and 38.27–55.61% on H22 hepatoma. The survival time was prolonged by 35.1–43.9% in mice bearing sarcoma 180. The antitumor activity was revealed to be mediated by increasing the indexes of the immune organs and the levels of IL-2 and TNFα in the serum.[2] The treatment with the extract could also promote the cell apoptosis and retard the growth of human prostate cancer cells (DU145 and PC3) *in vitro* and *in vivo*.[3] The dry matter of the culture broth from *P. igniarius* and its fraction-II were able to elicit tumor cell necrosis and to extend the life span of mice implanted with H22 hepatoma together with the decrease of Bcl-2 expression and the increase of Bax expression. When the extract (1000 mg/kg/day) or the fraction-II (360 mg/kg/day) is orally given to mice, the growth inhibitory rates were 33.5% and 40.3% against H22 hepatoma, respectively.[4]

The aqueous extracts of the fruiting bodies of *P. igniarius* (PI) and *P. linteus* (PL) also exhibited antimutagenic activity against indirect-acting mutagens (2-aminofluorene and BAP) and direct-acting mutagens (sodium azide and 4-nitro-*O*-phenylenediamine) on *Salmonella typhimurium* strains TA 98 and TA 100. Furthermore, both extracts from PI and PL were able to increase GST activities and GSH level in cultured murine Hepa1c1c7 hepatoma cells, suggesting that the herb Sang Huang has promising potential in the liver cancer chemoprevention.[5]

Antitumor Constituents and Activities

Pyranobenzopyrans

Phelligridins-A (**1**)–E isolated from the ethanolic extract of Sang Huang fruiting body exhibited a different degree of cytotoxicity (IC_{50}: 0.008–0.192 μM) against a small panel of human cancer cell lines such as MCF-7 (breast), BGC 823 (gastric), A549 (lung), Bel7402 (liver), Ketr3 (renal), and HCT-8 (colon) tumor cells *in vitro*.[6] Of these compounds, phelligridin-C (**2**) and phelligridin-D (**3**) selectively and significantly suppressed the proliferative of A549 and Bel-7402 cells with the highest IC_{50} values in range of 0.008–0.016 μM, while phelligridin-J (**4**) only exerted relatively lower antigrowth effect against A549 and Bel-7402 cell lines *in vitro* with the respective IC_{50} values of 4.2 and 9.2 μM. To human A2780 ovarian cancer and HCT-8 colon cancer cell lines, phelligridin-J (**4**) and phelligridin-G (**5**) showed moderate and selective cytotoxicity *in vitro* with IC_{50} values between 7.2 and 30.2 μM.[7,8] A pyranopyran derivative assigned as phelligridin-B

(**6**) was also effective in the *in vitro* experiment, and its best suppression was shown in the Bel-7402 hepatoma cells (IC_{50}: 0.050 μM).[6] Considering the structure and the bioactivity relationship in the Bel-7402 cells, a parahydroxystyryl moiety linked at a pyranone ring seems important for the antihepatoma potency.[6]

Additionally, the antineoplasm-related antioxidant activity such as inhibiting rat liver microsomal lipid peroxidation was observed after the treatment with phelligridin-G (**5**), phelligridin-H, phelligridin-I, and phelligridin-J (**4**), respectively, and their moderate IC_{50} values ranged from 3.7 to 8.2 μM. Both phelligridin-H and phelligridin-I were also reported as inhibitors of protein tyrosine phosphatase-1B.[7,8]

Furopyrans

Two isolated fyrapyran derivatives assigned as phelligridin-F (**7**) and inoscavin-A (**8**) demonstrated noticeable cytotoxic effect against the same panel of human neoplastic cell lines *in vitro*. In the Ketr3 renal cancer cells and the HCT-8 colon cancer cells, their suppressive degrees were in a similar level (IC_{50}: >0.104 versus >0.108 μM), but in the A549 lung cancer, MCF-7 breast cancer, and BGC 823 gastric cancer cell lines, the activities of phelligridin-F (**7**) were 1.17–1.28 times more potent than those of inoscavin-A (**8**) (IC_{50}: 0.084–0.095 versus >0.108 μM), and in the Bel-7402 hepatoma cells, both presented a similar level of inhibitory effect (IC_{50}: 0.046 versus 0.088 μM).[6]

Dihydroxystyryl Derivatives

Compared to (E)-4-(3,4-dihydroxyphenyl)but-3-en-2-one (**9**), hispolon (**10**) was more sensitive to MCF-7 breast cancer and Bel-7402 hepatoma cell lines with IC_{50} values of 0.025 and 0.038 μM, respectively. Both derivatives showed the similar degree of antiproliferative activities, and their IC_{50} values in the A549, BGC823, Ketr3, and HCT-8 cell lines ranged between 0.14 and >0.28 μM.[6–8] Hispolon (**10**) also exerted the inhibitory effect on the proliferation of various AML cell lines such as NB4 and HL-60 cells. In the NB4 cells, hispolon (**10**) induced G0/G1-phase arrest, associated with a marked decrease in the protein expression of p53, cyclin-D1, cyclin-E, and CDK-2 and CDK-4, with concomitant induction of p21waf1/Cip1 and p27Kip1. Hispolon (**10**) also promoted both extrinsic and intrinsic apoptotic pathways, such as activation of caspase-3, caspase-8, caspase-9, PARP, and Bax protein and increases of the levels of intrinsic related proteins (cytochrome c), the extrinsic apoptotic proteins (Fas and FasL), and the ratio of Bax/Bcl-2, in the NB4 cells.[9] Hispolon (**10**) induced the HL-60 cell apoptosis through JNK1/2-mediated activation of caspase-8, caspase-9, and caspase-3 plus PARP cleavage. The antileukemia activity was further demonstrated in mice with HL-60 tumor xenografts.[10]

In correlation with the induction of cell cycle arrest at S phase and apoptosis, the antiproliferative activity of hispolon (**10**) was elicited in human Hep3B hepatocellular carcinoma cells. The mechanistic exploration revealed that the S phase arrest by hispolon (**10**) was associated with a marked decrease in the expression of cyclin-A, cyclin-E, and CDK-2 proteins and the induction of p21waf1/Cip1 and p27Kip1, and the elicited apoptosis was evidenced by the upregulation of JNK, p38 MAPK, and ERK expressions, caspase activation, and PARP cleavage.[11] In two lung cancer cell lines (A549 and H661), hispolon (**10**) suppressed the cell viability and elicited G0/G1 cell cycle arrest and apoptosis via (1) increases of the expression of CDK inhibitor p21CIP1 and p27KIP1 and of p53; (2) decrease of the expression of cyclin-D1, cyclin-E, CDK2, CDK4, and CDK6; (3) loss of mitochondrial membrane potential and release of cytochrome c into the cytosol; and (4) cleavage of caspase-9, caspase-3, and PARP. However, the hispolon treatment was more effective on H661 cells than on A549 cells in inhibiting cell viability and inducing cell apoptosis.[12] Hispolon (**10**) was also capable of retarding the invasion, the motility, and the metastasis of human SK-Hep1 hepatoma cells in the absence of cytotoxicity. The antiinvasive and antimetastatic mechanism was found to be mediated by the reduced expression of MMP-2, MMP-9, and u-PA through the suppression of FAK signaling pathway and the activity of PI3K/Akt and RhoA.[13]

Accordingly, these findings evidenced that hispolon (**10**) may have the developmental potential to serve as a therapeutic adjuvant for the treatment of several types of neoplastic diseases and the prevention of cancer cell metastasis.

Triterpenoids

The total triterpenoid extract from *P. igniarius* displayed the suppressive effect against the proliferation of human U251 glioblastoma cells together with enhancing the apoptotic death of tumor cells.[14]

Polysaccharides

Polysaccharide components are the major contributors for the anticancer effect of Sang Huang (*P. igniarius* and *P. linteus*), which usually showed no direct repressive effect against the tumor cell growth, but they displayed obvious anticarcinoma effect in animal models. The oral administration of the polysaccharides (from the mycelium of *P. igniarius*) in dosages of 0.1–0.4 g/kg per day markedly inhibited the cell growth of entity sarcoma 180 by 31.8–53.13% in mice and prolonged the life duration of mice bearing ascites sarcoma 180.[15,16] The polysaccharides (from *P. linteus*) extended the survival time of mice bearing Ehrlich ascites carcinoma by 47.2–50.4% at an oral dose of 0.5–1.0 g/kg per day[16] and restrained the growth of murine H22 hepatoma and LLC *in vivo* at doses of 0.25–1.0 g/kg per day.[15–17] Simultaneously, the spleen index, the thyme index, and the interleukin-2 in tumor-bearing mice were significantly augmented, the macrophages activity and the phagocytosis ability were enhanced, and the secretion of TNFα from the macrophages was improved after the treatment with the polysaccharides.[15–19] The evidences clearly indicated that the neoplasm inhibition of Sang Huang polysaccharides is mainly attributed to their significant immunoregulative function. However, the polysaccharides extracted from *P. baumii* interestingly demonstrated direct *in vitro* inhibitory effect on sarcoma 180 cells through the direct induction of the tumor cell apoptosis and the G2/M cell cycle arrest.[20] *P. igniarius* polysaccharides also showed the *in vitro* inhibitory effect on the cell growth of human HepG2 hepetoma and MCF-7 breast cancer. The highest inhibitory rates on the HepG2 and MCF-7 cell lines were 59.18% and 55.39% at the half-suppressive concentrations of 196.9 and 162.5 μg/mL, respectively.[21]

The Sang Huang polysaccharides also exhibited remarkable anticarcinogenesis-related, antioxidative, and antimutagenic properties. These effects were principally associated with the marked activation of anticarcinogenic enzymes, such as SOD, GST, QR, and GSH, and notable reduction of MDA, LPO, and free radicals.[5,22] By means of micronucleus and sperm abnormality tests in mice, the *P. igniarius* polysaccharides were verified to have an ability to protect bone marrow polychromatic erythrocyte damaged from the mutation of CTX and to markedly reduce the frequency of abnormal sperms and micronucleus caused by CTX.[21] Based upon these data, the Sang Huang polysaccharides have been demonstrated to possess remarkable potential in the promotion of human immunoprotective system and the prevention of carcinogenesis.

A water-soluble anticancer active polysaccharide labeled PB (17 kDa) was prepared from the mycelia of *P. baumii*. The immunoregulatory activity of PB were shown in RAW264.7 macrophages *in vitro*, and the PB treatment exerted a significant increase of cellular proliferation rate, NO production, and expression levels of IL-1β, IL-18, IL-6, IL-12p35, and IL-12p40 genes. The exposure of HepG2 cells to PB (400 μg/mL) after 48 h resulted in the induction of S phase cell arrest and apoptotic death, leading to a marked inhibitory effect against the proliferation of the human hepatoma cells.[23] PL and PLP60-B1 are two polysaccharides obtained from two species of mushrooms *P. linteus* and *P. baumii*, respectively. Both showed similar S phase cell arrest-moderated antiproliferative, antiadhesive and antiinvasive activities on the HepG2 cells *in vitro* and immunoenhancing properties.[24,25] From the fruit bodies of *P. igniarius* produced in Korea and Japan, two individual polysaccharides were purified, exerting marked antigrowth effect in mice bearing sarcoma with the inhibitory rates of 52.36% and 72.64%, respectively. The polysaccharide from Japanese *P. igniarius* consisted of six monosaccharides (rhamnose, arabinose, xylose, glucose, mannose, and galactose), whereas the polysaccharide from Korean *P. igniarius* consisted of five monosaccharides (rhamnose, arabinose, glucose, mannose, and galactose).[26] From a water-soluble intracellular polysaccharides (IPS) extracted from the cultured mycelia of *P. igniarius*, four homogeneous polysaccharides, IPSW-1 (34.1 kDa), IPSW-2 (17.7 kDa), IPSW-3 (15.1 kDa), and IPSW-4 (21.7 kDa), were purified. IPSW-1, IPSW-2, and IPSW-3 only contained glucose, while IPSW-4 was composed of rhamnose, xylose, mannose, glucose, and galactose in a molar ratio of 1.29:1.21:1:43.86:1.86. All these IPSWs could dose-dependently retard the growth of human SW480 (colon) and HepG2 (liver) cancer cell lines, but the inhibitory potencies were IPSW1 > IPSW3 > IPSW2 > IPSW4.27. Hence, the polysaccharides of *P. igniarius* should be considered as a source of prospective anticancer agent.

Exopolysaccharide

An exopolysaccharise termed PIEP was prepared from *P. igniarius*, which exhibited antitumor- and LPO-resisting effects on HepG2 hepatoma and MCF-7 breast cancer. The IC_{50} values of PIEP were 194.42 and 261.56 μg/mL, and the *in vivo* inhibitory rates at doses of 300 and 600 mg/kg/day were 44.78% and 49.63%, respectively, in animal models transplanted with two tumors. Importantly, PIEP is capable of suppressing the gene mutation of body cells and germ cells induced by CTX. PIEP also markedly reduced the sperm abnormality frequency, distinctly increased the activity of SOD, and decreased the content of MDA in the serum and the liver of traumatic mice.[27] Therefore, PIEP is confirmed to be an antitumor immunostimulating and antioxidative agent similar to the Sang Huang polysaccharides.

Endo-Polysaccharide

PIE was an endo-polysaccharide purified from the submerged fermentation product of *Phellinus igniarius*, which was composed of mannose, xylose, fucose, glucose, and galactose with a molar ratio of 1:2.3:6.4:22.1:19.83. The oral administration of PIE characteristically inhibited the growth of sarcoma 180 and H22 hepatoma cells and prolonged the life span of mice. Simultaneously, the IL-2 and/or IL-18 concentrations were significantly augmented in the serum in doses of 500 and 250 mg/kg. The evidences implied that the antitumor effect of PIE should also be largely attributed to the immunostimulating potential.[28]

Heteropolysaccharide

P60W-1 (17.1 kDa) was extracted from the fruit bodies of Chinese *P. igniarius*, which consist of fucose, glucose, mannose, galactose, and 3-*O*-methylgalactose in a molar ratio 1:1:1:2:1. The treatment with P60W-1 in a dose of 100 mg/kg per day showed an *in vivo* antitumor effect, inhibiting the growth of hepatoma H22 and Lewis lung cancer cells in mice by 48% and 37%, respectively.[29]

Protein-Bound Polysaccharides

An isolated protein-bound polysaccharide (PL) significantly repressed the proliferation of human SW480 colon cancer cells *in vitro* and *in vivo*. After the treatment, the expressions of β-catenin and cyclin-D1 were diminished and the transcription activities of T cell factor and lymphocyte-enhancer binding factor were markedly reduced. Also, the HUVEC proliferation index, the capillary tube formation, and the MVD were notably lessened. These data suggest that PL is capable of suppressing tumor growth, invasion, and angiogenesis through the inhibition of Wnt/β-catenin signaling in the SW480 cell lines.[30]

P1, a proteoglycan purified from *Phellinus linteus*, showed an antiproliferative effect against four tested human neoplastic cell lines, HepG2 (liver), HT-29 (colon), NCI-H 460 (lung), and MCF-7 (breast), *in vitro*; especially, P1 was greatly effective in the suppression of HT-29 cells. Along with the blockage of Reg IV/EGFR/Akt signaling pathway and the activation of P27kip1-cyclin D1/E-CDK2 pathway, P1 promoted the HT-29 cells to apoptosis and induced S phase cell cycle arrest.[31,32] When *in vivo* treatment with P1 in a dose of 100 mg/kg is done, the indexes of the spleen and the thymus and the levels of plasmatic pIgR and IgA were significantly elevated as well in HT-29-bearing mice. These results evidenced that P1 played two potential roles in the anticancer effect, i.e., (1) directly suppressing the cancer cell growth and inducing the cell apoptosis, and (2) promoting the host immune functions partly by protecting T cells from escaping PGE2 attack and enhancing the mucosal IgA response.[31,32] Similarly, the S phase cell arrest was also caused by P1

(200 μg/mL) significantly in HepG2 hepatoma cells followed by the reduction of calreticulin expression and the augmentation of P27kipl-cyclin A/D1/E-CDK2 pathway, whose antihepatoma effect was further demonstrated in an animal model. The intragastrical administration of P1 in 200 mg/kg dose for 18 days significantly diminished the solid tumor volume and weight in nude mice implanted with HepG2 cells.[33]

Glycoprotein

A glycoprotein PLG-3 was isolated from the cultured mycelia of *Phellinus linteus* AML1101 with cold water, whose molecular weight is 2.5×10^4 Da. PLG-3 consisted of approximately 85.5% protein and 13.7% polysaccharide, and its polysaccharide portion is composed of mannose, xylose, arabinose, glucose, and galactose with a molar ratio of 7.74:2.22:1.46:1.29:0.61. PLG-3 exhibited moderate antiproliferative effect on A549 lung carcinoma cells and HepG2 hepatoma cells *in vitro* with IC_{50} values (at 72 h) of 16.54 and 18.30 μg/L, respectively.[34]

Enzyme

Sang Huang secretes a main lignolytic enzyme designated as a lignin peroxidase (molecular weight: 37 kDa). This lignin peroxidase could hydrolyze steam-exploded wood powder (*Quercus mongolica*) into small lignin molecules (ELg). The ELg displayed cytotoxicity against several cancer cell lines (such as HepG2 hepatoma, B16 melanoma, SK-N-SH neuroblastoma, and MBT-2 bladder cancer), but the cytotoxic effect of ELg on normal Chang liver cells was much less active than on the HepG2 and B16 cells. The finding suggested that the lignin peroxidase may be applied for the generation of valuable medical products by biodegradation from wood lignocellulose.[35]

Adjuvant Application

Sang Huang contains abundant biologically active and degradative enzymes. When soybeans or waxy brown rice are fermented with the fungus *P. igniarius*, more effective extract or polysaccharides could be artificially produced. The methanolic extracts derived from the fermentation of these materials with Sang Huang fungi exhibited notably enhanced inhibition of polyamine biosynthesis and activities of phase II and antioxidant enzymes, i.e., QR, GST, SOD, and GSH levels, in Hepalclc7 cells (murine hepatoma) *in vitro* and *in vivo*.[36–38] In general, the elevation of the phase II and the antioxidant enzyme activities was more pronounced in the liver and the kidney than in the lung, the stomach, and the colon.[36] The polysaccharides from soybeans after the fermentation with the fungi *P. igniarius* significantly diminished the tumor incidence in a two-stage skin carcinogenesis mouse model initiated by DMBA and promoted with TPA for 12 weeks. After the treatment, the numbers of skin tumors per mouse were repressed by 70–88%, and the percentage of mice with tumors was decreased by 30%–70%.[39]

The results suggested that the adjuvant application of Sang Huang may be useful to produce potential agents for cancer chemoprevention and polyamine metabolism inhibition in various target organs.

References

1. Wen, K. et al. 2002. Comparision of antitumor activity among four antitumor drugs including *Phellinus linteus*. *J. Jilin Univ. (Med. Edit.)* 38: 247–9.
2. Zhang, W. et al. 2011. Antitumor effect of *Phellinus linteus* and its mechanism. *Zhongcaoyao* 42: 2047–50.
3. Tsuji, T. et al. 2010. *Phellinus linteus* extract sensitizes advanced prostate cancer cells to apoptosis in athymic nude mice. *PLoS One* 5: e9885.
4. Geng, Y. et al. 2013. Effects of dry matter of culture broth from *Phellinus igniarius* submerged fermentation and its fractions on mice hepatoma 22. *Junwu Xuebao* 32: 1046–55.
5. Shon, Y. H. et al. 2001. Antimutagenicity and induction of anticarcinogenic phase II enzymes by basidiomycetes. *J. Ethnopharmacol.* 77: 103–9.
6. Mo, S. Y. et al. 2004. Phelligridins C-F: Cytotoxic pyrano[4,3-c][2]benzopyran-1,6-dione and furo [3,2-c]pyran-4-one derivatives from the fungus *Phellinus igniarius*. *J. Nat. Prod.* 67: 823–8.
7. Wang, Y. et al. 2007. Structures, biogenesis, and biological activities of pyrano[4,3-c]iso-chromen-4-one derivatives from the fungus *Phellinus igniarius*. *J. Nat. Prod.* 70: 296–99.
8. Wang, Y. et al. 2005. A unique highly oxygenated pyrano[4,3-c][2]benzopyran-1,6-dione derivative with antioxidant and cytotoxic activities from the fungus *Phellinus igniarius*. *Organic Lett.* 7: 1675–8.
9. Chen, Y. C. et al. 2013. Hispolon from *Phellinus linteus* induces G0/G1 cell cycle arrest and apoptosis in NB4 human leukaemia cells. *Am. J. Chinese Med.* 41: 1439–57.
10. Hsiao, P. C. et al. 2013. Hispolon induces apoptosis through JNK1/2-mediated activation of a caspase-8, -9, and -3-dependent pathway in acute myeloid leukemia (AML) cells and inhibits AML exnograft tumor growth in vivo. *J. Agric. Food Chem.* 61: 10063–73.
11. Huang, G. J. et al. 2011. Hispolon induces apoptosis and cell cycle arrest of human hepatocellular carcinoma Hep3B cells by modulating ERK phosphorylation. *J. Agric. Food Chem.* 59: 7104–13.
12. Wu, Q. G. et al. 2014. The anticancer effects of hispolon on lung cancer cells. *Biochem. Biophys. Res. Commun.* 453: 385–91.
13. Huang, G. J. et al. 2010. Hispolon suppresses SK-Hepl human hepatoma cell metastasis by inhibiting matrix metalloproteinase-2/9 and urokinase-plasminogen activator through the PI3K/Akt and ERK signaling pathways. *J. Agric. Food Chem.* 58: 9468–75.
14. Xie, J. N. et al. 2012. Extraction of total triterpenoids from *Phellinus igniarius* and evaluation its inhibitory activity on human glioblastoma U251 cells in vitro. *Zhongguo Shiyan Fangjixue Zazhi* 18: 24–6.
15. Yang, Q. et al. 2006. Study on antitumor effect of medicinal fungi *Phellinus igniarius* extracts. *Zhongguo Zhongyao Zazhi* 31: 1713–5.
16. Dong, W. et al. 2009. Tumor-inhibitory and liver-protective effects of *Phellinus igniarius* extracellular polysaccharides. *World J. Microbiol. Biotech.* 25: 633–8.
17. Zhang, J. et al. 2006. Studies of *Phellinus linteus* aboutantitumor activity and enhancing immune effect. *Chinese J. Integrated Tradit. Western Med.* 7: 1825–7.

18. Zhang, M. et al. 2006. Studies on the antitumor activity of *Phellinus linteus*. *Zhongyao Yaoli yu Linchunag* 22: 56–8.
19. Liu, H. Y. et al. 2006. Studies of the antitumor activities and effects on the immune function of Sang-Huang mushroom polysaccharides in mice. *J. Taishan Med. College* 27: 211–3.
20. Wu, W. W. et al. 2007. The direct repressive effect of polysaccharide from *Phellinus baumii* Piat on tumor cell line S180. *J. Liaoning Med. Univ.* 22–4.
21. Li, Y. M. et al. 2006. Inhibitory effect of polysaccharide from *Phellinus igniarius* on tumor growth in vitro and mutation induced by CP. *J. Zhongguo Univ. Tech.* 36: 700–4.
22. Zheng, L. J. et al. 2006. The antimutation and antioxidationeffects of *Phellinus igniarius* intracellular polysaccharide. *Carcinogenesis, Teratogenesis Mutagenesis* 18: 465–8.
23. Xue, Q. et al. 2011. Immunostimulatory and antitumor activity of a water-soluble polysaccharide from *Phellinus baumii* mycelia. *World J. Microbiol. Biotechnol.* 27: 1017–23.
24. Wang, G. B. et al. 2011. Inhibitory effects of *Phellinus baumii* polysaccharide on the proliferation and invasion of HepG2 cell. Junwu Xuebao 30: 288–94.
25. Wang, G. B. et al. 2012. Polysaccharides from *Phellinus linteus* inhibit cell growth and invasion and induce apoptosis in HepG2 human hepatocellular carcinoma cells. *Biologia* 67: 247–54.
26. Qin, J. Z. et al. 2009. Antitumor effect of polysaccharide from *Phellinus igniarius* fruit-body. *Shipin Keji* 204–7.
27. Zheng, L. J. et al. 2007. Preliminary study on pharmacological activities of exopolysaccharides of *Phellinus igniarius*. *Shipin Kexue* 28: 318–21.
28. Chen, L. et al. 2011. Endo-polysaccharide of *Phellinus igniarius* exhibited anti-tumor effect through enhancement of cell mediated immunity. *Intl. Immuno-pharmacol.* 11: 255–9.
29. Yang, Y. et al. 2008. Research on the structure and antitumor activity of polysaccharide P60W-1 isolated from fruiting bodies of *Phellinus igniarius*. *Mushroom Sci.* 17: 700–14.
30. Song, K. S. et al. 2011. Protein-bound polysaccharide from *Phellinus linteus* inhibits tumor growth, invasion, and angiogenesis and alters Wnt/β-catenin in SW480 human colon cancer cells. *BMC Cancer* 11: 307.
31. Li, Y. G. et al. 2011. Antitumor effects of proteoglycan from *Phellinus linteus* by immunomodulating and inhibiting Reg IV/EGFR/Akt signaling pathway in colorectal carcinoma. *Intl. J. Biol. Macromol.* 48: 511–7.
32. Zhong, S. et al. 2013. Activation of P27kipl-cyclin Dl/E-CDK2 pathway by polysaccharide from *Phellinus linteus* leads to S-phase arrest in HT-29 cells. *Chemico-Biological Interactions* 206: 222–9.
33. Li, Y. G. et al. 2013. Polysaccharide from *Phellinus linteus* induces S-phase arrest in HepG2 cells by decreasing calreticulin expression and activating the P27kipl-cyclin A/D1/E-CDK2 pathway. *J. Ethnopharmacol.* 150: 187–95.
34. Cui, F. J. et al. 2012. Anti-proliferative activity of glycoprotein PLG-3 from the submerged mycelia of *Phellinus linteus* AML1101 in vitro. *Adv. Mater Res.* 554–6 (Pt. 2, Advances in Chemistry Research II), 1140–7.
35. Lee, J. S. et al. 2004. Production of lignin peroxidase by *Phellinus igniarius* and cytotoxic effects of lignin hydrolysates derived from wood biomass on cancer cells. *J. Applied Pharmacol.* 12: 189–93.
36. Shon, Y. H. et al. 2000. Enhancement of phase II and antioxidant enzymes in mice by soybeans fermented with basidiomycetes. *J. Microbiol. Biotech.* 10: 851–7.
37. Shon, Y. H. et al. 2001. In vitro cancer chemopreventive activities of polysaccharides from soybeans fermented with *Phellinus igniarius* or Agrocybe cylindracea. *J. Microbiol. Biotech.* 11: 1071–6.
38. Park, K. B. et al. 2002. Induction of anticarcinogenic enzymes of waxy brown rice cultured with *Phellinus igniarius* 26005. *Microbiol.* 30: 213–8.
39. Shon, Y. H. et al. 2002. Cancer chemoprevention: Inhibitory effect of soybeans fermented with basidiomycetes on 7,12-dimethylbenz[a]anthracene/12-*O*-tetradecanoylphorbol-13-acetate-induced mouse skin carcinogenesis. *Biotechnol. Lett.* 24: 1005–10.

142 Qian Cao 茜草

Indian madder

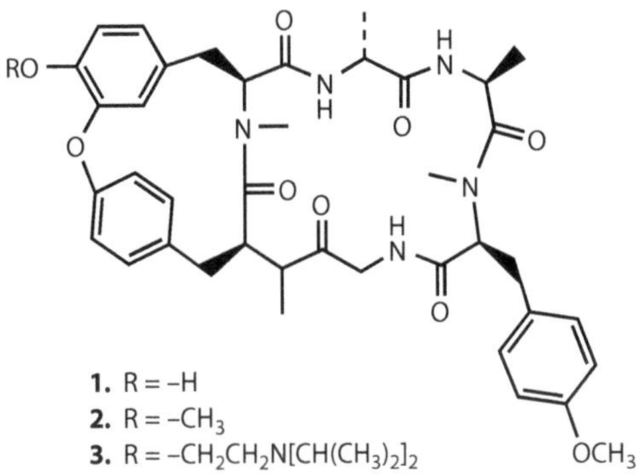

1. R = -H
2. R = $-CH_3$
3. R = $-CH_2CH_2N[CH(CH_3)_2]_2$

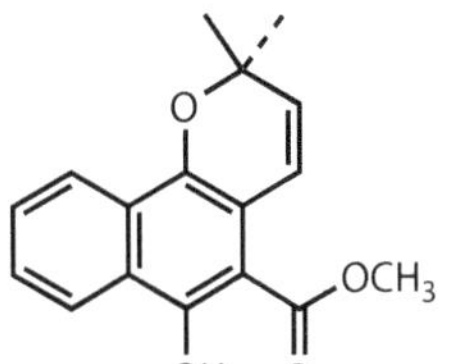

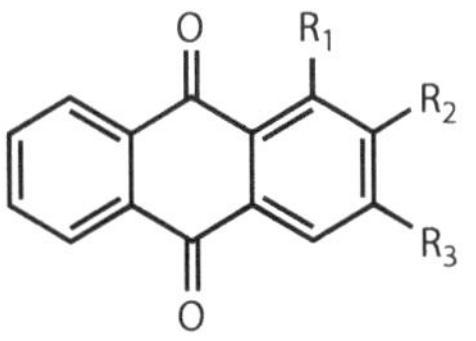

9. R_1 = $-OCOCH_3$, R_2 = -H, R_3 = $-OCH_3$
10. R_1 = -OH, R_2 = OCH_3, R_3 = -H
11. R_1 = -OH, R_2 = CH_3, R_3 = -H

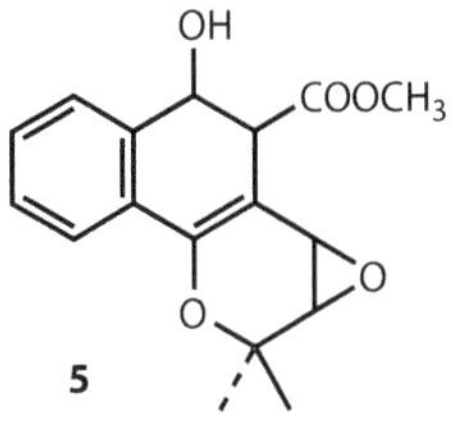

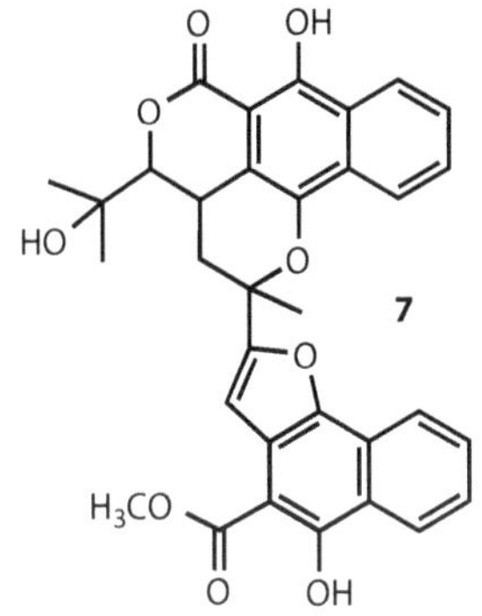

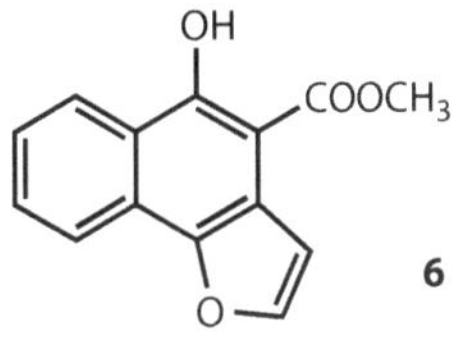

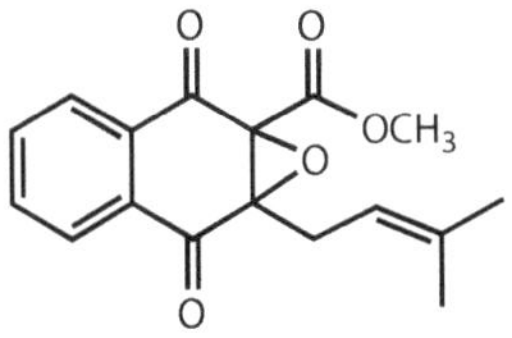

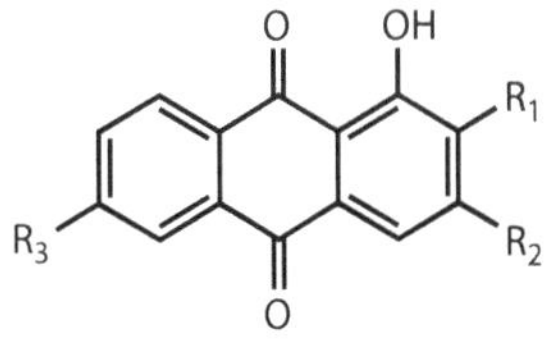

12. R_1 = $-CH_2OH$, R_2 = R_3 = -H
13. R_1 = $-CH_3$, R_2 = R_3 = -OH

Herb Origination

The herb Qian Cao (Indian madder) has a thousand-year history in China as a folk medicine. It was documented in two important Chinese ancient documents: *Huangdi-Neijing*, the first Chinese medicinal literature, and *Shennong Ben Cao Jing*, the first Chinese classic material medica. The herb origin is the roots of a Rubiaceae plant, *Rubia cordifolia* L. This perennial climber is widely distributed throughout Asiatic and African regions in the world. As a Chinese traditional herb, its roots are generally collected in November and dried in the sun.

Antitumor Constituents and Activities

Bicyclic Hexapeptides

Sixteen antineoplastic bicyclic hexapeptides and one dimer were discovered from the Qian Cao roots. These peptides showed the growth suppressive effect toward P388 and L1210 leukemia, B16 melanoma, Colon 38, Lewis lung carcinoma, and Ehrlich ascites carcinoma. Among these peptides, RA-VII (**1**) and RA-V (**2**) were the most potent tumor inhibitors.[1–4] The i.p. administration of the bicyclic hexapeptides to mice inhibited the growth of the P388 cells *in vivo*. The effective dose ranges were 0.01–4.0 mg/kg for RA-VII and 0.05–10.0 mg/kg for RA-V and RA-V-23. The minimum effective doses (*in vivo*) were 10 mg/kg for RA-IV and 0.05–0.5 mg/kg for RA-III.[5] The treatment of human DLD-1 colon cancer cells demonstrated that the cell growth inhibition induced by RA-VII was accompanied by a partial G1 phase arrest and a rapid decrease in the level of cyclin-D1 protein.[6] The *in vitro* and *in vivo* studies clearly confirmed that RA-VII (**1**) is an inhibitor of the protein synthesis in the neoplastic cells.[6] When RA-VII (**1**) was combined with RA-V-23, the anticancer activity was obviously enhanced in the i.p. injection to the tested mice.[5] RA-V (**2**) also demonstrated significant inhibitory effects against human KB nasopharynx carcinoma, mouse P388 leukemia, and mouse MM2 mammary carcinoma cells.[7] After the i.p. administration of RA-V in a dose of 10 mg/kg, the life duration of mice bearing P388 leukemia was prolonged by 187.4%.[8] At a dose of 3.13 mg/kg, the derivative (**3**) of RA-V and RA-VII (**1**) could reduce the volume of P388 leukemia in a mouse model. The derivative (**3**) exerted more promising antitumor activity than RA-VII (**1**) on P388 leukemia, adenocarcinoma 26, and colon B16 melanoma *in vitro*.[9–11] In recent years, more new bicyclopeptide of the RA-series, RA-XVIII, RA-XIX, RA-XX, RA-XXI, and RA-XXII, were isolated from the Qian Cao roots. Their cytotoxicities were tested by using murine P388 leukemia cell line *in vitro* to show the IC_{50} values in the range of 0.012–0.63 μg/mL.[12,13]

Naphthohydroquines

Mollugin (**4**), a major bioactive component present in Qian Cao roots, showed the antiproliferative activity against murine P388 leukemia *in vivo* and human Col2 colon cancer cells *in vitro*[14,15] as well as exerted apoptosis-inducing effect in human Jurkat leukemia T-cells via ER stress-mediated JNK activation and Bcl-xL-regulated caspase cascade activation.[16] By blocking the FAS gene expression through the inhibition of a HER2/Akt/SREBP-1c signaling pathway, mollugin (**4**) obstructed the cell proliferation and elicited the apoptotic death in HER2-overexpressing human

SKBR-3 (breast) and SKOV-3 (ovary) cancer cell lines in dose- and time-dependent manners without affecting the immortalized normal MCF-10A mammary epithelial cell line.[17] Both primary and metastatic human oral squamous cell carcinoma cells (OSCCs) could be induced to apoptotic death and sub-G1 phase arrest by mollugin (**4**). During the actions in the OSCC cells, mollugin suppressed the activation of NF-κB and NF-κB-dependent gene products related to antiapoptosis (Bcl-2 and Bcl-xL), angiogenesis (FGF-2 and VEGF), and invasion (MMP-9 and ICAM-1); induced the activations of p38, ERK, and JNK; and stimulated the expressions of HO-1 and Nrf2.[18] Moreover, mollugin (**4**) could induce both apoptosis and autophagy of tumor cells via PI3K/AKT/mTOR/p70S6K, and ERK signaling pathways.[19]

Importantly, mollugin (**4**) also was effective in the reversal of the drug resistance and the inhibition of drug-resistant MCF-7/Adm breast cancer cells due to the notable reduction of P-gp and MDR1 expressions, the blockage of CREB and NF-κB signaling pathway via AMPK activation, and the decrease of COX-2 expression.[20] However, mollugin (**4**) only exerted modest antiproliferative effects on human HepG2 hepatoma cells.[21] Its two derivatives, epoxymollugin (**5**) and furomollugin (**6**), exhibited more reduced inhibitory effect on HepG2 cells, MCF-7 cells or HT-29 cells.[21]

An isolated dimer of naphtha-hydroquinone designated as rubicordifolin (**7**) demonstrated both cytotoxic and antitumor properties. It obstructed the proliferation of mouse P388 leukemia, hamster V-79 lung carcinoma, and human KB nasopharynx carcinoma cell lines *in vitro* with IC_{50} values (μg/mL) of 4.7, 2.9, and 1.2, respectively, and inhibited the growth of mouse sarcoma 180 cells *in vivo* at a dose of 10 mg/kg.[22]

Naphthoquinone and Anthraquinones

In the *in vitro* assays, 2-carboxymethyl-3-prenyl-2,3-epoxy-1,4-naphthoquinone (**8**) showed antiproliferative effect against mouse P388 leukemia cells, hamster V-79 lung cancer cells, and human KB nasopharynx carcinoma cells with IC_{50} values of 1.7, 0.12, and 0.7 μg/mL, respectively, and at a dose of 5 mg/mL, it also repressed the growth of mouse sarcoma 180 cells *in vivo*.[17] But 2-carboxymethyl-3-prenyl-2,3-epoxy-1,4-naphthoquinone (**8**) exhibited moderate to weak antiproliferative effects when exposed to human HepG2 (liver), HT-29 (colon), and MCF-7 (breast) cancer cell lines with IC_{50} values of 40.5, 25.0, and 14.3 μM, respectively, whereas 1-acetoxy-3-methoxy-9,10-anthraquinone (**9**) displayed weak effect against the three cell lines (IC_{50}: 69.3–81.8 μM). The weak level of potency was also observed in the HT-29 cell line after being treated with alizarin 2-methylether (**10**) *in vitro*.[21] 1-Hydroxytectoquinone (**11**) exhibited marked cytotoxicity in human A375 melanoma cells,[23] and two other anthraquinones assigned as 1-hydroxy-2-hydromethyl-9,10-anthraquinone (**12**) and 2-methyl-1,3,6-trihydroxy-9,10-anthraquinone (**13**) displayed marked inhibitory effect on the V-79 cells *in vitro* (IC_{50}: 7.8 and 9.7 μg/mL, respectively).[22]

In addition, a mixture of anthraquinones prepared from the Qian Cao roots restrained the growth of human SMMC-7721 hepatoma cells and the activity of telomerase via the downregulation of hTERT gene.[24] Also, anthraquinones reduced SOD activity and augmented MDA activity in the SMMC-7721 cells, whose interactions might be involved in the antitumor and anticarcinogenic mechanism.[25] However, the suppressive potency of these nonbicyclepeptides was less than those of bicyclic hexapeptides RA-VII (**1**) and RA-V (**2**).

Other Bioactivities

The herb Qian Cao is used in Chinese medicine for treating arthritis, cough, bronchitis, dysentery, dysmenorrhea, uterine hemorrhage, inflammation of the joints, and stones in the kidney. In India, this plant has been used for the treatment of rheumatism, menstrual pain, and urinary disorders. Pharmacological studies already substantiated that Qian Cao exerts multiple biological activities, such as hemostatic, hematopoietic, expectorant, leukocytotic, antiplatelet aggregation, coronary flow-increasing, antitussive, myocardial-protecting, oxidation resistance and radical removal, phlegm removal, and antibacterial effects. Mollugin (**4**) and 3,4-dihydromollugin also possess biological properties including antiallergic and antiinflammatory activities.

References

1. Itokawa, H. et al. 2000. Antitumor compounds isolated from higher plants. *J. Biochem. Mol. Biol. Biophys.* 4: 213–22.
2. Itokawa, H. et al. 1986. Studies on antitumor cyclic hexapeptides RA obtained from Rubiae radix, Rubiaceae: VI. Minor antitumor constituents. *Chem. Pharm. Bull.* 34: 3762–8.
3. Hitotsuyanagi, Y. et al. 2000 and 2004. RA-dimer A, a novel dimeric antitumor bicyclic hexapeptide from *Rubia cordifolia* L. *Tetrahedron Lett.* 41: 6127–30; 45: 935–8.
4. Kato, T. et al. 1987. Antitumor activity and toxicity in mice of RA-700, a cyclic hexapeptide. *Anticancer Res.* 7(3 Pt B): 329–34.
5. Itokawa, H. et al. 1983. Studies on the antineoplastic cyclic hexapeptides obtained from Rubiae radix. *Proc. Intl. Congr. Chemother. 13th* 16: 284/110–284/113; 114–284/116.
6. Wakita, K. et al. 2001. Antitumor bicyclic hexapeptide RA-VII modulates cyclin D1 protein level. *Anti-Cancer Drugs* 12: 433–9.
7. Itokawa, H. et al. 1984. Cell growth-inhibitory effects of derivatives of antitumor cyclic hexapeptide RA-V obtained from Rubiae radix (V). *Gann.* 75: 929–36.
8. Itokawa, H. et al. 1989. Macrocyclic neoplasm inhibitor from *Rubia cordifolia. Jpn. Kokai Tokkyo Koho* JP 01230599 A 19890914.
9. Itokawa, H. et al. 1997. Preparation of cyclic hexapeptide compounds as antitumor agents. *PCT Int. Appl.* 12 pp. WO 96-JP2570.
10. Itokawa, H. et al. 1984. Isolation and antitumor activity of cyclic hexapeptides isolated from rubiae radix. *Chem. Pharm. Bull.* 32: 284–90.
11. Hitotsuyanagi, Y. et al. 1997. Studies on Rubia akane (RA) derivatives: II. Novel water-soluble analogs retaining potent antitumor activity of RA-VII, a cyclic hexapeptide from Rubia plants. *Bioorg. Med. Chem. Lett.* 7: 3125–8.
12. Lee, J. E. et al. 2008. A novel bicyclic hexapeptide, RA-XVIII, from *Rubia cordifolia*: Structure, semi-synthesis, and cytotoxicity. *Bioorg. Med. Chem. Lett.* 18: 808–11.

13. Lee, J. E. et al. 2008. Structures of cytotoxic bicyclic hexapeptides, RA-XIX, -XX, -XXI, and -XXII, from *Rubia cordifolia*. *Tetrahedron* 64: 4117–25.
14. Gutpa, P. P. et al. 1999. Biological activity of *Rubia cordifolia* and isolation of an active principle. *Pharm. Biol.* 37: 46–9.
15. Chang, L. C. et al. 2000. Rubiasins A-C, new anthracene derivatives from the roots and stems of *Rubia cordifolia*. *Tetrahedron Lett.* 41: 7157–62.
16. Kim, S. M. et al. 2009. Mollugin induces apoptosis in human Jurkat T cells through endoplasmic reticulum stress-mediated activation of JNK and caspase-12 and subsequent activation of mitochondria-dependent caspase cascade regulated by Bcl-xL. *Toxicol. Applied Pharmacol.* 241: 210–20.
17. Do, M. T. et al. 2013. Mollugin inhibits proliferation and induces apoptosis by suppressing fatty acid synthase in HER2-overexpressing cancer cells. *J. Cell. Physiol.* 228: 1087–97.
18. Lee, Y. M. et al. 2013. Involvement of Nrf2-mediated upregulation of heme oxygenase-1 in mollugin-induced growth inhibition and apoptosis in human oral cancer cells. *BioMed Res. Intl.* 210604, 14 pp.
19. Zhang, L. et al. 2014. Mollugin induces tumor cell apoptosis and autophagy via the PI3K/AKT/mTOR/p70S6K and ERK signaling pathways. Biochem. *Biophys. Res. Commun.* 450: 247–54.
20. Tran, T. et al. 2013. Reversal of P-glycoprotein-mediated multidrug resistance is induced by mollugin in MCF-7/adriamycin cells. *Phytomed.* 20: 622–31.
21. Son, J. K. et al. 2008. Anticancer constituents from the roots of *Rubia cordifolia* L. *Chem. Pharm. Bull.* 56: 213–6.
22. Ghosh, S. et al. 2010. Anti-inflammatory and anticancer compounds isolated from *Ventilago madraspatana* Gaertn., *Rubia cordifolia* Linn. and *Lantana camara* Linn. *J. Pharmacy Pharmacol.* 62: 1158–66.
23. Itokawa, H. et al. 1993. Anthraquinones, naphthohydroquinones and naphthohydroquinone dimers from *Rubia cordifolia* and their cytotoxic activity. *Chem. Pharm. Bull.* 41: 1869–72.
24. Wang, Y. S. et al. 2009. Inhibition of anthraquinones of *Rubia cordifolia on* liver carcinoma SMMC-7721 cells and its mechanism. *Shandong Yiyao* 49: 36–8.
25. Wang, Y. S. et al. 2010. Antioxidation of anthraquinones of *Rubia cordifolia* on hepatocellular carcinoma SMMC-7721. *Shandong Yiyao* 50: 45–6.

143 Juan Bai 卷柏

Resurrection fern or Little club moss

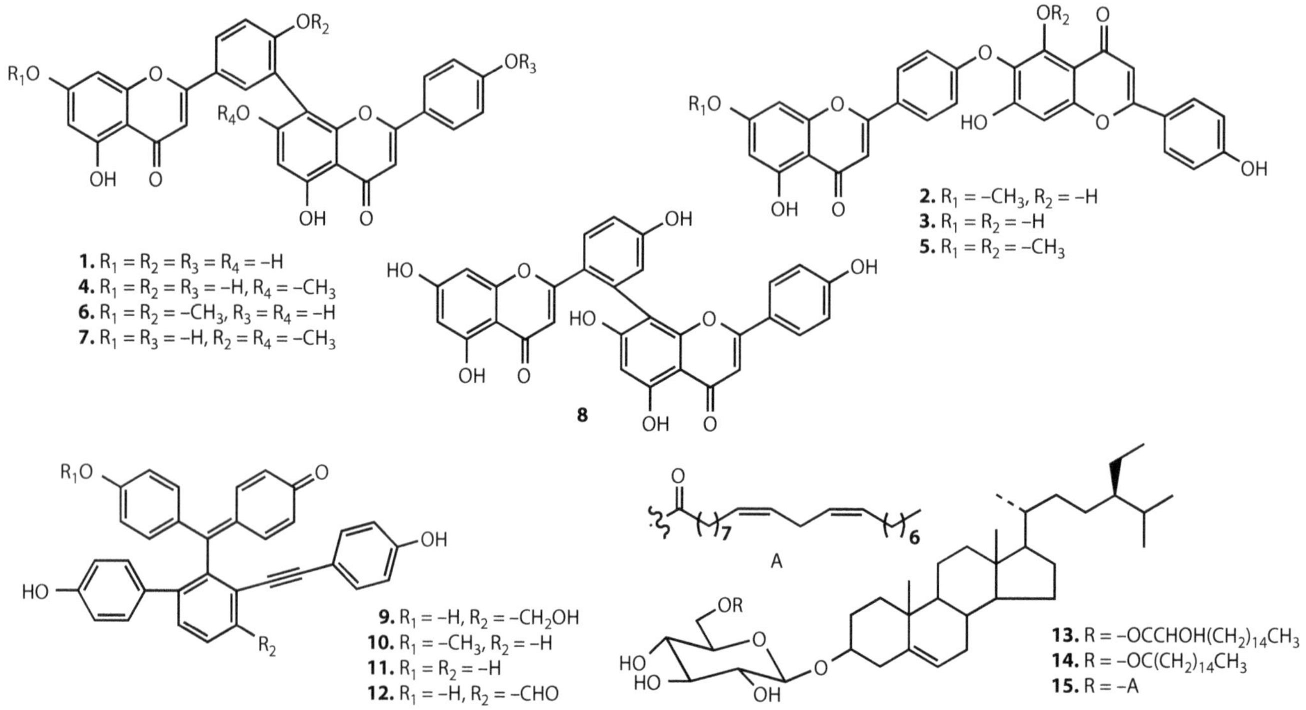

1. $R_1 = R_2 = R_3 = R_4 = -H$
4. $R_1 = R_2 = R_3 = -H, R_4 = -CH_3$
6. $R_1 = R_2 = -CH_3, R_3 = R_4 = -H$
7. $R_1 = R_3 = -H, R_2 = R_4 = -CH_3$

2. $R_1 = -CH_3, R_2 = -H$
3. $R_1 = R_2 = -H$
5. $R_1 = R_2 = -CH_3$

8

9. $R_1 = -H, R_2 = -CH_2OH$
10. $R_1 = -CH_3, R_2 = -H$
11. $R_1 = R_2 = -H$
12. $R_1 = -H, R_2 = -CHO$

A

13. $R = -OCCHOH(CH_2)_{14}CH_3$
14. $R = -OC(CH_2)_{14}CH_3$
15. $R = -A$

Herb Origination

The herb Juan Bai (Resurrection fern) originated from two species of *Selaginella* genus plants. The major source of the herb is a whole plant of *Selaginella tamariscina* (Selaginellaceae). Its distribution is broadly in the eastern and southern regions of Asia. The herb was recorded as a top-grade drug in the first Chinese classic of materia medica entitled *Shennong Ben Cao Jing*. The herb can be collected annually and dried in the sun for folk medical practice.

Antitumor Activities

The tumor inhibition and survival extension effects of Juan Bai were shown against mouse sarcoma 180 and Ehrlich ascites cancer in animal models in the early investigation. The inhibitory rates of its water and ethanolic extracts in mice were 61.2% and 18.6% against the S180, respectively.[1] The oral administration of the ethanol extract could provide marked inhibition of tumor growth in mice inoculated with Lewis lung carcinoma cells.[2] Feeding 1–5% Juan Bai extract to mice notably diminished MNNG-caused PCNA labeling index of the glandular stomach epithelium in mice, suggesting that Juan Bai has an ability for the chemoprevention of gastric carcinogenesis.[3] The treatment with the Juan Bai extract markedly promoted the apoptosis of HL-60 leukemia cells and further exerted cytotoxicity to HL-60 cells in a dose-dependent manner. The HL-60 cell apoptotic death induction was revealed to be mediated by a caspase activation pathway, including the specific proteolytic cleavage of PARP, the decrease of Bcl-2 expression, and the increase of proapoptotic Bax levels.[4]

Three fractions derived from Juan Bai by respective potations with chloroform, ethyl acetate, and n-butanol solvents showed cytotoxicity in human U937 histiocytic lymphoma cells and diminished the survival rates of murine P388 leukemia cells and human MKN45 gastric cancer cells but no effect on normal human lymphocytes under the same conditions. The tumoricidal effect of these fraction were found to be primarily mediated by p53 activation and G1 arrest in the cell cycle progression.[5,6] Moreover, the Juan Bai extracts also demonstrated notable inhibitory effect against the growth and the invasion of highly metastatic human A549 NSCLC cells and LLC cells *in vitro*, associated with decreases of MMP-2 and MMP-9 expressions and urokinase plasminogen activator dose-dependently. The antiinvasive and antimetastatic activities of Juan Bai extracts was demonstrated in the animal model implanted with Lewis lung carcinoma.[7] Similarly, the extract restrained the metastasis of U2OS human osteosarcoma cells, whose antimetastatic effect was revealed to be mediated by downregulating MMP-2 and MMP-9 secretions and increasing TIMP-1 and TIMP-2 expressions via p38- and AKT-dependent pathways.[8] The antimetastatic activity was also achieved by its 50% ethanolic extract on human nasopharyngeal carcinoma HONE-1 cells, whose effect may involve a Src/FAK/ERK1/2 pathway, including the blockage of ERK1/2 phosphorylation and MMP-9 expression.[9] Therefore, Juan Bai may be a potential candidate deserving further development as a preventive agent for carcinoma cell growth and metastasis.

Anticancer Constituents and Activities

Biflavonoids

Four biflavonoids, amentoflavone (**1**), cryptomerin-B, isocryptomerin, and 2′8″-biapigenin (**8**), were isolated from the EAF. The first three biflavonoids showed anticancer, immunosuppressive, and antiinflammatory activities.[10,11] Amentoflavone (**1**) lessened the survival of P388 cells dose-dependently, but it had no such effect on human MKN45 gastric cancer cells.[6] After the treatment with 100 μM amentoflavone (**1**), a dramatic suppression on the cell growth was observed on SK-BR-3 breast cancer cells *in vitro*, accompanied by apoptotic promotion and marked inhibition of fatty acid synthase (FASN) and fatty acid synthesis in FASN-overexpressed SK-BR-3 cells, evidencing that the breast cancer apoptosis induced by amentoflavone was partly associated with the blockage of fatty acid synthesis in the SK-BR-3 cells.[12] *In vitro* assays also displayed that amentoflavone (**1**) obviously restrained the proliferation of human BGC-823 gastric tumor cells (IC_{50}: 1.89 μg/mL) and weakly retarded human HL-60 (leukemic), HeLa (cervix), MCF-7 (breast), and BEL-7402 (liver) tumor cell lines (IC_{50}: 46.97–76.83 μM).[13,14] The inhibitory effect of amentoflavone (**1**) on the MCF-7 and HeLa cells was found to be mediated by increasing of phosphatase and tensin homolog (PTEN) expression levels due to hPPARγ activation.[15] After being treated with amentoflavone (**1**), the MCF-7 breast cancer cells showed a series of cellular alterations related to mitochondria-mediated apoptosis, including mitochondrial dysfunction, release of cytochrome c from the mitochondria, and activation of caspase-3.[16] Moreover, amentoflavone (**1**) also promoted the apoptosis and the sub-G1 cell arrest of both SiHa and CaSki cervical neoplastic cells through the mitochondria-emanated intrinsic pathways, i.e., up-expressing PPARγ/PTEN proteins and down-expressing human E7 papillomavirus protein.[17] At a concentration of 200 μM, amentoflavone (**1**) and its acetate derivative acted as inhibitors of human DNA Topo-I to display dose-dependent growth suppressive activity against Ehrlich carcinoma cells *in vitro* with IC_{50} values of about 26 μM for amentoflavone (**1**) and 10 μM for its acetate.[18]

More bioactive biflavonoids were isolated from Juan Bai and evaluated *in vitro* with three human cancer cell lines. The antiproliferative effect of hinokiflavone (**3**) was markedly shown in human Bel-7402 hepatoma and BGC-823 gastric cancer cell lines with IC_{50} values of 1.43 and 1.02 μg/mL, respectively.[14] Neocryptomerin (**2**) and hinokiflavone (**3**) showed moderate antiproliferative effect on HeLa cells (IC_{50}: 10.35 and 19.27 μg/mL), U251 glioma cells (IC_{50}: 19.05 and 29.81 μg/mL), and MCF-7 cells (IC_{50}: 30.09 and 39.32 μg/mL), respectively.[19] The inhibition of 7″-*O*-methylamentoflavone (**4**) (IC_{50}: 48.11–75.94 μg/mL) was much lower in these tumor cell lines as compared to those of bioflavonoids (**1–3**), implying that the methoxylation at C-7″ of amentoflavone (**1**) would notably weaken the antitumor function. Pulvinatabiflavone (**5**) was inactive in the U252 and MCF-7 cell lines, but it exerted the most potent inhibitory effect on the HeLa cells (IC_{50}: 2.36 μg/mL).[19] Ginkgetin (**6**) and isoginketin (**7**) were active in inhibiting the Bel7402 cells (IC_{50}: 5.00 and 6.01 μg/mL, respectively), and ginkgetin (**6**) was also effective in suppressing human A549 lung cancer cells (IC_{50}: 1.00 μg/mL).[14] In addition, 2′,8″-biapigenin (**8**), another biflavonoid constituent derived from Juan Bai, was able to block transactivations of iNOS and COX-2 through the inactivation of NF-κB by preventing the nuclear translocation of p65 in macrophages.[11] The findings suggested that these biflavonoids and the Juan Bai extract have developing potentials for the chemoprevention of carcinogenesis as well as for the treatment of inflammatory diseases.

Acetylenic Compounds

Six selaginellin derivatives isolated from the *S. tamariscina* were evaluated by a small panel of human tumor cell lines, including U251 glioma, HeLa cervical cancer, and MCF-7 breast neoplastic cells. Most of the selaginellins demonstrated medium suppressive effect against the three cancer cell lines. Among these acetylenic compounds, selaginellin-M (**9**) exerted relatively better antiproliferative effect. The IC_{50} values were 15.05, 16.61, and 24.49 μg/mL for selaginellin-M (**9**), 25.34, 22.51, and 33.84 μg/mL for selaginellin-N (**10**), and 27.35, 22.53, and 48.83 μg/mL for selaginellin-A (**11**), respectively, in U251, HeLa and MCF-7 cells.[19] The potent effect was achieved by selaginellin-M (**9**) in BGC-823 gastric cancer cells (IC_{50}: 1.86 μg/mL), and no activity was found in the A549 lung cancer and Bel-7402 hepatoma cell lines.[14] The moderate inhibition was also shown by selaginellin-O (**12**) in the HeLa cells.[20]

N,N-Dimethyltyramine Glycosides

From a 70% ethanolic extract of Juan Bai, two N,N-dimethyltyramine glycosides, hordenine-*O*-α-L-rhamnopyranoside(**13**) and hordenine-*O*-[(6″-*O*-*trans*-cinnamoyl)-4′-*O*-β-D-glucopyranosyl-α-L-rhamnopyranoside] (**14**) were discovered, which showed the dose-dependent antitumor metastatic activity on human mammary cancer MDA-MB-231 cells *in vitro*.[21]

Sterols

A bioassay-guided fractionation of the dichloromethane extract of Juan Bai led to the isolation of six sterols such as ergosta-4,6,8(14),22-tetraene-3-one, ergosterol endoperoxide, 7β-hydroxycholesterol, and 7β-hydroxysitosterol. The sterols were reported to have modest antiproliferative activity in five human tumor cell lines *in vitro*.[22]

Other Bioactivities

The whole plant of Juan Bai (Resurrection fern) has astringent and haemostatic properties. Its decoction is traditionally used in China for the treatment of traumatic bleeding, hemoptysis in pulmonary disease, gastrointestinal bleeding, hematuria, metrorrhagia, rectal prolapse, persistence of postpartum lochial discharge, leucorrhoea, and allergy. The herb is also used in therapeutic treatments of chronic trachitis and small intestine contraction in China. Modern pharmaceutical studies provided scientific evidences for Juan Bai having antibacterial and antigastric ulcer activities. The Juan Bai extract was also capable of relaxing smooth muscle of the ileum and antagonizing the excitation of the small intestine induced by acetylcholine or barium chloride. Amentoflavone (**1**) is known to possess antiinflammatory and antifungal benefits. In a single-dose acute toxicity test, the oral administration of the ethanolic extract of Juan Bai at a dose of 10,000 mg/kg did not cause any lethality in mice.[2]

References

1. Chan, M. Y. et al. 1987. *Kong-ai Bencao* (Chinese Anticancer Herbs), First Edition. Hunan Science and Technology Press, Changsha, p. 174.
2. Ha, L. M. et al. 2012. Toxicity and anticancer effects of an extract from *Selaginella tamariscina* on a mice model. *Nat. Prod. Res.* 26: 1130–4.
3. Lee, I. S. et al. 1999. Effects of *Selaginella tamariscina* on *in vitro* tumor cell growth, p53 expression, G1 arrest and in vivo gastric cell proliferation. *Cancer Lett.* 144: 93–9.
4. Ahn, S. H. et al. 2006. *Selaginella tamariscina* induces apoptosis via a caspase-3-mediated mechanism in human promyelocytic leukemia cells. *J. Med. Food* 9: 138–44.
5. Lee, I. S. et al. 1998. Molecular mechanisms of *Selaginella tamariscina* for antineoplastic activity in human leukemia cell line U937. *Animal Cell Technol: Basic Appl Aspects, Proc. Annual Meet. Japanese Assoc. Animal Cell Technol*, 9th, *Yokohama*, September 1–4, 1996, 83–9.
6. Lee, I. et al. 1992. Cytotoxicity of folk medicine in murine and human cancer cells. *Saengyak Hakhoechi* 23: 132–6.
7. Yang, S. F. et al. 2007. Antimetastatic activities of *Selaginella tamariscina* (Beauv.) on lung cancer cells in vitro and in vivo. *J. Ethnopharmacol.* 110: 483–9.
8. Yang, J. S. et al. 2013. *Selaginella tamariscina* (Beauv.) possesses antimetastatic effects on human osteosarcoma cells by decreasing MMP-2 and MMP-9 secretions via p38 and Akt signaling pathways. *Food Chem. Toxicol.* 59: 801–7.
9. Hsin, C. H. et al. 2013. *Selaginella tamariscina* extract suppresses TPA-induced invasion and metastasis through inhibition of MMP-9 in human nasopharyngeal carcinoma HONE-1 cells. *BMC Complem. Altern. Med.* 13, 234/1–234/11.
10. Kang, S. S. et al. 1998. Biflavonoids from *Selaginella tamariscina. Repub. Korea* KR 94–12693 19940607.
11. Woo, E. R. et al. 2006. Inhibition of nuclear factor-κB activation by 2′,8″-biapigenin. *Biol. Pharm. Bull.* 29: 976–80.
12. Lee, J. S. et al. 2009. Fatty acid synthase inhibition by amentoflavone induces apoptosis and anti-proliferation in human breast cancer cells. *Biol. Pharma. Bull.* 32: 1427–32.
13. Jing. Y. et al. 2010. Amentoflavone and the extracts from *Selaginella tamariscina* and their anticancer activity. *Asian J. Tradit Med.* 5: 226–9.
14. Cao, Y. et al. 2012. Cytotoxic Constituents from *Selaginella tamariscina. Nat. Prod. Res. Develop.* 24: 150–4.
15. Lee, E. J. et al. 2012. Cytotoxic activities of amentoflavone against human breast and cervical cancers are mediated by increasing of PTEN expression levels due to peroxisome proliferator-activated receptor γ activation. *Bull. Korean Chem. Soc.* 33: 2219–23.
16. Pei, J. S. et al. 2012. Amentoflavone induces cell-cycle arrest and apoptosis in MCF-7 human breast cancer cells via mitochondria-dependent pathway. *In Vivo* 26: 963–70.
17. Lee, S. J. et al. 2011. The biflavonoid amentoflavone induces apoptosis via suppressing E7 expression, cell cycle arrest at sub-G1 phase, and mitochondria-manated intrinsic pathways in Human cervical cancer cells. *J. Med. Food* 14: 808–16.
18. Grynberg, N. F. et al. 2002. DNA topoisomerase inhibitors: Biflavonoids from *Ouratea* species. *Braz. J. Med. Biol. Res.* 35: 819–22.
19. Zhang, G. G. et al. 2012. Isolation and cytotoxic activity of selaginellin derivatives and biflavonoids from *Selaginella tamariscina. Planta Med.* 78: 390–2.
20. Yang, C. et al. 2012. Bioactive selaginellins from *Selaginella tamariscina* (Beauv.) Spring. *Beilstein J. Org. Chem.* 8: 1884–9.
21. Qi, Y. et al. 2014. Antitumor metastatic constituents from *Selaginella tamariscina* (Beauv.) Spring. *Zhongchengyao* 36: 1682–7.
22. Roh, E. M. et al. 2010. Structural implication in cytotoxic effects of sterols from *Selaginella tamariscina. Archiv. Pharm. Res.* 33: 1347–53.

144 Jiu Lian 韭蓮

Rain lily

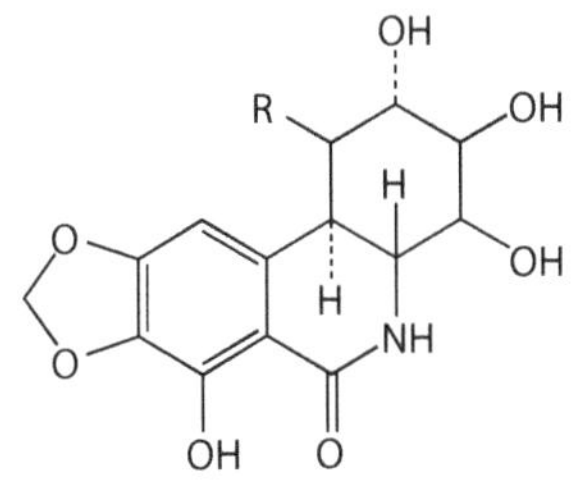

1. R = -OH
7. R = -OOC-$CH_2CH(OH)CH_3$
9. R = -OOC-Ph

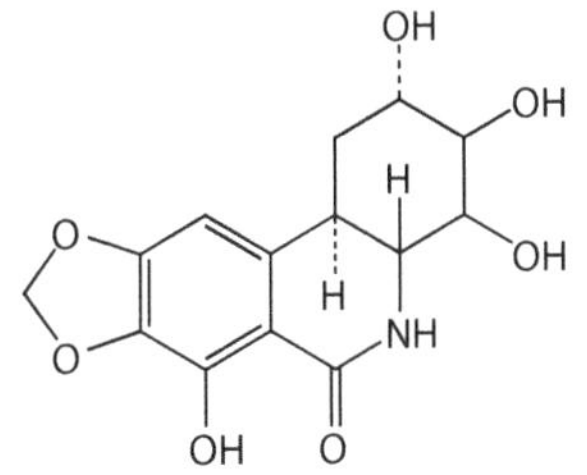

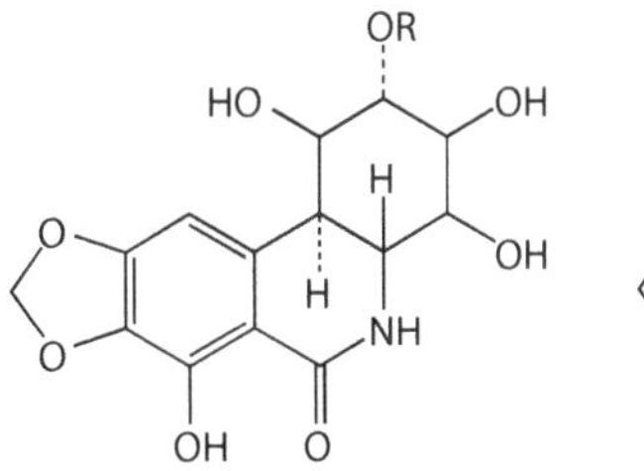

8. R = -beta-D-glucose

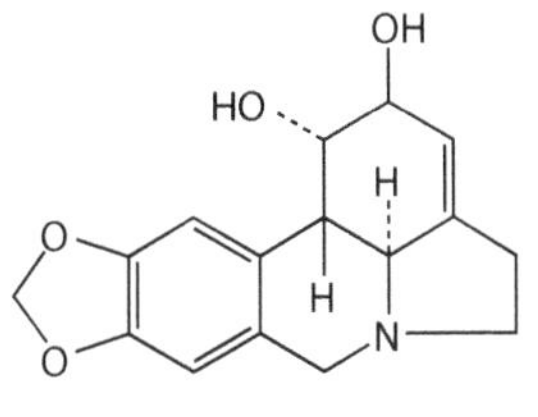

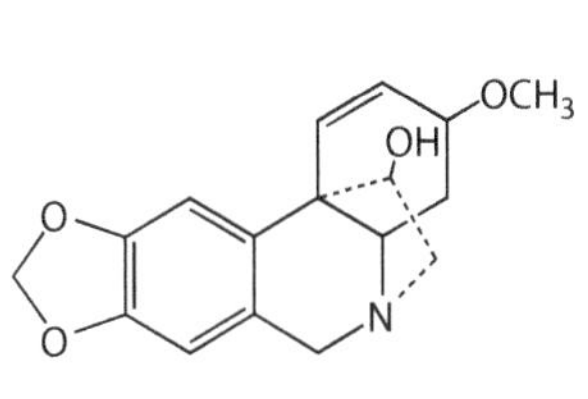

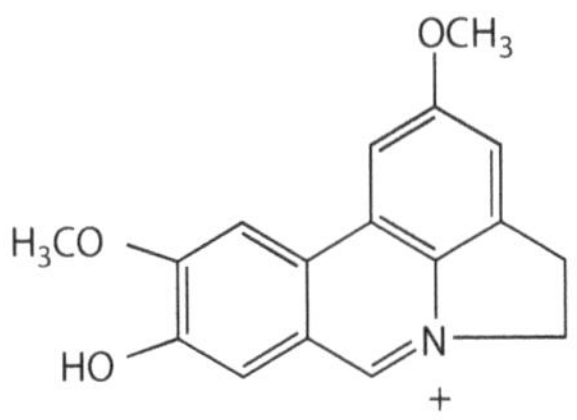

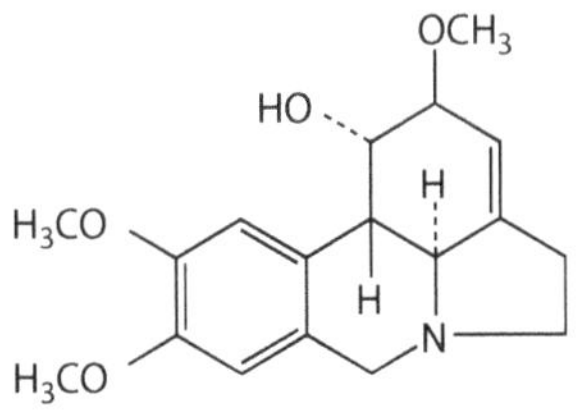

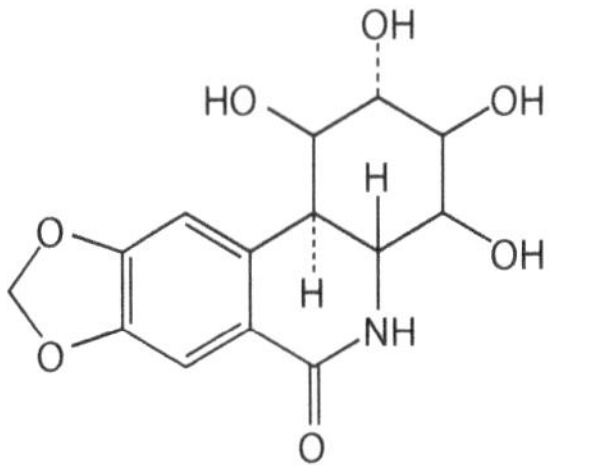

Herb Origination

The herb Jiu Lian (Rain lily) is an Amaryllidaceae plant, *Zephyranthes grandiflora*, whose plant native range is Central America from Mexico to Guatemala. The herbaceous perennial plant is naturalized in Yunnan province of China and cultured in many gardens of the world as an ornamental plant. The whole plant and bulbs are collected in summer and autumn and dried in the sun for Chinese folk medical practice.

Antitumor Constituents and Activities

The bioassay-directed fractionation of a butanolic extract from the bulbs of *Z. grandiflora* resulted in the isolation of two isocarbostyril alkaloids, pancratistatin (**1**) (see Section Shui Gui Jiao) and *trans*-dihydronarciclasine (**2**), as the major anticancer constituents in the herb. The potent inhibitory effect of pancratistatin (**1**) was demonstrated in the *in vitro* investigation with a panel of human neoplastic cell lines, BXPC-2 (pancreas), MCF-7 (breast), SF-268 (brain), NCI-H460 (lung), KM20L2 (colon) ,and Du-145 (prostate), showing IC_{50} values of 0.043–0.098 μM. Both alkaloids (**1** and **2**) displayed potent cytotoxicity against mouse P388 lymphocytic leukemia cells *in vitro* with ED_{50} values of 0.052 and 0.0032 μg/mL, respectively. The antileukemia effect of pancratistatin (**1**) was also observed in mice bearing P388 cells at doses of 0.75–6.0 mg/kg, showing T/C values of 138–165%. When the dose was raised to 12.5 mg/kg, the inhibitory effect was augmented with the T/C data of 206%. The *in vivo* anticancer effect of pancratistatin (**1**) was further shown in mouse models implanted with L1210 leukemia, B16 melanoma, or M-5076 ovarian sarcoma.[1–4]

Eight other types of alkaloids designated as lycorine (**3**), haemanthamine (**4**), zephgrabetaine (**5**), galanthine (**6**), lycoramine, hamayne, tortuosine, and ungeremine were also found from the isolation of the bulbs of *Z. grandiflora*. All the alkaloids exerted a dose-dependent cytotoxic effect on two neoplastic cell lines, rat C-6 glioma cells and CHO-K1 Chinese hamster ovary cells. Lycorine (**3**) and haemanthamine (**4**) showed the prominent cytotoxic activity among the alkaloids.[5]

Structural Modification

Because naturally occurring pancratistatin (**1**) has low aqueous solubility (~50 μg/mL), which limits its clinical evaluation in intravenous formulation, several phosphate prodrugs of pancratistatin (**1**) have been synthesized for the increase of the aqueous solubility. The free hydroxyl groups in positions at C-3, C-4, and C-7 of pancratistatin (**1**) were utilized to create mono- or cyclic phosphate derivatives. The pancratistatin prodrugs showed not only increase of water solubility but also effective release of the active form of pancratistatin (**1**) through the action of cellular phosphatases in human body.[6]

For the discovery of more active agents, pancratistatin (**1**) was utilized as a starting molecule for the synthesis different types of derivatives. A produced hydroxybutyril derivative (**7**) displayed the enhanced cytotoxicity on the P388 cells, being twofold greater than pancratistatin (**1**), whereas a β-D-glucoside derivative (**8**) exerted the same level of cytotoxic effect as pancratistatin (**1**) against the P388 cells. The cytotoxicity of pancratistatin-1-benzoate derivative (**9**) was 10 times more potent than that of its original molecule, and the IC_{50} values ranged from 0.00023 to 0.0044 μM *in vitro* in a panel of human BXPC-3 (pancreas), MCF-7 (breast), SF268 (CNS), NCI-H460 (lung-NSC), KM20L2 (colon), and Du-145 (prostate) neoplastic cell lines and mouse P388 leukemia cell lines. However, 7-deoxypancratistatin (**10**) exhibited 10- to 20-fold lower cytotoxicity than pancratistatin (**1**).[4]

References

1. Pettit, G. R. et al. 1984. Antineoplastic agents: 105. Zephyranthes. *J. Nat. Prod.* 47: 1018–20.
2. Pettit, G. R. et al. 1990. Antineoplastic agents: 162. *Zephyranthes grandiflora. J. Nat. Prod.* 53: 176–8.
3. Cragg, G. M. et al. 1997. Natural products in drug discovery and development. *J. Nat. Prod.* 60: 52–60.
4. Ingrassia, L. et al. 2008. Amaryllidaceae isocarbostyril alkaloids and their derivatives as promising antitumor agents. *Transl. Oncol.* 1: 1–13.
5. Katoch, D. et al. 2013. Zephgrabetaine: A new betaine-type amaryllidaceae alkaloid from *Zephyranthes grandiflora. Nat. Prod. Commun.* 8: 161–4.
6. Pettit, G. R. et al. 2004. Antineoplastic agents: 511. Direct phosphorylation of phenpanstatin and pancratistatin. *J. Nat. Prod.* 67: 322–7.

8

Anticancer Potentials of Expectorant, Antitussive, and Antiasthmatic Herbs

CONTENTS

145 Bai Qu Cai 白屈菜

Greater celandine or Tetterwort

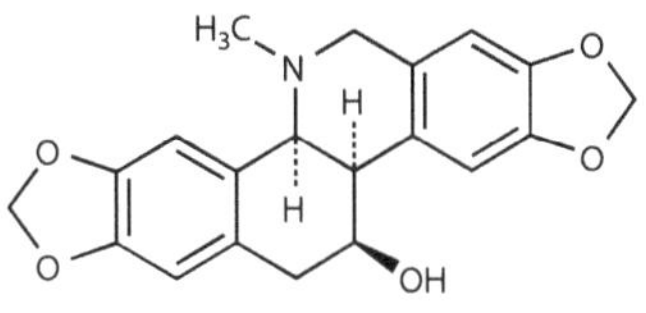

1 2 3 4 5

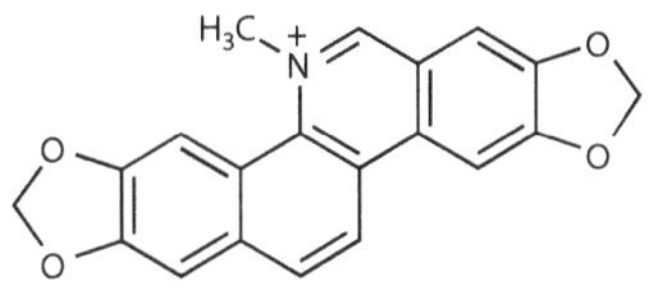

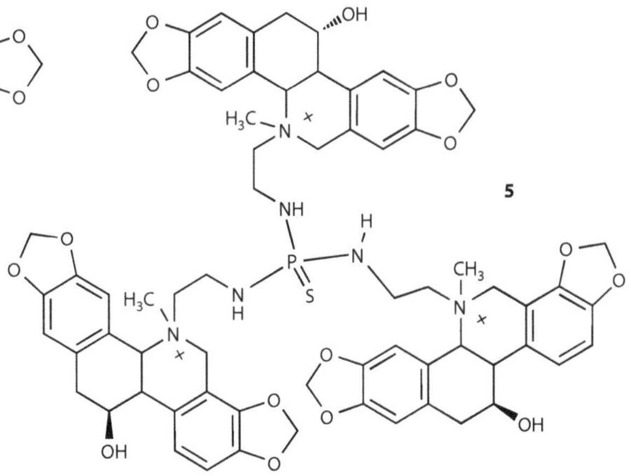

Herb Origination

The herb Bai Qu Cai (Greater celandine) is a widespread plant of *Chelidonium majus* L. (Papaveraceae), which is native to Europe, the Mediterranean basin, and western Asia. A varietal plant *C. majus* var. *asiaticum* is widely distributed in the temperate regions of eastern Asia. The two plants are the major sources for this herb, which has been used as a folk remedy for medicinal purposes in Asian countries for a long period. The herb used in China is normally collected during the flower-blooming season, which can be used as fresh and dried herb.

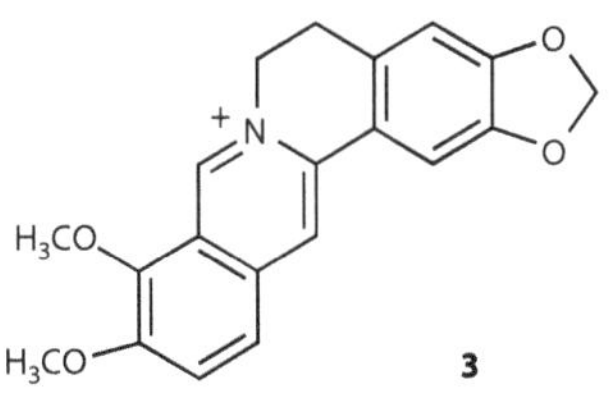

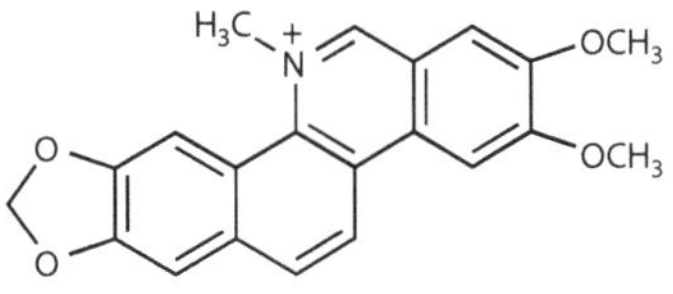

Antitumor Activities

Bai Qu Cai is extensively used in traditional systems of Chinese medicine against various liver ailments including hepatoma. *In vivo* multiple assays further corroborated its antitumor, antigenotoxic, anticlastogenic, and hepatoprotective properties against p-DAB-induced hepatocarcinogenesis. Bai Qu Cai even at microdoses was effective in combating hepatoma by modulating the activities of some functional enzymes in the liver.[1,2] Its methanolic extract also showed significant inhibitory activity toward mouse Ehrlich ascites tumor and sarcoma 180 *in vivo* and obvious cytotoxicity on human Eca-109 esophagus carcinoma cells *in vitro*. The treatment with 2 mg/mL concentration of the extract caused Eca-109 cells to completely lose their ability for propagation. When the concentration was raised to 5 mg/mL, 50% of the Eca-109 cells would be killed.[3] The Bai Qu Cai extract also exerted the suppressive effects on glandular stomach carcinogenesis induced by MNNG in rats.[4] By the treatment, the incidences of forestomach cancer lesions (papillomas and squamous cell carcinomas) showed a tendency for decrease.[5]

Antitumor Constituents and Activities

Phytochemical approaches led to the separation of different groups of chemical constituents from *C. majus*, such as alkaloids, polyphanols, carotenoids, flavonoids, hydroxycinnamic acids, and polysaccharides. The alkaloids showed multiple responses to the bioactivities of the herb. Protoberberines and benzophenanthridines are the major types of alkaloids discovered from Bai Qu Cai. Besides coptisine, the major alkaloids in the plant were identified as chelidonine (**1**), sanguinarine (**2**), berberine (**3**), and chelerythrine (**4**).

Alkaloids

The separated alkaloids exerted cytotoxic effect on human neoplastic cell lines *in vitro*. The IC_{50} values of (+)-chelidonine (**1**) were 8.3 and 5.9 μg/mL in MCF breast cancer cells and HT-29 colon cancer cells, while the values of (−)-stylopine were 16.6 and 13.9 μg/mL in the MCF cells and DU-145 prostate cancer cells, respectively. But no such effect was observed in A549 lung cancer cells after being treated with chelidonine.[6] Chelidonine (**1**) also completely blocked the growth of L1210 cells, although showed no significant cytotoxicity or DNA damage in both mouse leukemia L1210 cells and primary mouse spleen cells. Comparably, sanguinarine (**2**) and chelerythrine (**4**) exerted selective cytotoxic and DNA-damaging effects against the L1210 cells and primary mouse spleen cells in a dose-dependent manner.[7] When being treated with the alkaloids (**1–3**), the proliferation of human HeLa cervical cancer cells was obstructed with ED_{50} values of 0.27, 0.54, and >3.5 μg/mL, respectively.[3,8] More investigations revealed that chelidonine (**1**) efficiently promoted sub-G1 and G0/G1 cell cycle arrest and apoptosis of the HeLa cells through the alteration of p38-p53 and AKT/PI3 kinase signaling pathways, i.e., (1) increase of ROS generation and change in mitochondrial membrane potential; (2) up-expression of p38, p53, and other pro-apoptotic genes; and (3) down-expression of AKT, PI3K, JAK3, STAT3, E6, E7, and other antiapoptotic genes.[9] Likewise, the proapoptotic and DNA-damaging effects of chelidonine (**1**) and sanguinarine (**2**) in human MT-4 acute T lymphoblastic leukemia cells was mediated by the up-expression of pBax and the activation of caspase-9 and caspase-3. The chelidonine (**1**) concurrently induced the MT-4 cell cycle arrest at G2/M phase in the treatment.[10] In Dalton's lymphoma cell line, chelerythrine (**4**) induced ROS-dependent mitochondrial pathway to promote the cell apoptosis.[11]

Moreover, the chelidonine (**1**) and the total alkaloids of the herb could dose-dependently inhibit P-gp/MDR1 activity in Caco-2 (colorectal) and CEM/ADR5000 (leukemic) cancer cells to reverse the resistance to DOX. The treatment of Caco-2 cells with 50 μM chelidonine or 50 μg/mL alkaloids and for up to 48 h resulted in a marked decrease in mRNA levels of P-gp/MDR1, MRP1, BCRP, CYP3A4, GST, and hPXR. Concomitantly, chelidonine (**1**) and the alkaloids inhibited the activity of drug modifying enzymes CYP3A4 and GST and induced the apoptosis of the MDR cells via the activation of caspase-3, caspase-8, and caspase-6/9.[12] Thus, chelidonine (**1**) is a potential candidate for overcoming MDR and for enhancing cytotoxicity of chemotherapeutics. The findings disclosed that the antitumor activity is mediated by the different mechanisms and suggested that chelidonine (**1**) and sanguinarine (**2**) are the drug leads deserving of further investigation and development.

Semisynthetic Alkaloid

In Vitro *Anticancer Activities*

Ukrain (**5**), a semisynthetic thiophosphamide derived from the Bai Qu Cai alkaloids, displayed a selective cytotoxicity against tumor cells *in vitro* and *in vivo* and also exhibited its ability to modulate immunocyte functions in tumor-bearing organs. The exposure of Ukrain to human ME180 cervical epitheloid cancer cells and A431 epidermis cancer cells resulted in G2/M cell cycle arrest and apoptotic death of the cancer cells and selective inhibition of the growth of ME180 cells and A431 cells at a dose range of 3.5–7.0 μM.[13] Similarly, after 24 h of treatment with 3.5 μM of Ukrain, 73% human LNCaP prostate cancer cells were arrested at the G2/M phase and the apoptotic cells were steadily amplified in a dose-dependent manner.[14] Concurrently, the interactions related to the antitumor mechanism such as the regulation of p27 protein (a CDK inhibitor) and the decrease of CDK (CDK1 and CDK2) levels were observed in Ukrain (**5**)-treated A431 cells, LNCaP cells and ME180 cells, but there were no substantial changes in the expression of Bcl-2 and Bax proteins.[15] In the treatment of human PC3 prostate cancer cells, Ukrain markedly induced the apoptosis and diminished the survival of the AI prostate cancer cells by (1) obviously upregulating the proapoptotic mRNA expression of Bad, Bax, and FasL; (2) decreasing the cell survival protein p-Akt and the antiapoptotic protein Bcl-2; and (3) amplifying the levels of cleaved PARP and caspase-10.[16] Ukrain (**5**) also presented the anticancer effect in three pancreatic ductal adenocarcinoma cell lines (HPAF-II, HPAC, and PL45), where Ukrain (**5**) elicited abnormal mitosis in the tested cells by the alteration of mitotic spindle microtubule dynamics and stimulated the cell apoptosis through an extrinsic pathway.[17] After 48 h of exposure to murine (4T07 and TUBO) and human (SKBR-3) breast cancer cell lines, Ukrain (**5**) at a concentration of 50 μg/mL dose- and time-dependently enhanced >50% apoptotic death of the tested cells.[18] Ukrain (**5**) was also able to exert high suppressive activity against progressive human Ewing tumor.[19]

In Vivo *Anticancer Activities*

The *in vivo* experiments proved that Ukrain treatment was effective in the suppression of Ehrlich ascites and solid carcinomas, where the solid Ehrlich's carcinoma (ECA) cells showed more sensitivity to Ukrain than the ascites ECA cells.[18] The intravenous injection of Ukrain (**5**) in doses of 5 or 12.5 mg/kg markedly retarded the growth of 4T07 breast cancer cells by 60% and 40%, respectively. The *in vivo* treatment was capable of eliciting protective antitumor immunity following secondary challenge.[20] A monotherapy of Ukrain (**5**) and a combinational therapy with Ukrain (**5**) and RAM (pathogen-associated molecules) were performed in mice implanted with low- and high-metastasizing B16 melanomas. The results showed that both therapies with Ukrain exerted marked growth inhibition in melanoma-bearing mice, but the monotherapy with Ukrain (**5**) was more effective in mice with high-metastasizing tumors and a combined treatment with RAM and Ukrain (**5**) was more expressed in mice with low-metastasizing melanoma.[21] Moreover, the antimetastatic formation of Ukrain was demonstrated in an animal model with Lewis lung carcinoma and showed significant suppressive effect against the growth of existing tumor.[22,23]

Synergistic Anticancer Activity

When Ukrain (**5**) is combined with bortezomib (an anticancer drug), the inhibitory effect was achieved against mouse 4T1 breast cancer cells, where bortezomib synergistically potentiated the cell death elicited by Ukrain (**5**). However, no significant enhancement of cytotoxicity was observed against the 4T1 cells in the cotreatment of Ukrain (**5**) with cisplatin, etoposide, 5-FU, or quercetin.[24]

Immunostimulating Activity

As mentioned earlier, Ukrain (**5**) is also capable of significantly affecting the state of the immune system via the improvement of the endocrine thymic function and the antioxidation capability (AOC) in the spleen and the enhancement of the serum IFN level and the adhesion of peritoneal macrophages. Also, the Ukrain derivatives could enlarge the amounts of lymphocytes, monocytes, and blood glucose level (BGL) in the peripheral blood of mice bearing Lewis tumor.[22,23]

Ukrain Derivatives

Some derivatives were created from the Ukrain (**5**), whose derivatives could selectively arrest the cell cycle at the G2/M phase of leukemia cell lines (Jurkat and THP-1) and pancreatic cancer cell lines (MIA PaCa2, BxPC3, and AsPC1).[25] Because the Ukrain derivatives are inhibitors of mitochondrial monoamine oxidase,[26] the respiration of the mitochondria during the phosphorylation of exogenous ADP was highly enhanced by the derivatives in tumor-bearing mice, resulting in the significant obstruction of the growth and the lung metastasis of the primary melanoma.[27]

In summary, Bai Qu Cai alkaloids, Ukrains (**5**) and its derivatives, may be considered to have further developing potential to be chemotherapeutic agents, and the scientific evidences may also provide a positive hint into designing Ukrain-based drug development for the treatment of malignant tumor diseases.

Polyphenolic Extracts

The polyphenolic/flavonoid extracts prepared from Bai Qu Cai showed significant free radical-scavenging activities. Importantly, the free radical-scavenging activity usually showed a close relationship with anticarcinogenic effect. In the experiments with different ethanolic extracts, the extract of celandine roots strongly scavenged free hydroxyl radical and hypochlorite anion, whereas the extract of celandine flowers exerted the best ability to scavenge peroxyl radical and singlet oxygen. The superoxide anion and hydrogen peroxide were best scavenged by the ethanolic extract prepared from the celandine leaves.[28]

Polysaccharides

A polysaccharide component prepared from the herb Bai Qu Cai was discovered to possess antitumor activity in addition to the immunostimulation and the enhancement of hematopoietic function.[29] CM-Ala, a protein-bound polysaccharide, was isolated from the aqueous extract of Bai Qu Cai. By culturing with splenocytes for five days, CM-Ala augmented the cytotoxic rate from 0.88% to 34.18% against Yac-1 lymphoma cell line. CM-Ala also demonstrated mitogenic activities on both spleen cells and bone marrow cells and induced the proliferation of splenocytes by 84-fold and augmented GM-CFC by 1.48-fold over than the non-treated ones. Also, CM-Ala simultaneously enhanced the production of NO by twofold in the peritoneal macrophages, thereby exerting antitumor effect. All these results clearly confirmed that the CM-Ala has a possibility to be developed as an effective antitumor immunostimulator.[30]

Enzymes

From the fractionation of the fresh herb's milky sap, two nucleases CMN1 (20 kDa) and CMN2 (36 kDa) were separated. They exhibited the apoptotic activity in human HeLa cervical carcinoma cells but no effect in Chinese Hamster Ovary (CHO) tumor cells. The highest proapoptotic activity was elicited by CMN2 in a concentration of 13.3 ng/mL, leading 62% of the HeLa cells to apoptotic death.[31]

Nanoformulation

For efficiently delivering chelidonine (**1**) to the cancer cells, chelidonine-loaded poly(lactide-co-glycolide) (PLGA) nanoparticles were created by encapsulating chelidonine in biodegradable PLGA polymers. The nanochelidonine exerted stronger apoptotic and inhibitory efficacies against HepG2 hepatoma cells *in vitro* and *in vivo* without any toxicity. Also, the nanochelidonine presented well-improved bioavailabilities, such as rapid cellular uptake, better tissue distribution profile, and greater ability of prolonged and sustained release of chelidonine (**1**).[32] Besides, the nanochelidonine was found to permeated into the brain tissue, indicating that the nanoparticle has better potentials for brain carcinoma chemotherapy.[32]

Clinical Trials

Bai Qu Cai had been used in clinical trials to treat patients suffering from esophagus epitheloid carcinoma and prostomach carcinoma in China. It notably induced the degeneration of tumor tissue and the infiltration around the lymphocytes, whose results evidenced that the antitumor activity is mainly mediated by the stimulation of the immunorejection function.[33] An intravenous injection of Bai Qu Cai alkaloids to cancer patients in a dose of 10 mg per time and per three days potentiated the numbers of total T cells and supplementary T cells, lessened T suppressor cells, and amplified NK cells, whose data again confirmed Bai Qu Cai to be an antitumor immunoactivator.[34]

By randomized clinical trials, Ukrain (**5**) was demonstrated to have curative effects on a range of neoplasms. Thirty six patients with late-stage cancer had been treated with Ukrain (**5**) conjugated with thiophosphoric acid by intravenous injection every second day in a dose of 10 mg per administration, and each patient received 30 injections of this drug in the treatment period. The conjugated Ukrain (**5**) in a concentration not cytostatic in normal cells showed cytostatic and suppressive effects on the malignant tumor cells, together with marked immunopotentiating effect by regulating the T lymphocyte subsets.[35,36] Ukrain (**5**) has been now advertised as a promising chemotherapeutic agent for alternative cancer cures.[19]

Other Bioactivities

The herb Bai Qu Cai can be effectively used for the treatment of gall bladder, kidney, and liver diseases. Pharmacological researches established that the herb possesses analgesic, antispasmodic, antitussive, expectorant, antiasthmatic, antiviral, antiinflammatory, and antimicrobial properties. In addition, its fresh herb juice can be used for malignant skin disorders, corns, warts, and incurable herpes.

The studies in animal models afforded positive evidences for the isoquinoline alkaloids possessing analgesic, cholagogic, antimicrobial, CNS sedative, and immunostimulating properties. The whole plant extract in moderate doses showed toxicity due to containing isoquinoline alkaloids. The successful therapeutic treatment must be under the selected correct dosage.

References

1. Biswas, S. et al. 2002. Effect of a homeopathic drug, Chelidonium, in amelioration of p-DAB induced hepatocarcinogenesis in mice. *BMC Complem. Altern. Med.* 2: 4.
2. Biswas, S. et al. 2008. Efficacy of a plant extract (*Chelidonium majus* L.) in combating induced hepatocarcinogenesis in mice. *Food Chem. Toxicol.* 46: 1474–87.
3. Sokoloff, B. et al. 1968. The oncostatic and oncolytic factors present in certain plants. *Oncol.* 22: 49–60.
4. Zhang, Z. X. et al. (a) 1985. Effect of Chelidonium majus on human esophageal cancer cells in vitro. *J. Henan Med. Univ.* (4): 260; (b) 1999. *Chin. Materia Medica.* Vol. 3, 3–2230, 617. Shanghai Science and Technology Press, Shanghai, China.
5. Kim, D. J. et al. 1997. Chemopreventive effects of *Chelidonium majus* L. (Papaveraceae) herb extract on rat gastric carcinoma induced by N-methyl-N′-nitro-N-nitrosoguanidine (MNNG) and hypertonic sodium chloride. *J. Food Sci. Nutri.* 2: 49–54.
6. Lee, J. et al. 2005. Cytotoxic isoquinoline alkaloids from *Chelidonium majus* var. *asiaticum*. *Agricult. Chem. Biotechnol.* 48: 198–201.
7. Kaminskyy, V. et al. 2008. Differential effect of sanguinarine, chelerythrine and chelidonine on DNA damage and cell viability in primary mouse spleen cells and mouse leukemic cells. *Cell Biol. Intl.* 32: 271–7.
8. Hladon, B. et al. 1978. Cytotoxic activity of some alkaloids on human *Chelidonium majus* and animal tumor cell cultures in vitro. *Ann. Pharm.* (Poznan) 13: 61–8.
9. Paul, A. et al. 2012. Chelidonine isolated from ethanolic extract of *Chelidonium majus* promotes apoptosis in HeLa cells through p38-p53 and PI3K/AKT signalling pathways. *Zhongxiyi Jiehe Xuebao* 10: 1025–38.
10. Philchenkov, A. et al. 2008. Apoptogenic activity of two benzophenanthridine alkaloids from *Chelidonium majus* L. does not correlate with their DNA damaging effects. *Toxicol. in Vitro* 22: 287–95.
11. Kumar, S. et al. 2014. Chelerythrine induces reactive oxygen species-dependent mitochondrial apoptotic pathway in a murine T cell lymphoma. *Tumor Biol.* 35: 129–40.
12. El-Readi Mahmoud, Z. et al. 2013. Modulation of multidrug resistance in cancer cells by chelidonine and *Chelidonium majus* alkaloids. *Phytomed.* 20: 282–94.
13. Roublevskaia, I. N. et al. 2000. Bcl-2 overexpression protects human keratinocyte cells from Ukrain-induced apoptosis but not from G2/M arrest. *Druds under Exper. Clin. Res.* 26: 149–56.
14. Roublevskaia, I. H. et al. 2000. Induced apoptosis in human prostate cancer cell line LNCaP by Ukrain. *Druds under Exper. Clin. Res.* 26: 141–7.
15. Roublevskaia, I. H. et al. 2000. Induced G2/M arrest and apoptosis in human epidermoid carcinoma cell lines by the semisynthetic drug Ukrain. *Anticancer Res.* 20: 3163–7.
16. Venkatesh, K. et al. 2011. Effect of Ukrain on cell survival and apoptosis in the androgen-independent prostate cancer cell line PC3. *J. Envir. Pathol. Toxicol. Oncol.* 30: 11–9.
17. Gagliano, N. et al. 2012. Pancreatic cancer cells retain the epithelial-related phenotype and modify mitotic spindle microtubules after the administration of Ukrain in vitro. *Anti-Cancer Drugs* 23: 935–46.
18. Susak, Y. M. et al. 2010. Comparative investigation of the effect of Ukrain on growth of ascite and solid forms of Ehrlich's carcinoma. *Experim. Oncol.* 32: 107–10.
19. Lanvers-Kaminsky, C. et al. 2006. In vitro toxicity of Ukrain against human Ewing tumor cell lines. *Anti-Cancer Drugs* 17: 1025–30.
20. Bozeman, E. N. et al. 2012. Ukrain, a plant derived semisynthetic compound, exerts antitumor effects against murine and human breast cancer and induce protective antitumor immunity in mice. *Experim. Oncol.* 34: 340–7.
21. Skivka, L. M. et al. 2011. The effect of monotherapy and combined therapy with NSC-631570 (Ukrain) on growth of low- and high-metastasizing B16 melanoma in mice. *J. Oncol. Pharmacy Practice* 17: 339–49.
22. Shalimov, S. A. et al. 2001. Antitumor and immunomodulating effects of a drug composition based on thiophosphoric derivatives of celandine alkaloids. *Eksperimental'naya Onkologiya* 23: 282–6.

23. Shalimov, S. A. et al. 2003. Antimetastatic effect of the preparation of thiophosphorous acid and celandine alcaloids in vivo after removal of primary tumor. *Eksperimental'naya Onkologiya* 25: 152–4.
24. Savran, B. et al. 2014. Anticancer agent Ukrain and bortezomib combination is synergistic in 4T1 breast cancer cells. *Anti-Cancer Agents in Med. Chem.* 14: 466–72.
25. Ramadani, M. et al. 2000. Selective induction of apoptosis in pancreatic cancer cell lines by NSC-631570. *Chirurgisches Forum fuer Exper. Kinische Forschung* 79–83.
26. Yagodina, O. V. et al. 2003. Inhibition of the activity of mitochondrial monoamine oxidase by alkaloids isolated from *Chelidonium majus* and Macleaya, and by derivative drugs "Ukrain" and "Sanguirythrine." *Tsitologiya* 45: 1032–7.
27. Zemskov, S. V. et al. 1996. Antimetastatic effect of Ukrain and its influence on the oxygen and energy metabolism of mice with melanoma B16. *Eksperimental'naya Onkologiya* 18: 405–8.
28. Papuc, C. et al. 2012. Scavenging activity of reactive oxygen species by polyphenols extracted from different vegetal parts of celandine (*Chelidonium majus*). Chemiluminescence screening. *Revista de Chimie* 63: 193–7.
29. Kim, G. H. et al. 2000. Antitumor, immunity-reinforcing, and hematogenous polysaccharide composition extracted from *Chelidonium majus* linne herb. *Repub. Korean Kongkae Taeho Kongbo* KR2000065692 A 20001115.
30. Song, J. Y. et al. 2002. Immunomodulatory activity of protein-bound polysaccharide extracted from *Chelidonium majus*. *Archiv. Pharm. Res.* 25: 158–64.
31. Nawrot, R. et al. 2008. Nucleases isolated from *Chelidonium majus* L. milky sap can induce apoptosis in human cervical carcinoma HeLa cells but not in Chinese hamster ovary CHO cells. *Folia Histochemica et Cytobiologica* 46: 79–83.
32. Paul, A. et al. 2013. Cytotoxicity and apoptotic signalling cascade induced by chelidonine-loaded PLGA nanoparticles in HepG2 cells in vitro and bioavailability of nano-chelidonine in mice in vivo. *Toxicol. Lett.* 222: 10–22.
33. Xian, M. S. et al. 1989. Efficacy of traditional Chinese herbs on squamous cell carcinoma of the esophagus: Histopathologic analysis of 240 cases. *Acta Med. Okayama* 43: 345–51.
34. Nowicky, J. W. et al. 1991. Evaluation of thiophosphoric acid alkaloid derivatives from *Chelidonium majus* L. (Ukrain) as an immuno-stimulant in patients with various carcinomas. *Drugs Exp. Clin. Res* 17: 139–43.
35. Ernst, E. et al. 2005. Ukrain–a new cancer cure? A systematic review of randomized clinical trials. *BMC Cancer* 5: 69.
36. Nowicky, J. W. et al. 1992. Ukrain both as an anticancer and immunoregulatory agent. *Drugs Exp. Clin. Res.* 18(Suppl): 51–4.

146 Yun Zhi 雲芝

Turkey tail or Kawaratake

Herb Origination

The herb Yun Zhi (Turkey tail) is the fruit body of an inedible mushroom, *Coriolus versicolor* (= *Trametes versicolor*). The mushroom is a small, flexible polypore fungus with a wide variety of colors. The mushrooms generally grow on tree trunks and fallen logs in the woods throughout the world. Yun Zhi has been broadly used in herbal remedies throughout Asia for centuries. Traditionally, the mushroom is harvested, dried, ground to a powder, and then taken as a tea drink.

Antitumor Activities

The inedible mushroom Yun Zhi has been demonstrated to exert antitumor effects on various types of cancer cells. Its aqueous ethanolic extract was cytotoxic to HeLa cervical cancer and fibroblast cells *in vitro*. At the 10 μL treatment level, the cell growth inhibitory rates were 45% and 38%, respectively, on the two tumor cell lines.[1] The extract also markedly inhibited the proliferation of B cell lymphoma (Raji) cells and two promyelocytic leukemia (HL-60 and NB-4) cells in a dose-dependent manner *in vitro*. At 50–800 μg/mL concentration, its inhibition against the growth of these cancer cells could reach to 90%. The IC_{50} values were 147.3 μg/mL on HL-60 cells, 253.8 μg/mL on Raji cells, and 269.3 μg/mL on NB-4 cells, but it showed no obvious cytotoxic effect on normal liver WRL cells.[2] During the antitumor action on the HL-60, Raji, and NB-4 cells, the nucleosome productions were notably amplified and the cells were promoted to apoptosis by downregulating Bcl-2 expression and upregulating Bax expression. Also, cytochrome c was released from the mitochondria to the cytosol after the treatment (24 h) in HL-60 cells. The antitumor effect was further confirmed by using the athymic nude mouse xenograft model with HL-60 leukemia cells *in vivo*.[3] Also, the antiproliferative effects against lymphoma and leukemia cells were accompanied by the induction of apoptotic mitochondrial pathway. Moreover, the extract at the same time significantly augmented the proliferation of murine splenic lymphocytes in time- and dose-dependent manners and prominently accelerated the production of four T help 1-related cytokines, including IL-2, IL-12, IL-18, and IFN-γ.[4] The experiments proved that Yun Zhi has excellent capability to augment NK cell activity and T cell proliferation, and to enhance IFN and interleukin-2 responses. These immunoenhancing functions could also inhibit the tumor metastasis and counteract the depressive effect of chemotherapy on WBC counts. The Yun Zhi extract has been used in patients as an adjunct to conventional carcinoma treatments, and the marked increase of survival rates resulted.[4,5]

Antitumor Constituents and Activities

Polysaccharides and protein-bound polysaccharides were found to be the major anticarcinoma components in the fungi. These components were effective in the blockage of BAP binding to the DNA in mouse liver cells and the reduction of oxidative DNA damage and superoxide anion formation, exerting both antigenotoxic- and antitumor-promoting activities *in vitro*. The data demonstrated that the polysaccharides have great potential in the chemotherapy and chemoprevention of cancer.[5] PSK and PSP are the two most valuable polysaccharide-type agents prepared from Yun Zhi for cancer therapy clinics.

PSK

PSK, also known as krestin derived from the hot water extract of cultured Yun Zhi mycelia by Japanese researchers, is a unique protein-bound β-glucan. It is composed of 62% polysaccharide with (1–4) and (1–3) bonds and 38% protein. Its polysaccharide portion contains small amount of fucose but no arabinose and rhamnose. PSK has been used as a chemoimmunotherapy agent in the treatment of cancer patients along with several therapy protocols in Asia for over 30 years. Many clinical trials demonstrated that PSK could improve the quality of life after surgery or in chemotherapy, and it could extend the survival rates by 5–10 years, especially, for patients with colorectal and stomach cancers. In addition, it also has antiviral, cholesterol-regulating, and immunopotentiating properties.[6,7]

In vitro and *in vivo* studies have suggested that the efficacy of PSK is a biological response modifier (BRM), which potentially augments the ability of the host to defend itself from tumor progression via the increase of leukocyte activation and response through the upregulation of key immune cytokine expression, including the activation of NK cells and lymphocyte-activated killer (LAK) cells. Thus, PSK in combination with chemotherapy could remarkably enhance the anticancer effect of cisplatin against human cervical cancer and rat H4-II-E hepatoma *in vivo*.[8] In a dose of 250 mg/kg (twice a week for three weeks), PSK was effective in the prolongation of the survival period in rats bearing mammary adenocarcinoma and in the inhibition of tumor growth during the carcinogenesis.[9] When the cotreatment with an anticancer drug etoposide is done, PSK demonstrated synergistic apoptosis-inducing effects *in vitro* to enhance the chemotherapeutic potency.[10] In addition, PSK also could also regulate the cytokines related to differentiation and induce leukemic cell differentiation *in vitro*.[6]

Moreover, PSK has an antioxidant capacity to mimic SOD activity and to decrease lipid peroxide production, whose effects may enable PSK to defend the host from oxidative stress and to attenuate the carcinogenic incidences. When used in combination with chemotherapy and/or radiotherapy in cancer treatment, PSK might play roles not only as a normal tissue chemo- and radioprotector, but also as an inhibitor to prevent second primary carcinogenesis.[8]

Importantly, PSK is effective to both primary and metastatic carcinomas to prolong the survival periods.[11] The experiments in metastasis models revealed that PSK has the abilities to suppress the pulmonary metastasis of human DU145M prostate neoplastic cells and methylcholanthrene-induced sarcoma cells and to obstruct the lymphatic metastasis of mouse P388 leukemia cells and the metastasis of advanced human HCT-116 and SW480 colorectal cancer cells, whose antimetastatic effects were also observed in the treatment of rat AH60C hepatoma, mouse colon 26, and RL leukemia after being treated with PSK. The antimetastatic effect of PSK was found to closely correlate with the activation of macrophages and the enhancement of the antitumor immunocascade actions and to also associate with the inhibition of metalloproteinases and the regulation of MRP-3, lymphotactin, transgelin, and/or Pirin activities.[6,11,12] The antimetastasis elicited by PSK normally followed five main processes: (1) inhibiting the tumor cell invasion, adhesion, and matrix-degrading enzyme secretion; (2) repressing the tumor cell-induced platelet aggregation for the inhibition of tumor cells attached to endothelial cells; (3) blocking the tumor cell motility and migration; (4) suppressing the angiogenesis in tumor; and (5) reducing the free radical and superoxidant trapping for antitumor progression.[13]

Although PSK has few light side effects, it can be administered for long periods in cancer therapy clinics without toxicity, appearing to be a useful adjuvant agent for enhancing the effects of chemotherapy and radiotherapy, reducing current cancer treatment-caused side effects, and preventing the cancer cells to metastasis.

PSP

PSP, as a polysaccharopeptide, was prepared from the mycelial broth of Yun Zhi fungi COV-1 strain by Chinese researchers, which has been developed as an adjuvant in cancer chemotherapy in China. The molecule of PSP (26–100 kDa) contains a main chain of an α-(1–4) and β-(1–3) glucan and tightly bound polypeptides (15–38%). Its polysaccharide portion is composed of a small amount of xylose, galactose, mannose, arabinose, and rhamnose in addition to glucose and the peptide portion mainly consisted of aspartic acid and glutamic acid.[14–17]

PSP at the concentration of 1 mg/mL markedly inhibited the proliferation of some human tumor cell lines, such as SGC-7901 (stomach), SPC (lung), HepG2 (liver), SLY, and Mei cells *in vitro*, and showed significant inhibitory effect on sarcoma 180 and P388 leukemia *in vivo*.[18,19] The oral administration of PSP to mice at a dosage of 1–2 g/kg per day for 15–20 days or at a dosage of 2.5 g/kg per day for four weeks resulted in the growth inhibition on human lung adenocarcinoma and human nasopharyngeal cancer for 50–70%, and 63–77%, respectively.[20–22] The i.p. injection of PSP at a dose of 50 mg/kg/day to mice for about three weeks suppressed the growth of Lewis lung cancer cells by nearly 45%.[23] Normally, PSP does not exert a direct cytotoxic effect on tumor cells. However, a direct cytotoxicity by PSP was only observed on human SPC lung cancer cells *in vitro*.[18]

Similar to PSK, PSP can accelerate the apoptotic death of many carcinoma cells. For instance, the induction of apoptosis and the inhibition of MDA-MB-231 breast carcinoma cells were primarily mediated by the upregulation of p21 and the downregulation of cyclin-D1.[24] The HL-60 cell apoptosis elicited by PSP is commonly associated with a decrease of Bcl-2/Bax ratio, the drop of mitochondrial transmembrane potential, the release of cytochrome c, and the activation of caspase-3, caspase-8, and caspase-9. The apoptosis of human HL-60 promyelocytic leukemia cells promoted by PSP might be also mediated by the upregulation of early transcription factors, such as AP-1, EGR1, IER2, and IER5, and the downregulation of NF-κB transcription pathways. Simultaneously, several apoptotic and antiproliferation genes such as GADD45A/B and TUSC2 were appreciably increased, and the batch of phosphatase and kinase genes was decreased. PSP also altered some other carcinogenesis-related gene transcripts such as SAT, DCT, Melan-A, u-PA, and cyclin-E1 in the HL-60 cells. These gene expression events further stimulated the HL-60 cell apoptosis.[25,26] The apoptosis of human Molt-4 leukemia cells enhanced by PSP was accompanied by the cell cycle arrest at S phase.[27]

Besides the antitumor effects, PSP displayed potent immunostimulatory properties, such as the promotion of T cell and $CD4^+$ T helper cell proliferation, the activation of NK and LAK cells, the rise of the thymus weight, the enhancement of the macrophage activity in normal mice, and the improvement of the proliferation index of human normal peripheral blood mononuclear cells. It also increased serum C3 and IgG contents and promoted anticancer cytokine IL-2, IL-6, IFNγ, and TNFα production in tumor-bearing animals. The data designated that the *in vivo* suppression of tumor mass growth by PSP ought to be principally attributed to these remarkable immunopotentiating activities. Several randomized clinical trials have demonstrated that PSP has a great potential as an adjuvant agent in cancer chemotherapies and radiotherapies based upon the positive results such as the enhancement of anticancer activities and the improvement of life quality of the patients who have carcinoma in the stomach, the esophagus, the colon, the breast, and the lung.[6,13,27–30] The investigations also told us that PSP could minimize the toxicity and the side effects that were induced by chemotherapeutic drugs, such as DOX, CTX, etoposide, etc., and radiotherapy,[31–34] and it could potentiate the cytotoxicity of clinical chemodrugs and radiotherapy, via an effective enhancement of immune responsiveness protective effects.

Furthermore, PSP has a great capacity to suppress the vascular density in cancer tissue via a significant decrease of VEGF expression. The antiangiogenic property should be one of the pathways involved in the tumor inhibitory effect elicited by PSP.[35] In addition, due to having antioxidative function and inducing SOD, PSP could notably scavenge active oxygen and protect the cell damages from superoxide radical ($O^{2-\cdot}$), SOD abnormities, $O^{2-\cdot}$ overproduction.[36] The findings afforded more supports for the use of PSP to restrain the carcinogenesis.

Consequently, PSP is primarily considered as a BRM with potential cancer therapeutic applications. During 1991–1997, encapsulated PSP had been subjected tophase II and III clinical trials as an adjuvant for the treatment of stomach, primary lung, and esophagus carcinoma patients in Shanghai (China). The overall effective ratio was significantly increased from 42% to 85.8% with relatively low toxic side effects.[37]

VPS

VPS, a versicolor polysaccharide, is the third product prepared from Yun Zhi mushroom that is commercialized as a dietary supplement in the United States, which is also being studied for the cancer treatment *in vivo*. However, the VPS was reported to have no effect on colon carcinoma in mice, but it also enhanced the colon cancer development induced by a carcinogen 1,2-dimethylhydrazine dihydrochloride (1,2-DMH) *in vivo*.[6,38]

References

1. Uenyayar, A. et al. 1977. Evaluation of cytotoxic and mutagenic effects of *Coriolus versicolor* and *Funalia trogii* extracts on mammalian cells. *Drug Chem. Toxicol.* 29: 69–83.
2. Lau, C. B. S. et al. 2004. Cytotoxic activities of *Coriolus versicolor* (Yunzhi) extract on human leukemia and lymphoma cells by induction of apoptosis. *Life Sci.* 75: 797–808.
3. Ho, C. Y. et al. 2006. *Coriolus versicolor* (Yunzhi) extract attenuates growth of human leukemia xenografts and induces apoptosis through the mitochondrial pathway. *Oncol. Reports* 16: 609–16.
4. Ho, C. Y. et al. 2004. Differential effect of *Coriolus versicolor* (Yunzhi) extract on cytokine production by murine lymphocytes in vitro. *Intl. Immunopharmacol.* 4: 1549–57.
5. Kim, H. S. et al. 1999. In vitro chemopreventive effects of plant polysaccharides (Aloe barbadensis Miller, Lentinus edodes, *Ganoderma lucidum* and *Coriolus versicolor*). *Carcinogenesis* 20: 1637–40.
6. Fisher, M. et al. 2002. Anticancer effects and mechanisms of polysaccharide-K(PSK): Implications of cancer immunotherapy. *Anticancer Res.* 22: 1737–54.
7. Hobbs, C. R. et al. 2004. Medicinal value of Turkey tail fungus *Trametes versicolor* (L.Fr.) Pilat (*Aphyllophoromycetideae*). *Intl. J. Med. Mushrooms* 6: 195–218.
8. Kobayashi, Y. et al. 1994. Enhancement of anticancer activity of cisdiaminedichloroplatinum by the protein-bound polysaccharide of Coriolus versicolor QUEL (PSK) in vitro. *Cancer Biotherapy* 9: 351–8.
9. Fujii, T. et al. 1995. Prolongation of the survival period with the biological response modifier PSK in rats bearing N-methyl-N-nitrosourea-induced mammary gland tumors. *In Vivo* 9: 55–8.
10. Takahata, K. et al. 1999. Antitumor drugs containing apoptosis-inducing and -promoting agents. *Jpn. Kokai Tokkyo Koho* JP 97–250051 19970829.
11. Ebina, T. et al. 2003. Activation of antitumor immunity by intratumor injection of biological preparations. *Gan to Kagaku Ryoho* 30: 1555–8.
12. Yoshikawa, R. et al. 2004. Gene expression in response to antitumor intervention by polysaccharide-K (PSK) in colorectal carcinoma cells. *Oncol. Reports* 12: 1287–93.
13. Kobayashi, H. et al. 1995. Antimetastatic effects of PSK (krestin), a protein-bound polysaccharide obtained from basidiomycetes: An overview. 1995. *Cancer Epidemiol., Biomarkers Prevention* 4: 275–81.
14. Zhou, J. X. et al. 1988. The antitumor and immunomodulating activity of PSP in mice. *J. Shanghai Teachers Univ.* 17: 72–7.
15. Zhou, Y. L. et al. 1999. Active principles from Coriolus sp. In Yang, Q. Y. (ed.). *Int. Symp. Trad. Chin. Med. Cancer: Dev. Clin. Valid.—Adv. Res. in PSP 1999.* Hong Kong Association for Health Care Ltd, Hongkong, pp. 111–124.
16. Jong, S. C. et al. 1998. PSP—A powerful biological response modifier from the mushroom *Coriolus vesicolor.* In Yang, Q. Y. (ed.). *Int. Symp. Trad. Chin. Med. Cancer: Dev. Clin. Valid.—Adv. Res. in PSP 1999.* Hong Kong Association for Health Care Ltd, Hongkong, pp. 16–28.
17. Ng, T. B. et al. 1998. A review of research on the protein-bound polysaccharide (polysaccharo-peptide, PSP) from the mushroom Coriolus versicolor (Basidiomycetes: Polyporaceae). *General Pharmacol.* 30: 1–4.
18. Xu, L. Z. et al. 1989. Experimental research on the anticancer immunomodulative effect of the polysocoharibepeptide of *Coriolus versicolor. Chin. J. Cancer Res.* 1: 7–12.
19. Dong, Y. et al. 1996. Antitumor effects of a refined polysaccharide peptide fraction isolated from *Coriolus versicolor*: In vitro and in vivo studies. *Res. Comm. Mole. Pathol. Pharmacol.* 92: 140–8.
20. Zeng, S. et al. 1993. The anticancerous effects of Yun Zhi essence on human lung adenocarcinoma inoculated in nude mice. In Yang, Q. and Kwok, C. (eds.). *Proc. PSP Int. Symp. Fudan University Press*, Shanghai, pp. 97–103.
21. Wang, C. A. et al. 1993. The effect of Yun Zhi essence and schizophyllan in activating the lymphocytes of the peripheral blood to kill stomach liver and lung cancerous cells and leukocytes. *Proc. PSP Int. Symp.* Fudan University Press, Shanghai, pp. 139–142.
22. Zeng, S. J. et al. 1999. The anticancerous effects of PSP compound on human nasopharyngeal carcinoma inoculated on nude mice. In Yang, Q. Y. (ed.). *Int. Symp. Trad. Chin. Med. Cancer: Dev. Clin. Valid.—Adv. Res. PSP 1999.* Hong Kong Association for Health Care Ltd, Hongkong, p. 201.
23. Chu, K. K. W. et al. 2002. Coriolus versicolor: A medicinal mushroom with promising immunotherapeutic values. *J. Clin. Pharmacol.* 42: 976–84.
24. Chow, L. W. C. et al. 2003. Polysaccharide peptide mediates apoptosis by up-regulating p21 gene and down-regulating cyclin D1 gene. *Am. J. Chin. Med.* 31: 1–9.
25. Yang, X. T. et al. 2005. The cell death process of the anticancer agent polysaccharide-peptide (PSP) in human promyelocytic leukemic HL-60 cells. *Oncol. Report*s 13: 1201–10.
26. Zeng, F. Y. et al. 2005. Molecular characterization of *Coriolus versicolor* PSP-induced apoptosis in human promyelotic leukemic HL-60 cells using cDNA microarray. *Intl. J. Oncol.* 27: 513–23.
27. Li, X. Y. et al. 2000. Immunomodulating components from Chinese medicines. *Pharm. Biol.* 38(Suppl.): 33–40.
28. Lee, C. L. et al. 2006. The culture duration affects the immunomodulatory and anticancer effect of polysaccharopeptide derived from *Coriolus versicolor. Enzyme Microbial Technol.* 38: 14–21.
29. Li, X. Y. et al. 1999. Advances in immunomodulating studues of PSP. In Yang, Q. Y. (ed.). *Int. Symp. Trad. Chin. Med. Cancer: Dev. Clin. Valid.—Adv. Res. PSP 1999.* Hong Kong Association for Health Care Ltd, Hongkong, pp. 39–46.
30. Liu, W. K. et al. 1999. Evidence that *C. versicolor* polysaccharopeptide acts on tumor cells through an immunomodulatory effect on macrophages. In Yang, Q. Y. (ed.). *Int. Symp. Trad. Chin. Med. Cancer: Dev. Clin. Valid.—Adv. Res. PSP 1999.* Hong Kong Association for Health Care Ltd, Hongkong, pp. 187–91.
31. Mao, X. W. et al. 1996. Immunotherapy with low-dose interleukin-2 and a polysaccharopeptide derived from *Coriolus versicolor. Cancer Biother. Radiopharm.* 11: 393–403.
32. Hui, K. P. Y. et al. 2005. Induction of S phase cell arrest and caspase activation by polysaccharide peptide isolated from *Coriolus versicolor* enhanced the cell cycle dependent activity and apoptotic cell death of doxorubicin and etoposide, but not cytarabine in HL-60 cells. *Oncol. Reports* 14: 145–55.

33. Chan, S. L. et al. 2006. Effects of polysaccharide peptide (PSP) from *Coriolus versicolor* on the pharmacokinetics of cyclophosphamide in the rat and cytotoxicity in HepG2 cells. *Food Chem. Toxicol.* 44: 689–94.
34. Mao, X. W. et al. 2001. Evaluation of polysaccharopeptide effects against C6 glioma in combination with radiation. *Oncol.* 61: 243–53.
35. Ho, J. C. K. et al. 2004. Fungal polysaccharopeptide inhibits tumor angiogenesis and tumor growth in mice. *Life Sci.* 75: 1343–56.
36. Wu, F. L. et al. 1994. Inhibitory effect of PSP (polysaccharide-peptide from *Coriolus versicolor*) on human hepatoma explanted in nude mice. *J. Jinan Univ., Sci. Med. Edit.* 15: 1–5.
37. Liu, J. X. et al. 1999. Phase III clinical trial for Yun Zhi polysaccharopeptide (PSP) capsules. In Yang, Q. Y. (ed.). *Int. Symp. Trad. Chin. Med. Cancer: Dev. Clin. Valid.—Adv. Res. PSP 1999.* Hong Kong Association for Health Care Ltd, Hongkong, pp. 295–303.
38. Toth, B. et al. 2006. Effects of VPS extract of Coriolus versicolor on cancer of the large intestine using a serial sacrifice technique. *In Vivo* 20: 341–6.

147 Song Gan Lan 松橄欖

Volvate polypare or Cryptopori volvati

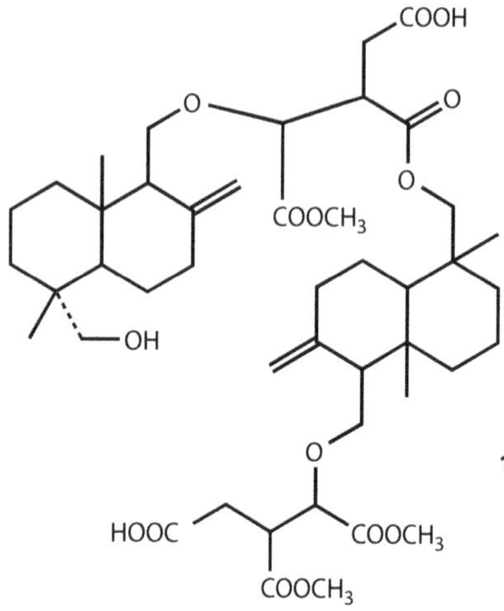

Herb Origination

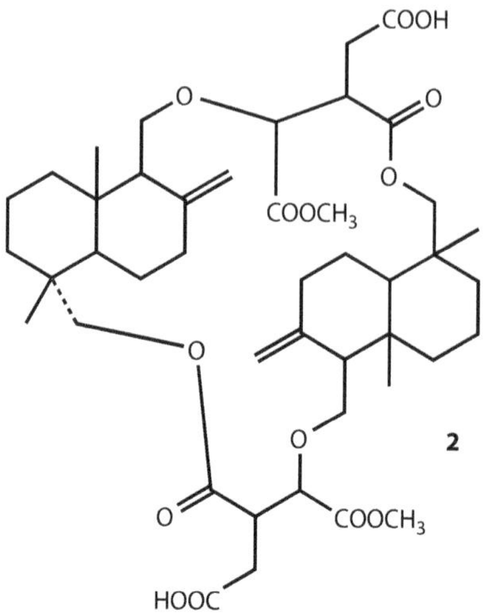

The herb Song Gan Lan (Volvate polypare) is the dried fruit body of a Polyporaceae fungi, *Cryptoporus volvatus*. The edible fungi typically grow on recently killed trees. The distribution of Song Gan Lan broadly ranged from the southern regions of China to Korea, Japan, and North America.

Antitumor Constituents and Activities

Both petrol ether and ethyl acetate extracts derived from Song Gan Lan demonstrated cytotoxicity against human carcinoma cell lines such as HeLa (cervix) and SMMC-7721 (liver) *in vitro*, but its methanol extract only showed weaker *in vitro* activity on the cancer cells, and its water extract displayed *in vivo* antineoplastic effect.[1,2] The aqueous extract from Song Gan Lan is rich in polysaccharides that have been proven to have antitumor and immunoregulatory properties.[3]

Cryptoporic Acids

Cryptoporic acids-A–G, seven bitter drimane-type sesquiterpenoids with an isocitric acid group were isolated from the fungi. These terpenoids strongly inhibited the release of superoxide anion radicals from guinea pig peritoneal macrophage and rabbit polymorphonuclear leukocyte, indicating that the cryptoporic acids have abilities to protect the LPO and to scavenge active oxygen free radicals, having potential benefits in the treatment of carcinogenesis, cancer development, as well as ulceration and inflammation.[4] However, the isolated cryptoporic acid B and cryptoporic acid-G, cryptoporic acid B methyl ester and, 1′,1″-dicarboxylic cryptoporic acid D showed weak cytotoxic activity (IC_{50}: >100 μmol/L) to human tumor cell lines (such as PC3, PANC-1, A549, and MCF-7).[5]

In vivo experiments confirmed that cryptoporic acid E (**1**) exhibited remarkable inhibitory effect against the carcinogenesis in the skin and the colon. It significantly reduced the incidences of colon carcinogenesis promoted by N-methyl-N-nitrosourea in rats and induced by 1,2-dimethylhydrazine in mice.[6] It also suppressed skin tumorigenesis initiated by DMBA and promoted by okadaic acid in mice.[7] Intrarectal deoxycholic acid-induced colonic mucosal ornithine decarboxylase activity was obviously diminished by the cryptoporic acid E (**1**).[6] However, cryptoporic acid D (**2**) could slightly enhance the tumor promotion and activate PKC. In comparison of the structure of cryptoporic acid E (**1**), the presence of a macrolide ring formed in cryptoporic acid D (**2**) is known, and only this structural difference totally altered their effect on the tumor cell growth.[8]

Polysaccharides

From a hot water extract of the fruiting bodies of Song Gan Lan, a water-soluble (1–6)-branched (1–3)-β-D-glucan (molecular weight: 4.4×10^5) termed H-3-B was isolated. Both H-3-B and its sonicated glucan (S-H-3-B; molecular weight: 1.37×10^5) exhibited the antitumor activity against the sarcoma 180 *in vivo*.[9] A protein–polysaccharide complex was prepared after dialysis and lyophilization of the water extract of Song Gan Lan, whose complex contains 18.2% protein and 55.3% polysaccharide and is composed of four types of monosaccharides and 18 kinds of amino acids. The i.p. injection of this protein–polysaccharide complex to tumor bearing mice for 10 days notably inhibited the growth of sarcoma 180 cells with the inhibitory rates of 80.4% in a high dose of 50 mg/kg/day and 70.3% in a low dose of 20 mg/kg/day.[2]

Other Bioactivities

The herb Song Gan Lan (Volvate polypare) has been reported to possess antiallergy, antiinflammation, and immunomodulatory activities besides the anticarcinoma and anticarcinogenesis.

References

1. Ren, G. et al. 2006. Evaluation of cytotoxic activities of some medicinal polypore fungi from China. *Fitoterapia* 77: 408–10.
2. Kim, B. K. et al. 1982. Antitumor components of *Cryptoporus volvatus*. *Han'guk Kyunhak-hoechi* 10: 111–7.
3. Xie, Q. M. et al. 2006. Effects of cryptoporus polysaccharide on rat allergic rhinitis associated with inhibiting eotaxin mRNA expression. *J. Ethnopharmacol.* 107: 424–30.
4. Masakazu, S. et al. 2000. Chemistry of cryptoporic acids having antitumor promotion activity. *Tennen Yuki Kagobutsu Toronkai Koen Yoshishu* 42nd, 751–6.
5. Wu, W. et al. Chemical constituents and cytotoxic activity on the fruiting bodies of *Cryptoporus sinensis*. *Zhongguo Yaowu Huaxue Zazhi* 21: 47–52.
6. Narisawa, T. et al. 1992. Inhibitory effect of cryptoporic acid E, a product from fungus *Cryptoporus volvatus*, on colon carcinogenesis induced with N-methyl-N-nitrosourea in rats and with 1,2-dimethylhydrazine in mice. *Jpn J. Cancer Res.* 83: 830–4.
7. Matsunaga, S. et al. 1991. Differential effects of cryptoporic acids D and E, inhibitors of superoxide anion radical release, on tumor promotion of okadaic acid in mouse skin. *Carcinogenesis* 12: 1129–31.
8. Asakawa, Y. et al. 1992. Cryptoporic acids A-G, drimane-type sesquiterpenoid ethers of isocitric acid from the fungus *Cryptoporus volvatus*. *Phytochem.* 31: 579–92.
9. Kitamura, S. et al. 1994. An antitumor, branched (1–3)-β-D-glucan from a water extract of fruiting bodies of *Cryptoporus volvatus*. *Carbohydr Res.* 263: 111–21.

148 Lan An 藍桉

Blue gum

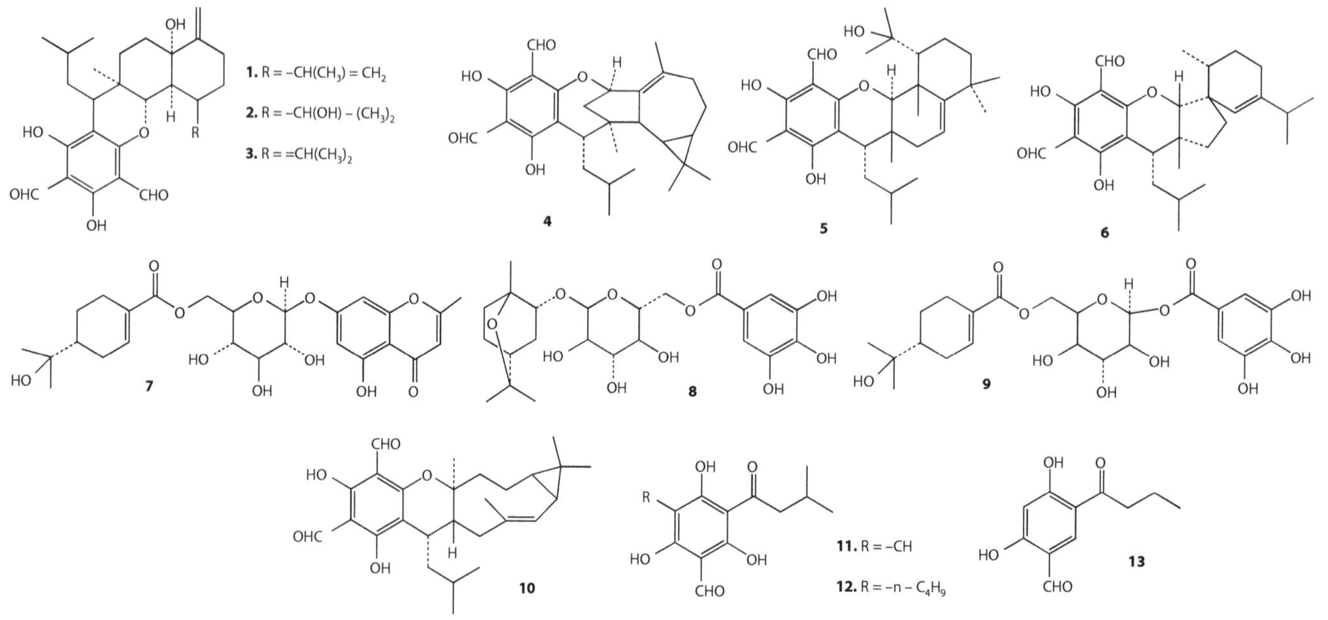

Herb Origination

Lan An (Blue gum) is a Myrtaceae tree, *Eucalyptus globulus*, which is one of the most widely cultivated trees native to Australia. This evergreen tree has been introduced to southern China for over 110 years. Its leaves and fruits are generally collected in autumn and dried in the sun for the application as Chinese herbs. The freshly collected herb is better for the medical practice.

Antitumor Constituents and Activities

Agents from the Fruits

The total triterpenoids derived from Lan An fruit demonstrated obvious inhibitory effect against the proliferation of a panel of human neoplastic cell lines. Its maximum inhibitory rates could reach to 87.25–95.12% on hepatoma cell lines (HepG2, SMMC-7721, BEL-7402, BEL-7404) with IC_{50} values of 8.84–11.5 μg/mL, 88.19–89.27% on gastric cancer cell lines (AGS, SGC-7901) with IC_{50} values of 6.61–7.08 μg/mL, and 88.08–93.05% on colon cancer cell lines (Caco-2, LS-174-T) with IC_{50} values of 7.24–9.55 μg/mL. It was also effective in the suppression of 786-0 renal cancer, A549 lung cancer, HeLa cervical cancer, MCF-7 breast cancer, Eca-109 esophageal cancer, and HO-8910 ovarian cancer cell lines, where their IC_{50} values were <20 μg/mL and the maximum inhibitions were over 85%, whose potencies were similar to those of 5-FU and VCR. But the total triterpenoids were also sensitive to K562 leukemia and DU-145 prostate cancer cell lines with 51.80% and 68.42% inhibitory rates, respectively. Phytochemical approaches revealed that the total triterpenoids from Lan An fruit are largely composed of ursolic acid (23.3%), betulonic acid (26.8%), betulinic acid (13.2%), and colosolic acid (10.3%).[1,2]

The separation of the Lan An fruit yielded eucalyptals-A–E (**1–5**) and euglobalin-3 (**6**), which are six cytotoxic sesquiterpenes coupled with 3,5-diformyl-isopentyl phloroglucinol. *In vitro* bioassay showed that eucalyptal-A–C (**1–3**) restrained the proliferation of human HL-60 leukemia cells and their IC_{50} values were 1.7, 6.8, and 17 μM, respectively.[3] Eucalyptal-D (**4**), eucalyptal-E (**5**), and euglobalin-3 (**6**) exhibited obvious *in vitro* cytotoxic activities against four human cancer cell lines. The IC_{50} values were 4.63–7.22 μM in KE-97 gastric cancer cells, 7.16–10.71 μM in Jurkat T lymphoma cells, 6.65–14.27 μM in BGC-823 gastric cancer cells, and 10.77–24.57 μM in Huh hepatoma cells.[4] Another isolated cypellocarpa-C (**7**) is a phenol glycoside acylated with (+)-oleuropeic acid, which showed potent *in vitro* short-term antitumor-promoting activity against EBV-EA activation promoted by TPA. It also remarkably suppressed a two-stage skin carcinogenesis induced by NO and TPA in mouse and reduced the percentage of tumor-carrying mice from 100% to 30% after a 10-week treatment.[5]

Agents from the Leaves

The treatment with 0.5 mL (50 mg/mL) aqueous extract of Lan An leaves significantly decreased the DNA quantities in various neoplastic cell lines, such as hepatoma, large cell lung cancer, renal cell carcinoma, colon adenocarcinoma, liposarcoma, craniopharyngioma, pineal parenchymal tumor, breast adenocarcinoma, meningioma, medulloblastoma, uterus adenosarcoma, heart sarcoma, gastric adenocarcinoma, Hodgkin's lymphoma, thymoma, leukemia, multiple myeloma, and rhabdomyoma.[6] Several gallic acid-conjugated monoterpene glycosides were isolated from the hot water extract of Lan An leaves. Globulusin-A (**8**) and globulusin-B, cypellocarpin-A, and eucaglobulin (**9**) showed antioxidant activity in scavenging DPPH free radicals. In association with concentration-dependent inhibition on inflammatory cytokines (such as TNFα and interleukin-1β), globulusin-A (**8**) and eucaglobulin (**9**) at 40 μM concentrations restrained the viability of human THP-1 myeloma cells by 71.4% and inhibited melanogenesis in murine B16F1 melanoma cells *in vitro*.[7]

From the leaves and the flower buds of *E. globulus*, many monoterpene-linked euglobals were isolated and showed their inhibitory effects on EBV-EA by a short-term *in vitro*. The results exhibited that most of the euglobals, such as euglobal-III (**10**) grandinol (**11**), homograndinols, and the relatives (**12** and **13**), exerted stronger inhibitory effects on EBV-EA, indicating antimelanoma-promoting potential. Euglobal-III (**10**) also exerted marked inhibition on mouse skin tumor promotion in an *in vivo* two-stage carcinogenesis test.[8,9]

Agents from Crown Gall

Crown gall is the plant tumor of *E. globulus* tree. The crown gall also exhibited the inhibitory effect on the TPA-induced EBV-EA activation. The 80% methanol and the acetone extracts of the plant tumor obstructed the EBV-EA activation by 68% and 65.3% at a concentration of 10 μg/mL, respectively, and by 100% at a concentration of 100 μg/mL (70% viability).[10]

Other Bioactivities

The fruits and the leaves of Lan An (Blue gum) have been used as traditional Chinese medicines to cure diseases such as flu, influenza, inflammation, dysentery, eczema, and scald. Pharmacological studies have proven that the herbs play important roles in antiinflammatory, antioxidant, hypoglycemic, aldose-inhibitory, and antimicrobial effects.

References

1. Wu, Y. T. et al. 2004. An extract from a eucalyptus plant and its medicinal usage. *China Patent* CN1521182 A, CN 03115235.
2. Ding, X. L. et al. 2008. The research progress of chemical components and pharmacology effects of the fruit of eucalyptus globules. *J. Jilin Med. College* (4): 53–5.
3. Wang, J. et al. 2012. Eucalyptals D and E, new cytotoxic phloroglucinols from the fruits of *Eucalyptus globulus* and assignment of absolute configuration. *Tetrahedron Lett.* 53: 2654–8.
4. Yin, S. et al. 2007. Eucalyptals A-C with a new skeleton isolated from *Eucalyptus globulus. Org. Lett.* 9: 5549–52.
5. Yang, X. W. et al. 2007. Intestinal permeability of antivirus constituents from the fruits of *Eucalyptus globulus* Labill. in Caco-2 cell model. *Bioorg. Med. Chem. Lett.* 17: 1107–11.
6. Bayazit, V. et al. 2005. Effects of DNA isolated, limonin, α-interferon, interleukin-2 and tamoxifen citrate, aqueous extract of Eucalyptus globulus leaves on amount of DNA in cancerous organs of female mice. *J. Chem. Soc. Pakistan* 27: 299–305.
7. Hasegawa, T. et al. 2008. Bioactive monoterpene glycosides conjugated with gallic acid from the leaves of *Eucalyptus globulus. Phytochem.* 69: 747–53.
8. Takasaki, M. et al. 1990. Inhibitors of skin-tumor promotion: VIII. Inhibitory effects of euglobals and their related compounds on Epstein-Barr virus activation. *Chem. Pharm. Bull.* 38: 2737–9.
9. Takasaki, M. et al. 1995. Structures of euglobals from Eucalyptus plants. *Tennen Yuki Kagobutsu Toronkai Koen Yoshishu* (37th), pp. 517–22.
10. Brantner, A. H. et al. 2003. Crown gall—A plant tumour with biological activities. *Phytother. Res.* 17: 385–90.

149 Xuan Fu Hua 旋覆花

Inula flower or Elecampane flower

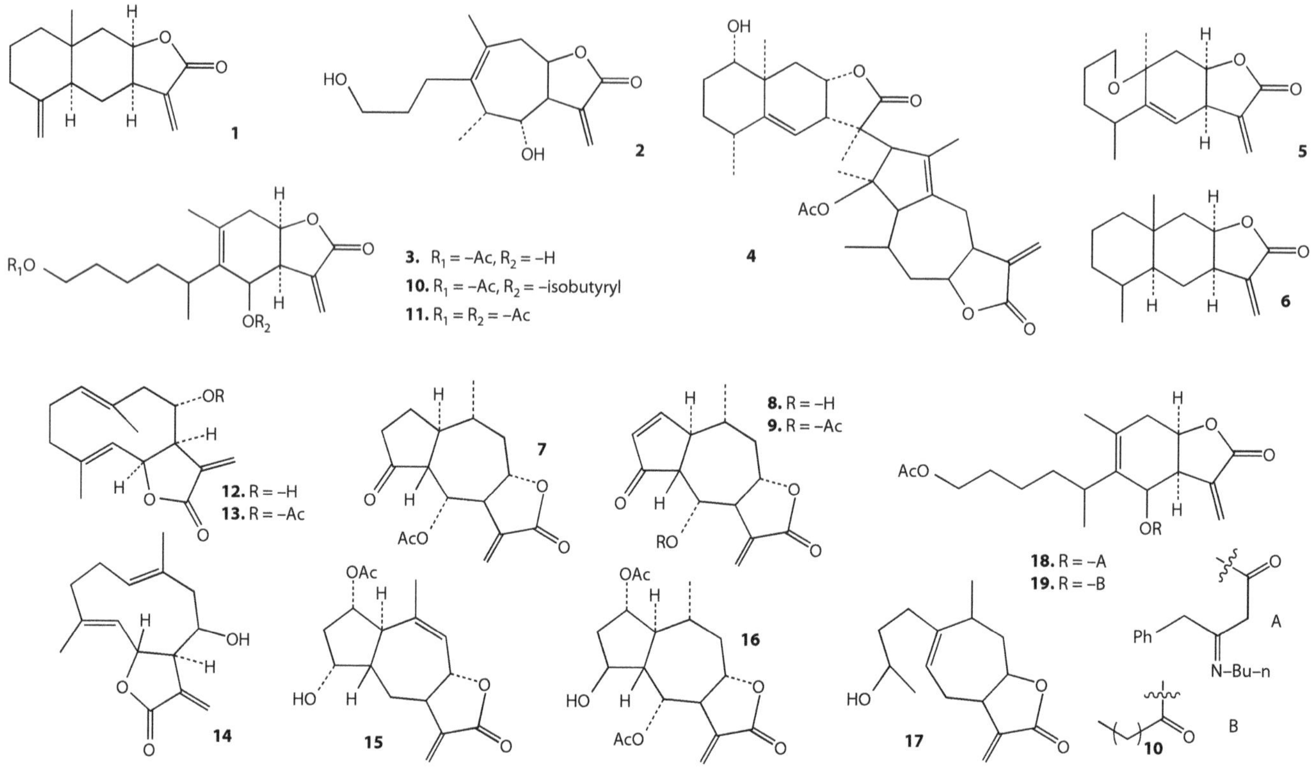

3. R_1 = –Ac, R_2 = –H
10. R_1 = –Ac, R_2 = –isobutyryl
11. R_1 = R_2 = –Ac

8. R = –H
9. R = –Ac

12. R = –H
13. R = –Ac

18. R = –A
19. R = –B

Herb Origination

The herb Xuan Fu Hua (Inula flower) is the dried flowers of two Compositae plants, *Inula japonica* (= *I. britannica* var. *chinensis*) and *I. britannica*. The former plant is extensively distributed in the northern, eastern, and middle regions of China as well as Korea and Japan, and the latter one is native to Europe and temperate Asia. The flowers are normally collected between July and October in China and dried in the sun. Xuan Fu Hua was one of folk herbs documented in the first Chinese classic of materia medica entitled *Shennong Beng Cao Jing* (approximately AD 220).

Anticarcinogenetic Constituents

The ethanolic extract of Xuan Fu Hua has been used as an agent for cancer prevention and treatment due to its activities in inducing the cytotoxicity and the apoptotic death of the cancer cells. Various sesquiterpene lactones from the herb were found to have cytotoxic properties, but they are not quite the same sesquiterpenes separated from the two herb origins.

Agents from the Flowers of I. japonica

Isohelenin (= Isoalantolactone) (**1**) is a major cytotoxic sesquiterpene found from this herb source, which displayed marked cytotoxicity against SMMC-7721 (liver) and HO-8910 (ovary) human cancer cells *in vitro* (respective IC_{50}: 6.21 and 5.28 μg/mL), whereas deacetylinulicin (**2**) only had moderate activity against the two carcinoma cell lines (respective IC_{50}: 52.22 and 21.32 μg/mL).[1] The antiproliferative effects of isoalantolactone (**1**) was also shown in many types of human cancer cell lines such as HLE (liver), MM1-CB (skin), KT (breast), HeLa (cervix), SHIN3, HOC-21 and HAC-2 (ovary), and U251SP (glioma) cells, concomitant with the increase of the apoptotic rates at a concentration of 12.5 μmol/L *in vitro*.[2,3] In an *in vivo* model, isoalantolactone (**1**) markedly suppressed the growth of sarcoma 180.[4] But 1-*O*-acetylbritannilactone (ABL) (**3**), and britannilactone showed weak or moderate antigrowth activities to HeLa, SHIN3, HOAC-21, HAC-2, U251SP, HLE, MM1-CB, and KT cell lines even in the concentration of 100 μmol/L.[2,3] ABL (**3**), which was also found in *I. Britannica*, also showed chemopreventive properties by inducing cell apoptosis in breast, ovarian, and colon cancers. By inducing G0/G1 cell cycle arrest and apoptosis, ABL (**3**) dose- and time-dependently suppressed the growth of HT-29 human colon cancer cells in association with the strong decrease of cyclin-E and CDK4 protein levels and the up-expression p21 and KLF4.[4] It was also capable of restraining the proliferation of vascular smooth muscle cells and neointima formation after a balloon injury in rats.[4] The analysis of the SARs demonstrated that the antitumor effects should be closely related to their structural characters, i.e., an α-exomethylene-γ-lactone ring is necessary for these activities and 1,10-seco of eudesmane sesquiterpene lactone reduces the antitumor activity.[2–5]

Twelve dimeric sesquiterpene lactones assigned as japonicones-A–L (comprised by guaiane and eudesmane skeletons) were discovered from the aerial part of *I. japonica*. Among these molecules, japonicone-A (**4**) showed the most potent cytotoxicity against four human cancer cell lines such as A549 (lung), LoVo (colon), MDA-MB-435 (breast), and CEM (T cell lymphoblastoid), and their IC_{50} values were 1.620, 0.256, 0.198, and 0.001 μg/mL, respectively, whose potencies were even stronger than doxycycline (an antitumor drug).[6] Burkitt lymphoma cells were particularly sensitive, but normal cells were resistive to japonicone-A (**4**). The treatment with japonicone-A (**4**) resulted in G2/M phase arrest and apoptotic death, thereby inhibiting the growth and the proliferation of Raji, BJAB, and NAMALWA lymphoma cells. In an *in vivo* model, japonicone-A (**4**) obstructed the local growth of lymphoma cells and blocked the dissemination of cancer cells to multiple organs. The noticeable anticancer effects on Burkitt lymphoma cells *in vitro* and *in vivo* were found to be mediated by targeting of NF-κB signaling cascade, i.e., downregulation of NF-κB target genes involved in the cell apoptosis (Bcl-2, Bcl-xL, XIAP, TRAF2) and in the cell cycle and growth (cyclin D, c-Myc).[7] The *in vitro* and *in vivo* experiments also revealed that the japonicine-A (**4**) exerted the antigrowth effects against NSCLC cells via mitochondria-mediated pathways and against breast cancer cells (MCF-7, MCF-7 p53-/-, and, MDA-MB-231) by targeting the NFAT1-MDM2-p53 pathway.[8,9] The results provide a basis for future preclinical and clinical evaluations of japonicone-A (**4**) as a chemotherapeutic agent for lymphoma and other solid tumors.

Eupatolide (**5**) is a cyclodeca[b]furan-type sesquiterpene lactone derived from *Inula japonica*, capable of sensitizing human breast cancer cells to TRAIL-induced apoptosis in MCF-7, MDA-MB-231, and MDA-MB-453 cell lines. Therefore, the cytotoxicity of TRAIL could be significantly enhanced in combination with a subtoxic dose of eupatolide (**5**) on the breast carcinoma cells. Also, eupatolide (**5**), by suppressing AKT phosphorylation and downregulating c-FLIP expression, exerted an ability to overcome TRAIL resistance in the breast carcinoma cell lines.[10]

Agents from the Flowers of I. britannica

More sesquiterpene lactones isolated from the flowers of *I. britannica* are principally responsible for the cytotoxicity on a variety of neoplastic cells. Britannilide (**6**) and eremobritanilin (**7**) restrained the proliferation of mouse P388 leukemia cells *in vitro*.[11] A group of other sesquiterpene lactones such as ergolide (**8**), 8-*epi*-helenalin (**9**), bigelovin (**10**), and 6α-isoseptuplinolide exhibited the suppressive effects against human HL-60 (promyelocytic leukemic), Malme-3M (skin), MCF-7 (breast), SKOV-3 (ovary), A549 (lung), and HCT-15 (colon) neoplastic cell lines *in vitro*. The ED_{50} values of ergolide (**8**) and bigelovin (**10**) were 2.7 and 5.6 μM, respectively, in HL-60 cells, which were the most potent in the assay results.[12] 1,6-*O,O*-Diacetylbritannilactone (ODABL) (**11**) significantly promoted the apoptosis and S phase cell cycle arrest of HL-60 cells, associated with the phosphorylation of Bcl-2 and Bid, the release of cytochrome c from the mitochondria, and the activation of caspases (caspase-8, caspase-9, and caspase-3). Also, the production of ROS and the activation of MAPK and c-Jun N-terminal kinase signaling pathways might play important roles in the ODABL (**11**)-provoked HL-60 cell apoptosis.[13] Besides the inhibition of human HL-60 and Molt-4 leukemia cell lines, ODABL (**11**), 6β-*O*-isobutyrylbritannilactone (**12**), hydroxylalantolactone, and 8-epi-ivangustin also displayed moderate suppressive effects against the growth of three human cell lines, A549 (lung cancer), Bel-7402 (hepatoma), and K562 (erythroleukemia), *in vitro*, with IC_{50} values of approximately 12.4–35.5 μM. The IC_{50} value of 12.4 μM achieved by ODABL (**11**) was on the K562 cells.[14] A separate treatment with ODABL (**11**) and 1-*O*-acetylbritannilactone (**3**) for 14 days markedly restrained the proliferation and the clonogenic growth of MCF-7 and T47D (breast), OVCAR and PA-1 (ovary), and Du-145 and DuPro-1 (prostate) human cancer cell lines *in vitro* (IC_{50}: 5–20 μM).[15] The induction of G2/M cell cycle arrest and apoptosis were observed in the inhibition of various cancer cells (breast, prostate, bladder, ovarian, colorectal, and lung) caused by ODABL (**11**).[13,15] The potent activity of OABL was revealed to be due to an acetyl group at 6-hydroxy position enhancing the lipophilicity, and the esterification of 6-OH and α-methylene-γ-lactone functionalities plays important roles in conferring cytotoxicity.[16]

Two other α-methylene-γ-lactone-bearing sesquiterpene lactones, neobritannilactone-B (**13**) and acetyl neobritannilactone-B (**14**) were isolated from this herb, exerting potent apoptosis-inducing effects in human HT-29 and Colo205 (colon), AGS (adenogastric), and HL-60 (leukemic) cancer cell lines *in vitro* in a dose-dependent manner. The percentages of apoptotic cells were amplified in Colo205, HT-29, HL-60, and AGS cells after 24 h of incubation with neobritannilactone-B (**13**) and acetyl neobritannilactone-B (**14**) (25 μM). Their IC_{50} values were in a range of 14.3–56.1 μM, and acetyl neobritannilactone-B (**14**) was more potent than ergolide (**8**) in the *in vitro* assays.[17] Both sesquiterpenes were found to be marked inducers of AGC cell apoptosis and notable inhibitors of AGC cell viability, and the IC_{50} values were 4.2 μM for acetyl neobritannilactone-B (**14**) and 7.6 μM for neobritannilactone-B (**13**).[17,18] Prominently, gaillardin (**15**), britannin (**16**), and 4H-tomentosin (**17**) exerted similar or better cytotoxic activity on drug-resistant cancer cell lines such as MRP1-overexpressed COR-L23/R (lung) cells and P-gp-overexpressed NCI-H460/R (lung), DLD1-TxR (colon), and U87-TxR (brain) cell lines and their drug-sensitive counterparts.[19] More data showed that the IC_{50} values of britannin (**16**) were 2.2, 5.9, 5.4, and 3.5 μg/mL in HepG2 (liver), MCF-7 (breast), MDBK (renal), and A549 (lung) carcinoma cell lines. Its antigrowth effect on MCF-7 and MDA-MB-468 breast cancer cells was mediated by the activation of the mitochondrial apoptotic pathway.[20,21]

Mechanism Studies

The mechanism for the anticancer property of ergolide (8) was found to be attributable to the induction of apoptosis by three signaling pathways, i.e., chromosome pathway, NF-κB signaling pathway, and JNK signaling pathway. The stimulation of Jurkat T cell apoptotic death by ergolide (8) was confirmed through a series of signal conductions i.e., Bax translocation, cleavage of PARP, cytochrome c release, caspase-3 activation, and DNA fragmentation. In parallel, the Bcl-2/NF-κB signaling pathway was significantly suppressed by the ergolide (**8**) in association with the downregulation of cell survival molecules such as X chromosome-linked inhibitor of apoptosis.[22] NF-κB was recognized to play important roles in the carcinogenetic and inflammatory signaling pathways. In RAW 264.7 macrophages, NF-κB inactivation by ergolide (**8**) might be attributed to the inhibition of nuclear translocation of NF-κB, whose interactions resulted from the blockage of IκB degradation and the direct modification of active NF-κB, leading to the inhibition of the expressions of iNOS and COX-2.[23]

Structure Modification

For the enhancement of biological activity, the molecular modification is always one of the best ways to reach the target. The introduction of an alkyl to the 6-hydroxyl of ABL (**3**) could augment the anti-growth effect against cancer cells. The most potent derivatives were 6-*O*-(2-*O*-benyloximene-3-phenyl)-propionyl-1-*O*-acetylbritannilactone (**18**) and 6-*O*-lauroyl-1-*O*-acetylbritannilactone (**19**). The IC_{50} values of 6-*O*-(2-*O*-benyloximene-3-phenyl)-propionyl-1-*O*-acetyl britannilactone (**18**) were 0.22 μg/mL in Bel-7402 cells and 3.8 μg/mL in HL-60 cells, and the IC_{50}s of 6-*O*-lauroyl-1-*O*-acetylbritannilactone (**19**) were 2.91–6.78 μM in HCT116, HEp-2, and HeLa cells. Compared to its parent compound, the derivatives presented the enhanced antitumor activities being comparable to those of etoposide (IC_{50}: 2.13–4.79 μM).[16,24,25]

Other Bioactivities

The herb Xuan Fu Hua (Inula flower) is used in Chinese medicine for the treatment of diverse diseases such as tracheitis, bronchitis, hepatitis, and alimentary tract neoplasm. The dried roots and leaves of this plant are used as other Chinese herbs to treat knife wounds, furunculosis, and cough. Pharmacological studies have proved that Xuan Fu Hua has diversified effects, such as antiasthmatic, antitussive, antidropsical, antioxidant, antidiabetes, antihepatitic, hypolipidemia, hepatoprotective, antiulcer, antifungal, and antibacterial properties.

References

1. Yang, C. et al. 2003. Sesquiterpenes and other constituents from the aerial parts of *Inula japonica*. *Planta Med.* 69: 662–6.
2. Yu, F. et al. 2010. Studies on the anti-growth activity of three sesquiterpene compounds to human tumor cell lines. *Tianran Chanwu Yanjiu Yu Kaifa* 22: 506–9.
3. Si, Y. R. et al. 2010. Study of the anti-proliferative activity and mechanism of three sesquiterpene compounds on gynecologic tumor cell lines. *Aibian, Jibian, Tubian* 22: 28–31.
4. Fang, X. M. et al. 2011. Acetylbritannilactone suppresses growth via upregulation of kruppel-like transcription factor 4 expression in HT-29 colorectal cancer cells. *Oncol. Reports* 26: 1181–7.
5. Li, Y. et al. 2012. Antitumour activities of sesquiterpene lactones from *Inula helenium* and *Inula japonica*. *Zeitschrift fuer Naturforschung, C: J. Biosci.* 67: 375–80.
6. Qin, J. J. et al. 2009. Japonicones A-D, bioactive dimeric sesquiterpenes from *Inula japonica* Thunb. *Bioorg. Med. Chem. Lett.* 19: 710–3.
7. Li, X. G. et al. 2013. Japonicone A suppresses growth of Burkitt lymphoma cells through its effect on NF-κB. *Clin. Cancer Res.* 19: 2917–28.
8. Du, Y. et al. 2015. Japonicone A inhibits the growth of non-small cell lung cancer cells via mitochondria-mediated pathways. *Tumour Biol.* 2015 Apr 25.
9. Qin, J. J. et al. 2015. Japonicone A as a novel anti-breast cancer therapeutic agent by targeting the NFAT1-MDM2-p53 pathway. *Cancer Res.* 75(15 Suppl.): 2434.
10. Lee, J. K. et al. 2010. The sesquiterpene lactone eupatolide sensitizes breast cancer cells to TRAIL through down-regulation of c-FLIP expression. *Oncol. Reports* 23: 229–37.
11. Bai, N. S. et al. 2003. Three new sesquiterpene lactones from *Inula britannica*. *ACS Symposium Series* (2003), 859 (Oriental Foods and Herbs), 271–8.
12. Park, E. J. et al. 1998. Cytotoxic sesquiterpene lactones from *Inula britannica*. *Planta Med.* 64: 752–4.
13. Pan, M. H. et al. 2007. Involvement of MAPK, Bcl-2 family, cytochrome c, and caspases in induction of apoptosis by 1,6-*O*,*O*-diacetyl-britannilactone in human leukemia cells. *Mol. Nutr. Food Res.* 51: 229–38.
14. Qi, J. L. et al. 2008. Sesquiterpene lactones and their antitumor Activity from the flowers of *Inula britannica*. *Letters in Drug Design Discovery* 5: 433–6.
15. Rafi, M. M. et al. 2005. A sesquiterpenelactone from *Inula britannica* induces antitumor effects dependent on Bcl-2 phosphorylation. *Anticancer Res.* 25: 313–8.
16. Dong, S. et al. 2014. Semisynthesis and in vitro cytotoxic evaluation of new analogues of 1-*O*-acetylbritannilactone, a sesquiterpene from Inula Britannica. *Eur. J. Med. Chem.* 80: 71–82.
17. Bai, N. S. et al. 2006. Sesquiterpene lactones from *Inula britannica* and their cytotoxic and apoptotic effects on human cancer cell lines. *J. Nat. Prod.* 69: 531–5.
18. Ho, C. T. et al. 2007. Antitumor neobritannilactone B and acetyl neobritannilactone B. *PCT Intl. Appl.* (2007), WO 2007109119 A2 20070927.
19. Fischedick, J. T. et al. 2013. Cytotoxic activity of sesquiterpene lactones from *Inula britannica* on human cancer cell lines. *Phytochem. Lett.* 6: 246–52.
20. Moghadam, M. H. et al. 2012. Anti-proliferative activity and apoptotic potential of britannin, a sesquiterpene lactone from Inula aucheriana. *Nat Prod Commun.* 7: 979–80.
21. Maryam, H. M. et al. 2015. Britannin, a sesquiterpene lactone, inhibits proliferation and induces apoptosis through the mitochondrial signaling pathway in human breast cancer cells. *Tumour Biol.* 36: 1191–8.
22. Song, Y. J. et al. 2005. Apoptotic potential of sesquiterpene lactone ergolide through the inhibition of NF-κB signaling pathway. *J. Pharmacy Pharmacol.* 57: 1591–7.
23. Whan, H. J. et al. 2001. Ergolide, sesquiterpene lactone from *Inula britannica*, inhibits inducible nitric oxide synthase and cyclooxygenase-2 expression in RAW 264.7 macrophages through the inactivation of NF-κB. *Br. J. Pharmacol.* 133: 503–12.
24. Liu, S. X. et al. 2004. Studies on 1-*O*-acetylbritannilactone and its derivative, (2-*O*-butyloxime-3-phenyl)-propionyl-1-*O*-acetylbritannilactone ester. *Bioorg. Med. Chem. Lett.* 14: 1101–4.
25. Liu, S. X. et al. 2005. Design, synthesis, and antitumor activity of (2-*O*-alkyloxime-3-phenyl)-propionyl-1-*O*-acetylbritannilactone esters. *Bioorg. Med. Chem.* 13: 2783–9.

150 Ting Li Zi 葶藶子

Pepperweed seed

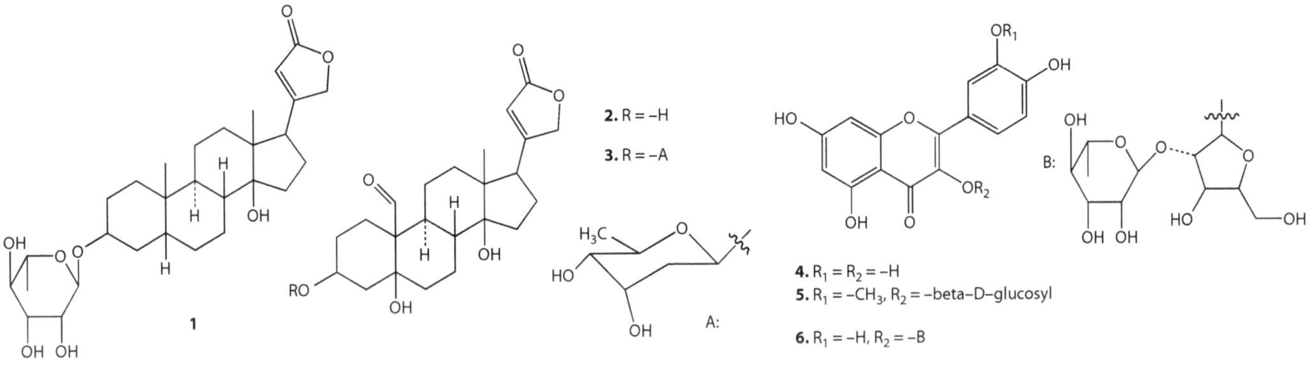

1

2. R = –H

3. R = –A

4. $R_1 = R_2 = –H$

5. $R_1 = –CH_3$, R_2 = –beta-D-glucosyl

6. $R_1 = –H$, $R_2 = –B$

Herb Origination

The herb Ting Li Zi (Pepperweed seed) is the dried matured seeds of three Brassicaceae plants, *Lepidium apetalum* (Pepperwort), *Lepidium virginicum* (Virgina pepperweed), and *Descurainia sophia* (Flixweed tansy mustard). The distribution of these annual or biennial plants is wide ranging in China, while the second origin is native to North America and the third origin is also grown in Europe. The seeds are collected in summer and dried in the sun for application in Chinese folk medicine.

Antitumor Activities

In the early investigations, Ting Li Zi showed the potent antitumor effect against human nasopharyngeal cancer and cervical carcinoma cell lines at a concentration of 20 μg/mL, and it also markedly retarded the growth of mouse EACs *in vivo* without obvious side effects.[1] An extract of the pulverizing parched *Lepidium apetalum* seeds displayed the obvious inhibitory effect against U251 (glioma), HepG2 (hepatoma), SGC (gastric cancer), MCF-7 (breast cancer), and small-cell lung cancer cell lines *in vitro*.[2,3] The methanolic extract of *L. apetalum* seeds was reported to have moderate suppressive activity against the proliferation of adult T cell leukemia/lymphoma cells (derived from a patient) and human T cell lymphotropic virus type I infected cells and against human SNU-1 (stomach), SNU-4 (colorectal), and SNU-354 (liver) neoplastic cell lines *in vitro*.[4,5] The 70% ethanolic extract, its n-butanolic partitioned fraction, and the volatile oil, which all were derived from *Descurainia sophia* seeds, demonstrated dose-dependent suppressive effect against the proliferation of human carcinoma cell lines, NCI-H460 (lung), SF-268 (CNS), and SGC-7901 (stomach) cells and showed significant suppression on the NCI-H460 cells by 78.1%, 76.27%, and 61.25%, respectively, at a 100 μg/mL concentration.[6] Through biphasic regulatory mechanism involving in the activation of signaling pathway, the treatment with the 80% ethanolic extract exerted a cytotoxic effect on four human lung cancer cell lines (A549, NCI-H23, NCI-H460, and NCI-H226) with IC_{50} values of 2.88, 6.60, 8.08, and 13.18 μg/mL at 48 h, respectively. But it also exhibited the inhibition on a normal human IMR-90 lung fibroblast cells (IC_{50}: 10.54 μg/mL, at 48 h).[7]

Additionally, two aqueous extracts, WELVL and WELVR, were respectively isolated from the leaves and the roots of *Lepidium virginicum*. The treatment of human colon carcinoma HCT116 cells with WELVL or WELVR resulted in the suppression of growth and induced apoptosis, where WELVR was greater than WELVL. The WELVR-enhanced apoptotic death of the HCT116 cells was found to be associated with (1) the up-expression of Fas ligand, Bax, and Bad; (2) the down-expression of Bcl-2, Bcl-xL, and Bid; (3) the reduction of mitochondrial membrane potential; (4) the downregulation of IAPs, such as XIAP, cIAP-1, and cIAP-2; and (5) the activation of caspase-3, caspase-8, and caspase-9 and the degradation of caspase-3 substrate proteins, such as PARP, β-catenin, and PLC-γ1.[8]

All the described findings may provide scientific evidences to elucidate the antitumor effect of the three origins of Ting Li Zi, and suggest that the bioactive constituents in Ting Li Zi are potential drug leads deserving further investigation in cancer chemotherapy and prevention.

Antitumor Constituents and Activities

Phytochemical studies of the herb have reported that Ting Li Zi contains various types of secondary metabolites, such as cardiac glycosides, flavonoids, lactones, lipids, sulfur glycosides, lignins/norlignans, and coumarins, showing biological properties. Of them, several constituents including cardenolid glycosides, flavonoids, and sulfur glycoside demonstrated different degrees of antiproliferative effect against human neoplastic cells *in vitro*. Evomonoside (**1**), a cardiac glycoside separated from *L. apetalum* seeds, played a cytotoxic role on three human cancer cell lines, SNU-1 (stomach), SNU-4 (colon), and SNU-354 (liver) cells, with IC_{50} values of 0.003, 0.03, and 1.24 μg/mL, respectively.[5] Strophanthidin (**2**) and its glycoside termed helveticoside (**3**) were obtained from the isolation of *D. sophia* seeds. The cytotoxic activity of strophanthidin (**2**) presented in the *in vitro* assays on human neoplastic cell lines, BGC-823 (stomach), MDA-MB-435 (breast), PC-3M-1E8 (prostate) Bel-7402 (liver), and HeLa (cervix), with IC_{50} values of 0.0225, 0.142, 4.48, 2.34, and 0.541 μg/mL, respectively,[9] whereas helveticoside (**3**) was potently effective in the inhibition of human cancer cell lines,

A549 (lung), HCT-116 (colon), SNU-638 (stomach), PC3 (prostate), SK-MEL-28 (skin), HepG2 (liver), and SKOV-3 (ovary), with IC_{50} values (μg/mL) of 0.034, 0.052, 0.069, 0.178, 0.538, 0.596, and 1.123, respectively.[10] The potency of helveticoside (**3**) on the cancer cell lines was found to be superior or similar to a well-known anticancer drug, DOX.[10]

The isolated antitumor flavonoids from *D. sophia* seeds were quercetin (**4**), isorhamnetine-3-*O*-β-glucoside (**5**), and artabotryside-A (**6**). In the *in vitro* assays, isorhamnetin-3-*O*-β-D-glucopyranoside (**5**) had moderate cytotoxicity only toward human HL-60 AML cells (IC_{50}: 2.24 μg/mL), while quercetin (**4**), a common flavone, showed marked to moderate suppressive effect against a group of human tumor cell lines.[9,10] The IC_{50} values of quercetin (**4**) were 0.651 μM in A549 cells, 0.743 μM in HCT-116 cells, 0.812 μM in SNU-638 cells, and 2.507–7.442 μM in SK-MEL-28, PC3 and HepG2 cells but no activity in SKOV-3 ovarian cancer cell cells.[10] Accompanied by the marked stimulation of apoptosis, G2/M cell arrest, and mitotic arrest, artabotryside-A (**6**) retarded the proliferation of human U87 glioma cells in dose- and time-dependent manners. During the apoptosis promoted by artabotryside-A (**6**), the increase of ROS level and the decrease of mitochondrial membrane potential were found to be involved in a caspase-dependent apoptotic pathway in U87 cells, but it was less toxic to normal mouse splenocytes and glial cells. The evidences highlighted that artabotryside-A (**6**) might be a safe candidate for the prevention and the treatment of gliomas.[11]

In addition, a group of glucosinolates were extracted and purified from the boiling water of the seeds of *D. sophia*. Among the glucosinolates, benzyl glucosinolate displayed anticancer activity.[12]

Other Bioactivities

According to traditional Chinese medicine, Ting Li Zi was known to have the ability to clear away heat from the lung and relieve asthma, promoting diuresis, and detumescence. Thus, it is used as a remedy for the treatment of sputum and phlegm turbidity in lungs, coughs and abundant sputum, inflated chest, throat disease, abdominal edema, measles, smallpox, and urinary obstruction. Modern pharmacological researches have shown that *Lepidium apetalum* seeds have cardiotonic, cholesterol level-regulating, antipigmentation, and oral cancer antagonism effects, whereas *Descurainia sophia* seeds possess antiasthmatic, antitussive, diuretic, and purgative properties. Also, both seeds showed cardiotonic acitivity.

References

1. Sun, K. et al. 2002. Progress in the studies on chemical constituents and pharmacological effect of *Semen lepidii* and *Semen descurainiae*. *Zhongcaoyao* 33: U003–U005.
2. Yu, J. N. et al. 2013. *Lepidium apetalum* seed extract containing antitumor bioactive component, and preparation method and application thereof. *Faming Zhuanli Shenqing* CN 103006741 A 20130403.
3. Yu, J. N. et al. 2013. Preparation method and application of antitumor effective component extract of parched *Lepidium apetalum* seed. *Faming Zhuanli Shenqing* CN 103120710 A 20130529.
4. Nakano, D. et al. 2011. Screening of promising chemotherapeutic candidates against human adult T-cell leukemia/lymphoma from plants: Active principles from *Physalis pruinosa* and structure-activity relationships with withanolides. *J. Nat. Med.* 65: 559–67.
5. Hyun, J. W. et al. 1995. Evomonoside: The cytotoxic cardiac glycoside from *Lepidium apetalum*. *Planta Med.* 61: 294–5.
6. Li, H. W. et al. 2013. Research progress in chemical constituents of *Lepidium apetalum* and *Descurainia sophia* and their pharmacological activities. *Drug Eval. Res.* 36: 235–40.
7. Kim, B. Y. et al. 2013. Gene expression profile of the A549 human non-small cell lung carcinoma cell line following treatment with the seeds of Descurainia sophia, a potential anticancer drug. *Evidence-based Complem. Altern. Med.* 2013: 584–604.
8. Chae, Y. H. et al. 2011. Induction of apoptosis in human colon carcinoma HCT116 cells using a water extract of *Lepidium virginicum* L. *Han'guk Sikp'um Yongyang Kwahak Hoechi* 40: 649–59.
9. Sun, K. et al. 2004. Two new lactones and one new aryl-8-oxabicyclo[3,2,1]oct-3-en-2-one from Descurainia sophia. *Chem. Pharm. Bull.* 52: 1483–6.
10. Lee, Y. J. et al. 2013. Cytotoxic and anti-inflammatory constituents from the seeds of Descurainia sophia. *Archiv. Pharm. Res.* 36: 536–41.
11. Khan, M. et al. 2012. Artabotryside A, a constituent from *Descurainia sophia* (L.) induces cell death in U87 glioma cells through apoptosis and cell cycle arrest at G2/M phase. *J. Med. Plants Res.* 6: 3754–65.
12. Chen, J. M. et al. 2006. Extraction and identification of several glucosinolates in *Descurainia sophia* seeds. *Xibei Zhiwu Xuebao* 26: 1231–5.

151 Tong Guang San 通光散

Rajmahal hemp

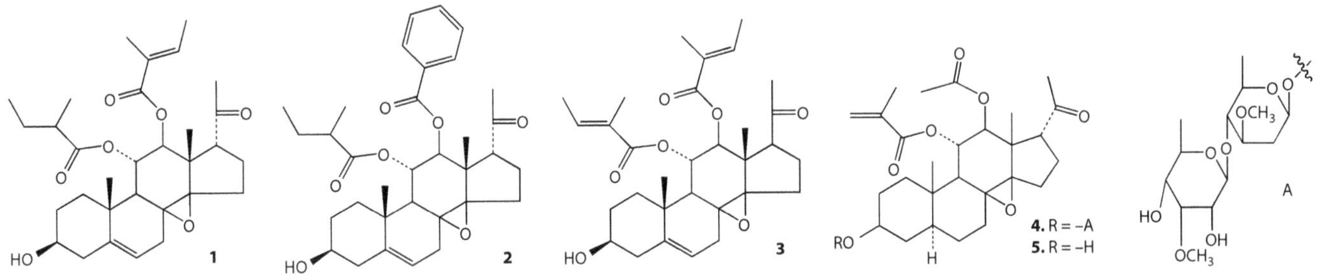

Herb Origination

The herb Tong Guang San (Rajmahal hemp) is the dried stems, roots, and leaves of an Asclepiadaceae plant, *Marsdenia tenacissima*. This perennial climber plant is only distributed in the Chinese provinces of Guizhou and Yunnan, as well as south Asian regions. Normally, its stems are collected in autumn and winter, and its roots and leaves are collected annually as a Chinese folk herb. Its stem is the major useful part for the medicinal practice.

Antitumor Activities

Effects from Tong Guang San

An intravenous injection prepared from Tong-Guang-San stem demonstrated marked antineoplastic property against a group of murine solid tumors, such as Ehrlich ascites cancer, sarcoma 180, U14 cervical cancer, HSC hepatoma, and Walker sarcoma 256, with the inhibitory range of 43.6–61.6% *in vitro*. The hypodermic administration of the injection to mice obstructed the cell growth of L1210 leukemia and reticulocyte sarcoma by 52.1% and 56.1%, respectively.[1,2] MTE, an extract prepared from Tong Guang Teng could time- and dose-dependently hinder the proliferation of human U937 lymphoma and HL-60 leukemia cancer cell lines. Also, in a concentration of 50 μg/mL, MTE promoted the apoptosis of U937 and HL-60 cells by decreasing the mitochondrial transmembrane potential and activating caspase-3.[3] The cotreatment of low cytotoxic dose of MTE (8 mg/mL) with gefitinib additively enhanced the growth inhibition and markedly prompted cell cycle arrest and apoptosis caused by gefitinib in both EGFR mutant (HCC827) and wild-type NSCLC cells (H292).[4] Likewise, low-dose MTE (5 g/kg) markedly augmented gefitinib efficacy in resistant H460 (K-ras mutant) and H1975 (EGFR T790M mutant) NSCLC xenografts in nude mice.[5] The combination also retarded the cross-linking between c-Met and EGFR and synergistically induced the apoptosis of the NSCLC cell lines by suppressing the phosphorylation of PI3K/Akt/mTOR and ERK1/2.[4,5] In the cotreatment of gefitinib-resistant NSCLC cells and hepatoma HepG2 cells, MTE also significantly diminished the intrinsic clearance of gefitinib (an EGFR inhibitor and an antitumor drug) via the down-expressions of cytochrome P450 (CYP) 3A4 and CYP2D6 enzymes to restore the sensitivity of gefitinib to tumor cells.[6] Therefore, the data implied that the Tong Guang San extract is a potential agent to clinically promote the efficacy of gefitinib in resistant NSCLC. Additionally, the Tong Guang San extract also exerted moderate antimutagenic and anticarcinogenic activities against BAP (an oncogene)-induced origins of tumor.[7,8]

Effects from Xiaoaiping

Xiaoaiping is a standard aqueous extract of Tong Guang San. Its treatment arrested the cell cycle progress at G0/G1 stage and retarded the proliferation of human EC-9706 esophageal carcinoma cells, whose antigrowth rates reached 90.15% and 68.02% after the exposure of Xiaoaiping on EC-9706 cells in 40 and 20 mg/mL concentrations, respectively.[9] An *in vivo* experiment further confirmed the antitumor activity of Xiaoaiping. The i.p. administration of Xiaoaiping to tumor-bearing mice for three weeks in different doses suppressed the growth of mouse H22 hepatoma cells, whose optimal dose was found to be 40 g/kg per day in the mouse model. The antihepatoma effect was found to be partly contributed by its angiogenesis-suppressive activity, where Xiaoaiping obstructed the VEGF and lessened the MVD of the tumor, thereby blocking the blood supply and hindered the growth of hepatoma.[10] During the treatment of human SGC-7901 gastric cancer cells *in vitro* and *in vivo*, Xiaoaiping exerted moderate antitumor activity and elicited the apoptosis and G1-cell cycle arrest of SGC-7901 cells in association with the decrease of Bcl-2 expression and the increase of Bax and caspase-3 expressions. In nude mice implanted with the SGC-7901 cancer cells, the inhibition rates of Xiaoaiping were 61.19% and 69.07% on the tumor weight and tumor volume in a mid-dose (200 mg/kg) and a high dose (400 mg/kg), respectively.[11] Furthermore, Xiaoaiping in a cotreatment was able to potentiate the chemotherapeutic effect of oxaliplatin in the promotion of tumor cell apoptosis and the inhibition of human Caov-3 ovarian cancer cells.[12]

Antitumor Constituents and Activities

Polyoxypregnane types of C21 steroids and glycosides were the major components isolated from Tong Guang San. The total C21 steroids and aglycones (ETA) showed the ability to sensitize KB-3-1, HeLa, HepG2, and K562 cell lines to paclitaxel treatment. The *in vivo* combination of paclitaxel and ETA significantly lessened the volume and the weight of HeLa cervical tumors and markedly inhibited the growth of KB-3-1 cervix tumors.[13] In the isolated aglycones, 11α-*O*-2-methylbutyryl-12β-*O*-tigloyl-tenacigenin-B (**1**), 11α-*O*-2-methylbutyryl-12β-*O*-benzoyltenacigenin-B (**2**), and 11α,12β-*O,O*-ditigloyl-17β-tenacigenin-B (**3**) exerted a cytotoxic effect against a multidrug-resistant human KB-VI nasopharyngeal cancer cells *in vitro* (ED_{50}: 2.5–4.1 μg/mL)[14] but showed lower activity during the glycosidation of the C21 steroids.[15] Importantly, tenacissimoside-A (**4**) and its aglycone assigned as 11α-*O*-benzoyl-12β-*O*-acetyltenacigenin-B (**5**) possess significant abilities in reversing MDR through the suppression of P-gp. By the interactions, the 21C-steroids potently augmented the sensitivity of P-gp-overexpressed HepG2/Dox cells to the antitumor drugs such as DOX, vinblastine, puromycin, and paclitaxel. 11α-*O*-Benzoyl-12β-*O*-acetyltenacigenin-B (**5**) (20 μg/mL) could enhance the sensitivity of HepG2/Dox cells to paclitaxel by 326-fold. A preliminary mechanistic exploration revealed that the suppression on P-gp-mediated MDR by the C21 steroid might be mediated by directly interacting with the P-gp substrate site.[16]

Likewise, tenacigenin-D was found to circumvent P-gp-mediated MDR through an inhibitory effect on P-gp with a similar potency to verapamil. Thus, tenacigenin-D potentiated the anticancer activity of erlotinib and gefitinib in EGFR/TKI-resistant NSCLC cells.[17] Tenacissoside-C exhibited obvious cytotoxicity on K562 leukemia cells *in vitro* and *in vivo* (IC_{50}: 15.1 μM for 72 h). Simultaneously, tenacissoside-C induced G0/G1 cell cycle arrest of K562 cells through the down-expression of cyclin-D1 and elicited apoptosis of K562 cells through a mitochondrial pathway. The *in vivo* antileukemia effect was also accompanied by a marked antiangiogenic effect in nude mice against K562 cells.[18] These results collectively indicated that some C21 steroids from the herb may be potential therapeutic candidates for the reversal of MDR in the cancer treatment.

Other Bioactivities

The herb Tong Guang San (Rajmahal hemp) has long been employed for the treatment of cancer and asthma in China. Pharmacological investigations have proven that the herb also exerts antiasthmatic and vasodilative effects besides anticancer.

References

1. State Administration of Traditional Chinese Medicine, 1999. *Chinese Materia Medica*, Vol. 6, 6–5704, 278. Shanghai Science Technology Express. Shanghai, China.
2. Ye, D. Q. et al. 1984. The meeting report for antitumor activity of *Marsdenia tenacissima. Yixue Yanjiu Tongxun* (7): 9.
3. Li, D. et al. 2008. Marsdensia tenacissima induces apoptosis of human U937, HL60 leukemic cells. *Chin. J. Biochem. Pharm.* 29: 33–7.
4. Han, S. Y. et al. 2014. Enhancement of gefitinib-induced growth inhibition by Marsdenia tenacissima extract in non-small cell lung cancer cells expressing wild or mutant EGFR. *BMC Complem. Altern. Med.* 14: 165/1–165/11.
5. Han, S. Y. et al. 2015. Marsdenia tenacissima extract enhances gefitinib efficacy in non-small cell lung cancer xenografts. *Phytomed.* 22: 560–7.
6. Han, S. Y. et al. 2014. Marsdenia tenacissima extract inhibits gefitinib metabolism in vitro by interfering with human hepatic CYP3A4 and CYP2D6 enzymes. *J. Ethnopharmacol.* 151: 210–7.
7. Lee, H. et al. 1988. Antimutagenic activity of extracts from anticancer drugs in Chinese medicine. *Mutation Res.* 204: 229–34.
8. Qian, J. et al. 2009. Progress on antitumor effects of *Marsdenia tenacissima. Zhongguo Zhongyao Zazhi* 34: 11–3.
9. Zhang, M. Z. et al. 2008. Studies on the effect of Xiaoaiping on EC-9706 esophageal cancer cells and the mechanism. *Lishizhen Med. Materia Medica Res.* 19: 1182–4.
10. Zhao, H. P. et al. 2012. Effect of Xiao'aipng on growth and angiogenesis of H22 hepatic carcinoma in mice. *Zhongliu Fangzhi Yanjiu* 39: 497–501.
11. Koumtebaye, E. et al. 2012. Antitumor activity of Xiaoaiping injection on human gastric cancer SGC-7901 cells. *Zhongguo Tianran Yaowu* 10: 339–46.
12. Wang, C. et al. 2012. Effect of Xiaoaiping injection sensitized oxaliplatin on inhibition of human ovarian cancer Caov-3 cells proliferation. *Cancer Res. on Prov. Treat.* 39: 780–3.
13. Zhu, R. J. et al. 2014. Total aglycones from *Marsdenia tenacissima* increases antitumor efficacy of paclitaxel in nude mice. *Mol.* 19: 13965–75.
14. Luo, S. Q. et al. 1993. Polyoxypregnanes from *Marsdenia tenacissima. Phytochem.* 34: 1615–20.
15. Zhang, H. et al. 2010. Five new C21 steroidal glycosides from the stems of *Marsdenia tenacissima. Steroids* 75: 176–83.
16. Hu, Y. J. et al. 2008. Tenacigenin B derivatives reverse P-glycoprotein-mediated multidrug resistance in HepG2/Dox cells. *J. Nat. Prods.* 71: 1049–51.
17. Yao, S. et al. 2014. Polyoxypregnane steroids from the stems of *Marsdenia tenacissima. J. Nat. Prod.* 77: 2044–53.
18. Ye, B. G. et al. 2014. In vitro and in vivo antitumor activities of tenacissoside C from *Marsdenia tenacissima. Planta Med.* 80: 29–38.

152 Mao Pao Tong 毛泡桐

Empress tree or Princess tree

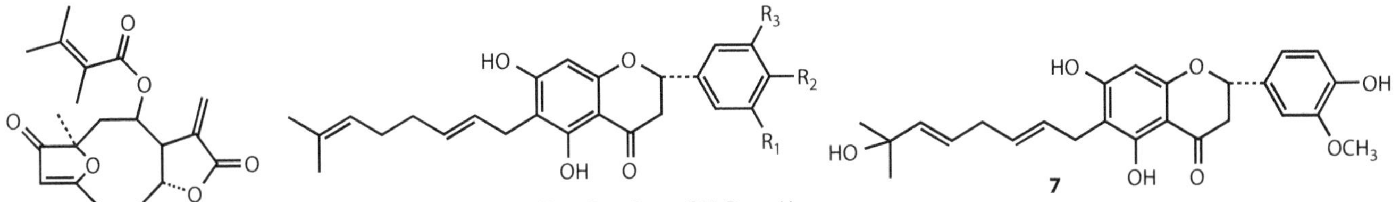

1

2. R_1 = -OCH_3, R_2 = -OH, R_3 = -H **4.** R_1 = R_2 = -OH, R_3 = -H
3. R_1 = -OCH_3, R_2 = R_3 = -OH **5.** R_1 = R3 = -H, R_3 = -OH

6. R_1 = -OCH_3, R_2 = -OH, R_3 = -H

7

Herb Origination

Mao Pao Tong (Empress tree) is a Scrophulariaceae plant, *Paulownia tomentosa*, whose tree is native to central and eastern China. It is also distributed in Korea and Japan and naturalized in the southeastern region of the United States. The tree is a source of Chinese herbs for a thousand years. Its flowers, fruits, roots, leaves, and stem skins can be used as Chinese folk herbs independently.

Antitumor Constituents and Activities

Sesquiterpenoid

A sesquiterpenoid constituent identified as isoatriplicolide tiglate (**1**) was isolated from the flowers and the leaves of Mao Pao Tong. The *in vitro* cytotoxicity of isoatriplicolide tiglate (**1**) was approved in a small panel of human cancer cell lines including A549 (lung), SKOV-3 (ovary), XF498 (brain), SK-Mel-2 (skin), and HCT15 (colon) cells with ED_{50} values in the range of 0.2–1.5 µg/mL, whose potency was comparable to a reference Adm (ED_{50}: 0.1–2.3 µg/mL).[1] Isoatriplicolide tiglate (**1**) also markedly repressed the proliferation of breast cancer cell lines (MCF7, HS578T, and T47D) and cervical cancer cell lines (HeLa, SiHa, and C33A). After the *in vitro* treatment, it could promote the S/G2 cell cycle arrest at <10 µg/mL concentrations and stimulate the caspase-dependent apoptosis at >50 µg/mL concentrations. The apoptotic death of human MDA-MB-231 breast carcinoma cells was significantly triggered by isoatriplicolide tiglate (**1**) through both extrinsic and intrinsic pathways.[2]

Flavonoids

From its fruits, many geranylated flavanones were separated, and some of them were demonstrated to have selective cytotoxicity on seven different human carcinoma cell lines. Schizolaenone-C (**2**), diplacone (**3**), and 3′-*O*-methyl-5′-*O*-hydroxydiplacone (**4**) displayed obvious cytotoxic effect on U266 multiple myeloma cells with EC_{50} values of 1.9–5.5 µM. T lymphoblastic leukemia (CEM) cells were sensitive to 3′-*O*-methyl-5′-*O*-hydroxydiplacone (**4**) (EC_{50}: 3.2 µM) and schizolaenone-C (**2**) (EC_{50}: 12.3 µM), wherein the cytotoxicity of 3′-*O*-methyl-5′-*O*-hydroxydiplacone (**4**) was greater than that of olomoucine-II (an anticancer agent), while monocytic leukemia THP-1 cells were only sensitive to schizolaenone-C (**2**) (ED_{50}: 8.5 µM). Diplacone (**3**) and schizolaenone-C (**2**) were the most cytotoxic to RPMI8226 multiple myeloma cells with the same EC_{50} values of 7.1 µM, being similar to olomoucine-II, and 3′-*O*-methyl-5′-*O*-hydroxydiplacone (**4**) was effective to the RPMI8226 cells as well with an EC_{50} value of 10 µM. The cell proliferation of HeLa cervical cancer was suppressed by schizolaenone-C (**2**), diplacone (**3**), and 3′-*O*-methyldiplacone (**5**) in the ED_{50} levels of 6.3–9.2 µM.[3] In an assay with K562 leukemia cells, diplacone (**3**) (IC_{50}: 4 µM) and 3′-*O*-methyl-5′-*O*-hydroxydiplacone (**4**) (IC_{50}: 6 µM) exerted greater cytotoxicity, whereas other isolated geranylated flavanones such as mimulone (**5**), 3′-*O*-methyldiplacone (**6**), 3′-*O*-methyldiplacol, 3′-*O*-methyl-5′-*O*-methyldiplacone, and isoacteoside exerted the moderate inhibitory effects (IC_{50}: 13–29 µM).[4] Mimulone (**5**) was also isolated from *P. tomentosa* fruits, which, in the *in vitro* assay, triggered the caspase-mediated apoptosis through an extrinsic pathway and induced autophagy through a p53-mediated AMPK/mTOR pathway in human A549 lung denocarcinoma cells, leading to the prevention of the cell proliferation in dose- and time-dependent manners. Also, the induced autophagy then amplified the cell apoptotic death,[5] whose finding strongly suggests that mimulone (**5**) is a potential agent for targeting both autophagy and apoptotic cell death in human lung cancer.

In ≥5 µM concentration, tomentodiplacone-B (**7**) directly suppressed the proliferation of human monocytic leukemia THP-1 cells together with the blockage of the cell cycle progression from G1 phase into DNA synthesis via the downregulation of CDK-2 activity and the decline of cyclin-E1 and cyclin-A2 protein levels.[6] But the treatment with schizolaenone-C (**2**), diplacone (**3**), and 3′-*O*-methyl-5′-*O*-hydroxydiplacone (**4**) also obviously restrained the proliferation of normal BJ human fibroblast cells (EC_{50}: 4.7–7.5 µM).[3]

Phenolic Glycosides

A phenolic glycoside identified as acteoside was another kind of active constituent isolated from the fruits of *P. tomentosa*. This compound exhibited moderate antiproliferative effect against human K562 leukemia cells in an *in vitro* model, and its IC_{50} value was 30 µM.[4]

References

1. Moon, H. -I. et al. 2001. Anticancer compound of *Paulownia tomentosa*. *Nat. Prod. Sci.* 7: 21–2.
2. Jung, S. et al. 2012. Inhibitory effect and mechanism on anti-proliferation of isoatriplicolide tiglate (PCAC) from *Paulownia coreana*. *Mol.* 17: 5945–51.
3. Smejkal, K. et al. 2010. Cytotoxic activities of several geranyl-substituted flavanones. *J. Nat. Prod.* 73: 568–72.
4. Smejkal, K. et al. 2008. Cytotoxic activity of C-geranyl compounds from *Paulownia tomentosa* fruits. *Planta Med.* 74: 1488–91.
5. An, H. K. et al. 2014. Mimulone-induced autophagy through p53-mediated AMPK/mTOR pathway increases caspase-mediated apoptotic cell death in A549 human lung cancer cells. *PLoS One* 9: e114607/1–e114607/20.
6. Kollar, P. et al. 2011. Geranylated flavanone tomentodiplacone B inhibits proliferation of human monocytic leukaemia (THP-1) cells. *Br. J. Pharmacol.* 162: 1534–41.

153 Luo Tuo Peng 駱駝蓬

Harmal or Syrian rue

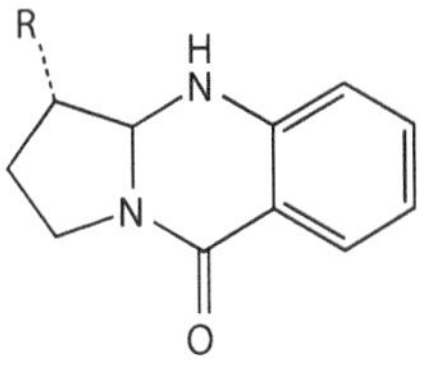

1. R = -OH
2. R = -H

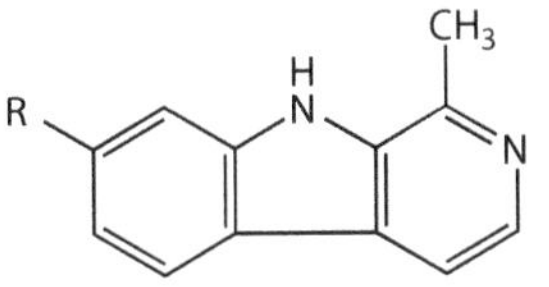

3. R = $-OCH_3$
5. R = -H

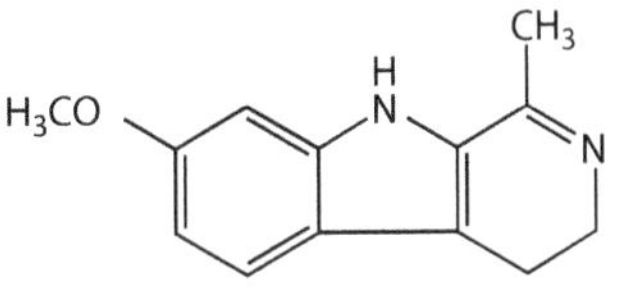

4

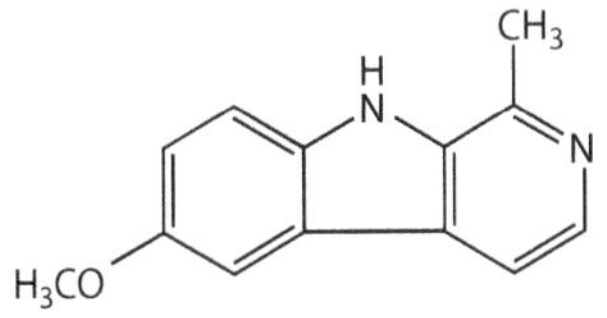

6

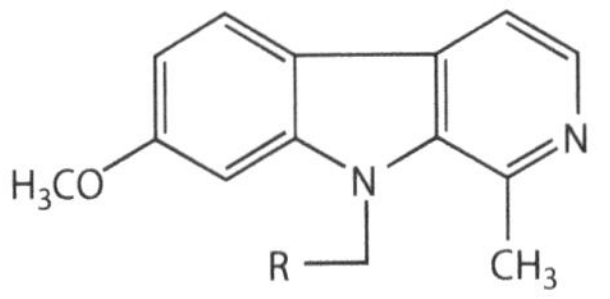

7. R = $-CH_3$
8. R = $-CH_2CH_3$
9. R = $-C_6H_5$

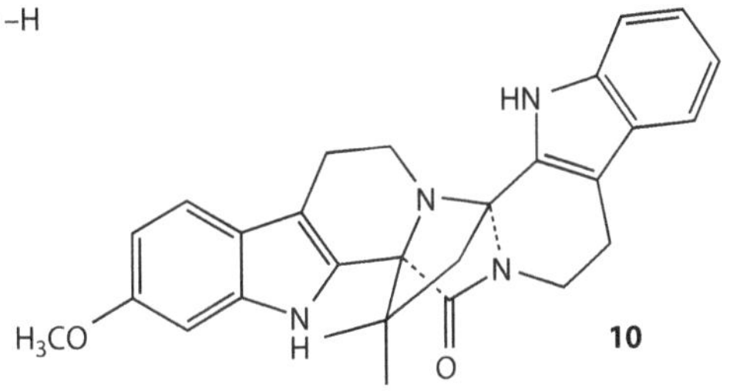

10

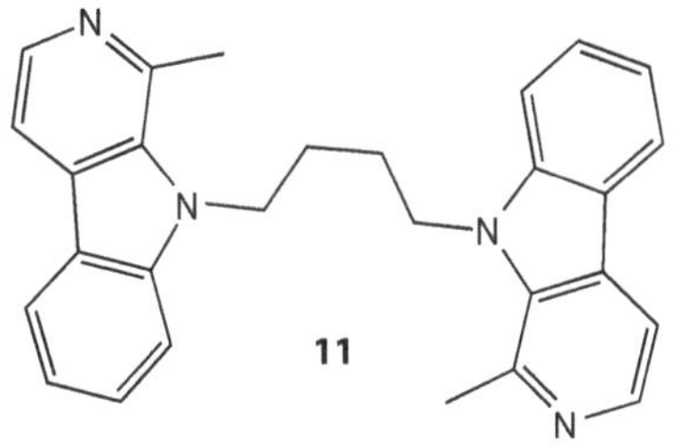

11

Herb Origination

The herb Luo Tuo Peng (Harmal or Syrian rue) is the dried plant *Peganum harmala* L. (Zygophyllaceae), which is native to the east Mediterranean area, east of India, and part of China. The plant has spread invasively to the salt desert shrub lands of western United States. In China, it is distributed in arid lands of the northwestern and northern areas. The whole plant is commonly collected in summer and autumn and dried in the sun for use in Chinese medicine. Its seeds are also separately collected to be used as another herb.

Antitumor Constituents and Activities

Alkaloids

The whole plant of Luo Tuo Peng and its seeds are abundant of β-carboline alkaloids. The total β-carboline alkaloid components derived from the plant aerial part exhibited the cell growth suppressive effect against L1210 leukemia and K562 erythroleukemia *in vitro*. By i.p. or oral administration, its extract obstructed the growth of mouse entity sarcoma 180 cells by >30% *in vivo*.[1] In the *in vitro* assays, the total alkaloids derived from its seeds obviously hindered the proliferation of various types of human tumor cell lines such as BEL-7402 and Hep3B (liver), MGC-803 (stomach), CNE-2 (nasopharynx), HeLa (cervix), JEG-3 (chorion), K562 and HL-60 (leukemia) cells, and mouse tumor cell lines (sarcoma 180 and L1210 leukemia) *in vitro*.[2–7] Also, the proliferation of the cancer cell lines (Med-mek and UCP-Med carcinoma and UCP-Med sarcoma and Sp2/O-Ag14 myeloma) was significantly diminished by the alkaloids in varying concentrations (10–120 μg/mL), and the complete cell death was progressed after the treatment for 48–72 h.[8,9] When human SORb50 Rb cells were incubated with 12 μg/mL of the seed alkaloids for 72 h, the inhibitory rate on the tumor cells reached to 96.60% (IC_{50}: 1.44 μg/mL).[8] The cell cycle arrest and the growth inhibition in JEG-3 choriocarcinoma cells were elicited by the alkaloids by upregulating the expression of GADD45α.[7] The noticeable antineoplastic activity of the seed alkaloids was also demonstrated in mouse models against Sp2/O myeloma, L2 reticulocyte sarcoma, and ascites hepatoma[8–12] and in nude mice against human Bel-7402 hepatoma and MGC-803 gastric cancer,[9] whose effect was accompanied by the induction of cell cycle arrest and supermicrostructure destruction (including damages of mitochondria, nucleus, and chromatin) and blockage of DNA Topos and DNA synthesis.[6–12] Moreover, the seed alkaloids in a cotreatment could enhance the cytotoxicity of cisplatin against Bel-7402 hepatoma cells xenografted in nude mice.[9]

The major β-carboline alkaloids with anticancer activity in Harmal were revealed to be deoxyvasicinone (**1**), vasicinonel (**2**), harmine (**3**), harmaline (**4**), harmane (**5**), and isoharmine (**6**). Harmine (**3**) and harmaline (**4**) are the dominant alkaloids of the plant extract with a relative abundance of 7% and 4.85% (wt./wt.), respectively.[13]

Harmines

Harmine (**3**) and its three derivatives (**7**, **8**, and **9**) demonstrated potent cytotoxicity on HepG2 hepatoma cells (IC_{50}: 0.011–0.021 μmol/mL) *in vitro*, concomitant with the induction of apoptosis and the up-expression of a death receptor Fas. The suppressive rate of harmine (**3**) in a 47–94 μg/mL concentration reached to 59–71.9% on the cultured HeLa cells.[14,15] The marked inhibitory activity was also proven in mice bearing LLC, sarcoma 180, or HepG2 hepatoma after the treatment of harmine (**3**) and its derivatives individually.[15] Moreover, the alkaloids such as harmine, harmalicidine, vasicinone, and peganine (vasicine) showed the inhibitory effect in varying degrees against human cancer cell lines (Med-mek and UCP-med carcinoma and UCP-med sarcoma and Sp2/O-Ag14 myeloma). Of the tested agents, harmine (**3**) was the most potent in inhibiting the growth (IC_{50}: 2.43–18.39 μg/mL) of the tested tumor cells, while peganine was the least active (IC_{50}: 50– >100 μg/mL). Sp2/O-Ag14 cells were the most sensitive to these alkaloids (IC_{50}: 2.43–19.20 μg/mL), and the UCP-med carcinoma was the least sensitive (IC_{50}: 13.83–59.97 μg/mL).[16] Furthermore, the approaches in the SAR indicated that both R3 and R9 substitutions at harmine (**3**) molecule would display higher antitumor effect and lower toxicity.[15]

Likewise, harmine (**3**) played the inhibitory role in highly metastatic murine B16F-10 melanoma cell invasion, migration, and angiogenesis. The apoptosis of B16-F10 melanoma cells was promoted by harmine (**3**) through both intrinsic and extrinsic pathways, i.e., activating Bax, caspase-3, caspase-9, and p53 and upregulating caspase-8 and Bid, thereby restraining the cell proliferation, the metastasis, and the tumor nodule formation in the lung tissue of the B16-F10 cells. The suppression of lung metastasis-related signaling pathways were found to closely correlate with the downregulation of ERK, VEGF, and MMP-9 expressions and the blockage of transcription factors and proinflammatory cytokines.[17,18] The i.p. injection of harmine (**3**) to mice in a dose of 10 mg/kg notably attenuated the B16-F10 melanoma-directed capillary formation and angiogenesis by decreasing the proliferation of vascular endothelial cells and reducing the expression of various proangiogenesis factors, for instance, suppressing the expressions of VEGF, NO, iNOS, COX-2, and proinflammatory cytokines; inhibiting transcription factors like NF-κB, CREB, and ATF-2; and augmenting antitumor factors like IL-2 and TIMP. Due to the important capacities, harmine (**3**) directly obstructed the microvessel outgrowth and the metastasis *in vivo*.[19] Also, harmine (**3**) induced the apoptotic death and inhibited the proliferation, the migration, and the invasion of human gastric cancer cells via the downregulation of COX-2 expression.[20] According to these evidences, harmine (**3**) is suggested as a potential drug lead for further development in anticancer, antiangiogenic, and antimetastatic therapies.

Additionally, two harmine derivatives were synthesized by conjugating 2-amino-2-deoxy-D-glucose and their difference was only at C-9 of harmine with ethyl or phenylpropyl. The derivation prominently enhanced the inhibitory rate on human HepG2 hepatoma cells and reduced the toxicity on normal L02 hepatic cells compared to harmine.[21]

Harmaline

Harmaline (**4**) at a 4.7 μg/mL concentration sensitively inhibited the proliferation of several human carcinoma cell lines such as Bcap-37 (breast), LoVo (colon), BGC-823 (stomach), and HeLa (cervix) cells.[18] Both harmaline (**4**) and harmine (**3**) were effective in the repression of human UACC-62 (skin), TK-10 (kidney), MCF-7 (breast), Hep3B (liver), and HL-60 and K562 (leukemic) neoplastic cell lines *in vitro*.[22–25] The daily i.p. administration of harmaline (**4**) to murine animals at doses of 22.5–45 μg/mL for eight days obstructed the cell growth of hepatoma, sarcoma 180, and L2 reticulosarcoma *in vivo*.[26] Harmaline (**4**) significantly caused the damage of the cell membrane and restrained the proliferation of Hep3B hepatoma cells, but it promoted the growth of human L02 hepatic cells even at a low concentration.[25] A *trans*-[Pd(harmaline-DMSO)Cl_2] complex, which was yielded by the reaction of harmaline (**4**) with *trans*-[Pd$(DMSO)_2Cl_2$] in 1:1 molar ratio, displayed marked cytotoxicity on several neoplastic cell lines (i.e., P388, L1210, K562, Raji, HeLa, RD, and HEp-2) *in vitro*, and the potencies could be compared to those of anticancer drugs (cisplatin, carboplatin, and 5-FU).[27]

Isoharmine and Others

The antiproliferative effect of isoharmine (**6**) was shown in HeLa cervical cancer cells and CNE-2 nasopharyngeal cancer cells with the inhibitory rates of 59% and 89.5%, respectively, at a 47 μg/mL concentration.[28] In addition, harmalol, a main metabolite of harmine (**3**) and harmaline (**4**), was able to restrain the activity of carcinogen (TCDD or dioxin)-induced enzyme CYP1A1 in both murine Hepa 1c1c7 hepatoma and human HepG2 hepatoma cell lines, whose effect was mediated by AhR-dependent transcriptional and posttranslational mechanisms. The anticarcinogenetic activity was also effective in hindering dioxin (an extensively spread environmental contaminant)-caused deleterious effect.[29–30] (S)-vasicinone-1-*O*-β-D-glucoside and (S)-vasicinone displayed weak suppressive activity against human MCG-803 gastric cancer cells.[31] Peganumine A (**10**), a dimeric β-carboline alkaloid with a unique 3,9-diazatetracyclo[6.5.2.01,9.03,8]pentadec-2-one scaffold, was isolated from the seeds of *P. harmala*. It showed selective cytotoxicity on HL-60 leukemia cells (IC_{50}: 5.8 μM) and moderate effect on MCF-7 (breast), PC3 (prostate), and HepG2 (liver) cancer cell lines (IC_{50}: 38.5, 40.2, and 55.4 μM, respectively).[32] B-9-3 (**11**), a semisynthesized dimeric β-carboline alkaloid, exerted a strong suppressive activity against human lung cancer, breast cancer, and colorectal cancer cell lines concomitant with induction of apoptosis and inhibition of cell migration. Also, B-9-3 (**11**) was able to block the tube formation in HUVEC, indicating an antiangiogenetic potential.[33]

Moreover, harmine (**3**), harmiline (**4**), and harmane (**5**) were inhibitors of DNA Topo-I and Topo-II, and the order of potencies were harmine harmine (**3**) > harmane (**5**) > harmaline (**4**).[34,35] The alkaloids could interact with the DNA of the tumor cells through both groove binding and intercalative modes, resulting in major changes in the DNA structure. The affinity of alkaloid–DNA binding for the β-carboline alkaloids was in the order of tryptoline < harmane (**5**) < harmaline (**4**) < harmalol < harmine (**3**).[12]

Proteins

A crude protein component was prepared from the seeds of Luo Tuo Peng by a treatment with 80% saturated ammonium sulfate solution. The protein component exhibited certain inhibition effect against three human cancer cell lines, HeLa (cervix), Eca-109 (esophagus), and BEL-7404 (liver) cells, *in vitro*, showing IC_{50} values of 72, 257, and 174 μg/mL, respectively. The protein could also significantly promote HeLa cell apoptosis in a dose-dependent manner.[36] From the crude protein component, two antiproliferative proteins designated as PhLTP (14.8 kDa) and PHP (16 kDa) were purified. PHP is an alkaline protein, which is stable in a 4–60°C temperature range, and in a 4–10 pH range. PHP was able to inhibit the proliferation of Eca-109 (esophageal), B16 (skin), HeLa (cervix), and MGC-7 (gastric) cancer cell lines with IC_{50} values (μM) of 0.7, 1.47, 2.74, and 3.13, respectively.[37] PhLTP presented its antiproliferative activity in human cancer cell lines (HeLa, Eca-109, MGC-9, and BEL-7404 cells).[38] Its recombinant PhLTP in a dosage of 25 mg/kg inhibited the growth of B16 murine melanoma cells by 71.7% and also restrained the tumor angiogenesis in C57BL/6J mice with no toxicity in the liver, the lung, and other organs.[39]

Other Medical Uses

The herb Luo Tuo Peng (Harmal or Syrian rue) has often been made into folk medicines in many countries, having a history dating back to thousands of years. The herb has been used to treat many healthy problems including asthma, infertility, menstrual problems, labor pain, wounds, and some others, and it has been used as analgesic, abortifacient, antiinflammatory, and anthelmintic agents. It can also reduce spermatogenesis and male fertility in rats, and it shows antibacterial activity against drug-resistant bacteria. The seeds can also be utilized to kill algae, bacteria, intestinal parasites, insects, and molds. Laboratory tests substantiated that harmaline (**4**) is a stimulant of the CNS and is a reversible inhibitor of MAO-A (a category of antidepressant). The PHP protein also displayed antifungal and anti-HIV-1 reverse transcriptase activities.[37]

References

1. Fan, Z. G. et al. 1993. Antitumor constituents of *Peganum harmala* L. (I) *J. Shenyang Univ. Pharm.* 10: 136.
2. Li, C. J. et al. 1987. Isolation and elucidation of anticancer constituents from *Peganum harmala* and the pharmacological experiments. *J. Xinjiang Med. Univ.* 10: 27–31.
3. Wang, X. H. et al. 1993. In vitro antitumor studies of harmaline. *J. China Med. Univ.* 22: 182–3.
4. Yang, X. P. et al. 1991. Inhibitory effect of total alkaloids from *Peganum harmala* against human liver and gastric cancer cells in vitro and in vivo. *Aizheng* 10: 463–5.
5. Jahaniani, F. et al. 2005. Xanthomicrol is the main cytotoxic component of *Dracocephalum kotschyii* and a potential anticancer agent. *Phytochem.* 66: 1581–92.
6. Shan, S. G. et al. 2012. Effects of total alkaloids of harmaline on LO2 and Hep3B cells. *Shizhen Guoyi Guoyao* 6: 1414–5.
7. Shan, S. G. et al. 2013. Effect and mechanism of *Peganum harmala* alkaloids on cell cycle of JEG-3 cells. *Shanxi Yiyao Zazhi* 42: 24–5.
8. Lamchouri, F. et al. 2000. In vitro cell-toxicity of *Peganum harmala* alkaloids on cancerous cell-lines. *Fitoterapia* 71: 50–4.
9. Lamchouri, F. et al. 1999. Antitumor principles from *Peganum harmala* seeds. *Therapie* 54: 753–8.
10. Jin, J. et al. 1990. Effects of harmaline and 5-FU on human retinoblastoma cell line SO-RB50. *Chin. J. Ophthalmol.* 54: 286–8.
11. Hu, H. T. et al. 1993. The effects of total alkaloids from *Peganum harmala* on hepatoma cell cytokinetic in mice. *Aizheng* 12: 489–91.
12. Shao, J. et al. 1993. The damage of the total alkaloids of hamaline on the ultrastructure of reticulum-cell sarcoma L2 cells in mice. *Aizheng* 12: 214–6.
13. Nafisi, S. et al. 2010. β-Carboline alkaloids bind DNA. *J. Photochem. Photobiol. B: Biology* 100: 84–91.
14. Yang, X. P. et al. 1986. In vitro inhibitory effect of harmine against human cervical cancer HeLa cells. *J. Zhongshan Med. Univ.* 7: 44.
15. Chen, Q. et al. 2005. Antitumor and neurotoxic effects of novel harmine derivatives and structure-activity relationship analysis. *Intl. J. Cancer* 114: 675–82.
16. Lamchouri, F. et al. Cytotoxicity of alkaloids isolated from *Peganum harmala* seeds. *Pakistan J. Pharm. Sci.* 26: 699–706.
17. Hamsa, T. P. et al. 2011. Harmine activates intrinsic and extrinsic pathways of apoptosis in B16F-10 melanoma. *Chin. Med.* 6: 11.
18. Hamsa, T. P. et al. 2011. Studies on anti-metastatic and anti-invasive effects of harmine using highly metastatic murine B16F-10 melanoma cells. *J. Envir. Pathol. Toxicol. Oncol.* 30: 123–37.
19. Hamsa, T. P. et al. 2010. Harmine inhibits tumour specific neo-vessel formation by regulating VEGF, MMP, TIMP and pro-inflammatory mediators both in vivo and in vitro. *Eur. J. Pharmacol.* 649: 64–73.
20. Zhang, H. et al. 2014. Harmine induces apoptosis and inhibits tumor cell proliferation, migration and invasion through down-regulation of cyclooxygenase-2 expression in gastric cancer. *Phytomed.* 21: 348–55.
21. Wang, A. et al. 2013. Novel 2DG-based harmine derivatives for targeted cancer therapy. *Proc. SPIE* 8582(*Biophotonics Immune Responses VIII*), 85820V/1–85820V/7. (February 21, 2013).
22. Zheng, T. et al. 1990. In vitro inhibitory activity of total alkaloids of harmaline on human cancer cell lines. *J. Beijing Med. Univ.* 22: 382.
23. Zaker, F. et al. 2007. A study on the antitumor and differentiation effects of *Peganum harmala* derivatives in combination with ATRA on leukaemic cells. *Archiv. Pharm. Res.* 30: 844–9.
24. Berrougui, H. et al. 2005. Cytotoxic activity of methanolic extract and two alkaloids extracted from seeds of *Peganum harmala* L. *J. Nat. Remedies* 5: 41–5.
25. Shan, S. G. et al. 2012. Effects of total alkaloid of Harmaline (TAH) on growth of L02 and Hep3B cells. *Shizhen Guoyi Guoyao* 23: 1414–5.
26. Xu, Z. D. et al. 1989. Anticancer effect of harmaline. *Aizheng* 8: 94–7.
27. Al-Allaf, T. A. K. et al. 1998. Palladium(II) complex derived from harmaline, an alkaloid isolated from *Peganum harmala* seeds: Synthesis, characterization and cytotoxic activity. *Asian J. Chem.* 10: 342–6.
28. Li, C. J. et al. 1984. Isolation of new anticancer compounds from *Peganum harmala* and the antitumor activity. *J. Xinjiang Med. College* 7: 294–5.
29. El Gendy, M. A. M. et al. 2010. *Peganum harmala* L. is a candidate herbal plant for preventing dioxin mediated effects. *Planta Med.* 76: 671–7.
30. El Gendy, M. A. M. et al. 2012. Harmaline and harmalol inhibit the carcinogen-activating enzyme CYP1A1 via transcriptional and post-translational mechanisms. *Food Chem. Toxicol.* 50: 353–62.
31. Wang, C. H. et al. 2015. Antitumor quinazoline alkaloids from the seeds of *Peganum harmala*. *J. Asian Nat. Prod. Res.* 17: 595–600.
32. Wang, K. B. et al. 2014. Peganumine A, a β-carboline dimer with a new octacyclic scaffold from *Peganum harmala*. *Organic Lett.* 16: 4028–31.

33. Daoud, A. et al. 2014. B-9-3, a novel β-carboline derivative exhibits anticancer activity via induction of apoptosis and inhibition of cell migration in vitro. *Eur. J. Pharmacol.* 724: 219–30.
34. Sobhari, A. M. et al. 2002. An in vitro evaluation of human DNA topoisomerase I inhibition by *Peganum harmala* L. seeds extract and its β-carboline alkaloids. *J. Pharm. Pharmace. Sci.* 5: 18–22.
35. Wang, C. H. et al. 2008. Inhibitory effects of *Peganum harmala* L. seeds extract and its β-carboline alkaloids on activity of DNA topo-isomerase II in vitro. *Zhongguo Linchuang Yaolixue Zazhi* 24: 422–5.
36. Luo, J. J. et al. 2010. Study on the antitumor activity of protein extracts of *Peganum harmala* seeds in vitro. *Shengw Jishu* 20: 32–4.
37. Ma, X. J. et al. 2013. Purification and characterization of a novel antifungal protein with antiproliferation and anti-HIV-1 reverse transcriptase activities from *Peganum harmala* seeds. *Acta Biochimica et Biophysica Sinica* 45: 87–94.
38. Ma, X. J. et al. 2012. Purification and identification of a novel protein with antitumor activity from *Peganum harmala* seeds. *Tianran Chanwu Yanjiu Yu Kaifa* 24: 1020–5.
39. Zhao, J. et al. 2013. The antitumor effects of recombinant *Peganum harmala* lipid transfer protein (rPhLTP) on the B16 solid tumor. *Shengwu Jishu* 23: 86–89.

154 Luo Tuo Hao 駱駝蒿

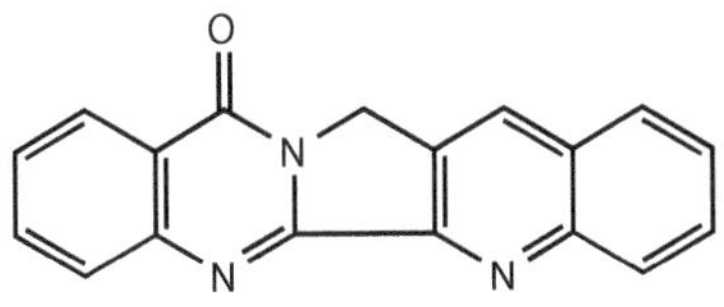

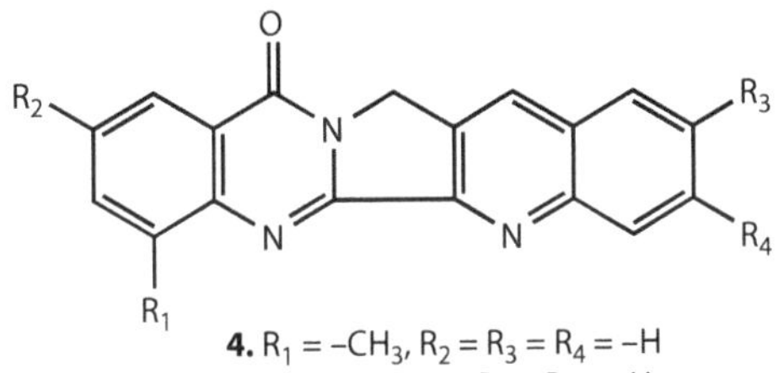

4. $R_1 = -CH_3, R_2 = R_3 = R_4 = -H$
5. $R_2 = -OH, R_1 = R_3 = R_4 = -H$
6. $R_1 = R_2 = -H, R_3 = R_4 = -OCH_3$

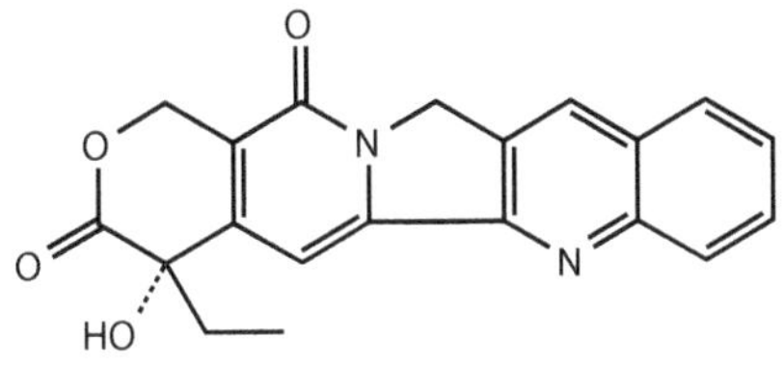

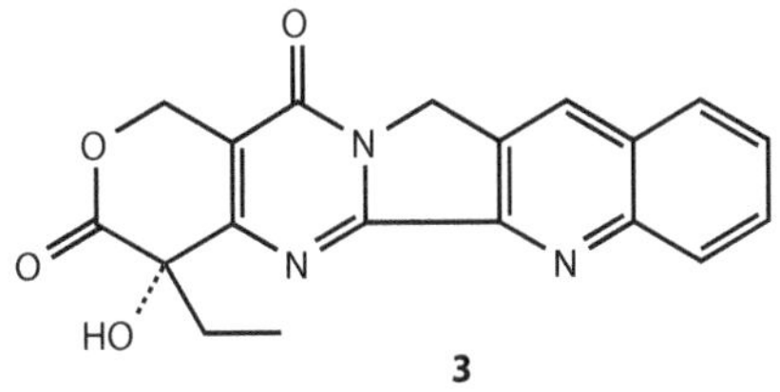

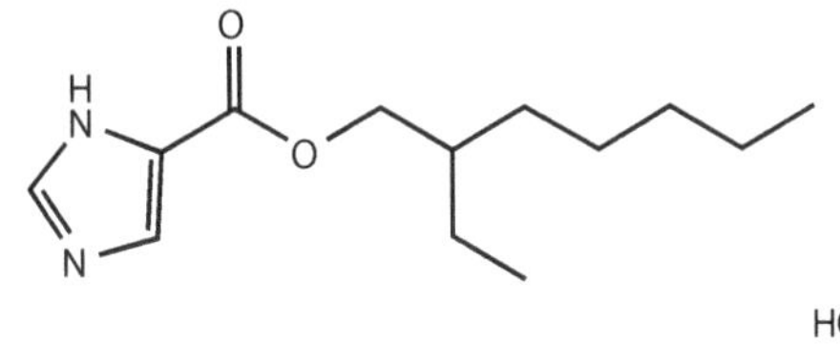

Herb Origination

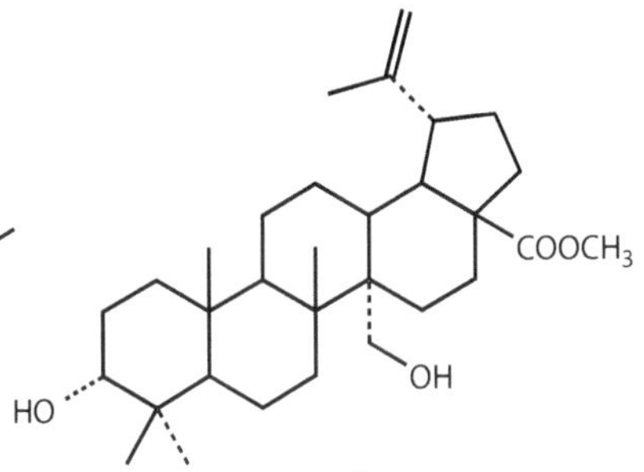

The herb Luo Tuo Hao is the dried whole plant of *Peganum nigellastrum* (Zygophyllaceae). The herbaceous plant distribution is broadly in the arid lands of northwestern China as well as Mongolia and eastern Siberia. In China, the herb is generally collected in summer and autumn and dried in the sun for the folk medicinal use.

Antitumor Activities and Constituents

The β-carboline-type alkaloids in Luo Tuo Hao are the major antitumor active substances similar in Luo Tuo Peng. After 24 h of incubation with ascitic hepatoma cells, 100 μg of the alkaloids significantly blocked the synthesis of the DNA and the protein and executed 50% of the tumor cells. The daily i.p. injection of the fat-soluble alkaloids in doses of 25 or 50 mg/kg for seven days demonstrated the anticarcinoma effect in mice implanted with the ascitic hepatoma cells as well as amplified the plasma cAMP by 43.3–91.5%.[1–3]

Six alkaloids assigned as luotonins-A–F were separated from the aerial parts of *P. nigellastrum*. Luotonin-A, luotonin-B, and luotonin-E were a group of unique alkaloids holding a pyrroloquinazolinoquinoline skeleton and having obvious structural similarities to camptothecin (**2**), an important chemotherapeutic agent. Of them, luotonin-A (**1**) exerted the most powerful cytotoxicity against murine P388 leukemia cells with an IC_{50} value of 1.8 μg/mL.[4,5] Luotonin-A (**1**) was also a significant inhibitor of Topo-I and Topo-II. It exerted Topo-I-dependent cytotoxic effect as its structurally related camptothecin (**2**) did.[6,7] Luo Tuo Hao also contains other types of antineoplastic alkaloids such as vasicinone, deoxyvasicinone, harmine, and harmaline (see Section Luo Tuo Peng).

A water-soluble derivative of luotonin-A and camptothecin, 14-azacamptothecin (**3**), was synthesized as a Topo-I inhibitor and an antitumor agent, but it was less active compared to camptothecin (**2**). Three analogous derivatives (**4–6**) were developed from the structural modification of luotonin-A (**1**), displaying better moderate cytotoxicity than the parent molecule on human H460 lung cancer cells *in vitro*. The IC_{50} values were 3.8 μM for **4**, 5.5 μM for **5**, 7.0 μM for **6**, and 7.7 μM for **1**.[7]

From Luo Tuo Hao, a different type of alkaloid, 2-ethylheptyl 1H-imidazole-4-carboxylate (**7**), was separated, demonstrating the inhibitory activity on EGFRs for 33.06% at a concentration of 10 μM to exert antiangiogenic potential.[8] In addition, several triterpenoids were isolated from the roots of Luo Tuo Hao. Only 3α,27-dihydroxylup-20(29)-en-28-oic acid methyl ester (**8**) in these triterpenoids noticeably suppressed the activity of human Topo-II with the IC_{50} value of 8.9 μM/mL.[9]

Other Medical Uses

The herb Luo Tuo Hao has been used in Chinese folk medicinal practice for the treatment of rheumatism, abscess, and inflammation.

References

1. Xiao, X. H. et al. 1988. Effect of alkaloids from *Paganum nigellastum* on mouse ascitic hepatoma and isolated cells. *Zhongguo Yaolixue yu Dulixue Zazhi* 2: 232–4.
2. Xie, J. C. et al. 2002. Affinitive separation and on-line identification of antitumor components from *Peganum nigellastrum* by coupling a chromatographic column of target analogue imprinted polymer with mass spectrometry. *Analytical Chem.* 74: 2352–60.
3. Xie, J. C. et al. 2002. Efficient separation and identification of active compounds from herb by combining molecular imprinting affinity chromatography with mass spectrometry. *Huaxue Xuebao* 60: 385–8.
4. Ma, Z. Z. et al. 2000. Alkaloids and phenylpropanoids from *Peganum nigellastrum*. *Phytochem.* 53: 1075–8.

5. Ma, Z. Z. et al. 1999. The structures of new alkaloid components from *Peganum nigellastrum*. *Tennen Yuki Kagobutsu Toronkai Koen Yoshishu* 41st 547–52.
6. Cagir, A. et al. 2003. Luotonin A. A naturally occurring human DNA topoisomerase I poison. *J. Am. Chem. Soc.* 125: 13628–9.
7. Ma, Z. Z. et al. 2005. Luotonin A: A lead toward anticancer agent development. *Heterocycles* 65: 2203–19.
8. Chen, R. et al. 2009. Extraction of 2-ethylheptyl 1H-imidazole-4-carboxylate as EGFR inhibitor for treatment of tumor. *Faming Zhuanli Shenqing Gongkai Shuomingshu* CN 101397274 A 20090401.
9. Ma, Z. Z. et al. 2000. Three new triterpenoids from *Peganum nigellastrum*. *J. Nat. Prods.* 63: 390–2.

155 Bai Su 白蘇

Perilla or Beefsteak plant

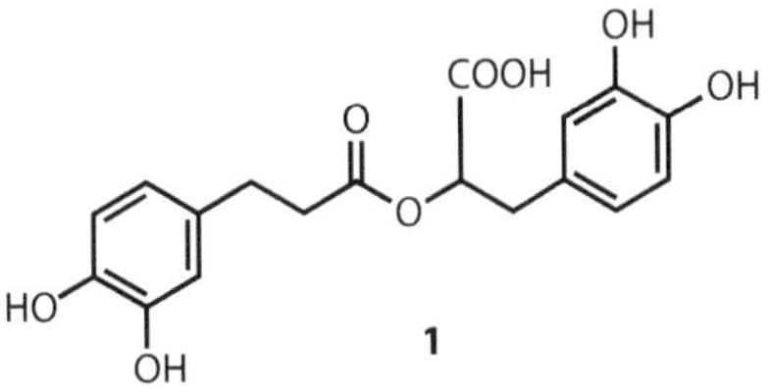

Herb Origination

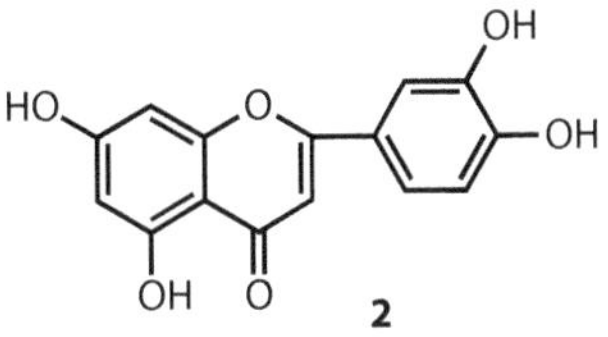

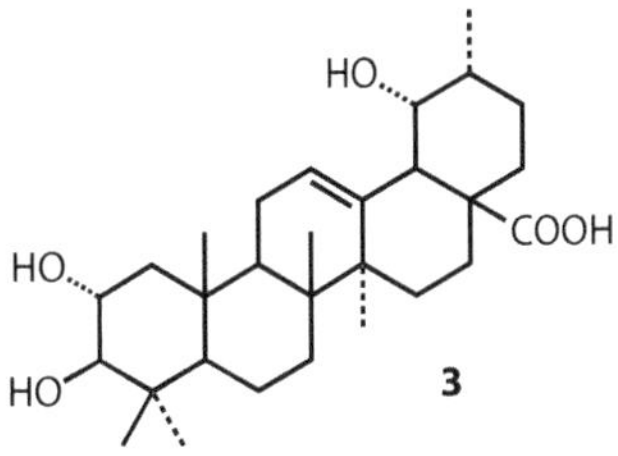

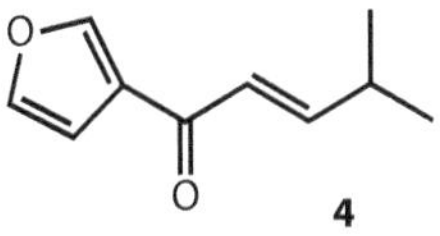

The herb Bai Su is an ornamental plant *Perilla frutescens* (Labiatae), which is native to east Asia. The plant has been used as a traditional Chinese herb for more than two thousand years and as a traditional crop of southern China, India, Thailand, Japan, Korea, and other Asian countries. Its leaves, stalks, and seeds can be used for purposes in both medicine and cuisine. Since the late 1800s, the annual plant was naturalized by Asian immigrants to the United States in the beginning, and it is widely spread in southeastern United States now. Normally, the leaves are collected in summer and autumn, and the stalks are collected after its fruits have ripened.

Antitumor Activities and Constituents

The Perilla leaf extract displayed an ability to suppress the viability of human HepG2 hepatoma cells and human HL-60 leukemia cells in a dose-dependent manner. The antiproliferative effect in HL-60 cells was found to be strictly related to the induction of p21-mediated G1 cell cycle arrest and apoptosis via combinational mitochondrial, death receptor-mediated, and ER pathways.[1,2] The methanolic extract of Perilla stalk could moderately inhibit the proliferation of human A549 NSCLC cells *in vitro*, but the extract showed to be more active as an antioxidant than its leaves and seeds.[3] The methanolic extract could also enhance the biological activities of phase II enzymes including QR, whose phase-II enzymes had been reported as anticarcinogenic marker enzymes associated with the protection of animals from neoplastic, mutagenic, and toxic effects of many oncogens.[4,5] A butanolic fraction prepared from Bai Su significantly exerted a suppressive effect against the growth of melanoma cells.[6] The results indicated that Bai Su may be employed as a potential source of natural antioxidant and anticarcinogenic and agent for healthcare.

Likewise, the treatment with the ethanolic extract of Perilla seed (PSE) dose-dependently inhibited the proliferation of HCT116 colorectal cancer cells and H1299 NSCLC cells by ~94% at a concentration range of ~350 μg/mL and completely abolished the colony formation at a concentration of 175 μg/mL. PSE at a concentration range of 87.5–350 μg/mL was also effective in inhibiting the migration of H1299 cells and in radical-scavenging antioxidation.[7]

Polyphenolic Component

Rosmarinic acid (**1**) and luteolin (**2**) isolated from Bai Su demonstrated marked suppressive effects DMBA-initiated and TPA-promoted skin papillomas in mice. Two polyphenolic components could remarkably diminish the incidence and the multiplicity of tumorigenesis by a topical application prior to the carcinogens inoculated, where the topical application of luteolin (**2**) resulted in a more potent preventive effect. The anticarcinogenic mechanism was found to be closely related to the significant inhibition toward COX-2 mRNA expression and inflammation and the enhancement of scavenging active oxygen species.[8,9] The antiproliferative activity was also observed in rosmarinic acid (**1**)-treated HepG2 cells, together with prominent apoptotic induction and apoptosis-related gene regulation.[1] In addition, rosmarinic acid (**1**) also exerted an inhibitory activity against an anticancer drug Adm-induced H9C2 cardiac muscle cell apoptosis by retarding ROS generation and reducing JNK and ERK activations. This result suggested that rosmarinic acid (**1**) may be a potential agent for the inhibition of cardiotoxicity in patients exposed to Adm, an anticancer drug.[10]

Methyl caffeate, a component derived from Bai Su, showed potent cytotoxic effects against human A549 lung cancer cells and human K562 leukemia cells *in vitro*. The methyl caffeate and di-Bu phthalate as well as the Bai Su methanol extract were capable of repressing the complex formation between the Fos–Jun dimer and the AP-1 binding site, whose action should be involved in the anticarcinoma mechanism.[11] Therefore, the polyphenols derived from the herb may provide a beneficial chemopreventive effect as a daily food supplement.

Triterpene Acids

Eight triterpene acids isolated from Bai Su exhibited inflammatory effects. Of the triterpene acids, ursolic acid, corosolic acid, 3-epi-corosolic acid, tormentic acid (**3**), and 3-epi-maslinic acid could potently suppress TPA-induced EBV-EA. Tormentic acid (**3**) also exerted strong antitumor-promoting activity in the two-stage mouse skin carcinogenesis caused by DMBA as an initiator and TPA as a promoter.[12] The three triterpene acids (ursolic acid, corosolic acid, and oleanolic acid) were the active principles responsible for the cytotoxicity on human HL-60 (leukemia), MCF-7 (breast cancer), and

HepG2 (hepatoma) cell lines *in vitro* with IC_{50} values in the range of 12–48 μM.[13]

Essential Oil

Perilla oil is rich in the n-3 polyunsaturated fatty acid such as α-linolenic acid, which demonstrated the inhibitory effect against colon carcinogenesis induced by N-ethyl-N-nitrosourea (2 mg × 3/week, two weeks) in rats while taking a diet containing 12% Perilla oil. Also, deoxycholic acid (a marker of tumor promotion)-enhanced colonic mucosal ornithine decarboxylase activity in intrarectal area was significantly lower in Perilla oil-fed rats.[14] The Perilla oil also retarded the breast carcinogenesis caused by the injection of DMBA or the transplant of subcutaneous tumor.[15] Moreover, a diet containing 5% Perilla oil could remarkably restrain the metastasis of ascites tumor to the lung and reduce the metastatic foci on the lung surface.[16] Isoegomaketone (**4**), a Bai Su essential oil component, could markedly inhibit the viability of human DLD1 colon cancer cells in a dose-dependent manner and promote the cell apoptosis of DLD1 cells through both caspase-dependent and caspase-independent pathways, including the cleavage of Bid and the translocation of Bax, the release of cytochrome c from the mitochondria to the cytoplasm, the cleavage of PARP, the activation of caspase-8, caspase-9, and caspase-3, as well as the translocation of AIF, a caspase-independent mitochondrial apoptosis factor, from the mitochondria into the nucleus.[17] Similarly, isoegomaketone (**4**) also effectively inhibited the growth of B16 melanoma cells and promoted the apoptosis via the activation of ROS-mediated, caspase-dependent, and caspase-independent pathways.[18] By blocking the P13K/Akt signaling pathway, the treatment with isoegomaketone (**4**) obstructed the proliferation of Huh-7 and Hep3B hepatoma cell lines *in vitro* and profoundly diminished the volume and the weight of Huh-7 tumor in a xenograft animal model.[19] Moreover, isoegomaketone (**4**), through the upregulation of DR5 via a ROS-independent pathway, could potentiate TRAIL-mediated apoptosis in TRAIL-resistant primary prostate cancer cells.[20]

Other Bioactivities

Bai Su (Perilla) has been used in oriental medicine for centuries as antiasthmatic, antipyretic, antidote, antiseptic, antispasmodic, antitussive, diaphoretic, aromatic, emollient, carminative, expectorant, tonic, restorative, pectoral, stomachic, antimicrobial, and antibacterial agents. Ongoing studies have suggested that this plant is useful in curing other various diseases and disorders including neoplasm. The Bai Su extract and its major constituent rosmarinic acid (**1**) were reported to lessen LPS-induced liver injury in D-galactosamine-sensitized mice. The protective activity in hepatocytes is largely attributed to its capacities in scavenging and reducing superoxide or peroxynitrite.[21]

References

1. Lin, C. S. et al. 2007. Growth inhibitory and apoptosis inducing effect of *Perilla frutescens* on human hepatoma HepG2 cells. *J. Ethnopharmacol.* 112: 557–67.
2. Kwak, C. S. et al. 2009. Perilla leaf, *Perilla frutescens*, induces apoptosis and G1 phase arrest in human leukemia HL-60 cells through the combinations of death receptor-mediated, mitochondrial, and endoplasmic reticulum stress-induced pathways. *J. Med. Food.* 12: 508–17.
3. Lin, E. S. et al. 2010. Antioxidant and antiproliferative activities of methanolic extracts of *Perilla frutescens*. *J. Med. Plants Res.* 4: 477–83.
4. Hong, E. Y. et al. 1997. Modulation of cellular quinone reductase inducibility by roasting treatment and acid hydrolysis of perilla. *Han'guk Sikp'um Yongyang Kwahak Hoechi* 26: 186–92.
5. Hong, E. Y. et al. 1997. Fractionation of anticarcinogenic enzyme inducer(s) from roasted Perilla. *Han'guk Sikp'um Yongyang Kwahak Hoechi* 26: 193–7.
6. Lee, K. N. et al. 1997. Development of anticancer agents from korean medicinal plants: Part 5. Cytotoxic activity of the butanol-soluble fraction of *Perilla frutescens* against human skin melanoma cells. *Saengyak Hakhoechi* 28: 264–70.
7. Kim, S. et al. 2015. Antioxidant activities of *Perilla frutescens* britton seed extract and its inhibitory effects against major characteristics of cancer cells. *Han'guk Sikp'um Yongyang Kwahak Hoechi* 44: 208–15.
8. Osakabe, N. et al. 2004. Rosmarinic acid inhibits epidermal inflammatory responses: Anticarcinogenic effect of *Perilla frutescens* extract in the murine two-stage skin model. *Carcinogen.* 25: 549–57.
9. Ueda, H. et al. 2003. Inhibitory effect of Perilla leaf extract and luteolin on mouse skin tumor promotion. *Biol. Pharm. Bull.* 26: 560–3.
10. Kim, D. D. et al. 2005. Inhibitory effects of rosmarinic acid on adriamycin-induced apoptosis in H9c2 cardiac muscle cells by inhibiting reactive oxygen species and the activations of c-Jun N-terminal kinase and extracellular signal-regulated kinase. *Biochem. Pharmacol.* 70: 1066–78.
11. Lee, S. P. et al. 2001. Inhibitory effect of methyl caffeate on Fos-Jun-DNA complex formation and suppression of cancer cell growth. *Bull. Korean Chem. Soc.* 22: 1131–5.
12. Banno, N. et al. 2004. Triterpene acids from the leaves of *Perilla frutescens* and their anti-inflammatory and antitumor-promoting effects. *Biosci. Biotech. Biochem.* 68: 85–90.
13. Akihisa, T. et al. 2006. Cytotoxic activity of *Perilla frutescens* var. *japonica* leaf extract is due to high concentrations of oleanolic and ursolic acids. *J. Nat. Med.* 60: 331–3.
14. Narisawa, T. et al. 1991. Inhibitory effect of dietary perilla oil rich in the n-3 polyunsaturated fatty acid α-linolenic acid on colon carcinogenesis in rats. *Jpn. J. Cancer Res.* 82: 1089–96.
15. Wang, S. L. et al. 1995. Perilla oil and α-linolenic acid. *J. Shenyang Univ. Pharm.* 12: 228.
16. Hori, T. et al. 1987. Effect of dietary essential fatty acids on pulmonary metastasis of ascites tumor cells in rats. *Chem. Pharm. Bull.* 35: 3925–7.
17. Cho, B. O. et al. 2011. Isoegomaketone induces apoptosis through caspase-dependent and caspase-independent pathways in human DLD1 cells. *Biosci. Biotechnol. Biochem.* 75: 1306–11.
18. Kwon, S. J. et al. 2014. Induction of apoptosis by isoegomaketone from *Perilla frutescens* L. in B16 melanoma cells is mediated through ROS generation and mitochondrial-dependent, -independent pathway. *Food Chem. Toxicol.* 65: 97–104.

19. Wang, Y. et al. 2013. Extract of *Perilla frutescens* inhibits tumor proliferation of HCC via PI3K/AKT signal pathway. *Afri. J. Tradit. Complem. Altern. Med.* 10: 251–7.
20. Lee, J. H. et al. 2014. Sensitization of tumor necrosis factor-related apoptosis-inducing ligand (TRAIL)-resistant primary prostate cancer cells by isoego-maketone from *Perilla frutescens. J. Nat. Prod.* 77: 2438–43.
21. Osakabe, N. M. et al. 2002. Rosmarinic acid, a major polyphenolic component of *Perilla frutescens,* reduces lipopolysaccharide (LPS)-induced liver injury in D-galactosamine (D-GalN)-sensitized mice. *Free Radical Biol. Med.* 33: 798–806.

156 Ye Gan Cao 野甘草

Sweetbroom or Broomweed

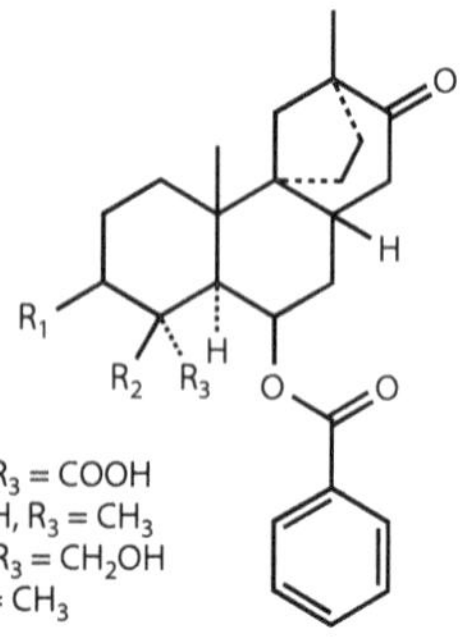

1. R_1 = H, R_2 = CH_3, R_3 = COOH
6. R_1 = H, R_2 = COOH, R_3 = CH_3
2. R_1 = H, R_2 = CH_3, R_3 = CH_2OH
4. R_1 = OH, R_2 = R_3 = CH_3

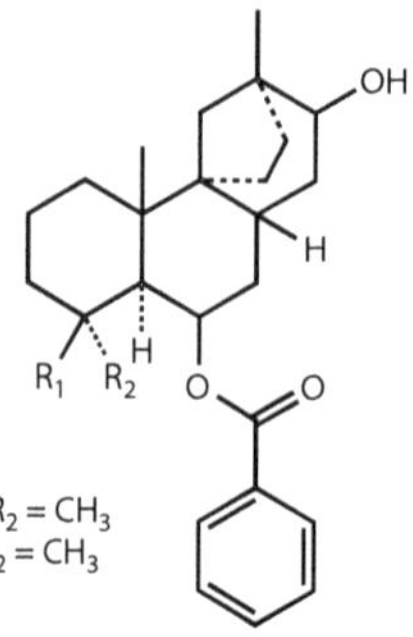

5. R_1 = CH_2OH, R_2 = CH_3
7. R_1 = COOH, R_2 = CH_3

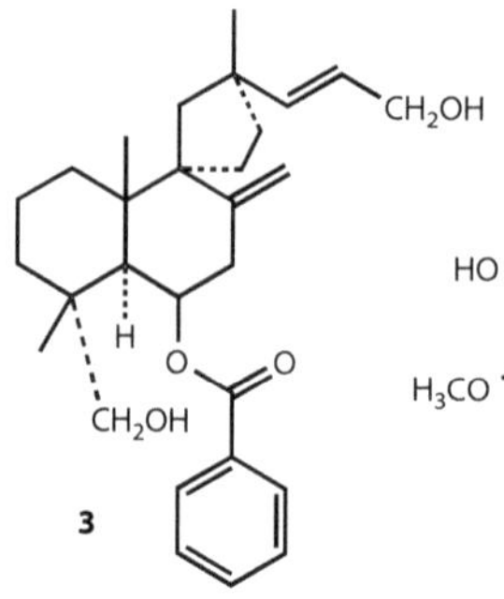

3

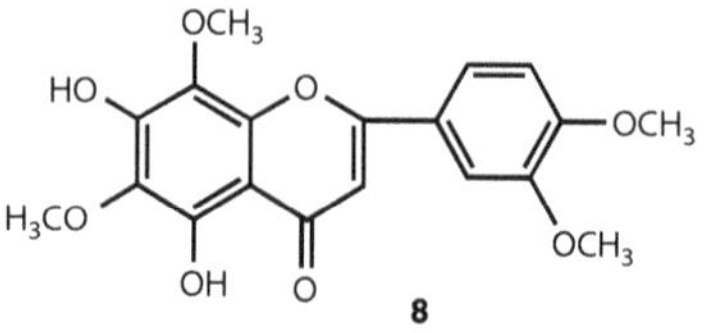

8

Herb Origination

The herb Ye Gan Cao (Sweetbroom) is a Scrophulariaceae plant, *Scoparia dulcis* L. This erect perennial herbaceous plant is widely distributed in the tropical and subtropical regions of Asia, Africa, and the Americas, including southern China. It is found in abundance in South America and the Amazon region. The entire plant can be collected annually and used as fresh and sun-dried herb for Chinese folk medical practice.

Antitumor Constituents and Activities

Diterpenoids

A group of labdane-derived diterpenoids was isolated from Ye Gan Cao, which was demonstrated to possess antineoplastic property. Scopadulcic acid-B (**1**) displayed potent cytotoxicity against various tumor cell lines with IC_{50} values of 0.068–0.076 μg/mL *in vitro*, but its cytotoxicity was also strong toward normal cells with an IC_{50} value of 0.097–0.245 μg/mL. The oral or i.p. administration of scopadulcic acid-B (**1**) at doses of 25–100 mg/kg per day prolonged the median survival time of mice bearing Ehrlich ascites tumor cells by 12–25% without body weight change over the treatment period.[1] Besides the anticancer effects, scopadulcic acid-B (**1**) also exerted antitumor promoting activities on skin tumor formation initiated with DMBA and promoted by TPA in mice, where the TPA-enhanced phospholipid synthesis was restrained.[2]

In an *in vitro* assay, other isolated diterpenoids such as scopadulciol (**2**) and scopadiol (**3**) suppressed the growth of a panel of human gastric cancer cell lines (SCL, SCL-6, SCL-37′6, SCL-9, NUGC-4, and Kato-3) with ED_{50} values in the range of 8.9–37.7 μM. Isodulcinol (**4**), dulcidiol (**5**), and 4-epi-scopadulcic acid-B (**6**) exhibited moderate to weak cytotoxicity against the first four or five stomach tumor cell lines with ED_{50} values of 19.5–71.7 μM.[3] In the treatment of the AGS gastric cancer cells, scopadulciol (**2**) also induced p53- and proteasome-dependent degradation of β-catenin to obstruct TCF/β-catenin transcription and to promote TNF-related apoptosis of TRAIL-resistant AGS when combined with TRAIL.[4] From the extract of *S. dulcis*, whose plant was collected in Vietnam, three cytotoxic diterpenoids identified as isodulcinol (**4**), dulcidiol (**5**), and 4-*epi*-scopadulcic acid-B (**6**) were isolated, showing the inhibition on human KB nasopharyngeal neoplastic cells (respective IC_{50}: 4, 2, and 2.5 μg/mL) and also the moderate inhibition on MDR-associated proteins (respective IC_{50}: 10, 30, and 15 μg/mL).[5]

Flavone

A flavone component, hymenoxin (**8**), separated from the herb Ye Gan Cao showed the same degree of cytotoxicity not only against cultured human tumor cell lines (HeLa-229, HeLa-S3, and HEp-2) but also against normal human tissues (FL, Chang liver, and intestine 407).[6]

Benzoxazinoid

Several benzoxazinoids were isolated from the aerial part of *S. dulcis*, but only 1-hydroxy-6-methoxy-2-benzoxazolinone (**9**) showed a moderate inhibition against the proliferation of human DU-145 prostate cancer cell line with an IC_{50} value of 65.8 μg/mL.[7]

Other Bioactivities

Fresh or dried Ye Gan Cao (Sweetbroom) has been traditionally used as remedies for hypotension, ailments in the gastrointestinal tract and the liver, bronchitis, and diabetes. Ye Gan Cao also has many other medical applications in the tropical countries such as abortifacient, contraceptive, expectorant, analgesic, antipyretic, emmenagogue, depurative, and diarrhea. It is used to treat dysmenorrhea, dysentery, kidney stone, fever, wounds, ulcer, and skin diseases.

Scopadulcic acid-B (**1**) and scopadulciol (**2**) were disclosed to have the inhibitory effects on porcine gastric H^+, K^+-ATPase, gastric proton pump, replication of (HSV-1, and bone resorption induced by parathyroid hormone.[8,9] Scopadulciol (**2**) exhibited stimulatory effects on the antiviral potency of acyclovir (ACV) or ganciclovir (GCV) by activating HSV-1 thymidine kinase and the cellular concentration of the active triphosphates of ACV or GCV.[10]

References

1. Hayashi, K. et al. 1992. Cytotoxic and antitumor activity of scopadulcic acid from *Scoparia dulcis* L. *Phytother. Res.* 6: 6–9.
2. Nishino, H. et al. 1993. Antitumor-promoting activity of scopadulcic acid-B, isolated from the medicinal plant *Scoparia dulcis* L. *Oncol.* 50: 100–3.
3. Ahsan, M. et al. 2003. Cytotoxic diterpenes from *Scoparia dulcis. J. Nat. Prods* 66: 958–61.
4. Fuentes, R. G. et al. 2015. Scopadulciol, isolated from *Scoparia dulcis*, induces β-catenin degradation and overcomes tumor necrosis factor-related apoptosis ligand resistance in AGS human gastric adenocarcinoma cells. *J. Nat. Prod.* 78: 864–72.
5. Phan, M. G. et al. 2006. Chemical and biological evaluation on scopadulane-type diterpenoids from *Scoparia dulcis* of vietnamese origin. *Chem. Pharm. Bull.* 54: 546–9.
6. Hayashi, T. et al. 1988. A cytotoxic flavone from *Scoparia dulcis* L. *Chem. Pharm. Bull.* 36: 4849–51.
7. Wu, W. H. et al. 2012. Benzoxazinoids from *Scoparia dulcis* (sweet broomweed) with antiproliferative activity against the DU-145 human prostate cancer cell line. *Phytochem.* 83: 110–5.
8. Riel, A. M. et al. 2002. Efficacy of scopadulcic acid A against *Plasmodium falciparum* in vitro. *J. Nat. Prod.* 65: 614–5.
9. Hayashi, T. 2000. Biologically active diterpenoids from *Scoparia dulcis* L. *Studies in Nat. Prod. Chem.*, 21(Bioactive Natural Products: Part B), 689–727.
10. Hayashi, T. et al. 2008. Studies on evaluation of natural products for antiviral effects and their applications. *Yakugaku Zasshi* 128: 61–79.

157 Gua Lou 栝樓

Snake gourd

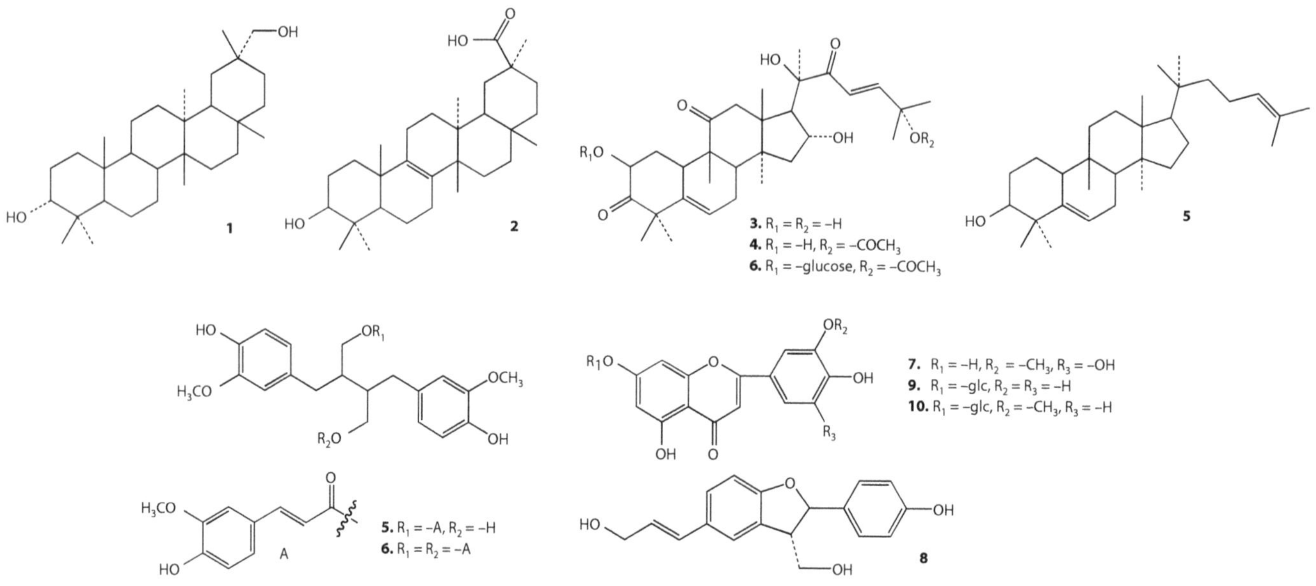

3. $R_1 = R_2 = -H$
4. $R_1 = -H, R_2 = -COCH_3$
6. $R_1 = -glucose, R_2 = -COCH_3$

7. $R_1 = -H, R_2 = -CH_3, R_3 = -OH$
9. $R_1 = -glc, R_2 = R_3 = -H$
10. $R_1 = -glc, R_2 = -CH_3, R_3 = -H$

5. $R_1 = -A, R_2 = -H$
6. $R_1 = R_2 = -A$

Herb Origination

The herb Gua Lou (Snake gourd) originated from a Cucurbitaceae plant of *Trichosanthes kirilowii* and *T. rosthornii*. The fruit, the seed, and the peel can be used individually as folk medicines in China. The Gua Lou fruit was documented in the first Chinese classic materia medica titled as *Shennong Ben Cao Jing* as one of the 50 fundamental herbs used in traditional Chinese medicine. The herb is mainly produced in Shandong, Anhui, and Henan provinces of China.

Antitumor Constituents and Activities

Multiflorane-Type Triterpenoids

Eleven multiflorane-type triterpenoids and 38 of their derivatives were isolated from Gua Lou seeds, and they demonstrated the inhibitory effect on Epstein-Barr virus early antigen (EBV-EA) activation induced by a tumor promoter TPA. Especially, karounidiol (**1**) and bryonolic acid (**2**) were revealed to possess remarkable antitumor promotion activity, whose potencies were either comparable to or stronger than that of glycyrrhetic acid, a known natural antitumor promoter. *In vivo* experiments exhibited that the treatment with karounidiol (**1**) in 2 μmol dose per mouse obviously retarded skin carcinogenesis initiated by 7,12-dimethylbenz(a)anthracene (DMBA) and promoted by TPA. Moreover, karounidiol (**1**) exhibited cytotoxic activity against many human cancer cell lines such as renal cancer (UO-31, ACHN, and SN12C) cells, leukemia (CCCF-CEM and SR) cells, NSCLC (A549/ATCC, NCI-H460, and NCI-H522) cells, colon carcinoma (HCT-116) cells, ovarian neoplastic (OVCAR-3 and OVCAR-6) cells, and brain cancer (U251) cells, with GI_{50} values in the range of 1.63–3.56 μM.[1,2]

Bryonolic acid (**2**) could also be highly yielded from the cultured Gua Lou hairy root cells with *Agrobacterium rhizogenes* (ATCC 15834). Bryonolic acid (**2**) was cytotoxic to various cancer cells *in vitro*, exhibiting stronger inhibitory effect toward the cancer cell growth compared to karasurin-A, an antitumor protein purified from Gua Lou roots. The IC_{50} values were 15, 24, and 20 μg/mL, respectively, against the cell growth of B16 melanoma, BeWo chorioepithelioma, and PLC/PRF-5 hepatoma. It also significantly retarded the proliferation of L1210 and CCER-CEM leukemia cells and LS174T colon cancer cells, and the potency of antileukemia in L1210 cells reached to an IC_{50} value of 0.024 μg/mL *in vitro*. The appearance of a DNA ladder was detected in the bryonolic acid-treated leukemia HL-60RG cells, implying that the cell apoptosis was triggered and normal rat hepatocytes were less sensitive to the bryonolic acid (**2**).[3–5] More bryonolic acid analogs were separated from the hairy roots, showing different degrees of the antitumor property as well.[6]

Cucurbitane-Type Triterpenoids

A group of cucurbitane triterpenes, namely cucurbitacin-D (**3**) and cucurbitacin-B (**4**), isocucurbitacin-B, 3-epi-isocucurbitacin-B, isocucurbitacin-D, dihydrocucurbitacin-B and dihydrocucurbitacin-E, and dihydroisocucurbitacin-B, were isolated from the roots of the Gua Lou plant. All these cucurbitacins were significantly cytotoxic to human A549 (lung), SKOV-3 (ovary), SK-MEL-2 (skin), XF-498 (brain), and HCT15 (colon) neoplastic cell lines *in vitro*.[7] Cucurbitacin-D (**3**) and 23,24-dihydrocucurbitacin-D notably inhibited the activity of tyrosinase in B16-F10 melanoma cells and promoted the apoptotic death through the activation of caspase-3 and the phosphorylation of JNK in hepatocellular carcinoma cells.[8,9] (see Section

Tian Gua Di). Two more active triterpenes, cucurbitadienol (**5**) and arvenin-I (**6**), were discovered from the *T. kirilowii* roots collected in Vietnam. Cucurbitadienol (**5**) showed obvious suppression against HT-29 (colon) and OVCAR (ovarix) human cancer cell lines (respective IC_{50}: 4.1 and 6.5 μM) and against A549 (lung) and MCF-7 (breast) cancer lines (respective IC_{50}: 11.3 and 17.3 μM), whereas arvenin-I (**6**) showed obvious suppression against A549 and OVCAR cells (IC_{50}: 15–17 μM) and against HT-29 and MCF-7 cells (IC_{50}: 42–50 μM).[10]

The antiproliferative effects of cucurbitacin-B (**4**) were also demonstrated in various leukemia and lymphoma cells *in vitro*, as well as in primary mononuclear bone marrow cells derived from patients with AML or myelodysplastic syndrome. After the cucurbitacin-B treatment, the myeloid leukemia cells displayed multiple changes such as significant S phase cell cycle arrest, enlargement of the cell size, multinucleation, and increase of monocytic- and granulocytic-specific CD11b expression.[11] Moreover, cucurbitacin-B (**4**) also exerted the antiproliferative effects against seven human pancreatic cancer cells, five human GBM cells, three breast cancer cells (T47D, SKBR-3, and MCF-7), and four cutaneous SCC (the second most common skin cancer with a substantial risk of metastasis) cell lines (SRB1, SRB12, SCC13, and COLO16) *in vitro*.[12–15] The clonogenesis of nearly all the GBM, cutaneous squamous cell carcinoma (CSCC), and pancreas carcinoma cell lines were obstructed by cucurbitacin-B (**4**) at 10^{-7} to 10^{-8} M concentrations.[12–15] An *in vivo* investigation showed that the growth inhibitory rate of cucurbitacin-B (**4**) was achieved by 69.2% in nude mice with pancreatic tumor xenografts.[14]

The mechanism-related investigations further revealed the characteristic pathways exerted by cucurbitacin-B (**4**) for its marked suppression on the different types of cancer cells. The suppressive effect of cucurbitacin-B (**4**), in the breast cancer cells, especially in estrogen receptor$^-$ SK-BR-3 cells, was found to be mediated by hindering telomerase and downregulating both hTERT and c-Myc expressions, whereas in the glioblastoma cell lines (U87 and T98G), by affecting the cytoskeleton and the microtubules via a JNK pathway.[12,13] The cucurbitacin-B treatment also caused the cell cycle G_2/M phase arrest and the apoptosis of pancreatic cancer cells dose- and time-dependently through the inhibition of JAK2/STAT3 pathway and the reduction of cyclin-A, cyclin-B1, and Bcl-xL expressions with subsequent activation of caspase-3 and caspase-9, but the elicited G2/M cell arrest of cutaneous SCC cell lines (SRB1 and SRB12) was associated with the decrease of CDC2 and cyclin-B1 levels.[14,15]

Importantly, cucurbitacin-B (**4**) synergistically potentiated the cytotoxicity of chemotherapeutic agents, cisplatin and gemcitabine, in the CSCC cell lines.[14–16] The synergistic efficacies in the growth inhibition, the G2/M cell arrest, and the apoptosis induction in HEp-2 laryngeal cancer cells *in vitro* and *in vivo* were found to closely correlate with the diminishment of p-STAT3, Bcl-2, and cyclin-B1 expressions.[16] Consequently, the affirmative evidences encouraged the use of cucurbitacins in clinical trials for the treatment of hematopoietic and solid malignancies and suggested that the combination of cucurbitacin-B (**4**) with clinical anticancer drugs may be a feasible strategy to improve chemotherapeutic results in patients.

Other Types of Molecules

Some other types of constituents derived from the Gua Lou seeds also demonstrated the antiproliferative property. Two lignans, hanultarin (**5**) and 1,4-*O*-diferuloyl-secoisolariciresinol (**6**), and one flavone, isoetin 5′-methyl ether 5,7,2′,4′-tetrahydroxy-5′-methoxyflavone (**7**), exerted marked cytotoxic effect against human A549 (lung) and SK-Mel-2 (skin) cancer cells and against mouse B16-F10 (skin) tumor cells (IC_{50}: 0.92–7.23 μg/mL for one flavone, isoetin 5′-methyl ether 5,7,2′,4′-tetrahydroxy-5′-methoxyflavone (**7**) and 3–13 μg/mL for hanultarin (**5**) and 1,4-*O*-diferuloyl-secoisolariciresinol (**6**)).[17,18] Interestingly, the lignan diester (**6**) was two to four times more potent than the lignan monoester (**5**) on all tested cell lines, implying that the simple covalent bonds between the ferulic acid and secoisolariciresinol can markedly augment the antitumor effect.[19] A lignan, trichobenzolignan (**8**), and two flavonoids, chrysoeriol-7-*O*-β-D-glucoside (**9**) and luteolin 7-*O*-β-D-glucoside (**10**), which were isolated from the roots of *T. kirilowii*, showed moderate to weak inhibitory effect against HT-29 (colon), OVCAR (ovary), A549 (lung), and MCF-7 (breast) human cancer cell lines *in vitro*, except luteolin 7-*O*-β-D-glucoside (**10**) exerted potent suppression on the A549 cells (IC_{50}: 2.7 μM).[10] In addition, the Gua Lou root also contain a kind of natural antiangiogenic component, which has been demonstrated in the *in vivo* and *in vitro* assays.[20,21]

Glycoprotein

Trichokirin, a glycoprotein with strong ribosome-inactivating activity, was also found to exert antitumor activity. When trichokirin was conjugated to a monoclonal antibody directed on a Thy 1.2 antigen, the created immunotoxin showed the selectivity for killing Thy 1.2 antigen-expressed leukemia cells.[22]

Polysaccharide

Snake gourd root polysaccharides exerted the antiproliferative effect against MCF-7 (breast) and HeLa (cervix) cancer cell lines *in vitro* at concentrations of 5.0, 10.0, and 20.0 mmol/L. The treatment with 10.0 μmol/L polysaccharide of Snake gourd root for two days promoted the apoptosis of MCF-7 cells concomitantly with the activation of intracellular caspase-3 and caspase-8. The polysaccharides were also capable of amplifying the proliferation of peripheral blood mononuclear cells.[23,24]

Other Bioactivities

Gua Luo (Snake gourd) is one of most popular herbal plants in east Asia, whose tuber has been prescribed for the treatment of patients with diabetes, breast abscesses, rigorous coughing, inflammatory, HIV-positive, and cancer-related symptoms, and it is also used as an abortifacient. Pharmacological evidences suggested that Gua Lou seed has purgative, antiplatelet aggregation, and coronary dilative properties, and the Gua Lou fruit possesses microcirculation-promoting, coronary dilative, antimyocardial ischemia, antiplatelet aggregation, antiarrhythmic, and antiulcerative activities.

Side Effects

An overdose of the Gua Lou seed extract causes side effects in the gastrointestinal area such as nausea, emetic, diarrhea, and purgative. The Gua Lou fruit and peel can also induce gastrointestinal upset, but the side effects are low.

References

1. Akihisa, T. et al. 2001. Antitumor promoting effects of multiflorane-type triterpenoids and cytotoxic activity of karounidiol against human cancer cell lines. *Cancer Lett.* 173: 9–14.
2. Yasukawa, K. et al. 1994. Inhibitory effect of karounidiol on 12-*O*-tetradecanoylphorbol-13-acetate-induced tumor promotion. *Biol. Pharm. Bull.* 17: 460–2.
3. Takeda, T. et al. 1994. Bryonolic acid production in hairy roots of *Trichosanthes kirilowii* Max. var. *japonica* Kitam. transformed with *Agrobacterium rhizogenes* and its cytotoxic activity. *Chem. Pharm. Bull.* 42: 730–2.
4. Kondo, T. et al. 1995. Cytotoxic activity of bryonolic acid isolated from transformed hairy roots of *Trichosanthes kirilowii* var. *japonica*. *Biol. Pharm. Bull.* 18: 726–9.
5. State of Administration in Chinese Medicine, *Chinese Materia Medica*, 1999, Vol. 5, 5–4661, 579. Shanghai Science and Technology Press. Shanghai, China.
6. Ogiwara, Y. et al. 1995. Antitumor agents containing pentacyclic triterpenoids. *Jpn. Kokai Tokkyo Koho* JP 07252141 A 19951003.
7. Ryu, S. Y. et al. 1994/1995. Antitumor activity of *Trichosanthes kirilowii*. *Archiv. Pharm. Res.* 17: 348–53; 18: 60.
8. Hyuncheol, O. et al. 2002. Cucurbitacins from *Trichosanthes kirilowii* as the inhibitory components on tyrosinase activity and melanin synthesis of B16/F10 melanoma cells. *Planta Med.* 68: 832–3.
9. Haritunians, T. et al. 2008. Cucurbitacin B induces differentiation, cell cycle arrest, and actin cytoskeletal alterations in myeloid leukemia cells. *Leukemia Res.* 32: 1366–73.
10. Minh, C. V. et al. 2015. Chemical constituents of *Trichosanthes kirilowii* and their cytotoxic activities. *Arch. Pharm. Res.* 38: 1443–8.
11. Takahashi, N. et al. 2009. Cucurbitacin D isolated from *Trichosanthes kirilowii* induces apoptosis in human hepatocellular carcinoma cells in vitro. *Intl. Immunopharmacol.* 9: 508–13.
12. Yin, D. et al. 2008. Cucurbitacin B markedly inhibits growth and rapidly affects the cytoskeleton in glioblastoma multiforme. *Intl. J. Cancer* 123: 1364–75.
13. Suwit, D. et al. 2010. Antiproliferative effects of cucurbitacin B in breast cancer cells: Down-regulation of the myc/hTERT/telomerase pathway and obstruction of the cell cycle. *Intl. J. Mol. Sci.* 11: 5323–38.
14. Thoennissen, N. H. et al. 2009. Cucurbitacin B induces apoptosis by inhibition of the JAK/STAT pathway and potentiates antiproliferative effects of gemcitabine on pancreatic cancer cells. *Cancer Res.* 69: 5876–84.
15. Chen, W. K. et al. 2010. Cucurbitacin B inhibits growth, arrests the cell cycle, and potentiates antiproliferative efficacy of cisplatin in cutaneous squamous cell carcinoma cell lines. *Intl. J. Oncol.* 37: 737–43.
16. Liu, T. Y. et al. 2008. Combined antitumor activity of cucurbitacin B and docetaxel in laryngeal cancer. *Eur. J. Pharmacol.* 587: 78–84.
17. Moon, S. et al. 2008. Hanultarin, a cytotoxic lignan as an inhibitor of actin cytoskeleton polymerization from the seeds of *Trichosanthes kirilowii*. *Bioorg. Med. Chem.* 16: 7264–9.
18. Rahman, M. et al. 2007. Isoetin 5′-methyl ether, a cytotoxic flavone from *Trichosanthes kirilowii*. *Bull. Korean Chem. Soc.* 28: 1261–4.
19. Lee, E. Y. et al. 2011. Synthesis and evaluation of cytotoxic effects of hanultarin and its derivatives. *Bioorg. Med. Chem. Lett.* 21: 6245–8.
20. Ke, Y. et al. 2002. Natural anti-angiogenic composition containing *Trichosanthes kirilowii* rhizome extracts. *PCT Int. Appl.* WO 2002053165 A1 20020711.
21. Wang, S. S. et al. 2004. Angiogenesis and anti-angiogenesis activity of Chinese medicinal herbal extracts. *Life Sci.* 74: 2467–78.
22. Casellas, P. et al. 1988. Trichokirin, a ribosome-inactivating protein from the seeds of *Trichosanthes kirilowii* Maximowicz. Purification, partial characterization and use for preparation of immune-toxins. *Eur. J. Biochem.* 176: 581–8.
23. Zhao, G. Z. et al. 2011. Effect of *Trichosanthes kirilowii* polysaccharides on peripheral blood mononuclear cell proliferation and cell proliferation inhibition of breast cancer and cervical carcinoma. *Shizhen Guoyi Guoyao* 22: 2140–2.
24. Cao, L. L. et al. 2012. Effects of snakegourd root polysaccharide on apoptosis of MCF-7 cells. *Zhejiang Daxue Xuebao, Yixueban* 41: 527–34.

158 Hong Che Zhou Cao 紅車軸草

Red clover

1. R = -H
2. R = $-CH_3$

3. R = -H
4. R = $-CH_3$

Herb Origination

The herb Hong Che Zhou Cao (Red clover) originated from a Leguminosae plant, *Trifolium pretense* L., which distributed in the northeastern and northern parts of China and part of the provinces from the east to the south. Also, the plant is wildly cultured in the country now. Its young twigs with flowers and leaves are collected in summer and dried without the sun for the folk medical use.

Anticarcinogenic Constituents and Activities

The water extract derived from Red clover inhibited the growth of sarcoma 45 cells in mice, but it is inactive on Ehrlich ascites neoplastic cells. Its ethanolic extract demonstrated the inhibitory effect against BAP-caused carcinogenesis *in vivo*. Two anticarcinogenic isoflavones such as genistein (**1**) and biochanin-A (**2**) were separated from the extract, and both inhibited the metabolic activation of BAP (an oncogen) by 54% and reduced the linkage of BAP to the DNA by 37%–50% at concentrations of 25 μg/mL, leading to the anticarcinogenic effect.[1,2] Biochanin-A (**2**) dose-dependently restrained the cell growth through the blockage of thymidine incorporation and the increase of DNA fragmentation and apoptosis in human LNCaP prostate adenocarcinoma cells *in vitro*, whose effect was also accompanied with induction of G0/G1 cell arrest and regulation of cyclin-B and p21 expressions. *In vivo* tests of LNCaP xenograft cancer in athymic mice further confirmed that biochanin-A (**2**) noticeably lessened the size of prostate cancer and declined the incidence of carcinogenesis.[3] In the presence of formononetin (**4**), the cell cycle of MCF-7 breast cancer was arrested at G0/G1 phase by inactivating IGF1/IGF1R-PI3K/Akt pathways and diminishing cyclin-D1 mRNA and protein expression, which data indicated the use in the prevention of breast carcinogenesis.[4] Moreover, formononetin (**4**) demonstrated the inhibitory effect on the migration and the invasion of MDA-MB-231 and 4T1 breast cancer cells *in vitro* and *in vivo*, despite no effective inhibition on the viability of MDA-MB-231 and 4T1 cells in 24 h with a concentration lower than 160 μmol/L, whose antiinvasive effect on the breast cancer cells was triggered by up-expressing TIMP-1 and TIMP-2 and down-expressing MMP-2 and MMP-9 through the PI3K/AKT signaling pathway.[5]

Moreover, biochanin-A (**2**) is an inhibitor of cytochrome P450 (CYP)-1A1 and cytochrome P450 (CYP)-1B1 enzymes. Because DMBA-caused carcinogenesis is dependent on the CYP1 enzymes, biochanin-A (**1**) markedly decreased the DMBA–DNA lesions to show the anticarcinogenesis effect through the inhibition of CYP1 enzyme activities. The results illustrated that the isoflavones such as genistein (**1**), biochanin-A (**2**), and daizein (**3**) are able to diminish the DNA damage caused by polycyclic aromatic hydrocarbon and to prevent the carcinogenesis.[6]

Red clover isoflavones (such as genistein, formononetin, biochanin, and daidzein) are inhibitors of COX. A high intake of dietary Red clover isoflavones could exert the anticarcinogenic effect via the suppression of COX activity.[5] Because Red clover isoflavones also possess photoprotective activity, the isoflavones were used to formulate a lotion for reducing the activity of ornithine decarboxylase and the contact hypersensitivity of solar-simulated UV radiation. When experimental mice were chronically irradiated by UV radiation (50 days), the daily application of the lotion of Red clover isoflavones markedly restrained the photosensitive carcinogenesis, exhibiting the chemopreventive function.[6]

In addition, biochanin-A (**2**) and formononetin (**4**) could be converted to produce more active genistein (**1**) and daidzein (**3**), respectively, by the bioreactions with human liver microsomes and cytochrome enzyme CYP1B1-catalyzed O-demethylation.[7]

References

1. Chae, Y. H. et al. 1991. Effects of synthetic and naturally occurring flavonoids on benzo(a)pyrene metabolism by hepatic microsomes prepared from rats treated with cytochrome P-450 inducers. *Cancer Lett.* 60: 15–24.
2. Cassady, J. M. et al. 1988. Use of a mammalian cell culture benzo(a)pyrene metabolism assay for the detection of potential anticarcinogens from natural products: Inhibition of metabolism by biochanin A, an isoflavone from *Trifolium pratense* L. *Cancer Res.* 48: 6257–61.
3. Rice, L. et al. 2002. Mechanisms of the growth inhibitory effect of the isoflavonoid biochanin A on LNCaP cells and xenografts. *Prostate* 52: 201–12.
4. Chen, J. et al. 2011. Formononetin induces cell cycle arrest of human breast cancer cells via IGF1/PI3K/Akt pathways in vitro and in vivo. *Horm Metab Res.* 43: 681–6.
5. Zhou, R. et al. 2014. Formononetin inhibits migration and invasion of MDA-MB-231 and 4T1 breast cancer cells by suppressing MMP-2 and MMP-9 through PI3K/AKT signaling pathways. *Horm Metab Res.* 46: 753–60.
6. Chan, H. Y. et al. 2003. The red clover (*Trifolium pratense*) isoflavone biochanin A modulates the biotransformation pathways of 7, 12-di-methylbenz[a]-anthracene. *Br. J. Nutr.* 90: 87–92.
7. Lam, A. N. C. et al. 2004. Effect of red clover isoflavones on Cox-2 activity in murine and human monocyte/macrophage cells. *Nutr. Cancer* 49: 89–93.

159 Du Jiao Lian 獨角蓮

Giant voodoo lily

Herb Origination

The herb Du Jiao Lian (Giant voodoo lily) originates from an Araceae plant, *Typhonium giganteum*, which is to China, and its distribution is broad in many Chinese provinces below 42° north latitude. Its tuber roots are usually collected in winter and processed for medicinal application.

Antitumor Activities and Constituents

The rhizome of Du Jiao Lian is one of the herbs commonly used in traditional Chinese medicine against cancer in clinics. *In vitro* investigations demonstrated that its aqueous extract could restrain the proliferation of human, SMMC-7721 (liver), MCF-7 (breast), and HeLa (cervix) cancer cell lines, concomitant with the induction of the cell apoptotic death. The extract also arrested the SMMC-7721 cell cycle progression at S phase.[1–3] Its 20% ethanolic extract showed certain inhibitory effect against the *in vitro* proliferation of four tested human tumor cell lines, MGC-803 (stomach), Hep-2 (liver), A549 (lung), and MCF-7 (breast) cells, where the 20% ethanolic extract was relatively sensitive to the MGC-803 cells for marked induction of the cell apoptosis.[4] The 70% ethanolic extract of the herb was effective in the proliferation delay and apoptosis promotion on human Bel-7402 hepatoma and human A549 NSCLC cells.[5] By down regulating Bcl-2 protein expression and upregulating Bax protein expression, Du Jiao Lian extracts induced the apoptosis of human SHG-44 glioma cells, exerting the antiproliferative effect.[6] A supercritical fluid extraction with CO_2 (SFE-CO_2) extract of the Du Jiao Lian tuber showed the antiproliferative effect *in vitro* against HCT-8 colon cancer, HO-8910 ovarian cancer, SGC-7901 gastric cancer, and SMMC-7721 hepatoma cells. Compared to other cell lines, SMMC-7721 cells were more sensitive to the SFE-CO_2 extract, where the SFE-CO_2 extract blocked the cell cycle in both S and G2/M phases and triggered the apoptosis of SMMC-7721 cells through a ROS-mediated mitochondrial signaling pathway, i.e., increase of intracellular calcium levels, upregulation of Bax expression, downregulation of Bcl-2 expression, loss of mitochondrial membrane potential, and activation of caspase-3 and caspase-9.[7,8]

The *in vivo* anticancer property of the Du Jiao Lian tuber has been demonstrated in mouse models. At doses of 25 and 125 mg/kg, the treatment with the herb extract suppressed the growth of sarcoma 180 by over 30% and prolonged the life span of mice bearing EAC by 40%. Simultaneously, the extract also enhanced the lymphocyte transformation and the indexes of the thymus and the spleen in S180-bearing mice, showing that the extract has an ability to enhance the host immune system.[9] To mice inoculated with ascites type of HcaF25/CL16A3 hepatoma, the gavage of the herb decoction for 15 days notably reduced the tumor weight and raised the spleen index in association with the downregulation of p53 expression in the tumor tissue.[10] The administration of the ethanolic extract to mice implanted with H22 hepatoma by gavage inhibited the tumor growth by 44.45% and increased the body weight by 37.20%, concomitant with the repressed PCNA and mutant p53 expressions and the enhanced antioxidative capability (such as increase of SOD activity and T-AOC level and decrease of MDA content).[11] The induction of H22 cell apoptotic death by the herb suspension was found to be also correlated with the inhibition of telomerase activity, the enhancement of p16 expression, and the downregulation of Bcl-2 expression.[12] During the treatment, the herb suspension obviously promoted the thymine function and enhanced the expressions of IL-2-included Th1-type cytokines in mice transplanted with H22 hepatoma.[13,14] Also, its alcohol extract could augment the serum IL-2 and TNFα levels of H22 liver cancer-bearing mice.[15] During immunoenhancing function *in vivo*, the extract of the Du Jiao Lian tuber was demonstrated to have marked capacities to amplify the proliferation and the cytotoxicity of T lymphocytes, to augment the activities of the macrophages and the NK cells to the cancer cells, and to increase the production of TNFα and IL-1 from the macrophages.[16] Moreover, the serum that was obtained from Du Jiao Lian treated mice also showed dose-dependent suppressive effect against the proliferation of human K562 leukemia cells *in vitro*, whose inhibitory rate reached its highest at 31.65% after 72 h of treatment. The Du Jiao Lian-contained serum could also promote the K562 leukemia cells to differentiation and to apoptosis in time- and concentration-dependent manners.[17]

Moreover, the expression of bFGF and its related angiogenesis factors could be notably diminished by the aqueous extract, implying the potential of the herb in the inhibition of vascular endothelial cell proliferation and angiogenesis.[18] Consequently, all these scientific evidences revealed that the anticarcinoma property of Du Jiao Lian is largely correlated with its five functions: (1) inhibiting tumor cells proliferation, (2) promoting cancer cell apoptosis and/or disturbing the cell cycle, (3) repressing angiogenesis in tumor tissue, (4) potentiating the host immune functions, and (5) enhancing the activity of SOD and blocking the oxidation and peroxidation, suggesting that Du Jiao Lian (Giant voodoo lily) may be a promising herbal drug in the chemotherapy of human neoplastic disease, especially hepatoma and lung malignant tumors.

Lignans and Sterol

The investigations further found that the isolated lignan components and β-sitosterol displayed the anticancer effect, and they were relatively sensitive to human SGC-7901 gastric cancer cells and human Bel-7402 hepatoma cells, respectively, *in vitro*.[19,20] By upregulating the expressions of TRAIL, TRAIL-R1, and TRAIL-R2 and lessening the expression of TRAIL-R4, the lignans provoked apoptosis-related signaling pathway in SGC-7901 cells.[20]

Polysaccharide

A polysaccharide component was extracted from *T. giganteum* tuber displaying antiproliferative effect in Bel-7402 (liver) and lung (A549) human neoplastic cell lines *in vitro*, whose cancer inhibition could be amplified in time- and concentration-dependent manners.[21]

References

1. Wang, S. Q. et al. 2006. Inference of the aqueous extract of *Typhonium giganteum* on the gene expression of hepatoma SMMC-7721 cells. *Zhongcaoyao* 37: 1384–7; 2003. Studies on the proliferation restrain of *Typhonium giganteum* Engl to hepatocarcinoma cell SMMC-7721. *Chin. J. Cell Biol.* 25: 185–8.
2. Wang, L. M. et al. 2009. Inhibition of proliferation and induction of apoptosis in MCF-7 cell by *Typhonium giganteum* Engl. *Shenyang Nongye Daxue Xuebao* 40: 174–7.
3. He, X. L. et al. 2011. Studies on the anti-proliferation and apoptosis-induction of HeLa cervical cancer cells in vitro. *Lishizhen Med. Materia Medica Res.* 22: 1620–1.
4. Duan, Y. M. et al. 2010. The in vitro anticancer activity of ethanolic extract of *Typhonium giganteum*. *Acta Chin. Med. Pharmacol.* 38: 20–3.
5. Song, Y. L. et al. 2012. Antitumor effects of *Typhonium giganteum* Engl, tuber extracts. *Intl. Conference on Biomed. Engin. Biotechnol.* p. 68.
6. Cao, Z. Y. et al. 2013. Proliferation inhibition and inducing apoptosis of *Rhizoma typhonii* extracts on glioma cells and their mechanisms. *Jilin Daxue Xuebao, Yixueban* 39: 649–52.
7. Li, Q. Y. et al. 2011. GC-MS analysis and in vitro antitumor activity of the extract from *Typhonium giganteum* Engl using supercritical fluid CO_2. *Zhiwu Yanjiu* 31: 113–6.
8. Li, Q. Y. et al. 2011. SFE-CO2 extract from *Typhonium giganteum* Engl. tubers, induces apoptosis in human hepatoma SMMC-7721 cells involvement of a ROS-mediated mitochondrial pathway. *Mol.* 16: 8228–43.
9. Ceng, Y. et al. 2005. Effect of *Typhonium giganteum* on mouse S180 in vivo. *Chin. J. Med.* 5: 02-0099-02.
10. Zhu, Y. H. et al. 2006. Studies on the anticancer activity of Baifuzi. *Pharmacol. Clin. Chin. Materia Medica* 22: 122–3.
11. Jiang, X. D. et al. 2012. Antioxidative and antitumor effects of *Typhonium giganteum* ethanol extracts on H22 xenograft mice. *Zhongguo Laonianxue Zazhi* 32: 1415–6.
12. Yu, X. H. et al. 2012. Study on correlation of Baifuzi suspension on mice p16, bcl-2 expression and telomerase activity. *Tianjin J. Tradit. Chin. Med.* 29: 166–8.
13. Yu, X. H. et al. 2011. Study on the inhibition of Baifuzi suspension against H22 tumor growth in mice and the influence on immune function. *J. Zhejiang Chin. Med. Univ.* (5): 735–6, 740.
14. Yu, X. H. et al. 2011. The immune adjustment mechanism of antitumor efficacy of SGTR on H22 tumor hearing mice. *Tianjin J. Tradit. Chin. Med.* 28: 23–4.
15. Huang, Z. et al. 2013. Effects of alcohol extracts of *Typhonium giganteum* Engl. on the serum IL-2 and TNFα levels of H22 liver cancer-bearing mice. *Zhongliu Yaoxue* 3: 432–5.
16. Shan, B. E. et al. 2001. Human T-Cell and monocyte modulating activity of *Rhizoma typhonii* in vitro. *Zhongguo Zhongxiyi Jiehe Zazhi* 21: 768–72.
17. Ke, R. et al. 2011. Inhibition of proliferation and induction of apoptosis by the herb serum containing HORN LIAN on K562 leukemia cells. *Acta Chin. Med. Pharmacol.* (2): 37–40.
18. Hua, D. et al. 2011. The study on the expression of HORN LIAN to angiogenic factor bFGF in the antitumor effect on H22 tumor-bearing mice. *Information on Tradit. Chin. Med.* 28: 97–9.
19. Gu, S. S. et al. 2013. The advanced researches in anticancer of Baifuzi. *China Cancer* 22: 38–40.
20. Ma, L. Y. et al. 2010. Study of lignans of *Rhizoma typhonii* on the expression of TRAIL and its receptors in gastric carcinoma cell line (SGC-7901). *Chin. J. New Drugs* 19: 225–8.
21. Du, X. C. et al. 2015. Extraction of polysaccharide from *Typhonium giganteum* Engl. and its anticancer activities in vitro. *Shenyang Huagong Daxue Xuebao* 29: 7–9, 27.

9

Anticancer Potentials of Tonic Herbs

CONTENTS

160 Ci Wu Jia 刺五加

Siberian ginseng

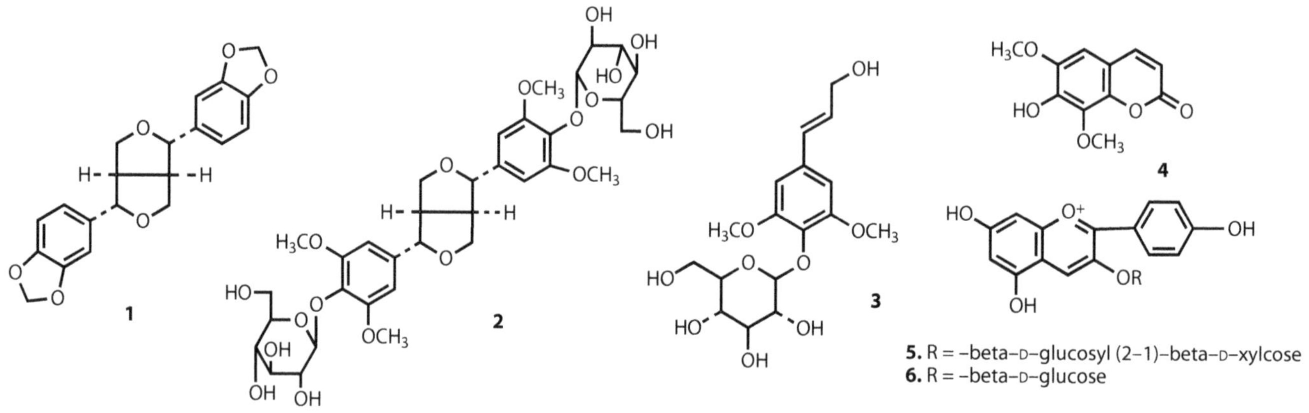

5. R = –beta-D-glucosyl (2–1)-beta-D-xylcose
6. R = –beta-D-glucose

Herb Origination

The herb Ci Wu Jia (Siberian ginseng) is a famous tonic herb in eastern Asia, which originated from an Araliaceae plant, *Acanthopanax senticosus* (= *Eleutherococcus senticosus*). This woody shrub is distributed in the northeastern region of Asia. The dried roots, stems, and leaves collected from the Ci Wu Jia plant have traditionally been used for enhancing human health in China, Russia, and Korea.

Antitumor Activities

In vivo experiments demonstrated that Ci Wu Jia extract was markedly effective in the suppression of tumor growth, carcinogenesis, and carcinoma metastasis, but it also exerted valuable immune-regulative benefits for the significant decrease of toxicity and side effects caused by chemotherapeutic treatments.[1] For example, the extract apparently reduced the incidence rate of lung carcinogenesis induced by urethane, inhibited 6-methylthiopyrimidine mutating rat goiter tumor, obstructed spontaneous leukemia and mouse myeloid leukemia caused by indole, and suppressed the growth of a variety of cancers (brain and spinal gliomas, peripheral neurinoma, and cervical/vaginal cancer) induced in rats by nitrosoethylurea or dimethylbenzanthracene.[1–3] If the tested murine animals are freely given drinking water containing its alcoholic extract, the metastasis of SSK sarcoma cells and Krukenberg's tumor cells in rats was obviously retarded and the time and the number of surviving animals were increased, and the toxic effects of anticancer drugs (cyclophosphane, benzotepa, and ethymidine) were lessened in mice with sarcoma 180 and in rats with Walker carcinoma.[4,5] The Ci Wu Jia extract also could elicit the apoptotic death and the blockage of DNA biosynthesis in Spc-A1 lung carcinoma cells *in vitro*.[6] The exposure of human KATO-III gastric cancer cells to the hot water extract of Ci Wu Jia stem bark (whose plant was collected in Hokkaido, Japan) elicited both growth inhibition and apoptotic death in concentration- and time-dependent manners.[7] When a Ci Wu Jia aqueous extract was combined with either cytarabine or N6-(δ2-isopentenyl)-adenosine, an additive antiproliferative effect could be achieved against murine L1210 leukemia.[8]

In experimental lung metastasis of 26-M3.1 colon carcinoma cells, the intravenous administration of the aqueous extract for two days before the tumor inoculation significantly displayed a therapeutic effect against the metastasis of 26-M3.1 cancer cells. Although the aqueous extract at >1 mg/mL concentration did not directly affect the growth of the 26-M3.1 cells, the peritoneal macrophages were stimulated by the extract to produce various cytokines such as IL-1β, TNFα, IL-12, and IFNγ, whose immunostimulation in turn markedly resulted in remarkable tumoricidal activity against the tumor cells.[9] The intravenous injection of the aqueous extract obviously augmented the natural killer (NK) cytotoxicity to Yac-1 murine T lymphoma cells.[9] In addition, both EtOAc and n-butanolic fractionations from Ci Wu Jia displayed strong antioxidant and DPPH free radical-scavenging effects, and EtOAc fractionation also exhibited high antilipid peroxidative activities in rat liver microsomes.[10] Based upon the encouraging evidences, Ci Wu Jia was demonstrated to possess antitumor potential in the inhibition of tumor cell growth and metastasis. The anticancer and anticarcinogenic effects were also largely associated with its notable immunostimulating and antioxidative properties. Therefore, Ci Wu Jia is recommended to be used prophylactically for the prevention of cancer formation, development, and metastasis.

Antitumor Constituents and Activities

By modern phytochemical approaches, a variety of active constituents was discovered from Ci Wu Jia, such as glycosides, flavonoids, coumarins, lignans, and polysaccharides. The multiple bioactivities of constituents have been established, including marked immunoregulating antitumor potential.

Macromolecules

Two types of macromolecules, polysaccharides and glycoproteins, were found to be the antineoplastic components in Ci Wu Jia with a wide spectrum of immunoregulatory functions. The IC_{50} values of the polysaccharides were 0.38 and 0.28 mg/mL, respectively, in murine sarcoma 180 cells and human K562 eryothroleukemia cells.[11] *In vivo* experiments revealed that the anticarcinoma effect was closely correlated with many characteristic changes of tumor cell membrane caused by Ci Wu Jia polysaccharides.[12] No direct cytotoxic effect was observed in mouse ascites hepatoma cells, but Ci Wu Jia polysaccharides could prolong the life span of mice bearing the ascites hepatoma. When hypodermic injection of the polysaccharides is done to mice in a dose of 0.34 g/kg for 10 successive days, the growth inhibition was induced against the S180 and S37 sarcomas *in vivo*.[13] The Ci Wu Jia polysaccharides also markedly lengthened the survival duration of mice implanted with Ehrlich ascites neoplasm, sarcoma 180, or L615 reticulocytic leukemia.[14] If an i.p. injection of the polysaccharides to mice in doses of 100 or 200 mg/kg for 10–20 days and the inoculation of the tumor cells at the fourth day are done, the polysaccharides obviously obstructed the growth of cancer cells and extended the life time of the mice. Simultaneously, the atrophy of the thymus and the adrenal gland atrophy in mice caused by the implanted cancer cells could be remarkably resisted by the polysaccharide treatment.[14,15]

The administration of a crude polysaccharide component EN-3 (50 μg/mouse) prepared from Ci Wu Jia resulted in a 66.1% therapeutic effect on the lung tumor metastasis. Moreover, EN-3 and GF-AS (a soluble protein layer from Ci Wu Jia), were capable of enhancing the proliferation of normal splenocyte and stimulating the activity of peritoneal macrophage and the production of various cytokines such as IL-1β, TNFα, IL-12, and IFNγ. By the intravenous injection of the EN-3 (4–100 μg/mouse), EN-3 significantly augmented the cytotoxicity of natural killer cells to YAC-1 lymphoma cells. In an experimental model, prophylactical intravenous administration of GF-AS, a crude glycolprotein from Ci Wu Jia, dramatically retarded the lung metastasis of 26-M3.1 colon carcinoma cells in a dose-dependent manner. From the GF-AS, an active glycolprotein fraction named EN-SP was purified, which exerted higher antimetastatic activity and more potent proliferation of splenocyte than GF-AS.[16,17]

Furthermore, a combinational treatment with cisplatin (10 μg) and EN-3 (5 μg) synergistically inhibited the growth of sarcoma 180 by >95% and prolonged the life span for >60 days in a mouse model and also effectively restrained the metastasis of 26-M3.1 colon cancer cells. Due to the remarkable nonspecifical stimulation of the immune system, these macromolecules including EN-3, GF-AS, and EN-SP exerted the efficient chemoimmunotherapeutic functions not only in promoting the antitumor activity and anticarcinogenic immunity but also in eliminating toxic and side effects caused by chemotherapy.[14–18]

Small Molecules

Two of the neoplastic lignans from the n-butanolic extract of Ci Wu Jia were identified as sesamin (**1**) and liriodendrin (**2**). Sesamin (**1**) in an *in vitro* assay suppressed the growth of human KATO-III gastric cancer cells and enhanced the cell apoptosis,[9] while liriodendrin (**2**) augmented an immunoenhancing benefit through the elevation of β-endorphin levels in the rat plasma.[19] An phenolic glucoside, syringin (**3**), demonstrated moderate antiproliferative effect on human HeLa (cervix), A549 (lung), MCF-7 (breast), and PC3 (prostate) cancer cell lines *in vitro*, with the IC_{50} values in the range of 14.42–32.96 μg/mL. The *in vivo* antitumor effect of syringin (**3**) was proven in a mouse model implanted with sarcoma 180, and the inhibitory rates were 25.89% in a low intravenous dose and 61.16% in a high intravenous dose for the same seven-day the treatment.[20] Isofraxidin (**4**), a major coumarine compound isolated from the Ci Wu Jia stem bark, was found to have antiinvasive activity in human HuH-7 and HepG2 hepatoma cell lines by repressing MMP-7 expression and ERK1/2 phosphorylation.[21]

In nude rats xenografts planted with human EC9706 esophageal cancer cells, Ci Wu Jia saponins (ASS) in doses of 50–150 mg/kg significantly diminished the tumor size without significant abnormality in the liver and the kidney tissues.[22] But ASS evidenced weak *in vitro* inhibition against the proliferation of human MCF-7 breast cancer cells in a dose-dependent manner.[23] The *in vitro* investigation also showed that ASS in concentrations of 250 and 500 μg/mL could lessen the expression of VEGF in human HepG2 hepatoma cells, implying that the antigrowth mechanism of ASS is probably related to its antiangiogenic property as well.[24] In addition, cyanidin-3-*O*-sambubioside (**5**), an anthocyanin isolated from the fruits of *A. senticosus*, showed moderate suppressive effect against the proliferation of LNCap (prostate), Molt-4F (leukemic), and ACHN (renal) human cancer cell lines (respective IC_{50}: 5.2, 11.2, and 22.5 μg/mL) and antioxidant effects against DPPH, ABTS, and hydroxyl radicals.[25] By the downregulation of MMP-9 expression and the reconstitution of extracellular matrix (Matrigel), cyanidin-3-*O*-sambubioside (**5**) inhibited the metastasis processes, such as angiogenesis and invasion, in human MDA-MB-231 breast cancer cells.[26] In both *in vitro* and *in vivo* assays, cyanidin-3-glucoside (**6**) exerted antitumor and apoptosis-inducing activities on human H1299 lung cancer cells (IC_{50}: 14.5 μg/mL) and human HO-8910PM ovarian cancer cell line (IC_{50}: 13.82 μg/mL), whose effects were correlated with the downregulation of XIAP and the upregulation of Smac protein in the H1299 cells and the downregulation of Mucin-4 protein in the HO-8910PM cells.[27,28] In addition, the pretreatment of cyanidin-3-glucoside (**6**) could play a marked protective role against oxidative stress and toxicity induced by acrylamide in the MDA-MB-231 cells, by reducing ROS generation, inhibiting GSH peroxidase (GSH-Px) and GST activities, recovering GSH depletion, enhancing expressions of GPx1, GSTP1 and γ-glutamyl cysteine synthase, and retarding cytochrome P 450 2E1 (CYP2E1) expression.[29] Therefore, the results suggested that the stem and the fruit of *A. senticosus* are the effective sources to be used for cancer prevention due to the anticarcinogenic, anticancer, and antioxidant properties.

Other Bioactivity

Ci Wu Jia (Siberian ginseng) is an adaptogen and a comprehensive tonic herb with a wide range of health benefits. Particular attention has been given to the herb for its antiinflammatory, antioxidative, antifatigue, antidiabetes, hypolipide, immunoprotecting and immunoregulating, antimicrobial, and antiviral activities besides its anticarcinogenesis. In China, Ci Wu Jia has been successfully utilized to reverse bone marrow inhibition caused by radiation and/or chemotherapy, and the polysaccharides of Ci Wu Jia can be used to protect the marrow and to increase the blood corpuscle production.[25] In addition, Ci Wu Jia exerted significant antidepressant effects in a rat model.[30]

References

1. Cao, X. L. et al. 1980. Review of the researches of *Acanthopanax senticosus* in overseas. *Zhongcaoyao* 11: 277–82.
2. Huang, L. et al. 2011. *Acanthopanax senticosus*: Review of botany, chemistry and pharmacology. *Pharmazie*. 66: 83–97.
3. Bespalov, V. G. et al. 1993. Inhibitory effect of *Acanthopanax senticosus* extract on the development of experimentally induced tumors of the nervous system, cervix uteri and vagina. *Khimiko-Farmatsevticheskii Zhurnal* 27: 63–5.
4. Malyugina, L. et al. 1964. Influence of drugs upon the metastasis of malignant tumors. *Acta Unio Internationalis Contra Cancrum* 20: 199–200.
5. Monakhov, B. V. et al. 1965/1967. Effect of *Eleutherococcus senticosus* on therapeutic activity of cyclophosphane, ethymidine, or benzotepa. *Voprosy Onkologii* 11: 60; 13: 94–7.
6. Zhang, M. Y. et al. 2002. Study on apoptosis of Spc-A1 cell induced by *Acanthopanax senticosus*. *J. Jilin Univ.* (*Med. Edit.*), 28: 37–9.
7. Hibasami, H. et al. 2000. Induction of apoptosis by *Acanthopanax senticosus* HARMS and its component, sesamin in human stomach cancer KATO III cells. *Oncol. Reports* 7: 1213–16.
8. Hacker, B. et al. 1984. Cytotoxic effects of *Eleutherococcus senticosus* aqueous extracts in combination with N6-(Δ2-isopentenyl)-adenosine and 1-β-D-arabinofuranosylcytosine against L1210 leukemia cells. *J. Pharm. Sci.* 73: 270–2.
9. Yoo, T. J. et al. 2004. Anti-metastatic activity of *Acanthopanax senticosus* extract and its possible immunological mechanism of action. *J. Ethnopharmacol.* 93: 247–53.
10. Yu, C. Y. et al. 2003. Intraspecific relationship analysis by DNA markers and in vitro cytotoxic and antioxidant activity in *Eleutherococcus senticosus*. *Toxicol. in Vitro* 17: 229–36.
11. Tong, L. et al. 1994. Effects of plant polysaccharides on cell proliferation and cell membrane contents of sialic acid, phospholipid and cholesterol in S 180 and K562 cells. *Zhongguo Zhongxiyi Jiehe Zazhi* 14: 482–4.
12. Dong, L. et al. 1994. Impact of three plant polysaccharides on the production of IL-2 in mouse spleen cells. *Zhongguo Yaolixue Tongbao* 10: 105.
13. Chen, X. J. et al. 1984. The antitumor and immunoenhancing activities of Siberian ginseng polysaccharides. *Aizheng* 3: 191–3.
14. Ji, Y. B. et al. 1994. An experimental study of the anticancer effect of compound herbal polysaccharide preparation. *Zhongguo Haiyang Yaowu* 13: 20–4.
15. Xie, S. S. et al. 1989. Immunoregulatory effect of polysaccharide of *Acanthopanax senticosus* (PAS) I. Immunological mechanism of PAS against cancer. *Zhonghua Zhongliu Zazhi* 11: 338–40.
16. Ha, E. et al. 2003. Immunostimulation activity of the crude polysaccharides fractionated from *Eleutherococcus senticosus*, and its application to prevent of tumor by combination therapy with cisplatin. *Yakhak Hoechi* 47: 159–66
17. Ha, E. et al. 2004. Anti-metastatic activity of glycoprotein fractionated from *Acanthopanax senticosus*, involvement of NK-cell and macrophage activation. *Archiv. Pharm. Res.* 27: 217–24.
18. Yoon, T. J. et al. 2007. Induction of enhancement of antitumor immunity by polysaccharides fractionated from *Acanthopanax senticosus*. *Saengyak Hakhoechi* 38: 117–22.
19. Nishibe, S. S. et al. 1997. Bioactive phenolic compounds for cancer prevention from herbal medicines, Editor(s): Ohigashi, H. *Food Factors for Cancer Prevention*, [International Conference on Food Factors: Chemistry and Cancer Prevention], Hamamatsu, Japan, Dec., 1995, pp. 276–9.
20. Wang, Z. et al. 2010. Extraction and antitumor effect of syringin in *Acanthopanax senticosus*. *Shizhen Guoyi Guoyao* 21: 752–3.
21. Yamazaki, T. et al. 2010. Isofraxidin, a coumarin component from *Acanthopanax senticosus*, inhibits matrix metalloproteinase-7 expression and cell invasion of human hepatoma cells. *Biol. Pharm. Bull.* 33: 1716–22.
22. Li, Y. L. et al. 2008. Antitumor effect of *Acanthopanax senticosus* saponin on EC9706 nude rat model of esophageal carcinoma. *Shandong Yiyao* 48: 49–50.
23. Sun, Y. F. et al. 2012. Anti-breast cancer cell activity of saponins in *Acanthopanax senticosus* (Rupr. et-Matrix.) Harms. *Shizhen Guoyi Guoyao* 23: 926–7.
24. Feng, J. D. et al. 2007. Inhibitory effect of *Acanthopanax senticosus* saponin on the expression of vascular endothelial growth factor in human HepG2 cell line. *Zhongyao Xinyao yu Linchuang Yaoli* 18: 339–41.
25. Lee, J. H. et al. 2013. Studies on the anthocyanin profile and biological properties from the fruits of *Acanthopanax senticosus* (Siberian ginseng). *J. Funct. Foods* 5: 380–8.
26. Lee, S. J. et al. 2013. Cyanidin-3-*O*-sambubioside from *Acanthopanax senticosus* fruit inhibits metastasis by downregulating MMP-9 in breast cancer cells MDA-MB-231. *Planta Med.* 79: 1636–40.
27. Lu, L. et al. 2012. Antitumor effect of cyanidin-3-glucoside on lung cancer in vitro and in vivo. *Zhonghua Linchuang Yishi Zazhi, Dianziban* 6: 1157–61.
28. Zeng, L. C. et al. 2012. Study on antitumor effect of cyanidin-3-glucoside on ovarian cancer. *Zhongguo Zhongyao Zazhi* 37: 1651–4.
29. Song, J. et al. 2013. Protection of cyanidin-3-glucoside against oxidative stress induced by acrylamide in human MDA-MB-231 cells. *Food Chem. Toxicol.* 58: 306–10.
30. Kwak, T. H. et al. 2003. Active fraction having anticancer and anti-metastasis isolated from Acanthopanax species and fruits. *PCT Int. Appl.* WO 2003099309 A1 20031204.

161 Huang Qi 黄芪

Milk vetch root or Astragalus

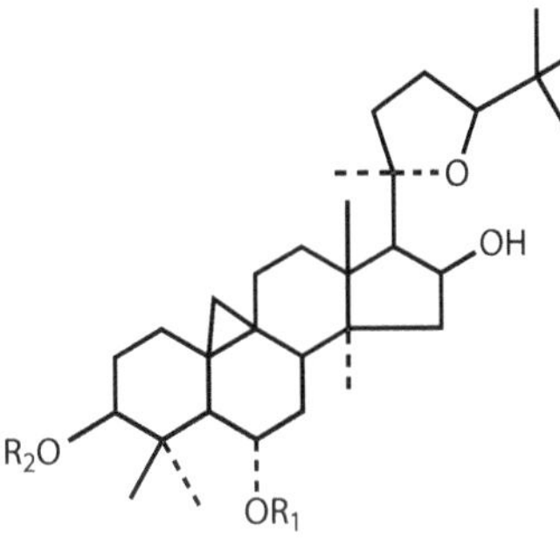

1. R_1 = -glc, R_2 = -xyl-2-Ac
2. R_1 = -H, R_2 = -glc-2-rham
3. R_1 = -H, R_2 = -glc-4-rham
4. R_1 = -xyl, R_2 = -rham
5. R_1 = -xyl, R_2 = -xyl
6. R_1 = -H, R_2 = -glc A-2-xyl-2-rham
7. R_1 = -xyl, R_2 = -xyl-4-OOCCH = CHCH$_3$
8. R_1 = -H, R_2 = -glc-4-rham

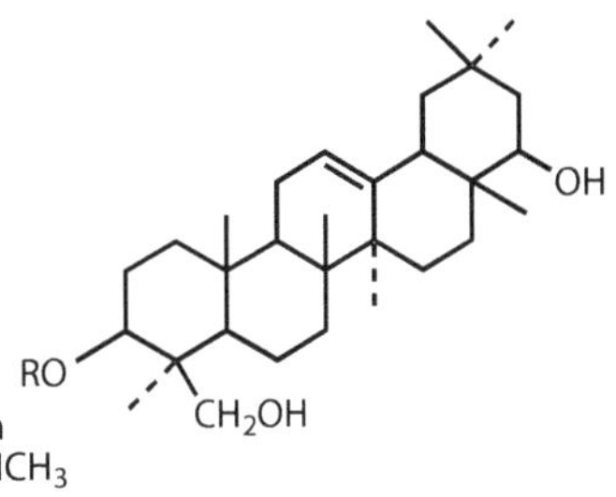

9. R = -glc A(-6-CH3)-2-glc-2-rham

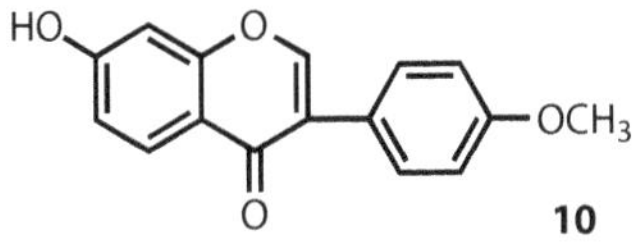

10

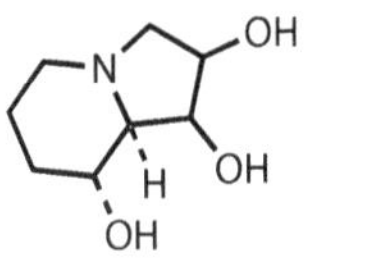

11

Herb Origination

The herb Huang Qi (Astragali radix) is an important traditional Chinese medicine, and it was recorded in *Shennong Ben Cao Jing*, the first Chinese classic of materia medica. The herb is the dried roots of two Leguminosae plants, *Astragalus membranaceus* (= *A. propinquus*) and *A. membranaceus* var. *mongholicus*. The plants are native to the northern and eastern areas of China as well as Mongolia and Korea. The herb is mainly produced in the northwestern provinces of China and cultivated in many places. The roots are usually harvested as the medicinal part from its four-year-old plants.

Anticarcinogenic Activities

Significant antineoplastic and antioxidative roles of Huang Qi extract were found *in vivo* in solid tumors such as in the lung, the liver, the gastrointestinal tract, the nasopharynx, and the breast.[1,2] Huang Qi extract inhibited the growth of gastric cancer cells *in vitro* mainly through it cytostatic effect via blockage of cell respiration and DNA synthesis but not cytotoxicity[1] and restrained the proliferation of HEp-2 laryngeal cancer cells in a dose-dependent manner by inducing G2/M cell cycle arrest and cell apoptosis.[3] In a physiological dose of 0.2 g/mL, a Hung Qi injection inhibited the proliferation and induced the cell cycle arrest and the apoptosis of hormone-sensitive MCF-7 breast cancer cells.[4] The injection, in the *in vitro* assay, inhibited the proliferation of U937 leukemia cells and induced the cell apoptosis via the down regulation of c-Myc expression and up regulation of p27 expression.[5] The *in vivo* antiproliferative and apoptosis-inducing effects of the Huang Qi injection was also established in a mouse model transplanted with H22 hepatoma. Concurrently, the indexes of the thymus and the spleen and the levels of IL-2 and TNFα were significantly augmented by the injection.[6] Moreover, the injection could induce lymphokine-activated killer-like activity toward WEHI-164 sarcoma cells *in vitro*, and the macrophage pretreated with the injection could increase the cytostatic effect toward MBL-2 lymphoid leukemia *in vitro* and *in vivo*.[7] Also, the *in vitro* experiment showed that Huang Qi injection could induce monocytic differentiation of both human and murine neoplastic cells.[7,8] Collectively, these results evidenced that Huang Qi is capable of exerting the antitumor effect that might be achieved primarily by activating the antitumor immunoregulating and immunorestorative mechanism in the host.

Moreover, Huang-Qi exerted notably suppressive effect against carcinogenesis caused by various mutagens. The daily intramuscular administration of the Huang Qi injection to rats markedly diminished the possibility of lung carcinogenesis induced by 3-methylcholanthrenelipiodol.[8] The treatment with Huang Qi extract by gavage in doses of 90 or 180 mg/kg for three to eight weeks effectively delayed DEN- and AAF (two oncogens)-provoked liver carcinogenesis in rats, whose inhibitory effect was correlated with the decrease of GST-P expression and GST-P-positive foci formation.[9] The injection of the Huang Qi extract in doses of 10–40 mg/kg/day together with N-butyl-N′-butanolnitrosoamine (BBN) (a mutagen) to mice obviously declined the rate of carcinogenesis in the bladder. The extract was also able to improve the cytotoxicity of lymphocytes against YAC-1 lymphoma cells and to protect the production of IFNγ and IL-2 in lymphocytes from the depression by BBN.[10] Therefore, it is clear that the Huang Qi extract plays an effective role of anticarcinogenesis notably through the activation of cytotoxic cytokines and increase of their production.

Immunoactivity in Cancer Patients

By augmenting the function of both lymphocytes and macrophages and improving reticulocyte and monocyte-macrophage, Huang Qi efficiently enhanced the marked cellular immune response in the cancer patients. Thus, the herb is able to modulate the myelosuppression from the impairment caused by chemotherapy and to overcome the toxicity/side effects of anticancer drugs to the hematopoietic system. Huang Qi combined with radiotherapy improved the life quality of cancer patients through the immunoenhancing functions besides the potentiation of the treatment and the reduction of the radiotoxicity.[11] In lung carcinoma cells that were directly collected from patients, the expression of IL-2 and IFNγ are negative, but the mRHA expression rates of IL-4, IL-6, and IL-10 in peripheral blood mononuclear cells (PBMCs) from patients are obviously higher than those from healthy controls. If these cells were treated with Huang Qi, the IFNγ and the IL-2 could be significantly activated in parallel with the decrease of IL-4, IL-6, and IL-10 expression.[12] The cotreatment of esophageal cancer cells with a combination of Huang Qi and cytokines (such as IL-2, IL-2 + IL-4, or IL-2 + TNFα) notably enhanced the proliferation-promoting and specific antitumor activities of tumor-infiltrating lymphocyte (TIL).[13] Similarly, the antitumor activity of TIL cells from patients with pulmonary carcinoma were markedly improved by the Huang Qi treatment.[14] The evidences further highlighted that the antineoplastic property of Huang Qi may be largely achieved by activating the antitumor immune mechanism in the host besides the suppression of tumor cell proliferation and the promotion of the cell apoptosis.

Antitumor Constituents and Activities

The biological activities of Huang Qi were believed to be principally contributed by its constituents, viz., saponins, isoflavonoids, alkaloids, aminobutyric acid, lectin, and polysaccharides, together with trace elements (iron, copper, selenium iron, magnesium, calcium, and zinc).

Saponins

Total triterpene saponins (AST) were extracted from Huang Qi as the major components, which displayed potential antitumor effects on various human cancer cell lines and tumor xenografts. When human HepG2 and Bel-7404 hepatoma cells are cultured with the AST (20–80 mg/L) for six days, the tumor cell apoptosis was promoted and the cell growth was markedly suppressed in a dose-dependent manner.[15] The mechanism for the growth inhibition and the apoptosis induction was involved in an ERK-independent nuclear factor-κB (NF-κB) signaling pathway, including (1) diminution of NF-κB/DNA-binding activity; (2) downregulation of antiapoptotic proteins Bcl-2 and Bcl-xL expressions; (3) augmentation of wtp53 and caspase expressions; and (4) reduction of α-fetoprotein (a hepatocellular tumor marker) expression.[16] The antigrowth activity of AST (60 μg/mL) was also demonstrated in HT-29 colon carcinoma cells in association with cell cycle G2/M arrest and a subsequent increase in apoptosis, whose mechanism was followed in both mTOR and ERK signaling pathways and concomitant with the regulation of p21 expression and the inhibition of CDK activity.[17,18] The reduction of the tumor size in HT-29 nude mice xenograft by the AST was comparable with an anticancer drug 5-FU.[18] By regulating calpain-mediated glucose-regulated protein expression and ER stress, AST triggered the cell apoptosis and obstructed the development of human colon tumor 116 (HCT116) colon cancer cells. The combination of calpain inhibitors and AST could promote more pronounced proapoptotic effect in the HCT 116 cells.[19] Based on the results, AST can be considered as a potential adjuvant in the combination with other orthodox chemotherapeutic drugs to treat patients suffering from hepatoma and colon carcinoma.

Astragaloside-II (**1**) isolated from both Chinese *A. membranaceus* and Egyptian *A. spinosus* exhibited marked inhibitory effects against the growth of many human tumor cells *in vitro*, such as colon cancer (Colo205, HCT-15, SW620), breast cancer (SF-539, U251), leukemia (HL-60, K562, RPM18226), melanoma (LOXIMVI, M14), small cell lung cancer (DMS114), and kidney cancer (786-0) cell lines. Among these cells, the SW620 cells and HL-60 cells were the most sensitive to astragaloside-II.[20] Astragaloside-II (**1**) also was able to enhance the T cell activation by regulating CD45 PTPase activity.[21] Astragaloside-IV (**3**) in the *in vivo* model suppressed progression of Lewis lung cancer by the down regulation of regulatory T cells (Tregs) and the up regulation of CTLs via the blockage of indoleamine 2,3-dioxygenase expression.[22] Eight more saponins elucidated as cycloaraloside-A (**2**), astraverrucin-IV (**3**), astraversianin-VI (**4**), astraversianin-X (**5**), astragaloside-VIII (**6**), kahiricoside-I (**7**), azukisaponin-V (**8**), and peregrinoside-I (**9**) were separated from three other Egyptian *Astragalus* plants (*A. olysaccha, A. kahiricus*, and *A. hamosus*), whose triterpene oligoglycosides exerted no significant cytotoxicity but could stimulate the proliferation of splenocytes in a mouse model.[23,24]

Isoflavonoids

Both formononetin (**10**) and isoliquiritigenin were isolated from Huang Qi. Both demonstrated anticarcinogenic and apoptosis-facilitating activities in human HCT116 colon carcinoma cells. The proapoptosis was associated with the down-expression of Bcl-2 and Bcl-xL, the activation of caspases, and the up-expression of NSAID-activated gene (NAG-1) and its upstream regulator in the drug-treated tumor cells.[25,26] The treatment of three types of human breast cancer cell lines (MDA-MB-468, MCF-7, and SK-BR-3) with formononetin (**10**) in a concentration of over 20 μM induced the cell cycle arrest at G1 stage and reduced the PCNA expression, thereby suppressing the proliferation of the breast tumor cells.[25,26] Both *in vitro* and *in vivo* experiments demonstrated that formononetin (**10**) dose-dependently suppressed the growth of PC3 prostate cancer cells and HeLa cervical cancer cells in association with the induction of G0/G1 cell cycle arrest via the inactivation of Akt/cyclin D1/CDK4 in the PC3 cells and the induction of apoptosis and the repression of AKT phosphorylation in the HeLa cells.[27,28] At a noncytotoxic concentration, formononetin (**10**) markedly restrained the migration and the invasion of MDA-MB-231 and 4T1 breast cancer cells *in vitro* and *in vivo* by diminishing MMP-2 and MMP-9 expression by suppressing PI3K/AKT signaling pathway.[29] Therefore, formononetin (**10**) may be used as a potential agent for te clinical treatment of carcinomas in the breast, the cervix, and the prostate. Additionally, isoliquiritigenin was capable of inducing G2 cell cycle arrest in the HCT116 cells.[25,26]

Moreover, Huang Qi flavonoids could elicit synergic antitumor effect with rIL-2 and enhance the cytotoxicity of lymphokine-activating killer (LAK) by 20-fold, revealing that the flavonoids also possess the immunoregulatory property that not only additively enhanced the anticancer effect but also attenuated toxic side effects in the cancer patients.[30] The cotreatment with the flavonoids and γ-ray radiation had greater inhibition on the proliferation of HepG2 cells than the γ-ray or the flavonoid treatment only, indicating that the flavonoids can enhance the radiation toxicity on the hepatoma cells.[31]

Alkaloids

Swainsonine (**11**) was an indolizine alkaloid extracted from Huang Qi roots, which acted as a potent inhibitor of Golgi α-mannosidase-II (an immunomodulator) and as a potential agent for chemotherapy. *In vitro* and *in vivo* experiments showed that it retarded the growth of C6 glioma cells and SGC-7901 gastric carcinoma cells with an IC_{50} value of 0.05 and 0.84 μg/mL (in 24 h), respectively. After the treatment with swainsonine (**11**) *in vivo*, the cell apoptosis was enhanced and the tumor weights declined, whose mechanism may correlate with the modulation of apoptosis-related gene expressions and the induction of overloading-[Ca^{2+}]i-induced ER stress.[32,33] During the *in vivo* treatment, it concurrently stimulated macrophages and restored bone marrow damage. Also, the alkaloid could markedly lessen DOX-caused toxicity in mice.[34–37] According to the findings, swainsonine (**11**) may be recommended as a potential adjuvant agent for further development to improve cancer chemotherapy.

Lectin

Two lectins assigned as AML and AMML were isolated from the herb, which are glycoproteins holding 10.7% and 19.6% neutral carbohydrate contents, respectively. The molecular mass of AML is 31.5 kDa and is stable at pH 5–12 conditions and <55°C temperature for 30 min, whereas AMML is composed of two identical subunits each with a molecular mass of 29.6 kDa and galactose specificity. An *in vitro* experiment demonstrated that AML and AMML were capable of inhibiting the proliferation of three human cancer cells, K562 (leukemia), MG63 (osteoma), and HeLa (cervix cancer). The maximum growth inhibition by AMML at a concentration of 80 mg/mL was 92% in HeLa cells, 84% on K562 cells, and 48% on MG63 cells. The morphological studies showed outstanding apoptosis characteristics and significant S cell arrest in the HeLa and K562 cell lines after the AMML treatment.[38–41] The investigations showed the value of the lectins that can be subjected to further development for chemoprevention.

Polysaccharides

The polysaccharides of Huang Qi are effective immunoregulators. Although the polysaccharide-homogeneous substances were obtained from different *Astragalus* species, they exhibited the almost the same kind of immunostimulating activity without toxic/side effects in different mammalian systems; however, the potency was different. In the *in vitro* assay, the polysaccharides suppressed the cellular proliferation activity and promoted the apoptotic death of KG-1a human acute myelocytic leukemia cells, whose effects were attributed to the inhibition of PTEN-PI3K-Akt signaling pathway.[42] The polysaccharides at higher doses (25 mg/mL) deceased more than 40.5% (24 h) and 67.3% (48 h) of HepG2 hepatoma cell viability and augmented 23.9% (24 h) and 38.2% (48 h) of cell apoptosis *in vitro*.[43] Also, Huang Qi polysaccharides exhibited the suppressive effect against MNU-induced mammary carcinoma in rats and virus-induced splenic lymphoma in mice.[44] Astragalus polysaccharides had no cytotoxicity on K562, SMMC-7721, A549, and HCT116 cell lines *in vitro* but displayed marked antitumor effect against mouse implanted with H22 hepatoma or sarcoma 180 *in vivo* with the inhibitory rates of 45.09–50.35% at a dose of 100 mg/kg; at the same time, both expression levels of IL-2 and TNFα were markedly enhanced.[45,46]

More experiments found that the polysaccharides are able to restore the cytokine balance in local microenvironments of the hepatoma cells, associated with the inhibition of FOXp3 expression and the blockage of immune suppressive effects of $CD4^+CD25^+$Treg cells. The results implied that the application of Huang Qi polysaccharides in the tumor microenvironment may exert the antitumor effects through the enhanced immune system and consequently prolong the survival rate *in vivo*.[47] Also, by modulating LMO2, Klf1, Klf3, Runx1, Sp1, and EphB4 genes and amplifying γ-globin expression and fetal hemoglobin synthesis, Huang Qi polysaccharides could exert potent activities on the erythroid differentiation in human K562 leukemia cells.[48]

APS

A water-soluble Huang Qi polysaccharide (APS) was elucidated as an α-(1–4)-D-glucan (≈3.6×10^4 Da) with a single α-D-glucose at the C-6 position on every an average of nine residues along the main chain.[49] APS is an inhibitor of P-gp efflux pump function and a stimulator of macrophage.[50,51] By diminishing the P-gp efflux pump function and downregulating MDR1 expression, APS dose-dependently augmented the sensitivity of anticancer drugs (such as cyclophosphamid, adriamycin, 5-FU, cisplatin, etoposide, and VCR) to a multidrug-resistant H22/Adm hepatoma *in vivo*, but APS had no direct antitumor activity on the cells *in vitro*.[51]

APS-I and ASP-II

APS-I and APS-II, two polysaccharides with respective molecular weights of 4.77×10^6 and 8.68×10^3 Da, were prepared from the herb. APS-I and APS-II were mainly composed of glucose and small amounts of arabinose and xylose, with their molar ratios of 18.14:0.54:1.0 and 29.39:0.23:1.0, respectively. Both have structurally similar main chains composed of major α-(1–3)-glucose and a few (1–4)-, (1–6)-glucoses, whereas the side chain contained arabinoses and xyloses. The *in vivo* inhibitory rates of APS-I and APS-II were 55.47% and 47.72%, respectively, against H22 hepatoma cells in mice.[52]

The i.p. injection of APS to mice bearing spontaneous B16 melanoma extended the life span for five to six days. If it is combined with IL-2 or LAK cells, the living days would be prolonged to nine days.[53] A clinical trial further demonstrated that the anticancer activities of IL-2 and LAK could be potentiated by the Huang Qi polysaccharides. When the cancer patients (one case of late-phase gastric cancer and two cases of ovarian cancer) are orally administered with APS in an empty stomach two times per day, the production of IL-2 accelerated, and then the IL-2 elicited the activation of lymphocytes (CTL) in the ascites. The activated CTL would be increased in the surroundings of tumor cells to induce the vascular degeneration of the tumor in the plasma and finally to promote the tumor cells to death.[54,55] Moreover, the APS could potentiate the activity of NK cells and enhance the TNF secretion from PBMCs collected either from cancer patients or from healthy people.[56]

F3

From Huang Qi, an immunostimulating polysaccharide named F3 was prepared, which consists of 99% carbohydrates and <1% protein. *In vitro* experiments indicated that F3 could enhance the ability of IL-2-induced lymphokine-activated killer cells in killing melanoma A-375P cells.[57]

PAMs

Antitumor immunomodulating active polysaccharides (PAMs) were prepared from the *A. membranaceus* roots collected from different geographic origins in inner Mongolia. The compositions of the monosaccharides and the amino acids were comparable among PAMs from five different habitats, but the amounts of selenium widely varied in the collections. The PAMs with different levels of selerium repressed the *in vivo* proliferation of transplanted H22 ascitic hepatoma and S180 sarcoma cells with low toxic impacts on tumor-bearing mice. The selenium-containing PAMs enhanced the cytotoxicities of NK and $CD8^+$ T cells through the amelioration of host $CD4^+$ T cell apoptosis and the serum cytokine dysregulation caused by tumor transplantation. The PAMs also selenium-dependently improved the phagocytotic function of intraabdominal macrophages and suppressed M2-like polarization of tumor-associated macrophages to contribute to the antitumor immunomodulation activities of PAMs.[58]

Taken together, the Huang Qi polysaccharide components have been comprehensively studied, especially with respect to the anticancer and immunoenhancing properties and the ability to counteract the side effects of chemotherapeutic drugs, strongly suggesting that Huang Qi polysaccharides may become an immunotherapeutic adjuvant for improving cancer chemotherapy and chemoprevention.

Protein

A protein called arabinogalactan (at least 100 kDa) was isolated from Huang Qi, which was reported to exert the interesting immunostimulating effects by upregulating the hematopoiesis, increasing the proliferation or the maturation of megakaryocytes, augmenting the productions of IL-1ρ, IL-6, TNFα, IFNγ, GM-CSF, or G-CSF and the activity of neutrophils, and accelerating the immune recovery activity to cytotoxic agents and radiation.[59]

Clinical Trials

One hundred thirty-six patients with histologically or cytologically confirmed NSCLC were treated with the combined cisplatin and APS. After three cycles of the treatment, APS markedly reduced the cisplatin-caused side effects and improved the life quality besides increasing of the patient's survival time compared to using cisplatin alone.[60] Likewise, a total of 30 cases of patients with advanced NSCLC were treated with APS (250 mg, once per day) and Iodine-125 (I125) brachytherapy for 42 days. The combinational treatment of advanced NSCLC could slightly augment the anticancer effect of I125 but largely improve the quality of life of the patients through the enhancement of immune functions.[61]

New Prescription

Sea pyrimidine (SP), a composition of Chinese–Western medicine, was prepared containing 5-FU, extracts of Huang Qi and Kushen (*Sophora flavescens* Ait.), and a certain seaweed. In the investigations, SP promoted the apoptosis of SGC-7901 gastric cancer cells by opening the calcium channel and releasing intracellular calcium to initiate the cellular degradation.[62,63]

Other Bioactivities

The herb Huang Qi has been commonly used in traditional Chinese medicine for thousands of years. The clinical uses confirmed that Huang Qi is helpful in strengthening the immune system, enhancing metabolism and digestion, improving the functioning of the lungs, the adrenal glands, and the gastrointestinal tract, protecting, the liver, etc. Thus, Huang Qi is often used in combination with other herbs in Chinese remedies. Modern investigations have shown that Huang Qi possesses antiaging, antianoxia, antifree radical oxidative, antioxidant, immunoregulaing, and antiinflammatory properties plus bidirectional regulation of blood sugar and blood pressure. By decreasing free radical release and damage, Huang Qi is potentially protective against cardiotoxicity and renal toxicity caused by antitumor agents such as DNR.[64] More data proved that astragaloside-IV (**3**) and ASP were also capable of repressing DOX-caused oxidative stress and apoptosis in cardiocytes and inhibiting DOX-mediated cardiotoxicity by regulating PI3k/Akt and/or p38MAPK pathways.[65,66]

References

1. Lin, J. et al. 2003. Effects of Astragali radix on the growth of different cancer cell lines. *World J. Gastroenterol.* 9: 670–3.
2. Peng, X. Z. et al. 2011. Evaluation of in vitro antioxidant and antitumour activities of *Astragalus membranaceus* aqueous extract. *J. Med. Plants Res.* 5: 6564–70.
3. Song, Y. et al. 2013. Effects of astragalus on cell proliferation and apoptosis in laryngeal carcinoma cell line. *Shiyong Yaowu Yu Linchuang* 16: 5–7.
4. Zhou, R. F. et al. 2009. Effect of Astragalus mongholicus injection on proliferation and apoptosis of hormone sensitive (MCF-7) breast cancer cell lines with physiological dose E2. *Zhongyaocai.* 32: 744–7.
5. Jia, X. H. et al. 2013. Effect of Astragalus injection on U937 leukemia cells proliferation and apoptosis and relevant molecular mechanisms. *Zhongguo Dangdai Erke Zazhi* 15: 1128–33.
6. Li, L. K. et al. 2011. Antitumor and immunomodulatory effects of astragalus injection on H22 bearing mice. *Sichuan J. Pharmacol. Sci.* 1: 14–6.
7. Cho, W. C. et al. 2007. *In vitro* and *in vivo* antitumor effects of *Astragalus membranaceus. Cancer Lett.* 252: 43–54.
8. Liu, M. Q. et al. 1992. Inhibitory effect of astragalus injection and Fuzheng extract on rat lung cancer. *Cancer Res. Prev. Treat.* 19: 133.
9. Cui, R. T. et al. 2003. Suppressive effect of *Astragalus membranaceus* Bunge on chemical hepatocarcinogenesis in rats. *Cancer Chemother. Pharmacol.* 51: 75–80.
10. Kurashige, S. et al. 1999. Effects of Astragali radix extract on arcinogenesis, cytokine production, and cytotoxicity in mice treated with a carcinogen, N-butyl-N-butanolnitrosoamine. *Cancer Investigation* 17: 30–5.
11. Ha, M. W. et al. 1997. Laboratory study on *Astragalus membranaceus* mistura in prophylaxis and treatment of myelosuppression caused by cancer chemotherapy. *J. China Med. Univ.* 26: 449–52.
12. Xiao, W. et al. 2001. Pattern of TH1/TH2 and regulation of astragalus in lung cancer. *J. Shangdong Med. Univ.* 39: 309–12.
13. Ren, D. L. et al. 2000. Study on effects of *Astragalus membranaceus* and *Rehmannia glutinosa* on proliferation and specific antitumor activities of tumor infiltrating lymphocyte from esophageal cancer. *Huaxi Yaoxue Zazhi* 15: 161–3.

14. Li, D. F. et al. 1997. Effects of ginsenoside and *Astragalus membranaceus* on antitumor activities of tumor infiltrating lymphocytes (TIL) from patients with pulmonary carcinoma. *Zhongguo Mianyixue Zazhi* 13: 296–8.
15. Yang, Y. et al. 2001. Effects of total astragalosides on hepatoma cells apoptosis and wtp53 expression. *Chin. Pharmacol. Bull.* 17: 447–51.
16. Auyeung, K. K. et al. 2009. Astragalus saponins induce apoptosis via an ERK-independent NF-κB signaling pathway in the human hepatocellular HepG2 cell line. *Intl. J. Mol. Med.* 23: 189–96.
17. Auyeung, K. K. et al. 2010. Astragalus saponins modulate mTOR and ERK signaling to promote apoptosis through the extrinsic pathway in HT-29 colon cancer cells. *Intl. J. Mol. Med.* 26: 341–9.
18. Tin, M. M. Y. et al. 2007. Astragalus saponins induce growth inhibition and apoptosis in human colon cancer cells and tumor xenograft. *Carcinogenesis* 28: 1347–55.
19. Wang, Y. et al. 2014. Astragalus saponins modulates colon cancer development by regulating calpain-mediated glucose-regulated protein expression. *BMC Complem. Altern. Med.* 14: 401/1–401/12.
20. Abdallah, R. M. et al. 1993. Astragalosides from Egyptian *Astragalus spanosus*. *Pharmazie* 48: 452–4.
21. Wan, C. P. et al. 2013. Astragaloside II triggers T cell activation through regulation of CD45 protein tyrosine phosphatase activity. *Acta Pharmacol Sin.* 34: 522–30.
22. Zhang, A. L. et al. 2014. Astragaloside IV inhibits progression of lung cancer by mediating immune function of Tregs and CTLs by interfering with IDO. *J. Cancer Res. Clin. Oncol.* 140: 1883–90.
23. Verotta, L. et al. 2001. Cycloartane saponins from *Astragalus peregrinus* as modulators of lymphocyte proliferation. *Fitoterapia* 72: 894–905.
24. Verotta, L. et al. 2002. Cycloartane and oleanane saponins from Egyptian Astragalus spp. as modulators of lymphocyte proliferation. *Planata Med.* 68: 986–94.
25. Auyeung, K. K. et al. 2010. Novel herbal flavonoids promote apoptosis but differentially induce cell cycle arrest in human colon cancer cells. *Investigational New Drugs* 28: 1–13.
26. Zhou, R. J. et al. 2013. Effects of formononetin on proliferation and cell cycle of different subtypes of breast cancer cell lines. *Zhongliu Fangzhi Yanjiu* 39: 1051–5.
27. Li, T. Y. et al. 2014. Formononetin promotes cell cycle arrest via downregulation of Akt/Cyclin D1/CDK4 in human prostate cancer cells. *Cell. Physiol. Biochem.* 34: 1351–8.
28. Jin, Y. M. et al. 2014. In vitro and in vivo anti-cancer activity of formononetin on human cervical cancer cell line HeLa. *Tumor Biol.* 35: 2279–84.
29. Zhou, R. et al. 2014. Formononetin inhibits migration and invasion of MDA-MB-231 and 4T1 breast cancer cells by suppressing MMP-2 and MMP-9 through PI3K/AKT Signaling Pathways. *Hormone Metab. Res.* 46: 753–60.
30. Zhong, M. et al. 2001. Effects of Astragalus polysaccharide (APS) and Astragalus flavonoids (AF) on the cytotoxicity of LAK and NK cells in normal and tumor bearing mice. *J. Sichuan Univ. (Sci. Edit.)* 38: 718–22.
31. Xu, Z. M. et al. 2012. Effects of total flavonoids of Astragalus on promotive apoptosis of radiated hepatoma cells. *Zhongguo Dangdai Yiyao* 19: 10–12.
32. Sun, J. Y. et al. 2009. Suppressive effects of swainsonine on C6 glioma cell in vitro and in vivo. *Phytomed.* 16: 1070–4.
33. Sun, J. Y. et al. 2007. Inhibition of the growth of human gastric carcinoma in vivo and in vitro by swainsonine. *Phytomed.* 14: 353–9.
34. Das, P. C. et al. 1995. Activation of resident tissue-specific macrophages by swainsonine. *Oncol. Res.* 7: 425–33.
35. Oredipe, O. A. et al. 2003. Mice primed with swainsonine are protected against doxorubicin-induced lethality. *Cell. Mol. Biol.* 49: 1089–99; 1037–48.
36. Oredipe, O. A. et al. 2003. Limits of stimulation of proliferation and differentiation of bone marrow cells of mice treated with swainsonine. *Intl. Immuno-pharmacol.* 3: 1537–47.
37. Klein, J. L. et al. 1999. Swainsonine protects both murine and human haematopoietic systems from chemotherapeutic toxicity. *British J. Cancer* 80: 87–95.
38. Yan, Q. J. et al. 2009. Antiproliferation and apoptosis of human tumor cell lines by a lectin (AMML) of *Astragalus mongholicus*. *Phytomed.* 16: 586–93.
39. Li, Y. X. et al. 2009. Antiproliferation and apoptosis of K562 cells by *Astragalus mongholicus* lectin. *Zhongguo Yaolixue Tongbao* 25: 904–7.
40. Yan, Q. J. et al. 2010. Characterisation of a novel monomeric lectin (AML) from *Astragalus membranaceus* with anti-proliferative activity. *Food Chem.* 122: 589–95.
41. Huang, L. H. et al. 2012. *Astragalus membranaceus* lectin (AML) induces caspase-dependent apoptosis in human leukemia cells. *Cell Proliferation* 45: 15–21.
42. He, M. H. et al. 2014. Astragalus polysaccharide induces apoptosis of human KG-1a cells through inhibiting PTEN-PI3K-Akt signaling pathway. *Baixuebing Linbaliu* 23: 219–22.
43. Wu, Y. J. et al. 2010. Inhibition of *Astragalus membranaceus* polysaccharides against liver cancer cell HepG2. *Afri. J. Microbiol. Res.* 4: 2181–3.
44. Verbiscar, A. J. et al. 1994. Astragalus polysaccharide immunomodulators. *PCI Int. Appl.* WO 9404162 A1 19940303.
45. Ren, M. P. et al. 2010. Antitumor activity of Astragalus polysaccharides. *Zhongguo Xinyao Zazhi* 19: 221–4.
46. Yang, B. et al. 2013. Antitumor and immuno-modulatory activity of *Astragalus membranaceus* polysaccharides in H22 tumor-bearing mice. *Intl. J. Biol. Macromol.* 62: 287–90.
47. Li, Q. et al. 2012. Inhibiting effect of Astragalus polysaccharides on the functions of $CD4^{+}CD25$ highTreg cells in the tumor micro-environment of human hepatocellular carcinoma. *Chin. Med. J.* 125: 786–93.
48. Yang, M. 2010. Effects of Astragalus polysaccharide on the erythroid lineage and microarray analysis in K562 cells. *J. Ethnopharmacol.* 127: 242–50.
49. Li, S. et al. 2009. Characterization and renal protective effect of a polysaccharide from *Astragalus membranaceus*. *Carbohydr. Polym.* 78: 343–8.
50. Zhao, L. H. 2011. Characterization of polysaccharide from Astragalus radix as the macrophage stimulator. *Cell Immunol.* 271: 329–34.
51. Tian, Q. E. et al. 2012. Effects of Astragalus polysaccharides on P-glycoprotein efflux pump function and protein expression in H22 hepatoma cells in vitro. *BMC Complem. Altern. Med.* 12: 94.
52. Zhu, Z. Y. et al. 2011. Structural analysis and antitumor activity comparison of polysaccharides from Astragalus. *Carbohydrate Polymers* 85: 895–902.
53. Wang, G. et al. 1994. Study of the antitumor effect with Astragalus polysaccharide and IL-2/LAK. *Zhongguo Mianyixue Zazhi* 10: 359–61.

54. Cheng, L. et al. 2012. Astragalus polysaccharides induced gene expression profiling of intraepithelial lymphocytes in immune-suppressed mice. *J. Med. Plants Res.* 6: 2504–13.
55. Zhao, K. S. et al. 1993. Huangqi polysaccharide enhances the production of tumor necrosis factor in human peripheral blood mononuclear cells. *Zhongguo Zhongxiyi Jiehe Zazhi* 13: 263–5.
56. Yang, H. X. et al. 1998. Death and apoptosis of LAK cell during immunologic assault and the rescuing effects of APS. *Zhongguo Zhongliu Linchang* 25: 669–72.
57. Chu, D. T. et al. 1990. Immunostimulant containing interleukin-2 and substance F3 from *Astragalus membranaceus* as activity enhancer. *Faming Zhuanli Shenqing Gongkai Shuomingshu* CN 1047296 A 19901128.
58. Li, S. et al. 2014. Selenium-dependent antitumor immunomodulating activity of polysaccharides from roots of *A. membranaceus. Intl. J. Biol. Macromol.* 69: 64–72.
59. An, J. H. et al. 2001. Hematopoietic arabinogalactan composition. *PCT Int. Appl* 46pp, WO 2001000682 A1 20010104.
60. Guo, L. 2012. Astragalus polysaccharide injection integrated with vinorelbine and cisplatin for patients with advanced non-small cell lung cancer: Effects on quality of life and survival. *Med. Oncol.* 29: 1656–62.
61. Sun, F. et al. 2014. Clinical study of Astragal polysaccharides combined with iodine-125 in treatment of advanced non-small cell lung cancer. *Zhongguo Shiyan Fangjixue Zazhi* 20: 189–92.
62. Li, Y. B. et al. 2001. Effect of Sea pyrimidine on apoptosis of human gastric cancer cell SGC-7901. *Zhongcaoyao* 32: 901–4.
63. Ji, Y. B. et al. 2002. Effect of Sea pyrimidine injection on apoptosis of human gastric cancer cell SGC-7901. *Zhongguo Haiyang Yaowu* 21: 13–7.
64. Luo, Z. G. et al. 2009. *Astragalus membranaceus* prevents daunorubicin-induced apoptosis of cultured neonatal cardiomyocytes: Role of free radical effect of *Astragalus membranaceus* on daunorubicin cardiotoxicity. *Phytother. Res.* 23: 761–7.
65. Jia, Y. Y. et al. 2014. Astragaloside IV inhibits doxorubicin-induced cardiomyocyte apoptosis mediated by mitochondrial apoptotic pathway via activating the PI3K/Akt pathway. *Chem. Pharm. Bull.* 62: 45–53.
66. Cao, Y. et al. 2014. Astragalus polysaccharide suppresses doxorubicin-induced cardiotoxicity by regulating the PI3k/Akt and p38MAPK pathways. *Oxid. Med. Cellular Longev.* 2014: 674219.

162 Bai Zhu 白術

White atractylodes

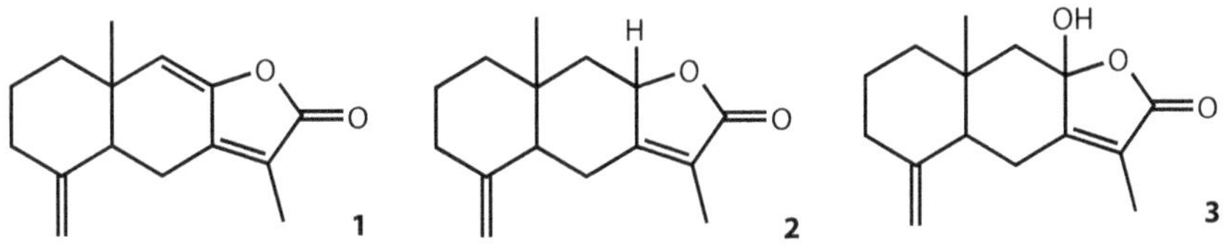

Herb Origination

The herb Bai Zhu (White atractylodes) is the dried rhizomes of a Compositae plant, *Atractylodes macrocephala*, whose plant is mainly cultivated in the Chinese provinces of Zhejiang and Anhui for traditional Chinese medicinal use. The rhizomes are collected in the winter when the aerial parts have withered and dried using stove heat.

Antitumor Activities and Constituents

Bai Zhu methanolic extract, in the *in vitro* assay, induced the apoptosis of human Jurkat lymphoma, U937, and HL-60 leukemia cell lines, whose apoptosis was triggered by the generation of intracellular ROS, especially hydrogen peroxide (H_2O_2) and superoxide anion (O^{2-}).[1] The treatment with Bai Zhu water extract at a dose of 0.5 g/mL for 10 days retarded the growth of tumor cells by 77.1% concomitant with the reduction of the content of TNFα in a serum and the increase of IL-2 level and thymus index in mice bearing sarcoma 180.[2] The *in vivo* experiment also evidenced that the Bai Zhu extract could restore the decreased immune function caused by radiation through notably improved T cell proliferation and markedly elevated IL-2 level in radiotherapy-treated mice bearing S180, indicating that Bai Zhu may be used to antagonize the immunosuppression caused by radiotherapy and tumor antigen.[3] The following approaches provided more chemical and pharmacological bases for the traditional application of Bai Zhu in cancer treatment and prevention.

Volatile Oil

An *in vitro* assay found that Bai Zhu volatile oil (BZVO) directly destroyed Ehrlich ascites carcinoma cells and retarded the mitosis of human Eca109 esophageal cancer cells. The BZVO displayed obvious inhibitory activities against the proliferation and the invasion of cancer cells in mice together with the amplification of the immune function of the host.[4] The i.p. injection with BZVO to tumor-bearing mice resulted in marked suppressive effect against the growth of Ehrlich ascites carcinoma and ascites lymphosarcoma at doses of 50 and 100 mg/kg. The survival duration of the tumor-bearing mice was prolonged by 197% after the administration of BZVO in a large dose of 150 mg/kg.[4] The *in vivo* oral treatment with BZVO at a dose of 250 mg/kg demonstrated 51.6% and 53.2% suppressive rates against mouse transplanted with H22 hepatoma and sarcoma 180, respectively.[5] Also, the lung metastasis of H22 cells by blood and lymphatic tracks was markedly retarded in mouse models by BZVO treatment, associated with the pointedly decreases of MMP-9 secretion and expression.[6] BZVO was also able to restrain the proliferation, the adhesion, and the invasion of human highly metastatic PG lung cancer cells.[7,8] In addition, Zbo-1 (a part extract with low polarity) prepared from BZVO exhibited the antitumor effect in mice bearing sarcoma 180 at a high dose of 200 mg/kg, and the growth inhibitory rate was 27.74%.[9] Butenolide-β, a nonsesquiterpenoid compound isolated from the BZVO, demonstrated the suppressive effect against the growth of sarcoma 180 *in vivo*, and its inhibitory rate was >30%.[10] Moreover, BVZO concurrently played another important role in the activation of host nonspecific immune functions by augmenting the macrophage activity during the cancer treatments *in vivo*.[11]

For testing the influence of unstableness and easy oxidation, the antitumor activity of BZVO has also been studied in the different oxidative conditions. The results showed that both predecomposed and postdecomposed BZVO could still obstruct the proliferation of human SKOV3 ovarian cancer cells and induce the cell apoptotic death and the cell cycle arrest in time- and dose-dependent manners. However, the predecomposed BZOV presented obviously higher antiproliferative activity than the postdecomposed BZVO. Both showed different process in the induction of apoptosis and cell cycle arrest. The apoptosis was mainly induced in the early stage by the predecomposed BZOV but in both early and late stages by the postdecomposed BZVO, while the cell cycle progression stopped by the predecomposed and postdecomposed BZVO was at G2/M phase and S phase, respectively.[12] Also, through the downregulation of serum TNFα and IL-6 to normal level and the elevation IL-2 level in serum, BZVO significantly improved the life quality of mice implanted with Lewis lung carcinoma and hindered tumor development.[13] Therefore, BZVO was demonstrated to possess multiple anticarcinoma activities, such as antiproliferation, antinvasion, antimetastasis, and immunostimulation, whose remarkable evidences provided a scientific basis for using Bai Zhu in cancer chemotherapy and rediotherapy.

Sesquiterpenoids

Four anticancer components identified as atractylenolide-I (**1**), atractylenolide-II (**2**), atractylenolide-III (**3**), and butenolide-B were discovered from the volatile oil. The three atractylenolides displayed antiproliferative effect against mouse CT26 colon cancer cells *in vitro* at concentrations of 50–200 μg/mL. At an optimal dose of 50 μg/mL and the best delivery time of 48 h, atractylenolide-II (**2**) exerted the highest suppressive effect on the CT26 cells.[14] Atractylenolide-I (**1**) showed dose-dependent cytotoxicity in human HL-60 promyeloleukemia cells (IC_{50}: 10.6 μg/mL at 12 h), but atractylenolide-III (**3**) was not active to

HL-60 cells.[15] The treatment with atractylenolide-I (**1**) markedly diminished the percentage of viability and promoted the apoptosis of human A549 and HCC827 lung cancer cell lines *in vitro* in a dose-dependent manner via a mitochondria-mediated apoptotic pathway, and the activities were further proven in nude mice transplanted with A549 cells.[16] Atractylenolide-I (**1**) was able to attenuate gastric CSC traits partly by inactivating Notch1, leading to the down-expression of its downstream targets Hes1, Hey1, and CD44 *in vitro*, and it also inhibited the self-renewal capacity of gastric stem-like cells by the repression of their sphere formation capacity and cell viability, implying the developing potential of atractylenolide-I in the treatment of gastric cancer.[17]

Similarly, atractylenolide-II (**2**) and atractylenolide-III (**3**) inhibited the cell growth and stimulated the cell cycle arrest and the apoptosis of B16 melanoma and A549 lung cancer cells *in vitro*.[18,19] The apoptotic mechanism was found to be correlated with the induced multiple interactions, i.e., increase of Bax expression, decrease of Bcl-2 and Bcl-xL expressions, cleavage of PARP, release of cytochrome c, and activation of caspase-3 and caspase-9.[17–19] Atractylenolides-II (**2**) could also p53-dependently elicit the activation of p38 and the inactivation of ERK and Akt in the induction of B16 melanoma cell apoptosis, and atractylenolide-III (**3**) has an ability to suppress angiogenesis-related HUVEC proliferation and capillary tube formation.[18,19] Moreover, atractylenolide-I (**1**) was capable of significantly sensitizing the response of MyD88-positive human epithelial ovarian cancer (EOC)cells to paclitaxel through the blockage of MD-2-mediated TLR4/MyD88 signaling and decrease of the protein expressions of IL-6, VEGF, and survivin, thereby eliciting early apoptosis and growth inhibition of the MyD88$^+$-EOC cells. The results evidenced that the combinational therapy with atractylenolide-I (**1**) and paclitaxel may be a promising strategy for the treatment of MyD88-positive EOC.[20]

Polysaccharides

A. macrocephala polysaccharides stimulated C6 glioma cell apoptosis *in vitro* via a mitochondrial pathway, i.e., loss of mitochondrial membrane potential, release of cytochrome c to cytosol, activation of caspase-3 and caspase-9, and cleavage of PARP, thereby obviously inhibiting the proliferation of C6 cells in a concentration-dependent manner.[21] AMP-1, a Bai Zhu polysaccharide, is composed of galactose and mannose in a molar ratio of 1.0:1.9 with a molecular weight of 3.8×10^3. The structure of AMP-1 was formed with a backbone of β-(1–2)-D-galactose residues with branches of single β-D-mannose residue at C-6. An *in vivo* assay displayed that AMP-1 could restrain the cell growth of sarcoma 180 and Lewis pulmonary cancer in mice and simultaneously promote the immune functions. The increase of immunoregulation by Bai Zhu polysaccharides prominently contributed to the tumor inhibitive activity and the decrease of invasion of tumor tissue.[22,23]

Other Bioactivities

The herb Bai Zhu is widely used in Chinese medicine prescription to be combined with other herbs. Pharmacological studies confirmed that Bai Zhu has multiple medical properties such as hepatoprotective, choleretic, diuretic, antiulcerative, hypoglycemic, anticoagulant, immunoenhancing, radical-scavenging, antioxidative, vasodilative, and antibacterial. *In vitro* and *in vivo* treatments with atractylenolide-I (**1**) potently inhibited the angiogenesis in chronic inflammation by the downregulation of NO, TNFα, IL-1β, IL-6, VEGF, and placenta growth factor (PIGF).[24]

References

1. Huang, H. L. et al. 2005. Reactive oxygen species mediation of baizhu-induced apoptosis in human leukemia cells. *J. Ethnopharmacol.* 97: 21–9.
2. Zhu, Q. J. et al. 2006. Study on antitumor effect and mechanism of extract of largehead atractylodes rhizome. *J. Shandong Univ. TCM* 30: 69–71.
3. Yao, S. J. et al. 2006. Studies of reducing poison and increasing effect of *Atractylodes macrocephala* on immune function of tumor-bearing mice after chemotherapy. *Chin. J. Primary Med. Pharm.* 13: 74–5.
4. Zhang, Z. et al. 2007. Research about the antitumor function of *Atractylodes macrocephala* volatile oil. *Cancer Res. Clinic* 18: 799–800.
5. Wang, X. et al. 2002. Inhibitory activity of volatile oil from *Atractylodes macrocephala* parenchymatous tumor in mice. *Chin. Remedies Clinics* 2: 239–40.
6. Wang, Y. J. et al. 2009. Studies on the antimetastasis effect and mechanism of Baizhu volatile oil in mice implanted H22 hepatoma. *Shaani Zhongyi* 30: 735–6.
7. Yang, E. et al. 2012. Advance on the chemical constituents and pharmacological effects of *Atractylodes macrocephala* Koidz. *Guangdong Yaoxueyuan Xuebao* 28: 218–21.
8. Xiang, X. Q. et al. 2013. Research progress and application in antitumor effects of *Atractylodes macrocephala* Koidz. *Zhongguo Shiyan Fangjixue Zazhi* 19: 367–70.
9. Shen, G. Q. et al. 2009. Chemical compositions and antitumor test of volatile oil from rhizoma *Atractylodis macrocephalae. J. Beijing Univ. TCM* 32: 413–5.
10. Tang, D. F. et al. 1984. Constituents of the essential oil from rhizome of *Atractylodes macrocephala* produced in Pingjiang [China] and their antitumor effect. *Yaoxue Tongbao* 19: 555–8.
11. Guan, X. H. et al. 2001. Effect of atractylodes macrocephala-koidz on immune function of mice. *J. Beihua Univ. (Sci. Edit.)* 2: 122–4.
12. Yan, K. L. et al. 2011. Effects of pre- and post-decomposed Rhizoma *Atractylodis macrocephalae* volatile oil on apoptosis induction and cell cycle arrest in human epithelial ovarian cancer cell line SKOV-3. *Chin. Med. Clinics* 11: 1375.
13. Qiu, G. Q. et al. 2006. Experimental studies on the inference of volatile oil from Atractylodes 27: 477–9.
14. Gao, X. L. et al. 2013. Atractylenolide II significantly reduces proliferation of mouse colon cancer cells. *Shijie Huaren Xiaohua Zazhi* 21: 2690–3.
15. Wang, C. C. et al. 2006. Pro-oxidant and cytotoxic activities of atractylenolide I in human promyeloleukemic HL-60 cells. *Food Chem. Toxicol.* 44: 1308–15.
16. Liu, H. Y. et al. 2013. Antitumor effects of atractylenolide I isolated from *Atractylodes macrocephala* in human lung carcinoma cell lines. *Mol.* 18: 13357–68.
17. Ma, L. et al. 2014. Atractylenolide I-mediated Notch pathway inhibition attenuates gastric cancer stem cell traits. *Biochem. Biophys. Res. Commun.* 450: 353–9.
18. Ye, Y. et al. 2011. Atractylenolide II induces G1 cell-cycle arrest and apoptosis in B16 melanoma cells. *J. Ethnopharmacol.* 136: 279–82.

19. Kang, T. H. et al. 2011. Atractylenolide III, a sesquiterpenoid, induces apoptosis in human lung carcinoma A549 cells via mitochondria-mediated death pathway. *Food Chem. Toxicol.* 49: 514–9.
20. Huang, J. M. et al. 2014. Atractylenolide-I sensitizes human ovarian cancer cells to paclitaxel by blocking activation of TLR4/MyD88-dependent pathway. *Scientific Reports* 4: 3840.
21. Li, X. J. et al. 2014. *Atractylodes macrocephala* polysaccharides induces mitochondrial-mediated apoptosis in glioma C6 cells. *Intl. J. Biol. Macromol.* 66: 108–12.
22. Tian, G. Y. et al. 2003. *Atractylodes macrocephala* polysaccharide used as antitumor agent and immunoregulator and its production and its uses. *Faming Zhuanli Shenqing Gongkai Shuomingshu* CN 2002–111279 20020405.
23. Shan, J. J. et al. 2003. Structural elucidation and antitumor activity of polysaccharide AMP-1 from *Atractylodes macrocephala* K. *Chin. J. Chem.* 21: 87–90.
24. Wang, C. H. et al. 2009. Inhibitory effect of atractylenolide I on angiogenesis in chronic inflammation in vivo and in vitro. *Eur. J. Pharmacol.* 612: 143.

163 Shan Hai Luo 山海螺

Bonnet bellflower

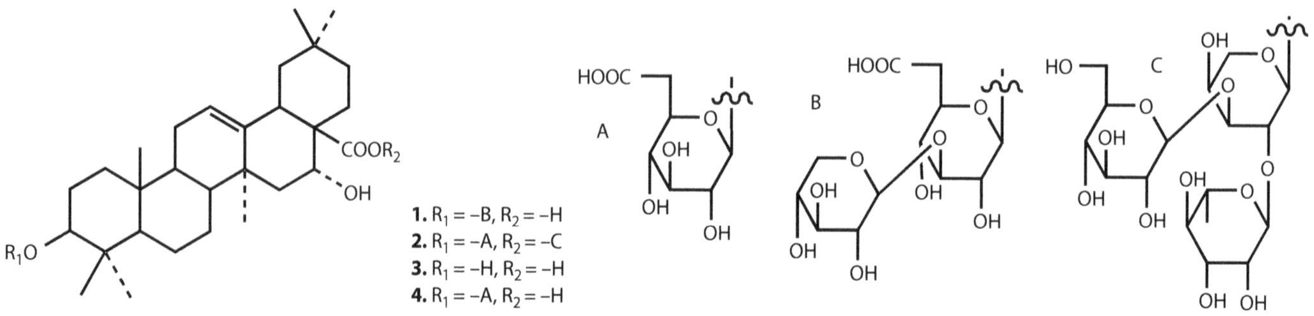

Herb Origination

The herb Shan Hai Luo (Bonnet bellflower) is the roots of a climber plant, *Codonopsis lanceolata* (Campanuculaceae). The perennial vine plant is widely distributed from China to Korea and Japan, and it has been used as a traditional medicine for a long time. Its roots are collected in July and August and dried in the sun for folk medical practices. The herb also can be used fresh.

Antitumor Activities

The cytotoxic activity of Shan Hai Luo 70% ethanol extract and its EAF were demonstrated in four human cancer cell lines, HeLa (cervix), HepG2 (liver), MCF-7 (breast), and A549 (lung), *in vitro*. The treatment with the fraction in a dose of 1 mg/mL resulted in significant cytotoxicity (74.5%, 70.7%, and 80.3%, respectively) on the HeLa, MCF-7, and A549 cells and lower cytotoxicity (<31%) on a normal human embryo kidney cell line (293). In an *in vivo* test, the EAF at a dose of 50 mg/kg achieved marked inhibitory effect against the growth of sarcoma 180 cells at 56.4%.[1] The 70% ethanolic (EtOH) extract and its EAF also displayed strong antimutagenic effects against the mutation caused by 4-nitroquinoline-l-oxide (4NQO) and MNNG.[1] Its n-butanolic fraction significantly obstructed the proliferation of human HT-29 colon cancer cells in dose- and time-dependent manners by inducing G0/G1 phase arrest and apoptosis. The critical roles of ROS generation and polyamine depletion were established to be involved in the HT-29 cell apoptotic death induced by the extract together with the increase of Bax/Bcl-2 ratio, the activation of caspase-3 and p53, and the decrease of survivin expression.[2]

Antitumor Constituents and Activities

Triterpenoids and Saponins

The major components in Shan Hai Luo were found to be triterpenoid saponins assigned as codonoposides. Most of the codonoposides displayed low antitumor effects, but only codonoposide-1c (**1**) and lancemaside-D (**2**) were demonstrated as inhibitors against the proliferation of cancer cells *in vitro*. Codonoposide-1c (**1**) could facilitate the apoptotic death of human HL-60 promyelocytic leukemia cells through Bax reduction in the cytosol, Bid cleavage and translocation to the mitochondria, release of cytochrome c and Smac/DIABLO, and activation of caspase-8, caspase-9, and caspase-3, leading to the inhibitory activity on the HL-60 cells.[3] The treatment with lancemaside-D (**2**) in a 25 mg/L concentration for 48 h restrained the proliferation of human HepG2 hepatoma cells by 67.75% and caused the G0/G1 cell cycle arrest and the DNA metabolism disturbance in the HepG2 cells.[4]

Complete acidic hydrolysis of the codonoposides produced echinocystic acid (**3**), and partial acidic hydrolysis afforded two prosapogenins (**1** and **4**). The codonoposide-1c (**1**) and echinocystic acid 3-O-glucuronoside (**4**) demonstrated greater inhibitory effect against the proliferation of cancer cells than echinocystic acid (**3**). The IC_{50} values were 0.015, 0.030, and 0.040 mM for **1**; 0.159, 0.061, and 0.107 mM for **4**; and >0.3, 0.185, and 0.160 mM for **3**, respectively, on U937 lymphoma, HL-60 leukemia, and 3LL lung cancer cell lines. This result suggested that the glycoside linkage of a glucuronic acid at C-3 of echinocystic acid (**3**) could enhance the cytotoxic effect such as echinocystic acid 3-O-glucuronoside (**4**), and an additive glycosylation of a xylose to the sugar part of echinocystic acid (**3**) strongly augmented the cytotoxicity such as echinocystic acid 3-O-glucuronoside (**4**).[5]

Polysaccharides

A bioactive polysaccharide CLP isolated from Shan Hai Luo demonstrated the suppressive effect against sarcoma 180 in rats. The inhibitory rates of CLP were 15–54% in the treatment with doses of 0.5–2.0 g/kg for 10 days.[6] Further separation of the crude polysaccharide afforded five fractions labeled as Fr-I–Fr-V. Both Fr-I and Fr-II contain protein and phenolic units in their polysaccharide molecules. Fr-I (molecular weight: <1000) displayed marked growth inhibitory activity against two human neoplastic cell lines, SNU-1 (stomach) and HeLa (cervix), *in vitro*, and Fr-II (molecular weight: 1000–3000) showed the similar properties on the same cell lines but less active than Fr-I.[7]

Other Bioactivities

The herb Shan Hai Luo (Bonnet bellflower) decoction is used in the treatment of lung abscesses, amenorrhea, milk flow obstruction, acute and inflamed boils and abscesses, and lymphadenopathy.

Pharmacological studies proved that Shan Hai Luo possesses sedative, hypotensive, antioxidative, anticonvulsant, analgesic, and antibacterial activities. The herb was reported to be able to restore weak memory induced by drugs. In addition, the polysaccharide Fr-I also exerted DPPH radical-scavenging effect and an inhibitory effect on angiotensin-converting enzyme (ACE), while Fr-II showed no effect on ACE.[7]

References

1. Kim, S. Y. et al. 2009. Antimutagenic and antitumor effects of *Codonopsis lanceolata* extracts. *J. Korean Soc. Food Sci. Nutr.* 38: 1295–301.
2. Wang, L. et al. 2010. Codonopsislanceolata extract induces G0/G1 arrest and apoptosis in human colon tumor HT-29 cells-involvement of ROS generation and polyamine depletion. *Food Chem. Toxicol.* 49: 149–54.
3. Lee, K. W. et al. 2005. β-D-xylopyranosyl-(1–3)-β-D-glucuronopyranosyl echinocystic acid isolated from the roots of *Codonopsis lanceolata* induces caspase-dependent apoptosis in human acute promyelocytic leukemia HL-60 cells. *Biol. Pharm. Bull.* 28: 854–9.
4. Yu, X. et al. 2012. Effects of lancemaside D on time effect of proliferation and cell cycle of HepG-2 cells. *Jilin Daxue Xuebao, Yixueban* 38: 236–9.
5. Lee, K. T. et al. 2002. Structure of a new echinocystic acid bisdesmoside isolated from *Codonopsis lanceolata* roots and the cytotoxic activity of prosapogenins. *J. Agricul. Food Chem.* 50: 4190–3.
6. Han, C. J. et al. 2000. Inhibitory effects of *Codonopsis lanceolata* polysaccharide for sarcocarcinoma S180 of mice. *J. Yanbian Univ. (Med. Edit.)*, 23: 249–50.
7. Kim, D. S. et al. 2006. Physiological activities of different molecular weight fractions of crude polysaccharides from dodok (*Codonopsis lanceolata*). *J. Food Sci. Nutr.* 11: 261–7.

164 Dong Chong Xia Cao 冬虫夏草

Cordyceps

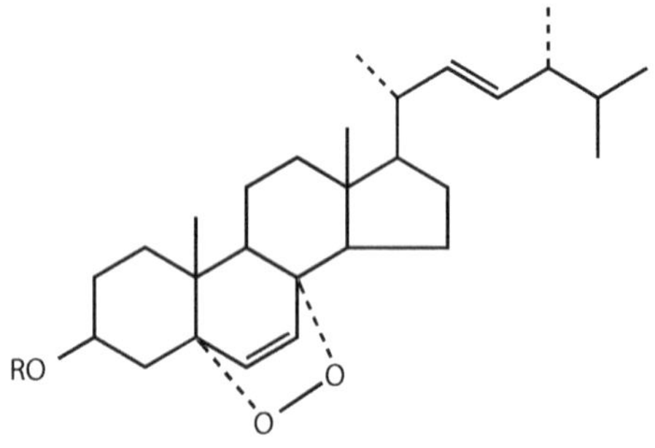

Herb Origination

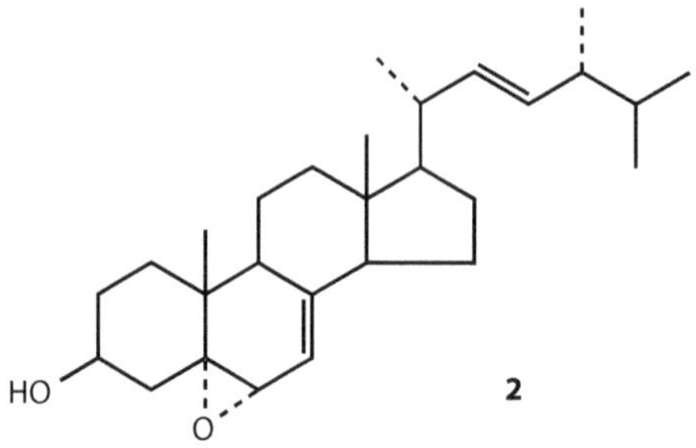

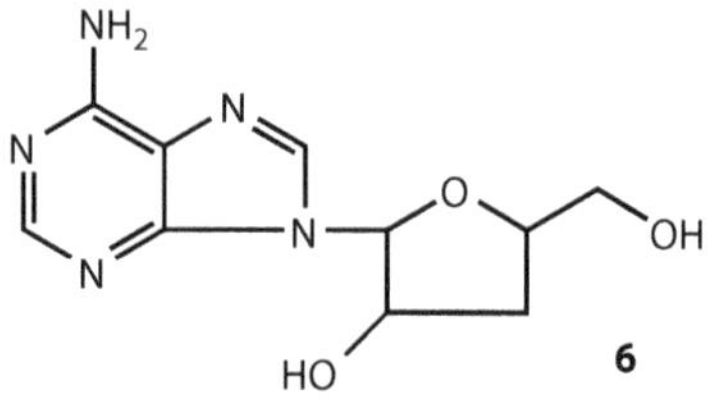

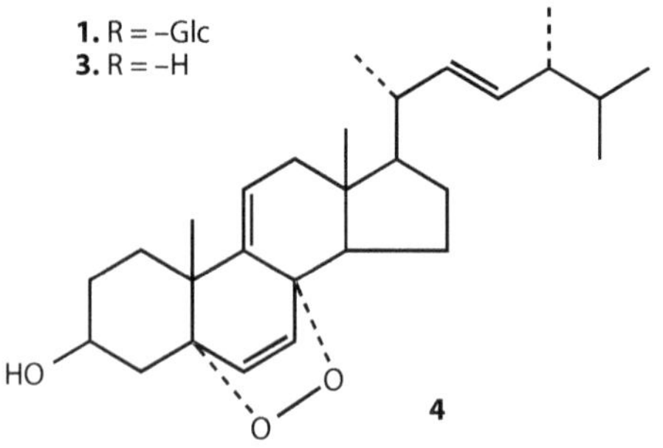

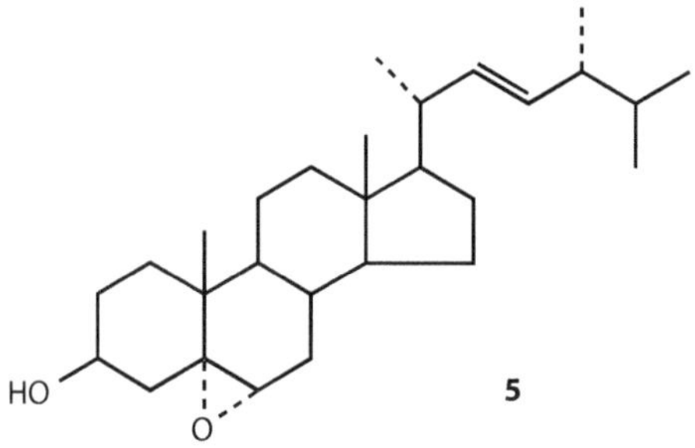

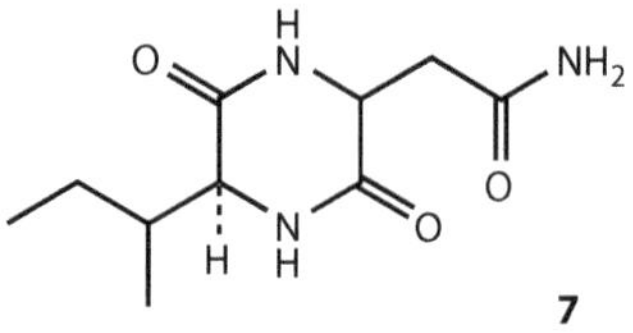

The herb Dong Chong Xia Cao (Cordyceps) is one of the most famous Chinese tonic medicines, whose herb is the dried complex of stroma and sclerotia (larvae corpse) of fungi *Cordyceps sinensis* (Clavicipitaceae). Cordyceps was firstly documented as Yartsa gunbu in the Tibetan pharmacopeia in the fifteenth century. The fungi parasites in Hepialus larvae lived in alpine meadow environments. The herb is usually collected in early summer and is primarily produced in the border of the Chinese provinces of Qinghai, Tibet, Sichuan, and Yunnan.

Antitumor Activities

Extracts from the Herb

The crude methanolic extract derived from Cordyceps significantly suppressed the growth of human K562 leukemia, Raji Burkitt's lymphoma, Calu-1 lung cancer, amnion-derived Wish, and African green monkey kidney Vero cell lines *in vitro*.[1] The oral administration of the extract led to a reduction of the tumor size and a prolongation of the host survival time in mice implanted with EL-4 lymphoma. Simultaneously, the treatment also augmented the T-independent antibody responses and the activity of peritoneal macrophages, but both were diminished by EL-4 leukemia transplantation and/or CTX treatment in tumor-bearing mice.[2] Thus, the evidences clearly revealed that the anticancer effect of Cordyceps extract may be mediated through its remarkable immunomodulating actions.

The treatment with a warm water extract (ECS) prepared from the dried Cordyceps increased the median survival durations of mice bearing EAC by 316% or Meth-A fibrosarcoma by 312%.[3] When ECS is combined with MTX, the survival time of tumor-bearing mice was markedly lengthened against B16 melanoma with no significant decrease of body weight. The extract at a concentration of 100 μg/mL also induced B16 melanoma cell apoptosis *in vitro* after 48 h of exposure.[4] But no cytotoxic effect was found for ECS on either EAC cells and Meth-A cells *in vitro*.[3] Furthermore, 2′-deoxy-coformycin (an adenosine deaminase inhibitor) could exert a remarkable reinforcement effect on the antitumor activity of the water extract.[5]

Four fractions labeled as R, F1, F2, and F3 were obtained from EtOH extract of Cordyceps by SC-CO2 fluid extractive fractionation. These fractions were effective in inhibiting the cell proliferation and the colony formation of human HT-29 and HCT-116 colorectal and Hep3B and HepG2 hepatocellular carcinoma cell lines together with the induction of apoptosis and sub-G1 cell arrestment. The fractions also markedly enhanced the activity of scavenging free radicals at a 2 mg/mL concentration with the effective rates for R (93%), F1 (75%), E (66%), F2 (47%), and F3 (27%). The R-fraction had no effect on the growth of normal dividing human PBMCs.[6] Therefore, the Cordyceps may be biologically beneficial to the cancer chemotherapy as an adjuvant agent.

Extracts from Its Mycelia or Parasitic Fungi

For finding potential herb sources of Cordyceps, the cultivated fungi mycelium has been comprehensively studied. Compared to the natural herb Cordyceps, the cultivated mycelium has similar contents of protein and carbohydrate components but has much higher contents of polysaccharide, adenosine, and cordycepin.[7] The cultivated fungi exhibited stronger antitumor activity than then natural Cordyceps against human MCF-7 breast cancer, HepG2 hepatoma, HL-60 premyelocytic leukemia cell lines, and mouse B16 melanoma cells *in vitro*.[8] The mycelium also suppressed the cell proliferation of MA-10 mouse Leydig tumor and promoted the MA-10 cells to apoptosis by downregulating NF-κB expression and activating caspase-8-dependent/caspase-9-independent pathways.[9] The apoptotic death of the HL-60 cells induced by the mycelium (at 25 μg/mL) was found to be mediated by a mitochondrial pathway rather than a death receptor pathway, such as the decrease of Bcl-2 expression, the augmentation of Bax expression, the release of cytochrome c into the cytoplasm, the loss of MTP, and the activation of caspase-2, caspase-3, and caspase-9.[10]

All organic solvent extracts from the cultivated mycelium demonstrated a dose-dependent inhibitory effect on the proliferation of human MCF-7 breast cancer, HL-60 leukemia, and HepG2 hepatoma cell lines and mouse B16 melanoma cells. In particular, its EtOAc extract exhibited the highest effect against all four tested cell lines *in vitro* with IC_{50} values between 12 and 45 μg/mL. In contrast, it had much lower cytotoxicity against normal mouse bone marrow cells. In an *in vivo* test, the EtOAc extract caused 60% decrease of B16 melanoma size in mice after 27 days treatment. The EtOAc extract was found to contain carbohydrates, adenosine, ergosterols, and trace amount of cordycepin. Among these components, ergosterols and its analogs were identified as major bioactive constituents in the extract contributing to the *in vitro* cytotoxicity.[11] At large i.p. doses (50 and 100 mg/kg) for nine consecutive days, the EtOH extract of the mycelium significantly extended the life span and markedly reduced the tumor weights and volumes in mice inoculated with sarcoma 180 cells. The EtOH extract of the mycelium was also able to potentiate phagocytosis and immunostimulating function.[12] Moreover, WECS, a hot water extract from cultured fruit body of *C. sinensis*, in association with the significant increase of TIMP-1 secretion, could reduce the number of metastatic nodule of B16-F0 melanoma cells in the liver of C57BL/6 mice and obviously prolong the survival time of the mice.[13] Based upon the given evidences, the cultivated fungi have been established to be an effective and economical substitute of the wild herbal *C. sinensis* for the healthcare application.[7]

Antitumor Constituents and Activities

Ergosterols

The bioactivity-directed isolation led to the separation of two antineosplatic ergosterol analogs from the methanolic extract and elucidated as 5α,8α-epidioxy-24(R)-methylcholesta-6,22-dien-3β-D-glucopyranoside (**1**) and 5,6-epoxy-24(R)-methylcholesta-7,22-dien-3β-ol (**2**). This ergosterol glucoside (**1**) at a concentration of 10 μg/mL displayed a greater suppressive effect against the proliferation of K562, Jurkat, and HL-60 leukemias, WM-1341 melanoma, and RPM1-8226 multiple myeloma cell lines with the inhibitory rates of 10–40%.[14] From the EAF of the cultivated mycelium, five steroids designated as 5α,8α-epidioxy-22E-ergosta-6,22-dien-3β-ol (**3**), 5α,8α-epidioxy-22E-ergosta-6,9(11),22-trien-3β-ol (**4**), 5α,6α-epoxy-5α-ergosta-7,22-dien-3β-ol (**5**), sitosterol, and ergosterol were isolated. Compounds 5α,8α-epidioxy-22E-ergosta-6,22-dien-3β-ol (**3**), 5α,8α-epidioxy-22E-ergosta-6,9(11),22-trien-3β-ol (**4**), and 5α,6α-epoxy-5α-ergosta-7,22-dien-3β-ol (**5**)holding a peroxide ring or an epoxide ring demonstrated substantial cytotoxic activity against HL-60 leukemia cells *in vitro* at concentrations of 10–20 μg/mL together with the promotion of the HL-60 cells to apoptosis, and their IC_{50} values were 7.3–7.8 μg/mL, whereas sitosterol and ergosterol displayed only moderate antitumor activity on the HL-60 cells.[15]

Cordycepin

Cordycepin (**6**) (see Section Yong Cao) displayed moderate suppressive effects against the proliferation of mouse B16-BL6 melanoma cells and Lewis lung carcinoma cells (IC_{50}: 39 and 48 μM, resppectively) *in vitro*, accompanied by the stimulation of adenosine A3 receptors in the tumor cells.[16] The mechanism in the B16-BL6 cells was associated with the stimulation of adenosine A3 receptors followed by a Wnt signaling pathway, including GSK-3β activation and cyclin-D1 inhibition.[17] The oral administration of cordycepin (**6**) in a dose of 15 mg/kg per day for two weeks significantly reduced the wet weight of primary tumor lump by 36% without systemic toxicity or any loss of body weight.[18] The unique nucleoside (**6**) also showed remarkable ability to provoke cell apoptosis and cell cycle arrest in human OSCC lines (OEC-M1, KB, and HSC3).[19,20] Through an adenosine 2A receptor-p53-caspase-7-PARP pathway and increase of p53 protein levels and phosphorylated p53 in tumor cells, cordycepin (**6**) promoted the apoptosis of rat C6 glioma cells.[21] The apoptosis of CGTH W-2 thyroid carcinoma cells induced by cordycepin (**6**) was mediated by a calcium-calpain-caspase-7-PARP pathway and the expression of adenosine receptors.[22] The i.p. administration of cordycepin (**6**) to the spleen of mice inoculated with B16-F0 melanoma cells resulted in notably lower serum alanine aminotransferase levels, prevention of tumor metastasis from the spleen to the liver of mice, and longer survival times in mice.[23] Collectively, cordycepin, an active component of Cordyceps, may be a candidate anticancer agent, but it needs more support from *in vivo* experiments and pharmacokinetic evaluation.

Cyclodipeptide

A cyclodipeptide designated as cordycedipeptide-A (**7**) was discovered from the cultivated liquid of Cordyceps mycelium, demonstrating cytotoxicities to human neoplastic cell lines such as A375 melanoma, L-929 acrobatma, and HeLa cervical cancer *in vitro*.[24]

Exopolymers

An exopolymer (EPS) was prepared from the broth of cultivated *C. sinensis*. In a mouse model, prophylactical intravenous injection of EPS significantly suppressed the metastasis of 26-M3.1 colon cancer cells by stimulating the innate immune system and augmenting the macrophage and NK cell activities.[25]

Polysaccharides

Several specific polysaccharide components having both tumor-inhibiting and immunoenhancing activities have been isolated from Cordyceps and its cultivated fungi.

PSCS

A polysaccharide fraction (PSCS) of Cordyceps displayed the antineoplastic activity against sarcoma 180 *in vivo* and the protective activity against radiation-caused damage and chemodrug (such as cortisone and CTX)-induced side effects in mice. PSCS also have capabilities to activate the phagocytotic function of reticuloendothelial system and the macrophages in the abdominal cavity, to stimulate lymphocyte transformation, to augment blood serum Immunoglobulin G (IgG), and plasma corticosterone levels, and to increase the spleen weight *in vivo*.[26] PSCS (10 μg/mL)-stimulated blood mononuclear (PSCS-MNC-CM) cells demonstrated significant suppressive effect against the proliferation of U937 lymphoma cells, resulting in growth inhibition rates of 78–83%. The treatment with the PSCS-MNC-CM complex could also induce about 50% of U937 cell differentiation into mature monocyte macrophages to express the nonspecific esterase activity and the surface antigens of CD11β, CD14, and CD68. The differentiated U937 cells exhibited the functions of phagocytosis and superoxide production. The tumoricidal and differentiating effects of PSCS-MNC-CM were further revealed to be largely contributed by the elevated cytokines, especially, IFNγ and TNFα.[27] Moreover, PSCS was able to augment T cell immunoresponse and to enhance immune functions on bone marrow-derived DCs from patients with CML.[28]

EPSF

An exopolysaccharide fraction (EPSF), which was derived from the cultivated fungi, could obviously enhance the phagocytosis of peritoneal macrophages and the proliferation of spleen lymphocytes at doses of 60 and 120 mg/kg in mice transplanted with B16 melanoma. The metastasis of B16 cells to the lungs and the livers was also notably blocked by EPSF at a dose of 120 mg/kg. During the antitumor action, EPSF decreased the expressions of Bcl-2, c-Myc, c-Fos, and VEGF in the lungs and the livers of mice implanted with B16 melanoma. The results clearly proved that EPSF possesses remarkable immunopotentiation-related anticancer and antimetastatic activities, suggesting that EPSF may be a potential adjuvant for improving cancer chemotherapy.[29,30]

CSP-1

CSP-1 was a polysaccharide (210 kDa) prepared from the cultured mycelia, which is composed of glucose, galactose, and mannose in a ratio of 10:7.5:6, displaying strong antioxidation and hypoglycemic properties.[31] In addition, in a test with rat PC12 pheochromocytoma cells, CSP-1 protected the PC12 cells from further injury from H_2O_2 and elevated the survival of the PC12 cells by over 60%, together with lessened activities of GSH-Px and SOD in a dose-dependent manner, indicating the potential of CSP-1 in the treatment of Alzheimer's disease.[32] CME-1 was a polysaccharide (27.6 kDa) from the mycelia of *C. sinensis*, which contained 95% carbohydrates and had a mannose/galactose/glucose composition ratio of 39.1:59.2:1.7. Its structure consist of a backbone possessing (1–4)-linked mannose and galactose branches attached to O-6 of the mannose. CME-1 inhibited MMP-1 expressions in B16-F10 melanoma cells via the downregulation of NF-κB or ERK/p38 MAPK, thereby inhibiting the migration of B16-F10 cells.[33]

WIPS and AIPS

Two polysaccharides, WIPS (1180 kDa) and AIPS (1150 kDa), were fractionated from hot water and alkaline extracts of *C. sinensis* mycelial biomass (strain Cs-HK1), respectively. Both were glucan, but WIPS was characterized as α-D-glucans with a backbone of (1–4)-linked α-D-Glcp (>60%) and a short branch of (1–6)-linked α-D-Glcp (~14%), and AIPS was a linear glucan. In the mouse models, AIPS exhibited more significant antitumor and immunostimulatory effects than WIPS against the growth of melanoma cells.[34]

Cordyglucan and CSPS-1

Cordyglucan was derived from herb Cordyceps, whose structure holds (1–3)-β-D-glucan main linkages with (1–6)-linked β-D-glucosyl branches.[35] CSPS-1 (1.17×10^5 Da) was extracted from mycelia of *C. sinensis* obtained by solid-state culture, which was mainly composed of (1–6)-linked α-D-Glc and α-D-Gal, with minor β-(1–4)-D-Xyl and β-(1–4)-D-Man residues probably located in the side chains with a trace amount of α-(1–3)-L-Rha residue. In biological assays, cordyglucan showed suppressive effect against the growth of sarcoma 180 *in vivo* without toxicity,[35] whereas CSPS-1 exerted dose-dependent antiproliferative and proapoptotic effects on sarcoma 180 cells *in vitro*.[36]

PS and a Mannoglucan

PS (derived from Cordyceps strain G1) is a complex of polysaccharide (80.11%) and protein (13.79%). Similarly, PS demonstrated remarkable antioxidative activity, e.g., activation of SOD and GSH-Px and reduction of the level of MDA in the liver and the brain of tumor-bearing mice. The suppression of SOD and GSH-Px activities and the decrease of MDA were largely found in response to the inhibitory effect against the growth of H22 hepatoma and brain cancer cell lines.[37] A neutral mannoglucan (7.7 kDa) purified from the Cordyceps mycelium has α-D-glucan backbone with (1–4)- and (1–3)-linkages and α-D-Man branched at C-6 of the α-(1–3)-Glc residues, wherein the molar ratio of the residues of mannose and glucose was 1:9. In the *in vitro* tests, the mannoglucan exerted moderate cytotoxic effect on human SPC-1 lung cancer cells with IC_{50} value of 63 μg/mL, but it had weak antigrowth activity against SW480 colorectal cancer cells and BCAP37 breast cancer cells.[38]

Cordysinocan and Others

Cordysinocan (~82 kDa) was isolated from a strain of *C. sinensis* (UST 2000), whose exopolysaccharide is composed of glucose, mannose, galactose in a ratio of 2.4:2:1. Through the induction of cell proliferation and secretion of IL-2, IL-6, and IL-8, cordysinocan activated the immune responses in T lymphocytes and macrophages, thereby triggering immune responses.[39] Also, a polysaccharide-rich fraction prepared from the herb was able to enhance cisplatin cytotoxicity in human H157 NSCLC cell line, concomitant with the significant reduction of VEGF and bFGF protein expressions.[40] The Cordyceps polysaccharides might offer photoprotection on UVB-induced cyclobutane–pyrimidine dimers and DNA damage to human skin cells to lessen the risk of basal cell carcinoma.[41]

Other Bioactivities

The herb Dong Chong Xia Cao (Cordyceps) has been demonstrated to possess broad healthy benefits such as tonic, antiaging, immunomodulating, male hormone–like, hypoglycemic, hypolipidemic, antioxidant, free radicals-scavenging, antiinflammatory, anticonvulsion, expectorant, hypocholesterolemic, and sedative properties according to pharmacological investigations.

References

1. Kuo, Y. C. et al. 1994. Growth inhibitors against tumor cells in *Cordyceps sinensis* other than cordycepin and polysaccharides. *Cancer Investig.* 12: 611–5.
2. Yamaguchi, N. et al. 1990. Augmentation of various immune reactivities of tumor-bearing hosts with an extract of *Cordyceps sinensis. Biotherapy* 2: 199–205.
3. Yoshida, J. et al. 1989. Antitumor activity of an extract of *Cordyceps sinensis* (Berk.) Sacc. against murine tumor cell lines. *Jpn. J. Exper. Med.* 59: 157–61.
4. Nakamura, K. et al. 2003. Combined effects of *Cordyceps sinensis* and methotrexate on hematogenic lung metastasis in mice. *Receptors Channels* 9: 329–34.
5. Yoshikawa, N. et al. 2007. Reinforcement of antitumor effect of *Cordyceps sinensis* by 2′-deoxy-coformycin, an adenosine deaminase inhibitor. *In Vivo* 21: 291–5.
6. Wang, B. J. et al. 2005. Free radical scavenging and apoptotic effects of *Cordyceps sinensis* fractionated by supercritical carbon dioxide. *Food Chem. Toxicol.* 43: 543–52.
7. Leung, P. H. et al. 2006. Mycelium cultivation, chemical composition and antitumour activity of a Tolypocladium sp. fungus isolated from wild *Cordyceps sinensis. J. Applied Microbiol.* 101: 275–83.
8. Zhang, Q. X. et al. 2005. Comparison of antitumor effect of extracts in cultivated *Cordyceps sinensis* fungus HK-1 and natural *Cordyceps sinensis. Zhongcaoyao* 36: 1346–9.
9. Yang, H. Y. et al. 2006. *Cordyceps sinensis* mycelium induces MA-10 mouse Leydig tumor cell apoptosis by activating the caspase-8 pathway and suppressing the NF-κB pathway. *Archiv. Androl.* 52: 103–10.
10. Zhang, Q. X. et al. 2007. *Cordyceps sinensis* mycelium extract induces human premyelocytic leukemia cell apoptosis through mitochondrion pathway. *Experimental Biol. Med.* (Maywood, NJ, USA) 232: 52–7.
11. Wu, J. Y. et al. 2007. Inhibitory effects of ethyl acetate extract of *Cordyceps sinensis* mycelium on various cancer cells in culture and B16 melanoma in C57BL/6 mice. *Phytomed.* 14: 43–9.
12. Shin, K. et al. 2003. Antitumour and immuno-stimulating activities of the fruiting bodies of *Paecilomyces japonica*, a new type of Cordyceps spp. *Phytotherapy Res.* 17: 830–3.
13. Kubo, E. et al. 2012. Effect of *Cordyceps sinensis* on TIMP-1 secretion from mouse melanoma cells. *Central Eur. J. Biol.* 7: 167–71.
14. Bok, J. W. et al. 1999. Antitumor sterols from the mycelia of *Cordyceps sinensis. Phytochem.* 51: 891–8.
15. Matsuda, H. et al. 2009. Apoptosis-inducing effects of sterols from the dried powder of cultured mycelium of *Cordyceps sinensis. Chem. Pharm. Bull.* 57: 411–4.
16. Nakamura, K. et al. 2006. Antitumor effect of cordycepin (3′-deoxyadenosine) on mouse melanoma and lung carcinoma cells involves adenosine A3 receptor stimulation. *Anticancer Res.* 26: 43–7.
17. Yoshikawa, N. et al. 2008. Cordycepin (3′-deoxyadenosine) inhibits the growth of B16-BL6 mouse melanoma cells through the stimulation of adenosine A3 receptor followed by glycogen synthase kinase-3β activation and cyclin D1 suppression. *Naunyn-Schmiedeberg's Archives of Pharmacol.* 377: 591–5.
18. Yoshikawa, N. et al. 2004. Antitumor activity of cordycepin in mice. *Clin. Experim. Pharmacol. Physiol.* 31(Suppl. 2): S51–53.
19. Wu, W. C. et al. 2007. The apoptotic effect of cordycepin on human OEC-M1 oral cancer cell line. *Cancer Chemother. Pharmacol.* 60: 103–11.
20. Lee, J. H. et al. 2011. Anticancer effects of Cordycepin on oral squamous cell carcinoma proliferation and apoptosis in vitro. *J. Cancer Therapy* 2: 224–34.
21. Chen, Y. et al. 2014. Cordycepin induces apoptosis of C6 glioma cells through the adenosine 2A receptor-p53-caspase-7-PARP pathway. *Chemico-Biol. Interactions* 216: 17–25.
22. Chen, Y. et al. 2010. Cordycepin induces apoptosis of CGTH W-2 thyroid carcinoma cells through the calcium-calpain-caspase 7-PARP pathway. *J. Agricult. Food Chem.* 58: 11645–52.
23. Sato, A. et al. 2013. Inhibitory effect of cordycepin on experimental hepatic metastasis of B16-F0 mouse melanoma cells. *In Vivo* 27: 729–32.
24. Jia, J. M. et al. 2005. Cordycedipeptide A, a new cyclodipeptide from the culture liquid of *Cordyceps sinensis* (Berk.) Sacc. *Chem. Pharm. Bull.* 53: 582–3.
25. Yoon, T. J. et al. 2008. Innate immune stimulation of exopolymers prepared from *Cordyceps sinensis* by submerged culture. *Applied Microbiol. Biotechnol.* 80: 1087–93.
26. Zang, Q. Z. et al. 1985. Pharmacological action of the polysaccharide from cordyceps (*Cordyceps sinensis*). *Zhongcaoyao* 16: 306–11.
27. Chen, Y. J. et al. 1997. Effect of *Cordyceps sinensis* on the proliferation and differentiation of human leukemic U937 cells. *Life Sci.* 60: 2349–59.
28. Huang, Z. L. et al. 2011. The immunomodulatory effects of *Cordyceps sinensis* on dendritic cells derived from chronic myelogenous leukemia (CML). *J. Med. Plants Res.* 5: 5925–32.
29. Yang, J. Y. et al. 2005. Effects of exopolysaccharide fraction (EPSF) from a cultivated *Cordyceps sinensis* fungus on c-Myc, c-Fos, and VEGF expression in B16 melanoma-bearing mice. *Pathol. Res. Practice* 201: 745–50.
30. Zhang, W. Y. et al. 2005. Immunomodulatory and antitumour effects of an exopolysaccharide fraction from cultivated *Cordyceps sinensis* (Chinese caterpillar fungus) on tumour-bearing mice. *Biotechnol. Applied Biochem.* 42: 9–15.
31. Li, S. P. et al. 2006. Hypoglycemic activity of polysaccharide, with antioxidation, isolated from cultured Cordyceps mycelia. *Phytomed.* 13: 428–33.
32. Li, S. P. et al. 2003. A polysaccharide isolated from *Cordyceps sinensis*, a traditional Chinese medicine, protects PC12 cells against hydrogen peroxide-induced injury. *Life Sci.* 73: 2503–13.
33. Jayakumar, T. et al. 2014. Anticancer effects of CME-1, a novel polysaccharide, purified from the mycelia of *Cordyceps sinensis* against B16-F10 melanoma cells. *J. Cancer Res. Therap.* 10: 43–9.

34. Yan, J. K. et al. 2011. Physiochemical properties and antitumor activities of two α-glucans isolated from hot water and alkaline extracts of Cordyceps (Cs-HK1) fungal mycelia. *Carbohydrate Polymers* 85: 753–8.
35. Wu, Y. L. et al. 2005. Structure analysis and antitumor activity of (1–3)-β-D-glucans (cordyglu-cans) from the mycelia of *Cordyceps sinensis*. *Planta Med.* 71: 381–4.
36. Mei, Y. X. et al. 2014. Isolation, characterization, and antitumor activity of a novel heteroglycan from cultured mycelia of *Cordyceps sinensis*. *Planta Med.* 80: 1107–12.
37. Chen, J. P. et al. 2006. Morphological and genetic characterization of a cultivated *Cordyceps sinensis* fungus and its polysaccharide component possessing antioxidant property in H22 tumor-bearing mice. *Life Sci.* 78: 2742–8.
38. Wu, Y. L. et al. 2007. Isolation and characterization of a mannoglucan from edible *Cordyceps sinensis* mycelium. *Carbohydrate Res.* 342: 870–5.
39. Cheung, J. K. H. et al. 2009. Cordysinocan, a polysaccharide isolated from cultured Cordyceps, activates immune responses in cultured T-lymphocytes and macrophages: Signaling cascade and induction of cytokines. *J. Ethnopharmacol.* 124: 61–8.
40. Ji, N. F. et al. 2011. Polysaccharide of *Cordyceps sinensis* enhances cisplatin cytotoxicity in non-small cell lung cancer H157 cell line. *Integrative Cancer Therapies* 10: 359–67.
41. Wong, W. C. et al. 2011. Photoprotective potential of Cordyceps polysaccharides against ultraviolet B radiation-induced DNA damage to human skin cells. *British J. Dermatol.* 164: 980–6.

165 Gan Cao 甘草

Liquorice root or Licorice roots

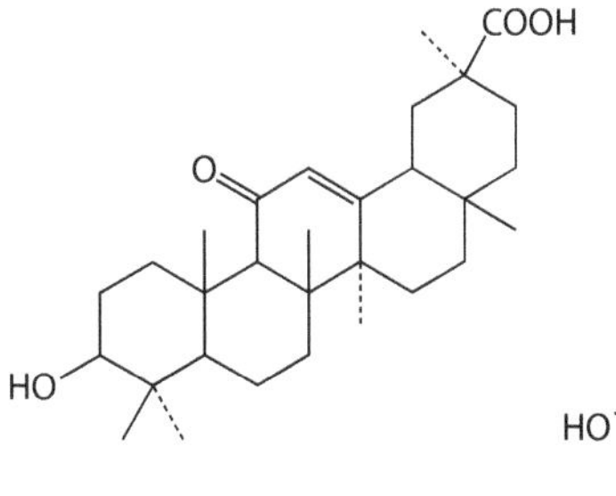

1. R = -alpha-D-GlcA-2-beta-D-GlcA
2. R = -H

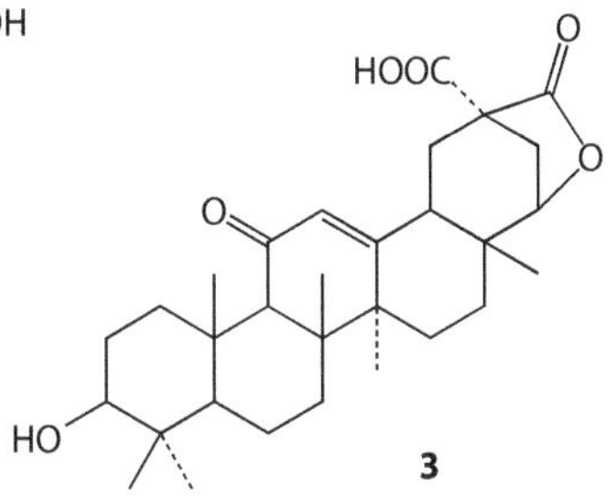

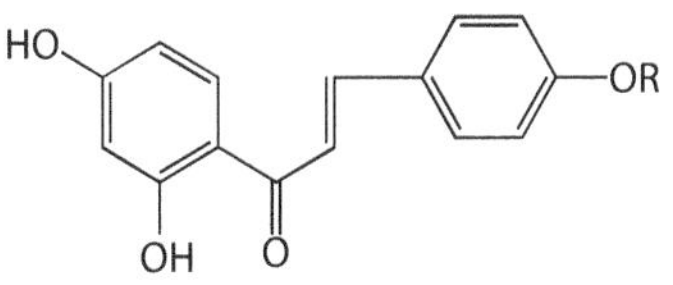

9. R = -H
10. R = -beta-D-glucose

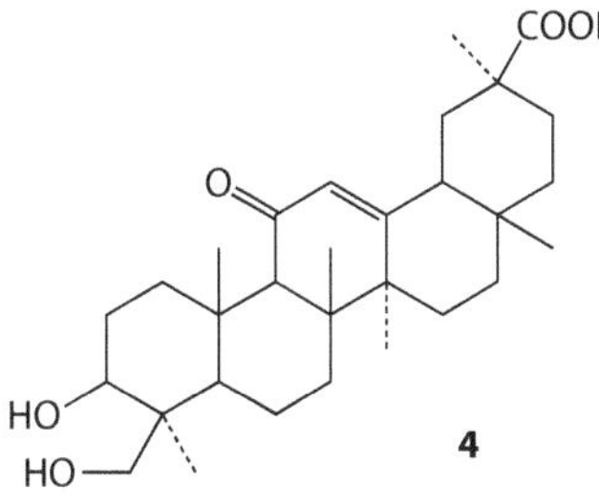

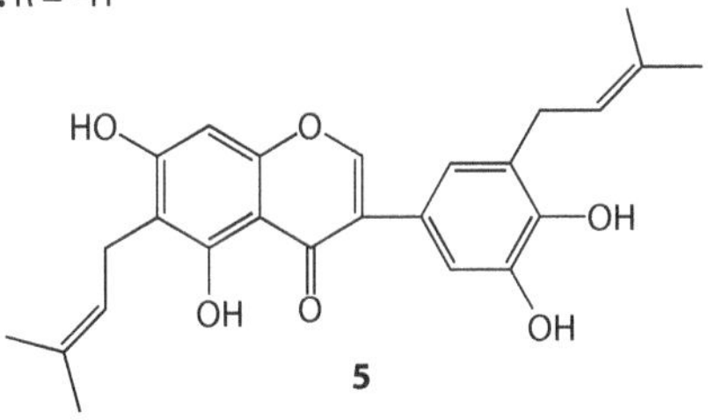

Herb Origination

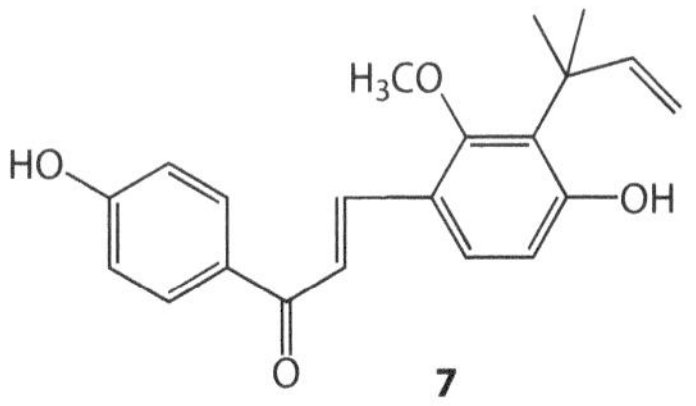

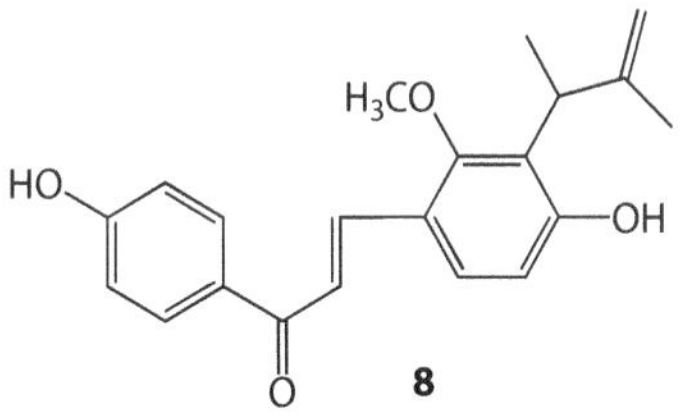

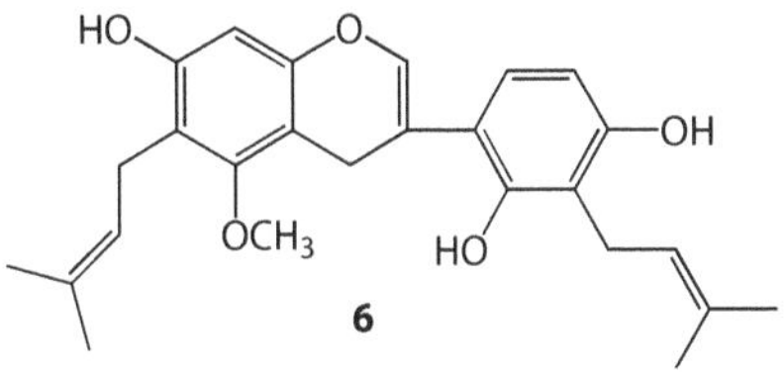

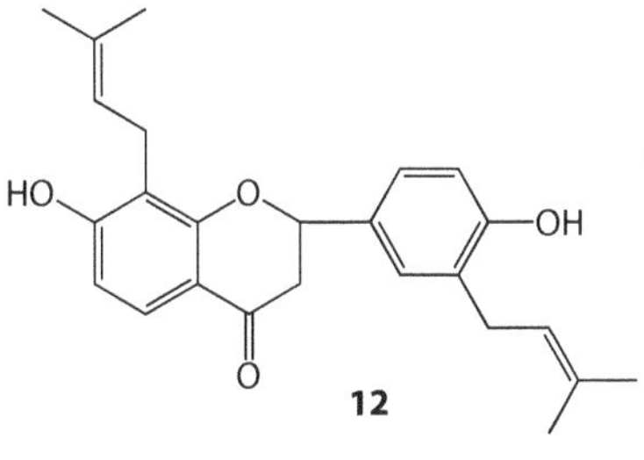

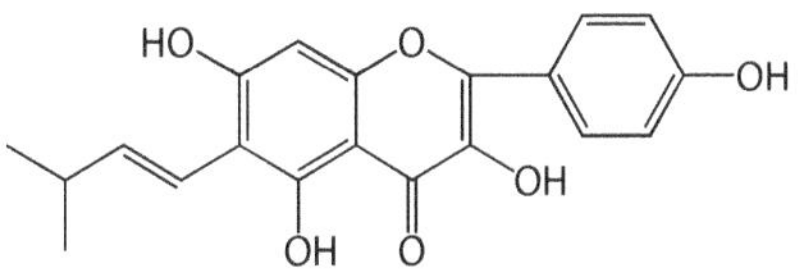

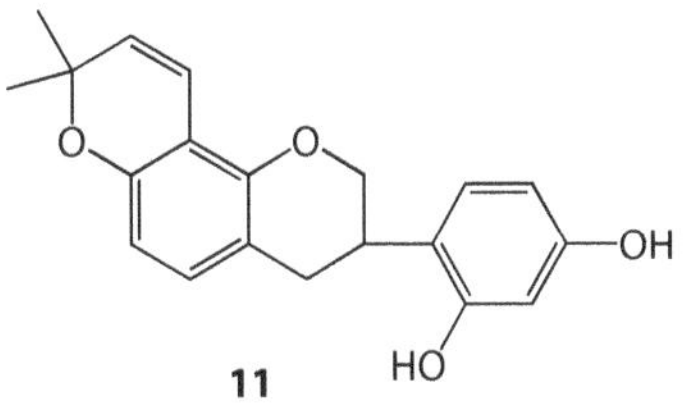

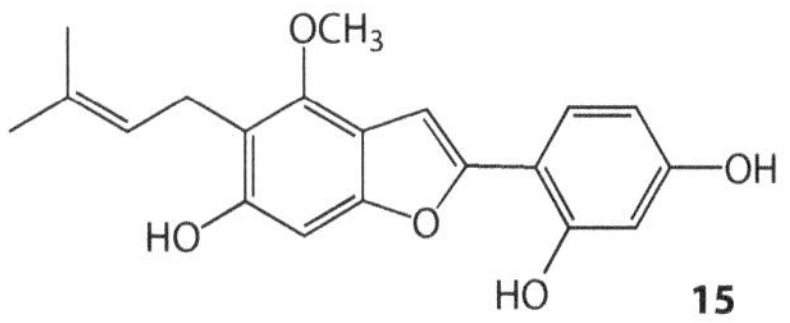

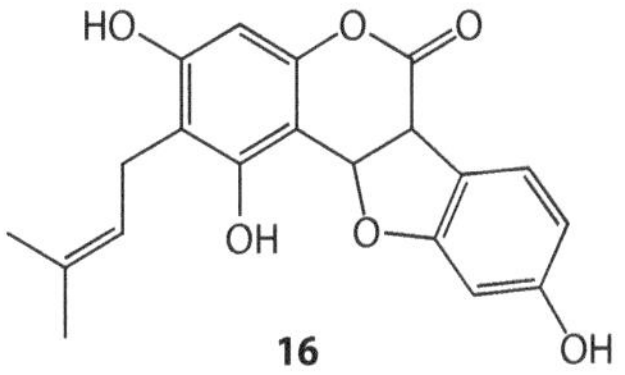

The herb Gan Cao (Liquorice root) is one of the most frequently prescribed traditional Chinese medicines, which was documented in the first Chinese materia medica entitled *Shennong Ben Cao Jing*. Its origin is the rhizomes of three Leguminosae plants, *Glycyrrhiza uralensis*, *G. inflata*, and *G. glabra*. Most of these plants grow in the semiarid sand lands of northwestern China. Autumn is the best season for the harvest of the herb, and the best quality of Gan Cao is produced in the provinces of inner Mongolia and Xinjiang.

Antitumor Constituents and Activities

Saponins, triterpenoids, and flavonoids are the major constituents isolated from Gan Cao. Some of them have been extensively explored for their biological properties, particularly, anticancer-related potentials. Due to the gentle anticarcinogenic and antitumor activities, Gan Cao and its active constituents were suggested to be used as an adjuvant agent in therapeutic prescriptions and cancer prevention.

Saponins

Glycyrrhizic acid (**1**) (= Glycyrrhizin) is one of the major saponins in Gan Cao, which showed broad anticarcinogenic, antimutational, and antineoplastic functions in *in vivo* and *in vitro* experiments. The treatment with glycyrrhizic acid (**1**) was capable of suppressing various carcinogenesis *in vivo*, such as DMBA plus phorbol 12-myristate 13-acetate (PMA)-elicited melanoma, dimethylhydrazine-caused mouse carcinoma, and MNNG-induced duodenal adenocarcinoma in mouse models.[1] A daily diet containing glycyrrhizic acid (**1**) to rats notably restrained AFB1-induced and diacetamidofluorene-promoted hepatomagenesis via the inhibition of AFB1-induced oxidative stress, the reduction of metabolic activation of hepatotoxin, and the enhancement of detoxifier enzyme activities to protect the hepatocytes.[1,2] Similarly, glycyrrhizic acid (**1**) also suppressed the hepatomagenesis initiated by diethylnitrosamine and promoted by diacetamidofluorene and protect the hepatocytes from the hepatotoxicity and carcinogenesis caused by polyoxidated biphenyls and methylaminoazobenzene, *in vivo*. At its best dose of 432 mg/kg, the incidence of hepatomagenesis was lessened by glycyrrhizic acid (**1**) from 64% to 21%. Concurrently, the level of v-glutamyltranspetidase increased in the liver by the oncogens was obviously diminished and the damaged DNA was restored to normal level by the treatment.[1]

The antineoplastic activity of glycyrrhizic acid (**1**) has been confirmed by various *in vitro* and *in vivo* assays against several carcinoma cells such as human lines, MCF-7 (breast), SGC-7901 (stomach), PGCL3 (lung), LNCaP, and DU-145 (prostate), and mouse lines: B16 melanoma and submaxillary gland fibrosarcoma, in concentration- and/or time-dependent manner.[1] At a concentration of 1 mg/mL, glycyrrhizic acid (**1**) exerted noticeable antitumor effect on human HeLa (cervix), Bcap-37 (breast), and MGC-803 (stomach) neoplastic cell lines with inhibitory rates of 79.71%, 76.37%, and 71.06%, respectively, but only 24.29% on Bel-7404 hepatoma cells.[3–5] The treatment with glycyrrhizic acid (**1**) not only inhibited the proliferation of the Bel-7402 cells *in vitro* with IC_{50} 3.94 mM but also induced the cell apoptosis and the differentiation at its 5 mM concentration.[6] The treatment could trigger a protective autophagy by the activation of ERK in HepG2 hepatoma, which might attenuate the anticancer effects of glycyrrhizic acid (**1**).[7] Moreover, 0.5 and 1 mM concentrations of glycyrrhizic acid (**1**) could elicit both apoptosis and differentiation of PGCL3 lung carcinoma cells, and it also restrained the invasion of PGCL3 cells.[5] The apoptosis of MCF-7 cells induced by a 7.5 mM concentration of glycyrrhizic acid (**1**) was found to be mediated by marked decrease of intracellular Ca^{2+} level.[8] In the B16 cells and submaxillary gland fibrosarcoma cells, their cell cycle progression was arrested from G1 phase to S phase, thereby exerting antiproliferative effect after being treated with glycyrrhizic acid (**1**).[9] Giving glycyrrhizic acid (10 mg/kg) to tumor-bearing mice four times every two days obviously attenuated the pulmonary metastasis of B16-F10 cells, where the effect was found to be regulated by counteracting tumor-associated T helper-type 2 cells and activating $CD4^+$, $CD28^+$, and $TCR\alpha/\beta^+$ T cells.[10] Moreover, glycyrrhizic acid (**1**) could reduce Kaposi sarcoma-associated herpes virus latency and terminate the latent KSHV infection in transformed B lymphocytes, then it enhanced G1 cell arrest and apoptotic death of the KSHV-infected tumor cells concomitant with the descent of LANA levels and the stimulation of p53 activation, ROS increase and mitochondrial dysfunction.[4]

Additionally, glycyrrhizic acid (**1**) is a marked immunoregulator, being able to provoke the production of IFN and $CD4^+$ T cells and to enhance the activities of NK cells and macrophage, thereby augmenting the host immune system.[11] Therefore, by prominent immunoregulation, glycyrrhizic acid (**1**) potentiated the activity of anticancer drugs and attenuated the toxic/side effects caused by these drugs. Continuous gavage of glycyrrhizic acid (**1**) in doses of 50 and 100 mg/kg to mice prolonged the lifetime of mice implanted with ascites hepatoma cells, diminished the tumor weight of mice transplanted with entity solid hepatoma, and also notably potentiated the activities of VCR and CTX. Simultaneously, it enhanced the hematopoietic recovery that was damaged by CTX.[12] The studies also demonstrated that glycyrrhizic acid (**1**) was capable of increasing the level of cisplatin in multidrug-resistant hepatoma Huh-7 cells, thereby reversing the cisplatin-caused drug resistance and inhibiting the viability of Huh-7 cells.[13]

Two salts of the major saponin, i.e., diammonium glycyrrhizinate and monoammonium glycyrrhizinate, are commercially employed in pharmaceutical industry and clinics. Both were reported to have the antiproliferative activity against several neoplastic cells in the investigations.

Triterpenoids

Glycyrrhetinic acid (**2**) is the aglycone of glycyrrhizic acid (**1**), which has two isomers, i.e., 18β-glycyrrhetinic acid (**2a**) and 18α-glycyrrhetinic acid (**2b**). By the same mechanism as glycyrrhizic acid (**1**), glycyrrhetinic acid (**2**) exerted the antiproliferative effect against the Bel-7402 and PGCL3 cells, but the effect was much greater than that of glycyrrhizic acid (**1**).[5] By blockage of the cell cycle progression from G1 to S phase and augmentation of melanogenesis, glycyrrhetinic acid (**2**) retarded the growth of B16 melanoma cells.[9] Similarly, by eliciting of G0/G1 cell arrest by activating p21 and p27 expressions, 18β-glycyrrhetinic acid (**2a**) was effective in the suppression of human BGC-823 gastric cancer and human HT-29 colon carcinoma.[14,15] Also, glycyrrhetinic acid (**2**) demonstrated the inhibitory effect against human K562 and HL-60 leukemia cells and SK-MEL-1 melanoma cells *in vitro* and against rat myeloma *in vivo*.[16,17] The antileukemia activity in the K562 cells was found to be associated with the blockage of a linkage between ATP and angiotensin-II.[18,19] The proliferation of AD human LNCap prostate cancer cells could be repressed by glycyrrhetinic acid (**2**), but it was not effective to AI human PC3 and DU145 prostate cancer cell lines.[20]

Moreover, through multiple pathways, glycyrrhetinic acid (**2**) could enhance the apoptosis of various tumor cells. 18β-Glycyrrhetinic acid (**2a**) dose-dependently augmented the apoptosis of Bel-7402 and HepG2 hepatoma cells and PGCL3 lung cancer cells.[6,21,22] The apoptosis of MCF-7 breast cancer cells elicited by 18β-glycyrrhetinic acid (**2a**) was trigged by the largely increased Ca^{2+} level in the cells.[23] The increase of ROS level was an important step in the apoptotic progression of four types of human tumor cell lines (HLE hepatoma, HL-60 leukemia, KATO-III gastric cancer, and SiHa cervical cancer) induced by glycyrrhetinic acid (**2**).[24–26] By associating the inactivation of MMP-2 and MMP-9, it was able to restrain the invasion of SK-MEL-1 melanoma cells and K562 and HL-60 leukemia cells.[16,17] Similarly, 18β-glycyrrhetinic acid (**2a**) declined cathepsin-B secretion to obstruct the adhesion, the migration, and the invasion of highly metastasized PGCL3 lung cancer cells.[22] The P-gp in human KB-C2 oral epithelial carcinoma was also lessened by glycyrrhetinic acid (**2**). The inactivation of P-gp and MRP-1 by glycyrrhetinic acid (**2**) augmented the levels of chemotherapeutic drugs in the neoplastic cells, thereby overcoming the MDRs.[27] Moreover, 18β-glycyrrhetinic acid (**2a**) and glycyrrhetinic acid (**2**) also has the ability to elicit the differentiation of Bel-7402 cells and K562 cells.[3,28]

In recent years, several triterpenoid glucuronides were separated from Gan Cao (*G. uralensis*). They showed no cytotoxicity on the tested cancer cell lines, but four aglycones derived from the three saponins exerted selective and moderate inhibitory effect against human HeLa cervical carcinoma and MCF-7 breast cancer cell lines *in vitro*. One of the aglycones was identified as glycyrrhetinic acid (**2**), which displayed moderate suppressive effect against the HeLa and MCF-7 cells *in vitro* with IC_{50} values of 15.5 and 11.4 μM, respectively, but other two, 29-carboxylglabrolide (**3**) and 24-glycyrrhetic acid (**4**) showed lower activities on Hela cells (IC_{50}: 35.3 and 19.9 μM) and MCF-7 cells 38.5 and 20.5 μM), respectively.[29] Furthermore, a PEG derivative of 18β-glycyrrhetinic acid was synthesized through its C-20 carboxyl group that was coupled with $PEG\text{-}NH_2$ by an amide bond. This derivative, having 280 times higher water solubility than its parent molecule, displayed the equal potency in the inhibition of B16 melanoma cells.[30] Sodium glycyrrhetinate was demonstrated to be greater than other chemotherapeutic drugs (VCR and MTX) with no serious side effect in the suppression of colorectal cancer, cervical cancer, and bladder cancer.[30,31] Thus, sodium glycyrrhetinate is employed as an antitumor agent in Chinese clinics.

Moreover, glycyrrhetinic acid (**2**) showed great chemopreventive effect against the carcinogenesis caused by various chemical oncogens and promoters.[32,33] DMBA plus TPA-caused skin carcinogenesis in a mouse model was inhibited by 60% and 80%, respectively, after being treated with 18β-glycyrrhetinic acid (**2a**) and 18α-glycyrrhetinic acid (**2b**) for 16 weeks.[10] In addition, a different type of triterpene termed betulinic acid was isolated from the roots of *G. uralensis*, which exhibited moderate suppressive effect against SKOV-3 (ovary), A498 (kidney), A549 (lung), and HCT15 (colon) cancer cell lines (IC_{50}: 2.7–4.8 μM).[34]

Flavonoid Extracts

The total flavones of Gan Cao at a 200 μg/mL concentration demonstrated obvious inhibitory effect on four kinds of human neoplastic cell lines, Bcap-37 (breast), HeLa (cervix), Bel-7404 (liver), and MGC-803 (stomach) cells, *in vitro*, together with the induction of the cell apoptosis. Its inhibitory rates were 79.55%, 79.98%, 67.91%, and 37.86%, respectively.[3] The administration of Glycyrrhiza flavonoids to tumor-bearing mice at a dose of 11.25 mg/kg obviously restrained the duplication and the synthesis of DNA and RNA in sarcoma 180 cells and H22 hepatoma cells.[35] A total flavonoid extract (LTFs) of *G. inflate*, which was obtained by an ultrasonic wave method, exerted *in vitro* inhibitory effect on human SiHa cervical cancer cells.[36] Additionally, G9315 was a six flavonoid complex extracted from *G. inflate*. At a dose of 2 mg, G9315 exerted noticeable antipromoting effect on two-stage mouse skin carcinogenesis induced by DMBA and promoted by croton oil *in vivo*, whereas at a 10 μg/mL dose, it restrained croton oil-caused chemiluminescence of polymorphonuclear leukocyte in Wistar rats. G9315 could also repress TPA-enhanced 32Pi incorporation into phospholipid fraction in the HeLa cells and markedly obstruct cytoxan-caused micronucleus formation of the mouse bone marrow. Moreover, G9315 at its doses of 10–20 μg/mL inhibited the LPO of mouse liver mitochondria induced by croton oil and of liver microsome induced by CCl4. These evidences proved that the G9315 and the Glycyrrhiza flavonoids may be used as antimutagenic, anticarcinogenic, and antioxidant agents for the prevention of malignant tumorigenesis.[37–39] Phytochemistry studies combined with biological activity have further revealed that chalcones and isoflavones are two important types of Glycyrrhiza flavonoids being responsible for antitumor and antitumorigenic activities.

Isoflavones

HEGU was an extract of Gan Cao, which contained isoangustone -A (**5**), licorcidin (**6**), and other isoprene-linked isoflavones or isoflavans, but it had no detectable glycyrrhizic acid. In *in vitro* models with human DU-145 prostate cancer cells or mouse 4T1 breast tumor cells, HEGU and isoangustone-A (**5**) dose-dependently diminished DNA synthesis and induced G1 phase arrest via the reduction of the levels of CDK2 and CDK4 and the decline the levels of cyclin-D1 and cyclin-A. During the induction of apoptosis of androgen-insensitive DU-145 cells by isoangustone-A (**5**), the expressions of Fas, DR4, cleaved caspase-8, and Mcl-1S were augmented, the mitochondrial membrane depolarization and the cytochrome c release were elicited, and caspase-9, caspase-7, caspase-3, and PARP were activated, showing that these events are involved in the intrinsic apoptosis pathway and the DR4 activation importantly contributing to the apoptotic promotion.[40,41] In SW480 human colorectal adenocarcinoma cells, isoangustone-A (**5**) promptly inhibited the cell viability in time- and concentration-dependent manners and activated caspase-dependent apoptosis by disrupting mitochondrial functions.[42] Isoangustone-A (**5**) significantly blocked cell cycle progression at G1 phase in human SK-MEL-28 melanoma cells via the down-expression of G1 phase regulatory proteins (cyclin-D1 and cyclin-E) and suppressed the cell proliferation by targeting PI3K, MKK4, and MKK7 in both cultured and xenograft mouse models.[43]

Furthermore, in the association with a series of events such as marked retardation of the secretion and activation of MMP-2 and MMP-9, reduction of TIMP-1 and integrin-α2 protein level, and up-expression of TIMP-2, HEGU exerted the dose-dependent inhibitory effect against basal and epidermal growth factor-induced cell migration, invasion, and adhesion of the DU-145 cells.[44] Lupiwighteone, another isolated isoflavonoid from Gan Cao, showed the antigrowth effect against human DU-145 prostate carcinoma cells and HUVECs in dose- and time-dependent manners, whose effect was accompanied by the induction of cell cycle arrest and apoptosis. The data proved the anticancer and antiangiogenesis potentials of Lupiwighteone.[45]

Chalcones

In Gan Cao, chalcones were the second most important components for the anticancer properties. Several chalcones were separated from the herb and were evaluated in the *in vitro* models for its anticancer-related activities. Laicochalcone-A (**7**) and laicochalcone-E (**8**) separated from the LTFs acted as inhibitors of Topo-I to exert moderate inhibition against different human A549 and Calu-1 (lung), HCT-15 (colon), SKOV-3 (ovary), SK-MEL-2 (skin) carcinoma cell lines, and HT1080 fibrosarcoma cells.[46–48] The treatment of human PC3 AI prostate cancer cells with licochalcone-A (**7**) elicited the G2/M-arrest of cell cycle progression in correlation with the reticence of cyclin-B1 and CDC2 activities and then induced modest level of apoptosis.[49] Licochalcone-A (**7**) induced intrinsic and extrinsic apoptoses of FaDu HNSCCs via ERK1/2 and p38 phosphorylation-mediated TRAIL expression[50] and elicited the apoptosis of HepG2 human hepatoma cells through ER stress via phospholipase Cγ1-, Ca^{2+}-, and ROS-dependent pathways.[51] Through the downregulation of Sp1 expression and the subsequent regulation of Sp1 downstream proteins such as p27, p21, cyclin-D1, Mcl-1, and survivin, licochalcone-A (**7**) enhanced the apoptotic death of oral squamous cell carcinoma cell lines (NH22 and HSC4).[52] The antiinvasive and antimetastatic effects of licochalcone-A (**7**) were demonstrated in human A549 and H460 (lung) and SCC-25 (oral) cancer cells, whose mechanisms were revealed to be mediated by the inactivation of Akt signaling pathway with the down-expression of MMP-1 and MMP-3 in the A549 cells and by the down-expression of MMP-2, NF-κB, and N-cadherin and the up-expression of TIMP-2 and E-cad in the SCC-25 cells.[53,54] The oral gavage of licochalcone-E (**8**) in doses of 7 or 14 mg/kg per day for 25 days repressed the growth and the lung metastasis of 4T1 mammary orthotopic cancer cells with stimulated apoptosis, whose effects in the 4T1 cells were found to be associated by multiple pathways: (1) reduction of the expressions of Ki67, cyclins, and CDKs; (2) decrease of Bcl-2 expression and increase of Bax expression and cleaved caspase-3; (3) decline of VEGF-A and VEGF -C, VEGFR-2, and lymphatic vessel endothelial receptor-1 expressions; (4) reduction of CD31, CD45, COX-2 levels, iNOS, and HIF-α activities. Concurrently, the levels of proinflammatory cytokines and angiogenesis/metastasis-related proteins were attenuated in the lung tissues as well.[55] The migration and the invasion of human MDA-MB-231 breast carcinoma cells were also dose-dependently obstructed by licochalcone-E (**8**), whose effects was found to be associated with (1) inhibited MMP-9 secretion, urokinase-type plasminogen activator, and VEGF-A; (2) stimulated secretion of tissue inhibitor of MMP-2; and (3) obstructed the tube formation of vascular endothelial cells.[55] Similarly, the *in vitro* and *in vivo* tests with HUVECs and CT-26 colon carcinoma revealed that the antitumor effect of licochalcone-A (**7**) may be attributed, in part, to the decrease of angiogenesis by the blockage of VEGF/VEGFR-2 signalings.[56]

Isoliquiritigenin (**9**), another bioactive chalcone isolated from Gan Cao, showed prominent suppressive effects against various cancer cells. It was capable of reducing the proliferation of human DU-145 and LNCap (prostate), HeLa, SiHa, and CaSki (cervix), and A549 and NCI-H187 (lung) cancer cell lines in a dose-dependent manner.[58–60] The IC_{50} values in the CaSki and NCI-H187 cells were 19.3 μmol/L and 16.6 μg/mL, respectively, whose potencies were greater than in the HeLa and SiHa cells. The inhibitory effect on CaSki cells was found to be accompanied by the induction of S and G2/M cell cycle arrest via the decreases of P34cdc2 phosphorylation and cyclin-B1 expression and of caspase-dependent apoptosis via the down-expression of HPV16 E6 and the increase of p53 and p21 levels.[61,62] Besides the blockage of the cell cycle progression at G2/M stage, isoliquiritigenin (**9**) also elicited the A549 cell apoptosis to exert its antiproliferative effect.[63] The apoptosis and the cell cycle arrest of human hepatoma HepG2 cells were promoted by isoliquiritigenin (**9**) via a p53-dependent pathway.[64] Through the downregulation of the arachidonic acid metabolic network and the deactivation of PI3K/Akt, isoliquiritigenin (**9**) induced growth inhibition and apoptosis in human MCF-7 and MDA-MB-231 breast cancer cels.[65] Notably, the antigrowth and proapoptotic effects were confirmed in nude mice xenografted with MDA-MB-231 breast cancer, together with lessened intratumoral levels of eicosanoids and phospho-Akt (Thr308).[65] The treatment of with isoliquiritigenin (**9**) amplified the apoptotic rates in human MGC-823 gastric cancer cells and human uterine leiomyoma cells, thereby retarding the cell proliferation.[66,67] COX-2 was found to play an important role for the induction of apoptosis in the isoliquiritigenin (**9**)-treated colorectal cancer cells.[68] Moreover, the isoliquiritigenin (**9**) treatment was able to hinder the pulmonary metastasis of mouse renal cancer cells *in vivo* without any weight loss or leukocytopenia and also to prevent severe leukocytopenia caused by 5-FU.[69] More evidences further proved isoliquiritigenin (**9**) to have obvious abilities in the activation of macrophages and the facilitation of cytotoxicity of lymphocytes.[69] Due to the immunopotentiating properties, isoliquiritigenin (**9**) could prevent the toxicity caused by chemotherapeutic agents in the kidney and the liver in an animal model implanted with colon cancer.[70]

Furthermore, the four flavonoids from Glycyrrhiza i.e., isoliquiritigenin (**9**), isoliquiritin (**10**), liquiritigenin, and liquiritin were investigated for their antimigration and antiangiogenesis. In a same concentration of 60 μM, all the flavonoids restrained the cell migration via diminished MMP-2 and VEGF secretions, where the contribution for the antiangiogenesis and the antimigration was isoliquiritigenin (**9**) $\gg$ liquiritigenin > isoliquiritin (**10**) > liquiritin, and the IC_{50} value of isoliquiritigenin (**9**) was 40.3 μM.[71]

Flavanes

Glabridin (**11**), a major active flavonoid in *G. glabra*, is a phytoestrogen. It can bind to the human estrogen receptor and exert estrogen-like functions. Thus, at concentrations of >15 μM, glabridin (**11**) inhibited the proliferation of breast cancer cells in an estrogen receptor-independent manner, but at concentrations of <10 μM, it exhibited estrogen receptor-dependent growth-promoting effect.[72] More evidences disclosed that glabridin (**11**) was able to attenuate the tumor growth, the mesenchymal characteristics, and the CSC-like properties in the breast cancer cells via demethylation-activated miR-148a.[73] In four AML cell lines (HL-60, MV4-11, U937, and THP-1), glabridin (**11**) obviously obstructed the cell proliferation and induced the apoptosis of HL-60 cells in dose- and time-dependent manners via p38 MAPK and JNK1/2 pathways, caspases activation, and PARP cleavage.[74] The studies also demonstrated that glabridin (**11**) at a 10 μM concentration had no inference on the cell viability, but it could repress the cell migration and the invasion of human A549 NSCLC cells, human MDA-MB-231 breast cancer cells and HUVECs *in vitro*. By inhibiting the FAK/rho signaling pathway, glabridin (**11**) in a 10 μM concentration effectively retarded the angiogenesis of A549 cancer and MDA-MB-231 cancer in both cell culture and nude mice models.[75,76] Moreover, glabridin (**11**), at a concentration range of 25–250 μg/mL, showed significant inhibitory effect on the proliferation of human Bel-7402 hepatoma cells, whose maximum inhibitory rate was up to 90.11%.[77] Glabridin (**11**) was also able to inhibit the migration/invasion capacities of hepatoma cell lines (Huh7 and Sk-Hep-1), even if it had low cytotoxicity *in vitro* at high concentrations, whose antiinvasive effect was associated with the down-expression of MMP-9, the inhibition of NF-κB and AP-1 signaling pathways and ERK1/2 and JNK1/2 phosphorylations, and the up-expression of TIMP-1. An *in vivo* experiment further confirmed that the administration of glabridin effectively suppressed the hepatoma formation.[78] Therefore, glabridin (**11**) may be a potential agent, which is beneficial to the treatment and the prevention of lung cancer, breast cancer, and hepatoma in three ways i.e., inhibition of migration, invasion, and angiogenesis.

Moreover, icoricidin (**6**) as well as 5,7,4′-trihydroxy-6,8-diprenylisoflavone, which were isolated from the EtOAc extract of Gan Cao, were also active in inhibiting mouse LA795 lung adenocarcinoma cells *in vitro*.[79] Glabridin (**11**) as well as 18β-glycyrrhetinic acid (**2a**) are also potent antioxidants. Both were reported to show protective activity against direct and indirect oxidative DNA fragmentations caused by UVB radiation to avoid the apoptosis increase of human keratinocyte, evidencing that both molecules are capable of reducing sunlight-induced skin cancer.[80]

Flavones

Two prenylated flavones, glabrol (**12**) and licoflavonol (**13**), were discovered from the fractionation of *G. uralensis* roots. Both, in an *in vitro* assay, moderately obstructed the proliferation of SKOV-3 (ovary), A498 (kidney), A549 (lung), and HCT15 (colon) cancer cell lines (respective IC_{50}: 2.8–4.8 μM and 9.3–12.3 μM), whose activities of glabrol (**12**) were greater than those of the isolated isoflavones and chalcones, such as isoangustone-A (**5**) (IC_{50}: 7.7–10.9 μM), licochalcone-A (**7**) (IC_{50}: 2.8–8.1 μM), isoliquiritigenin (**9**) (IC_{50}: 8.4–18.1 μM) and phaseoluteone (IC_{50}: 3.4–8.7 μM), but similar to those of betulinic acid (**14**) (IC_{50}: 2.7–4.8 μM), on the four human cancer cell lines.[34]

Coumarine

A 70% methanol soluble fraction derived from the acetone extract of *G. glabra* exhibited the inhibitory activity against the proliferation of human U937 monoblastic leukemia cells together with the promotion of apoptosis. High performance liquid chromatography (HPLC) separation led to finding a bioactive coumarine identified as licocoumarone (**15**), which was found to have the ability to stimulate the apoptotic death of U937 cells *in vitro*.[81] By the induction of G0/G1 cell cycle arrest, apoptosis, and defective autophagy, the isolated glycyrol (**16**) showed moderate cytotoxic effect against AGS (gastric) and HCT116 (colon) human colon cell lines (IC_{50}: 23.0 and 21.0 μM, respectively). But it was inactive or weak to MDA-MB-231, MCF-7, and T47D human breast cancer cell lines, Chang human normal hepatic cells, and MRC5 human normal lung fibroblast cells. The proapoptotic mechanism in the AGS and HCT116 cells was revealed to be mediated by both extrinsic and intrinsic pathways including JNK/p38 MAPKs and AMRP activations and caspase activation. The *in vivo* anticancer activity of glycyrol (**16**) was further proven in a nude mice model xenografted HCT 116 cells. The treatment with 10 mg/kg glycyrol lessened the tumor volume and the tumor weight without obvious toxicology and body weight change.[82]

Polysaccharides

The Glycyrrhiza polysaccharide component is mainly composed of glucan, rhamnose, arabinose, and galactose, but its backbone structure has not been finally determined. The polysaccharides showed no *in vitro* suppression on human SGC-7901 gastric cancer cells, but it could lengthen the life duration of mice bearing ascites tumor and restrain the growth of solid tumor cells *in vivo*. Glycyrrhiza polysaccharide was also demonstrated to have prominent immunoregulative functions such as the activation of macrophage, the augmentation of NK cell activity, the induction of IL-1 and IFN secretion, the increase of lymphocyte proliferation, etc. The treatment with the polysaccharides in a large dose provoked sarcoma 180 cell degeneration and necrosis in the tumor marginal division.[83,84] By influencing P53/PI3K/AKT pathways, the polysaccharides dose-dependently promoted the apoptosis of hepatoma cells *in vivo* and inhibited the proliferation of Bel7402 hepatoma cells *in vitro* in a dose-dependent manner.[85] According to the affirmative results, Glycyrrhiza polysaccharides may be recommended to be used as a supplement for synergistical suppression of tumor cells, reduction of chemotherapy-caused toxicity, and improvement of patient's life quality and survival time.

Other Medical Uses

The herb Gan Cao (Liquorice root) is utilized in various Chinese herb prescriptions for the treatment of many ailments including asthma, canker sores, chronic fatigue, depression, emphysema, gingivitis, gout, HIV and viral infections, fungal infections, ulcers, liver problems, menopause, psoriasis, tendinitis, prostate enlargement, tuberculosis, and arthritis. However, the administration of Gan Cao with large doses in short terms or normal doses in long terms would cause some side effects, leading to hypokalemia and serious increases in blood pressure. Thus, Gan Cao must be used carefully for aged patients and patients suffering angiocardiopathy and/or renal disease.

References

1. Zhang, M. F. et al. 2010. Antitumor activity of Glycyrrhizic acid. *Shanghai Med.* 31: 492–5.
2. Chan, H. T. et al. 2003. Inhibition of glycyrrhizic acid on aflatoxin B1-induced cytotoxicity in hepatoma cells. *Toxicol.* 188: 211–7.
3. Huang, W. et al. 2003. Studies on differentiation and apoptosis of human hepatocarcinoma cells induced by all trans-retinoic acid, 18β-glycyrrhetinic acid and Glycyrrhizin. *Chin. J. Integr. Tradit. Western Med. on Liver Diseases* 13: 148–50.
4. Ma, M. et al. 2008. Comparison in anti-proliferative effects of active components from *Glycyrrhiza uralensis* on four kinds of human cancer cells. *Shizhen Guoyi Guoyao* 19: 9–11.
5. Curreli, F. et al. 2005. Glycyrrhizic acid alters Kaposi sarcoma-associated herpesvirus latency, triggering p53-mediated apoptosis in transformed B lymphocytes. *J. Clin. Investigation* 115: 642–52.
6. Huang, W. et al. 2003. Studies on mechanism of proliferative and invasive inhibition of glycyrrhizin on human lung cancer cells. *J. Modern Clin. Med. Bioengin.* 9: 174–6.
7. Tang, Z. H. et al. 2014. Glycyrrhetinic acid triggers a protective autophagy by activation of extracellular regulated protein kinases in hepatocellular carcinoma cells. *J. Agricul. Food Chem.* 62: 11910–6.
8. Zhang, Z. L. et al. 2004. Proliferative inhibition and apoptotic induction effect of glycyrrhizin on human breast carcinoma cells. *Practical J. Cancer* 19: 16–18.
9. Chen, X. M. et al. 2006. Study on relationship between glycyrrhizin-induced apoptosis and intracellular Ca^{2+} concentration in human breast carcinoma cells. *China J. Modern Med.* 16: 3729–32.

10. Kobayashi, M. et al. 2002. Inhibitory effect of Glycyrrhizin on experimental pulmonary metastasis in mice inoculated with B16 melanoma. *Anticancer Res.* 22: 4053–8.
11. Wang, Z. Y. et al. 1991. Inhibition of mutagenicity in *Salmonella typhimurium* and skin tumor initiating and tumor promoting activities in SENCAR mice by glycyrrhetinic acid: Comparison of 18α- and 18β-stereoisomers. *Carcinogen.* 12: 187–92.
12. Li, C. X. et al. 1996. Antitumor activity of Glycyrrhizin and its toxicity. *J. Guiyang Med. College* 21: 183–5.
13. Wakamatsu, T. et al. 2007. The combination of Glycyrrhizin and lamivudine can reverse the cispatin resistance in hepatocellular carcinoma cells through inhibition of multidrug resistance-associated proteins. *Intl. J. Oncol.* 31: 1465–72.
14. Wang, Y. H. et al. 2007. Inhibition of 18β-glycyrrhetinic acid on proliferation of human BGC823 gastric carcinoma cell line. *J. Jiangsu Univ.* (Med. Edit.), 17: 251–3.
15. Ge, Y. et al. 2008. Study on inhibition of 18β-glycyrrhetinic acid on proliferation of human colon cancer HT29 cells. *Lishizhen Med. Materia Med. Res.* 19: 143–4.
16. Zhang, J. L. et al. 2008. Effect of glycyrrhetinic acid on invasive capacity of leukemic cells and activity of gelatinase. *Chin. J. Integrated Tradit. Western Med.* 28: 903–6.
17. Wang, Y. et al. 2009. The influence of glycyrrhitic acid on the invasiveness and expression of gelatinase in melanoma cells. *Chin. J. Dermatovenereol.* 23: 207–10.
18. Fujita, M. et al. 2002. Blockade of angiotensin AT1a receptor signaling reduces tumor growth, angiogenesis, and metastasis. *Biochem. Biophys. Res. Commun.* 294. 441–7.
19. Liu, X. Y. et al. 2005. Mechanism of inhibition of K562 leukemia cells proliferation by glycyrrhetinic acid. *Chin. J. Hospital Pharmacy* 25: 315–8.
20. Hawthorne, S. et al. 2008. Effects of glycyrrhetinic acid and liquorice extract on cell proliferation and prostate-specific antigen secretion in LNCaP prostate cancer cells. *J. Pharm. Pharmacol.* 60: 661–6.
21. Satomi, Y. et al. 2005. Glycyrrhetinic acid and related compounds induce G1 arrest and apoptosis in human hepatocellular carcinoma HepG2. *Anticancer Res.* 25: 4043–7.
22. Huang, W. et al. 2003. Studies on differentiation and apoptosis of human lung carcinoma cells induced by all trans-retinoic acid, 18β-glycyrrhetinic acid and glycyrrhizin. *China Cancer* 12: 665–7.
23. Huang, W. et al. 2006. 18β-glycyrrhetinic acid-induced apoptosis and changed intracellular Ca^{2+} concentration in human breast carcinoma cells. *China Oncol.* 16: 102–6.
24. Hibasami, H. et al. 2006. Glycyrrhetic acid induces apoptosis in human hepatoma, promyelotic leukemia and stomach cancer cells. *Intl. J. Mol. Med.* 17: 215–9.
25. Makino, T. et al. 2006. Generation of reactive oxygen species and induction of apoptosis of HL-60 cells by ingredients of traditional herbal medicine, Sho-saiko-to. *Basic Clin. Pharmacol. Toxicol.* 98: 401–5.
26. Lee, C. S. et al. 2008. 18β-Glycyrrhertinic acid induces apoptosis cell death in SiHa cells and exhibits a synergistic effect against antibiotic anticancer drug toxicity. *Life Sci.* 83: 481–9.
27. Yuan, L. B. et al. 2008. Effects of glycyrrhetinic acid on proliferation and differentiation of K562 leukemia cells. *Zhejiang Medical J.* 30: 463–5.
28. Nabekura, T. et al. 2008. Inhibition of P-glycoprotein and multidrug resistance protein 1 by dietary phytochemicals. *Cancer Chemother. Pharmacol.* 62: 867–73.
29. Zheng, Y. F. et al. 2010. Oleanane-type triterpene glucuronides from the roots of *Glycyrrhiza uralensis* Fischer. *Planta Med.* 76: 1457–63.
30. Hong, W. et al. 2006. Synthesis of a conjugate of 18β-glycyrrhetinic acid and polyethylene glycol and its in vitro antitumor activity. *J. East China Univ. of Sci. Tech.* 32: 415–7.
31. Shen, X. P. et al. 2007. Research and application of Radix Glycyrrhizae. *Asian J. Pharmacodyn. Pharmacokin.* 7: 181–200.
32. Nishino, H. et al. 1986. Glycyrrhetic acid inhibits tumor-promoting activity of teleocidin and 12-*O*-tetradecanoylphorbol-13-acetate in two-stage mouse skin carcinogenesis. *Jpn. J. Cancer Res.* 77: 33–8.
33. Agarwal, M. K. et al. 2005. Inhibiting effect of 18β-glycyrrhetinic acid in 12-*O*-tetradecanoylphorbol-13-acetate induced cutaneous oxidative stress and tumor promotion in mice. *Redox Rep.* 10: 151–7.
34. Lee, J.-E. et al. 2015. Two minor chalcone acetylglycosides from the roots extract of *Glycyrrhiza uralensis. Archiv. Pharm. Res.* 38: 1299–303.
35. Ji, Y. B. et al. 2005. Effect of Glycyrrhiza flavonoids on DNA and RNA in tumor cell of S180 and H22 tumor-bearing mice. *Zhongcaoyao* 36: 1518–20.
36. Guo, X. et al. 2013. Anticancer activity of flavonoids from Xinjiang *Glycyrrhiza inflata* Licorice on proliferation, cytotoxicity and apoptosis in cervical carcinoma cells. *J. Med. Plants Res.* 7: 173–8.
37. Fu, N. W. et al. 1995. Anti-promoting and anti-mutagenic action of G9315. *Zhongguo Yixue Kexueyuan Xuebao* 17: 349–52.
38. Fu, N. W. et al. 1995. Anti-promoting, antimutagenic and antioxidant action of Glycyrrhiza flavonoids. *Tianran Chanwu Yanjiu Yu Kaifa* 7: 29–34.
39. Fu, N. W. et al. 1995. Antipromoting tumor and antioxidant actions of G9315. *Zhongcaoyao* 26: 411–3, 422.
40. Seon, M. R. et al. 2012. Hexane/ethanol extract of *Glycyrrhiza uralensis* and its active compound isoangustone A induce G1 cycle arrest in DU145 human prostate and 4T1 murine mammary cancer cells. *J. Nutr. Biochem.* 23: 85–92.
41. Seon, M. R. et al. 2010. Isoangustone A present in hexane/ethanol extract of *Glycyrrhiza uralensis* induces apoptosis in DU145 human prostate cancer cells via the activation of DR4 and intrinsic apoptosis pathway. *Mol. Nutr. Food Res.* 54: 1329–1339.
42. Huang, W. et al. 2014. Isoangustone A induces apoptosis in SW480 human colorectal adenocarcinoma cells by disrupting mitochondrial functions. *Fitoterapia* 94: 36–47.
43. Song, N. R. et al. 2013. Isoangustone A, a novel licorice compound, inhibits cell proliferation by targeting PI3K, MKK4, and MKK7 in human melanoma. *Cancer Prev. Res.* (Phila). 6: 1293–303.
44. Park, S. Y. et al. 2010. Hexane-ethanol extract of *Glycyrrhiza uralensis* containing licoricidin inhibits the metastatic capacity of DU145 human prostate cancer cells. *British J. Nutr.* 104: 1272–82.
45. Ren, J. et al. 2015. Isoflavone lupiwighteone induces cytotoxic, apoptotic, and antiangiogenic activities in DU-145 prostate cancer cells. *Anti-Cancer Drugs* 26: 599–611.

46. Yoon, G. et al. 2007. Topoisomerase I inhibition and cytotoxicity of licochalcones A and E from Glycyrrhiza inflate. *Archiv. Pharm. Res.* 30: 313–6.
47. Han, L. Z. et al. 2013. Preparation and antitumor activities in vitro of total flavonoids from residues of Glycyrrhiza inflata and licochalcone A. *Xiandai Yaowu Yu Linchuang* 28: 668–72.
48. Yoon, G. et al. 2005. Cytotoxic allyl retrochalcone from the roots of Glycyrrhiza inflate. *Chem. Pharm. Bull.* 53: 694–5.
49. Fu, Y. et al. 2004. Licochalcone-A, a novel flavonoid isolated from licorice root (Glycyrrhiza glabra), causes G2 and late-G1 arrests in androgen-independent PC3 prostate cancer cells. *Biochem. Biophys. Res. Commun.* 322: 263–70.
50. Park, M. R. et al. 2015. Licochalcone-A induces intrinsic and extrinsic apoptosis via ERK1/2 and p38 phosphorylation-mediated TRAIL expression in head and neck squamous carcinoma FaDu cells. *Food Chem. Toxicol.* 77: 34–43.
51. Choi, A. Y. et al. 2014. Licochalcone A induces apoptosis through endoplasmic reticulum stress via a phospholipase Cγ1-, $Ca2^{+}$-, and reactive oxygen species-dependent pathway in HepG2 human hepatocellular carcinoma cells. *Apoptosis* 19: 682–97.
52. Cho, J. J. et al. 2014. Licochalcone A, a natural chalconoid isolated from Glycyrrhiza inflata root, induces apoptosis via Sp1 and Sp1 regulatory proteins in oral squamous cell carcinoma. *Intl. J. Oncol.* 45: 667–74.
53. Huang, H. C. et al. 2014. Licochalcone A inhibits the migration and invasion of human lung cancer cells via inactivation of the Akt signaling pathway with downregulation of MMP-1/-3 expression. *Tumor Biol.* 35: 12139–49.
54. Shen, H. et al. 2014. Antimetastatic effects of licochalcone A on oral cancer via regulating metastasis-associated proteases. *Tumor Biol.* 35: 7467–74.
55. Soo, J. K. 2013. Licochalcone E present in licorice suppresses lung metastasis in the 4T1 mammary orthotopic cancer model. *Cancer Prevention Res.* 6: 603–13.
56. Kim, Y. H. et al. 2010. Antiangiogenic effect of licochalcone A. *Biochem. Pharmacol.* 80: 1152–9.
57. Zhang, J. et al. 2004. Preparation of isoliquiritigenin liposome and its depressive effect on proliferation of human cervical cancer cells in vitro. *Chin. J. Clin. Pharmacol. Ther.* 9: 1268–72.
58. Kanazawa, M. et al. 2003. Isoliquiritigenin inhibits the growth of prostate cancer. *Eur. Urol.* 43: 580–6.
59. Li, T. et al. 2004. Induction of cell cycle arrest and p21 (CIPI/WAF1) expression in human lung cancer cells by isoliquiritigenin. *Cancer Lett.* 207: 27–35.
60. Khamsan, S. et al. 2012. The isolation of bioactive flavonoids from *Jacaranda obtusifolia* H. B. K. ssp. rhombifolia (G. F. W. Meijer) Gentry. *Acta Pharm.* 62: 181–90.
61. Zhang, J. et al. 2005. Inhibiting effect of isoliquiritigenin on proliferation of human cervical cancer cells in vitro and in vivo. *Chin. J. Pharmacol. Toxicol.* 19: 436–42.
62. Hirchaud, F. et al. 2013. Isoliquiritigenin induces caspase-dependent apoptosis via downregulation of HPV16 E6 expression in cervical cancer Ca Ski cells. *Planta Med.* 79: 1628–35.
63. Hsu, Y. L. et al. 2004. Isoliquiritigenin inhibits the proliferation and induces the apoptosis of human non-small cell lung cancer A549 cells. *Clin. Exp. Pharmacol. Physiol.* 31: 414–8.
64. Ya, L. H. et al. 2005. Isoliquiritigenin induces apoptosis and cell cycle arrest through p53-dependent pathway in HepG2 cells. *Life Sci.* 77: 279–92.
65. Li, Y. et al. 2013. Isoliquiritigenin induces growth inhibition and apoptosis through downregulating arachidonic acid metabolic network and the deactivation of PI3K/Akt in human breast cancer. *Toxicol. Applied Pharmacol.* 272: 37–48.
66. Kim, D. C. et al. 2008. Induction of growth inhibition and apoptosis in human uterine leiomyoma cells by isoliquiritigenin. *Reprod. Sci.* 15: 552–8.
67. Ma, J. et al. 2001. Apoptosis induced by isoliquiritigenin in human gastric cancer MGC-803 cells. *Planta Med.* 67: 754–7.
68. Tetsuyuki, T. et al. 2006. Cyclooxygenase-2 plays suppressive role for induction of apoptosis in isoliquiritigenin-treated mouse colon cancer cells. *Cancer Lett.* 231: 319–25.
69. Yamazaki, S. et al. 2002. Isoliquiritigenin suppresses pulmonary metastasis of mouse renal cell carcinoma. *Cancer Lett.* 183: 23–30.
70. Lee, C. K. et al. 2008. Isoliquiritigenin inhibits tumor growth and protects the mouse xenograft model of colon carcinoma. *J. Pharmacol. Sci.* 106: 444–51.
71. Liu, J. H. et al. 2010. Antitumor angiogenesis of four different active ingredients from Glycyrrhiza. *Xiandai Shengwuyixue Jinzhan* 10: 2731–4.
72. Tamir, S. et al. 2000. Estrogenic and antiproliferative properties of glabridin from licorice in human breast cancer cells. *Cancer Res.* 60: 5704–9.
73. Jiang, F. et al. 2015. Glabridin inhibits cancer stem cell-like properties of human breast cancer cells: An epigenetic regulation of miR-148a/SMAd2 signaling. *Mol. Carcinogenesis* 15 May 2015, DOI: 10.1002/mc.22333.
74. Huang, H. L. et al. 2014. Glabridin mediate caspases activation and induces apoptosis through JNK1/2 and p38 MAPK pathway in human promyelocytic leukemia cells. *PLoS One* 9: e98943/1-e98943/8.
75. Tsai, Y. M. et al. 2011. Glabridin inhibits migration, invasion, and angiogenesis of human non-small cell lung cancer A549 cells by inhibiting the FAK/rho signaling pathway. *Integr. Cancer Ther.* 10: 341–9.
76. Hsu, Y. L. et al. 2011. Glabridin, an isoflavan from licorice root, inhibits migration, invasion and angiogenesis of MDA-MB-231 human breast adenocarcinoma cells by inhibiting focal adhesion kinase/Rho signaling pathway. *Mol. Nutr. Food Res.* 55: 318–27.
77. Mourboul, A. et al. 2013. Anticancer activity of flavonoids from Xinjiang Glycyrrhiza glabra in human Bel-7402 hepatocarcinoma cell line. *Xinjiang Yike Daxue Xuebao* 36: 1744–8.
78. Hsieh, M. J. et al. 2014. Glabridin inhibits migration and invasion by transcriptional inhibition of matrix metalloproteinase 9 through modulation of NF-κB and AP-1 activity in human liver cancer cells. *British J. Pharmacol.* 171: 3037–50.
79. Yang, L. et al. 2009. Studies on the anticancer constituents in *Glycyrrhiza uralensis* Fisch. *Tianran Chanwu Yanjiu Yu Kaifa* 21: 438–40, 448.
80. Veratti, E. et al. 2011. 18β-glycyrrhetinic acid and glabridin prevent oxidative DNA fragmentation in UVB-irradiated human keratinocyte cultures. *Anticancer Res.* 31: 2209–15.

81. Watanabe, M. et al. 2002. Identification of licocoumarone as an apoptosis inducing component in licorice. *Biol. Pharm. Bull.* 25: 1388–90.
82. Xu, M. Y. et al. 2014. Antitumor activity of glycyrol via induction of cell cycle arrest, apoptosis and defective autophagy. *Food Chem.* 74. 311–9.
83. Xie, H. L. et al. 2011. Study progress on the pharmacological action of glycyrrigan. *Value Engineering* 30: 285.
84. Liu, S. X. 2013. Research progress in pharmacological effects of glycyrrhiza polysaccharide. *Chin. J. Veteri. Drug* 47: 64–7.
85. Chen, J. Y. et al. 2013. Glycyrrhiza polysaccharide induces apoptosis and inhibits proliferation of human hepatocellular carcinoma cells by blocking PI3K/AKT signal pathway. *Tumor Biol.* 34: 1381–9.

166 Ling Zhi 靈芝

Ganoderma or Reishi

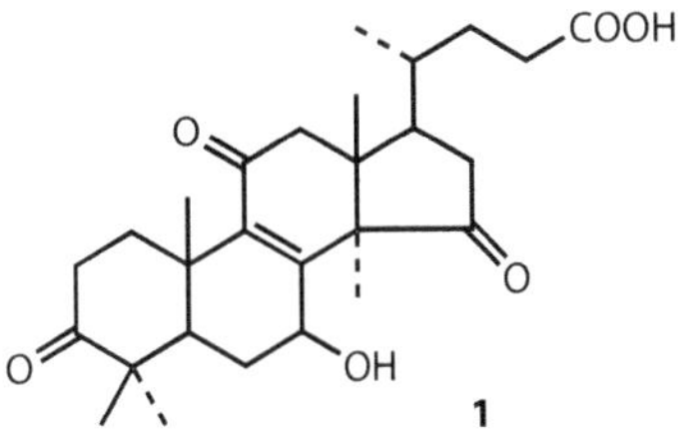

Herb Origination

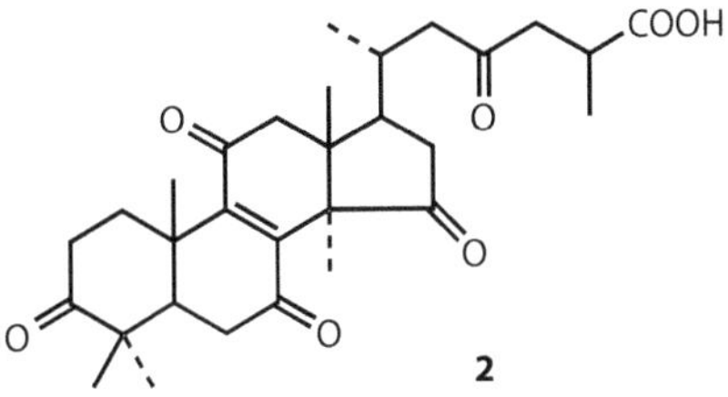

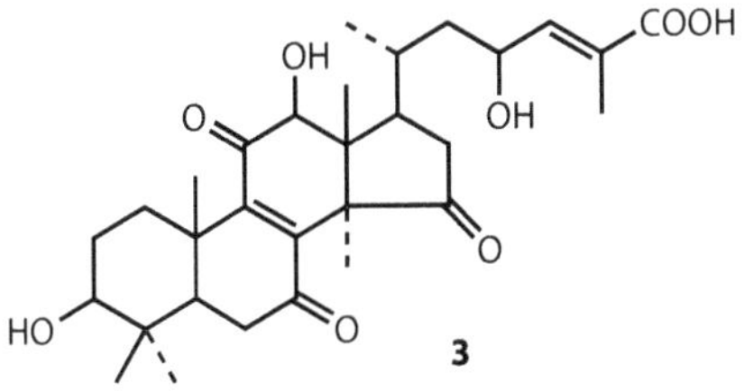

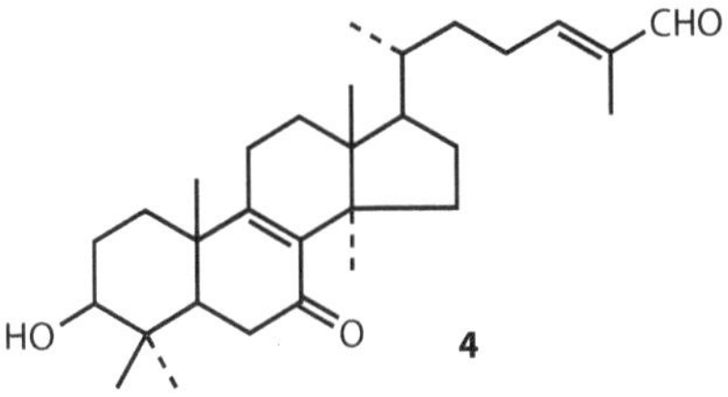

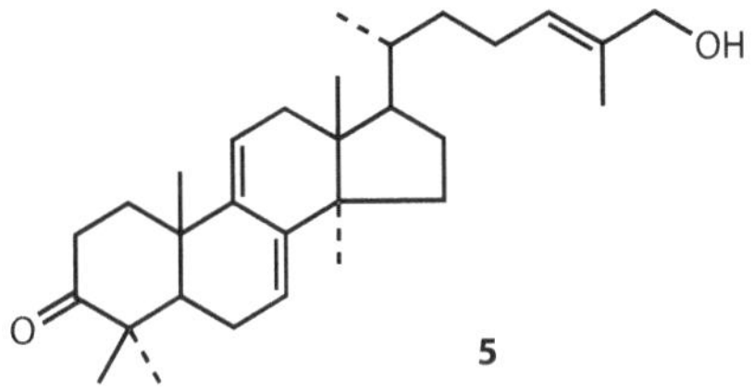

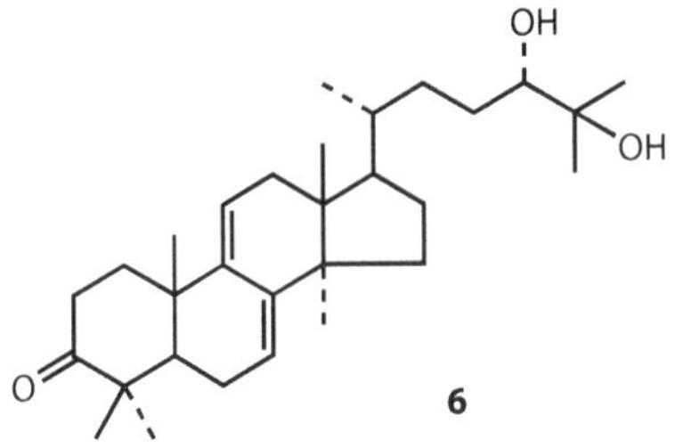

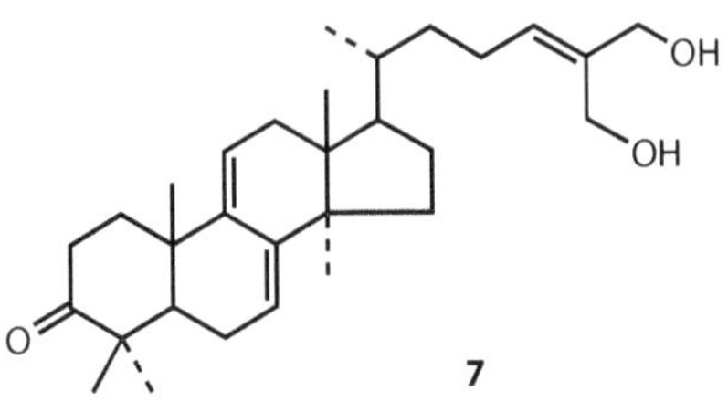

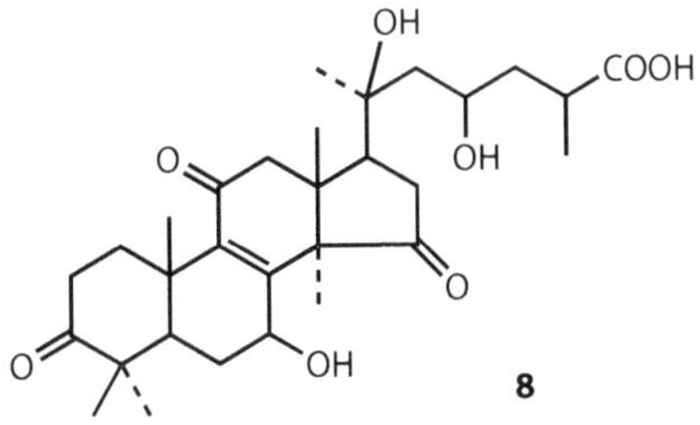

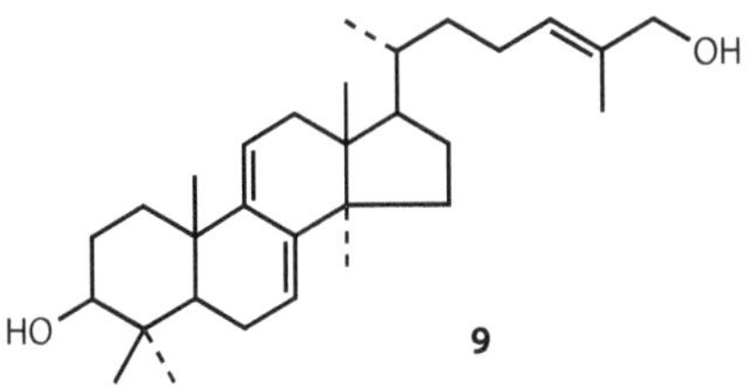

The herb Ling Zhi enjoys special veneration in east Asia for more than 4000 years, where it has been recognized as powerful medicinal fungi with remarkable health properties. Ling Zhi in today's China originated from two major Ganoderma mushrooms, *G. lucidum* and *G. sinense* (Polyporaceae). The fungi parasitize on the roots of oak and other hardwoods and appear to be kidney-shaped or circular with shiny painted purple brown color. The artificial cultivation of a variant form of Ling Zhi is used in recent years due to its bioeffects shown to be similar to those of natural Ling Zhi.

Antitumor Activities

The biological activities of Ling Zhi have been fully investigated by bioassays *in vitro* and *in vivo*, suggesting that the cancer preventive and tumoricidal properties of Ling Zhi were primarily contributed by eliciting a series of anticancer-related interactions, i.e., (1) potentiation of the host's immune functions (such as increase T and B lymphocytes, macrophages, NK cells, and antigen-presenting cells); (2) direct antiproliferation and induction of cell cycle arrest and apoptosis; (3) antiangiogenesis; (4) scavenging radicals and antioxidant; (5) induction of the cell differentiation; (6) detoxification of carcinogens and inhibition of cancer metabolic activation; and (7) activation of phase II-metabolizing enzymes.[1–3]

To human breast carcinoma cells, Ling Zhi markedly retarded the proliferation of estrogen-dependent MCF-7 cells and estrogen-independent MDA-MB-231 cells by different pathways. The effect on MDA-MB-231 cells was mainly mediated by the moderation of Akt/NF-κB signaling, i.e., inhibiting the phosphorylation of Akt on Ser473, downregulating the expressions of Akt and cyclin-D1, which were controlled by NF-κB, and reducing the activities of NF-κB and CDK4.[4] The inhibitory mechanism in MCF-7 cells was revealed to be based on the modulation of an ER-involved paythway, by downregulating c-Myc and cyclin-D1 expressions, augmenting p21/Waf1 activity and pro-apoptotic Bax expressions, directly promoting the cells to apoptosis, and restraining the growth of MCF-7 cells.[5,6] Reishi was also effective in the inhibition of inflammatory SUM-149 breast cancer cells, whose mechanism was correlated with (1) reduced expression of genes related to cell survival and proliferation (TERT, PDGFB), (2) inhibited expression of genes related to anti-apoptosis (Bcl-2, Bcl-xL, c-Myc) and enhanced IL8 expression, and (3) suppressed the expression of genes related to adhesions (E-cadherin, eIF4G), invasion and metastasis (MMP-9).[7] Also, an ethanol-soluble and acidic component (ESAC) from *G. lucidum* could exert the anti-proliferative effects on human MCF-7 and MDA-MB-231 breast cancer cell lines in both time- and concentration-dependent manners together with induction of DNA damage, G1 cell cycle arrest and apoptosis.[8] The findings substantiated Ling Zhi as a suitable herb for chemoprevention and chemotherapy of breast cancer.

Similarly, the inhibition of Ling Zhi against the proliferation and the viability of human PC3 and LNCaP prostate cancer cells was accompanied by the promotion of cell cycle arrest and apoptosis. The apoptosis of LNCaP cells was notably accelerated through an extrinsic pathway, i.e., upregulation of Bax expression, activation of caspase-8 and caspase-3, and decrease of cyclin-D1 expression, resulting in the antiproliferative effect against the LNCaP cells by the Ling Zhi.[9,10] In the PC3 cells, Ling Zhi diminished the expressions of Cdc2, cyclin-B and cyclin-D1 and upregulated p21 expression, leading the cell cycle arrest at G2/M phase.[9,10] Ling Zhi simultaneously interfered with the AR function via the competition with the natural ligand dihydrotestosterone and suppression of AR/androgen response element complex formation. By these events, Ling Zhi displayed the antiproliferative effect against the PC3 cells. Ling Zhi also exerted the inhibitory effect against prostate cancer-dependent angiogenesis in the PC3 cells as well as against morphogenesis of the human aortic endothelial cells, by modulating MAPK and Akt signaling, diminishing the secretion of VEGF and transforming growth factor (TGF)-β1 and the phosphorylation of Erk1/2 and Akt kinases, and reducing AP-1 activity.[10] Furthermore, due to its inhibitory effects on angiogenesis and NF-κB-regulated u-PA and u-PA receptor, Ling Zhi was also capable of repressing the cell migration of these highly invasive human breast and prostate cancer cells.[9,11,12]

Both the unboiled aqueous extract and the methanol extract/semipurified fraction from Reishi demonstrated cytotoxic and caspase-3-involved apoptosis-inducing effects in an *in vitro* model with IL-3-dependent lymphoma cells (DA-1).[13] The ethanol-soluble and acidic component of Ling Zhi suppressed the growth of human BEL-7402 hepaoma cells, showing an IC_{50} value of 12.4 μg/mL.[14] Although Ling Zhi showed no cytotoxicity on human HT-29 colonic carcinoma cells at doses less than 10 mg/mL, it could induce the apoptosis of HT-29 cells by increasing caspase-3 activity at doses of 0.5–5 mg/mL and decreasing COX-2 mRNA expression at a 5 mg/mL concentration, as well as increasing NO production and decreasing the expressions of IL-8, macrophage inflammatory protein 1δ, VEGF and platelet-derived growth factor. The results implied that Ling Zhi only has proapoptotic and antiinflammatory activities during the early inflammation in the colon carcinoma cells.[15] Moreover, the *in vitro* antitumor property of Ling Zhi was proven in animal models with low toxicity. The growth inhibitory rates on the BEL-7402 hepatoma cells were 43.9% in a dose of 20 mg/kg/day and 74.9% in a dose of 5 mg/kg/day by peritoneal injection of the ethanol-soluble and acidic component of Ling Zhi.[14] The chloroform extract and the EtOAc extract of Sunrecome (a Ling Zhi product) could suppress the growth of MGC-803 gastric carcinoma cells by 83.1% at a concentration of 0.125 mg/mL *in vivo*.[16] The growth inhibition on murine WEHI-3 leukemia cells by Ling Zhi *in vivo* was accompanied by the increase of CD3 and CD19 levels, the decrease of Mac-3 and CD11b markers, and the promotion of activities of NK and macrophage from PBMC.[17]

Importantly, Ling Zhi demonstrated equal cytotoxicity to both drug-sensitive and drug-resistant small-cell lung carcinoma cells *in vitro*. By the elicitation of cell cycle arrest/apoptosis and the activation of caspase-3 and caspase-9, Ling Zhi significantly augmented the antiproliferative activities of chemotherapeutic agents (such as etoposide and DOX).[18] Clinical approaches further demonstrated that the life quality of 65% lung cancer patients was improved with the coadministration of Ling Zhi.[19] In a combinational therapy with cisplatin, the methanolic extract of Ling Zhi at doses of 250 and 500 mg/kg additively augmented the antitumor activity of cisplatin and also rendered notable preventive effect synchronously against cisplatin-induced nephrotoxicity and LPO through the reduction of the GSH level and the restoration of cisplatin-reduced renal antioxidant defense enzyme systems (such as SOD, catalase, GSH-Px).[20] Consequently, all these positive results substantiated that Ling Zhi and its products are helpful and promising adjuvants in the treatment of diverse forms of leukemia and solid carcinoma.

Antitumor Constituents and Activities

Two major constituents, oxygenated lanostanoid-type triterpenes and β-D-glucan-type polysaccharides discovered from Ling Zhi, were principally responsible for the significant inhibitory effect of Ling Zhi against the growth and the proliferation of neoplastic cells.

Triterpenoids

Both total triterpenoids and acidic triterpenoids prepared from the methanolic extract of Ling Zhi fruit body could restrain the growth of B16 mouse melanoma cells *in vitro* and *in vitro*, whereby the total triterpenoids exhibited stronger effect against rat C6 astrocytoma and mouse L929 fibrosarcoma cell lines, whose mechanism comprised the suppression of cell proliferation and the induction of caspase-dependent apoptosis that was mediated by upregulated p53 and downregulated Bcl-2 expressions.[21] The triterpenoid fraction also displayed the inhibitory effect against primary solid tumor growth in the spleen and against liver metastasis and secondary metastatic Lewis lung carcinoma in mice at doses of 100 and 200 mg/kg.[22] The triterpenoids markedly diminished the tumor size in nude mice implanted with human Hep3B/T2 hepatoma cells.[23] The triterpenoid fraction at 800 μg/mL concentration also inhibited Matrigel-induced angiogenesis by the repression of heparin and VEGF in an *in vivo* model, signifying that the anticarcinoma and antimetastatic effects were importantly correlated to the inhibition of angiogenesis.[22] Moreover, the triterpenoid extract derived from Ling Zhi mycelium effectively inhibited human HL-60 acute promyelocytic leukemia cell proliferation, together with the arrest of cell cycle and the induction of apoptosis,[24] and strongly restrained the growth of human Huh-7 hepatoma cells by causing a rapid decrease of PKC activity and augment of JNK and p38 MAPKs in the *in vitro* experiments.[25]

Up to now, over 120 species of oxygenated triterpenoids were discovered from the fruit body, the mycelium, and the spores of Ling Zhi. Many of the triterpenoids have been proven to possess antineoplastic and anticarcinogenic activities. Lucidenic acid A (**1**), ganoderic acid E (**2**), and lucidenic acid N exerted significant cytotoxicity against HepG2 and HepG2,2,15 hepatoma cells and P388 leukemia cells *in vitro*.[26] Lucidenic acid A (**1**) and lucidenic acid B, ganoderic acid θ (**3**) and ganoderic acid G, and ganodermanontriol noticeably suppressed the growth LLC and Meth-A fibrosarcoma cells *in vitro* (ED_{50}: 2.3–20 μg/mL),[27] whereas ganoderenic acid D was cytotoxic in HepG2, HeLa, and Caco-2 cancer cell lines (IC_{50}: 0.14–0.26 mg/mL), and ganoderic acid B exhibited 40.3% inhibition against human SKBR3 breast cancer cells at 20 μmol/L.[28,29] The cytotoxic activitiy of lucialdehyde-B and lucialdehyde-C (**4**), ganodermenonol (**5**), and ganodermanondiol (**6**) were observed in the tested tumor cells (sarcoma 180, LLC, T-47D, and Meth-A) *in vitro*.[30] Among them, the most potent cytotoxic agent was lucialdehyde-C (**4**) against the four cancer cell lines, and its ED_{50} values were 10.7, 4.7, 7.1, and 3.8 μg/mL, respectively.[30] Ganoderiol-F (**7**) markedly inhibited the growth of Lewis lung cancer cells in mice without side effect on the PBMCs,[31] and it also promoted the growth arrest of HepG2 and Huh7 hepatoma and K562 leukemia cell lines *in vitro*.[32] Ganodermenonol (**5**) and ganoderic acids displayed the inhibitory rates of as high as 64% and 70% on BEL-7402 hepatoma cells *in vitro* at doses of 1.5 and 5.0 μg/mL, respectively, and had no toxicity to normal live cells.[33–35] Compared to NCI-H460, HeLa, and U937 cell lines, 23-dihydroganoderic acid N (**8**) was rather sensitive to MCF-7 breast cancer cells *in vitro*.[17,36] The major components of Sunrecome (a Ling Zhi product) are two triterpenoric acids assigned as 3β-hydroxy-4,4,14-trimethyl-7,11,15-trioxochol-8-en-24-oic acid, and 3β-hydroxy-7,11,12,15,23-pentaoxolanost-8-en-26-oic acid. Their moderate IC_{50} values were 18.0 and 9.85 μM in P388 leukemia, 12.70 and 17.10 μM in HeLa cervical cancer, 22.0 and 51.0 μM in BEL-7402 hepatoma, and 1.5 and 42 μM in SGC-7901 gastric cancer, respectively.[37] Moreover, ganoderol-B (**9**) could repress the growth of androgen-positive human LNCaP prostate cancer cells in a murine animal model through the downregulation of AR signaling pathway as an important mechanism similar to a 5α-reductase inhibitor, which has an ability to bind to the AR to the prostate.[38]

Besides *in vitro* or *in vivo* evidences on the proliferative inhibition against tumor cells (SW620, LLC, LS180, S180) and on the mitochondria apoptosis induction in the lung cancer cells, the ganoderic acids and the methyl ester of ganoderic acid also displayed the antitumor-related immunoenhancing effect through the increase of IL-2 and NK cells to suppress the growth and the metastasis of Lewis lung carcinoma cells *in vivo*.[35,39–42] Moreover, the antitumor-promoting and antiinflammatory effects of Ling Zhi triterpenoid fraction were shown in the EBV-EA in Raji cells, and the suppressive ratios of many Ling Zhi triterpenoids reached to 94–100% against EBV-EA.[43,44] Some Ling Zhi triterpenoids such as 20-hydroxylucidenic acid N also displayed remarkably inhibitory effect against a two-stage mouse skin carcinogenesis initiated by DMBA and promoted by TPA in an *in vivo* test.[45]

Based upon the summarization, the oxygenated triterpenoids is demonstrated as one type of the major active components in Ling responsible for the antineoplastic, anticarcinogenic, and immunoenhancing activities of Ling Zhi against malignant tumor initiation and progression.

Polysaccharides

Various polysaccharides derived from Ling Zhi, in particular β-D-glucans and glycoproteins, were found to be the major active components responsible for the antineoplastic, chemopreventive and immunoenhancive activities. Although 10 mg/mL of an aqueous polysaccharide fraction of Ling Zhi showed no direct antiproliferation as evaluated *in vitro* using MCF-7 (breast), SPC-A (lung), and SMMC-7721 (liver) cancer cell lines,[46] but it caused significant *in vitro* cytotoxic effects in human tumor cell lines (CaSki, SiHa, Hep3B, HepG2, HCT116, HT-29) and promoted the apoptotic death of CaSki, HepG2, and HCT116 cells.[47] *G. lucidum* polysaccharides (GLP) could elicit the apoptosis of human acute promyelocytic leukemia NB4 cells *in vitro* via the up-expression of Egr-1, thereby restraining the proliferation of NB4 cells.[48] Two homogeneous polysaccharides (GLPL1 and GLPL3) with small molecular weights of 4100 and 5700, respectively, were prepared from the Ling Zhi fruit body. GLPL1 was composed of only glucose, while GLPL3 was composed of glucose and galactose. *In vitro* experiments exhibited that GLPL1 and GLPL3 remarkably retarded the growth of KB nasopharyngeal cancer cells, and GLPL3 also restrained the proliferation of BGC (gastric) and Caco (colon) cancer cells.[49] GLPH1, another homogeneous polysaccharide composed of glucose, galactose, and traces of mannose and fucose with a molecular weight of 45,000, was purified from the crude polysaccharides of Ling Zhi. Its suppressive effect was demonstrated *in vitro* against the growth of KB, BGC, and B16 cells.[50]

The notable *in vivo* antitumor activity of Ling Zhi polysaccharides was primarily presented in the prolongation of the life span and the inhibition of the tumor cell growth against various cancers in animal models, for instance, against P388, L1210, K562 and HL-60 leukemia, U937 and L929 lymphoma, sarcoma 180, and Lewis lung carcinoma.[51–56] The treatment of mice with the polysaccharides at doses of 20–100 mg/kg for 10 days significantly reduced the size of sarcoma 180 dose-dependently with the inhibitory rates of 32.3–84.9%.[48] The polysaccharides could also induce the apoptosis and the differentiation of U937 lymphoma cells and HL-60 leukemia cells in mice and inhibit the metastasis of fibrosarcoma to the lung.[54] Moreover, the polysaccharides could markedly potentiate the therapeutic effects in the combination with chemotherapeutic drugs (Adm, 5-FU, MTX, thioguanine, and cisplatin) or a synthetic immunomodulator (imexon).[54]

Furthermore, the antineoplastic activity of Ling Zhi polysaccharides was found to be principally attributed to the immunopotentiating responses in the host, which includes (1) activation of immune effectors (such as T cells and B cells, NK cells, spleen lymphocyte, and macrophages), (2) enhancement of phagocytic activity of primary neutrophils, and (3) promotion of biological response by binding to the membrane complement receptor-3 on immune effector cells, together with the apoptosis promotion through the increase of p38 MAPK activity and mitogenicity. These immune interactions significantly augmented the levels and the activities of cytokines (such as ILs, IFNs, TNFα, and macrophage colony-stimulating factor) and enhanced the cytotoxicities of NK cells and T lymphocyte. The simulated TNFα and IFNγ further accelerated the apoptosis of tumor cells.[46,57–66] Ling Zhi polysaccharides also inhibited the adhesion of fibrinogen to B16 and A375 melanoma cells and then enhanced the NK cytotoxicity on the melanoma cells.[67] The immunosuppression of B16-F10 melanoma cell culture supernatant (B16-F10-CS) on lymphocytes could be fully or partially antagonized by the polysaccharides, where B16-F10-CS elevated the levels of immunosuppressive IL-10, TGF-β1, and VEGF were downregulated by the treatment with polysaccharides.[68] Gl-PS, a *G. lucidum* polysaccharides, had been used in lung cancer patients, where the patient plasma-caused lymphocyte inhibition could be reversed by GI-PS.[69] Accordingly, the Ling Zhi polysaccharides were considered to have a capability to strengthen the beneficial remedy and the prevention in humans through the activation of a defense system.

In addition, a selenium-containing polysaccharide, SeGLP-1, was prepared from Ling Zhi cultured in a selenium-rich condition. SeGLP-1 not only significantly obstructed the growth of mouse Hca-f hepatoma cells *in vivo* with 44% maximal inhibition rate, but also markedly improved the activities of SOD and GSH-Px and reduced the MDA content of the blood and the liver. The antigrowth activity of SeGLP-1 in tumor-bearing mice was found to also largely correlate to its enhanced antioxidative capacity.[70,71] SCGLP1, a chemically sulfated Ling Zhi polysaccharide, could significantly obstruct the proliferation and the viability of human MG63 osteosarcoma cells in dose- and time-dependent manners and cause apoptotic death of MG63 cells through an increase in G0/G1 phase arrest, but it had minor cytotoxic effect on human normal osteoblast cells.[72]

Glycopeptites

A polysaccharide peptide designated as GLPP was prepared from Ling Zhi, which contains 10.6% protein and holds an average molecular weight of 6600 Da. Its polysaccharide potion is composed of mannose, glucose, and galactose in a molar ratio of 0.9:15:1, respectively. The oral administration of the GLPP at doses of 100 and 300 mg/kg/day to tumor-bearing mice notably repressed the cell proliferation of sarcoma 180, hepatoma, and EAC and dose-dependently enhanced the phagocytic coeffective and index.[73] In dosages of 50–200 mg/kg, the inhibitory ratio of GLPP was 35.2–61.9% against sarcoma 180 in mice. Despite no direct action against human PG lung carcinoma cells *in vitro*, the treatment with GLPP-treated serum in doses of 50–200 mg/kg could greatly inhibit the xenograft PG cancer in nude mice by 46.0–55.5% and retard the PG cell proliferation *in vitro* by 22.5–30.3%.[74] Moreover, GLPP at 300 mg/kg per day was able to restore ^{60}Co radiation and CTX diminished the indexes of the thymus and the spleen and the levels of WBCs and bone marrow karyotes. The results evidenced that the potential anticancer activity of GLPP was largely dependent on its immunopotentiating property,[73,74] although the anticancer-related antigrowth, antiangiogenesis, and antioxidation were observed in the GLPP treatment. The antiangiogenic activity of GLPP was evidenced by the dose-dependent inhibition against HUVECs,[74,75] and the antioxidant property of GLPP was presented in the scavenging free radicals *in vivo* and *in vitro*.[76]

GLIS was a proteopolysaccharide separated from Ling Zhi, which demonstrated similar immunoenhancing property, including the activation of the immune system by the increase of macrophages and bone marrow macrophages and the modulation of cytokine production (IL-1β, IL-12p35, and IL-12p40), as well as the significant promotion of NO production.[77] A fucose-containing glycoprotein fraction (F3) isolated from the water-soluble extract of Ling Zhi was also found to have a notable ability to stimulate the spleen cell proliferation and cytokine expressions (such as IL-1, IL-6, IL-12, IFNγ, TNFα, granulocyte-macrophage colony-stimulating factor [GM-CSF], granulocyte-colony stimulating factor [G-CSF], and macrophage colony-stimulating factor [M-CSF]) in mouse. The mechanism of F3 on macrophages was figured out, where F3 binds to TLR4 receptor and activated ERK, c-Jun N-terminal kinase, and p38 to induce IL-1 expression. When human umbilical cord blood monocytes were treated with the F3 (10–100 μg/mL) for seven days, the population of $CD14^+CD26^+$ monocyte/macrophage, $CD83^+CD1a^+$ dendritic cells, and $CD16^+$ $CD56^+$ NK cells were 2.9, 2.3, and 1.5 times augmented, respectively, and the NK cell-mediated cytotoxicity was also significantly enhanced by 31.7%, demonstrating that F3 is capable of eliciting remarkable immunomodulating antineoplastic therapeutic activity *in vivo*.[78–80] In addition, the F3 was able to accelerate the apoptosis of human THP-1 leukemia cells, whose action was proposed to be through death receptors, DR3 and DR4/5.[81]

Proteins

Three kinds of bioactive proteins named LZP-1, LZP-2, and LZP-3 were isolated from the fruit body and the spore of Ling Zhi with average molecular weights of 67.0, 43.0, and 45.7 ku, respectively. These proteins, in assays, demonstrated obvious mitogenic and immunomodulating activities, whose effects are closely related to the potential value of anticancer therapeutic treatment and prevention.[82]

Taken together, these positive research results clearly evidenced that these triterpenoids, glycol peptides, polysaccharides, and proteins were the important components in the synergistical response of the anticancer and immunoregulating effects of Ling Zhi, and suggested that Ling Zhi and its products are promising agents in clinical usage for the improvement of chemotherapy and radiotherapy.

Nanoformulation

In order to enhance the bioavailability, an oral nanoemulsion of Ling Zhi polysaccharides was created, which is composed of 18.9–78.6% of oil phase, 0.1–2.2% of polysaccharide from *G. lucidum* fruit body, 19.9–76.6% of surfactant and cosurfactant, and the balance of distilled water. The oral nanoemulsion of Ling Zhi polysaccharides has been proven to have lymphatic affinity and to have ability in lessening drug the degradation from gastrointestinal acid and enzymes, leading to prolongation of the drug half-life and improvement of absorption rate and bioavailability.[83] The nanoemulsion for direct oral administration, or filled into hard gelatin capsules or soft gelatin capsules or hard gelatin capsules or enteric soft gelatin capsule, has been prepared for oral preparation.

Other Bioactivities

The herb Ling Zhi has been reported to have a wide range of pharmacological effects, including sedative, anticonvulsion, hypotensive, hypoglycemic, antiplatelet aggregation, antithrombotic, hepatoprotective, coronary dilative, immunomodulation, antioxidant, radical-scavenging, antiaging, antiradiation, antiatherosclerotic, hypolipidemic, analgesic, antiandrogenic, antiulcer, antifibrotic, antidiabetic, chemo- and radioprotective, sleep-promoting, anti-inflammatory, antiviral, anti-HIV, and antibacterial properties. Based upon the described health benefits earlier, Ling Zhi and its related products are often selected in clinical treatment of various diseases including hepatitis and diabetes as an adjuvant.

References

1. Lin, Z. B. et al. 2004. Antitumor and immunoregulatory activities of *Ganoderma lucidum* and its possible mechanisms. *Acta Pharmacol. Sinica* 25: 1387–95.
2. Gao, Y. H. et al. 2004. Chemopreventive and tumoricidal properties of Ling Zhi mushroom *Ganoderma lucidum* (W.Curt.:Fr.) Lloyd (Aphyllophoromycetideae): Part II. Mechanism considerations (review). *Intl. J. Med. Mushrooms* 6: 219–30.
3. Lin, Z. B. et al. 2994. Antitumor and immunoregulatory activities of *Ganoderma lucidum* and its possible mechanisms. *Acta Pharmacol. Sinica* 25: 1387–95.
4. Jiang, J. H. et al. 2004. *Ganoderma lucidum* suppresses growth of breast cancer cells through the inhibition of Akt-NF-κB signaling. *Nutr. Cancer* 49: 209–16.
5. Jiang, J. H. et al. 2006. *Ganoderma lucidum* inhibits proliferation of human breast cancer cells by downregulation of estrogen receptor and NF-κB signaling. *Intl. J. Oncol.* 29: 695–703.
6. Hu, H. B. et al. 2002. *Ganoderma lucidum* extract induces cell cycle arrest and apoptosis in MCF-7 human breast cancer cell. *Intl. J. Cancer* 102: 250–3.
7. Martinez-Montemayor, M. et al. *Ganoderma lucidum* (Reishi) inhibits cancer cell growth and expression of key Mmolecules in Inflammatory Breast Cancer. *Nutr. Cancer* 63: 1085–94.
8. Wu, G. S. et al. 2012. *Ganoderma lucidum* extract induces G1 cell cycle arrest, and apoptosis in human breast cancer cells. *Am. J. Chin. Med.* 40: 631–42.
9. Stanley, G. et al. 2005. *Ganoderma lucidum* suppresses angiogenesis through the inhibition of secretion of VEGF and TGF-β1 from prostate cancer cells. *Biochem. Biophys. Res. Commun.* 330: 46–52.
10. Zaidman, B. Z. et al. 2007. Androgen receptor-dependent and -independent mechanisms mediate *Ganoderma lucidum* activities in LNCaP prostate cancer cells. *Intl. J. Oncol.* 31: 959–67.
11. Jiang, J. H. et al. 2004. *Ganoderma lucidum* inhibits proliferation and induces apoptosis in human prostate cancer cells PC3. *Intl. J. Oncol.* 24: 1093–9.
12. Liu, G. Q. et al. 2005. Mechanisms of the anticancer action of *Ganoderma lucidum* (Leyss. ex Fr.) Karst: A new understanding. *J. Integrative Plant Biol.* 47: 129–35.
13. Calvino, E. et al. 2011. Cytotoxic action of *Ganoderma lucidum* on interleukin-3 dependent lymphoma DA-1 cells: Involvement of apoptosis proteins. *Phytother. Res.* 25: 25–32.
14. Huang, S. M. et al. 2004. Antitumor activity of ethanol-soluble and acidic components from *Ganoderma lucidum*. *Tianran Chanwu Yanjiu Yu Kaifa* 16: 146–8
15. Hong, K. J. et al. 2004. Effects of *Ganoderma lucidum* on apoptotic and anti-inflammatory function in HT-29 human colonic carcinoma cells. *Phytother. Res.*18: 768–70.
16. Weng, X. C. et al. 2006. Research on tumor inhibitory action of triterpenoid compound (Sunrecome). *Zhonghua Yiyao Zazhi* 6: 248–252.
17. Chang, Y. S. et al. 2009. *Ganoderma lucidum* extracts inhibited leukemia WEHI-3 cells in BALB/c mice and promoted an immune response *in vivo. Biosci. Biotech. Biochem.* 73: 2589–94.
18. Sadava, D. et al. 2009. Effect of Ganoderma on drug-sensitive and multidrug-resistant small-cell lung carcinoma cells. *Cancer Lett.* 277: 182–9.
19. Yuen, J. W. M. et al. 2005. Anticancer effects of *Ganoderma lucidum*: A review of scientific evidence. *Nutr. Cancer* 53: 11–17.
20. Sheena, N. et al. 2003. Prevention of nephrotoxicity induced by the anticancer drug cisplatin, using *Ganoderma lucidum*, a medicinal mushroom occurring in South India. *Current Sci.* 85: 478–82.
21. Trajkovic, L. M. et al. 2009. Anticancer properties of *Ganoderma lucidum* methanol extracts in vitro and in vivo. *Nutr. Cancer* 61: 696–707.
22. Kimura, Y. et al. 2002. Antitumor and antimetastatic effects on liver of triterpenoid fractions of *Ganoderma lucidum*: Mechanism of action and isolation of an active substance. *Anticancer Res.* 22: 3309–18.
23. Shiao, M. S. et al. 2004. Pharmacological and genomic studies on the medicinal fungus *Ganoderma lucidum. Abstracts of Papers, 227th ACS National Meeting, Anaheim, CA, United States,* March 28-April 1, (2004), AGFD-130.
24. Yang, X. T. et al. 2005. Comparison study of the in vitro anticancer activity and mechanism of ethanol extracts from mycelia of different *Ganoderma lucidum* strains. *Junwu Xuebao* 24: 251–8.
25. Lin, S. B. et al. 2003. Triterpene-enriched extracts from *Ganoderma lucidum* inhibit growth of hepatoma cells via suppressing protein kinase C, activating mitogen-activated protein kinases and G2-phase cell cycle arrest. *Life Sci.* 72: 2381–90.
26. Wu, T. S. et al. 2001. Cytotoxicity of *Ganoderma lucidum* triterpenes. *J. Nat. Prod.* 64: 1121–2.
27. Min, B. S. et al. 2000. Triterpenes from the spores of *Ganoderma lucidum* and their cytotoxicity against Meth-A and LLC tumor cells. *Chem. Pharm. Bull.* 48: 1026–33.
28. Ruan, W. M. et al. 2014. Extraction optimisation and isolation of triterpenoids from *Ganoderma lucidum* and their effect on human carcinoma cell growth. *Nat. Prod. Res.* 28: 2264–72.
29. Dong, H. L. et al. 2013. Triterpenoid acids from sporophore of *Ganoderma lucidum* and their inhibition on proliferation of SKBR3 human breast cancer cells. *Xiandai Yaowu Yu Linchuang* 28: 132–7.
30. Gao, J. J. et al. 2002. New triterpene aldehydes, lucialdehydes A-C, from *Ganoderma lucidum* and their cytotoxicity against murine and human tumor cells. *Chem. Pharm. Bull.* 50: 837–40.
31. Gao, J. J. et al. 2006. In vivo antitumor effects of bitter principles from the antlered form of fruiting bodies of *Ganoderma lucidum. J. Nat. Med.* 60: 42–8.
32. Chang, U.-M. et al. 2006. Ganoderiol F, a ganoderma triterpene, induces senescence in hepatoma HepG2 cells. *Life Sci.* 79: 1129–39.
33. Yang, H. L. et al. 2005. Ganoderic acid produced from submerged culture of *Ganoderma lucidum* induces cell cycle arrest and cytotoxicity in human hepatoma cell line BEL7402. *Biotechnol. Lett.* 27: 835–8.
34. Min, B. S. et al. 2004. Chemical and biological evaluation of germinated and mature antler-shaped fruiting bodies of *Ganoderma lucidum. J. Nat. Med.* (Tokyo, JPN) 58: 91–7.
35. Weng, C. J. et al. 2008. Lucidenic acid inhibits PMA-induced invasion of human hepatoma cells through inactivating MAPK/ERK signal transduction pathway and reducing binding activities of NF-κB and AP-1. *Carcinogenesis* 29: 147–56.

36. Kang, K.-A. et al. 2006. Anticancer effects of 23-Dihydroganoderic acid N. *Environ. Mutagens Carcinog.* 26: 116–8.
37. Guan, S. H. et al. 2006. Two new lanostanoid triterpenes from the fruit body of *Ganoderma lucidum*-the major component of sunrecome. *Nat. Prod. Commun.* 1: 177–81.
38. Liu, J. et al. 2007. The anti-androgen effect of ganoderol B isolated from the fruiting body of *Ganoderma lucidum. Bioorg. Med. Chem.* 15: 4966–72.
39. Zhou, C. Y. et al. 2004. Antitumor effect of ganoderic acid from *Ganoderma lucidum. Junwu Xuebao* 23: 275–9.
40. Wang, G. et al. 2007. Enhancement of IL-2 and IFN-γ expression and NK cells activity involved in the antitumor effect of ganoderic acid Me in vivo. *Intl. Immunopharmacol.* 7: 864–70.
41. Tang, W. et al. 2006. Ganoderic acid T from *Ganoderma lucidum* mycelia induces mitochondria mediated apoptosis in lung cancer cells. *Life Sci.* 80: 205–11.
42. Li, C. H. et al. 2004. Ganoderic acid X, a lanostanoid triterpene, inhibits topoisomerases and induces apoptosis of cancer cells. *Life Sci.* 77: 252–65.
43. Iwatsuki, K. et al. 2003. Lucidenic acids P and Q, methyl lucidenate P, and other triterpenoids from the fungus *Ganoderma lucidum* and their inhibitory effects on Epstein-Barr virus activation. *J. Nat. Prod.* 66: 1582–5.
44. Akihisa, T. et al. 2006. Prophylactic antitumor agents containing *Ganoderma lucidum* triterpenes or sterols. *Jpn. Kokai Tokkyo Koho* JP 2004–199471 20040706.
45. Akihisa, T. et al. 2007. Anti-inflammatory and antitumor-promoting effects of triterpene acids and sterols from the fungus *Ganoderma lucidum. Chem. Biodiver.* 4: 224–31.
46. Ooi, L. S. M. et al. 2002. Induction of gene expression of immunomodulatory cytokines in the mouse by a polysaccharide from *Ganoderma lucidum* (Curt.: Fr.) P. Karst. *Intl. J. Med. Mushrooms* 4: 27–35.
47. Gao, Y. H. et al. 2005. Antitumor activity and underlying mechanisms of Ganopoly, the refined polysaccharides extracted from *Ganoderma lucidum*, in mice. *Immunol. Investigations* 34: 171–98.
48. Li, G. Y. et al. 2013. Effect of *Ganoderma lucidum* polysaccharides on apoptosis and Egr-1 expression in NB4 cells. *Zhongyao Xinyao Yu Linchuang Yaoli* 24: 476–9.
49. Zhao, S. H. et al. 2003. Isolation, purification, characterization and anti-tumor activities of Ganoderma Lucidum polysaccharide. *Zhongguo Shenghua Yaowu Zazhi* 24: 173–6.
50. Huang, C. et al. 2005. Isolation, purification, composition and activity of *Ganoderma lucidum* polysaccharide. *Zhongguo Shenghua Yaowu Zazhi* 26: 221–3.
51. Lee, K. H. et al. Pharmacological, toxicological studies of antitumor polysaccharides obtained from *Ganoderma lucidum* IY 009. *Sanop Misaengmul Hakhoechi* 22: 182–9.
52. Zhang, J. S. et al. 2004. Comparison of bioactivity of fruiting body and mycelia of *Ganoderma lucidum* and their purified fractions. *Junwu Xuebao* 23: 85–92.
53. Min, B. S. et al. Chemical and biological evaluation of germinated and mature antler-shaped fruiting bodies of *Ganoderma lucidum. J. Nat. Med.* 58: 91–7.
54. Lee, S. S. et al. 2003. Antitumor effects of polysaccharides of *Ganoderma lucidum* (Curt.:Fr.) P. Karst. (Ling Zhi, Reishi mushroom) (Aphyllophoromycet-ideae). *Intl. J. Med. Mushrooms* 5: 1–16.
55. Cheng, K. C. et al. 2007. *Ganoderma lucidum* polysaccharides in human monocytic leukemia cells: From gene expression to network construction. *BMC Genomics* 8, 411.
56. Jiang, Y. et al. 2005. Chemistry of polysaccharide Lzps-1 from *Ganoderma lucidum* spore and antitumor activity of its total polysaccharides.*Yaoxue Xuebao* 40: 347–50.
57. Zhou, S. F. et al. 2002. The immunomodulating effects of *Ganoderma lucidum* (Curt.: Fr.) P. Karst. (Ling Zhi, reishi mushroom) (Aphyllophoromycetideae). *Intl. J. Med. Mushrooms* 4: 1–11.
58. Hsu, M. J. et al. 2003. Signaling mechanisms of enhanced neutrophil phagocytosis and chemotaxis by the polysaccharide purified from *Ganoderma lucidum. British J. Pharmacol.* 139: 289–98.
59. Zhang, Q. H. et al. 1999. The antitumor activity of *Ganoderma lucidum* (Curt.:Fr.)P. Karst. (Ling Zhi) (Aphyllophoromycetideae) polysaccharides is related to tumor necrosis factor-α and interferon-γ. *Intl. J. Med. Mushrooms* 1: 207–15.
60. Mojadadi, S. et al. 2006. Immunomodulatory effects of *Ganoderma lucidum* (W. Curt.:Fr.) P. Karst. (Aphyllophoromycetideae) on $CD4^+/CD8^+$ tumor infiltrating lymphocytes in breast-cancer-bearing mice. *Intl. J. Med. Mushrooms* 8: 315–20.
61. Zhu, X. L. et al. 2005. Effects of *Ganoderma lucidum* polysaccharides on proliferation and cytotoxicity of cytokine-induced killer cells. *Acta Pharmacol. Sinica* 26: 1130–7.
62. Gao, Y. H. et al. 2007. Mechanisms for the antitumor effect of the refined polysaccharides extracted from *Ganoderma lucidum* in mice. *Recent Progress in Medicinal Plants* 17: 221–47.
63. Zhu, X. L. et al. 2006. Modulation of cytokines production, granzyme B and perforin in murine CIK cells by *Ganoderma lucidum* polysaccharides. *Carbohydrate Polymers* 63: 188–97.
64. Liu, G. Q. et al. 2006. Structure-activity relationship and anticancer mechanisms of *Ganoderma lucidum* polysaccharides. *Junwu Xuebao* 25: 430–8.
65. Miura, N. et al. 2000. Studies on *Ganoderma lucidum* II-the antitumor effect of the water-soluble extract from the antler-shape fruiting body of *Ganoderma lucidum. Res. Commun. Pharmacol. Toxicol.* 5: 191–3.
66. Tang, Q. J. et al. 2004. Activation of mouse macrophages by the alkali-extracted polysaccharide from spore of *Ganoderma lucidum. Xibao Yu Fenzi Mianyixue Zazhi* 20: 142–4.
67. Zheng, S. et al. 2012. *Ganoderma lucidum* polysaccharides eradicate the blocking effect of fibrinogen on NK cytotoxicity against melanoma cells. *Oncol. Lett.* 3: 613–6.
68. Sun, L. X. et al. 2011. *Ganoderma lucidum* polysaccharides antagonize the suppression on lymphocytes induced by culture supernatants of B16F10 melanoma cells. *J. Pharm. Pharmacol.* 63: 725–35.
69. Sun, L. X. et al. 2014. Protection against lung cancer patient plasma-induced lymphocyte suppression by *Ganoderma lucidum* polysaccharides. *Cellular Physiol. Biochem.* 33: 289–99.
70. Shang, D. J. et al. 2002. Study on antioxidative and antitumor effect of selenium containing polysaccharide in *Ganoderma lucidum* in mice. *Yingyang Xuebao* 24: 249–51.
71. Li, X. L. et al. 2007. Inhibition of *Lycium barbarum* polysaccharides and *Ganoderma lucidum* polysaccharides against oxidative injury induced by γ-irradiation in rat liver mitochondria. *Carbohydrate Polymers* 69: 172–8.

72. Sun, Z. C. et al. 2014. A chemically sulfated polysaccharide derived from *Ganoderma lucidum* induces mitochondrial-mediated apoptosis in human osteo-sarcoma MG63 cells. *Tumor Biol.* 35: 9919–26.
73. Pang, X. et al. 2007. Potential of a novel polysaccharide preparation (GLPP) from anhui-grown *Ganoderma lucidum* in tumor treatment and immuno-stimulation. *J. Food Sci.* 72: S435–S442.
74. Cao, Q. Z. et al. 2004. Antitumor and anti-angiogenic activity of *Ganoderma lucidum* polysaccharides peptide. *Acta Pharmacol. Sinica* 25: 833–838.
75. Cao, Q. Z. et al. 2006. *Ganoderma lucidum* polysaccharide peptide inhibits the growth of vascular endothelial cell and the induction of VEGF in human lung cancer cell. *Life Sci.* 78: 1457–63.
76. Lin, Z. B. et al. 2002. Progress of studies on the antitumor activity and immunomodulating effect of Ganoderma. *J. Beijing Univ. Med. Edit.* 34: 493–8.
77. Ji, Z. et al. 2007. Immunomodulation of RAW264.7 macrophages by GLIS, a proteopolysaccharide from *Ganoderma lucidum*. *J. Ethnopharmacol.* 112: 445–50.
78. Wang, Y. Y. et al. 2002. Studies on the immuno-modulating and antitumor activities of *Ganoderma lucidum* (Reishi) polysaccharides: Functional and proteomic analyses of a fucose-containing glycoprotein fraction responsible for the activities. *Bioorg. Med. Chem.* 10: 1057–62.
79. Chien, C. C. M. et al. 2004. Polysaccharides of *Ganoderma lucidum* alter cell immunophenotypic expression and enhance CD^{56+} NK-cell cytotoxicity in cord blood. *Bioorg. Med. Chem.* 12: 5603–9.
80. Chen, H. S. et al. 2004. Studies on the immuno-modulating and antitumor activities of *Ganoderma lucidum* (Reishi) polysaccharides. *Bioorg. Med. Chem.* 12: 5595–601.
81. Cheng, K. C. et al. 2007. *Ganoderma lucidum* polysaccharides in human monocytic leukemia cells: From gene expression to network construction. *BMC genomics* 8: 411.
82. Ye, B. P. et al. 2002. Isolating of proteins from Lingzhi and study on its immune activity. *Yaowu Shengwu Jishu* 9: 150–2.
83. Yu, R. M. et al. 2011. *Ganoderma lucidum* polysaccharide oral nanoemulsion, its preparation method and medical application. *Faming Zhuanli Shenqing* CN 102058530 A 20110518.

167 Jiao Gu Lan 絞股蘭

Gynostemma

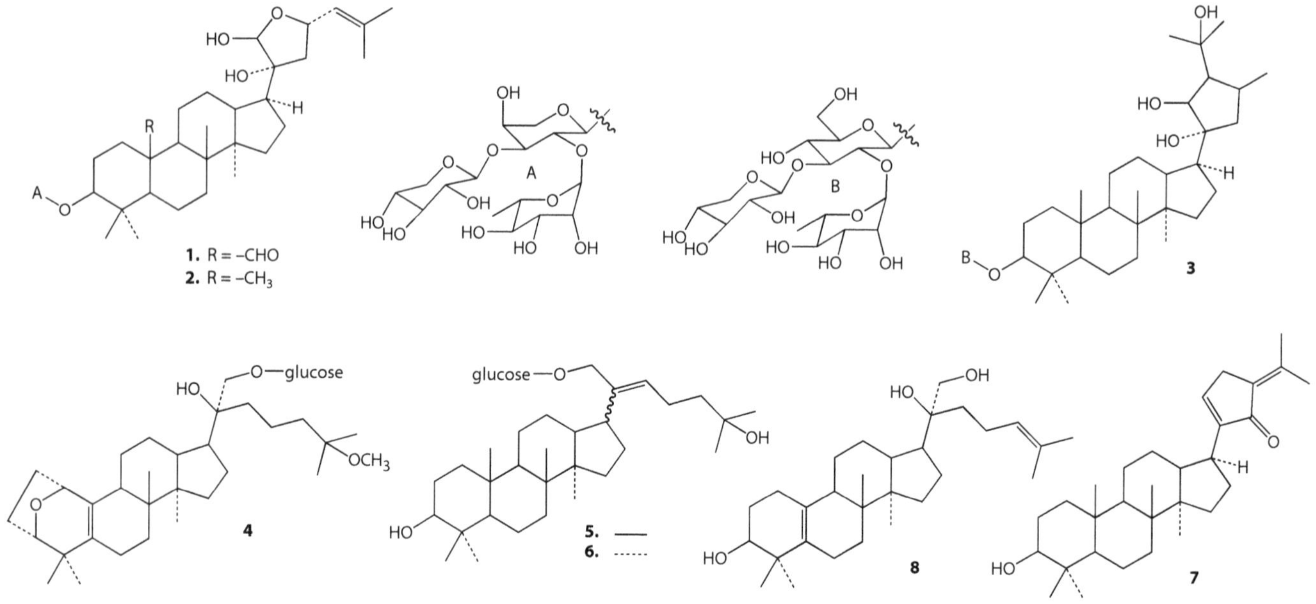

Herb Origination

The herb Jiao Gu Lan is the dried whole vine plant of *Gynostemma pentaphyllum* (Cucurbitaceae). The plant is grown in the most temperate climates and is widely distributed in southern area of the Yangtze River and the provinces of Shaanxi and Gansu in China as well as in southern Korea, Japan, and other parts of Asia. The herbaceous vine is commonly collected in summer and autumn and then dried in the sun for Chinese folk medicinal use.

Antitumor Activities

The oral administration of the Jiao Gu Lan decoction or the aqueous extract of its fresh cultured tissues to mice every day could prolong the life span of mice bearing Ehrlich ascites cancer or L615 leukemia, but it is invalid to transplanted hepatoma in mice.[1,2] Free drinks of 2% Jiao Gu Lan decoction for 18 weeks could delay the initiation of esophageal epithelial papilloma induced by the injection of methyl-n-amyl nitrosamine in rats.[3] The hot water extract of Jiao Gu Lan showed DT-diaphorase-inducing activity in murine hepatoma (Hepa1c1c7) cell line. Its antimutagenic properties mostly presented in the mutations induced by AFB1, Glu-P-1, Glu-P-2, Trp-P-1, Trp-P-2, 2-amino-3-methylimidazo[4,5-f]quinoline, or BAP. But it showed no such effect in 2-(2-Furyl)-3-(5-nitro-2-furyl) acryl-amide-caused mutation, and it even enhanced the mutagenicity of 2-aminoanthracene and MNNG.[4] The administration of the Jiao Gu Lan extract to hamsters for four to eight weeks also reduced the incidence of leukoplakia mutation caused by dimethylbenzanthracene.[5,6] In the Jiao Gu Lan extract, the most potent anticarcinogenic components were identified to be triterpenoid saponins with free hydroxyl at C-20.[5,6] The ethanol extract exerted antiproliferative and apoptosis-inducing effects on C-6 glioma cells, whose apoptotic promotion was associated with the increase of SOD activity, the rise the H_2O_2 concentration to a toxic level, and the activation of caspase-3.[7]

Antitumor Constituents and Activities

The major components in Jiao Gu Lan are triterpenoid saponins which primarily contributed to the multiple health benefits including the antineoplastic and anticarcinogenic properties. Other types of components such as flavonoids, carotenoids, chlorophylls, and polysaccharides prepared from the herb were also found to partially show the growth inhibition of tumors.

Total Saponin Components

Antiproliferative and Apoptosis-Inducing Effects

The total saponins designated as gypenosides (GPs) from Jiao Gu Lan were proven to possess tumoricidal effect by *in vitro* and *in vivo* experiments. When cultured with tumor cells, the 0.55% concentration of GPs could directly kill sarcoma 180 cells by 82.7%.[8] The daily oral administrations of GPs in 50 mg/kg dose for seven days minimized the tissue size of mouse sarcoma 180 by 40%.[9] In concentrations of 0.5–2.0 mg/mL, the GPs exhibited suppressive effect against the proliferation of human SMMC-7721 hepatoma cells *in vitro* by blocking the incorporation of TdR, UR, and Leu into the DNA and retarding the synthesis of DNA and RNA.[10] Through the upregulation of Bax, Bak, and Bad and the downregulation of Bcl-2 and Bcl-xL, the GPs elicited the apoptosis of human hepatoma cell lines (Huh-7, Hep3B, and HA22T). Also, the treatment caused mitochondrial cytochrome c release to the cytosol, activation of caspases, and cleavage of PARP, whose interactions are closely involved in the apoptosis-enhancing mechanism in these hepatoma cell lines.[11] The inhibitory effect of GPs was obviously more potent in the growth of human lung cancer cell lines (A549, Calu, and 592/9) than in HeLa-S3 cervical cancer and Colo205 colon cancer cell lines in concentrations of 1–10 μg/mL.[12] The viabilities of A549 lung cancer cells, SCC4 tongue cancer cells, and Colo205 colon cancer cells were reduced, and the cell apoptosis and the cell cycle arrest were elicited after the GP treatment.[13–15] During the treatment, p16, p21, p27, and p53 proteins were increased in the A549 cells, ROS and Ca^{2+} were overproduced in Colo205 cells, Huh-7 cells, and SCC4 cells to cause dysfunction of the mitochondria and apoptosis.[13–16] Similarly, GPs induced necrosis and apoptosis in human HepG2 hepatoma cells through a sustained increase of $[Ca^{2+}]i$ level, and Ca^{2+}-implicated ER stress and mitochondria-dependent pathways.[17] In human SAS oral cancer cells, GPs induced DNA damage and G0/G1 cell arrest and resisted DNA repair-associated gene expressions, then elicited the cell apoptotic death through caspase-dependent and caspase-independent apoptotic signaling pathways. The anticancer effect in human HeLa cervical cancer cells was correlated with the down-expression of cytosolic N-acetyl-transferase and the decrease of DNA-2-aminofluorene adduct formation levels.[18–20] Through the elevation of intracellular ROS level and oxidative stress and the induction of mitochondria-dependent cell apoptosis, GPs inhibited the cell proliferation and the migration in SW620 and SW480 (colon) and Eca-109 (esophagus) human cancer cell line in dose- and time-dependent manners.[21,22] The results provide mechanistic insight into the rational basis of GPs in the treatment of solid tumor diseases and indicated that the cytotoxic mechanism of GPs should be different based upon the variety of cancer cells.

The significant antileukemia effect of GPs was demonstrated in murine L1210 lymphocytic leukemia cells and WEHI-3 myelomonocytic leukemia cells *in vitro*. After the treatment in a 350 μg/mL concentration for 4 h, GPs stimulated the production of ROS to the highest level, obviously decreased the membrane potential, and enhanced DNA damage and morphological changes, finally eliciting the growth inhibition of L1210 cells.[23] In a mouse model, the oral consumption of GPs inhibited the growth of WEHI-3 cells and augmented the survival rate of mice implanted with WEHI-3 leukemia cells. The GP treatment augmented the ROS and Ca^{2+} levels, induced the depolarization of mitochondrial membrane potential, increased Bax level and reduced Bcl-2 level, and stimulated the releases of cytochrome c, AIF, and endonuclease-G from the mitochondria, whose series of events then triggered the cell cycle arrest and the apoptosis of WEHI-3 cells.[24]

Antimetastasis Effect

In the *in vitro* studies, the GPs inhibited the migration and then invasion of human SCC4 tongue cancer cells and human SAS oral carcinoma cells in dose- and time-dependent responses. During the treatment, GPs diminished the key protein expressions such as RAS, NF-κB, COX2, ERK1/2, MMP-9, and MMP-2 and restrained SOS, u-PA, FAK, and RAC-alpha serine/threonine-protein kinase (Akt), thereby obstructing the invasion and the metastasis of SAS cells and SCC4 cells.[25,26] The blockage of NF-κB and MMPs signal pathways was found to be involved in the mechanisms that correlates to the GP-inhibited cancer cell invasion and migration.[26] The results evidenced the potential capacity of GPs for treatment of the metastatic and invasive oral carcinoma.

Antimultidrug Resistance Effect

In anti-MDR studies, GPs diminished the overexpression of P-glycoprotein (P-gp and then reversed the colchicine resistance by approximately 15-fold in a highly multidrug-resistant leukemia subline (CCRF-CEM/VLB100) at a concentration of 0.1 mg/mL. But GPs showed no such MDR reversal effect in the tumor cells treated with taxol and vinblastine.[27]

Antitumorigenic Effect

The GPs also displayed remarkable antitumorigenic activity besides the anticancer property. GPs at 1.5 g/kg or 0.488 g/kg doses were orally administrated to mice for 14 continuous days, resulting in obviously declined incidence of hepatomagenesis caused by an oncogene DEN *in vivo*.[28]

Immunostimulating Effect

GPs in 1–10 μg/mL concentrations were capable of enhancing the proliferation of normal human mix lymphocytes. The oral administration of 3 mg of GPs per day for seven days was able to largely potentiate the activated levels of spleen cells, peripheral blood cells, T cells, and B cells and to elevate the levels of Immunoglobulin M (IgM) and IgG in mice. These findings demonstrated that GPs also play an important role in the potentiation of host immunological function.[12,29,30]

Individual Saponins

Several separated GPs were demonstrated to have moderate antitumor activities. GPs-VN1–VN7 moderately suppressed the growth of four human adenocarcinoma cell lines, A549 (lung), HT-29 (colon), MCF-7 (breast), and SK-OV-3 (ovary), *in vitro*, but GP-VN1, GP-VN5, and GP-VN6 were weakly effective in hindering human HL-60 promyelocytic leukemia cells.[31] Three other GPs ((23S)-3β,20ξ,21ξ-trihydroxy-19-oxo-21,23-epoxydammar-24-ene 3-O-[α-L-rhamnopyranosyl(1-2)][β-D-xylopyranosyl(1-3)]-α-L-arabinopyranoside(**1**); (23S)-21ξ-O-ethyl-3β,20ξ,21-trihydroxy-19-oxo-21,23-epoxydammar-24-ene 3-O-[α-L-rhamnopyranosyl(1-2)][β-D-xylopyranosyl(1-3)]-α-L-arabinopyranoside (**2**); (20S)-3β,20,21ξ,25-tetrahydroxy-21,24ξ-cyclodammarane 3-O-{[α-L-rhamnopyranosyl(1-2)][β-D-xylopy ranosyl(1-3)]-β-D-6-O-acetylglucopyranoside (**3**)) demonstrated the antiproliferative effect against human SGC-7901 gastric cancer cells and BEL-7402 hepatoma cells. At a 100 mm concentration, the GPs (**1–3**) restrained the growth of SGC-7901 and BEL-7402 cells by 21% and 77%, 93% and 92%, and 8% and 40%, respectively.[32] The studies also revealed that the GPs with free hydroxyl groups at C-21 and C-20 generally exerted marked contribution to the antiproliferative effect on lung cancer, cervical carcinoma, and melanoma cell lines but no influences to normal cell proliferation.[33]

Both vascular cell adhesion molecules (VCAM) and NF-κB are the important targets for cancer growth inhibition, and the tissue factor (TF) is also an attractive target involved in tumor cell proliferation, metastasis, and angiogenesis. GP-XLIX is an NF-κB inhibitor and a selective activator for peroxisome proliferator-activated receptor-α, able to restrain a cytokine TNFα-induced VCAM-1 overexpression and hyperactivity in human endothelial cells and also to inhibit TF overexpression in human THP-1 monocytic cells by a PPARα-dependent pathway.[34–36] These findings established that GP-XLIX has a potential for the chemoprevention of neoplastic disease. Likewise, more cancer inhibitory dammarane-type triterpene saponins have been discovered from the herb in recent years. They similarly displayed moderate to weak cytotoxic effects on the A549, HepG2, or HL-60 cell lines.[37–40]

Sapogenins

Several triterpene sapogenins were isolated from a hydrolyzate of Jiao Gu Lan total saponins and were identified as gypensapogenins-H–L. Gypensapogenin-H (**4**), gypensapogenin-I, and gypensapogenin-L possessed an unusual unprecedented ring-A. In the *in vitro* assay, gypensapogenin-H (**4**), gypensapogenin-J, (**5**) and gypensapogenin-K (**6**) showed moderate to weak antiproliferative effects on MCF-7 (breast), HCT-116, and HT-29 (colon) human neoplastic cell lines, whereas gypensapogenin-I and gypensapogenin-L were only moderately active to the MCF-7 and HT-29 cell lines. However, these sapogenins were inactive to BGC-823 gastric cancer cells and MCF-10a breast surface epithelial cells. Among them, the strongest inhibition was achieved by gypensapogenin-H (**4**) on the MCF-7 cells (IC_{50}: 6.85 μM), which could significantly trigger the ROS-involved apoptotic death of MCF-7 cells.[41] Other hydrolyzates of GPs assigned as gypensapogenin-C (**7**) exhibited marked inhibitory activity toward A549 (lung) and U87 (brain) human cancer cell lines (respective IC_{50}: 0.11 and 0.58 μM), whereas gypensapogenin-A was weak to A549 (lung) and Hep3B (liver) cancer cell lines.[42] 20S-Dammar-24-en-2α,3β,12β,20-tetrol also exerted the antiproliferative activity against the A549 cells (IC_{50}: 12.54 μg/mL).[37] H6 (**8**), a GP aglycon, displayed a similar level of suppression on drug-resistant KB/VCR and MCF-7/Adm cell lines and their parental cells. Its anti-MDR mechanism was revealed to be mediated by repressions of P-gp RNA transcript level by stimulating the P-gp ATPase activity and of MRP1 and BCRP by the blocking STAT3 phosphorylation.[43] Based on the findings, H6 (**8**), a multitarget MDR-reversal agent with no obvious toxic effect, was suggested to have a potential to circumvent P-gp- and MRP1-mediated drug resistance.

Flavonoid Glycosides

A flavonoid fraction derived from Jiao Gu Lan was mainly composed of quercetin- and kaempferol-glycosides. The fraction was moderately effective in inhibiting the growth of PC3 (prostate) Hep3B (liver) human cancer cell lines *in vitro*. After the treatment with the flavonoid fraction, the PC3 cell cycle was arrested at both S and G2/M phases by modulating the expression of G2 and M checkpoint regulators (cyclin-A and cyclin-B), and the PC3 cell apoptosis was promoted through an intrinsic mitochondrial pathway. However, the cell cycle progression of Hep3B hepatoma cells was arrested at G0/G1 stage by the flavonoid fraction.[43,44]

Carotenoid and Chlorophyll Fractions

Both carotenoid and chlorophyll fractions prepared from the herb were effective at a 50–100 μg/mL concentration against human Hep3B hepatoma cells with a dose-dependent response. The two fractions promoted the cell cycle arrest and elicited the necrosis and/or the apoptosis of Hep3B cells. The antihepatoma activity of the carotenoid fraction was more potent than that of the chlorophyll fraction. Moreover, the carotenoid fraction was found to be composed of all *trans*- and all *cis*-isomers of lutein, α-carotene, β-carotene, as well as epoxy-containing carotenoids, whereas the chlorophyll fraction consisted of chlorophyll-a and chlorophyll-b and their derivatives.[45]

Polysaccharides

A water-soluble nonstarch polysaccharide (PSGP) was isolated from the Jiao Gu Lan tea, which is composed of glucose (23.2%), galactose (18.9%), arabinose (10.5%), rhamnose (7.7%), galacturonic acid (4.7%), xylose (3.9%), mannose (3.1%), and glucuronic acid (1.2%). The PSGP is capable of stimulating the peritoneal macrophages to release NO, ROS, and TNFα significantly in a dose-dependent manner. The PSGP-stimulated macrophage markedly inhibited the proliferation of human HT-29 and SW-116 colon carcinoma cells.[46] Another polysaccharide extract was isolated from Jiao Gu Lan, showing the similar degree of suppressive effect against the growth and the DNA synthesis of Hce 8693 colon cancer cell as that of GPs.[47]

From the separation of Jiao Gu Lan water extract, an acidic polysaccharide GP-B1 (79 kDa) and a native polysaccharide GPP2 were obtained. The *in vivo* treatment with GP-B1 exerted a significant inhibitory effect on the growth of B16 melanoma dependent of the immune stimulation, i.e., augmentation of splenocyte proliferation and spleen weight, elevation of TNFα, IFNγ, and IL-12 levels in the serum, and reduction of IL-10 production.[48] However, GPP2 showed no effect related to the antitumor, but the sulfated GPP2 with an average molecular mass ranging from 8.64 to 11.2 Da could restrain the growth of HepG2 and HeLa cell lines and significantly induce the cell cycle arrest at S phase *in vitro* with low toxicity.[49]

A neutral polysaccharide (CGPP) was extracted from *G. pentaphyllum* by water and ethanol, whose CGPP was mainly composed of mannose, glucose, arabinose, rhamnose, galactose, and glucuronic acid in molar ratios of 2.0:2.2:1.3:2.2:1.2:2.5. The treatment with CGPP (50 and 200 mg/kg) effectively inhibited the growth of H22 hepatoma in Imprinting Control Region (ICR) mouse. The *in vivo* antitumor activity of CGPP was at least partly contributed by CGPP-improved immune responses of the host organism, such as augmentation of the spleen/thymus indexes and splenocytes proliferation and marked promotion of the levels of cytokines such as IL-2, TNFα, and IFNγ, as well as activation of NK cells and CTL in the tumor-bearing mice.[50]

From the research results, the Jiao Gu Lan polysaccharides are considered as safe and effective supplementary agents for the treatment of carcinomas of the colon, the liver, and others.

Other Bioactivities

The herb Jiao Gu Lan (Gynostemma) has been used in Chinese herbal medicine for centuries with a cure-all reputation. Scientific studies found out that Jiao Gu Lan has disease prevention and therapeutic features, including antiplatelet aggregation, immunepotentiating, and antithrombotic properties. Also, it optimizes lipid metabolism and promotes the healthy functions in the cardiovascular system and the CNS. As an adaptogen and antioxidant, it is effective in regulating blood pressure, lowering cholesterol, and improving endurance. According to the remarkable biological activities, the alcoholic extract of Jiao Gu Lan and its capsule or pill form are now available in Chinese clinics, and Jiao Gu Lan tea is marketed in the United States under the trade names Panta tea or Penta tea.

References

1. Wang, Z. J. et al. (a) 1990. *Zhongliu* 10: 246; (b) 1999. *Chinese Materia Medica*. Vol. 5, 5–4609, 534–35. Shanghai Science and Technology Press, Shanghai, China.
2. Wei, S. L. et al. 1988. Inhibition of *Gynostemma pentaphyllum* against tumor translated in mouse. *Diyi Junyi Daxue Xuebao* 8: 333–4.
3. Wang, C. J. et al. 1995. A preliminary observation of preventive and blocking effect of *Gynostemma pentaphyllum* (Thunb) Makino on esophageal cancer in rats. *J. Huaxi Med. Univ.* 26: 430–2.
4. Kulwat, C. et al. Antimutagenicity and DT-diaphorase inducing activity of *Gynostemma pentaphyllum* Makino extract. *J. Med. Investig.* 52: 145–50.
5. Zhou, Z. T. et al. (a) 2000. Effect of *Gynostemma pentaphyllum* Mak on point mutation of Ha-ras oncogene in blocking leukoplakia from carcinogenesis. *Zhonghua Kouqiang Yixue Zazhi* 35: 91–4; (b) 1996. The effect of *Gynostemma pentaphyllum* mak (GP) on carcinogenesis of the golden hamster cheek pouch induced by DMBA. *Zhonghua Kouqiang Yixue Zazhi* 31: 267–70.
6. Zhou, Z. T. et al. 1998. Effect of *Gynostemma pentaphyllum* mak on carcinomatous conversions of golden hamster cheek pouches induced by dimethyl-benzanthracene: A histological study. *Chin. Med. J.* 111: 847–50.
7. Schild, L. et al. Selective induction of apoptosis in glioma tumour cells by a *Gynostemma pentaphyllum* extract. *Phytomed.* 17: 589–97.
8. Wang, Y. Q. et al. 1988. Antitumor effect of total saponin from *Gynostemma pentaphyllum*. *Zhongxiyi Jiehe Zazhi* 8: 286.
9. Arichi, S. et al. 1985. Saponins of *Gynostemma pentaphyllum* as neoplasm inhibitors. *Jpn. Kokai Tokkyo Koho* JP 60105627 A 19850611.
10. Chen, W. et al. 1993. Effect of total gypenosides on nucleic acid and protein synthesis of cultured hepatoma cells. *J. Xi'an Med. Univ.* 14: 14–6.
11. Wang, Q. F. et al. 2002. Regulation of Bcl-2 family molecules and activation of caspase cascade involved in gypenosides-induced apoptosis in human hepatoma cells. *Cancer Lett.* 83: 169–78.
12. Liu, H. et al. 1994. Inhibitory effect of total gypenosides on lung cancer cells in vitro. *J. Xi'an Med. Univ.* 15: 346–8.
13. Lu, H. F. et al. 2008. Gypenosides induced G0/G1 arrest via inhibition of cyclin E and induction of apoptosis via activation of caspases-3 and -9 in human lung cancer A549 cells. *In Vivo* 22: 215–22.
14. Chen, J. C. et al. 2006. Gypenosides induced apoptosis in human colon cancer cells through the mitochondria-dependent pathways and activation of caspase-3. *Anticancer Res.* 26: 4313–26.
15. Chen, J. C. et al. 2009. Gypenosides induced G0/G1 arrest via CHk2 and apoptosis through endoplasmic reticulum stress and mitochondria-dependent pathways in human tongue cancer SCC-4 cells. *Oral Oncol.* 45: 273–83.
16. Wang, Q. F. et al. 2007. Gypenosides induce apoptosis in human hepatoma Huh-7 cells through a calcium/reactive oxygen species-dependent mitochondrial pathway. *Planta Med.* 73: 535–44.
17. Sun, D. P. et al. 2013. Gypenosides induce apoptosis by Ca^{2+} overload mediated by endoplasmic-reticulum and store-operated Ca^{2+} channels in human hepatoma cells. *Cancer Biother.Radiopharm.* 28: 320–6.
18. Chiu, T. H. et al. 2004. Gypenosides inhibited N-acetylation of 2-aminofluorene, N-acetyltrans-ferase gene expression and DNA adduct formation in human cervix epithelioid carcinoma cells (HeLa). *Res. Commun. in Mol. Pathol. Pharmacol.* 115–116: 157–74.
19. Lu, K. W. et al. 2010. Gypenosides causes DNA damage and inhibits expression of DNA repair genes of human oral cancer SAS cells. *In Vivo* 24: 287–92.
20. Lu, K. W. et al. 2012. Gypenosides suppress growth of human oral cancer SAS cells in vitro and in a murine xenograft model: The role of apoptosis mediated by caspase-dependent and caspase-independent pathways. Integrative Cancer Therapies 11: 129–40.
21. Yan, H. et al. 2014. Antiproliferation and anti-migration induced by gypenosides in human colon cancer SW620 and esophageal cancer Eca-109 cells. *Human Experim. Toxicol.* 33: 522–33.
22. Yan, H. et al. 2014. Anticancer effect and the underlying mechanisms of gypenosides on human colorectal cancer SW480 cells. *PLoS One* 9: e95609/1–e95609/10.
23. Yang, J. et al. 2010. Suppressive effect of gypenosides on murine leukemia L1210 cell lines. *Zhongyaocai* 33: 1588–92.
24. Hsu, H. Y. et al. 2011. An experimental study on the antileukemia effects of gypenosides in vitro and in vivo. *Integr. Cancer Therapies* 10: 101–12.
25. Lu, K. W. et al. 2008. Gypenosides inhibited invasion and migration of human tongue cancer SCC4 cells through downregulation of NF-κB and matrix metalloproteinase-9. *Anticancer Res.* 28: 1093–100.
26. Lu, K. W. et al. 2011. Gypenosides inhibits migration and invasion of human oral cancer SAS cells through the inhibition of matrix metalloproteinase-2, -9 and urokinase-plasminogen by ERK1/2 and NF-κB signaling pathways. *Human Experim. Toxicol.* 30: 406–15.
27. Huang, T. H. W. et al. 2007. Specific reversal of resistance to colchicine in CEM/VLB100 cells by *Gynostemma pentaphyllum* extract. *Phytomed.* 14: 830–9.
28. Wang, H. Y. et al. 2004. Quantitative evaluation of the influences from glycyrrizin and pypenosides on the precancerous lesions of rat hepatoma. *J. Zhongshan Med. Univ.* 15: 37–40.
29. Wan, J. J. et al. 1993. Effects of *Gynostemma pentaphyllum* on tumor cell proliferation and immune function. *J. Fujian College TCM* 3: 159–61.
30. Xu, C. F. et al. 2002. Inhibitory effects of total Gypenosides on sarcoma 180 cells and K562 cells. *J. Xi'an Med. Univ.* 23: 217–9.
31. Ky, P. T. et al. 2010. Dammarane-type saponins from *Gynostemma pentaphyllum*. *Phytochem.* 71: 994–1001.
32. Yin, F. et al. 2006. Nine new dammarane saponins on *Gynostemma pentaphyllum*. *Chem. Biodiver.* 3: 771–82.

33. Chen, Y. et al. 1986. The studies of *Gynostemma pentaphyllum* in Japan. *Zhejiang Yyaoxue* 3: 33–6.
34. Huang, T. H. W. et al. 2007. Gypenoside XLIX, a naturally occurring PPAR-α activator, inhibits cytokine-induced vascular cell adhesion molecule-1 expression and activity in human endothelial cells. *Eur. J. Pharmacol.* 565: 158–65.
35. Huang, T. H. W. et al. 2006. Gypenoside XLIX isolated from *Gynostemma pentaphyllum* inhibits NF-κB activation via a PPAR-α dependent pathway. *J. Biomed. Sci.* 13: 535–48.
36. Huang, T. H. W. et al. 2007. Gypenoside XLIX, a naturally occurring gynosaponin, PPAR-α dependently inhibits LPS-induced tissue factor expression and activity in human THP-1 monocytic cells. *Toxicol. Applied Pharmacol.* 218: 30–6.
37. Chen, D. J. et al. 2014. Cytotoxic activity of gypenosides and gynogenin against non-small cell lung cancer A549 cells. *Bioorg. Med. Chem. Lett.* 24: 186–91.
38. Shi, L. et al. 2015. In vitro inhibitory activities of six gypenosides on human liver cancer cell line HepG2 and possible role of HIF-1α pathway in them. *Chemico-Biol. Interactions* 238, 48–54.
39. Piao, X. L. et al. 2014. Novel dammarane saponins from *Gynostemma pentaphyllum* and their cytotoxic activities against HepG2 cells. *Bioorg. Med. Chem. Lett.* 24: 4831–3.
40. Shi, L. et al. 2012. Two new triterpene saponins from *Gynostemma pentaphyllum. J. Asian Nat. Prod. Res.* 14: 856–61.
41. Zhang, X. S. et al. 2015. Novel dammarane-type triterpenes isolated from hydrolyzate of total *Gynostemma pentaphyllum* saponins. *Bioorg. Med. Chem. Lett.* 25: 3095–9.
42. Li, N. et al. 2012. Triterpenes possessing an unprecedented skeleton isolated from hydrolyzate of total saponins from *Gynostemma pentaphyllum. Eur. J. Med. Chem.* 50: 173–8.
43. Zhu, H. R. et al. 2012. Reversal of P-gp and MRP1-mediated multidrug resistance by H6, a gypenoside aglycon from *Gynostemma pentaphyllum*, in vincristine-resistant human oral cancer (KB/VCR) cells. *Eur. J. Pharmacol.* 696: 43–53.
44. Cheng, T. C. et al. 2011. Antiproliferation effect and apoptosis mechanism of prostate cancer Cell PC3 by flavonoids and saponins prepared from *Gynostemma pentaphyllum. J. Agricult. Food Chem.* 59: 11319–29.
45. Tsai, Y. C. et al. 2010. Preparative chromatography of flavonoids and saponins in *Gynostemma pentaphyllum* and their antiproliferation effect on hepatoma cells. *Phytomed.* 18: 2–10.
46. Tsai, Y. C. et al. 2010. Preparation of carotenoids and chlorophylls from *Gynostemma pentaphyllum* (Thunb.) Makino and their anti-proliferation effect on hepatoma cells. *J. Med. Food* 13: 1431–42.
47. Yang, X. B. et al. 2008. Isolation and characterization of immunostimulatory polysaccharide from an herb tea, *Gynostemma pentaphyllum* Makino. *J. Agricul. Food Chem.* 56: 6905–9.
48. Jin, M. et al. 1992. Effect of a Jiao-Gu-Lan extract on colon cancer cell growth. *Xiandai Yinyong Yaoxue* 9: 49–52.
49. Li, X. L. et al. 2012. Isolation and antitumor activities of acidic polysaccharide from *Gynostemma pentaphyllum* Makino. *Carbohydrate Polymers* 89: 942–47.
50. Chen, T. et al. 2011. Catalytic synthesis and antitumor activities of sulfated polysaccharide from *Gynostemma pentaphyllum* Makino. *Carbohydrate Polymers* 83: 554–60.

168 Ren Shen 人参

Ginseng

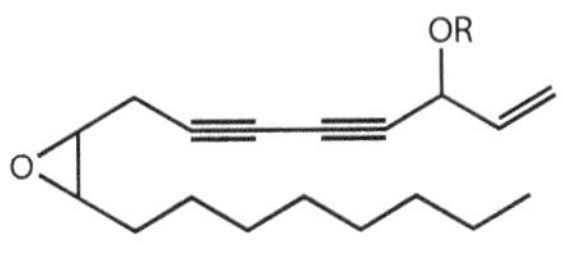

1. R = H
2. R = -OCCH$_3$

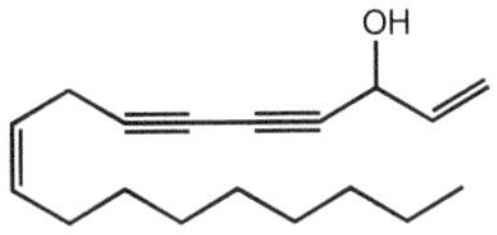

3

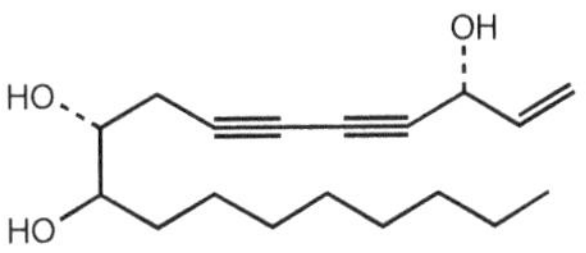

4

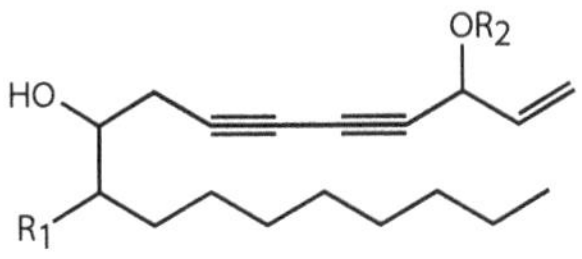

5. R$_1$ = -Cl, R$_2$ = -H
6. R$_1$ = -I, R$_2$ = -OCCH$_3$

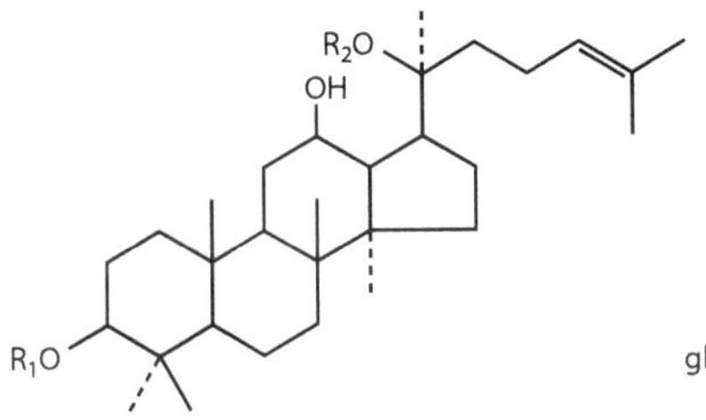

7. R$_2$ = - glc-(2-1)-glc, R$_2$ = -H
8. R$_1$ = -glc, R$_2$ = -H
9. R$_1$ = -H, R$_2$ = -glc
10. R$_1$ = -R$_2$ = -H

glc = D-beta-glucopyranosyl

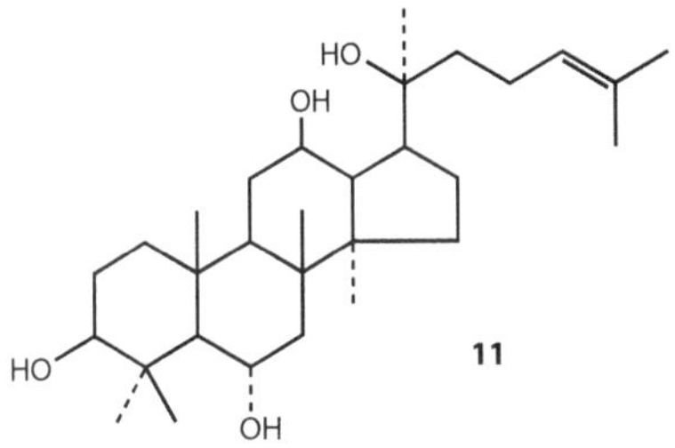

11

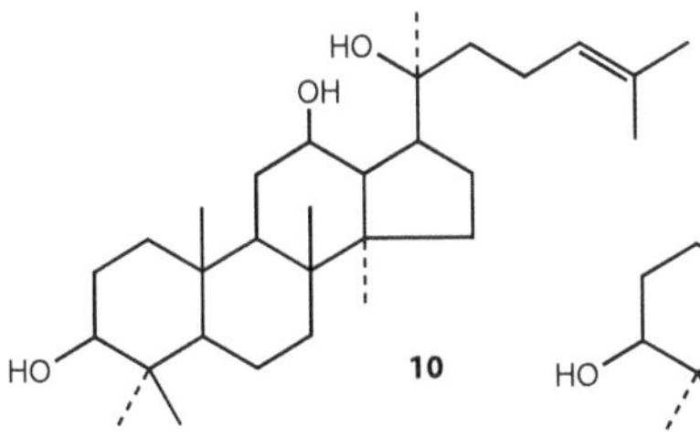

10

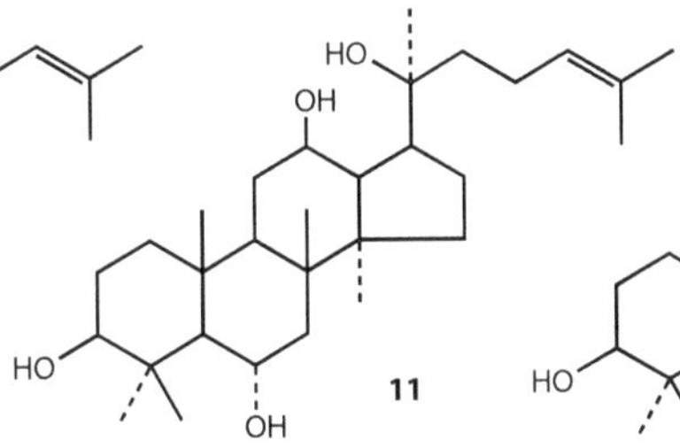

11

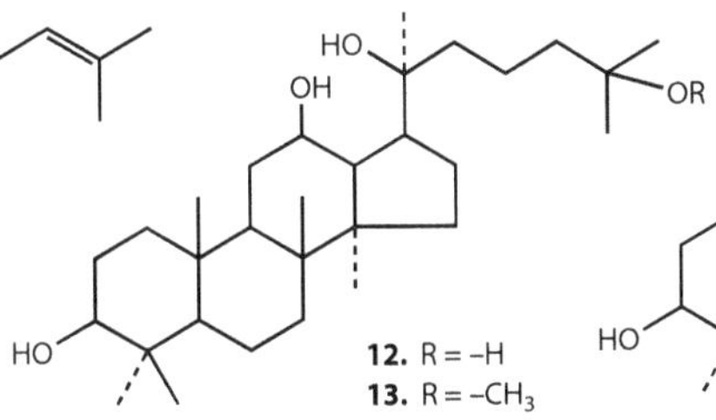

12. R = -H
13. R = -CH$_3$

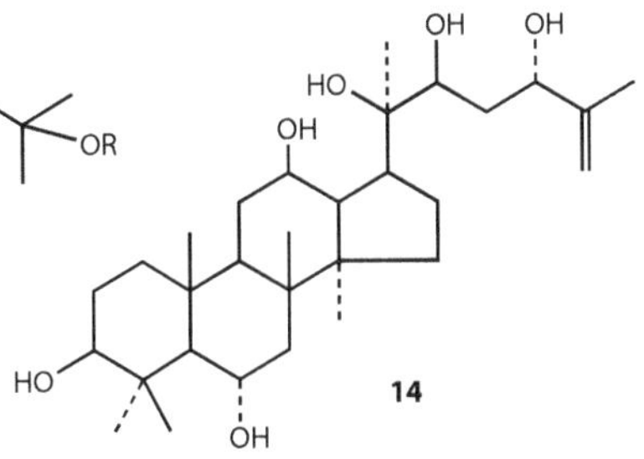

14

Herb Origination

Ren Shen (Ginseng) is the dried rhizomes and roots of an Araliaceae perennial plant, *Panax ginseng*, which is referred to as one of the most famous tonic herbs in the world. It is mostly distributed in the regions of the Changbai Mountains and southeast Xiao Xing'an Ling Mountains in northeast China as well as Korea. Ren Shen has been used for a thousand years in Chinese systems of medicine. The first Chinese herbal classic titled as *Shennong Ben Cao Jing* recorded it as a drug in the top grade. The Ginseng plants are cultivated in the Changbai Mountain range of China and Korea. The famous northeast Ginseng and Korean Ginseng originated from the same species of plants that are grown in the similar natural environment. But according to the different processes, Ginseng has many market specifications, which can be mainly classified to two forms, namely white Ginseng (air-dried in the sun) and red Ginseng (steamed and dried).

Antitumorigenetic Activities

Ren Shen has been widely used as a traditional oriental medicine for its broad spectrum of biological effects. Its antimutagenic, antitumorigenic, and antitumor activities were demonstrated by extensive *in vitro* and *in vivo* studies. The powders and the extracts of the five- and six-year-old white Ginsengs and four- to six-year-old red Ginseng exerted significant anticarcinogenic effects in mice models with pulmonary carcinoma. The prolonged administration of red Ginseng extract was able to significantly inhibit the carcinogenesis in the liver and the lung that was induced by carcinogens (AFB1 or urethane and BAP, respectively), and it also exerted protective and antioxidant effects on AFB1-caused hepatotoxicity.[1–5] The intake of Ginseng could reduce the risk of gastric tumor and the incidence of papillomas and restrain the development of mammary tumors induced by N-methyl-N-nitrosourea and brain and spinal cord tumor development induced by N-ethyl-N-nitrosourea. It also inhibited DMBA-caused carcinogenesis in the uterus, the cervix, and the vagina and effectively diminished the occurrence of UVA-induced skin neoplasm.[4–7] Also, the Ginseng treatment efficiently enhanced the ^{60}Co γ radiotherapy against human PC3 prostate carcinoma cells in nude mice xenograft.[4–8] During the suppression of the tumorigenesis of BAP, DMBA, and/or croton oil, Ginseng significantly diminished the frequencies of chromosomal aberrations and micronuclei, whose interactions are closely involved in its antimutagenic and anticarcinogenic mechanism.[4,9]

In addition to the chemopreventive activities, Ginseng also exerted remarkable potentials in antitumor immunostimulation and antioxidation. In the animal models, Ginseng prominently enhanced the cytotoxicity of macrophages and the formation of T lymphocyte rosette and stimulated the production of thyroid hormones and the activation of NK cells.[9,10] The i.p. injection of the red Ginseng extract in a dose of 200 mg/kg significantly decreased GST-P-formed positive foci caused by 0.01% acetyl-amino-fluorene in the rat hepatocarcinogenesis.[11] The methanolic extract derived from heat-processed Ginseng exhibited notable abilities to scavenge superoxides generated by xanthine–xanthine oxidase and to attenuate the LPO in rat brain homogenates. The antioxidative effects by Ginseng also protected the skin from TPA-induced tumor promotion after the topical application of the same extract onto the shaven backs of mice.[12] Due to the remarkable antitumor immunostimulation and antioxidation, Ginseng was capable of synergistically improving the anticancer effect of chemotherapeutic drugs in a combinational treatment. At a concentration of 0.3 mg/mL, the red Ginseng and white Ginseng extracts significantly potentiated the antigrowth effects of 5-FU and promoted the cell cycle arrest of human HCT-116 colorectal cancer cells.[13] Additionally, the research results proved that the products from the tissue culture of the Ginseng root also has marked growth inhibitory effect against various of human neoplastic cells including MKN-74 (stomach), SW620 (colon), and PC3 (prostate) cell lines.[14]

These solid evidences truly corroborated that the carcinogenic inhibitory property of Ginseng should be mostly contributed by its immunoenhancing, chemopreventing, and antioxidant activities. Hence, Ginseng and its products may be considered as a promising adjuvant agent for the prevention and the clinical treatment of malignant tumor.

Antitumor Constituents and Activities

Numerous studies in chemical biology have revealed that three major types of bioactive components in Ginseng, i.e., polyacetylenes, triterpenoid saponins, and polysaccharides, are responsible for most of Ginseng's medicinal properties, including the anticarcinogenic and anticancer activities.

Polyacetylene

A petroleum ether extract derived from Ginseng contains rich polyacetylenes, which displayed significant growth inhibition against HepG2 hepatoma and L929 fibroblast cell lines *in vitro*.[15] But some polyacetylenes exerted marked cytotoxicity in the bioassay against L1210 (leukemia), DT (renal), HeLa (cervix), T24 (bladder), and MCF-7 (breast) malignant cell lines and NIH/3T3 fibroblast cells, whose potencies were greater than those of 5-FU and cisplatin chemotherapeutic drugs.[16] Of the active polyacetylenes, panaxydol (**1**) displayed more prominence, and its IC_{50} values were 0.65 μM in DT cells, 0.19 μM in L1210 cells, and 1.3 μM in NIH/3T3 cells.[16] In the experiments, either panaxydol (**1**) or panaxynol (**2**) induced the cell cycle arrest of human SK-MEL-1 melanoma cells at G1 phase by reducing CDK2 expression and upregulation p27KIP1 and p21WAF1 protein expressions, thereby markedly restraining the cell proliferation.[17,18]

Panaxytriol (**3**) demonstrated significant inhibitory effect against the cell growth and the DNA syntheses in the various tested tumor cells. The cytotoxicity of panaxytriol (**3**) on mouse P388D1 lymphoma cells was in both time- and dose-dependent manners with IC_{50} value of 3.1 μg/mL. The treatment of P388D1 cells with 5 μg/mL of panaxytriol (**3**) for 24 and 36 h promoted the cell cycle arrest at G2/M phase *in vitro*.[19] The intramuscular administration of panaxytriol (**3**) in a dose of 40 mg/kg resulted in a significant antigrowth effect in mice transplanted with B16 melanoma.[20] Also, the cellular accumulation of mitomycin-C (MMC) could be augmented in human MK-1 gastric cancer cells by panaxytriol (**3**), achieving synergistic antitumor effect.[21] More evidences demonstrated that the inhibitory effects of panaxydol (**1**), panaxynol (**2**), and panaxytriol (**3**) were closely dependent on their concentration, i.e., they are cytotoxic at a high concentration, but they are cytostatic at a low concentration.[22]

Moreover, two polyacetylenes, panaxacol and dihydropanaxacol, isolated from the callus cells of Ginseng, exerted the inhibitory rates of up to 95% and 80%, respectively, against the growth of Yoshida sarcoma cells at a 10 μg/mL concentration *in vitro*.[23] Other polyacetylene such as 3-acetylpanaxydol (**4**), chlorohydrin (**5**), panaxydol (**1**), 10-acetylpanaxytriol, panaxyne, panaxyne epoxide, chloropanaxydiol, panaxydol linoleate, and ginsenoyne-A linoleate can be also produced by tissue culture techniques. These polyacetylenes were effective in the inhibition of murine L1210 leukemia cells,[24–26] and the ED_{50} values of 3-acetylpanaxydol (**4**), 10-acetylpanaxytriol, and panaxydol chlorohydrin (**5**) were 0.52, 1.2, and 0.50 μg/mL, respectively.[27–29] More approaches clearly indicated that the cytotoxic activity of panaxydol (**1**) and panaxytriol (**3**) on the L1210 cells would be diminished by acetylization.[28] When the structure of panaxydol (**1**) was modified by esterification, hydroiodination, and methylation, the resulted derivative (**6**) would display greater cytotoxicity on L1210 cells and HeLa cells with IC_{50} values (μg/mL) of 0.06 and 12.7, respectively.[30]

Total Saponins

Ginsenosides, the triterpenoid saponins derived from Ginseng, are the principal constituents responsible for the biological effects of Ginseng. The anticancer activity of total saponins of Ginseng (TSPG) was proven in three types of human leukemia cell lines, HL-60 (promyelocytic), K562 (chronic myelocytic), and KG1α (acute myelocytic), together with the inductive effect of apoptosis.[31–34] Compared to its nonheat-processed crude saponins, the heat-processed crude saponins showed more potent inhibition in the proliferation of human HCT-15 colorectal cancer cells and the promotion of apoptosis by a mitochondrial pathway.[35] Furthermore, the genotoxicity caused by CTX in peripheral lymphocyte cells and bone marrow cells could be significantly reduced, and the CTX-induced bone marrow cell apoptosis could be restrained in the presence of TSPG. The CTX-reduced enzymatic antioxidant (T-SOD, GPx, and catalase [CAT]) activities were recovered, and the contents of the nonenzymic antioxidant (GSH) were raised during the TSPG treatment.[36] These findings evidenced that the tonic and antioxidative properties of TSPG may be used not only for obviously suppressing the cancer growth and development but also for effectively enhancing the efficacy of chemotherapeutic agents and reducing the side effects of chemotherapy to protect cancer patients.[31,32]

Likewise, the medicinal chemistry studies also afforded some important evidences, revealing that anticarcinogenicity is more prominent in red Ginseng made by heat treatment and steaming. The result indicated that various steaming temperature and time treatments of the Ginseng herbs may partly stepwise deglycosylate Ginseng saponins to yield less glycosylated ginsenosides, such as Rg2, 20R-Rg2, Rg3, Rh1, and Rh2, and decrease others (Rb1, Rb2, Rb3, Rc, Rd, Re ,and Rg1).[37] The heat process, i.e., deglycosylation, is able to enhance the role of Ginseng in the inhibition of cancer growth and carcinogenesis. Also, utilizing the enzyme reactions and structural modifications could transform the ineffective ginsenosides (Rb1, Rb3, Rd, and Re) to active saponins such as M1 and monoesters of ginsenosides (DM1, PM1, and SM1).[38] These deglycosylated saponins showed the considerable cytotoxicity against human cancer cell lines, such as MCF-7 (breast), SK-MEL-2 (skin), and B16 (ovary), and moderate effects on COR-L23 lung carcinoma cells *in vitro*.[38]

Moreover, protopanaxadiol (PPD) class ginsenosides present to be 2.5 times higher in the red Ginseng than in the white Ginseng. Normally, the PPD ginsenosides showed more cytotoxicity and more efficient cellular uptake in the tumor cells, especially in MCF-7 breast cancer cells, compared to protopanaxatriol (PPT) class ginsenosides.[39] Additionally, only a few oleanane-type saponins exist in Ginseng, and they only showed anticarcinogenic activity against two-stage skin cancer-promotion *in vitro* and *in vivo*.[40]

Individual Saponins

Up to now, over 30 ginsenosides were isolated from Ginseng roots and leaves, such as ginsenosides (Rg3, Rh1, Rh2, Rg1, Rg5, Rk1, Ro, F1, L8, F3, and Rf). Comprehensively, the three less glycosylated ginsenosides, Rg3 (**7**) (20R- or 20S-), Rh2 (**8**) (20R- or 20S-), and M1 (**9**), are very useful as potential candidates for the prevention and the treatment of malignant tumor cell initiation, growth, and metastasis. The Rg3 (**7**) was already used in clinical treatment as an adjuvant anticancer agent in China. The following summarized scientific data has provided the solid evidences for further development and application.

Ginsenoside-Rg3

Rg3 (**7**), Rh2 (**8**), and Rg5 were able to notably decrease the incidence of BAP-induced mouse lung carcinogenesis.[40,41] The pretreatment of Rg3 (**7**) to mice obviously repressed TPA-induced skin cancer promotion and carcinogenesis of human breast epithelial MCF-10A cells by inhibiting the activities of COX-2 and epidermal ornithine decarboxylase and lessening the expressions of NF-κB and ERK.[12] Similarly, Rg3 (**7**) in 25–100 μM concentrations dose-dependently inhibited the growth of human SW620 and HCT116 colon cancer cell lines via the decrease of NF-κB activity and the induction of apoptosis.[42,43] A 28-day oral treatment with Rg3-fortified Red ginseng preparation (100 mg/kg) remarkably suppressed the growth of human H460 NSCLC cells, leading to the decrease of the tumor volume and weight by 30–31% in nude mice concomitant with the facilitated splenocyte proliferation and the enhanced carbon particle phagocytic index of blood macrophages *in vivo*.[45] By significantly inducing DNA double-strand breaks and damage, ginsenoside Rg3 (**7**) dose-dependently exerted the cytotoxicity on four human osteosarcoma cell lines (MG-63, OS732, U-2OS, and HOS), and the MG-63 and U-2OS cells were the most sensitive to Rg3.[46] By impacting the cell cycle and the cell apoptosis, Rg3 (**7**) markedly inhibited the proliferation of Eca9706 esophageal cancer cells.[47] The proapoptotic effect was also observed in liver carcinoma cells after the Rg3 treatment *in vitro* and *in vivo*.[48] The administration of Rg3 (5 mg/kg) by gastrogavage once a day for four weeks, combined with 5-FU (20 mg/kg) by i.p. injection once every four days for four weeks, significantly inhibited the growth of transplanted human hepatocellular carcinoma and obviously reduced intratumoral MVD by inhibiting the angiogenesis of malignant tumor in nude mice.[49] Similarly, when Rg3 (50 μM) is combined with an anticancer drug such as docetaxel (DOC) (5 nM), paclitaxel (10 nM), cisplatin (10 μM), or DOX (2 μM), the cotreatments were more effective in inducting apoptosis and inhibiting colon cancer cells, whose synergistic effects were mediated by up-expressions of apoptotic proteins (Bax, caspase-3, and caspase-9) and down-expressions of antiapoptotic genes and proliferation marker genes (Bcl-2, IAP, COX-2, c-Fos, c-Jun, and cyclin-D1).[43] The synergistic antitumor effect of Rg3 and cisplatin was also observed in cisplatin-resistant T24R2 bladder cancer cells.[50] In the cotreatment, Rg3 (**7**) was able to sensitize human A549 and H1299 nonNSCLC cell lines to γ-radiation by suppressing NF-κB activity and NF-κB-regulated gene products, leading to the inhibition of tumor progression. The augmentation of the radiation therapy by Rg3 (**7**) was further proven in C57BL/6 mice model bearing a Lewis lung carcinoma.[51] Rg3 (**7**), in addition, was found to have the inhibitory properties against the invasion, the metastasis, and the angiogenesis of cancer cells.[40]

Actually, Rg3 (**7**) has two epimers, i.e., 20(S)-Rg3 and 20(R)-Rg3, whose epimerization is produced by steam process. The apoptosis of human HT-29 colon cancer cells was promoted by 20(S)-Rg3 via an AMPK signaling pathway.[44] The growth inhibition of human U87-MG glioma cells by 20(S)-Rg3 was found to be also mediated by the suppression of voltage-gated K^+ channels concomitant with the induction of G2/M cell arrest and apoptosis of U87-MG cells.[52] 20(S)-Rg3 also stimulated the apoptosis of humanAGS gastric cancer cells through the activation of caspase-3, caspase-8, and caspase-9 and the moderation of Bcl-2 and Bax expressions.[53] 20(R)-Rg3, but not 20(S)-Rg3, could suppress the migration, the invasion, and the anoikis resistance of A549 lung cancer cells by inhibiting TGF-β1-induced epithelial–mesenchymal transition (EMT) and TGF-β1-regulated MMP-2 and repressing Smad2 and p38-MAPK.[54] Similarly, 20(S)-Rg3 potently blocked the hypoxia-induced EMT of ovarian cancer cells *in vitro* and *in vivo*, where the HIF-1α expression was induced by 20(S)-Rg3 to trigger the anticancer effects.[55] In addition, Rg3 (**7**) also reduced the extent of MNNG-induced DNA damage and apoptosis in a normal human fibroblast cell line to exert the protective and anticarcinogenic activities.[46]

Ginsenoside-Rh2

Rh2 (**8**) exhibited various anticarcinoma-related properties. In the *in vitro* experiments, Rh2 (**8**) significantly inhibited the cell growth and induced the apoptosis of many types of human tumor cell lines, including A375-S2 (skin), HeLa (cervix), RM-1 (prostate), HepG2 and Hep-A-22 (liver), HL-60 (leukemic), A549 and A549/DDP (lung), and SK-N-BE2 (brain) cells.[56–68] In nude mice models, the significant suppressive activity were further confirmed against the growth of human carcinoma cells of the ovary and the prostate.[56,69] The apoptotic mechanism of Rh2 was revealed to correlate with the reduction of Bcl-2 expression, the upregulation of Bax expression, the activation of p53 and caspase cascade, and the arrest of cell cycle.[60–63] But the apoptosis in HeLa cells was mainly associated with ROS- and Ca^{2+}-mediated c-Jun NH2-terminal kinase-1 activations, and the A549 cell death process was critically dependent on the increase of DR4 death receptor expression in the Rh2 treatments.[57,60] In comparison with other ginsenosides, Rh2 (**8**) and Rh1 were able to diminish the thymidine incorporation into the tumor cells, and Rh2 (**8**) exhibited the strongest inhibition on DNA synthesis.[59] Likewise, Rh2 (**8**) blocked the cell cycle progression at G1 phase in HL-60 leukemia cells via the downregulations of CDK-4, CDK-6, cyclin-D1, cyclin-D2, cyclin-D3, and cyclin-E and the upregulation of CDK inhibitors (such as p21CIP1/WAF1 and p27KIP1). By increasing the TGF-β production, Rh2 elicited the differentiation of HL-60 cells.[70] Moreover, by repressing the activation of p38 MAPK, ERK, and JNK, Rh2 (**8**) exerted significant inhibitory effect on MMPs in human astroglioma cells, leading to the marked obstruction of the cell invasion.[71] The administration of Rh2 (5–20 mg/kg) markedly potentiated the cytotoxicity of CTX in mice bearing B16 melanoma cells or Lewis lung carcinoma cells and greatly enhanced the apoptotic effect of cisplatin in PC3M prostatic cancer cells *in vivo*. At the same time, the genotoxic effect of the anticancer drugs could be notably attenuated in the combined treatments.[72,73] The synergistic activity of Rh2 (**8**) is also considerable for improving cancer chemotherapy.

Ginsenoside M1

Actually, ginsenoside-M1, ginsenoside-K, and ginsenoside-IH-901 are the same saponin (= 20-*O*-β-D-glucosyl-20(S)-protopanaxadiol), which can be transformed from ginsenoside-Rd1 by intestinal bacteria hydrolyzation.[72,73] The broad spectrum of cancer cell inhibition of M1 (**9**) has been confirmed in many neoplastic cells *in vitro*, including HL-60 and K562 myeloid leukemias, PC-14 pulmonary adenocarcinoma, HepG2, SMMC7721 and BEL-7402 hepatomas, 95-D high-metastatic lung cancer, MKN-45 gastric cancer, B16-BL6 high-metastatic melanoma, and a cancer cell subline resistant to cisplatin (PC/DDP).[74–79] The treatment with the M1 (**9**) to mice obviously reduced the number of aberrant crypts induced by 1,2-dimethyl hydrazine and azoxymethane (AOM), sufficiently prevented the colon carcinogenesis by 80%, concomitantly lessened the cell growth, and increased apoptosis through significant decrease of EGFR and ErbB2 activation and Cox-2 expression.[73,80] In association with upregulating p53 activity and Bax and caspase expressions, M1 (**9**) markedly promoted the apoptosis and the G0/G1 cell cycle arrest of human SMMC7721 hepatoma cells.[81] Ginsenoside-K (**9**) enlarged the intracellular ROS generation, which then triggered the apoptosis of human HT-29 colon cancer cells through the modulation of mitochondria-dependent apoptotic pathway and MAPK pathway.[82] M1 (**9**) was also effective in the suppression of migration and invasion in association with the diminution of TNFα-induced NF-κB activation and MMP-9 secretion/expression. By the noticeable effects, the M1 (**9**) obstructed the migration/invasion of human astroglioma cells and markedly lessened the lung and liver metastases of colon neoplastic cells and lung metastasis of B16-BL6 melanoma cells.[81–84]

Other Ginsenosides

Besides Rg3 (**7**), Rh2 (**8**), and M1 (**9**), other Ginseng saponins also displayed various degrees of anticancer effects against some types of cancer cells. For instance, Pk1 markedly restrained human HepG2 hepatoma cells in coordination with the inhibition of telomerase and the induction of apoptosis via (1) obvious decrease of both hTERT and c-Myc expressions, (2) upregulation of caspase-8 and caspase-3, and (3) activation of ERK.[85] The suppression of Rg1 was also present in the two-stage mouse skin carcinogenesis and in the proliferation of human MG-63 osteosarcoma cells.[86,87] In both anchorage-independent and -dependent manners, the proliferation and the colony formation of breast cancer cells could be obstructed by Rp1 concomitant with the promotion of cell cycle arrest and apoptosis by declining the stability of the IGF-1R protein.[88] The ginsenosides (such as Ro, Rh1, Rh2, F1, L8, Rg1, F3, and Rf) could exert the antiproliferative effect against human U2OS osteosarcoma cells through the increase of G0/G1 cell cycle arrest and/or cell death induction.[87,89] Two other saponins, 3,6,20(S)-trihydroxy-12,23-epoxydammar-24-ene-6,20-di-*O*-β-D-glucoside and 3β,12β,20-trihydroxydammar-24-en-3-yl-3-*O*-β-D-6′-acetyl glucoside, which were isolated from the leaves of *P. ginseng*, showed moderate inhibition against U937 lymphoma cells, HeLa cervix cancer cells, and HepG2 hepatoma cells *in vitro*.[67]

Furthermore, several ginsenosides with protopanaxatriol aglycone, such as Rb1, Rb2, Rc, Rg1, and Re, were found to exert chemosensitizing effect in multidrug-resistant tumor cells by directly repressing P-gp expression, leading to the elevation of the intracellular accumulation of antitumor drugs. Thus, this group of saponins was capable of markedly reversing the resistances of DNR and DOX in AML-2/D100 and AML-2/DX100 cells, to augment the anticancer activity.[89–91]

Triterpenoids

The majority of triterpenoids present in Ginseng can release their aglycones by the metabolization or the deglycosylation of intestinal bacteria after oral administration. 20(S)-Protopanaxadiol (20(S)PPD) (**10**) and 20(S)-protopanaxatriol (20(S)PPT) (**11**) are the main sapogenin metabolites from PPD ginsenosides (e.g., Rg3 and Rh2) and PPT ginenosides (e.g., Re and Rg1), respectively, which have been well characterized to possess the pleiotropic anticancer capabilities on various neoplastic cells. For instance, the total prosapogenins obtained from acid hydrolyzation displayed cytotoxicity against A549 (lung), SKOV-3 (ovary), SK-MEL-2 (skin), and P388, L1210, and K562 (leukemic) tumor cell lines *in vitro*.[92] PPD (**10**) and PPT (**11**) have been identified to have a significant effect in reducing the cell viability and inducing the apoptosis of two Int-407 and Caco-2 intestinal cancer cells and leukemia THP-1 cells.[93–95] The IC_{50} values in the THP-1 cells were in the range of 13–19 μg/mL for PPD, PPT, as well as PPD-related ginsenoside Rh2.[95] The PPD and PPT ruled in two different apoptosis-inducing pathways in Caco-2 cells, i.e., PPD did not change caspase-3 activity, while PPT augmented caspase-3 activity, but PPD exerted significantly higher effect in the promotion of Caco-2 cell apoptosis.[93,94] The growth of two human Reh and RS4, and 11 acute lymphoblastic leukemia cell lines was obstructed by PPD (**10**) together with the induction of cell cycle arrest and cell differentiation but no apoptosis. It also showed little toxicity to PBMCs.[96] The investigations further demonstrated that PPD (**10**)-type sapogenins usually display greater anticarcinogenetic and anticancer activities than PPT (**11**)-type ones because PPD derivatives have more lipophilic structures to confer more potent cytotoxicity.

Moreover, *in vitro* and *in vivo* experiments demonstrated that PPD (**10**) could suppress the growth of human SMMC-7721 hepatoma, SF188, and U87MG gliomas cell lines. Interestingly, PPD activated caspase-3, caspase-8, caspase-7, and caspase-9 only in the SF188 cells within 3 h but did not activate any caspases in the U87MG cells during the apoptotic promotion, revealing that PPD induced different forms of programmed cell death, i.e., apoptosis and autophagy by both caspase-dependent and caspase-independent mechanisms.[97–99] The antigrowth activity of PPD was confirmed against hepatoma-22 cells, Lewis lung cancer cells, and B16 melanoma cells *in vivo* in doses of 25–100 mg/kg, and the anticancer effect was found to be also contributed by its immunepotentiating property (such as significantly increasing the activity of body immunity, improving the lymphocyte transformation, enhancing natural killer cell activity, and increasing the contents of IL-2).[100]

Likewise, a derivative of PPD, 25-hydroxyprotopanaxadiol (**12**) (25-OH-PPD) (isolated from the fruits of *P. ginseng*), demonstrated significant dose-dependent inhibitory effects on the proliferation of human LNCaP and PC3 prostate cancer cell lines, correlating with the induction apoptosis and G1 cell cycle arrest. In nude mice bearing PC3 prostate tumor xenograft, 25-OH-PPD (**12**) repressed the tumor growth dose-dependently, and it safely improved the anticancer potencies of chemotherapeutic agents (taxotere and gemcitabine) and radiotherapy.[101,102] 20(S)-25-Methoxyprotopanaxadiol (**13**) (20(S)-25-OMe-PPD), discovered from the leaves of Tian Qi and Ren Shen, was capable of repressing the proliferation of 12 human cancer cell lines *in vitro*. The suppressive potencies of 20(S)-25-OMe-PPD (**13**) were greater than those of 20(S)-PPD (**10**) by 5- to 15-fold and of ginsenoside-Rg3 (**7**) by 10- to 100-fold on most tested cell lines.[103] These results highlighted some SARs of the PPD-type sapogenins, which may provide valuable clues to modify PPD analogs for more active potentials.

Normally, PPT (**11**) displayed less inhibitory effect on the growth of tumor cells in comparison to PPD (**10**). PPT (**11**) was effective in the inhibition of human U2OS osteosarcoma cells through the increase of the cell cycle arrest at G0/G1 phase and the cell apoptosis.[87] PPT (**11**) also exerted dose-dependent inhibitory effects against the growth, invasion, and migration of murine B16-BL6 melanoma cells and human HT1080 fibrosarcoma cells *in vitro*. Either oral administration or intravenous injections of PPT resulted in significant repressive effect against the growth and the lung metastasis of melanoma B16-BL6 cells *in vivo*. The antitumor and antimetastatic activities of PPT (**11**) were usually more potent than those of PPT ginsenosides in most the cases, implying that the glycosylation may reduce the potency of PPT ginsenosides. The *in vivo* antimetastatic effect of PPT ginsenosides were mediated by the intestinal bacterial metabolites after oral administration.[104] Moreover, PPT (**11**) could be rapidly esterified with fatty acids, and the esterified PPT did not directly affect the tumor growth *in vitro*, but it showed an ability to enhance the cytotoxicity of splenic NK cells to neoplastic cells and to augment the NK cell-mediated tumor cell lysis.[105,106] In addition, a PPT-type analog, 20(R),22(ξ),24(S)-dammar-25(26)-ene-3β,6α,12β-20,22,24-hexanol (**14**), which was isolated from the leaves of *P. ginseng*, exhibited the moderate inhibition against human HepG2 hepatoma cells concomitant with p53-mediated cell cycle arrest and caspase-activated apoptosis, with the IC_{50} value of 20.1 μM.[64]

Using biotransformation techniques may change the bioprofile of PPT (**11**) and make it sensitive to other specific carcinoma cells. When PPT (**11**) was cultivated with a fungus, *Mucor spinosus*, seven cytotoxic metabolites such as 29-hydroxyl-20(S)-protopanaxatriol, 27-hydroxyl-20(S)-protopanaxatriol, 28-hydroxyl-20(S)-protopanaxatriol, 2-oxo-20(S)-protopanaxatriol, 12-oxo-27-hydroxyl-20(S)-protopanaxatriol, 12-oxo-26-hydroxyl-20(S)-protopanaxatriol, and 12-oxo-15α-hydroxyl-20(S)-protopanaxatriol were constructed, whose metabolites exhibited the potent inhibitory effects against human HL-60 leukemia cells *in vitro*.[107,108]

Polysaccharides

Polysaccharides are another biologically active components prepared from Ginseng, which exhibited tumoricidal activity against a wide range of tumor cells. *In vivo* studies with carcinomas such as K562, HL-60, and KG1α cells revealed that Ginseng polysaccharides (GPSs) had no direct effect on killing tumor cells, but they induced peritoneal macrophage-mediated cytotoxic activity toward the neoplasm. The phagocytic activity could be notably stimulated in the GPS treatment accompanied by the increase of CD68, asparagus polysaccharide (ACP), and α-ANE expressions, the elevation of TNFα, IL-1, and IL-6 levels, and the enhancement of NO production.[108] From the GPS, three polysaccharides labeled as ginsan, GR-5N, and RGAP were separated, which all displayed immune modulatory property.[109]

Ginsan, an acidic polysaccharide, with a molecular weight of 150,000 Da, is composed of 47.1% glucose and galactose, 43.1% galacturonic acid, and 3.7% protein, which is an ideal nontoxic antineoplastic immunostimulator. By remarkably activating multiple immune systems, ginsan exerted obvious *in vivo* suppressive effects against the growth of B16 melanoma and the pulmonary metastasis of B16-F10 melanoma and against BAP-induced autochthonous lung carcinogenesis without a major histocompatibility restriction. The antitumor immunotherapeutic modality was found to be parallel to its capabilities in (1) endogeneously inducing the proliferation of spleen cells and cytotoxic T cells and B cells, (2) increasing the blastogenesis of T cells and lymphokine-activated killer cells, (3) stimulating the Th1-type cytokine expression (such as IL-2 and IFNγ) and the macrophage-type cytokine expression (such as IL-1α and GM-CSF from Th1 cells), and (4) enhancing the proliferation of macrophages and lymphocytes. The ginsan could also activate macrophages to produce reactive nitrogen intermediates.[110–112]

RGAP is an acidic polysaccharide isolated from the red Ginseng, which is composed of arabinose, glucose, glucuronic acid, and galacturonic acid in the ratio of 1.0:3.2:32.4:16.3. RGAP markedly increased the production of NO and TNFα and enhanced the tumoricidal activity of NK cells. The RGAP-treated peritoneal macrophages that contain high levels of NO and TNFα exerted the tumoricidal effect against P815 mastocytoma cells and WEHI-164 fibrosarcoma cells.[113,114] The inhibition ratios of RGAP in mice implanted with sarcoma 180, 3LL lung carcinoma, or JC adenocarcinoma were 26.8–31.6%, after being treated with RGAP (300 mg/kg).[102] The i.p. administration of RGAP in doses of 100 or 300 mg/kg to B16-F10 melanoma-bearing mice notably obstructed the lung metastasis.[115] The immunomodulatory antitumor activity of RGAP was further evaluated by combinational treatments with anticancer agents (such as CTX, paclitaxel, and 5-FU) in the experimental tumor models. RGAP (25–100 mg/kg) not only demonstrated a synergistic antitumor effect in mice transplanted with sarcoma 180, B16 melanoma, or LL/2 lung carcinoma with prolonged survival rates, but also obviously diminished toxic and side effects caused by the chemotherapeutic drugs by restoring splenocyte proliferation and NK cell activity, augmenting CD11b^{+} cell- and B cell-specific mitogenic activities, and inducing IL-6 secretion in the spleen cells.[116,117]

A glucan named as GR-5N with a molecular weight of 25,000 Da was isolated from white Ginseng, which is composed of only glucose with a 1–4 glycosyl linkage main chain and 1–6-linked branch chain. The administration of the GR-5N in a daily dose of 100 mg/kg to mice markedly prolonged the life span of tumor-bearing mice by 46.8%.[118] PSG, another Ginseng polysaccharides, displayed antitumorigenic and radioprotective effects. The treatment with PSG markedly increased the percentage of T lymphocytes in the peripheral blood of the tested animals and elongated the survival rate of mice receiving X-ray (7.5–8.5 Gy) exposure.[119]

PGP2a (3.2×10^4 Da) and PGPW1 (3.5×10^5 Da) were the two homogeneous polysaccharides prepared from the roots of *Panax ginseng*. PGP2a was an acidic protein–polysaccharide consisted of galactose, arabinose, glucose, and galacturonic acid in a molar ratio of 3.7:1.6:0.5:5.4, while PGPW1 consisted of glucose, galactose, mannose, and arabinose in a molar ratio of 3.3:1.2:0.5:1.1. PGP2a and PGPW1 showed potent anti-growth effect on human HGC-27 gastric cancer cells in a dose-dependent fashion in association with causing G2/M cell arrest and cell apoptosis through the down-expressions of Twist and AKR1C2 proteins and the up-expression of NF1 protein.[120,121] PGPW1 also lessened the migration and the invasion of HGC-27 cells by regulating Twist, AKR1C2, NF1, E-cad, vimentin, and N-cadherin expressions.[120] In the assay with human T24 bladder cancer cells, PGPW1 dose-dependently displayed potent antiproliferative and antimetastatic activities. The down-expression of M3 muscarinic receptor on T24 cell surface by PGPW1 was found to contribute to the antitumor functions.[122] Likewise, GLCP, a crude polysaccharide from Ginseng leaves, could significantly reduce cell viability, augment apoptosis-related proteins expression, and promote cell apoptosis and autophagy in human SMMC-7721 hepatoma cells at concentrations of 1.5–2 mg/mL, whose mechanism may be associated with the downregulation of caveolin-1 protein, an essential structural molecule of caveolae.[123]

All these findings highly suggest that the bioactive polysaccharides may be used as an adjuvant in cancer chemotherapeutic and radiotherapeutic applications to improve the quality of carcinoma clinical treatment.

Glycolipoproteins

Gintonin is a hydrophobic amino acid-rich glycolipoprotein (≈67 kDa), which exists in at least six different forms. Its main carbohydrates are glucose and glucosamine, whereas its lipid components contain linoleic, palmitic, oleic, and stearic acids. Gintonin was able to transiently increase the intracellular free Ca^{2+} concentration ($[Ca^{2+}]i$) for exerting the antitumor effect against mouse EACs.[124]

Nanoformulation

Rg3 (**7**) has been formulated to an immune nanoemulsion (VRIN). VRIN could inhibit the growth and the lymphatic metastasis of human gastric cancer cell transplantation tumor in nude mice, whose model was developed by surgical orthotopic implantation of red fluorescent protein-expression NUGC-4 tumor. In a dose of 1 mg/kg, VRIN reduced the tumor weight by 72.9% and diminished the metastasis ratio of the lymph nodes by 87.5%. The inhibition of the tumor lymphangiogenesis was mediated by downregulating VEGF-C expressions. The anticancer and antimetastatic activities of VRIN in the dose of 1 mg/kg were superior to those of 5-FU in a dose 20 mg/kg in the *in vivo* experiment.[125] In addition, Rg3-liposome (L-Rg3) was developed for the optimization of the anticancer effects of Rd3 (**7**). The cytotoxicity and the tumor inhibition of L-Rg3 were significantly enhanced against human A549 lung cancer *in vitro* and *in vivo* and against human HepG2 hepatoma *in vitro* compared to those of Rg3.[126]

Other Bioactivities

Extensive epidemiological studies have shown that Ginseng as a traditional tonic medicine also possesses broad pharmacological potencies for human health, for instance, CNS-modulating, memory-enhancing, immunopotentiating, leucocyte-restoring, cardiovascular-positive, antishock, adaptogenic, antioxidative, hormonal system-strengthening, haematogenesis-simulating, endocrine system-improving, radiation-protecting, antiaging, protein and nucleic acid synthesis-enhancing, and metabolism-promoting activities.

References

1. Yun, T. K. et al. 2001. Anticarcinogenic effect of *Panax ginseng* C.A. Meyer and identification of active compounds. *J. Korean Med. Sci.* 16(Suppl.): S6–S18.
2. Yun, T. K. et al. 1998. Nontoxic and nonorgan specific cancer preventive effect of *Panax ginseng* C. A. Meyer. *ACS Symposium Series, (Functional Foods for Disease Prevention II: Medicinal Plants and Other Foods)*, 702: 162–77.
3. Bespalov, V. G. et al. 2001. Chemoprevention of mammary, cervix and nervous system carcinogenesis in animals using cultured *Panax ginseng* drugs and preliminary clinical trials in patients with precancerous lesions of the esophagus and endometrium. *J. Korean Med. Sci.* 16(Suppl.): S42–S53.
4. Panwar, M. et al. 2005. Inhibition of benzo(a)pyrene induced lung adenoma by *Panax ginseng* extract, EFLA400, in Swiss albino mice. *Biol. Pharm. Bull.* 28: 2063–7.
5. Kim, Y. S. et al. 2011. Protective effect of Korean red ginseng against aflatoxin B1-induced hepatotoxicity in rat. *J. Ginseng Res.* 35: 243–9.
6. Lee, H. J. et al. 2009. Photoprotective effect of red ginseng against ultraviolet radiation-induced chronic skin damage in the hairless mouse. *Phytother. Res.* 23: 399–403.
7. Panwar, M. et al. 2005. Evaluation of chemopreventive action and antimutagenic effect of the standardized panax ginseng extract, EFLA400, in Swiss albino mice. *Phytother. Res.* 19: 65–71.

8. Hur, J. M. et al. 2011. The ethanol extract of red ginseng enhances antitumor effects using Co60 gamma irradiation. *J. Applied Biol. Chem.* 54: 15–20.
9. Panwar, M. et al. 2005. Evaluation of chemopreventive action and antimutagenic effect of the standardized panax ginseng extract, EFLA400, in Swiss albino mice. *Panwar, Meenakshi; Phytother. Res.* 19: 65–71.
10. Yun, Y. S. et al. 1987. Effect of red ginseng on natural killer cell activity in mice with lung adenoma induced by urethane and benzo(a)pyrene. *Cancer Detect. Prevent.* (Suppl.1) (Immunobiol. Cancer AIDS), 301–9.
11. Kang, K. S. et al. 1997. Involvement of the enhancement of natural killer cell activity on the anticancer effect of Red Ginseng during rat hepatocarcinogenesis. *Korean J. Toxicol.* 13: 23–37.
12. Surh, Y. J. et al. 2001. Molecular mechanisms underlying antitumor promoting activities of heat-processed *Panax ginseng* C.A. Meyer. *J. Korean Med. Sci.* 16(Suppl.): S38–S41.
13. Fishbein, A. B. et al. 2009. Asian ginseng enhances the antiproliferative effect of 5-fluorouracil on human colorectal cancer: Comparison between white and red ginseng. *Archiv. Pharm. Res.* 32: 505–13.
14. Park, J. S. et al. 2009. Cell growth inhibitiory effect of tissue cultured root of wild *Panax ginseng* C.A. Mayer extract on various cancer cell lines. *Nat. Prod. Sci.* 15: 1–7.
15. Kim, I. W. et al. 1993. Cytotoxic activity of polyacetylene of ginseng against HepG2 (hepatoma) and L929 cells, in vitro. *Koryo Taehakkyo Uikwa Taehak Nonmunjip* 30: 35–52.
16. Hirakura, K. et al. 2000. Cytotoxic activity of acetylenic compounds from *Panax ginseng. Nat. Med.* (Tokyo, Jpn) 54: 342–5.
17. Cho, H. K. et al. 1999. Molecular mechanism of the antiproliferative effect of ginseng panaxynol on a human malignant melanoma cell line, SK-MEL-1. *J. Ginseng Res.* 23: 190–7.
18. Moon, J. et al. 2000. Induction of G1 cell cycle arrest and p27KIP1 increase by panaxydol isolated from *Panax ginseng. Biochem. Pharmacol.* 59: 1109–16.
19. Kim, J. Y. et al. 2002. Inhibitory effect of tumor cell proliferation and induction of G2/M cell cycle arrest by panaxytriol. *Planta Med.* 68: 119–22.
20. Katano, M. et al. 1990. Cell growth inhibitory substance isolated from *Panax ginseng* root: Panaxytriol. *Gan to Kagaku Ryoho* 17: 1045–9.
21. Matsunaga, H. et al. 1994. Potentiation of cytotoxicity of mitomycin C by a polyacetylenic alcohol, panaxytriol. *Cancer Chemother. Pharmacol.* 33: 291–7.
22. Matsunaga, H. et al. 1990. Cytotoxic activity of polyacetylene compounds in *Panax ginseng* C.A. Meyer. *Chem. Pharm. Bull.* 38: 3480–2.
23. Fujimoto, Y. et al. 1987. Acetylenes from the callus of *Panax ginseng. Phytochem.* 26: 2850–2.
24. Fujimoto, Y. et al. 1988. A new cytotoxic chlorine-containing polyacetylene from the callus of *Panax ginseng. Chem. Pharm. Bull.* 36: 4206–8.
25. Kim, S. I. et al. 1989. Panaxyne epoxide, a new cytotoxic polyyne from *Panax ginseng* root against L1210 cells. *Archiv. Pharm. Res.* 12: 48–51.
26. Kim, S. I. et al. 1989. Panaxyne, a new cytotoxic polyyne from *Panax ginseng* root against L1210 cell. *Saengyak Hakhoechi* 20: 71–5.
27. Ahn, B. Z. et al. 1989. Acetylpanaxydol and panaxydol chlorohydrin, two new polyines from Korean ginseng with cytotoxic activity against L1210 cells. *Archiv der Pharmazie* (Weinheim, Germany) 322: 223–6.
28. Kim, S. I. et al. 1989. 10-Acetyl panaxytriol, a new cytotoxic polyacetylene from *Panax ginseng. Yakhak Hoechi* 33: 118–23.
29. Hirakura, K. et al. 1994. Acetylnic compounds of *Panax ginseng* and neoplasm inhibitors containing them. *Jpn. Kokai Tokkyo Koho* Application: JP 92-82700 19920304.
30. Hirakura, K. et al. 1992. Isolation of acetylene compounds from *Panax ginseng* C.A. Meyer and preparation of their derivatives as antitumor agents. *Jpn. Kokai Tokkyo Koho* JP 91-45503 19910219.
31. Chen, T. M. et al. 2003. Experimental study on effect of apoptosis of K562 cells treated with TSPG. *Zhongcaoyao* 34: 235–7.
32. Chen, T. M. et al. 2007. Influences of total saponins of *Panax ginseng* on Fas, sFas and FasLin human chronic myelocytic leukemia K562 cells. *Zhongcaoyao* 38: 418–20.
33. Fang, X. M. et al. 2010. Effect of total saponins of *Panax ginseng* on caspase-3 and Fas genes expression in apoptosis of HL-60 cells. *Zhejiang Yixue* 32: 1021–4, 1027.
34. Liu, X. Y. et al. 2010. Total saponins of *Panax ginseng* suppress proliferation and improve apoptosis of leukemia KG1α cells. *Di-San Junyi Daxue Xuebao* 32: 2599–603.
35. Kim, J. Y. et al. 2011. Increased expression of apoptotic genes in cancer cells by heat-processed crude saponin. *Mol. Cell. Toxicol.* 7: 7–13.
36. Zhang, Q. H. et al. 2008. Protective effects of total saponins from stem and leaf of *Panax ginseng* against cyclophosphamide-induced genotoxicity and apoptosis in mouse bone marrow cells and peripheral lymphocyte cells. *Food Chem. Toxicol.* 46: 293–302.
37. Chen, C. F. et al. 2008. Comparison of the pharmacological effects of *Panax ginseng* and *Panax quinquefolium. Acta Pharmacol. Sinica* 29: 1103–8.
38. Lei, J. et al. 2007. Isolation, synthesis and structures of cytotoxic ginsenoside derivatives. *Mol.* 12: 2140–50.
39. Lee, J. I. et al. 2011. Cellular uptake of ginsenosides in Korean white ginseng and red ginseng and their apoptotic activities in human breast cancer cells. *Planta Med.* 77: 133–40.
40. Shibata, S. 2001. Chemistry and cancer preventing activities of ginseng saponins and some related triterpenoid compounds. *J. Korean Med. Sci.* 16(Suppl.): S28–S37.
41. Yun, T. K. et al. 2001. Cancer chemopreventive compounds of red ginseng produced from *Panax ginseng* C.A. Meyer. *J. Ginseng Res.* 25: 107–11.
42. Kim, S. M. et al. 2009. Inhibition of NF-κB by ginsenoside Rg3 enhances the susceptibility of colon cancer cells to docetaxel. *Archiv. Pharm. Res.* 32: 755–65.
43. Luo, X. J. et al. 2008. Characterization of gene expression regulated by American ginseng and ginsenoside Rg3 in human colorectal cancer cells. *Intl. J. Oncol.* 32: 975–83.
44. Yuan, H. D. et al. 2010. 20(S)-ginsenoside Rg3-induced apoptosis in HT-29 colon cancer cells is associated with AMPK signaling pathway. *Mol. Med. Reports* 3: 825–31
45. Park, D. S. et al. 2011. Immunopotentiation and antitumor effects of a ginsenoside Rg3-fortified red ginseng preparation in mice bearing H460 lung cancer cells. *Envirim. Toxicol. Pharmacol.* 31: 397–405.

46. Zhang, Y. H. et al. 2014. Ginsenoside Rg3 induces DNA damage in human osteosarcoma cells and reduces MNNG-induced DNA damage and apoptosis in normal human cells. *Oncol. Reports* 31: 919–25.
47. Yin, S. G. et al. 2014. Ginsenoside Rg3 inhibiting human esophageal carcinoma Eca9706 cells growth through affecting on cell cycle and cell apoptosis. *Zhongyao Yaoli Yu Linchuang* 30: 48–50.
48. Ma, Y. et al. 2014. Effect of ginsenoside Rg3 on inducing apoptosis of hepatocellular carcinoma in mice. *Zhongguo Yaoye* 23: 21–3.
49. Chen, Y. L. et al. 2012. Antitumor effects of 5-fluorouracil combined with ginsenoside Rg3 in nude mice hepatocellular carcinoma. *Zhongguo Xiandai Yixue Zazhi* 22(19): 29–31.
50. Lee, Y. J. et al. 2014. Synergistic antitumor effect of ginsenoside Rg3 and cisplatin in cisplatin-resistant bladder tumor cell line. *Oncol. Reports* 32: 1803–8.
51. Wang, L. et al. 2015. Ginsenoside Rg3 sensitizes human non-small cell lung cancer cells to γ-radiation by targeting the nuclear factor-κB pathway. *Mol. Med. Reports* 12(1, Pt. A), 609–14.
52. Ru, Q. et al. 2014. 20(S)-ginsenoside Rg3 inhibits human glioma cell growth through the suppression of voltage-gated K^+ channels. *Adv. Mater. Res. Adv. Appli. Sci. Eng. Technol.* 998–999 (2), 160–3.
53. Park, E. H. et al. 2014. Stereospecific anticancer effects of ginsenoside Rg3 epimers isolated from heat-processed American ginseng on human gastric cancer cells. *J. Ginseng Res.* 38: 22–7.
54. Kim, Y. J. et al. 2014. Stereospecific effects of ginsenoside 20-Rg3 inhibits TGF-β1-induced epithelial-mesenchymal transition and suppresses lung cancer migration, invasion and anoikis resistance. *Toxicol.* 322: 23–33.
55. Liu, T. et al. 2014. Ginsenoside 20(S)-Rg3 targets HIF-1α to block hypoxia-induced epithelial-mesenchymal transition in ovarian cancer cells. *PLoS One* 9: e103887.
56. Yun, T. K. 2003. Experimental and epidemiological evidence on non-organ-specific cancer-preventive effect of Korean ginseng and identification of active compounds. *Mutat. Res.* 523–524: 63–74.
57. Ham, Y. M. et al. 2006. Ginsenoside-Rh2-induced mitochondrial depolarization and apoptosis are associated with reactive oxygen species- and Ca^{2+}-mediated c-Jun NH2-terminal kinase 1 activation in HeLa cells. *J. Pharmacol. Experim. Therap.* 319: 1276–85.
58. Zhou, D. B. et al. 2005. Study on apoptosis of human lung adenocarcinoma cell line A549/DDP induced by ginsenoside Rh2 in vitro. *Zhongguo Feiai Zazhi* 8: 257–60.
59. Byun, B. Y. et al. 1995. Antiproliferative effects of *Panax ginseng* ginsenosides on DNA synthesis in cultured mouse fibroblasts. *Koryo Insam Hakhoechi* 19: 114–6.
60. Cheng, C. C. et al. 2005. Molecular mechanisms of ginsenoside Rh2-mediated G1 growth arrest and apoptosis in human lung adenocarcinoma A549 cells. *Cancer Chemother. Pharmacol.* 55: 531–40.
61. Kim, Y. S. et al. 2004. Ginsenoside Rh2 induces apoptosis via activation of caspase-1 and -3 and upregulation of Bax in human neuroblastoma. *Archiv. Pharm. Res.* 27: 834–9.
62. Fei, X. F. et al. 2003. Ginsenoside Rh2 showing ability to induce apoptosis in HeLa cells. *J. Chem. Res. in Chin. Univ.* 19: 49–53.
63. Fei, X. F. et al. 2002. Apoptotic effects of ginsenoside Rh2 on human malignant melanoma A375-S2 cells. *Acta Pharmacol. Sinica* 23: 315–22.
64. Hou, Y. J. et al. 2008. Effect of ginsenoside-Rh2 on apoptosis in myeloid leukemia cell strain in dose- and time-dependent manners. *Zhongguo Zuzhi Gongcheng Yanjiu Yu Linchuang Kangfu* 12: 2331–4.
65. He, J. C. et al. 2007. Apoptosis of RM-1 prostatic cancer cells induced by ginsenoside Rh2. *J. Jilin Univ.* (*Med. Edit.*), 33: 655–7.
66. Shin, H. J. et al. 2004. Enhancement of antitumor effects of paclitaxel (taxol) in combination with red ginseng acidic polysaccharide (RGAP). *Planta Med.* 70: 1033–8.
67. Huang, J. et al. 2008. A new triterpenoid from *Panax ginseng* exhibits cytotoxicity through p53 and the caspase signaling pathway in the HepG2 cell line. *Archiv. Pharm. Res.* 31: 323–9.
68. Zhou, H. H. et al. 2010. Preparation and inhibitory effects of 20(S)-ginsenoside Rh2 on Hep-A-22 cells. *Chem. Res. in Chin. Univs.* 26: 567–71.
69. Kong, F. L. et al. 2006. Inhibitory effects of ginsenoside Rh2 on prostatic cancers in vivo. *J. Beihua Univ.* (*Sci. Edit.*), 7: 321–3.
70. Chung, K. S. et al. 2013. Ginsenoside Rh2 induces cell cycle arrest and differentiation in human leukemia cells by upregulating TGF-β expression. *Carcinogenesis* 331–40.
71. Kim, S. Y. et al. 2007. Repression of matrix metalloproteinase gene expression by ginsenoside Rh2 in human astroglioma cells. *Biochem. Pharmacol.* 74: 1642–51.
72. Wang, Z. H. et al. 2006. Ginsenoside Rh2 enhances antitumour activity and decreases genotoxic effect of cyclophosphamide. *Basic Clinical Pharmacol. Toxicol.* 98: 411–5.
73. Meng, Y. et al. 2003. Ginsenoside Rh2 enhances the apoptotic effect of cisplatin on PC-3M prostatic cancer cells. *Zhongguo Bingli Shengli Zazhi* 19: 689–92
74. Lee, J. Y. et al. 2005. Antitumor promotional effects of a novel intestinal bacterial metabolite (IH-901) derived from the protopanaxadiol-type ginsenosides in mouse skin. *Carcinogenesis* 26: 359–67.
75. Zhou, W. et al. 2006. Studies on the preparation, crystal structure and bioactivity of ginsenoside compound K. *J. Asian Nat. Prod. Res.* 8: 519–27.
76. Lee, S. J. et al. 1999. Antitumor activity of a novel ginseng saponin metabolite in human pulmonary adenocarcinoma cells resistant to cisplatin. *Cancer Lett.* (Shannon, Ireland) 144: 39–43.
77. Ming, Y. L. et al. 2007. Apoptosis induced by a novel intestinal metabolite of ginseng saponin in human hepatocellular carcinoma BEL-7402 cells. *Zhongcaoyao* 38: 1511–4.
78. Ming, Y. L. et al. 2007. Anti-proliferation and apoptosis induced by a novel intestinal metabolite of ginseng saponin in human hepatocellular carcinoma cells. *Cell Biol. Intl.* 31: 1265–73.
79. Cho, S. H. et al. 2009. Compound K, a metabolite of ginseng saponin, induces apoptosis via caspase-8-dependent pathway in HL-60 human leukemia cells. *BMC Cancer* 18: 449.
80. Dougherty, U. et al. 2011. American ginseng suppresses Western diet-promoted tumorigenesis in model of inflammation-associated colon cancer: Role of EGFR. *BMC Complem. Altern. Med.* 11: 111.

81. Suda, K. et al. 2000. An intestinal bacterial metabolite (M1) of ginseng protopanaxadiol saponins inhibits tumor-induced neovascularization. *Wakan Iyakugaku Zasshi* 17: 144–50.
82. Lee, I. K. et al. 2010. Compound K, a metabolite of ginseng saponin, induces mitochondria-dependent and caspase-dependent apoptosis via the generation of reactive oxygen species in human colon cancer cells. *Intl. J. Mol. Sci.* 11: 4916–31.
83. Choo, M. K. et al. 2008. A ginseng saponin metabolite suppresses tumor necrosis factor-α-promoted metastasis by suppressing nuclear factor-kappaB signaling in murine colon cancer cells. *Oncol. Reports* 19: 595–600.
84. Jung, S. Y. et al. 2005. Ginseng saponin metabolite suppresses phorbol ester-induced matrix metalloproteinase-9 expression through inhibition of activator protein-1 and mitogen-activated protein kinase signaling pathways in human astroglioma cells. *Intl. J. Cancer* 118: 490–7.
85. Kim, Y. J. et al. 2008. Antitumor activity of the ginsenoside Rk1 in human hepatocellular carcinoma cells through inhibition of telomerase activity and induction of apoptosis. *Biol. Pharm. Bull.* 31: 826–30.
86. Konoshima, T. et al. 1997. Antitumor-promoting activities of ginsenoside Rg1 and Panax notoginseng. *Food Factors for Cancer Prevent. International Conference on Food Factors: Chemistry and Cancer Prevention, Hamamatsu, Japan*, 235–9.
87. Li, Q. F. et al. 2008. Anticancer effects of ginsenoside Rg1, cinnamic acid, and tanshinone IIA in osteosarcoma MG-63 cells: Nuclear matrix downregulation and cytoplasmic trafficking of nucleophosmin. *Intl. J. Biochem. Cell Biol.* 40: 1918–29.
88. Kang, J. H. et al. 2011. Ginsenoside Rp1 from *Panax ginseng* exhibits anticancer activity by downregulation of the IGF-1R/Akt pathway in breast cancer cells. *Plant Foods for Human Nutr.* 66: 298–305.
89. Zhang, Y. W. et al. 2001. Effect of ginsenosides from *Panax ginseng* on proliferation of human osteosarcoma cell U2OS. *Zhongcaoyao* 32: 232–5.
90. Wang, L. B. et al. 2008. A new compound with cytotoxic activities from the leaves of *Panax ginseng* C.A. Meyer. *Chin. Chem. Lett.* 19: 837–40.
91. Choi, C. H. et al. 2003. Reversal of P-glycoprotein-mediated multidrug resistance by proto-panaxatriol ginsenosides from Korean red ginseng. *Planta Med.* 69: 235–40.
92. Baek, N. I. et al. 1995. Cytotoxicities of ginseng saponins and their degradation products against some cancer cell lines. *Archiv. Pharm. Res.* 18: 164–8.
93. Popovich, D. G. et al. 2004. Mechanistic studies on protopanaxadiol, Rh2, and ginseng (*Panax quinquefolius*) extract induced cytotoxicity in intestinal Caco-2 cells. *J. Biochem. Mol. Toxicol.* 18: 143–9.
94. Popovich, D. G. et al. 2004. Ginsenosides 20(S)-protopanaxadiol and Rh2 reduce cell proliferation and increase sub-G1 cells in two cultured intestinal cell lines, Int-407 and Caco-2. *Can. J. Physiol. Pharmacol.* 82: 183–90.
95. Popovich, D. G. et al. 2002. Structure-function relationship exists for ginsenosides in reducing cell proliferation and inducing apoptosis in the human leukemia (THP-1) cell line. *Archiv. Biochem. Biophys.* 406: 1–8.
96. Sun, L. H. et al. 2011. Anticancer effects of 20(S)-protopanoxadiol on human acute lymphoblastic leukemia cell lines Reh and RS4;11. *Med. Oncol.* (NY, U.S.) 28: 813–21.
97. Zhang, R. et al. 2008. Effect of 20(S)-protopanaxadiol on SMMC-7721 human liver cancer in vivo and in vitro. *Zhongguo Yaolixue Tongbao* 24: 1504–8.
98. Liu, G. Y. et al. 2007. 20S-Protopanaxadiol-induced programmed cell death in glioma cells through caspase-dependent and -independent pathways. *J. Nat. Prod.* 70: 259–64.
99. Chen, M. X. et al. 2007. Studies on effect of 20(S)-protopanaxadiol on anti-tumor and immune regulation. *Zhongguo Yaoshi* 10: 1165–8.
100. Wang, W. et al. 2007. In vitro anticancer activity and structure-activity relationships of natural products isolated from fruits of *Panax ginseng*. *Cancer Chemotherapy Pharmacol.* 59: 589–601.
101. Wang, W. et al. 2008. Experimental therapy of prostate cancer with novel natural product anticancer ginsenosides. *Prostate* 68: 809–19.
102. Zhao, Y. et al. 2007. Isolation, structural determination, and evaluation of the biological activity of 20(S)-25-methoxyl-dammarane-3β,12β,20-triol [20(S)-25-OCH_3-PPD], a novel natural product from Panax notoginseng. *Med. Chem.* 3: 51–60.
103. Wakabayashi, C. et al. 1997. Expression of in vivo anti-metastatic effect of ginseng protopanaxatriol saponins is mediated by their intestinal bacterial metabolites after oral administration. *Wakan Iyakugaku Zasshi* 14: 288–9.
104. Hasegawa, H. et al. 2002. Prevention of growth and metastasis of murine melanoma through enhanced natural-killer cytotoxicity by fatty acid-conjugate of protopanaxatriol. *Biol. Pharm. Bull.* 25: 861–6.
105. Wakabayashi, C. et al. 1997. The expression of in vivo anti-metastatic effect of ginseng protopanaxatriol saponins is mediated by their intestinal bacterial metabolites after oral administration. *Wakan Iyakugaku Zasshi* 14: 180–5.
106. Zhang, J. et al. 2007. Biotransformation of 20(S)-protopanaxatriol by Mucor spinosus and the cytotoxic structure activity relationships of the transformed products. *Phytochem.* 68: 2523–30.
107. Tian, Y. et al. 2005. Microbial transformation of 20(S)-protopanaxatriol by Mucor spinosus. *J. Nat. Prod.* 68: 678–80.
108. Wang, J. et al. 2010. Induction of tumoricidal activity in mouse peritoneal macrophages by ginseng polysaccharide. *Intl. J. Biol. Macromol.* 46: 389–95.
109. Lee, Y. S. et al. 1997. Activation of multiple effector pathways of immune system by the antineoplastic immunostimulator acidic polysaccharide ginsen isolated from *Panax ginseng*. *Anticancer Res.* 17(1A): 323–31.
110. Kim, K. W. et al. 1998. Acidic polysaccharide from *Panax ginseng*, ginsan, induces Th1 cell and macrophage cytokines and generates LAK cells in synergy with rIL-2. *Planta Med.* 64: 111–15.
111. Kim, K. W. et al. 1997. Preclinical evaluation of polysaccharides extracted from Korean red-ginseng as an antineoplastic immune-stimulator. *Koryo Insam Hakhoechi* 21: 78–84.
112. Kim, K. W. et al. 1998. The pattern of cytokine mRNA expression induced by polysaccharide from *Panax ginseng* C.A. Meyer. *J. Ginseng Res.* 22: 324–30.
113. Kim, Y. S. et al. 2002. Anticancer activities of red ginseng acidic polysaccharide by activation of macrophages and NK cells. *Yakhak Hoechi* 46: 113–9.

114. Kwak, Y. S. et al. 2003. Isolation of immunomodulatory antitumor active polysaccharide (RGAP) from red ginseng byproduct and its physicochemical properties. *Han'guk Sikp'um Yongyang Kwahak Hoechi* 32: 752–7.
115. Shin, H. J. et al. 2004. A further study on the inhibition of tumor growth and metastasis by red ginseng acidic polysaccharide (RGAP). *Nat. Prod. Sci.* 10: 284–8.
116. Shin, H. J. et al. 2004. Enhancement of antitumor effects of paclitaxel (taxol) in combination with red ginseng acidic polysaccharide. *Planta Med.* 70: 1033–8.
117. Kwak, Y. S. et al. 2003. Anticancer activities by combined treatment of red ginseng acidic polysaccharide (RGAP) and anticancer agents. *J. Ginseng Res.* 27: 47–51.
118. Fu, P. P. et al. 1994. Chemical properties and antitumor activity of polysaccharides from roots of *Panax ginseng*. *J. Baiqiuen Med. Univ.* 20: 39–41.
119. Li, J. C. et al. 1988. Effect of polysaccharides in roots of *Panax ginseng* on radiation-protective and immune functions in mice exposed to x-rays. *J. Baiqiuen Med. Univ.* 14: 296–9.
120. Cai, J. P. et al. 2013. *Panax ginseng* polysaccharide suppresses metastasis via modulating Twist expression in gastric cancer. *Intl. J. Biol. Macromol.* 57: 22–5.
121. Li, C. et al. 2014. *Panax ginseng* polysaccharide induces apoptosis by targeting Twist/AKR1C2/NF-1 pathway in human gastric cancer. *Carbohydrate Polymers* 102: 103–9.
122. Li, C. et al. 2012. Purification, characterization and anticancer activity of a polysaccharide from *Panax ginseng*. *Intl. J. Biol. Macromol.* 51: 968–73.
123. Fu, X. Z. et al. 2014. Anticancer effect of ginseng leaves crude polysaccharides on human hepatoma cell SMMC-7721. *Chin. Med.* 5: 87–93.
124. Pyo, M. K. et al. 2011. Novel glycolipoproteins from ginseng. *J. Ginseng Res.* 35: 92–103.
125. Dai, X. .J et al. 2014. Effect of ginsenoside Rg3 immune-nanoemulsion on growth and lymphangiogenesis of human gastric cancer cell transplantation tumor in nude mice. *Zhonghua Zhongliu Fangzhi Zazhi* 21: 1935–9.
126. Yu, H. et al. 2013. Development of liposomal Ginsenoside Rg3: Formulation optimization and evaluation of its anticancer effects. *Intl. J. Phaem.* 450: 250–8.

169 Xi Yang Shen 西洋参

American ginseng

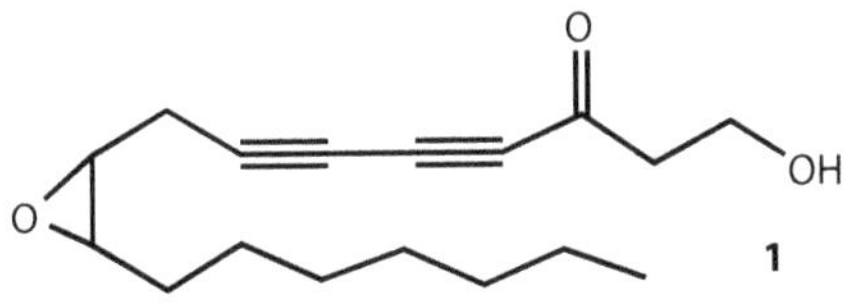

Herb Origination

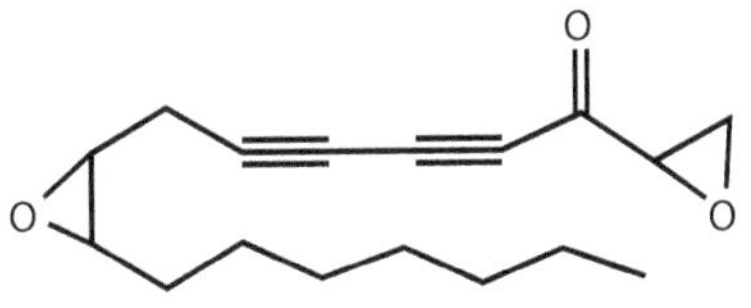

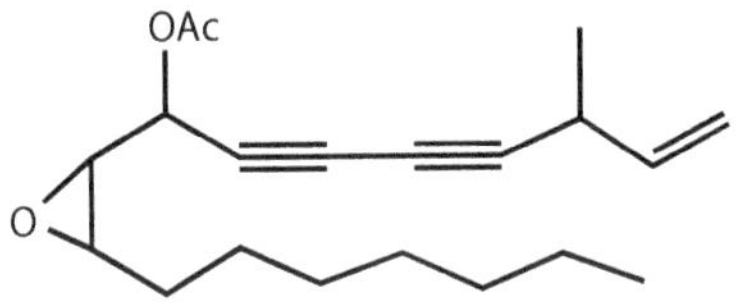

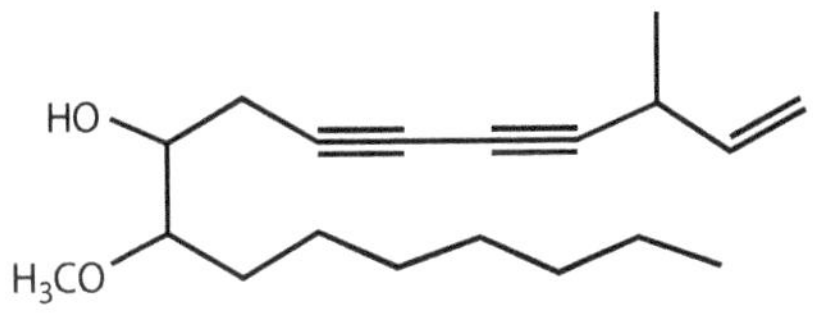

The herb Xi Yang Shen (American ginseng) is the dried rhizomes of an Araliaceae plant *Panax quinquefolium* L. This plant's rhizomes and leaves were one of the most sacred herbs traditionally used by Native American Indians for medicinal purposes. The plant was formerly widespread in the Appalachian and Ozark regions of the United States, and now it commercially grows in Wisconsin and Minnesota in the United States and in British Columbia and Ontario in Canada. Since the nineteenth century, the dried rhizomes and roots were introduced to Chinese markets.

Anticarcinogenesis and Constituents

Similar to Ginseng, the antineoplastic constituents in Xi Yang Shen were also found to be 20(S)-protopanaxadiol-type saponins, 20(S)-protopanaxatriol-type saponins, polyacetylenes, and polysaccharides.

Saponins

Xi Yang Shen has increased contents of ginsenoside-Rh2 and ginsenoside-Rg3, two anticancer saponins (see Ren Shen), by steam process, although it contains considerably less varieties of the saponins compared to those in Ginseng.[1–3] The 2 h or the 4 h steamed Xi Yang Shen exerted obvious antigrowth effect against human MCF-7 and MDA-MB-231 breast cancer cells and human HCT-116 and SW-480 colorectal carcinoma cells *in vitro*.[2–6] Similarly, the steamed Xi Yang Shen berry extract, in which the number of ginsenoside-Rg3 was increased, showed the augmented antiproliferative effects against human colorectal cancer HCT-116, SW-480 and HT-29 cell lines. In xenograft nude mice, 50 mg/kg of the extract markedly suppressed the growth of HCT-116 cells *in vivo* and significantly induced the apoptosis and the G1 cell cycle arrest.[7] The apoptotic mechanisms were found to be involved in an Ephrin receptor pathway plus the cell cycle arrest in the HCT-116 cells and to follow a mitochondrial pathway triggered by ROS increase in the SW-480 cells.[2–6] The anticarcinoma effect on the SW-480 cells could also be enhanced by the antioxidants and the inhibitors of the NF-κB pathway.[5] The inhibitory mechanism in MCF-7 and MDA-MB-231 breast cancer cells was revealed to closely correlate with the transcriptional activation of p21 independent of p53, then markedly leading to blockage of the tumor cell cycle proliferative phase.[8] When combined with antitumor drugs, Xi Yang Shen synergistically and remarkably potentiated the antigrowth activity against the MCF-7 cells.[9] When the patients with breast cancer undergoing radiotherapy were administered with panaxatriol (a secondary sapogenin derived from the acidic hydrolysis of Ren Shen/Xi Yang Shen saponins), the treated group showed higher percentages of CD^{8+} and CD^{25+} T lymphocytes in peripheral blood, indicating that the panaxatriol could promote cellular immune function in the patients.[10] Likewise, in a mice model, Xi Yang Shen saponins are capable of enhancing IL-3- and IL-6-like substances produced from the splenocytes and partially restoring the proliferation of bone marrow stem cells and splenocyte, which were depressed by CTX, leading antagonization of the toxic/side effects caused by the chemotherapeutic agents.[11]

Both saponins of the American ginseng and the Ginseng had been reported to have an ability to lessen the incidence of DMBA-induced tumorigenesis in mice together with dose-dependent inhibition of DMBA-activating cytochrome P450 enzymes (such as CYP1A1, CYP1A2, and CYP1B1). American ginseng was 45-fold more potent than Ginseng in inhibiting CYP1A2, and it also repressed 7-ethoxyresorufin O-dealkylation activity preferentially in human liver microsomes.[12] Additionally, 20(S)-protopanaxadiol, an aglycone of ginsenoside, showed antiproliferative effect on human A549 NSCLC cells by triggering mitochondria-mediated apoptosis in A549 cells by inhibiting PI3K/Akt signaling pathway[13] (see Section Ren Shen).

Polyacetylenes

Besides the ginsenosides, polyacetylenes also acted as the tumor inhibitors. Eight polyacetylenes isolated from Xi Yang Shen exerted obvious cytotoxic effect on mouse L1210 leukemia cells. Among them, PG-7 (**1**) exhibited the highest potency of antileukemia effect (IC_{50}: 0.1–0.5 μg/mL). The IC_{50} values of panaquinquecol-4 (**2**) and panaquinquecol-6 (**3**) were the same as 0.5 μg/mL, while that of PG-1–3 were between 0.5 and 1.0 μg/mL on the L1210 cells.[14–17] PG-1 (**4**) at a 10 μg/mL concentration completely inhibited the proliferation of L1210 cells *in vitro*.[17] Moreover, the isolated natural polyacetylenes, i.e., PQ-1 (**4**, 3R,9R,10R), panaxydiol (3R,10S), panaxytriol (3R,9R,10R), acetylpanaxydol (3R,9R,10S), and panaxydol (3R,9R,10S), showed the IC_{50} values of 0.1–1.0 μg/mL in the L1210 cells (see Ren Shen). Their corresponding (3*S*)-isomers were synthesized, and they showed 10 times more potent effect on the L1210 cells (IC_{50}: 0.01–0.1 μg/mL).[18]

Polysaccharides

A homogeneous glucogalactan (PPQ) (54kDa) was purified from American ginseng, which is composed of glucose and galactose in a molar ratio of 2.1:1. An *in vivo* test with a Lewis lung carcinoma model displayed that PPQ not only inhibited the growth of lung tumor, but also enhanced the indexes of the thymus and the spleen and elevated the levels of IFNγ, IL-10, and IL-2, indicating that PPQ has a possible therapeutic potential for cancer treatment and prevention.[19]

Other Bioactivities

Besides antineoplastic and anticarcinogenetic activities, pharmacological evidences have proven that Xi Yang Shen (American ginseng) possesses hypnosis, anticonvulsive, antiarrhythmic, memory-enhancing, immunoincremental, and cardiovascular functional protective properties.

References

1. Popovich, D. G. et al. 2004. Mechanistic studies on protopanaxadiol, Rh2, and ginseng (*Panax quinquefolius*) extract induced cytotoxicity in intestinal Caco-2 cells. *J. Biochem. Mol. Toxicol.* 18: 143–9.
2. Luo, X. J. et al. 2008. Characterization of gene expression regulated by American ginseng and ginsenoside Rg3 in human colorectal cancer cells. *Intl. J. Oncol.* 32: 975–83.
3. Wang, C. Z. et al. 2009. The mitochondrial pathway is involved in American ginseng-induced apoptosis of SW-480 colon cancer cells. *Oncol. Reports* 21: 577–84.
4. King, M. L. et al. 2010. Role of cyclin inhibitor protein p21 in the inhibition of HCT116 human colon cancer cell proliferation by American ginseng (*Panax quinquefolius*) and its constituents. *Phytomed.* 17: 261–8.
5. Li, B. H. et al. 2010. Antioxidants potentiate American ginseng-induced killing of colorectal cancer cells. *Cancer Lett.* 289: 62–70.
6. Wang, C. Z. et al. 2008. Chemopreventive effects of heat-processed *Panax quinquefolius* root on human breast cancer cells. *Anticancer Res.* 28: 2545–51.
7. Xie, J. T. et al. 2009. In vitro and in vivo anticancer effects of American ginseng berry: Exploring representative compounds. *Biol. Pharm. Bull.* 32: 1552–8.
8. Zhang, D. J. et al. 1992. Effects of *Panax quinquefolia* saponins on hematopoietic growth factor in cyclophosphamide depressed mice. *J. Baiqiu'en Med. Univ.* 18: 412–4.
9. Duda, R. B. et al. 2001. American ginseng transcriptionally activates p21 mRNA in breast cancer cell lines. *J. Korean Med. Sci.* 16(Suppl): S54–S60.
10. Duda, R. B. et al. 1999. American ginseng and breast cancer therapeutic agents synergistically inhibit MCF-7 breast cancer cell growth. *J. Surgical Oncol.* 72: 230–9.
11. Wang, C. G. et al. 2005. Effects of panaxatriol from *Panax quinquefolium* leaf (PQL) on levels of immunoglobulins, complements C3 and C4 and expressions of CD4, CD8 and CD25 in peripheral blood lymphocytes of patients with breast carcinoma undergoing radiotherapy. *Jilin Daxue Xuebao, Yixueban* 31: 287–9.
12. Chang, T. K. H. et al. 2002. In vitro effect of standardized ginseng extracts and individual ginsenosides on the catalytic activity of human CYP1A1, CYP1A2, and CYP1B1. *Drug Metabol. Dispos.* 30: 378–84.
13. Zhang, Y. L. et al. 2013. 20(S)-Protopanaxadiol triggers mitochondrial-mediated apoptosis in human lung adenocarcinoma A549 Cells via inhibiting the PI3K/Akt signaling pathway. *Am. J. Chin. Med.* 41: 1137–52.
14. Fujimoto, Y. S. et al. (a) 1992. Acetylenes from *Panax quinquefolium*. *Phytochem.* 31, 3499-501; (b) 1994. Polyacetylenes from *Panax quinquefolium* 35: 1255–7.
15. Fujimoto, Y. et al. 1994. Panaquinquecols of *Panax quinquefolium* and their use as anticancer agents. *Jpn. Kokai Tokkyo Koho* JP 06009418 A 19940118.
16. Fujimoto, Y. et al. 1991. Cytotoxic acetylene from *Panax quinquefolium*. *Chem. Pharm. Bull.* 39: 521–3.
17. Fujimoto, Y. et al. 1992. Heptadecenediynol compounds from *Panax quinquefolium* and neoplasm inhibitors containing them. *Jpn. Kokai Tokkyo Koho* JP 04018046 A 19920122.
18. Satoh, Y. et al. 2007. Studies on Panax acetylenes: Absolute structure of a new Panax acetylene, and inhibitory effects of related acetylenes on the growth of L1210 cells. *Chem. Pharm. Bull.* 55: 561–4.
19. Zhu, W. J. et al. 2012. Immunoregulatory effects of a glucogalactan from the root of *Panax quinquefolium* L. *Carbohydrate Polymers* 87: 2725–9.

170 Hong Jing Tian 紅景天

Golden root or Roseroot or Arctic root

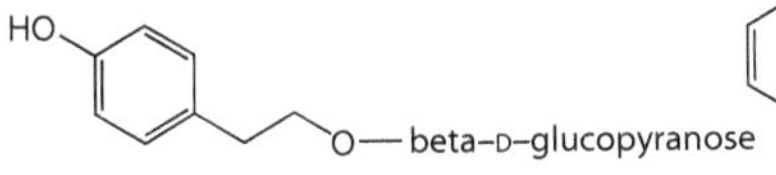

HO — O— beta-D-glucopyranose **1**

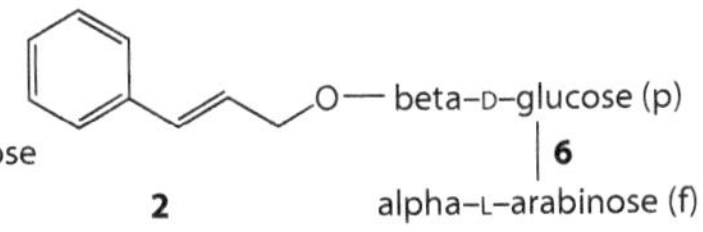

O— beta-D-glucose (p) | 6 alpha-L-arabinose (f) **2**

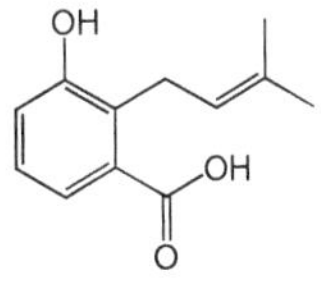

OH, OH, O **3**

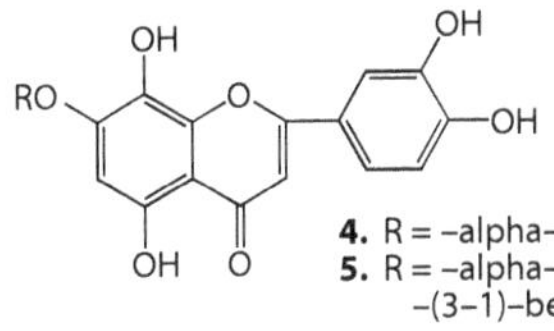

RO, OH, OH, O, OH, OH

4. R = -alpha-L-rhamnose (p)
5. R = -alpha-L-rhamnose (p) -(3-1)-beta-D-glucose (p)

Herb Origination

The herb Hong Jing Tian (Golden root) is the dried whole plants and/or roots of several Rhodiola genus plants (Crassulaceae) such as *R. rosea*, *R. algida*, *R. sachalinensis*, *R. dumulosa*, *R. crenulata*, and *R. imbricate*. These perennial plants generally grow in high-altitude and cold regions (over 2280 m elevation) of China. *R. rosea* is now also cultivated in Europe and North America, and it came to the market as a dietary supplement for tonic. In China, the best quality of Hong Jing Tian is traditionally collected in autumn and dried in the sun or on a stove under 70°C.

Antitumor Activities

The herb Hong Jing Tian has been widely used in clinical practice in recent years for its remarkable property in cancer prevention and treatment. The *in vitro* researches demonstrated that the extract of *R. rosea* rhizomes inhibited the division of human HL-60 myeloid leukemia cells and elicited the G2/M cell cycle arrest, apoptosis, and necrosis, thereby notably restraining the survival of HL-60 cells.[1] Its antitumor and antimetastatic activities were established in murine animal models with transplantable NK/Ly tumor, Ehrlich's adenocarcinoma, B16 melanoma, or Lewis lung tumor.[2] The extract of *R. algida* var. *tangutica* showed its cytostatic and antiproliferative effects on human MCF-7 breast cancer cells together with the increase of apoptotic body and the decrease of the division of the MCF-7 cells.[3] *In vitro* and *in vivo* studies also revealed that the treatment with Hong Jing Tian extract downregulated the expression of VEGF and upregulated the expression of Duffy antigen receptor for chemokines (DARC), then exerted the antiagiogenetic potential in the breast adenocarcinoma.[4] The treatment with the aqueous extract of *R. imbricata* at 100 and 200 μg/mL concentrations *in vitro* significantly diminished the proliferation of human K562 erythroleukemic cells in association with the induction of G2/M cell cycle and apoptotic death via the increase of intracellular ROS generation.[5] When tested in concentrations of over 250 μg/mL, the extract of *R. sachalinensis* dose-dependently restrained the growth of T241 fibrosarcoma cells *in vitro*. The daily *in vivo* administration of the extract to tumor-bearing mice for 21 days resulted in a significant suppression against the growth of primary T241 fibrosarcoma with the inhibitory rate of 70.9%. However, its anticancer effect on T241 tumor was found to be also caused by an immune-activated indirect cytotoxicity of the extract.[6] Moreover, a phenol-enriched extract from *R. crenulata* was able to suppress the proliferation, the motility, and the invasion of aggressive human MDA-MB-231 and mouse V14 breast carcinoma cell lines and also the effect on normal human mammary epithelial cells. An *in vivo* experiment showed that the dietary intake of the extract was effective in preventing the tumor initiation and slowing down the tumor development in mice bearing tumor, proving its possible potential for the treatment of the breast cancer progression and metastasis.[7] The extract of *R. rosea* could also enhance the anticarcinoma and antimetastatic effects of the treatment in combination with CTX and reduce the antitumor drug-induced toxicities. Similarly, the extract improved the inhibition of tumor dissemination and prevented liver toxicity when combined with Adm.[8]

Moreover, 130 breast cancer patients in Huaxi Hospital of Sichuan University of China were recruited between 2006 and 2007. The treatment with the extract of *R. algida* markedly augmented the immunity of the patients who received the chemotherapy postmastectomy, such as promotion of the proliferation of lymphocytes, increase of the levels of IL-2, IL-4, and GM-SCF, and augmentation of the mRNA content of these cytokines, eventually leading to cancer cell death. Correspondingly, the WBC levels of the patients were elevated to normal range, and the quantity of oral ulcers were attenuated after the treatment.[9] The aqueous extract of *R. imbricata* was also reported to have significant ability to enhance the cytotoxic activity of NK cells.[5]

According to the evidences, the Hong Jing Tian (Golden root) extract may be considered to have the potential to be used as an adjuvant concurrently with chemotherapy for the improvement of the anticancer activity and the occurrence of side effects from clinical anticancer drugs.[10]

Antitumor Constituents and Activities

Up to now, about 140 compounds were identified from the subterranean portion of *R. rosea*, revealing that the Rhodiola roots contain multiple constituents such as phenols, organic acids, phenolcarbonic acids, terpenoids, flavonoids, alkaloids, and polysaccharides. The antineoplastic-related activities of Hong Jing Tian were found to be primarily contributed by its phenols, flavonoids, and polysaccharides.

Phenylpropanoid Glycosides

Salidroside (**1**) is the major constituent in Hong Jing Tian for inhibiting the proliferation of neoplastic cell lines such as H22 and Hepal-6 hepatoma, W256 sarcoma, sarcoma 180, SGC-7902 gastric cancer, and SACC-2 saliva adenoid cystic carcinoma.[11,12] The treatment with salidroside (**1**) arrested the cell cycle progression at G0/G1 stage and notably suppressed the growth of human A549 NSCLC cells, whose effect was correlated with the marked downregulation of c-Myc expression and the activation of p21 protein. Also, salidroside (**1**) was capable of inhibiting the expression of HIF-α in the A549 cells, whose HIF-α was reported to play an important role in the inhibition of tumor growth, angiogenesis, and lymph node metastasis of the NSCLC.[13,14] The treatment of human UMUC3 bladder transitional cancer cells with salidroside (**1**) caused an enlarged percentage of cells undergoing autophagy through the decrease of 4E-BP1 phosphorylation and the increases of AMPK-α phosphorylation and 4E-BP1 binding to m7 GTP, implying that salidroside (**1**) has a potential in the chemoprevention of bladder carcinogenesis.[15] Salidroside (**1**) could inhibit the formation and the growth of human U251 glioma cells and arrest the cell cycle *in vivo* and *in vitro*, concomitant with the improvement of the tumor microenvironment via the inhibition of oxidative stress and astrocytes.[16] Also, salidroside (**1**) acted as an antioxidant dose-dependently inhibiting the intracellular ROS formation and markedly reducing wound closure areas of human fibrosarcoma HT1080 cells, thereby suppressing the tumor cell invasion and metastasis. The antiinvasive and antimetastatic activities of salidroside (**1**) were revealed to be associated with the inhibition of ROS-initiated PKC-ERK1/2 signaling pathway, i.e., attenuated the activities of PKC, MMP-2, and MMP-9, increased TIMP-2 expression, and repressed ERK1/2 phosphorylation.[17] Similarly, by interfering intracellular ROS generation and downregulating ROS-phospho-p38 signaling pathway, salidroside (**1**) significantly induced the cell cycle arrest in G0/G1 phase and promoted the apoptotic death of human A549 alveolar adenocarcinoma cells, thereby restraining the proliferation and the metastasis of the A549 cells.[18]

Moreover, salidroside (**1**) and rosavin (**2**) demonstrated marked antiangiogenesis activity. Daily feeding of salidroside (**1**) or rosavin (**2**) to mice grafted with syngeneic L-1 sarcoma cells in doses of 4 or 8 μg highly decreased the neovascular reaction on the skin and significantly obstructed tumor-induced angiogenesis after 72 h.[8,19] Through the downregulation of c-Myc expression, salidroside (**1**) was capable of inducing the differentiation of human hepatoma SMMC-7721 cells as well *in vitro*.[20] Both aqueous and 50% hydroalcoholic extracts in daily doses of 100–400 μg could exert the similar degree of antiangiogenetic effect in the *in vivo* experiments.[8,11]

In addition, salidroside (**1**) was also able to protect rat adrenal gland pheochromocytoma PC12 cells against glutamate excitotoxic-caused injuries by decreasing $[Ca^{2+}]i$ of PC12 cells and suppressing the excessive entry of Ca^{2+} and the calcium stores release.[21] The pretreatment of SH-SY5Y human neuroblastoma cells with salidroside (**1**) markedly attenuated H_2O_2-induced cell viability loss and apoptosis and restored H_2O_2-induced loss of mitochondrial membrane potential and the elevation of intracellular calcium level in a dose-dependent manner, whose mechanism in the protection of neuron cells from oxidative stress was correlated with the induction of several antioxidant enzymes, thioredoxin, heme oxygenase-1 and peroxiredoxin-I; the upregulation of antiapoptotic Bcl-2 and Bcl-xL; and the inhibition of proapoptotic Bax. The findings indicated that salidroside (**1**) has a protective function against oxidative stress-induced brain cell apoptosis and suggested that salidroside (**1**) might be a potential agent for preventing neurodegenerative diseases implicated with oxidative stress.[22]

Phenolics and Phenolic Glycosides

Nineteen phenolics and phenolic glycosides were isolated from the EtOAc extract of *R. imbricata* roots. Some of them exerted weak suppressive effect against MCF-7 (breast) and A549 (lung) human cancer cell lines in the *in vitro* assay (IC_{50}: 70–90 μM). Only 3-hydroxy-2-(3-methyl-2-buten-1-yl)-benzoic acid (**3**) exhibited the moderate effect on the MCF-7 cells (IC_{50}: 28.7 μM).[23] In addition, gallic acid separated from *R. cremulata* showed a quite high *in vitro* activity for inducing the apoptosis and inhibiting the proliferation of human MGC80–3 gastric cancer cells.[24]

Flavonoid Glycosides

The bioactivity-directed fractionation of a 95% EtOh extract from the stems of *R. rosea* led to the isolation of several flavonoids. Among them, gosypetin-7-*O*-α-L-rhamnopyranoside (**4**) and rhodioflavonoside (**5**) displayed moderate inhibitory activity against human PC3 prostate carcinoma cell line, and the IC_{50} values were 50 and 80 μg/mL, respectively.[25]

Polysaccharides

An injection prepared from Rhodiola polysaccharides with a molecular weight of 20,000–80,000 Da were reported to possess marked antitumor, immunoenhancing, hypoglycemic, and hypolipidemic activities.[26] A homogeneous polysaccharide termed RRP-ws was isolated from the *R. rosea* roots, which contains 95.14% total carbohydrate, 2.08% protein, and no sulfate. Its saccharide portion was composed of glucose, galactose, mannose, and rhamnose with a relative molar ratio of 4.2:2.4:1.6:1.0. In an *in vitro* assay, RRP-ws exerted a direct cytotoxic effect against the growth of sarcoma 180 cell line. In a mouse model, RRP-ws suppressed the growth of sarcoma 180 and also augmented the spleen/thymus indexes and the body weight. Simultaneously, RRP-ws amplified the production of IL-2, TNFα, and IFNγ in a serum and elevated the ratio of $CD4^+/CD8^+$ on peripheral blood T lymphocyte in mice bearing tumor. The solid evidences recommended that RRP-ws can be employed as a promising immunotherapeutic agent for improving cancer therapy.[27]

Other Bioactivities

Hong Jing Tian is a medicinal plant having stimulating and adaptogenic properties, and it is often used in Chinese medicine for treating cancer, tuberculosis, and diabetes; preventing cold and flu, aging, and liver damage; improving hearing; strengthening the nervous system; and enhancing immunity. Salidroside (**1**) and rosavin (**2**), as the major agents from Hong Jing Tian, are responsible for neuroprotective, antidepressant, and anxiolytic effects besides anticarcinogenesis and immunoregulation. Normally, salidroside (**1**) may be more effective than rosavin (**2**).

References

1. Majewska, A. et al. 2006. Antiproliferative and antimitotic effect, S phase accumulation and induction of apoptosis and necrosis after treatment of extract from *Rhodiola rosea* rhizomes on HL-60 cells. *J. Ethnopharmacol.* 103: 43–52.

2. Dement'eva, L. A. et al. 1987. Effect of a Rhodiola extract on the tumor process in an experiment. *Voprosy onkologii* 33: 57-60.
3. Lu, D. X. et al. 2011. The study of cytostatic effect on MCF-7 cells of the alcohol extract of *Rhodiola algida* var. *tangutica*. *Procedia Envir.l Sci.* 8: 615–9.
4. Qie, W. L. et al. 2007. Study of growth and invasiveness inhibition by Rhodiola in human breast cancer cells. *Zhonghua Zhongliu Fangzhi Zazhi* 14: 1292–5.
5. Mishra, K. P. et al. 2008. Aqueous extract of *Rhodiola imbricata* rhizome inhibits proliferation of an erythroleukemic cell line K562 by inducing apoptosis and cell cycle arrest at G2/M phase. *Immunobiol.* 213: 125–31.
6. Zhao, X. et al. 2008. *Rhodiola sachalinensis* suppresses T241 fibrosarcoma tumor cells proliferation in vitro and growth in vivo. *Zhongyaocai* 31: 1377–80.
7. Tu, Y. F. et al. 2008. *Rhodiola crenulata* induces death and inhibits growth of breast cancer cell lines. *J. Med. Food* 11: 413–23.
8. Skopinska-Rozewska, E. et al. 2008. The influence of *Rhodiola rosea* extracts and rosavin on cutaneous angiogenesis induced in mice after grafting of syngeneic tumor cells. *Central Eur. J. Immunol.* 33: 102–7.
9. Loo, W. T. Y. et al. 2010. *Rhodiola algida* improves chemotherapy-induced oral mucositis in breast cancer patients. *Expert Opinion on Investigational Drugs* 19(S1): S91–S100.
10. Kelly, J. G. et al. 2010. Rhodiola and related plants: A role in cancer prevention and therapy. *Bioactive Foods and Extracts, Cancer Treatment and Prevention*, Ross, R. and Preedy, V. R. (eds.), pp. 37–45.
11. Zhu, Y. J. et al. 2012. Effect of salidroside on proliferation of carcinoma cell and angiogenesis of zebrafish. *J. Modern Oncol.* 20: 2239–43.
12. Li, M. H. et al. 2007. Study on salidroside inhibiting SACC-2 cell proliferation of parotid carcinoma cell in vitro. *J. Oral Sci. Res.* 23: 386–7.
13. Li, B. et al. 2012. Salidroside decrease expression of hypoxia-inducible factor-1α in cultured human lung cancer cells. *Afri. J. Pharmacy Pharmacol.* 6: 2526–30
14. Yao, Y. Y. et al. 2012. The effects of salidroside on transcription factors and cell growth inhibition in human lung adenocarcinoma epithelial cells. *Afri. J. Pharmacy Pharmacol.* 6: 893–8.
15. Liu, Z. B. et al. 2012. *Rhodiola rosea* extracts and salidroside decrease the growth of bladder cancer cell lines via inhibition of the mTOR pathway and induction of autophagy. *Mol. Carcinogen.* 51: 257–67.
16. Zhang, Y. S. et al. 2013. Effects of salidroside on glioma formation and growth inhibition together with improvement of tumor micro-environment. *Chin. J. Cancer Res.* 25: 520–26.
17. Sun, C. et al. 2012. Salidroside inhibits migration and invasion of human fibrosarcoma HT1080 cells. *Phytomed.* 19: 355–63.
18. Wang, J. et al. 2014. Anticancer effect of salidroside on A549 lung cancer cells through inhibition of oxidative stress and phospho-p38 expression. *Oncol. Lett.* 7: 1159–64.
19. Skopińska-Rózewska, E. et al. 2008. The influence of *Rhodiola quadrifida* 50% hydro-alcoholic extract and salidroside on tumor-induced angiogenesis in mice. *Pol. J. Vet. Sci.* 11: 97–104.
20. Xie, F. W. et al. 2005. Reverse effects of salidroside on expression of c-myc in SMMC-7721 cell line in vitro. *Xinan Guofang Yiyao* 15: 613–5
21. Cao, L. L. 2005. The effect of salidroside on cell damage induced by glutamate and intracellular free calcium in PC12 cells. *J. Asian Nat. Prod. Res.* 8: 159–65.
22. Zhang, L. et al. 2007. Protective effects of salidroside on hydrogen peroxide-induced apoptosis in SH-SY5Y human neuroblastoma cells. *Eur. J. Pharmacol.* 564: 18–25.
23. Choudhary, A. et al. 2015. Isolation and characterization of phenolic compounds from *Rhodiola imbricata*, a Trans-Himalayan food crop having antioxidant and anticancer potential. *J. Funct. Foods* 16: 183–93.
24. Nie, Y. Y. et al. 2011. Structural identification and biological activity of *Rhodiola crenulata* extract. *Shizhen Guoyi Guoyao* 22: 1962–5.
25. Ming, D. S. et al. 2005. Bioactive compounds from *Rhodiola rosea* (Crassulaceae). *Phytother. Res.* 19: 740–3.
26. Zhang, H. F. 2995. Rhodiola polysaccharides injection preparation and its preparation method. *Faming Zhuanli Shenqing Gongkai Shuomingshu* CN 1686157 A 20051026.
27. Cai, Z. B. et al. 2012. Antitumor effects of a purified polysaccharide from *Rhodiola rosea* and its action mechanism. *Carbohydrate Polymers* 90: 296–300.

171 Dang Gui 當歸

Chinese angelica

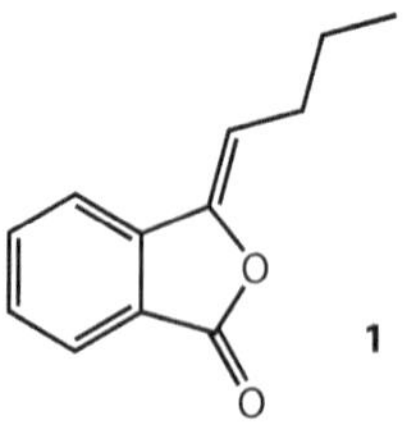

Herb Origination

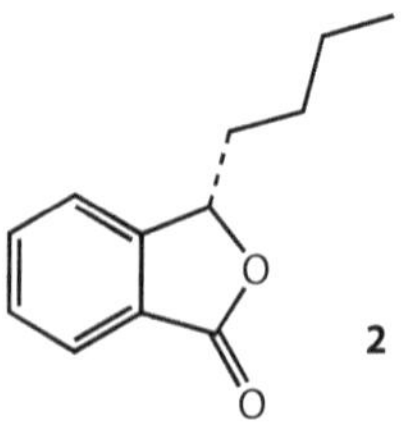

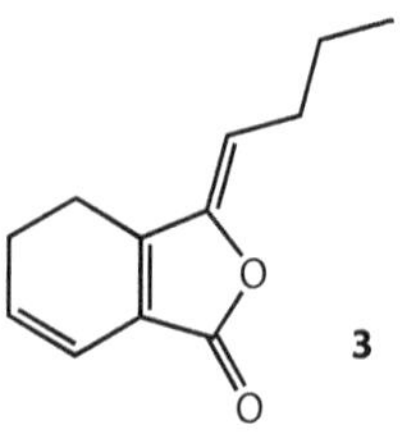

The herb Dang Gui (Chinese angelica) is one of the most popular traditional Chinese herbs used for thousands of years in China, Korea, and Japan. Dang Gui was documented in *Shengnong Ben Cao Jing*, the first Chinese classic of materia medica. It originated from the dried roots of an Umbelliferae plant, *Angelica sinensis*. The herb is primarily produced in the regions of western China. Its roots are collected in late autumn and dried with wood fume and mild heat for the medicinal application.

Antitumor Activity and Constituents

AS-AC, a Dang Gui acetone extract, exerted dose-dependent antiproliferative activity against human A549 (lung), HT29 (colon), DBTRG-05MG (brain), and J5 (liver) neoplastic cell lines (IC_{50}: 35–50 μg/mL, 24 h). The treatment with AS-AC on the A549 cells resulted in the down-expression of Bcl-2, the decrease of CDK4 protein level, and the activation of caspase-9 and caspase-3, finally leading to the cell cycle arrest at G0/G1 phase, chromatin changes and the cell apoptotic death.[1] A chloroform extract (AS-CH) of Dang Gui displayed potency in suppressing the cell growth of malignant glioblastoma multiform *in vitro* and *in vivo* without cytotoxicity to the fibroblasts, whose antigrowth effect was found to be closely accompanied by the induction of cell cycle arrest and apoptosis. The resulted G0/G1 cell cycle arrest in DBTRG-05MG and RG2 brain cancer cell lines by AS-CH were associated with the up-expression of CDK inhibitors (such as p21) and decreased the phosphorylation of Rb proteins. Concurrently, the apoptosis-associated proteins were dramatically activated by AS-CH in rat RG2 cells and human DBTRG-05MG cells, then triggering both p53-dependent and p53-independent pathways for the apoptotic death.[2] Either AS-AC or AS-CH at a lower (50 μg/mL) and a higher (100 μg/mL) concentrations significantly obstructed the proliferation of GBM8401 brain astrocytoma cells *in vitro* by 30–50% and downregulated the expressions of cathepsin-B and VEGF). In a nude mice model transplanted with the brain tumor, the microvessel formation was prominently blocked by the two lipid-soluble extracts. These findings recommended that Dang Gui has the important potential for improving the chemotherapy of high-grade astrocytomas.[3] When the EtOH extract of AS was complexed with 2-hydroxypropyl-β-cyclodextrin (a cyclic oligosaccharide) in a weight ratio of 1:5, the antihepatoma activity could be augmented to 94% from 68% of the AS extract.[4]

Dang Gui was also found to diminish the adhesive, invasive, and migratory abilities of human A549 lung adenocarcinoma cells through a lower antiproliferative effect on the A549 cells at a high concentration *in vitro*. The assays with animal models also corroborated the suppression of lung metastasis in nude mice at a high dose of the Dang Gui extract, whose effects on the lung cancer cells were found to correlate with decreases of MMP-2, MMP-9, TGF-β1, and TIMP-1 activities and increase of TIMP-2 function.[5] In addition, SFE-AS, a supercritical extract from *A. sinensis* showed a preventive effect on AOM/dextran sodium sulfate-induced colorectal carcinoma associated with the inflammation in a mice model, whose activity might be related with the significant reduction of PCNA, COX-2, and iNOS expressions.[6]

Antitumor Constituents and Activities

Phthalides

Three phthalides assigned as n-butylidenephthalide (**1**), senkyunolide-A (**2**), and z-ligustilide (**3**) were isolated from a chloroform extract of Dang Gui. Their cytotoxicities and antiproliferative effects were shown in human HT-29 colon cancer cells in a dose-dependent fashion. The potencies of n-butylidenephthalide (**1**) and senkyunolide-A (**2**) were almost four times greater than that of z-ligustilide (**3**).[7] n-Butylidenephthalide (**1**) was also effective in the growth inhibition of two human hepatoma cells (HepG2 and J5) and two glioblastoma multiform cells (DBTRG-05MG and RG2) *in vitro* and *in vivo*.[8,9] The Per os (p.o.) administration of z-ligustilide (**3**) in doses of 5, 20, and 80 mg/kg/day for seven days inhibited the growth of H22 hepatoma in tumor-bearing mice and also obviously amplified thymus and spleen indexes, serum hemolysin concentration, macrophage phagocytosis, spleen lymphocyte proliferation, and CTL and NK cell activities in normal ICR mice, where z-ligustilide (**3**) at a dose of 20 mg/kg exerted the best boosted immune system and tumor inhibition, compared to its 5 and 80 mg/kg doses.[10]

The apoptosis induced by the 25 μg/mL concentration of n-butylidenephthalide (**1**) in the HepG2 cells and J5 cells was found to be associated with the induction of Nur77 translocation from the nucleus to the cytosol, the release of cytochrome c, and the caspase-3 activation. cAMP-response element-binding protein pathway was also partly involved in the hepatoma cell apoptosis.[8] By upregulating the expression of cyclin kinase inhibitors (including p21 and p27), increasing apoptosis-associated proteins, diminishing Rb proteins phosphorylation, and downregulating the cell cycle regulators, n-butylidenephthalide (**1**) elicited human DBTRG-05MG glioma cells and rat RG2 glioma cells to G0/G1 cell arrest and apoptotic death.[9] All these data encouraged the further development of the n-butylidenephthalide (**1**) as a potential agent for clinically improving the chemotherapies of brain neoplasm and hepatocellular carcinoma.

z-Butylidenephthalide (Bdph), as an isomer isolated from the chloroform extract of Dang Gui, also exerted the antineoplastic effect. When z-butylidenephthalide (Bdph) was incorporated into p(CPP-SA), a Bdph-Wafer polymer (a biodegradable polyanhydride) was generated. The subcutaneous injection of the Bdph-Wafers could deliver a sufficient concentration of Bdph to the cancer cell site and effectively reduce the size of glioblastoma multiform in a dose-dependent manner in two xenograft animal models implanted with RG2 cells and DBTRG-05MG cells, respectively. The antiglioma effect of Bdph on the RG2 cells was found to be mediated by the inhibition of a PKC pathway to upregulate Nurr77 and to promote its translocation from the nucleus to the cytoplasm.[11]

Total Polysaccharide Components

Polysaccharide components are one of the major inhibitors in response of the anticancer property of Dang Gui, exerting marked inhibitory effect against the growth of Ehrlich tumor, hepatoma, sarcoma 180, Lewis lung cancer, and B16 melanoma cells. The life span of mice bearing cancer was significantly extended without toxic/side effects, implying that it may be used in a long-term administration.[12] The i.p. injection of the total polysaccharide (AP-0) at doses of 30–300 mg/kg per day for 10 days significantly reduced the production of ascitic liquids and prolonged the life survival time of mice bearing Ehrlich ascites cancer or L1210 leukemia but no obvious effect against sarcoma 180. *In vitro* experiments on the invasion and the metastasis of human hepatoma (HCC) showed that AP-0 as well as its subfractions (AP-1, AP-2, and AP-3) restrained the adhesion of HCC to extracellular matrix proteins (fibronectin and Matrigel) at different degrees. Among them, only AP-3 showed significant blocking effect on the adhesion of HCC to the fibronectin with an inhibitory rate of 30.3%, whereas AP-0 and AP-2 remarkably retarded the invasion of HCC into the Matrigel-reconstituted basement membrane with the inhibitory rates of 56.4% and 68.3%, respectively. The treatment with AP-0, AP-1, or AP-3 also partially obstructed the chemotactic migration abilities of HCC.[13]

Likewise, the presence of *A. sinensis* polysaccharides not only repressed the proliferation of human K562 erythroleukemia cells but also elicited the differentiation of K562 cells to erythrocyte and granulocyte series.[14] *A. sinensis* polysaccharides showed remarkable dose-dependent inhibition of proliferation of human-derived $CD34^+CD38^-$ leukemia stem cells (LSCs) *in vitro*, where *A. sinensis* polysaccharides induced the senescence of human-derived leukemia bone marrow $CD34^+CD38^-$ LSC by regulating the cell telomere system after being treated with 40 μg/mL of *A. sinensis* polysaccharides for 48 h.[15] The *A. sinensis* polysaccharides treatment also obviously inhibited human KG1α AML cell proliferation and blocked the cell cycle at G0/G1 phase, concomitant with marked up-expression of aging-related proteins (P16 and RB).[16] In mice implanted with K562 cells, the i.p. injection of *A. sinensis* polysaccharides (200 mg/kg/day) for 14 days obviously reduced the amount of peripheral blood WBC, the percentage of neutrophiles, and the number of femur bone marrow mononuclear cells (BMMCs), as well as up-expressed the aging-related proteins of P16, Rb, CDK4, and cyclin-D1, to effectively inhibit the proliferation of the BMMCs of the human leukemia mouse model.[17] The effects of *A. sinensis* polysaccharides on KG1α *in vitro* and on K562 cells *in vivo* could be augmented by the cotreatment with cytarabine (2.5 mg/kg/day).[16,17] Also, *A. sinensis* polysaccharides inhibited the proliferation of human MCF-7 breast cancer cells *in vitro*, and the *A. sinensis* polysaccharides after sulfated modification showed obviously enhanced anticancer effect on the MCF-7 and K562 cell lines.[18]

Moreover, *A. sinensis* polysaccharides were capable of augmenting the releases of NO, TNFα, and ROS from macrophages and improving the activities of iNOS and lysozyme in macrophages, suggesting that the antitumor role of *A. sinensis* polysaccharides is also indirectly mediated by its immunoregulations, i.e., increasing macrophages to produce TNFα and stimulating lymphocyte function.[19,20] Therefore, *A. sinensis* polysaccharides could prominently recover the damaged lymphocyte and reduce the toxic/side effects caused by chemotherapy and radiotherapy after the cotreatment besides augmenting the tumor inhibitory activity synergistically.[19–21] A polysaccharide-rich extract of Dang Gui exerted the synergistic effect on CTX in the treatment concomitant with an obviously decrease of lectin and DNA polymerase and a remarkable increase of SOD. The extract also significantly diminished the chemotherapeutic toxicity and protected hematopoietic and gastrointestinal tissues from the cytotoxic activity of CTX.[22,23]

Homogeneous Polysaccharides

Four purified polysaccharides, APS-1d, APS-2a, APS-3b, and APS-3c, have been reported to have anticarcinoma and immunopotentiating properties. APS-1d showed cytotoxicity toward several neoplastic cell lines; especially, it was effective in the suppression of human HeLa cervical cancer cells *in vitro* and *in vivo*. The antiproliferative and apoptotic effects were mostly triggered by the activation of the intrinsic mitochondrial pathway.[24] APS-2a, APS -3b, and APS -3c significantly inhibited the growth of sarcoma 180 and extended the life span of mice transplanted with S180.[25,26] APS-3c (1.4×10^4 Da) also exerted the antiproliferative effect on human HL-60 myeloblastic leukemia cells and human SW1116 colon cancer cells.[27] Moreover, APS-2a showed its immunoenhancing ability to augment the thymus indexes and the spleen indexes in mice, whereas APS-3b and APS-3c were able to dose-dependently enhance the proliferation of the splenocytes, upregulate the expressions of IFNγ, IL-2, and IL-6 mRNA in the splenocytes, and stimulate the productions of NO and TNFα in the peritoneal macrophages.[25,26] These evidences clearly demonstrated that the Dang Gui polysaccharides may be helpful in cancer chemoprevention and chemotherapy as a dietary supplement.

Oligosaccharide–Protein Complex

An oligosaccharide–protein complex with low molecular weight (approximately 3000) was isolated from Dang Gui, which consists of protein (4.73%), carbohydrate (85.85%), and uronic acid (5.2%). The oligosaccharide–protein complex displayed both remarkable antigrowth and immunoenhancing activities in mice bearing Ehrlich ascites carcinoma *in vitro* and *in vivo*.[28]

Other Bioactivities

The herb Dang Gui (Chinese angelica) has a long history in Chinese medicine as remedies for women's disorders, gynecological ailment, and gastrointestinal disorders. The herb is also broadly used to treat cardiovascular and cerebrovascular diseases in China. Pharmacological experiments have proven that Dang Gui possesses multiple health benefits such as vasodilative, antithrombotic, antiatheroscherosis, hepatoprotective, hypolipidemic, coronary flow-increasing, antiplatelet aggregation, antiinflammatory, choleretic, antioxidation, free radical-scavenging, antiradiation, lymphocyte- and phagocyte-activating, hemoglobin- and erythrocyte-growing, and immunoenhancing properties. The Dang Gui extract is able to elicit a typical cardioprotective effect and to diminish DOX-induced oxidative stress and cardiac toxicities.[29] However, the herb is not recommended during pregnancy due to possible hormonal, anticoagulant, and antiplatelet properties.

References

1. Cheng, Y. L. et al. 2004. Acetone extract of *Angelica sinensis* inhibits proliferation of human cancer cells via inducing cell cycle arrest and apoptosis. *Life Sci.* 75: 1579–94.
2. Tsai, N. M. et al. 2005. The antitumor effects of *Angelica sinensis* on malignant brain tumors in vitro and in vivo. *Clin. Cancer Res.* 11: 3475–84.
3. Lee, W. H. et al. 2006. Biological inhibitory effects of the Chinese herb danggui on brain astrocytoma. *Pathobiol.* 73: 141–8.
4. Hsu, C. M. et al. 2014. Inhibitory effect of *Angelica sinensis* extract in the presence of 2-hydroxypropyl-β-cyclodextrin. *Carbohydrate Polymers* 114: 115–22.
5. Gao, M. et al. 2012. *Angelica sinensis* suppresses human lung adenocarcinoma A549 cell metastasis by regulating MMPs/TIMPs and TGF-β1. *Oncol. Reports* 27: 585–93.
6. An, J. et al. 2014. Chemo-preventive effect of *Angelica sinensis* supercritical extracts on AOM/DSS-induced mouse colorectal carcinoma associated with inflammation. *Zhongguo Zhongyao Zazhi* 39: 1265–9.
7. Kan, W. L. T. et al. 2008. Study of the anti-proliferative effects and synergy of phthalides from *Angelica sinensis* on colon cancer cells. *J. Ethnopharmacol.* 120: 36–43.
8. Chen, Y. L. et al. 2008. The induction of orphan nuclear receptor Nur77 expression by n-butylenephthalide as pharmaceuticals on hepatocellular carcinoma cell therapy. *Mol. Pharmacol.* 74: 1046–58.
9. Tsai, N. M. et al. 2006. The natural compound n-butylidenephthalide derived from *Angelica sinensis* inhibits malignant brain tumor growth in vitro and in vivo. *J. Neurochem.* 99: 1251–62.
10. Long, R. et al. 2012. Effects of ligustilide on tumor growth and immune function in institute of cancer research mice. *Tropical J. Pharm. Res.* 11: 421–8.
11. Harn, H. et al. 2011. Local interstitial delivery of z-butylidenephthalide by polymer wafers against malignant human gliomas. *Neuro Oncol.* 13: 635–48.
12. Zheng, Z. J. et al. (a) 1994. *Guowai Yixue, Yaoxue Fence* 16: 254; (b) 1999. *Chinese Materia Medica.* Vol. 5, 5–5092, 898. Shanghai Science and Technology Press, Shanghai, China.
13. Shang, P. et al. 2003. Experimental study of antitumor effects of polysaccharides from *Angelica sinensis. World J. Gastroenterol.* 9: 1963–7.
14. Zheng, M. et al. 2002. Experimental study on effect of Angelica polysaccharide in inhibitory proliferation and inducing differentiation of K562 cells. *Zhongguo Zhongxiyi Jiehe Zazhi* 22: 54–7.
15. Li, C. P. et al. 2014. Study on mechanism of telomere system regulation and senescence induction of leukemia stem cells by *Angelica sinensis* polysaccharide. *Zhongcaoyao* 45: 2364–9.
16. Xu, C. Y. et al. 2014. Experimental study on aging effect of *Angelica sinensis* polysaccharides combined with cytarabine on human leukemia KG1α cell lines. *Zhongguo Zhongyao Zazhi* 39: 1260–4.
17. Xu, C. Y. et al. 2014. Effects of combined injection of *Angelica sinensis* polysaccharide and cytarabine on bone marrow mononuclear cells of transplanted human leukemia mice. *Zhongcaoyao* 45: 3418–23.
18. Wu, S. Z. et al. 2013. Sulfated modification and antitumor activity of polysaccharide from *Angelica sinensis. Zhongguo Yiyuan Yaoxue Zazhi* 33: 1832–5.
19. Sun, Y. L. et al. 2006. Effect of angelica sinensis polysaccharide on peripheral blood lymphocyte of radiation damage rats. *Zhonghua Fangshe Yixue yu Fanghu Zazhi* 26: 369–70.
20. Yang, X. B. et al. 2004. Role of Angelica polysaccharides in inducing effector molecule release by peritoneal macrophages. *Xibao yu Fenzi Mianyixue Zazhi* 20: 747–9.
21. Cheng, G. Q. et al. (a) 1986. *Gansu Yiyao* 5: 3; (b) 1999. *Chinese Materia Medica.* Vol. 5, 5-5092, 898. Shanghai Science and Technology Press, Shanghai, China.
22. Gao, G. Y. et al. 1997. Synergistic effect of *Angelica sinensis* on cyclophosphamide in treating transplanted tumors of mice. *Zhongguo Yiyuan Yaoxue Zazhi* 17: 304–5.
23. Hui, M. K. C. et al. 2006. Polysaccharides from the root of *Angelica sinensis* protect bone marrow and gastrointestinal tissues against the cytotoxicity of cyclophosphamide in mice. *Intl. J. Med. Sci.* 3: 1–6.
24. Cao, W. et al. 2010. A novel polysaccharide, isolated from *Angelica sinensis* (Oliv.) Diels induces the apoptosis of cervical cancer HeLa cells through an intrinsic apoptotic pathway. *Phytomed.* 17: 598–605.
25. Cao, W. et al. 2010. Characterizations and antitumor activities of three acidic polysaccharides from *Angelica sinensis* (Oliv.) Diels. *Intl. J. Biol. Macromol.* 46: 115–22.
26. Cao, W. et al. 2008. Structural analysis and antitumor activity in vivo of polysaccharide APS-2A from *Angelica sinensis. Zhongyaocai* 31: 261–6.
27. Cao, W. et al. 2008. Physicochemical properties and Antitumor activity in vitro of polysac-charide APS-3c from *Angelica sinensis* (Oliv.) diels. *Tianran Chanwu Yanjiu Yu Kaifa* 20: 217–22.
28. Choy, Y. M. et al. 1994. Immunopharmacological studies of low molecular weight polysaccharide from *Angelica sinensis. Am. J. Chin. Med.* 22: 137–45.
29. Xin, Y. F. et al. 2007. *Angelica sinensis*: A novel adjunct to prevent doxorubicin-induced chronic cardiotoxicity. *Basic Clin. Pharmacol. Toxicol.* 101: 421–6.

172 Bai Shou Wu 白首烏

Bunge swallowwort

1. R = -Cym1-(4-1)-Ole-(4-1)-Cym1-(4-1)-Cym2-(4-1)-Glc
2. R = -Cym1-(4-1)-Dig1-(4-1)-Ole-(4-1)-Cym1-(4-1)-Glc
3. R = -Cym1-(4-1)-Ole-(4-1)-Cym1-(4-1)-Glc
4. R = -Cym1-(4-1)-Dig2-(4-1)-Cym1
5. R = -H

Cym1: beta-D-Cymaropyranosyl
Cym2: alpha-L-Cymaropyranosyl
Ole: beta-D-Oleandropyranosyl
Dig1: beta-D-Digitoxopyranosyl
Dig2: alpha-L-Diginopyranosyl
Glc: beta-D-glucopyranosyl

Herb Origination

The herb Bai Shou Wu originated from the dried roots of two Asclepiadaceae climbing vines, *Cynanchum auriculatum* and *C. bungei*. The former plant is distributed in China, Bhutan, North India, Kashmir, Nepal, and Pakistan. The two sources of the herb are mainly produced in the Chinese provinces of Jiangsu and Shandong. As a Chinese herb, the roots are collected between late autumn and early spring traditionally and dried in the sun for the medicinal purpose. The herb also can be used fresh.

Antitumor Activities and Constituents

The EtOh extract from the root tuber of Bai Shou Wu and its four fractions exhibited cytotoxic activity against human K562 erythroleukemia, SHG44 glioma, HCT-8 colon carcinoma, A549 lung cancer, and PC3 prostate cancer cell lines *in vitro* and exerted the growth inhibition against sarcoma 180 *in vivo*.[1]

C21 Steroidal Glycosides

The antineoplastic principles in Bai Shou Wu were demonstrated to be a group of C21 steroidal glycosides, exerting direct cytotoxicity against mouse Ehrlich ascites cancer, ascites sarcoma 180, and rat C6 glioma cells *in vitro* by inhibiting the DNA biosynthesis and inducting the apoptosis and cell cycle arrest.[2,3] The total glycosides moderately restrained the growth of human K562 (leukemic), PC3 (prostate), HeLa (cervix), MCF-7 (breast), BEL-7402 (liver), and SGC-7901 (gastric) cancer cell lines.[4–6] Intraperitoneal injection of the total C21 steroidal glycosides in doses of 25–250 mg/kg to mice bearing Ehrlich ascites cancer or sarcoma 180 markedly repressed the tumor cell growth and prolonged the animal survival duration. The steroidal glycosides in a dose of 225 mg/kg was injected (IP) to mice implanted with Lewis lung cancer resulted in 38.68% inhibition.[2,6,7] Simultaneously, it showed moderate effect of inhibiting the vascular growth in tumor tissues.[6] Treatment with the glycosides notably augmented the suppressive effect of CTX.[2,7] Moreover, the C21 steroidal glycosides were found to be more sensitive to mouse H22 hepatoma cells, causing the hepatoma cell to swell, and vacuolization even caused the membrane to be broken.[8] The cytotoxic effect of the steroidal glycosides on HeLa tumor cells was accompanied by the dramatic morphological alterations, cell membrane shrinkage, and nuclear pyknosis.[9] Also, the C21-sterols of Bai Shou Wu in doses of 10, 20, 40 mg/kg per day for nine days significantly diminished the cell viability by 34.79%, 47.08%, and 50.23%, respectively, in a transplanted mouse model with hepatoma substantiality.[10]

Over 10 cytotoxic C21-steroidal glycosides have been isolated from Bai Shou Wu, showing great potential for further preclinical investigation. Auriculoside-A (**1**) and auriculoside-B (**2**) displayed potent cytotoxicity on all four tested human solid tumor cell lines (Hce-8693 cecum adenoma, PC3 prostate cancer, HeLa cervical cancer, and PAA lung carcinoma) *in vitro*.[11,12] When the treatment of the cancer cells is done separately, auriculoside-A (**1**) and cynanauriculoside-A (**3**) restrained the growth of MCF-7 breast cancer cells, HO-8910 ovarian cancer cells, and Bel-7402 hepatoma cells *in vitro* and repressed the growth of mouse sarcoma 180 cells *in vivo*. The exposure of the two pregnant glycosides to MCF-7 cells notably promoted the apoptosis and the cell cycle arrest of breast tumor cells.[13,14] Also, the serum after auriculoside-A (**2**) biotransformed in the body still showed the antitumor effect and the ability of apoptosis-inducing.[15] Wilfoside-C1N, wilfoside-C3N, and wilfoside-K1N separated from the herb demonstrated moderate dose-dependent inhibitory effect against the proliferation of human A549 lung cancer cells with disturbed cell cycle.[16] The wilfoside-C3N (**4**), one of the most abundant C21 steroidal glycoside in the herb, also moderately inhibited the proliferation of human ECA109 esophageal carcinoma cells *in vitro* in dose- and time-dependent manners. By a mitochondrial pathway (dependent on caspase-2, caspase-3, caspase-9 and mitochondria and independent of Fas-FasL and caspase-8), wilfoside-C3N (**4**) elicited the apoptosis of Eca-109 cells.[17] Several other C21 steroidal glycosides isolated from Bai Shou Wu, such as caudatin-2,6-dideoxy-3-*O*-methy-β-D-cymaroside, caudatin-3-*O*-β-cymaroside, kidjoranin-3-*O*-β-digitoxoside, and kidjoranin-3-*O*-α-diginosyl-(1–4)-β-cymaroside were demonstrated to possess modest anticarcinoma and apoptosis-inducing properties in human SMMC-7721 hepatoma cells *in vitro*.[18–19] Among the four pregnane glycosides, the SMMC-7721 cells were more sensitive to caudatin-3-*O*-β-cymaroside with an IC_{50} value of 8.6 μM, whereas the IC_{50} values of three other were in the range of 13.49–19.6 μM.[16–23] The last three glycosides plus kidjoranin-3-*O*-β-cymaroside also displayed moderate effect in the inhibition of human HeLa cervical carcinoma cells *in vitro*.[18,22] Caudatin (**5**), a C21 sterol aglycone in Bai Shou Wu, could induce cell cycle arrest at G0/G1 or G2 phase and promote apoptosis of SMMC7721 and HepG2 cells via the decrease of cyclin-D1 expression, the increase of p21 and p53 levels, and the activation of ERK and JNK, finally achieving the suppression of cell proliferation.[24–26] Similarly, caudatin-induced time- and dose-dependent growth inhibitions against U251 and U87 human glioma cells were mainly achieved by the induction of DNA damage-mediated G0/G1 and S phase cell arrest via the promotion of p53, p21, and histone phosphorylation, the activation of ERK, and the inactivation of cyclin-D1 and AKT pathway.[27] Furthermore, the treatment with caudatin also obstructed the metastatic capability of SMMC-7721 cells by blocking GSK3β/β-catenin pathway and inhibiting Wnt signaling pathway targeted genes (such as MMP-2, MMP-9, and COX-2), with a concomitant VEGF reduction.[25] The C21 steroidal glycosides could stimulate bone marrow cells to proliferate and relieve marrow depression induced by chemotherapy of CTX in mice transplanted with hepatoma cells.[28]

Other Bioactivities

The herb Bai Shou Wu has been demonstrated to possess hypolipidemic, immunomodulation, and antioxidant properties by the pharmacological researches. The C21 steroidal glycosides obviously inhibited the contraction of myocardial cells.

References

1. Lei, S. et al. 2005. Antitumor activity of crude extract and fractions from root tuber of *Cynanchum auriculatum* Royle ex Wight. *Phytother. Res.* 19: 259–61.
2. Zhao, J. et al. 1988. Effects of total glucose extracted from *Cynanchus auriculatus* (CA) in inhibiting tumors. *Zhongguo Yiyao Xuebao* 3: 109–12.
3. Wang, Y. Q. et al. 2011. Inhibitive effect of C-21 steroidal glycosides of *Cynanchum auriculatum* on rat glioma cells in vitro. *J. Zhejiang Univer.* (*Med. Edit.*), 40: 402–7.
4. Li, N. et al. 2010. In vitro antitumor activity of glycosides from total steroidal glycosides of Radix *Cynanchi auriculati. Yiyao Daobao* 29: 582–4.
5. Zheng, W. et al. 2012. Studies on PC3 cell apoptosis-inducing effect of C21 steroidal glycosides from Radix Cynanchi auriculati by high performance centrifugal partition chromatography. *Zhongguo Yiyao Daobao* 9: 22–3, 27.
6. Ji, J. N. et al. 2011. Studies on the antitumor activity of C21 steroidal glycosides in *Cynanchum auriculatum. Zhonghua Zhongyiyao Xuekan* 29: 1055–7.
7. Gu, L. G. et al. 1987. Antitumor effect of C21-steroidal glycosides from *Cynanchum auriculatum. Zhongguo Yiyao Xuebao* 2: 281–2.
8. Gu, L. G. et al. 1991. The antitumor effect of steroidal glycosides from *Cynanchum auriculatum. J. Beijing College TCM* 14: 32–3.
9. Zhang, R. S. et al. 2000. Antitumor activity of total steroid glycosides from the roots of *Cynanchum auriculatum. Zhongcaoyao* 31: 599–601.
10. Wang, D. Y. et al. 2007. Apoptosis induced by the C21 sterols in Baishouwu and its mechanism of action in hepatoma. *Yaoxue Xuebao* 42: 366–70.
11. Zhang, R. S. et al. 2000. Two new cytotoxic C21 steroidal glycosides from the root of *Cynanchum auriculatum. Tetrahedron* 56: 3875–9.
12. Zhang, R. S. et al. 2000. Studies on cytotoxic constituents of *Cynanchum auriculatum* Royle ex Wight. *Yaoxue Xuebao* 35: 431–7.
13. Wang, Y. Q. et al. 2009. Antitumor activity of cynanauriculoside A and its effect on apoptosis induction in tumor cells. *Zhongcaoyao* 40: 920–4.
14. Zhang, R. S. et al. 2007. Cytotoxic and apoptosis-inducing properties of auriculoside A in tumor cells. *Chem. Biodiver.* 4: 887–92.
15. Tao, F. et al. 2013. Research on inhibition effect of auriculoside A-containing serum on cancer cell lines. *Zhonghua Zhongyiyao Xuekan* 31: 2247–8.
16. Yao, N. et al. 2009. Effects of three C21 steroidal saponins from *Cynanchum auriculatum* on cell growth and cell cycle of human lung cancer A549 cells. *Zhongguo Zhongyao Zazhi* 34: 1418-21.
17. Liu, K. Y. et al. 2010. Antitumor effects by Wilfoside C3N treatment in ECA109 cells. *Anti-Cancer Drugs* 21: 625–31.
18. Xu, F. et al. 2007. Application of kidjoranin 3-*O*-β-cymaropyranoside from *Cynanchum auriculatum. Faming Zhuanli Shenqing Gongkai Shuomingshu* CN 2007–10021374 20070410.
19. Ye, L. F. et al. 2013. Cytotoxic and apoptosis-inducing properties of a C21-steroidal glycoside isolated from the roots of *Cynanchum auriculatum. Oncol. Lett.* 5: 1407–11.
20. Peng, Y. R. et al. 2011. Caudatin-2,6-dideoxy-3-*O*-methy-β-D-cymaropyranoside 1 induced apoptosis through caspase 3-dependent pathway in human hepatoma cell line SMMC7721. *Phytother. Res.* 25: 631-7.
21. Xu, J. L. et al. 2010. Studies on the chemistry and antieoplastic activities in the root of *Cynanchum auriculatum. Zhonghua Zhongyiyao Xuekan* 28: 416–8.
22. Li, Y. B. et al. 2008. Two new cytotoxic pregnane glycosides from *Cynanchum auriculatum. Planta Med.* 74: 551–4.
23. Peng, Y. R. et al. 2008. Antitumor activity of C21 steroidal glycosides from *Cynanchum auriculatum* Royle exWight. *Phytomed.* 15: 1016–20.
24. Peng, Y. R. et al. 2008. Apoptosis induced by caudatin in human hepatoma cell line SMMC7721. *Zhongguo Tianran Yaowu* 6: 210–3.
25. Luo, Y. et al. 2013. Caudatin inhibits human hepatoma cell growth and metastasis through modulation of the Wnt/β-catenin pathway. *Oncol. Reports* 30: 2923–8.
26. Fei, H. R. et al. 2012. Caudatin induces cell cycle arrest and caspase-dependent apoptosis in HepG2 cells. *Mol. Biol. Reports* 39: 131–8.
27. Fu, X. Y. et al. 2015. Caudatin inhibits human glioma cells growth through triggering DNA damage-mediated cell cycle arrest. *Cell. Mol. Neurobiol.* 35: 953–9
28. Wang, D. Y. et al. 2014. Antitumor effect of C21 steroidal glycosides in radix *Cynanchi bungei* on Heps rats and its influence on hematopoiesis. *Shiyong Linchuang Yiyao Zazhi* 18: 6–8, 22.

173 Liu Huang Jun 硫黄菌

Sulfur shelf

1. R_1 = –H, R_2 = –CH_3
2. R_1 = R_2 = –H
3. R_1 = –glucose, R_2 = –CH_3

Herb Origination

The herb Liu Huang Jun (Sulfur shelf) is the dried fruit body of mushroom *Laetiporus sulphureus* (Polyporaceae). The sulfur-to-fresh orange colored fungi parasitically grow on a wide range of coniferous and deciduous hosts such as the black locust tree. The edible mushrooms distributed over the world can be collected annually and then dried in the sun for medicinal use.

Antitumor Constituents and Activities

Three benzofurans identified as egonol (**1**), demethoxyegonol (**2**), and egonol glucoside (**3**) were isolated from the fruit body of Liu Huang Jun, showing moderate cytotoxicity against human Kato-III gastric cancer cells *in vitro*, with respective IC_{50} values of 28.8, 27.7, and 24.9 μg/mL.[1] A cytostatic (±)-laetirobin (**4**) discovered from the fungus was capable of rapidly entering tumor cells, stopping the cell division at a late stage of mitosis, and accelerating the cell apoptotic death.[2] From the cultures of *L. sulphureus*, several mycophenolic acid derivatives and terpenoids were separated and evaluated by the *in vitro* assays. 6-((2E,6E)-3,7,11-Trimethyldedoca-2,6,10-trienyl)-5,7-dihydroxy-4-methylphtanlan-1-one (**5**) and eburicoic acid (**6**) showed moderate to weak cytotoxicity against human A549 (lung), SMMC-7721 (liver), and HL-60 (leukemic) cancer cell lines with IC_{50} values of 27.4–39.1 μM for 6-((2E,6E)-3,7,11-trimethyldedoca-2,6,10-trienyl)-5,7-dihydroxy-4-methylphtanlan-1-one (**5**) and 14.8–37.5 μM for eburicoic acid (**6**). The two were also effective in inhibiting MCF-7 breast cancer cells (IC_{50}: 35.7 μM) and SW-480 colon cancer cells (IC_{50}: 36.1 μM), respectively.[3,4]

Significant amounts of protein–polysaccharides fractions (PPF) were prepared from Liu Huang Jun, showing both cytostatic and immunostimulating properties *in vitro*. The intravenous administration of the PPF to tumor-bearing mice significantly suppressed the growth of sarcoma 180 cells and prolonged the life span of the tested mice, achieving a higher antitumor effect and a lower toxicity. Furthermore, PPF was able to increase the number of plaque-forming cells in the spleen of mice and to immunize sheep red blood cells, evidencing that PPF is an immunopotentiator.[5,6]

References

1. Yoshikawa, K. et al. 2001. A benzofuran glycoside and an acetylenic acid from the fungus *Laetiporus sulphureus* var. *miniatus*. *Chem. Pharm. Bull.* 49: 327–9.
2. Lear, M. J. et al. 2009. Laetirobin from the parasitic growth of *Laetiporus sulphureus* on *Robinia pseudoacacia*. *J. Nat. Prods.* 72: 1980–7.
3. Fan, Q. Y. et al. 2014. Mycophenolic acid derivatives from cultures of the mushroom *Laetiporus sulphureu*. *Chin. J. Nat. Med.* 12: 685–8.
4. He, J. B. et al. Seven new drimane-type sesquiterpenoids from cultures of fungus *Laetiporus sulphureus*. *Fitoterapia*. 2015 102: 1–6.
5. Gasiorowski, K. et al. 1994. Polysaccharides from *Laetiporus sulphureus* (Basidiomycetes): II. Evaluation of immunostimulative and antitumor activity. *Bull. Polish Academy of Sciences: Biol. Sciences* Volume Date 1993, 41: 347–52.
6. Kang, C. Y. et al. 1982. Studies on constituents of higher fungi of Korea: XLV. An antitumor component of *Laetiporus sulphureus* and its immunostimulating activity. *Archiv. Pharm. Res.* 5: 39–43.

174 Tian Men Dong 天門冬

Chinese asparagus

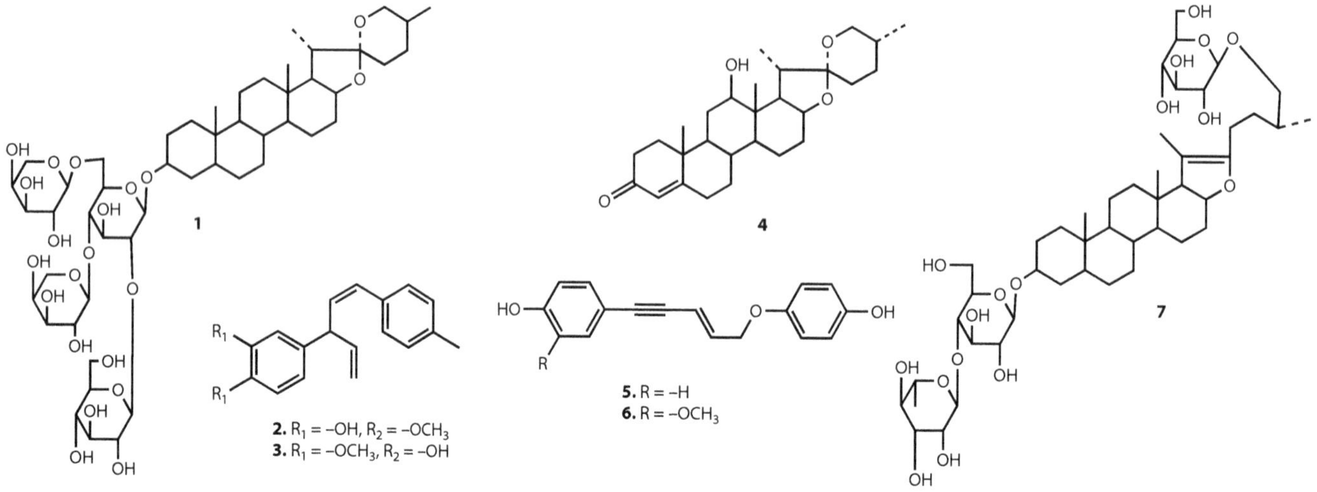

2. R_1 = –OH, R_2 = –OCH$_3$
3. R_1 = –OCH$_3$, R_2 = –OH

5. R = –H
6. R = –OCH$_3$

Herb Origination

The herb Tian Men Dong (Chinese asparagus) is the dried root tuber of a Liliaceae plant, *Asparagus cochinchinensis.* The perennial plant mostly grows in Eastern Asia regions such as China, Japan, and Korea. After being collected during autumn and winter, the roots are steamed or boiled thoroughly and then dried by oven. Since being documented in the first Chinese classic of materia medica titled as *Shennong Ben CaoJing*, the herb has been used in traditional Chinese medicine for over 2000 years.

Antitumor Constituents and Activities

Small Molecules

The bioassay-directed separation of the herb Tian Men Dong led to the discovery of several bioactive constituents. The total saponin extracted from Asparagi Radix, in an *in vitro* assay, exerted dose-dependent antiproliferative and proapoptotic effects against human HL-60 promyelocytic leukemia cell line.[1] Two spirostanol saponins, 25(S)-5β-spirostan-3β-ol-3-*O*-α-L-rhamnosyl-(1–4)-β-D-glucoside and asparacoside (**1**), and two phenolic components, 3′-hydroxy-4′-methoxy-4′-dehydroxynyasol (**2**) and 3″-methoxynyasol (**3**), displayed moderate cytotoxicities in a panel of human cancer cell lines, KB (nasopharynx), Col-2 (colon), Lu-1 (lung), LNCaP (prostate), as well as HUVECs *in vitro*, with IC_{50} values in the range of 4–16 μg/mL.[2,3] Also, a C-27 spirosteroid elucidated as asparacosin-A (**4**) and two acetylenic derivatives elucidated as asparenydiol (**5**) and 3″-methoxyasparenydiol (**6**) showed moderate antigrowth effect against the KB cells *in vitro* (IC_{50}: 10.7, 2.4, and 12.0 μg/mL, respectively).[2] A furostanol saponin identified as aspacochioside-C (**7**) exerted marked cytotoxic activity against human A549 lung cancer cells (IC_{50}: 3.87 μg/mL).[4] In addition, an isolated common flavone termed quercetin exhibited strong to moderate cytotoxic activities against human HeLa (cervix), NCI-H460 (lung), HepG2 (liver), and MCF-7 (breast) cancer cell lines with IC_{50} values of 5.78, 12.57, 20.58, and 31.04 μg/mL, respectively.[5]

Macromolecules

ACP exhibited the suppressive activity against three human neoplastic cell lines, MCF-7 (breast), KB (nasopharynx) and SMMC-7721 (liver), *in vitro,* and exerted the inhibitory effect on murine Lewis lung tumor *in vivo.* During the promotion of SMMC-7721 cells to apoptosis, ACP downregulated the Bcl-2 expression, upregulated the Bax expression, and arrested the cell cycle at S phase. The backbone of ACP1 (a purified ACP) is composed of eight β-(1–4) linked D-galactosidic and six α-(1–6) linked D-glucosidic linkages, with glucosyl branches attached at C3 of a galactosyl residue of the main chain. ACP1 showed the distinctive effect of antioxidant besides antitumor. Four separated individual polysaccharides, ACP-A, ACP-B, ACP-C, and ACP-D, were obtained from the separation of ACP. The oral administration of these polysaccharides to mice reduced the cell growth of sarcoma 180 by approximately 25–50% *in vivo.*[6–9]

Other Medical Uses

The herb Tian Men Dong (Chinese asparagus) has been used as Chinese medicine for its pharmacological functions including cough-relieving, antipyretic, antiseptic, antitussive, phlegm-removing, asthma-relieving, antiinflammation, diurectic, immunoregulating, digestive system-enhancing, and nervine activities. Nyasol and 1,3-bis-di-p-hydroxyphenyl-4-penten-1-one were the two constituents isolated from the herb, and both demonstrated moderate anti-HIV activities with IC_{50} values of 11.7 and 20.0 μg/mL, respectively.[3]

References

1. Huang, Y. et al. 2014. Inhibitory effect of total saponins in Guizhou's asparagi radix on the human promyelocytic leukemia HL-60 cells. *Shiyan Fangjixue Zazhi* 20: 137–9.
2. Xu, C. L. et al. 2005. Studies on the active constituents of Asparagi radix. *Tianran Chanwu Yanjiu Yu Kaifa* 17: 128–30.
3. Zhang, H. J. et al. 2004. Bioactive constituents from *Asparagus cochinchinensis*. *J. Nat. Prod.* 67: 194–200.
4. Shen, Y. et al. 2011. A new furostanol saponin from *Asparagus cochinchinensis*. *Archiv. Pharm. Res.* 34: 1587–91.
5. Son, H. L .et al. 2013. Phytochemical composition, in vitro antioxidant and anticancer activities of quercetin from methanol extract of Asparagus cochinchinensis (LOUR.) Merr. Tuber. *J. Med. Plants Res.* 7: 3360–6.
6. Li, Z. X. et al. 2000. Studies on chemical structure and antitumor activity of galactoglucan from *Asparagus cochinchinensis*. *J. Lanzhou Univ.* (*Sci. Edit.*), 36: 77–81.
7. Li, Z. X. et al. 2000. The chemical structure and antioxidative activity of polysaccharide from *Asparagus cochinchinensis*. *Yaoxue Xuebao* 35: 358–62.
8. Du, X. H. et al. 1990. Exploitation of antitumor medicinal plants: IV. Studies on the isolation of antitumor active constituents of polysaccharides from Chinese herb *Asparagus cochinchinensis* (Lour.) Merr. *J. Shenyang Pharm. College* 7: 197–201.
9. Zhang, M. G. et al. 2011. Effect of *Asparagus cochinchinensis* polysaccharide on human liver cancer SMMC-7721 cells and its mechanism. *Zhonghua Shiyan Waike Zazhi* 28: 1997–8.

175 Shi Hu 石斛

Dendrobii or Dendrobe

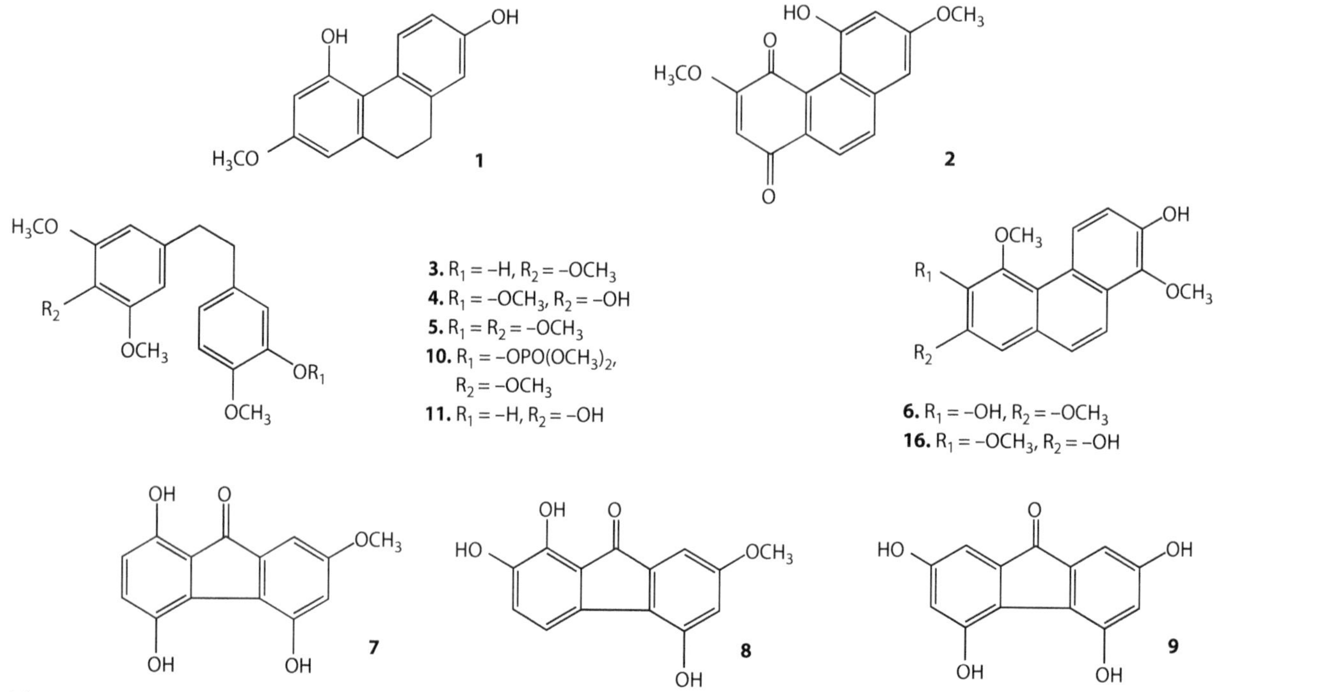

3. R_1 = –H, R_2 = –OCH_3
4. R_1 = –OCH_3, R_2 = –OH
5. R_1 = R_2 = –OCH_3
10. R_1 = –$OPO(OCH_3)_2$, R_2 = –OCH_3
11. R_1 = –H, R_2 = –OH

6. R_1 = –OH, R_2 = –OCH_3
16. R_1 = –OCH_3, R_2 = –OH

(a)

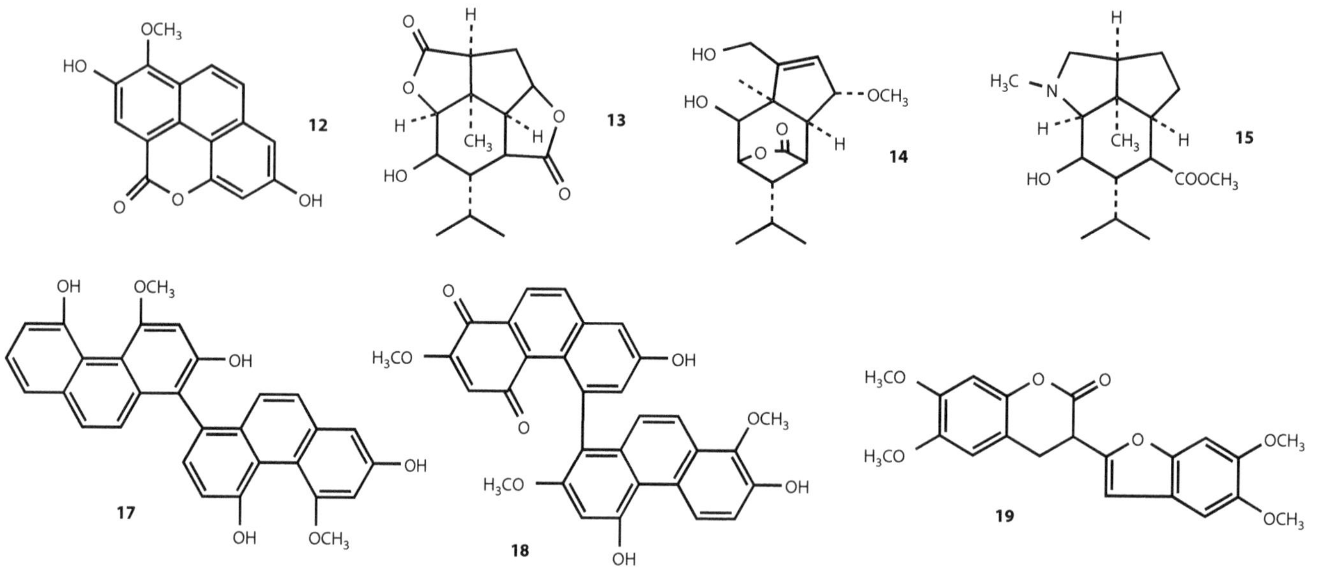

(b)

Herb Origination

The herb Shi Hu (Dendrobii) is the dried or fresh stems of five Orchidaceae plants, *Dendrobium nobile*, *D. chrysotoxum*, *D. loddigesii*, *D. fimbratum*, and *D. candidum*, which are all distributed in south and southwest China. The herb was documented as a top-grade drug in the first Chinese herbal classic entitled *Shennong Ben Cao Jing*, whose book has been used in Chinese medicine for over two thousand years.

Antitumorigenetic Constituents and Activities

In the phytochemical investigations, several types of antitumor agents were found from the five origin plants of the herb, but these were different based upon the plant source.

Agents from D. nobile

From a major source of the herb (*D. nobile*), two phenanthrenes assigned as 4,7-dihydroxy-2-methoxy-9,10-dihydrophenanthrene (**1**) and denbinobin (**2**) were isolated, demonstrating cytotoxicity on several human cell lines, such as A549 lung cancer, SKOV-3 ovarian cancer, and HL-60 promyelocytic leukemia cells, *in vitro*.[1] Denbinobin (**2**) also markedly suppressed the cell viability and promoted the apoptosis of another panel of human cell lines such as K562 (leukemia), BxPC-3 (pancreatic cancer), and Colo205 and HCT-116 (colon cancer) *in vitro* in a concentration-dependent manner, and the IC_{50} value was 1.84 μM in K562 cells.[2–8] The antineoplastic effect in the treatment with ≤20 μM of denbinobin (**2**) was revealed to be associated with augmenting tubulin polymerization, arresting cell cycle progression, and promoting apoptosis via multiple signaling mechanisms such as (1) deregulation of Bcr-Abl and inhibition of NF-κB; (2) activation of p53 tumor suppressor; (3) upregulation of downstream effectors (p21WAF1/CIP1, Bax, NOXA, and PUMA); (4) increase of ROS generation and decrease of LPO (6) release of AIF and inactivation of Akt and activation of Bid; and (7) activation of caspase-3, caspase-8, and caspase-9.[2–8]

The suppressive activity of denbinobin (**2**) on the cell growth was further demonstrated by *in vivo* experiments with nude mice xenografted with Colo205 or HCT-116 carcinoma.[4,5] When the i.p. administration of denbinobin (**2**) in a dose of 50 mg/kg is done to nude mice, the Colo205 colon cancer cells were significantly repressed up to 68%.[4] Denbinobin (**2**) also dose-dependently suppressed the cell invasion and elicited the apoptosis in highly invasive human SNU-484 gastric cancer cells, whose antiinvasive effect was attributed to its significant inhibitory properties against MMP-2 and MMP-9 expressions. The findings highlighted the application of denbinobin (**2**) for the chemoprevention of invasion and carcinogenesis in the colon and the stomach.[9] More evidences indicated that denbinobin (**2**) could prevent CXCL12-induced PC3 cell migration and metastasis by inhibiting Rac1 activity, wherein CXCL12 is preferentially expressed in the bone and is targeted by the prostate cancer cells.[10] Also, a synergistic effect could be obviously achieved in the inhibition of human BxPC-3 pancreatic cancer cells by the cotreatments of 3 μmol/L denbinobin (**2**) with a soluble FasL at low concentrations of 10–50 ng/mL or a membrane-bound FasL, whose effect was correlated with an increase of caspase-independent apoptosis and a decrease DcR3 levels that played a major role in this synergistic effect.[11]

Agents from D. chrysotoxum

Three types of antineoplastic agents, including a phenanthrene (confusarin (**6**)), three dihydrostilbene derivatives (erianin (**3**), chrysotoxine (**4**), and chrysotobibenzyl (**5**)), and three fluorenones (1,4,5-trihydroxy-7-methoxy-9H-fluoren-9-one (**7**), dendroflorin (**8**), and denchrysan-A (**9**)), were isolated from Shi Hu (*D. chrysotoxum*). The first three agents (erianin (**3**), chrysotoxine (**4**), and chrysotobibenzyl (**5**)) demonstrated significant cytotoxic effect on human K562 leukemia cells *in vitro* with IC_{50} values of 0.0065, 5.43, and 0.32 μg/mL, respectively[12] whereas the three fluorenones (1,4,5-trihydroxy-7-methoxy-9H-fluoren-9-one (**7**), dendroflorin (**8**), and denchrysan-A (**9**)) displayed selective cytotoxic effect against human BEL-7402 hepatoma cells (respective IC_{50}: 1.49, 0.97, and 1.38 μg/mL) and almost no activity on human cancer cell lines such as K562 and HL-60 (leukemia), SGC-7901 (stomach), and A549 (lung).[13]

The treatment with erianin (**3**) in concentrations of 20–81.9 nmol/L could arrest the cell cycle at G2/M phase and significantly repress the proliferation of human HL-60 leukemia cells (IC_{50}: 38 nmol/L, in 24 h), being more potent than VCR (IC_{50}: 101 nmol/L).[14] The suppressive ratios of erianin (**3**), chrysotoxine (**4**), and confusarin (**6**) were 29.1–50.82% against mouse HepA hepatoma cells and 51.96–62.25% against mouse ESC cells, respectively.[15] Similarly, associated with the induced apoptosis and G2/M cell cycle arrest, erianin (**3**) moderately restrained the proliferation of Huh7 hepatoma cells in dose- and time-dependent manners, mechanistically associated with the downregulation of the expressions of Akt and Mcl-1 and the activation of PARP cleavage.[16] *In vivo* experiments with xenografted hepatoma BEL-7402 cells or melanoma A375 cells further proved the growth inhibitory activity of erianin (**3**) on the neoplastic cells.[17] After the intravenous injection of erianin fat emulsion to beagle dogs, the cancer inhibitory effect was notably achieved.[18] Erianin (**3**) also obstructed the proliferation of HUVEC by disrupting the endothelial tube formation and abolishing the migration across the collagen and the adhesion to the fibronectin, suggesting that erianin (**3**) exerted antiangiogenic activity as well. Therefore, erianin (**3**) could rapidly shutdown the vascular formation in the hepatoma and melanoma models *in vivo* and *in vitro*.[17]

Importantly, erianin (**3**) and chrysotoxine (**4**) were able to reverse the MDR and to amplify the accumulation of a chemotherapeutic drug Adm in a drug-resistant murine B16/h MDR-1 melanoma cells (B16 cells transfected with human MDR-1 gene).[19] Moreover, the preparation of erianin (**3**) to a phosphate predrug (**10**) not only significantly augmented the solubility but also enhanced the antitumor potency. The inhibitory ratio of the predrug (**10**) was notably upgraded to 99–100% against HL-60 leukemia cells *in vitro*.[20,21]

Agents from D. loddigesii *and* D. fimbriatum

Moscatilin (**11**) is a *cis*-dihydrostilbene, which was isolated from Shi Hu (*D. loddigesii*). The treatment of HCT-116 colorectal cells with moscatilin (**11**) *in vitro* and *in vivo* time-dependently arrested the cell cycle at G2/M stage and induced DNA damage, tubulin depolymerization, and apoptosis through the activation of c-Jun NH_2-terminal protein kinase and mitochondria-involved intrinsic apoptotic pathway, finally leading to the suppression on the cancer cell growth.[22,23] In association with the induction of apoptosis and mitotic catastrophe, the exposure of moscatilin (**11**) restrained the growth of both human esophageal SCC cells and adenocarcinoma cells dose- and time-dependently.[24] The nontoxic concentrations of moscatilin (**11**) were still able to inhibit the motility and the invasion of human H23 NSCLC cells accompanied by the attenuation of endogenous ROS, the downregulation of activated FAKs (phosphorylated FAK, Tyr 397) and the enhancement of ATP-dependent tyrosine kinases (phosphorylated Akt, Ser 473).[25] Usually, the transcriptional factors inducing epithelial–mesenchymal transition such as Twist, Snail, and Akt play key roles in cancer cell migration and metastasis. Moscatilin (**11**) could significantly block the migration of human MDA-MB-231 breast carcinoma cells via Akt- and Twist-dependent inhibitory pathways but not the inference of Snail, and subsequently inhibiting N-cadherin expression. Corresponding to the *in vitro* results, the *in vivo* treatment with moscatilin (100 mg/kg) significantly restrained the breast cancer metastasis to the lungs and reduced the numbers of metastatic lung nodules and lung weight without causing any toxicity in the MDA-MB-231 metastatic animal model.[26] The evidences demonstrated a promising antimetastatic potential of moscatilin (**11**) for the prevention of human breast cancer and human lung cancer metastasis. In addition, fimbriatone (**12**) was isolated from Shi Hu (*D. fimbriatum*) as an agent showing a potential inhibitory effect *in vitro* on human gastric cancer cell line.[27]

Agents from Other Dendrobium Plants

The attempt of searching novel bioactive agents from the same genus plants has been ongoing. The investigations expanded the Shi Hu source to other *Dendrobium* plants, which had not been used as Chinese folk medicines before. The alkaloids extracted from fresh *D. candidum* obviously inhibited the growth of transplanted Lewis tumor *in vivo*. The anticancer mechanism was related to the improvement of the spleen index and the regulation of TNFα and IL-2 expressions.[28] Two picrotoxinin-type sesquiterpenes, termed flakinin-A (**13**) and flakinin-B (**14**), and one dendrobine-type sesquiterpene alkaloid, called mubironine-C (**15**), were separated from Snowflake Red Star, a whole plant of *Dendrobium sp.* The three sesquiterpenes exhibited obvious cytotoxic effect on murine L1210 leukemia cells *in vitro* with IC_{50} values of 4.0, 8.5, and 2.6 μg/mL, respectively.[29] Four known bibenzyls assigned as chrysotoxine (**4**), chrysotobibenzyl (**5**), moscatilin (**11**), and crepidatin were separated from the stem of *D. pulchellum*, displaying the abilities to obstruct the growth and the metastasis of lung cancer cells in anchorage-independent condition.[30] From the separation of *D. thyrsiflorum* stems (a herb distributed in Laos, Thailand, Vietnam, and Hainan and Xishuangbanna of China), three phenanthrenes, termed denthyrsinin (**16**), denthyrsinol (**17**), and denthyrsinone (**18**), and one coumarinbenzofuran, named denthyrsin (**19**), were discovered to have antiproliferative activity against human HeLa (cervical), K562 (leukemic), and MCF-7 (breast) cancer cell lines *in vitro*, with IC_{50} value in a range of 0.45–18.1 μM.[31]

Polysaccharides

Several antitumor polysaccharides have been prepared from the plant sources of Shi Hu. Two polysaccharides labeled as DNP-W1 and DNP-W3, derived from the stems of *D. nobile*, displayed high inhibitory activities against sarcoma 180 *in vivo* and HL-60 leukemia *in vitro*. DNP4-2, a water-soluble polysaccharide fraction prepared from the same plant collected in Africa, exhibited immunoregulatory activity such as notable increases of the immune index and the secretion of IL-2, TNFα, and IFNγ, and it also reduced the concentration of MDA in the blood serum besides exerting tumor inhibition.[32,33] SDP is a water-soluble *D. candidum* polysaccharide, exerting the inhibitory effect against the growth of human SMMC27721 hepatoma cells *in vitro* and in a mice model with implanted sarcoma 180. Besides the apoptosis of human SH2SY5Y neuroblastoma cells significantly promoted by the SDP *in vivo*, the indexes of the thymus and the spleen and the levels of IL-2 and TNFα in mouse serum were effectively increased, the SOD activity was augmented, and the MDA level was diminished,[34,35] proving the SDP exerted both antigrowth and immunostimulating functions.

From suspension-cultured protocorms of *D. candidum*, a single homogeneous polysaccharide named DCPP1a-1 (189 kD) was prepared, composed of mannose and glucose in a molar ratio of 7.015:1 with α-glycosidic linkages. At a dose of 50, 150, and 250 mg/kg, DCPP1a-1 demonstrated the suppressive effect against the growth of murine H22 hepatoma cells by 28.6%,19.3%, and 15.7%, respectively, in mice. Concurrently, it significantly raised the thymus and spleen indexes and augmented the antioxidant effect such as marked free radical scavenging.[36] Similarly, a polysaccharide component from fresh *D. candidum* exerted obvious antigrowth effect against Lewis lung tumor *in vivo* in association with the improvement of the spleen index and the TNFα and IL-2 expressions.[28] Hence, the antitumor mechanism of the polysaccharides from *D. candidum* and *D. nobile* were known to be largely attributed to the promotion of immune organ function and/or the induction of oxidative resistance.

Other Bioactivities

According to numerous research results, Shi Hu (Dendrobii) was found to be capable of promoting the secretion of gastric juice, digestion, phagocytosis, and metabolism and restoring immune function, and it possesses antimutagenic, antioxidant, and antiaging properties.

References

1. Lee YH et al. 1995. In vitro and in vivo antitumoral phenanthrenes from the aerial parts of *Dendrobium nobile*. *Planta Med.* 61: 178–80.
2. Huang YC et al. 2005. Denbinobin-mediated anticancer effect in human K562 leukemia cells: Role in tubulin polymerization and Bcr-Abl activity. *J. Biomed. Sci.* 12: 113–21.
3. Sanchez-Duffhues G et al. 2009. Denbinobin inhibits nuclear factor-κB and induces apoptosis via reactive oxygen species generation in human leukemic cells. *Biochem. Pharmacol.* 77: 1401–9.
4. Yang KC et al. 2005. Molecular mechanisms of denbinobin-induced anti-tumorigenesis effect in colon cancer cells. *World J. Gastroenterol.* 11: 3040–5.
5. Chen TH et al. 2008. Denbinobin induces apoptosis by apoptosis-inducing factor releasing and DNA damage in human colorectal cancer HCT-116 cells. *Naunyn-Schmiedeberg's Arch. Pharmacol.* 378: 447–57.
6. Kuo CT et al. 2008. Denbinobin induces apoptosis in human lung adenocarcinoma cells via Akt inactivation, Bad activation, and mitochondrial dysfunction. *Toxicol. Lett.* 177: 48–58.
7. Kuo CT et al. 2009. Apoptosis signal-regulating kinase 1 mediates denbinobin-induced apoptosis in human lung adenocarcinoma cells. *J. Biomed. Sci.* 16: 43.
8. Devi PU et al. 2009. Antitumor and antimicrobial activities and inhibition of in-vitro lipid peroxidation by *Dendrobium nobile*. *Afri. J. Biotechnol.* 8: 2289–93.

9. Song JI et al. 2012. Denbinobin, a phenanthrene from *Dendrobium nobile*, inhibits invasion and induces apoptosis in SNU-484 human gastric cancer cells. *Oncol. Reports* 27: 813–8.
10. Lu TL et al. 2014. Denbinobin, a phenanthrene from *Dendrobium nobile*, impairs prostate cancer migration by inhibiting Rac1 activity. *Am. J. Chin. Med.* 42: 1539–54.
11. Yang CR et al. 2009. Combined treatment with denbinobin and Fas ligand has a synergistic cytotoxic effect in human pancreatic adenocarcinoma BxPC-3 cells. *British J. Pharmacol.* 157: 1175–85.
12. Wang TS et al. 1997. In vitro inhibition of leukemia K562 cells growth by constituents from *Dendrobium chrysotoxum*. *Tianran Chanwu Yanjiu Yu Kaifa* 9: 1–3.
13. Chen YG et al. 2008. 1,4,5-Trihydroxy-7-methoxy-9H-fluoren-9-one, a new cytotoxic compound from *Dendrobium chrysotoxum*. *Food Chem.* 108: 973–6.
14. Li YM et al. 2011. Erianin induced apoptosis in human leukemia HL-60 cells. *Acta Pharmacol. Sinica* 22: 1018–22.
15. Ma GX et al. 1994. Inhibitory effects of *Dendrobium chrysotoxum* and its constituents on the mouse HePA and ESC. *Zhongguo Yaoke Daxue Xuebao* 25: 188–9.
16. Su P et al. 2011. Inhibitory effect of erianin on hepatocellular carcinoma (HCC) Huh7 cells. *Yingyong Yu Huanjing Shengwu Xuebao* 17: 662–5.
17. Gong YQ et al. 2004. In vivo and in vitro evaluation of erianin, a novel anti-angiogenic agent. *Eur. J. Cancer* 40: 1554–65.
18. Zhou HH et al. 2009. Liquid chromatographic-mass spectrometry analysis and pharmacokinetic studies of erianin for intravenous injection in dogs. *Arzneimittel-Forschung* 59: 141–5.
19. Ma GX et al. 1998. The activity of erianin and chrysotoxine from *Dendrobium chrysotoxum* to reverse multidrug resistance in B16/h MDR-1 cells. *J. Chin. Pharm. Sci.* 7: 142–6.
20. Li YP et al. 2007. Preparation of erianin phosphates and sulfates as antitumor agents. *PCT Int. Appl.* WO 2006-CN1918 20060801.
21. Zou Y et al. 2005. Preparation of 2-methoxy-5-[2-(3,4,5-trimethoxyphenyl)ethyl]-phenol phosphates as antitumor agents. *Faming Zhuanli Shenqing Gongkai Shuomingshu* CN 2005-10034460 20050430.
22. Chen TH et al. 2008. Moscatilin induces apoptosis in human colorectal cancer cells: A crucial role of c-Jun NH2-terminal protein kinase activation caused by tubulin depolymerization and DNA damage. *Clin. Cancer Res.* 14: 4250–8.
23. Ho CK et al. 2003. Moscatilin from the orchid *Dendrobium loddigesii* is a potential anticancer agent. *Cancer Investig.* 21: 729–36.
24. Chen CA et al. 2013. Moscatilin induces apoptosis and mitotic catastrophe in human esophageal cancer cells. *J. Med. Food* 16: 869–77.
25. Kowitdamrong A et al. 2013. Moscatilin inhibits lung cancer cell motility and invasion via suppression of endogenous reactive oxygen species. *BioMed Res. Intl.* 2013: 765894.
26. Pai HC et al. 2013. Moscatilin inhibits migration and metastasis of human breast cancer MDA-MB-231 cells through inhibition of Akt and Twist signaling pathway. *J. Mol. Med.* (Heidelberg, Germany) 91: 347–56.
27. Bi ZM et al. 2003. Studies on the chemical constituents of *Dendrobium fimbriatum*. *Acta Pharm. Sinica* 38: 526–9.
28. Wang J et al. 2014. Study on the mechanism of extracts from fresh *Dendrobium candidum* against Lewis lung cancer. *Zhongguo Xiandai Yingyong Yaoxue* 31: 953–7.
29. Morita H et al. 2000. New Picrotoxinin-type and dendrobine-type sesquiterpenoids from Dendrobium Snowflake "Red Star." *Tetrahedron* 56: 5801–5805.
30. Chanvorachote P et al. 2013. Anti-metastatic activities of bibenzyls from *Dendrobium pulchellum*. *Nat. Prod. Commun.* 8: 115–8.
31. Zhang GN et al. 2005. Bi-bicyclic and bi-tricyclic compounds from *Dendrobium thyrsiflorum*. *Phytochem.* 66: 1113–20.
32. Wang JH et al. 2010. Comparison of antitumor activities of different polysaccharide fractions from the stems of *Dendrobium nobile* Lindl. *Carbohydrate Polymers* 79: 114–8.
33. Luo AX et al. 2011. Immune stimulating activity of water-soluble polysaccharide fractions from *Dendrobium nobile* Lindl. *Afri. J. Pharm. Pharmacol.* 5: 625–31.
34. Jin LH et al. 2010. The antitumor effect and mechanism of soluble polysaccharides from *Dendrobium candidum*. *Jiankang Yanjiu* 30: 167–70.
35. Jin LH et al. 2010. Experimental study on antitumor effect of *Dendrobium candidum* polysaccharides. *Zhongguo Yaoxue Zazhi* 45: 1734–7.
36. He TG et al. 2007. Physicochemical properties and antitumor activity of polysaccharide DCPP 1a-1 from suspension-cultured protocorms of Dendrobium candidum. *Tianran Chanwu Yanjiu Yu Kaifa* 19: 578–83.

176 Mo Han Lian 墨旱蓮

False daisy

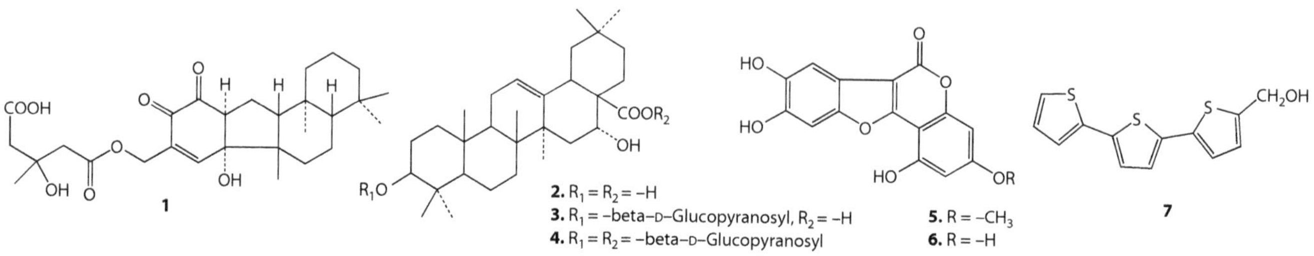

2. $R_1 = R_2 = -H$
3. R_1 = -beta-D-Glucopyranosyl, R_2 = -H
4. $R_1 = R_2$ = -beta-D-Glucopyranosyl

5. R = $-CH_3$
6. R = -H

Herb Origination

The herb Mo Han Lian (False daisy) originated from the whole plant *Eclipta prostrata* (= *Eclipta alba* and *Verbesina prostrata*) (Compositae). This annual plant is broadly distributed in China, Korea, Japan, and Southeast Asian countries as well as in Australia and Brazil. The herb is mainly produced in the eastern provinces in China, and it is normally collected in spring and autumn and dried in the sun for folk medicinal practice. The herb Mo Han Lian can be collected anytime when used fresh for treatment needs.

Antimutation Activities

The herb water decoction exhibited moderate tumoricidal activity against human Eca-109 esophageal cancer cells *in vitro*.[1] A hydroalcoholic extract prepared from Mo Han Lian displayed moderate cytotoxic effects *in vitro* against two human tumor cell lines (HepG2 hepatoma and A498 renal cancer) and a rat C6 glioma cell line with IC_{50} values of about 22, 25, and 50 μg/mL, respectively. The effects were associated with DNA damage and apoptotic induction, as well as the downregulation of MMPs (MMP-2 and MMP-9) and NF-κB expressions.[2] The *in vivo* antitumor effect was observed in mice implanted with EAC when the methanolic extract at doses of 250 and 500 mg/kg/day is orally administered for 10 consecutive days. The life span of EAC-bearing mice was prolonged, and the hematological parameters were obviously improved during the treatment.[3] The aqueous extract of Mo Han Lian markedly inhibited the growth of solid sarcoma 180 cells in mice with the inhibitory rates of 42.94–52.06% at different dosages, and it also enhanced the immune system after intra-astric administration *in vivo*.[4]

Moreover, the fresh juice of Mo Han Lian was demonstrated to have the antiinvasive and antimigration activities in some types of carcinoma cells *in vitro* with IC_{50} values of 31–70 μg/mL without affecting the cell adhesion.[5] In correlation with the inhibition of MDR1 and P-gps, 10 and 20 μg/mL of the hydroalcoholic extract could significantly retard the proliferation of multidrug-resistant hepatocellular carcinoma DR-HepG2 cells.[6] The Mo Han Lian juice showed an ability to inhibit angiogenesis as well in an *in vivo* model.[5] Additionally, either oral or i.p. administration of the aqueous extract in doses of 7.5–30 g/kg to mice obviously protected the myeloid chromosome and polychromatic erythrocyte from chemotherapeutic damage.[7]

Antitumor Constituents and Activities

Triterpenoids

From the plant leaves, an anticancer active triterpenoid designated as dasyscyphin-C (**1**) was isolated, and it exerted 52% inhibitory effect against the growth of human HeLa cervical cancer cells *in vitro* (IC_{50}: 50 μg/mL), while 5-FU, an antitumor drug, elicited 57.5% HeLa cell death (IC_{50}: 36 μg/mL). The treatment with 50 μg/mL of dasyscyphin-C (**1**) resulted in moderate antiproliferative effect on human HepG2 hepatoma cells *in vitro* (IC_{50}: 23.5 μg/mL).[8,9] Also, several oleanolic acid-type triterpenoids were found in the herb. Echinocystic acid (**2**), eclalbasaponin-II (**3**), and echinocystic acid 3-*O*-(6-*O*-acetyl)-β-D-glucoside were effective in the inhibition of human SKOV-3 ovarian cancer cells (IC_{50}: 39.03–40.84 μM). The antihepatoma activity of eclalbasaponin-I (**4**) was weak on human SMMC-7721 hepatoma cells (IC_{50}: 111.17 μg/mL) but was better than that of 5-FU (IC_{50}: 195.31 μg/mL) and lower than that of its 30% EtOh fraction (IC_{50}: 74.24 μg/mL).[10,11] Also, echinocystic acid (**2**) and eclalbasaponin-II (**3**) displayed the suppressive effect against the proliferation of rat hepatic stellate cells in dose- and time-dependent manners *in vitro*,[12] implying the antihepatomagenetic potential.

Coumestans

Two coumestans assigned as wedelolactone (**5**) and demethylwedelolactone (**6**) were naturally occurring in the plant *E. alba*, which have abilities to not only obstruct the growth of human MDA-MB-231 breast cancer cells anchorage-independently but also suppress the cell motility and the invasion of the breast cancer cells via a marked decrease of MPP activities and the blockage of IκBα/NF-κB and MEK/ERK signaling pathways. The antiinvasive effect of dimethylwedelolactone (**6**) was further confirmed in an *in vivo* test with nude mice, where it obstructed the metastasis and the lung colonization of the breast cancer cells.[9]

Terthiophenes

Several unique terthiophenes were discovered from Mo Han Lian, and they showed different degree of inhibitory activities on human endometrial cancer (Hec1A and Ishikawa) and/or human ovarian cancer (SKOV-3) cell lines. Among them, α-terthienylmethanol (**7**) exhibited the most potent cytotoxicity against Hec1A and Ishikawa cell lines (IC_{50}: <0.4 μM) and against SKOV-3 cells (IC_{50}: 7.73 μM), which were stronger than cisplatin (IC_{50}: ~11.25 μM).[13,14] The growth inhibitory effect of α-terthienylmethanol in the endometrial cancer cells was mediated by the induction of apoptosis associated with the increase of intracellular ROS level via NADPH oxidases, the activation of caspase, the release of decreased cytochrome c, and the accumulation of sub-G1.[13]

Nanoformulation

For the development of better tolerated anticancer drugs, silver nanoparticles (AgNPs) were rapidly synthesized using the aqueous leaf extract of *E. alba*. The physiochemical structural analysis showed that obtained AgNPs were crystal in nature. The AgNPs in nanomolar concentrations exerted significant antiproliferation effect against tested human cancer cell lines (MCF-7 and Caco-2).[15] A simple and inexpensive approach was followed for the synthesis of zinc oxide nanoparticles (ZnO-NPs) using the aqueous leaf extract of *E. prostrata*. The synthesized ZnO-NPs shaped with an average size of 29 nm at a 100 mg/mL concentration exhibited significant cytotoxic and proapoptotic effects on HepG2 human hepatoma cells together with the induction of caspase-3 activation and DNA fragmentation.[16] The marked outcome of the studies would help formulate value-added herbal-based nanomaterials in biomedical and nanotechnological industries.

Other Bioactivities

Mo Han Lian (False daisy) is useful in the treatment of inflammations, hernia, eye diseases, bronchitis, asthma, lencoderma, anemia, heart and skin diseases, syphilis, etc. in the folk medicinal practice. Pharmacological studies already characterized the herb as responsible for multiple health benefits such as analgesic, hepatoprotective, antivenomous, antiinflammatory, hypolipdimeic, antihyperglycement, coronary flow-enhancing, hair growth-promoting, immunopotentiating, antiaggressive, and antimicrobial properties. For its marked antihepatotoxic activity, Mo Han Lian is beneficial for the care of infectious hepatitis, liver cirrhosis, and liver and spleen enlargement.

References

1. Chen, K. J. et al. 1989. *Anticancer Chinese Traditional Medicines*, First Edition, p. 289, Chinese Publications of Ancient Medical Books, Beijing.
2. Chaudhary, H. et al. 2011. Evaluation of hydro-alcoholic extract of *Eclipta alba* for its anticancer potential: An in vitro study. *J. Ethnopharmacol.* 136: 363–7.
3. Gupta, M. et al. 2005. Anticancer activity of *Indigofera aspalathoides* and *Wedelia calendulaceae* in swiss albino mice. *Iran. J. Pharma. Res.* 6: 141–5.
4. Zheng, H. et al. 2008. Antitumor effect of aqueous extract from herba *Eclipta prostrata* on S180 solid tumor in mice. *Herald Med.* 12: 1438–9.
5. Lirdprapamongkol, K. et al. 2008. Juice of *Eclipta prostrata* inhibits cell migration *in vitro* and exhibits anti-angiogenic activity *in vivo*. *In Vivo* 22: 363–8.
6. Chaudhary, H. et al. 2013. Evaluation of hydro-alcoholic extract of *Eclipta alba* for its multidrug resistance reversal potential: An In Vitro Study. *Nutr. Cancer* 65: 775–80.
7. Zhou, Y. B. et al. 1986. The efficacy of Eclipta in treatment of coronary heart disease. *Tianjing Yiyao* 14: 490.
8. Khanna, V. G. et al. (a) 2009. Anticancer-cytotoxic activity of saponins isolated from the leaves of *Gymnema sylvestre* and *Eclipta prostrata* on HeLa cells. *Intl. J. Green Pharmacy* 3: 227–9; (b) 2010. Non-proliferative activity of saponins isolated from the leaves of *Gymnema sylvestre* and *Eclipta prostrata* on HepG2 cells-in vitro study. *Intl. J. Pharm. Sci. Res.* 1: 38–42.
9. Lee, Y. J. et al. 2012. Demethylwedelolactone derivatives inhibit invasive growth in vitro and lung metastasis of MDA-MB-231 breast cancer cells in nude mice. *Eur. J. Med. Chem.* 56: 361–7.
10. Liu, Q. M. et al. 2012. Eclipta prostrata L. phytochemicals: Isolation, structure elucidation, and their antitumor activity. *Food Chem. Toxicol.* 50: 4016–22.
11. Lee, J. S. et al. 2015. α-Terthienylmethanol, isolated from *Eclipta prostrata*, induces apoptosis by generating reactive oxygen species via NADPH oxidase in human endometrial cancer cells. *J. Ethnopharmacol.*169: 426–34.
12. Lee, M. K. et al. 2008. Antiproliferative activity of triterpenoids from *Eclipta prostrata* on hepatic stellate cells. *Phytomed.* 15: 775–80.
13. Lee, J. S. et al. 2015. α-Terthienylmethanol, isolated from *Eclipta prostrata*, induces apoptosis by generating reactive oxygen species via NADPH oxidase in human endometrial cancer cells. *J. Ethnopharmacol.* 169: 426–34.
14. Kim, H. Y. et al. 2015. Constituents of the aerial parts of *Eclipta prostrata* and their cytotoxicity on human ovarian cancer cells in vitro. *Archiv. Pharmacal Res.* 38: 1963–9.
15. Premasudha, P. et al. 2015. Biological synthesis and characterization of silver nanoparticles using *Eclipta alba* leaf extract and evaluation of its cytotoxic and antimicrobial potential. *Bull. Materials Sci.* 38: 965–73.
16. Chung, I.-M. et al. 2015. An investigation of the cytotoxicity and caspase-mediated apoptotic effect of green synthesized zinc oxide nanoparticles using *Eclipta prostrata* on human liver carcinoma cells. *Nanomaterials* 5: 1317–30.

177 Bei Sha Shen 北沙参

Radix glehniae

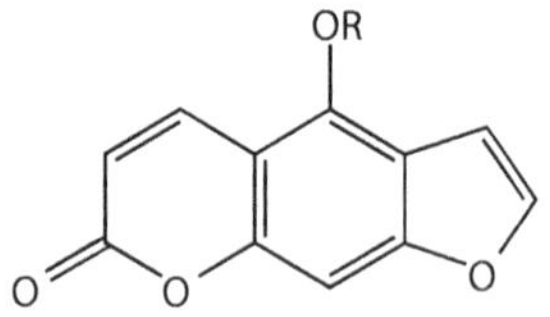

1. R = $-CH_2-CH=(CH_3)_2$
4. R = $-CH_3$

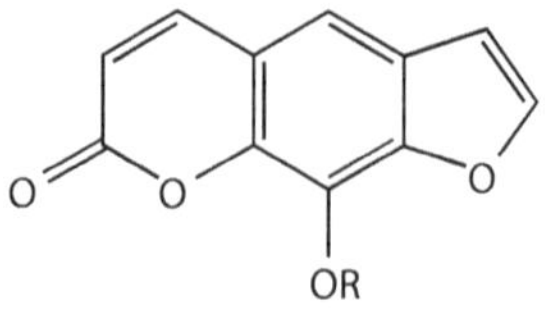

2. R = $-CH_2-CH=(CH_3)_2$
3. R = $-CH_3$

Herb Origination

The herb Bei Sha Shen is the dried roots of an Umbelliferae plant, *Glehnia littoralis*. This perennial plant grows on the sandy beaches of eastern Asia and western North America. It can be cultivated in fertilized loose sandy soil. For traditional Chinese medical use, its roots are better collected in autumn, and its skin is removed and then dried in the sun or by oven.

Antitumor Activities

Three extracts were obtained from Bei Sha Shen treated by water and alcohol, showing the inhibitory effect against the proliferation of human A549 (lung) and Hep (live) neoplastic cell lines but not sensitive to SGC gastric cancer cells.[1] The crude extracts and a solvent-partitioned fraction from *G. littoralis* demonstrated different degrees of antiproliferative effects against human HT1080 (fibrosarcoma), HT-29 (colon cancer), AGS (gastric cancer), and U937 (lymphoma) cell lines. Especially, its n-hexane and 85% aqueous methanol fractions exerted comparatively greater antiproliferative effects. During the suppression on the human cancer cell lines, the mRNA expressions of iNOS, COX-2, and Bcl-2 genes in the tumors were responsibly diminished in a concentration-dependent manner.[2,3] All the extracts of n-hexane, ether, and ethyl acetate displayed *in vitro* inhibitory effect on TPA-stimulated ^{32}P-incorporation into the phospholipids of human HeLa cervical cancer cells, indicating that they are cytotoxic to the HeLa cells.[4] In addition, the water and alcoholic extracts of Bei Sha Shen could also restrain the mutation caused by 2-acetylaminofluorene, 2,7-diacetylaminofluorene, or sodium azide, implying that the extracts contains the antimutant components.[5] These scientific evidences suggest that *G. littoralis* may possibly be used as a valuable chemopreventive agent or food supplement for reducing cancer risk and cell mutation.

Antitumor Constituents and Activities

The systematic separation of the solvent-partitioned fractions led to finding four furanocoumarins and two polyacetylenic alcohols having suppressive activities against the proliferation of human cancer cells and the expressions of MMP-2 and MMP-9 in HT1080 fibrosarcoma cells.[3] The major furanocoumarins assigned as isoimperatorin (**1**), imperatorin (**2**), and xanthotoxol (**3**) played a marked role in the antigrowth effect against seven human tumor cell lines such as SMMC-7721 and HepG2 (liver), A549 (lung), MKN-45 (stomach), HeLa (cervix), and MCF-7 and MDA-MB-231 (breast) in an *in vitro* assay. The IC_{50} values ranged from 0.39 to 4.11 μg/mL for isoimperatorin (**1**), from 0.58 to 5.38 μg/mL for imperatorin (**2**), and from 1.36 to 7.39 μg/mL for xanthotoxol (**3**). The HepG2 hepatoma cells were greatly sensitive to these furanocoumarins (IC_{50}: 0.84–1.36 μg/mL), but the MCF-7 breast cancer cells were greatly responsible for the treatment with isoimperatorin (**1**) (IC_{50}: 0.39 μg/mL) and imperatorin (**2**) (IC_{50}: 0.58 μg/mL).[6] An *in vitro* experiment also displayed that isoimperatorin (**1**) and imperatorin (**2**) were effective in the suppression of four Mo-Han-Lian human cancer cell lines, SKOV-3 (ovary), SK-MEL-2 (skin), XF-498 (brain), and HCT-15 (colon) cells. Their ED_{50} values were 6.8–12.2 and 12.3–19.4 μg/mL, respectively.[7] Bergapten (**4**) is also a bioactive furanocoumarin from the herb, which at a 100 μg/mL concentration exerted the highest inhibitory rates of 95.0% on the HepG2 cells and 79.6% on SGC-7901 gastric cancer cells *in vitro*.[8]

Other Bioactivities

The herb Bei Sha Shen (Radix Glehnia) has been used as a tonic, antiphlogistic, and mucolytic herb for the treatment of respiratory and gastrointestinal disorders. Pharmacological investigation has proven that Bei Sha Shen possesses systematically immunoenhancing, liver-protective, and lung-protective properties. The polysaccharides of Bei Sha Shen can directly scavenge free radicals, playing an antiaging effect.

References

1. Liu, X. L. et al. 2009. Study on antitumor effect in vitro of different extractions by water from roots of *Glehnia littoralis*. *J. Anhui Agricul. Sci.* 37: 9481–2, 9490.
2. Seo, Y. W. et al. 2010. *Glehnia littoralis* extracts for preventing and treating cancer. *Repub. Korean Kongkae Taeho Kongbo* KR 2010037781 A 20100412.
3. Kong, C. S. et al. 2010. Constituents isolated from *Glehnia littoralis* suppress proliferations of human cancer cells and MMP expression in HT1080 cells. *Food Chem.* 120: 385–94
4. Okuyama, E. et al. 1990. Studies on the antitumor-promoting activity of naturally occurring substances: II. Inhabition of tumor-promoter-enhanced phospholipids metabolism by umbelliferous materials. *Chem. Pharm. Bull.* 38: 1084–6.
5. Wang, Z. M. et al. 1993. Antimutant effect of Beishashen. *Shanghai Zhongyiyao Zazhi* (5): 47–8.
6. Wang, M. et al. 2012. Study on activity of five furanocoumarins from the root bark of *Changium smyrnioides* in vitro. *Chin. J. Exp. Trad. Med. Formulae* 18: 203–5.
7. Kim, Y. K. et al. 2007. Antiproliferative effect of furanocoumarins from the root of *Angelica dahurica* on cultured human tumor cell lines. *Phytother Res.* 22: 288–90.
8. Dong. F. et al. 2010. Isolation and identification of bergapten in dry root of *Glehnia littoralis* and preliminary determination of its antitumor activity in vitro. *Zhiwu Ziyuan Yu Huanjing Xuebao* 19: 95–6.

178 Nü Zhen Zi 女貞子

Glossy privet

Herb Origination

The herb Nü Zhen Zi (Glossy privet) is the dried ripe fruit of *Ligustrum lucidum* (Oleaceae). This shrub plant is native to the southern area of the Yangtze River in China, but its cultivation broadly spread worldwide, even to the southeastern United States. Its fruits are normally collected in the late winter and dried in the sun for Chinese medicinal practice. As a valuable Chinese herb used for over 1000 years, Nü Zhen Zi was documented in the first Chinese classic material medica entitled *Shennong Ben Cao Jing*.

Antitumor Relative Activities and Constituents

The exposure of the fruit methanolic extract to human U87MG glioma cells at a 5 mg/mL concentration could force the cells to apoptotic death and loss of viability through the downregulation of an Akt/mTOR/survivin pathway *in vitro*. The daily oral gavage of the extract at doses of 50 and 100 mg/kg in U87MG xenograft nude mice model for nine weeks inhibited the glioma cell growth and reduced the tumor volume with no obvious toxicity.[1] The crude aqueous extract of Nü Zhen Zi demonstrated the growth inhibitory activity on five human carcinoma cell lines and three murine carcinoma cell lines representing different tissues (breast, lung, pancreas, and prostate).[2] The aqueous extract also enhanced the sensitivity of DLD-1 colon cancer cells to DOX-induced apoptosis through the activation of tumor inhibitor genes p14 and p53 and the repression of Tbx3 expression.[3] Also, the Nü Zhen Zi extract serves as a mutagenetic inhibitor, exerting the protection against the mutagenesis caused by cyclophosphamine and urethane.[4]

Moreover, the cancer cells are known to induce hurtful factors suppressing macrophage function and splenocyte activity leading to the blockage of IL-2 production. The extract of Nü Zhen Zi showed an ability to reverse the repressed macrophage chemiluminescent oxidative burst in two murine urological neoplasms, i.e., renal cell cancer (Renca) and bladder tumor (MBT). A 10-day experiment in mice bearing Renca cells demonstrated that the treatment of Nü Zhen Zi extract potently restored the depression of macrophages and splenocytes via the augmentation of phagocyte and LAK cell activities, with the cure rates in a range of 57–100%.[5,6] The results highlighted that Nü Zhen Zi possesses remarkable immunopotentiating antitumor activity.

An antitumor polysaccharide was prepared from Nü Zhen Zi, which exhibited no direct suppressive effect on the proliferation of human SMMC-7721 hepatoma cells *in vitro*, but it obviously restrained the growth and the formation of the tumor and diminished the tumor weight in mice transplanted with entity type of murine H22 hepatoma and sarcoma 180 and prolonged the life duration of mice bearing EAC carcinoma.[7] A combinational treatment of Nü Zhen Zi polysaccharides with a safe phytochemical drug (BDI) and oleanolic acid was able to improve the hemopoiesis of both leukemia patients and healthy volunteers, accompanied by the elevated IL-2 level and augmented G-CSF and TNFα.[8] Consequently, Nü Zhen Zi polysaccharides can be considered as a potential supplement for amplifying the immune function and attenuating the side effects of chemotherapy and radiotherapy. In addition, six secoiridoid glucosides isolated from Nü Zhen Zi demonstrated significant anticarcinogenesis-related antioxidative activity.[9]

Other Bioactivities

The herb Nü Zhen Zi (Chinese privet) has been used as an important traditional Chinese medicine since ancient China. Modern investigations have established that Nü Zhen Zi possesses antidiabetic, hepatoprotective, leukocytotic, antiinflammatory, antimutagenic immunoincremental, hypolipidemic, hypoglycemic, lipid metabolism-promoting, and antiallergic properties.

References

1. Rittenhouse, J. R. et al. 1991. Chinese medicinal herbs reverse macrophage suppression induced by urological tumors. *J. Urol.* 146: 486–90.
2. Lau, B. H. et al. 1994. Chinese medicinal herbs inhibit growth of murine renal cell carcinoma. *Cancer Biother.* 9: 153–61.
3. Jeong, J. C. et al. 2011. *Fructus ligustri lucidi* extracts induce human glioma cell death through regulation of Akt/mTOR pathway in vitro and reduce glioma tumor growth in U87MG xenograft mouse model. *Phytother. Res.* 25: 429–34.
4. Shoemaker, M. et al. 2005. In vitro anticancer activity of twelve Chinese medicinal herbs. *Phytother. Res.* 19: 649–51.
5. Zhang, J. F. et al. 2011. Aqueous extracts of *Fructus ligustri lucidi* enhance the sensitivity of human colorectal carcinoma DLD-I cells to doxorubicin-induced apoptosis via Tbx3 suppression. *Integr. Cancer Therapies* 10: 85–91.
6. Wang, Z. X. et al. (a) 1991. *J. Fujian College TCM* (3): 50; (b) 1999. *Chinese Materia Medica*. Vol. 6, 6-5496, 185. Shanghai Science and Technology Press, Shanghai, China.
7. Li, L. et al. 2008. The study on the antitumor effect of LLP in vitro and in vivo. *Zhongguo Yaolixue Tongbao* 24: 1619–22.
8. Liu, Y. G. et al. 2002. Botanical drug for increasing immunity and decreasing side effects of chemotherapy. *U.S. Pat. Appl. Publ.* US 2001–798047, 20010305.
9. Ma, S. C. et al. 2001. In vitro evaluation of secoiridoid glucosides from the fruits of *Ligustrum lucidum* as antiviral agents. *Chem. Pharm. Bull.* 49: 1471–3.

179 Gou Qi Zi 枸杞子

Wolfberry or Fructus lycii

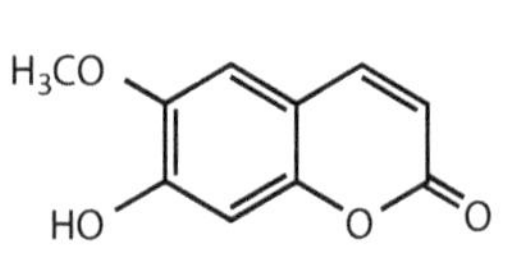

Herb Origination

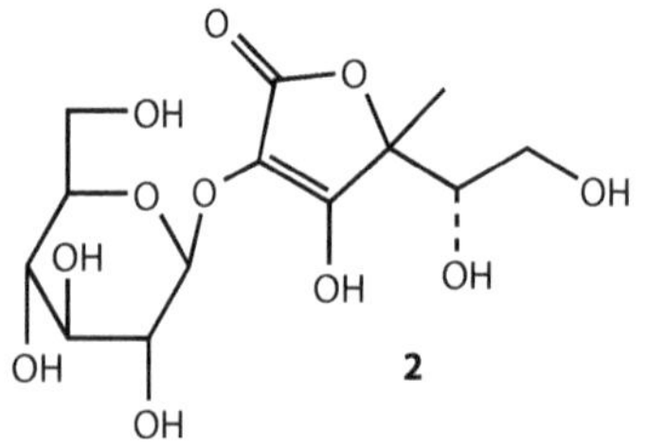

The herb Gou Qi Zi (Wolfberry) is the dried fruits of *Lycium barbarum* L. (Solanaceae), which is one of the famous herbs documented as a top-grade drug in *Shennong Ben Cao Jing*, the first Chinese classic of materia medica. This deciduous woody perennial plant is broadly native to southeastern Europe and Asia. In China, it is distributed in the northwestern and northern regions. The herb is produced by both wild growing and cultivation, but the best quality of the herb is produced in Ningxia province.

Antitumor Activity and Constituents

Scientific investigations showed that the fruit juice and the fruit powder could enhance the cytotoxicity of the mouse splenocyte to inhibit the growth of sarcoma 180 cells. The fruits, the fruit stems, and the leaves of Gou Qi Zi demonstrated significant inhibitory effects against human KATO-III gastric carcinoma and HeLa cervical cancer cell lines *in vitro* concomitant with the blockage of DNA synthesis and mitosis.[1,2] A Gou Qi Zi injection had been tried in the treatment of patients suffering from breast cancer in China, leading to the notable potentiation of the cytotoxicity of the lymphocyte from the breast cancer patients.[2,3] All the research results recommended that Gou Qi Zi may be a potential dietary supplement and anticancer agent aimed at the prevention and the treatment of carcinogenesis.

Polysaccharides

Antitumor Activity

The major antitumor component in Gou Qi Zi was identified to be polysaccharides (LBP). *In vitro* assays revealed that LBP is capable of retarding the proliferation of multiple neoplastic cell lines. In 0.02–1.0 mg/mL concentration, LBP induced the cell apoptosis of human HL-60 leukemia cells after 48 h of exposure and dose-dependently obstructed the growth of leukemia cells.[4,5] LBP elicited the antiproliferation of human MCF-7 breast cancer cells and arrested the cell cycle in S phase by activating ERK.[6] Similarly, the proliferation of human QGY7703 hepatoma cells was suppressed by LBP together with the stimulation of cell cycle arrest at S phase and apoptosis. Concurrently, the amount of RNA and the intracellular Ca^{2+} concentration were enlarged in QGY7703 cells, implying that the obvious increases of Ca^{+} may play an important role for the apoptotic initiation.[7] After being treated with LBP in doses of 0.1–1 mg/mL for approximately eight days, the cell cycle of human SW480 and Caco-2 colon cancer cell lines was arrested at G0/G1 stage by repressing the cell cycle-associated proteins (cyclins and CDKs), and the proliferation of SW480 and Caco-2 cells was significantly restrained.[8,9] LBP also effectively retarded the growth of human Eca-109 esophageal carcinoma cells and human A549 lung adenocarcinoma cells and induced the apoptosis through the downregulation of survivin mRNA expression.[10] The inhibitory effect of LBP on the proliferation of human HeLa cervical cancer cells was elicited by stimulating apoptotic death via a mitochondrial pathway.[11] More *in vitro* results showed that LBP markedly enhanced both PC3 and DU-145 prostate cancer cells to apoptosis and inhibited the growth of PC3 and DU-145 cells in dose- and time-dependent relationships. The significant inhibitory effect on the PC3 carcinoma was further proven in a nude mouse model.[12,13] The marked antigrowth effect of LBP was also demonstrated in nude mice implanted with SKOV-3 ovarian cancer xenograft, whose effect was found to be mediated by the increase of IGFBP-1 level and the decline of the neoplasm-increased IGF-I and IGFR levels.[14] In a dose of 20 mg/kg per day, LBP obviously exerted the depressant effects on the volume and the weight of hepatoma in mice with 42.23% inhibitory rate. Concurrently, LBP repressed the hTERT expression and the telomerase activity.[15] LBP also exerted antiangiogenic effects against MCF-7 breast carcinoma cells in association with the blockage of PI3K/HIF-1α/VEGF signaling pathways and the inhibition of IGF-1-involved angiogenesis.[16] The combination of the polysaccharides with carboplatin more easily inhibited the cell growth and induced the apoptosis of human U251 glioma cells.[17]

By using an ultrafiltration membrane method, LBP was separated into several fractions. Of them, fractions LBP-a8, LBP-a3, LBP-a1, and LBP-a4 showed the antiproliferative effect on human SMMC-7721 hepatoma cells in time- and dose-dependent manners. LBP-a4 (10.2 kDa), which consists of 11.5% uronic acid, 0.34% protein, and 39.02% neutral sugar, that could arrest the SMMC-7721 cells at G0/G1 phase and accumulate the intracellular Ca^{2+} concentration significantly. However, LBP-p8 fraction promoted the growth of SMMC-7721 cells in the assay, but LBP-p8 did not influence the cell cycle progression and the Ca^{2+} concentration in cytoplasm. The LBP-p8 has a larger molecule (6.5×10^3 kDa) consisted of 13.4% uronic acid, 4.77% protein, and 26.26% neutral sugar.[18]

Immunoenhancing Activities

Besides the direct antigrowth activity, LBP also possesses immunostimulating properties. The treatment of sarcoma 180 *in vivo* with LBP promoted a series of immune characters (such as thymus index, splenocyte production, T lymphocyte proliferation index, TNFβ levels, macrophage phagocytic function, NK cytotoxicity, CTL activity, and anti-SRBC antibody secretion) and markedly lessened LPO in mice, implying that the antitumor effect of LBP was also attributed to its remarkable enhancement of the immune function.[19,20] In H22 ascites hepatoma-bearing mice, the antitumor effect of LBP was found to also correlate with augmenting the number of $CD4^{+}$ and $CD8^{+}$ T cells in TIL to relieve the tumor-caused immunosuppression and enhancing the antineoplastic function of the immune system.[21] LBP could also protect the thymus gland cells and decrease the levels of serum VEGF and TGF-β1 in mice bearing H22 hepatoma.[22] LBP had no effects on the proliferation of T-activated killer cells (T-AK), but in the presence of anti-CD3 antibody (CD3McAb) and rIL-2, the polysaccharide could increase the IL-2R expression in the T-AK cells by 21–68% and subsequently reinforce the proliferation of T-AK cells and enhance the tumoricidal effects of T-AK cells against Raji and L1210 leukemia cells.[23] By significant immunoenhancing function, LBP combination with 5-FU lessened the immune system damage induced by 5-FU.[24]

At doses of 100 or 200 mg/kg, LBP was effective on peripheral red blood cells and platelet counts to recover MMC-induced myelosuppression in mice.[25] Due to the properties in the augmentation of spleen CTL and NK cells, the administration of LBP could partially or completely reverse the immunosuppressive effect of an antitumor agent CTX (Cy).[26,27] During the period of 1991–1993, 171 cancer patients were involved in the investigation regarding T lymphocyte blastogenetic rate (LBR) and phagocytosis rate of macrophages (PRM). The results corroborated that LBP was capable of significantly promoting the immune responses by restoring T3, T4, and T4/T8 ratio and raising the LBR and PRM levels, which were notably declined by radiotherapy and chemotherapy.[28] In addition, the Gou Qi Zi polysaccharide could decrease the frequency of the sister chromatid exchange caused by MMC in the lymphocyte, suggesting that LBP can be used to protect genetic damage caused by mutagenic and genotoxic agents.[29] LBP exerted a typical protective effect as well on DOX-induced cardiotoxicity by inhibiting the oxidative stress.[29,30] Consequently, the Gou Qi Zi polysaccharides lead to a potential use in China as a supplement for anticarcinogenesis, antitumor, and immunopotentiation to prevent the adverse effects of chemotherapy and radiotherapy.[31]

Polysaccharide–Protein Complex

LBP3p and LBPF4 are anticancer active polysaccharide-protein complexes isolated from Gou Qi Zi. The treatment with LBP3p (5–20 mg/kg, Per os [p.o.] per day) for 10 days obviously retarded the growth of transplantable sarcoma 180 and enhanced the function of the immune system (including macrophage phagocytosis, spleen lymphocyte proliferation, CTL activity, IL-2 mRNA expression, and the form of antibody secreted by spleen cells) in mice, and it reduced the LPO.[32] The administration of LBP3p also dose-dependently potentiated the expressions of IL-2 and TNFα in human PBMCs.[33] LBPF4 has a glycan portion called as LBPF4-OL, which plays an important role in the immunosimulative effects, such as markedly inducing the spleen cell proliferation, enhancing the production of IL-6, IL-8, IL-10, and TNFα in the spleen cells, and greatly strengthening macrophage to release TNFα and IL-1β.[34] The approaches revealed that LBP3p and LBPF4-OL may be used to enhance immune responses and potential therapeutic efficacy for the improvement of cancer treatment.

Small Molecules

The total flavonoids from Lycium barbarum (TFL) derived from Gou Qi Zi exhibited scavenging effect on active oxygen species, which might be related to the anticarcinogenic potential. TFL-scavenged O^{2-} in a xanthine/xanthine oxidase system reached 51%, and the scavenged OH^- produced a Fenton reaction to 20–72% dose-dependently. TFL at its concentrations of 1.0–5.0 mg/mL was able to promote normal polymorphonuclear neutrophil (PMN) energy metabolism and to completely block the heat output from phorbol myristate acetate-stimulated PMN, leading to the decline of the heat output of murine L1210 leukemia cells *in vitro*, whose evidences confirmed that TFL is a potent scavenger for free oxygen species.[35] Scopoletin (**1**), a coumarin component isolated from Gou Qi Zi, displayed marked suppressive effect against the proliferation of human PC3 prostatic cancer cells *in vitro*.[36]

2-*O*-β-D-Glucopyranosyl-L-ascorbic acid (AA-2G) (**2**), a natural glycoside of vitamin C (L-ascorbic acid), is one of the main biologically active components in Gou Qi Zi. The cytotoxic and antigrowth activities of AA-2G were shown in human HeLa cervical cancer cell lines in a cell type-, time-, and dose-dependent behavior. Similar to vitamin C, the growth suppressive effect of AA-2G on HeLa cells was accompanied by the induction of apoptosis and cell cycle arrest through a mechanism of stabilizing p53 protein. Also, AA-2G (**2**) and vitamin C possess similar hydroxyl radical-scavenging and antioxidant capabilities. *In vitro* radical scavenging assays demonstrated that AA-2G (**2**) was able to scavenge 1,1-diphenyl-2-picrylhydrazyl and hydroxyl peroxide but was incapable of scavenging superoxide anion radicals. Also, its capacity to scavenge nitrite (NO^{2-}) was lower than that of vitamin C. *In vivo* studies further confirmed that AA-2G was able to protect the liver from carbon tetrachloride-induced acute liver injury in mice, and it could repress H_2O_2-induced hemolysis.[37,38] Therefore, these findings showed that AA-2G (**2**) is an active antioxidant agent, which may be cooperative for the prevention of carcinogenesis.

Other Bioactivities

As a recognized traditional Chinese medicine, Gou Qi Zi (wolfberries) exhibited significant multiple biological activities, including hypoglycemic, hypolipidemic, immunostimulatory, antiaging, antioxidant, hepatoprotection, and cytoprotection. Also, Gou Qi Zi is often added to rice congee and almond jelly as a nutritional food, and it is often used in Chinese tonic soups, in combination with chicken or pork, vegetables, and other herbs. Gou Qi Zi contains carotenoids.[39] Gou Qi Zi polysaccharides were found to have various important biological properties, such as antioxidant, hepatoprotection, immunoregulation, antiosteoporosis, antidiabetes, antifatigue, neuroprotection, and radioprotection.

References

1. Hu, Q. H. et al. 1984. Effect of Ningxia wolfberry on cultured cancer cells. *Ningxia Yixueyuan Xuebao* 1: 37–8.
2. Cao, J. G. 1997. Research progress in the increase of leukocyte by the ingredients of Chinese herbs. *J. Jiangxi TCM College* 9: 45–6.
3. Wang, X. F. et al. 1997. Effect of seven varieties of medicinal herbs of minor molecule substance on cytotoxic activity. *Zhonghua Weishengwuxue he Mianyixue Zazhi* 17: 446–8.
4. Gan, L. et al. 2001. Inhibition on the growth of human leukemia cells by *Lycium barbarum* polysaccharide. *Weisheng Yanjiu* 30: 333–5.
5. Gan, L. et al. 2001. Effect of *Lycium barbarum* polysaccharide on apoptosis of human leukemia cells. *Yingyang Xuebao* 23: 220–4.

6. Shen, L. L. et al. 2012. *Lycium barbarum* polysaccharide stimulates proliferation of MCF-7 cells by the ERK pathway. *Life Sci.* 91: 353–7.
7. Zhang, M. et al. 2005. Effect of *Lycium barbarum* polysaccharide on human hepatoma QGY7703 cells: Inhibition of proliferation and induction of apoptosis. *Life Sci.* 76: 2115–24.
8. Mao, F. et al. 2011. Anticancer effect of *Lycium barbarum* polysaccharides on colon cancer cells involves G0/G1 phase arrest. *Med. Oncol.* 28: 121–6.
9. Xiao, L. et al. 2011. Effects of LBP on human lung adenocarcinoma A549 cell apoptosis and expressions of surviving. *Shizhen Guoyi Guoyao* 22: 2917–8.
10. Yang, S. L. et al. 2010. *Lycium barbarum* polysaccharide on inhibition and apoptosis of human esophageal carcinoma cell Eca-109. *Zhiye Yu Jiankang* 26: 2407–9.
11. Zhu, C. P. et al. 2013. *Lycium barbarum* polysaccharide inhibits the proliferation of HeLa cells by inducing apoptosis. *J. Sci. Food Agricul.* 93: 149–56.
12. Luo, Q. et al. 2009. *Lycium barbarum* polysaccharides induce apoptosis in human prostate cancer cells and inhibits prostate cancer growth in a xenograft mouse model of human prostate cancer. *J. Med. Food* 12: 695–703.
13. Xiang, C. Y. et al. 2013. Effects of *Lycium barbarum* polysaccharide on proliferation and apoptosis of human prostate carcinoma DU-145 cells in vitro. *Yingyang Xuebao* 35: 489–91, 495.
14. Wei, M. et al. 2011. *Lycium barbarum* polysaccharides on interfering IGF-I, IGFR and IGFBP-1 levels of human ovarian carcinoma in nude mice. *J. Hunan Univ. TCM* 31: 19–22.
15. Zhang, M. H. et al. 2012. Effects of *Lycium barbarum* polysaccharides on telomerase activation and hTERT expression on portability liver cancer in mice. *Shizhen Guoyi Guoyao* 23: 2438–40.
16. Huang, X. et al. 2012. Polysaccharides derived from *Lycium barbarum* suppress IGF-1-induced angiogenesis via PI3K/HIF-1α/VEGF signaling pathways in MCF-7 cells. *Food Chem.* 131: 1479–84.
17. Liu, W. B. et al. 2013. Glioma U251 cell growth inhibition and apoptosis effect of *Lycium barbarum* polysaccharide combined with carboplatin. *Jiefangjun Yixueyuan Xuebao* 34: 179–80, 188.
18. Zhang, M. et al. 2013. Characterization of *Lycium barbarum* polysaccharide and its effect on human hepatoma cells. *Intl. J. Biological Macromol.* 61: 270–5.
19. Liu, J. L. et al. 1996. Tumor-inhibition of *Lycium barbarum* polysaccharide on S180-bearing mice. *Zhongguo Mianyixue Zazhi* 12: 115–7.
20. Gan, L. et al. 2003. Effect of *Lycium barbarum* polysaccharide on antitumor activity and immune function. *Yingyang Xuebao* 25: 200–2, 214.
21. He, Y. L. et al. 2005. Effects of *Lycium barbarum* polysaccharide on tumor microenvironment T-lymphocyte subsets and dendritic cells in H22-bearing mice. *Zhongxiyi Jiehe Xuebao* 3: 374–7.
22. He, Y. L. et al. 2005. Effect of *Lycium barbarum* polysaccharide on immunosuppressive factors VEGF and TGF-β1 in H22-bearing mice. *Zhongyao Xinyao yu Linchuang Yaoli* 16: 172–4.
23. Wei, H. L. et al. Enhancement of proliferation and tumoricidal activities of T-AK cells by plant polysaccharides. *Zhongcaoyao* 33: 140–3.
24. Li, X. B. et al. 2013. Antitumor and immunomodulatory function of *Lycium barbarum* polysaccharides in combination with 5-fluorouracil. *Zhongguo Gonggong Weisheng* 29: 1463–5.
25. Gong, H. Y. et al. 2004. Therapeutic effects of *Lycium barbarum* polysaccharide (LBP) on mitomycin C-induced myelosuppressive mice. *J. Experim. Therap. Oncol.* 4: 181–7.
26. Wang, B. K. et al. 1990. Effect of *Lycium barbarum* polysaccharides on the immune responses of T, CTL and NK cells in normal and cyclophosphamide-treated mice. *Zhongguo Yaolixue Yu Dulixue Zazhi* 4: 39–43.
27. Wang, B. K. et al. 1988. Effect of *Lycium barbarum* polysaccharides (LBP) on immune function of S180-bearing mice and their antitumor activity. *Zhongguo Yaolixue yu Dulixue Zazhi* 2: 127–31.
28. Liu, J. N. et al. 1996. Effect of Lycium polysaccharide on immune responses of cancer patients following radiotherapy. *Zhonghua Fangshe Yixue Yu Fanghu Zazhi* 16: 18–20.
29. Zhou, G. L. et al. 2011. Protective effect of *Lycium barbarum* polysaccharides to doxorubicin-induced cytotoxicity in cardiac myoblasts H9c2. *Zhonghua Zhongyiyao Xuekan* 29: 1500–2.
30. Xin, Y. F. et al. 2011. Electrocardiographic and biochemical evidence for the cardioprotective effect of antioxidants in acute doxorubicin-induced cardiotoxicity in the beagle dogs. *Biol. Pharm. Bull.* 34: 1523–6.
31. Tao, M. X. et al. 1992. Effect of *Lycium barbarum* polysaccharide against genetic damage in vitro. *Zhongcaoyao* 23: 474–6.
32. Gan, L. et al. 2004. Immunomodulation and antitumor activity by a polysaccharide-protein complex from *Lycium barbarum*. *Intl. Immuno-pharmacol.* 4: 563–9.
33. Gan, L. et al. 2003. A polysaccharide-protein complex from *Lycium barbarum* upregulates cytokine expression in human peripheral blood mononuclear cells. *Eur. J. Pharmacol.* 471: 217–22.
34. Zhang, X. R. et al. 2011. Macrophages, rather than T and B cells are principal immuno-stimulatory target cells of *Lycium barbarum* L. polysaccharide LBPF4-OL. *J. Ethnopharmacol.* 136: 465–72.
35. Huang, Y. Q. et al. 1998. Scavenging effect of total flavonoids of *Lycium barbarum* L. on active oxygen radicals and inhibitory effects on heat output from L1210 cells. *Weisheng Yanjiu* 27: 109–11.
36. Liu, X. L. et al. 2000. Extraction and isolation of active component in fruit of *Lycium barbarum* for inhibiting PC3 cell proliferation in vitro. *Zhongguo Zhongyao Zazhi* 25: 481–3.
37. Zhang, Z. P. et al. 2011. Comparative evaluation of the antioxidant effects of the natural vitamin C analog 2-*O*-β-D-glucopyranosyl-L-ascorbic acid isolated from Goji berry fruit. *Archiv. Pharm. Res.* 34: 801–10.
38. Zhang, Z. P. et al. 2011. Selective suppression of cervical cancer Hela cells by 2-*O*-β-D-glucopyranosyl-L-ascorbic acid isolated from the fruit of *Lycium barbarum* L. *Cell Biol, Toxicol.* 27: 107–21.
39. Lu, H. M. et al. 2005. Resolution of carotenoid isomers in *Lycium barbarum* L. by heuristic evolving latent projection. *Sepu* 23: 415–7.

180 Yong Cao 蛹草

Cordyceps militaris

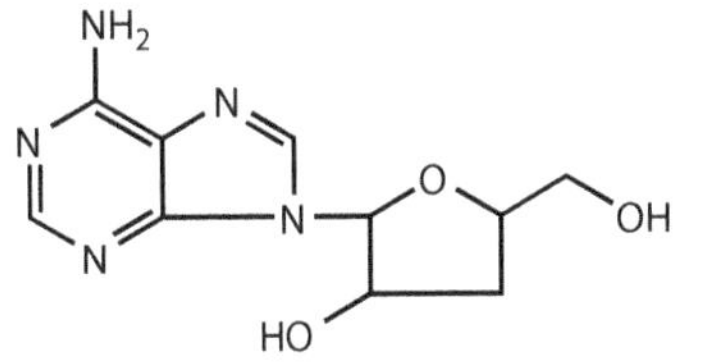

Herb Origination

The herb Yong Cao is the dried sclerotium and stroma of Clavicipitaceae fungi, *Cordyceps militaris*. The fungi mycelia are parasites in the insect pupae or larvae of Diptera, Lepidoptera, and Coleoptera, and then they are completely absorbed into the body of the pupae and the larvae as a nutritive matter to form a complex of the fungi and the dead body. The herb is largely produced in the Chinese provinces of Jilin, Hebei, Shaanxi, and Fujian, as well as commonly in the uplands of northern Ireland.

Antitumor Activities

The extract of Yong Cao demonstrated a significant suppressive effect against the growth of sarcoma 180 cells and Lewis pneumonic carcinoma cells in mice. It also prolonged the survival period of mice implanted with S180 and inhibited the metastasis of Lewis lung cancer cells.[1,2] The water-soluble extract/fraction of Yong Cao displayed the inhibition against the proliferation of seven human carcinoma cell lines, MDA-MB-231 (breast), A549 (lung) SNH-1 (stomach), SNU-C4 (colorectal), and Hep3B and SNH-354 (liver), and a laryngeal cancer cell lines *in vitro*.[3,4] The antiproliferative effect exerted by the extract on Hep3B and MDA-MB-231 cell lines was primarily associated with caspase-3-activated apoptotic promotion.[5,6] It also amplified the populations of apoptotic sub-G1 phase and concomitantly degraded PARP and β-catenin proteins in the Hep3B cells,[5] and it restrained the Akt activation, altered the mitochondrial membrane permeability, and diminished the telomerase activity in the MDA-MB-231 cells.[6] The growth inhibition and the apoptosis induction in the A549 cells by the treatment with its water extract should be correlated with multiple interactions involved in the antineoplastic mechanism, i.e., (1) downregulation of Bcl-2 expression; (2) upregulation of Bax protein and induction of Fas; (3) catalytical activation of caspase-8; and (4) dose-dependently inhibition of telomerase activity via the inhibition of hTERT, c-Myc, and Sp1 expressions.[7]

The anticarcinoma effect of Yong Cao has been further confirmed in clinical treatments of several carcinomas (including in the stomach, the liver, the nose and the pharynx, and others).[8] Moreover, the water extract could profoundly potentiate the cytotoxicity of specific CTL induced by DCs and augment the expression of CD40, CD54, CD80, CD86, and MHC class-II in murine bone marrow-derived myeloid DCs.[9] The DC maturation induced by Yong Cao can play a critical role in the improvement of the immunoregulatory function in patients with impaired host defense.[9] The extract could also enhance the activities of SOD, GSH-Px, and catalase in the serum and increase SOD and GSH-Px in the liver of mice bearing H22 tumor.[10] The findings substantiated that the extract of Yong Cao possesses immunoregulatory and antioxidant activities *in vitro* and *in vivo*, whose effects must contribute to its antineoplastic property.

When adding Radix astragali as a medium for culturing *C. militaris*, the broth of fermentation exhibited an enhanced antineoplastic activity. It moderately inhibited the growth of two human cancer cells such as MCF-7 (breast) and HepG2 (liver) and a murine CT26 colorectal adenocarcinoma cells. The oral administration of the broth in dosages of 100 or 200 mg/kg per day to rats implanted with CT26 cells significantly reduced the tumor volume by 43.81% and 48.89% and decreased the tumor weight by 31.21% and 39.48%, respectively.[11] These evidences indicated that the broth of Yong Cao fermentation may be a potential source for the development of antitumor agents. Moreover, both *in vitro* and *in vivo* experiments demonstrated the antiagiogenic and proapoptotic properities of *C. militaris* extract in human melanoma cells, whose effects were mediated by the mitigation of Akt1 and GSK-3β activation, the increase of p38α phosphorylation, and the downregulation of VEGF expression.[12]

Antitumor Constituents and Activities

Nucleoside

A unique nucleoside cordycepin (**1**) is the major carcinoma inhibitor discovered in Yong Cao and Dong Cong Xia Cao, which exhibited strong anticancer activity on human solid tumor cell lines such as A549 (lung), SKOV-3 (ovary), SK-MEL-2 (skin), XF-498 (CNS), HCT-15 (colon), and 5637 and T24 (bladder) *in vitro*.[13] The highest inhibitory rate of cordycepin (**1**) in a concentration of 100 μg/well was 90.0% against the growth of A549 cells *in vitro*, whereas the least cytotoxicity was only 11.3% on human normal 293 cells.[14] The treatment of the two bladder carcinoma cell lines (5637 and T24) with cordycepin (**1**) at a dose of 200 μM significantly arrested the cell cycle at G2/M phase and dose-dependently retarded the cancer cell growth in association with the upregulation of p21WAF1 expression and p53-independent pathway.[15] Cordycepin (**1**) elicited the cell cycle arrest of human HT-29 colon cancer cells at sub-G1 and G2/M phases at a 100 μM concentration and increased the G1 phase arrest at ≥200 μM. During the treatment, cordycepin (**1**) also dose-dependently promoted the HT-29 cell apoptosis through a DR3 signaling pathway where DR3, caspase-8, and caspase-1 were activated and the cleaved caspase-3 and cleaved PARP expressions were augmented along with the increase of p53 and Bax expressions. Therefore, cordycepin (**1**) significantly inhibited the viability and the proliferation of HT-29 cells in dose and time-dependent manners.[16] Cordycepin (**1**) could also improve the sensitivity of human Hep3B hepatoma cells to TRAIL-mediated apoptosis by inactivating JNK signaling pathway including the decline of Bcl-2 family protein expression and the activation of caspase cascade.[17] An *in vivo* test of cordycepin (**1**) was performed in a mouse model implanted with Ehrlich ascites tumor. In a daily dosage of 150 mg/kg for five days, the cordycepin (**1**) treatment obviously extended the life span of the tumor-bearing mice with antigrowth effect.[18] Moreover, in association with tightening of tight junctions, reducing MMP-2 and MMP-3 activities, and augmenting TIMP-1 and TIMP-2 levels, cordycepin (**1**) time-dependently restrained the motility and the invasion of human LNCaP prostate cancer cells, whose effects were also related to the inactivation of PI3K/Akt pathway in LNCaP cells.[19]

The antimutagenic activity of cordycepin (**1**) was proven by using *Salmonella typhimurium* strains TA98 and TA100. At a concentration of 100 μg/plate, cordycepin (**1**) suppressed the mutagenesis induced by 4NQO, BAP) 3-amino-1,4-dimethyl-5H-pyrido [4,3-b] indol (Trp-P-1), or MNNG.[15] Moreover, cordycepin (**1**) was able to remarkably attenuate the expressions of COX-2 and iNOS in RAW 264.7 macrophage cells and to restrain NO production by retarding NF-κB activation and Akt and p38 phosphorylation. In addition, the *in vivo* antitumor capacity of cordycepin (**1**) was also found to be partially attributed to its immunoenhancing activity.[20] JLM0636, a cordycepin-enriched *C. militaris* extract, could exert sevenfold higher antitumor and immunomodulatory effects on FM3A breast tumor-bearing mice than the *C. militaris* extract after daily feeding in a dose of 7.42 mg/g (dry weight). During the effects, JLM0636 augmented tumor-specific IFNγ-expressing $CD8^+$ T cell responses.[21] Taken together, these findings evidenced that cordycepin (**1**) may provide potential therapeutic and chemoprotective benefits for carcinogenesis-related inflammation and cancer immunotherapy.

Ergosterols and Others

The isolated ergosterols, palmitic acid, and 3,4-*O*-isopropylidene-D-mannitol only showed moderate to weak antiproliferative effect on a small panel of human cancer cell lines. The IC_{50} values of ergosterol (**2**) were 35.6 μg/mL in PC3 prostate carcinoma cells and 61.5 μg/mL in HepG2 hepatoma cells, and the IC_{50} values on the colon 205 cells and the PC3 cells were 62.4 and 59.5 μg/mL for ergosterol palmitate (**3**) and 66.8 and 75.1 μg/mL for palmitic acid (**4**). The lower inhibitory effect was also exerted by ergosterol peroxide and 3,4-*O*-isopropylidene-D-β-mannitol in the colon 205 and PC3 cell lines (IC_{50}: 75.5–95.8 μg/mL).[22]

Polysaccharide

A polysaccharide was prepared from Yong Cao, which is composed of galactose, mannitose, and glucose (3.8:35:10). The polysaccharide could potentiate the cellular immune function by augmenting splenic T cells and IL-1 activities, promoting lymphocyte transformation, and increasing serum IgG antibodies, whose immunoenhancing function is probably helpful for the prevention of carcinogenesis and the treatment of malignant diseases.[23] In the *in vitro* assay, the *C. militaris* polysaccharide could trigger apoptosis and G0/G1 cell arrest in human SMMC-7721 (liver), BGC-823 (stomach), and MCF-7 (breast) cancer cell lines, thereby restraining the cell proliferation.[24]

CMP-1 is a polysaccharide isolated from the cultured *Cordyceps militaris* with a low molecular weight (4.3 kDa), whose backbone is composed of (1–4)-linked α-D-glucopyranosyl, (1–6)-linked β-D-glucopyranosyl, and (1–4)-linked β-D-glucopyranosyl residues, which branched at O-6. The branches consisted of (1–3)-linked α-Lrhamnopyranosyl terminated with (1-)-linked α-D-glucopyranosyl residues. Its proliferation-inhibitory effect presented in four test human cancer cell lines, such as HP-29 (colon), HrLa (cervix), HepG2 (liver), and K562 (leukemia), *in vitro*. CMP-1 also has significant abilities to stimulate mouse splenocyte proliferation and to free radical scavenging.[25]

Peptide and Protein

Cordymin, a peptide with a molecular mass of 10,906 Da and an N-terminal amino acid sequence, was purified from the *Cordyceps militaris*. Cordymin was effective in the antiproliferative action on human MCF-7 breast tumor cells when its concentration is up to 1 mM, but it showed no inference on HT-29 colon cancer cells and immune function.[26] Cordyceps protein extract demonstrated noticeable *in vitro* antiproliferative effect against three tested human solid tumor cell lines, A549 (lung), HepG2 (liver), and MCF-7 (breast), and the IC_{50} values were 8, 10, and 14 μg/mL, respectively.[27]

Other Bioactivities

Pharmacological evidences demonstrated that the bioactive principles of Yong Cao are beneficial to act as neuroprotective, male hormone–like, immunomodulatory, hepatoprotective, renoprotective, pneumoprotective, larvicidal, antioxidant, antiaging, antiinflammatory, steroidogenic, hypoglacaemic, hypolipidaemic, antidiabetic, anti-HIV, antiinfection, antifibrotic, antifatigue, and insecticidal agents. These remarkable properties let it be marketable as over-the-counter medicine.[28,29]

References

1. Liu, J. et al. 1997. Anticarcinogenic effect and hormonal effect of *Cordyceps militaris* Link. *Zhongguo Zhongyao Zazhi* 22: 111–3.
2. Liu, J. et al. 1992. Studies on the antitumor effect of *Cordyceps militaris* Link. *J. Norman Bethune Univ. Med. Sci.* 18: 423–5.
3. Lim, H. W. et al. 2004. Antitumor activity of *Cordyceps militaris* on human cancer cell lines. *Saengyak Hakhoechi* 35: 364–7.
4. Liu, F.-A. et al. 1995. Comparative studies on the rule of anti-laryngeal activity of *Cordyceps militaris* and *Cordyceps senensis*. *J. Norman Bethune Univ. (Med. Sci.)* 21: 39–40.
5. Kim, K. M. et al. 2008. Induction of apoptotic cell death by aqueous extract of *Cordyceps militaris* through activation of caspase-3 in human hepatocarcinoma Hep3B cells. *Han'guk Sikp'um Yongyang Kwahak Hoechi* 37: 714–20.
6. Jin, C. Y. et al. 2008. Induction of apoptosis by aqueous extract of *Cordyceps militaris* through activation of caspases and inactivation of Akt in human breast cancer MDA-MB-231 cells. *J. Microbiol. Biotechnol.* 18: 1997–2003.
7. Park, S. E. et al. 2009. Induction of apoptosis and inhibition of telomerase activity in human lung carcinoma cells by the water extract of *Cordyceps militaris*. *Food Chem. Toxicol.* 47: 1667–75.
8. Yang, Q. Z. et al. 1995. Primary clinical studies on the anticancer effect of *Cordyceps militaris*. *Zhongchengyao* 17: 22–3.
9. Kim, G. et al. 2006. Water extract of *Cordyceps militaris* enhances maturation of murine bone marrow-derived dendritic cells in vitro. *Biol. Pharm. Bull.* 29: 354–60.

10. Zhang, X. J. et al. 2008. Effect of extract from *Cordyceps militaris* on antioxidation of mice bearing H22 tumor cells. *Shizhen Guoyi Guoyao* 19: 943–4.
11. Lin, Y. W. et al. 2008. Antitumor activity of the fermentation broth of *Cordyceps militaris* cultured in the medium of Radix astragali. *Process Biochem.* 43: 244–50.
12. Ruma, I. M. W. et al. 2014. Extract of *Cordyceps militaris* inhibits angiogenesis and suppresses tumor growth of human malignant melanoma cells. *Intl. J. Oncol.* 45: 209–18.
13. Ahn, Y. et al. 2001. Anticancer agent cordycepin extracted from *Cordyceps militaris* and producing method thereof. *Repub. Korean Kongkae Taeho Kongbo* KR 99-54999 19991204.
14. Cho, M.-A. et al. 2003. Antimutagenicity and cytotoxicity of cordycepin isolated from *Cordyceps militaris. Food Sci. Biotechnol.* 2: 472–5.
15. Lee, S. J. et al. 2009. Cordycepin causes p21WAF1-mediated G2/M cell-cycle arrest by regulating c-Jun N-terminal kinase activation in human bladder cancer cells. *Archiv. Biochem. Biophysics* 490: 103–9.
16. Lee, S. Y. et al. 2013. Anticancer effect and apoptosis induction of cordycepin through DR3 pathway in the human colonic cancer cell HT-29. *Food Chem. Toxicol.* 60: 439–47.
17. Lee, H. H. et al. 2013. Cordycepin increases sensitivity of Hep3B human hepatocellular carcinoma cells to TRAIL-mediated apoptosis by inactivating the JNK signaling pathway. *Oncol. Reports* 30: 1257–64.
18. Jagger, D. V. et al. 1961. Inhibition of Ehrlich mouse ascites tumor growth by cordycepin. *Cancer Res.* 21: 216–20.
19. Jeong, J. W. et al. 2012. Inhibition of migration and invasion of LNCaP human prostate carcinoma cells by cordycepin through inactivation of Akt. *Intl. J. Oncol.* 40: 1697–704.
20. Kim, H. Y. et al. 2006. Cordycepin inhibits lipopolysaccharide-induced inflammation by the suppression of NF-κB through Akt and p38 inhibition in RAW 264.7 macrophage cells. *Eur. J. Pharmacol.* 545: 192–9.
21. Jeong, M. H. et al. 2013. Cordycepin-enriched *Cordyceps militaris* induces immunomodulation and tumor growth delay in mouse-derived breast cancer. *Oncol. Reports* 30: 1996–2002.
22. Rao, Y. K. et al. 2010. Constituents isolated from *Cordyceps militaris* suppress enhanced inflammatory mediator's production and human cancer cell proliferation. *J. Ethnopharmacol.* 131: 363–7.
23. Wu, G. H. et al. 2007. Separation, purification and immunoregulation effect of polysaccharides in cultured *Cordyceps militaris. Zhongguo Tianran Yaowu* 5: 73–6.
24. Chen, C. et al. 2015. *Cordyceps militaris* polysaccharide triggers apoptosis and G0/G1 cell arrest in cancer cells. *J. Asia-Pacific Entomol.* 18: 433–8.
25. Jing, Y. S. et al. 2014. Elucidation and biological activities of a new polysaccharide from cultured *Cordyceps militaris. Carbohydrate Polymers* 102: 288–96.
26. Wong, J. H. et al. 2011. Cordymin, an antifungal peptide from the medicinal fungus *Cordyceps militaris. Phytomed.* 18: 387–92.
27. Zhao, S. et al. 2013. Preparation method of protein extracts with antitumor efficacy from edible fungi. *Faming Zhuanli Shenqing* CN 103285043 A 20130911.
28. Ng, T. B. et al. 2005. Pharmacological actions of Cordyceps, a prized folk medicine. *J. Pharmacy Pharmacol.* 57: 1509–19.
29. Das, S. K. et al. 2010. Medicinal uses of the mushroom *Cordyceps militaris*: Current state and prospects. *Fitoterapia* 81: 961–8.

181 Xu Duan 續斷

Chinese teasel

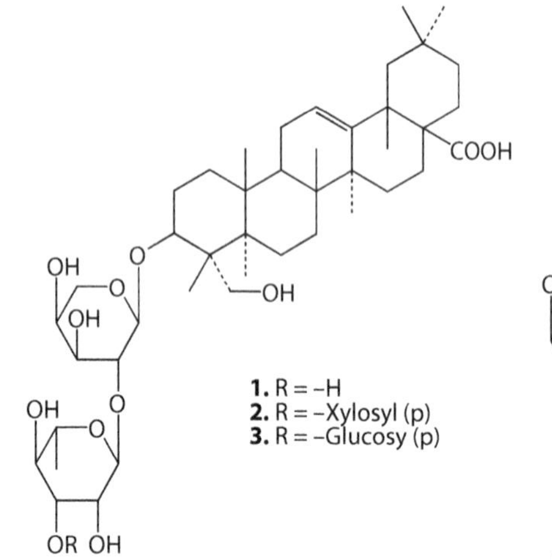

1. R = -H
2. R = -Xylosyl (p)
3. R = -Glucosy (p)

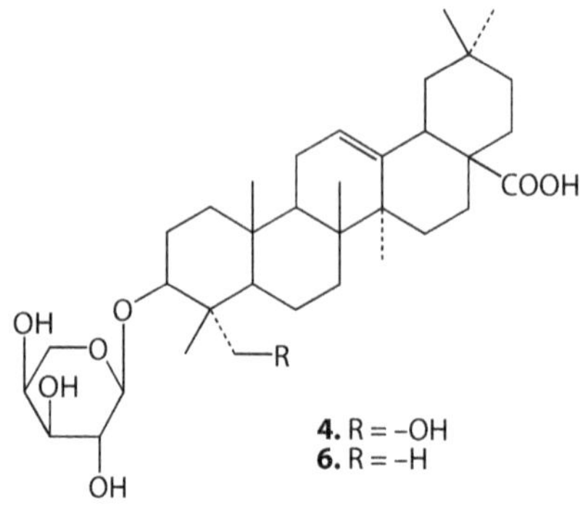

4. R = -OH
6. R = -H

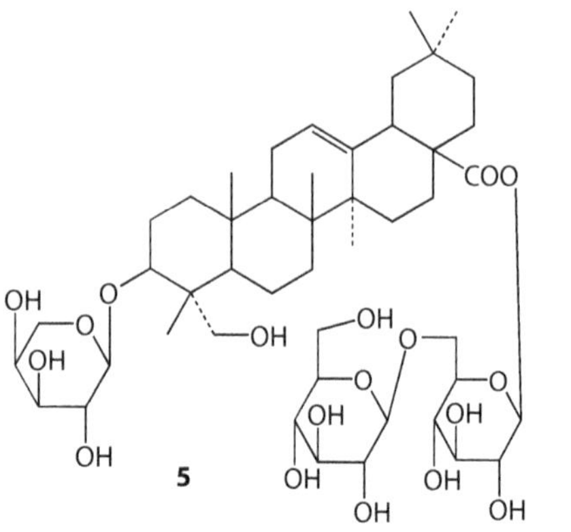

5

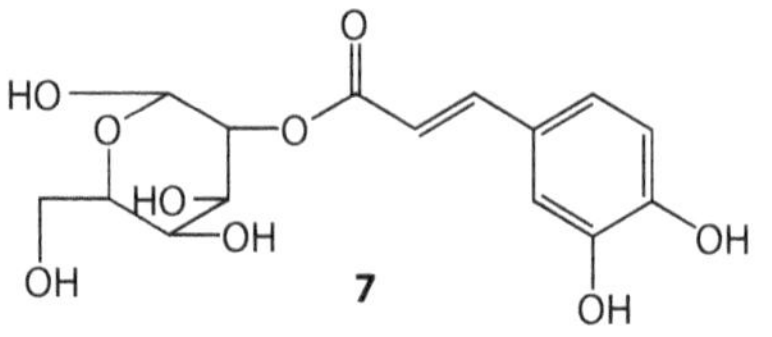

7

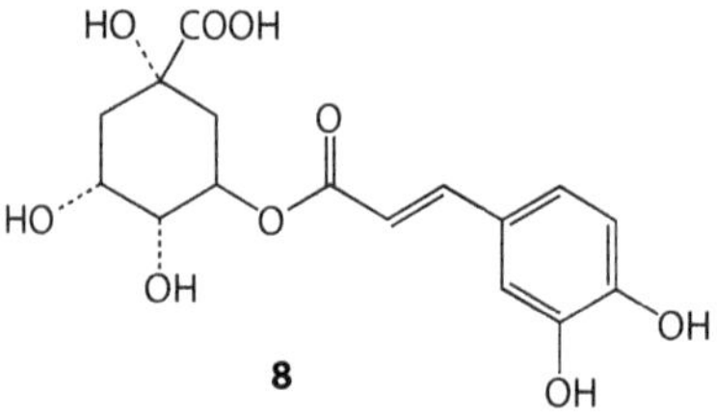

8

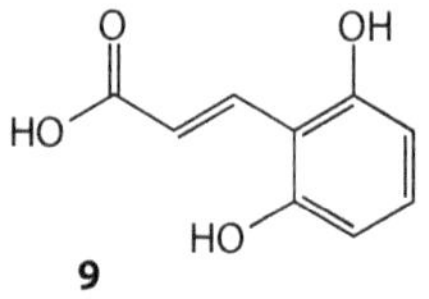

9

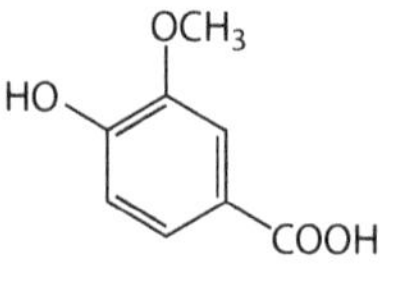

10

Herb Origination

The herb Xu Duan (Chinese teasel) is the dried roots of a Dipsacaceae plant, *Dipsacus asperoids* (= *Dipsacus asper*). This perennial plant is distributed in the southwestern and south-central regions of China. Its roots are generally collected in autumn and dried by oven for application as traditional Chinese medicine.

Antitumor Constituents and Activities

In *in vitro* assays, the EtOh extract of Xu Duan showed cytotoxic effect on human A549 (lung), Bel-7402 (liver), BGC-823 (stomach), HCT-8 (colon), A2780 (ovary) neoplastic cell lines, and mouse Neuro-2 neuroblastoma cells, while its methanolic extract promoted the apoptosis of human U937 histiocytic lymphoma cells.[1–3] In the phytochemical studies, dozens of constituents, including triterpene saponins, iridoids, phenolics, and alkaloids, have been isolated from Xu Duan. Some of the isolated saponins, phenolics, and polysaccharides were found to possess tumoricidal, cytotoxic, and osteoprotective properties by pharmacological experiments, whereas iridoid derivatives exhibited no such antineoplastic activity.

Saponins

Several triterpene saponins isolated from Xu Duan were demonstrated to have marked to moderate antiproliferative activity against the tested cancer cells. Three hederagenin glycosides termed 3-*O*-α-L-rhamnopyranosyl-(1–2)-α-L-arabinopyranosyl hederagenin (**1**), 3-*O*-β-D-xylopyranosyl-(1–3)-α-L-rhamnopyranosyl-(1–2)-α-L-arabinopyranosyl hederagenin (**2**), and 3-*O*-β-D-glucopyranosyl-(1–3)-α-L-rhamnopyranosyl-(1–2)-α-L-arabinopyranosyl hederagenin (**3**) showed obvious suppressive effect against two leukemia cell lines (L1210 and HL-60) *in vitro*, giving the IC_{50} values in the range of 4.7–8.7 μg/mL. The three saponins also efficiently retarded the growth of human SKOV-3 ovarian carcinoma cells with IC_{50} values of 6.3, 5.2, and 22.5 μg/mL, respectively.[4] Akebia saponin-PA (**4**) was effective in the inhibition of three human gastric cancer cell lines (MKN-45, SNU-638, and KATO-III cells), showing its IC_{50} values between 24.1 and 36.5 μM. During the antitumor action, akebia saponin-PA (**4**) elicited the apoptosis and the autophagy of the gastric cancer cells in correlation with the activation of caspase-3 and the formation of cytoplasmic vacuoles and microtubule-associated protein-1 light chain-3II (LC3-II) conversion. Furthermore, the akebia saponin-PA (**4**) activated p38/c-Jun N-terminal kinase, and the induced autophagy also promoted MAPK-mediated apoptosis, indicating that autophagy plays the additive role in akebia saponin-PA (**4**)-induced cell death of gastric cancer.[5] By chiefly activating the NO and apoptosis-related p53 and Bax expressions, akebia saponin-D (**5**) obviously increased the sub-G1 cell population and elicited the apoptosis of human U937 leukemic monocyte lymphoma cells, leading to exertion of the antileukemia effect.[3]

Ten other isolated triterpene saponins, including asperosaponins-A–C and akebia saponin-D (**5**), akebia saponin-PA (**4**), and akebia saponin-X, displayed no cytotoxic activity against three human A549, Bel-7402 and BGC-823 cancer cell lines *in vitro*. Only asperosaponin-C (**6**) and akebia saponin-PA (**4**) exerted moderate suppressive effect against the three tumor cell lines (IC_{50}s: 30–60 μM).[6] Moreover, asperosaponins-A–C, akebia saponin-D (**5**) and akebia saponin-PA (**4**), dipsacus saponin-A, HN-saponin-F, and 3-*O*-α-L-arabinopyranosyl oleanolic acid 28-*O*-β-D-glucopyranosyl-(1–6)-β-D-glucopyranoside showed significantly protective effects in PC12 rat pheochromocytoma cells against the Aβ(25–35)-elicited cytotoxic effect at a concentration of 100 μM.[6] Based upon these scientific evidences, the saponins isolated from Xu Duan were known to have a potential to be a supplement and an alternative medicine for the prevention and the treatment of neoplastic and Alzheimer's diseases.

Polyphenolics

During the screening of the herb extracts, the 95% EtOh extract of Xu Duan markedly retarded the proliferation of five human tumor cell lines. Bioassay-guided studies of the extract led to the separation of the main cytotoxic components, such as caffeic acid, vanillic acid, 2,6-dihydroxycinnamic acid, 2′-*O*-caffeoyl-D-glucopyranoside ester, and caffeoylquinic acid. In the *in vitro* models, 2′-*O*-caffeoyl-D-glucopyranoside ester (**7**) and caffeoylquinic acids (**8**) exerted the growth inhibition against the five human cancer cell lines such as A549 (lung), Bel-7402 (liver), HCT-8 (colon), BGC-823 (gastric), and A2780 (ovary) cells, giving IC_{50} values between 5.37 and 6.68 μg/mL. Vanillic acid (**9**) was effective in suppressing the growth of Bel-7402, HCT-8 and A2780 cell lines (IC_{50}: 5.22–7.40 μg/mL), while 2,6-dihydroxycinnamic acid (**10**) was active to the A549, Bel-7402, and BGC-823 cell lines (IC_{50}: 3.88–7.35 μg/mL).[2]

Alkaloids

The total alkaloids are one of the main ingredients of *D. asperoides*, which exhibited suppressive effects on the growth of human SaOS-2 osteosarcoma cells *in vitro*. If the concentration is increased, the gene expression of VEGF showed a decreasing trend.[7]

Polysaccharides

ADAPW, a water-soluble polysaccharide with an average molecular weight of 16 kDa, was purified from Xu Duan by alkaline extraction, whose ADAPW was composed of glucose, rhamnose, arabinose, and mannose in a molar ratio of 8.54:1.83:1.04:0.42. An *in vitro* assay exhibited that ADAPW restrained the proliferation of human HOS osteosarcoma cells in a dose-dependent manner and enhanced the cell apoptotic death. Its apoptosis-enhancing mechanisms were revealed to be mainly associated with ROS increase-prompted mitochondrial dysfunction and inhibition of PI3K/Akt signaling pathway. From the results, ADAPW can be considered to be potentially beneficial for the cancer prevention against human osteosarcoma.[8]

Other Bioactivities

The herb Xu Duan has been used in traditional Chinese medicine for hundreds of years as a tonic, antiosteoporosis, and antiaging agent for the therapy of low back pain, traumatic hematoma, threatened abortion, and bone fractures. Pharmacological tests proved that Xu Duan possesses antioxidant, anticomplementary, antiinflammatory, antinociceptive, osteoprotective, and cardioprotective properties. In recent reports, the extract of Xu Duan was found to reduce the cognitive deficits and the overexpression of β-amyloid protein induced by aluminum exposure and to inhibit Alzheimer's disease. The treatment with dipsacus saponin-XII and dipsacus saponin-X in a concentration of 4 μM stimulated the proliferation of rat UMR106 osteoblastic cells and augmented alkaline phosphatase activities simultaneously.[9]

References

1. Mazzio, E. A. et al. 2009. In vitro screening for the tumoricidal properties of international medicinal herbs. *Phytother. Res.* 23: 385–98.
2. Tian, X. Y. et al. 2007. On the chemical constituents of *Dipsacus asper*. *Chem. Pharm. Bull.* 55: 1677–81.
3. Jeong, S. I. et al. 2008. Apoptosis-inducing effect of akebia saponin D from the roots of *Dipsacus asper* Wall in U937 cells. *Archiv. Pharm. Res.* 31: 1399–404.
4. Hung, T. et al. 2005. Cytotoxic saponins from the root of *Dipsacus asper* Wall. *Archiv. Pharmacol. Res.* 28: 1053–6.
5. Xu, M. Y. et al. 2013. Akebia saponin PA induces autophagic and apoptotic cell death in AGS human gastric cancer cells. *Food Chem. Toxicol.* 59: 703–8.
6. Ji, D. et al. 2012. Triterpene saponins from the roots of *Dipsacus asper* and their protective effects against the Aβ(25–35) induced cytotoxicity in PC12 cells. *Fitoterapia* 83: 843–8.
7. Dai, J. H. et al. 2015. Total alkaloids in *Dipsacus asperoides* and their effects on proliferation of osteosarcoma SaOS-2 cell lines and gene expression of VEGF. *Biomed. Res.* 26: 37–42.
8. Chen, J. et al. 2013. *Dipsacus asperoides* polysaccharide induces apoptosis in osteosarcoma cells by modulating the PI3K/Akt pathway. *Carbohydrate Polymers* 95: 780–4.
9. Liu, J. J. et al. 2011. Triterpenoid saponins from *Dipsacus asper* and their activities in vitro. *J. Asian Nat. Prod. Res.* 13: 851–60.

182 Ku Gua Zi 苦瓜子

Bitter melon seed

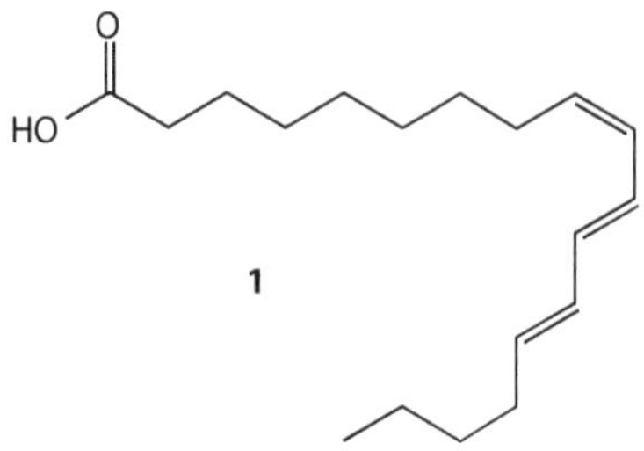

1

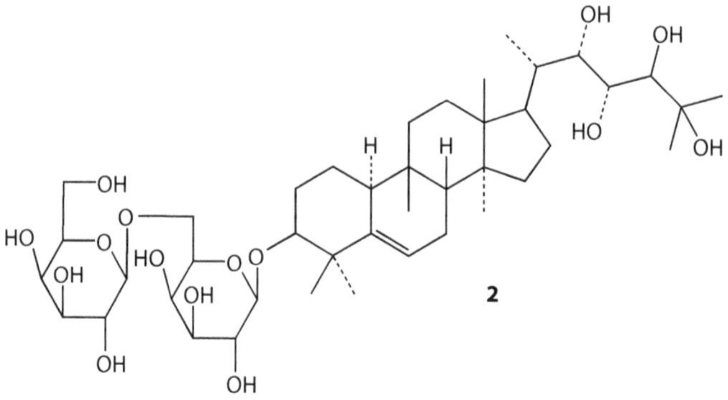

2

Herb Origination

The herb Ku Gua Zi (Bitter melon seed) is the dried seeds of a Cucurbitaceae plant, *Momordica charantia* L. The plant is extensively cultivated in many tropical and subtropical places of the world, especially in Asia, Africa, and the Caribbean. The edible fruits are one of the most common vegetables in south and east Asian countries.

Antitumor Constituents and Activities

The health benefits of *M. charantia* seeds and fruits have been broadly investigated, and many types of biological constituents have been discovered exerting cancer inhibitory potentials. The positive results obtained from the studies revealed that Ku Gua Zi seeds and fruits are valuable sources of food and alternative herb responsible for the antineoplastic and antiviral activities for therapeutic and preventive applications.

Free Fatty Acids

Ku Gua Zi oil contains 9-*cis*,11-*trans*,13-*trans*-conjugated linolenic acid (9*c*,11*t*, 13*t*-CLN) at a high level of more than 60–70%. The n-hexane extract of pulverized Ku Gua Zi oil was hydrolyzed with NaOH–EtOH to give free fatty acids, which at 50 μM showed 65% inhibition on the growth of human HT-29 colon cancer cells.[1] The free fatty acids and the purified 9*c*,11*t*,13*t*-CLN remarkably reduced the viability of Caco-2 colon cancer cells by promoting the cell apoptotic death in a dose-dependent manner, where GADD45 and p53 play a key role in the apoptosis-inducing pathways. Both GADD45 and p53 were remarkably activated and PPARγ mRNA and protein were upregulated in the treated Caco-2 cells.[2] *In vivo* experiments demonstrated that the dietary supplementation with 0.01% Ku Gua Zi oil markedly attenuated azoxymethane-induced colon carcinogenesis by 47% in correlation with the increase of PPARγ protein expression in the colon mucosa and the alteration of lipid composition in the colon and the liver.[3]

α-Eleostearic acid (**1**), a major conjugated linolenic acid in the bitter gourd seeds, was found to have strong suppressive effect against the growth of HL-60 leukemia, HT-29 colon carcinoma, and fibroblast cells. α-Eleostearic acid (**1**) and its analog (15,16-dihydroxy α-eleostearic acid) were the major inducers of apoptosis in the HL-60 cells.[4] The anti-breast-cancer effect of α-eleostearic acid (**1**) was shown in both estrogen receptor+ MDA-ERα-7 cells and estrogen receptor− MDA-MB-231 cells via an oxidation-dependent mechanism. At a concentration of 40 μmol/L, α-eleostearic acid (**1**) promoted the estrogen receptor-independent apoptosis in the MDA-MB-231 cells and MDA-ERα7 cells together with a G2/M block in the cell cycle.[5]

Ribosome-Inactivating Proteins

Momorcharins

Two ribosome-inactivating glycoproteins named momorcharin-α and momorcharin-β were purified from Ku Gua Zi, exerting suppressive effect against the growth of tumor cells. At dosages of 1.2 and 0.8 mg/kg, momorcharin-α could obstruct the growth of human MDA-MB-231 and MCF-7 breast tumor cells *in vitro* and *in vivo* with the induction of G0/G1 or G2/M cell cycle arrest and cell apoptosis. The IC_{50} values were 15.07, 33.66, and 42.94 μg/mL in the MDA-MB-231, MCF-7, and MDA-MB-453 breast cancer cell lines, respectively.[6] But, both momorcharins showed toxicity on the immunofunction in both tumor-bearing mice and normal mice. Momorcharin-α at the dose of 1.2 mg/kg showed minimal toxicity in mice.[6]

MCL

MCL is a D-galactose-specific lectin prepared from *Momordica charantia* seeds. In the *in vitro* study, MCL inhibited the growth of EAC cells by 8–23% at concentrations of 6–24 μg/mL. When MCL is administered in a dose of 2.8 mg/kg/day by i.p. injection for five days, the growth inhibitions by MCL could reach to 75% against the EAC cells in mice.[7]

Momordin-2

Momordin-2 is an immunotoxin extracted from the seeds of Ku Gua Zi. In the *in vitro* assays, it inhibited the protein synthesis in rabbit reticulocyte lysate and showed relatively low toxicity to Molt-4 leukemia cells. When the momordin-2 was conjugated to H65 monoclonal antibody that recognized human T lymphocyte CD5 surface antigen, the produced immunotoxin showed a potent specific cytotoxic effect to target Molt-4 cells and human peripheral blood T lymphocyte but no effect on human hematopoietic cells. The administration of the immunotoxin (i.p. administration to each mice is 10 μg at 48 h intervals) could suppress the tumor cell growth *in vivo*.[8]

MAP30

As a momordica anti-HIV protein, MAP30 (30 kDa) was purified to homogeneity from Ku Gua Zi seed and fruit. In addition to anti-HIV-1 infection and replication, MAP30 also exhibited antitumor activity as well as DNA Topo poison-like effect and cell-free ribosome inactivation.[9] According to the results of NCI's anticancer drug screening, MAP30 was found to have potent antitumor activity against certain human tumor cell lines. The most sensitive cell lines that responded to MAP30 were the neoplastic cells of renal, nonsmall cell lung, and breast with GI_{50} values ranging from 0.01 to 10 μg/mL.[10] The proliferation of human BGC-823 gastric carcinoma cells was moderately retarded *in vitro* by MAP30 (IC_{50}: 51.67 μg/mL) together with the cell proapoptosis.[11] The suppressive effect of MAP30 toward these types of carcinomas might be also affected by targeting immunofusions.[10]

The *in vitro* treatment of estrogen-independent and highly metastatic MDA-MB-231 breast cancer cells with MAP30 resulted in the cell growth inhibition along with the reduction of HER2 gene expression. The injection with MAP30 at a 10 μg dose to mice bearing the metastasis-developed MDA-MB-231 cells significantly prolonged the survival rate by 10 times, and 20–25% of the treated mice could remain tumor free for 96 days.[12] MCP30 was able to induce apoptosis of PIN prostate intraepithelial neoplasia cells and PCa prostate cancer cells *in vitro* and to restrain the growth of PC3 prostate cancer cells *in vivo* without any effect on normal prostate cells. In the PIN cells and he PCa cells, MCP30 mechanistically (1) inhibited histone deacetylase-1 activity, (2) increased PTEN expression and promoted histone-3 and histone-4 protein acetylation, (3) decreased the levels of c-Myc and cyclin-D1 and repressed Akt phosphorylation, and (4) inhibited Wnt signaling activity through the reduction of nuclear accumulation of β-catenin.[13,14] MAP30 was also effective in suppressing the HBeAg expression in HBV-DNA-transfected hepatocarcinoma 2.2.15 cells.[8] In association with the activation of caspase-8-regulated extrinsic and caspase-9-regulated intrinsic caspase cascades, MAP30 elicited the apoptosis of human HepG2 cells and exerted the anti-hepatoma effect *in vitro* and *in vivo*.[15] The antiproliferative effect of recombinant MAP30 was shown *in vitro* against human esophagus carcinoma 1.71 (EC-1.71) cells.[16] These findings clearly designated that MAP30 derived from Ku Gua Zi is a relatively safe agent having potential for the prevention and the treatment of cancer.

Methoxy-Ph Oxime

BMSE-W is an aqueous extract (ethanol/water 1:1) from the bitter melon seed, exhibiting marked cytotoxic activity toward human embryonic kidney 293T and HCT116 cells *in vitro*. GC-MS and HPLC analyses identified methoxy-Ph oxime (MPO) as a major active component in the BMSE-W. Increased PARP and β-actin cleavage and induced chromatin condensation were observed in the tumor cells after being treated with MPO, suggesting the apoptotic death as a plausible cause for the cytotoxicity.[17]

Triterpenoid

A triterpenoid established as momorcharaside-A (**2**) was separated from the seed of *M. charantia*, which exhibited obvious inhibition of DNA and RNA biosyntheses in mouse sarcoma 180 cells by 58% and 55% at a 100 μg/mL dose, respectively.[18]

References

1. Fujimoto, K. et al. 2002. Preparation of truncated *Momordica charantia* anti-HIV and anti-tumor MAP-30 or GAP-31 proteins. *Jpn. Kokai Tokkyo Koho* (2002), 5 pp. JP 2001–2239.
2. Yasui, Y. et al. 2005. Bitter gourd seed fatty acid rich in 9c,11t,13t-conjugated linolenic acid induces apoptosis and upregulates the GADD45, p53 and PPARγ in human colon cancer Caco-2 cells. *Prostaglandins Leukotrienes Essent. Fatty Acids* 73: 113–9.
3. Kohno, H. et al. 2004. Dietary seed oil rich in conjugated linolenic acid from bitter melon inhibits azoxymethane-induced rat colon carcinogenesis through elevation of colonic PPAR-γ expression and alteration of lipid composition. *Intl. J. Cancer* 110: 896–901.
4. Kobori, M. et al. 2008. α-Eleostearic acid and its dihydroxy derivative are major apoptosis-inducing components of bitter gourd. *J. Agricul. Food Chem.* 56: 10515–20.
5. Grossman, M. E. et al. 2009. Eleostreatic acid inhibits breast cancer proliferation by means of an oxidation-dependent mechanism. *Cancer Prev. Res.* 2: 879–86.
6. Cao, D. L. et al. 2015. α-momorcharin (α-MMC) exerts effective anti-human breast tumor activities but has a narrow therapeutic window in vivo. *Fitoterapia* 100: 139–49.
7. Kabir, S. R. et al. 2015. Momordica charantia seed lectin: Toxicity, bacterial agglutination and antitumor properties. *Applied Biochem. Biotechnol.* 175: 2616–28.
8. Wang, R. H. et al. 1992. In vitro cytotoxicity and in vivo antitumor activity of single chain immunotoxin. *Zhongguo Mianyixue Zazhi* 8: 356–60.
9. Lee-Huang, S. et al. 2000. Inhibition of MDA-MB-231 human breast tumor xenografts and HER2 expression by antitumor agents GAP31 and MAP30. *Anticancer Res.* 20(2A): 653–9.
10. Rybak, S. M. et al. 1994. In vitro antitumor-activity of the plant ribosome-inactivating proteins MAP-30 and GAP-31. *Intl. J. Oncol.* 5: 1171–6.
11. Xue, Y. J. et al. 2012. Effect of recombinant momordica anti-HIV protein of 30 kD on proliferation and apoptosis of human gastric carcinoma BGC-823 cells. *Jiangsu Yiyao* 38: 765–7.
12. Wang, J. P. et al. 2003. Inhibition of momordica anti-HIV protein of MAP30 on HBeAg expression by laser scanning confocal microscopy. *Xibao Yu Fenzi Mianyixue Zazhi* 19: 183–4.
13. Xiong, S. D. et al. 2009. Ribosome-inactivating proteins isolated from dietary bitter melon induce apoptosis and inhibit histone deacetylase-1 selectively in premalignant and malignant prostate cancer cells. *Intl. J. Cancer* 125: 774–82.
14. Lee-Huang, S. et al. 2003. Preparation of truncated *Momordica charantia* anti-HIV and anti-tumor MAP-30 or GAP-31 proteins. *U.S.* 22 pp. US 2000–645603, 20000825.
15. Fang, E. F. et al. 2012. The MAP30 protein from bitter gourd (*Momordica charantia*) seeds promotes apoptosis in liver cancer cells in vitro and in vivo. *Cancer Lett.* 324: 66–74.
16. Xue, Y. J. et al. 2011. Effects of recombinant MAP30 on cell proliferation and apoptosis of human esophageal carcinoma EC-1.71 cells. *Afri. J. Pharmacy Pharmacol.* 5: 2680–8.
17. Chipps, E. S. et al. 2012. Cytotoxicity analysis of active components in bitter melon (*Momordica charantia*) seed extracts using human embryonic kidney and colon tumor cells. *Nat. Prod. Commun.* 7: 1203–8.
18. Zhu, Z. J. et al. 1990. Bioactive constituents from bitter melon seed. *Yaoxue Xuebao* 25: 898–903.

183 Bu Gu Zhi 補骨脂

Scurfpea seeds or Babchi

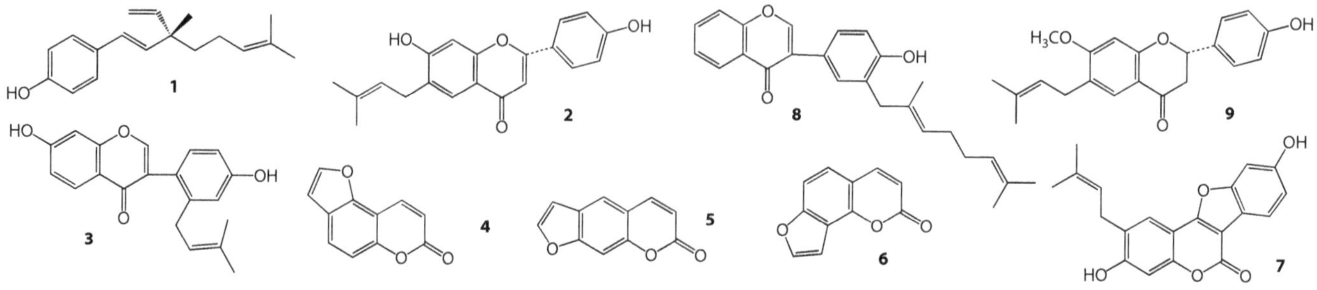

Herb Origination

The herb Bu Gu Zhi (Babchi) is the seeds of a Leguminosae plant, *Psoralea corylifolia* L. This erect annual plant is an endangered and medicinally important herb source in China, India, Europe, and others. The plant is indigenous to tropical and subtropical regions of the world. The herb is mainly produced in the Chinese provinces of Shanxi, Shaanxi, Anhui, Henan, and Sichuan, as well as in India. The normal collection season of the seeds is autumn when the fruit ripens.

Antitumor Activities

Bu Gu Zhi contains several antineoplastic components, and even its volatile oil shows antitumor activity. An active fraction AF derived from Bu Gu Zhi was examined by gas-chromatographic technique was determined to be a mixture of fatty glyceride. At a dose of 100 mg/kg, AF delayed the induction of papilloma and inhibited the growth of papilloma initiated by dimethylbenz(a) anthracene and promoted by croton oil in mice. The oral administration of the AF to mice significantly suppressed the cell growth of the soft tissue fibrosarcoma induced by subcutaneous injection of 20-methylcholanthrene.[1] An EtOh extract of Bu Gu Zhi exhibited cytotoxicity on L929 fibroblast cells *in vitro* and obstructed DNA replication enzymes and DNA polymerase concurrently.[2] Bu Gu Zhi extract not only inhibited the EAC ascitic tumor growth, but was also effective in the stimulation of immune system and NK cells in mice. It notably augmented antibody-dependent cellular cytotoxicity, antibody-forming cells, and antibody complement-mediated cytotoxicity.[3] Through a mitochondrial pathway, the extract promoted the apoptosis of MCF-7 breast cancer cells and dose-dependently diminished the proliferation of MCF-7 cells.[4] Moreover, an effective component extracted from the herb was patented, which could exert an interesting effect on the reversal of the tumor MDR. The active component can be made into conventional dosage forms such as tablet, capsule, oral liquid, and granule for clinical treatment cancer of patients.[5]

Antitumor Constituents and Activities

Activity-directed fractionation led to the discovery of a group of DNA polymerase inhibitors, such as bakuchiol (**1**), corylifolin (**2**), neobavaisoflavone (**3**), bakuchicin (**4**), resveratrol, and daidzein. Daidzein and bakuchicin (**4**) are also suppressors of Topo-II.[2,6]

Bakuchiol

Bakuchiol (**1**) and bakuchicin (**4**) exhibited obvious cytotoxicity on human HepG2 hepatoma cells *in vitro* and also possess hepatoprotective activity.[7] Bakuchiol (**1**) demonstrated moderate cytotoxic effect on a panel of human cancer cell lines, such as A549 (lung), SKOV-3 (ovary), SK-MEL-2 (skin), XF498 (brain), HCT15 (colon), and HEp-2 (larynx) cells, *in vitro*,[8,9] and exerted a prominent cytotoxic effect on murine L929 aneuploid fibrosarcoma cells through a mechanism in an injury of cell membrane and hemolytic activity.[6] When it was radiolabeled with I^{125}, the antigrowth activity of bakuchiol (**1**) was markedly potentiated. In murine LS-A lymphosarcoma cells and both ascitic and solid barcl-95 radiation-induced thymic lymphoma cells, the I^{125}-bounded bakuchiol (**1**) accomplished marked greater inhibitory effect than with the bakuchiol (**1**) alone.[10]

Neobavaisoflavone

In both *in vitro* and *in vivo* experiments, neobavaisoflavone (**3**) restrained the proliferation of prostate cancer cells and sensitized human LNCaP prostate cancer cells and human U373MG glioma cells to TRAIL-mediated apoptosis and growth suppression. Thus, the cotreatment of TRAIL and neobavaisoflavone (**3**) effectively reversed the resistance of carcinoma cells to TRAIL, whose effect was found to be correlated with the increase of Bid cleavage and BAX expression, the upregulation of DR5 expression, and the activation caspase-3, caspase-8, and caspase-9. The elicitation of TRAIL-mediated apoptosis in the glioma cells was also accompanied with the suppression of the migration and the invasion and the inhibition of the anoikis resistance. These findings recommended that the combination of TRAIL and neobavaisoflavone (**3**) may be an active therapeutic strategy for treating TRAIL-resistant glioma cells.[11]

Psoralen

In human BGC-823 gastric cancer cells *in vitro*, psoralen (**5**) displayed marked inhibitory effect (IC_{50}: 5.82 μg/mL), and its potency was stronger than that of isopsoralen (**6**) by over 25 times.[12] The daily i.p. injection of 10 μg of psoralen (**5**) to mice suppressed the growth of Ehrlich ascites cancer by 68%, sarcoma 180 by 40.2%, and H22 hepatoma by 20.5%. If psoralen (**5**) was subcutaneously injected to mice bearing one of the three types of tumors, respectively, the maximum inhibitory rates reached to 98–100%.[13] In nude mice implanted with MEC-1 human mucus epithelial carcinoma cells, the psoralen treatment retarded the cell growth by 79.1% and prolonged the life duration by 112%.[14] If combined with IFNα, the treatment could be remarkably improved with the evidences of better body conditions of MEC-1 tumor-bearing animals and life prolongation.[13] Both *in vitro* and *in vivo* experiments with EMT 6 mammary cancer cells demonstrated that psoralen (**5**) reduced the DNA content and caused the degeneration of the mitochondria, exerting marked antineoplastic effect with an IC_{50} value of 2.23 μg/mL.[15] Psoralen (**5**) was also able to suppress the growth of SMMC-7721 hepatoma cells in dose- and time-dependent manners and induced the cell apoptosis via the mechanism that involves caspase-3, p53, Bax, and Bcl-2 pathway.[16] In an *in vivo* experiment, psoralen (**5**) inhibited metastasis of the breast cancer to the bone, whose activity was due to psoralen inhibiting the growth of breast cancer cells in the bone microenvironment and regulating the function of osteoblasts and osteoclasts in tumor-bearing mice.[17]

Moreover, through the induction of Ca^{2+}-involved apoptosis, psoralen (**5**) obstructed the proliferation of human promyelocytic leukemia HL-60 cells.[18] Similarly, in correlation with the modulation of Ca^{2+}-dependent K^+ channels, 8-methoxypsoralen played an antiproliferative role on two human melanoma cell lines (SK-MEL-28 and C32TG).[19,20] Structurally modified derivatives from psoralen (**5**) remarkably potentiated the antigrowth effect against human HeLa cervical cancer cells. They were 8- to 22-fold more potent than 8-methoxypsoralen in the HeLa cells, but the derivatives were nearly invalid on the HL-60 cells.[21] Additionally, psoralen (**5**) is an activator of QR and an inhibitor of ornithine decarboxylase, exerting the inhibition on TPA-induced tumor promotion in mouse JB6 epidermal cells with an IC_{50} value of 17.1 μg/mL.[22]

Psoralen (**5**) is also a photosensitizing activator. With UV light irradiation (10 min), the photoactivated psoralen remarkably destroyed the K562, HL-60, NB4, and Raji leukemia cells *in vitro* and prolonged the life span of mice bearing L615 leukemia by 189.62% *in vivo*. But it showed low influence on the hemopoietic stem cells in mice bearing L615 leukemia.[23–25] The alteration of the Fas/FasL system was found to be one of the pathways for the increase of NB4 cell apoptosis under the UV radiation.[21] When activated by black light (3.650 Å) or laser light (4.416 Å), the phototoxicity of psoralen conjugated with the formation of DNA adduct, the damage of DNA, and the blockage of DNA synthesis in mouse sarcoma 180 cells, resulting in highly efficient killing of S180 cells.[26] Moreover, the treatment with psoralen (**5**) (40–80 mg/L) plus UVA (360 nm) irritation for 10–15 min prominently induced the apoptosis and the necrosis of three types of human *myeloid* leukemia cell lines (NB4, K562, and HL-60) and then remarkably obstructed the leukemias.[27,28] The proliferation and the colony of K562 cells could be killed by both previously and late photoactivated psoralen.[29] Also, two psoralen heterodimers were synthesized, which exhibited greater phototoxic activity against several cancer cell lines including A375 melanoma cells compared to their intrinsic cytotoxic effect.[30] The findings evidenced that the photosensitivity of psoralens can be promisingly used in clinical photochemotherapy.

Likewise, the proliferation and the metastasis of Mc3 mucoepidermoid carcinoma cells could be suppressed by psoralen (**5**) and 8-methoxypsoralen in association with the prominent activation of wild-type p53.[18] The capability of reversing the MDR of psoralen was proven in DOC-resistant A549 cells (A549/D16), whose MDR reversal was mediated by inhibiting ABCB1 gene and protein expression and decreasing ABCB1 activity and anticancer drug efflux, thereby sensitizing the drug-resistant cells to death in combination with chemotherapeutic drugs.[31]

Psoralidin

Another active constituent in Bu Gu Zhi is psoralidin (**7**), which obstructed the growth of human HT-29 (colon) and MCF-7 (breast) cancer cell lines *in vitro* (IC_{50}: 0.3–0.4 μg/mL), while psoralen (**5**) and isopsoralen (**6**) were weakly active on the two cell lines.[32,33] Psoralidin (**7**) also exerted considerable inhibitory effect against AI prostate cancer cells *in vitro* and *in vivo*,[34] but it had lower cytotoxicity to SNU-1 and SNU-16 gastric carcinoma cells and invalid to A541 (lung) and HepG2 (liver) human cancer cells *in vitro*.[32,33] Through the induction of autophagy but not apoptosis, which was mediated by inducing ROS production, psoralidin (**7**) the proliferation of A549 lung adenocarcinoma cells.[35] Psoralidin (**7**), similar to neobavaisoflavone (**3**), also displayed an ability to sensitize TRAIL-resistant cells and to markedly augment TRAIL-mediated apoptosis and cytotoxicity in human LNCaP prostate cancer cells. In the cotreatment of LNCaP cells with 50 μM of psoralidin (**7**) or 50 μM of neobavaisoflavone (**3**) on a 100 ng/mL TRAIL, the apoptotic percentages were raised to 64.4% or 77.5%, respectively.[36] Psoralidin (**7**) enhanced TRAIL-induced apoptosis in HeLa cervical cancer cells via the up-expression of TRAIL-R2 death receptor and the depolarization of mitochondrial membrane potential.[37] In addition, psoralidin (**7**) as well as an EAF from Bu Gu Zhi methanolic extract were found to have marked ability to activate QR), a protective phase II enzyme on mutagens and carcinogens, in murine Hepa 1c1c7 hepatoma cells.[38] SAR studies have been performed for psoralidin (**7**). The results indicated that a prenyl group is very important for the antitumor activity of psoralidin (**7**), and the location of hydroxyl group influences the activity.[34] Based on the evidences, several more potent and soluble psoralidin derivatives were synthesized for further investigation.[34]

Other Flavonoids

Corylifol-A and bavachinin are antitumor flavonoids isolated from the herb. Corylifol-A (**8**) displayed IC_{50} values of 4.6 and 13.5 μg/mL, respectively, against HepG2 and Hep3B human hepatoma cell lines.[39] *In vivo* studies showed that injecting bavachinin (**9**) thrice weekly for four weeks significantly reduced tumor volume and CD31 expression in nude mice with KB cancer xenografts. Bavachinin (**9**) was also an inhibitor of HIF-1α in human KB carcinoma and human HOS osteosarcoma cell lines. By the inhibition of HIF-1α, bavachinin (**9**) decreased HIF-1α-regulated transcription of genes associated with angiogenesis and energy metabolism, such as VEGF, Glut 1, and Hexokinase 2, exerting antiangiogenic activity. Bavachinin (**9**) obstructed the tube formation in HUVECs as well as the migration of KB cells *in vitro*.[40] These data evidenced that bavachinin (**9**) may be used as a therapeutic agent for inhibiting tumor angiogenesis. Additionally, the leaves of Bu Gu Zhi plant were reported to contain a large amount of anticancer agent assigned as genistein, which was also found in a number of plants such as soybeans, lupin, fava beans, kudzu, and coffee.[41]

Toxicity

Because bakuchiol (**1**) possesses certain toxicity on the kidney, it should be used very carefully in readministration. When associated with UV irradiation, a large dose of psoralen-type substance will cause light fatty degeneration in the liver, the genitalia, and the suprarenal cortex and cause testicle atrophy and weight lost.

Other Bioactivities

The herb Bu Gu Zhi (Babchi) has been extensively reported in traditional Chinese medicine, Indian pharmaceutical codex, pharmacopoeias of the British and the Americans, as well as in different traditional systems of medicine. The herb is valued in China as a tonic remedy to improve general vitality and to treat skin disorders such as vitiligo and psoriasis. Various biological benefits of the seeds (Bu Gu Zhi) were confirmed by the pharmacological investigations, having anthelmintic, astringent, antibacterial, aphrodisiac, cardiac, deobstruent, diaphoretic, stomachic, stimulant, diuretic, and tonic effects. Furthermore, the extract of Bu Gu Zhi (Babchi) demonstrated potent antioxidant effect, whose potencies are in the following order: psoralidin (**7**) > bakuchiol (**1**) > isopsoralen (**6**) > psoralen (**5**).[42]

References

1. Latha, P. G. et al. 1999. Inhibition of chemical carcinogenesis by *Psoralea corylifolia* seeds. *J. Ethnopharmacol.* 68: 295–8.
2. Sun, N. J. et al. 1998. DNA polymerase and topoisomerase II inhibitors from *Psoralea corylifolia. J. Nat. Prods.* 61: 362–6.
3. Latha, P. G. et al. 2000. Immunomodulatory and antitumor properties of *Psoralea corylifolia* seeds. *Fitoterapia* 71: 223–31.
4. Vasumathy, R. et al. 2014. Mechanism of cytotoxicity by *Psoralea corylifolia* extract in human breast carcinoma cells. *J. Environm. Pathol. Toxicol. Oncol.* 33: 265–77.
5. Cai, Y. et al. 2008. Effective component extracted from *Psoralea corylifolia* for reversing tumor multidrug resistance, and its preparation method and use. *Faming Zhuanli Shenqing Gongkai Shuomingshu* CN 101167792 A20080430.
6. Kubo, M. et al. 1989. Cytotoxicity of *Corylifolia fructus*: I. Isolation of the effective compound and the cytotoxicity. *Yaku Gaku Zasshi* 109: 926–31.
7. Cho, H. et al. 2001. Bakuchiol: A hepatoprotective compound of *Psoralea corylifolia* on tacrine-induced cytotoxicity in HepG2 cells. *Planta Med.* 67: 750–1.
8. Ryu, S. Y. et al. 1992. Antitumor activity of *Psoralea corylifolia. Archiv. pharm. Res.* 15: 356–9.
9. Whelan, L. C. et al. 2003. Ethanolic extracts of *Euphorbia* and other ethnobotanical species as inhibitors of human tumor cell growth *Phytomed.* 10: 53–8.
10. Bapat, K. et al. 2005. Preparation and in vitro evaluation of radioiodinated bakuchiol as an antitumor agent. *Applied Radiat. Isotopes* 62: 329–93.
11. Kim, Y. J. et al. 2014. Neobavaisoflavone sensitizes apoptosis via the inhibition of metastasis in TRAIL-resistant human glioma U373MG cells. *Life Sci.* 95: 101–7.
12. Guo, J. N. et al. 2003. Studies on extraction and isolation of active constituents from *Psoralea corylifolia* L. and the antitumor effect of the constituents *in vitro. Zhongyaocai* 26: 185–7.
13. Yang, Y. C. et al. (a) 1983. *Shanxi Xinyixue* 12: 49; (b) 1999. *Chinese Materia Medica.* Vol. 4, 4–3348, 605. Shanghai Science and Technology Press, Shanghai, China.
14. Li, Z. et al. 2007. Antitumor mechanism and application prospect of psoralen. *J. Mountain Agricul. Biol.* 26: 255–60.
15. Isoldi, M. C. et al. 2004. The role of calcium, calcium-activated K^+ channels, and tyrosine/kinase in psoralen-evoked responses in human melanoma cells. *Braz. J. Med. Biol. Res.* 37: 559–68.
16. Jiang, Z. Y. et al. 2014. Induction of apoptosis in human hepatocarcinoma SMMC-7721 cells in vitro by psoralen from *Psoralea corylifolia. Cell Biochem. Biophys.* 70: 1075–81.
17. Wu, C. Y. et al. 2013. Psoralen inhibits bone metastasis of breast cancer in mice. *Fitoterapia* 91: 205–10.
18. Wu, J. Z. et al. 2000. Effects of psoralen and 8 methoxypsoralen on the proliferation and metastatic potential of mucoepidermoid carcinoma Mc3 cells. *Disi Junyi Daxue Xuebao* 21: 911–4.
19. Wu, S. H. et al. 1998. In vitro and in vivo anticancer activity of psoralen. *Zhongguo Zhongyao Zazhi* 23: 303–5.
20. Cai, Y. et al. 2006. Apoptosis of HL-60 cell line induced by psoralen and its effect on intracellular Ca^{2+} concentration. *Zhongguo Zhongliu Linchuang* 33: 64–6.
21. Via, D. L. et al. 2004. Methyl derivatives of tetracyclic psoralen analogues: Anti-proliferative activity and interaction with DNA. *ARKIVOC* (5): 131–46.
22. Lee, S. J. et al. 2011. Effects of psoralen from *Psoralea corylifolia* on quinone reductase, ornithine decarboxylase, and JB6 cells transformation promotion. *Archiv. Pharm. Res.* 34: 31–6.
23. Lu, Z. H. et al. 1993. Inhibitory effects of psoralen plus ultraviolet irradiation on human leukemia cell lines. *Zhongguo Yaoli Xuebao* 14(suppl.): S028–S030.
24. Lu, Z. H. et al. 1991. The killing effects of psoralen plus ultraviolet irritation on mouse L615 leukemia cells. *Xueyexue Zazhi* 12: 637–9.
25. Xiang, Y. et al. 2010. Effect of combined application of psoralen and ultraviolet A for inducing NB4 cell apoptosis and its impact on Fas/FasL gene expressions. *Zhongguo Zongxiyi Jiehe Zazhi* 30: 45–7.
26. Cui, X. Q. et al. 1994. The killing effects of psoralen plus long wave UV irritation on leukemia cells. *Linchuang Xueyexue Zazhi* 7: 166–7.
27. Xiang, Y. et al. 2006. Effect of psoralen plus ultraviolet A on NB4 and K562 leukemia cell lines. *Disi Jundaxue Xuebao* 27: 609–11.
28. Zhang, C. et al. 2011. Effects of psoralen plus ultraviolet A on primary human myeloid leukemia cells. *Linchuang Junyi Zazhi* 39: 1–2.
29. Huang, Y. Z. et al. 2004. Inhibitive effect of previously activated psoralens on K562 cell proliferation. *J. Experim. Hematol.* 12: 568–71.
30. Ropp, S. et al. 2004. Synthesis and photocytotoxic activity of new α-methylene-γ-butyrolactonepsoralen heterodimers. *Bioorg. Med. Chem.* 12: 3619–25.

31. Hsieh, M. J. et al. 2014. Psoralen reverses docetaxel-induced multidrug resistance in A549/D16 human lung cancer cells lines. *Phytomed.* 21: 970–7.
32. Yang, Y. M. et al. 1996. The cytotoxicity of psoralidin from *Psoralea corylifolia. Planta Med.* 62: 353–4.
33. Mar, M. C. et al. 2001. Cytotoxic constituents of *Psoralea corylifolia. Archiv. Pharm. Res.* 24: 211–3.
34. Pahari, P. et al. 2010. Synthesis and structure-activity relationship (SAR) study of psoralidin derivatives, an anticancer natural product. *Abstracts of Papers, 239th ACS Natl* Meet., San Francisco, March 21–5, 2010. ORGN-291.
35. Hao, W. H. et al. 2014. Psoralidin induces autophagy through ROS generation which inhibits the proliferation of human lung cancer A549 cells. *Peer J.* e555/1–e555/13.
36. Szliszka, E. et al. 2011. Enhanced TRAIL-mediated apoptosis in prostate cancer cells by the bioactive compounds neobavaisoflavone and psoralidin isolated from *Psoralea corylifolia. Pharmcol. Rep.* 63: 139–48.
37. Bronikowska, J. et al. 2012. The coumarin psoralidin enhances anticancer effect of tumor necrosis factor-related apoptosis-inducing ligand (TRAIL). *Mol.* 17: 6449–64.
38. Lee, S. J. et al. 2009. Induction of quinone reductase activity by psoralidin isolated from *Psoralea corylifolia* in mouse hepa 1c1c7 cells. *Archiv. Pharm. Res.* 32: 1061–5.
39. Song, P. et al. 2013. Cytotoxic constituents from *Psoralea corylifolia. J. Asian Nat. Prod. Res.* 15: 624–30.
40. Nepal, M. et al. 2012. Anti-angiogenic and antitumor activity of bavachinin by targeting hypoxia-inducible factor-1α. *Europ. J. Pharmacol.* 691: 28–37.
41. Kaufman, P. B. et al. 1997. A comparative survey of leguminous plants as sources of the isoflavones, genistein and daidzein: Implications for human nutrition and health. *J. Altern. Complem. Med.* 7: 7–12.
42. Guo, J. et al. 2005. Antioxidants from Chinese medicinal herb-*Psoralea corylifolia* L. *Food Chem* 91: 287–92.

184 Xue Lian Hua 雪蓮花

Snow lotus

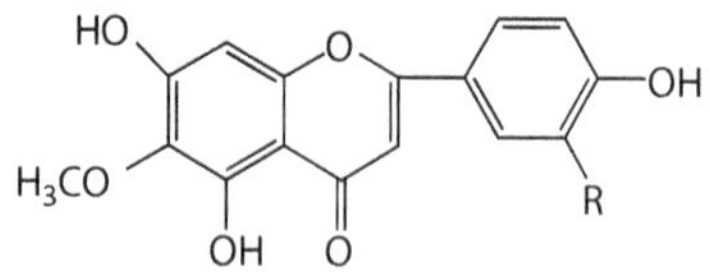

1. R = $-CH_3$
2. R = -H

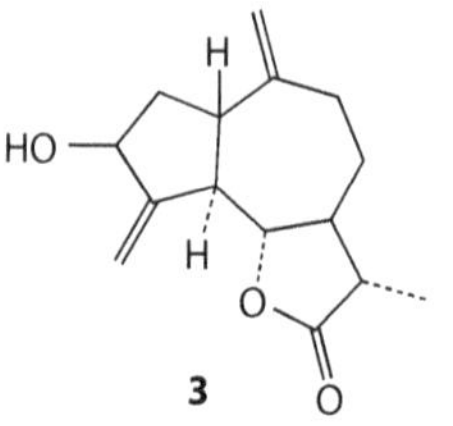

3

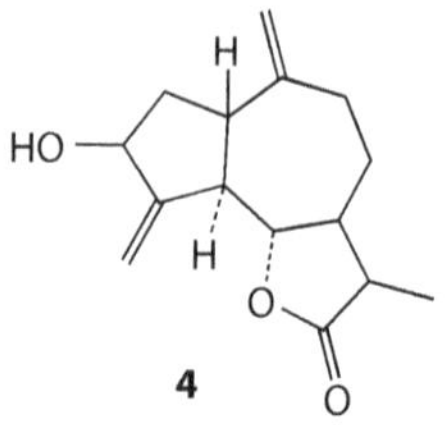

4

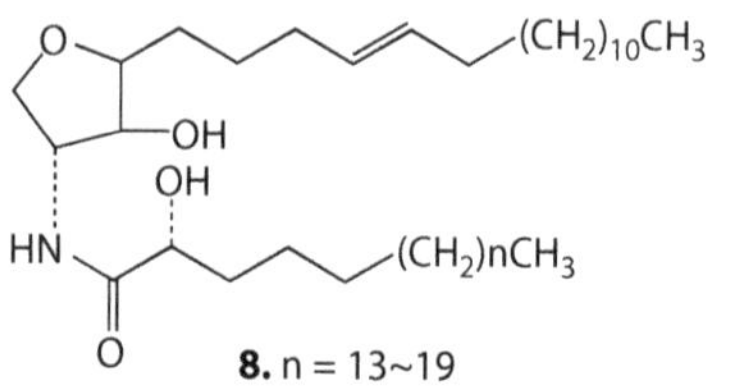

8. n = 13~19

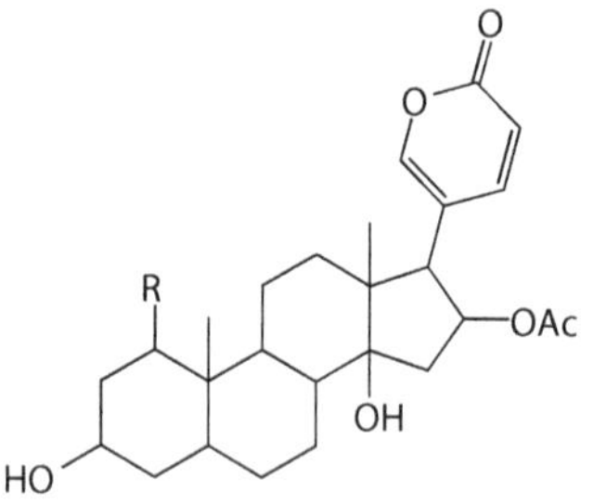

5. R = -H
5d. R = -OH

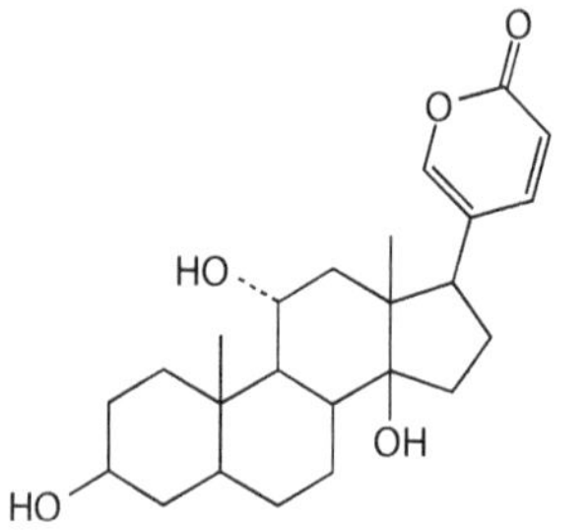

6

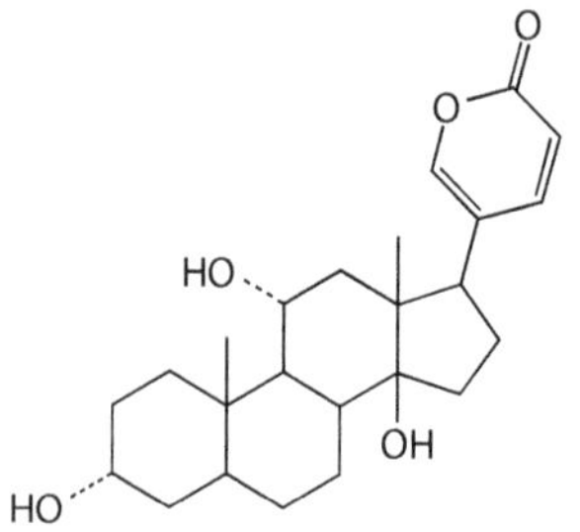

6a

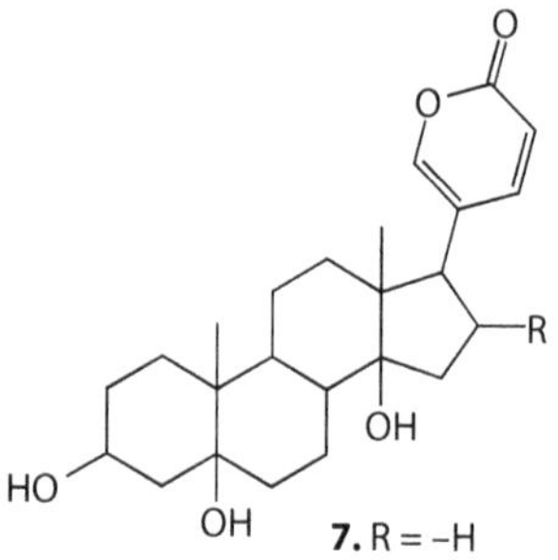

7. R = -H
5e. R = -OAc

Herb Origination

The herb Xue Lian Hua (Snow lotus) is the dried whole plant or the aerial parts with flowers of *Saussurea involucrate* (Compositae). The perennial herbaceous plant is distributed in the Chinese provinces of Xinjiang, Qinghai, Gansu, and Tibet, growing above the snow line in the mountains. June and July are the best time to collect the Snow lotus when they are in full blossom, and then the herb is dried in shade for medicinal utilization.

Antitumor Constituents and Activities

The EtOAc extract (SI-2) of the Snow lotus exhibited the most bioactive extract compared to others. The treatment with SI-2 resulted in significant and time-dependent growth inhibition and elicitation of G1 phase cell cycle arrest and apoptosis in human PC3 hormone-resistant prostate cancer cells *in vitro* and *in vivo*. The mechanism was found to associate with (1) inhibiting EGFR phosphorylation and reducing AKT and STAT3 activation, (2) strongly up-expressing p21WAF1/CIP and p27KIP1 (p53-independent pathway) and down-expressing cyclin-D1 and CDK4, and (3) activating Bax and caspase-3.[1] Its EtOh extract (SIE) showed cytotoxic and apoptotic effects on human HepG2 hepatoma cells, whose mechanism might be associated with the inhibition of DNA synthesis and the induction of G1 cell cycle G1 arrest and the apoptosis via the up-expression of caspase-3, caspase-9, and p21, the degradation of PARP, and the down-expression of CDK2 and XIAP.[2,3] The incubation of SK-Hep1 human hepatoma cells with SIE significantly inhibited cell adhesion to the gelatin-coated substrate and cell migration/invasion via the inhibition of MMP-2/-9 and MT1-MMP mRNA levels and the stimulation of TIMP-1.[4] These results proved that the extract of the Snow lotus is a potential agent for cancer treatment and prevention. Six types of components (such as alkaloids, sesquiterpene lactones, bufadienolides, flavones, and ceramides) isolated from the Snow lotus were reported to be responsible for the anticarcinoma property.

Alkaloids and Flavonoids

The total alkaloid in Xue Lian Hua presented the inhibition of DNA, RNA, and protein synthesis in mouse leukemia 7712 cells in vitro through the damage of the DNA template.[5] Also, the flavones, jaceosidin (**1**) and hispidulin (**2**) derived from Xue Lian Hua, blocked DNA synthesis in mouse sarcoma 180 cells and ascites hepatoma cells *in vitro* (IC_{50}: 70.8–116 μg/mL).[6] Moreover, the flavones could also stimulate the cytotoxicity of human PBMCs against the myelocytic leukemia K562 cells and Raji Burkitt lymphoma cells *in vitro*, showing obvious immunoregulating antitumor property, whose maximum response appeared at a 0.6 μg/mL concentration.[7]

Sesquiterpene Lactones

Two sesquiterpene lactones assigned as sausinlactone-A (**3**) and sausinlactone-B (**4**) demonstrated marked cytotoxicities against human A549 lung adenocarcinoma cells *in vitro* with IC_{50} values of 0.01 and 2.89 μg/mL, respectively.[8]

Bufadienolides

Three bufadienolides assigned as bufotalin (**5**), gamabufotalin (**6**), and telocinobufagin (**7**) exerted significant growth inhibitory effect against human HepG2 (liver) and MCF-7 (breast) cancer cell lines *in vitro*. The IC_{50} values were 0.05–0.07 μM for bufotalin (**5**), 0.05–0.06 μM for gamabufotalin (**6**), and 0.11–0.16 μM for telocinobufagin (**7**). The biotransformation of the three bufadienolides by cell suspension cultures yielded 11 products, viz., 3-epi-bufotalin (**5a**), 3-epi-desacetylbufotalin (**5b**), 3-epi-bufotalin 3-*O*-β-D-glucoside (**5c**), 1β-hydroxybufotalin (**5d**), and 5β-hydroxybufotalin (**5e**), yielded from bufotalin (**5**); 3-epi-gamabufotalin (**6a**), 3-dehydro-gamabufotalin (**6b**), and 3-dehydro-Δ1-gamabufotalin (**6c**), yielded from gamabufotalin (**6**); and 3-dehydroscillarenin (**7a**), 3-dehydrobufalin (**7b**), and 3-epi-telocinobufagin (**7c**), yielded from telocinobufagin (**7**). The bufadienolides **5a**, **5d**, **5e**, **5c**, **6a**, **7a**, and **7c** were effective in the inhibition on the HepG2 cells (IC_{50}: 0.09–0.41 μM), and **5a**, **5d**, **5e**, **6a**, and **7a** were also active in the MCF-7 cells (IC_{50}: 0.13–0.45 μM).[9] The most effective bufotalin analogs were 1β-hydroxybufotalin (**5d**) and 3-epi-gamabufotalin (**6a**) in the HepG2 cells (IC_{50}: 0.09 μM) and 3-epi-bufotalin 3-*O*-β-D-glucoside (**5c**), 5β-hydroxybufotalin (**5e**), and 3-epi-gamabufotalin (**6a**) in the MCF-7 cells (IC_{50}: 0.13–0.16 μM).[9] Additionally, an isolated mixture of ceramides (**8**) accomplished appreciable cytotoxic effect against three human cancer cell lines including HL-60 promyelocytic leukemia, A375-S2 melanoma, and HeLa cervical cancer.[10]

Other Bioactivities

The herb Xue Lian Hua (Snow lotus) has been used in traditional Chinese medicine to relieve colds and cough, to regulate the menstrual function, to stop bleeding, and even to treat rheumatoid arthritis. The major constituents in the herb possess the important biological activities, such as antiinflammatory, analgesic, antifatigue, antirheumatic, antifree radical, antiradiation, spasmolytic, and cardiovascular system-regulating effects.

References

1. Way, T. et al. 2010. Inhibition of epidermal growth factor receptor signaling by *Saussurea involucrata*, a rare traditional Chinese medicinal herb, in human hormone-resistant prostate cancer PC3 cells. *J. Agricul. Food Chem.* 58: 3356–65.
2. Byambaragchee, M. et al. 2014. Anticancer potential of an ethanol extract of *Saussurea involucrata* against hepatic cancer cells in vitro. *Asian Pac. J. Cancer Prev.* 15: 7527–32.
3. Byambaragchaa, M. et al. 2012. *Saussurea involucrata* extract induces cell cycle arrest and apoptosis in HepG2 human hepatocarcinoma cells. *The FASEB J.* 26: 1037.6.
4. Byambaragchee, M. et al. 2013. Anti-metastatic potential of ethanol extract of *Saussurea involucrata* against hepatic cancer in vitro. *Asian Pac. J. Cancer Prev.* 14: 5397–402.
5. Xiao, X. H. et al. 1986. Effect of the total alkaloid from *Saussurea involucrata* on metabolism of DNA, RNA, and protein in leukemia 7712 cells. *J. Lanzhou Univ.* (*Sci. Edit.*), 22: 102–5.
6. Liu, L. S. et al. 1985. Effect of flavones from *Saussurea involucrata* on DNA synthesis by cancer cells. *J. Lanzhou Univ.* (*Sci. Edit.*), 21: 80–3.
7. Ma, H. J. et al. 1998. Effect of *Saussurea involucrata* flavone on human peripheral blood mononuclear cells. *J. Xi'an Med. Univ.* 19: 168–9.
8. Xiao, W. et al. 2011. Sesquiterpene lactones from *Saussurea involucrata*. *Fitoterapia* 82: 983–7.
9. Zhang, X. et al. 2011. Biotransformation of bufadienolides by cell suspension cultures of *Saussurea involucrate*. *Phytochem.* 72: 1779–85.
10. Wu, W. et al. 2009. Novel ceramides from aerial parts of *Saussurea involucrata* Kar. et. Kir. *Archiv. Pharm. Res.* 32: 1221–5.

185 Hu Lu Ba 葫蘆巴

Fenugreek seed

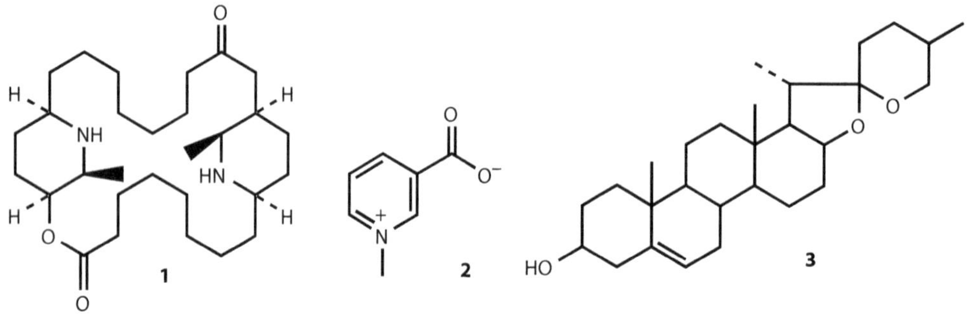

Herb Origination

The herb Hu Lu Ba (Fenugreek seed) is the dried seeds of a Leguminosae plant, *Trigonella foenum-graecum* L. This annual herbal is one of the oldest medicinal plants dating back to the ancient Egyptians, Greeks, and Romans. It has been naturalized worldwide as a semiarid crop. The seeds were used as an herb in traditional Chinese medicine since the late era of the Tang Dynasty. Today, the plant distribution is broad in China, and the herb is mainly produced in the provinces of Anhui, Sichuan, and Shaanxi.

Antitumor Activities

In vitro assays showed that the water extract of the Fenugreek seeds has a selective cytotoxicity against cancer cell lines such as T cell lymphoma, B cell lymphomas, thyroid papillary carcinoma, and MCF-7 breast cancer but is inactive on normal human lymphocytes and meningioma cells. The T cell lymphoma and breast cancer cell lines were highly apoptotic following the treatment.[1] The treatment with the methanolic extract from the Fenugreek seeds for 48 h showed a cytotoxic effect against HepG2 hepatoma cells and an apoptosis induction via the activation of p53, Bax, and PCNA in a caspase-3-dependent manner.[2] Similarly, its EtOh extract (10–15 μg/mL) was used to treat the cancer cell lines for 72 h, resulting in the inhibitory effects on breast (MCF-7, T47D, SKBR3, and MDA-MB-231), pancreatic (Pancl, MiaPaCa, HS766T, L3.6PL, and BXPC3), and prostate cancer (DU-145, LNCaP, and PC3) cell lines. The order of anticancer potencies was pancreatic cancer > prostate cancer ≫ breast cancer. The antiproliferative effect in the prostate cancer cell lines was mediated by the induction of cell cycle arrest and apoptotic death in association with the upregulation of p21 and the inhibition of TGFβ-induced phosphorylation of Akt in PC3 cells and the downregulation of mutant p53 in DU-145 cells.[3]

The i.p. administrations of the alcoholic extract to mice before or after the inoculation of tumor cells demonstrated >70% inhibition against the growth of EAC cells, whose effect was partially attributed to the extract-enhanced counts of peritoneal exudate cells and macrophage cells.[4] The inclusion of Fenugreek in the diet (2 g/kg, per day) not only significantly diminished the activities of β-glucuronidase and mucinase in various tissues but also notably attenuated the possibility of LPO with the simultaneous enhancement of circulating antioxidants, displaying the chemopreventive effect against the colon carcinogenesis.[5,6] In addition, the aqueous extract of Hu Lu Ba exerted beneficial impacts to reduce Adm-induced hepatotoxicity and to ameliorate the cytotoxicity of Adm in albino rats, whose effects were ascribable to its remarkable antioxidant responses.[7,8]

Antitumor Constituents and Activities

The GC-MS analysis of the methanolic extract showed the presence of 14 bioactive compounds including the main components, squalene (27.71%), naringenin (24.05%), tricin (6.98%), and kaempferol (6.77%). Squalene and naringenin were reported to have anticancer activity in primary tumor prevention.[2] The incubation of Jurkat human T lymphoma cells with the 50% EtOh extract of Fenugreek at concentrations of 30–1500 μg/mL for three days resulted in cell death in dose- and time-dependent manners, whose cell death was preceded by the appearance of multiple large vacuoles, membrane disintegration, and transcriptional upregulation of LC3, implying that the extract induced autophagy and autophagy-associated death of Jurkat cells.[9] The GC-MS analysis showed the 50% EtOh extract containing gingerol (4.82%), cedrene (2.91%), zingerone (16.5%), vanillin (1.52%), and eugenol (1.25%).[9] However, the alkaloid and steroidal components in Hu Lu Ba have been paid more attention for the anticancer effects.

Alkaloids

Hu Lu Ba contains two antineoplastic alkaloids assigned as carpaine (**1**) and trigonelline (**2**). Carpaine (**1**) exhibited the inhibitory effect against the proliferation of murine L1210 and P388 leukemia cells, where carpaine (**1**) was more sensitive to L1210 cells than to P388 cells. A 12.5 mg/kg dose of trigonelline (**2**) could prolong the life span of mice bearing P388 leukemia by 31%.[10]

Steroids

The isolated main steroidal components showed antitumor activity. *In vitro* experiments confirmed that diosgenin (**3**) (a steroidal compound from Hu Lu Ba) dose-dependently inhibited the cell growth and induced the apoptotic death of HT-29 (colon),

A431, and Hep2 (squamous) human cancer cell lines.[11–13] The mechanism in the A431 and Hep2 cells was correlated with (1) increasing sub-G1 population, LIVE/DEAD cytotoxicity, chromatin condensation, DNA laddering and TUNEL-positive cells, and Bax/Bcl-2 ratio; activating caspases and cleavage of PARP; and inhibiting Akt and JNK phosphorylations.[14] During the treatment, diosgenin (**3**) suppressed pAkt expression and Akt kinase activity and inhibited its downstream targets (NF-κB, Bcl-2, survivin, and XIAP) and repressed a Raf/MEK/ERK pathway in estrongen receptor$^+$ breast cancer cells, and induced G1 cell cycle arrest by down-expressing cyclin D1, CDK2 and CDK4 in both estrongen receptor$^+$ and estrongen receptor$^-$ breast cancer cells resulting in the inhibition of cell proliferation and induction of apoptosis.[14] The diosgenin treatment inhibited the telomerase activity by downregulating hTERT gene expression in the A549 lung cancer cell line.[15] An *in vivo* study proved that diosgenin (**3**) markedly inhibited the tumor growth in both MCF-7 and MDA-231 breast cancer xenografts in nude mice.[14,15] The migration and the invasion of PC3 prostate cancer cells were also obstructed by reducing MMP-2, MMP-9, and MMP-7 expressions and inhibiting ERK, JNK, and PI3K/Akt signaling pathways as well as NF-κB activity, showing the potential for diosgenin in antimetastatic therapy.[16] In addition, dietary 1% Hu Lu Ba powder or 0.05% or 0.1% diosgenin significantly inhibited the formation of mutagen azoxymethane-induced total colonic aberrant crypt foci and multicrypt foci in a dose-dependent manner.[12] Therefore, the diosgenin (**3**) showing obvious cytotoxicity to cancer cells points to the potential usefulness of Fenugreek in the prevention and the treatment of cancer.

Steroidal Saponins

Protodioscin, a steroidal saponin separated from Hu Lu Ba, displayed strong growth inhibitory effect against human HL-60 leukemia cells and increased the cell apoptotic death in time- and dose-dependent fashions. The apoptosis (hypodiploid phase) of HL-60 cells could be promoted by 75.2–100% after a three-day treatment with protodioscin (2.5–10 μM). But protodioscin exhibited only weak effect against KATO-III gastric cancer cells with no impact on the cell apoptosis.[11] The isolated dioscin was cytotoxic to five different human cancer cell line cells such as HCT116, HT-29, and Caco-2 (colon), A549 (lung), and HepG2 (liver) cancer cells *in vitro*, whose IC_{50} values ranged from 0.72 to 3.22 μM and from 2.88 to 8.53 μM in 2% and 10% fetal bovine serum (FBS) (vol./vol.) containing media, respectively. After the treatment with dioscin above 7.5 μM, the HT-29 cells were killed immediately.[17]

Polysaccharides

From the Fenugreek seeds, a polysaccharide termed PS2, was isolated and partially purified. The treatment with PS2 directly retarded the cell proliferation of human HCT-16 colon cancer cells and elicited a higher percentage of cell death *in vitro*. An *in vivo* experiment showed the inhibitory activity of PS2 against chemically induced colorectal cancer in rats with a marked reduction in the levels of MDA and LDH, as well as ALP and ALT.[13] Thus, the findings indicated that PS2 has a promising antitumorigenic property.

Other Bioactivities

The herb Hu Lu Ba (Fenugreek) is used as both herbs (the seeds and the leaves) and a spice (e.g., the seed is frequently used in curry). As a natural medicine, Fenugreek displays multiple biological activities such as antifertilic, hypotensive, antimale hormone, and vasodilative in the small intestine, the kidney, and the coronary besides the anticarcinogenesis. The Fenugreek seed is widely used by nursing mothers to increase inadequate breast milk supply, whose effect has been proven by modern studies. The seed can potently stimulate breast milk production as much as 900%, so that its capsule form is commercially available in many health food stores in some areas. Its encapsulated forms are being prescribed as dietary supplements for the control of hypercholesterolemia and diabetes due to its marked ameliorative effect on most metabolic symptoms associated with type I and type II diabetes in humans by improving glucose tolerance and reducing serum glucose. Also, Fenugreek and diosgenin (**3**) inhibited LXRα activity in HepG2 cells and decreased plasma and hepatic triglycerides in obese diabetic mice, indicating that the herb may be useful for the management of diabetes-related hepatic dyslipidemias.[18]

References

1. Abdulaziz, A. et al. 2014. The selective cytotoxic anticancer properties and proteomic analysis of *Trigonella foenum-graecum*. *BMC Complem. Altern. Med.* 14: 114.
2. Mahmoud, I. M. K. et al. 2015. *Trigonella foenum* (Fenugreek) induced apoptosis in hepatocellular carcinoma cell line, HepG2, mediated by upregulation of p53 and proliferating cell nuclear antigen. *BioMed Res. Intl.* Article ID 914645.
3. Shabbeer, S. et al. 2009. Fenugreek: A naturally occurring edible spice as an anticancer agent. *Cancer Biol. Ther.* 8: 272–8.
4. Sur, P. et al. 2001. *Trigonella foenum graecum* (fenugreek) seed extract as an antineoplastic agent. *Phytother. Res.* 15: 257–9.
5. Devasena, T. et al. 2002. Enhancement of circulatory antioxidants by fenugreek during 1,2-dimethylhydrazine-induced rat colon carcinogenesis. *J. Biochem. Mol. Biol. Biophysics* 69: 289–92.
6. Devasena, T. et al. 2003. Fenugreek affects the activity of β-glucuronidase and mucinase in the colon carcinogenesis. *Phytother. Res.* 179: 1088–91.
7. Sakr, S. A. et al. 2011. Effect of fenugreek seed extract on adriamycin-induced hepatotoxicity and oxidative stress in albino rats. *Toxicol. Industrial Health* 28: 876–85.
8. Sakr, S. A. et al. 2012. Aqueous fenugreek seed extract ameliorates adriamycin-induced cytotoxicity and testicular alterations in albino rats. *Reproduct. Sci.* 19: 70–80.
9. Al-Daghri, N. M. et al. 2012. Fenugreek extract as an inducer of cellular death via autophagy in human T lymphoma Jurkat cells. *BMC Complement. Altern. Med.* 12: 202.
10. Jing, Y. et al. 2003. Progress in studies on chemical constituents and pharmacological effect of *Trigonella foenum-graecum*. *Zhongcaoyao* 34: 1146–9.
11. Raju, J. et al. 2004. Diosgenin, a steroid saponin of *Trigonella foenum-graecum* (Fenugreek), Inhibits azoxymethane-induced aberrant crypt foci formation in F344 rats and induces apoptosis in HT-29 human colon cancer cells. *Cancer Epidemiol. Biomakers Preven.* 13: 1392–8.

12. Hibasami, H. et al. 2003. Protodioscin isolated from Fenugreek (*Trigonella foenum-graecum* L.) induces cell death and morphological change indicative of apoptosis in leukemic cell line HL-60, but not in gastric cancer cell line KATO III. *Intl. J. Mol. Med.* 11: 23–6.
13. Jwanny, E. E. et al. 2009. Effect of two polysaccharides on chemically-induced colorectal cancer in rats. *Adv. Food Sci.* 31: 202–9.
14. Srinivasan, S. et al. 2009. Diosgenin targets Akt-mediated prosurvival signaling in human breast cancer cells. *Intl. J. Cancer* 125: 961–7.
15. Rahmati-Yamchi, M. et al. 2014. Fenugreek extract diosgenin and pure diosgenin inhibit the hTERT gene expression in A549 lung cancer cell line. *Mol. Biol. Reports* 41: 6247–52.
16. Chen, P. S. et al. 2011. Diosgenin, a steroidal saponin, inhibits migration and invasion of human prostate cancer PC3 cells by reducing matrix metallo-proteinases expression. *PLoS One* 6: e20164.
17. Yum, C. H. et al. 2010. Cytotoxicity of dioscin and biotransformed fenugreek. *J. Korean Soc. for Applied Biol. Chem.* 53: 470–7.
18. Uemura, T. et al. 2010. Diosgenin, the main aglycon of fenugreek, inhibits LXRα activity in HepG2 cells and decreases plasma and hepatic triglycerides in obese diabetic mice. *J. Nutr.* 141: 17–23.

10

Anticancer Potentials of Purgative and Diuretic Herbs

CONTENTS

186 Lu Hui 蘆薈

Aloe

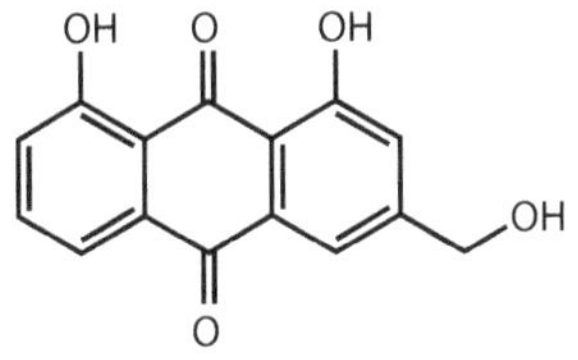

Herb Origination

The herb Lu Hui (Aloe) is the fresh and dried leaf juices of three Liliaceae plants, *Aloe vera*, *A. ferox*, and *A. vera* var. *chinensis*. The first two Aloes are imported from the islands in South America and South Africa, respectively, and the third one called Chinese Aloe is cultivated in the southern region of China.

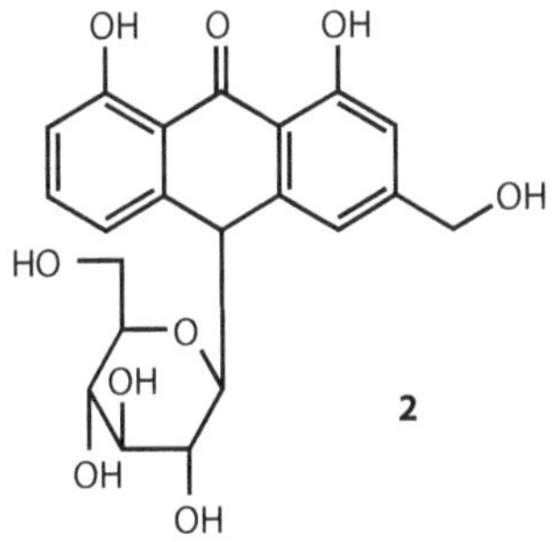

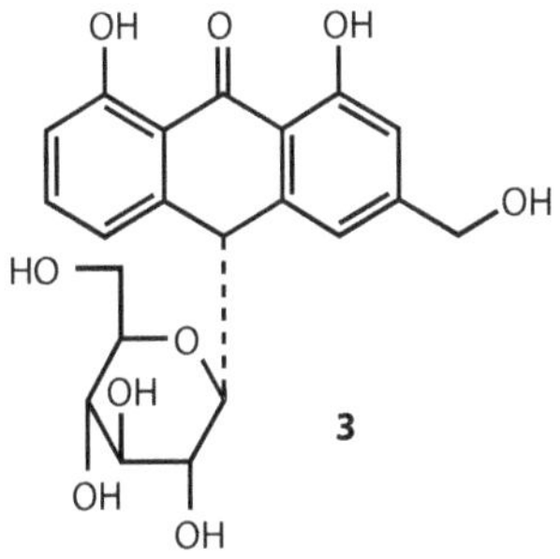

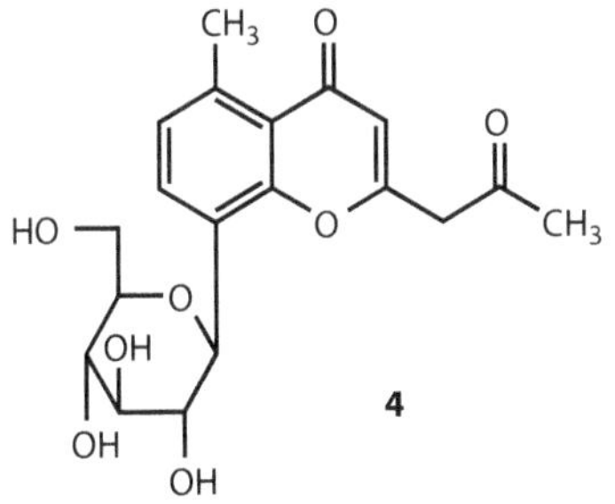

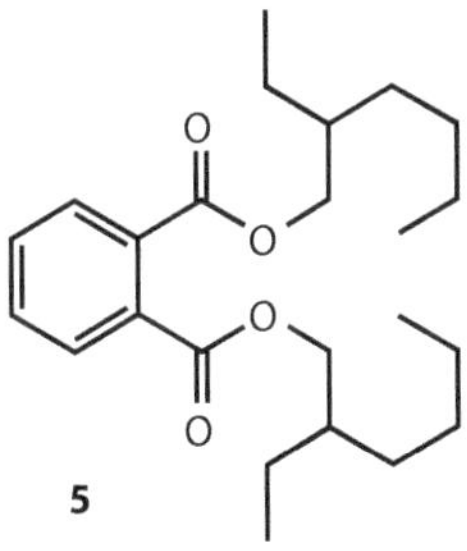

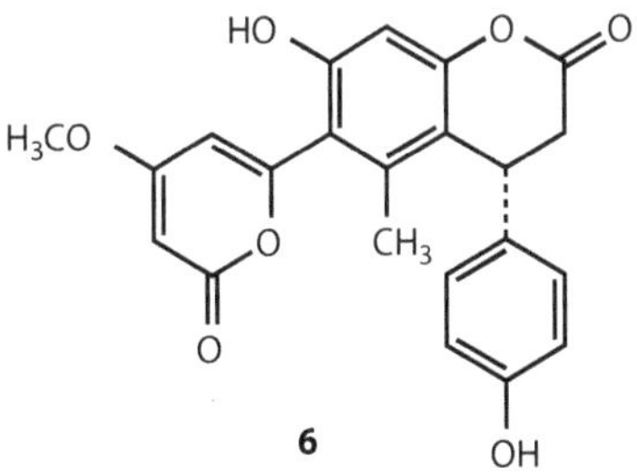

Antitumor Activity

Lu Hui (Aloe) presented attractive anti-neoplastic, radical-scavenging, and immunoenhancing characters *in vitro* and *in vivo*. A methanolic extract in concentrations of 0.25–5.0 mg/mL showed dose-dependent cytotoxicity against murine P388 and L1210 leukemia cell lines and human HCT-15 (colon) and SK-HepG-1 (liver) cell lines.[1] The extract exerted <33% growth inhibition against three types of human tumor cell lines, such as A549 (lung), LnCaP (prostate), and MG63 (osteosarcoma), at a 100 μg/mL concentration, and enhanced radical-scavenging effect by 47% at a concentration of 500 μg/mL.[2] *In vivo* experiments proved the antitumor property in rats bearing Yoshida AH-130 ascites hepatoma and in mice bearing sarcoma 180, Ehrlich ascites tumor, HepA ascites hepatoma, HepS hepatoma, or B16 melanoma.[3–5] Moreover, the extract promoted the proliferation of splenocytes and leucocytes and enhanced the lymphoid hyperplasia in the thymus and the spleen, indicating that the tumor preventive and the therapeutic effect of Aloe was partially attributed to its immunoenhancing function.[1,6] However, the extract showed the inhibition on C3H10T1/2 embryonic cells at the initiation stage of the transformation as well.[7]

In the tests, the synergistic effect of Aloe was also impressively observed. The daily gavage of the extract with a 670 μL/kg dose combined with a honey solution to rats implanted with Walker 256 sarcoma suppressed the tumor growth by reducing the proliferation and increasing the apoptosis susceptibility.[8] When the Aloe extract was combined with anticancer drugs (5-FU, mitomycin-C, or cisplatin), the cytotoxicity of the drugs was augmented on the P388, L1210, HCT-15, and SK-HepG-1 cancer cell lines and the toxicity of these drugs on the normal mouse splenocytes was reduced.[1] Importantly, preliminary clinical studies were performed on 50 patients suffering from advanced solid carcinomas (lung cancer, gastrointestinal tract tumors, brain glioblastoma, or breast cancer), whose results demonstrated that a therapy with pineal immunomodulating hormone melatonin (20 mg/day) plus the Aloe extract at least stabilized the disease and prolonged the survival.[9]

The antitumor-promoting activity of the Aloe extract was demonstrated in the suppression of two-stage skin carcinogenesis induced by DMBA and promoted by croton oil. The oral administration of the extract at a dose of 1000 mg/kg per day or the Aloe gel treatment at a dose of 1 mL/cm^2/mouse per day for 16 weeks in mice were found to be effective in lessening the number and the size of the papillomas, significantly reducing the LPO levels in the skin of the mice and declining the incidence of melanomagenesis.[10,11] Moreover, the treatment with two doses (30 or 60 μL/mice daily for 14 days) of the Aloe extract diminished the formation of MDA and the activity of lactate dehydrogenase in the liver, implying that it plays a role in the protection against prooxidant-induced membrane and cellular damages.

Taken together, the experiments provided solid evidences for Aloe possessing antitumor, antitumor-promoting, immunoregulating, and antioxidant functions, which are propitious to the prevention of carcinogenesis. Furthermore, the Aloe extract also markedly augmented the activities of GST, DT-Diaphorase (DTD), SOD, and catalase (CAT) in extrahepatic organs and obviously reduced the levels of cytochrome P450 and cytochrome b5. Thus, the Aloe extract acted as an inducer of phase II enzyme system to maintain the health of the organs (lung, kidney and fore-stomach) by detoxification of the reactive metabolites (including chemical carcinogens and drugs).[12]

Antitumor Constituents and Activity

Bioorganic chemists never missed searching for cancer inhibitors from the Aloe extract. In the continuous efforts, two major constituents, anthraquinones derivatives and polysaccharides, were found to be responsible for the bioactivities of Aloe.

Anthraquinones Derivatives

The anthracene derivatives from Aloe were effective in killing tumor cell lines (GM803, Y99, L929, and Meth-A) *in vitro*. Even at a concentration of 0.3 μg/mL, the cytotoxic rates on L929 and Y99 cell lines were >50%.[13] Bioactive anthracene derivatives such as Aloe emodin, chrysophanol, physcion, and aloin (barbaloin) were obtained from the systemic separation of the Aloe leaves. Especially, Aloe emodin and aloin acted as cancer inhibitors in the assays.

Aloe Emodin

Tumor Suppression via the Induction of Apoptosis and Cell Cycle Arrest As a typical anthraquinone in the Aloe, Aloe emodin (**1**) exhibited remarkable anticarcinoma effects on many tumor cells. Both brain glia cells (SVG) and glioma cells (U-373MG) were highly sensitive to Aloe emodin (**1**) concomitant with the inhibition of protein kinase C (PKC) activity and the reduction of the protein content of PKC isoenzymes. A 40 μM concentration of Aloe emodin could delay the number of cells entering and exiting DNA synthesis (S phase) in the SVG cells and the U-373MG cells, leading Aloe emodin (**1**) to arrest the cell cycle S phase progression and to minimize the brain tumor proliferation.[14] Aloe emodin (**1**) also displayed time- and dose-dependent proliferative suppressions in human SCC-4 tongue squamous carcinoma and U87 malignant glioma cell lines, via the induction of mitochondria-related apoptosis and cell cycle arrest at S phase.[15,16] The cell cycle arrest in the SCC-4 cells was correlated with the activation of p53, p21, and p27 and the decline of cyclin-A, cyclin-E, thymidylate synthase, and CDC25A, whereas the apoptosis of SCC-4 cells was triggered by augmenting the release of AIF, endonuclease-G, procaspase-9, and cytochrome c from the mitochondria via a loss of mitochondrial membrane potential and the increases of Bax/Bcl-2 ratio and caspase-9 and caspase-3 activation.[16]

Through a similar pathway, Aloe emodin (**1**) promoted the apoptotic death and restrained the proliferation of three human colon cancer cell lines (DLD-1, WiDr, and HT2) and two distinct human gastric carcinoma cell lines (AGS and NCI-N87) *in vitro* in dose- and time-dependent manners.[17–19] Notably, the WiDr cells were more sensitive to Aloe emodin (**1**) than the DLD-1 cells, while the AGS cells were more sensitive than the NCI-N87 cells. During the exposure in the cancer cells of the colon and the stomach, Aloe emodin (**1**) also retarded the casein kinase II activity and lessened the phosphorylation of Bid and the downstream substrate of casein kinase II.[17,18] In association with the decrease of the expressions of PKC and c-Myc and the blockage of cell cycle progression, Aloe emodin (**1**) exert a long-term antiproliferation effect and antimigration effect on human MGC-803 and SGC-7901 gastric cancer cells.[20] Similarly, the proliferation of human T24 bladder cancer and human nasopharyngeal cancer (NPC) cell lines could be markedly restrained by Aloe emodin (**1**) with promoted G2/M cell arrest and cell apoptosis.[21,22] The mechanisms in the T24 cells was correlated with increasing the levels of Weel and CDC25c, reducing the levels of CDK-1 and cyclin-B1, repressing Bcl-2 expression, and activating the expressions of p53, p21, Bax, caspase-3, and Fas/APO-1 receptor,[21] whereas in the NPC cells, it was mediated by increasing cyclin-B1 bound to CDC2 and augmenting caspase-8-activated mitochondrial death pathway.[22] In addition, both Aloe emodin (**1**) and emodin at concentrations of 5 or 10 μg/mL exerted marked inhibitory effect against human K252 leukemia cells.[19]

The apoptosis-inducing mechanisms by Aloe emodin (**1**) were observed to be unique in human H460 NSCLC cells and human Huh-7 hepatoma cells. The apoptosis of H460 cells was triggered by increasing the ER stress (i.e., activation of HSP70, 150 kDa oxygen-regulated protein, and protein disulfide isomerase) and the caspase-3 apoptotic pathway.[23] Through a special mechanism, i.e., downregulation of calpain-2 and ubiquitin-protein ligase E3A, the Aloe emodin (**1**) treatment stimulated Huh-7 cell apoptosis and exerted both dose- and time-dependent antiproliferative effects.[24] Also, a specific cytotoxicity of Aloe emodin (**1**) was present in neuroectodermal tumor cells (including Merkel cell cancer cells) *in vitro* but noninhibitions for normal cells (such as fibroblast and hemopoietic progenitor cells), where the cytotoxic effect was found to be parallel with the promotion of apoptosis, and the selectivity on neuroectodermal tumor cells was associated with a specific energy-dependent pathway of Aloe emodin incorporation.[25,26] In the presence of Aloe emodin (**1**), the anchorage-independent growth of human PC3 prostate cancer cells was inhibited by binding with mTORC2 in cells and retarding its kinase activity.[26,27] The *in vivo* antitumor activity was proven in athymic nude mice implanted with neuroectodermal tumor or PC3 tumor without any appreciable toxic effects.[25–27]

Induction of Tumor Cell Differentiation The treatment of human MGC-803 gastric cancer cells with Aloe emodin (**1**) dose-dependently inhibited the growth of cancer cells by means of cell cycle interruption and differentiation as well as repression of alkaline phosphatase activity.[28] Aloe emodin (**1**) also promoted the growth arrest and the differentiation of human U937 monoblastic leukemia cells to functionally mature monocyte, associated with a noticeable rise in transglutaminase activity.[29] Both mouse B16 melanoma cells and human A375 melanoma cells are sensitive to the Aloe emodin (**1**), where Aloe emodin (**1**) induced the differentiation of B16 cells toward melanocytes but elicited the massive apoptosis of A375 cells. The differentiation of B16 cells was found to be mediated by H_2O_2 production synchronized with rapid p53 accumulation and enhanced cyclin-D1 and cyclin-D3 expression.[30]

Metastasis and Angiogenesis Inhibitory Potentials An *in vitro* experiment demonstrated that Aloe emodin (**1**) notably inhibited the invasion, migration, and adhesion capacities of human HO-8910PM ovarian cancer cells. More studies revealed that its antimetastatic potential was principally parallel with the down-expression of FAK by Aloe emodin (**1**).[31] At a nontoxic concentration, Aloe emodin (**1**) obstructed the PMA-induced angiogenesis, migration, and invasion of WiDr colon cancer cells in association with the downregulation of MMP-2, MMP-9, RhoB, and VEGF expressions and the reduction of the DNA binding activity of NF-κB.[32] Aloe emodin (**1**) was also able to repress the proliferation of endothelial cells by inhibiting two main targets, i.e., urokinase secretion and tubule formation of endothelial cells, indicating that Aloe emodin (**1**) can behave as an antiangiogenic agent besides an antitumor.[33]

Drug Resistance-Reversing Effect In some cases, the antitumor effect of Aloe emodin (**1**) was more pronounced in the multidrug-resistant and P-gp-overexpressing cell lines than in their parent cells. In contrast to its IC_{50} value of 29 μM in human K562 leukemia cells *in vitro*, the suppressive effect of Aloe emodin (**1**) on K562/R MDR variant cells was more active with the IC_{50} value of 10.5 μM.[34]

Based on the scientific data, Aloe emodin (**1**) could be expected as a safe chemopreventive agent extensively used in the early stage of anticarcinogenesis. However, Aloe emodin (**1**) has been reported to dose-dependently rescue both B16 and A375 melanoma cells from DOX- or paclitaxel-induced killing, implying that a caution is warranted when Aloe emodin (**1**) is administrated to the melanoma patients with conventional chemotherapy.[33]

Aloin

The cytotoxicity of aloin (**2**, **3**), a pair of anthracycline-C-glocosides derived from the Aloe plant, was confirmed against human MCF-7 and SKBR-3 breast cancer cells *in vitro*. At higher concentrations, the aloin blocked the proportion of cells undergoing mitosis of the MCF-7 and SKBR-3 cells and induced apoptosis via the downregulation of cyclin-B1 and Topo-IIα protein expressions. The MCF-7 cells without erbB-2-topo-IIα coamplification were more sensitive to aloin than SKBR-3 cells with erbB-2-topo-IIα coamplification.[35] Both aloin and Aloe emodin (**1**) markedly promoted HeLaS3 cervical cancer cells to apoptosis and S phase cell cycle arrest.[35] The treatment of human leukemic cells with aloin (100 μg/mL) or Aloe emodin (**1**), respectively, resulted in significant cytotoxicity to AML cells and ALL cells.[36] An *in vivo* investigation also proved that the antineoplastic potency of aloin was greater than that of Aloe emodin (**1**) in mice implanted with Ehrlich ascites cancer cells due to the evidences in the growth suppression and the life span prolongation of the tested mice. In addition, both aloin and Aloe emodin (**1**) markedly elevated the activities of key antioxidant enzymes (SOD, GST, tGPx, and lactate dehydrogenase [LDH]).[36] Aloin at the concentration of 20–100 μM resulted in remarkable changes in the activity of almost all antioxidant enzymes, i.e., MnSOD activity was increased manyfold, whereas iNOS and CuZnSOD activities were decreased, and exerted the moderate antiproliferative effect.[36] These findings highlighted that aloin (**2**, **3**) may show its anticarcinogenic and chemopreventive effects by modulating the active levels of antioxidant and detoxification enzymes besides the apoptosis-induction and anti-proliferation activities.

Other Types of Constituents

Aloesin (**4**) was a C-glucosylchromone separated from Aloe leaves. The daily i.p. administration of aloesin (**4**) in 50 mg/kg dose to mice for 7–10 days suppressed the cell growth of sarcoma 180, Erhrich ascites carcinoma, and Heps hepatoma by 42.9–52.3%.[5] *In vivo* tests also confirmed that aloesin (**4**) extended the survival time of mice bearing leukemia and obstructed the growth of H22 hepatoma cells.[37] Furthermore, aloesin (**4**) exhibited a preventive effect on the UVB-induced immune suppression via the inhibition of tyrosine hydroxylase and dihydroxyphenylalanine oxidase.[38] Diethylhexylphthalate (**5**) (DEHP) is a potent antileukemia component. DEHP at a 10 μg/mL concentration could induce the apoptosis of human leukemic cell lines (K562,

HL-60, and U937) and significantly inhibit the leukemic cells by 74–83%, but DEHP was weak on normal MDBK cells even at the concentration of <50 μg/mL. DEHP (**5**) also showed antimutagenic activity in the assay by using *Salmonella typhimurium* TA98 and TA100.[39]

A dihydrocoumarin derivative designated as (R)-7-hydroxy-4-(4-hydroxyphenyl)-6-(4-methoxy-6-oxo-6H-pyran-2-yl)-4,5-dimethyl-3,4-dihydrochromen-2-one (**6**) derived from Aloe gel, was reported to possess the activities of anticancer, immunoregulation, and antioxidant. This coumarin (**6**) evidently depressed the oxidative activity of superoxide and hydroxyl radicals and remarkably modulated immune functions in relation to increasing the phagocytic activity and stimulating the production of superoxide anions, whose interactions is responsible for cancer prevention.[40,41]

Polysaccharides

Aloe polysaccharides (APs) were proven to have many pharmacological effects such as antitumor, antimutation, antiirradiation damage, immunity regulation, antisenescence, antigastric ulcer, antiendotoxin, etc.[42] The AP treatment in a 180 μg/mL concentration markedly obstructed the formation of BAP–DNA adduct in mouse and rat hepatocytes and obviously reduced the oxidative DNA damage induced by 8-hydroxydeoxyguanosine.[43] The AP was able to repress the activities of tyrosine kinase in human leukemic cells and to depress ornithine decarboxylase and superoxide anion formations. These approvals confirmed that the AP is a potential agent for both antitumor and antigenotoxic promotions.[43,44]

Moreover, in the studies regarding the influence on the activity of the immune-regulating factor in erythrocytes of mice bearing sarcoma 180, AP was demonstrated to have an ability to obviously improve red cell immune function by increasing receptor rosette-forming excited rate (RFER) and decreasing receptor rosette-forming inhibitory rate (RFIR) in the serum[45] and to inhibit the activities of Na^+- and K^+-ATPase in the tumor cell membrane, leading to the decline of the malignant grade of tumor cells.[46] The results revealed that the anticarcinoma effect of AP was closely attributed to the immunoregulatory function and the changes of the balance and the energy in the tumor cell membrane. By the continuing efforts, several individual AP were purified and evaluated in the assays.

Acemannan and CARN750

Acemannan is a major carbohydrate fraction obtained from the gel of the Aloe leaves. Its structure consists of a long chain of polydispersed β-(1,4)-linked mannan polymers with random *O*-acetyl groups. Acemannan was able to stimulate macrophage cytokines (such as IL-6, IL-1, and TNFα) production, surface antigen expression, NO release, and cell morphologic changes in RAW 264.7 macrophage cells *in vitro*, whose stimulation effect could be enhanced by a mixture of acemannan and IFNγ. The i.p. injection of acemannan to female mice bearing murine sarcoma caused vascular congestion, edema, polymorphonuclear leukocyte infiltration, and central necrosis foci with hemorrhage and peripheral fibrosis, leading to the immune attack to sarcoma in mice to necrosis and regression.[47,48] CARN750, a polydispersed β-(1,4)-linked acetylated mannan was found to have antineoplastic and macrophage-enhancing activities. Impressively, the daily administration of 1 mg/animal of CARN750 also displayed the greatest stimulatory hematopoietic activity in myelosuppressed mice.[49]

PAC-I, PAC-II, and PAC-III

PAC-I, PAC-II, and PAC-III (molecular weight: 10,000 kDa, 1300, and 470 kDa, respectively) are three purified APs. PAC-I and PAC-II, which both shared the same β-(1–4)-D-linked mannose with C-6 acetylation at mannosyl in the structures, displayed potent indirect tumoricidal response in a murine model with no toxicity, and both also stimulated the proliferation of peritoneal macrophages and splenic T and B cells, and activated these cells to secrete TNFα, IL-1β, IFNγ, IL-2, and IL-6. When treated by PAC-I *in vitro*, the peritoneal macrophage notably augmented the expression of FcγR and MHC-II and enhanced endocytosis, phagocytosis, NO production, and TNF-α secretion to serve the cytotoxic effect on the tumor cells. The administration of PAC-I into allogeneic mice dose-dependently potentiated the systemic TNFα production and prolonged the survival of tumor-bearing mice. PAC-I was, therefore, considered to be a valuable and potential therapeutic agent in the antineoplastic immunotherapy.[50,51]

PAVL, PAAM, and PAC

Three APs, assigned as PAVL, PAAM, and PAC, also demonstrated antitumor and immunoregulating effects in mice bearing entity sarcoma 180, and the tumor inhibitory rates were 50.58%, 43.51%, and 40.13%, respectively, in an oral dose of 100 mg/kg. PAVL and PAC markedly prolonged the survival times of mice implanted with H22 hepatoma. Compared to PAC and PAAM, PAVL exerted greater activity on the antitumor effects and the immunoregulating function on the carcinoma-bearing mice.[52]

AVP

A polysaccharide AVP was isolated from the Aloe gel-lyophilized powder with a molecular weight of 86,000, which consists of D-mannose and D-glucose (10.3:1.0). An *in vitro* assay showed that AVP could moderately restrain the growth of three human cancer cell lines, such as SMMC-7721 (liver), BGC-823 (stomach), and A549 (lung) cells.[53]

AP11, AP12, and AP13

AP11, AP12, and AP13, three Aloe polysaccharides, showed no obvious effect on the growth of HepG2 hepatoma cells but pointedly promoted the growth of PBMCs and augmented the PBMC activity on home body primary hepatoma cells *in vitro*. The AP11-interfered PBMC could inhibit the growth of hepatoma cells, indicating that the antitumor activity of AP11, AP12, and AP13 should be attributed to the interaction with PBMC and the regulation of the immune system.[54,55]

MAP

MAP is a structurally modified Aloe polysaccharide, which was prepared from partial breakdown of AP with cellulose. MAP having a molecular weight between 400 Da and 5 kDa displays the most potent macrophage-activating effect in a mouse macrophage RAW 264.7 cells *in vitro* and in mouse implanted with sarcoma 180 cells *in vivo*. The antitumor-related immunoregulatory activity was found to be correlated to the increases of NO release, surface molecule expression, cytokine secretion, and phagocytic activity.[56]

Aloe Lectins

Aloe leaf lectins (53 kDa) were mainly composed of D-mannose, D-glucose, and N-GlcNAc, exerting the inhibitory effect against the growth of colon cancer cell lines (HCT-15, HT-29, and SW-620) and a lung cancer cells (HOP-62) *in vitro*. The antitumor effect of Aloe lectins was also proven by *in vivo* tests, especially in displaying preventive effect against the tumor cell invasion by activating the immune system.[57,58] Three individual Aloe lectins, Lecl, Lec2, and Lec3, were purified, showing the molecular weights of Lec2 and Lec3 as 26,000, and 23,000, respectively. The proliferation of human K562 leukemia cells could be retarded by the Aloe lectins. The IC_{50} data were 1.418 mg/mL for Lec3, 2.305 mg/mL Lec2, and 4.193 mg/mL for Lecl.[59]

Octapeptide

An N-terminal octapeptide was derived from verectin, which is a bioactive 14 kDa glycoprotein, present in *A. vera*. The treatment of human AML cell line with the octapeptide (100 μg/mL) stimulated the cell apoptosis and hindered the proliferation of AML cells, but its activity was less than that of Aloe emodin (**1**), aloin (**2**, **3**) and aloesin (**4**). The octapeptide exhibited marked prolongation of the life duration in mice implanted with Ehrlich ascites carcinoma cells *in vivo*, whose potency was less than that of aloin (**2**, **3**) but greater than that of Aloe emodin (**1**) and aloesin (**4**).[36]

Other Activities

The herb Lu Hui (Aloe), in the pharmacological assays, demonstrated antibacterial, hepatoprotective, skin-protective, antiirradiation damage, antigastric ulcer, antitissue damage, antisensecence, immunoregulative, antimutation, antiendotoxin, and purgative effects.[60]

References

1. Pyo, M. Y. et al. 1999. Effects of *Aloe vera* on the cytotoxicity of anticancer drugs in vitro. *Yakhak Hoechi* 43: 104–10.
2. Masaldan, S. et al. 2011. Antioxidant and antiproliferative activities of a methanolic extract of *Aloe vera* leaves in human cancer cell lines. *J. Pharmacy Res.* 4: 2791–6.
3. Corsi, M. M. et al. 1998. The therapeutic potential of *Aloe vera* in tumor-bearing rats. *Intl. J. Tissue React.* 20: 115–8.
4. Jeong, H. Y. et al. 1994. Anticancer effects of aloe on sarcoma 180 in ICR mouse and on human cancer cell lines. *Yakhak Hoechi* 38: 311–21.
5. Li, W. F. et al. 1991. Antitumor activity and alcohol extract of Aloe and aloesin. *Zhongguo Zhongyao Zazhi* 16: 688.
6. Akev, N. 2007. Effect of *Aloe vera* leaf pulp extract on Ehrlich ascites tumours in mice. *Europ. J. Cancer Prev.* 16: 151–7.
7. Yamaguchi, I. et al. 1993. Components of the gel of *Aloe vera* (L.) Burm. f. *Biosci. Biotechnol. Biochem.* 57: 1350–2.
8. Lissoni, P. et al. 1998. Biotherapy with the pineal immunomodulating hormone melatonin versus melatonin plus *Aloe vera* in untreatable advanced solid neoplasms. *Nat. Immunity* 16: 27–33.
9. Tomasin, R. et al. 2011. Oral administration of *Aloe vera* and honey reduces Walker tumor growth by decreasing cell proliferation and increasing apoptosis in tumour tissue. *Phytother. Res.* 25: 619–23.
10. Chaudhary, G. et al. 2007. Chemopreventive potential of *Aloe vera* against 7,12-dimethybenz(a)anthracene induced skin papillomagenesis in mice. *Integrative Cancer Therapies* 6: 405–12.
11. Saini, M. et al. 2010. Antitumor activity of *Aloe vera* against DMBA/croton oil-induced skin papilla-magenesis in Swiss albino mice. *J. Environ. Pathol. Toxicol. Oncol.* 29: 127–35.
12. Singh, R. P. et al. 2000. Chemomodulatory action of *Aloe vera* on the profiles of enzymes associated with carcinogen metabolism and antioxidant status regulation in mice. *Phytomed.* 7: 209–19.
13. Xie, G. L. et al. 1998. Anticancerous activity of anthracene derivatives from aloe. *J. Zhongguo Med. Univ.* 27: 571–3.
14. Acevedo-Duncan, M. et al. 2004. Aloe-emodin modulates PKC isozymes, inhibits proliferation, and induces apoptosis in U-373MG glioma cells. *Int. Immunopharmacol.* 4: 1775–84.
15. Ismail, S. et al. 2013. Enhanced induction of cell cycle arrest and apoptosis via the mitochondrial membrane potential disruption in human U87 malignant glioma cells by aloe emodin. *J. Asian Nat. Prod. Res.* 15: 1003–12.
16. Chiu, T. H. et al. 2009. Aloe-emodin induces cell death through S-phase arrest and caspase-dependent pathways in human tongue squamous cancer SCC-4 cells. *Anticancer Res.* 29: 4503–11.
17. Lin, K. Y. et al. 2010. Aloe-emodin, an anthraquinone, in vitro inhibits proliferation and induces apoptosis in human colon cancer cells. *Oncol. Lett.* 1: 541–7.
18. Chen, S. H. et al. 2007. Aloe-emodin-induced apoptosis in human gastric carcinoma cells. *Food Chem. Toxicol.* 45: 2296–303.
19. Li, T. D. et al. 2009. Antitumor active components from *Aloe vera* var. chinensis Berg. *Shizhen Guoyi Guoyao* 20: 2397–8.
20. Guo, J. M. et al. 2008. Suppression of C-myc expression associates with anti-proliferation of aloe-emodin on gastric cancer cells. *Cancer Investig.* 26: 369–74.
21. Lin, J. G. et al. 2006. Aloe-emodin induces apoptosis in T24 human bladder cancer cells through the p53 dependent apoptotic pathway. *J. Urol.* 175: 343–7.
22. Lin, M. L. et al. 2010. Aloe-emodin induces apoptosis of human nasopharyngeal carcinoma cells via caspase-8-mediated activation of the mitochondrial death pathway. *Cancer Lett.* 291: 46–58.
23. Lai, M. Y. et al. 2007. Chaperones are the target in aloe-emodin-induced human lung non-small carcinoma H460 cell apoptosis. *Eur. J. Pharmacol.* 573: 1–10.
24. Jeon, W. et al. 2012. Apoptosis by aloe-emodin is mediated through down-regulation of calpain-2 and ubiquitin-protein ligase E3A in human hepatoma Huh-7 cells. *Cell Biol. Intern.* 36: 163–7.
25. Wasserman, L. et al. 2002. The effect of aloe-emodin on the proliferation of a new merkel carcinoma cell line. *Am. J. Dermatopathol.* 24: 17–22.
26. Pecere, T. et al. 2000. Aloe-emodin is a new type of anticancer agent with selective activity against neuroectodermal tumors. *Cancer Res.* 60: 2800–4.
27. Liu, K. D. et al. 2012. Aloe-emodin suppresses prostate cancer by targeting the mTOR complex 2. *Carcinogenesis* 33: 1406–11.

28. Guo, J. M. et al. 2007. Growth inhibitory effects of gastric cancer cells with an increase in S phase and alkaline phosphatase activity repression by aloe-emodin. *Cancer Biol. Therapy* 6: 85–8.
29. Tabolacci, C. et al. 2011. Aloe-emodin as antiproliferative and differentiating agent on human U937 monoblastic leukemia cells. *Life Sci.* 89: 812–20.
30. Radovic, J. et al. 2012. Cell-type dependent response of melanoma cells to aloe emodin. *Food Chem. Toxicol.* 50: 3181–9.
31. He, T. P. et al. 2008. Inhibitory effect of aloe-emodin on metastasis potential in HO-8910PM cell line. *J. Asian Nat. Prod. Res.* 10: 383–90.
32. Suboj, P. et al. 2012. Aloe-emodin inhibits colon cancer cell migration/angiogenesis by downregulating MMP-2/9, RhoB and VEGF via reduced DNA binding activity of NF-κB. *Eur. J. Pharm. Sci.* 45: 581–91.
33. Cardenas, C. et al. 2006. Evaluation of the anti-angiogenic effect of aloe-emodin. *Cell. Mol. Life Sci.* 63: 3083–9.
34. Grimaudo, S. et al. 1997. Effects of highly purified anthraquinoid compounds form *Aloe vera* on sensitive and multidrug-resistant leukemia cells. *Oncol. Reports* 4: 341–3.
35. Esmat, A. Y. et al. 2006. Cytotoxicity of a natural anthraquinone (aloin) against human breast cancer cell lines with and without ErbB-2-topoisomerase IIα coamplification. *Cancer Biol. Ther.* 5: 97–103.
36. El-Shemy, H. A. et al. 2010. Antitumor properties and modulation of antioxidant enzymes activity by *Aloe vera* leaf active principles isolated via supercritical carbon dioxide extraction. *Current Med. Chem.* 17: 129–38.
37. Wang, L. Q. et al. 2003. Tumor-inhibition rate of aloesin and its effects on survival-extending rate in tumor or leukemia bearing mice. *Zhongguo Yiyuan Yaoxue Zazhi* 23: 77–9.
38. Yagi, A. et al. 2003. Anti-inflammatory constituents, aloesin and aloemannan in Aloe species and effects of tanshinone VI in *Salvia miltiorrhiza* on heart. *Yakugaku Zasshi* 123: 517–32.
39. Lee, K. H. et al. (a) 2000. Induction of apoptosis in human leukemic cell lines K562, HL60 and U937 by diethylhexylphthalate isolated from *Aloe vera* L. *J. Pharmacy Pharmacol.* 52: 1037–41; (b) 2000. Anti-leukaemic and anti-mutagenic effects of di(2-ethylhexyl) phthalate isolated from *Aloe vera* Linne. *J. Pharmacy Pharmacol.* 52: 593–8.
40. Liu, Y. et al. 2006. Isolation and application of dihydrocoumarin derivatives extracted from Aloe. *Faming Zhuanli Shenqing Gongkai Shuomingsu* 12 pp., CN 1007-996, 20040806.
41. Zhang, X. F. et al. 2006. Isolation, Structure elucidation, antioxidative and immunomodulatory properties of two novel dihydrocoumarins from *Aloe vera*. *Bioorg. Med. Chem. Lett.* 16: 949–53.
42. Ji, Y. B. et al. 2003. Research on aloe polysaccharide. *Harbin Shangye Daxue Xuebao, Sci. Edit.* 19: 377–81.
43. Kim, H. S. et al. 1997. Inhibition of benzo(a)pyrene-DNA adduct formation by Aloe barbadensis Miller. *Carcinogenesis* 18: 771–6.
44. Kim, H. S. et al. 1999. In vitro chemopreventive effects of plant polysaccharides. *Carcinogenesis* 20: 1637–40.
45. Jia, S. H. et al. 2004. Study on influence of polysaccharides of *Aloe vera* L. on activity of immune regulate factor in erythrocytes of mice bearing S180. *Harbin Shangye Daxue Xuebao, Sci. Edit.* 20: 135–7.
46. Peng, H. S. et al. 2003. Effect of aloe polysaccharide on activities of Na^+, K^+-ATPase in tumor cell membrane of mice bearing tumor. *Harbin Shangye Daxue Xuebao, Sci. Edit.* 19: 6–7, 39.
47. Zhang, L. et al. 1996. Activation of a mouse macrophage cell line by acemannan: The major carbohydrate fraction from *Aloe vera* gel. *Immunopharmacol.* 35: 119–28.
48. Peng, S. Y. et al. 1991. Decreased mortality of Norman murine sarcoma in mice treated with the immunomodulator, Acemannan. *Mol. Biother.* 3: 79–87.
49. Egger, S. F. et al. 1996. Studies on optimal dose and administration schedule of a hematopoietic stimulatory β-(1,4)linked mannan. *Intl. J. Immunopharmacol.* 18: 113–26.
50. Leung, M. Y. K. et al. 2004. Chemical and biological characterization of a polysaccharide biological response modifier from *Aloe vera* L. var. *chinensis* (Haw.) Berg. *Glycobiol.* 14: 501–10.
51. Liu, C. et al. 2006. Macrophage activation by polysaccharide biological response modifier isolated from *Aloe vera* L. var. *chinensis* (Haw.) Berg. *Intl. Immunopharmacol.* 6: 1634–41.
52. Zou, X. et al. 2004. Study on antitumor effects of three kinds of aloe polysaccharides. *Harbin Shangye Daxue Xuebao, Sci. Edit.* 20: 14–7.
53. Pi, W. X. et al. 2007. Purification process of Aloe polysaccharide and its antitumor activity in vitro. *Zhongguo Tianran Yaowu* 5: 425–7.
54. Miao, Y. Y. et al. 2009. Effect of *Aloe vera* polysaccharide at different molecular weight and concentration on the growth of PBMC and HepG2. *Zhongguo Xiandai Zhongyao* 11: 24–7.
55. Miao, Y. Y. et al. 2010. Effect of PBMC on homebody primary hepatoma cells and intervention of *Aloe vera* polysaccharide. *Shizhen Guoyi Guoyao* 21: 801–3.
56. Im, S. A. et al. 2005. Identification of optimal molecular size of modified Aloe polysaccharides with maximum immunomodulatory activity. *Int. Immuno-pharmacol.* 5: 271–9.
57. Akev, N. et al. 2007. Tumour preventive effect of *Aloe vera* leaf pulp lectin (Aloctin I) on Ehrlich ascites tumours in mice. *Phytother. Res.* 21: 1070–5.
58. Kaur, M. et al. 2011. Purification and characterization of a lectin from leaf pulp of *Aloe vera* (L.) BURM.F. *J. Pharmacy Res.* 4: 2441–6.
59. Tian, B. et al. 2002. Characterization of lectins from Aloe species and their influences on growth of animal cells. *Xiandai Huagong* 22: 33–7.
60. Kumar, S. et al. 2014. Ethnobotanical and pharmacological properties of *Aloe vera*: A review. *J. Med. Plants Res.* 8: 1387–98.

187 He Zi Cao 合子草

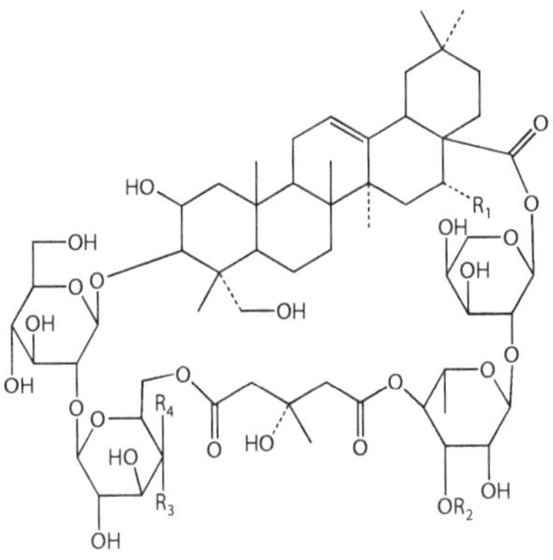

1. $R_1 = R_2 = R_4 = -H$, $R_3 = vOH$
2. $R_1 = R_3 = -H$, $R_4 = -OH$, R_2 = -D-beta-glucose
3. $R_1 = -OH$, $R_3 = -OH$, $R_4 = -H$, R_2 = -D-beta-glucose
4. $R_1 = -OH$, $R_3 = -OH$, $R_4 = -H$, R_2 = -D-beta-xylose
5. $R_1 = -H$, $R_3 = -OH$, $R_4 = -H$, R_2 = -D-beta-xylose
6. $R_1 = R_3 = -OH$, $R_2 = R_4 = -H$

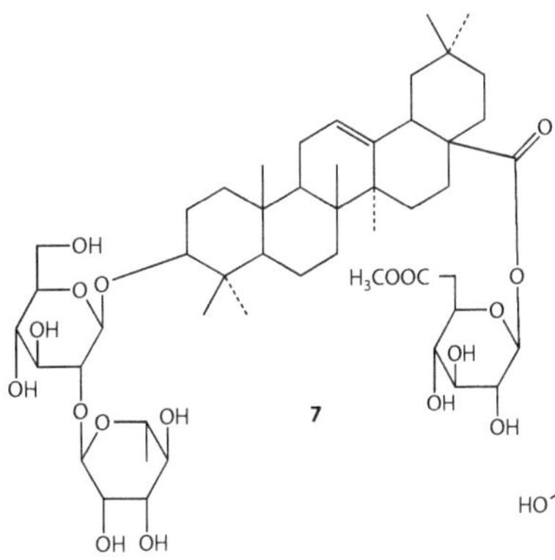

Herb Origination

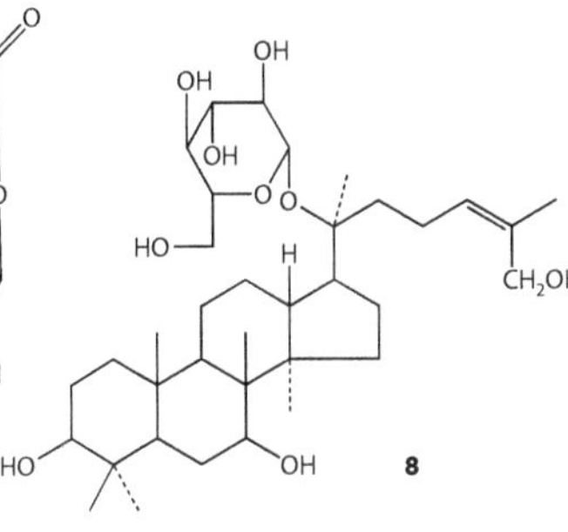

The herb He Zi Cao is the dried whole plant of *Actinostemma lobatum* (= *Actinostemma tenerum*) (Cucurbitaceae), but its seeds are used as folk medicines as well. This annual herbaceous vine generally grows in riverside and swamp-side, and it is broadly distributed in Southeast Asian countries. As Chinese herbs, the whole plant is collected in summer and autumn, whereas the seed is harvested when the seed is ripe at autumn.

Antitumor Activities and Constituents

Triterpenoid Saponins

The methanolic extract of He Zi Cao displayed moderate cytotoxicity (ED_{50}: <20 μg/mL) on the tested tumor cell lines *in vitro.* In continuing efforts, a group of saponins including cyclic bisdesmosides, noncyclic bisdesmosides, and dammarane-type saponins were isolated from the herb. The evaluation by a panel of NCI-60 human cancer cell lines *in vitro* revealed that the cyclic bisdesmosides possessed obvious cytotoxicity. The marked cytotoxic effects of lobatoside-B (**1**) are nonselectively exhibited in the NCI-60 cell lines (GI_{50}: 1.15–4.79 μM), whereas the cytotoxicity of lobatosides-C--F shown in 11 cell lines such as A549 (lung), SK-MEL-5 and SK-MEL-5 (skin), SF-295 (CNS), SW-620 and HCC-2998 (colon), UO-31 (renal), OVCAR-5 (ovary), PC3 and MDA-MB-435 (prostate), and HL-60 (leukemic) cancer cells (GI_{50}: 0.14–9.33 μM). Especially, A549/ATCC (NSCLC), SK-MEL-5 (melanoma), and SW-620 (colon cancer) cell lines were sensitive to lobatoside-E (**2**) (GI_{50}: 0.14, 0.14, and 0.36 μM, respectively). Lobatoside-C and lobatoside-D were relatively selective to HL-60 leukemia cells and SK-MEL-28 melanoma cells (GI_{50}: 1.78–1.94 μM) but less potent than lobatoside-B (**1**) and lobatoside-E (**2**). Lobatoside-E (**2**) also presented the cytotoxic effect against HeLa cervical cancer cells.[1,2]

In the detail fractionation, five more cytotoxic cyclic bisdesmosides were obtained from the herb, which were determined to be lobatoside-L (**3**), lobatoside-M, tubeimoside-III (**4**), tubeimoside-V (**5**), and dexylosyltubeimoside-III (**6**).[2] The last three saponins had been reported from the isolation of Tu Bei Mo (*Bolbostemma paniculatum*) as cancer inhibitors.[3] These saponins exhibited moderate or weak cytotoxic effect against all tested human ECA109 (esophagus), MGC-803 (stomach), and A549 (lung) cancer cell lines *in vitro.* The IC_{50} values of lobatoside-L (**3**) and tubeimoside-III (**4**) were 8.25 and 3.71 μM in ECA-109 cells, respectively, whose activities were 1.8- and 4-fold greater than that of an anticancer agent cisplatin (IC_{50}: 15.34 μM).[2] Lobatoside-C, lobatoside-D, lobatoside-G, lobatoside-N and tubeimoside-II showed marked cytotoxic effects in a dose-dependent manner against HCT-116 and HT-29 (colon), MCF-7 (breast), and A549 (lung) human cancer cell lines. Especially, one of them exhibited stronger activities (IC_{50}: 0.88 and 0.98 μM) on HT-29 and A549 cell lines than cisplatin.[4] If the treatment with 0.5% KOH is done, the cyclic bisdesmosides were converted to noncyclic bisdesmosides and the anticancer activities would be reduced.[1] Therefore, a cyclo-bridge with 3-hydroxy-3-methylglutarate in these cyclic bisdesmosides was recognized to be an essential region for cancer cell inhibition and apoptosis-induction. However, a noncyclic bisdesmoside termed lobatoside-*O* (**7**), which has a β-D-glucuronic acid linked at a carbonyl of C-28, displayed a similar level of antiproliferative effects on the MCF-7, HCT-116, HT-29, and A549 cell lines (IC_{50}: 7.58–18.72 μmol/mL) as those of cisplatin (IC_{50}: 8.97–17.56 μmol/mL).[5]

In addition, a dammarane-type triterpene saponin assigned as actinostemmoside-B (**8**) showed antiproliferative effect against FXF-393 (renal cancer) and RPMI-8226 (leukemia) cell lines (GI_{50}: 3.47 and 5.37 μM, respectively). When a methyl group at C-8 in the aglycone of actinostemmoside-B (**8**) was replaced with a hydroxylmethyl group ($-CH_2OH$), the antitumor activity would be abortive.[2]

Overall, the *in vitro* scientific evidences demonstrated that the cyclic bisdesmosides, especially lobatoside-E (**2**) and lobatoside-L (**3**) were deemed to be the cytotoxic principals of He Zi Cao. The results also supported the herb deserving continuous research *in vivo* and further development in cancer chemotherapy and prevention.

Flavonoids

Moreover, an extract of the whole plant of He Zi Cao was found to have marked anticarcinogenesis-related radical-scavenging activity. The bioactivity-guided fractionation of the extract led to the isolation of four flavonoids such as kaempferol-3-*O*-α-L-rhamnosyl

(1–6)-β-D-glucoside, quercetin-3-*O*-β-L-rhamnosyl (1–6)-β-D-glucoside, quercetin-3-*O*-β-D-glucoside, and quercetin. They showed significant antioxidative effects during the tests of free radical-scavenging and superoxide quenching-activities, whose effects might closely contribute to the anticarcinogenesis.[6] Also, at high doses (8.75 and 12.5 g/kg), the aqueous extract of He Zi Cao showed antimutant activity in a mouse model, but its alcohol extract had no such activity.[7]

Other Medical Uses

The herb He Zi Cao has been traditionally used in China as a diuretic for treating ascites swelling and nephrotic edema, as a medicine for expelling pathogenic cold and dampness, and as an antidote for poisonous snakebites. A butanolic fraction from He Zi Cao was reported to possess antithrombotic activity, and the He Zi Cao extract was shown to have immunopotentiating activity.[8–10] A toxicological experiment showed that the LD_{50} values were 132.34 g/kg for the herb decoction and 7.17 g/kg for the total saponin component.[9,10]

References

1. Fujiola, T. et al. 1996. Antitumor agents: 171. Cytotoxicities of lobatosides B, C, D and E, cyclic Bisdesmosides isolated from *Actinostemma lobatum* Maxim. *Bioorg. Med. Chem. Lett.* 6: 2807–10.
2. Li, W. et al. 2012. Cyclic bisdesmosides from *Actinostemma lobatum* Maxim (Cucurbitaceae) and their in vitro cytotoxicity. *Fitoterapia* 83: 147–52.
3. Cheng, G. et al. 2006. Tubeimoside V, a new cyclic bisdesmoside from tubers of *Bolbostemma paniculatum*, functions by inducing apoptosis in human glioblastoma U87MG cells. *Bioorg. Med. Chem. Lett.* 16: 4575–80.
4. Cao, J. Q. et al. 2015. A new cyclic bisdesmoside from *Actinostemma lobatum* Maxim. *Pharmazie* 70: 347–50.
5. Cao, J. Q. et al. 2015. Three new triterpene saponins from *Actinostemma lobatum* Maxin and their cytotoxicity in vitro. *Phytochem. Lett.* 11: 301–5.
6. Kim, D. K. 2010. Antioxidative constituents from the whole plant of *Actinostemma lobatum* Maxim. *J. Korean Soc. for Applied Biol. Chem.* 53: 746–51.
7. Wu, P. N. et al. 2002. Study on the anti-mutagenic effect of *Actinostemma lobatum*. *Chin. Archiv. Tradit. Chin. Med.* 20: 729–30.
8. Kim, K. H. et al. 2008. Blockade of glycoprotein IIb/IIIa mediates the antithrombotic activity of butanol fraction of *Actinostemma lobatum* Maxim. *J. Ethnopharmacol.* 116: 431–8.
9. Ni, P. et al. 2001. Pharmacological and toxicological research on Hezicao (*Actinostemma lobatum*). *Primary J. Chin. Materia Med.* 16: 14–5.
10. Yue, W. W. et al. 2013. Advances in studies on chemical constituents and pharmacological activities of *Actinostemma lobatum* Maxim. *Shenyang Yaoke Daxue Xuebao* 30: 484–8.

188 Zhu Ling 豬苓

Polyporus

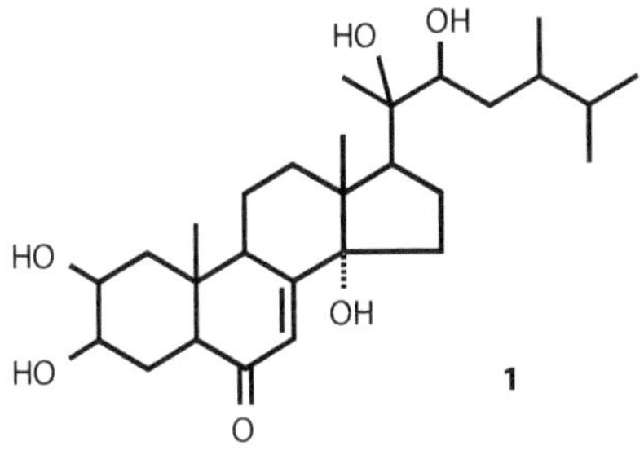

Herb Origination

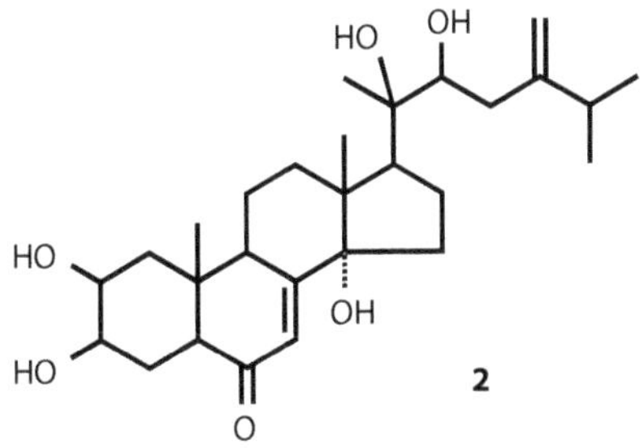

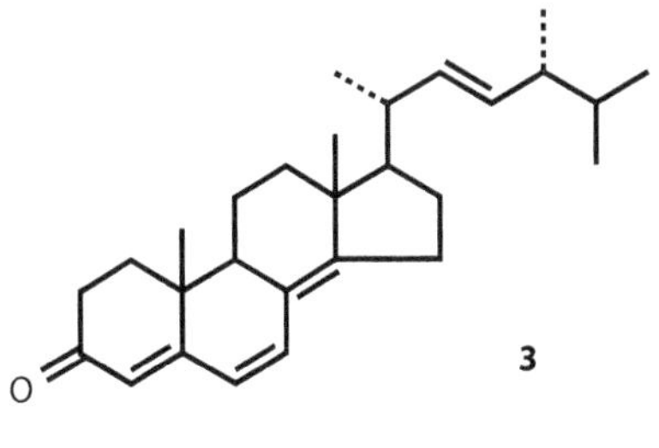

The herb Zhu Ling (Polyporus) is the dried sclerotium of fungi *Polyporus umbellatus*. This Polyporaceae fungus is distributed in many places of China as well as in the northern part of North America as growing near the bases of the roots of hardwoods. The herb is predominantly produced in the Chinese provinces of Shaanxi and Yunnan. The earliest document of Zhu Ling as an herb is in the first Chinese classic materia medica titled *Shennong Beng Cao Jing*.

Antitumor Activities

In the preliminary studies, the Zhu Ling extract displayed *in vivo* antitumor effect against murine sarcoma 180, U14 cervical cancer, and H22 hepatoma but not on leukemia.[1,2] The extract not only increased the intracellular levels of cAMP and cAMP/cGMP ratio, but also inhibited the activity of cAMP phosphodiesterase and affected the activities of four lysosomal enzymes (acid phosphatase, DNase, RNase, and cathepsin-D) in the H22 cells *in vivo*. The Zhu Ling extract could also restore the levels of glycogen, glucose-6-phosphate, and fructose-1,6-diphosphate in the liver, increase the liver catalase and succinic dehydrogenase, and decrease the oxygen consumption in mice bearing the H22 hepatoma.[3] These results designated that the Zhu Ling extract has marked immunostimulating and hepatoprotecting activities, leading to the exertion of the antihepatoma effect. The oral administration of the extract to mice implanted with sarcoma 180 lengthened the survival duration by 71.6%. When combined with mitomycine-C, the extract could augment the cytotoxicity to S180 cells and improve the life span of tumor-bearing mice by up to 119.9%. The *in vivo* antitumor effect was found to be largely associated with the increase of lymphocytes infiltrated and surrounded tumor cells and the inhibition of the synthetic rates of DNA, RNA, and protein in the S180 cells.[4]

Antitumor Constituents

Sterones

A group of ergone-type sterone derivatives with anticancer property were isolated from Zhu Ling. Polyporusterone-A (**1**), polyporusterone-B (**2**), and polyporusterone-C--G demonstrated moderate cytotoxicity against the proliferation of murine L1210 leukemia cells *in vitro*.[5,6] Another sterone analog assigned as ergosta-4,6,8(14),22-tetraen-3-one (**3**) isolated from Zhu Ling also exhibited the cytotoxic activities on human cancer cell lines *in vitro*.[7]

Polysaccharides

The major neoplasm inhibitor in Zhu Ling is the polysaccharide components (PUPS), which display only *in vivo* anticancer effect. The treatment with PUPS (200 mg/kg, per two day, by i.p. administration) for eight days could reduce the number of tumor cells by 39% in mice bearing H22 hepatoma.[8] PUPS did not show the growth inhibition against Lewis lung tumor, but it could obstruct the spontaneous tumor metastasis.[9] By reducing the expressions of N-ras and c-Myc, PUPS suppressed the growth of HepA hepatoma cells.[10] Although only weak suppressive effect against U14 uterine cancer cell growth is shown *in vitro*, the intramuscular (i.m.) injection of PUPS in a dose of 50 mg/kg effectively promoted the antigrowth activity of chemotherapeutic drugs (such as CTX, amethopterin, and mitomycin) in mice bearing U14 cervical cancer cells.[9] In a butyl(butyl)nitrosamine (BBN)-induced rat bladder cancer model, the Polyporus polysaccharide (PU-PPS) and the herb exerted antitumor effect by potentiating the host immune function *in vivo*, whose mechanism is largely due to their positive effects on the thymus and spleen indexes, the lymphocytic infiltration, and the CD86 expression.[11] From these evidences, the antineoplastic potential of Zhu Ling polysaccharides was confirmed to be principally attributed to their marked immunoenhancing property.

Moreover, the Zhu Ling polysaccharides were capable of reversing the immunosuppression caused by sarcoma 180, ^{60}Co irradiation and CTX via downregulated secretion of immunosuppressive substances, upregulated proliferation of mouse splenocytes, and production of IL-2 and augmented activity of NK cells, etc.[12] Similarly, the *in vitro* treatment with PUPS could diminish the immunosuppressions of Colon26 tumor cells in association with notable lessening of the secretions of five immunosuppressors (TGF-β1, VEGF, IL-4, IL-6, and IL-10). The inhibition of immunosuppressors is considered as one of the antitumor effects of Zhu Ling polysaccharides.[13] Also, the immunopotentiating activity of PUPS could be pointedly augmented when combined with IL-2 in the treatment, where the cytotoxicities of NK cells and LAK cells were more stimulated and the levels of TNF and IFN were more elevated.[14]

Through the up-expressions of CD86, CD40, and TLR4/CD14, the treatment with PPS and Bacille Calmette–Guerin (BCG) synergistically obstructed the development and the invasion of bladder cancer cells in model rats and reduced the BCG-caused side effects.[15]

Exo-Biopolymers

A protein–polysaccharide component isolated from Zhu Ling was composed of 78.2% polysaccharide and 16.8% protein. The protein–polysaccharide component demonstrated the suppressive effect against the viability of L1210 and K562 leukemia cells *in vitro* by 47.4% and 45.0%, respectively, at concentrations of 50–400 μg/mL. The *in vivo* anticancer effects of the protein–polysaccharide component was demonstrated in mice implanted with solid sarcoma 180 cells at doses of 20–160 mg/kg/day, but the growth inhibition might not be related to the tumor cell apoptosis.[13] In addition, the protein–polysaccharide component also possesses antimutagenic property. The treatment with 2.5–10.0% of the protein–polysaccharide component could diminish mutagenicity evoked by 2-nitrofluorene and sodium azide in *Salmonella typhimurium* strains TA 98 and TA 100.[16]

Other Bioactivities

Pharmacological investigations have revealed that Zhu Ling (Polyporus) has diuretic, hepatoprotective, immunostimulating, antioxidative, and antibacterial properties.

References

1. Institute of Materia Medica, Chinese Academy of Medical Sciences. 1978. *Zhongcaoyao Tongxun* (8): 372; (b) 1999. *Chinese Materia Medica*, Vol. 1, 1-0227, 551–4. Shanghai Science and Technology Press, Shanghai, China.
2. Institute of Chinese Materia Medica, China Academy of Traditional Chinese Medicine. 1979. *Xinyiyao Zazhi* (2): 15, 73.
3. Wu, G. L. et al. 1982. Biochemical actions of some anticancer agents. *J. Beijing Normal Univ. Sci. Edit.* (2): 57–66.
4. You, J. S. et al. 1994. Combined effects of chuling (*Polyporus umbellatus*) extract and mitomycin C on experimental liver cancer. *Am. J. Chinese Med.* 22: 19–28.
5. Murayama, M. et al. 1992. Makisterone derivatives as anticancer agents. *Jpn. Kokai Tokkyo Koho* JP 90–125552 19900517.
6. Ohsawa, T. et al. 1992. Studies on constituents of fruit body of *Polyporus umbellatus* and their cytotoxic activity. *Chem. Pharm. Bull.* 40: 143–7.
7. Lee, W. Y. et al. 2005. Cytotoxic activity of ergosta-4,6,8(14),22-tetraen-3-one from the sclerotia of *Polyporus umbellatus*. *Bull. Korean Chem. Soc.* 26: 1464–6.
8. Wei, Q. et al. 1983. Effects of *Polyporus umbellatus* polysaccharides on liver carbohydrate metabolism and adrenocortical function of mice bearing hepatoma H22. *Zhongguo Yaoli Xuebao* 4: 52–4.
9. Wang, D. C. et al. 1983. Some pharmacological effects of Grifola polysaccharide. *Zhongcaoyao* 14: 267–8.
10. Song, G. C. et al. 2008. Effect of *Ganoderma applanatum* polysaccharides GF on N-ras and C-myc oncogene expressions in HepA tumor cells. *J. Tongji Med. Univ., Med. Edit.* 29: 45–7, 52.
11. Li, C. X. et al. 2012. Effects of *Polyporus umbellatus* and Polyporus polysaccharide on thymus index, spleen index and CD86 expression in rat bladder cancer. *Mianyixue Zazhi* 28: 116–9.
12. Yang, L. J. et al. 2004. Effect of *Polyporus umbellatus* polysaccharide on the immune-suppression property of culture supernatant of sarcoma 180 (S180) cells. *Xibao yu Fenzi Mianyixue Zazhi* 20: 234–7.
13. Cui, C. et al. 2009. In vitro effects of *Polyporus umbellatus* polysaccharide on immunosuppressions of Colon26 tumor cells. *Mianyixue Zazhi* 25: 650–4.
14. Xu, H. W. et al. 1998. Study on cytotoxicity of *Polyporus umbellatus* polysaccharide and IL-2 activated peripheral blood monocytes on tumor cells. *Zhongguo Mianyixue Zazhi* 14: 109–11.
15. Zhang, G. W. et al. 2015. Efficacy of Zhuling polyporus polysaccharide with BCG to inhibit bladder carcinoma. *Carbohydr. Polym.* 118: 30–5.
16. Lee, J. W. et al. 2004. Antitumor and antimutagenic effect of the protein polysaccharides from *Polyporus umbellatus*. *Han'guk Sikp'um Yongyang Kwahak Hoechi* 33: 475–9.

189 Fu Ling 茯苓

Poria, Tuckahoe, or Hoelen

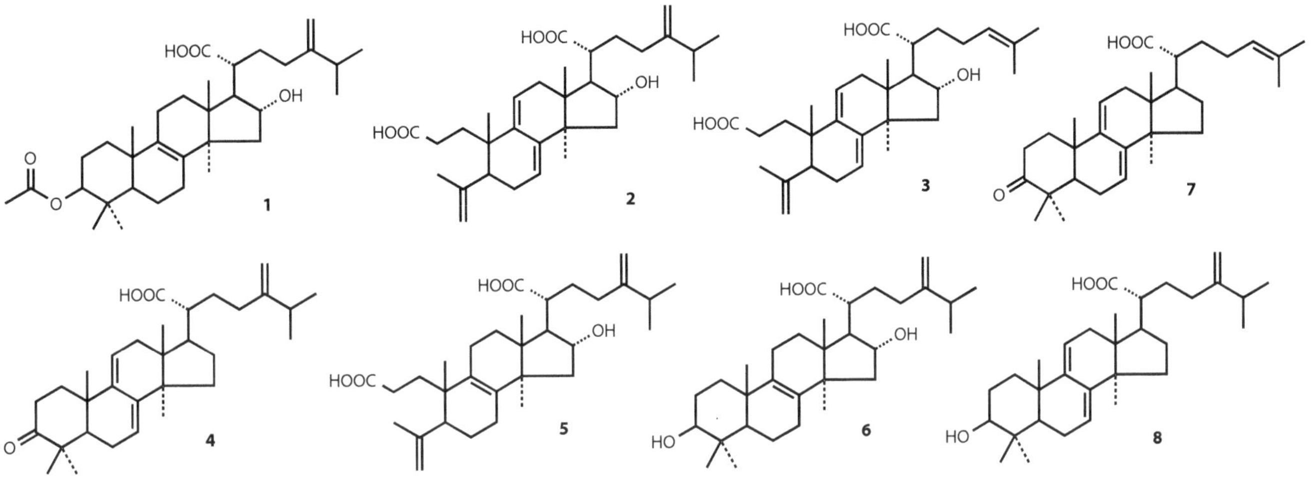

(a)

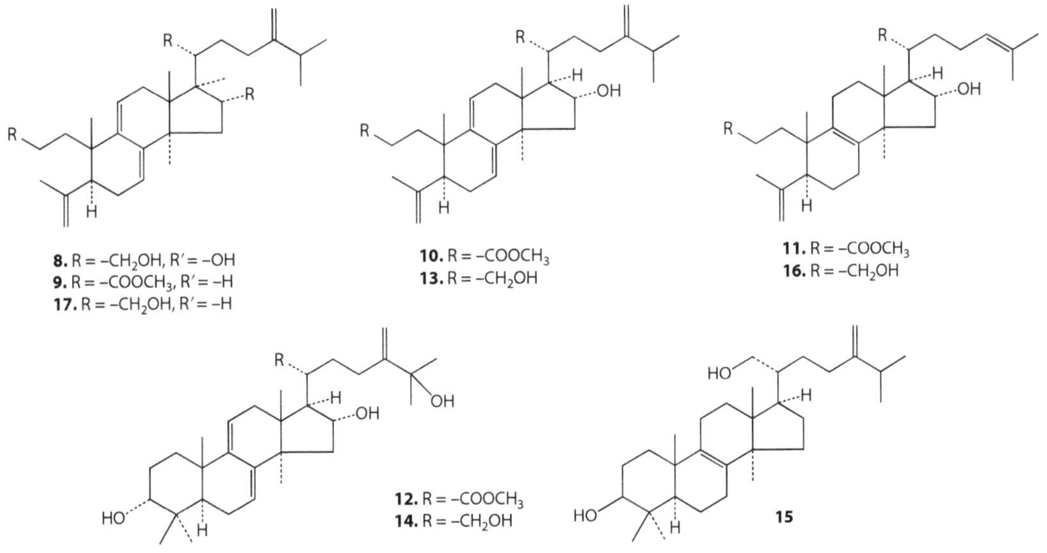

8. R = $-CH_2OH$, R′ = $-OH$
9. R = $-COOCH_3$, R′ = $-H$
17. R = $-CH_2OH$, R′ = $-H$

10. R = $-COOCH_3$
13. R = $-CH_2OH$

11. R = $-COOCH_3$
16. R = $-CH_2OH$

12. R = $-COOCH_3$
14. R = $-CH_2OH$

(b)

Herb Origination

The herb Fu Ling (Poria) is derived from the sclerotium of a Polyporaceae fungus, *Poria coco* (= *Pachyma cocos* Fr.). The fungi grow around the roots of old or dead pine trees. The fungi are commonly used as a Chinese herbal medicine in east Asia for centuries. The herb is collected from July to September and dried in the shade for the application as traditional medicine. The Chinese provinces of Yunnan, Anhui, and Hubei are the main producers of this herb.

Antitumor Constituents and Activity

Pharmacology combined with phytochemistry studies revealed the antineoplastic and anticarcinogenetic effects of Fu Ling were principally contributed from its two types of bioactive constituents, triterpenoids and polysaccharides.

Triterpenoids

Fu Ling presents to be rich in triterpenoid components. Many lanostane-type triterpene acids were separated from the fungus sclerotium and assayed for their anticancer and anticarcinogenetic activities. A triterpenoid fraction derived from the methanolic extract of the cultivated *P. cocos* could restrain the cell growth of various solid cancers such as in the lung, the ovary, the skin, the CNS, the rectum, etc.[1] The lanostane-type and 3,4-*seco*-lanostane-type triterpene acids separated from the fungi also showed potent inhibitory effects against a tumor promoter TPA induced EBV-EA activation in Raji cells, implying that the Fu Ling triterpene acids possess valuable antitumor-promoting properties.[2–5] Moreover, others such as pachymic acid (**1**), poricoic acid A (**2**), poricoic acid B (**3**), poricoic acid C, dehydropachymic acid, 16-deoxyporicoic acid B, dehydroeburiconic acid (**4**), 3-*O*-acetyl-16α-hydroxytrametenolic acid, and 25-methoxy-poricoic acid A demonstrated prominent suppressive effect against DMBA-initiated and TPA-promoted mouse skin two-stage carcinogenesis *in vivo*.[3–7] The investigations regarding the SAR disclosed that the triterpene acids having hydroxylation at C-16α or C-25 and cleavage of ring-A to form 3,4-*seco*-3-oic acid exerted enhanced antitumor-promoting effect.[2–5]

The evaluation of the cytotoxicities of poricoic acid A (**2**) and poricoic acid G (**5**) on the NCI panel of 60 human cancer cell lines revealed that poricoic acid G (**5**) had significant cytotoxicity to HL-60 leukemia cells (GI_{50}: 39.3 nM) and moderate cytotoxic to the other tumor cell lines (GI_{50}: >22 μM), whereas poricoic acid A (**2**) displayed the modest cytotoxicity (GI_{50}: 15–30 μM) to all the 60 human cancer cell lines tested.[2] Sixteen other lanostane-type triterpene acids and a diterpene acid assigned as 7-oxo-15-hydroxydehydrodroabietic acid from Fu Ling displayed dose-dependent cytotoxicity on two *in vitro* human cell lines, HL-60 (leukemia) and CRL1579 (melanoma). Among these terpenoids, the potency of 16α,25-dihydroxyeburiconic acid (IC_{50}: 28.7 μM) on the CRL1579 melanoma cells was almost comparable to that of cisplatin (IC_{50}: 21.1 μM), whereas dehydroeburiconic acid (**4**) and 25-hydroxy-3-epi-dehydrotumulosic acid exerted weak inhibitory effect on the CRL1579 cells.[4] The higher growth inhibitory effect was achieved by dehydroeburiconic acid (**4**) on PANC-1 pancreatic cancer cells and SK-BR-3 breast cancer cells (IC_{50}: 5.5 and 12.2 μM, respectively) and by 25-hydroxy-3-epidehydrotumulosic acid on OVCAR-3 ovarian cancer cells (IC_{50}: 9.5 μM). Among these cell lines, A549 lung cancer cells were sensitive to 25-hydroxy-3-epidehydrotumulosic acid, dehydroeburiconic acid (**4**), and poricoic acid A (**2**) (IC_{50}: 4.0, 10, 27 μM, respectively), and Du-145 prostate cells was only temperately sensitive to poricoic acidsA (**2**) (IC_{50}: 14.5 μM), which was less active than cisplatin (IC_{50}: 9.2 μM).[8] The moderate cytotoxicities was also observed in the *in vitro* treatment with ehydropachymic acid, pachymic acid (**1**), and tumulosic acid (**6**) on HT-29 colon cancer cells (IC_{50}: 10.4–29.1 μM)[9] and poricoic acid C, dehydroeburiconic acid (**4**), poricoic acid G (**5**), poricoic acid H, and 25-hydroxy-3-epidehydro-tumulosic acid on the HL-60 leukemic cells (IC_{50}: 25.9–38.0 μM).[8] The proliferation of human pancreatic cancer cell lines (Panc-1, MiaPaca-2, AsPc-1, and BxPc-3) was inhibited when it is exposed to pachymic acid (**1**), polyporenic acid C and dehydropachymic acid, but pachymic acid (**1**) demonstrated the strongest activity against BxPc-3 cells with an IC_{50} value of 0.26 μM (in 24 h) together with arrested G0/G1 cell cycle.[10] By inducing the ER stress via the up-expression of XBP-1s, ATF4, Hsp70, CHOP, and phospho-eIF2α, pachymic acid (**1**) elicited apoptotic death in gemcitabine-resistant pancreatic cancer cells (Panc-1 and MiaPaca-2) and significantly suppressed the growth of Mia Paca-2 tumor *in vivo* without toxicity in a dose of 25 mg/kg.[11] Pachymic acid (**1**) was also able to markedly repress the invasive behavior of BxPc-3 cells through Matrigel and reduction of MMP-7 expression.[10] In addition, seven other triterpene acids from Fu Ling were cytotoxic to human DU-145 (prostate) and A549 (lung) cancer cell lines *in vitro*. Apparently, the inhibitory potency toward A549 cells was greater than on Du-145 cells.[12]

Pachymic acid (**1**) was also found to have the abilities to significantly suppress the cell proliferation and to promote the apoptosis in dose- and time-dependent fashions on two human prostate cancer cell lines *in vitro*. Its antigrowth potency on androgen-insensitive DU145 cells was greater than on androgen-responsive LNCaP cells, whose antiprostate cancer mechanism was further revealed to correlate with (1) elevation of p21 expression, (2) increase of Bcl-2 phosphorylation and decrease of Bad phosphorylation, and (3) reduction of prostaglandin synthesis and AKT activity and activation of caspase-9 and caspase-3. Pachymic acid (**1**) provoked the cell apoptosis and the induction of the mitochondria dysfunction largely through the blockage of the AKT signal pathway.[13] The induction of EJ bladder cancer cell apoptosis was revealed to be mediated by (1) up-generation of ROS and upregulation of DR5; (2) down-expression of Bcl-2 and Bcl-xL and up-expression of Bax and Bad; (3) loss of mitochondrial membrane potential, release of cytochrome c, and activation of caspase-3, caspase-8. and caspase-9; and (4) subsequent cleavage of PARP and suppressed IAP family proteins, signifying both intrinsic and extrinsic pathways involved in the proapoptosis.[14] Likewise, both dehydroebriconic acid (**4**) and dehydrotrametenonic acid (**7**) could dose-dependently halt the cell cycle of human NUGC-3 gastric cancer at G1 phase and moderately repress the cell proliferation with LD_{50} values of 63.6 and 38.4 μM, respectively,[15,16] whereas dehydrotrametenolic acid (**8**) selectively restrained the proliferation of H-ras-transformed rat2 fibroblast cells (GI_{50} 40 μM) together with the promotion of G2/M cell arrest and cell apoptosis, whose apoptotic mechanism of dehydrotrametenolic acid (**8**) was revealed to be associated with the degradation of PARP and lamin A/C, the diminution of the expressions of H-ras, Akt, and Erk, and the activation of caspase-3.[17,18]

In addition, pachymic acid (**1**), tumulosic acid (**6**), polyporenic acid C, dehydropachymic acid, and others were found to be inhibitors of both DNA topoisomerases Topo-I and Topo -II.[9] The IC_{50} values of dehydroebriconic acid (**4**) and dehydrotrametenonic acid (**7**) were 4.6 and 37.5 μM, respectively, against Topo-II activity. Dehydroebriconic acid (**4**) not only potently inhibited Topo-II but also moderately repressed mammals DNA polymerases (α, β, γ, δ, ε, η, ι, and λ).[15] Dehydrotrametenonic acid (**7**) is the moderate inhibitors of bovine thymus DNA polymerase-α and recombinant rat DNA polymerase-β as well.[16] These evidences corroborated that the inhibitory effects against DNA polymerases and DNA Topo by these triterpane acids from Fu Ling might partially be involved in their antitumor and anticarcinogenetic mechanisms.

Simply Modified Triterpenoids

Six lanostane-type triterpene acids isolated from *Poria cocos* were simply modified to produce their methyl esters and hydroxyl derivatives. The cytotoxicity of these derivatives was evaluated by an *in vitro* assay by using eight human neoplastic cell lines, showing nine compounds possessing notably improved inhibitory activity with IC_{50} values of <10 μM against the some tumor cell lines. Poricotriol-A (**8**), a hydroxy derivative of poricoic acid A, exerted potent cytotoxicities on human tumor cell lines, and its IC_{50} values of 1.2–5.5 μM were present on the six tested cell lines, HL-60 (leukemic), CRL1579 (skin), AZ521 (stomach), A549 (lung), OVCAR-3 (ovary), and SK-BR-3 (breast) cancer cells. Moreover, the most potent effect on HL-60 cells was achieved by the methyl esters dimethyl poricoate C (**9**); dimethyl poricoate H (**10**); dimethyl poricoate G (**11**); methyl 25-hydroxy-3-epidehydrotumulosate (**12**) (IC_{50}: 2.4, 3.6, 8.8, and

6.9 μM, respectively) and the hydroxyl derivatives poricotriol-A (**8**), poricotriol H (**13**); 25-hydroxy-3-epidehydrotumulosol (**14**); dehydroeburicol (**15**); poricotriol G (**16**) (IC_{50}: 1.9, 2.9, 2.5, 6.7, and 7.5 μM, respectively). The strongest antitumor compounds on SK-BR-3 cells was poricotriol-A (**8**) and dimethyl poricoate G (**11**) (IC_{50}: 1.2 and 4.3 μM, respectively) and on AZ521 cells was poricotriol-A (**8**) (IC_{50}: 1.4 μM). Poricotriol-A (**8**) and dehydroeburiconic acid hydroxyl derivative (**15**) also displayed the highly enhanced inhibitory effect on A549, CRL1579, and OVCAR-3 cells with IC_{50} values of 4.2 and 4.0 μM, 5.5 and 2.8 μM, and 2.2 and 6.4 μM, respectively. Particularly, the cytotoxic activities of poricotriol-A (**8**) against the A549, CRL1579, OVCAR-3, SK-BR-3, and AZ521 cell lines, dehydroeburiconic acid hydroxyl derivative (**15**) against the A549, CRL1579, and OVCAR-3 cell lines, and poricoic acid H-hydroxyl derivative (**13**) against the CRL1579 cells were superior to those of two reference agents (cisplatin and/or 5-FU), tested in the same assay. In addition, the DU-145 prostate cancer cells was less resistant to these tested derivatives as compared to other cell lines. The derivatives poricotriol-A (**8**), dimethyl poricoate H (**10**), methyl 25-hydroxy-3-epidehydrotumulosate (**12**), and poricoic acid C (**17**) showed moderate cytotoxicities in DU-145 cells, (IC_{50}: 14.5–28.9 μM) but are less active than cisplatin (IC_{50}: 9.2 μM).[8]

Poricotriol-A (**8**) was selected for the evaluation of apoptosis-inducing activity and mechanism exploration. The obtained data suggested that the apoptosis of HL-60 cells promoted by poricotriol-A (**8**) was mediated by both mitochondrial and death receptor pathways including the increase of Bax/Bcl-2 ratio and the activation of caspase-3, caspase-8, and caspase-9. However, poricotriol-A (**8**)-stimulated A49 cell apoptotic death was processed by a caspase-independent mitochondrial pathway with AIF translocation.[8] Based upon these results, poricotriol-A (**8**) can be considered as a potential therapeutic agent for further development in cancer treatment.

Polysaccharides

A group of diverse polysaccharides was prepared from the herb, the mycelia, and the cultured fungi of Fu Ling and were further demonstrated to possess immunopotentiating antitumor properties. A Fu Ling polysaccharide derived from the fungi but with no specific name was reported in the beginning of 2010. The polysaccharide was composed of xylose, galactose, arabinose, ribose, mannose, and glucose in the molar percentages of 0.54%, 1.01%, 1.09%, 1.6%, 11.3%, and 85.9%, respectively. Feeding the polysaccharide for seven weeks to tested mice markedly suppressed the growth of tumor cells and increased the activities of SOD, CAT, and GPx, indicating that the polysaccharide is an important member of the antitumor immunopromoter in Fu Ling.[19]

PCME

PCME are polysaccharides fractionated from the mycelia of Fu Ling. I.p. injection of PCME could restrain the growth of sarcoma 180 and Ehrlich carcinoma in mice and prolong the lifespan of mice inoculating with IMC breast cancer or sarcoma 180. However, PCME was non-active on L1210 and P388 leukemias and B16 melanoma *in vivo*. The anti-neoplastic spectrum of PCME was similar to other polysaccharides such as PSK or lentinan but it was more effective than Krestin (PSK).[20]

PCM3-II

A water-soluble β-glucan PCM3-II, composed mainly of (1–3)- and (1–4)-linked glucoses, was purified from the mycelia of Fu Ling. PCM3-II could dose-dependently reduce the proliferation and the viability of human MCF-7 breast cancer cells by 50% at its concentration of 400 μg/mL. After 72 h of treatment with PCM3-II, the cell cycle was time-dependently arrested at G1 phase followed by the downregulation of the expressions of cyclin-D1 and cyclin-E in the breast carcinoma cells. The apoptosis in the MCF-7 cells was also promoted by PCM3-II in association with the reduction of the antiapoptotic Bcl-2 protein.[21]

PC-PS

PC-PS is a neutral polysaccharide fraction (molecular weight: ≈160 kDa) isolated from Fu Ling, effectively acting as a potent biological response modifier on the antiproliferation and the differentiation of human U937 and HL-60 leukemia cell lines *in vitro*. When human blood mononuclear cells were stimulated by PC-PS for five days, the produced and modified cells (PC-PS-MNC-CM5) demonstrated potent suppressive effect against the growth of U937 and HL-60 cells by 87.3% and 74.7%, respectively. PC-PS-MNC-CM5 was also able to differentiate about 66.6% of the U937 cells and 49.4% of the HL-60 cells into mature monocytes/macrophages, correlating with the marked expressions of the surface antigens of CD11b, CD14, and CD68. Antibody neutralization tests with the PC-PS-MNC-CM5 clearly revealed that the tumor growth inhibitory and the differentiation-inducing activities were primarily due to the cytokines of IFNγ and TNFα, which were notably augmented by PC-PS-MNC-CM5.[22]

H11

An antitumor polysaccharide assigned as H11 (molecular weight: 5×10^6) was isolated from the mycelia of Fu Ling, which is a β-D-glucan consisted of (1–3)- and (1–6)-components in 4:1 ratio. H11 exhibited no direct antitumor activity *in vitro* but displayed potent *in vivo* inhibition against neoplasm growth through host-mediated immune events as usual. At daily doses of 4 or 8 mg/kg for 10 times, the antigrowth effect of H11 could almost reach to 100% against entity sarcoma 180 cells *in vivo*, but it had no such effect on the ascites sarcoma 180 at doses of 2–20 mg/kg.[23,24]

PC3 and PC4

From the mycelia of Fu Ling, two special glucans designated as PC3 and PC4 were isolated, which are a linear β-(1–3)-D-glucan and a β-(1–3)-D-glucan with a few glucuronic acid and branches, respectively. Their potent antineoplastic effects appeared only after their structures were modified by borohydride reduction and then by partial hydrolysis. The growth inhibition of the degraded β-D-glucans could reach to 96.88% in animal models transplanted with sarcoma 180 or EAC *in vivo*.[25]

Modification of (1–3)-D-Glucans

Sulfated (1–3)-D-Glucans

Several water-insoluble (1–3)-β-D-glucans and (1–3)-α-D-glucans were obtained from the mycelia of Fu Ling and were devoid of antitumor activity. When the glucans were reacted with dimethyl sulfoxide, the sulfate substitution mainly occurred on the C-6 position and secondly on the C-4 and C-2 positions. The derivatives with better water solubility and higher molecular weight exhibited significant antiproliferative effect against human HepG2 hepatoma, MKN-45, and SGC-7901 gastric carcinoma cells *in vitro* and against murine S180 cells *in vivo*. The sulfated glucans could enhance the apoptosis of sarcoma 180 cells dose- and time-dependently by the upregulation of Bax and the down-regulation of Bcl-2, and they could also reduce the toxicity of anticancer agent 5-FU.[26–30]

PCS3-II was a (1–3)-β-D-glucan prepared from fresh sclerotium of *P. cocos*, and its sulfated product termed S-PCS3-II (molecular weight: 3.8 × 10^4) was water insoluble. S-PCS3-II demonstrated its antiproliferative effect against human gastric adenocarcinoma cell lines (MKN-45, SGC-7901, and MKN-28) *in vitro*, whereas PCS3-II, its native β-glucan, showed no such activity. The *in vivo* antitumor effect of S-PCS3-II was demonstrated in nude mice implanted with human MKN-45 low differentiation gastric adenocarcinoma cells. Its growth inhibitory rate could reach 47.9% at a high dose of S-PCS3-II, implying that it may be a potential agent for therapy and prevention of the gastric cancer.[31,32]

Carboxymethylated (1–3)-β-D-Glucan

PCS3-II was derived from fresh sclerotium of *P. cocos*. The introduction of carboxymethylated groups into the water-insoluble PCS3-II obviously increased the water solubility, chain stiffness, and antigastric adenocarcinoma activity. The carboxymethylated β-D-glucan named C-PCS3-II (molecular weight: 18.9 × 10^4) exerted significant suppressive effect against the proliferation of human gastric adenocarcinoma cell lines (MKN-45, SGC-7901, and MKN-28) in an *in vitro* assay.[31]

Carboxymethylated-Sulfated (1–3)-β-D-Glucan

A carboxymethylated-sulfated (1–3)-β-D-glucan assigned as CS-PCS3-II was chemically synthesized from a (1–3)-β-D-glucan called PCS3-II. CS-PCS3-II contained sulfate and carboxymethyl groups with a degree of substitution of 0.36 and 1.05, respectively, and it existed as an extended flexible chain. An *in vivo* experiment exhibited that CS-PCS3-II significantly restrained the growth of mouse sarcoma 180 cells together with appeared signs of necrosis and apoptosis. The inhibitory rate of CS-PCS3-II was obviously higher than that of PCS3-II. Also, the CS-PCS2-II was capable of remarkably augmenting the indexes of the phagocyte and the thymus, the spleen index, the hemolytic activity, the spleen antibody production, and the delayed type of hypersensitivity (DTH), resulting in significant immunopotentiation in mice. More data suggested that the introduction of the carboxymethyl and sulfate groups to PCS3-II markedly improved its possible contact with the receptors of immune cells through hydrogen binding and electrostatic attraction, leading to stronger immunological responses that augment the inhibition of tumor cell proliferation.[33] S-CMP was a carboxymethylated-sulfated (1–3)-β-D-glucan derived from the sclerotium of *P. cocos* by another research group. Similarly, S-CMP displayed marked *in vivo* immunological activities and inhibition rate against HepG2 hepatoma in mice, with significant increases in serum hemolysin antibody titer, spleen antibody production, and DTH.[34]

Phosphorylated (1–3)-β-Glucan

When (1–3)-β-glucans prepared from the fungi were phosphorylated to have the extended chain conformation, the modified polysaccharides were phosphorylated (1–3)-β-glucans with relatively high molecular weight ranging from 2.6 × 10^4 to 2.68 × 10^5, which could augment the host immune system and exert potent *in vivo* anticancer activities at low dosages. Some phosphorylated (1–3)-β-glucans demonstrated relatively strong inhibition against sarcoma 180 cells *in vitro* and *in vivo*.[35]

Partially Depolymerized β-Glucan

A water-insoluble polysaccharide (PCS) obtained by alkaline extraction from *P. cocos* sclerotium was partially depolymerized by ultrasonication for 90 min to give PCS90. PCS90 (43 kDa) had a linear (1–3)-β-D-glucan and improved water solubility. In a mouse model implanted with SW620 colorectal cancer, PCS90 showed inhibitory effects toward the cell proliferation (IC_{50}: 32.2 μg/mL), whose activity was 5.26-fold greater than that of untreated β-D-glucan. The finding suggested that the ultrasonic treatment might be an effective method for promoting the properties of water-insoluble homoglycans.[36]

Heteropolysaccharides

Two water-soluble heteropolysaccharides designated as Pi-PCM1 and Pi-PCM2 were extracted from the *P. cocos* mycelia produced in fermentation with 0.9% NaCl or hot water, respectively. An extracellular heteropolysaccharide called Pi-PCM0 was obtained by supersonic extraction of the culture media. The three heteropolysaccharides are primarily composed of galactose, glucose, and mannose in their saccharide potions, and Pi-PCM1 and Pi-PCM2 existed as a compact random coil in an aqueous solution, close to a global shape. All three heteropolysaccharides demonstrated antitumor activities against mouse solid sarcoma 180 cells *in vivo* and against human HL-60 leukemia cells *in vitro*.[37–39] But the heteropolysaccharides prepared from Fu Ling mycelia cultured with the wild strain in a medium containing corn steep liquor exerted the highest antitumor activities against sarcoma 180 *in vivo*.[40]

Other Bioactivities

Fu Ling (Poria) is a commonly used herb in tradition Chinese medicinal practive. It demonstrated multiple therapeutic functions including diuretic, antigastric ulcer, hepatoprotective, immunoenhancing, sedative, hypoglycemic, antiaging, lithiasis-preventing, and leukocyte-raising properties besides anticancer and anticaricinogenesis.

References

1. Kwon, M. S. et al. 1999. Antimicrobial and antitumor activity of triterpenoids fraction from *Poria cocos* Wolf. *Han'guk Sikp'um Yongyang Kwahak Hoechi* 28: 1029–33.
2. Ukiya, M. et al. 2002. Inhibition of tumor-promoting effects by poricoic acids G and H and other lanostane-type triterpenes and cytotoxic activity of poricoic acids A and G from *Poria cocos*. *J. Nat. Prods.* 65: 462–5.

3. Akihisa, T. et al. 2007. Triterpene acids from *Poria cocos* and their antitumor-promoting effects. *J. Nat. Prods.* 70: 948–53.
4. Akihisa, T. et al. 2009. Antitumor-promoting effects of 25-methoxyporicoic acid A and other triterpene acids from *Poria cocos. J. Nat. Prods.* 72: 1786–92.
5. Akihisa, T. et al. 2007. Triterpene acids from *Poria cocos* and their anti-tumor-promoting effects. *J. Nat. Prods.* 70: 948–53.
6. Kaminaga, T. et al. 1996. Inhibitory effects of lanostane-type triterpene acids, the components of *Poria cocos*, on tumor promotion by 12-*O*-tetradecanoyl-phorbol-13-acetate in two-stage carcinogenesis in mouse skin. *Oncol.* 53: 382–5.
7. Kaminaga, T. et al. 1995. Inhibitory effect of triterpenes of *Poria cocos* on tumor promotion in mouse skin two-stage carcinogenesis. *Wakan Iyakugaku Zasshi* 12: 444–5.
8. Kikuchi, T. et al. 2011. Cytotoxic and apoptosis-inducing activities of triterpene acids from *Poria cocos. J. Nat. Prod.* 74: 137–44.
9. Li, G. et al. 2004. Cytotoxicity and DNA topoisomerases inhibitory activity of constituents from the sclerotium of *Poria cocos. Archiv. Pharm. Res.* 27: 829–33.
10. Cheng, S. J. et al. 2013. Triterpenes from *Poria cocos* suppress growth and invasiveness of pancreatic cancer cells through the downregulation of MMP-7. *Intl. J. Oncol.* 42: 1869–74.
11. Cheng, S. J. et al. 2015. Pachymic acid inhibits growth and induces apoptosis of pancreatic cancer in vitro and in vivo by targeting ER stress. *PLoS One* 10: e0122270/1-20.
12. Zhou, L. et al. 2008. Cytotoxic and antioxidant activities of lanostane-type triterpenes isolated from *Poria cocos. Chem. Pharma. Bull.* 56: 1459–62.
13. Gapter, L. L. et al. 2005. Induction of apoptosis in prostate cancer cells by pachymic acid from *Poria cocos. Biochem. Biophys. Res. Commun.* 332: 1153–61.
14. Jeong, J. W. et al. 2015. Pachymic acid induces apoptosis of EJ bladder cancer cells by DR5 up-regulation, ROS generation, modulation of Bcl-2 and IAP family members. *Phytother. Res.* 29: 1516–24.
15. Mizushina, Y. et al. 2004. A novel DNA topoisomerase inhibitor: Dehydroebriconic acid, one of the lanostane-type triterpene acids from *Poria cocos. Cancer Sci.* 95: 354–60.
16. Akihisa, T. et al. 2005. Dehydrotrametenonic acid, and DNA polymerase and DNA topo-isomerase inhibitors containing it. *Jpn. Kokai Tokkyo Koho* JP 2003–197516 20030716.
17. Kang, H. M. et al. 2006. Dehydrotrametenolic acid selectively inhibits the growth of H-ras transformed rat2 cells and induces apoptosis through caspase-3 pathway. *Life Sci.* 78: 607–13.
18. Kwon, B. M. et al. 2006. Anticancer composition comprising 3β-hydroxylanosta-7,9(11), 24-trien-21-oic acid isolated from *Poria cocos* for inhibiting expression of oncogenes. *Repub. Korean Kongkae Taeho Kongbo* KR 2004-69077 20040831.
19. Ke, R. D. et al. 2010. Analysis of chemical composition of polysaccharides from *Poria cocos* Wolf and its antitumor activity by NMR spectroscopy. *Carbohydr. Polym.* 80: 31–4.
20. Kanayama, H. et al. 1986. Studies on the antitumor active polysaccharides from the mycelia of *Poria cocos* Wolf. III. Antitumor activity against mouse tumors. *Yakugaku Zasshi* 106: 307–12.
21. Zhang, M. et al. 2006. Growth-inhibitory effects of a β-glucan from the mycelium of *Poria cocos* on human breast carcinoma MCF-7 cells: Cell-cycle arrest and apoptosis induction. *Oncol. Reports* 15: 637–43.
22. Chen, Y. Y. et al. 2004. Antiproliferative and differentiating effects of polysaccharide fraction from fu-ling (*Poria cocos*) on human leukemic U937 and HL-60 cells. *Food Chem. Toxicol.* 42: 759–69.
23. Kanayama, H. et al. 1986. Studies on the antitumor active polysaccharides from the mycelia of *Poria cocos* Wolf. II. Structural of antitumor polysaccharide H11. *Yakugaku Zasshi* 106: 206–11.
24. Kanayama, H. et al. 1983. A new antitumor polysaccharide from the mycelia of *Poria cocos* Wolf. *Chem. Pharm. Bull.* 31: 1115–8.
25. Ding, Q. et al. 1998. Influence of molecular weight and periodate modification of β-D-glucans from *Poria cocos* sclerotium on antitumor activities. *Chin. J. Polymer Sci.* 16: 62–6.
26. Wang, Y. F. et al. 2004. Correlation of structure to antitumor activities of five derivatives of a β-glucan from *Poria cocos* sclerotium. *Carbohydrate Res.* 339: 2567–74.
27. Wang, Y. F. et al. 2005. Chemical structure and antitumor activity of sulfated derivatives of water-insoluble polysaccharide isolated from *Poria cocos. Polym. Preprints (Am. Chem. Soc., Div. Polym. Chem.)* 46: 605–6.
28. Wang, Y. F. et al. 2007. Solution properties of antitumor sulfated derivatives of β-D-glucan from *Poria cocos. Abstracts of Papers, 233rd ACS Natl. Meet., Chicago, IL*, March 25–29, POLY-513.
29. Huang, Q. L. et al. 2006. Evaluation of sulfated α-glucans from *Poria cocos* mycelia as potential antitumor agent. *Carbohydr. Polym.* 64: 337–44.
30. Lin, Y. L. et al. 2004. Molecular mass antitumor activities of sulfated derivatives of α-glucan from *Poria cocos* mycelia. *Intl. J. Biol. Macromol.* 34: 289–94.
31. Li, Y. Q. et al. 2012. Correlation between structure and anti-gastric adenocarcinoma activity of β-D-glucan isolated from *Poria cocos* sclerotium. *Shijie Huaren Xiaohua Zazhi* 20: 1277–83.
32. Li, Y. Q. et al. 2012. The inhibition effect study of sulfated derivatives polysaccharides from sclerotium of *Poria cocos* for nude mice gastric adenocarcinoma. *Shiyong Linchuang Yiyao Zazhi* 16: 1–4.
33. Chen, X. Y. et al. 2010. Immunopotentiation and antitumor activity of carboxymethylated-sulfated β-(1–3)-D-glucan from *Poria cocos. Intl. Immunopharmacol.* 10: 398–405.
34. Wang, H. L. et al. 2015. In vivo immunological activity of carboxymethylated-sulfated (1–3)-β-D-glucan from sclerotium of *Poria cocos. Intl. J. Biol. Macromol.* 79: 511–7.
35. Chen, X. Y. et al. 2009. Chain conformation and antitumor activities of phosphorylated (1–3)-β-D-glucan from *Poria cocos. Carbohydr. Polym.* 78: 581–7.
36. Chen, J. L. et al. 2015. Preparation and structural characterization of a partially depolymerized β-glucan obtained from *Poria cocos* sclerotium by ultrasonic treatment. *Food Hydrocoll.* 46: 1–9.
37. Huang, Q. L. et al. 2007. Structure, molecular size and antitumor activities of polysaccharides from *Poria cocos* mycelia produced in fermenter. *Carbohydr. Polym.* 70: 324–33.
38. Zhang, L. N. et al. 2005. Effect of molecular mass on antitumor activity of heteropolysaccharide from *Poria cocos. Biosci. Biotech. Biochem.* 69: 631–4.
39. Huang, Q. L. et al. 2007. Structure, molecular size and antitumor activities of polysaccharides from *Poria cocos* mycelia produced in fermenter. *Carbohydr. Polym.* 70: 324–33.
40. Jin, Y. et al. 2003. Antitumor activities of heteropolysaccharides of *Poria cocos* mycelia from different strains and culture media. *Carbohydrate Res.* 338: 1517–21.

190 Yuan Hua 芫花

Lilac daphne

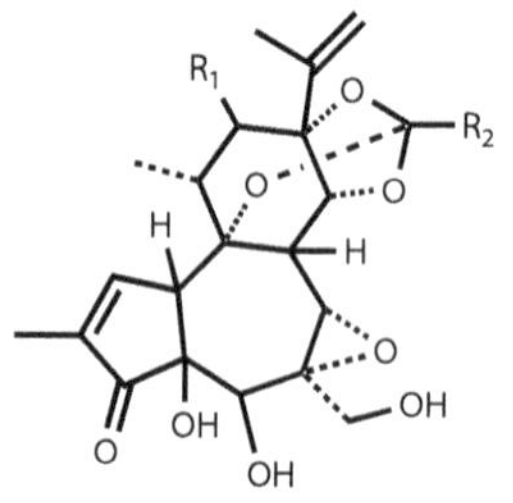

1. R_1 = -OOCPh, R_2 = -A
2. R_1 = -OAc, R_2 = -A
3. R_1 = $-OOCCH_2CH_3$, R_2 = -A
4. R_1 = $-OOCCH_2CH_2CH_3$, R_2 = -A
7. R_1 = -OOCPh, R_2 = -Ph
A = $-CH=CHCH=CHCH_2CH_2CH_2CH_2CH_3$

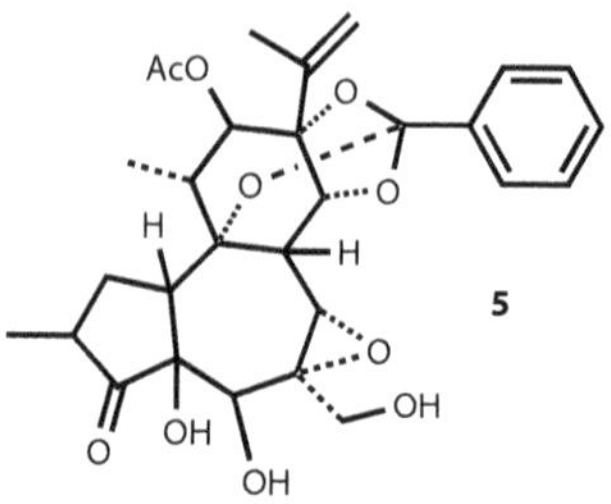

Herb Origination

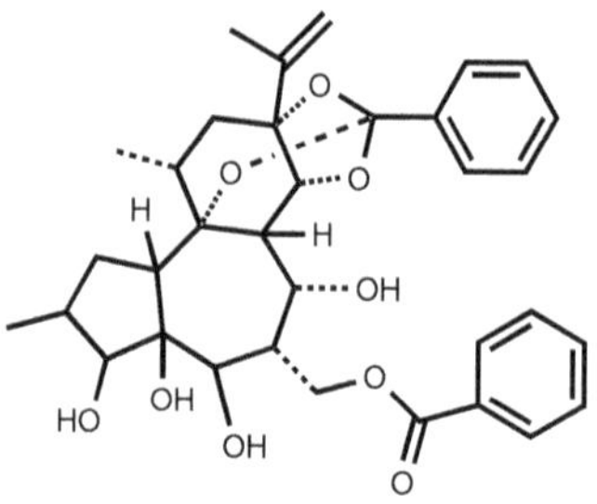

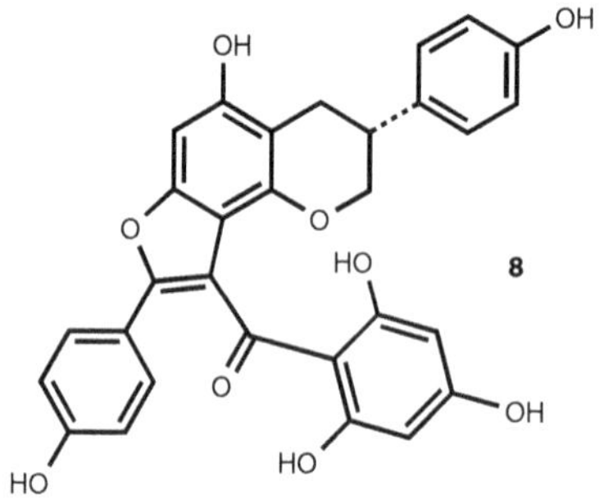

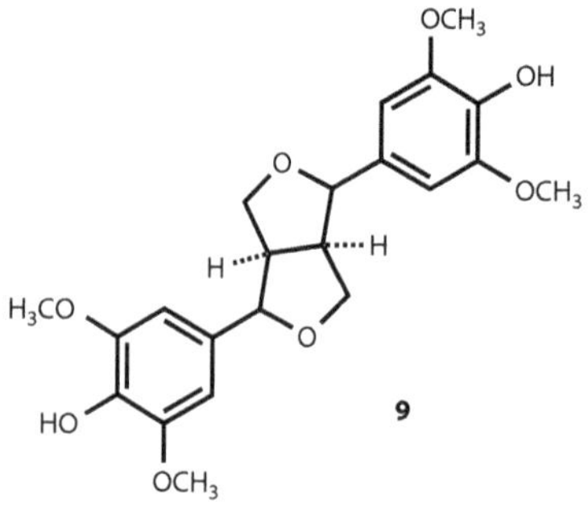

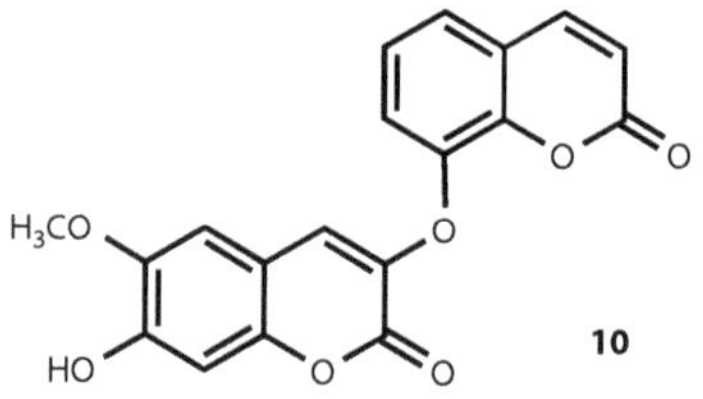

The herb Yuan Hua (Lilac daphne) is the dried flower bud of a Thymelaeaceae shrub, *Daphne genkwa* Sieb. et Zucc. The poisonous plant is native to the east Asian region (China, Korea, and Japan). In China, it is widely distributed in the regions of the Yangtze and Yellow Rivers. The buds are collected in spring before the flowers bloom and dried in the sun for the folk medical practice. Its root is commonly used as another herb in Chinese natural remedy.

Antitumor Constituents and Activity

Both the flower bud and the root of Yuan Hua are poisonous but were used in the treatment of carcinoma diseases in the last decade. The constituents in *Daphne genkwa* were found to be diterpenes, flavonoids, coumarins, chlorogenic acids, and lignans. The isolated daphnane-type diterpene esters are the major bioactive constituents in response to the antineoplastic property. Several flavonoid and lignan components derived from the plant were also reported to display moderate inhibitory effect against some carcinoma cell lines.

Diterpene Esters

By the extensive approaches, more than 23 daphnane-type diterpenes were discovered in Yuan Hua, and most of these diterpene esters were cytotoxic to carcinomas. By high performance liquid chromatography (HPLC) analysis, yuanhuacine (**1**) and yuanhuadine (**2**) were identified to be the principal diterpenoids, whose average content rates were 0.0020% and 0.0078% in its flower buds and 0.0151% and 0.0033% in its roots, respectively.[1] In the earlier *in vitro* studies, yuanhuacine (**1**) (= gnidilatidin) had been shown to possess potent suppressive activity against P388 and L1210 (leukemic), A549 (lung), KB (nasopharynx), and A375 (skin) cancer cell lines, whereas yuanhuadine (**2**), genkwanine-B and genkwanine-D were markedly effective in the inhibition of P388 leukemia cells (IC_{50}: 0.15–8.4 μM), whose mechanisms were correlated with the blockage of DNA and protein synthesis and the attenuation of DNA Topo activity.[2,3]

All the 23 isolated diterpenoids displayed the inhibitory effect on HT-1080 fibrosarcoma cells. Yuanhuadine (**2**), yuanhuapine (**5**), genkwadaphnine (**7**), simplexin, yuanhuafine, and genkwanine-M exerted the strongest effect on the HT-1080 cells (IC_{50}: <0.1 μM) and genkwadane-B, genkwadane-D, pimelotide-A, yuanhuacine (**1**), and yuanhuaoate-B were cytotoxic to the cells at the respective IC_{50} levels of 9.56, 7.71, 4.55, 0.83, 2.02, and 0.59 μM, compared with 5-FU (IC_{50}: 35.62 μM). Especially, yuanhuatine, yuanhuaoate-B, pimelotide-C, yuanhuadine (**2**), yuanhuacine (**1**), and genkwadaphnine (**7**) were cytotoxic to MCF-7 breast cancer cells (IC_{50}: 0.37–7.36 μM),[4] whereas yuanhuacine (**1**) and isoyuanhuadine exerted the inhibition on the HeLa cells (IC_{50}: 5.56 and 0.64 μM, respectively). The *in vitro* assay also showed that yuanhuacine (**1**), yuanhuatine, and genkwanine-M obviously retarded the growth of A375-S2 melanoma cells (IC_{50}: 3.62–9.31 μM), and yuanhuacine (**1**) exerted antihepatoma effect against HepG2 cells (IC_{50}: 8.04 μM).[4] The antigrowth effects were further shown in other human solid cancer cell lines, giving the IC_{50} values of yuanhuadine (**2**) as 7.4 μM in PC3 (prostate) cells, 10.2 and 11.8 μM in HCT-116 and SW480 (colon) cells, 2 μg/mL in Colo205 (colon) cells, 12.7 μM in T47D (breast) cells, 12.9 μM on SKHEP-1 (liver), >20 μM in SNU-638 (gastric) cells, and 10–19 μg/mL in HT-29, MDA-MB-231, Huh 7, AGS, A2058, and B16 cells,[5] and the IC_{50} values of yuanhuacine (**1**) were 3 μg/mL in Colo205 cells and 15–23 μg/mL in HT-29, MDA-MB-231, A2058, AGS, and B16 cells.[6] By upregulating p21 expression via a p53 protein-independent cascade, yuanhuacine (**1**) arrested the cell cycle of T24T (bladder) and HCT116 (colon) human cancer cells at G2/M stage.[7] In human squamous cell carcinoma (SCC12 and SCC13) cells, genkwadaphnin (**7**) triggered ROS-mediated apoptosis through the activation of JNK/p38 MAPK pathways.[8]

More assays confirmed that yuanhuadine (**2**), yuanhuahine (**3**), yuanhualine (**4**), yuanhuapine (**5**), yuanhuagine, yuanhuafine, genkwanine-D, genkwanine-H, and genkwanine-J, exerted moderate cytotoxicity on human A549 lung cancer cells (IC_{50}: 12–53 nM) but relatively noncytotoxic on human MRC-5 normal lung epithelial cells.[9] In the treated A549 cells, the diterpenoids (yuanhuadine (**2**), yuanhuahine (**3**), yuanhualine (**4**), and yuanhuapine) markedly promoted the apoptotic death in association with the suppression of Akt/mTOR and EGFR signaling pathways and caused the cell cycle arrest at G0/G1 and G2/M phases in association with the activation of p21 and p53 and the decline of cyclin-A, cyclin-B1, and cyclin-E, CDK-2 and CDK-4, Rb phosphorylation, and c-Myc expressions. The diterpenoids (yuanhuadine (**2**), yuanhuahine (**3**), yuanhualine (**4**), and yuanhuapine) also blocked the signal transduction in the A549 cells via the inhibition of Akt, STAT3, and Src, thereby restraining the proliferation of A549 cells.[5,10] The anti-growth effect of yuanhuadine (**2**) was also observed in other human NSCLC cell lines (IC_{50}: <1–9.1 μM). Specifically, the NSCLC cell lines (A549, H292, H1993, and SK-MES-1) were more sensitive to yuanhuadine (**2**) than other NSCLC cell lines (H1299 and H358).[5] *In vivo* experiments correspondingly confirmed the anticancer effect of yuanhuadine (**2**). The oral administration of yuanhuadine (**2**) in a dose of 0.5 mg/kg/day for 14 days markedly inhibited the tumor growth in athymic xenograft nude mice implanted with the A549 lung cancer, without overt toxicity.[5] The i.p. injection of yuanhuacine (**1**) and genkwadaphnin (**7**) to Lewis lung carcinoma-inoculated mice at a dose of 0.5 mg/kg/day, respectively, resulted in the growth suppressive rates of 45.8% and 63.1%.[11] Moreover, through its antiEGFR effect, yuanhuadine (**2**) was also able to overcome the drug resistance and to augment the cytotoxic effect of anticancer drugs on gemcitabine- or gefitinib-resistant A549 lung cancer cells and gefitinib- or erlotinib-resistant H292 lung mucoepidermoid carcinoma cells.[5,10] Similarly, the synergistic inhibition was achieved by yuanhualine (**4**) when combined with gemcitabine, gefitinib, or erlotinib on the A549 cells.[12]

The antileukemia effect was accomplished by yuanhuacine (**1**), genkwanin-I (**6**), and genkwadaphnin (**7**). The diterpenoids moderately restrained the growth of human HL-60 promyelocytic leukemia cells at the IC_{50} levels of 11.74–12.90 μM. Both yuanhuacine (**1**) and genkwadaphnin (**7**) demonstrated the capacity to activate the apoptotic process via the cleavage of procaspase-3 and PARP into active forms and the decrease of Bcl-2 and Bcl-xL expressions and the increase of Bax expression in the HL-60 cells.[10,11] Both diterpenes (yuanhuacine (**1**) and genkwadaphnin (**7**)) also obstructed the syntheses of DNA and protein and exerted significant antileukemic activity at a low dose against P388 and L1210 leukemia cells *in vitro*.[13,14] Genkwadane-D exerted the antileukemia effect on K562 cells (IC_{50}: 5.11 μM).[4] Recently, more highly oxygenated daphnane-type diterpene esters have been discovered from the flower buds of *D. genkwa*. Genkwanine N 20-palmitate exhibited cytotoxic activity against A549 (lung) and HepG2 (liver) neoplastic cell lines, whereas neogenkwanines-C–E exerted the growth inhibitory effects on Hep3B hepatoma cells (IC_{50}: 7.61–8.35 μM), HL-60 leukemia cells (IC_{50}: 10.07–11.17 μM), and U87 cells (IC_{50}: 27.11–47.60 μM).[15,16]

The remarkable findings suggest that the daphnane-type diterpenoids might be chemotherapeutic drug leads for the development and the design of novel agents to fight human malignant tumors. However, yuanhuacine (**1**), yuanhuadine (**2**), and genkwanine-D, genkwanine-H, and genkwanine-J, exhibited notable inhibition on normal human mammary epithelial cells (IC_{50}: 2.9–15.0 μM) and had no such effect on normal human MRC-5 lung epithelial cells.[3,9]

Relationship of Structure–Activity

The analysis of the data obtained from the cytotoxicity of the 23 daphnane-type diterpenes in 10 human neoplactic cell lines figured out the structure–bioactivity-related informatics showed the following: (1) the presence of a 1,10 double bond will reduce the anticancer activity; (2) opening of the 6,7-epoxide group is detrimental to the inhibitory activity; (3) replacing an aromatic group with an unsaturated alkyl group in an orthoester chain enhances the anticancer activity; and (4) the benzoyl moiety is an important pharmacophore of inhibitory activity.[4] A systematic investigation demonstrated that most of the daphnane-type diterpenes restrained the four tumor cell lines (HL-60, A549, Hep3B, and U87).[17] Because genkwanines-A–I have the same basic backbone with an orthoester group, their effects on the tumor cells and the endothelium cells were revealed to be obviously related to the acyloxyl groups at some specific locations, such as (1) acyloxyl groups at C-3/C-20 are necessary for the cytotoxicity on tumor cells and the inhibitory effect on endothelium cells; (2) a benzoyloxy group at C-3/C-20 shows better inhibitory effect than a fatty acyloxy group, and the fatty acyloxy group with less unsaturation markedly attenuates the antitumor activity; (3) the absence of an orthoester group is detrimental to the antitumor activity; and (4) the molecules with a 6,7-epoxyl group show more potent anticancer activity, but a long-chain fatty orthoester group showed more cytotoxicity against human normal mammary endothelium cells.[3]

In addition, five daphnane-type diterpene esters such as yuanhuacine (**1**), yuanhuadine (**2**), yuanhuapine (**5**), yuanhuajine, and yuanhuagine are also inhibitors of DNA Topo-I at the IC_{50} levels of 38.0–53.4 μM. The orthoester group in these structures seems to be necessary for the inhibitory activity against the DNA Topo-I and the DNA Topo-I inhibitory property involved in the antitumor mechanisms of the daphnane-type diterpene esters.[18] Taken together, the scientific data provide valuable information for the design and the semisynthesis of drug candidates on the basis of the daphnane-type diterpenes for cancer therapy.

Flavonoids

The total flavonoids from the roots of *D. genkwa* were demonstrated to possess anticarcinoma, antimetastasis, and immunostimulating properties in the *in vitro* experiments. The oral administration of the total flavonoids to tumor-bearing mice for 14 days resulted in a considerable suppression against the growth of S180 sarcoma in doses of 25–75 mg/kg/day and an inhibition on the growth and metastasis of Lewis lung cancer in doses of 40–80 mg/kg/day for 14 days. Simultaneously, the *in vivo* treatment significantly enhanced lymphocyte proliferation and the cytolytic activity of NK cells and protected host immunocyte viability and peripheral lymphocytes from tumor-induced reduction. HPLC analysis revealed the total flavonoids contain daphnodorin-B, daphnodorin-G, and daphnodorin-H, daphnodorin-G 3′-methyl ether, daphnodorin-H 3′-methyl ether, and its 3-methyl ether, genkwanol-A, genkwanin, and yuenkani, and daphnodorin-B (**8**). But the separated flavonoids only had weak cytotoxicity on the tumor cell lines (S180, LLC, HeLa, HA-116, and MCF-7) *in vitro*. According to the results, the immunoenhancing activity of the total flavonoids was considered to be mostly responsible for the *in vivo* antitumor and antimetastasis effects.[19–21]

Lignans

A furofuran-type lignan identified as (−)-syringaresinol (**9**) was isolated from the dried flower buds of *D. genkwa*, which inhibited the proliferation of human HL-60 promyelocytic leukemia cells (IC_{50}: 5.8 μM). By amplifying the expressions of CDKi proteins (such as p21cip1/waf1 and p27kip1) with a simultaneous decrease of the expressions of CDK-2, CDK-4, CDK-6, cyclin-D1, cyclin-D2, and cyclin-E, it arrested the cell cycle of HL-60 cells at G1 phase. The proapoptotic process by syringaresinol (**9**) was correlated with a series of morphological changes such as cytochrome c release, activation of caspases, and PARP cleavage. The evidences indicated that (−)-syringaresinol (**9**) is one of the contributors for the cancer suppressive property of Yuan Hua.[22]

Coumarins

Daphnoretin (**10**) is a *bis*-coumarin derivative isolated from the herbal plant. Its antitumor activity was confirmed in the *in vitro* and *in vivo* models with Ehrlich ascites carcinoma. Dosing daphnoretin (**10**) for three days at 6 mg/kg per day could markedly diminish the cell number per milliliter by 60% along with blockage of the synthesis of the protein and the DNA in the Ehrlich cells.[23–25] Along with the induction of G2/M cell arrest and apoptosis, daphnoretin (**10**) exerted the antiproliferative effect against human osteosarcoma cells (IC_{50}: 3.89 μM, 72 h). The G2/M phase arrest was mediated by the downregulation of CDC2, cyclin-A, and cyclin-B1 expressions, and the apoptosis was followed by caspase-3-activating pathway including decrease of Bcl-2 expression and increase of Bax level and release of mitochondrial cytochrome c.[25] In addition, daphnoretin (**10**) was also able to retard the hepatitis B surface antigen expression in human Hep3B hepatoma cells.[26]

Other Medicinal Uses

The herb Yuan Hua (Lilac daphne) is a Chinese herbal medicine that has been traditionally used as the agents for analgesic, anti-inflammation, anticonvulsion, diuretic, antitussive, expectorant, anthelminthic, and abortifacient purposes.

References

1. Zhang, S. X. et al. 2007. Evaluation of *Daphne genkwa* diterpenes: Fingerprint and quantitative analysis by high performance liquid chromatography. *Phytochem. Analysis* 18: 91–7.
2. Hall, I. H. et al. 1986. The effects of genkwadaphnin and gnidilation on the growth of P388, L1210 leukemia and KB carcinoma cells in vitro. *Eur. J. Cancer Clin. Oncol.* 22: 45–51.
3. Zhan, Z. J. et al. 2005. Novel diterpenoids with potent inhibitory activity against endothelium cell HMEC and cytotoxic activities from a well-known TCM plant *Daphne genkwa*. *Bioorg. Med. Chem*, 13: 645–55.
4. Li, F. F. et al. 2013. Daphnane-type diterpenes with inhibitory activities against human cancer cell lines from *Daphne genkwa*. *Bioorg. Med. Chem. Lett.* 23: 2500–4.
5. Hong, J. Y. et al. 2011. Growth inhibition of human lung cancer cells via down-regulation of epidermal Growth factor receptor signaling by Yuanhuadine, a daphnane diterpene from *Daphne genkwa*. *J. Nat. Prod.* 74: 2102–8.
6. Li, S. et al. 2013. Isolation of anticancer constituents from flos genkwa (*Daphne genkwa* Sieb.et Zucc.) through bioassay-guided procedures. *Chem. Central J.* 7: 159/1–9.
7. Zhang, R. W. et al. 2014. The Chinese herb isolate yuanhuacine (YHL-14) induces G2/M arrest in human cancer cells by up-regulating p21 protein expression through an p53 protein-independent cascade. *J. Biol. Chem.* 289: 6394–403.
8. Li, Z. J. et al. 2014. Genkwadaphnin induces reactive oxygen species (ROS)-mediated apoptosis of squamous cell carcinoma (SCC) cells. *Biochem. Biophy. Res. Commun.* 450: 1115–9.
9. Hong, J. Y. et al. 2010. Daphnane diterpene esters with anti-proliferative activities against human lung cancer cells from *Daphne genkwa*. *Chem. Pharm. Bull.* 58: 234–7.
10. Jo, S. K. et al. 2012. Anticancer activity of novel daphnane diterpenoids from *Daphne genkwa* through cell-cycle arrest and suppression of Akt/STAT/Src signalings in human lung cancer cells. *Biomol. Therap.* 20: 513–9.
11. Park, B. Y. et al. 2007. Daphnane diterpene esters isolated from flower buds of *Daphne genkwa* induce apoptosis in human myelocytic HL-60 cells and suppress tumor growth in Lewis lung carcinoma (LLC)-inoculated mouse model. *J. Ethnopharmacol.* 111: 496–503.
12. Li, L. Z. et al. 2010. A novel daphnane-type diterpene from the flower bud of *Daphne genkwa*. *Chem. Nat. Compds.* 46: 380–2.
13. Liou, Y. F. et al. 1982. Antitumor agents LVI: The protein synthesis inhibition by genkwadaphnin and yuanhuacine of P388 lymphocytic leukemia cells. *J. Pharm. Sci.* 71: 1340–4.
14. Kasai, R. J. et al. 1981. Antitumor agents: Part 40. Genkwadaphnin, a potent antileukemic diterpene from *Daphne genkwa*. *Phytochem.* 20: 2592–4.
15. Jiang, H. L. et al. 2015. A new highly oxygenated daphnane diterpene esters from the flower buds of *Daphne genkwa*. *Nat. Prod. Res.* 29: 1878–83.

16. Li, L. Z. et al. 2015. Neogenkwanines A–H: Daphnane-type diterpenes containing 4,7 or 4,6-ether groups from the flower bud of *Daphne genkwa*. *RSC Adv*. 5: 4143–52.
17. Li, F. F. et al. 2012. Systematic studies on chemical constituents from *Daphne genkwa*. *Planta Med. (11th Annual Oxford Int. Conf. Sci. Bot.)* 78: P59.
18. Zhang, S. X. et al. 2006. Preparation of yuanhuacine and relative daphne diterpene esters from *Daphne genkwa* and structure–activity relationship of potent inhibitory activity against DNA topoisomerase I. *Bioorg. Med. Chem*. 14: 3888–95.
19. Zheng, W. F. et al. 2007. Total flavonoids of *Daphne genkwa* root significantly inhibit the growth and metastasis of Lewis lung carcinoma in C57BL6 mice. *Intl. Immunopharmacol*. 7: 117–27.
20. Zheng, W. F. et al. 2007. Antitumor activity of daphnodorins from *Daphne genkwa* roots. *Intl. Immunopharmacol*. 7: 128–34.
21. Wei, Z. W. et al. 2008. Antitumor activities of total flavonoids from the roots of *Daphne genkwa*. *Pharm. J. Chinese People's Liberation Army* 24: 116–20.
22. Park, B. Y. et al. 2008. (-)-Syringaresinol inhibits proliferation of human promyelocytic HL-60 leukemia cells via G1 arrest and apoptosis. *Intl. Immunopharmacol*. 8: 967–73.
23. Diogo, C. V. et al. 2009. Mitochondrial toxicity of the phyotochemicals daphnetoxin and daphnoretin-relevance for possible anticancer application. *Toxicol. in Vitro* 23: 772–9.
24. Hall, I. H. et al. 1982. Antitumor agents LIII: The effects of daphnoretin on nucleic acid and protein synthesis of Ehrlich ascites tumor cells. *J. Pharma. Sci*. 71: 741–4.
25. Gu, S. B. et al. 2012. Daphnoretin induces cell cycle arrest and apoptosis in human osteosarcoma (HOS) cells. *Mol*. 17: 598–612.
26. Chen, H. C. et al. 1996. Identification of a protein kinase C activator, dephnoretin, that suppresses hepatitis B virus gene expression in human hepatoma cells. *Biochem. Pharmacol*. 52: 1025–32.

191 Ze Qi 澤漆

Sun spurge

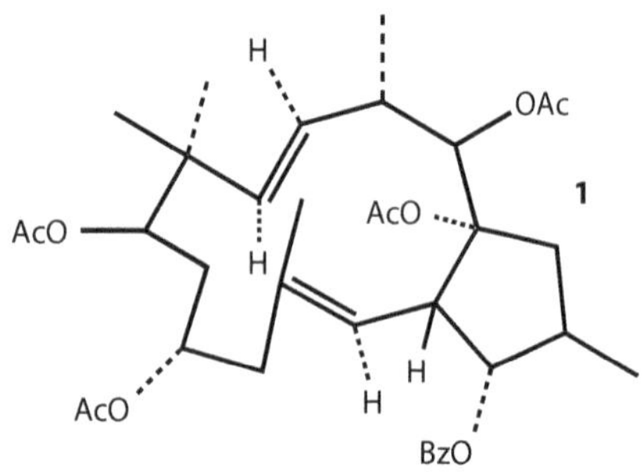

Herb Origination

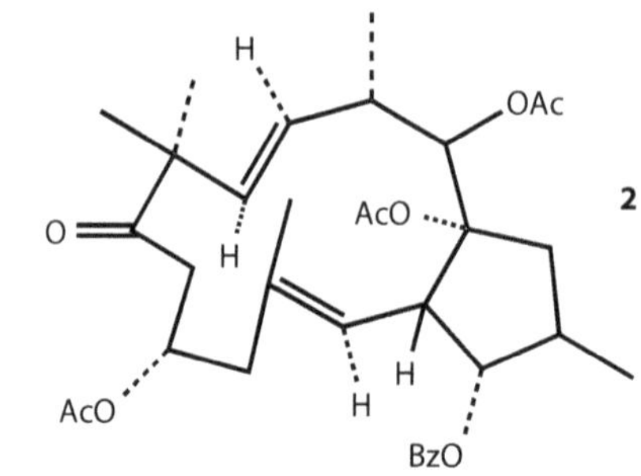

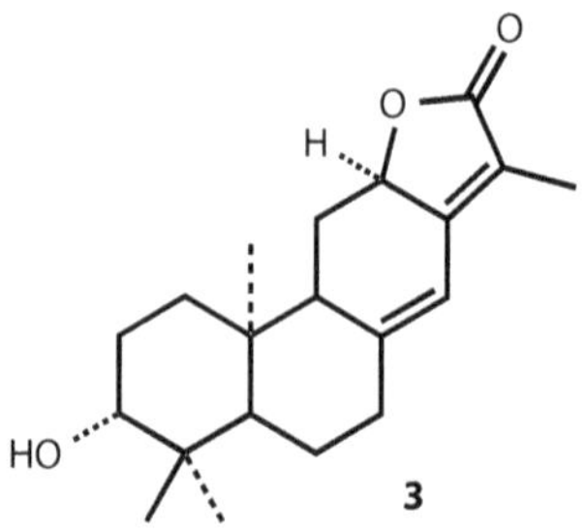

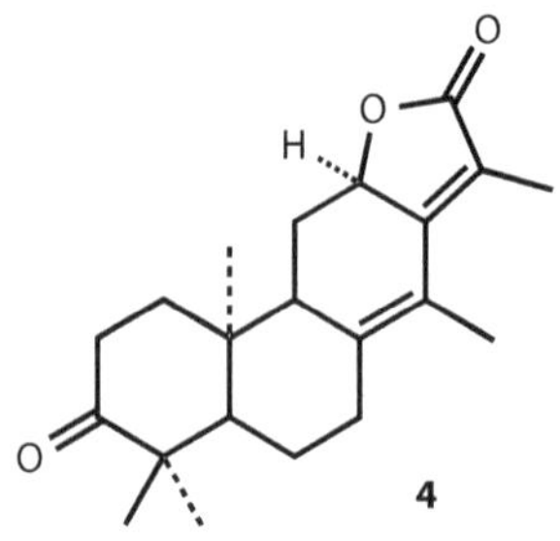

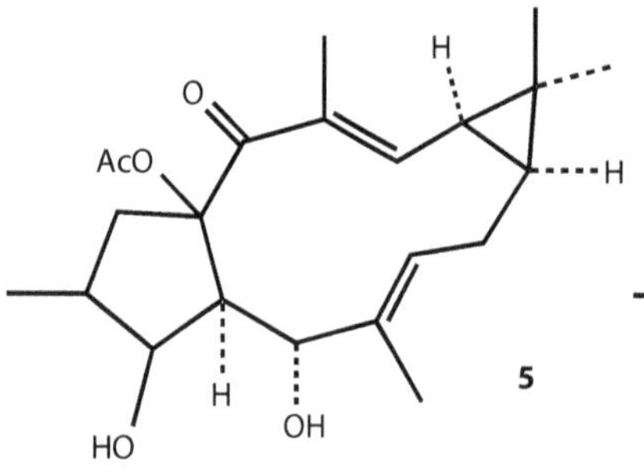

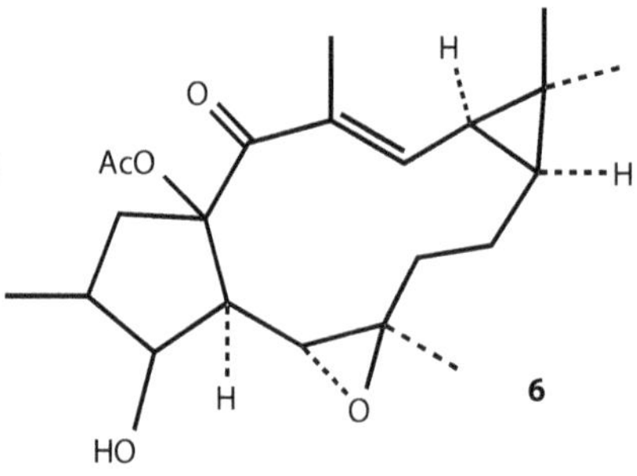

The herb Ze Qi (Sun spurge) originated from the entire plant *Euphorbia helioscopia* L. (Euphorbiaceae). This annual herbaceous plant is native to most of Europe, northern Africa, and eastward through most of Asia. Its distribution is very wide in China except for the Tibet province. The plant is collected during the flower season of April and May and dried in the sun.

Antitumor Activities

Early studies showed that the Ze Qi extract inhibited the growth of mouse L160 leukemia, sarcoma 180, and sarcoma 37 cell lines.[1] An aquatic extract derived from the Ze Qi roots was shown to have the suppressive effect on three neoplastic cell lines *in vitro*. The antigrowth rates after being treated with 4 mg/mL of the aquatic extract were 59.8%, 66.4%, and 70.5% on human SMMC-7721 (liver), HeLa (cervix), and MKN-45 (stomach) neoplastic cell lines, respectively.[2] Its EtOAc extract (EAE) at concentrations of 100–200 μg/mL elicited the G1 cell cycle arrest and the apoptosis of the SMMC-7721 cells, thereby markedly suppressing the proliferation of hepatoma cells in time- and dose-dependent manners. The EAE was also found to have an ability to exert dose-dependent suppressive effect on cancer cell invasion and MMP-9 expression. According to the high performance liquid chromatography-mass spectrometry (HPLC-MS) analyzed data, the major constituents of the EAE was revealed to be flavonoids.[3]

Additionally, a water extract of *E. helioscopia* not only restrained the growth of sarcoma 180 in mice but also elevated the indexes of the spleen and the thymus, the activation of SOD, and the reduction of MDA content in the serum, indicating that the antitumor activity was also closely associated with its abilities in inhibiting LPO, scavenging free radicals, and enhancing the immune system.[4]

Antitumor Constituents and Activities

Diterpenoids

From the Ze Qi extract, several cytotoxic macrocyclic diterpenoids were discovered. Euphornin (**1**) was cytotoxic to mouse LA795 lung adenocarcinoma cells *in vitro*, whereas euphornin-L (**1**) and euphoscopin-F (**2**) showed marked antiproliferative effect on human HL-60 leukemia cells (IC_{50}: 2.7 and 9.0 μM, respectively).[5,6] A jatrophane-type diterpenoid elucidated as helioscopinolide-A (**3**) as well as euphornin exerted the cytotoxic effect in HeLa (cervix) and MDA-MB-231 (breast) cancer cell lines *in vitro*. The respective IC_{50} values were 0.11 and 3.1 μM in the HeLa cells and 2.1 and 13.4 μM in the MDA-MB-231 cells.[7] Helioscopinolide-A and helioscopinolide-B also moderately restrained the growth of MCF-7 (breast), NCI-H460 (lung), and SF-268 (brain) human tumor cell lines *in vitro*.[8] Moreover, some of the diterpenoids isolated from Ze Qi were found to have notable capability to reverse MDR via the inhibition of the transport activities of P-gp and MRP1. Helioscopinolide-A (**3**), helioscopinolide-B, helioscopinolide-E (**4**), and helioscopinolide-F in a concentration range of 4–40 μg/mL exerted a dose-dependent anti-MDR effect in MRP1 gene-transfected mouse lymphoma cells,[9,10] and helioscopinolide-E (**4**) showed a selectivity toward a drug-resistant EPG85-257RD gastric cell line (IC_{50}: 4.4 μM).[11] Both helioscopinolide-B and helioscopinolide-E (**4**) were also found to be the effective inhibitors of P-gp-mediated transport of rhodamine 123 in multidrug-resistant mouse T lymphoma cells.[9,10] Furthermore, three isolated macrocyclic diterpenoids assigned as piscatoriol-A (**5**) and piscatoriol-B and 15-acetoxy-5,6-epoxylathyr-12-en-3-ol-14-one (**6**) were able to synergistically enhance the antiproliferative activity of DOX in human MDR1 gene-transfected mouse L5178Y T lymphoma cells, whose MDR-reversal effect was mediated by P-gp-independent cellular pathways responsible for MDR1.[11]

Phenolic Components

A group of commonly occurring phenolic compounds was isolated from the 50% acetone extract of *E. helioscopia*. Of them, gallic acid, methyl gallate, and ethyl gallate showed the antitumor metastasis activity (IC_{50}: 0.48, 4.57, and 4.61 μmol/L, respectively).[12]

Other Medicinal Uses

The herb Ze Qi (Sun spurge) demonstrated multiple pharmacological effects in the experimental studies. It was utilized in China for the clinical treatment of ascites, edema, tuberculosis, lymphoid, asthma, and tinea.

References

1. Qian, B. W. 1977. *Clinic Use of Chinese Folk Anticancer Drugs*, First Edition, pp. 1464. Shanghai People's Publisher, Shanghai, China.
2. Cai, Y. et al. 1999. Antitumor activity of the root of *Euphorbia helioscopia* in vitro. *Zhongyaocai* 22: 85–7.
3. Wang, Z. Y. et al. 2012. Anticancer potential of Euphorbia helioscopia L extracts against human cancer cells. *Anatomical Record* 295: 223–3.
4. Hu, Z. Z. et al. 2013. Antitumor effect of Euphorbia helioscopia extraction. *Food and Drug* 28: 330–1.
5. Chen, H. X. et al. 2012. Analysis of euphornin in Euphorbia helioscopia L. and its cytotoxicity to mice lung adenocarcinoma cells (LA795). *Nat. Prod. Res.* 26: 2112–6.
6. Tao, H. W. et al. 2008. Cytotoxic macrocyclic diterpenoids from *Euphorbia helioscopia*. *Archiv. Pharm. Res.* 31: 1547–51.
7. Lu, Z. Q. et al. 2008. Cytotoxic diterpenoids from *Euphorbia helioscopia*. *J. Nat. Prods.* 71: 873–6.
8. Valente, C. et al. 2004. Bioactive diterpenoids, a new jatrophane and two ent-abietanes, and other constituents from *Euphorbia pubescens*. *J. Nat. Prod.* 67: 902–4.
9. Ferreira, M. J. U. et al. 2005. Inhibition of P-glycoprotein transport activity in a resistant mouse lymphoma cell line by diterpenic lactones. *Anticancer Res.* 25: 3259–62.
10. Wesolowska, O. et al. 2007. Inhibition of MRP1 transport activity by phenolic and terpenic compounds isolated from Euphorbia species. *Anticancer Res.* 27: 4127–34.
11. Reis, M. A. et al. 2014. Diterpenes from *Euphorbia piscatoria*: Synergistic interaction of lathyranes with doxorubicin on resistant cancer cells. *Planta Med.* 80: 1739–45.
12. Yao, X. J. et al. 2013. Chemical constituents in *Euphorbia helioscopia* and their antitumor metastasis activities. *Xiandai Yaowu Yu Linchuang* 28: 826–9.

192 Gan Sui 甘遂

Kansui

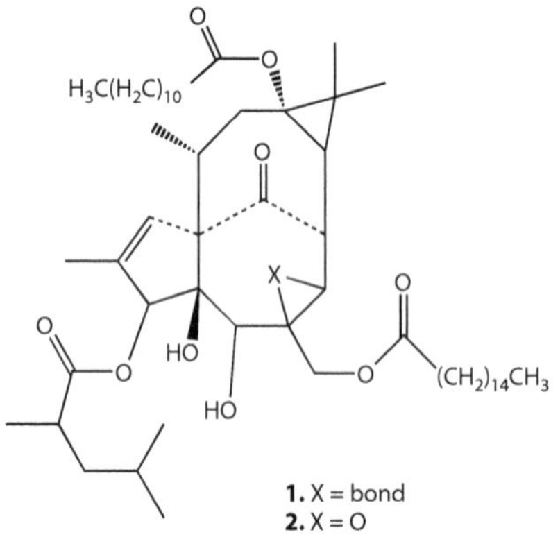

1. X = bond
2. X = O

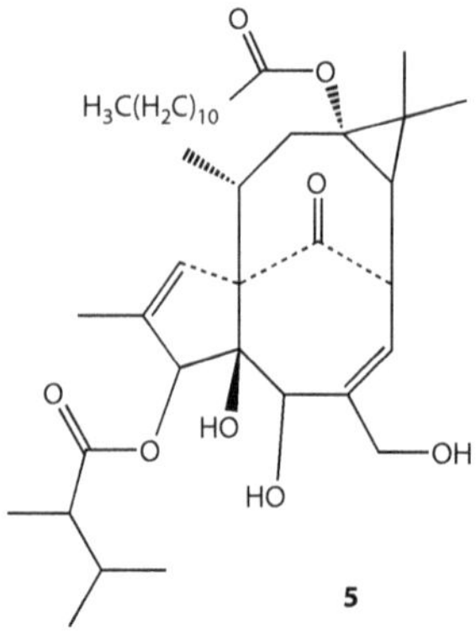

5

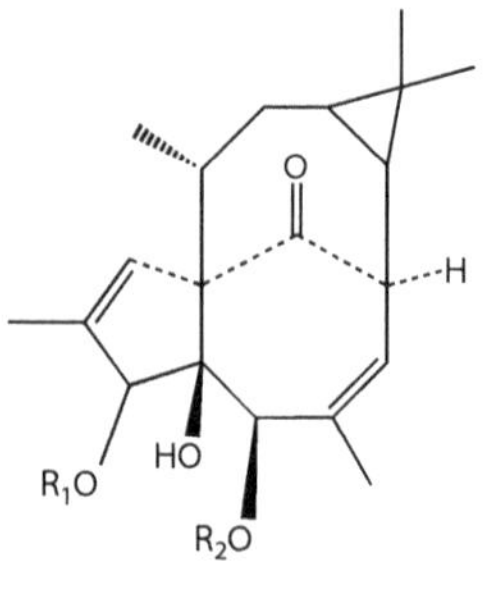

3. R_1 = Ac, R_2 = Bz
4. R_1 = Bz, R_2 = Ac
Bz: benzoyl

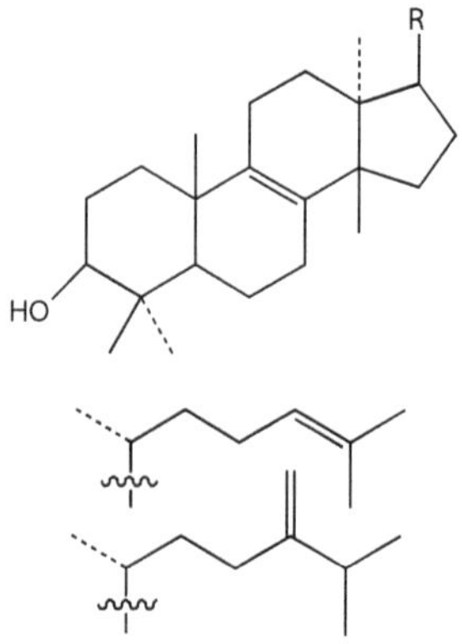

6. R =
7. R =

Herb Origination

The herb Gan Sui (Kansui) is one of the traditional Chinese drugs with a long medicinal history, which was documented in the first Chinese classic of materia medica titled as *Shennong Ben Cao Jing*. The herb is the dried root tuber of a Euphorbiaceae plant, *Euphorbia kansui*. This Chinese characteristic plant is primarily distributed in some of the north and west provinces of China. The roots are generally collected in spring just before flowering or in autumn when the aerial part is withered.

Antitumor Constituents and Activities

Gan Sui is a terpene-rich plant. Especially, diterpenoids are the major constituents in the herb, which are primarily responsible for the biological activities of Gan Sui. A few other components such as triterpenes and fatty acids from the herb also showed the antitumor potential.

Diterpenoids

Several anticancer ingenol-type diterpene esters including kansuiphorines-A–D were isolated from Gan Sui, which elicited the tumor growth inhibition, associated with the blockage of cell division and the induction of apoptosis in a variety of tumor cells.[1–5] Kansuiphorin-A (**1**) and kansuiphorin-B (**2**) displayed potent antileukemic activity in mice transplanted with P388 leukemia with T/C data greater than or equal to 176–177% at doses of 0.1 and 0.5 mg/kg. The cytotoxic effect of kansuiphorin-A (**1**) was also shown in a panel of human carcinoma cell lines, including leukemia (Molt-4, HL-60, TB, and K562), NSCLC (H-322 and HOP-62), melanoma (SK-MEL-5, RPMI-7951, and Maime-3M), kidney cancer (A498, A-704, and SN-12 K1), and colon cancer (SW-620), *in vitro*.[1,2] The ED_{50} values of kansuiphorine-C (**3**) and kansuiphorine-D (**4**) were 2.1–5.8 µg/mL in murine P388 and L1210 leukemia cells but were invalid to human A549 lung cancer, KB nasopharyngeal carcinoma, and HCT-8 colon cancer cell lines.[5] More isolated ingenol-type diterpenoids such as 5-*O*-(2′E,4′E-decadienoyl)-20-*O*-acetylingenol, 5-*O*-(2′E,4′Z-decadienoyl)-20-*O*-acetyl-ingenol, 20-*O*-(2′E,4′E-decadienoyl)-20-*O*-acetylingenol, and 3-*O*-(2,3-dimethylbutanoyl)-13-*O*-dodecanoylingenol (**5**) exhibited moderate cytotoxicities on BGC-823 and SGC-7901 (stomach), Bel-7402 (liver), and/or Bel-7402/5FU (drug-resistant) neoplastic cell lines, where the IC_{50} values of **5** were 0.84, 2.37, 9.58, and 1.95 µM, respectively. Interestingly, the antihepatoma activity on the drug-resistant Bel-7402/5FU cells was 4.7-fold more potent than on the Bel-7402 cells.[6]

Moreover, kansuinin-B, 20-OD-ingenol-Z, and 20-OD-ingenol-E exerted marked suppressive effect against the proliferations of isolated embryonic cell lines including murine MMT breast cancer, LC-549 testicular tumor, and 3T3 Swiss albino fibroblast cells.[7] 20-O-Ingenol-EZ has the abilities to restrain the proliferation of MMT-cells and arrest the cell cycle at G2/M stage.[8,9] The antiproliferative effect 3EZ,20Ac-ingenol on DT40 chicken-B cells was mediated by eliciting G2/M cell arrest and apoptosis via the decrease of p-Akt expression, the breakage of DNA double-strand, and the activation of caspase-3.[10] Some of the diterpenoids effectively obstructed the proliferation of human SGC-7901 gastric cancer cells by blocking the cell cycle at G1 phase *in vitro*.[3] Additionally, many of the diterpenoids in Gan Sui are Topo-II inhibitors.[8,9] All these discoveries may provide the useful information for the design and the development of anticancer drug candidates and the application of Gan Sui diterpenoids in the cancer treatment.

Triterpenoids

The triterpenoid constituents including euphol (**6**) were separated from the herb, showing the inhibitory effect against skin carcinogenesis on the shaved backs of mice. The typical application of euphol (**8**) (2.0 µM) markedly suppressed the tumor-promoting effect of TPA in mouse melanona initiated by DMBA.[11] α-Euphorbol (**7**) showed the cytotoxic effect on some tumor cell lines.[12]

Fatty Acids

An octadecenoic acid mixture prepared from Gan Sui, which mainly contained oleic acid and linoleic acid, was demonstrated to exert cytotoxic and antitumor activities on BEL-7402 (liver), SGC-7901 (gastric), and HL-60 (leukemic) human cancer cell lines *in vitro* where the octadecenoic acid mixture functionally and structurally induced the damage of cell membrane and cell ultrastructures and promoted G0/G1 cell cycle arrest and apoptosis/necrosis, finally resulting in the dose-dependent diminution of the tumor size, whose inhibitory potencies may be comparable with or greater than those of 5-FU (a chemotherapeutic agent).[13]

Toxicity

Gan Sui shows some toxicity. The LD_{50} value of the 50% ethanolic extract was about 346 mg/kg by i.p. injection to mice. The intravenous injection of the Gan Sui extract in a 10 mg/kg dose to rabbits for seven continuous days caused some toxicity in the head, the liver, and the kidney. Also, Gan Sui has obvious toxicity toward the embryo but no influence to the health of mother parent.

Other Bioactivities

In general, Gan Sui is used to purge severe fluid accumulation and kill bowel helminthes in Chinese medicine. It may be selected to treat acute symptoms attendant to liver cirrhosis, hydrothorax, dysuria, constipation, pleurisy, ascites, and lymphatic node inflammations. However, because the herb initiates both strong effects and side effects, exercise and care are necessary when in the treatment. Researchers have substantiated the herb to possess purgative, pregnancy-terminating, and immunosuppressive properties. Euphol (**5**) can excite the cervix to induce abortion. Thus, the herb is prohibited to be used in pregnant women and patients who are weak.

References

1. Wu, T. S. et al. 1991. Antitumor agents: 119. Kansuiphorins A and B, two novel anti-leukemic diterpene esters from *Euphorbia kansui*. *J. Nat. Prod.* 54: 823–9.
2. Kitanaka, S. et al. 2003. Diterpenes from *Euphorbia kansui* and compositions containing them as antiinflammatory or antitumor agents. *Jpn. Kokai Tokkyo Koho* JP 2003171349 A 20030620.
3. Yu, F. R. et al. Isolation and characterization of methyl esters and derivatives from *Euphorbia kansui* (Euphorbiaceae) and their inhibitory effects on the human SGC-7901 cells. *J. Pharmacy Pharm. Sci.* 8: 528–35.
4. Kitanaka, S. et al. 2005. Diterpenes having cell division-inhibiting activity derived from *Euphorbia kansui*. *Jpn. Kokai Tokkyo Koho* JP 2005041800 A 20050217; 2005. Ingenol-type diterpene esters as cell division inhibitors. *Jpn. Kokai Tokkyo Koho* JP 2005041799 A 20050217.
5. Pan, D. J. et al. 1991. Kansuiphorin C and D, cytotoxic diterpenes from *Euphorbia kansui*. *Phytochem.* 30: 1018–20.
6. Wang, H. Y. et al. 2012. Bioactivity-guided isolation of antiproliferative diterpenoids from *Euphorbia kansui*. *Phytother. Res.* 26: 853–9.
7. Miyata, S. et al. 2004. Selective inhibition of the growth of cancer cells by diterpenes selected with embryonic cells of Xenopus. *Cell Biol. Intl.* 28: 179–84.
8. Miyata, S. et al. 2006. Inhibition of cellular proliferation by diterpenes, topoisomerase II inhibitor. *Bioorg. Med. Chem.* 14: 2048–51.
9. Yoshida, C. et al. 2010. Analysis of inhibition of topoisomerase IIα and cancer cell proliferation by ingenol EZ. *Cancer Sci.* 101: 374–8.
10. Fukuda, Y. et al. 2013. 3EZ,20Ac-ingenol, a catalytic inhibitor of topo-isomerases, downregulates p-Akt and induces DSBs and apoptosis of DT40 cells. *Archiv. Pharm. Res.* 36: 1029–38.
11. Yasukawa, K. et al. 2000. Inhibitory effect of euphol, a triterpene alcohol from the roots of *Euphorbia kansui* on tumor promotion by 12-*O*-tetradecanoylphorbol-13-acetate in two-stage carcinogenesis in mouse skin. *J. Pharmacy Pharmacol.* 52: 119–24.
12. Zheng, W. F. et al. 1998. Cytotoxicity and antiviral activity of the compounds from *Euphorbia kansui*. *Planta Med.* 64: 754–6.
13. Yu, F. R. et al. 2008. Cytotoxic activity of an octadecenoic acid extract from *Euphorbia kansui* on human tumor cell strains. *J. Pharmacy Pharmacol.* 60: 253–9.

193 Lang Du 狼毒

Chinese chellera

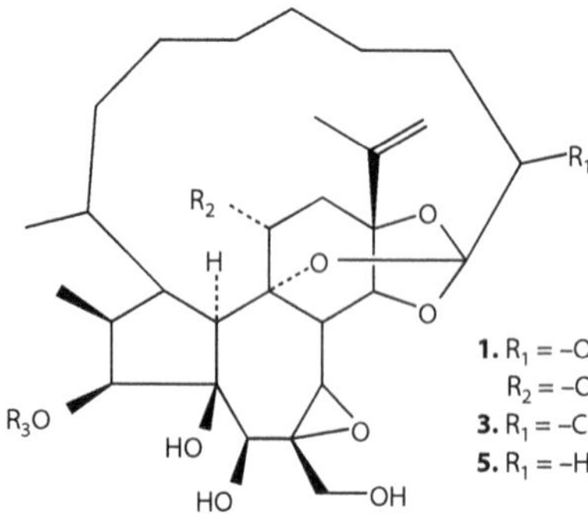

1. R_1 = –OH, R_3 = –Bz, R_2 = –OOCC$_6$H$_6$
3. R_1 = –CH$_3$, R_2 = –OBz, R_3 = –H
5. R_1 = –H, R_2 = –OCH$_3$, R_3 = –Bz

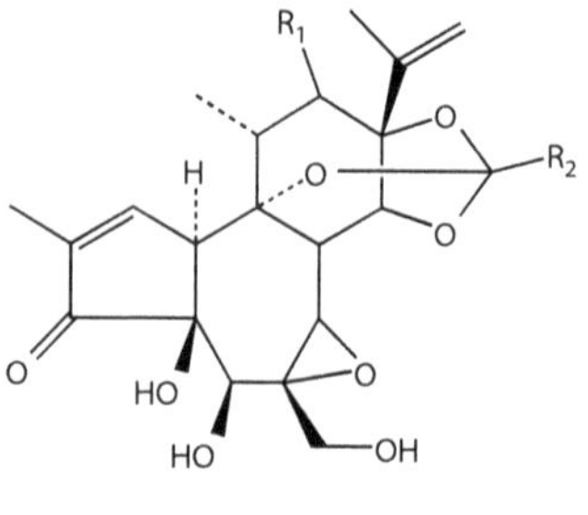

4. R_1 = –OH, R_2 = –A
6. R_1 = –H, R_2 = –A
7. R_1 = –H, R_2 = –B
11. R_1 = –OAc, R_2 = –A

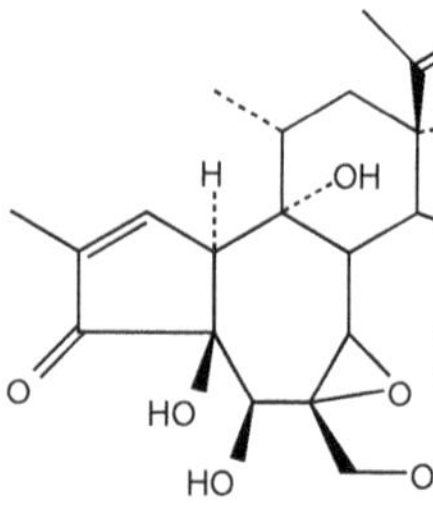

9. R_1 = –H, R_2 = –A
10. R_1 = –A, R_2 = –H

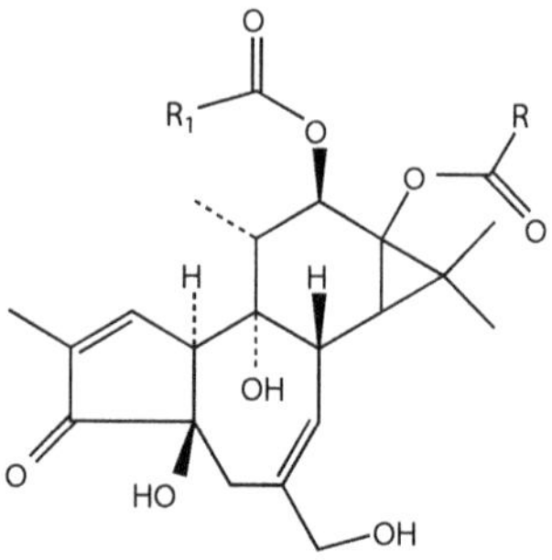

12. R_1 = –C$_6$H$_6$, R_2 = –(CH$_2$)$_3$CH$_3$
13. R_1 = R_2 = –CH$_3$
14. R_1 = CH$_3$, R_2 = –C$_6$H$_6$

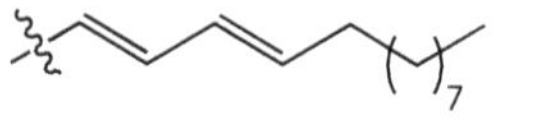

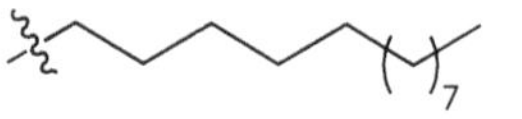

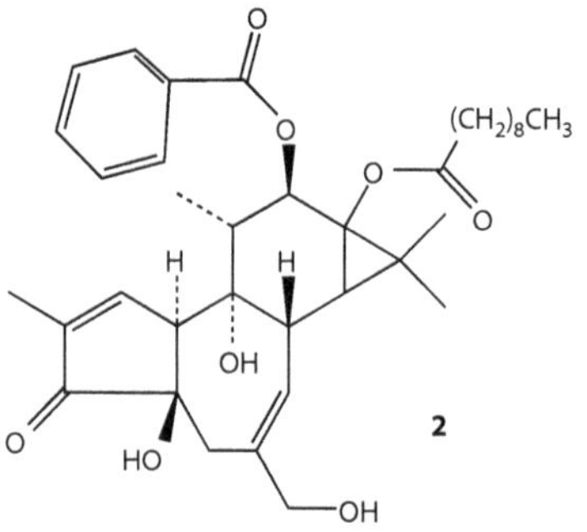

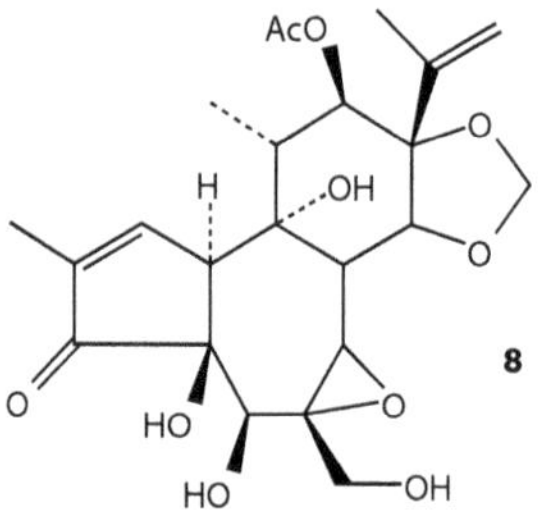

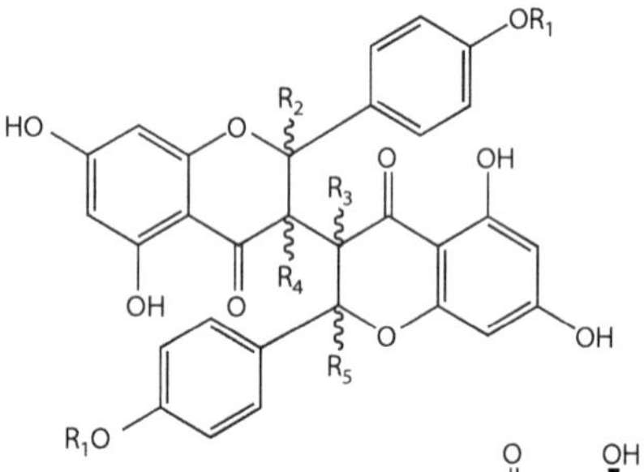

15. R_1 = –H, R_2 = R_5 = –H, R_3 = R_4 = –H
16. R_1 = –CH$_3$, R_2 = R_3 = –H, R_4 = R_5 = –H
17. R_1 = –CH$_3$, R_2 = R_3 = R_4 = R_5 = –H
18. R_1 = –CH$_3$, R_2 = R_3 = R_4 = –H, R_5 = –H
19. R_1 = –H, R_2 = R_3 = –H, R_4 = R_5 = –H
20. R_1 = –H, R_2 = R_5 = –H, R_3 = R_4 = –H

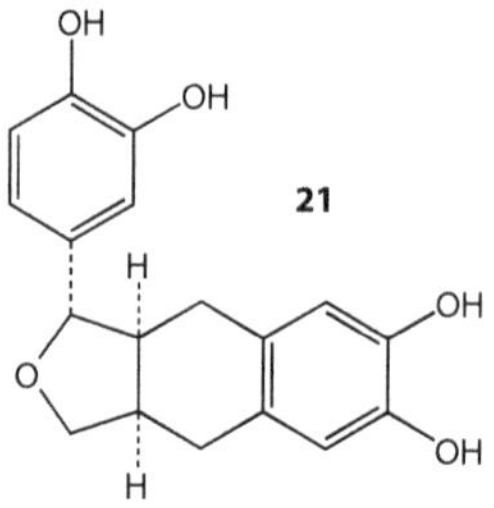

Herb Origination

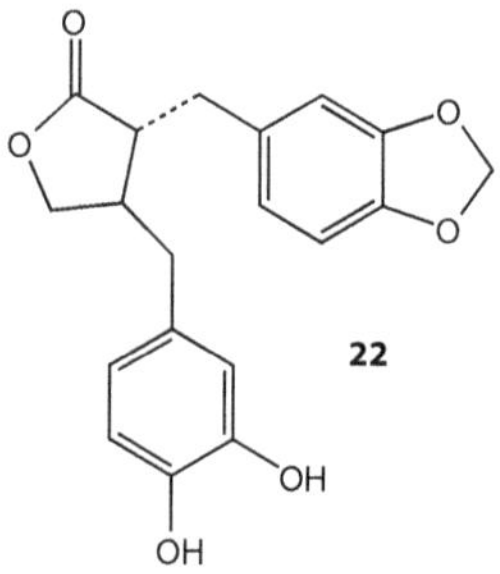

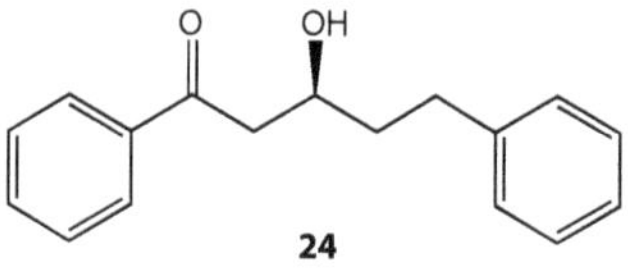

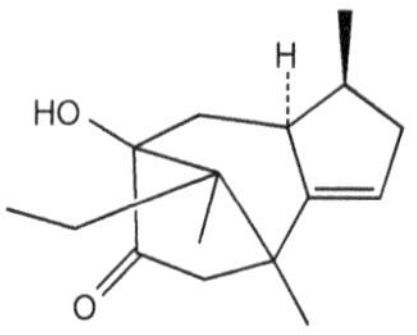

The herb Lang Du (Chinese chellera) originated from the roots of a Thymelaeaceae plant *Stellera chamaejasme* L. This perennial plant is distributed in northern and southwestern China as well as Nepal, Bhutan, Mongolia, and part of Russia. As a Chinese herb, the root is collected in autumn and used in both conditions of fresh and sun-dried.

Antitumor Activities

The Lang Du petroleum ether extract and chloroform extract exerted strong inhibition against the proliferation of human cancer cells, such as HL-60 (leukemic), BEL-7402 (liver), and SGC-7901 (stomach) cell lines in a significant dose-dependent response, while its n-butanolic extract and methanolic extract exhibited low activity in the *in vitro* assay.[1] However, the i.p. administration of its alcoholic extract in a dose of 80.66 mg/kg or its aqueous extract in a dose of 10.48 g/kg to tumor-bearing mice restrained the growth of lung carcinoma cells by 70% and 59.91%, respectively.[2] The *in vivo* inhibitory rates of its aqueous extract toward the growth of hepatoma cells and cervical cancer U14 cells were 36.7% and 50.5%, respectively.[2] ESC, ESC-1, and ESC-2, which were three fractions derived from the alcoholic extract (the two latter were isolated from ESC), displayed obvious effect on NCI-H460 (lung), and BEL-7402 and SK-HEP-1 (liver) human cancer cell lines, *in vitro*, in association with apoptosis induction, whose inhibitory rates were between 64.82% and 92.27% in concentrations of 100 and 200 mg/L (72 h), and the order of the antitumor effects of ESCs was ESC-2 > ESC >

ESC-1.[3] The antiproliferative effect of methanolic extract was further confirmed on K562 leukemia, sarcoma 180, and YAC-1 lymphoma cells *in vitro* and on murine P388 leukemia and H22 hepatoma *in vivo*.[4–6] The apoptosis and the G0/G1 phase cell arrest of K562 cells were remarkably increased by the treatment, where the activity of p53 was substantially amplified and the expressions of Bcl-2 and c-Myc were obviously lessened.[4,5] Also, the daily administration of the methanolic extract in a dose of 5 μg/kg improved the immune function in sarcoma 180-bearing mice besides inhibiting the tumor growth. The immunoenhancing property of the methanolic extract was remarkable in the normal animal model as well. A 0.1–10 μg/mL of the methanolic extract could stimulate normal mouse splenocytes to proliferate and transform and enhance splenocyte NK activity *in vitro*. Therefore, the scientific data demonstrated the extracts of Lang Du to be a potential adjuvant in the cancer prevention and treatment.[5]

Moreover, the serum of tumor-bearing mice after the i.p. injection with Lang Du extract also exerted the remarkable cytotoxic property. The exposure of the activated serum to exponentially growing tumor cells presented the suppressive effect against the proliferation of human HL-60 leukemia and SGC-7901 gastric adenocarcinoma cell lines[7] and against the DNA synthesis of mouse L1210 leukemia cells.[8] Also, the serum containing Lang Du could significantly enhanced the antigrowth effects of chemotherapeutic drugs VP-16 and DOX against BEL-7402 hepatoma cells. In the treated BEL-7402 cells, 50 mg/mL of the serum combined with VP-16 (1 μM/L) promoted the G2/M cell cycle arrest by 68.2% and augmented the apoptosis by 100.0%; concurrently, the Bcl-2 expression was lessened from 45.6% to 23.9%. These results demonstrated that the potent anticancer activity of Lang Du presented not only in the inhibition of various neoplastic cells but also in the potentiation of chemotherapeutic agents synergistically in the cancer treatment.[9]

Antitumor Constituents and Activities

Phytochemical researches revealed that Lang Du has extensive types of constituents, including alkaloids, flavonoids, diterpenoids, lignans, coumarins, and proteins. All the components showed different degrees of inhibitory effects in the *in vitro* or *in vivo* assays, but the diterpenoids and the bioflavonoids from Lang Du were demonstrated as the major cancer inhibitors.

Diterpenoids

The major anticancer components in Lang Du were found to be diterpenoids including gnidimacrin (**1**), stellerarin (**2**), stelleramacrin-A (**3**), stelleramacrin-B (**4**), and pimeleafactor-P2 (**5**). The diterpenoids displayed potent cytotoxic and antitumor activities against P388, L1210, and K562 leukemia cells *in vivo* and *in vitro*. An *in vitro* assay also showed the potent antigrowth effects of gnidimacrin (**1**) against human leukemia cell lines (HL-60 and CCRF-CEM).[10–13] At an i.p. dosages of 0.02–0.03 mg/kg of gnidimacrin (**1**), the prolongation of the life span was 70% and 80% in mice implanted with leukemia P388 or L1210, respectively.[11] Gnidimacrin (**1**) was also sensitive to K562 erythroleukemia cells accompanied by the induction of the bubbles in cell surface and the G1 cell cycle arrest via the reduction of CDK2 and CDC25A activities at a growth-inhibitory concentration (0.0005 μg/mL). Likewise, gnidimacrin (**1**) directly affected the PKC activity and inhibited a carcinoma-promoting agent phorbol-12,13-dibutyrate binding to the K562 cells. But, when its concentration was over 0.05 μg/mL, both PKC and anticancer-related activities were obviously inhibited, indicating that PKC (particularly PKC-βII) is one of the major determinants of the cell's ability to respond to gnidimacrin (**1**).[13–16] The obstruction of the L1210 cell division by gnidimacrin (**1**) was also concomitant with the enlargement of the cell size and the increase of the multinuclear cells.[9] The proliferation of the human stomach carcinoma cell lines (Kato-III, MKN-28, and MKN-45) was potently obstructed by the gnidimacrin treatment (IC_{50}: 0.007–0.00012 μg/mL).[11–14] Gnidimacrin (**1**), even at a low concentration (10^{-5} to 10^{-6} μM), still suppressed the proliferation NSCLC cells, and at 10^{-1} to 10^{-2} μM concentrations, it inhibited H69 small cell lung cancer cells and HLE hepatoma cells.[14] Moreover, gnidimacrin (**1**) was shown to suppress the growth of murine solid tumor cells such as Lewis lung tumor, colon cancer 26, and B16 melanoma *in vivo* with lifetime extension of 40–49% in doses of 0.01–0.02 mg/mL.

Likewise, more bioactive daphnane diterpenoids were discovered in Lang Du. Huratoxin (**6**), 12β-acetoxyhuratoxin (**7**), simplexin (**8**), wikstroelide-J (**9**), and its analog (**10**), in the *in vitro* assay with human A549 NSCLC cells, displayed significant cytotoxicity with IC_{50} values in ranging from 0.3 to 24 nM.[17,18] Huratoxin (**6**) and subtoxin-1 (**11**) significantly suppressed the growth of P388 leukemia cells in mice, and other diterpenoids (**12**, **13**, and **14**) obstructed the proliferation of leukemia adult T cell line *in vitro*.[13]

Flavonoids

Total flavonoid component was obtained from the herb by ultrasonic extraction, which showed the antiproliferative effect on human A549 lung carcinoma cells in dose- and time-dependent manners together with the induction of G1 cell cycle arrest and apoptotic death.[19] The total flavonoids also exerted marked antitumor activity against SGC-7901, BEL-7402, and HL-60 cell lines *in vitro* and against transplanted mouse S180 and H22 solid tumor *in vivo* with a lower acute toxicity, whose antitumor potencies were greater than those of VCR on the *in vitro* cancer cell lines.[20] Several biflavonoids were separated from the roots of *S. chamaejasme* as tumor growth inhibitors, whose cytotoxic effect of bioflavonoids on the tumor cells was largely attributed to the blockage of β-tubulin deploymerization. A separated chamaejasmine (**15**) showed more prominent anticancer activity *in vitro* against all tested human MCF-7 (breast), HCT-8 (colon), A549 (lung), SGC-7901 (stomach), HepG2 (liver), HO-4980, HeLa (cervix), and LNCap and PC3 (prostate) cancer cell lines. Chamaejasmine (**15**) showed more potent cytotoxicity than taxol against the PC3, MCF-7, A549, and HO-4980 cancer cell lines (IC_{50}: 2.28–5.31 μM), but less cytotoxicity than taxol (an antitumor drug) against normal Vero and MDCK cell lines.[21] Also, chamaejasmine (**15**) augmented G2/M cell cycle arrest and cell apoptosis by a ROS-mediated and mitochondria-dependent mechanism, thereby restraining the growth of A549 cells in time- and dose-dependent manners,[22] while exerting the profound antiproliferative and proapoptotic effects via the activation of p21 and p53, the down-expression of Bcl-2, and the increase of Bax and caspase-3 activities in human MG63 osteosarcoma cells.[23] These evidenced recommended that chamaejasmine (**15**) may be a candidate agent for cancer chemoprevention.

The anticancer activity of chamaejasmin-A (**16**) was demonstrated by using *in vitro* models with four human tumor cell lines such as CAL-27 (oral), UMSCC-1 (oral cavity), UMSCCG19, and HEp-2 (larynx) cells. The IC_{50} values ranged from 3.48 to 12.09 μM, and its higher cytotoxicity presented in HEp-2 cells (IC_{50}: 3.48 μM). The growth inhibitory effect of chamaejasmin-A (**16**) was further confirmed in mice with gavage intake. Similarly, its antigrowth activity was accompanied by the inhibition of β-tubulin deploymerization as chamaejasmine (**15**).[24] Moreover, both chamaejasmenin-B (**17**) and neochamaejasmin-C (**18**) exerted the potent antiproliferative effects in human HepG2 and SMMC-7721 hepatoma, MG63, U2OS, and KHOS osteosarcoma, A549 NSCLC, HeLa cervical cancer, and HCT-116 colon cancer cell lines, *in vitro*, where the A549 and KHOS cell lines were more sensitive to bioflavonoids (**17** and **18**), and chamaejasmenin-B (IC_{50}: 1.08–10.8 μmol/L) was slightly more effective than neochamaejasmin-C (IC_{50}: 3.07–15.97 μmol/L). The antitumor effect by the bioflavonoids was mediated by the elicitation of apoptosis and G0/G1 phase arrest, whose mechanism was characterized in the up-expression of γ-H2AX (a DNA damage marker).[25] Also, chamaejasmenin-B (**17**) acted as an inhibitor of P-gp in MDCK-hMDR1 cells, and it obstructed the P-gp-mediated efflux in a concentration-dependent manner.[26]

Likewise, the treatment of the LNCaP cells with low doses of neochamaejasmin-A (**19**) (≤6.25 μg/mL) caused the G1 cell cycle arrest with the decrease of the cyclin-D expression. By reducing the cellular thymidine incorporation and the DNA-binding abilities of NF-κB and AP-1, neochamaejasmin-A (**19**) retarded the proliferation of human LNCaP prostate cancer cells. When neochamaejasmin-A (**19**) is exposed with higher doses (≥12.5 μg/mL), the LNCaP cell apoptosis was elicited by p21 activation and ultimately promotion of Fas-caspase-8 and caspase-3 apoptotic machinery pathways.[27] Isochamaejasmin (**20**) was found to retard the proliferation of human HeLa cervical cancer cells (EC_{50}: 3.23 μM) by stimulating the expression of NF-κB-directed reporter gene and potentiating time-dependent phosphorylation of MAPK ERK 1/2 and p38. Moreover, a methyl derivative and two stereoisomers of isochamaejasmin from the herb showed more cytotoxicity on the HeLa cells than isochamaejasmin (**20**) but have no ability to activate NF-κB-directed reporter gene.[28]

According to the prominent results, the chamaejasmine-type bioflavonoids may be recommended as potential sources of anticancer agents for the development in chemotherapy and prevention and in the pharmaceutical industry.

Other Types of Constituents

Other types of components in Lang Du also demonstrated the biological potentials in the suppression of cancer cell growth and induction of apoptotic death. Its total alkaloid, whose content was 68.24% in Lang Du, displayed marked *in vitro* antiproliferative effect on, SGC-7901 (stomach), BEL-7402 (liver), and HL-60 (leukemia) human tumor cell lines, associated with the promotion of G0/G1 cell arrest and apoptosis.[29] The total lignan was isolated from the Lang Du, exerting significant inhibition on the proliferation and the clone formation of human neoplastic cell lines such as SGC-7901, BEL-7402, or HL-60 cell lines *in vitro*.[30] Two separated lignans assigned as (–)-haplomyrfolin (**21**) and stelleralignan (**22**) and one sesquiterpene termed chamaejasmone-D (**23**) showed the inhibitory effect against the proliferation of A549 lung cancer cells (respective IC_{50}: 0.27, 1.53, and 1.95 μM).[18] (+)-3-Hydroxy-1,5-diphenyl-1-pentanone (**24**), a bicoumarin, displayed both effects in immunomodulation and anticarcinoma.[31]

Additionally, a total protein component and six purified proteins were separated from Lang Du. The proteins B, C, D, and F and the total proteins exerted antitumor function, but the proteins A, C, and D and the total proteins were also toxic to normal cells.[32]

Other Bioactivities

The herb Lang Du (Chinese chellera) has been used to treat solid tumors, tuberculosis, and psoriasis. The decoction of Lang Du also exerted analgesic, antiviral, anticonvulsive, immunoregulatory, and antibacterial effects. The isolated constituents such as gnidimacrin (**1**) and eudesmin also exhibited anti-HIV activity.[33]

Toxic and Side Effects

Most ancient materia medica books in China recorded Lang Du to be toxic. The overdose of Lang Du may cause stomachache and diarrhea, so it has to be carefully administered orally.

References

1. Wang, B. et al. 2004. The antitumor activities of the extracts from *Stellera chamaejasme* L. in vitro by means of systematic solvent extraction. *Zhongyaocai* 27: 355–7.
2. Yang, B. Y. et al. 1986. Antitumor effects of *Stellera chamaejasme. Zhongxiyi Jiehe Zazhi* 6: 532.
3. Liu, X. N. et al. (a) 2010. Antitumor effect of alcohol extract of *Stellera chamaejasme* in vitro. *Zhongguo Zhongyao Zazhi* 35: 3048–51; (b) 2014. Antitumor pharmacological evaluation of extracts from *Stellera chamaejasme* L based on hollow fiber assay. *BMC Complem. Altern. Med.* 14: 116/1–8.
4. Feng, W. J. et al. 1997. Antitumor principles of *Stellera chamaejasme* L. *Chin. J. Cancer Res.* 9: 89–95.
5. Zhang, K. J. et al. 2003. Study on the antitumor mechanisms of the methanol extract of *Stellera chamaejasme. Zhonghua Weishengwuxue He Mianyixue Zazhi* 23: 734–8.
6. Mei, A. M. et al. 2006. Effects of the extracts of *Stellera chamaejasme* on the cell cycle of mice liver cancer H22 cells. *Zhongguo Xiandai Yixue Zazhi* 16: 3709–11.
7. Jia, Z. P. et al. 2001. *Stellera chamaejasme* induced apoptosis of HL-60 cells and regulated expression of bcl-2 protein in SGC-7901 cells. *Zhongcaoyao* 32: 1097–101.
8. Jia, Z. P. et al. 2001. Effect of serum of mice taken *Stellera chamaejasme* extract on proliferation, clonal formation and DNA synthesis of mouse L1210 leukemic cells. *Zhongcaoyao* 32: 807–9.

9. Fan, J. J. et al. 2001. Synergistic anti-hepatoma effect and its mechanism of *Stellera chamaejasme* mouse drug-serum with cytotoxic chemotherapeutic agents in vitro. *Shijie Huaren Xiaohua Zazhi* 9: 1008–12.
10. Feng, W. J. et al. 1992. Studies on antitumor active compounds of *Stellera chamaejasme* L. and their mechanism of action. *Toho Igakkai Zasshi* 38: 896–909.
11. Ikekawa, T. et al. 1993. Carcinostatic compounds and production thereof. *PCT Int. Appl.* WO 9303039 A1 19930218.
12. Feng, W. J. et al. 1991. Studies on antitumor Chinese medicines (II). Antitumor constituents of *Stellera chamaejasme* L. *Wakan Iyaku Gakkaishi* 8: 96–101.
13. Ikekawa, T. et al. 1996. Extraction of antitumor diterpenes from *Stellera chamaejasme*. Jpn. Kokai Tokkyo Koho JP 08310993 A 19961126; 1996. *Jpn. Kokai Tokkyo Koho* JP 95-144190.
14. Feng, W. J. et al. 1995. The antitumor activities of gnidimacrin isolated from *Stellera chamaejasme* L. *Zhonghua Zhongliu Zazhi* 17: 24–6.
15. Yoshida, M. et al. (a) 1996. Antitumor activity of daphnane-type diterpene gnidimacrin isolated from *Stellera chamaejasme* L. *Intl. J. Cancer* 66: 268–73; (b) 2001. Antitumor action of the PKC activator gnidimacrin through cdk2 inhibition, 94: 348–52.
16. Yoshida, M. et al. (a) 1998. Mechanism of antitumor action of PKC activator, gnidimacrin. *Intl. J. Cancer* 77: 243–50; (b) 2003. Involvement of PKC βII in anti-proliferating action of a new antitumor compound gnidimacrin, *Intl. J. Cancer* 105: 601–6.
17. Liu, L. P. et al. 2014. Topoisomerase II inhibitors from the roots of *Stellera chamaejasme* L. *Bioorg. Med. Chem.* 22: 4198–203.
18. Pan, G. F. et al. 2007. Advances of studies on antitumor mechanism of *Stellera chamaejasme* L. *Zhonghua Zhongyiyao Zazhi* 22: 873–5.
19. Duan, X. et al. 2012. Influence of total flavonoid extract of *Stellera chamaejasme* on cell proliferation and cell cycle of lung carcinoma. *Hebei Yike Daxue Xuebao* 33: 308–10.
20. Wang, M. et al. 2005. The antitumor effects of total-flavonoid from *Stellera chamaejasme*. *Zhongguo Zhongyao Zazhi* 30: 603–6.
21. Fang, W. et al. 2011. Anticancer activity of chamaejasmine: Effect on tubulin protein. *Mol.* 16: 6243–54.
22. Yu, H. et al. 2011. Chamaejasmine induces apoptosis in human lung adenocarcinoma A549 cells through a Ros-mediated mitochondrial pathway. *Mol.* 16: 8165–80.
23. Yang, D. W. et al. 2015. Apoptosis induced by chamaejasmine in human osteosarcoma cells through p53 pathway. *Tumor Biol.* 36: 5433–9.
24. Zhao, Y. et al. 2012. Inhibitory action of chamaejasmin A against human HEp-2 epithelial cells: effect on tubulin protein. *Mol. Biol. Reports* 39: 11105–12.
25. Zhang, C. et al. 2013. In vitro anticancer activity of chamaejasmenin B and neochamaejasmin C isolated from the root of *Stellera chamaejasme* L. *Acta Pharmacologica Sinica* 34: 262–70.
26. Pan, L. Y. et al. 2015. Inhibitory effects of neochamaejasmin B on P-glycoprotein in MDCK-hMDR1 cells and molecular docking of NCB binding in P-glycoprotein. *Mol.* 20: 2931–48.
27. Liu, W. K. et al. 2008. Involvement of p21 and FasL in induction of cell cycle arrest and apoptosis by neochamaejasmin A in human prostate LNCaP cancer cells. *J. Nat. Prods.* 71: 842–6.
28. Tian, Q. H. et al. 2005. Stereospecific induction of nuclear factor-κB activation by isochamaejasmin. *Mol. Pharmacol.* 68: 1534–42.
29. Wang, M. et al. 2010. Antitumor activity of *Stellera chamaejasme* alkaloids and its mechanism. *Zhongyaocai* 33: 1919–22.
30. Wang, B. et al. 2008. Antitumor activities in vitro of total-lignan from *Stellera chamaejasme* L. in vitro. *J. Lanzhou Univ.* (*Science Edition*), 44: 63–5.
31. Xu, Z. H. et al. 2001. A new bicoumarin from *Stellera chamaejasme* L. *J. Asian Nat. Prod. Res.* 3: 335–40.
32. Bo, Y. K. et al. 2010. Study on in vitro activity of protein site from *Stellera chamaejasme* L. *Shizhen Guoyi Guoyao* 21: 2262–4.
33. Ikekawa, T. et al. (a) 1996. Extraction of antitumor diterpenes from *Stellera chamaejasme*. *Jpn. Kokai Tokkyo Koho* JP 08310993 A 19961126; (b) 1996. Extraction of anticancer and antiviral substances from *Stellera chamaejasme* for therapeutic use. *Jpn. Kokai Tokkyo Koho* JP 08092118 A 19960409.

194 Zi Shan 紫杉

Taxane or Yew

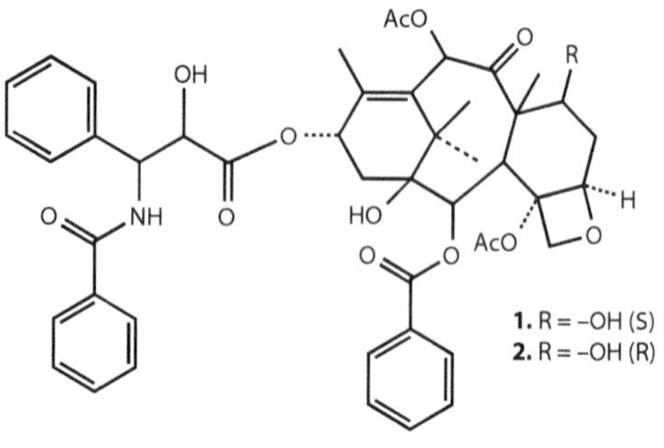

1. R = -OH (S)
2. R = -OH (R)

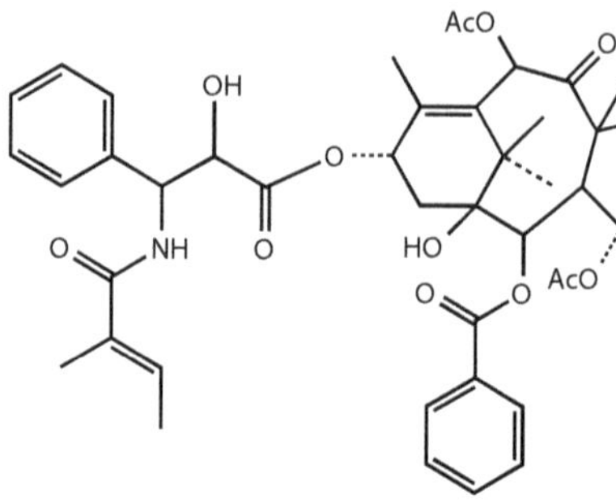

Herb Origination

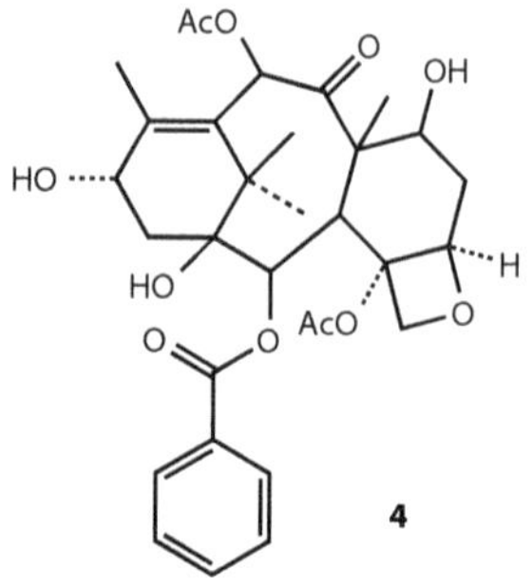

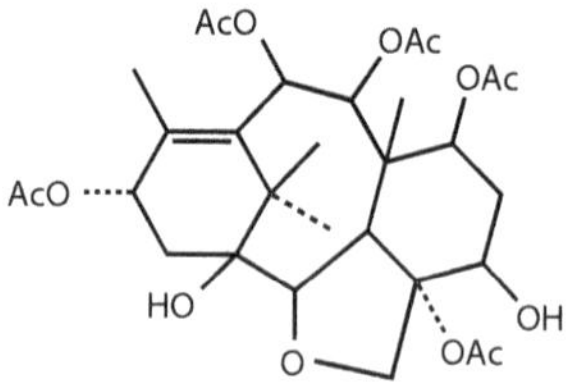

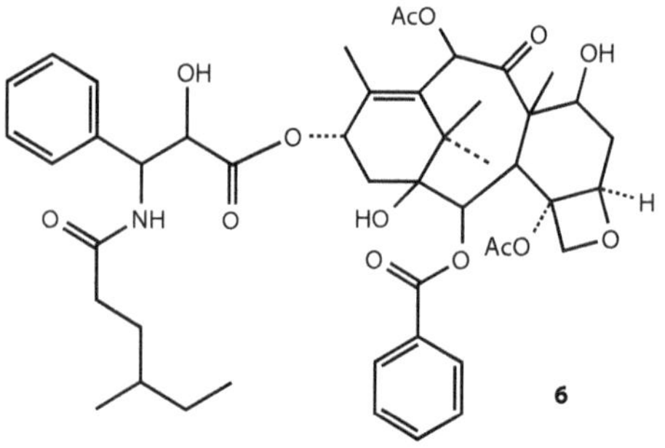

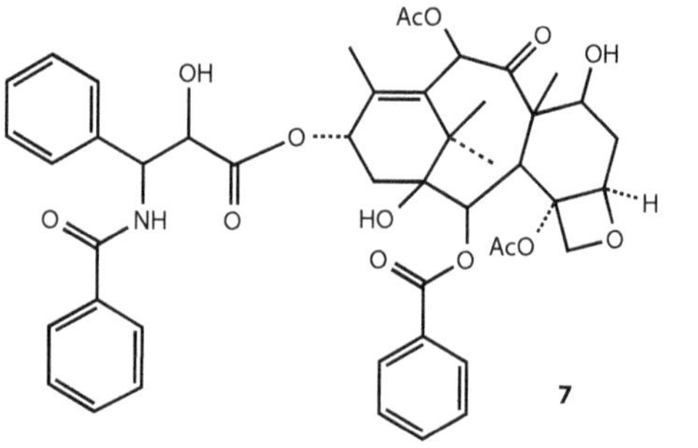

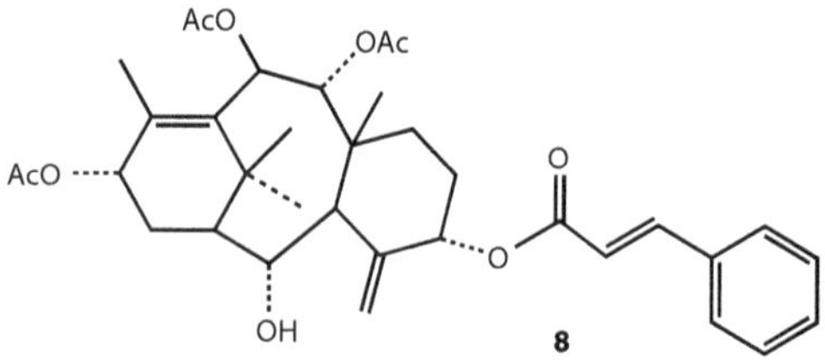

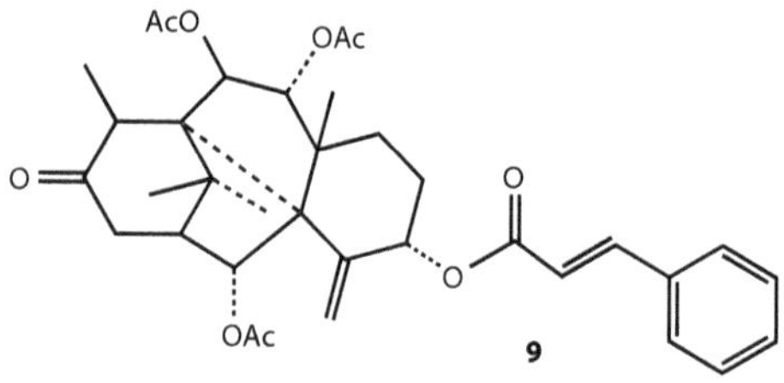

The herb Zi Shan is also named as Hong Dou Shan in China, which is an evergreen yew, *Taxus cuspidate* (Taxaceae). This yew tree species is mainly distributed in the northeast region of China as well as Korea and Japan. Since a famous anticancer drug taxol (paclitaxel) was successfully discovered and developed from the bark of a Pacific yew tree (*T. brevifolia*), the different Taxus species in the world were paid more attention as valuable sources for the preparation of taxol and the isolation of new taxane diterpenoids from various species of yews. Other species of taxane trees (such as *T. chinensis*, *T. yunnanensis*, *T. mairei*, and *T. wallichiana*) in China were also extensively studied for the development of taxoid type of diterpenoids as antineoplastic agents.[1]

Antitumor Constituents and Activities

The ethanolic extract from the Chinese yew (*T. cuspidate*) not only notably suppressed the cell growth of sarcoma 180 and truly extended the life span of mice implanted with L615 leukemia but also accelerated lymphocytes in the body surrounding the tumor tissue, inducing the cancer cell necrosis and reducing the tumor size.[2] The ethanolic extract from Yunnan yew (*T. yunnanensis*) demonstrated remarkable antitumor effects against murine P388 leukemia with 52.7% of inhibitory rate and 84% of life extension in murine animals bearing Lewis lung carcinoma.[3] Both taxane trees had been confirmed as a valuable source that contain the powerful cytotoxic agents taxol and taxoids.

Antitumor Activity of Taxol

Taxol (**1**) exhibited potent and broad spectral activity against the growth of various human neoplastic cell lines and murine tumor cell lines (such as L1210 and P1534 leukemias and Walker 256 sarcoma). The IC_{50} values were 1.9 ng/mL for KB epidermoid cancer and HCT-8 colon cancer, 3.6 ng/mL for A2780 ovarian cancer, 5 ng/mL for MGC-803 gastric cancer, 10 ng/mL for MCF-7 breast cancer, 0.05 μg/mL for A549 lung epithelial cancer, and 0.07 μg/mL for Bel-7402 hepatoma.[4–6] When using taxol (**1**) in a concentration of 10^{-7} mol/L to treat four types of human colon carcinoma cell lines (CCL-187, CX-1, CCL-229, and Clone-A), the suppressive rates were 34.54%, 67.40%, 58.71%, and 70.87%, respectively. Relatively, the stronger cytotoxicities were observed in CX-1 cells and Clone-A cells with IC_{50} values of 9×10^{-10} and 4×10^{-9} mol/L, respectively, after 72 h of treatment.[7]

The inhibitory effect of taxol (**1**) on SMMC-7721 hepatoma cells and A549 and H1299 lung cancer cells were revealed to correlate with the arrest of the cell growth period at G2/M phase and the induction of the apoptosis.[8–10] Taxol (**1**) could also specifically bind to the β-subunit of tubulin in the cancer cells and induce the microtubule breakdown. In KB epidermoid carcinoma cells and L1210 leukemia cells, taxol (**1**) exerted greater suppressive effect compared to VCR and colchicines.[5,6] Meaningfully, taxol (**1**) was also remarkably effective in the inhibition of VCR-resistant KB/VCR cells and HCT-8/VCR cells with IC_{50} values of 0.2 and 0.11 μg/mL, respectively.[4]

The antitumor property of taxol (**1**) was also further demonstrated in animal models, where taxol was significantly effective toward three types of leukemia (L1210, P1534, and P388), B16 melanoma, W256 sarcoma, sarcoma 180, and Lewis lung cancer in mice and toward many types of human solid carcinomas in the breast, the ovary, the lung, the brain, the endometrial, and the tongue (recurrent) in nude mice [2,3,6] but no activity on colon 38 cancer and breast CD8F cancer.[11] At present, taxol (**1**) is extensively used clinically for the chemotherapy of patients suffering from ovarian cancer, NSCLC, head and neck cancer, breast cancer, and advanced forms of Kaposi's sarcoma.

Antimetastatic Activity of Taxol

Moreover, the antimetastatic potential of taxol (**1**) has also been investigated. In an *in vivo* melanoma spontaneous metastasis model, the metastatic formation in the pulmonary of mice was significantly inhibited by the i.p. injection of taxol at a dose of 5 mg/kg/day for three weeks. During the treatment, taxol amplified the expressions of metastatic suppressor gene nm23 mRNA and E-cad to exert the antigrowth and antimetastatic effects on the melanoma cells and reduced the expression of VEGF to block the angiogenesis in the melanoma tissue.[12] These evidences provided the scientific suggestion for the use of taxol as a chemotherapuetic drug to suppress an early stage of melanoma metastases.[12]

Anticancer Mechanism of Taxol

Extensively studies on taxol (**1**) revealed that the antitumor effect was principally attributed to two major mechanisms. In the first, taxol (**1**) induced the microtubule breakdown by specifically binding to the β-subunit of tubulin and enhancing the additional microtubule assembly. When the complexes of microtubule/paclitaxel are formed, the microtubule losses the disassemble ability and the tumor cells are destroyed during the cell division. In addition to stabilizing the microtubules, taxol effectively sequestered the free tubulin and depleted the cells supply of tubulin monomers and dimers, and then triggered the tumor cells to apoptosis.[13,14]

However, the apoptotic-inducing mechanisms of taxol (**1**) in some other different types of cancer cell lines displayed their own characteristic pathways. For example, the treatment of human SKOV-3 ovarian cancer cells with taxol elicited the translocation of AIF from the mitochondria to the cytosol to provoke caspase-independent and AIF-dependent apoptosis.[15] The taxol-induced apoptosis of human HeLa ovarian carcinoma cells was found to correlate with the activation of MAPKs.[16] In human CCRF-HSB-2 lymphoblastic leukemia cells, the FAS-associated death domain protein-dependent apoptosis was promoted by taxol (**1**) primarily through the cleavage of Bcl-2 and the activation of caspase-10.[17]

Synergistic Effects of Taxol

Pyrazolotriazolopyrimidine derivatives (PTP-ds) were known to have an ability to elevate the sensitivity of malignant melanoma cells to chemotherapeutic drugs by inhibiting MDR-associated ATP-binding cassette drug transporter. The combination of taxol (**1**) with PTP-d could greatly promise the treatment of human A375 melanoma cells.[18] Also, an *in vivo* experiment had been used to further investigate the synergistic effect of taxol (**1**) in combination with a bioreductive agent NLCQ-1 in the murine tumor models (EMT6/BALB/c and SCCVII/C3H), where NLCQ-1 could markedly potentiate the antineoplastic potency of taxol (**1**) against solid tumors possessing hypoxic regions.[19] The cotreatment of taxol with suitable agents could be suggested as a useful strategy for further development of efficient chemotherapies.

Antitumor Activity of Other Taxoids

In the three recent decades, numerous taxoids were discovered from various taxian trees in different areas of the world. The new members of taxoids hold taxol-type diterpenoid skeleton similarly displaying a variety of suppressive effect on the growth of carcinoma cells. Among a group of taxoids isolated from the needles and the twigs of Chinese yew (*T. cuspidate*), 7-Epitaxol (**2**), 7-epicephalomannine (**3**), taxinine NN-6, taxine NA-2, taxagifine, and taxuspine-H were inhibitory active on human fibroblast cells (WI-38)-induced malignant tumor VA-13 cells, and 7-epitaxol (**2**), 7-epicephalomannine (**3**), taxinine NN-1, taxagifine, and 9,10-deacetyltaxinine were also effective in the decrease of human HepG2 hepatoma cell survival. 2,9-Diacetyl-5-cinnamoyl-phototaxicin-II, 10-acetyltaxuspine-B, and 5-acetyltaxuspine-W were suppressive against the proliferation of breast carcinoma cells *in vitro*. Moreover, five taxoids, i.e., taxine NA-8, taxine NA-2, taxinine NN-1, and 5-cinnamoyl-10-acetyltaxicin-II, demonstrated significant reversal activity against VCR-resistant human ovarian cancer 2780AD cells, whose activity was stronger than a chemotherapeutic agent verapamil. The antitumor effect of 7-epicephalomannine was found to be the same as taxol, acting on the tubulin as a specific molecular target.[20–22]

From the Japanese yew (*T. cuspidate*), over 125 taxoids have been discovered to date. Among them, taxuspine-E (**4**) displayed potent cytotoxicity against human KB epidermoid carcinoma cells and murine L1210 leukemia cells with IC_{50} values of 0.08 and 0.27 μg/mL, respectively, whereas taxuspine-K (**5**) and taxuspine-M showed moderate cytotoxic activity against L1210 cells (IC_{50}: 1.2–10 μg/mL) and KB cells (IC_{50}: 4.5–8.8 μg/mL).[23,24] But because taxuspine-E (**4**) has no C-13 side chain in its structure, its suppressive effect on KB cells was 1700-fold less than taxol.[25] Several other toxoids such as taxuspinanane-A (**6**) and taxuspinanane-I (**7**), were found from a variation of Japanese yew (*T. cuspidata* var. *nana*), possessing the remarkable cell growth-inhibitory activity against murine P388 leukemia cells (IC_{50}: 0.01 and 0.17 μg/mL, respectively). The cytotoxicity of taxuspinanan-A (**6**) was fourfold greater than that of taxol (IC_{50}: 0.04 μg/mL) in the P388 cells.[26,27]

Anti-MDR Activity of Other Taxoids

Some nontaxol-type taxoids derived from yew and its callus cultures were found to have remarkable modulating ability for reversing the MDR in tumor cells as potent as verapamil, whereas taxol and taxol-type compounds did not show such effect.[28–37] The MDR reversal activity of taxine NA-8, taxine NA-2, taxinine NN-1 (**8**), and 5-cinnamoyl-10-acetyltaxicin-II were more potent than that of verapamil. Taxuspine-C (**9**), taxezopidine-G, taxezopidine-H, 5-*O*-phenylpropionylated taxinine-A, and other taxoids could amplify the cellular accumulation of VCR in the multidrug-resistant tumor cell lines (such as P388 cells and 2780AD cells) to markedly improve the chemotherapeutic effect of VCR in mice.[31,33,38,39] 5-*O*-Benzoylated taxinine-K (BTK), 2-desacetoxytaxinine-J, taxuspine-C (**9**), and 2′-desacetoxyaustrospicatine could efficiently reverse the MDR in KB-8-5 and KB-C2 cells caused by chemotherapeutic drugs such as taxol, VCR, DOX (Adm), or colchicine. The anti-MDR mechanism were found to be related to the competitive inhibition of azidopine binding to the P-P-gp and the direct reduction of the overexpressed P-gp.[32,40] Moreover, BTK also moderately reversed another type of resistance to the Adm of KB/MRP cells where MRP is overexpressed. BTK showed no direct inhibition on the transporting activity of MRP, but the anti-MDR effect of BTK was achieved by shifting the distribution of Adm from the punctate cytoplasmic compartments to the nucleoplasm and the cytoplasm in the KB/MRP cells by inhibiting acidification of cytoplasmic organelles.[40] The investigations suggested that some nontaxol-type taxoids may be potential drug candidates that will be useful for overcoming the MDR in clinical chemotherapy of malignant diseases.[31]

References

1. Shi, Q. W. et al. 1998. Taxoids from the bark and needles of Chinese yew, *Taxus mairei*. *Tennen Yuki Kagobutsu Toronkai Koen Yoshishu* 40: 347–52.
2. Yuan, C. S. et al. 1993. The pharmaceutical studies on the antitumor activity of *Taxus cuspidata* Sieb. et Zucc. *Zhongyiyao Xuebao* (6): 38–9.
3. Chen, W. M. et al. 1991. Studies on the antitumor constituents of *Taxus yunnanensis*. *Yaoxue Xuebao* 26: 747–54.
4. Han, R. et al. 1996. Pharmacological and pharmacokinetic studies on the antitumor effect of paclitaxel. *Zhongguo Xinyao Zazhi* 5: 248–51.
5. Cragg, G. M. et al. 1993. The taxol supply crisis. New NCI policies for handling the large-scale production of novel natural product anticancer and anti-HIV agents. *J. Nat. Prod.* 56: 1657–68.
6. He, X. W. et al. 1994. New anticancer drug taxol. *Zhongguo Xiandai Yingyong Yaoxue* 11: 7–9.
7. Fang, J. et al. 1999. Cytotoxicity of taxol against human colorectal cancer cell lines in vitro. *J. Zhongguo Univ. Pharm.* 28: 241–2.
8. Zhao, S. Y. et al. 2002. Apoptosis-inducing effect of taxol on hepatoma SMMC-7721 cells. *Zhonghua Zhongliu Fangzhi Zazhi* 9: 257–9.
9. Yuan, J. H. et al. 2000. Anti-hepatoma activity of taxol in vitro. *Acta Pharmacol. Sinica* 21: 450–4.
10. Das, G. C. et al. 2001. Taxol-induced cell cycle arrest and apoptosis: Dose–response relationship in lung cancer cells of different wild-type p53 status and under isogenic condition. *Cancer Lett.* 165: 147–53.
11. Han, R. et al. 1993. The advanced approaches on taxus and taxol. *Guowai Yixue, Cancer section* 20: 207–10.
12. Wang, F. et al. 2003. Taxol inhibits melanoma metastases through apoptosis induction, angiogenesis inhibition, and restoration of E-cadherin and nm23 expression. *J. Pharmacol. Sci.* 93: 197–203.
13. Schiff, P. B. et al. 1980. Taxol stabilizes microtubules in mouse fibroblast cells. *Proc. Natl. Acad. Sci. U.S.A.* 77: 1561–5.
14. Schiff, P. B. et al. 1981. Taxol assembles tubulin in the absence of exogenous guanosine 5′-triphosphate or microtubule-associated proteins. *Biochem.* 20: 3247–52.
15. Ahn, H. J. et al. 2004. Mechanism of taxol-induced apoptosis in human SKOV3 ovarian carcinoma cells. *J. Cell. Biochem.* 91: 1043–52.
16. Kim, S. S. et al. 1999. Taxol-induced apoptosis and nuclear translocation of mitogen-activated protein (MAP) kinase in HeLa cells. *J. Biochem. Mol. Biol.* 32: 379–84.
17. Park, S. J. et al. 2004. Taxol induces caspase-10-dependent apoptosis. *J. Biol. Chem.* 279: 51057–67.
18. Stefania, M. et al. 2003. Pyrazolotriazolopyrimidine derivatives sensitize melanoma cells to the chemotherapeutic drugs: Taxol and vindesine. *Biochem. Pharmacol.* 66: 739–48.
19. Maria, P. et al. 2002. Synergistic enhancement of the antitumor effect of taxol by the bioreductive compound NLCQ-1, in vivo: Comparison with tirapazamine. *Oncol. Res.* 13: 47–54.
20. Wang, L. Y. et al. 2008. The polar neutral and basic taxoids isolated from needles and twigs of *Taxus cuspidat*a and their biological activity. *J. Wood Sci.* 54: 390–401.
21. Tong, X. J. et al. 1994. Chemical constituents of leaves and twigs of *Taxus cuspidata*. *Yaoxue Xuebao* 29: 55–60.
22. Wang, J. H. et al. 2008. Effects of 3 taxanes from *Taxus cuspidate* on inhibiting proliferation of cultured breast cancer cells in vitro. *Zhongyao Yaoli yu Linchuang* 24: 27–8.
23. Wang, X. X. et al. 1996. Taxuspines K, L, and M, new taxoids from Japanese yew *Taxus cuspidata*. *Tetrahedron* 52: 2337–42.
24. Kobayashi, J. et al. 1995. Taxuspines E apprx. H and J, new taxoids from the Japanese yew *Taxus cuspidata*. *Tetrahedron* 51: 5971–8.
25. Kobayashi, J. et al. 1995. Taxuspines A-E, new taxoids from Japanese yew, *Taxus cuspidata* inhibiting drug transport activity of P-glycoprotein on multidrug-resistant cells. *Tennen Yuki Kagobutsu Toronkai Koen Yoshishu* 37th, pp. 192–7.
26. Morita, H. et al. 1997. Taxuspinananes A and B, new taxoids from *Taxus cuspidata* var. *nana*. *J. Nat. Prods.* 60: 390–2.
27. Morita, H. et al. 1998. Taxoids from *Taxus cuspidata* var. *nana*. *Phytochem.* 48: 857–62.
28. Dai, J. G. et al. 2006. A new taxoid from a callus culture of *Taxus cuspidata* as an MDR reversal agent. *Chem. Pharm. Bull.* 54: 306–9.
29. Kobayashi, J. et al. 1998. Effects of taxoids from *Taxus cuspidata* on microtubule depolymerization and vincristine accumulation in MDR cells. *Intl. Congress Series, 1157 (Towards Natural Medicine Research in the 21st Century)*, pp. 185–95.

30. Hideyuki, S. et al. 2004. Biological activity and chemistry of taxoids from the Japanese yew, *Taxus cuspidata*. *J. Nat. Prods.* 67: 245–56.
31. Kobayashi, J. et al. 1997. Effects of taxoids from *Taxus cuspidata* on microtubule depolymerization and vincristine accumulation in MDR cells. *Bioorg. Med. Chem. Lett.* 7: 393–8.
32. Kobayashi, J. et al. 2000. Multidrug resistance reversal activity of taxoids from *Taxus cuspidata* in KB-C2 and 2780AD cells. *Jpn J. Cancer Res.* 91: 638–42.
33. Sakai, J. et al. 2001. Two taxoids from *Taxus cuspidata* as modulators of multidrag resistant tumor cells. *Heterocycles* 54: 999–1009.
34. Bai, J. et al. 2004. Production of biologically active taxoids by a callus culture of *Taxus cuspidata*. *J. Nat. Prod.* 67: 58–63.
35. Bai, J. et al. 2005. Taxoids and abietanes from callus cultures of *Taxus cuspidata*. *J. Nat. Prod.* 68: 497–501.
36. Kosugi, K. et al. 2000. Neutral taxoids from *Taxus cuspidata* as modulators of multidrug-resistant tumor cells. *Phytochem.* 54: 839–45.
37. Kobayashi, J. et al. 1998. Modulation of multidrug resistance by taxuspine C and other taxoids from Japanese yew. *Bioorg. Med. Chem. Lett.* 8: 1555–8.
38. Sako, M. et al. 1999. Highly increased cellular accumulation of vincristine, a useful hydrophobic antitumor-drug, in multidrug-resistant solid cancer cells induced by a simply reduced taxinine. *Bioorg. Med. Chem. Lett.* 9: 3403–6.
39. Okumura, H. et al. 2000. Reversal of P-glycoprotein and multidrug-resistance protein-mediated drug resistance in KB cells by 5-*O*-benzoylated taxinine K. *Mol. pharmacol.* 58: 1563–9.
40. Okumura, H. et al, 2000. Reversal of P-glycoprotein and multidrug-resistance protein-mediated drug resistance in KB cells by 5-O-benzoylated taxinine *K. Mol. pharmacol.* 58: 1563-9.

11

Anticancer Potentials of Hard Lump-Resolving and Swelling-Reducing Herbs

CONTENTS

195 Tu Bei Mu 土貝母

Bulbus bolbostemmae

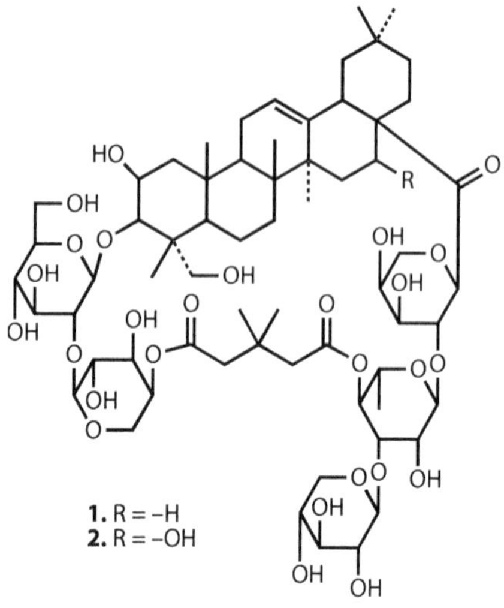

1. R = –H
2. R = –OH

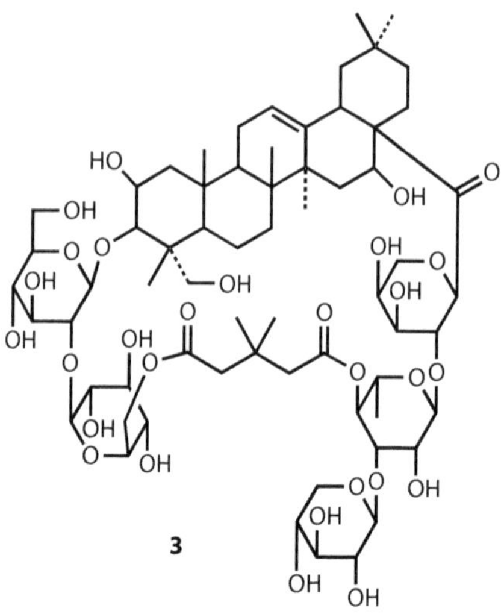

3

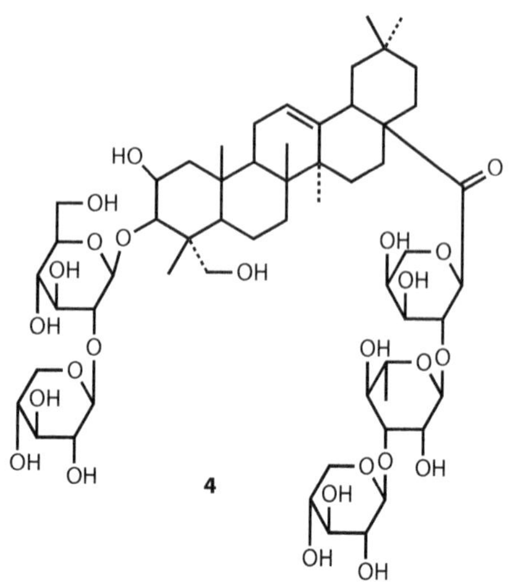

4

Herb Origination

The herb Tu Bei Mu is the dried bulbs and tubers of a Cucurbitaceae plant, *Bolbostemma paniculatum*. This plant is distributed in central China as well as Sichuan and Shandong provinces, and it is widely cultured in China. As a Chinese folk herb, the bulb is traditionally collected in late autumn and winter and dried in the sun after being fully steamed.

Antitumor Activities and Constituents

The impressive constituents discovered from the herb are the oleanane-type triterpene saponins with a unique cyclic structure between the aglycone and the saccharide. These agents were demonstrated to be primarily responsible for the antitumor activity and toxicity of the herb.

Cucurbitacine Triterpenoids

Four cucurbitacines such as cucurbitacin-E (**3**), 23,24-dihydrocucurbitacin-E (**4**), isocucurbitacin-B (**1**), and 23,24-dihydroisocucurbitacin-B (**2**) were separated from the EtOAc and n-BuOH extracts of the bulb of *B. paniculatum*. The *in vitro* assay showed significant to weak suppressive activities against HeLa (cervix) and HT-29 (colon) human cancer cell lines. The IC_{50} values were 0.93 and 2.63 μM for 23,24-dihydrocucurbitacin-E (**4**), 4.92 and 7.30 μM for cucurbitacin-E (**3**), 7.21 and 9.73 μM for isocucurbitacin-B (**1**), and 34.61 and 23.11 μM for 23,24-dihydroisocucurbitacin-B (**2**), respectively, in the HeLa and HT-29 cells. The activities of 23,24-dihydrocucurbitacin-E (**4**), cucurbitacin-E (**3**), and isocucurbitacin-B (**1**) on the two cell lines were more potent than those of 5-FU (an anticancer drug), but they were inactive on MCF-7 and BCG-823 breast cancer cell lines.[1] Cucurbitacin-E (**3**) also demonstrated the cytotoxic activity against malignant glioma GBM 8401 cells and induced cell cycle G2/M arrest in the cells via the upregulation of GADD45 γ and binding with CDC2.[2]

Triterpenoid Saponins

The three unique saponins designated as tubeimoside-I (**1**), tubeimoside-II (**2**), and tubeimoside-III (**3**) were separated from Tu Bei Mu as inhibitors of neoplastic growth, tumorigenesis, and inflammation. Their activities were normally tubeimoside-III > tubeimoside-II > tubeimoside-I, and their toxicities were tubeimoside-III > tubeimoside-I > tubeimoside-II.[3] Among them, tubeimoside-I (**1**) has been paid more attention for extensive investigations. The sensitivities of different types of cancer cell lines to tuneimoside-I (**1**) were found as glioblastoma > neuroblastoma > pancreas cancer > colon cancer > cervical cancer > gastric cancer.[4,5] An *in vitro* assay showed the inhibitory activity of tubcimoside-1 (**1**) on human malignant tumor cell lines, such as A549 (lung), Colo320DM (colon), BGC-823 and HGC-27 (stomach), and A-172, GOTO and PANC-1 (pancreas) cells, *in vitro*. The IC_{50} values ranged between 0.15 and 0.43 μM for the last four cell lines.[6–9] Besides the obvious growth inhibitory effect, the exposure of the tubeimoside-I (**1**) induced G2/M cell cycle arrest of HeLa cervical cancer cells via the decrease of the levels of cyclinB1, CDC25C and CDC2 and increase of Chk2 phosphorylation and promoted the apoptosis of HeLa cells via two pathways of mitochondrial dysfunction and ER stress cell death.[10–12] The apoptotic mechanism of tubeimoside-I (**1**) in human nasopharyngeal cancer CNE-2Z cells was associated with the downregulation of Bcl-2, the activation of Bax, and the increase of cytosolic tubulin proportion and microtubular network disruption, whose interactions led to the apoptosis-inducing and antigrowth effects in the CNE-2Z cells (IC_{50}: 16.7 μM, 72 h).[13,14] Similarly, by downregulating Bcl-2 and upregulating Fas and p53, tubeimoside-I (**1**) and tubeimoside-III (**3**) promoted the apoptotic death of human SW480 rectal cancer cells.[14]

Moreover, tubeimoside-I (**1**) dose- and time-dependently inhibited the proliferation of both human HepG2 hepatoma and L-02 normal live cell lines, but the HepG2 cells appeared to be more sensitive to the agent. The apoptotic mechanisms in the HepG2 cells were followed to be both extrinsic and intrinsic pathways, by which tubeimoside-I (**1**) induced ROS accumulation, mitochondrial membrane disruption, nuclear condensation, release of cytochrome c from the mitochondria, activation of caspase-3 and caspase-9, as well as blockage of the signaling regulations by TNFα, NF-κB, p53, and JNK, thereby exerting the antihepatoma effect.[16–18] The G2/M cell arrest and the apoptosis provoked by tubcimoside-1 (**1**) in human SKOV-3 ovarian cancer cells were correlated with activation of ERK signal transduction and a caspase-dependent mitochondrial pathway plus the increase of intracellular Ca^{2+} level.[19] The treatment of human JEG-3 choriocarcinoma cells with tubeimoside-I (**1**) elicited significant apoptosis and G2 cell arrest via the regulation of p38/MAPK, ERK1/2 and PI3K/Akt signaling pathways and the induction of mitochondrial dysfunction.[20] The apoptotic promotion in U251 glioma cells was elicited by amplifying Bax expression, attenuating Bcl-2 expression, and initiating ROS/cytochrome c/caspase-3 pathway.[21] These evidences revealed that the anticancer mechanisms of tubeimoside-I (**1**) were normally characteristic to the different types of neoplastic cell lines.

In vivo experiments in mice further confirmed that the tubeimoside-I (**1**) was capable of obstructing the tumor cell growth and inducing the cell apoptosis to prolong the life span of tumor-bearing mice. The daily intraperitoneal (i.p.) administration of tubeimoside-I (**1**) in a 3 mg/kg dose to mice for 16 continuous days resulted in the growth inhibition on sarcoma 180 by 71.5% and lifetime prolongation of mice bearing Ehrlich ascites cancer or sarcoma 180. When the tumor-bearing mice was injected 4 mg/kg of tebeimoside-I (**1**) per day for two weeks, the growth of murine H22 hepatoma cells was suppressed by 64%.[6,7] Furthermore, an advanced analysis armed at structure–bioactivity relationship between tubeimoside-I (**1**) and tubeimoside-II (**2**) disclosed that a C-16 hydroxyl group of tubeimoside-II plays an important role in the enhancement of the biological activity and the reduction of its toxicity. Therefore, tubeimoside-II (**2**) exhibited the relatively lowest acute toxicity in the tubeimosides.[2]

Tubeimoside-III (**3**) also demonstrated the cell-killing effects against various neoplastic cell lines in the bladder, the stomach, the liver, the ovary, the lung, and the kidney, as well as AML and erythroleukemia by inducing apoptosis and affecting cell lipid metabolism, with low toxic side effects.[22,23] The cytotoxic activities of tubeimoside-III (**3**) and dexylosyltubeimoside-III on HT-29, MCF-7, BGC-823, and HeLa human cancer cell lines were 3- to 16-fold that of 5-FU (IC_{50}: 1.30–3.42 versus 11.61–23.08 μM), whereas those of lobatoside-C, tubeimoside-V, and tubeimoside-I (**1**) on the four cell lines were better than or comparable to that of 5-FU.[1] Tubeimoside-V was also obviously effective in the antiproliferative effect on human U87MG glioblastoma cells in time- and dose-dependent fashions (IC_{50}: 3.6 μM). During the effect, tubeimoside-V promoted the prominence of cell cycle arrest and suggestive of apoptosis together with decreased Bcl-2 expression and increased Bax expression.[24]

Besides exerting the antileukemia effect, tubeimoside-I (**1**) and tubeimoside-III (**3**) also exerted an ability to provoke the differentiation of human K562 erythroleukemia cells, associated with the decrease of c-Myc expression, increase of c-fos expression, and induction of hemoglobin production.[25,26] In *in vitro* and *in vivo* experiments, tubeimoside-I (**1**) and tubeimoside-III (**3**) showed a potent antitumor-promoting effect on TPA-promoted two-stage carcinogenesis of mouse skin after topical application. However, if administered orally, tubeimoside-III (**3**) had no activity in the inhibition of tumor promotion, which was an important difference in bioactivities between tubeimoside-I (**1**) and tubeimoside-III (**3**).[23,27] In addition, a different type of saponin designated as bisdesmoside-1 (**4**) was separated from the herb, which does not have a cyclic connection in its saccharide potion, but it also displayed obvious cytotoxic effect against human K562 leukemia and BEL-7402 hepatoma cell lines and showed no hemolytic activity to erythrocytes in rabbits.[28]

Overall, all these evidences demonstrate that tubeimosides are efficient agents for suppressing the neoplastic cell growth and tumor promotion, having a great potential for further development in the clinical treatment of cancer.

Other Bioactivities

Pharmacological investigations have proven that tubeimoside-I (**1**), tubeimoside-II (**2**), and tubeimoside-III (**3**) have antiinflammatory, antiplatelet aggregation, antihemopexis, and antifibrin-dissolving activities. More research results evidenced that tubeimosides may be also developed into new drugs for the clinical treatment of infections from virus and acquired immune deficiency syndrome (AIDS).

References

1. Tang, Y. et al. 2015. Bioassay-guided isolation and identification of cytotoxic compounds from *Bolbostemma paniculatum*. *J. Ethnopharmacol.* 169: 18–23.
2. Hsu, Y. C. et al. 2014. Inducement of mitosis delay by cucurbitacin E, a novel tetracyclic triterpene from climbing stem of *Cucumis melo* L., through GADD45γ in human brain malignant glioma (GBM) 8401 cells. *Cell Death Disease* 5: e1087.
3. Yu, T. X. et al. 2001. Structure–activity relationship of tubeimosides in anti-inflammatory, antitumor, and antitumor-promoting effects. *Acta Pharmacol. Sinica* 22: 463–8.
4. Peng, J. P. et al. 1996. Anti-blood coagulation and cytotoxic effects of compounds from Chinese plants used for thrombosis-like diseases. *Nat. Med.* 50: 358–62.
5. Yang, P. et al. 2002. Cell cycle arrest and apoptosis induced by tubeimoside in HeLa cells. *Aizheng* 21: 346–50.
6. Ma, R. D. et al. 1992. Potent inhibitory effects of tubeimoside 1 isolated from the bulb of *Bolbostemma paniculatum* (Maxim) Franquet on inflammatory ear edema and tumor promotion in mice. *Chin. Sci. Bull.* 37: 602–6.
7. Yu, L. J. et al. 1994. Potent antitumor activity and low toxicity of tubeimoside 1 isolated from *Bolbostemma paniculatum*. *Planta Med.* 60: 204–8.
8. Zhang, Y. et al. 2011. Tubeimoside-1 inhibits proliferation and induces apoptosis by increasing the Bax to Bcl-2 ratio and decreasing COX-2 expression in lung cancer A549 cells. *Mol. Med. Reports* 4: 25–9.
9. Zhang, Y. et al. 2013. Effects of tubeimoside-1 on the proliferation and apoptosis of BGC823 gastric cancer cells in vitro. *Oncol. Lett.* 5: 801–4.
10. Xu, Y. et al. 2009. Tubeimoside-1 exerts cytotoxicity in HeLa cells through mitochondrial dysfunction and endoplasmic reticulum stress pathways. *J. Proteome Res.* 8: 1585–93.

11. Wang, F. et al. 2006. Role of mitochondria and mitochondrial cytochrome c in tubeimoside I-mediated apoptosis of human cervical carcinoma HeLa cell line. *Cancer Chemother. Pharmacol.* 57: 389–99.
12. Xu, Y. et al. 2011. Multiple pathways were involved in tubeimoside-1-induced cytotoxicity of HeLa cells. *J. Proteomics* 75: 491–501.
13. Ma, R. D. et al. 2008. Anti-microtubule activity of tubeimoside I and its colchicine binding site of tubulin. *Cancer Chemother. Pharmacol.* 62: 559–68.
14. Weng, X. Y. et al. 2004. Apoptosis of human nasopharyngeal carcinoma CNE-2Z cells induced by tubeimoside I. *Aizheng* 22: 806–11.
15. Yu, C. et al. 2006. Mechanisms of apoptosis induced by tubeimosides in human rectal cancer cell line SW480 in vitro. *Zhongguo Yaolixue Tongbao* 22: 880–4.
16. Wang, Y. S. et al. 2011. Natural plant extract tubeimoside I promotes apoptosis-mediated cell death in cultured human hepatoma (HepG2) cells. *Biol. Pharm. Bull.* 34: 831–8.
17. Yin, Y. et al. 2011. NF-κB, JNK and p53 pathways are involved in tubeimoside-1-induced apoptosis in HepG2 cells with oxidative stress and G2/M cell cycle arrest. *Food and Chemical Toxicol.* 49: 3046–54.
18. Huang. Y. S. et al. 2011. Natural plant extract tubeimoside I induces cytotoxicity via the mitochondrial pathway in human normal liver cells. *Mol. Med. Reports* 4: 713–8.
19. Chen, W. J. et al. 2012. Tubeimoside-1 induces G2/M phase arrest and apoptosis in SKOV-3 cells through increase of intracellular Ca^{2+} and caspase-dependent signaling pathways. *Intl. J. Oncol.* 40: 535–43.
20. Huang, P. et al. 2011. Cytotoxicity of tubeimoside I in human choriocarcinoma JEG-3 cells by induction of cytochrome c release and apoptosis via the mitochondrial-related signaling pathway. *Intl. J. Mol. Med.* 28: 579–87.
21. Jia, G. et al. 2015. Tubeimoside-1 induces glioma apoptosis through regulation of Bax/Bcl-2 and the ROS/Cytochrome C/Caspase-3 pathway. *Onco. Targer Ther.* 8: 303–11.
22. Yu, C. et al. 2005. *Faming Zhuanli Shenqing Gongkai Shuomingshu.* 12 pp. CN 1002–843, 20040215.
23. Yu, L. J. et al. 1995. Inhibition of the tumor promoting action of 12-*O*-tetradecanoylphorbol-13-acetate by tubeimoside III isolated from *Bolbostemma paniculatum. Carcinogenesis* 16: 3045–8.
24. Cheng, G. et al. 2006. Tubeimoside V, a new cyclic bisdesmoside from tubers of *Bolbostemma paniculatum*, functions by inducing apoptosis in human glioblastoma U87MG cells. *Bioorg. Med. Chem. Lett.* 16: 4575–80.
25. Yu, C. et al. 2007. Extraction of tubeimosides from *Bolbostemma paniculatum* and their effects on human erythroleukemia K562. *Xinan Daxue Xuebao, Ziran Kexueban* 29: 89–95.
26. Liu, J. Y. et al. 2006. Differentiation-inducing activity of tubeimoside I in human erythroleukemic K562 cells. *Zhongguo Linchuang Yaolixue yu Zhiliaoxue* 11: 743–7.
27. Yu, L. J. et al. 1992. Potent anti-tumorigenic effect of tubeimoside 1 isolated from the bulb of *Bolbostemma paniculatum* (Maxim) Franquet. *Intl. J. Cancer* 50: 635–8.
28. Tang, H. F. et al. 2006. Isolation and structural elucidation of a bioactive saponin from tubers of *Bolbostemma paniculatum. Zhongguo Zhongyao Zazhi* 31: 213–7.

196 Chan Su 蟾酥

Toad venom

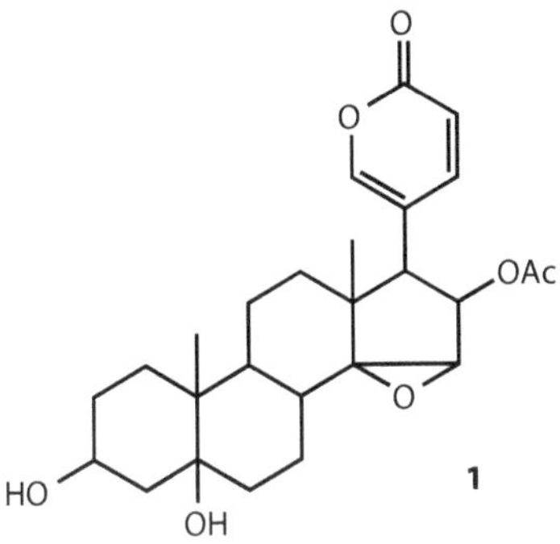

HO OH OAc O O O 1

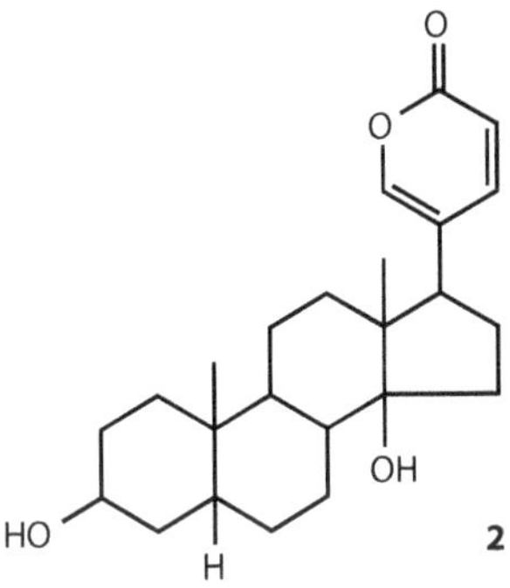

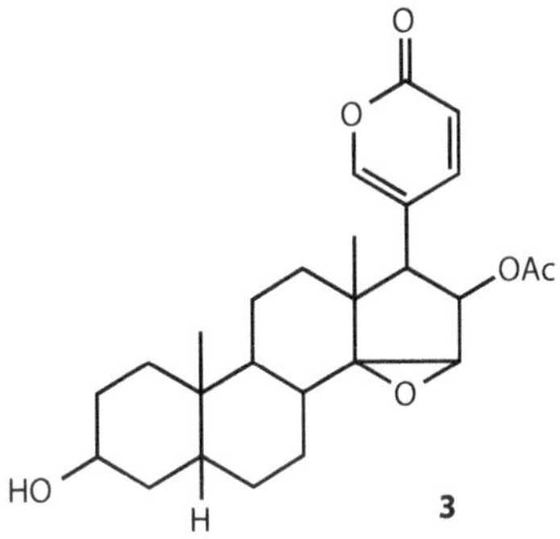

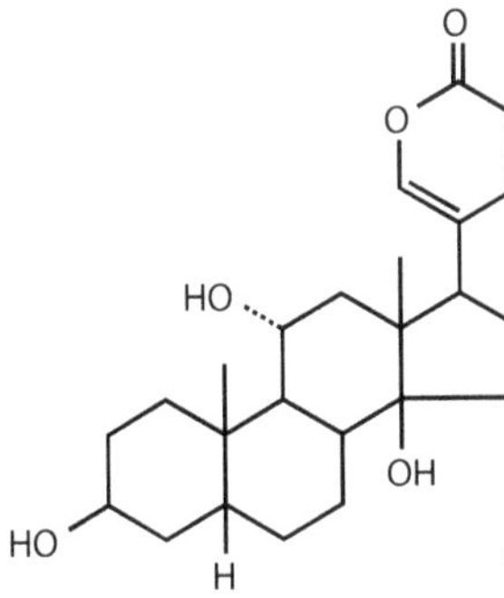

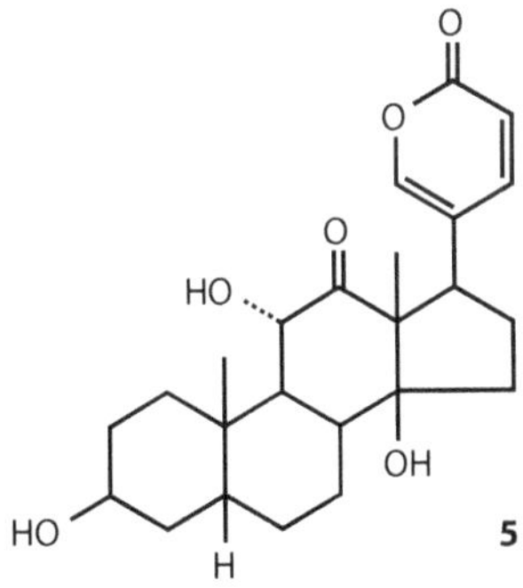

HO H OH O O 2

HO H OAc O O O 3

HO HO H OH O O 4

HO HO H OH O O O 5

HO H O O O O 6

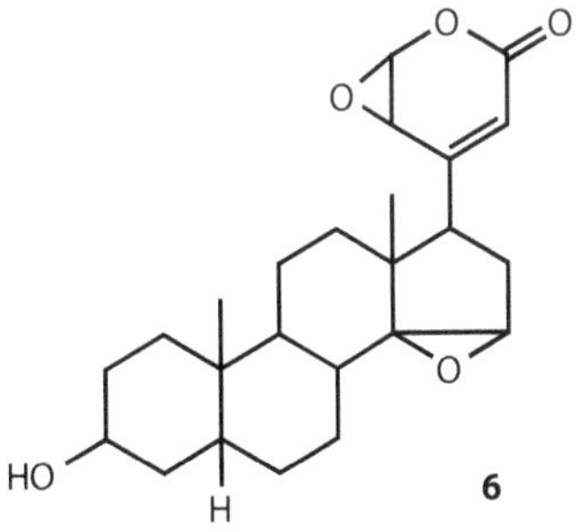

Herb Origination

The herb Chan Su (Toad venom) is the dried glandular secretion of a white serous, which is collected from the auricular and skin glands of toads, *Bufo bufo gargarizans* Cantor and *Bufo melanostictus* Schneider (Bufonidae). The former species of toad is distributed in the northern region of China as well as in the Sichuan province, and the latter one is distributed in the southern area of the Yangtze River as well as in Southeast Asia. The dried toad skin called Chan Pi is also used in traditional Chinese medicines.

Antitumor Activities

In recent years, the products containing or made from toad skin or Chan Su have been used in the treatment of cancer patients in China, exhibiting significant therapeutic results.[1] The Chan Su extracts have been indeed investigated in both *in vitro* and *in vivo* models. It markedly suppressed the proliferation of human leukemia cell lines followed by the promotion of the G2/M cell arrest and apoptosis.[2,3] By the treatment with Chan Su extract, the viability of human T24 bladder cancer cells was concentration-dependently suppressed and the apoptosis was enhanced in association with a series of interactions such as down-expression of antiapoptotic Bcl-2 and Bcl-xs/L and up-expression of proapoptotic Bax, concomitant with the degradation of PARP and β-catenin protein and the proteolytic activation of caspase-3 and caspase-9. Also, the Chan Su extract diminished COX-2 expression levels through an inhibition in prostaglandin-E2 synthesis.[4]

Cinobufacini is a traditional Chinese medicinal preparation widely used in clinics for the treatment of various cancers in China, which is the aqueous extract from the dried toad skin of *B. bufo gargarizans*, containing over 50% contents of water-soluble peptides. The clinical data proved that cinobufacini may have an effective chemotherapeutic potential to improve the life quality of cancer patients with low toxicity and few side effects.[5] *In vitro* experiments in two human hepatocellular cell lines (HepG2 and Bel-7402) demonstrated that cinobufacini significantly obstructed cell proliferation and induced apoptosis, whose mechanism was mediated by mitochondria- and Fas-involved caspase-dependent pathways, i.e., increase of Bax/Bcl-2 ratio, loss of mitochondrial membrane potential, release of cytochrome c, degradation of PARP, upregulation of Fas expression, and activation of caspases.[6] At a 50 μg/mL concentration, cinobufacini obviously inhibited the proliferation of human MDA-MB-231 breast cancer cells followed by the damage of the cell membrane structure and cytoskeleton networks and the increase of apoptosis and S phase cell cycle arrest.[7] The antigrowth effect of cinobufacini was also moderately demonstrated in human tumor cell lines such as BGC823 and MCG803 (stomach), DLD-1 and HT-29 (colon), and MIAPACA-2 (pancrease) with the IC_{50} values ranging from 25 to 123 μg/mL.[8]

TSE, an extract of the toad skin (*B. melanostictus*) collected in India was found as a potent antitumor agent having antiproliferative, cytotoxic, and apoptogenic activities against U937 and K562 myeloid leukemia cells.[9] At its IC_{50} dose, TSE restrained the proliferating cell nuclear antigen expression and arrested the cell cycle at G1 phase together with induction of apoptosis in both leukemia cells, but its cytotoxic potency on human normal PBMCs was less than on the U937 and K562 cells.[9] Also, an *in vivo* experiment revealed that *Bufonis venenum* had therapeutic effects on L7212 leukemia by inducing apoptosis and improving the immune system.[10]

In addition, the toad coat is another officinal part of *B. bufo gargarizans* for the antitumor and immunity activities. A great dosage of the toad coat (16 g/kg, per day) fed to mice inoculated with sarcoma 180, H22 hepatoma, or Lewis lung cancer cells could remarkably reduce the tumor weight and enhance the activities of both T lymphocyte and NK cells *in vivo*.[11]

Antitumor Constituents and Activities

Bufotoxins

Bufadienolides, a group of cardiotonic steroids with A/B *cis* and C/D *cis* structure as well as a ring of α-pyrone at the C-17 position, were isolated from Chan Pi and Chan Su. The approaches proved that the bufotoxins possess a broad spectrum of anticancer activity, which was evidenced by the inhibition of cell proliferation, the promotion of apoptosis, the disruption of cell cycle, the induction of cell differentiation, the repression of tumor angiogenesis, the reversal of cell MDR, and the stimulation of the immune response in the treatment of a variety of tumor cells with bufotoxins.[5] Cinobufagin (**1**), bufalin (**2**), and cinobufotalin (**3**) are the prominent bufotoxic steroids in these two herbs. The three major constituents play critical roles in the growth suppression of different types of neoplastic cells as well as antiinflammation.

Antileukemia Effect

Cinobufagin (**1**) was marked effective in the growth inhibition of human HL-60 and NB4 promyelocytic leukemia cells *in vitro*, and its IC_{50} value in the HL-60 cells was 1.25 ng/mL. It significantly restrained the cell proliferation and evidently induced the cells to apoptosis, including change of organelle structure such as swelling of the ER and the mitochondria and increase of lysosome. During the interactions, cinobufagin (**1**) also blocked the DNA synthesis and arrested the cell cycle at S phase in HL-60 cells and reduced Bcl-2 expression and increased Fas mRNA level in the NB4 cells.[12,13] Bufalin (**2**) is an apoptotic promoter in many human leukemia cells such as Molt-3 lymphoblastic cells, THP-1 monocytic cells, and HL-60 promyelocytic cells, but not in normal human leukocytes.[14,15] The HL-60 cell apoptosis enhanced by bufalin (**2**) correlated with the activation of Racl, PAK, and JNK pathways, including decrease of Bcl-2 and survivin expressions, mitochondrial release of Smac/DIABLO, and activation of caspase-3, and its IC_{50} value at 72 h in the HL-60 cells was 2.1 nmol/L.[15–17] As an inhibitor of Topo-II and Na^+-/K^+-ATPase, bufalin (**2**) concurrently reduced the amount and the activity of Topo-II and especially changed the intracellular concentration of Na^+ ions, which acts upstream of the Bcl-2 expression in human leukemia cells.[8,12] Besides the inhibitory activity, bufalin (**2**) also demonstrated strong differentiation-inducing activity in four human leukemia-derived cells (U937 monoblastic, K562 erythroleukemia, HL-60 promyelocytic, and ML1 myeloblastic) at a concentration of as low as 10 nM,[18,19] and it displayed modest functional and morphological differentiations of leukemia cells from AML patients in primary culture.[19] When bufalin (**2**) is combined with all-*trans*-retinoic, a synergistic differentiation could be effectively achieved in the treatment of acute promyelocytic leukemia cells.[20]

Antisexual Organ Cancer Effect

Cinobufagin (**1**) and bufalin (**2**) demonstrated a significant suppressive effect against the proliferation of prostate carcinoma cell lines (LNCaP, DU145, and PC3) after two to four days of *in vitro* culture at doses of 0.1–10 μM. The increased intracellular calcium ($[Ca^{2+}]i$) concentration by both cinobufagin and bufalin provoked the apoptosis of the three prostate cancer cells followed by caspase-3 activation in the DU145 and PC3 cells and caspase-9 activation in the LNCaP cells.[16,20] The marked cytotoxic activity of cinobufagin (**1**), bufalin (**2**), and cinobufotalin (**3**) was also demonstrated in human HeLa cervical cancer cells *in vitro*,[17,21] whose HeLa cell apoptosis could be accelerated by bufalin (**2**) in a concentration of 10^{-8} M in association with the augmentation of Tiam1 (a downstream mediator for the apoptosis) expression.[17] The proliferation of human MCF-7 breast cancer cells could be significantly diminished by the treatment of cinobufotalin (**3**) *in vitro* at concentrations of 0.4 and 0.2 g/mL.[22]

Antihepatoma Effect

Even at a low concentration, cinobufagin (**1**) and bufalin (**2**) still remarkably inhibited the growth of human SMMC-7721, BEL-7402, and HepG2 hepatoma cells *in vitro*, and the IC_{50} value of cinobufagin (**1**) in the SMMC-7721 cells was 2.72 ng/mL, whose antineoplastic effects were stronger than mitomycin-C at the same concentration, and the effect of bufalin (**2**) was more potent than that of cinobufagin (**1**). During the antigrowth action in the hepatoma cells, the cell cycle was arrested at G2/M phase and the cell apoptotic death was accelerated followed by the upregulation of Bax expression. The apoptosis-inducing effect of cinobufagin (**1**) and bufalin (**2**) in hepatoma HepG2 cells was found to be elicited by Fas- and mitochondria-mediated pathways and Fas-mediated caspase-10-dependent pathway. Furthermore, both cinobufagin (**1**) and bufalin (**2**) at a high dose could demolish the tumor cell membrane effectively.[23,24] The remarkable antihepatoma effect was also demonstrated in murine animal models with xenografts or homografts.[25–27] Besides the antiproliferative effect on HCCLM3 and HepG2 cell lines, bufalin (**2**) could also inhibit the hepatoma cell migration, invasion, and adhesion via the suppression of AKT/GSK3β/β-catenin/E-cad signaling pathway, i.e., significantly declined the levels of pAKT, pGSK3β, MMP-9, and MMP-2; amplified the levels of GSK3β and E-cad; and obstructed the nuclear translocation of β-catenin.[28] Similarly, by inhibiting MMP-2 and MMP-9 and involving PI3K/AKT and NF-κB pathways, bufalin (**2**) inhibited the migration and the invasion of human SK-Hepl hepatocellular carcinoma cells to prevent the metastasis of malignant liver tumor.[29] The evidences suggested that bufalin (**2**) may be a potential therapeutic candidate for the treatment of hepatoma.

Moreover, more than 25 cardiotonic steroids isolated from the herbs were exhibited to possess significant cytotoxicity against human SMMC-7721 hepatoma cells *in vitro*. The most potent components were gamabufutalin (**4**) and arenobufagin (**5**) with the IC_{50} values of 0.1 and 0.03 μg/mL, respectively. Others demonstrated their IC_{50} values in the range of 0.12–4.72 μg/mL.[30,31]

Antigastrointestinal Cancer Effect

The marked cytotoxic effect of cinobufagin (**1**) and cinobufotalin (**3**) was demonstrated *in vitro* against human gastrointestinal cancer cell lines such as HCT-8 (colon) and BGC (stomach).[21] Bufalin (**2**) effectively promoted the apoptosis of human Colo320DM colon adenocarcinoma cells[17] and significantly caused G2/M cell cycle arrest of human MGC-803 gastric carcinoma cells in association with the upregulation of p16, p21, and pRb protein expressions, resulting in the notable growth inhibition on the tumor cells. The IC_{50} of bufalin (**2**) at 72 h was 0.036 μmol/L on the MGC-803 cells *in vitro*.[32] Moreover, by the treatment of cinobufagin (**1**) combined with an anticancer drug 5-FU, the antineoplastic effect was synergistically potentiated against the BGC823 gastric carcinoma cells.[33]

Antimelanoma Effect

The treatment with cinobufagin (**1**) at concentration of 10^{-4} M for six days resulted in a stimulatory effect on the melanin synthesis of mouse melanoma B16-F10 cells.[34] Bufalin (**2**) also increased the cellular melanin content and stimulated the tyrosinase activity for exerting the antiproliferative effect against the melanoma B16-F10 cells.[35]

Antisarcoma Effect

An *in vitro* assay showed that bufalin (**2**) significantly inhibited the cell proliferation and induced the G2/M cell arrest and the apoptosis of both methotrexate 300-sensitive and methotrexate 300-resistant human U-2OS osteosarcoma cells, via the increase of Bax/Bcl-2 protein ratio and the augmentation of cancer-suppressor protein p53 expression.[36] The suppressive effect of bufalin (**2**) against the tumor cell growth was also found to be related to its clear inhibition of Topo-II catalytic activity.[36] *In vivo* studies confirmed the cell growth inhibitory effect of cinobufagin (**1**) against mouse sarcoma 180 and L6 reticulosarcoma cells. The *in vivo* inhibitory rates was over 30% by the oral administration in a dose of 20 g/kg, but it had no obvious antitumor activity if its dose was below 8 g/kg.[21,25]

Other Anticancer Effect

The marked cytotoxic activity of cinobufagin (**1**) and cinobufotalin (**3**) was also observed in other types of human malignant tumor cell lines such as KB nasopharynx and BIU bladder cancer cells *in vitro*. Cinobufotalin (**3**) in its dosages (i.p.: 8–12.5 g/kg) exerted the antigrowth effect against Lewis lung cancer cells and prolonged the survival time of mice. However, it had obvious toxicity and no effect on the metastasis of Lewis lung cancer.[37] Cinobufagin (**1**) could act as a potent inhibitor against human U266 multiple myeloma cells, whose effects were associated with ROS-mediated activation of ERK, JNK, and p38 MAPK leading to the activation of caspase-3 in U266 cells.[38] By eliciting interplay between apoptosis and autophagy via the stimulation of the ER stress, bufalin (**2**) significantly obstructed the growth of malignant glioma cells.[39] Bufalin (**2**) was also effective in inhibiting the proliferation of human MG-63 osteosarcoma cells and inducing the cell apoptosis in dose- and time-dependent manners by targeting mitochondrial-dependent signaling pathway such as downregulation of Bcl-2/Bax, upregulation of ROS and apoptotic protease activating factor-1 (Apaf-1), disruption of mitochondrial transmembrane potential, activation of caspase-3 and caspase-9, and cleavage of PARP.[40]

Antiangiogenic Effect

Angiogenesis is crucial for carcinogenic and cancer growth-developing processes. Arenobufagin (**5**) was capable of obstructing the VEGF-induced viability, migration, invasion, and tube formation in HUVECs *in vitro* and inhibiting the sprouting formation from VEGF-treated aortic rings in an *ex vivo* model. Moreover, arenobufagin (**5**) inhibited the activities of VEGFR-2-mediated signaling cascades and restrained VEGF-induced VEGFR-2 autophosphorylation. The evidences clearly demonstrated that arenobufagin (**5**) is a specific inhibitor of VEGF-mediated angiogenesis,[41] whose property should be beneficial for chemotherapy in the treatment of cancer development.

Peptides

Two antimicrobial peptide termed buforin-I and buforin-II were generated by pepsin-directed proteolysis in the cytoplasm of the gastric gland cells of toad *B. bufo gargarizans*. Buforin-I was composed of 39-amino acid units, whereas buforin-II is a 21-amino acid peptide that can be derived from buforin-I. Both peptides share a complete sequence identity with the N-terminal region of histone H2A that directly interacts with nucleic acids. The buforins were demonstrated to possess antiendotoxin and anticancer activities, and both were also capable of enhancing the innate immune system and the innate host defense, shown to be as an attractive application in the cancer therapy.[42] Two *Bufo gargarizans* antimicrobial peptides, BG-CATH37 and BG-CATH(5-37), were also reported to have the advantages of significant antimicrobial and antitumor effects.[43]

TSP, an antitumor peptide isolated from the toad skin (*B. bufo gargarizans*), strongly inhibited the proliferation and the viability of human HepG2 hepatocarcinoma cells but had little toxicity to normal liver L-02 cells. At a 50 μg/mL concentration, TSP primarily arrested the HepG2 cell cycle at G1 phase and promoted the HepG2 cells to apoptosis. The cytotoxicity of 5-FU (a chemotherapeutic drug) could be synergistically enhanced by the TSP treatment.[44]

Proteins

BMP1 is a protein (79 kDa) separated from the aqueous extract of the toad skin (*B. melanostictus*). It could exert antiproliferative and apoptogenic activities against EAC cells with limited toxicity. The i.p. administration of BMP1 in doses of 0.5 and 1.0 mg/kg per day for three days significantly diminished the tumor cell viability, thereby obviously prolonging the life period of mice bearing EAC with no obvious hematological side effects.[45] The anticancer activity of BMP1 was also proven in an *in vitro* assay with human U937 and K562 leukemic cells and human HepG2 hepatoma cells. The growth of U937 cells and K562 cells were moderately restrained by the BMP1 treatment with IC_{50} values of 49 and 30 μg/mL, respectively. The antigrowth effect in the three cancer cell lines was accompanied by Sub-G1 and/or G1 cell cycle arrest through the increase of CDKIs (p21cip1 and p27kip1) expressions and the decrease of CDK2 and PCNA expressions. In parallel, the Bax and p53 expressions were upregulated and caspase-3 and caspase-9 were activated, leading the HepG2 cells to apoptosis. The BMP1 also displayed low immunogenic properties with minimum toxicity against normal PBMCs.[46]

Structure–Activity Relationship

The cytotoxicities of the 30 bufadienolides were investigated by using an *in vitro* bioassay of four human carcinoma cell lines (BGC823, HeLa, HL-60, and Bel-7402). The results suggested that 3-OH glucosylation or hydroxylation at C-1β or C-12 positions might be promising designs for more polar bufadienolides with enhanced cytotoxicities. For example, 1β-hydroxylbufalin and 12β-hydroxylbufalin showed potent cytotoxicities against BGC-823 gastric cancer cells and HeLa cervical carcinoma cells with IC_{50} values of 10^{-5} to 10^{-6} mol/mL. Both molecules were more active than their parent bufalin (**2**). However, the activity would be significantly reduced when the hydroxylation is at 15α-, 15β-, or 16α-positions and 14β/15β-epoxy ring at bufalin (**2**).[47] Also, the bufalin derivatives were normally more active than their corresponding cinobufagin (**1**) analogs.

12α-Hydroxylated cinobufagin (**1**) was about 10 times more active than its 12β-OH epimer, implying that the 16-acetoxyl group was essentially important for the cytotoxicity of cinobufagin (**1**) analogs. The 3-OH glucosylated cinobufagin (**1**) was two times more active than its origin compound against all the four test cancer cell lines, whereas the glucosylation of 16-OH could not improve the activity. All the deacetylation at cinobufagin (**1**) obviously reduced the cytotoxicities.[47] Moreover, cinobufotalin (**3**) and cinobufagin (**1**) exhibited marked cytotoxic activity on human carcinoma cells such as HCT-8, KB, BGC, and BIU cells *in vitro*. However, the oral administration of these agents showed no/less suppressive effect on the tumor cell growth, whose reason was found to be that cinobufagin (**1**) and cinobufotalin (**3**) could be converted to non-anticancer active metabolites, namely, deacetylcinobufagin and deacetyl-cinobufotalin, respectively, by the deactivation of human intestinal bacteria during the drug through gastrointestinal tract.[21]

Furthermore, 80 natural and synthetic derivatives of bufadienolides were applied to study the SARs. The assays of primary PLC/PRF/5 hepatoma cells confirmed that most important factors for the cytotoxicity were α-pyrone ring, 14β-OH or 14α,15α-epoxy, 19-CHO, 11α-OH, and 16β-OAc groups, and the D-ring structure and the 3-substituent structure also contributed to the activity. The molecules with an aldehyde group at C-19, a hydroxyl group at C-11, or acetate demonstrated stronger activity, and the 14β-hydroxy derivatives were generally more potent than the 14,15-epoxy analogs and the opened α-pyrone ring compounds.[48,49] The bufenolides having an oxo group at C-3 position and an epoxy at C-20 and C-21 positions were found to exert significant inhibitory effect against human MH-60 leukemia cells and KB oral epidermoid carcinoma cells *in vitro*. But, according to SAR studies, 20,21-epoxybufenolides generally displayed less and/or different activity than the parent bufadienolide system. 3-Formates of the 20,21-epoxy bufenolides were inactive against the KB and MH-60 carcinoma cell lines.[50] The 20β,21β-epoxyresibufogenin (**6**) and its responding formate possess potent inhibitory activity on the growth of IL-6-dependent MH-60 cells but not on the IL-6-independent growth of MH-60 cells. The evidences given earlier indicated that the epoxide groups at the 14,15- and/or 20,21-positions were required to exert the cytotoxic effect. In addition, the introduction of an acetyl group to C-3 position demonstrated considerable growth inhibition toward the IL-6-dependent MH-60 cells, but 16-OH acetylation would reduce the suppressive rate.[51]

Clinical Practices

The herbs Chan Su and Chan Pi had been clinically explored in the treatment of some cancers in China, because it does not only inhibit and kill some types of cancer cells, especially hepatoma, but is also satisfactorily effective in treating patients with neoplasm either when applied alone or together with interventional therapy.

1. A phase 1 trial was designed for 15 patients with advanced cancer, including NSCLC (2 cases), hepatocellular cancer (11 cases), and pancreatic cancer (2 cases), by the Chan Su treatment. Five intravenous doses (10–90 mL/m^2) of Chan Su were administered for 14 days followed by 7 days off as a cycle treatment. The patients without significant adverse events or progressive disease continued with the treatment beyond two cycles. Six cases (40%) had stable results or minor tumor shrinkage. Eleven patients had no drug-related toxicity, and their quality of life was improved obviously. One patient with hepatocellular cancer had 20% regression (life duration of 11 months) in a dose of 10 mL/m^2.[52]
2. One hundred patients with moderate and advanced primary hepatoma were randomly divided into cinobufacini injection-treated group (50 patients) and control group (50 patients). The cancer progressive rate of the drug-treated group (18%) was lower than that of the control group (32%). The survival rate of >12 months of the drug-treated group (30%) was higher than that of the control group (18%). The patients' liver function such as serum total bilirubin and alanine transaminase were obviously decreased in the drug-treated group but increased a lot in the control group.[53]
3. Sixty-two cases with advanced NSCLC were divided into two groups. Thirty patients in the test group were treated with a combination of huachansu (cinobufotalin) injection and chemotherapy, and 32 patients in the control group only received chemotherapy. The total efficiency rates in the two groups after two cycles of treatment were 53.50% and 43.80%. The combined treatment with chemotherapy can improve the curative effect of NSCLC and the life quality of patients as well as reduce the side effects and enhance the immune function.[54]
4. Toad rice wine (15 gutted toads in 1.5 L of rice wine were steamed for 2 hours) was prepared for the treatment of 32 cases of leukemia patients, including acute histiocytic leukemia (5 cases), lymphoblastic leukemia (9 cases), chronic lymphoblastic leukemia (1 case), acute granulocyte leukemia (4 cases), chronic granulocyte leukemia (3 cases), promyelocyte leukemia (4 cases), erythroleukemia (3 cases), and preleukemia (3 cases). Each adult patient drank the toad rice wine (15–30 mL, three times per day) for over 20 days. The total remission rate resulted to 75%, while the complete remission rate was 25%. The treatment markedly prolonged the survival rate of patients and the most extended life duration reached to 71 months. The toad rice wine seems sensitive to ALL and less responsive to promyelocyte leukemia and histiocytic leukemia.[55]

5. Eighty-four cases of confirmed advanced primary hepatoma were randomly and equally allocated into two groups. Group A was given transcather arterial chemoembolization (TACE) combined with cinobufotain, whereas group B was only given TACE. The effective rate and the survival rate in group A are much higher than those in group B. The activity of NK, CD3, CD4, CD8, and CD4/CD8 were much improved in group A, but it decreased in group B after the treatment. The clinical trial suggested that cinobufotain is a beneficial agent for augmenting the antihepatoma effect and the immunologic function after TACE.[56]
6. Eighty-nine cases of lung cancer hydrothorax among elderly patients were randomly divided into a combination group (46 cases) and a chemotherapy group (43 cases). The combination group received cinobufacini injection (80–100 mL) combined with staphylococcin (20 mL) and cisplatin (10–15 mg/m^2), and the chemotherapy group received only cisplatin (40–50 mg/m^2). Both groups were treated for one month by intrapleural administration. The resulted efficiency of the combination group and the chemotherapy group were 76.1% and 63.5%, respectively, implying that the combined treatment might be generalized in clinics for elderly patients with lung cancer hydrothorax.[57]

Many clinical investigations had been preceded in China by using cinobufacini in the treatment of cancer patients.[58–61] Based upon the positive results, the three kinds formulations of cinobufacini (injection, oral liquid, and capsule) were utilized for clinical cancer therapy in China. The drugs showed great potential for the treatment of gastric cancer, lung carcinoma, colon cancer, esophagus carcinoma, pancreatic cancer, and acute leukemia. When combined with standard chemotherapy and radiotherapy, the drugs can exert significant synergic effect and reduced the toxic and side effects cause by chemotherapy and radiotherapy.

Other Bioactivities

The herbs Chan Su and Chan Pi display cardiotonic, artery pressure-stimulating, antishock, antimyocardial ischemia, antiplatelet aggregation, immunoenhancing, smooth muscle-exciting, antiinflammatory, and antibacterial effects. Both herbs also possess local narcotic and anti-HBV activities.[62]

Because Chan Pi, Chan Su and their products have toxicity, the dosage must be carefully calculated in clinical use. The toxicity of cinobufagin (**1**) is relatively lower in comparison with other cardiotonic steroids. The i.p. injection of cinobufagin to rats in dose of 4 or 20 mg/kg (responding to the clinical dosage of 100-fold or 500-fold) per a couple days for 20 continuous days showed no significant toxic reaction.

References

1. Feng, G. X. 2002. Prospect of anticancerous natural products from animals. *J. Hubei Univ. for Nationalities, Science Edit.* 20: 45–8.
2. Jin, B. et al. 2004. Partial purification and antileukemia effect of toad toxication. *J. China Med. Univ.* 33: 517–9.
3. Lu, X. L. et al. 2003. Effect of toad toxication on proliferation and progression of cell cycle in cultured leukemia K562 cells. *J. China Med. Univ.* 32: 19–20.
4. Ko, W. S. et al. 2005. Induction of apoptosis by Chan Su, a traditional Chinese medicine, in human bladder carcinoma T24 cells. *Oncol. Reports* 14: 475–80.
5. Qi, F. H. et al. 2011. Antitumor activity of extracts and compounds from the skin of the toad *Bufo bufo gargarizans* Cantor. *Int. Immuno-pharmacol.* 11: 342–9.
6. Qi, F. H. et al. 2012. Induction of apoptosis by cinobufacini preparation through mitochondria- and Fas-mediated caspase-dependent pathways in human hepatocellular carcinoma cells. *Food Chem. Toxicol.* 50: 295–302.
7. Ma, L. N. et al. 2012. Cinobufacini induced MDA-MB-231 cell apoptosis-associated cell cycle arrest and cytoskeleton function. *Bioorg.Med. Chem. Lett.* 22: 1458–63.
8. Xu, W. et al. 2012. In vitro anti-proliferation effect of peptides from cinobufacini injection. *Yaoxue Xuebao* 47: 822–6.
9. Giri, B. et al. 2006. Antiproliferative, cytotoxic and apoptogenic activity of Indian toad (*Bufo melanostictus* Schneider) skin extract on U937 and K562 cells. *Toxicon* 48: 388–400.
10. Xiao, Y. et al. 2014. Research on therapeutic effects of *Bufonis venenum* on L7212 leukemia and its mechanism. *Zhongyaocai* 37: 199–201.
11. Miao, Z. L. et al. 2010. Studies on antitumor and enhancing immunity activity of toad coat. *Zhongguo Zhongyao Zazhi* 35: 211–4.
12. Zhao, J. B. et al. 2001. Experimental study on anticancer action of cinobufagin in vitro. *Disi Junyi Daxue Xuebao* 22: 1504–7.
13. Wang, Y. et al. 2005. Study on apoptosis of NB4 cells induced by cinobufagin and its mechanism. *Zhongliu* 25: 534–7.
14. Kawazoe, N. et al. 1999. Induction of apoptosis by bufalin in human tumor cells is associated with a change of intracellular concentration of Na^+ ions. *J. Biochem.* 126: 278–86.
15. Tian, X. et al. 2006. Downregulation of bcl-2 and survivin expressions and release of Smac/DIABLO involved in bufalin-induced HL-60 apoptosis. *Zhonghua Xueyexue Zazhi* 27: 21–4.
16. Hashimoto, S. et al. 1997. Bufalin reduces the level of topoisomerase II in human leukemia cells and affects the cytotoxicity of anticancer drugs. *Leukemia Res.* 21: 875–83.
17. Cao, H. et al. 2007. Involvement of Tiam1 in apoptosis induced by bufalin in HeLa cells. *Anticancer Res.* 27: 245–50.
18. Zhang, L. S. et al. 1991. Bufalin as a potent inducer of differentiation of human myeloid leukemia cells. *Biochem. Biophys. Res. Commun.* 178: 686–93.
19. Zhang, L. S. et al. 1992. Induction by bufalin of differentiation of human leukemia cells HL-60, U937, and ML1 toward macrophage/monocyte-like cells and its potent synergistic effect on the differentiation of human leukemia cells in combination with other inducers. *Cancer Res.* 52: 4634–41.
20. Yamada, K. et al. 1998. Enhancement by bufalin of retinoic acid-induced differentiation of acute promyelocytic leukemia cells in primary culture. *Leukemia Res.* 22: 589–95.
21. Yang, X. W. et al. 2001. Studies on metabolism of cinobufagin and cinobufotalin by human intestinal bacteria. *J. Beijing Univ. Med. Edit.* 33: 199–204.
22. Wang, S. J. et al. 2006. Experimental study of triptolide only or combined with cinobufotalin on MCF-7 growth of breast cancer. *Xiandai Zhongxiyi Jiehe Zazhi* 15: 573–4, 642.

23. Wang, D. L. et al. 2010. Apoptosis-inducing activity of compounds screened and characterized from cinobufacini by bioassay-guided isolation. *Mol. Med. Reports* 3: 717–22.
24. Qi, F. H. et al. 2011. Bufalin and cinobufagin induce apoptosis of human hepatocellular carcinoma cells via Fas- and mitochondria-mediated pathways. *Cancer Sci.* 102: 951–8.
25. Gu, W. et al. 2007. Inhibitory action of bufalin on human transplanted hepatocellular tumor and its effects on expressions of Bcl-2 and Bax proteins in nude mice. *Zhongxiyi Jiehe Xuebao* 5: 155–9.
26. Su, Y. H. et al. 2003. Inhibition effects of three kinds of bufotoxins on human SMMC-7721 and BEL-7402 hepatoma cells lines. *Dier Junyi Daxue Xuebao* 24: 393–5.
27. Yin, C. N. et al. 1993. Anticancer effect of cinobufotanin oral liquid. *Guangzhou Yiyao* 24: 19.
28. Qiu, D. Z. et al. 2013. Bufalin, a component in Chansu, inhibits proliferation and invasion of hepatocellular carcinoma cells. *BMC Complem. Alternat. Med.* 13, 185: 11 p.
29. Chen, Y. Y. et al. 2015. Bufalin inhibits migration and invasion in human hepatocellular carcinoma SK-Hepl cells through the inhibitions of NF-κB and matrix metalloproteinase-2/-9-signaling pathways. *Environmental Toxicol.* 30: 74–82.
30. Wu, F. K. et al. 2011. Cytotoxic constituents from the skin of the toad *Bufo bufo gargarizans. J. Asian Nat. Prod. Res.* 13: 111–6.
31. Zhao, H. Y. et al. 2010. Studies on cytotoxic constituents from the skin of the toad *Bufo bufo gargarizans. J. Asian Nat. Prod. Res.* 12: 793–800.
32. Yue, Y. et al. 2005. Effect of bufalin on cell cycle arrest of gastric cancer MGC-803 cells. *Zhongliu Fangzhi Zazhi* 12: 409–12.
33. Fang, Q. X. et al. 2004. Interaction between 5-fluorouracil and cinobufagin on human gastric carcinoma cell line. *Zhongguo Yiyuan Yaoxue Zazhi* 24: 616–7.
34. Zhang, L. S. et al. 1992. Stimulation of melanin synthesis of B16-F10 mouse melanoma cells by bufalin. *Life Sci.* 51: 17–24.
35. Yin, J. Q. et al. 2007. Bufalin induces apoptosis in human osteosarcoma U-2OS and U-2OS methotrexate 300-resistant cell lines. *Acta Pharmacologica Sinica* 28: 712–20.
36. Pastor, N. et al. 2002. A comparative study of genotoxic effects of anti-topoisomerase II drugs ICRF-193 and bufalin in Chinese hamster ovary cells. *Mutat. Res. Genet. Toxicol. Environ. Mutagen.* 515: 171–80.
37. Lin, Y. et al. 2003. Experimental study on anticancer action of cinobufotalin injection for pulmonary carcinoma. *J. Zhongyiyao Univ.* 20: 69–71.
38. Baek, S. H. et al. 2015. Cinobufagin exerts anti-proliferative and pro-apoptotic effects through the modulation ROS-mediated MAPKs signaling pathway. *Immunopharmacol. Immunotoxicol.* 37: 265–73.
39. Shen, S. Y. et al. 2014. Bufalin induces the interplay between apoptosis and autophagy in glioma cells through endoplasmic reticulum stress. *Intl. J. Biol. Sci.* 10: 212–24.
40. Wang, D. W. et al. 2014. Bufalin inhibited the growth of human osteosarcoma MG-63 cells via down-regulation of Bcl-2/Bax and triggering of the mitochondrial pathway. *Tumor Biol.* 35: 4885–90.
41. Li, M. M. et al. 2012. Arenobufagin, a bufadienolide compound from toad venom, inhibits VEGF-mediated angiogenesis through suppression of VEGFR-2 signaling pathway. *Biochem. Pharmacol.* 83: 1251–60.
42. Cho, J. Y. et al. 2009. Buforins: Histone H2A-derived antimicrobial peptides from toad stomach. *Biochimica et Biophysica Acta, Biomembranes* 1788: 1564–9.
43. Gao, Y. Y. et al. 2015. Bufo gargarizans antimicrobial peptides BG-CATH37 and BG-CATH(5-37), and coding genes and application thereof. *Faming Zhuanli Shenqing* CN 104530209 A 20150422.
44. Lu, C. X. et al. 2011. Anticancer peptide from Chinese toad (*Bufo bufo gargarizans*) skin enhanced sensitivity to 5-Fu in hepato-carcinoma cells (HepG2). *Clinical Oncol. Cancer Res.* 8: 149–54.
45. Bhattacharjee, P. et al. 2011. Apoptogenic activity and toxicity studies of a cytotoxic protein (BMP1) from the aqueous extract of common Indian toad (*Bufo melanostictus* Schneider) skin. *Toxicon* 57: 225–36.
46. Gomes, A. et al. 2011. Anticancer activity of a low immunogenic protein toxin (BMP1) from Indian toad (*Bufo melanostictus* Schneider) skin extract. *Toxicon* 58: 85–92.
47. Ye, M. et al. 2004. Novel cytotoxic bufadienolides derived from bufalin by microbial hydroxylation and their structure-activity relationships. *J. Steroid Biochem. Mol. Biol.* 91: 87–98.
48. Kamano, Y. et al. 1998. Structure-cytotoxic activity relationship for the toad poison bufadienolides. *Bioorg. Med. Chem.* 6: 1103–15.
49. Kamano, Y. et al. 1996. Structures and antineoplastic activity of the toad poison bufadienolides. *Tennen Yuki Kagobutsu Toronkai Koen Yoshishu* 38th, 9–354.
50. Kamano, Y. et al. 2002. Isolation and structure of a 20,21-epoxybufenolide series from "Ch'an Su" *J. Nat. Prod.* 65: 1001–5.
51. Enomoto, A. et al. 2004. Inhibitory effects of bufadienolides on interleukin-6 in MH-60 cells. *J. Nat. Prod.* 67: 2070–2.
52. Meng, Z. Q. et al. 2009. Pilot study of huachansu in patients with hepatocellular carcinoma, non-small-cell lung cancer, or pancreatic cancer. *Cancer* 115: 5309–18.
53. Chen, Z. et al. 2003. Clinical observation of cinobufacini injection used to treat moderate and advanced primary liver cancer. *J. Chinese Integrative Med.* 1: 184–6.
54. Li, X. Q. et al. 2009. Clinical research of combined huachansu injection with chemotherapy on advanced non -small cell lung cancer. *Modern Oncol.* 17: 60–1.
55. Qian, J. M. et al. 1984. Chemotherapy of 32 cases of leukemia with a Chinese herb Chanchu rice-wine. *Liaoning Zhongyi Zazhi* 4: 18.
56. Liu, X. H. et al. 2009. Clinical effect of cinobufotain on patients with liver malignancy after transcather arterial chemoembolization. *Chinese J. Modern Drug Application* 23: 134–5.
57. Gao, Y. X. et al. 2012. 89 Cases of lung cancer hydrothorax among elderly patients in the treatment with cinobufacini injection combined with staphylococcin and cisplatin. *Contemporary Med.* (Chinese) 18: 139–40.
58. Niu, J. X. et al. 2008. Clinical effect of cinobufacini injection in treating advanced malignant tumor of digestive tract in 30 patients. *J. Tianjin Univ. TCM.* 2: 105–7.
59. Lu, H. et al. 2009. The research progress in the anticarcinoma with cinobufacini. *J. Youjiang Med. College for Nationalities* 5: 895–6.
60. Zuo, X. D. et al. 2003. The clinical investigation of cinobufacini in cancer therapy. *Chinese Cinical Oncol.* 8: 232–5.
61. Peng, B. et al. 2011. Progress in study on basic and clinical application in treating liver cancer by cinobufagin injection. *Yaowu Pingjia Yanjiu* 34: 63–6.
62. Wang, D. L. et al. 2011. Chemical constituents and bioactivities of the skin of *Bufo bufo gargarizans* Cantor. *Chem. Biodivers.* 8: 559–7.

197 Tian Gua Di 甜瓜蒂

Melon pedicle

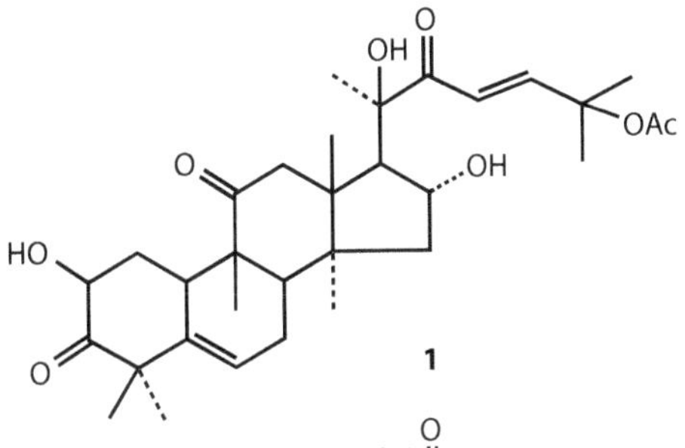

Herb Origination

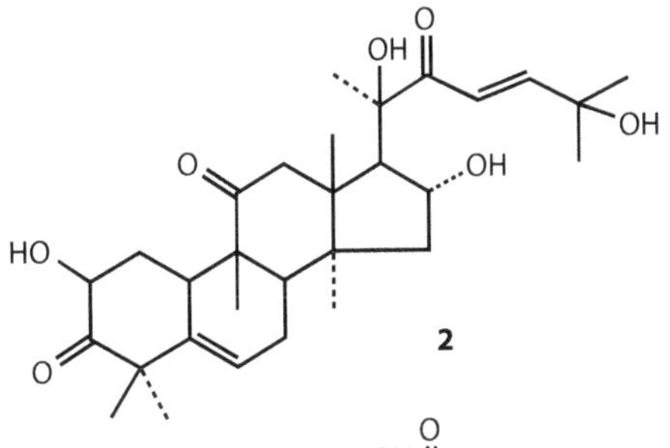

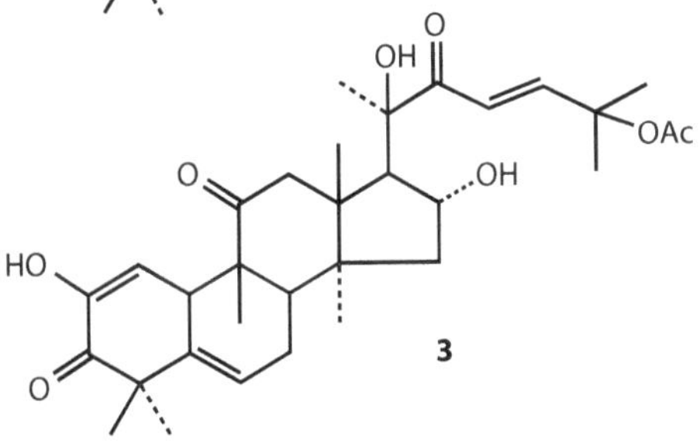

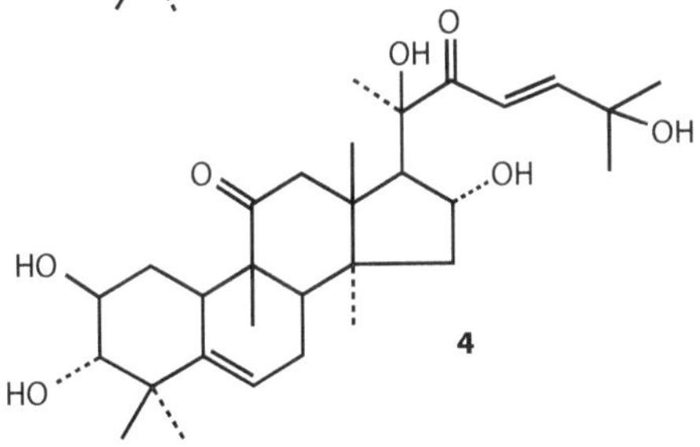

The herb Tian Gua Di (Melon pedicle) is the dried fruit peduncle of a Cucurbitaceae plant, *Cucumis melo* L. The melon is widely naturalized in many places of the world as one of the favorable fruits. As a Chinese herb, its peduncle is collected when the melon fruit is ripe at autumn and dried for folk medicinal use.

Antitumor Activities and Constituents

According to the phytochemical discoveries, cucurbitacin type of triterpenoids were known to be the characteristic and major constituents in many Cucurbitaceae plants, which were in charge of the multiple biological activities of the herb. Most of them showed the significant cytotoxic effect.

Cucurbitacins

Cucurbitacin-B (**1**), cucurbitacin-D (**2**), cucurbitacin-E (**3**), and isocucurbitacin-B as well as cucurbitacin-B-2-*O*-glucoside were found from Tian Gua Di with relatively higher contents. The growth inhibitory effect was truly achieved by many cucurbitacins such as cucurbitacin-B (**1**), cucurbitacin-D (**2**), cucurbitacin-E (**3**), cucurbitacin-F, 23,24-dihydrocucurbitacin-B, 23,24-dihydrocucurbitacin-E, isocucurbitacin-B, isocucurbitacin-D, dihydrocucurbitacin-B, and 3-epoxycucurbitacin-B against several human carcinoma cells such as A549 (lung), SKOV-3 (ovary), XF-498 (brain), SK-MEL-2 (skin), HCT-15 (colon), and BEL7402 (liver) cells, *in vitro*.[1,2] The growth of HCT-116 colon carcinoma cells was suppressed by 77–81.5%, and the proliferation of MCF-7 breast cancer cells was obstructed by 66.5–87% in the respective treatment with cucurnitacin-B (**1**), cucurnitacin-D (**2**), cucurnitacin-E (**3**) at a concentration of 0.4 μM.[3] The *in vitro* assay also showed the remarkable cytotoxicity of cucurnitacin-B (**1**), cucurnitacin-D (**2**), cucurnitacin-E (**3**), and cucurnitacin-I on human KB nasopharyngeal carcinoma and HeLa cervical cancer cell lines with ED_{50} values of 0.01–0.005 μg/mL.[4] Cucurbitacin-A, cucurbitacin-B (**1**), and cucurbitacin-E (**3**) were effective in the inhibition of the proliferation of both HeLa and HepG2 cell lines. Their IC_{50} values were 0.176, 0.18, and 2.32 μg/mL in HeLa cells and 0.216, 0.176, and 2.37 μg/mL in HepG2 cells, respectively.[5]

The inhibitory rates achieved by cucurnitacin-B (**1**) were 96% on NCI-H460 lung cancer cells at a 0.1 μM dose and 92% on SF-268 CNS cells at a 0.05 μM dose.[3] The cytotoxicity of cucurbitacin-B (**1**) was 10 times more potent than that of cucurbitacin-D (IC_{50}: 0.003 versus 0.04 μg/mL) on PC3 prostate carcinoma cells and similarly potent to those of cucurbitacin-D on Meth-A fibrosarcoma cells (IC_{50}: 0.15 versus 0.65 μg/mL) and 3T3 embryoblastoma cells (IC_{50}: 1.8 versus 2.75 μg/mL).[6] The anticancer property of cucurbitacin-B (**1**) and cucurbitacin-D (**2**) were demonstrated in mice implanted with sarcoma 180 or Ehrlich ascites cancer.[4,7] Cucurbitacin-B (**1**) also suppressed the cell growth of Walker sarcoma, sarcoma 37, and Lewis lung cancer in murine animal models.[8,9] By inhibiting JAK2/STAT3 signaling and enhancing IFNγ-related STAT1 activation, cucurnitacin-B (**1**) augmented the sensitivity of 16HBE/BPDE cells (Benzo(a) pyrene-trans-7,8-dihydrodiol-9,10-epoxide [BPDE]-transformed human 16HBE bronchial epithelial cells) to p53-specific cytotoxic T lymphocytes by inhibiting the JAK2/STAT3 activation and enhancing the IFNγ-related STAT1 activation in the 16HBE/BPDE cells, by which the interactions of cucurnitacin-B elicited the differentiation of immature myeloid DCs and augmented the antitumor immunity in patients with lung cancer.[10]

The cucurbitacin-D (**2**) treatment could promote the apoptosis of T cell leukemia cells both *in vitro* and *in vivo* via the decrease of the proteasome activity, and it could also obstruct the growth of human chronic lympholeukemia cells and lymphosarcoma cells *in vitro*, whose cytotoxicity was fivefold higher than of normal lymphocytes.[6,11] When the double bond at C-23/24 of cucurbitacin-D (**2**) was hydrogenated, the antitumor potency would be attenuated 10 times, but its growth inhibition on KB nasopharynx cancer cells had almost no change (IC_{50}: 0.021 μg/mL).[6] In a cotreatment, low doses of cucurbitacin-D (**2**) could synergistically potentiate the antiproliferative effects of VPA, a histone deacetylase inhibitor.[12]

Cucurbitacin-E (**3**) was relatively paid more attention by researchers in the investigation. It was sensitive to HOP-P2 NSCLC, SF-539 and T-47D breast cancers, LOXIMVI and SK-MEL-2 melanomas, RXF-393, CAKI-1, and A498 kidney carcinomas so that it displayed strong cytotoxicity.[13] Cucurbitacin-E (**3**) also exerted its potent growth inhibitory effect against prostate cancer cells (IC_{50} 7–50 nM in two to six day of exposures), melanoma cells (IC_{50}: 0.87 μM) and breast tumor cells (IC_{50}: 1.95 μM) *in vitro*.[14,15] In association with inducing the cell cycle G2/M arrest and apoptosis, cucurbitacin-E (**3**) markedly suppressed the proliferation of T24 (bladder), Pang-1 (pancreas), ES-2 (ovary), and HL-60 and Jurkat (leukemic) human tumor cell lines *in vitro*.[16–18] By the upregulation of GADD45-γ and binding with CDC2, cucurbitacin-E (**3**) arrested cell cycle at G2/M phase and exerted the antiproliferative effect against human glioma GBM 8401 cells.[19,20] Compared with cucurbitacin-I (a deactyl derivative), the cytotoxicity of cucurbitacin-E (**3**) was greater in human U937 and HL-60 leukemia and HT1080 fibrosarcoma cell lines.[21] Moreover, by the cotreatment, cucurbitacin-E (**3**) was able to significantly reduce the efflux of (DOX in M5076 ovarian sarcoma cells, resulting in the enhancement of the antitumor activity of DOX.[22]

Moreover, the significant cytotoxicity of cucurbitacin-A was present in A549/ATCC lung cancer cells and BEL-7402 hepatoma cells *in vitro*.[21] The acetylation at C-25 of cucurbitacin-F (**4**) could augment the cytotoxicity (ED_{50}: 10^{-2} μg/mL) by over 10 times against A549 lung carcinoma cells, MCF-7 breast cancer cells, and HT-29 colon neoplastic cells compared to that of the basic cucurbitacin.[23] In addition, from a fully ripened Japanese pickling melon (*C. melo* var. *conomon*), 3-methylthiopropionic acid ethyl ester was discovered by bioassay-directing separation, which also exists in many fruits. This agent showed an ability to augment the differentiation of human RCM-1 colon cancer cells at a dose range of 0.25–2 mM but no cytotoxic effects. Its colon cancer cell differentiation-enhancing action was achieved by stimulating the ducts formation and alkaline phosphatase (ALPase) activity, which are characteristic marks for neoplastic cell differentiation.[24]

Consequently, the impressive cytotoxic, apoptosis-, and differentiation-inducing activities strongly demonstrated that the cucurbitacins, especially, cucurbitacin-B (**1**), cucurbitacin-D, (**2**) and cucurbitacin-E (**3**), are the promising cancer inhibitors and drug leads that deserve for further development in preclinical investigation.

Mechanism Exploration

The anticancer mechanism of cucurbitacins have been explored, revealing that cucurbitacin-B (**1**) and cucurbitacin-E (**3**) are capable of influencing multiple pathways, including (1) marked disruption of the action in cytoskeleton and direct disruption of F-actin cytoskeleton, (2) induction of cell cycle arrest via STAT3/p53/p21 signaling and decline of CDK1 and cyclin-B activities, (3) promotion of apoptotic death, and (4) blockage of blood supply and new vessel formation.[12–25] The apoptosis-promoting mechanism was disclosed to be mediated by multiple interactions, i.e., (1) decrease of the expressions of antiapoptotic proteins, XIAP, myeloid cell leukemia-1(Mcl-1), and survivin and increase of the level of proapoptotic protein Bax; (2) release of Apaf-1 and AIF and activation of caspase-8, caspase-9, and caspase-3; (3) enhancement of eIF2α phosphorylation (such as in leukemia cells); (4) increase of mitochondria-dependent apoptosis through the inhibition of Fas/CD95 or JAK/STAT3 signaling (such as in T24 cells); and/or (5) blockage of cofilin-dephosphorylation-dependent pathway (such as in U937 cells).[16–30] By restraining p38 MAPKs and suppressing VEGFR-2-mediated JAK/STAT3 signaling pathway, cucurbitacin-E (**3**) obstructed tumor angiogenesis in a xenograft human prostate tumor model besides the growth inhibition.[26] By the treatment of prostate cancer cells with cucurbitacins, the resulting intracellular action of rhodamine–phalloidin binding caused an inappropriate increase in the filamentous or the polymer actin fraction in the tumor cells, leading to the sensitive growth inhibition.[14] Likewise, cucurbitacin-E (**3**) was able to enhance the immunoregulating effect in peripheral lymphocytes concurrently, and the amplified lymphocyte could exert cytotoxicity against the cancer cells.[27]

All these findings not only evidenced the inhibitory and apoptosis-inducing mechanisms but also confirmed that cucurbitacins also possess antiangiogenic and immunoenhancing potentials, intensely providing the scientific basis for cucurbitacins, the promising candidates, facing the next step development.

Clinical Trials

A tablet of cucurbitacins prepared from Tian Gua Di has been tried for the treatment of patients suffering from primary hepatoma in China and showed more encouraging results in the patients of early and middle phases compared to 5-FU (an anticancer drug). The clinical trial exhibited total effective rates of 80% on simple hepatoma, 65% on sclerotic hepatoma, but invalid on inflammatory hepatoma. The best dose was found to be 1.8 mg per day. If the dose was up to 2.1 mg per day, the side effects in the gastrointestinal tract would appear. Normally, the symptoms such as abdominal distention, liver area pain, and cancer size were lessened along with the significant improvement of appetite, immune functions, physical recovery, and life span after the treatment.[28–30]

Cucurnitacin-B (**1**) is a selective inhibitor of JAK2/STAT3 signaling, which had been used to treat 12 patients with advanced lung cancers by daily oral administration for seven consecutive days. The frequency of Lin-DR$^+$CD33$^+$ was significantly increased by cucurnitacin-B (**1**), but the frequency of Lin-DR$^-$CD33$^+$ was reduced in patients with the lung cancers. It also was able to enhance BPDE-transformed human bronchial epithelial cells to p53-specific cytotoxic T lymphocytes. These clinical findings revealed that cucurnitacin-B (**1**) may have a possibility to promote immature myeloid DCs to differentiation and to improve antitumor immunities.[10]

Other Bioactivities

The herb Tian Gua Di (Melon pedicle) plays multiple pharmacological roles in immunopotentiating, hepatoprotective, and capillary permeability-enhancing effects besides anticancer in the pharmacological investigations. Currently, the cucurbitacins are used in the treatment of chronic hepatitis and primary liver cancer in China.

Side Effects

Cucurbitacins showed certain toxicity in clinical application. The overdosed oral administration of cucurbitacins can cause violent vomiting via the stimulation of the vomiting center. But the hypodermic and intravenous injections of the same dose have no such problem. The toxic symptoms in large doses are also able to induce anemia and hepatic damage. Because the antineoplastic effective dose is close to 50% of the lethal dose (LD_{50}), the administration of cucurbitacins must be done carefully.[31]

References

1. Kim, D. K. et al. 1997. Cytotoxic constituents of *Sorbaria sorbifolia* var. *stellipila*. *Archiv. Pharm. Res.* 20: 85–7.
2. Ryu, S. Y. et al. 1994. Antitumor activity of *Trichosanthes kirilowii*. *Archiv. Pharm. Res.* 17: 348–53.
3. Jayaprakasann, B. et al. 2003. Anticancer and antiinflammatory activities of cucurbitacins from *Cucurbita andreana*. *Cancer Lett.* 189: 11–6.
4. Konopa, J. et al. 1974. Cucurbitacins, cytotoxic and antitumor substances from *Bryonia alba* L: Part II. Biological studies. *Arzneimittelforsch./Drug Res.* 24: 1741–3.
5. Tang, L. et al. 2012. Studies on the separation of cucurbitacins from the fruit base of *Cucumis melo* L. and their antitumor activities. *Zhejiang Gongye Daxue Xuebao* 40: 388–91, 449.
6. Frei, B. et al. 1998. Phytochemical and biological investigation of *Begonia heracleifolia*. *Planta Med.* 64: 385–6.
7. Stuppner, H. et al. 1989. New cucurbitacin glycosides from *Picrorhiza kurrooa*. *Planta Med.* 55: 559.
8. Kupchan, C. et al. 1967. Tumor inhibitors. XXIII.1, The cytotoxic principles of *Marah oreganus* H. *J. Med. Chem.* 10: 337–40.
9. Liu, C. X. et al. (a) 1985. Cucurbitacin analogs protect HepG2 and HSC-T6 liver cell lines against cytotoxicity and proliferation. *Abst. 231st ACS Nat. Meeting*, Atlanta, GA, US, March 26–30, 2006, MEDI-025; (b) 1999. *Chinese Materia Medica*. Vol. 5, 5–4580, 516. Shanghai Science Technology Press, Shanghai, China.
10. Lu, P. et al. 2012. Cucurbitacin B regulates immature myeloid cell differentiation and enhances antitumor immunity in patients with lung cancer. *Cancer Biother. Radiopharm.* 27: 495–503.
11. Shohat, B. et al. 1967. Action of elatericin A on human leukemic and normal lymphocytes. *J. Nat. Cancer Ins.* 38: 1–9.
12. Ding, N. et al. 2011. Apoptosis induction through proteasome inhibitory activity of cucurbitacin D in human T-cell leukemia. *Cancer* 117: 2735–46.
13. Richard, W. F. et al. 1994. Cucurbitacins: Differential cytotoxicity, dereplication and first isolation from *Gonystylus keithii*. *J. Nat. Prod.* 57: 1442–5.
14. Duncan, K. L. K. et al. 1996. Cucurbitacin E-induced disruption of the actin and vimentin cytoskeleton in prostate carcinoma cells. *Biochem. Pharm.* 52: 1553–60.
15. Attard, E. et al. 2004. Cytotoxicity of cucurbitacin E extracted from *Ecballium elaterium* and anticancer agents in vitro. *J. Nat. Remedies* 4: 137–42.
16. Huang, W. W. et al. 2012. Cucurbitacin E induces G2/M phase arrest through STAT3/p53/p21 signaling and provokes apoptosis via Fas/CD95 and mitochondria-dependent pathways in human bladder cancer T24 cells. *Evidence-Based Complem. Altern. Med.* 2012: 952762.
17. Li, Y. et al. 2010. The induction of G2/M cell-cycle arrest and apoptosis by cucurbitacin E is associated with increased phosphorylation of eIF2α in leukemia cells. *Anti-Cancer Drugs* 21: 389–400.
18. Sun, C. Y. et al. 2010. Inhibitory effect of cucurbitacin E on pancreatic cancer cells growth via STAT3 signaling. *J. Cancer Res. Clin. Oncol.* 136: 603–10.
19. Shan, X. L. et al. 2010. Inhibitory effect and mechanism of cucurbitacin E on the proliferation of ovarian cancer cells. *Chin. J. Cancer* 29: 20–4.
20. Hsu, Y. C. et al. 2014. Inducement of mitosis delay by cucurbitacin E, a novel tetracyclic triterpene from climbing stem of *Cucumis melo* L., through GADD45γ in human brain malignant glioma (GBM) 8401 cells. *Cell Death Disease* 5: e1087.
21. Nakashima, S. C. et al. 2010. Cucurbitacin E as a new inhibitor of cofilin phosphorylation in human leukemia U937 cells. *Bioorg. Med. Chem. Lett.* 20: 2994–7.
22. Sadzuka, Y. et al. 2010. Enhancement of doxorubicin concentration in the M5076 ovarian sarcoma cells by cucurbitacin E co-treatment. *Intl. J. Pharm.* 383: 186–91.
23. Mata, R. et al. 1990. Cytotoxic constituents of *Exostema mexicanum*. *Planta Med.* 56: 241.
24. Nakamura, Y. et al. 2008. 3-Methylthiopropionic acid ethyl ester, isolated from Katsurauri enhanced differentiation in human colon cancer cells. *J. Agricul. Food Chem.* 56: 2977–84.
25. Chen, C. et al. 2009. Cucurbitane-type triterpenoids from the stems of *Cucumis melo*. *J. Nat. Prod.* 72: 824–29.
26. Dong, Y. M. et al. 2010. Cucurbitacin E, a tetracyclic triterpenes compound from Chinese medicine, inhibits tumor angiogenesis through VEGFR2-mediated Jak2-STAT3 signaling pathway. *Carcinogenesis* 31: 2097–104.
27. Attard, E. et al. 2005. Immunomodulatory activity of cucurbitacin E isolated from Ecballium elaterium. *Fitoterapia* 76: 439–41.
28. Chen, X. L. et al. 1984. Clinical treatment of 50 cases of primary liver cancer with cucurbitacin. *Xinyao Yu Linchuang* 3: 21–2.
29. Ren, F. B. et al. 1986. Current studies of studies of cucurbitacin in treatment of hepatitis and primary hepatoma in pharmacology and clinics. *Zhongxiyi Jiehe Zazhi* 6: 633–5.
30. Chen, J. C. et al. 2005. Cucurbitacins and cucurbitane glycosides:structures and biological activities. *Nat. Prod. Reports* 22: 386–99.
31. Bartalis, J. et al. 2002. Echinacea: Antioxidant, anti-hyaluronidase and cytotoxic activities. *Abst. 223rd ACS Nat. Meeting*, Orlando, FL. pp. 199.

198 Xi Shu 喜樹

Happy tree

1. $R_1 = R_2 = R_3 = -H$
2. $R_1 = -OH, R_2 = R_3 = -H$
3. $R_1 = -A, R_2 = -H, R_3 = -CH_2CH_3$
4. $R_1 = -OH, R_2 = -CH_2N(CH_3)_2, R_3 = -H$
5. $R_1 = R_3 = -H, R_2 = -NO_2$
6. $R_1 = R_3 = -H, R_2 = -NH_2$

Herb Origination

The herb Xi Shu (Happy tree) originated from a Nyssaceae tree, *Camptotheca acuminata*, whose plant is distributed only in southern and southeast areas of China. Its roots, root barks, and fruits are collected and dried in the sun for medicinal use, especially for anticancer treatment.

Antitumor Activities and Constituents

Both alcoholic extracts from the roots and the fruits of Xi Shu exhibited suppressive effect on transplanted carcinoma cells in animal models.[1] The Xi Shu leaves could also inhibited the cell growth of KB nasopharyngeal cancer, Hep3B, and HCC3b hepatocellular carcinoma *in vitro*.[2] The phytochemistry approaches lead to the discovery of a group of potent anticancer principles camptothecin (CPT) (**1**) and its derivatives from various parts of the plant such as its roots, stem barks, fruits, and leaves. CPT (**1**) was the most important constituent isolated from Xi Shu with high quantity.[3] These Xi Shu alkaloid components were also potent inhibitors of DNA Topo-I.

Camptothecin

CPT (**1**) displayed a strong suppressive effect against a number of human neoplastic cell lines such as small cell lung cancer, colon and rectal carcinomas, pancreas and stomach cancers, ovarian, breast and cervical cancers, and mouse carcinoma cell lines such as L1210 leukemia, B16 melanoma, Lewis lung cancer, B22 brain tumor and Ehrlich ascites cancer, and rat W256 walker sarcoma and Yoshita sarcoma, *in vitro*. The IC_{50} value toward the L1210 cells was impressive to be 1.36×10^{-4} μg/mL.[4–6] The daily i.p. injection with CPT (**1**) of 0.25–25 mg for 7–10 continuous days extended lifetime of mice bearing L1210, L5178Y, K1946, or P388 leukemia cells by 200%[6,7] and prolonged the life span of mice bearing multidrug-resistant L1210 or P388 leukemia cells.[7] The biosynthesis of DNA and RNA in HeLa cervical carcinoma cells and L5178 leukemia cells could be obstructed by CPT (**1**) at a 1 mg/mL concentration but no inference to the mitochondria in the liver and the brain of normal rats.[8] Further studies revealed that a unique mechanism also largely involved in the antitumor activity of CPT (**1**), where CPT obstructed intranuclear enzyme Topo-1, leading to the blockage of DNA replication, the damage of DNA structure, and the disturbance of cell cycle proceeding in the tumors.[4,9]

Also, a water solubility-improved CTP sodium salt exerted the significant suppressive effect against the cell growth of sarcoma 180 and Heps hepatoma by 52–53% and the life extension in mice implanted Ehrlich ascites cancer by 54%.[10] When CTP (**1**) was prepared as a polyliposome, its antiproliferative effect on mouse hepatoma cells could be remarkably enhanced *in vivo*, and the inhibitory rates against DNA and RNA biosynthesis in the hepatoma cells were 73.7% and 82.9%, respectively.[11] In the *in vivo* models, the CTP polyliposome restrained the growth of sarcoma 180 cells and ascetic hepatoma cells by 74% and 82%, respectively, and also extended the life duration of mice bearing Ehrlich ascites cancer by 126%.[10]

In an attempt to improve the poorly aqueous solubility and the unpredictable toxicities of CPT (**1**), a number of analogs have been discovered and/or synthesized.

10-Hydroxycamptothecin

10-Hydroxycamptothecin (HCPT) (**2**) is another bioactive alkaloid isolated from Xi Shu, exhibiting a broad anticancer spectrum *in vitro* and *in vivo*, whose activity was found to be related to its inhibitory effect on Topo-I. The treatment of murine ascites hepatoma cells with HCPT (**2**) markedly diminished the DNA preparation and inhibited the phosphorylation in histone H1 and H3 in a time-dependent manner, indicating that HCPT-induced tumor cell killing was partly associated with the suppression of histone H1 and H3 phosphorylation.[12] Moreover, HCPT (**2**) at an optimal concentration of 0.1 μg/mL displayed significant suppressive inhibitory effect on three human hepatoma cells (HepG2 and Bel-7402). The growth inhibition in the HepG2 cells dose- and time-dependently was accompanied by apoptotic changes and cell cycle disturbance at G2/M phase (at low dose) or S phase (at high dose).[13] Also, HCPT reduced the activity of the nuclear RNA polymerase-II and polymerase-I of murine hepatoma cells and retarded the DNA replication.[14] The i.p. administration of HCPT (10 mg/kg, four times a day for three days) to mice bearing hepatoma could elevate the intracellular levels of cAMP and adenylate cyclase by 67% and 82%, respectively, exerting antihepatoma effect.[15] Similarly, by the elicitation the Topo-I inhibition and protein-associated DNA strand breaks, the proliferation of human HL-60 promyelocytic leukemia cells and HL-60/m-AMSA (m-AMSA-resistant mutant) cells were dose-dependently obstructed by HCPT (**2**).[16] By the induction of G2 cell arrest and apoptosis via a caspase-3-dependent pathway, HCPT (**2**) significantly restrained the proliferation of Colo 205 cells *in vitro* at a low concentration (5–20 nM) and potently restrained the growth of colon cancer with no acute toxicity in nude mice xenografts after being orally administered with

HCPT in doses of 2.5–7.5 mg/kg for two days.[17] *In vivo* experiments also fully confirmed the antineoplastic activity of HCTP (**2**). The daily i.p. administration of HCTP to mice and rats at 1–2 mg/kg dose for seven to nine days obviously prolonged the life span of murine animals implanted with L1210 or P388 leukemia, ascites hepatoma, Ehrlich ascites tumor, ascitic reticulocyte sarcoma, or Yoshita sarcoma by ~280%. HCTP (**2**) also obstructed the growth of several murine entity tumor cells such as sarcoma 180, sarcoma 37, U14 cervical carcinoma, and rat W256 walker sarcoma *in vivo*.[18,19]

Based upon preclinical studies of pharmacokinetics, tissue distribution, metabolism, and elimination in rats, HCPT (**2**) was found to broadly distribute on various tissues including the enterohepatic system, the kidney, and the bone marrow through its metabolism *in vivo*. No obvious toxicity was observed at its doses of 1 or 3 mg/kg but its dose-dependent toxicity was observed with intravenous administration. Polyuria and hematuria happened only during the initial 3 h after dosing of HCPT (**2**) at 10 mg/kg.[20] In the treatment with higher doses of HCPT, the chromosomal aberrations was initiated in Chinese hamster ovary cells and the micronucleus formation in mouse bone marrow.[21] Due to having the more potent antitumor activity and less toxicity, HCPT (**2**) have been selected to undergone clinical use in China.

Irinotecan and SN-38

Irinotecan (CPT-11) (**3**), is a water-soluble semisynthetic derivative of CPT, which has higher therapeutic efficacy and less toxicity. CPT-11 demonstrated broad *in vitro* and *in vivo* cancer inhibitions against various gastrointestinal malignancies (in the esophagus, the stomach, the pancreas, or the biliary tract), pediatric or adult CNS tumors, as well as other cancers with MDR expression. CPT-11 (**3**) and its active metabolite SN-38 exerted the suppressive effect on DNA Topo-I and the growth of neoplastic cells. The activation of interleukin-1β-converting enzyme and the elevation of its mRNA level were found to be partially involved in the mechanism of CPT-11 inducing the apoptosis of human K562 erythroleukemia cells.[22,23]

The studies in athymic nude mice showed that a combination of CPT-11 (**3**) with chemotherapeutic agents temozolomide or 1,3-bis(2-chloroethyl)-1-nitrosourea potentiated the growth inhibitory effect on human glioma cells.[24] CPT-11 also exhibited the synergistic activity against esophageal carcinoma in combination with 5-FU or cisplatin and in combinations of cisplatin/irinotecan/taxol or cisplatin/irinotecan/5-FU. The preliminary clinical data recommended the combinational chemotherapies for the treatment of upper gastrointestinal malignancies. No irreversible or unusual toxicities were observed with irinotecan (**3**) in animal toxicity studies.[22,25] The optimal dose of CPT-11 (**3**), which can be safely combined with cisplatin (80 mg/m^2), was found to be 60 mg/m^2.[26] Thirty-three patients with recurrent malignant glioma had been treated with the maximum tolerated daily dose of irinotecan (350–550 mg/m^2) plus temozolomide (150 mg/m^2) for 5 days from days 1 to 5 every 28 days, resulting in 25.8% response to the treatment, and 35.48% of the patients remained stable.[27] Moreover, concurrent administrations of CYP450 enzyme-inducing antiepileptic drugs could augment the irinotecan clearance and influence its active metabolite SN-38 disposition. Furthermore, SN-38 also exhibited antimetastasis potential in colorectal adenocarcinoma but its limiting toxicities are myelotoxicity and essentially late diarrhea.[28]

Other CPT Analogs

The wide-ranging structural modifications were approached in the A, B, C, D, and E rings of CPT (**1**). A number of water-soluble CPT analogs such as irinotecan (**3**), topotecan (**4**), rubitecan (**5**), diflomotecan (BN80915), 9-aminocamptothecin (**6**), and exatecan (DX-8951) have been proven for the cancer therapeutic activity against diverse cancer types including different leukemia and lymphoma, NSCLC and small cell lung carcinomas, colon and rectal cancers, carcinoma of the CNS, renal cell carcinoma, and ovarian and breast carcinomas in humans.[29–34] The broad spectrum of antitumor activity was proven to be also attributed to the unique mechanism of Topo-I inhibition with the lack of clinical cross-resistance.[35] For that reason, these water-soluble semisynthetic derivatives have undergone extensive evaluation and have been employed in a wide spectrum of clinical trials in patients with metastatic cancers.[29–34]

Further investigations on their SAR indicated that a lactone ring in these molecules is necessary for the activity, but the lactone is easily hydrolyzed into the less active hydroxyl carboxylic acid. Actually, irinotecan (**3**) is a prodrug that can be cleaved in the gastrointestinal tract by a carboxylesterase-converting enzyme to form an active metabolite SN-38, but both molecules kept the active lactone form.[36] 7-Tertbutyldimethylsilyl-10-hydroxycamptothecin (DB-67) is a novel lipophilic CPT derivative, which exhibited the growth inhibitory action in two NSCLC cell lines (A549 and H460) *in vitro*, however, the A549 cells were more resistant to the DB-67 than the H460 cells. After 8–18 h of exposure to DB-67, the Topo-I levels significantly decreased in both A549 and H460 cells. Dosing the DB-67 once every 48–72 h may maximize the interaction of the agent with Topo-I, indicating that the DB-67 has a long-acting benefit for easier use.[36] Also, the preclinical studies of several other CPT derivatives such as grimatecan (ST1481), diflomotecan (BN80915), and lurtotecan (OSI-201) are undergoing clinical trials.[34,37]

Other Bioactivities

Besides the potent antineoplastic property, CPT (**1**) is also capable of exerting immunosuppressive, pregnancy-terminating, and antiherpes activities. Because CPT obstructs the proliferation of fibrocytes, it may be used in the treatment of psoriasis and skin warts.

References

1. Beijing Institute of Medicine. 1979. Review of the researches on Chinese herbal medicines in China for 30 years. *Yaoxue Xuebao* 14: 746.
2. Lorence, A. et al. 2004. Camptothecin: Over four decades of surprising findings. *Phytochem.* 65: 2735–49.
3. Lerchen, H.-G. et al. 2002. Milestones in camptothecin research. *Drugs of the Future* 27: 869–78.
4. Gallo, R. C. et al. 1971. Studies on the antitumor activity, mechanism of action, and cell cycle effects of camptothecin. *J. Nat. Cancer Inst.* 46: 789–95.

5. Cai, J. C. et al. 1973. Review of the foreign research in anticancer camptothecin. *Yiyao Gongye* 4: 789.
6. Ulukan, H. et al. 2002. Camptothecins: A review of their chemotherapeutic potential. *Drugs*, 62(14), 2039–57.
7. Hellwig, V. et al. 2002. New drugs with Chinese medicine. *Chemie in Unserer Zeit* 36: 22–8.
8. Shamma, M. et al. 1974. Camptothecin. *J. Pharm. Sci.* 63: 163–83.
9. Sriram, D. et al. 2005. Camptothecin and its analogues: A review on their chemotherapeutic potential. *Nat. Prod. Res.* 19: 393–412.
10. State Administration of Traditional Chinese Medicine, 1999. Chinese Materia Medica. Vol. 5, 5–4911, 731. Shanghai Science Technology Press, Shanghai, China.
11. Li, M. et al. 1988. Studies on the tumor cell kinetics and molecular pharmacology of camptothecin polyphase liposome. *J. Shenyang Pharm. Univ.* 5: 161.
12. Ling, Y. H. et al. 1993. Hydroxycamptothecin as a DNA topoisomerase-I inhibitor inhibited histone H1 and H2 in mouse ascites hepatoma. *Acta Pharmacol. Sinica* 14: 546–54.
13. Zhang, X. W. et al. 1999. Apoptosis induction and cell cycle perturbation in human hepatoma Hep G2 cells by 10-hydroxycamptothecin. *Anti-Cancer Drugs* 10: 569–76.
14. Xu, B. et al. 1985. The effect of hydroxycamptothecin in the activity of RNA and DNA polymerases prepared from murine hepatoma cells. *Am. J. Chin. Med* 13: 23–31.
15. Ling, Y. H. et al. 1982. Influerence of hydroxycamptothexin on the activity of adenylate cyclase in mouse hepatoma cells. *Acta Pharmacol. Sinica* 3: 264.
16. Ling, Y. H. et al. 1990. DNA topoisomerase I as a site of action for 10-hydroxycamptothecin in human promyelocytic leukemia cells. *Cancer Biochem. Biophys.* 11: 23–30.
17. Ping, Y. H. et al. 2006. Anticancer effects of low-dose 10-hydroxycamptothecin in human colon cancer. *Oncol. Rep.* 15: 1273–9.
18. Wall, M. E. et al. (a) 1998. Camptothecin and taxol: Discovery to clinic. *Med. Res. Reviews* 18: 299–314.
19. Shanghai Institute of Materia Medica. (a) 1978. *Zhonghua Yixue Zazhi* 58: 598; 1999. (b) *Chinese Materia Medica.* Vol. 5, 5–4911, 731. Shanghai Science Technology Press, Shanghai, China.
20. Zhang, R. W. et al. 1998. Preclinical pharmacology of the natural product anticancer agent 10-hydroxyl-camptothecin, an inhibitor of topoisomerase I. *Cancer Chemother/Pharmacol.* 41: 257–67.
21. Tu, Z. H. et al. 1990. Effect of hydroxycamptothecin on induced chromosomal aberrations in Chinese hamster ovary cells and micronucleus formation in mouse bone marrow and fetal liver. *Acta Pharmacol. Sinica* 11: 378–81.
22. Robert, J. et al. 1998. Pharmacology of irinotecan. *Drugs of Today* 34:777–803.
23. Shibata, Y. et al. 1996. Stimulation of interleukin-1-convertng enzyme activity during growth inhibition by CPT-11 in the human myeloid leukemia cell line K562. *Biochem. Mol. Med.* 57: 25–30.
24. Friedman, H. S. et al. 2003. The emerging role of irinotecan (CPT-11) in the treatment of malignant glioma in brain tumor. *Cancer* 97(Suppl.): 2359–62.
25. O'Reilly, E. M. et al. 2001. Cisplatin and irinotecan in upper gastrointestinal malignancies. *Oncol.* 15(Suppl. 5): 42–5.
26. Ardizzoni, A. et al. 1995. Camptothecin analogues in the treatment of non-small cell lung cancer. *Lung Cancer* 12 (Suppl. 1): S177–85.
27. Loghin, M. E. et al. 2007. Phase I study of temozolomide and irinotecan for recurrent malignant gliomas in patients receiving enzyme-inducing antiepileptic drugs. *Clin. Cancer Res.* 13: 7133–8.
28. Torck, M. et al. 1996. Camptothecin and derivatives: A new class of antitumor agents. *J. de pharmacie de Belgique* 51: 200–7.
29. Yang, S. S. et al. 2001. *Drug Discovery and Traditional Chinese Medicine.* Lin, Y. (ed.). *First Int. Conf. Trad. Chin. Med.*, College Park, MD, p. 61.
30. Burris, H. A. et al. Phase II trial of oral rubitecan in previously treated pancreatic cancer patients. *Oncologist* 10: 183–90.
31. Zamboni, W. C. et al. 2005. Relationship between plasma exposure of 9-nitrocamptothecin and its 9-aminocamptothecin metabolite and antitumor response in mice bearing human colon carcinoma xenografts. *Clin. Cancer Res.* 11: 4867–74.
32. Miller, D. et al. 2005. Phase II evaluation of 9-aminocamptothecin (9-AC, NSC #603071) in platinum-resistant ovarian and primary peritoneal carcinoma. *Gynecol. Oncol.* 96: 67–71.
33. Leguizamo, J. et al. 2003. A phase I study of 9-aminocamptothecin as a colloidal dispersion formulation given as a fortnightly 72-h infusion. *Cancer Chemother. Pharmacol.* 52: 333–8.
34. Glaberma, U. et al. 2005. Alternative administration of camptothecin analogues. *Expert Opinion on Drug Delivery* 2: 323–33.
35. Rothenberg, M. L. et al. 1997. Topoisomerase I inhibitors: Review and update. *Oncology/ESMO* 8: 837–55.
36. Abang, A. M. et al. 1998. The clinical pharmacology of topoisomerase I inhibitors. *Seminars in Hematol.* 35(Suppl 4): 13–21.
37. Seiden, M. V. et al. 2004. A phase II study of liposomal lurtotecan (OSI-211) in patients with topotecan resistant ovarian cancer. *Gynecol. Oncol.* 93: 229–32.

199 Mao Ci Gu 毛慈菇

Cremastra

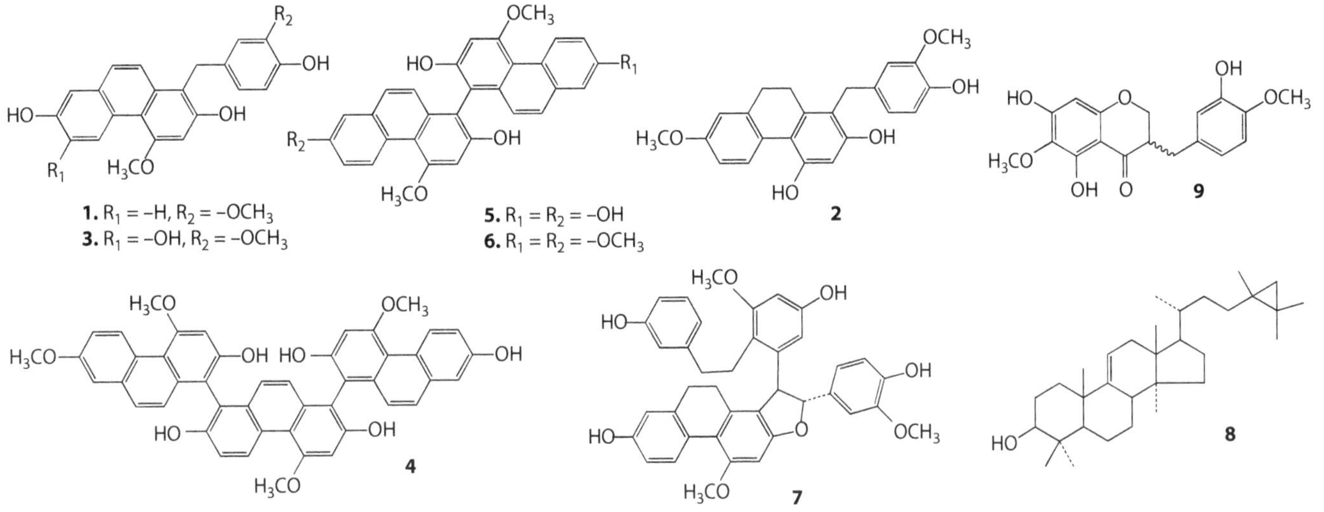

1. R_1 = -H, R_2 = -OCH_3
3. R_1 = -OH, R_2 = -OCH_3

5. R_1 = R_2 = -OH
6. R_1 = R_2 = -OCH_3

Herb Origination

The herb Mao Ci Gu is the dried tuber rhizomes of an Orchidaceae plant, *Cremastra appendiculata*. This evergreen orchid widely spreads in most woodland at elevations of 1300 to 2300 m throughout east Himalaya, China, Korea, Japan, Kuril Islands, and Southeast Asian countries. Commonly, its tubers are collected in summer and autumn, and then steamed and dried for Chinese folk medical practice. Due to the greatly increased use of *C. appendiculata*, the herb has become difficult to collect in the wild, and its supply is now carried out by cultivation.

Antitumor Activities and Constituents

Mao Ci Gu has a great reputation in China for its anticancer potential because it is often used in Chinese medicine to treat cancer patients with esophageal cancer. In recent years, a group of phenanthrenes was discovered from the herb as its major constituents.

Phenanthrenes

In the exploration of anticancer constituents in Mao Ci Gu, several isolated phenanthrenes displayed moderate or weak cytotoxic effect against human cancer cell lines *in vitro*. Two phenanthrenes, i.e., 1-(30-methoxy-40-hydroxy-benzyl)-4-methoxyphenanthrene-2, 7-diol (**1**) and 1-(30-methoxy-40-hydroxybenzyl)-7-methoxy-9,10-dihydrophen-anthrene-2,4-diol (**2**), displayed the inhibitory effect on the proliferation of MDA-MB-231 breast cancer cells (IC_{50}: 10.42–11.92 μmol/L). 1-(30-Methoxy-40-hydroxybenzyl)-4-methoxyphenanthrene-2,6,7-triol (**3**) was effective on HCT-116 colon cancer cells (IC_{50}: 14.22 μmol/L). But the three phenanthrenes were less active or inactive to A549 (lung), HepG2 (liver), and MCF-7 (breast) human cancer cell lines.[1] A triphenanthrene, 2,7,2′,7′,2″-pentahydroxy-4,4′,4″,7″-tetramethoxy-1,8,1′,1″-triphenanthrene (**4**), and two biphenanthrenes, cirrhopetalanthrin (**5**) and 2,2′-di-hydroxy-4,7,4′,7′-tetramethoxy-1,1′-biphenanthrene (**6**), exerted nonselective moderate cytotoxicity against A2780 (ovary), Bel-7402 (liver), BGC-823 and MCF-7 (breast), HCT-8 (colon), and A549 (lung) human cancer cell lines (IC_{50}: 8.0–17.8 μM). Of these phenanthrenes, the strongest cytotoxicity was achieved by the triphenanthrene (**4**) on the first five cancer cell lines (IC_{50}: 8.0–8.4 μM).[2] Another isolated biphenanthrene named (2,3-*trans*)-3-[2-hydroxy-6-(3-hydroxyphenethyl)-4-methoxybenzyl]-2-(4-hydroxy-3-methoxyphenyl)-10-methoxy-2,3,4,5-tetrahydrophenanthro-[2,1-b]furan-7-ol (**7**) was shown to have a moderate effect in the inhibition of A549 lung carcinoma cells (IC_{50}: 16.0 μM).[3] However, the three multiphenanthrenes (**4–6**) were also cytotoxic to a human normal epithelial WISH cell line, and the biphenanthrene (**6**) was the most cytotoxicity on WISH cells (IC_{50}: 5.0 μM).[2]

Triterpenoid and Flavanone

Moreover, an isolated triterpenoid elucidated as (+)-24,24-dimethyl-25,32-cyclo-5α-lanosta-9(11)-en-3β-ol (**8**) was found to have *in vitro*-selective cytotoxicity against human MCF-7 breast cancer cell line (IC_{50}: 3.18 μM).[4] Besides the antiproliferative effect, a potent angiogenesis inhibitor was discovered from the isolation of Mao Ci Gu, whose structure was determined as 5,7-dihydroxy-3-(3-hydroxy-4-methoxybenzyl)-6-methoxychroman-4-one (**9**). This homoisoflavanone (**9**) could suppress bFGF-induced angiogenesis and invasion of HUVECs (IC_{50}: 0.5 μg/mL) *in vitro* and restrain the angiogenesis of the chorioallantoic membrane of a chick embryo *in vivo* without showing any toxicity.[5]

Other Medical Uses

The herb Mao Ci Gu has a long history of medicinal utilization in mainland China for the treatment of carbuncle and furuncle, scrofulous phlegm nucleus, lymphoid tuberculosis, and snakebite.

References

1. Liu, L. et al. 2013. Three new phenanthrenes from *Cremastra appendiculata* (D. Don) Makino. *Chin. Chem. Lett* 24: 737–9.
2. Xue, Z. et al. 2006. Mono-, bi-, and triphenanthrenes from the tubers of *Cremastra appendiculata*. *J. Nat. Prod.* 69: 907–13.
3. Wang, Y. et al. 2013. Phenanthrenes, 9,10-dihydrophenanthrenes, bibenzyls with their derivatives, and malate or tartrate benzyl ester glucosides from tubers of *Cremastra appendiculata*. *Phytochem.* 94: 268–76.
4. Li, S. et al. 2008. Terpenoids from the tuber of *Cremastra appendiculata*. *J. Asian Nat. Prod. Res.* 10: 677–83.
5. Shim, J. S. et al. 2004. Anti-angiogenic activity of a homoisoflavanone from *Cremastra appendiculata*. *Planta Med.* 70: 171–3.

200 Huang Yao Zi 黄藥子

Air potato

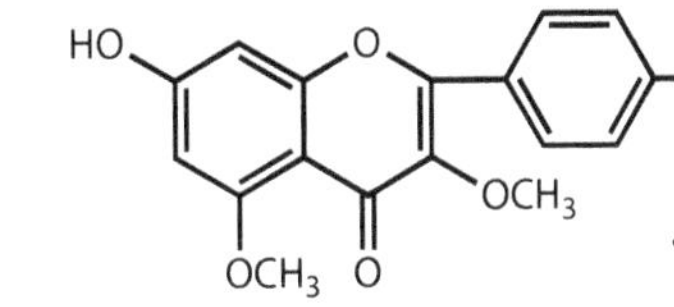

1

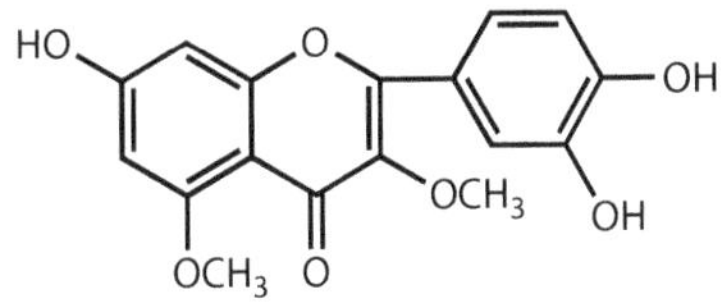

2

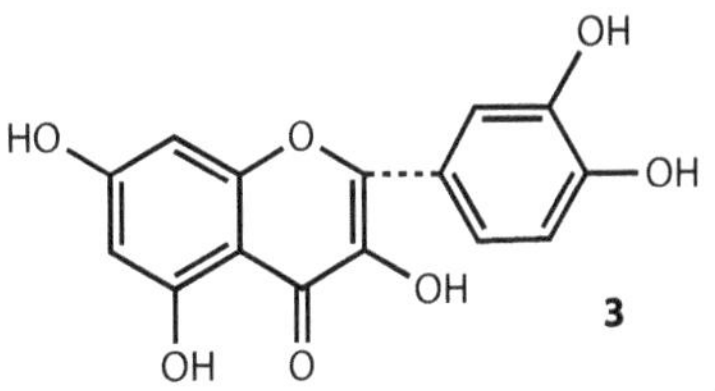

3

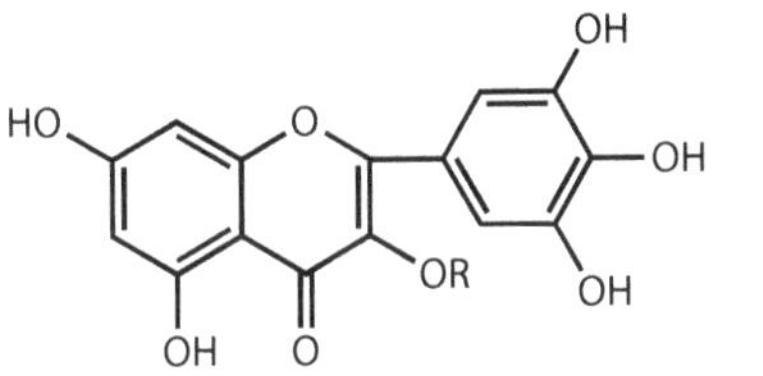

4. R = -H
6. R = -Gal
7. R = -Glu

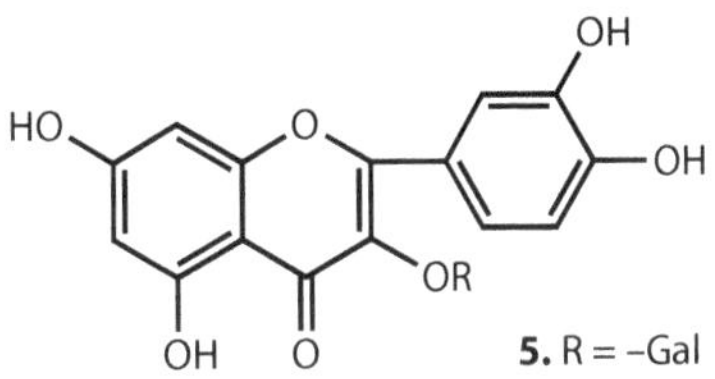

5. R = -Gal

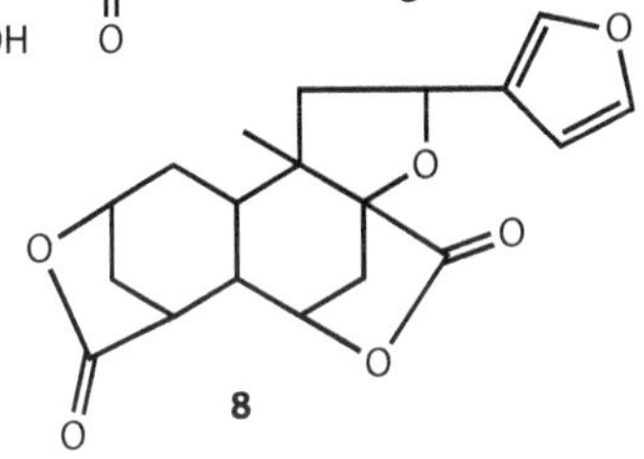

8

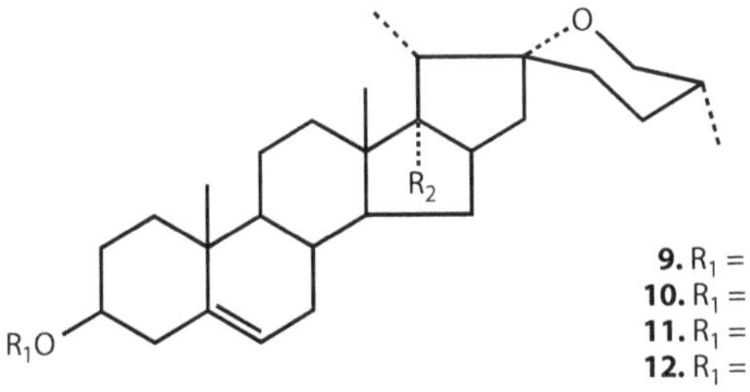

9. R_1 = -A, R_2 = -OH
10. R_1 = -B, R_2 = -OH
11. R_1 = -A, R_2 = -H
12. R_1 = -B, R_2 = -H

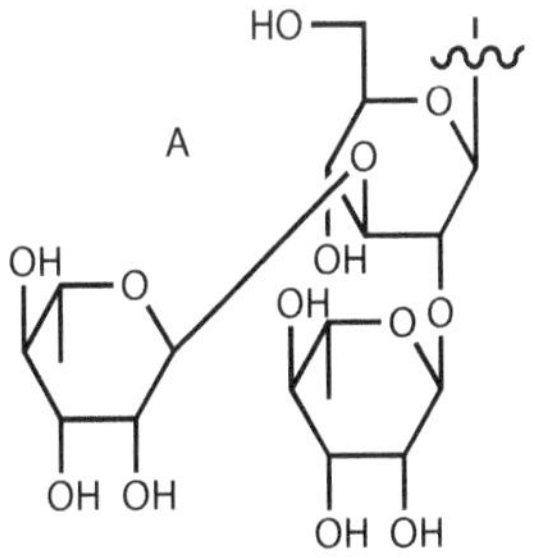

A

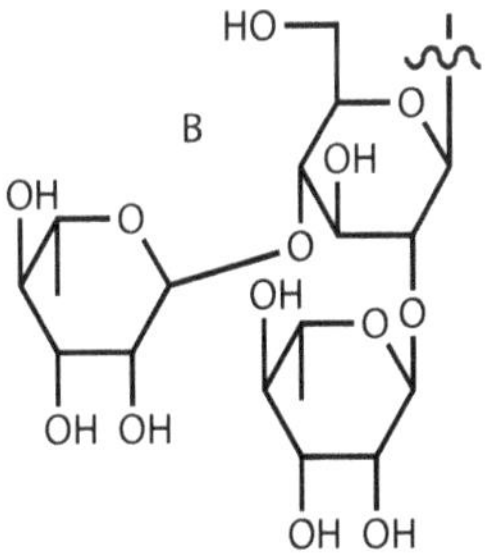

B

Herb Origination

The herb Huang Yao Zi (Air potato) is the dried rhizomes of a Dioscoreaceae vine plant, *Dioscorea bulbifera* L. This perennial plant is widely distributed in the eastern and southern regions of China as well as many tropical areas in the world, including Florida and Texas in the United States as an invasive species. The rhizomes are collected in winter and dried in the sun for the preparation of the herb, but it can also be used fresh for folk remedy.

Antitumor Activities

Huang Yao Zi is often used for the treatment of tumor, lymphoid tuberculosis, and thyromegaly in Chinese folk medicine. The petroleum ether extract derived from Huang Yao Zi showed strong anticancer activity. The formation of ascites volume and the viability of HepA hepatoma cells were markedly inhibited by the petroleum ether extract *in vivo.* The treatment with 100 mg/kg of the extract prolonged the life span of mice bearing the HepA ascites.[1] The ethanolic extract of Huang Yao Zi could notably restrain the proliferation and the angiogenesis of Ehrlich ascite tumor cells, choriocarcinoma cells, breast cancer cells, glioblastoma cells, and endothelial cells *in vitro* in a dose-dependent manner.[2] The methanolic fraction and the EAF derived from its 75% ethanolic extract could reduce the weights of sarcoma 180 and hepatoma H22 in mice and display the suppressive effect against TPA-promoted mouse epidermal tumor JB6 (Cl-22 and Cl-41) cells. The EAF could also augment the weights of the spleen and the thymus and amplify the amounts of total leukocytes, lymphocytes, and neutrophils in the tumor-bearing mice.[1–4]

Antitumor Constituents and Activities

As one of the Dioscoreaceae plants, the steroidal glycosides are the major constituents in the rhizomes of *D. bulbifera.* Several steroidal glycosides and flavonoids isolated from the herb were shown to be moderate inhibitors of cancer proliferation and tumor promotion. Up to now, no potent cancer inhibitors have been found from the herb.

Flavonoids

The separation of the EAF gave eight antitumor-promoting flavonoids, which were identified as kaempferol-3,5-dimethyl ether (**1**), caryatin (**2**), (+)-catechin (**3**), myricetin (**4**), quercetin-3-*O*-galactoside (**5**), myricetin-3-*O*-galactoside (**6**), and myricetin-3-*O*-glucoside (**7**), whose structures possessing two hydroxyl groups at C-7 and C-4′ displayed the important inhibitory effect on the tumor cells, but the flavonol aglycones and the flavonol glycosides showed different degrees of the tumor suppression. Compared to (−)-epicatechin, the (+)-catechin (**3**) demonstrated a much stronger inhibitory activity, which indicated that stereochemistry of the flavonoids also affect the inhibitory efficiency.[2–5]

Diterpene Lactone

Only one tumor suppressive diterpene lactone was isolated from the herb, and it was identified as diosbulbin-B (**8**). As a major active constituent in the herb, diosbulbin-B (**8**) moderately restrained the tumor-promoting activity and dose-dependently exerted the antitumor effects at dosages of 2–16 mg/kg *in vivo* with no significant liver toxicity.[5]

Steroids and Their Glycosides

Four steroidal sapogenin 3-*O*-trisaccharides isolated from the rhizomes were evaluated in two human hepatoma cell lines (Bel-7402 and SMMC7721) *in vitro*. Spiroconazole-A (**9**) and pennogenin-3-*O*-α-L-rhamnosyl-(1–4)-[α-L-rhamnosyl-(1–2)]-β-D-glucoside (**10**) markedly obstructed the SMMC7721 cells by 99.1% and 92.6% (IC_{50}: 4.54 and 4.85 μM, respectively).[6] Diosgenin-3-*O*-α-L-rhamnosyl-(1–2)-[α-L-rhamnosyl-(1–3)]-β-D-glucoside (**11**) and diosgenin-3-*O*-α-L-rhamnosyl-(1–2)-[α-L-rhamnosyl-(1–4)]-β-D-glucoside (**12**) displayed moderate cytotoxic effect against both SMMC7721 (IC_{50}: 3.89–7.47 μM) and Bel-7402 cells (IC_{50}: 10.87–19.10 μM).[7] In an *in vitro* assay with ECV-304 urinary bladder neoplastic cells, spiroconazole-A (**9**), pennogenin-3-*O*-α-L-rhamnosyl-(1–4)-α-L-rhamnosyl-(1–4)-[α-L-rhamnosyl-(1–2)]-β-D-glucoside, and 26-*O*-β-D-glucosyl-(25R)-5-en-furost-3β,17α,22α,26-tetraol-3-*O*-α-L-rhamnosyl-(1–4)-α-L-rhamnosyl-(1–4)-[α-L-rhamnosyl-(1–2)]-β-D-glucoside, which were separated from the flowers of *D. bulbifera*, displayed a moderate cytotoxicity on the ECV-304 cells with IC_{50} values of 8.5, 14.3, and 5.8 μg/mL (8.3, 11.8, and 6.6 μM), respectively.[8]

Polysaccharides

DBLP, which is a crude polysaccharide prepared from *D. bulbifera*, could restrain the growth of U14 cervical carcinoma cells and promote the tumor cell apoptosis in a mouse model. Simultaneously, DBLP augmented the thymus weight and decreased the apoptosis of the thymus and the spleen. Furthermore, DBLP also has the abilities to reduce the ratio of $CD4^+/CD8^+$ T lymphocyte in the peripheral blood according to the CTX-treated group. The results proved that the anticancer effect on the cervical carcinoma was mediated by not only the apoptotic induction of tumor tissue but also the regulation of immune response in the tumor-bearing mice.[9]

Other Bioactivities

Huang Yao Zi (Air potato) has been utilized as a folk remedy to treat conjunctivitis, diarrhea, and dysentery. Huang Yao Zi is an iodine-rich herb (14.3 mg/kg), which can be used to treat goitrous diseases induced by lack of iodine. Also, the Huang Yao Zi extract has been shown to exert antihypoglycemic, antidiabetic, antiviral, antigoitrogenic, and antibacterial effects.

References

1. Yu, Z. L. et al. 2004. Anticancer effects of various fractions extracted from *Dioscorea bulbifera* on mice bearing HepA. *Zhongguo Zhongyao Zazhi* 29: 563–7.
2. Kaveri, K. et al. 2012. Evaluation of antiangiogenic and antiproliferative potential in ethanolic extract of *Dioscoria bulbifera* L. *Current Trends in Biotechnol. Pharmacy* 4: 930–42.
3. Gao, H. Y. et al. 2002. Antitumor-promoting constituents from *Dioscorea bulbifera* in JB6 mouse epidermal cells. *Biol. Pharm. Bull.* 25: 1241–3.
4. Wang, J. M. et al. 2012. Antitumor activity of *Dioscorea bulbifera* L. rhizome in vivo. *Fitoterapia* 83: 388–94.
5. Gao, H. Y. et al. 2007. Constituents from antitumor-promoting active part of *Dioscorea bulbifera* L. in JB6 mouse epidermal cells. *Asian J. Tradit. Med.* 2: 104–9.
6. Liu, H. et al. 2009. Steroidal sapogenins and glycosides from the rhizomes of *Dioscorea bulbifera*. *J. Nat. Prod.* 72: 1964–8.
7. Liu, H. et al. 2011. Steroidal saponins from the rhizomes of *Dioscorea bulbifera* and their cytotoxic activity. *Planta Med.* 77: 845–8.
8. Tapondjou, L. A. et al. 2013. Steroidal saponins from the flowers of *Dioscorea bulbifera* var. *sativa*. *Phytochem.* 95: 341–50.
9. Cui, H. X. et al. 2012. Antitumor activity and possible mechanism of crude polysaccharides from *Discorea bulbifera* L. on the mice bearing U14 cervical carcinoma. *Adv. Materials Res.* 560–561: 374–9.

201 Ru Jiang Da Ji 乳浆大戟

Leafy spurge

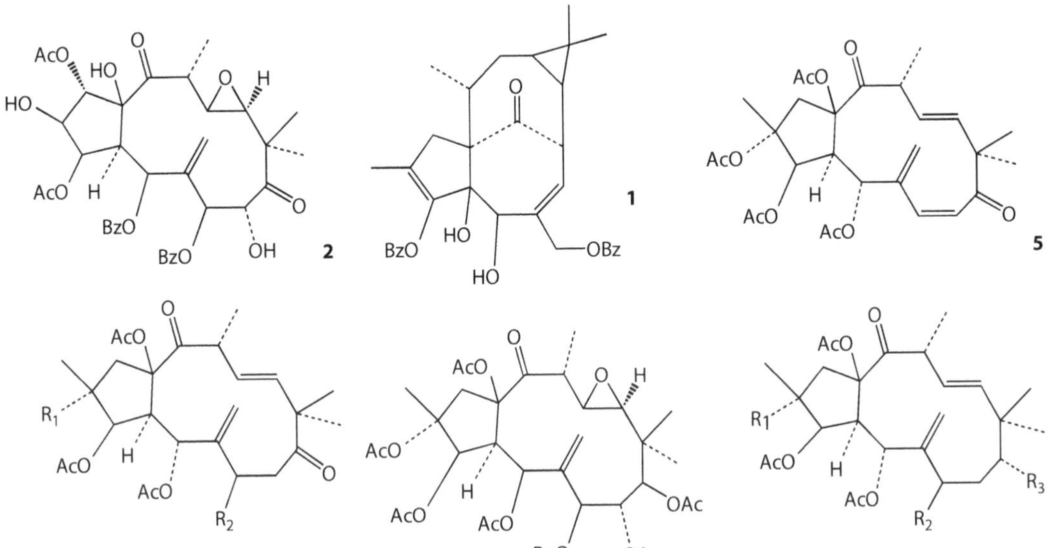

3. R_1 = –H, R_2 = –OBu
6. R_1 = –OBz, R_2 = –OAc
7. R_1 = –OAc, R_2 = –OAc

8. R_1 = –H, R_2 = –OBu, R_3 = –ONic
9. R_1 = R_2 = R_3 = –OAc

Bz: benzoyl

Bu: isobutyryl

Nic: nicotinoyl

Herb Origination

The herb Ru Jiang Da Ji (Leafy spurge) originated from an Euphorbiaceae plant, *Euphorbia esula* L., whose herbal plant is native to central and southern Europe and eastward through most of Asia, north of the Himalaya, to Korea and eastern Siberia. This perennial plant spread quickly in Northern America since the early 1800s and was classified as an invasive species. Leafy spurge now grows throughout the world except in Australia. In China, the herbaceous plant is collected in spring and summer; it can be used fresh or sun-dried herb for Chinese folk medicinal practice.

Tumor-Related Activity and Constituents

By phytochemical investigations, Ru Jiang Da Ji was recognized to be a rich source of jatrophane diterpenoids. Many diterpenoids have been separated from the herb and showed antitumor and anticarcinogenic activities.

Antitumor Diterpenoids

In the early studies, an isolated diterpenoid diester termed ingenol 3,20-dibenzoate (**1**) exerted the anticancer activity on murine P388 lymphocytic leukemia in mice.[1] Later, a series of macrocyclic jatrophane diterpenoids have been discovered from the Leafy spurge and demonstrated interesting cytotoxicity against the proliferation of cancer cells. 1α,2β-Diacetoxy-5α,7β-dibenzoyloxy-9,14-dioxo-11β,12α-epoxy-2α,8α,15β-trihydroxy-13βH-jatropha-6(17)-ene (**2**) displayed noticeable cytotoxic activity against B16 melanoma cells (IC_{50}: 1.81 μg/mL).[2] Fourteen jatrophane diterpenes had been evaluated in a set of human gynecological origin neoplastic cell lines such as MCF-7 (breast), Ishikawa (endometrial), and HeLa (cervix). Esulatin-J (**3**), esulatin-A (**4**), and esulatin -E (**5**) were the most effective to all three of cells; especially, esulatin-J (**3**) displayed higher cell growth inhibitory activity on Ishikawa cells (98.4%) and MCF-7 cells (81.4%), whereas esulatin-I (**6**) and esulatin-B (**7**) exhibited obvious inhibition on MCF-7 cells (60.1% and 43.3%, respectively) at the same concentration (30 μg/mL). Chemical esulatin-J (**3**), esulatin-E (**5**), esulatin-I (**6**), and esulatin-B (**7**) are tetra- or pentaesters of jatrophane polyols all having a keto group at C-9, and esulatin-A (**4**) contains an epoxy group at C-11–C-12. Preliminary analysis of the relationships in the structure–activity presented that these structural characteristics might be closely related to the antigrowth function in the cancer cell lines mentioned earlier.[3]

Moreover, the MDR-reversing activities of these jatrophane diterpenes were proven in L5178 mouse lymphoma cells transfected with the pHa MDR1/A retrovirus DNA. Esulatin-J (**3**) and esulatin-M (**8**) were found to be the most powerful inhibitors of efflux pump activity of P-gp in the tumor cells, whose efficacy was two- to fivefold higher than that of verapamil (a standard agent). Therefore, esulatin-J (**3**) and esulatin-M (**8**) were considered to have the important potential to overcome the MDR of cancer cells.[3] Other jatrophane diterpenes such as esulatin-A (**4**), esulatin-B (**7**), and esulatin-D (**9**) showed weak reversing effect on mouse multidrug-resistant lymphoma cells.[4]

Tumorigenic Diterpenoids

An acetyl acetate extract separated from the aerial parts of Ru Jiang Da Ji was found to have an ability to promote the skin carcinogenesis caused by dimethylbenzoanthracene. From the extract, ingenol 6-dodecanoate and its three analogs (euphorbia factor E1, E2, and E3) were separated but were determined to possess weak tumorigenic activity.[5] Interestingly, their structures are quite similar to the tumor-inhibitory ingenol 3,20-dibenzoate (**1**) having the same ingenol skeleton when compared with these molecules. But the structural differences were only at the varieties and the numbers of side chain connected with the basic skeleton. Only such differences unbelievably determined the totally different bioactivities related to the inhibitor or the promoter of neoplasm.

References

1. Kupchan, S. M. et al. 1976. Antileukemic principles isolated from Euphorbiaceae plants. *Sci.* 191: 571–2.
2. Liu, L. G. et al. 2002. New macrocyclic diterpenoids from *Euphorbia esula. Planta Med.* 68: 244–8.
3. Vasas, A. et al. 2011. Jatrophane diterpenes from *Euphorbia esula* as antiproliferative agents and potent chemosensitizers to overcome multidrug resistance. *J. Nat. Prod.* 74: 1453–61.
4. Hohmann, J. et al. 2002. Discovery and biological evaluation of a new family of potent modulators of multidrug resistance: Reversal of multidrug resistance of mouse lymphoma cells by new natural Jatrophane diterpenoids isolated from Euphorbia species. *J. Med. Chem.* 45: 2425–31.
5. Seip, E. H. et al. 1982. Skin irritant ingenol esters from *Euphorbia esula. Planta Med.* 46: 215–8.

202 Lang Du Da Ji 狼毒大戟

Fischer euphorbia

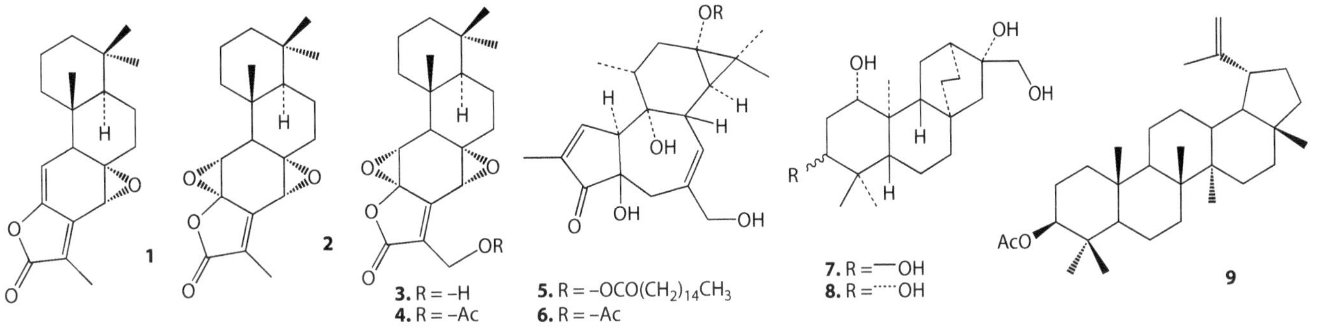

3. R = -H
4. R = -Ac
5. R = $-OCO(CH_2)_{14}CH_3$
6. R = -Ac
7. R = —OH
8. R = ·····OH

Herb Origination

The herb Lang Du Da Ji (Fischer euphorbia) is the dried roots of a Euphorbiaceae plant, *Euphorbia pallasii* (= *E. fischeriana*). The distribution of this perennial herbaceous plant ranged in the northeast and north of China. Its roots are usually collected in spring or autumn and dried in the sun for application in traditional Chinese medicine.

Antitumor Activities

In vivo experiments demonstrated the anticancer activity of Lang Du Da Ji, but the potency was dependent upon different routes of administration. Normally, i.p. and intravenous injections exhibited better tumoricidal effect than oral administration. Daily 10–15 mL/kg dose of 10% Lang Du Da Ji intravenous injection to tumor-bearing mice resulted in 43.8–52.43% inhibition against entity hepatoma cells for 8–9 continuous and 37–45% inhibition against sarcoma 180 by either i.p. or intravenous injection for 9–10 successive days, and it was inactive in oral administration at the same dose level.[1] By daily oral administration of its water extract or its alcohol extract in large doses (5–15 g/kg) for 7 days to mice bearing Lewis lung cancer, the suppressive rates were up to 30.56–61.11%. But no significant activity was observed in the same dose on sarcoma 180, ascites hepatoma, and gastric carcinoma *in vivo*.[2] Fraction-B derived from the herb obviously obstructed the growth of Ehrlich entity neoplasm, Walker sarcoma 256, and Lewis lung carcinoma by i.p. injection, whereas it was invalid to mouse L1210 and P388 leukemia.[3]

Moreover, the aqueous extract displayed strong inhibition on the proliferation of mouse L615 T lymphocyte leukemia cells *in vivo* by intragastric (i.g.) administration of 3 g/kg/day for seven days. Concurrently, typical DNA apoptotic fragments were remarkably increased, and the c-Myc/ras gene expressions were diminished in a dose-dependent manner, implying that the apoptotic promotion was accompanied by the antitumor effect on L615 leukemia.[4,5] In addition to attacking the L615 leukemia cells, the decreased activities of GSH-Px and SOD were also significantly recovered by the aqueous extract.[6]

Antitumor Constituents and Activities

Eight anticancer terpenes were discovered from the Lang Du Da Ji, namely, diterpenoids (jolkinolides-A (**1**) and -B (**2**), 17-hydroxyjolkinolide-B (**3**), 17-acetoxyjolkinolide-B (**4**), and 16-hydroxypseudojolkinolide-B),[7] diterpenoids (12-deoxyphorbol-13-decanoate (**5**) and prostratin (**6**)), and a triterpenoid (lupeol-3-acetate (**7**)).[8]

Diterpenoid Lactones

Jolkinolide-B (JB) (**2**) exhibited moderate to weak inhibitory activity on LNCaP (prostate), Eca-109 (esophagus), and HepG2 (liver) human cancer cell lines (IC_{50}: 12.5, 23.7 and >50 μg/mL, respectively) *in vitro*.[9,10] It was reported to block bromodeoxyuridine incorporation into the LNCaP cells and diminished the DNA synthesis in a concentration-dependent manner.[9] The treatment of the LNCaP cells with 25 μg/mL of JB (**2**) could elicit the cycle G1 phase arrest and neuronendocrine differentiation by upregulating the activities of neuroendocrine markers, keratin 8/18, and neuron-specific enolase. When the concentration was over 25 μg/mL, JB (**2**) caused DNA fragmentation and apoptotic death of the LNCaP cells.[11] JB (**2**) and 16-hydroxypseudojolkinolide-B also markedly suppressed the proliferation of human K562 CML and CNE2 nasopharyngeal cancer cells. The IC_{50} value of JB (**2**) on the K562 cells was 12.1 μg/mL, and the cytotoxic potency of 16-hydroxypseudojolkinolide-B on the two neoplastic cells was near to those of Adm (an anticancer agent).[12] In the JB (**2**) treatment, the viability of human leukemia U937 cells was dose- and time-dependently declined and the apoptotic death was enhanced by downregulating PI3K/Akt and IAP family proteins and triggering caspase-3 and caspase-9 activations.[13] Similarly, through the inhibition of PI3K/Akt/mTOR signaling pathway, JB (**2**) induces apoptosis in MDA-MB-231 and MCF-7 breast cancer cell lines. The treatment with JB (**2**) restrained the MCF-7 cell growth with cell cycle S arrest and diminished the MCF-7 tumor volume and weight in nude mice.[14,15] Moreover, JB (**2**) also acted as an inhibitor of VCAM-1 formation (IC_{50}: 0.2 μg/mL), suggesting that the diterpenoid lactone is able to play an important role in the antiangiogenesis besides the antigrowth activity.[12]

17-Acetoxyjolkinolide-B (AJB) (**4**) is a novel-type inhibitor on the NF-κB pathway. The effect of AJB on the induction of tumor cell apoptosis was closely correlated with its effective inhibition against TNFα-induced NF-μB activation and NF-κB-related gene expressions, but it had no effects on other kinases such as p38, p44/42, and JNK and no effects in the binding of TNFα to its receptor or binding of NF-κB to the DNA. AJB directly targeted the Inhibitor of kappa B kinase (IκK) and kept the IKK in its phosphorylated form irreversibly, leading to the blockage of NF-κB nuclear translocation, which is a unique mechanism to strongly induce the tumor cell apoptosis.[16] In further investigations, AJB (**4**) presented a potential as a novel-type anticancer drug candidate. Both AJB (**4**) and 17-hydroxyjolkinolide-B (HJB, **3**), whose structures only showed one different substitution at C-17, exerted similar apoptotic pathways as a STAT3 signaling inhibitors, where they strongly obstructed the constitutive STAT3 activation and directly inactivated the JAK family kinases (such as JAK1, JAK2, and TYK2) by covalently cross-linking with JAKs.[17]

Diterpenoids

Two tigliane-type diterpenoids, assigned as 12-deoxyphorbol-13-decanoate (**5**) and prostratin (**6**), as well as AJB (**4**), demonstrated potent cytotoxic activity to human Burkitt's lymphoma Ramos B cells *in vitro* with IC_{50} values of 0.023, 0.0051, and 0.056 μg/mL, respectively.[8] Prostratin (**6**) also exerted a certain degree of antitumor activity on HepG2 (liver) and MCF-7 (breast) cancer cell lines, while langduin-A had the antitumor effect to SGC-7901 and MCF-7 cancer cell lines, and 13-*O*-acetylphorbol had the effect on MCF-7 cells.[18] The *in vitro* and *in vivo* assays proved the antigrowth effect of 12-deoxyphorbol-13-palmitate on BGC823 gastric cancer cells concomitant with the induction of G2/M cell cycle arrest and apoptosis.[19] Two isolated ent-atisane diterpenoids, ent-1β,3β,16β,17-tetrahydroxyatisane (**7**) and ent-1β,3β,16β,17-tetrahydroxyatisane (**8**), showed the inhibitory effects against MCF-7 cells (respective IC_{50}: 23.21 and 15.42 μM).[20]

Triterpenoid

Lupeol-3-acetate (**9**) markedly retarded a two-stage carcinogenesis *in vivo* in mouse skin provoked by DMBA as an initiator and TPA as a promoter,[21] but it showed weak cytotoxicity on human A2780 ovarian cancer cells *in vitro*.[22]

Polysaccharides

EFP-AW1 was a polysaccharide component extracted from *E. fischeriana*, which in a mouse model with sarcoma 180 significantly amplified the T lymphocyte proliferation and the number of $CD8^{+}T$ lymphocytes in the peripheral blood and reduced the TGF-β1 secretion, leading to the enhancement of the immune response function and to the inhibition of tumor cell metastasis and recurrence.[23]

Elements

The herb was identified to be abundant in K, Mg, Fe, and Zn, which may be involved in the anticarcinoma activity and regulation of the human body's immunity function in certain complex forms with the active molecules.[24]

Toxicity

The herb Lang Du Da Ji (Fischer euphorbia root) exhibited certain toxicity. The LD_{50} values of its water extract and alcoholic extract by i.p. injection were 275.9 and 171.9 g/kg, respectively. The daily i.p. (20g) or oral (125 g) administration of the water extract as well as the oral (50 g) administration of the alcoholic extract for 10–14 continuous days resulted in no significant toxicity and side effects. However, overdosed administration will cause some side effects.

References

1. Yang, B. Y. et al. 1984. Inhibition of *Euphorbia fischeriana* on the growth of tumor cells transplanted in mice. *Hebei Zhongyi* 3: 23.
2. Shen, Z. Q. et al. 1984. Antineoplastic effect of *Euphorbia fischeriana* Steud on mice with implanted tumor. *Zhongxiyi Jiehe Zazhi* 4: 46–7.
3. Lu, B. F. et al. 1986. Experimental antitumor action of *Euphorbia fischeriana*. *J. Herbin Med. Univ.* 20: 90–3.
4. Cui, X. et al. 2002. Apoptosis in L615 T-lymphocytic leukemia cells mediated by extract of *Euphorbia fischeriana* Stead. *J. Shandong Med. Univ.* 40: 37–9.
5. Yao, P. et al. 2003. Effects of *Euphorbia fischeriana* stead on leukemia caused by retrovirus. *Zhonghua Weishengwuxue yu Mianyixue* 23: 183–7.
6. Cui, X. et al. 1998. Inhibition of L615 leukemia cell proliferation and recovery of GSH-Px and sod activation in L615 mice *Euphorbia fischeriana* Steud. *J. Shandong Med. Univ.* 36: 289–92.
7. Liu, G. F. et al. 1987/1988. Isolation and identification of antitumor constituents of diterpenoids lactone in *Euphorbia fischeriana* Steud. *Zhongyao Tongbao* 12: 484; 13: 291–2.
8. Wang, Y. B. et al. 2006. Diterpenoids from the roots *of Euphorbia fischeriana*. *J. Nat. Prod.* 69: 967–70.
9. Liu, W. K. et al. 2002. Jolkinolide B induces neuroendocrine differentiation of human prostate LNCaP cancer cell line. *Biochem. Pharmacol.* 63: 951–7.
10. Luo, H. Y. et al. 2006. Induction of apoptosis in K562 cells by jolkinolide B. *Canadian J. Physiol. Pharmacol.* 84: 959–65.
11. Liu, W. et al. 2000, Studies on *Euphorbia fischeriana* diterpenoid lactones inhibitory effect on human tumor cells in vitro. *Zhongyaocai* 23: 623–5.
12. Kamimura, D. et al. 1995. Vascular cell adhesion molecule-1 formation inhibitors containing jolkinolide B or benzenepropanamide derivative. *Jpn. Kokai Tokkyo Koho* JP 94–96237, 19940510.
13. Wang, J. H. et al. 2011. Jolkinolide B from *Euphorbia fischeriana* Steud induces apoptosis in human leukemic U937 cells through PI3K/Akt and XIAP pathways. *Mol. Cells* 32: 451–7.

14. Lin, Y. et al. 2012. Jolkinolide B induces apoptosis in MDA-MB-231 cells through inhibition of the PI3K/Akt signaling pathway. *Oncol. Reports* 27: 1976–80.
15. Xu, H. Y. et al. 2013. Jolkinolide B induces apoptosis in MCF-7 cells through inhibition of the PI3K/Akt/mTOR signaling pathway. *Oncol. Reports* 29: 212–8.
16. Yan, S. S. et al. 2008. 17-Acetoxyjolkinolide B irreversibly inhibits IκB kinase and induces apoptosis of tumor cells. *Mol. Cancer Therap.* 7: 1523–32.
17. Wang, Y. et al. 2009. 17-Hydroxyjolkinolide B inhibits signal transducers and activators of transcription 3 signaling by covalently cross-linking janus kinases and induces apoptosis of human cancer cells. *Cancer Res.* 69: 7302–10.
18. Wang, M. et al. 2013. Antitumor activity of tigliane type diterpene from *Euphorbia fischeriana* Steud. *Zhongyiyao Xuebao* 41: 11–4.
19. Xu, H. Y. et al. 2013. 12-Deoxyphorbol 13-palmitate mediated cell growth inhibition, G2-M cell cycle arrest and apoptosis in BGC823 cells. *Eur. J. Pharmacol.* 700: 13–22.
20. Wang, M. et al. 2016. Two new ent-atisanes from the root of *Euphorbia fischeriana* Steud. *Nat. Prod. Res.* 30: 144–9.
21. Yasukawa, K. et al. 1995. Some lupane-type triterpenes inhibit tumor promotion by 12-*O*-tetrade-canoylphorbol-13-acetate in two-stage carcinogenesis in mouse skin. *Phytomed.* 1: 309–13.
22. Chaturvedula, V. S. P. et al. 2002. Two new triterpene esters from the twigs of *Brachylaena ramiflora* from the Madagascar rainforest. *J. Nat. Prods.* 65: 1222–4.
23. Cui, L. R. et al. 2013. *Euphorbia fischeriana* polysaccharide regulates immune function in S180 tumor-bearing mice. *Zhongguo Shiyan Fangjixue Zazhi* 19: 255–8.
24. Liu, W. Z. et al. 2002. Determination of trace elements in *Euphorbia fischeriana* Steud. *Guangdong Weiliang Yuansu Kexue* 9: 56–8.

203 Teng Huang 藤黄

Gamboge

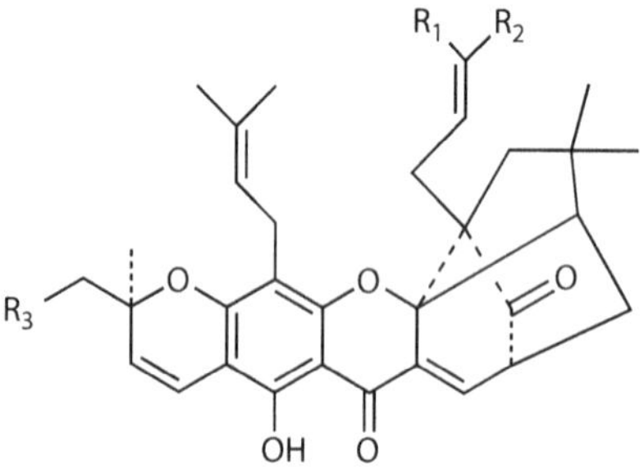

Gambogic acid (**6**)	$R_1 = -COOH$, $R_2 = -CH_3$, R_3 = prenyl
Isomorellin	$R_1 = -CH_3$, $R_2 = -CH_3$, $R_3 = -H$
Morellic acid (**7**)	$R_1 = -COOH$, $R_2 = -CH_3$, $R_3 = -H$
Desoxymorellin (**1**)	$R_1 = -CH_3$, $R_2 = -CH_3$, $R_3 = -H$
Gambogin	$R_1 = -CH_3$, $R_2 = -CH_3$, R_3 = prenyl
Morellin di-Me acetal (**3**)	$R_1 = -CH(OCH_3)_2$, $R_2 = -CH_3$, $R_3 = -H$
Isogambogic acid (**10**)	$R_1 = -CH_3$, $R_2 = -COOH$, R_3 = prenyl
Isomorellinol (**8**)	$R_1 = -CH_3$, $R_2 = -COOH$, $R_3 = H$

Prenyl = $-CH_2CH_2CH{=}C-(CH_3)_2$

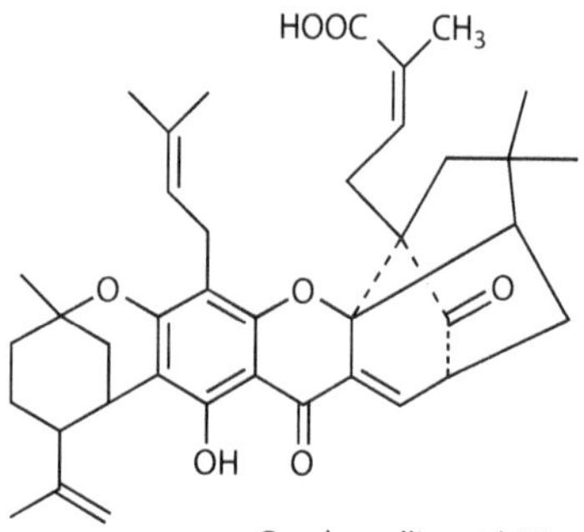

Gambogellic acid (**5**)

Gambogenic acid	$R_1 = -COOH$, $R_2 = -CH_3$
Gambogenin	$R_1 = -CHO$, $R_2 = -CH_3$
Isogambogenin (**4**)	$R_1 = -CH_3$, $R_2 = -CHO$
Desoxygambogenin (**2**)	$R_1 = R_2 = -CH_3$

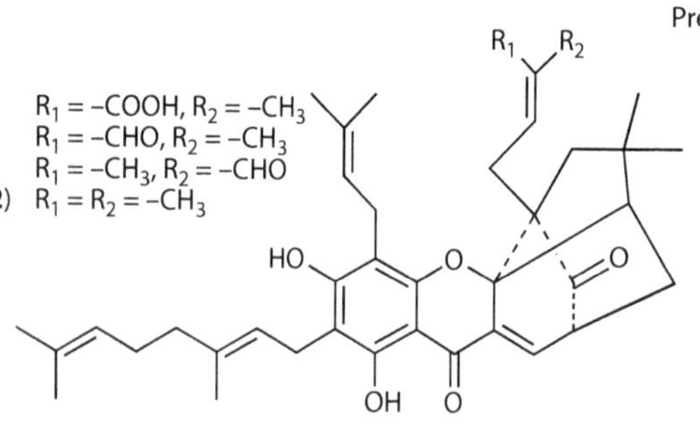

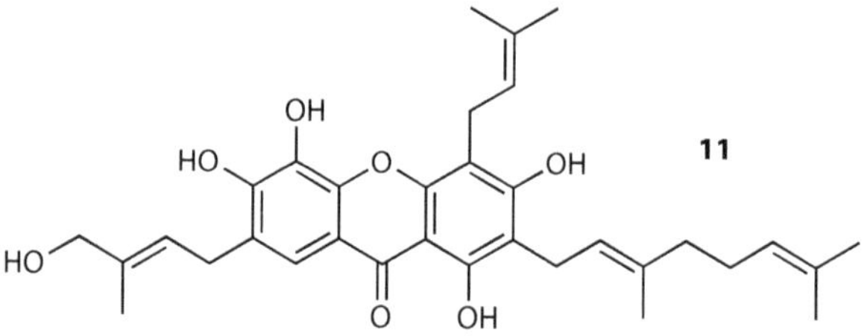

11

Herb Origination

The herb Teng Huang (Gamboge) is a brownish dried resin, which is exuded from the stems of a tropical tree, *Garcinia hanburyi* (Guttiferae). The plant is distributed throughout south Asian countries, and it is cultivated in southern Chinese provinces now. The resin has been collected for application as a folk medicine and a dye for over a thousand years.

Antitumor Activities

In vitro and *in vivo* pharmacological investigations demonstrated that the Teng Huang resin possesses selective antitumor activity. In *in vitro* models, the resin exerted remarkable suppressive and murderous effects against human cell lines such as HeLa (cervical cancer), K562 (entry leukemia), and BEL-7402 and SMMC-7721 (hepatomas). The inhibitory activity was further demonstrated in animal models implanted with murine neoplasms including Ehrlich ascites carcinoma, sarcoma 180, sarcoma 37, Walker sarcoma 256, U14 cervical carcinoma, MA737 breast cancer, and ARA4 and ARS carcinomas, in dose- and time-dependent manners.[1–6] If the resin was protreated by steam at 126°C for 30 min, its anticarcinoma potency would be maximized.[7,8] Compared to some chemotherapeutic drugs such as camptothecine, lycorine-betaine, and pretazetine, the Teng Huang resin demonstrated more potent tumoricidal effect.[6]

Antitumor Constituents and Activities

The molecules with a caged xanthone skeleton are the major constituents discovered from the Teng Huang resin by the phytochemical approaches. The xanthones were demonstrated to be responsible for the biological functions of Gamboge, including the anticancer activity, although the isolated minority of components showed some bioactivities.

Xanthones

Up to now, over 50 xanthones have been discovered from the resin, and these xanthones demonstrated different degrees of inhibition against the growth of neoplastic cells. Of them, desoxymorellin (**1**) and desoxygambogenin (**2**) exerted the highest antigrowth effect toward human HeLa cervical cancer and HEL erythroleukemia cell lines *in vitro*. Morellin dimethyl acetal (**3**), isogambogenin (**4**), and gambogellic acid (**5**) displayed stronger inhibitory effect on these tumor cells than gambogic acid (**6**).[9,10] Many of the xanthones such as morellic acid (**7**) markedly retarded the growth of various human cancer cell lines, such as HeLa (cervix), COL-2 (colon), KB (nasopharynx), BCA-1 and T47D (breast), SMMC-7721 (liver), LU-1 (lung), BGC-823 and SGC-7901 (stomach), HEL, K562 and HL-60 (leukemic) cells, murine P388 leukemia, and ASK glioma cells, *in vitro*.[9–23] Most of the 16 tested xanthones were effective in the inhibition of A549 (lung), HCT116 (colon), and MDA-MB-231 (breast) human cancer cell lines, where isogambogic acid, isomorellic acid, and gambogellic acid (**5**) showed marked activities against the three cell lines (IC_{50}: 0.08–0.80 μM). The strongest suppressive effect was achieved by gambogellic acid (**5**) in the HCT116 cells (IC_{50}: 0.08 μM). The higher effects were shown by gambogellic acid, isomorellic acid, 30-isogambogenic acid, and hydroxylepigambogic acid on the MDA-MB-231 cell line (IC_{50}: <0.5 μM), whereas by isogambogenic acid, formoxanthone-J and 22,23-dihydroxydihydrogambogenic acid on the HCT116 cells (IC_{50}: <0.7 μM).[24] Gambogic acid (**6**), isomorellinol (**8**) isomorellin (**9**), and forbesione dose-dependently displayed the potent growth inhibition on KKU-100 and KKU-M156 cholangiocarcinoma cell lines *in vitro*.[14] Through the mitochondrial-dependent pathway and the extrinsic death receptor pathway, gambogic acid (**6**) induced p53-independent apoptotic death in HepB3 and Huh7 hepatoma cell lines, thereby exerting the antiproliferative effect (IC_{50}: 1.8 and 2.2 μM, 24 h).[25] The cytotoxic effect of gambogic acid (**6**) on SH-SY5Y human neuroblastoma cells was associated with the induction of apoptosis via an intrinsic mitochondrion-dependent caspase pathway (IC_{50}: 1.28 μM, 6 h).[26] Moreover, a highly rearranged and pentaprenylated xanthonoid, gamboketanol, and two other xanthonoids, gambogefic acid A and gambogellic acid A, showed modest inhibitory effect on HeLa cells.[23] An isolated xanthone (**11**) exerted remarkable antitumor effects against various human cancer cells in the lab experiments. The IC_{50} values of xanthone (**11**) were 1.14–2.72 μg/mL in U251 (brain), Bel-7402 and HepG2 (liver), CNE (nasopharyngus), and HeLa-229 (cervix) tumor cell lines. The *in vivo* effect of xanthone (**11**) was demonstrated in nude mice implanted with NCI-H460 human lung cancer xenografts.[27] A Teng Huang amide derived from the reaction of gambogic acid (**6**) and piperidine was able to promote the apoptosis of cancer cells via significant activation of caspases. Its GI_{50} and LD_{50} values were 50 nm on the proliferation of human T47D breast cancer cells.[15]

Moreover, some caged xanthones such as gambogic acid (**6**), 30-hydroxygambogic acid, and their (2S)-epimers also interestingly have the abilities to reverse the drug resistance and to exert cytotoxic effect against DOX-resistant human K562 erythroleukemia cells.[17,18] Gambogic acid (**6**), isomorellinol (**8**), and isogambogic acid (**10**) were directly cytotoxic to drug-resistant KV-V1 cancer cells, and a gambogic aldehyde was cytotoxic to both drug-sensitive and drug-resistant mouse leukemia cell lines (P388 and P388/ADR).[19,28] Likewise, gambogic acid (**6**) at concentrations of >0.6 μM not only reduced the proliferation in SK-HEP1 hepatoma cells but also suppressed the migration and the invasion of SK-HEP1 cells via the down-expression of integrin β1/rho family GTPase signaling pathway, the inhibition of actin cytoskeleton, and the migration and the decreases of MMPs and NF-κB expressions, indicating an antimetastatic potential of gambogic acid for the treatment of hepatoma.[29] The antiinvasive and antimetastatic activities of gambogic acid (**6**) were attributed to RECK upregulation at both protein and mRNA levels.[30] Gambogic acid (**6**), morellic acid (**7**), gambogenin, and isogambogenic acid were found to be inhibitors of angiogenesis evidenced by *in vitro* HUVEC cell migration assay and *in vivo* zebrafish model.[31] Besides the growth inhibition, gambogic acid (**6**) was also able to promote the differentiation of U937 and HL-60 cells together with the up-expression of p21waf1/cip1.[32] Furthermore, the antitumor effects of gambogic acid (**6**) were confirmed by the *in vivo* experiments. The i.p. injection of gambogic acid (**6**) at a dose of 5 mg/kg to tumor-bearing mice established the significant inhibitory effect on Ehrlich ascites cancer and ascites sarcoma 180 concomitant with the reduction of ascites and the increase of nudinuclear cells; however, gambogic acid (**6**) was inactive in oral administration.[11]

SAR Investigation

The exploration of relationships between the structures and the cytotoxicities disclosed that α,β-unsaturated ketone was essential for the growth inhibition in all tested tumor cell lines. The electrophilic property of the conjugated carbonyl group in the xanthones might act in the corresponding targets leading to apoptotic acceleration. When the α,β-unsaturated ketone moiety in the structures was deficient, the cytotoxicities would be obviously diminished.[22–34] The data provided a noticeable clue for the establishment of more attractive anticancer agents.

Triterpenoids

2α-Hydroxy-3β-*O*-acetyllup-20(29)-en-28-oic acid (**12**) and 3-*O*-(4′-*O*-acetyl)-α-L-arabinopyranosyloleanolic acid (**13**) were isolated from a chloroform extract of the resin. The two triterpenoids displayed moderate antiproliferative and apoptosis-inducing effects against four human leukemia cell lines (HL-60, NB4, U937, and K562) *in vitro*, where the second triterpenoid was more potent than the first one, and its IC_{50} values were in a range of 2.45–4.15 μM.[35] The *in vitro* assay also demonstrated the antiproliferative effect of 2α-hydroxy-3β-*O*-acetyllup-20(29)-en-28-oic acid (**12**) in MGC-803 and SGC-7901 (stomach), A549 (lung), SPC-1 (pancreas), and HO-8910 (cervix) human cancer cell lines (IC_{50}: 1.86–3.47 μg/mL) and of 3-*O*-(4′-*O*-acetyl)-α-L-arabinopyranosyloleanolic acid (**13**) in Bxpc-3 (pancreas), CNE (nasopharyngus), and Bcap-37 and MCF-7 (breast) human cancer cell lines (IC_{50}: 1.85–4.25 μg/mL).[36] Both triterpenoids (2α-hydroxy-3β-*O*-acetyllup-20(29)-en-28-oic acid (**12**) and 3-*O*-(4′-*O*-acetyl)-α-L-arabinopyranosyloleanolic acid (**13**)) were further evaluated in NCI-H460 human lung cancer xeaografts in nude mice. The intravenous administration of 2α-hydroxy-3β-*O*-acetyllup-20(29)-en-28-oic acid (**12**) or 3-*O*-(4′-*O*-acetyl)-α-L-arabinopyranosyloleanolic acid (**13**) in a dose of 3 mg/kg could obstruct the growth of NCI-H460 cells with T/C data of 79.46% and 70.05%, respectively.[36]

Exploration of Mechanism

The potent xanthones have attracted scientists to explore the mechanism by employing modern techniques especially developed in recent years. As a major xanthone constituent found from the resin, gambogic acid (**6**), has always been used for the mechanistic studies. The antitumor potency of gambogic acid has been demonstrated to be selectively correlated with its abilities in (1) promoting the cancer cells to apoptosis and cell cyclic period arrest, (2) suppressing DNA synthesis, (3) devastating microtubule by depolymerization, and (4) obviously repressing NF-κB effects and NF-κB connected antiinflammatory activities.

The apoptosis-stimulating effect in the neoplasm including SMMC-7721 hepatoma, Raji Burkitt's lymphoma, and multiple myeloma cell lines was revealed to be principally mediated by STAT3-involved and/or mitochondria-dependent signaling pathways, i.e., (1) downregulation of antiapoptotic proteins (Bcl-2, Bcl-xL, Mcl-1, and surviving); (2) upregulation of Bax and AIF proteins; (3) decrease of both inducible and constitutive STAT3 activation; (4) reduction of cyclin-D1 and VEGF expressions; (5) release of cytochrome c and AIF from the mitochondria; (6) loss of the mitochondrial membrane potential; and (7) activation of caspases and induction of DNA fragmentation, leading to the acceleration of apoptosis and the sensitization of carcinoma cells.[14,37–40] In addition, ROS accumulation played an important role in the signaling pathways of SMMC-7721 cell apoptosis. The downstream effect of ROS elicited p38 activation and JNK phosphorylation and downregulated hTERT transcription and c-Myc expression, consequently leading to the ultimate reduction of telomerase activity and to cancer inhibition.[38,41,42]

Moreover, the microtubule cytoskeleton disruption and microtubule depolymerization occurred in human MCF-7 breast cancer cells after the treatment with 2.5 μM gambogic acid (**6**).[43] In gambogic acid-treated human BGC-823 gastric cancer cells, CDC2/p34 kinase was inactivated, but CDK7 activity markedly declined, whose events were responsible for the irreversible G2/M phase cell cycle arrest and proliferative inhibition of BGC-823 cells.[44] The antiproliferative effect of gambogic acid (**6**) on the HeLa cervical carcinoma cells was primarily followed by blocking the DNA synthesis and interfering the proceeding of the cell cyclic period.[45]

The decreases of NF-κB activation and NF-κB-dependent reporter gene expression were also found to be involved in the apoptosis acceleration in human leukemia cells treated by gambogic acid (**6**). Concurrently, a series of NF-κB-regulated gene products, including antiapoptotic genes (IAP1 and IAP2, Bcl-2, Bcl-xL, and TRAF1), proliferative genes (c-Myc and cyclin-D1), invasive factors (COX-2 and MMP-9), angiogenic factor (VEGF), and inflammation-related factors (TNFR1, TRADD, TRAF2, NIK, IKKβ, and TAK1/TAB1), were markedly downregulated, and the nuclear translocation and phosphorylation of p65 and IκBα were lessened.[46] More studies have confirmed that the antitumor activity of gambogic acid (**6**) was mediated by the ligation of TfR1 as well in some cases.[47,48]

Importantly, gambogic acid (**6**) exerted the antiinvasive and antimetastatic properties against highly metastatic cells. In the *in vivo* treatment of MDA-MB-435 breast cancer cells, the xanthone dose-dependently repressed the cell invasion through the Matrigel and significantly inhibited lung metastases, whose effects were found to be attributed to its abilities in the blockage of PKC signaling pathway and the reduction of MMP-2 and MMP-9 expression levels.[48] The *in vitro* and *in vivo* explorations further elucidated that gambogic acid (**6**) was able to reduce the possibility of tumor cell adhesion by diminishing integrin-β1 abundance and cholesterol content and to inhibit the function of membrane lipid raft-associated integrin.[49] Reversion-inducing-cystein-rich (RECK) protein was found to play a key role in gambogic acid (**6**)-induced antiinvasion in A549 human lung cancer cells, where gambogic acid (**6**) effectively suppressed HDAC1/Sp1 binding and Sp1 phosphorylation and blocked ERK signaling pathway, leading to the upregulation of RECK.[30] All the results regarding the anticancer mechanisms of Teng Huang xanthones provided broad theoretic evidences and scientific bases for the further development of the agents to clinical applications.

Clinical Trial

The Teng Huang resin had been applied for clinical trials in China. Forty-one cases of skin cancer were treated with the oral administration of Teng Huang resin tablets in doses of 60–90 mg/kg three times per day or the drop intravenous administration of the resin injection of 100–200 mg mixed with 5% glucose solution twice per week, while the 5% Teng Huang resin solution was daubed on the melanoma area per day or every two days. The obtained total effective rate was up to 71%.[50] As a result, the support for the xanthones was positively afforded to serve as a promising therapeutic candidate in the treatment of skin neoplastic diseases.

Toxicity

Teng Huang (Gamboge) resin is usually utilized in traditional Chinese medicine for internal purgative and externally infected wounds because the resin and the xanthones are toxic. The toxic symptoms display the inhibitions at nerve centralism and respiration. The overdose of xanthones for a long time will lead to swelling or cell deformity of the heart, the liver, and the kidney and induce hepatanecrosis and scleroma at the subcutaneous tissue. But at normal doses, the resin and the xanthones do not influence the function of the heart, the liver, and the kidney, and it had almost no suppressive toxic on the marrow.[51]

Other Bioactivity

Some xanthones isolated from the resin, such as gambogic acid (**6**), morellic acid (**7**), desoxymorellin (**1**), hanburin (**11**) dihydroisomorellin, forbesione, and 8,8α-epoxymorellic acid, demonstrated anti-HIV-1 activity in reverse transcriptase assay, while desoxygambogenin (**2**) and dihydroisomorellin were found to be moderately active in the syncytium assay.[22]

References

1. Chen, B. R. et al. 1980. Separation and structure elucidation of gambogic acid. *J. Jiangxi Med. College* 20: 1–7.
2. Lei, Q. M. et al. 1985. Studies on antitumor of gamboge. *Zhonghua Zhongliu Zazhi* 7: 282.
3. Lei, Q. M. et al. 2003. Retrospect and prospect of anticancer efficacy of gamboge. *Zhongliu Fangzhi Zazhi* 10: 216–9.
4. Cao, J. M. et al. 1980. Inhibitory effect of Gamboge extract (736–1) on human hepatoma cell cline. *Jiangxi Yiyao* 3: 1–2.
5. Cao, W. D. et al. (a) 1982. *Zhongcaoyao* 13: 170; (b) 1999. *Chinese Materia Medica.* Vol. 3, 3–2196, 590. Shanghai Science Technology Press, Shanghai, China.
6. Chan, L. F. et al. (a) 1982. *Zhongyaocai Keji* 3: 32; 1999. *Chinese Materia Medica.* Vol. 3, 3–2196, 590. Shanghai Science Technology Press, Shanghai, China.
7. Lu, Y. M. et al. 1996. Comparison of cytotoxicity of different processed products of gamboge on K562 tumor cells. *Zhongguo Zhongyao Zazhi* 21: 90–91.
8. Ye, D. J. et al. 1996. Selection of technology for processing steamed *Garcinia hanburyi* with high pressure by using orthogonal experiment design. *Zhongguo Zhongyao Zazhi* 21: 472–3.
9. Asano, J. et al. 1996. Cytotoxic xanthones from *Garcinia hanburyi. Phytochem.* 41: 815–20.
10. Tao, S. J. et al. 2009. Cytotoxic polyprenylated xanthones from the resin of *Garcinia hanburyi. J. Nat. Prods.* 72: 117–24.
11. Cao, Y. C. et al. 1981. Antitumor activity of gambogic acid on sarcoma 180. *Jiangxi Yixueyuan Xuebao* 21: 13.

12. Feng, F. et al. 2007. Five novel prenylated xanthones from Resina Garcinia. *J. Asian Nat. Prods. Res.* 9: 735–41.
13. Han, Q. B. et al. 2006. Cytotoxic polyprenylated xanthones from the resin of *Garcinia hanburyi. Chem. Pharm. Bull.* 54: 265–7.
14. Hahnvajanawong, C. et al. 2010. Apoptotic activity of caged-xanthones from *Garcinia hanburyi* in cholangiocarcinoma cell lines. *World J. Gastroenterol.* 16: 2235–43.
15. Cai, S. X. et al. 2000. Synthesis of gambogic acid analogs and derivatives as activators of caspases and inducers of apoptosis. *PCT Int. Appl.* WO 2000044216 A2 20000803.
16. Xie, H. et al. 2009. GA3, a new gambogic acid derivative, exhibits potent antitumor activities in vitro via apoptosis-involved mechanisms. *Acta Pharmacol. Sinica* 30: 346–54.
17. Han, Q. B. et al. 2006. A pair of novel cytotoxic polyprenylated xanthone epimers from gamboges. *Chem. Biodiv.* 3: 101–5.
18. Han, Q. B. et al. 2006. Gambogic acid and epigambogic acid, C-2 epimers with novel anticancer effects from *Garcinia hanburyi. Planta Med.* 72: 281–4.
19. Lin, L. J. et al. 1993. Isogambogic acid and isomorellinol from *Garcinia hanburyi. Magn. Resonance Chem.* 31: 340–7.
20. Guo, Q. L. et al. 2004. Gambogic acid inducing apoptosis in human gastric adenocarcinom SGC-7901 cells. *Tianran Yaowu Zazhi* 2: 106–10.
21. Liu, J. B. et al. 2005. Experimental research of anti-pancreatic cancer with gambogic acid. *Linchuang Zhongliuxue Zazhi* 10: 274–7.
22. Reutrakul, V. et al. 2007. Cytotoxic and anti-HIV-1 caged xanthones from the resin and fruits of *Garcinia hanburyi. Planta Med.* 73: 33–40.
23. Zhang, H. Z. et al. 2004. Discovery, characterization and SAR of gambogic acid as a potent apoptosis inducer by a HTS assay. *Bioorg. Med. Chem.* 12: 309–17.
24. Deng, Y. X. et al. 2013. Three new xanthones from the resin of *Garcinia hanburyi. Planta Med.* 79: 792–6.
25. Lee, P. N. H. et al. 2013. Antiproliferative activity of gambogic acid isolated from *Garcinia hanburyi* in Hep3B and Huh7 cancer cells. *Oncol. Reports* 29: 1744–50.
26. Rahman, A. et al. 2013. Cytotoxic effect of gambogic acid on SH-SY5Y neuroblastoma cells is mediated by intrinsic caspase-dependent signaling pathway. *Mol. Cell. Biochem.* 377: 187–96.
27. Xiao, W. et al. (a) 2014. Antineoplastic compound extracted from cambogia and preparation method and application of antineoplastic compound. *Faming Zhuanli Shenqing* CN 103724313 A 20140416; (b) 2009. Two new compounds, 2α-hydroxy-3β-acetoxy-lup-20(29)-en-28-oic acid and 10α-hydroxyepigambogic acid, from *Garcinia hanburyi*, their preparation method and medical application. *Faming Zhuanli Shenqing* CN 101607978 A 20091223.
28. Wang, L. L. et al. 2008. A new cytotoxic caged polyprenylated xanthone from the resin of *Garcinia hanburyi. Chin. Chem. Lett.* 19: 1221–3.
29. Park, M. S. et al. 2015. Antimetastatic effects of gambogic acid are mediated via the actin cytoskeleton and NF-κB pathways in SK-HEP1 cells. *Drug Develop. Research* 76: 132–42.
30. Qi, Q. et al. 2015. Involvement of RECK in gambogic acid induced anti-invasive effect in A549 human lung carcinoma cells. *Mol. Carcinogen.* 54(S1): E13–E25.
31. Yang, J. H. et al. 2013. In vitro and in vivo antiangiogenic activity of caged polyprenylated xanthones isolated from *Garcinia hanburyi* Hook. *Mol.* 18: 15305–13.
32. Chen, Y. et al. 2014. Gambogic acid induces growth inhibition and differentiation via upregulation of p21waf1/cip1 expression in acute myeloid leukemia cells. *J. Asian Nat. Prod. Res.* 16: 1000–8.
33. Tao, S. J. et al. 2010. A highly rearranged pentaprenyl xanthonoid from the resin of *Garcinia hanburyi. Helv. Chim. Acta* 93: 1395–400.
34. Zhang, H. Z. et al. 2004. Discovery, characterization and SAR of gambogic acid as a potent apoptosis inducer by a HTS assay. *Bioorg. Med. Chem.* 12: 309–17.
35. Zhang, Q. G. et al. 2009. Gambogic acid induces Raji cell apoptosis in vitro and its mechanism. *Baixuebing Linbaliu* 18: 643–6, 653.
36. Xiao, W. et al. 2014. Antitumor compound extracted from *Garcinia hanburyi* Hook f., its preparation method and application. *Faming Zhuanli Shenqing* CN 103665089 A 20140326.
37. Nie, F. F. et al. 2009. Reactive oxygen species accumulation contributes to gambogic acid-induced apoptosis in human hepatoma SMMC-7721 cells. *Toxicol.* 260: 60–7.
38. Yang, Y. et al. 2007. Differential apoptotic induction of gambogic acid, a novel anticancer natural product, on hepatoma cells and normal hepatocytes. *Cancer Lett.* 256: 259–66.
39. Prasad, S. et al. 2011. Gambogic acid inhibits STAT3 phosphorylation through activation of protein tyrosine phosphatase SHP-1: Potential role in proliferation and apoptosis. *Cancer Preven. Res.* 4: 1084–94.
40. Zhang, Q. et al. 2009. Gambogic acid induces Raji cell apoptosis in vitro and its mechanism. *Baixuebing Linbaliu* 18: 643–6, 653.
41. Guo, Q. L. et al. 2006. Inhibition of human telomerase reverse transcriptase gene expression by gambogic acid in human hepatoma SMMC-7721 cells. *Life Sci.* 78: 1238–45.
42. Chen, J. et al. 2008. Microtubule depolymerization and phosphorylation of c-Jun N-terminal kinase-1 and p38 were involved in gambogic acid induced cell cycle arrest and apoptosis in human breast carcinoma MCF-7 cells. *Life Sci.* 83: 103–9.
43. Yu, J. et al. 2007. Gambogic acid-induced G2/M phase cell-cycle arrest via disturbing CDK7-mediated phosphorylation of CDC2/p34 in human gastric carcinoma BGC-823 cells. *Carcinogenesis* 28: 632–8.
44. Qiu, X. H. et al. 1986. Influence of gambogic acid on the cell cycle of HeLa cells. *Zhongyao Tongbao* 11: 627–9.
45. Pandey, M. K. et al. 2007. Gambogic acid, a novel ligand for transferrin receptor, potentiates TNF-induced apoptosis through modulation of the nuclear factor-κB signaling pathway. *Blood* 110: 3517–25.
46. Palempalli, U. D. et al. 2009. Gambogic acid covalently modifies IκB kinase-β subunit to mediate suppression of lipopolysaccharide-induced activation of NF-κB in macrophages. *Biochem. J.* 419: 401–9.
47. Wang, L. L. et al. 2008. Two novel triterpenoids with antiproliferative and apoptotic activities in human leukemia cells isolated from the resin of Garcinia hanburyi. *Planta Med.* 74: 1735–40.

48. Qi, Q. et al. 2008. Involvement of matrix metalloproteinase 2 and 9 in gambogic acid induced suppression of MDA-MB-435 human breast carcinoma cell lung metastasis. *J. Mol. Med.* 86: 1367–77.
49. Li, C. L. et al. 2011. Gambogic acid inhibits tumor cell adhesion by suppressing integrin β1 and membrane lipid rafts-associated integrin signaling pathway. *Biochem. Pharmacol.* 82: 1873–83.
50. Jiangxi Tenghuang Kangai Research Group. (a) 1986. *Chin. J. Dermatol.* 19: 31; (b) 1999. *Chinese Materia Medica.* Vol. 3, 3–2196, 590. Shanghai Science Technology Press, Shanghai, China.
51. Qi, Q. et al. 2008. Studies on the toxicity of gambogic acid in rats. *J. Ethnopharmacol.* 117: 433–8.

204 Bi Hu 壁虎

Gecko

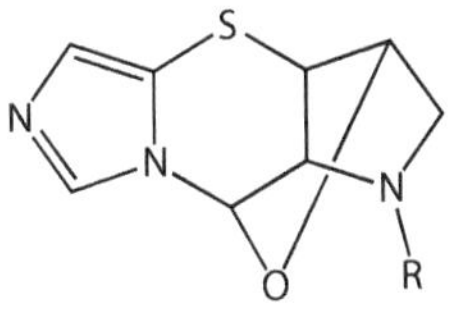

1. R = -H
2. R = $-COOCH_3$
3. R = $-COOCH_2CH_3$

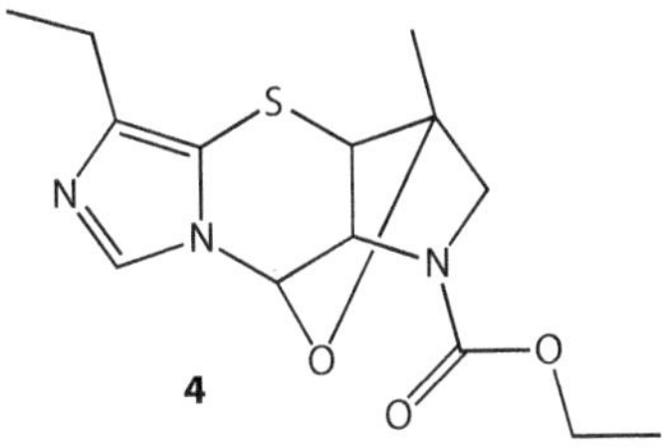

Herb Origination

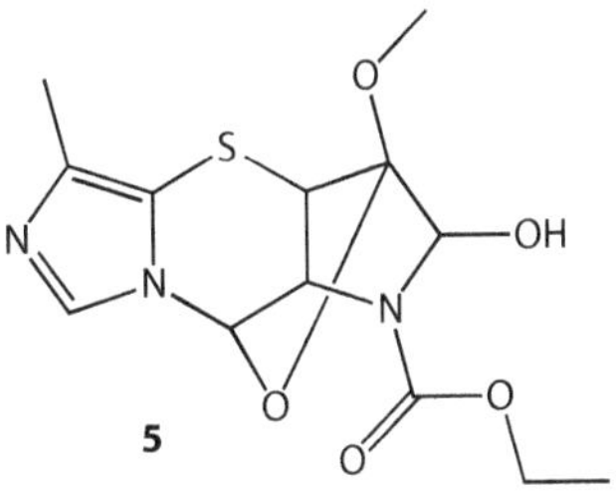

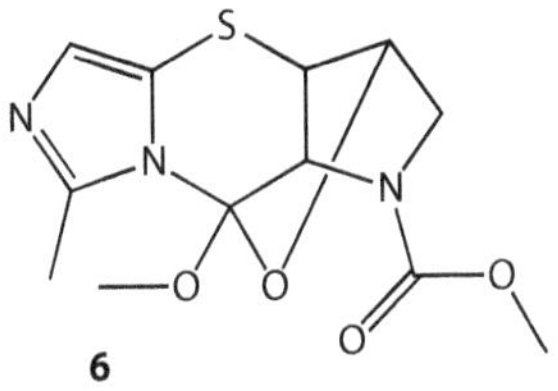

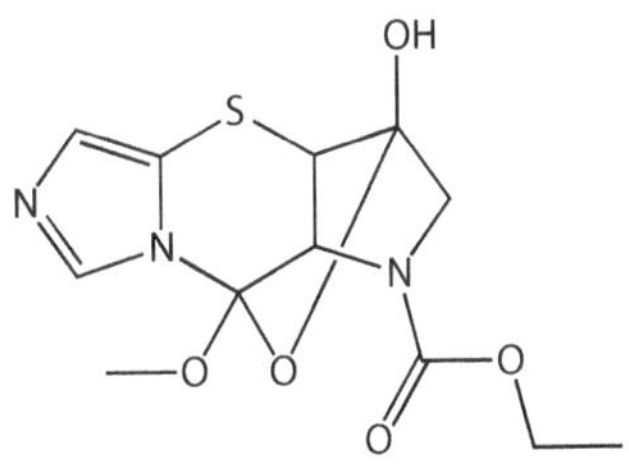

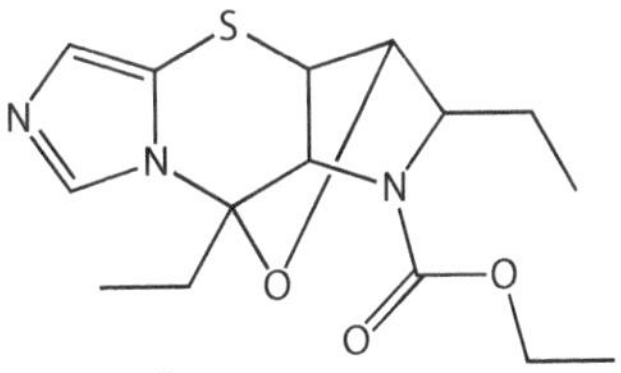

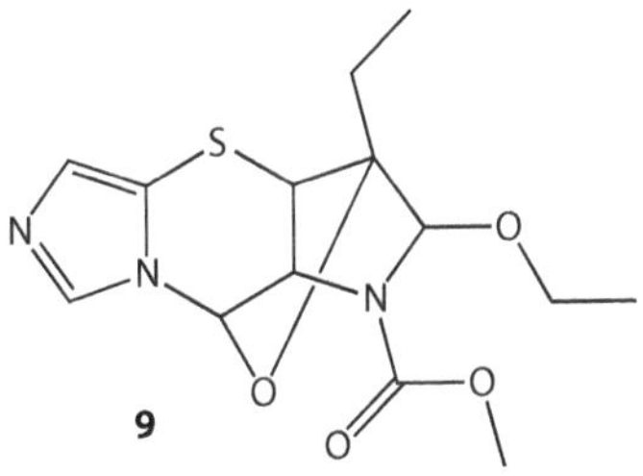

The herb Bi Hu (Gecko) has been used in traditional Chinese medicine for over a thousand years, whose herb originates from three Gekkonidae animals, *Gekko swinhonis* Guenther, *G. japonicus* (Dumeril et Bibron), and *G. subpalmatus* Guenther. As a traditional Chinese medicine, the Gecko is collected in spring and autumn, and its whole body without the internal organs is dried in the sun or by oven.

Antitumor Activities

Bi Hu has been employed in Chinese medicine prescriptions for the treatment of tumor-related diseases. The scientific investigations of Bi Hu have been established in 10 recent years targeting its antineoplastic potentials. FGFP and DGFP are the dried Bi Hu powders (freeze-dried powders from fresh or dried Bi Hu homogenized supernatants, respectively). Both powders and Bi Hu alcohol extract demonstrated notable *in vivo* suppressive effect against the growth of sarcoma 180 and H22 hepatoma in mice xenotransplant models. The daily gavage of dried Bi Hu powder to tumor-bearing mice for 14 days in doses of 13.5, 9, and 4.5 g/kg restrained the sarcoma 180 by 49.8%, 52.8%, and 43.1%, respectively.[1–7] The alcohol extract exerted better effect on sarcoma 180 *in vivo* with inhibitory rates of 63.94% and 69.53%, respectively, in doses of 1.2 and 2.4 g/kg.[1–3] When combined with CTX in the *in vivo* experiment, the alcohol extract could attenuate the negative effect of CTX and enhance the curative effect of CTX in depressing sarcoma 180.[8] At high doses, the antigrowth effect of FGFP, DGFP, alcohol extract, fresh, and processed Bi Hu could reach 47.4%–55.25% in mice implanted with H22 hepatoma.[4–7] The *in vivo* antitumor activity of FGFP on C6 glioma predominantly was present in the prolongation of the tested mouse life duration and the reduction of the tumor volume.[9,10] During the *in vivo* treatment, the expressions of bFGF and VEGF were diminished in the tumor tissue, implying that Bi Hu has an ability to diminish the formation of vessel tube. The antiangiogenesis potential of FGFP was also proven in a mouse model implanted with H22 hepatoma, where the oral administration of FGFP (1.2 g/kg, per day) for 20 times obviously attenuated the MVD in the liver tumor tissue.[7] Also, the *in vivo* FGFP treatment obstructed the formation of lymphangion in the tumor tissue together with its antiangiogenesis.[11]

The powders and the extracts prepared from Bi Hu as well as the Bi Hu-treated serum also exerted *in vitro* suppressive effect against human EC1 and EC9706 esophageal carcinoma cells, human C6 glioma cells, human HepG2 and Bel-7402 hepatoma cells, and mouse H22 hepatoma cells, and they induced the apoptotic death of these neoplastic cell lines in time- and concentration-dependent manners. The increased Bax/Bcl-2 ratio and Bax expression were found to be mechanistically involved in the tumor cell apoptosis induced by the Bi Hu powder and extracts.[3–9] Moreover, the water extract of Bi Hu usually showed greater inhibitory activity than the alcohol extract against the proliferation of carcinoma cells.[12] The enzymatic hydrolysates of Bi Hu (by pepsin, trypsase, or biomimetic enzyme) demonstrated more significant antitumor effect than the Bi Hu powders and extracts but no obvious influence on the indexes of the thymus and the spleen in both mouse models implanted with sarcoma 180 or H22 hepatoma.[13]

Furthermore, various components have been processed from different materials of Bi Hu displaying more marked and selective antitumor activity. GSAAC is a *G. swinhonis* anticancer active component, which significantly inhibited the proliferation and the migration of human hepatoma HepG2 cells *in vitro* in association with the blockage of cell cycle progression to G2 phase from S phase and the induction of early apoptosis.[14] An active component prepared from the freeze-dried powder of fresh *G. swinhonis* could efficiently repress the proliferation and induce the apoptosis of human Bel-7404 hepatoma cell line.[15]

Another component of fresh Bi Hu, which was obtained by using 85% ethanol plus ultrasound extraction, was effective in the suppression of the growth of mouse CT-26 colon carcinoma cells *in vitro* and *in vivo*. Its liposome formulation, which was formed by rotary membrane ultrasound method, showed increased antigrowth effect in the same dose compared to the original component. The i.p. administration of the liposome at a high dose of 10 mg/kg per day to mice for 14 days resulted in marked growth inhibition against CT-26 cells for 52.17%.[16,17]

In addition, the Southern gecko extract was reported to have anticarcinogenic activity against diethylnitrosamine-induced hepatic precancerous lesions in rats. The suppression of Ki-67 and EGFR might be an important event in the hepatocarcinogenesis inhibited by the Southern gecko extract.[18]

Antitumor Constituents and Activities

The focus on the discovery of antineoplastic constituents is the main topic in the current studies of Gecko. Up to now, no pure inhibitor has been reported from the separation of Gecko, but some cancer-suppressive components such as polysaccharides, polysaccharide–protein complexes, glycopeptides, and imidazole derivatives have been fractionated from Gecko.

Polysaccharides

The Gecko-sulfated polysaccharide designated as gepsin could markedly obstruct the proliferation of SMMC-7721 and Bel-7402 hepatocarcinoma cells and induce the differentiation of hepatocarcinoma cells but showed no toxicity to L-20 normal liver cells when exposed to gepsin (100 or 10 μg/mL) to the tested cells. During the *in vitro* treatment, gepsin did not induce the apoptosis of Bel-7402 cells and did not inhibit the viability of SMMC-7721 cells but blocked the cell cycle at G2/M phase. In the gepsin-treated hepatoma cells (100 μg/mL), the AFP secretion was decreased, while the ALB secretion was markedly increased and TGF-β1 level was significantly augmented, indicating that the differentiation of the hepatoma cells was induced in correlation with the upregulation of TGF-β1 level.[19,20] The activation of the Gecko polysaccharide to the lymphocyte proliferation in human PBMCs was also established in the *in vitro* investigations, whose evidence suggested that the Gecko polysaccharide may hold an ability to enhance the cytotoxicity of lymphocytes.[21] A polysaccharide isolated from the *G. swinhonis* by another research group was demonstrated having a similar degree of in *vitro* antihepatoma activity against H22 hepatoma cell line, whose highest growth inhibitory rate could reach to 79.1%. However, an *in vivo* experiment result showed that the polysaccharide has no obvious activity on the inhibition of H22 tumor cells, and its suppressive rate in a high dose was only 8.8%.[22] This result doubted the reported antihepatoma activity of gepsin, suggesting that it is necessary to confirm the antitumor effect of gepsin *in vivo* in animal models.

Polysaccharide–Protein Complex

An anticancer active sulfated polysaccharide–protein complex (GSPP) has been separated from *G. swinhonis*, whose structure was characterized having *O*-glycopeptide linkages. An *in vitro* assay revealed that GSPP suppressed the proliferation of SMMC-7721 cells together with the blockage of the S phase cell cycle and directly inhibited the migration of hepatoma cells via the decrease of intracellular calcium.[23] GSPP could also partially restore the defective biorheological characteristics of DCs by modifying the tumor microenvironment and decreasing the secretion of IL-10 of DCs.[24]

Glycopeptides

Gecko crude peptides significantly inhibited the growth of HepG2 hepatoma cells *in vitro* and promoted typical apoptotic morphological features by increasing Bcl-2/Bax ratio in dose- and time-dependent manners. It could also restore the WBC count and the indexes of the thymus and the spleen in nude mice xenograft model with H22 hepatoma besides the antitumor effect. Simultaneously, the crude peptides significantly decreased the VEGF protein expression levels in the xenograft tumors and reduced the levels of TNFα and IL-6 in the serum, implying that the peptides repress the angiogenesis in the tumor.[25] Continuing the separation of the Gecko-sulfated polysaccharide–protein complex led to obtaining a Gecko-sulfated glycopeptide-α, which demonstrated the suppressive effect against the proliferation and the migration of SMMC-7721 cells. The antimigration in SMMC-7721 cells was probably found by reducing the secretion of IL-8 and the concentration of the intracellular calcium and regulating the reorganization of cytoskeleton.[26] In addition, another sulfated glycopeptide obtained from the separation of *G. swinhonis* also displayed antiangiogenesis and antigrowth activities against hepatoma *in vitro* and *in vivo*, whose angiogenesis-suppressive effect might be mediated by blocking bFGF production, releasing from the extracellular matrix, and obstructing bFGF binding to its low affinity receptor, heparin/heparan sulfate.[27]

Imidazole Derivatives

The MTT-guided isolation led to obtaining anticancer active imidazole derivatives from the extract of fresh *G. swinhonis*, whose imidazole derivatives obviously restrained the proliferation of human Bel-7402 hepatoma cells *in vitro*. The inhibitory rates in the first three days were 71.24%, 91.37%, and 94.45%, respectively.[28] The medical application of nine Gecko imidazols (**1–9**) have been reported to claim that may be used as antitumor agents for treating gastric cancer, lung cancer, colon cancer, breast cancer, leukemia, tumor of the reproductive system, etc.[29] In order to augment the cancer-suppressive potency, an imidazole alkaloid liposome with highly entrapped efficiency and stability was prepared. Both Gecko imidazole alkaloids and imidazole alkaloid liposomes dose- and time-dependently suppressed the proliferation of CT-26 colon tumor cells *in vitro* and *in vivo*, but the imidazole alkaloid liposomes showed more significant antitumor potency.[30]

References

1. Jang, J. X. et al. 2007. Study on antitumor effect of dry and fresh *Gekko swinhonis* freeze-dried powders on mice sarcoma S180 and acute toxicity testing of two powders. *Zhongguo Zhongyao Zazhi*. 32: 238–41.

2. Liu, F. et al. (a) 2008. The inhibitory effect of dried Gecko esophageal cancer and sarcoma 180. *Zhongyaocai* 31: 1304–7; (b) 2008. Antitumor effect and mechanism of Gecko on human esophageal carcinoma cell lines in vitro and xenografted sarcoma 180 in Kunming mice. *World J. Gastroenterol.* 14: 3990–6.
3. Wang, X. L. et al. 2010. Effect of gecko alcohol extract on human esophageal squamous carcinoma cell line EC9706 and antitumor activity in vivo. *Zhongguo Zhongyao Zazhi* 35: 2175–9.
4. Luo WJ et al, 2012. Study on the antitumor effect of Gecko alcohol effect against H22 hepatoma. *Lishizhen Med. Materia Medica Res.* 23: 650-1.
5. Hou, X. N. et al. 2008. Comparative research on anticancer activity between fresh and processed *Gekko subpalmatus. Zhongyaocai* 31: 957–9.
6. Yang, J. X. et al. 2007. Antitumor effects of dry and fresh *Gekko swinhonis* Gunther freeze-dried powders on mouse H22 hepatocellular carcinoma in vivo and in vitro. *World Chin. J. Digestrol.* 15: 157–60.
7. Song, P. et al. 2006. Experimental study on mechanisms of lyophilized powder of fresh *Gekko chinenis* in inhibiting H22 hepatocarcinoma angiogenesis. *Zhongguo Zhongxiyi Jehe Zazhi* 26: 58–62.
8. Wang, X. L. et al. 2010. Study on the antitumor effects and synergism and attenuation effects of gecko alcohol extract. *Zhongyaocai.* 33: 1213–6.
9. Xie, S. et al. 2003. Effects of natural extraction of gecko in inducing apoptosis and antiproliferation of C6 glioma cells. *Cancer Res. on Prev. Treat.* 30: 458–61.
10. Song, P. et al. 2004. Study on sero-pharma-cology of fresh *Gekko swinhonis* Gunther freeze-dried powder in inducing cell apoptosis of C6 glioma cells in mice. *Zhongguo Zhongxiyi Jiehe Zazhi* 24: 919–21.
11. Zhang, F. C. et al. 2011. Study of the inhibition of Gecko lyophilized powder on tumor lymphangiogenesis. *Hebei J. TCM* 9: 1383–4.
12. Kang, D. et al. 2012. Effects on tumor activity of aqueous and ethanol extracts from *Gekko swinhonis* Gunther. *China Pharmacy* 3268–70.
13. Li, J. Q. et al. 2010. The antitumor activity of Gecko extraction with different processes. *Lishizhen Med. Materia Medica Res.* 21: 1629–30.
14. Xie, B. et al. 2012. Effects of the *Gekko swinhonis* anti-neoplasm active component on the proliferation, migration and apoptosis of HepG2 cells. *Zhongguo Yaolixue Tongbao* 28: 101–5.
15. Lu, H. J. et al. 2013. Impact of fresh Gecko active component on proliferation and apoptosis of human hepatocellular carcinoma cell line BEL-7404. *Chin. J. Oncol. Prev. Treat.* 5: 28–31.
16. Kang, J. G. et al. 2007. Experimental study of the effects of fresh *Gekko swinhonis* anti-neoplasm active component on inhibiting CT-26 tumor growth. *Chin. J. Hospital Pharmacy* 27: 441–4.
17. Li, Y. H. et al. 2009. Extraction of anti-neoplasmactive component from *Gekko swinhonis* and its inhibitory effectson CT-26 murine colon carcinoma. *J. Fourth Mil. Med. Univ.* 30: 1103–6.
18. Wang, X. J. et al. 2010. Effects of Southern Gekko on diethylnitrosamine-induced hepatic precancerous lesions in rats. *Chin. J. Cancer Prev. Treat.* 17: 1718–21.
19. Wu, X. Z. et al. 2006. Effects of Gekko sulfated polysaccharide on the proliferation and differentiation of hepatic cancer cell line. *Cell Biol. Int.* 30: 659–64.
20. Xin, L. et al. 2011. Effects of Gekko sulfated polysaccharide on the differentiation of hepatic cancer cell line SMMC-7721. *Tianjin Yiyao* 39: 1123–6.
21. Yan, Z. C. et al. 2007. Influences of *Gekko swinhonis* polysaccharides on lymphocyte proliferation and cytotoxicity. *Zhongcaoyao* 38: 1230–3.
22. Yang, L. H. et al. 2008. In vivo and in vitro research on antitumor effects of Gekko polysaccharide on murine H22 hepatoma. *Tianjin J. TCM* 25: 494–6.
23. Chen, D. et al. 2010. Effects of Gekko sulfated polysaccharide–protein complex on human hepatoma SMMC-7721 cells: Inhibition of proliferation and migration. *J. Ethnopharmacol.* 127: 702–8.
24. Chen, D. et al. 2012. Effects of Gekko sulfated polysaccharide-protein complex on the defective biorheological characters of dendritic cells under tumor microenvironment. *Cell Biochem. Biophys.* 62: 193–201.
25. Song, Y. et al. 2012. Gecko crude peptides induce apoptosis in human liver carcinoma cells in vitro and exert antitumor activity in a mouse ascites H22 xenograft Model. *J. Biomed. Biotech.* ID 743573.
26. Wu, X. Z. et al. Anti-migration effects of Gekko sulfated glycopeptide on human hepatoma SMMC-7721 cells. *Mol.* 16: 4958–70.
27. Zhang, S. X. et al. 2012. Gekko-sulfated glycopeptide inhibits tumor angiogenesis by targeting basic fibroblast growth factor. *J. Biol. Chem.* 287: 13206–15.
28. Gao, L. J. et al. Experimental study of separating *Gekko swinhonis* active constituent using MTT method in vitro. *J. Weifang Med. College* 31: 32–5.
29. Zhang, S. Z. et al. 2010. Purification and characterization of antitumor compounds extracted from gecko. *Faming Zhuanli Shenqing* CN 101875661 A 20101103.
30. Kang, J. G. et al. 2009. Preparation of fresh *Gekko swinhonis* antitumor active component alkaloid liposomes and its quality evaluation. *Chin. J. New Drugs* 18: 1453–9.

205 Gou Wen 鉤吻

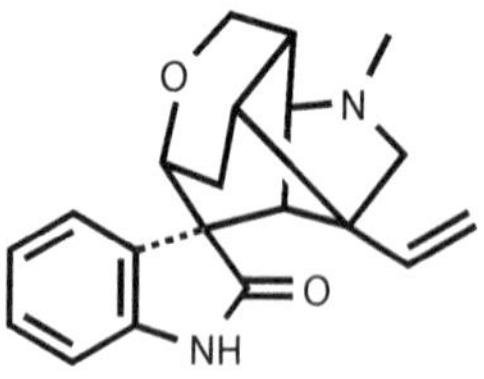

1

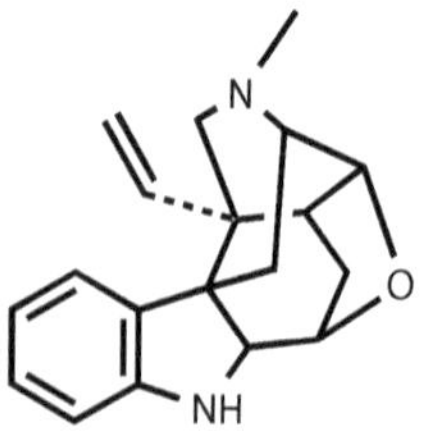

2

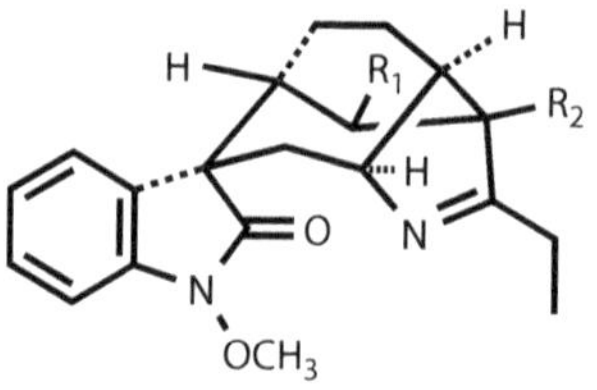

3. R_1 = -OAc, R_2 = -H
4. R_1 = R_2 = -OH

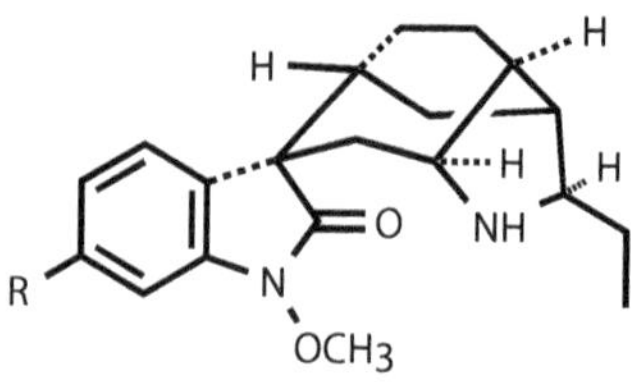

5. R = -H
6. R = -OCH_3

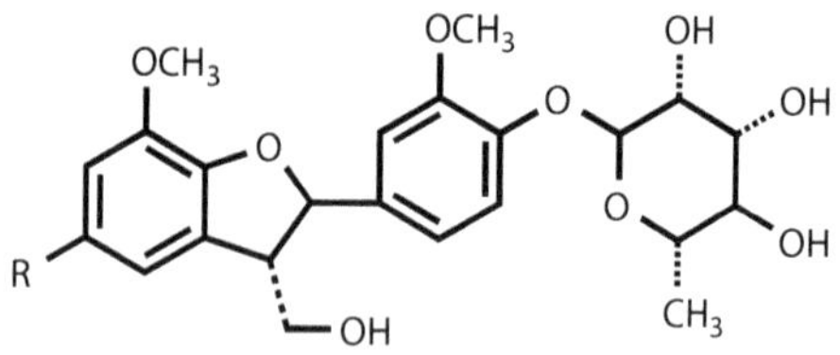

8. R = -CH = CH-COOH
9. R = -COOH

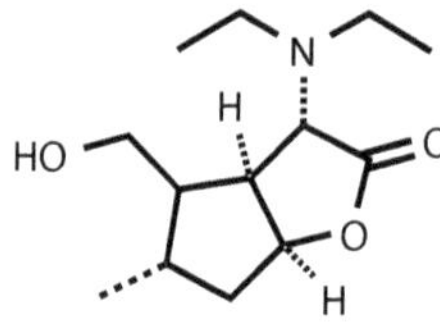

7

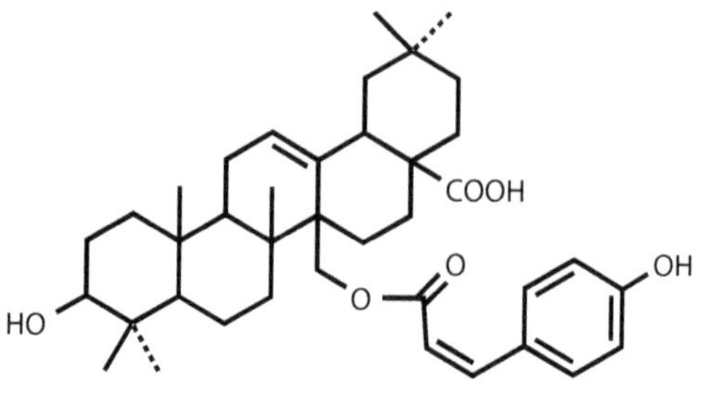

10

Herb Origination

The herb Gou Wen originated from a Loganiaceae plant, *Gelsemium elegans*. The plant, which possesses marked toxicity, is indigenous to southeastern Asia, especially, the southern region of the Yangtze River in China. Generally, the whole plant can be collected annually and can be used fresh and as dried herb for folk medicinal proposes.

Antitumor Activities and Constituents

The methanolic extract of Gou Wen exhibited cytotoxicity against human CaOV-3 ovarian cancer cells *in vitro* with an IC_{50} value of 5 μg/mL after 96 h of incubation but displayed lower inhibitory effect on the growth of human estrogen-receptor$^-$ MDA-MB-231 breast cancer cells with an IC_{50} value of 40 μg/mL.[1] Biology-related phytochemical investigations led to the discovery of alkaloids, lignans, and triterpenoids from the herb. The major constituents were assigned as indole alkaloids, which acted as the most important cancer inhibitors in Gou Wen.

Alkaloids

Approximately 120 alkaloids have been found from *Gelsemium* plants, with the predominant indole alkaloids including gelsemine, koumine, gelsemicine, gelsenicine, gelsedine, sempervirine, koumidine, koumicine, and humantenine. Koumine and gelsemine are the most and second most dominant alkaloids in *G. elegans*, and some of the alkaloids showed moderate anticancer activity. A Gou Wen injection of the total alkaloids has been clinically applied for the treatment of terminal esophageal cancer and hepatoma in China.[2,3] According to the structures, the alkaloids are classified into five types, i.e., gelsemine, gelsedine, koumine, humantenine, and sarpagine. The most active anticancer alkaloids in Gou Wen was identified as gelsemine (**1**), which displayed the antiproliferative effect against human adenocarcinoma cell lines such as Sc-823 (stomach) and AGZY-83-a (lung) *in vitro*, where it obstructed the growth of cancer cells and elicited the cell cycle arrest and the apoptosis. Gelsemine (**1**) in a concentration of 40 mg/mL promoted the death indexes and diminished the growth indexes in the Sc-823 and AGZY-83-a cells. Compared to the AGZY-83-a cells, gelsemine (**1**) was more sensitive to Sc-823 gastric carcinoma cells.[4] 21-Oxogelsemine and 4-N-demethylgelsemine, which are two metabolites of gelsemine (**1**), exerted the proliferative effect on HepG2 hepatoma cells for 67% and 48.1% and on HeLa cervical cancer cells for 28.3% and 24%, respectively, at the same concentration of 160 μmol/L, but the parent molecule had no such activity at that concentration.[5] The treatment with gelsenicine for 48 h showed significant inhibition against the proliferation of HepG2 cell and induced S cell arrest and cell apoptosis in HepG2 cells.[6]

Without obvious inhibition on the immune system, koumine (**2**) obviously suppressed the tumor growth and promoted the apoptosis of LoVo (colon) and MCF-7 (breast) human neoplastic cell lines *in vitro* and mouse H22 hepatoma cells *in vivo*. It also obstructed the DNA synthesis of the LoVo cells, thereby remarkably blocking the cell cycle progression from G1 to S phase, and it elicited the cell cycle arrest of the MCF-7 cells at G2/M phase.[7–10] N-4-Demethyl-21-dehydrokoumine displayed the inhibitory effect not only against the proliferation of HL-60 (leukemic), A549 (lung), SMMC-7721 (liver), SW480 (colon), and MCF-7 (breast) human tumor cell lines (IC_{50}: 4.6–9.3 μM) but also against BEAS-2B human bronchial epithelial cells (IC_{50}: 8.6 μM).[11] Four gelsedine-type alkaloids, i.e., 14-acetoxygelsenicine (**3**), 14,15-dihydoxygelsenicine (**4**), gelsedine (**5**), and gelsemicine (**6**), were shown to be more cytotoxic to human A431 epidermoid carcinoma cells *in vitro* (EC_{50}: 0.25–1.3 μM), compared to cisplatin (EC_{50}: 3.5 μM).[12] An isolated norhumantenine-A exerted moderate antiproliferative effect on A549 (lung), HL-60 (leukemic), and SMMC-7721 (liver) cancer cell lines (IC_{50}: 7.3–9.3 μM) in the *in vitro* assay,[10] while gelsochalotine showed weak cytotoxic effect on BEL-7420 (liver) and MDA-MD-435 (breast) human cancer cell lines.[13] In addition, gelsebamine (**7**), an artificial alkaloid derived from the extraction, selectively suppressed the proliferation of A549 lung adenocarcinoma cells,[14] and geleganidine-B and geleganidine-C inhibited the proliferation of MCF-7 human breast cancer cells (IC_{50}: 38.41 μM) and rat PC12 pheochromocytoma cells (IC_{50}: 16.10 μM), respectively.[15]

Other Components

Some nonalkaloid components from the Gou Wen were found to exert *in vitro* and *in vivo* antitumor effect and immune function-enhancing property.[16] Two benzofuran lignan glycosides, assigned as gelsemiunoside-A (**8**) and gelsemiunoside-B (**9**), were effective in the inhibition of the proliferation of human A375-S2 melanoma cells.[17] Uncarinic acid E (**10**), a triterpenoid, was isolated from the Gou Wen, presenting both time- and dose-dependent suppressive and apoptosis-eliciting effects against the growth of human HepG2 hepatoma cells, whose mechanism in HepG2 cells was associated with the accumulation of p53, the increase of Bax/Bcl-2 ratio, the activation of caspases, and the release of cytochrome c from the mitochondria, where the upregulation of p53 expression plays a pivotal role in the initiation of HepG2 cell apoptosis induced by uncarinic acid E (**10**).[18]

Other Bioactivities

The herb Gou Wen has been used in Chinese folk medicine as analgesic, immunoenhancement, and antispasmodic agents in clinics besides as an antitumor remedy. The total alkaloids were found to be responsible for the bioactivities related to the anti-inflammatory, analgesic, and sedative effects, which are also able to potentiate the phagocytosis of the macrophage and inhibit the contractibility of the cardiac muscle. Gelsemine (**1**) could effectively suppress cisplatin-induced renal injury, whose nephroprotective effect is mediated by the attenuation of oxidative stress.[19] However, the toxicity of Gou Wen is intensive so that the dose must be carefully controlled when in clinical application.

References

1. Abdul, W. K. et al. 2004. A study of the in vitro cytotoxic activity of *Gelsemium elegans* using human ovarian and breast cancer cell lines. *Trop. Biomed.* 21: 139–44.
2. Dai, R. H. et al. 1993. Preparation of Gouwen injection. *Zhongcaoyao* 24: 471–2.
3. Yang, K. Z. et al. Treatment of primary hepatocellular carcinoma with Gouwen: Report of 8 cases survived more than two years. (a) 1981. *Acta Guangxi Med. College* 3: 66–8; (b) 1999. *Chinese Materia Medica*. Vol. 6, 6–5530, 215. Shanghai Science Technology Press, Shanghai, China.
4. Liu, G. L. et al. 1992. Inhibitory effect of gelsemine injection on the proliferation of tumor cells. *Junshi Yixue Kexueyuan Yuankan* 16: 79.
5. Zhao, Q. C. et al. 2010, Antitumor activity of two gelsemine metabolites in rat liver microsomes. *J. Asian Nat. Prods. Res.*12: 731–9.
6. Gao, M. Y. et al. 2012. Anti-proliferation activity and the mechanisms of alkaloid monomers. *Zhongyaocai* 35: 438–42.
7. Chi, D. B. et al. 2003. Study of koumine-induced apoptosis of human colon adenocarcinoma LoVo cells in vitro. *Diyi Junyi Daxue Xuebao* 23: 911–3.
8. Lai, K. D. et al. 2004. Results in the study of chemical composition and biological activity of Vietnamese *Gelsemium elegans*. Part II. *Tap Chi Hoa Hoc* 42: 199–204.
9. Cai, J. et al. 2009. Antineoplastic effect of koumine in mice bearing H22 solid tumor. *J. Nanfang Med. Univ.* 29: 1851–2, 1856.
10. Zhang, X. H. et al. 2015. Apoptotic effect of koumine on human breast cancer cells and the mechanism involved. *Cell Biochem. Biophys.* 72: 411–6.
11. Xu, Y. K. et al. 2015. Koumine, humantenine, and yohimbane alkaloids from *Gelsemium elegans*. *J. Nat. Prod.* 78: 1511–7.
12. Kitajima, M. et al. 2006. Isolation of gelsedine-type indole alkaloids from *Gelsemium elegans* and evaluation of the cytotoxic activity of Gelsemium alkaloids for A431 epidermoid carcinoma cells. *J. Nat. Prod.* 69: 715–8.
13. Liang, S. et al. 2013. Gelsochalotine, a novel indole ring-degraded monoterpenoid indole alkaloid from *Gelsemium elegans*. *Tetrahedron Lett.* 54: 887–90.
14. Xu, Y. K. et al. 2006. Alkaloids from *Gelsemium elegans*. *J. Nat. Prod.* 69: 1347–50.
15. Zhang, W. et al. 2015. Geleganidines A-C, unusual monoterpenoid indole alkaloids from *Gelsemium elegans*. *J. Nat. Prod.* 78: 2036–44.
16. Zhao, M. H. et al. 2006. Comparative study on the antineoplastic effect of non-alkaloid components from *Gelsemium elegans* Benth in vitro and in vivo. *Zhongguo Yaofang* 17: 1776–8.
17. Hua, W. et al. 2008. Two new benzofuran lignan glycosides from *Gelsemium elegans*. *Chin. Chem. Lett.* 19: 1327–9.
18. Zhao, M. H. et al. 2006. The course of uncarinic acid E-induced apoptosis of HepG2 cells from damage to DNA and p53 activation to mitochondrial release of cytochrome c. *Biol. Pharm. Bull.* 29: 1639–44.
19. Lin, L. et al. 2015. Nephroprotective effect of gelsemine against cisplatin-induced toxicity is mediated via attenuation of oxidative stress. *Cell Biochem. Biophys.* 71: 535–41.

206 Shi Suan 石蒜

Red spider lily

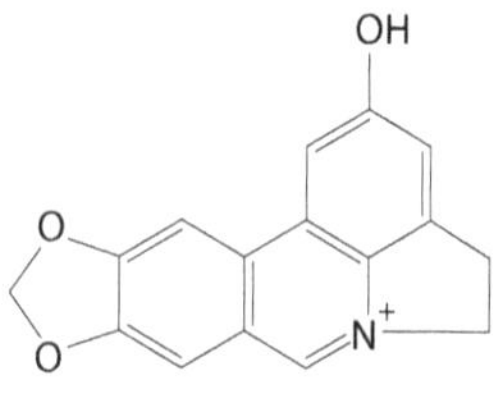

Herb Origination

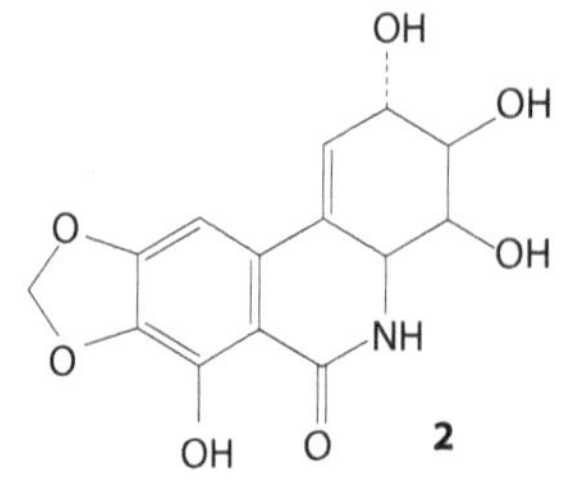

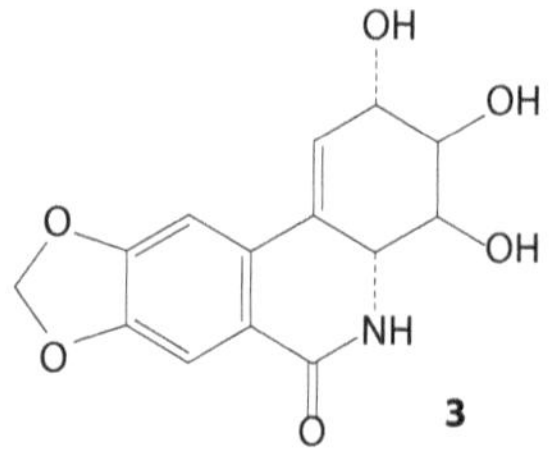

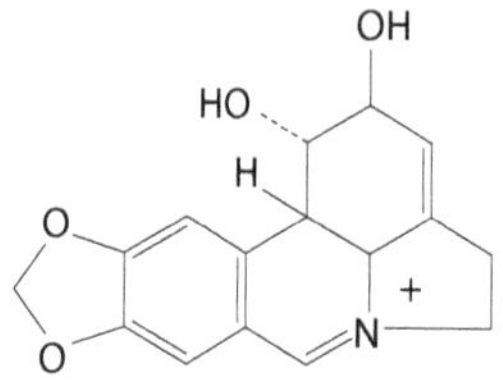

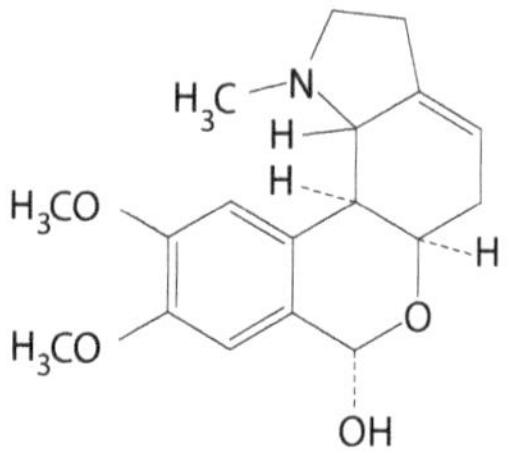

The herb Shi Suan (Red spider lily) originates from two perennial Amaryllidaceae plants, *Lycoris radiate* and *L. chinensis.* The former plant is native to southeast and southwest China, and it is distributed in Vietnam, Malaysia, and other Southeast Asian regions and has also been introduced in Japan and from there to the United States and elsewhere. The latter plant is native to a part of east China. Both plant bulbs are collected in autumn and dried for folk medical practice. The freshly collected bulbs can also be used in the Chinese remedies.

Antitumor Activity and Constituents

In the *in vitro* experiments, the ethanolic extract of *L. radiate* dose-dependently diminished the survival of B16-F10 melanoma cells and retarded the cell growth, accompanied by the elicitation of the G1 cell cycle arrest and the apoptosis through the pathways of p38 and AP-1 activation and caspase-3 stimulation.[1] Phytochemical approaches disclosed that the *L. radiate* bulbs are rich in alkaloid components, which mostly contribute to the cancer growth inhibitory effect of Shi Suan. The alkaloids also acted as an inhibitor of antiapoptosis factor Mcl-1, implying that the alkaloid component may be a potential agent for treating abnormal expression of Mcl-1–associated carcinoma and autoimmune diseases.[2]

A group of alkaloids has been isolated from the plant, and several of them exhibited antineoplastic, immunoenhancing, antiviral, and antimalarial activities. Lycorine, a phenanthridine alkaloid, is the major active compound isolated from the herb, which exerted obvious cytotoxic effect on several cancer cells *in vitro*; for instance, it retarded the proliferation of human Molt4 leukemia cells (ED_{50}: 0.4 μg/mL), human HepG2 hepatoma cells (ED_{50}: 1.3 μg/mL), and mouse P388 leukemia cells.[3–5] Lycobetaine (**1**), a betaine derivative of lycorine, exhibited significant inhibitory effect against the growth of human tumor xenografts tested within its concentrations between 0.002 and 27.5 μM (IC_{50}: 3.3 μM). It exerted the significant suppressive activity on GXF214 and GXF251 gastric cancers, LXFL529 large cell lung carcinoma, LXFS538 small cell lung cancer, CXF280 colon cancer, OVXF1023 ovarian cancer, and PAXF546 pancreatic cancer cell lines and obvious growth inhibition on BXF1299 and BXF1301 bladder cancers, MEXF989 melanoma, and RXF944LX renal carcinoma cell lines. Similar results were obtained for the xenograft-derived LXFL529L large cell lung cancer cell line (IC_{50}: 1.2 μM) and four leukemia cell lines (HL-60, Molt4, K562, and U937) with IC_{50} values of 0.7, 0.8, 1.3, and 2.5 μM, respectively. However, MX1 and MCF7X mammary carcinoma cell lines and LXFA289 and LXFA526 lung adenocarcinoma cell lines appeared to be more resistant to the lycobetaine (**1**).[4–6] The marked antineoplastic activity was also proven in mice/nude mice models implanted with mouse Ehrlich ascites tumor cells and human GXF251 gastric tumor xenograft.[4–6] Moreover, the studies in the SAR disclosed that the betaine skeleton and a methylenedioxy group in lycobetaine (**1**) are critical for the antitumor activity.[7]

Narciclasine (**2**) and lycoricidine (**3**) were evaluated *in vitro* with a panel of 60 cancer cell lines by the NCI, displaying significant cytotoxic, antiproliferative, and proapoptotic effects with IC_{50} values ranging from 0.046 to 0.33 μM.[8] Narciclasine (**2**) triggered an apoptotic process in human MCF-7 breast and PC3 prostate carcinoma cells by activating the initiator caspases of a death receptor pathway and eliciting caspase-8 interacting with Fas and DR4 receptors. But the narciclasine-induced downstream apoptotic pathways in MCF-7 cells diverged from those in the PC3 cells. In the MCF-7 cells, the apoptosis was elicited by mitochondria-dependent amplification with Bid processing, release of cytochrome c, and caspase-9 activation, whereas in the PC3 cells, the caspase-8 directly activated the caspase-3 in the absence of any release of mitochondrial proapoptotic effectors.[9] *In vivo* experimental models further showed that narciclasine (**2**) displayed marked anticancer activity against the growth and the metastases of brain cancer with no toxic side effects. The antiglioma activity was found to be involved in an impairment of actin cytoskeleton organization by targeting GTPases, including RhoA and eEF1A.[10] *In vivo* chronic treatments with narciclasine (**2**) in a dose of 1 mg/kg significantly augmented the survival of nude mice xenografted with highly invasive human glioblastoma and restrained several apoptosis-resistant brain metastases, such as melanoma and NSCLC-induced brain metastases.[10] Hence, narciclasine (**2**) was demonstrated as a promising agent for the treatment of primary brain cancers and various brain metastases.

Moreover, more minor alkaloids have been isolated from the herb and evaluated in eight human tumor cell lines: BEN-MEN-1 (meningioma), CCF-STTG1 (astrocytoma), CHG-5 (glioma), SHG-44 (glioma), U251 (glioma), HL-60 (myeloid leukemia), SMMC-7721 (hepatoma), and W480 (colon cancer), *in vitro*. A lycorine-type alkaloid, (+)-5,6-dehydrolycorine (**4**), showed higher cytotoxic effect against these tumor cell lines except for BEN-MEN-1 cells (IC_{50}: 9.4–11.6 μM), whereas three crinine-type alkaloids, (+)-3α,6β-diacetylbulbispermine, (+)-3α-hydroxy-6β-acetyl-bulbispermine, and (+)-3α-methoxy-6β-acetylbulbispermine, exhibited the similar degree of cytotoxicities against the HL-60 cells (IC_{50}: <10 μM) but only moderate against the CHG-5, SHG-44, CCF-STTG1, and U251 cells (IC_{50}: 10–30 μM).[11] The isolated homolycorine-type alkaloids had almost no activity on these cell lines (IC_{50}: >80 μM).[11] In addition, lycorenine (**5**) could selectively suppress the proliferation of human HepG2 hepatoma cells in an *in vitro* assay with an ED_{50} value of 1.2 μM.[3]

Clinical Studies

A clinic trial of lycobetaine (**1**) had been performed in China to treat 522 cases of malignant tumor in mid–late phases. The results showed a 42.1% total effective percentage and appeared to have greater effect in the treatment of patients with ovarian cancer in the late stage and gastric cancer in the mid–late phase.[12]

Other Bioactivities

Accumulated evidences proved that the major alkaloid lycorine possesses remarkable pharmacological effects on many diseases, including antiinflammation, antimalaria, antileukemia, immunostimulatory, antiviral, and antibacterial activities. It also exerts many other biological functions, such as suppression of acetylcholinesterase and Topo, inhibition of ascorbic acid biosynthesis, and control of circadian period length.

References

1. Son, M. S. et al. 2010. Ethanol extract of *Lycoris radiata* induces cell death in B16F10 melanoma via p38-mediated AP-1 activation. *Oncol. Reports* 24: 473–8.
2. Jiang, J. K. et al. 2009. Medical application of *Lycoris radiata* alkaloids as tumor anti-apoptosis factor Mcl-1 inhibitor. *Faming Zhuanli Shenqing* CN 101352437 A 20090128.
3. Weniger, B. et al. 1995. Cytotoxic activity of Amaryllidaceae alkaloids. *Planta Med.* 61: 77–9.
4. Owen, T. et al. 1976. A new antitumor substance-lycobetaine (AT-1840). *Kexue Tongbao* 21: 285–7.
5. Zhang. S. Y. et al. 1987. Inference of lycobetaine (AT-1840) on ultrastructure of mouse Ehrlich ascites tumor cells. *Zhongliu* 6: 249–50, 285–90.
6. Barthelmes, H. U. et al. 2001. Lycobetaine acts as a selective topoisomerase II beta poison and inhibits the growth of human tumour cells. *British J. Cancer* 85: 1585–91.
7. He, U. M. et al. 1989. Structure–activity-relationship study of the new anticancer drug lycobetaine (AT-1840). *Yaoxue Xuebao* 24: 302–4.
8. Ingrassia, L. et al. 2008. Amaryllidaceae isocarbostyril alkaloids and their derivatives as promising antitumor agents. *Transl. Oncol.* 1: 1–13.
9. Dumont, P. et al. 2007. The Amaryllidaceae isocarbostyril narciclasine induces apoptosis by activation of the death receptor and/or mitochondrial pathways in cancer cells but not in normal fibroblasts. *Neoplasia* 9: 766–76.
10. Goietsenoven, G. V. et al. 2013. Narciclasine as well as other *Amaryllidaceae isocarbostyrils* are promising GTPase targeting agents against brain cancers. *Med. Res. Reviews* 33: 439–55.
11. Hao, B. et al. 2013. Cytotoxic and antimalarial Amaryllidaceae alkaloids from the bulbs of *Lycoris radiate. Mol.* 18: 2458–68.
12. Cao, Z. F. 2013. Multiple biological functions and pharmacological effects of lycorine. *Sci. China Chem.* 56: 1382–91.

207 Ban Mao 斑蝥

Mylabris or Chinese blister beetle

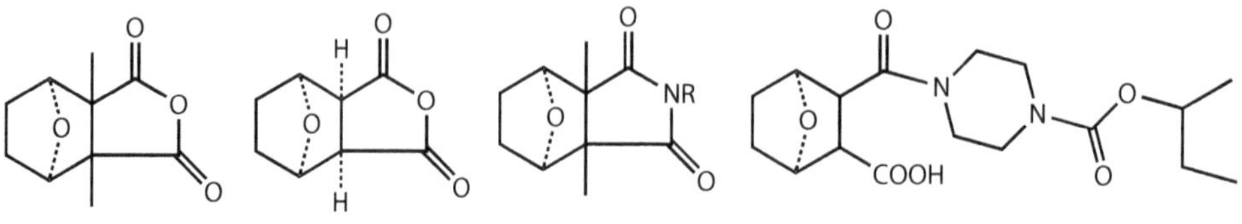

1 2 3. R = -H 5. R = -OH 4

Herb Origination

The herb Ban Mao is the dried blister beetle *Mylabris phalerata* and *M. cichorii* (Coleoptera), which are distributed in most places in China. The best collecting season for Ban Mao is between June and August. The insect herb has been used in traditional Chinese medicine for a thousand years; it was one of the Chinese medicinal drugs documented in the first Chinese classic materia medica entitled *Shengnong Ben Cao Jing.*

Antitumor Constituents and Activities

A butanolic fraction of Ban Mao was found to possess cytotoxic activity on human U937 monocytic leukemic cells *in vitro* (IC_{50}: 140 μg/mL). At a concentration of 31.25 μg/mL, the fraction effectively elicited the morphological changes of apoptosis in the U937 cells through cleavages of Bid, release of cytochrome c from the mitochondria into the cytosol, and activation of caspase cascade (caspase-8, caspase-9, and caspase-3). But over 500 μg/mL of the fraction was also active on peripheral blood mononuclear lymphocytes.[1]

Its major principle isolated from the dried body of Ban Mao was identified as cantharidin (**1**), which is largely responsible for the bioactivity of the herb Ban Mao. However, the existence of cantharidin (**1**) in the body of Ban Mao is normally in a bound form with magnesium or calcium.

Cantharidin

Cantharidin (**1**) displayed antineoplastic and apoptosis-inducing activities on many types of malignant tumor cells. Stomach/esophageal carcinoma cells and hepatoma cells are the most sensitive neoplasm for cantharidin (**1**), but it exhibited inactive/weak effect toward L615 leukemia, sarcoma 180 and AK sarcomas, L2 reticulosarcoma, W256 sarcoma, and Ehrlich ascites carcinoma *in vitro.*[2–5] The cantharidin treatment could cause acute and lethal toxic effects on hepatoma cells, i.e., inhibited mitochondria energy system and protein synthesis and indirectly retarded nucleic acid synthesis, blocked all phases of the hepatoma cell cycle progression, compelled the cells to necrosis, and atrophied the hepatoma tissue.[4] The i.p. administration of cantharidin (**1**) in doses of 0.7–1.25 mg/kg to tumor-bearing mice significantly restrained the growth of ascites hepatoma cells *in vivo*, but it also showed cytotoxicity against normal liver cells.[5] The IC_{50} values were 2.2 and 30.2 μM for 36 h, respectively, on Hep3B hepatoma cells and normal Chang liver cells *in vitro*, whose data mean there is no large difference.[4] The cytotoxicity of cantharidin (**1**) was also demonstrated on three other human tumor cell lines: KB (nasopharynx), DU-145 (prostate), and HeLa (cervix) *in vitro.*[5] By increasing ROS and Ca^{2+} production and mitochondria-dependent pathways, i.e., the up-expression of caspase-3, caspase-8, and caspase-9, cytochrome c, Bax, Bid, Endo G, and AIF and the down-expression of Bcl-2 and Bcl-x, cantharidin (**1**) elicited the cell apoptosis and the growth inhibition in human A375.S2 (skin) and H460 (lung) cancer cell lines. Simultaneously, cantharidin (**1**) induced the expressions of ER stress-related proteins such as GRP78, IRE1α/IRE1β, ATF6α, and caspase-12/-4 in the two cell lines and promoted the expression of calpain 2 and XBP-1 in H460 cells.[6,7] The cantharidin treatment in murine Dalton's lymphoma cells provoked ultrastructural and biochemical changes in the mitochondria leading to apoptosis and necrosis and exerting an anticancer effect.[8] Also, cantharidin (**1**) was capable of impairing the migration and the invasion of A375.S2 cells by suppressing MMP-2 and MMP-9 through PI3K/NF-κB signaling pathways.[9] Furthermore, compared to cantharidin (**1**), the bound cantharidin displayed more effective inhibitory effect against the proliferation of human PLC/PRF/5 and BEL-7404 (liver), HT-29 (colon), and SGC-7901 (stomach) cancer cell lines in a dose-dependent manner with IC_{50} values (μmol/L) of 86.77, 21.27, 28.51, and 10.86, respectively, implying that the bound cartharidin has greater bioavailability.[10,11]

Further studies revealed that cantharidin (**1**) is a selective inhibitor of PP1 (protein phosphatase-1) and PP2A. The cytotoxicity of cantharidin (**1**) was reported to be necessary in association with the inhibition of PP1 and PP2A activities.[5] Cantharidin (**1**), a potent PP2A inhibitor, could exert an oxidative stress-independent growth inhibition on pancreatic cancer cells together with the elicitation of G2/M cell cycle arrest and apoptosis.[12] Moreover, the *in vivo* treatment with cantharidin (**1**) extended the life span of mice implanted with ARS reticulosarcoma by 56%.[13] Based on the observations, cantharidin (**1**) was known as an anticancer lead for the development of a chemotherapeutic drug. Actually, cantharidin (**1**) has been employed as a clinical drug in China to treat hepatoma and esophageal carcinoma for a long time. But due to its highly toxic nature and severe side effects, its clinical application was limited.

Formulation of Cantharidin

Cantharidin (**1**) has been entrapped by nonionic surfactant vesicles to produce a new formulation labeled as CTD-NSVs. An *in vitro* assay showed that CTD-NSVs could induce more significant cell cycle arrest in the G0/G1 phase and higher apoptotic rates, thereby significantly enhancing the cytotoxic effect against human breast cancer MCF-7 cells. An *in vivo* treatment of mouse sarcoma 180 with CTD-NSVs at a dose of 1.0 mg/kg resulted in more enhanced antitumor activity with an inhibition rate of 52.76%, which was better than that of CTX (35 mg/kg, 40.23%) and free cantharidin (1.0 mg/kg, 31.05%). Also, the encapsulation of cantharidin into the nonionic surfactant vesicles distinctly reduced the acute toxicity and the liver toxicity from the free cantharidin (**1**) and prominently improved the antitumor potency.[14]

Peptides

Cantharis peptides were prepared from Mylabris by a bionic enzymolysis approach. Its suppressive effects on the proliferation of neoplastic cells were tested in mouse models. The inhibitory rates of cantharis peptide were 12.54% on human Bel-7402 hepatoma and 5.93% on mouse sarcoma 180, whose activities were apparently lower than those of cantharidin (**1**). But cantharis peptides showed no immunosuppression and negative influence on the growth of the thymus and the spleen.[15]

Structural Modification

In order to optimize the anticarcinoma agent with less toxicity, the numerous cantharidin analogs have been explored. Norcantharidin (NCTD) (**2**), a demethylated cantharidin, exerted better antihepatoma activity with little to no urinary irritation, indicating that the two methyl groups of cantharidin are not the main functional groups for the cytotoxicity but are associated with urinary irritation.[19–28] NCTD (**2**), which is a PP1 and a PP2A inhibitor with similar potency level to cantharidin (**1**), suppressed the cell growth by inducing apoptosis and/or blocking the cell cycle progression in various cancer cells,[19] exerting better anticancer spectrum and lower toxicity compared to cantharidin (**1**). But NCTD (**2**) showed the different targets on a variety of cancer cells in its inhibitory mechanisms. The antiproliferative activity of NCTD (**2**) on human HepG2 hepatoma cells was closely correlated to its ability of accelerating the apoptosis mediated by ROS generation and mitochondrial pathway.[20–22] Clinical evidences further substantiated that the antihepatoma effectiveness sequentially increased from cantharidin to disodium cantharidate, then to norcantharidin.[18,23] By alternating the activities of mitogen-activated kinases, transcription activators, and signal transducers, NCTD (**2**) promoted the mitotic arrest and apoptosis in human SKOV-3 ovarian neoplastic cells and breast cancer cells. NCTD (**2**) induced the cell cycle arrest at both G2/M and M phases of the ovarian cancer cells through restrained tubulin polymerization and mitotic spindle assembly, and it disturbed the cell cycle progression of the breast carcinoma cells through p53- and Chk-mediated pathways.[22–26] The proliferation of human GBC-SD gallbladder carcinoma could be suppressed by NCTD (**2**) via the decrease of the expressions of PCNA and Ki-67.[27] The induction of cell cycle arrest and the inhibition of human leukemic Jurkat T cells by NCTD (**2**) should be involved in MAPK-mediated regulation of IL-2 production.[28] The apoptosis of human melanoma A375-S2 cells was processed by the activation of caspase and mitochondrial pathways after NCTD (**2**) treatment.[29]

Moreover, the investigation has confirmed that NCTD (**2**) not only induced apoptosis, but also served as an antimetastasis agent in certain malignant cells.[30] By inhibiting MMP-9 and u-PA expressions via the phosphorylation of ERK1/2 and NF-κB signaling pathway, NCTD (**2**) acted as an inhibitor on the invasion and the metastasis of hepatoma cells.[31,32] It markedly diminished the MMP-9 expression by inhibiting Sp1 transcriptional activity and restraining several cadherin–catenin adhesion molecules and also exerted antiangiogenic activity in CT26 colorectal cancer cells.[33] The i.p. injection of NCTD (**2**) at a dose of 2 mg/kg/day to mice bearing CT26 tumor lessened both the growth and the pulmonary metastatic capacity of the CT26 cells and prolonged the survival duration of the tested mice.[34–36] At a 100 μM concentration, NCTD (**2**) dose-dependently retarded the cell growth, arrested the cell cycle at G2/M phase, enhanced the apoptosis, and even reduced the cell migration in the treatment of human NSCLC cell lines (A549 and PC9). Moreover, NCTD (**2**) was able to augment the anticancer potency of chemotherapeutic agents gefitinib and cisplatin.[37,38] Through induced transcriptional repression of Mcl-1, NCTD (**2**) could enhance ABT-737-induced apoptosis and cell viability inhibition in multiple hepatocellular carcinoma cells. The enhancement of ABT-737-mediated apoptosis by NCTD (**2**) was associated with the activation of mitochondrial apoptosis signaling pathway, which involved cytosolic release of cytochrome c, cleavage of caspase-9 and caspase-3.[39] The results therefore suggest that the combination treatment with NCTD (**2**) may overcome drug resistance and augment chemotherapeutic efficacy in treating human malignant tumor diseases, especially hepatoma.

Furthermore, the strategy of structural modification has also been focused in the introduction of nitrogen to the molecule. When an anhydride oxygen atom in cantharidin (**1**) was replaced by nitrogen to derive cantharimide (**3**), the toxicity was relatively reduced to the nonmalignant hematological disorder of the bone marrow cells. Based upon these data, the structural modification of cantharidin (**1**) has been concentrated on the substitution of various heterocyclic moieties to this amide atom.[38–43] Thus, several amide derivatives of cantharidin have been synthesized. Among them, N-benzylcantharidinamide (**4**) was able to suppress the expression of MMP-9 and invasive potentials in highly metastatic Hep3B hepatoma cell by inhibiting cytosolic translocation of HuR.[44] A cantharidin derivative, LB1 (**5**), was created from the opening of the anhydride and the linkage of a piperazine unit. It showed significant effect in the inhibition of PP2A without apparent toxicity. LB1 (**5**) could greatly enhance the effectiveness of DOX in the xenograft growth inhibition and prevent the lung metastases of an aggressive sarcoma derived from transformed mesenchymal stem cells in syngeneic rats.[45] For lowering the toxicity to the discovery of pharmaceutically valuable drug candidates, the attempt of structural modification starting from the cantharidin molecule has been continued.

Clinical Studies

In the 1970s, cantharidin (**1**) and its few derivatives had been subjected to clinical trials in China, receiving some positive results and experiences. However, since cantharidin (**1**) has strong toxicity on the liver, the renal system, and the gastrointestinal system, the administration of Ban Mao and cantharidin (**1**) in clinics must be particularly carefully done on its dose control. Overdoses may cause burning sensation in the throat and the mouth, dizziness, digestive disorder, and pollakiuria, etc. Patients who have cardiorenal disease and serious alimentary tract ulcer as well as pregnant woman should be prohibited from using Ban Mao and cantharidin (**1**) for treatment.

1. Over 300 cases of patients suffering from primary hepatoma were treated in clinical trial by using a cantharidin tablet (0.25 mg, per tablet). The starting oral dose was one tablet, two times per day, then it is gradually increased to three to six, three times per day. The total effective rate resulted to be 65%.[46]
2. Several dose programs were used to treat 27 patients with primary hepatoma in phase II or phase III. The oral dose of cantharidin (**1**) was 0.50 mg, once per day, then it is gradually increased to three to four times per day, or by daily slow intravenous injection of cantharidin (0.50 mg) with 50% glucose fluid (40 mL), then it is gradually increased to 1 mg per day. The average total cantharidin used for each patient was around to 82.15 mg, and the total effective rate was received as 51.8%.[47] Strong side effects in urological and digestive systems were observed during the treatment with cantharidin.
3. One hundred forty-two cases of primary hepatoma received treatment using N-hydroxycantharidinimide (**6**). The doses used in the period were daily oral administration of 25 mg N-hydroxycantharidinimide (**6**), three times per day, then it is gradually increased to 50–100 mg, three times per day, or daily slow intravenous injection of N-hydroxycantharidinimide in a dose 80 mg with 50% glucose fluid (20 mL). The total effective rate reached to 56.3%.[48]

Other Bioactivities

The herb Ban Mao displayed antiinflammatory, antivirus, antifungal, antibacterial, and gynecogen-like effects in the pharmacological investigations. Cantharidin (**1**) and most of its derivatives were able to promote leukocyte elevation, IL-1 production from spleen leukocyte, and IL-2 secretion.[49,50] The derivatives such as disodium cantharidate, methyl cantharidinimide, and N-hydroxycantharidinimide, etc., showed less urinary irritation than cantharidin (**1**).

References

1. Huh, J.-E. et al. 2003. *Mylabris phalerlata* induces apoptosis by caspase activation following cytochrome c release and Bid cleavage. *Life Sci.* 73: 2249–62.
2. Li, D. H. et al. 1980. Pharmacological study on new antitumor agent hydroxyl cantharidinimide. *Zhonghua Yixue Zazhi* 60: 410–3.
3. Wang, G. S. et al. 1980. Application and development of anticancer cantharidin. *Yaoxue Tongbao* 15: 23–6.
4. Wang, C. C. et al. 2000. Cytotoxic effects of cantharidin on the growth of normal and carcinoma cells. *Toxicol.* 147: 77–87.
5. Liu, D. W. et al. 2009. The effects of cantharidin and cantharidin derivates on tumor cells. *Anti-Cancer Agents in Med. Chem.* 9: 392–6.
6. Hsiao, Y. P. et al. 2014. Cantharidin induces G2/M phase arrest by inhibition of Cdc25c and cyclin A and triggers apoptosis through reactive oxygen species and the mitochondria-dependent pathways of A375.S2 human melanoma cells. *Intl. J. Oncol.* 45: 2393–402.
7. Hsia, T. C. et al. 2014. Cantharidin induces apoptosis of H460 human lung cancer cells through mitochondria-dependent pathways. *Intl. J. Oncol.* 45: 245–54.
8. Prasad, S. B. et al. 2013. Cantharidin-mediated ultrastructural and biochemical changes in mitochondria lead to apoptosis and necrosis in murine Dalton's lymphoma. *Microsc. Microanal.* 19: 1377–94.
9. Ji, B. C. et al. 2015. Cantharidin impairs cell migration and invasion of A375.S2 human melanoma cells by suppressing MMP-2 and -9 through PI3K/NF-κB signaling pathways. *Anticancer Res.* 35: 729–38.
10. Li, X. F. et al. 2013. Comparative study on anti-tumor effect of cantharidin and bound cantharidin from Meloidae. *Shizhen Guoyi Guoyao* 24: 535–8.
11. Li, X. F. et al. 2013. Inhibitory effect of bound cantharidin extracted from *Mylabris cichorii* on the proliferation of gastric carcinoma cell SGC-7901. *Tianran Chanwu Yanjiu Yu Kaifa* 25: 963–6.
12. Li, W. et al. 2010. Cantharidin, a potent and selective PP2A inhibitor, induces an oxidative stress-independent growth inhibition of pancreatic cancer cells through G2/M cell-cycle arrest and apoptosis. *Cancer Sci.* 101: 1226–33.
13. Chen, R. T. et al. 1977. Pharmacological study on cantharidin. *Zhonghua Yixue Zazhi* 57: 475–8.
14. Han, W. et al. 2012. Non-ionic surfactant vesicles simultaneously enhance antitumor activity and reduce the toxicity of cantharidin. *Intl. J. Nanomed.* 8: 2187–96.
15. Liao, X. Y. et al. 2013. Comparative study of antitumor activity of cantharidin and cantharis peptides. *Zhongyaocai* 36: 1566–9.
16. Hill, T.-A. et al. 2008. Norcantharidin analogues: Synthesis, anticancer activity and protein phosphatase 1 and 2A inhibition. *Chem. Med. Chem.* 3: 1878–92.
17. Wang, G. S. et al. 1987. Norcantharidin elevates white blood cells. *Yaoxue Tongbao* 22: 517.
18. Wang, G. S. et al. 1989. Medical uses of mylabris in ancient China and recent studies. *J. Ethno. Pharmacol.* 26: 147–62.
19. Hill, T.-A. et al. 2007. Heterocyclic substituted cantharidin and norcantharidin analogues—Synthesis, protein phosphatase (1 and 2A) inhibition, and anticancer activity. *Bioorg. Med. Chem. Lett.* 17: 3392–7.
20. Chang, C. et al. 2010. Involvement pf mitochondrial pathway in NCTD-induced cytotoxicity in human hepG2 cells. *J. Exp. Clin. Cancer Res.* 29: 145–53.
21. Chang, C. et al. 2011. The anti-proliferative effects of norcantharidin on human HepG2 cells in cell culture. *Mol. Biol. Rep.* 38: 163–9.
22. Chen, Y. N. et al. 2002. Effect mechanisms of norcantharidin-induced mitotic arrest and apoptosis in human hepatoma cells. *Intl. J. Cancer* 100: 158–65.
23. Wang, Z. T. et al. 1983. Studies on the antitumor drugs of cantharidin derivatives: I. Crystal, molecular, and electronic structure of N-hydroxy-cantharidinimide. *Fenzi Kexue Yu Huaxue Yanjiu* 3: 25–34.

24. Yang, P. J. et al. 2011. Norcantharidin induces apoptosis of breast cancer cells: Involvement of activities of mitogen activated protein kinases and signal transducers and activators of transcription. *Toxicol. In. Vitro* 25: 699–707.
25. Hong, X. F. et al. 2012. Inhibitory effect of norcantharidin on tubulin polymerization in vitro Inhibitory effect of norcantharidin on tubulin polymerization in vitro. *Chinese J. Pharmacol. Toxicol.* 26: 630–4.
26. Li, R. Q. et al. 2013. Norcantharidin induced mitotic arrest and apoptosis in human ovarian cancer SK-OV-3 cells. *Chinese J. Pharmacol. Toxicol.* 27: 180–6.
27. Fan, Y. Z. et al. 2007. Influence of norcantharidin on proliferation, proliferation-related gene proteins proliferating cell muclear antigen and Ki-67 of human gallbladder carcinoma GBC-SD cells. *Hepatobiliary Pancreat Dis. Int.* 6: 72–80.
28. Liao, H. F. et al. 2011. Norcantharidin induces cell cycle arrest and inhibits progression of human leukemic Jurkat T cells through mitogen-activated protein kinase-mediated regulation of interleukin-2 production. *Toxicol, In. Vitro* 25: 206–12.
29. An, W. W. et al. 2004. Norcantharidin induces human melanoma A375-S2 cell apoptosis through mitochondrial and caspase pathways. *J. Korean Med. Sci.* 19: 560–6.
30. Huang, Y. et al. 2009. Suppression of growth of highly-metastatic human breast cancer cells by norcantharidin and its mechanisms of action. *Cytotechnol.* 59: 201–8.
31. Yeh, C. B. et al. (a) 2012. Antimetastatic effects of norcantharidin on hepatocellular carcinoma by transcriptional Inhibition of MMP-9 through modulation of NF-kB activity. *PLoS One* 7: e31055; (b) 2010. Therapeutic effects of cantharidin analogues without bridging ether oxygen on human hepatocellular carcinoma cells. *Eur. J. Med. Chem.* 45: 3981–5.
32. Chen, Y. J. et al. 2009. A small-molecule metastasis inhibitor, norcantharidin, downregulates matrix metallo-proteinase-9 expression by inhibiting Spl transcriptional activity in colorectal cancer cells. *Chem. Biol. Interact.* 181: 440–6.
33. Chen, Y. J. et al. 2005. Inhibitory effect of norcantharidin, a derivative compound from blister beetles, on tumor invasion and metastasis in CT26 colorectal adenocarcinoma cells. *Anticancer Drugs* 16: 293–9.
34. Peng, F. et al. 2002. Induction of apoptosis by norcantharidin in human colorectal carcinoma cell lines: Involvement of the CD95 receptor/ligand. *J. Cancer Res. Clin. Oncol.* 128: 223–30.
35. Yang, P. Y. et al. 2010. Involvement of caspase and MAPK activities in norcantharidin-induced colorectal cancer cell apoptosis. *Toxicol. In. Vitro* 24: 766–75.
36. Kok, S. H. L. et al. 2007. Synthesis and structure evaluation of a novel cantharimide and its cytotoxicity on SK-Hep-1 hepatoma cells. *Bioorg. Med. Chem. Lett.* 17: 1155–9.
37. Luan, J. L. et al. 2010. Inhibitory effects of norcantharidin against human lung cancer cell growth and migration. *Cytotechnol.* 62: 349–55.
38. Lee, Y. H. et al. 2013. Norcantharidin suppresses cell growth and migration with enhanced anticancer activity of gefitinib and cisplatin in human non-small cell lung cancer cells. *Oncol. Reports* 29: 237–43.
39. Zhang, S. J. et al. 2012. Norcantharidin enhances ABT-737-induced apoptosis in hepatocellular carcinoma cells by transcriptional repression of Mcl-1. *Cellular Signalling* 24: 1803–9.
40. Lin, L. H. et al. 2004. Effects of cantharidinimides on human carcinoma cells. *Chem. Pharm. Bull.* 52: 855–7.
41. Kok, S. H. L. et al. 2006. Induction of apoptosis on carcinoma cell by two synthetic cantharidin analogues. *Int. J. Mol. Med.* 17: 151–7.
42. Lin, P. Y. et al. 2001. Synthesis of novel N-pyridylcantharidinimides by using high pressure. *J. Chinese Chem. Soc.* (Taiwan) 48: 49–53.
43. Zhou, Z. H. et al. 2000. Synthesis of glycerophospholipid conjugates of cantharidin andilts analogues. *Synthetic Commun.* 30: 3527–33.
44. Lee, J. Y. et al. 2014. A novel cantharidin analog N-Benzylcantharidinamide reduces the expression of MMP-9 and invasive potentials of Hep3B via inhibiting cytosolic translocation of HuR. *Biochem. Biophys. Res. Commun.* 447: 371–7.
45. Zhang, C. et al. 2010. A synthetic cantharidin analog for the enhancement of doxorubicin suppression of stem cell-derived aggressive sarcoma. *Biomaterials* 31: 9535–43.
46. Yi, S. N. et al. 1988. Preliminary study on the mechanism of increasing leukemia count induced by sodium norcantharidate. *J. Hunan Med. College* 327–30.
47. Shanghai Pujiang Hospital. (a) 1975. *Zhonghua Yixue Zazhi* 503; (b) 1999. *Chinese Materia Medica*. Vol. 9, 9–8120, 199–202. Shanghai Science Technology Press, Shanghai, China.
48. Dian, X. H. et al. 1981. Treatment of 27 cases of primary hepatoma with cantharidin. *Guizhou Yiyao* 37–9.
49. Zhou, A. R. et al. 1987. Influences of norcantharidin and dehydronorcantharidin on DNA synthesis in mouse morrow cells. *Yaoxue Tongbao* 22: 427.
50. Zhang, J. J. et al. 1992. Effects of cantharidin on interleukin-2 and interleukin-1 production in mice in vivo. *Zhongguo Yaoli Xuebao* 13: 263–5.

208 Shui Xian 水僊

Chinese sacred lily

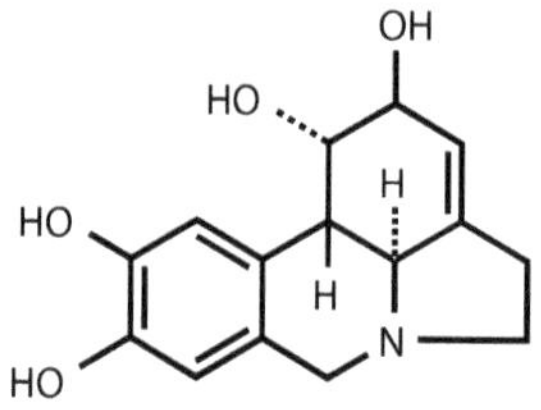

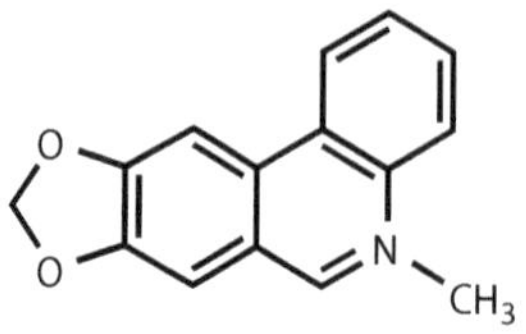

2. $CH_3O{-}SO_3^-$

3. $HOOCCH(OH)CH_2COO^-$

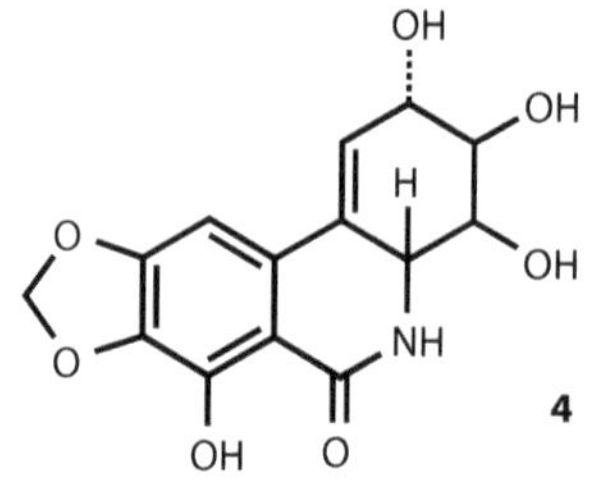

Herb Origination

Shui Xian (Chinese daffodil) is an Amaryllidaceae plant, *Narcissus tazetta* var. *chinensis*. Its flowers are very famous in the early spring. The flora plant was introduced to China more than 1000 years ago through the silk route and the Persian/Arab sea trade route. The plant is widely cultivated in southern China as an ornamental and is also used as an herb in China. Its flowers and bulbs were employed as medicinal parts in Chinese folk herbs.

Antitumor Constituents and Activities

In vitro assays showed that the treatment with the extracts of Shui Xian strongly lessened the survival rate of leukemia cells (HL-60, K562, KT1/A3, and A3R) and had less effect on noncancer cells lines (NHBE and NIH3T3). The extract could promote the apoptosis of HL-60 cells through both mitochondrial pathway and cell death receptor pathway.[1] The extract from the after-flowering bulbs of *N. tazetta* exhibited cytotoxic activity against HCT116 (colon) and HepG2 (liver) human cancer cell lines (IC_{50}: 4.2 and 2.2 μg/mL, respectively).[2] As an Amaryllidaceae plant, the Chinese daffodil is rich in the alkaloid component, which was shown to be primarily responsible for the bioactivities of Shui Xian.

Alkaloids

The i.p. injection of the total alkaloid extract in doses of 20–30 mg/kg to mice demonstrated significant inhibitory effect against the cell growth of Jensen sarcoma in rats and Ehrlich ascites tumor and Crocker sarcoma in mice.[3] The major alkaloid constituent assigned as pseudolycorine (**1**) displayed the growth suppression against W256 sarcoma in rats but did not show such effect on hepatoma, Ehrlich ascites, and sarcoma 180 in mice.[4] The separation of an ethanolic extract of the fresh flowers led to obtaining two quaternary alkaloids with a phenanthrene skeleton, which were assigned as N-methyl-8,9-methylenedioxyphenantridinium methylsulfate (**2**) and N-methyl-8,9-methylenedioxyphenantridinium malate (**3**), which both exhibited the cytotoxicity on a panel of neoplastic cell lines.[5] Narciclasine (**4**) isolated from the secreted mucilage of *N. tazetta* bulbs has been known to display cytotoxic activity against a panel of 60 cancer cell lines (mean IC_{50}: 47 nM) and to exert potent antiproliferative and proapoptotic effects on carcinoma cells. It stimulated the cancer cell apoptosis by activating the death receptor and/or mitochondrial pathways and impairing the organization of actin cytoskeleton. Importantly, the suppressive effect was demonstrated in both apoptosis-sensitive cancer cells and apoptosis-resistant cancer cells.[6]

Macromolecules

Nartazin, a glutamine-rich antifungal peptide (7.1 kDa), purified from the bulbs of Shui Xian, could restrain the proliferation of murine L1210 leukemia cells *in vitro* and also stimulate the proliferation of mouse splenocytes and bone marrow cells, implying that nartazin possesses both immune-enhancing and antileukemia properties.[7] Likewise, a water-soluble glycoprotein (2.6–4.2 kDa) prepared from the herb was found to obstruct the neoplastic cells.[8]

Toxicities

The i.p. LD_{50} value of Shui Xian was 110 mg/kg in rats. The acute i.p. of LD_{50} value of the total alkaloids was 182 mg/kg in mice, and its subacute LD_{50} values (after i.p. administration ×10 times) were 59 mg/kg/day in mice and 23 mg/kg/day in rats. The total alkaloids cause emesis in dogs after two to three injections and might produce leukocytosis for about a month of treatment at dose levels of ≤16 mg/kg.[3]

Other Bioactivities

The herb Shui Xian (Chinese daffodil) was reported to exert antibacterial and antifungal effects. Pseudolycorine (**1**) has hypotensive, nausea, vomiting, and anorexia activities.[4]

References

1. Liu, J. et al. 2006. Apoptosis of HL-60 cells induced by extracts from *Narcissus tazetta* var. *chinensis*. *Cancer Lett.* 242: 133–40.
2. Shawky, E. et al. 2015. In vitro cytotoxicity of some Narcissus plants extracts. *Nat. Prod. Res.* 29: 363–5.
3. Wu, T. C. et al. 1965. Antitumor drugs: XX. Therapeutic effect and toxicity of the total alkaloids from *Narcissus tazetta*. *Yaoxue Xuebao* 12: 31–5.

4. Pan, Q. C. et al. 1979. Antitumor and pharmacological studies on pseudolycorine. *Yaoxue Xuebao* 14: 705–9.
5. Youssef, D. T. A. et al. 2001. Cytotoxic quaternary alkaloids from the flowers of *Narcissus tazetta*. *Pharmazie* 56: 818–22.
6. Ji, Y. B. et al. 2013. Narciclasine—A potential anticancer drug. *Applied Mechanics and Materials* 411–414: 3154–7.
7. Chu, K. T. et al. 2004. First report of a glutamine-rich antifungal peptide with immunomodulatory and anti-proliferative activities from family Amaryllidaceae. *Biochem. Biophysical Res. Commun.* 325: 167–73.
8. Wang, G. et al. 2003. Glycopeptide of Narcissus tazetta seed and its application. *Faming Zhuanli Shenqing Gongkai Shuomingshu* CN 2002-110170 20020311.

209 Ku Zhi 苦蘵

Mullaca, Camapu, Fisali, or Ciplukan

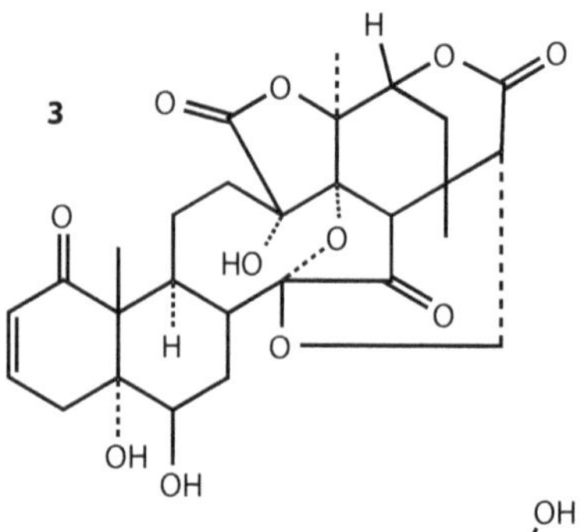

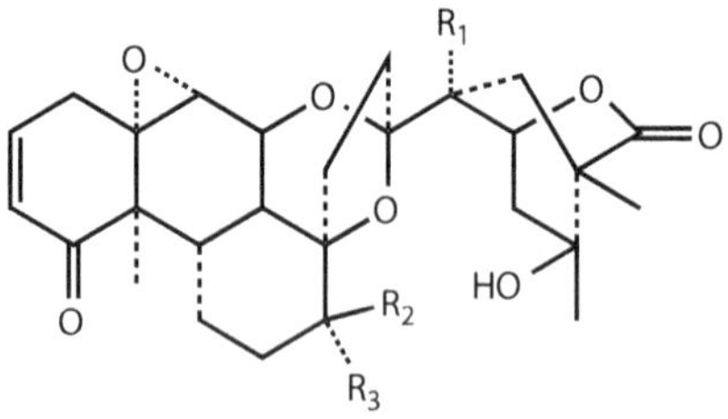

4. R_1 = -OH, R_2 = -H, R_3 = -CH_3
5. R_1 = -H, R_2 = -CH_3, R_3 = -OH
6. R_1 = -H, R_2 = -OH, R_3 = -CH_3

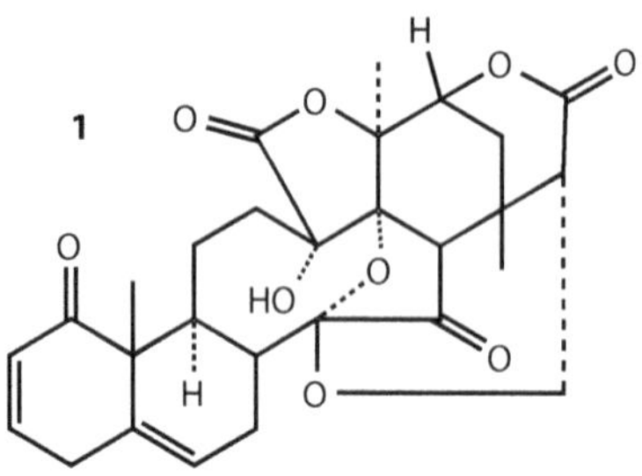

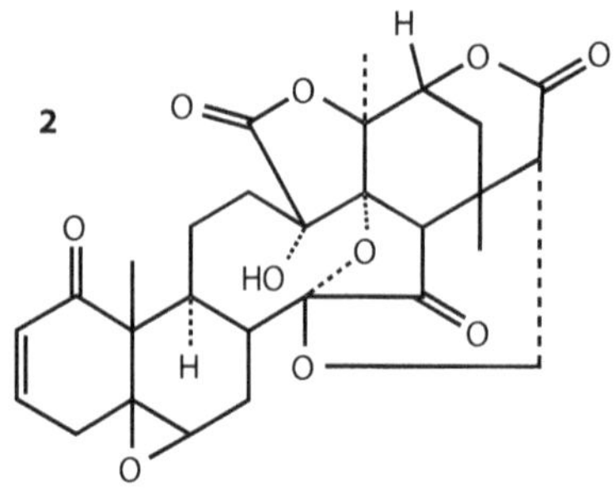

Glc: beta-D-glucopyranosyl
Rham: alpha-L-rhamnopyranosyl

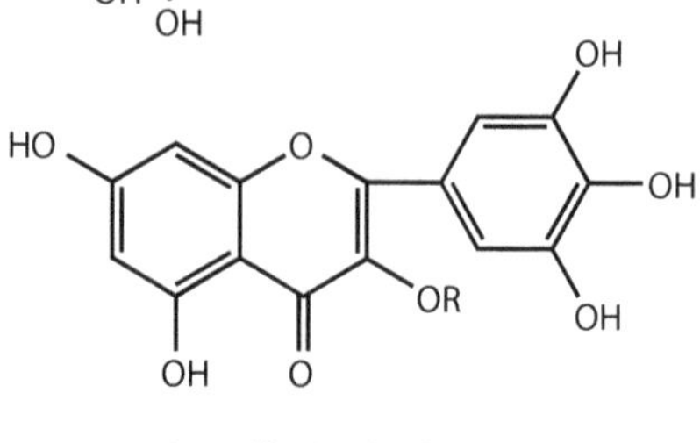

10. R = -Glc-(2-1)-Rham

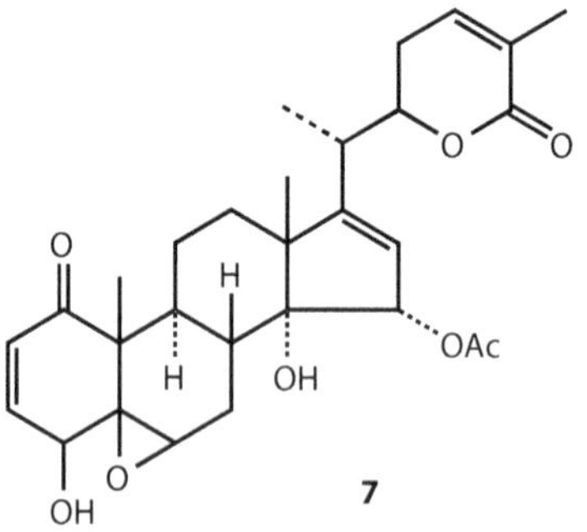

Herb Origination

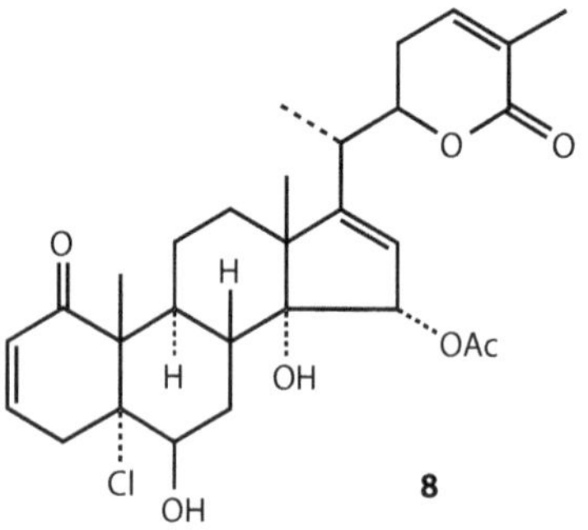

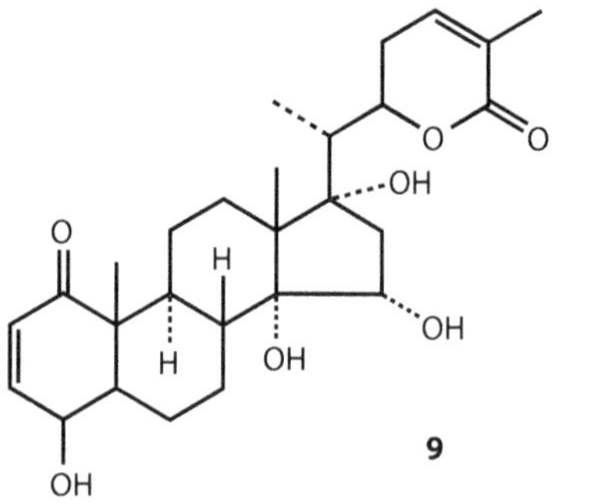

The herb Ku Zhi (Mullaca) originated from a whole herbaceous plant, *Physalis angulata* (Solanaceae). The annual plant is widely distributed in subtropical and tropical regions throughout the world. In China, the whole plant is normally collected in summer and autumn and dried in the sun for the medicinal practice, which can also be used fresh. Its edible fruits, roots, and epigeal parts are taken as traditional medicines as well as tea or infusion.

Antitumor Activities

An ethanolic extract of Ku Zhi showed marginal cytotoxic activity against human T47D ductal breast epithelial cancer cells *in vitro*, but the extract (80 μg/mL) synergistically augmented the chemotherapeutic effect of DOX (2–8 nM) in a combined treatment of the T47D cells.[1] In association with the induction of G2/M arrest and apoptosis, a methanolic extract of Ku Zhi exerted suppressive effect against the proliferation of human MCF-7 and MAD-MB-231 breast cancer cell lines, whose G2/M arrest of MDA-MB 231 cells was mediated by the activation of Chk2 and the increase of phosphorylated/inactivated Cdc25C levels, partially, via p21waf1/cip1 and P27kip1 (CDK inhibitors) pathways.[2] The exposure of human HSC-3 oral cancer cells to an EtOAc extract of Ku Zhi caused reactive oxygen stress and augmented oxidative stress markers, heme oxygenase-1, SOD, HSP70, and caspase-4, subsequently initiating the cell apoptosis.[3] Impressively, the EtOAc extract in a concentration range of 5–15 μg/mL obviously inhibited the migration and the invasion of the highly metastatic HSC-3 cells, associated with inhibition of MMP-9 and MMP-2 activities and u-PA in HSC-3 cells. The inhibitory effect was also present in VEGF-induced proliferation and migration/invasion of HUVECs *in vitro*. Consequently, the evidences corroborated the antiproliferative, antimetastatic and antiangiogenic activities of Ku Zhi that may be deserving of the development to prevent carcinoma cell metastasis and proliferation.[4] In addition, the capsules made of Ku Zhi fruits significantly restrained the growth of mouse lymphoma by 97% and murine Ehrlich cancer by 93%.[5]

Antitumor Constituents and Activities

Two kinds of unique constituents, a group of unusual 13,14-seco-16,24-cyclosteroids (i.e., physalins) and two groups of withanolide type of steroidal δ-lactones with ergosterol skeleton (i.e., physangulidines and withangulatins), were discovered from Ku Zhi in phytochemical researches. These atypical steroids as the major constituents in the herb were extensively evaluated by both *in vitro* and *in vivo* experiments. Some of them acted as inhibitors against cancer cell proliferation and viability, showing further developing potential.

Physalins

Physalin-B (**1**), physalin-D (**2**), and physalin-F (**3**) exerted significant cytotoxicity against various human solid tumor cell lines, such as KB (nasopharyngeal cancer), A431 (EGFR overexpressing skin cancer), PC3 (AR^- prostate cancer), ZR751 (ER^+ breast cancer), HCT-8 (colon cancer), and A549 (lung cancer), with EC_{50} values in the range of 0.3–5.9 μg/mL. They also restrained the growth of KB-VIN cells (a multidrug-resistant cancer cell subline).[6,7] Physalin-F (**3**) displayed relatively greater antiproliferative activity and also demonstrated the obvious cytotoxicity *in vitro* on other human tumor cell lines, HA22T (liver), HeLa (cervix), Colo-205 (colon), HEp2 (laryngeal), Calu-1 (lung), A498, ACHN, and UO-31 (kidney) cells, and two murine tumor cell lines, H1477 (melanoma) and 8401 (glioma). In the assays, the hepatoma cells were the most sensitive, and the cervical cancer cells was the next sensitive to physalin-F (**3**).[8] The apoptosis of A498 cells could be promoted by physalin-F (**3**) by augmenting a ROS-increased mitochondrial pathway and suppressing NF-κB activation.[8] Also, in the *in vivo* experiments, physalin-F (**3**) noticeably inhibited the growth of murine P388 lymphocytic leukemia, and physalin-B (**1**) and physalin-D (**2**) exerted the antitumor activity against sarcoma 180 in mice.[9,10] Moreover, a moderate inhibitory effect of physalin-U was observed in the panel of human cancer cell assay (EC_{50}: 11.1–20.0 μg/mL),[6,7] and the antiproliferative effect of physalin-W was shown in human 1A9 ovarian cancer cells (EC_{50}: 9.2 μM) *in vitro*.[1]

Moreover, in the continuing investigation, physalin-B (**1**) and physalin-F (**3**) were found to be also effective in the suppression of several human leukemia cell proliferation *in vitro* such as CTV1 (acute monocytic leukemia), HL-60 (acute promyelocytic leukemia), KG-1 (AML), B cell (acute B lymphoid leukemia), APM1840 (acute T lymphoid leukemia), and K562 (erythroleukemia), where the antileukemia activity of physalin-F (**3**) was stronger than that of physalin-B (**1**), and it was especially sensitive on the AML (KG-1) and the acute B lymphoid leukemia (B-cell).[11] Physalin-B (**1**) and physalin-F (**3**) at concentrations of 8 and 16 μM could promote the apoptotic death of human Jurkat T cell leukemia cells concomitant with the reduction of NF-κB activity.[12] The cytotoxicity of physalin-B (**1**) was also clearly demonstrated in v-raf murine sarcoma viral oncogene homolog-B1 (BRAF)-mutated melanoma A375 cells and A2058 cells (IC_{50}: <4.6 μg/mL). Concurrently, physalin-B (**1**) enhanced the apoptosis of the melanoma cancer cells by triggering NOXA, caspase-3, and mitochondria-mediated pathways, but it had no inference on human myoblastic cells and skin fibroblast cells.[13] Analyzing the structures of physalins to the corresponding antitumor activity indicated that the cytotoxic potency of physalins is probably contributed by the conjugated cyclohexanone moiety and the presence of an oxygen located at both C-5 and C-6.[14] In addition, physalin-B (**1**), physalin-F (**3**), and physalin-G but not physalin-D (**2**) were also reported to possess potent immunoregulative benefit.[15] These data prominently demonstrated that the physalins, especially physalin-B (**1**) and physalin-F (**3**), have the potential to be developed as effective drug leads for the treatment of malignant tumor diseases.

Physangulidines

Physangulidine-A (**4**), physangulidine-B (**5**), and physangulidine-C (**6**), three withanolides with an unusual carbon framework were discovered by a bioassay-directed isolation of the herb. The withanolides exerted moderate antiproliferative activity not only against human DU145 prostate carcinoma cells (respective GI_{50}: 3.56, 6.8, and 6.0 μM) but also against RWPE-1 normal prostate epithelial cells (respective GI_{50}: 2.4, 6.0, and 6.6 μM), where physangulidine-A (**4**) was the most active and abundant constituent. Physangulidine-A (**4**), was also effective in the inhibition of five other human cell lines: HT-29 (colon cancer), NCI-H460 (large cell lung cancer), HuTu 80 (duodenum cancer), M-14 (amelanotic melanoma), and MCF-7 (breast cancer) *in vitro*, with GI_{50} values of 2.73–5.26 μM. The inhibitory activities of physangulidine-A (**4**) were 2-fold and 11-fold greater than those of 5-FU (an anticancer drug) in HT-29 colon cancer cells and K562 leukemia cells, respectively, and were similar to those of 5-FU in other tested cancer cell lines, but it had less activity on mouse nonmalignant 3T3 cells.[16] Moreover, the studies further revealed that physangulidine-A (**4**) also induced defective mitosis and cell cycle arrest at G2/M phase and stimulated the apoptosis of human DU145 prostate cancer cells,[17] implying that the antimitotic and proapoptotic effects of physangulidine-A (**4**) may significantly contribute to the anticancer mechanism.

Withangulatins

Withangulatin-A (**7**) demonstrated the antiproliferative effect on human AGS (gastric) and Colo205 (colon) cancer cell lines, *in vitro* (IC_{50}: 1.8 and 16.6 μM, respectively), while withangulatin-I had lower activity.[18] The treatment with withangulatin-A (**7**) and physagulin-B (**8**) markedly obstructed the growth of human NCI-H460 lung cancer cells (IC_{50}: 1.4–1.6 μM) and human HCT-116 ileocecal carcinoma cells (IC_{50}: 0.43–2.11 μM).[19] The cytotoxic effect of withangulatin-B (**9**) was demonstrated in human DU-145 (AR^- prostate), LNCAP (AR^+ prostate), 1A9 (ovary), and HCT-116 (ileocecal) neoplastic cell lines (EC_{50}: 0.2–1.3 μg/mL) *in vitro*. Withanolide-C and withanolide-H, which both hold a 5,6-epoxide but lack a 2-in-1 system in its A-ring, exhibited moderate cytotoxicity against the 1A9, HCT-116, and LNCAP cancer cell lines, whereas withangulatin-G with 5α,6β-diol after cleavage of the epoxide ring presented a decreased suppression.[7] In addition, withangulatin-A (**7**) is a Topo-II inhibitor as well, being able to elicit Topo-II-mediated DNA damage and to block general protein synthesis.[20]

Flavonoid

Myricetin 3-*O*-neohesperidoside (**10**), a biologically active flavonoid glycoside, was isolated from Ku Zhi, showing remarkable cytotoxicity *in vitro* against P388 leukemia cells, KB-16 nasopharynx epidermoid carcinoma cells, and A549 lung adenocarcinoma cells with ED_{50} values of 0.048, 0.50, and 0.55 μg/mL, respectively.[21]

Structure–Activity Relationship

The further investigations of withangulatins as well as physalins afforded several SAR clues: (1) α,β-unsaturated ketone moiety in ring-A and/or 5β,6β-epoxy in ring-B appears to be necessary for the significant cytotoxicity; (2) cleavage of the epoxide ring to form 5α,6β-diol reduces the potency of anticancer; (3) no double bond at C2 exhibits decreased cytotoxicity (except of withangulatin-B); (4) 4β-hydroxy group is a cytotoxicity contributor; (5) presence of 4-oxo group in ring-A induces a decrease in the cytotoxicity; (6) different stereochemistry of the 5,6-epoxide ring displays no cytotoxicity; (7) an oxygenated substituent at the C5-OH appears to lose the antitumor activity; and (8) replacement of the C5-OH group by a Cl-atome will enhance the cytotoxic activity.[7,18] All this molecular bioinformation provided valuable and important clues for the discovery of clues for structural design and modification to discover more potential agents.

Other Medicinal Uses

The herb Ku Zhi (Mullaca) is broadly used in various countries as a popular medicine for the treatment of a variety of pathologies such as malaria, hepatitis, dermatitis, diuretic, liver problems, diabetes, asthma, and rheumatism, and it is used as an antimycobacterial, antipyretic, and immunomodulatory agent besides anticancer.

References

1. Armandari, I. et al. 2010. Synergistic combination of ciplukan (*Physalis angulata*) herbs ethanolic extract and doxorubicin on T47D breast cancer cells. *Indones. J. Cancer Chemoprev.* 1: 26–31.
2. Hsieh, W. T. et al. 2006. *Physalis angulata* induced G2/M phase arrest in human breast cancer cells. *Food Chemical Toxicol.* 44: 974–83.
3. Lee, H. Z. et al. 2009. Oxidative stress involvement in *Physalis angulata*-induced apoptosis in human oral cancer cells. *Food Chem. Toxicol.* 47: 561–70.
4. Hseu, Y. C. et al. 2011. Inhibitory effects of *Physalis angulata* on tumor metastasis and angiogenesis. *J. Ethnopharmacol.* 135: 762–71.
5. Ribeiro, I. M. et al. 2002. *Physalis angulata* L. antineoplasic activity, in vitro, evaluation from its stems and fruit capsules. *Rev. bras. de farmacogn.* 12(Suppl.): 21–3.
6. Kuo, P. C. et al. 2006. Physanolide A, a novel skeleton steroid, and other cytotoxic principles from *Physalis angulata. Org. Lett.* 8: 2953–6.
7. Damu, A. G. et al. 2007. Isolation, structures, and structure–cytotoxic activity relationships of withanolides and physalins from *Physalis angulata. J. Nat. Prod.* 70: 1146–52.
8. Wu, S. Y. et al. 2012. Physalin F induces cell apoptosis in human renal carcinoma cells by targeting NF-κB and generating reactive oxygen species. *PLoS One* 7: e40727.
9. Chiang, H. C. et al. 1992. Antitumor agent, physalin F from *Physalis angulata* L. *Anticancer Res.* 12: 837–43.
10. Magalhaes, H. I. F. et al. 2006. In-vitro and in-vivo antitumour activity of physalins B and D from Physalis angulata. *J. Pharmacy Pharmacol.* 58: 235–41.
11. Chiang, H. C. et al. 1992. Inhibitory effects of physalin B and physalin F on various human leukemia cells in vitro. *Anticancer Res.* 12: 1155–62.
12. Nadia, J. J. H. et al. 2006. Physalins from witheringia solanacea as modulators of the NF-κB cascade. *J. Nat. Prod.* 69: 328–31.
13. Hsu, C. C. et al. 2012. Physalin B from *Physalis angulata* triggers the NOXA-related apoptosis pathway of human melanoma A375 cells. *Food Chem. Toxicol.* 50: 619–24.
14. Magalhaes, H. I. F. et al. 2006. Preliminary investigation of structure-activity relationship of cytotoxic Physalis. *Letters in Drug Design Discov.* 3: 9–13.
15. Soares, M. B. P. et al. 2003. Inhibition of macrophage activation and lipopolysaccaride-induced death by seco-steroids purified from *Physalis angulata* L. *Eur. J. Pharmacol.* 459: 107–12.
16. Jin, Z. et al. 2012. Physangulidines A, B, and C: Three new antiproliferative withanolides from *Physalis angulata* L. *Org. Lett.* 14: 1230–3.
17. Reyes-Reyes, E. M. et al. 2013. Physangulidine A, a withanolide from *Physalis angulata* Perturbs the cell cycle and induces cell death by apoptosis in prostate cancer cells. *J. Nat. Prod.* 76: 2–7.
18. Lee, S. W. et al. 2008. Withangulatin I, a new cytotoxic withanolide from *Physalis angulata. Chem. Pharm. Bull.* 56: 234–6.
19. He, Q. P. et al. 2007. Cytotoxic withanolides from *Physalis angulata* L. *Chem. Biodiv.* 4: 443–9.
20. Juang, J. K. et al. 1989. A new compound, withangulatin A, promotes type II DNA topoisomerase-mediated DNA damage. *Biochem. Biophys. Res. Commun.* 159: 1128–34.
21. Ismail, N. et al. 2001. A novel cytotoxic flavonoid glycoside from Physalis angulata. *Fitoterapia* 72: 676–9.

210 Tian Nan Xing 天南星

Green dragon

Herb Origination

The herb Tian Nan Xing (Green dragon) is the dried bulb of an Araceae plant, *Pinellia pedatisecta*. This perennial herbaceous plant is broadly distributed in China except in the northwest and northeast regions. Its bulbs are generally collected in October and dried in the sun after its skin is removed. As one of the basic traditional Chinese medicines, Tian Nan Xing was recorded in the first Chinese classic of material medica entitled *Shennong Ben Cao Jing*, but it was classified as a low-grade drug due to its toxic property.

Antitumor Activities

The alcoholic extract of Tian Nan Xing demonstrated 45.8–53.7%, 37.1–53.4%, and 61.7–84.8% suppressions against the growth of sarcoma 180, HCA entity tumor, and U14 cervical carcinoma in murine animal models, respectively.[1] The EtOAc extract from Tian Nan Xing could dose-dependently obstruct the growth of human hepatoma Bel-7402 cells and promote the S cell cycle arrest and the caspase-3-activated apoptosis.[2] A lipid-soluble extract (PE) of Tian Nan Xing inhibited the growth of human CaSki and HeLa cervical cancer cells *in vitro* in time- and dose-dependent manners, but it had no such effect on human HBL-100 breast cancer cells except at a high dose (500 μg/mL), and it had little side effect on normal cells.[3,4] In the CaSki and HeLa cells treated with PE for 24 h, both mRNA and protein of HPV E6 and Bcl-2 were significantly lessened, and caspase-8 and caspase-3, Bax, p53, and p21 were amplified, thereby eliciting both cells to apoptosis. The results confirmed that PE acted as a growth inhibitor and an apoptosis inducer of the cervical cancer cells, whose mechanism was mediated by mitochondria-dependent and death receptor-dependent apoptotic pathways, and HPV E6 may be the key target of its action against the cervical cancer cells.[3,4]

In the 1970s, the Tian Nan Xing extract had been utilized to treat 157 cases of cervical cancer with different phases in a clinical trial in China. The positive and significant results were established, and the effective rate reached to 81.53%.[5] In addition, the Sansheng injection (a Chinese clinically therapeutic medicine) is composed of Tian Nan Xing as a major component. It directly obstructed/killed three tested human solid cancer cells (lung, liver, and stomach) *in vitro*.[6] The *in vivo* antineoplastic property of this injection was proven in mouse models transplanted with Ehrlich ascites tumor, Lewis lung tumor, or sarcoma 180. It was also effective in the growth inhibition of both types of ascites and entity mouse hepatoma cells.[6]

Antitumor Constituents and Activities

By the bioactivity-integrated phytochemical approaches, the antitumor activity of Tian Nan Xing has been revealed to be primarily contributed by its components of lectin, protein, and polysaccharide. β-Sitosterol, its major ingredient with small molecule, might partially participate in the antitumor effect of the Tian Nan Xing extract.

Lectins

A lectin component (molecular weight: 9067.5 U) was purified from Tian Nan Xing, but it contained no sugar chain. It inhibited the proliferation of sarcoma 180 cells *in vitro* but showed only 11.55% antitumor rate *in vivo* with no obvious effect on the cell cycle phase distribution and the immunity.[7] *P. pedatisecta* agglutinin (PPA), which is a specific mannose-binding lectin prepared from the herb, could elicit cytotoxicity to cancer cells and hinder the proliferation of cancer cells by targeting the methylosome.[8] The results suggested that the PPA may be developed into a novel agent for cancer gene therapy.

Proteins

Total protein derived from Tian Nan Xing probably contains only 1% sugar moiety but no phosphorus or lipoprotein. It displayed significant antitumor activity against mouse sarcoma 180 cells and human SKOV-3 ovarian cancer cells; however, it had no such effect on human SiHa cervical cancer cells. The growth of sarcoma 180 cells was inhibited by 58.3% in the treatment with the protein. At concentrations of 0.10–0.50 mg/mL the protein significantly inhibited the SKOV-3 cell growth in correlation with the induction of the cell proteomics changes.[9–12] The antitumor activity of the protein was also demonstrated in the inhibition of drug-resistant OVCAR human ovarian cancer cells line, although the inhibitory rate was lower than that in the drug-sensitive SKOV3 cells. There was also no negative effect of the protein on human umbilical cord blood hematopoietic cells.[13]

Polysaccharide

A water-soluble polysaccharide termed RAP-W1 (molecular weight: ≈57 kDa) was purified from Tian Nan Xing, which has 95.9% total carbohydrate content with no protein. Its saccharide composition is rhamnose, fucose, arabinose, mannose, galactose, and glucose in a ratio of 5:3:6:9:53. After the treatment of tumor-bearing mice for 14 days, RAP-W1 significantly suppressed the growth of human MCF-7 breast cancer cells and increased the body weight and the spleen index, as well as enhanced the activity of cytotoxic T lymphocytes. At the same time, the level of Th1 cytokines (INFγ and IL-2) in the serum of tumor-bearing mice was augmented, and Th2 cytokine (IL-10) secretion was dramatically reduced. The findings evidenced that the *in vivo* tumor inhibitory effect should be largely attributed to RAP-W1-activated T cells and immune functions.[14]

β-Sitosterol

Because β-sitosterol is one of the major small molecules in the Tian Nan Xing, it was used to assay the inhibitory effect on human SiHa cervical cancer cell line *in vitro*. At a 20 μmol/L concentration, the treatment of β-sitosterol could obviously inhibit the viability of SiHa cells in time- and dose-dependent manners. Simultaneously, the cell cycle of SiHa cells was accumulated in the S phase, and the percentage of apoptotic and necrotic death was augmented. The result endorsed that β-sitosterol might be a prospective safe adjuvant with low toxicity for cervical cancer treatment.[11]

Other Bioactivities

The poisonous bulbs/tubers of Tian Nan Xing have been used in Chinese medicine for the treatment of tetanus, infantile convulsion, cough with profuse sputum, limb paralysis, hemiplegia, scrofula, carbuncle, and venomous snakebite. A pharmacological investigation has shown that Tian Nan Xing possesses biological activities such as anticonvulsive, sedative, analgesia, expectorant, and antioxidant besides antitumor.

References

1. Li, J. et al. 2009. Antitumor activities of extracts from the medicinal plants *Pinellia ternata* and *Pinellia pedatisecta. ICBBE 2009 Third Int. Conf. Bioinformatics and Biomedical Engineering*, June 11–3, 2009.
2. Li, G. L. et al. 2010. Mechanisms of apoptosis induction effect of *Pinellia pedatisecta* Schott extract on CaSki cell lines of cervical cancer cultured in vitro. *Zhonghua Zhongyiyao Zazhi* 25: 449–52.
3. Li, G. L. et al. 2010. HPV E6 downregulation and apoptosis induction of human cervical cancer cells by a novel lipid-soluble extract (PE) from *Pinellia pedatisecta* Schott in vitro. *J. Ethnopharmacol.* 132: 56–64.
4. Li, G. L. et al. 2012. Effects of Pinellia extract fraction on expressions of HPVE6 and p53 genes in cervical cancer cell lines. *Zhonghua Zhongyiyao Zazhi* 27: 110–3.
5. Li, C. J. et al. 1978. The therapeutic studies on the cervical cancer patients treated by Huzhang. *Shanghai Med.* 1: 13–6.
6. Hong, Y. K. et al. 1986. An antitumor drug-complex Sansheng injection. *Xinyao yu Linchuang* 5: 127.
7. Zhu, L. et al. 2009. Isolation and purification of *Pinellia pedatisecta* lectin and its effects on mouse sarcoma S180 cells in vivo and in vitro. *J. Wuhan Univ.* (*Med. edit.*) 30: 10–5.
8. Lu, Q. et al. 2012. *Pinellia pedatisecta* agglutinin interacts with the methylosome and induces cancer cell death. *Oncogenesis* 1(Oct.): e29/1-e29/7.
9. Sun, G. X. et al. 1992. The extraction and chemical analysis of proteins from Pinellia pedatisecta and their inhibitory effects on the mouse sarcoma-180. *J. Shanghai Med. Univ.* 19: 17–20.
10. Chen, X. Y. et al. 2011. Proteomics study of total protein of *Pinellia pedaisecta* Schott effect on human ovarian cancer of cells. *Zhongguo Zhongxiyi Jiehe Zazhi* 31: 1651–6.
11. Wang, L. et al. 2009. Inhibitory effects of Pinellia's ingredients on the growth of cervical cancer cell lines. *J. Fudan Univ.* (*Med. Edit.*), 36: 675–80.
12. Zhou, L. et al. 2010. Alteration of protein profiles in human ovarian cancer cell line SKOV3 treated with protein of *Pinellia pedatisecta* Schott. *Zhonghua Zhongyiyao Xuekan* 28: 789–92.
13. Zhu, M. W. et al. 1999. The inhibitory effects of total proteins from *Pinellia pedatisecta* on the ovarian cancer cells and human umbilical cord blood hematopoietic cells. *J. Shanghai Med. Univ.* 26: 455–7.
14. Chen, G. et al. 2012. Characterization and antitumor activities of the water-soluble polysaccharide from Rhizoma Arisaematis. *Carbohydrate Polymers* 90: 67–72.

211 Xia Ku Cao 夏枯草

Selfheal

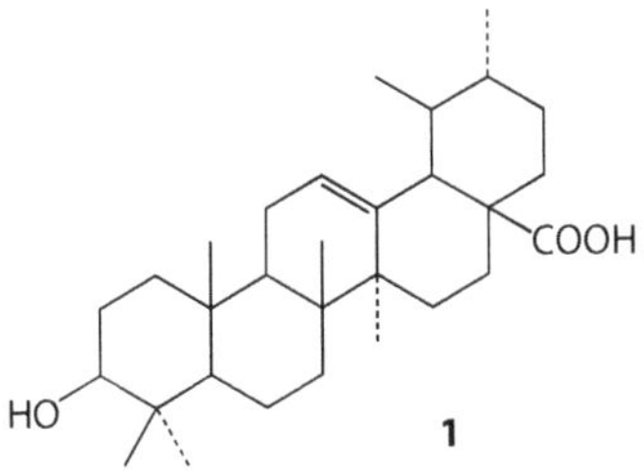

HO COOH 1 HO HO COOH 2 HO HO COOH 3 HO COOH 4

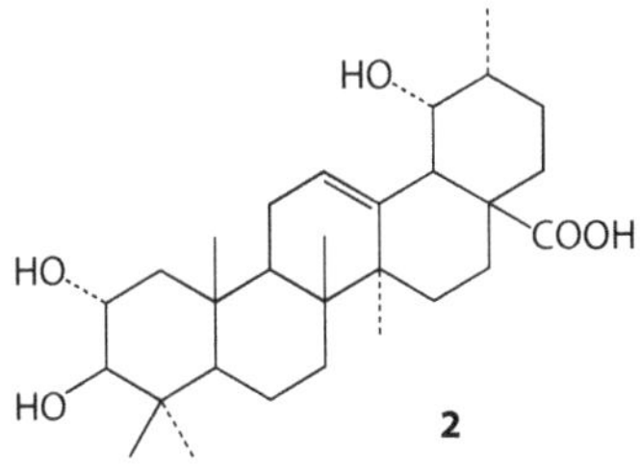

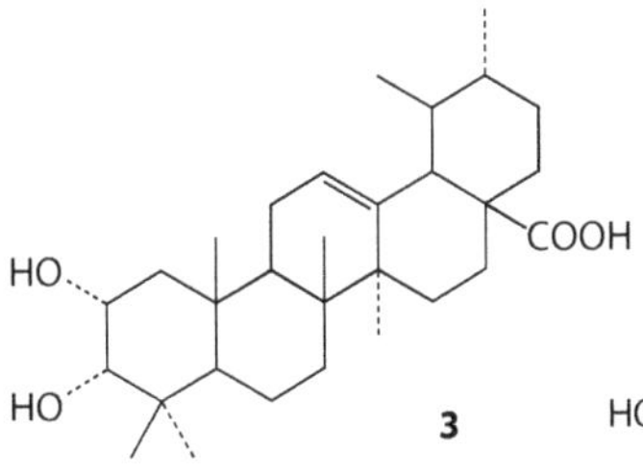

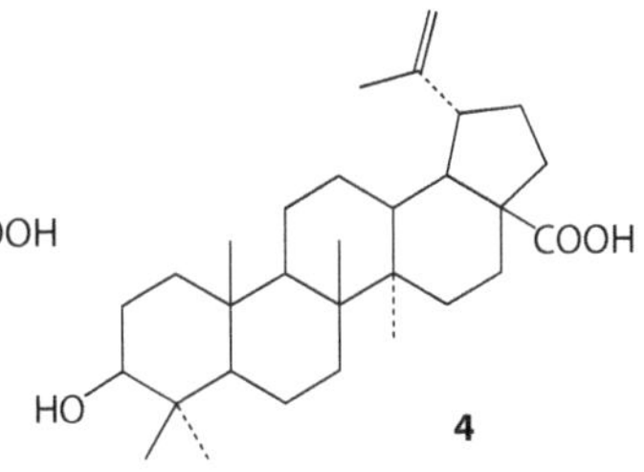

Herb Origination

The origin of herb Xia Ku Cao (Selfheal) is two perennial Labiatae plants, *Prunella vulgaris* and *P. asiatica*, whose herb was documented in the first Chinese classic of materia medica entitled *Shennong Ben Cao Jing*. The former plant is widely distributed in Europe, Asia, and North America, as well as most regions with temperate climates. In China, its dried brown fruit spikes are collected in May and June for folk medicinal purpose.

Antitumor Constituent and Activities

The extract of Prunellae spikes displayed moderate inhibitory effect against the proliferation of human cancer cell lines such as T lymphoma Jurkat cells, Burkitt lymphoma Raji cells, and HT-29 colon carcinoma cells, in dose- and time-dependent manners, as evidenced by its induced cell apoptotic or proteomic changes and reduced cell viability. The IC_{50} values in the Jurkat and Raji cell lines ranged between 18 and 20 μg/mL, whose pro-apoptotic mechanism was found to be closely correlated with the enlargement of p53 activity and Bax/Bcl-2 ratio, the collapse of mitochondrial membrane potential, and the activation of caspase-9 and caspase-3.[1–5] The ethanol extract of *P. vulgaris* var. *lilacina*, in the *in vitro* assay, induced significant antioxidant effect and cytotoxicity on various human cancer cell lines, such as HepG2, HT-29, A549, MKN45, and HeLa cancers.[6] *In vivo* experiments demonstrated that the extract in a dose of 200 mg/kg exerted an obvious inhibition against the growth of sarcoma 180 and in a dose of 100 mg/kg efficiently enhanced the cytotoxicity of cisplatin (DDP).[7] Moreover, the Xia Ku Cao ethanolic extract exerted the inhibition on HUVEC proliferation, migration, and tube formation by obstructing the expression of VEGF-A and VEGFR-2. The ethanolic extract also diminished the VEGF-A expression in human HT-29 colon cancer cells.[8] The evidences established the antiangiogenic property of Xia Ku Cao ethanolic extract.

A Xia Ku Cao injection had been clinically used in China to treat 78 cases of lung carcinoma with hydrothorax. The results showed that the injection was more effective than the chemotherapeutic drugs, cisplatin and VP16, and the side effects of the Xia Ku Cao extract was notably less than those of the anticancer agents.[9]

Triterpenoids

Ursolic acid (**1**) and its derivatives are the antitumor components in Xia Ku Cao. The ursolic acids (**1**) exerted the inhibitory activity against the growth of murine P388 and L1210 leukemia cells and human A549 lung cancer cells *in vitro*. But the activity was marginal toward human KB nasopharyngeal cancer cells, HCT-8 colon carcinoma, and MCF-7 breast neoplastic cells.[10] Rosmarinic acid (**2**) has been proven to have anticarcinogenetic activity.[11] 2α,3α-Dihydroxyurs-12-en-28-oic acid (**3**) isolated from the dried spikes of *P. vulgaris* var. *lilacina* exerted the cytotoxic and apoptosis-inducing effects against human acute leukemia Jurkat T cells, but it was less potent on normal peripheral T cells.[12] In addition, rosmarinic acid (**2**) as well as an EAF of Xia Ku Cao in the dose range of 0.005–0.05 mg/mL also showed a dose-dependent cytoprotective effect on DOX-induced oxidative stress in rat cardiomyocytes.[11] By retarding ERα expression, ursolic acid (**1**) and betulinic acid (**4**) inhibited estrogen signaling, demonstrating the potential use of ursolic acid (**1**) and betulinic acid (**4**) as therapeutic agents against estrogen-dependent tumors.[13]

Polysaccharides

The systematic researches discovered several polysaccharides from a water-soluble extract of Xia Ku Cao. But only polysaccharide P32 was reported to show antilung cancer activity in a mouse model with LLC *in vivo* and also immunomodulation effects such as increase of the thymus index and the spleen index in the tumor-bearing mice.[14] The separated neutral polysaccharides, acidic polysaccharides, and a sulfated glycoprotein-type polysaccharide displayed potent antioxidant property, especially, free radical-scavenging activity.[15–17] A neutral polysaccharide PP2 has the ability to prevent the membrane lipid from peroxidation and to reduce the hemolysis of red cells.[12] PVP was an ultrasonic extracted of *P. vulgaris* polysaccharides, which consists of 28.2% arabinose, 38.5% xylose, 16.5% galactose, 11.0% mannose, 3.0% glucose, and 2.8% rhamnose with 1- and 1–6 glycosidic linkages (48.0%), 1–3 glycosidic linkages (43.9%) and 1–2 and 1–4 glycosidic linkages (8.1%). Besides showing marked antioxidant and radical-scavenging activities, PVP at a 2.0 mg/mL concentration restrained the proliferation of HepG2 (liver), SGC7901 (gastric), and MCF-7 (breast) human cancer cells by 51.2%, 35.2%, and 31.8%, respectively, but exhibited no cytotoxicity on normal liver L02 cells.[18] *P. vulgaris*-sulfated polysaccharide at 200 μg/mL inhibited bFGF secretion *in vitro* and at 200 mg/kg, reduced MVD in tumor tissue sections *in vivo*, indicating the antiangiogenetic potential in the hepatoma.[19,20] These results demonstrated that polysaccharides isolated from *P. vulgaris* may be propitious to the cancer prevention.

Other Bioactivities

Xia Ku Cao (Prunella fruiting spikes) has long been used as an important component in formulated prescriptions of Chinese medicines to treat various health problems, such as blood stasis, edema, scrofula, lymphatic tuberculosis, acute conjunctivitis, thyromegaly, mammary gland hyperplasia, acute mastitis, and hypertension. Pharmacological studies disclosed that the Prunella fruiting spikes have hypotensive, antiinflammatory, hypoglycemic, heat-clearing, detoxifying, immunosuppressive, antivirus, and antibacterial properties and showed promising therapeutic effect for AIDS and diabetes. Its saponin components in Xia Ku Cao have significant anti-HIV activity.[21,22]

References

1. Chen, C. Y. et al. 2009. The effects and mechanism of action of *Prunella vulgaris* l extract on Jurkat human T lymphoma cell proliferation. *Chinese-German J. Clin. Oncol.* 8: 426–9.
2. Zhang, M. Z. et al. 2009. Study on proteomics of Jurkat cells treated with the extracts from *Prunella vulgaris. Zhongyaocai* 32: 917–22.
3. Zheng, L. P. et al. 2011. Spica Prunellae extract promotes mitochondriondependent apoptosis in human colon carcinoma cell line. *Afri. J. Pharmacy Pharmacol.* 5: 327–35.
4. Fu, X. R. et al. 2008. Effect and mechanism of *Prunella vulgaris* L extract on proliferation of human Burkitt lymphoma cell line Raji. *Shandong Medical J.* 24.
5. Li, J. et al. 2011. Apoptosis of human lymphoma Raji induced by *Prunella vulgaris* and its mechanism. *Zhongguo Laonianxue Zazhi* 31: 2528–9.
6. Hwang, Y. J. et al. 2013. In vitro antioxidant and anticancer effects of solvent fractions from *Prunella vulgaris* var. lilacina. *BMC Complem. Alternat. Med.* 13 310/1–310/9.
7. Zhu, N. et al. 2009. Synergistic antitumor effect of extract of *Prunella vulgaris* L and cisplatin in vivo. *Chin. J. Ethnomed. Ethnopharm.* 24: 20–2.
8. Lin, W. et al. 2011. Anti-angiogenic effect of Spica prunellae extract in vivo and in vitro. *Afri. J. Pharmacy Pharmacol.* 5: 2647–54.
9. Zhou, R. Y. et al. 2001. Clinical and experimental observations of hydrothorax in lung cancer cases treated with closed drainage and injection of selfheal Spike injection. *Zhejiang Zhongxiyi Jiehe Zazhi* 11: 5–8.
10. Lee, K. H. et al. 1988. The cytotoxic principles of *Prunella vulgaris, Psychotria serpens*, and *Hyptis capitata*: Ursolic acid and related derivatives. *Planta Med.* 54: 308–11.
11. Psotova, J. et al. 2005. Cytoprotectivity of *Prunella vulgaris* on doxorubicin-treated rat cardiomyocytes. *Fitoterapia* 76: 556–61.
12. Woo, H. J. et al. 2011. Apoptogenic activity of 2α,3α-dihydroxyurs-12-ene-28-oic acid from *Prunella vulgaris* var. *lilacina* is mediated via mitochondria-dependent activation of caspase cascade regulated by Bcl-2 in human acute leukemia Jurkat T cells. *J. Ethnopharmacol.* 135: 626–35.
13. Kim, H.-I. et al. 2014. Inhibition of estrogen signaling through depletion of estrogen receptor alpha by ursolic acid and betulinic acid from *Prunella vulgaris* var. lilacina. *Biochem. Biophys. Res. Commun.* 451: 282–7
14. Zhang, D. H. et al. 2006. Isolation, purification and antioxidant activity the polysaecharide of *Prunella vulgaris* (Labiatae). *Yunnan Plant Res.* 28: 410–24.
15. Wei, M. et al. 2010. Isolation and antioxidant activity of water-soluble acidic polysaccharide from *Prunella vulgaris* Linn. *Food Sci.* 31: 91–4.
16. Xi, Y. B. et al. 2010. Study on isolation and antioxidant activity of the polysaccharide from *Prunella vulgaris* L. *J. Guangdong Pharm. College* 26: 594–8.
17. Xiong, S. L. et al. 2010. Isolation and antioxidant activity of acidic polysaccharide with water-solubility from *Prunella vulgaris* Linn. *Fourth Int. Conf. on Bioinformatics and Biomedical Engineering (iCBBE)*, June 18–20, 2010.
18. Li, C. et al. 2015. Ultrasonic extraction and structural identification of polysaccharides from *Prunella vulgaris* and its antioxidant and antiproliferative activities. *Europ. Food Res. Technol.* 240: 49–60.
19. Wu, X. Z. et al. 2011. Effects of sulfated polysaccharide extracted from *Prunella vulgaris* on endothelial cells. *J. Med. Plants Res.* 5: 4218–23.
20. Wang, Y. N. et al. 2014. Effect and mechanism of *Prunella vulgaris* sulfated polysaccharide on angiogenesis in hepatocellular carcinoma. *Zhongguo Zhongliu Linchuang* 41: 758–61.
21. Liu, Y. et al. 2003. Advances in the study on the chemical constituents and biological activities of *Prunella vulgaris. J. Shenyang Pharm. Uni.* 20: 55–9.
22. Sun, W. G. et al. 2003. Advances in the study on the chemical constituents and pharmacological action of *Prunella vulgaris. Chin. J. Infor. Tradit. Chin. Med.* 10: 86–8.

212 Tian Pao Zi 天泡子

Sunberry or Wild cape gooseberry

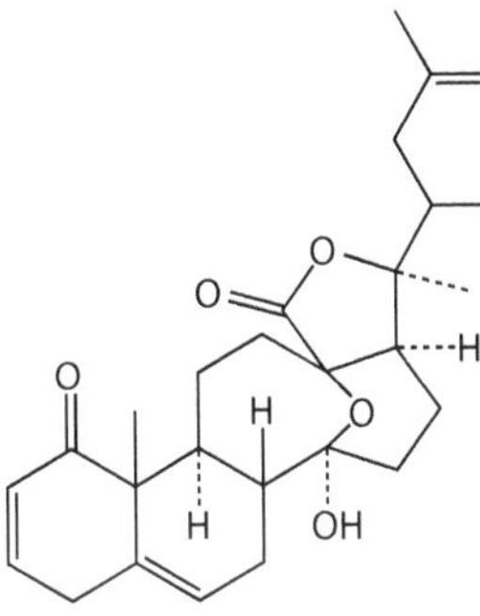

Herb Origination

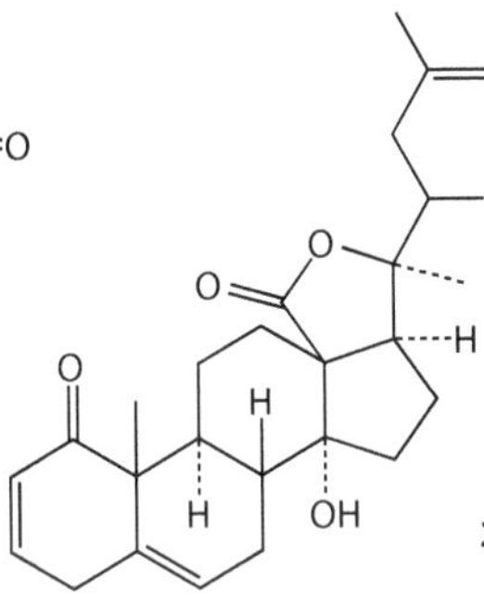

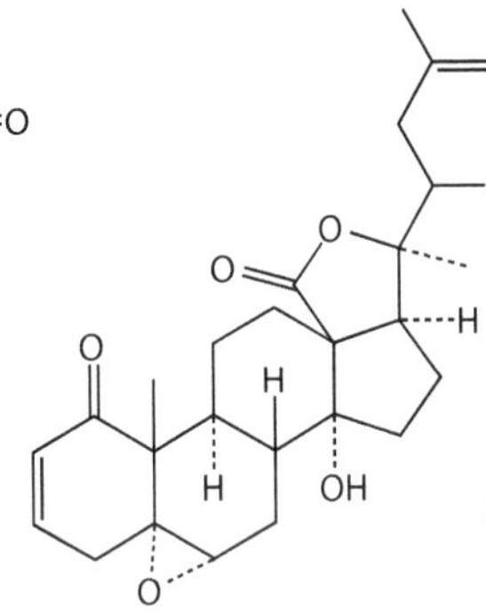

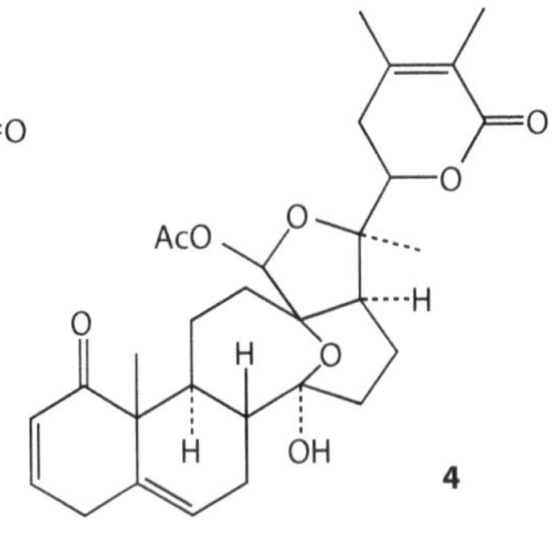

The origin of herb Tian Pao Zi (Sunberry) is a Solanaceae plant, *Physalis minima* L. This branched annual plant is native to pantropical regions from Southeast Asia into northern Australia. It is widely distributed throughout tropical and subtropical regions in the world. As a Chinese herb, the plant fruits and the whole plant with the fruits are generally collected between June and July and dried in the sun for folk medicinal use. The herb can also be used fresh.

Antitumor Activity and Constituents

The decoction of Tian Pao Zi demonstrated *in vitro* cytotoxicity against human NCI-H23 (lung), CORL23 (lung), and MCF-7 (breast) tumor cell lines. A chloroform extract derived from the herb exerted the growth suppressive effect against human T-47D breast cancer cells and human Caov-3 ovarian cancer cells *in vitro* with an EC_{50} value of 3.8 μg/mL in the T-47D cells. The extract markedly induced the T-47D and Caov-3 cells to programmed cell death via c-Myc-, p53-, and caspase-3-dependent pathways in lines, but the inhibition of Caov-3 cells was found to be mainly mediated by a combination of apoptotic and autophagic cell death mechanisms.[1,2]

A group of cytotoxic withanolides with unique structures has been discovered from Tian Pao Zi (*P. minima*). Withaphysalin-C (**1**) and withaphysalin-A (**2**), 5α,6α-epoxy-withaphysalin-A (**3**), and 18-*O*-acetylwithaphysalin-C (**4**) showed the moderate cytotoxicity toward human HCT-116 colorectal cancer cells and human NCI-H460 NSCLC cells *in vitro*, where the highest antiproliferative activity was achieved by withaphysalin-C (**1**) (IC_{50}: 14.0–15.3 μM) among the withanolides.[3] However, a major cytotoxic component in *P. minima*, which were collected from Malaysia and Thailand was assigned as physalin-F (see Section Ku Zhi), which notably restrained the proliferation of CORL23 lung cancer cells and MCF-7 breast cancer cells (IC_{50}: 0.4–0.59 μM, 48 h),[4] and remarkably inhibited the growth of T-47D breast cancer cells (EC_{50}: 3.6 μg/mL). Through the activation of caspase-3 and c-Myc pathways, physalin-F showed a dose-dependent apoptosis-triggering effect in the T-47D cells. Additionally, the two cytotoxic physalin-B and physalin-F could be produced by the cultures of the plant's hairy roots.[5]

Likewise, an earlier study had reported a minimal alkaloid component isolated from the fruits of Tian Pao Zi exhibited cytotoxicity against mouse ascites sarcoma 180 cells *in vitro* with significant inhibition of DNA synthesis, but it might cause bone marrow inhibition at the high concentration.[6]

Other Bioactivities

The herb Tian Pao Zi (Sunberry) was claimed to have anti-inflammatory, diuretic, laxative, and pregnancy-terminating properties. The analgesic and antiinflammatory properties have been shown in animal models.

References

1. Leong, O. K. et al. 2010. Growth arrest and induction of apoptotic and non-apoptotic programmed cell death by *Physalis minima*, L. chloroform extract in human ovarian carcinoma Caov-3 cells. *J. Ethnopharmacol.* 128: 92–9.
2. Leong, O. K. et al. 2010. Apoptotic effects of *Physalis minima* L. chloroform extract in human breast carcinoma T-47D cells mediated by c-myc-, p53-, and caspase-3-dependent pathways. *Integr. Cancer Therapies* 9: 73–83.
3. Ma, L. et al. 2007. Cytotoxic withaphysalins from *Physalis minima*. *Helv. Chim. Acta* 90: 1406–19.
4. Azlan, G. J. et al. 2002. Establishment of *Physalis minima* hairy roots culture for the production of physalins. *Plant Cell, Tissue and Organ Culture* 69: 271–8.
5. Lee, C. C. et al. 2005. Cytotoxicity of plants from Malaysia and Thailand used traditionally to treat cancer. *J. Ethnopharmacol.* 100: 237–43.
6. Ma, F. W. et al. 1991. Inhibitory effect of the *Physalis minima* alkaloid on DNA synthesis of S180 ascitic tumor cells of mice in vitro. *Shaanxi Yixue Zazhi* 20: 689–91.

213 Mao Zhua Cao 猫爪草

Catclaw buttercup

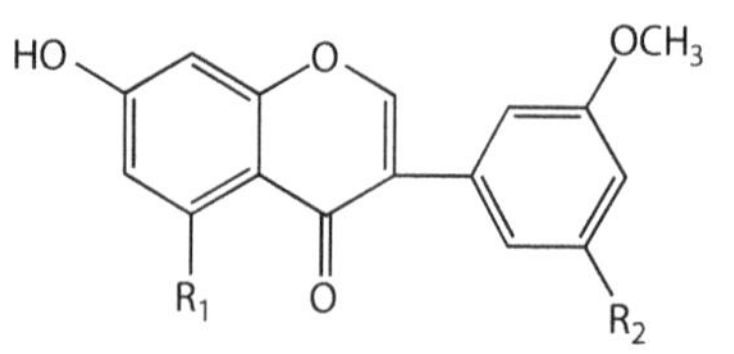

1. R_1 = –OH, R_2 = –OCH_3
2. R_1 = –OH, R_2 = –H
3. R_1 = –H, R_2 = –OH

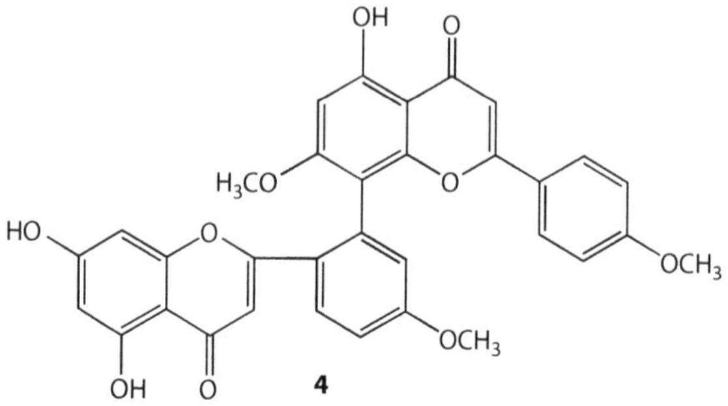

4

Herb Origination

The herb Mao Zhua Cao (Catclaw buttercup) is the dried roots of a Ranunculaceae plant, *Ranunculus ternatus*. The distribution of Mao Zhua Cao is generally around the lower and middle reaches of the Yangtze River, from south of Henan province to north of Guangxi province. The herb collection is traditionally done in early spring or late autumn. Its whole plant is also used as the Chinese herb.

Antitumor Activities and Constituents

In recent years, Mao Zhua Cao has been extensively used in Chinese clinics combined with other Chinese herbs for the treatment of a variety of cancers. The extract of Mao Zhua Cao roots demonstrated *in vitro* suppressive effect against the growth of human A549 lung adenocarcinoma, NCI-H460 large cell lung cancer, and MCF-7 breast cancer cell lines.[1,2] The extract was also able to amplify the nonspecial immune function of normal mice via the enhancement of the proliferation of lymphocytes and the potentiation of the cytotoxicity of NK cells and lymphocytes.[2]

Saponins

Saponins prepared from the herb were effective in the inhibition of S180, EAC, MCF-7, and BGC-823 cancer cell lines *in vitro*.[3,4] The *in vitro* assay also showed that the saponin dose-dependently restrained the proliferation and the colony formation of human HepG2 hepatoma cell line.[5] The Mao Zhua Cao saponins markedly inhibited the growth of human LoVo colon neoplastic cells, accompanied by the blockage of the cell cycle progression and the increase of the apoptosis. The downregulations of Bcl-2 expression and the upregulations of Bax expression and caspase-3 activity should be involved in a Ca^{2+}-involved apoptotic mechanism induced by the saponins.[6] The MCF-7 cell apoptosis induced by the saponins in a high concentration of 100 mg/L was found to be mediated by obviously promoting the expression of mfn2 gene.[7] In association with the induction of apoptosis and the blockage of cell cycle in the G0/G1 phase, the saponins obstructed the proliferation of two human NSCLC cell lines (A549 and NCI-H460).[8,9] Moreover, the saponins also displayed the suppressive effect on the growth of HCCLM3 and MHCC97-H high metastatic hepatocellular carcinoma cell lines.[10]

Flavonoids

Three isolated isoflavonoids assigned as ternatin-A (**1**), mutabilein (**2**), and 7,3′-dihydroxyl-5′-methoxyisoflavone (**3**) exhibited moderate cytotoxicity against four tested human cancer cell lines (HeLa, MCF-7, PANC-1, and HepG-2) with IC_{50} values ranging from 11.8 to 52.6 μg/mL. In contrast, kayaflavone (**4**), an isolated biflavonoid from the herb, displayed obvious inhibitory effect on HeLa (cervix) and HepG-2 (liver) cancer cell lines (respective IC_{50}: 3.26 and 8.67 μg/mL) and moderate effect on Panc-1 (pancreas) and MCF-7 (breast) cancer cell lines (respective IC_{50}: 16.44 and 12.64 μg/mL).[11]

Polysaccharides

The polysaccharides of Mao Zhua Cao were reported to be effective in the inhibition of S180, EAC, MCF-7, and BGC-823 carcinoma cells and to have significant abilities to augment phagocytosis percentage and phagocytic index of peritoneal macrophages and to promote plaque formation, hemolysin formation, and lymphocyte transformation in a mouse immunosuppressive model caused by CTX.[4,12] The polysaccharides in the *in vitro* assay also exerted proapoptotic effect on human MCF-7 breast cancer cells and thereby achieving growth inhibitory effect.[13] The immunoenhancing function of the polysaccharides are considered to be helpful for potentiating the anticancer treatment and lowering the toxicity of chemotheraphy.[12] A polysaccharide–protein complex designated as RTG-III was purified from the aqueous extraction of Mao Zhua Cao. Its molecular weight was about 2.3 × 10^4, and its contents of saccharide and protein were 80.1% and 12.6% respectively. The protein portion consisted of glutamic acid, glutamine and 16 other kinds of amino acids, while the saccharide portion consisted of rhamnose, glucose, arabinose, galactose, and mannose in the molar ratio of 1.0:1.17:51.71:2.16:0.46, whose protein and saccharide portions were linked through a non-*O*-glycosidic bond. RTG-III exerted marked inhibitory effect against human promyelocytic leukemia HL-60 cells in *vivo* by potentiating the immunological activity.[14]

Consequently, the results provided scientific evidences to support the use of Mao Zhua Cao in the prescriptions for the treatment and the prevention of malignant tumors.

Other Bioactivities

Pharmacological investigations substantiated Mao Zhua Cao (Catclaw buttercup) to have significant antitubercule bacillus, antibacterial, and antiinflammatory properties. The herb is often clinically used in folk medicine to treat tuberculosis, scrofula, cervical adenitis, sphagitis, thyromegaly, etc.

References

1. Tong, Y. L. et al. 2012. Application of *Ranunculus ternatus* extract in preparation of drugs for preventing and/or treating lung cancer. *Faming Zhuanli Shenqing* CN 102805768 A 20121205.
2. Yin, C. P. et al. 2008. Inhibiting effect of extracts in radix *Ranunculi ternati* on growth of human breast cancer cells in vitro. *Chin. J. Hosp. Pharm.* 28: 93–6.
3. Wang, A. W. et al. 2004. Study on antitumor effects in vitro of different extracts in Radix *Ranunculus ternate. Tianran Chanwu Yanjiu Yu Kaifa* 16: 529–31.
4. Niu, L. D. et al. 2013. Inhibitory effect of saponins and polysaccharides from Radix *Ranunculi ternati* on human gastric cancer BGC823 cells. *Afri J. Tradit. Complem. Altern. Med.* 10: 561–6.
5. Chen, X. et al. 2013. The study on effect of radix *Ranunculus ternate* saponins on the activity of human hepatocarcinoma cell line HepG2. *China Modern Doctor* 51: 3–5.
6. Zhou, Q. A. et al. 2009. Effect of radix *Ranunculus ternate* saponins on apoptosis and mitochondria membrane potential in human colon carcinoma LoVo cells. *Zhonghua Zhongyiyao Xuekan* 27: 1079–81.
7. Meng, Q. H. et al. 2011. Mechanism study of mfn2 gene in radix *Ranuncoli ternati* saponins and red clover Isoflavone-treated breast cancer. *China Pharmasit* 14: 1243–6.
8. Tong, Y. L. et al. 2013. In vitro study of Radix *Ranunculus ternati* saponins against A549 cell activity of non-small cell lung cancer. *Zhonghua Zhongyiyao Xuekan* 31: 2181–3.
9. Shan, Y. L. et al. 2013. Study on the in vitro activity of *Ranunculus ternati* radix saponins on non-small cell lung cancer cell of NCI-H460. *Zhongguo Xiandai Yingyong Yaoxue* 30: 1182–6.
10. Liu, S. et al. 2015. Inhibition of extracts in Radix *Ranunculi ternati* on cell HCCLM3 and MHCC97-H of liver cancer metastasis. *Shandong Yiyao* 55: 8–10.
11. Shen, H. et al. 2014. Cytotoxic metabolites from the roots of *Ranunculus ternatus. Chem. Nat. Compd.* 50: 621–3.
12. Hu, Z. K. et al. 2010. Effects of Radix *Ranunculi ternati* polysaccharide on immunological function of the immunosuppressional model mice induced by cyclophosphamide. *Zhongguo Xiandai Yingyong Yaoxue* 27: 89–91.
13. Sun, D. L. et al. 2013. A study on the inhibitory effect of polysaccharides from Radix *Ranunculus ternati* on human breast cancer MCF-7 cell lines. *Afr. J. Tradit. Complem. Alternat. Med.* 10: 439–43.
14. Chen, Y. et al. 2004. Purification and properties of a polysaccharide RTG-III from *Ranunculus ternali. Zhongguo Yaoxue Zazhi* 39: 339–42.

214 Liao Ge Wang 了哥王

Tie bush or Bootlace bush

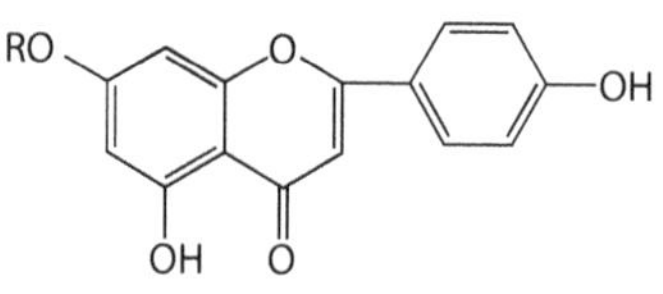

1. R = -CH$_3$ 2. R = -H

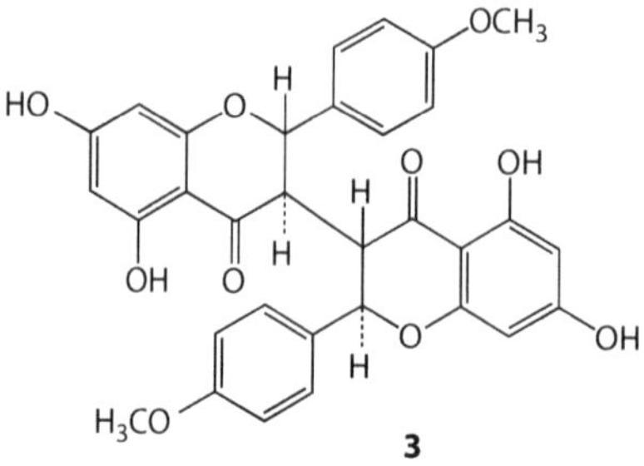

3

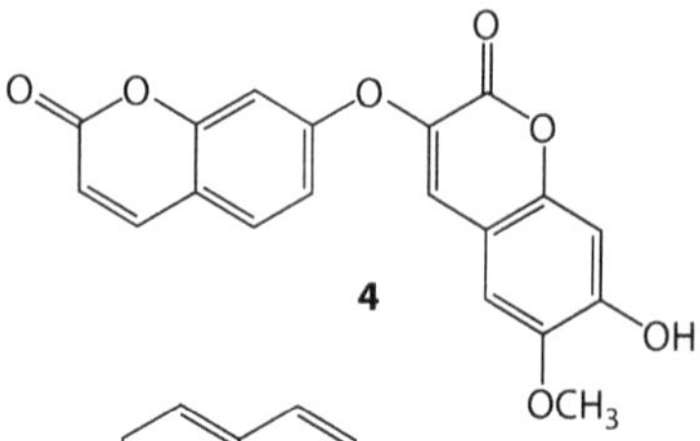

4

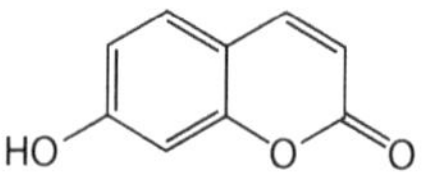

5

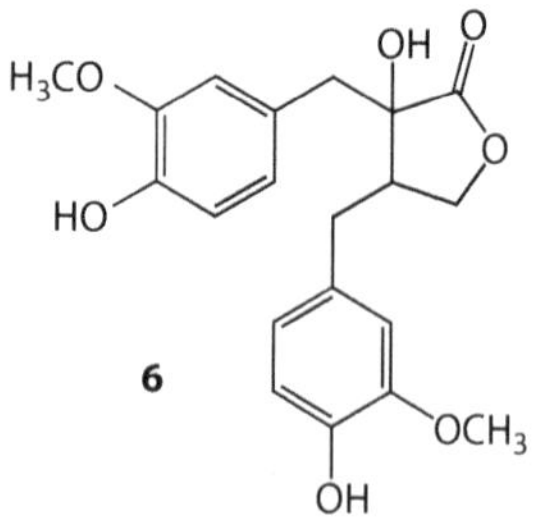

6

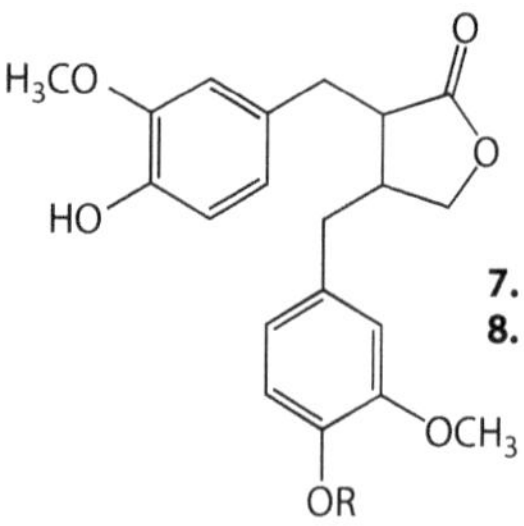

7. R = -OH 8. R = -CH$_3$

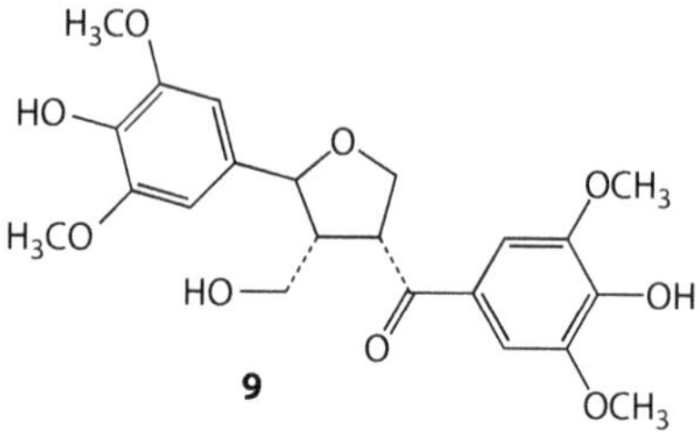

9

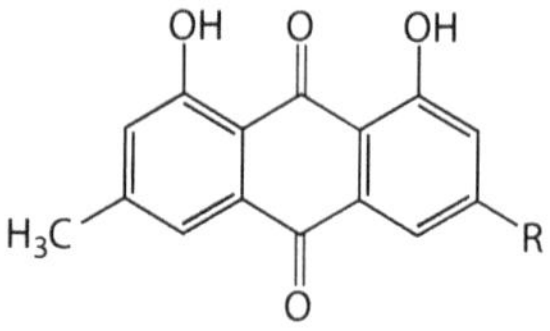

10. R = -OCH$_3$ 11. R = -H

Herb Origination

The herb Liao Ge Wang (Tie bush) originated from a Thymelaeaceae plant, *Wikstroemia indica*. This bush grows in forests and on rocky, shrubby slopes in central and southeastern China, Vietnam, India, and the Philippines. Its roots, stems, leaves, and fruits can be used separately in the Chinese medicines.

Antitumor Activity

The antitumor activity of the methanol extract of Liao Ge Wang was shown in Ehrlich ascites tumor implanted in mice with 97% inhibitory rate and in P388 lymphocytic leukemia with a T/C value of 180% after the i.p. injection to mice in a dose of 50 mg/kg/day.[1] Its 95%, 75%, and 50% ethanolic extract and water extract were sensitive to human HeLa (cervix) and SGC-7901 (stomach) cancer cell lines but insensitive to Bel-7402 hepatoma cells *in vitro*. The organic solvent partition fractions such as petroleum ether and chloroform exhibited antitumor activity against the three cell lines, the EAF showed a concentration-dependent antitumor activity against HeLa and SGC-7901 cells, and the n-butanol fraction had no activity.[2] The petroleum ether fraction showed moderate cytotoxic activity on the HeLa and SGC-7901 cell lines *in vitro* with CC_{50} values of 64.3 and 37.8 μg/mL, respectively.[3] A processed *W. indica* extract showed marked cytotoxicity in human breast cancer and drug-resistant breast cancer cell lines and mouse breast cancer cells, indicating that the extract is a potential agent in clinics for treating breast cancer and relieving inflammation and pain.[4]

Antitumor Constituents and Activities

The activity-guided fractionation of the extracts from the stems and the roots of *W. indica* resulted in the isolation of many bioactive constituents including flavonoids, biflavonoids, coumarins, lignans, anthraquinones, volatile oils, polysaccharides, etc. Most of them demonstrated different degrees of anticancer and anticarcinogenic activities, although no prominent cancer inhibitor was discovered from Liao Ge Wang.

Flavonoids

In the early researches, tricin and kaempferol-3-*O*-β-D-glucopyranoside derived from the methanolic extract of *W. indica* stems were shown to have the inhibitory activity against the growth of P388 lymphatic leukemia cells.[1] Kaempferol (**1**) and apigenin (**2**) are common flavones found in the fruit and other plants, which were shown to be a modulator in inflammatory diseases and also have a potential in anticarcinogenesis. In association with eliciting the tumor cell apoptosis, kaempferol (**1**) exerted the antiproliferative effect on multiple types of human tumor cell lines, such as H460 (lung), MDA-MB-231 and BT-549 (breast), MCF-7 (breast), PC3 (prostate), MIA PaCa-2 and Panc-1 (pancreas), OVCAR-3 (ovary), A2780/CP70 and A2780/wt (ovary), and HL-60 (leukemic) cell lines.[5] By the promotion of cell cycle arrest and apoptosis, apigenin (**2**) exerted moderate antitumor activity toward many human cancer cell lines, such as SK-BR-3 (breast), HepG2 and Huh7 (liver), HeLa (cervix), A2780 (ovary), BxPC-3 and PANC-1 (pancreas), and K562 (leukemic) cells.[5–7] The investigations revealed that the characteristic pathways were involved in the apoptosis-increasing mechanisms in the different types of malignant cells. By the suppression of Akt and NF-κB activities, apigenin (**2**) augmented the antigrowth and apoptosis-inducing activities of gemcitabine (an anticancer drug) against AsPC-1 and MiaPaca-2 pancreatic carcinoma cells *in vitro* and *in vivo*.[8] The antihepatoma effect of apigenin (**2**) on Huh7 cells was demonstrated in a nude mice xenograft model treated by a daily dose of 50 μg/mouse.[8,9] Due to the decline of COX-2 expression in MCF-7 breast cancer cells and MCF-10A breast epithelial cells, apigenin (**2**) showed a suppressive potential against the breast carcinogenesis.[9,10]

Several biflavonoids were isolated from the herb, demonstrating some interesting chemotherapeutic potential. Chamaejasmenin-A (**3**) exhibited obvious antiproliferative effect against the HeLa and HepG2 cell lines in a concentration-dependent manner and moderate cytotoxic effect against Bel-7402 hepatoma, MCF-7 breast cancer, and SGC-7901 gastric cancer cell lines.[5] A pair of bioflavonoid enantiomers, wikstaiwanone-A and wikstaiwanone-B, and a flavone glycoside, isorhamnetin-3-*O*-robinobioside, which were isolated from the rhizomes of *W. indica*, were effective in moderately retarding SW480 and SW620 human colon neoplastic cell lines.[11] Other isolated biflavonoids such as genkwanol-A, wikstrol-A, wikstrol-B, and daphnodorin-B did not show the anticancer activity but were found to have antimitosis, antifungal, and anti-HIV-1 activities.[12,13]

Coumarins

Daphnoretin (**4**), a biscoumarin derivative, extracted in good amounts from the root barks of *W. indica*, was found to have marked anticancer spectrum. It blocked the synthesis of nucleic acid and protein, leading to the suppression of the growth of Ehrlich ascites tumor cells.[1,14] *In vitro* experiments demonstrated that daphnoretin (**4**) markedly obstructed CNE brain cancer cells and HeLa cervical cancer cells at concentrations from 15.6 to 125 μg/mL and obviously restrained AGZY-83-a lung cancer cells, HEp2 laryngeal cancer cells, and HepG2 hepatoma cells (IC_{50}: 8.73, 9.71, and 31.34 μg/mL, respectively).[14,15] The obvious increase of intracellular calcium was found to be involved in the antigrowth mechanism in the AGZY-83-a, HEp2, and HepG2 cell lines.[14,15] By exciting a mitochondria-mediated pathway, daphnoretin (**4**) elicited the HeLa cells to apoptosis and then inhibited the viability and the proliferation of HeLa cells.[16] Daphnoretin was also observed to induce the cell apoptosis and the growth-inhibition in A549 lung cancer cells in a concentration- and/or a time-dependent manner.[17] In a toxic experiment, daphnoretin (**4**) appeared to have mitochondrial toxicity in its high concentrations in the tested mouse K1735-M2 metastatic melanoma cells, human MDA-MB-231 breast cancer cells, and mouse H9c2 myoblast cells, exerting the antiproliferative effect on the cancer cells.[18] Daphnoretin (**4**) also showed an ability to restrain the expression of hepatitis-B surface antigen in human Hep3B hepatoma cells.[19] In addition, another isolated coumarin compound assigned as umbelliferone (**5**) displayed the inhibitory effect against human EJ bladder cancer and KB nasopharyngeal carcinoma cell lines *in vitro* (IC_{50}: 1.3×10^{-6} and 3.2×10^{-6} mol/L, respectively).[20,21]

Lignans

(+)-Nortrachelogenin (**6**) was isolated from the methanolic extract of *W. indica* stems as a major antileukemia agent active in a mouse P388 cell assay.[1] Matairesinol (**7**) and arctigenin (**8**), two bioactive lignans derived from the herb, exhibited a dose-dependent inhibitory activity against human AGS gastric cancer cells and mouse Hepa 1c1c7 hepatoma cells *in vitro*, and both lignans also acted as an inducer of QR (a phase II detoxification enzyme) in the Hepa 1c1c7 cells. At a 200 μmol/L concentration, arctigenin (**8**) elicited an apparent apoptosis and cell cycle arrest of the AGS gastric cancer cells.[22] The antileukemia activity of arctigenin (**8**) was observed in two kinds of human leukemia cells (HL-60 and K562) *in vitro*. The apoptosis stimulated by arctigenin (**8**) in the HL-60 and K562 cells was associated to the increase of Bax/Bcl-2 ratio and the activation of caspase-3.[23] In addition, an *in vivo* test proved that arctigenin (**8**) has an ability to restrain the tumor promotion caused by chemical agents.[22,23] Five more anticancer lignans identified as matairesinol (**7**), ciwujiatone (**9**), wikstromol, syringaresinol, and pinoresinol were isolated from the rhizomes of *W. indica*, which all exhibited different inhibitions against human colon cancer cell lines (SW480 and SW620), and ciwujiatone (**9**) exerted the most prominent activities against the two cell lines among the lignans.[11]

Anthraquinones

The isolation of Liao Ge Wang also led to obtaining two anticancer active anthraquinones identified as phscion (**10**) and chrysophanol (**11**). *In vitro* experiments proved that both phscion (**10**) and chrysophanol (**11**) were effective in the suppression of K562 erythroleukemia cells, A431 epidermoid carcinoma cells, and PC3 prostate neoplastic cells. Moreover, phscion (**10**) and chrysophanol (**11**) exerted efficient antiproliferative effect against human MCF-7 breast cancer cells and human HL-60 promyelocytic leukemia cells, respectively. The IC_{50} value of chrysophanol (**11**) was 52.5 μg/mL in the K562 cells.[5,24]

Volatile Oils

The volatile compounds in the petroleum ether fraction displayed moderate or weak cytotoxicity on HeLa cervix carcinoma cells and HEp-2 laryngeal neoplastic cells with CC_{50} values of 64.3 and 37.8 μg/mL, respectively. By GC-MS analysis, the fraction was revealed to be mainly composed of fatty acids, unsaturated fatty acids, and their methyl esters, such as palmitic acid, oleic acid, stearic acid, methyl oleate, methyl palmitate, methyl stearate, etc. The unsaturated acids exhibited moderate cytotoxicity against the HeLa cells (CC_{50}: 74.3 μg/mL) and the HEp-2 cells (CC_{50}: 36.9 μg/mL).[3]

Other Medical Uses

The herb Liao Ge Wang (Tie bush) has long been employed as antipyretics, detoxicants, expectorants, vermifuges, as well as aborticides in clinical practice for the treatment of various diseases, such as arthritis, whooping cough, and syphilis, besides tumor. The antiinflammatory, antibacterial, antifertility, antiviral, and analgesic activities have been proven by pharmacological researches.[25] However, Liao Ge Wang causes toxic side effects; thus, the safety and the rationality must be ensured in the clinics. Furthermore, a biflavonoid, assigned as 4′-methoxydaphnodorin-E, was isolated from its antiviral fraction, displaying potent effect against respiratory syncytial virus with an IC_{50} value of 2.8 μM and a selective index value of 5.4.[26]

References

1. Lee, K. H. et al. 1981. Antitumor agents: 49. Tricin, kaempferol-3-O-β-D-glucopyranoside and (+)-nortrachelogenin, antileukemic principles from Wikstroemia indica. *J. Nat. Prod.* 44: 530–5.
2. Chen, Y. et al. 2008. Preliminary study on antitumor effect of extracts of *Wikstroemia indica. Chin. Archives of TCM* 26: 2520–2.
3. Wu, P. et al. 2010. Cytotoxicity and constituents of radix *Wikstroemiae indicae. Zhongyaocai* 33: 590–2.
4. Shen, Z. B. et al. 2012. *Wikstroemia indica* extract, its preparation method and application. *Faming Zhuanli Shenqing* CN 102344454 A 20120208.
5. Sun, L. X. et al. 2012. Cytotoxic constituents from *Wikstroemia indica. Chem. Nat. Compd.* 8: 493–7.
6. Johnson, J. L. et al. 2013. Flavonoid apigenin modified gene expression associated with inflammation and cancer and induced apoptosis in human pancreatic cancer cells through inhibition of GSK-3β/NF-κB signaling cascade. *Mol. Nutr. Food Res.* 57: 2112–7.
7. Cong, Y. et al. 2009. Chemical constituents and antitumor activity on leukemia K562 cell of *Leonurus heterophyllus. Zhongguo Zhongyao Zazhi.* 34: 1816–8.
8. Lee, S. Y. et al. 2008. Enhanced antitumor effect of combination therapy with gemcitabine and apigenin in pancreatic cancer. *Cancer Lett.*, 259: 39–49.
9. Lau, Y. G. et al. 2010. The dietary flavonoid apigenin blocks phorbol 12-myristate 13-acetate-induced COX-2 transcriptional activity in breast cell lines. *Food Chem. Toxicol.* 48: 3022–7.
10. Cai, J. et al. 2011. Apigenin inhibits hepatoma cell growth through alteration of gene expression patterns. *Phytomed.* 18: 366–73.
11. Shao, M. et al. 2014. Phenolic constituents from rhizome of *Wikstroemia indica* and their antitumor activity. *Tianran Chanwu Yanjiu Yu Kaifa* 26: 851–5, 875.
12. Wang, H. K. et al. 1998. Antitumor agents: 179. Recent advances in the discovery and development of flavonoids and their analogs as antitumor and anti-HIV agents. *Advances in Experim. Med. Biol.* 439: 191–225.
13. Hu, K. et al. 2000. Antifungal, antimitotic and anti-HIV-1 agents from the roots of *Wikstroemia indica. Planta Med.* 66: 564–7.
14. Yang, Z. Y. et al. 2014. Daphnoretin-induced apoptosis in HeLa cells: A possible mitochondria-dependent pathway. *Cytotechnol.* 66: 51–61.
15. Lu, C. L. et al. (a) 2010. Extraction optimisation of daphnoretin from root bark of *Wikstroemia indica* and its antitumor activity tests. *Food Chem.* 124: 1500–6; (b) 2012. Chemical compositions extracted from *Wikstroemia indica* and their multiple activities. *Chem. Pharm. Biol.* 50: 225–31.
16. Yang, Z. Y. et al. 2008. Study on extraction, isolation and antitumor activity of daphnoretin from *Wikstroemia indica. Tianran Chanwu Yanjiu Yu Kaifa* 20: 522–6.
17. Jiang, H. F. et al. 2014. Effect of daphnoretin on the proliferation and apoptosis of A549 lung cancer cells in vitro. *Oncol. Lett.* 8: 1139–42.
18. Diogo, C. V. et al. 2009. Mitochondrial toxicity of the phytochemicals daphnetoxin and daphnoretin-relevance for possible anticancer application. *Toxicol in Vitro.* 23: 772–9.
19. Chen, H. C. et al. 1996. Identification of a protein kinase C (PKC) activator, daphnoretin, that suppresses hepatitis B virus gene expression in human hepatoma cells. *Biochem Pharmacol.* 52: 1025–32.
20. Yang, X. W. et al. 2007. Inhibitory effects of 11 coumarin compounds against growth of human bladder carcinoma cell line E-J in vitro. *J. Chin. Integr. Med.* 5: 56–60.
21. Yang, X. W. et al. 2006. Inhibitory effects of 40 coumarins compounds against growth of human nasopharyngeal carcinoma cell line KB and human leukemia cell line HL-60 in vitro. *Zhongguo Xiandai Zhongyao* 8: 8–13.
22. Kang, K. S. et al. 2007. The chemo-preventive effects of *Saussurea salicifolia* through induction of apoptosis and Phase II detoxification enzyme. *Biol. Pharm. Bull.* 30: 2352–9.
23. Wang, L. 2008. Induction of apoptosis of human leukemia cells by arctigenin and its mechanism of action. *Acta Pharm. Sin.* 43: 542–7.
24. Liu, R. et al. 2005. Chemical constituents of *Schefflera venulosa* and their antitumor activities. *Zhongcaoyao* 36: 328–32.
25. Li, Y. T. et al. 2011. Reviews on chemical constituents and pharmacological action of *Wikstroemia indica. Zhongguo Shiyan Fangjixue Zazhi* 17: 252–5.
26. Huang, W. H. et al. 2012. A new biflavonoid with antiviral activity from the roots of *Wikstroemia indica. J. Asian Nat. Prod. Res.* 14: 401–6.

12

Anticancer Agents from Antispasmodic Chinese Herbs

CONTENTS

215 Quan Xie 全蠍

Scorpion

Herb Origination

The herb Quan Xie (scorpion) is the entire dried insect of *Buthus martensii* (= *Mesobuthus martensii*) (Buthidae). The insect is mostly found in north central and northeast of China as well as Korea, Japan, and Mongolia. The first documentation of this herb was in *Shu Ben Cao*, a local pharmacopeia in the Sichuan province between AD 935–960.

Antitumor Activities

The anticancer components of Quan Xie (scorpion) are briefly in its venom, which is a rich resource of neurotoxic proteins/peptides specifically interacting with various ionic channels in excitable membranes. *In vitro* and *in vivo* studies proved that the scorpion venom possesses marked cytotoxicity on mouse sarcoma 180, Ehrlich ascites carcinoma, human colon carcinoma, and U251-MG malignant glioma cells. The venom could cause morphological changes and vacuolar degeneration of the colon cancer cells, then force it to death, and it could induce U251-MG glioma cells to apoptosis through the inhibition and/or the modulation of various ion channels in the glioma cells.[1–5] The broad spectrum of antiproliferative and apoptosis-inducing effects was also evidenced in many types of human Yac-1 (lymphoma), Raji, HL-60 and K562 (leukemia), HeLa (cervix), Eca-109 (esophagus), and BEL-7402 (liver) malignant tumor cell lines as well as mouse B16 melanoma cells *in vitro*. The concentration of a water extract of scorpion with venom that caused all the tested tumor cells to die in 48–72 h was 10 mg/mL against BEL-7402 hepatoma cells and was 0.1 mg/mL against HeLa cervical cancer cells.[4,6] The venom could induce 100% death of cultured human cervical carcinoma cells at concentrations of 1–10 μg/mL and induce both apoptosis and necrosis of HeLa cells *in vitro* in association with the increase of p21 protein expression.[5,7] The marked antigrowth effect of the scorpion extract was also demonstrated in *in vivo* models implanted with murine lung adenocarcinoma, murine reticulosarcoma, or breast adenocarcinoma.[5]

The fractionation of the venom by chromatographies gave three components (SVC-I, SVC-II, and SVC-III). The assay resulted in the marked cytotoxic activity of SVC-II on three human neoplastic cell lines: Eca-109 (esophageal), HEp-2 (larynx), and C1184 (colorectal) in 4–20 μg/mL concentrations and showed the direct tumor-killing effect of SVC-III on Eca-109 cells *in vitro*.[8–11] The LD_{50} values of SVC-II and SVC-III were 8.0 and 4.5 μg/mL, respectively, on the Eca-109 cells.[12–14] By restraining the NF-κB signaling pathway, SVC-III suppressed the proliferation of human THP-1 leukemia cells and Jurkat cells together with the G1 cell cycle arrest by repressing the expression of cell cycle regulatory protein cyclin-D1 in a dose-dependent manner.[15] The obvious cytotoxic and antiformation activities of SVC-III were also demonstrated in human LoVo colon carcinoma cells.[16] Moreover, the scorpion venom holds a capability to reverse the MDR of MCF-7/Adm breast cancer cells. In 100–350 mg/L concentrations, the venom could enhance the sensitivities of the MCF-7/Adm cells to Adm and increase the intracellular Adm content in the MCF-7/Adm cells.[17] All these findings suggested that the scorpion venom has further developing potential for the treatment of malignancies, alone or in combination with other agents.

Antitumor Constituents and Activities

Over the past few decades, dozens of novel proteins/polypeptides in the scorpion venom (BMV) have been identified, cloned, and investigated for clinical applications including antitumor treatment.

Polypeptides

An anticancer polypeptide (APBMV) was discovered from the scorpion venom, which exhibited *in vitro* tumoricidal effect on five human tumor cell lines: SMMC-7721 hepatoma, HL-60 leukemia, Eca-109 esophageal cancer, MGD-803 gastric cancer, and CAN-2Z poor differential nasopharyngeal cancer at different concentrations of 4–16 μg/mL, and moderate inhibitory effect against SGC-7901 gastric cancer cells, LoVo, and HT-29 colon cancer cells.[18–21] The IC_{50} values were 8.07 μg/mL (at 96 h) in SMMC-7721 cells, 9.90 μg/mL (at 48 h) in HL-60 cells, and 0.024 μg/mL in Eca-109 cells. The CNE-2Z nasopharyngeal cancer cells treated with APBMV (16 μg/mL) for 48 h induced the cell cycle resistant at G1 and G2 phases, associated with the obvious decrease of p53 gene expression. The APBMV also reduced the CNE-2Z cell membrane potential and interfered with cell proliferation, colony formation, and mitosis, exerting the distinct cytotoxicity.[18–20] APBMV in a low concentration could enhance the cytotoxic activity of various chemotherapeutic drugs against LoVo colon neoplastic cells and promote the LoVo cells to apoptosis.[22]

Moreover, the treatment with the polypeptide at the concentrations of 400–800 mg/L significantly obstructed the growth of HO-8910 ovarian carcinoma cells by 47.93–66.92%.[23] Through strongly promoted expression of p27, decreased cyclin-E (one of the cyclins involved in G1 progression), and increased proapoptotic protein Bax, the polypeptide at a concentration of 40 μg/mL arrested the cell cycle and elicited the apoptosis of human DU-145 and PC3 prostate carcinoma cells, resulting in significant antigrowth effect against the two types of prostate cancer by 30.5% and 33.1%, respectively. When raising the concentration to 200 mg/L, the prostate cancer cell growth would be 100% obstructed.[24,25] The proliferation of human SKOV-3 ovarian cancer cells was notably restrained by 34.66% after the polypeptide treatment at the same concentration of 40 mg/L together with the increase of cell cycle arrest and apoptosis through the decline of surviving protein level and the upregulation of p27 protein and caspase-12 expression.[26] At a concentration of 15 μg/mL, the polypeptide could evidently depress the adhesion and the invasion of human leukemic primary cells and obviously interfere the leukemic cell extramedullary infiltration by over 50%.[27]

The i.p. injection of APBMV in a dose 0.04 mg/kg or 0.06 mg/kg to tumor bearing mice for 7–10 days resulted in the growth inhibitory rates of >30% on H22 hepatoma cells and 40.07–44.58% on B16 melanoma cells, compared to that of the anticancer drug 5-FU as 33.55% on B16 cells and 47.81% on H22 cells. At the same time, APBMV remarkably enhanced the NK cell activity and the hemolysin level of the peripheral blood and increased the transforming rate of lymphocytes and the WBC count of the peripheral blood, as well as promoted the proliferation of lymphocytes. The evidences clearly validated that APBMV has the capacity to strengthen the immunity function and to antagonize or recover the immunodeficiency caused by chemotherapies.[28–32] APBMV also resisted LPO injury and reduced the hematological system injury caused by radiotherapy. When the radiotherapy combined with APBMV for the treatment of H22-bearing mice, the tumor inhibitory rate was elevated to 70.45–78.29% in association with the increase of SOD activity and the decrease of LPO level. By the interactions, the radiation-caused hematological system injury was obviously diminished.[33–35] APBMV at concentrations of 10.83 and 0.0023 μg/mL could retard the colony formation of SMMC-7721 cells and Eca-109 cells *in vivo*, respectively.[36–38] The *in vivo* investigation further demonstrated that APBMV was capable of restraining the expressions of VEGF and bFGF to markedly suppress the angiogenesis and the angiogenesis-dependent tumor growth in mice transplanted with sarcoma 180 or hepatoma H22.[39] Probably based on the antiangiogenic property plus the abilities of inhibiting MMP-9 and COX-2 expressions, APBMV significantly obstructed tumor cell invasion and liver metastasis by 70% in nude mice implanted with a highly metastatic Mia-Paca2.3 pancreatic cancer cells.[40]

Accordingly, these researches evidently proved that the APBMV possesses potent direct tumoricidal property and provided a strong rationale for future studies to evaluate the prevention or/and intervention strategies by using APBMV in preclinical cancer models. Several purified polypeptides have been reported to possess diverse bioactivities including cancer suppression.

APs

Further separation of APBMV derived three homogeneity polypeptides, AP-I, AP-II, and AP-III. The AP-III was shown to be representative of the antineoplastic activity of APBMV.[41,42] But the toxicity of these purified polypeptides was higher than that of APBMV. The LD_{50} values in mice are 1.118 mg/kg for AP-I, 1.145 mg/kg for AP-III, and 1.386 mg/kg for APBMV.[43] Other research groups reported that an anticancer peptide fraction III dose-dependently promoted the endothelial apoptosis of HepG2 hepatoma cells via the downregulation of Bcl-2 and the activation of caspase-3 pathways, and a separated peptide fraction AP-III-1 could distinctly inhibit the growth of human tumor cell lines: SMMC-7721 (liver), HL-60 (leukemia), BGC (stomach), and A549 (lung) cells.[44,45]

ANTP

An anticancer peptide labeled as ANTP was prepared from the venom of Chinese scorpion, whose relative molecular mass was 6280 with rich glycine but no histidine and threonine. The cancer growth inhibitory effect of ANTP was demonstrated in mouse sarcoma 180 and Ehrlich ascites tumor models *in vivo*.[46]

Antigliomatin

Antigliomatin is a specific polypeptide extract prepared from the venom of Chinese scorpion *B. martensii*, which could diminish chloride channel currents on rat C6 glioma cells and exert specific toxicity against the glioma cells.[47] Catilan is an active component of the antigliomatin, which acted with the same effect as antigiomatin to specifically bind to the glioma cell surface as a specific chloride channel blocker and then destroy the tumor cells. Catilan could also delay the rectifier potassium channels. This neurotoxin has been clinically used to treat glioma and to reduce adverse drug reactions in China.[48]

BmK AGAP-SYPU2

By bioassay-driven chromatographic separation, a scorpion neurotoxin peptide with both analgesic and antitumor activities was isolated and designated BmK-AGAP-SYPU2. In the *in vivo* models, BmK-AGAP-SYPU2 exhibited antitumor activity against Ehrlich ascites tumor and S180 fibrosarcoma.[49] Moreover, the recombinant techniques have been used for producing the bioacitive peptide. The formed rBMK-AGAPs, such as rAGAP, CHis6-rAGAP, rBMK-CTa, and rpEGFP-N1-BmK CT, demonstrated the inhibitory activities *in vitro* or *in vivo* against C6 or SHG-44 glioma, SW480 colon cancer, Hep3B hepatoma, A549 lung cancer, or HuCC-T1 cholangiocarcinoma cells.[50–56]

Other Bioactivities

The herb Quan Xie (scorpion), especially its tail part, has been clinically used in traditional Chinese medicine for more than

2000 years to treat various neuronal problems such as chronic pain, rheumatism pain, migraine, facial paralysis, apoplexy, and epilepsy. Pharmaceutical approaches have proven that Quan Xie possesses anticonvulsant, antiepilepsy, antithrombotic, vessel-contracting, and analgesic properties.

References

1. Zhu, D. Y. et al. 1990. Inhibitory effect of scorpion extract on sarcoma 180 in mice. *Jiangsu Yiyao* 16: 513.
2. Dong, W. H. et al. 1993. Antitumor activity of Scorpion venom cruds (*Buthus martensii*) against Ehrlich ascites carcinoma in mice and HeLa cell line. *J. Henan Med. Univ.* 28: 298.
3. Wu, B. P. et al. 1993. Scorpion venom cruds (*Buthus martensii*) obstructs human colon cancer HR8348 cells in vitro. *Zhongguo Gangchangbing Zazhi* 13: 3.
4. Zhang, P. T. et al. A preliminary research of the antineoplasia effects induced by *Buthus martensii* of Chinese drug. *Wannan Yike Daxue Xuebao* (1987), 6: 1–5; (1989), 8: 77–79; (1990), 9: 1–3.
5. Wang, W. X. et al. 2005. Scorpion venom induces glioma cell apoptosis in vitro and inhibits glioma tumor growth in vivo. *J. Neuro-Oncol.* 73: 1–7.
6. Zhang, H. M. et al. 2006. Research progress in the antitumor effect of scorpion and scorpion veno. *J. Shenyang Pharm. Univ.* 23: 401–6.
7. Wang, Z. et al. 2012. Effects of *Buthus martensii* Karsch venom on cell proliferation and cytotoxicity in HeLa cells. *Adv. Mater. Res.* 345: 393–8.
8. Fu, S. B. et al. 2004. Inhibitory effects of scorpion venom and its separated components on growth of B16 melanoma cells. *J. Jilin Univ., (Med. Edit.)* 30: 178–81.
9. Jia, L. et al. 2001. Studies of BMK on inhibition of cell growth and induction of apoptosis in Yac-1 cell line. *J. Dalian Med. College* 23: 7–9.
10. Jia, L. et al. 2001. Inhibitory effect of *Buthus martensii* Karsch on human leukemia cell lines. *J. Dalian Med. College* 23: 15–6, 21.
11. Jia, L. et al. 2001. Studies of BMK on inhibition of cell growth and induction of apoptosis in leukemia Raji cell line. *J. Leukemia Lymphoma* 10: 205–7.
12. Dong, W. H. et al. 1995. The lethal and growth-inhibiting effects of the toxins existed in the scorpion venom (*Buthus martensii* karshi) on Eca109 cells. *Chinese J. Pathophysiol.* 11: 251–5.
13. Dong, W. H. et al. 1995. The effect of the component II in scorpion venom crude extracted from *buthus martensii* karsch (SVC II) on the human rectum adenocarcinoma C1184 cell line. *Cancer Res. Prev. Treat.* 22: 150–2.
14. Dong, W. H. et al. 1994. Toxicity study of Scorpion venom component II on human laryngo-carcinoma cells. *China J. Tradit. Chin. Med. Pharm.* (4): 9–11.
15. Song, X. F. et al. 2012. Scorpion venom component III inhibits cell proliferation by modulating NF-κB activation in human leukemia cells. *Experim. Therap. Med.* 4: 146–50.
16. Shen, D. H. et al. 2005. Inhibitory effect of antineoplastic polypeptide from *Buthus martensii* venom on transplanted tumors and H22 cells. *Practical J. Med. Pharm.* 22: 39–41.
17. Yu, L. J. et al. 2004. Study on effect of BMK scorpion venom on reversal of multidrug resistance in MCF-7/ADM cell line. *J. Jilin Univ., (Med. Edit.)* 30: 239–41.
18. Dong, W. H. et al. 2001. Effect of APBMV on cell cycle migration and expression of p53 gene of CNE-2Z cells. *J. Henan Med. Univ.* 36: 650–2.
19. Kong, T. H. et al. 2001. Effect of APBMV on membrane potential of CNE-2Z cells. *J. Henan Med. Univ.* 36: 653–5.
20. Kong, T. H. et al. 2004. Inhibitory effect of polypeptide from *Buthus martensii* Karsch on neoplasm cells. *Chin. J. Pathophysiol.* 20: 968–72.
21. Wang, X. L. et al. 2003. Antitumor effect of polypeptide from *Buthus martensii* venom: Experiment in vivo. *J. Prac. Med. Pharm.* 20: 124–6.
22. Wang, X. L. et al. 2003. Effect of APBMV on LoVo cells and its synergy with chemotherapy drugs. *Zhongguo Binli Shengli Zazhi* 19: 1324, 1336.
23. Qi, Q. H. et al. 2008. Inhibitory effects of polypeptide from *Buthus martensii* venom on growth of HO-8910 ovarian carcinoma cells. *Guangzhou Med. J.* 39: 7–10.
24. Zhang, Y. Y. et al. 2009. Anti-proliferation effect of polypeptide extracted from Scorpion venom on human prostate cancer cells in vitro. *J. Clinical Med. Res.* 1: 24–31.
25. Wang, Z. P. et al. 2006. Inhibition of polypeptide extract from scorpion venom (PESV) against proliferation of prostate cancer androgen-independent cell lines in vitro. *Chin. Pharmacol. Bull.* 22: 938–42.
26. Song, X. Y. et al. 2012. Inhibitory effect of polypeptide extracts from scorpion venom on proliferation of ovarian cancer SKOV3 cells. *Chin. J. New Drug* 21: 257–61.
27. Yang, W. H. et al. 2009. Experimental study of effect of peptide extract from scorpion venom in interference in leukemic cell extramedullary infiltration. *Chin. J. Clin. Pharmacol.* 242–5.
28. Dong, W. H. et al. 1999. Inhibitory effect of antineoplastic polypeptide from *Buthus martensii* venom on transplanting tumors. *J. Henan Med. Univ.* 34: 61–3.
29. Dong, W. H. et al. 1999. Influence of antineoplastic polypeptide from *Buthus martensii* venomon immune system function of hepatoma H22-bearing mice. *J. Henan Med. Univ.* 34: 67–70.
30. Kong, T. H. et al. 1999. Comparable study on antineoplastic and immunostimulant effects in mice of three preparations of antineoplastic polypeptide from *Buthus martensii* venom. *J. Henan Med. Univ.* 34: 55–8.
31. Li, X. W. et al. 2000. Inhibitory effect of different preparations of antineoplastic polypeptide from *Buthus martensii* venom on hepatoma-22 and influence of APBMV on the immune function of tumor-bearing mice. *J. Henan Med. Univ.* 35: 291–3.
32. Yang, J. B. et al. 2000. Effect of anticancer polypeptide from *Buthus martensii* venom on immune function of the H22-bearing mice. *Zhongguo Zhongyao Zazhi* 25: 736–9.
33. Kong, T. H. et al. 2000. Primary observation on effect of APBMV on tumor weight and general physical condition of hepatoma 22-bearing mice after radiotherapy. *Zhonghua Fangshe Yixue Yu Fanghu Zazhi* 20: 313–6.
34. Wei, L. et al. 2001. Effect of APBMV on tumor weight and lipid peroxidation of H22-bearing mice after radiotherapy. *J. Henan Med. Univ.* 36: 655–8.
35. Wei, L. et al. 2002. Influence of antineoplastic polypeptide from *Buthus martensii* venom on tumor weight and hematological system of hepatoma-bearing mice after radiotherapy. *Zhongliu Fangzhi Zazhi* 9: 147–50.

36. Dong, W. H. et al. 1999. Effect of antineoplastic polypeptide from *Buthus martensii* venom on four kinds of human tumor cell lines. *J. Henan Med. Univ.* 34: 52–5.
37. Han, X. F. et al. 1999. Inhibitory effect of antineoplastic polypeptide from *Buthus martensii* venom on human poor differentiation nasopharyngeal carcinoma cell line. *J. Henan Med. Univ.* 34: 58–60.
38. Yang, J. B. et al. 1999. Effect of anticancer polypeptide from *Buthus martensii* venom (APBMV) on Eca 109 cells and HeLa cells. *Zhongguo Bingli Shengli Zazhi* 15: 1116–9.
39. Zhang, W. D. et al. 2005. Polyptide extract from scorpion venom inhibits. *Chin. Pharmacol. Bull.* 21: 708–11.
40. Cui, Y. Z. et al. 2009. Polypeptide extract from Scorpion venom in inhibits liver metastasis in pancreatic cancer. *J. Shandong Univ. (Health Sci.)* 47: 20–3.
41. Kong, T. H. et al. 2000. Isolation and purification of anti-neoplastic polypeptide-III from APBMV. *J. Henan Med. Univ.* 35: 282–5.
42. Han, X. F. et al. 2000. Inhibitory effect of antineoplastic polypeptide-III (AP-III) from *Buthus martensii* venom on transplanting hepatoma-22 and influence of AP-III on thymus gland weight of tumor-bearing mice. *J. Henan Med. Univ.* 35: 288–90.
43. Han, X. F. et al. 2001. Observation of the toxicity of APBMV and AP-I, AP-III from APBMV. *J. Henan Med. Univ.* 36: 659–61.
44. Zhao, C. G. et al. 2006. Inhibitory effects of Scorpion venom and its components on four kinds of tumor cell lines. *J. Guangzhou Med. College* (1).
45. Li, J. W. et al. 2006. Effects of anticancer peptide fraction III from *Buthus martensii* Karsch on apoptosis of human liver cancer cells. *J. Jilin Univ. (Med. Edit.)* 32: 625–8.
46. Liu, Y. F. et al. 2002. Isolation, purification, and N-terminal partial sequence of an antitumor peptide from the venom of the Chinese scorpion *Buthus martensii* Karsch. *Preparative Biochem. & Biotechnol.* 32: 317–27.
47. Wang, Z. et al. 2011. Effects of antigliomatin from the scorpion venom of *Buthus martensii Karsch* on chloride channels on C6 glioma cells. *Neural Regen. Res.* 6: 1365–9.
48. Li, M. X. et al. 2011. Extract from *Buthus martensii Karsch* is associated with potassium channels on glioma cells. *Neural Regen. Res.* 6: 1147–50.
49. Shao, J. H. et al. 2014. Purification, characterization, and bioactivity of a new analgesic-antitumor peptide from Chinese scorpion *Buthus martensii* Karsch. *Peptides* 53: 89–96.
50. Liu, Y. F. et al. 2009. Production and antitumor efficacy of recombinant *Buthus martensii* Karsch AGAP. *Asian J. Tradit. Med.* 4: 228–33.
51. Zhang, J. H. et al. 2002. Purification of an analgesic antitumor peptide from Scorpion venom and its recombinant preparation method. *Faming Zhuanli Shenqing Gongkai Shuomingshu* CN 2001-128235 20010930.
52. Fu, Y. J. et al. 2007. Therapeutic potential of chlorotoxin-like neurotoxin from the Chinese scorpion for human gliomas. *Neuroscience Lett.* 412: 62–7.
53. Cao, Q. X. et al. 2015. In vitro refolding and functional analysis of polyhistidine-tagged *Buthus martensii* Karsch antitumor-analgesic peptide produced in Escherichia coli. *Biotechnol. Lett.* 37: 2461–6.
54. Ge, X. X. et al. 2013. Effects of recombinant analgesic-antitumor peptide on the inhibition of cholangiocarcinoma cell line HuCC-T1. *Yixue Yanjiusheng Xuebao* 26: 343–7.
55. Fu, Y. J. et al. 2013. pEGFP-N1-mediated BmK CT expression suppresses the migration of glioma. *Cytotechnol.* 65: 533–9.
56. Gu, Y. et al. 2013. Analgesic-antitumor peptide induces apoptosis and inhibits the proliferation of SW480 human colon cancer cells. *Oncol. Lett.* 5: 483–8.

216 Di Long 地龍

Earthworm

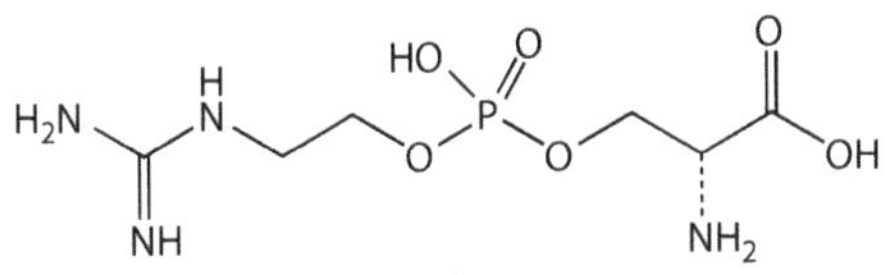

1

Herb Origination

The herb Di Long (earthworm) originates from a kind of tube-shaped and segmented worm commonly living in soil all over the world; this herb has been widely used in east Asia for a thousand years and was documented in the first Chinese materia medica entitled *Shennon Ben Cao Jing*. Traditionally, four kinds of Oligochaeta earthworm, *Pheretima aspergillum*, *P. guillelmi*, *P. vulgaris*, and *P. pectinifera*, are collected and their carcasses are processed to Di Long. The first earthworm species is broadly distributed in the southeast region of China, and the three latter are in eastern China. According to the scientific records, there are over 200 different earthworms living in East Asia.

Antitumor Activities

Great attention has been paid to the anticancer effect of earthworm by Chinese researchers. *In vivo* experiments confirmed that the Di Long extract significantly suppressed the growth of sarcoma 180 cells and H22 hepatoma cells transplanted in mice and prolonged the life span of mice.[1,2] The treatment of human HEp-2 laryngeal carcinoma cells *in vitro* by either using the Di Long extract alone or combining it with a radioactive-promoting agent AK2123 markedly inhibited the tumor proliferation.[3,4] An earthworm extract-II at concentrations of 0.45 and 0.9 mg/mL exerted marked suppressive effect against the proliferation of human Eca-109 (esophagus), HeLa (cervix), and K562 (leukemia) neoplastic cell lines *in vitro*. The gavage of the extract-II in doses (mL) of 300 and 600 to mice obviously retarded the growth of sarcoma 180 cells. The extract-treated HeLa cells showed the promotion of apoptosis and G0/G1 cell cycle arrest to reduce DNA synthesis.[5] Also, *in vivo* tests demonstrated that the extract could augment the radioactive-promoting and anticancer effects of AK2123.[3] When combined with 5-FU (an anticancer drug), the extract synergistically repressed the growth of MA737 breast adenoma cells and sarcoma 180 cells and promoted the cell necrosis to prolong the survival time of experimented animals bearing the tomurs.[6,7] In the integration with heat-therapy, the extract significantly exerted the anti-growth effect in mice bearing the entity EMT6 tumor. The synergetic action also occurred in association with IL-2 to suppress the growth of sarcoma 180 cells *in vivo*.[3]

Also, the Di Long extract demonstrated immunopotentiating effect such as promoting lymphocyte convertibility, enhancing phagocytic activity of macrophages, and enhancing NK cell activity and antibody-dependent mediated cytotoxicity (ADCC). These positive immune actions were further demonstrated by *in vivo* experiments in either normal or sarcoma 180 tumor-bearing mice and in human clinical trials.[8,9] The administration of the Di Long extract was also able to restore the lower active levels of ADCC NK and spleen IL-2 in mice caused by the tumor or the X-ray deep radiation treatment.[9,10] If esophageal cancer patients were treated with the Di Long extract (150 mg) two times per day successively during the treatment of ^{60}Co radiotherapy, the decrease of leukocytes would be effectively restricted, whose activity was better than an immunoenhancing agent polyactin-A.[11] The neoplasm normally diminished the functions of antitumor and antioxidant-related enzymes in the serum (such as SOD, hydroperoxidase, glutathioreductase and GSH peroxidase); however, the earthworm extract remarkably augmented these enzyme functions, reduced LPO, as well as scavenged free radicals.[6,12] Consequently, the tumor cell inhibitory activity of the earthworm is usually accompanied by the close relations with its immunoenhancing and antioxidation possessions.

Antitumor Components and Activities

A penetrated fraction of Di Long demonstrated the suppressive effects against sarcoma 180 and EMT6 entity tumor in mice and against the incorporation of thymidinie into MGC803 gastric cancer cells obviously, but its antitumor activity will disappear after being heated at 100°C for 20 min.[13,14] However, the Di Long contains some anticancer components that are resistant of heat.[14,15] Earthworm coelomocytes (leukocytes) have been reported to possess cytotoxicity at significantly high levels against various human leukemia cell lines including NK-sensitive K562 (erythromyeloid leukemia) and NK-resistant CEM (CD4/T cell leukemia), U937 (monoblastic/monocytic leukemia), and BSM (EBV-transformed B cell leukemia) cell lines.[16,17] The coelomic fluid could elicit the tumor cell apoptosis and inhibit the growth of Siha (cervical cancer), SW480 and Colo205 (colon cancer), Cos7 (kidney fibroblast), and PC12 (pheochromocytoma) cell lines markedly *in vitro*.[18] The cytotoxicity was also observed in HeLa cells, colon cancer cells, WBC malignant tumor cells, and brain tumor cells in the presence of the coelomic fluid of *E. eugeniae*.[19] At a 100 μL/mL concentration, the coelomic fluid could induce necrosis and inhibit the SiHa cells by 78.52% in 48 h. The apoptosis of SiHa cell was elicited at >20 μL/mL concentrations, and the apoptotic rate was elevated along with the increased incubation period.[20] The coelomic fluid obtained from other earchworm (such as *Eisenia foetida*) was also found to be capable of lysing different mammalian tumor cells *in vitro*, whose cytolytic activity was different from TNF-mediated lysis and was also not due to proteolysis.[21]

Enzymes

Earthworm fibrinolytic enzyme (EFE) is a complex protein enzyme, which is widely distributed in the earthworm's digestive cavity, possessing strong protein hydrolysis activity. EFE prepared from Di Long inhibited the growth of human BGC823 gastric cancer and B37 breast cancer in nude mice in a dose-dependent manner when administered by intragastric (i.g.) at 200–1000 mg/kg per day for 15–17 days, showing the high efficiency in preventing and treating tumors without obvious side effects. But there was no *in vitro* inhibition on the proliferation of human cancer cells such as BGC823 (stomach), MCF-7 (breast),

HCT-8 (colon), A549 (lung), and BEL-7402 (liver) at 50 μg/L of EFE.[22,23] During *in vitro* treatment at 9 uku/mL concentration, EFE showed antiproliferative effect on the cancer cell lines, MGC803 and SGC-7901 (stomach), Eca-109 (esophagus), SW1990 (colon), HeLa (cervix), and K562 (leukemia) cells, *in vitro*. The highest inhibition was observed in the MGC803 cells with 94.5% inhibitory rate with the IC_{50} value of 2.79 uku/mL. At the same concentration, the inhibition of the K562 cells reached to 87.2%.[22] The treatment with EFE suppressed the proliferation of four hepatoma cell lines (HLE, Huh7, PLC/PCF/5, and HepG2) together with eliciting apoptosis and restraining MMP-2 expression. The IC_{50} values were 2.11 uku/mL in HLE cells, 5.87 uku/mL in Huh7 cells, 17.30 uku/mL in HepG2 cells, and 25.29 uku/mL in PLC/PCF/5 cells. After the oral administration of EFE for four weeks, the growth of tumor xenograft of Huh7 cells was significantly obstructed in nude mice. The inhibitory rates in doses of 500 uku/kg/day and 1000 uku/kg/day were 46.08% and 57.52%, respectively.[24] The antihepatoma effect of EFE was also achieved in nude mice models with xenografted SMMC-7721 hepatoma cells.[25,26] EFE also exerted the effects on counteracting the adhesion and the metastasis of hepatoma SMMC-7721 cells and bladder cancer ECV-304 cells by depressing FAK and β1-integrin expression and inhibiting CD44v6 expression.[26,27] Furthermore, a synergistic antihepatoma activity with 5-FU was observed in the treatment with EFE *in vivo*.[26] Similarly, in association with lowering the CD44v6 expression, a dose-dependent inhibitory effect of EFE was noticed against the proliferation of human MGC803 gastric carcinoma cells and the adhesion of vascular endothelial cells.[28] These evidences designated that EFE should be one of the important components of Di Long, having indeed potential for further investigation in the antineoplastic therapy.

Proteins

A tumor cell-inhibiting active protein (42.2 kDa) was isolated from the earthworm (*Eisenia foetida*), which is composed of two subunits (33 and 10 kDa). The active protein displayed marked inhibitory effect against the proliferation of human Bel-7402 hepatoma cells and HeLa cervix carcinoma cells and promoted the cells to apoptotic death.[29] A group of antitumor protein components (EE) was reported in the isolation of the same earthworm (*E. foetida*) by another research group, which contains about 60.43% of protein and rich trace elements (such as Zn, Cu, Fe, and Se) with unstable nature in higher temperature. EE displayed moderate inhibitory effect against the growth of human carcinoma cell lines (such as HCT-116, SY5Y, K562, MGC803, and HeLa) *in vitro* with GI_{50} values between 60 and 110 μg/mL. The i.p. administration of EE in doses of 28 and 36 mg/kg obviously prolonged the survival time of mice bearing ascites sarcoma 180 by 135.3% and 123.5%, respectively, and even improved their physical conditions with low toxicity.[30]

ECFP is an earthworm protein prepared from the coelomic fluid of the earthworm (*E. foetida*), whose molecular weight is ~38.6 kDa. An *in vitro* assay displayed that ECFP time- and dose-dependently inhibited the proliferation of HeLa cervical cancer cells (IC_{50}: 77 μg/mL) and LTEP-A2 lung adenocarcinoma cells (IC_{50}: 126 μg/mL). But ECFP has marked hemolytic activity to chicken red blood cells, and its minimal hemolytic concentration is 0.39 μg/mL.[31] EFE6, a tumor antigrowth protein, was originally derived from an earthworm (*Metaphire guillelmi*) and was produced by using recombinant techniques. The antigrowth activity of EFE6 protein or polypeptide was demonstrated against several human tumor cell lines including SMCC7721 and HepG2 (liver), SW620 (colon), HO8910 (ovary), A549 (lung), BCAP-37 (breast), BGC823 (stomach), HeLa (cervix), and T24 (bladder) cells.[32] Also, these described earthworm proteins possess esterase and fibrinolysis activities. Therefore, the tumor suppressive proteins derived from the earthworm may have a potential pharmaceutical application in the future for treating tumor and other medical problems.

Glycoprotein

CCF-1 is a 42 kDa coelomic cytolytic factor derived from *E. foetida*, which is a protein binding β-1,3-glucan and LPS, having trypanolytic activity. Because CCF-1 has an ability to resemble TNFα activity, the CCF-1 may be functional in the tumor therapy or immunological treatment.[20,33] From the separation of the earthworm (*E. foelidea*) extract, a glycoprotein component named QY-1 (mol.wt. 63,000) was purified, which contains 2% saccharides and 16 kinds of amino acids with no Typ and Cys. *In vivo* studies exhibited that QY-1 not only obviously restrained the growth of mouse H22 hepatoma cells and prolonged the life span by 65.4% but also significantly enhanced the indexes of the thymus and the spleen and the function of macrophages and the increase of the activities of CAT, SOD, and GSH-Px in serum, indicating that the antitumor effect of QY-1 is principally attributed to its capacities in immunostimulation, radical scavenging, and anti-LPO.[34,35]

Guanidine Compound

D-Lombricine (**1**) extracted from the earthworm was found to suppress the growth of spontaneous mammary tumors of mice. Further approaches in bioactivity and structure relationship revealed that the existence and the length of the ethylene group in the guanidino compounds are important to the suppressive potency, and the guanidinoethyl group is the site of antitumor action. The results also revealed that subcutaneous administration is more effective than intragastrical adminstration.[36]

Other Bioactivities

The herb Di Long (earthworm) is historically used for the therapy of many diseases such as hypertension, bleeding, ulceration, burned and scalded wounds, epilepsy, and so on. Pharmacological studies demonstrated that the Di Long possesses anticoagulant, antithrombotic, antiarrhythmia, hypotensive, anticonvulsant, antiasthmatic, and antipyretic properties, besides its antineoplastic and immunoenhancing activities. But the herb should be used with caution during pregnancy because it can stimulate the uterus.

References

1. Wang, K. W. et al. 1991. Tumor inhibition of earthworm extract in mice. *Zhongguo Zhongliu Linchuan* 18: 133–4.
2. Wang, K. W. et al. 1991. Inhibitory activity of long treatment with 912 against tumor transplanted in mice. *Zhongguo Zhongliu Linchuan* 18: 143.

3. Zhu, M. S. et al. 1991. Radio-sensitizing effect of 912 and AK2123 on HEp-2 cancer cells. *Zhongguo Zhongliu Linchuan* 18: 141–2.
4. Zhang, F. K. et al. 1991. 912 suppressed HEp-2 cancer cells. *Zhongguo Zhongliu Linchuan* 18: 142–3.
5. He, D. W. et al. 2005. Study on the anti-tumor effects of earthworm extracts both in vivo and in vitro. *Zhongguo Shenghua Zazhi* 26: 353–5.
6. Zhang, Z. Z. et al. 912 and AK2123 ehance anntitumor activity of FU. *Zhongguo Zhongliu Linchuan* 18: 140–1.
7. Mao, H. S. et al. 1991. Oral administration of 912 treated 359 cases of malignant tumor. *Zhongguo Zhongliu Linchuan* 18: 166–70.
8. Tian, Q. et al. 912 and AK2123 augment the transformation of mouse spleen lymphocytes. *Zhongguo Zhongliu Linchuan* 18: 146–8; 156–8.
9. Ju, G. Z. et al. 1991. Regulation of 912 on the immune-repression induced by radiation. *Zhongguo Zhongliu Linchuan* 18: 174.
10. Zhang, Z. P. et al. 1991. Effect of 912 on human immune function. *Zhongguo Zhongliu Linchuan* 18: 184.
11. Xu, D. M. et al. 1991. Radiosensitizer 912 and immunostimulator polyactin A can be used to enhance the radiotherapy as an adjacent treatment. *Zhongguo Zhongliu Linchuan* 18: 154–5.
12. Sun, S. F. et al. 1991. Effect of earthworm extract on laser anticancer sensitizing effect of hematoporphyrin and its mechanism. *Disi Junyi Daxue Xuebao* 12: 141–4.
13. Li, Y. R. et al. 1991. Inhibitory effect of 912 dialysate against transplanted tumor in mice. *Zhongguo Zhongliu Linchuan* 18: 151–2.
14. Han, W. et al. 1991. First fraction from gel filtration of 912 inhibited MGC-803 gastric cancer cells. *Zhongguo Zhongliu Linchuan* 18: 135–6; 152–3.
15. Han, W. et al. 1991. Anticancer effects of fractions derived from gel filtration of earthworm extract on MGC-803 gastric cancer cells. *Disi Junyi Daxue Xuebao* 12: 409–10.
16. Zhu, F. R. et al. 2005. Review on the antitumor effect of the active substances from earth-worm. *Yaowu Shengwu Jishu* 12: 278–80.
17. Cossarizza, A. et al. 1996. Earthworm leukocytes that are not phagocytic and cross-react with several human epitopes can kill human tumor cell lines. *Experim. Cell Res.* 224: 174–82.
18. Wang, J. H. et al. 2011. Study on antineoplastic effect of earthworm coelomic fluid in vitro. *Zhonghua Shiyan He Linchuang Bingduxue Zazhi* 24: 409–11.
19. Dinesh, M. S. et al. 2013. Anticancer potentials of peptides of coelomic fluid of earthworm *Eudrilus eugeniae*. *Biosci. Biotech. Res. Asia* 10: 601–6.
20. Jaabir, M. S. et al. 2011. Evaluation of the cell-free coelomic fluid of the earthworm *Eudrilus euginiae* to induce apoptosis in SiHa cell line. *J. Pharmacy Res.* 4: 3417–20.
21. Bilej, M. et al. 1995. Identification of a cytolytic protein in the coelomic fluid of *Eisenia foetida* earthworms. *Immunol. Lett.* 45: 123–8.
22. Zhang, Z. G. et al. 2006. Application of earthworm fibrinolytic enzyme in preventing and treating tumors. *Faming Zhuanli Shenqing Gongkai Shuomingshu* CN 1004–988 20050712. Separation and research on antitumor components in earthworm 389–91.
23. Li, H. Y. et al. 2004. Antitumor activity of earthworm fibrinolytic enzyme. *Zhongguo Yaolixue Tongbao* 20: 908–10.
24. Chen, H. et al. 2007. Earthworm fibrinolytic enzyme: Antitumor activity on human hepatoma cells in vitro and in vivo. *Chin. Med. J.* 120: 898–904.
25. Shen, S. S. et al. 2008. Effects of EFE on adhesion of liver cancer cells. *Jiangsu Zhongyiyao* 40: 80–3.
26. Wang, J. et al. 2009. Effect of earthworm fibrinolytic enzyme on growth of xenografted tumor of hepatocellular carcinoma (HCC) and expression of CD44v6. *Zhongliu Fangzhi Yanjiu* 36: 375–9.
27. Chang, C. X. et al. 2009. Anti-metastasis activity of earthworm fibrinolytic enzyme on hepatoma cell in vivo. *Zhongyao Xinyao Yu Linchuang Yaoli* 20: 520–4.
28. Chen, H. et al. 2007. Earthworm fibrinolytic enzymes lowering of gastric cancer and vascular endothelial cell adhesion and CD44v6 expression. *Zhonghua Xiaohua Zazhi* 27: 682–4.
29. Jia, H. M. et al. 2003. A preliminary study on isolation of a tumor cell inhibiting active component from earthworm and its mechanism. *Zhongliu* 23: 481–5.
30. Xie, J. B. et al. 2003. Extraction and isolation of the antitumor protein components from earthworm (*Eisenia foetida* and *rei*). *Zhongguo Shengwu Huaxue Yu Fenzi Shengwu Xuebao* 19: 359–66.
31. Hua, Z. et al. 2011. Purification of a protein from coelomic fluid of the earthworm *Eisenia foetida* and evaluation of its hemolytic, antibacterial, and antitumor activities. *Pharm. Biol.* (London, UK) 49: 269–75.
32. Liu, X. L. et al. 2007. Sequence of tumor cell growth-inhibiting protein EFE6 from earthworm. *Faming Zhuanli Shenqing* CN 1990504 A 20070704.
33. De Baetselier, P. et al. 1999. Earthworm coelomic cytolytic factor CCF-1 and treatment of cancer and trypanosomal or bacterial infection. *PCT Intl. Appl.* WO 98-EP8169 19981216.
34. Lin, S. Q. et al. 2000. Studies on the antitumor active composition from earthworm. *Strait Pharm. J.* 12: 59–61.
35. Lin, S. Q. et al. 2002. Affecting tumorigenic mouse immune function and antioxidase of QY-I from earthworm. *Strait Pharm. J.* 14: 10–2.
36. Tsunoda, S. et al. 1997. Inhibition by guanidine compounds of the growth of spontaneous mammary tumours in SHN mice. *Anticancer Res.* 17: 3349–53.

217 Wu Gong 蜈蚣

Centipede

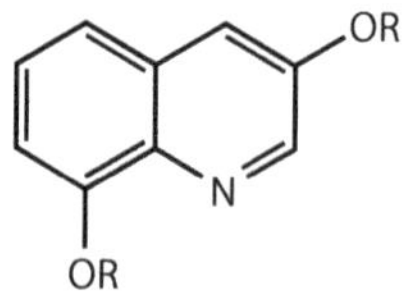

1. R = –H
2. R = $-CH_3$
3. R = –Ac

Herb Origination

The herb Wu Gong (centipede) is the roasted dry centipede *Scolopendra subspinipes mutilans* and *S. subspinipes mutidens* (Scolopendridae). The centipedes are widely distributed from east Asia to Australasia. The documentation of Wu Gong as a Chinese herb was in *Shennong Ben Cao Jing*, the first Chinese classic materia medica. The herb has been used for cancer treatment in traditional Chinese medicine for hundreds of years.

Antitumor Activities

The nonpolar solvent soluble extract of Wu Gong showed significant antineoplastic activity. The i.p. injection of the ester-soluble extract in doses of 140–150 mg/kg to tumor-bearing mice and rats markedly suppressed the cell growth of mouse sarcoma 180, U14 cervical cancer, B16 melanoma, ARS reticulosarcoma, and rat W256 carcinosarcoma with inhibitory rates of 25.9–61.8%. Its ether-soluble extract demonstrated more potent *in vivo* suppressive effects against the growth of the five types of tumor cells mentioned earlier with the inhibitory rates of 30.8–43.0% in doses of 25–50 mg/kg by i.p. injection and of 39.1% on sarcoma 180 in a dose of 25 mg/kg by oral administration. The methanolic extract of Wu Gong displayed lower antitumor activity against murine P388 leukemia and W256 sarcoma,[1] but an EAF from its 80% ethanolic extract exhibited the potent inhibitory activity (about 80%) against the proliferation of human HL-60 leukemia cells at a concentration of 50 μg/mL. The EAF simultaneously promoted the HL-60 cells into apoptosis by gradually lessening the expression of antiapoptotic Bcl-xL, activating caspase-3 and caspase-9, and cleaving of PARP.[2]

The venom of the centipedes was also found to have the inhibitory activity against the growth of human K562, U937 and HL-60 myelogenous leukemia cell lines in a dose-dependent manner with IC_{50} values of 20, 30, and 200 μg/mL, respectively. The treatment of K562 cells with the venom could elicit the cell cycle arrest at S phase and the apoptotic death in association with the activation of caspase-2, caspase-3, caspase-6, caspase-8, and caspase-9.[3]

Antitumor Constituents and Activities

According to scientific reports, the anticarcinoma and anticarcinogenic activities of Wu Gong (centipede) are considered to be contributed by three types of constituents, i.e. alkaloids, polysaccharides, and polysaccharide–protein complex.

Alkaloids

Jineol (**1**), a quinoline alkaloid found from the ethanolic extract of Wu Gong, exerted strong cytotoxic activities *in vitro* against five human neoplastic cell lines such as A549 NSCLC, SKOV-3 ovarian cancer, SK-Mel-2 melanoma, XF-498 CNS cancer, and HCT-15 colon carcinoma cells with ED_{50} values (μg/mL) of 5.8, 4.5, 5.6, 10, and 1.9, respectively. The methylation and the acetylation of 3-hydroxyl group in jineol (**1**) could obviously decrease the tumor inhibitory effect as compared to jineol.[4,5]

Polysaccharide

PSSM (33.1 kDa), a polysaccharide component prepared from *S. subspinipes mutilans*, obviously restrained the proliferation of human HeLa cervical carcinoma cells by 60.8% at its concentration of 3.13 μg/mL, but it had no effect on the human Eca-109 esophageal squamous cancer cells. The inhibitory effect of PSSM on the HeLa cells was found to be dependent to its ability to promote the G2/M cell cycle arrest and apoptosis.[6,7]

Polysaccharide–Protein Complex

A polysaccharide–protein complex (SPPC) was derived from *S. subspinipes mutilans*, which exerted significant *in vivo* antineoplastic property in mouse models. It inhibited the growth of sarcoma 180 transplanted in mice and prolonged the survival time of H22-bearing mice. In S180-bearing mice, it displayed an ability to promote specific and nonspecific immune response as evidenced by enhancing the activities of CTL, NK cells and the ratio of Th1/Th2 cytokines and increasing the percentages of $CD4^+$ T cells, B cells, and NK cells. But it also significantly suppressed the mRNA expression and the production of the immune-suppressive cytokines (IL-10 and TGF-β) and diminished arachidonic acid (AA)-metabolizing enzymes (COX-2 and CYP4A) and their products (PGE2 and 20-HETE) in tumor-associated macrophages (TAMs). The findings implied that the SPPC is an immunoregulatory antitumor agent, whose *in vivo* antigrowth effect should be mediated by improving antitumor immune responses at least partly by downregulating the AA-metabolic pathways in the TAMs.[8]

Protein

A bioactive protein component prepared from *S. subspinipes mutilans* displayed the antiproliferative effect against human Tea-8113 tongue carcinoma cell line *in vitro*, whose antiproliferative potency on the Tea-8113 cells could be gradually increased along with increasing the drug concentration and the effective time.[9] Another antitumor active protein (20 kDa) was isolated from Centipede, which showed obvious suppressive effect against human cancer cell lines such as A549 (lung), LoVo (colon), HepG2 (liver) and MCF-7 (breast), *in vitro*.[9]

Other Bioactivities

The herb Wu Gong has been traditionally employed to treat spasm, childhood convulsion, seizure, poisonous nodules, and diphtheria. Wu Gong also showed vasodilative, hypotensive, anticonvulsion, platelet aggregation-inducing, immunopotentiating, and antibacterial properties. The crude venom of Wu Gong displayed a medium toxicity in mice with LD_{50} value of 22.5 mg/kg (i.p.). A cardiotoxic protein designated as Toxin-S (60 kDa) was purified from Wu Gong. Its LD_{50} was 41.7 µg/kg (intravenous) in male mice.[10,11]

References

1. State Administration of Traditional Chinese Medicine. 1999. *Chinese Materia Medica*, 9: 143–6. Shanghai Science and Technology Press, Shanghai, China.
2. Kim, K. N. et al. 2008. Induction of apoptosis by *Scolopendra subspinipes mutilans* in human leukemia HL-60 cells through Bcl-xL regulation. *Han'guk Sikp'um Yongyang Kwahak Hoechi* 37: 1408–14.
3. Xu, S. Y. et al. 2013. The venom of the centipede *Scolopendra subspinipes mutilans* inhibits the growth of myelogenous leukemia cell lines. *Letters in Drug Design & Discovery* 10: 390–5.
4. Moon, S. et al. 1996. Jineol, a cytotoxic alkaloid from the centipede *Scolopendra subspinipes*. *J. Nat. Prod.* 59: 777–9.
5. Lee, H. S. et al. 1998. Quinoline compound extracted from Scolopendra subspinipes and its derivatives as anticancer agents. *U.S.* US 97-865126 19970530.
6. Li, X. N. et al. 2009. Study on purification and property of polysaccharide from *Scolopendra subspinipes mutilans*. *Zhongyaocai* 32: 846–8.
7. Li, X. N. et al. 2009. Effects of polysaccharide from *Scolopendra subspinipes mutilans* on proliferation of HeLa cells. *Shizhen Guoyi Guoyao* 20: 1571–3.
8. Zhao, H. X. et al. 2012. Antitumor and immunostimulatory activity of a polysaccharide-protein complex from *Scolopendra subspinipes mutilans* L. Koch in tumor-bearing mice. *Food Chem. Toxicol.* 50: 2648–55.
9. (a) Liu, B. et al. 2013. Inhibitory effect of active protein from *Scolopendra subspinipes mutilans* to human tongue cancer cell line Tea-8113. *Shizhen Guoyi Guoyao* 24: C3–C4; (b) Kong, Y. et al. 2010. An antitumor active protein prepared from Centipede. China Patent, CN 101747423 A, CN 201010104825.
10. Wang, Y. et al. 1985. Biological activities of centipede crude venom. *Kexue Tongbao* 30: 1102–5.
11. Gomes, A. et al. 1983. Isolation, purification and pharmacodynamics of a toxin from the venom of the centipede *Scolopendra subspinipes dehaani* Brandt. *Ind. J. Experimental Biol.* 21: 203–7.

218 Jiang Can 僵蠶

Batryticated silkworm or Bombyx batryticatus

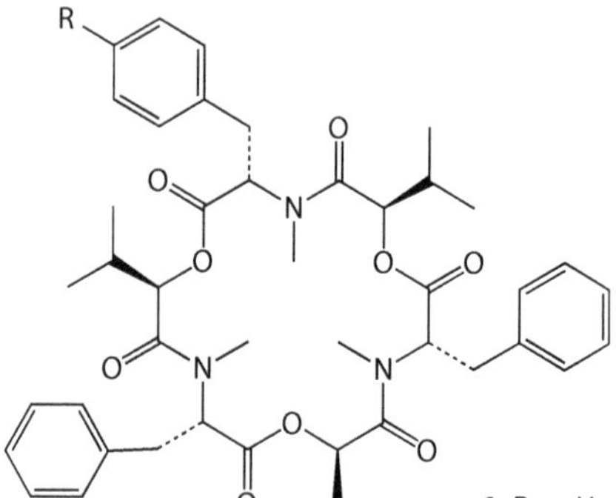

1. R = -H
2. R = -OH

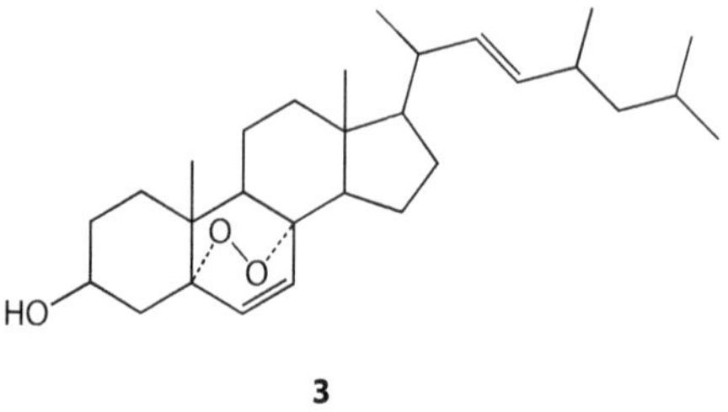

3

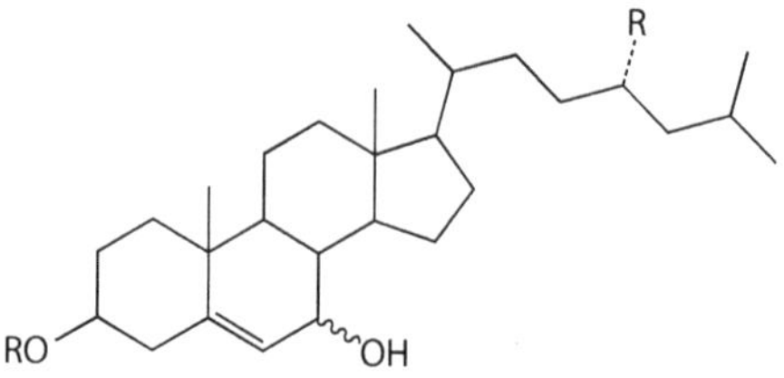

4. R = -H
5. R = $-CH_3$

Herb Origination

The herb Jiang Can (batryticated silkworm) is the dried larva of silkworm *Bombyx mori* L., which larva is died by naturally infection by a fungus *Beauveria bassiana* before its spitting silk. The herb Jiang Can is chiefly produced in the Zhejiang, Jiangsu, and Sichuan provinces of China, where it is collected and dried for folk medicinal use. Jiang Can was documented in the Chinese first classic of materia medica entitled *Shennong Ben Cao Jing*. In addition, the batryticated silkworm pupa called Jiang-Yong can also be utilized in Chinese folk medicines, sometime as a succedaneum of Jiang Can.

Antitumor Constituents and Activities

The daily intragastric administration of a 50% decoction of Jiang-Yong to tumor-bearing mice in a dose of 0.2 mL per mouse resulted in the growth suppression against sarcoma 180 cells. The inhibitory rate of Jiang Can ethanolic extract on Ehrlich entity tumor reached to 36% in a mouse model. *In vitro* tests showed that the Jiang Can extract was able to restrain the respiration of human hepatoma cells and to diminish the adenocarcinoma type of human rectum polyp.[1,2] The clinics in China proved that the Chinese medicinal proscriptions including Jiang Can are obviously effective in the suppression of tumor cells, the reduction of tumor size, and the improvement of symptoms.[3–6]

Cyclodepsipeptide

Several cyclodepsipeptides were separated from the *Bombyx batryticatus*. But only beauvericin (**1**) was reported to have a broad spectrum of cytotoxic effect *in vitro*. It showed marked to moderate cytotoxicity against human A549 and NCI-H460 (nonsmall cell lung), NCI-H187 (small cell lung), HeLa (cervix), MCF-7 (breast), KB (oral epidermal), MIA-PaCa2 (pancreas), SF-268 and XF498 (brain), SK-MEL-2 (skin), SKOV-3 (ovary), and HCT-15 and Caco-2 (colon) tumor cell lines[7–11] and had moderate to weak inhibitory effect on human PC3 (prostate) and PANC-1 (pancreas) tumor cell lines.[10] The cytotoxicity was also obviously observed in normal Vero kidney epithelial cells of an African green monkey.[9] Beauvericin-J (**2**), an analog of beauvericin (**1**), has only one more hydroxyl group in an amino acid unit compared to beauvericin (**1**). But the antiproliferative activity of beauvericin (**1**) was stronger than that of 7β-hydroxycampesterol (**5**) by 2–12 times in the same assay used with the NCI-H187, MCF-7, KB, and Vero cell lines, implying that the introduction of a hydroxyl group to the p-position of a benzene ring in beauvericin (**1**) world reduce the antitumor potency markedly.[9]

The cytotoxic effect of beauvericin (**1**) was further proven to be largely correlated with the promotion of tumor cells to apoptosis, whose mechanisms were revealed to be characteristically mediated by (1) stimulating oxidative stress-involved and mitochondria-dependent apoptosis together with loss of mitochondrial membrane potential, increase in LPO level, and G2/M cell arrest, in dose and time-dependent manners (such as in human Caco-2 colon adenocarcinoma cells)[12]; (2) enhancing apoptosis through the upregulation of Bax, Bak, and p-Bad expressions and the downregulation of Bcl-2 but no effect on the levels of Bcl-XL or Bad proteins in association with the significant reduction of mitochondrial membrane potential, the release of mitochondrial cytochrome c, and the activation of caspase-3 (such as in human NSCLC A549 cells)[13]; and (3) eliciting Ca^{2+}-actuated apoptotic death pathway including the increase of cytochrome c release and the augmentation of caspase-3 activity (such as in human CCRF-CEM ALL cells).[14]

Furthermore, the investigations demonstrated the potential of beauvericin (**1**) in the suppression of directional cell migration (haptotaxis) and angiogenesis as well. The beauvericin (**1**) treatment at concentrations ranging from 2.0 to 2.5 μM and 3.0 to 4.0 μM, respectively, obstructed the migration of both metastatic human cancer cell lines such as PC-3M (prostate) and MDA-MB-231 (breast). The IC_{50} values for anti-migration in PC-3M and MDA-MB-231 cells were 3.0 and 5.0 μM, respectively. Also, beauvericin (**1**) at a concentration of 3.0 μM could completely disrupt HUVEC-2 endothelial cell network formation *in vitro*, signifying the antiangiogenic activity. According to the relationship between the tested concentration and the activities, it is known that beauvericin (**1**) at sublethal doses is capable of retarding the migration of both metastatic cancer cells and the angiogenesis of HUVEC-2 cells.[11,15]

Sterols

Three sterols were isolated from the batryticated silkworm and were elucidated as ergosterol peroxide (**3**), 7β-hydroxycholesterol (**4**), and 7β-hydroxycampesterol (**5**). All three sterols were cytotoxic to HTC and ZHC hepatoma cell lines at a 33 μg/mL concentration. However, ergosterol peroxide (**3**) also exhibited the cytotoxicity on normal 3T3 mouse fibroblast cells at a 20 μg/mL concentration, whereas two other sterols had no such inhibition on the 3T3 cells.[16]

Oligosaccharides

Two antitumor active oligosaccharides assigned as BBPW-1 and BBPW-2 were isolated and purified from *Bombyx batryticatus* with molecular weights of 3.67×10^6 Da and 2.0×10^3 Da, respectively. Both polysaccharides showed direct cytotoxic effect against human HeLa cervical carcinoma cells and human HepG2 hepatoma cells, but they had no influence on normal human HEK293 embryonic kidney cells and murine RAW264.7 macrophages.[17–19] BBPW-2 also exerted long-term antiproliferative effect on human MCF-7 breast cancer cells *in vitro*. Apoptotic and cell cycle analysis revealed that BBPW-2 could elicit the cell cycle disruption of HeLa cells in G0/G1 and G2/M phases accompanied by an impressive increment of early apoptotic cells and late apoptotic and necrotic cells.[17] Chemical structural determination established that the BBPW-2 consisted of β-D-(1–2,6)-glucopyranosyl and β-D-(1–2,6)-mannosyl units serving as a backbone, α-D-(1–2)-galactopyranose and α-D-(1–3)-mannosyl units as branches, and α-D-mannopyranose and β-D-glucopyranose as its terminals.[17] These findings provided a scientific support for the oligosaccharides that may be a potential chemotherapeutic and preventive agent for cancer chemotherapies.

Other Bioactivities

The herb Jiang Can (batryticated silkworm) has been proven by pharmacological experiments possessing anticoagulant, hypnotic, anticonvulsion, hypoglycemic, and antibacterial properties, whereas beauvericin (**1**) has anticonvulsion, antiarrhythmia, antimalarial, sedation, and antitubercular activities. In mouse and rat models, the i.p. injection of the Jiang Can extract in doses ranging from 0.5 to 5 g/kg showed no toxicity reaction. However, a small number of patients complained about dry mouth and throat, nausea, reduced appetite, and lassitude after the administration of the herb. Therefore, caution should be taken by people with thrombocytopenia, coagulation disorders, and bleeding tendency and by patients with hepatic coma.

References

1. Wang, J. X. et al. 1999. The pharmacological research and clinical application of jiangcan and jiangyong. *Lishizhen Med. Material Medica Res.* 10: 637–9.
2. Wang, J. H. et al. 2003. The pharmacological research and clinical application on batryticated silkworm and muscardine pupae. *Lishizhen Med. Material Medica Res.* 14: 492–4.
3. Song, D. C. et al. 2014. Anticancer active traditional Chinese medicines. *Faming Zhuanli Shenqing* CN 103565961 A 20140212.
4. Li, S. S. et al. 2013. Traditional Chinese medicine formulation for treating cancer and rheumatism. *Faming Zhuanli Shenqing* CN 103330921 A 20131002.
5. Shi, Y. J. et al. 2013. Traditional Chinese medicine composition for preventing cancer and pain. *Faming Zhuanli Shenqing* CN 103239519 A 20130814.
6. Gu, H. T. et al. 2009. Traditional Chinese medicinal preparation for treating carcinoma and formulation thereof. *Faming Zhuanli Shenqing* CN 101530589 A 20090916.
7. Deng, C. M. et al. 2013. Secondary metabolites of a mangrove endophytic fungus *Aspergillus terreus* (No. GX7-3B) from the South China Sea. *Marine Drugs* 11: 2616–24.
8. Kwon, A. et al. 2000. Cytotoxic cyclodepsipeptides of *Bombycis corpus* 101A. *Yakhak Hoechi* 44: 115–8.
9. Isaka, M. et al. 2011. Cyclohexdepsi-peptides from Acremonium sp. BCC 28424. *Tetrahedron* 67: 7929–35.
10. Wang, Q. X. et al. 2011. Chemical constituents from endophytic fungus *Fusarium oxysporum*. *Fitoterapia* 82: 777–81.
11. Zhan, J. X. et al. 2007. Search for cell motility and angiogenesis inhibitors with potential anticancer activity: Beauvericin and other constituents of two endophytic strains of *Fusarium oxysporum*. *J. Nat. Prod.* 70: 227–32.
12. Prosperini, A. et al. 2013. Beauvericin-induced cytotoxicity via ROS production and mitochondrial damage in Caco-2 cells. *Toxicol. Lett.* 222: 204–11.
13. Lin, H.-I. et al. 2005. Involvement of Bcl-2 family, cytochrome c and caspase 3 in induction of apoptosis by beauvericin in human non-small cell lung cancer cells. *Cancer Lett.* (Amsterdam) 230: 248–59.
14. Jow, G. M. et al. 2004. Beauvericin induces cytotoxic effects in human acute lymphoblastic leukemia cells through cytochrome c release, caspase 3 activation: The causative role of calcium. *Cancer Lett.* 216: 165–73.
15. Xu, Y. Q. et al. 2007. Cytotoxic and antihaptotactic beauvericin analogues from precursor-directed biosynthesis with the insect pathogen *Beauveria bassiana* ATCC 7159. *J. Nat. Prod.* 70: 1467–71.
16. Cheng, K. P. et al. 1977. Chemistry and biochemistry of Chinese drugs: Part I. Sterol derivatives cytotoxic to hepatoma cells, isolated from the drug *Bombyx cum Botryte*. *J. Chem. Res., Synopses* (9): 217.
17. Jiang, X. et al. 2014. Structural elucidation and in vitro antitumor activity of a novel oligosaccharide from *Bombyx batryticatus*. *Carbohydrate Polymers* 103, 434–441.
18. Shi, L. G. et al. 2013. Method for preparing anticancer polysaccharide BBPW-1 from batryticated silkworm by separation and purification. *Faming Zhuanli Shenqing* CN 103265643 A 20130828.
19. Shi, L. G. et al. 2013. Method for preparing anticancer polysaccharide BBPW-2 from white silkworm. *Faming Zhuanli Shenqing* CN 103265644 A 20130828.

13

Anticancer Potentials of Anthelmintic Herbs

CONTENTS

219 Bing Lang 檳榔

Betel nut or Areca nut

Herb Origination

The herb Bing Lang (Betel nut) is the fruits of a Palmaceae plant, *Areca catechu* L., whose plant is domesticated in Malaysia and cultivated in southern China. Its seed nut, fruit cover, and male flower bud are individually used as folk medicines in China.

Antitumor Constituents and Activities

Six polyphenolic substances labeled as NF-86I, NF-86II, NPF-86IA, NPF-86IB, NPF-86IIA, and NPF-86IIB were isolated from Betel nuts and found to be inhibitors of neoplasm and 5′-nucleotidase. The average relative molecular masses of NPF-86IA, NPF-86IB, NPF-86IIA, and NPF-86IIB were 5620, 5000, 29,400, and 8610, respectively. These inhibitors demonstrated a moderate cytotoxic effect to Ehrlich ascites carcinoma, HL-60 leukemia cells, and HeLa cervical cancer *in vitro* but not effective on mouse L1210 leukemia cells. The *in vivo* therapeutic activity of these polyphenolic compounds was demonstrated on Ehrlich ascites carcinoma by i.p. administration (10 mg/kg) to mice.[1–3] An isolated antioxidant phenolic compound assigned as jacareubin (**1**) displayed a significant cytotoxicity against human hepatoma cells and human gastric carcinoma cells.[4] Arecoline (**2**), an alkaloid isolated from an Areca nut, was able to block the intermediate conductance calcium-activated potassium channels in human glioblastoma cell lines (U373 and U87MG), whose activity may potentiate the efficacy of cytotoxic drugs for the management of malignant gliomas.[5]

Tumorigenesis

Betel quid chewing is a major risk factor of OSCC. HSP47 expression was significantly upregulated in the Betel quid chewing-developed OSCCs, indicating that HSP47 can be clinically used as a marker for the lymph node metastasis of oral carcinogenesis. Experiments also showed that vitamin C, GSH, and N-acetyl-L-cysteine could potentially prevent Betel nut chewing-caused oral mucosal lesions.[6,7] Cetuximab-based therapy was recommended as an effective and safe treatment choice for recurrent/metastatic head and neck squamous cell carcinoma in areas where Betel nut chewing is popular.[8] Also, the Areca nut exposure could stimulate the secretion of tumor-promoting cytokines in gingival fibroblasts by blocking ROS generation that trigger DNA damage in oral keratinocytes.[9] *Panax notoginseng* (Tian Qi) saponins were reported to have the ability to inhibit Areca nut extract-induced oral submucous fibrosis *in vitro*.[10]

Nanoformulation

An aqueous extract of the Betel nuts was used to biomimetically formulate AgNPs. The AgNPs not only exerted a higher level of cytotoxicity on DAL cells in a mice model, leading to the decrease of tumor volume and the notable increase of life span of the tumor-induced mice,[11] but also exhibited efficient scavenging of stable or harmful free radicals including DPPH, NO, and OH. Moreover, the synthesized AgNPs were revealed to have potent catalytic activity in the degradation of organic pollutants (eosin yellowish, 4-nitrophenol, methylene blue, and methyl orange), whose function may have applications in the environmental field.[12]

References

1. Matsuo, T. et al. (a) 1988. Novel antitumor substances from betel nut. *Jpn. Kokai Tokkyo Koho* JP 87-233246, 19870917; (b) 1989. An anticancer agent containing extract of seed of *Areca catechu* L. belonging to Palmaceae. *Jpn. Kokai Tokkyo Koho* JP 01261403 A 19891018.
2. Uchino, K. et al. 1988. New 5′-nucleotidase inhibitors, NPF-86IA, NPF-86IB, NPF-86IIA, and NPF-86IIB from *Areca catechu*: Part I. Isolation and biological properties. *Planta Med.* 54: 419–22; 422–5.
3. Iwamoto, M. et al. 1988. New 5′-nucleotidase inhibitors, NPF-86IA, NPF-86IB, NPF-86IIA, and NPF-86IIB from *Areca catechu*: Part II. *Planta Med.* 54: 422–5.

4. Zhang, X. et al. 2010. Antioxidant and cytotoxic phenolic compounds of areca nut (*Areca catechu*). *Chem. Res. in Chinese Univ.* 26: 161–4.
5. So, E. C. et al. 2015. Arecoline inhibits intermediate-conductance calcium-activated potassium channels in human glioblastoma cell lines. *Eur. J. Pharmacol.* 758: 177–87.
6. Chang, M. C. et al. 2002. Prevention of the areca nut extract-induced unscheduled DNA synthesis of gingival keratinocytes by vitamin C and thiol compounds. *Oral Oncol.* 38: 258–65.
7. Lee, S. S. et al. 2011. Heat shock protein 47 expression in oral squamous cell carcinomas and upregulated by arecoline in human oral epithelial cells. *J. Oral Pathol. Med.* 40: 390–6.
8. Chang, M. H. et al. 2010. Cetuximab-based therapy in recurrent/metastatic head and neck squamous cell carcinoma: Experience from an area in which betel nut chewing is popular. *J. Chinese Med. Asso.* 73: 292–9.
9. Illeperuma, R. P. et al. 2015. Areca nut exposure increases secretion of tumor-promoting cytokines in gingival fibroblasts that trigger DNA damage in oral keratinocytes. *Intl. J. Cancer* 137: 2545–57.
10. Dai, J. P. et al. 2014. Panax notoginseng saponins inhibit areca nut extract-induced oral submucous fibrosis in vitro. *J. Oral Pathology Med.* 43: 464–70.
11. Sukirtha, R. et al. 2011. *Areca catechu* Linn.-derived silver nanoparticles: A novel antitumor agent against Dalton's ascites lymphoma. *Intl. J. Green Nanotechnol.* 3: 1–12.
12. Rajan, A. et al. 2015. Catalytic and antioxidant properties of biogenic silver nanoparticles synthesized using Areca catechu nut. *J. Mol. Liquids* 207: 231–6.

220 Gui Jian Yu 鬼箭羽

Winged euonymus

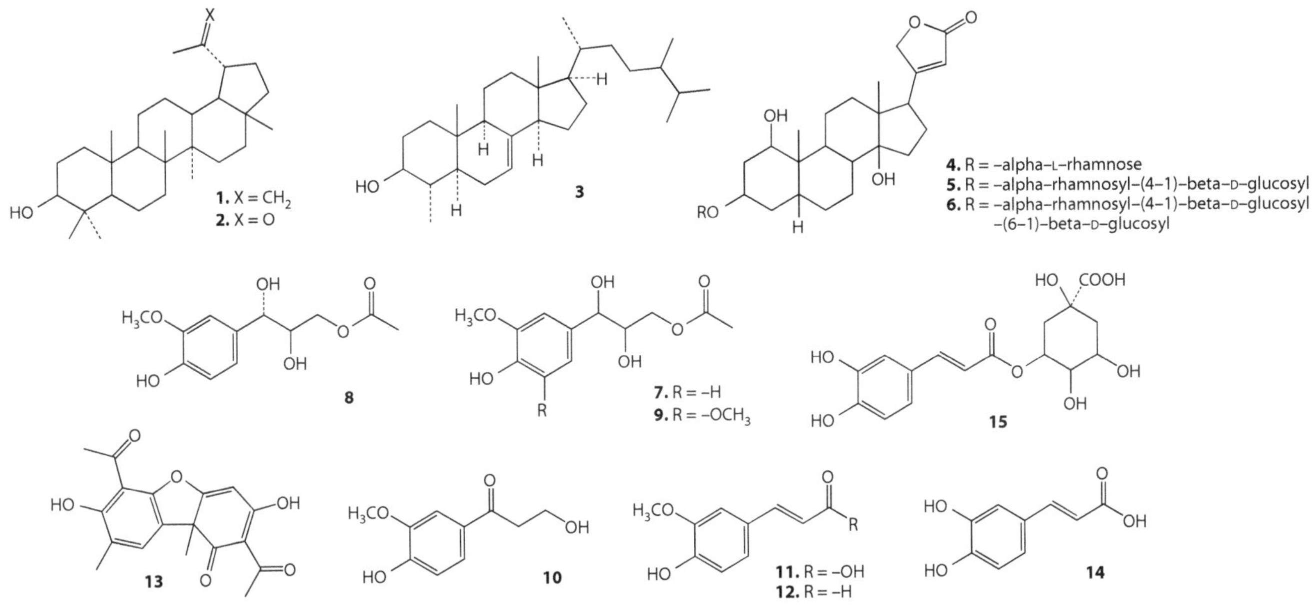

1. X = CH_2
2. X = O

4. R = –alpha-L-rhamnose
5. R = –alpha-rhamnosyl-(4–1)-beta-D-glucosyl
6. R = –alpha-rhamnosyl-(4–1)-beta-D-glucosyl –(6–1)-beta-D-glucosyl

7. R = –H
9. R = –OCH_3

11. R = –OH
12. R = –H

Herb Origination

The herb Gui Jian Yu (Winged euonymus) originates from the winged branches of a Celastraceae bush, *Euonymus alatus*, whose plant is native to northeastern Asia. Its distribution is broadly in central and northern China, Japan, and Korea. The plant was introduced to the United States around 1860 as an ornamental plant used in landscaping. In China, the winged branches are collected annually and dried in the sunlight for folk medical application.

Antitumor Constituents and Activities

The water-soluble extract of Gui Jian Yu showed certain anticancer activity, and it was reported to be used as a functional health herb for the prevention and the treatment of cancers.[1] In *in vitro* assays, the methanolic extract exerted marked cytotoxicity against human KB mouth epidermal cancer cells with an ED_{50} value of 3.08 μg/mL,[2] and the n-butanolic and chloroform fractions, which were derived from the methanolic extract of Gui Jian Yu, displayed moderate to weak cytotoxic activity against human Hep3B hepatoma cell line with IC_{50} values of 65 and 85 μg/mL, respectively.[3]

Triterpenoids and Steroids

Several triterpenoids and cardenolides isolated from the herb were evaluated *in vitro* with human promyelocytic leukemia HL-60 cells *in vitro*, Lupeol (**1**) and 3β-hydroxy-30-norlupan-20-one (**2**) demonstrated moderate growth inhibitory effects against the HL-60 cells (IC_{50}: 26.19–32.22 μM).[4] 24R-Methyllophenol (**3**) exhibited moderate to weak cytotoxic effect on HeLa (cervix), MCF-7 (breast), and HL-60 and Jurkat-T (leukemic) human cancer cell lines, (respective IC_{50}: 15.45, 15.14 21.72, and 63.31 μM).[5] Three cytotoxic cardenolides designated as acovenosigenin-A 3-*O*-α-L-ramnopyranoside (**4**), euonymoside-A (**5**), and euonymusoside-A (**6**) significantly obstructed the growth of HL-60 (leukemic), A549 (lung), and HeLa (cervix) human cancer cell lines. The IC_{50} values were 0.02–0.20 μg/mL for acovenosigenin-A 3-*O*-α-L-ramnopyranoside (**4**), 0.20–0.25 μg/mL for euonymoside-A (**5**), and 1.0–1.63 μg/mL for euonymusoside-A (**6**).[2] β-Sitosterol (a common sterol in numerous plants), in addition, was obtained in the fractionation of *E. alatus* cork, which showed moderate cytotoxicity on the HL-60 cells in the *in vitro* assay (IC_{50}: 6.22 μM).[5]

Phenolic Components

A bioassay-guided isolation of the methanolic extract from *E. alatus* twigs resulted in the discovery of 11 phenolic components. Of them, alatusol-A (**7**), alatusol-B (**8**), alatusol-C (**9**), 3-hydroxy-1-(3-methoxy-4-hydroxyphenyl)propan-1-one (**10**), (E)-ferulic acid (**11**), and (E)-coniferyl aldehyde (**12**) displayed the antiproliferative effect against A549 (lung), SK-MEL-2 (skin), SKOV-3 (ovary), and HCT-15 (colon) carcinoma cell lines with IC_{50} values of 15.20–29.81 μM.[6] Also, (+)-usnic acid (**13**) was effective in inhibiting the proliferation of HL-60 leukemia cells *in vitro* (IC_{50}: 27.78 μM).[4]

Moreover, the methanolic extract and an n-butanolic fraction were capable of significantly inhibiting the activity of MMP-9 in a concentration-dependent manner. The assay-guided fractionation led to the isolation of caffeic acid (**14**) and chlorogenic acid (**15**) from the extract. Both acted as inhibitors of MMP-9 (IC_{50}: 10–20 nM), indicating that the two compounds might be potential agents for antiinvasive and antimetastatic activities.[3,7,8]

Taken together, these results evidenced a possible value of Gui Jian Yu in cancer chemoprevention and cancer treatment and also suggested that the useful cancer chemopreventive effects can be further investigated by combinations of *in vivo* models.

Other Bioactivities

Pharmacological investigations have proven that Gui Jian Yu (Winged euonymus) possesses hypoglycemic, lipometabolism-moderating, and atherosclerosis-reducing potentials.

References

1. Lee, J. H. et al. 2004. Water soluble extract of euonymus alatus sieb having anticancer activity and the use thereof as functional health food. *Repub. Korean Kongkae Taeho Kongbo* KR 2004097446 A 20041118.
2. Kitanaka, S. et al. 1996. Cytotoxic cardenolides from woods of *Euonymus alata*. *Chem. Pharm. Bull.* 44: 615–7.
3. Cha, B. Y. et al. 2003. Inhibitory effect of methanol extract of *Euonymus alatus* on matrix metalloproteinase-9. *J. Ethnopharmacol.* 85: 163–7.
4. Fang, Z. F. et al. 2008. Studies on chemical constituents from *Euonymus alatus* II. *Zhongguo Zhongyao Zazhi* 33: 1422–4.
5. Jeong, S. Y. et al. 2013. Cytotoxic and antioxidant compounds isolated from the cork of *Euonymus alatus* Sieb. *Nat. Prod. Sci.* 19: 366–71.
6. Kim, K. H. et al. 2013. Phenolic constituents from the twigs of *Euonymus alatus* and their cytotoxic and anti-inflammatory activity. *Planta Med.* 79: 361–4.
7. Jin, U. H. et al. 2005. A phenolic compound, 5-caffeoylquinic acid (chlorogenic acid), is a new type and strong matrix metalloproteinase-9 inhibitor: Isolation and identification from methanol extract of *Euonymus alatus*. *Life Sci.* 77: 2760–9.
8. Park, W. W. et al. 2005. A new matrix metalloproteinase-9 inhibitor 3,4-dihydroxycinnamic acid (caffeic acid) from methanol extract of *Euonymus alatus*: Isolation and structure determination. *Toxicol.* 207: 383–90.

221 Si Gua Zi 絲瓜子

Luffa seed

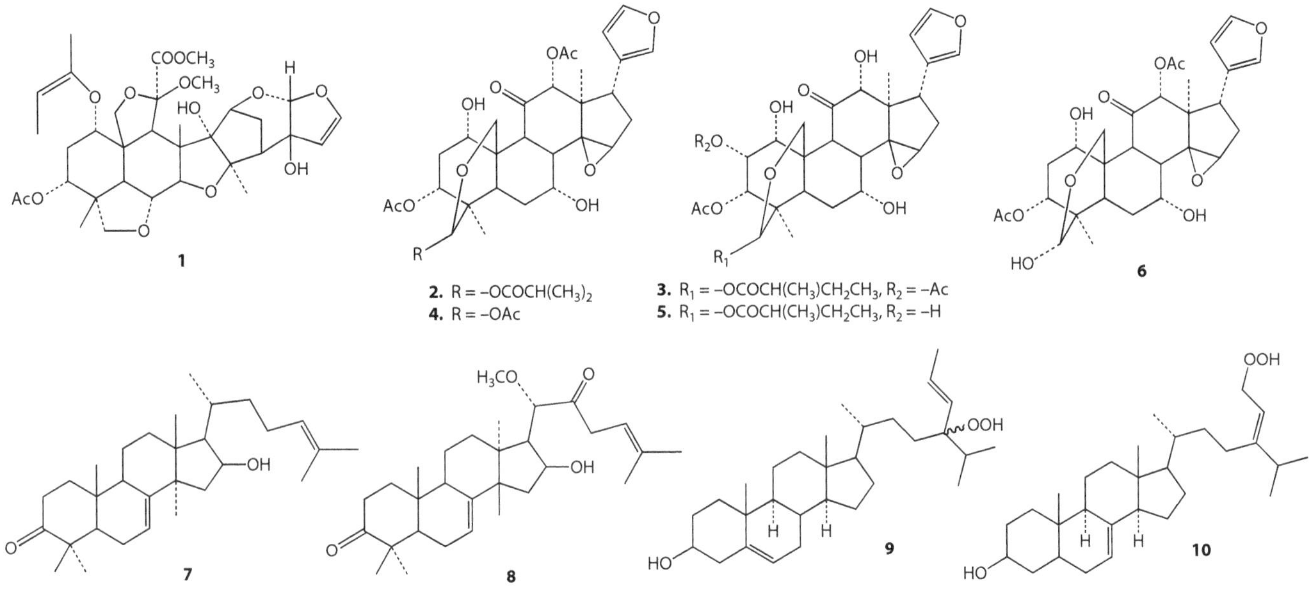

2. R = $-OCOCH(CH_3)_2$
4. R = $-OAc$

3. $R_1 = -OCOCH(CH_3)CH_2CH_3$, $R_2 = -Ac$
5. $R_1 = -OCOCH(CH_3)CH_2CH_3$, $R_2 = -H$

Herb Origination

The herb Si-Gua (Luffa) is a common vegetable crop originated from *Luffa cylindrical* (L.) Roem. and *L. acutangula* (Cucurbitaceae). The two gourd plants are native to tropical Asia, and are now commercially cultivated in China, Korea, Japan, and Central America. The Luffa seeds called Si Gua Zi are normally used as a folk medicine in China.

Antitumor Activities and Constituents

Luffin-A and Luffin-B

Luffin-A and luffin-B are two plant single-chain ribosome-inactivating proteins (RIPs) with cytotoxicity, which were separated from the seeds of *L. acutangula*. The two proteins differed in the contents of aspartic acid, threonine, proline, and alanine but were otherwise similar in amino acid composition. The luffins demonstrated both cytotoxic and inhibitory effects on cell proliferation in human metastatic melanoma cells and murine Ehrlich ascites tumor cells but displayed approximately 10 times greater potency in the Ehrlich cells than in the melanoma cells. The luffins were also found to increase DNA fragmentation and cytosolic oligonucleosome-bound DNA in both melanoma and Ehrlich cells. The increase of cytosolic nucleosomes could be supportive of the apoptosis induced by the luffins.[1] *In vitro* assays proved that both proteins restrained the growth of both melanotic and amelanotic human melanoma cells and inhibited the thymidine uptake by human choriocarcinoma cells.[2–4]

A luffin-A–immunotoxin-conjugated complex was created exhibiting greater growth inhibitory effect against M21 human melanoma cells *in vitro*.[5] Another immunotoxin complex was constructed with luffin-B and Ng76 (a monoclonal antibody to M23 human melanoma cells). The luffin-B–Ng76 complex displayed to be 4000-fold more cytotoxic to the M23 cells than free luffin-B. The IC_{20} values of luffin-B–Ng76 complex were 2.5×10^{-11} mol/L in melanoma M23 cells and 3.0×10^{-8} mol/L in nontarget HeLa cervical carcinoma cells *in vitro*.[6] In addition; the luffins were also incorporated into lecithin/cholesterol or lecithin/cholesterol/dicetyl phosphate to form negatively charged liposomes. The exposure of melanoma cells to the two types of liposomes resulted in the significant inhibition of protein synthesis and tumor cell growth. TUNEL reaction and quantitative determination of cytosolic oligonucleosome-bound DNA also confirmed that the luffin liposomes were capable of inducing tumor cell apoptotic death. The cytotoxic activity of the encapsulated luffins varied with the lipid composition of the vesicles, and the strongest effect was observed in the treatment with the luffins-lecithin/cholesterol liposomes.[7] According to these evidences, the liposome-incorporated luffins can be considered as an alternative to immunotoxins to be useful for the treatment of human melanoma in situ.

Luffaculin-1 and Luffaculin-2

Two other RIPs termed luffaculin-1 and luffaculin-2 were also isolated and purified from the seeds of *L. acutangula*. The molecular mass of luffaculin-1 and luffaculin-2 was estimated to be about 28 kDa. The cytotoxicities of luffaculin-1 and luffaculin-2 were demonstrated in human K562 leukemia cells *in vitro* with IC_{50} values of 1.1×10^{-6} and 2.0×10^{-7} mol/L, respectively.[8] Luffaculin-1 also exerted the antitumor activity on B16, MGC, and Bel neoplastic cell lines, giving IC_{50} values of 1.78×10^{-7}, 2.11×10^{-7}, and 4.21×10^{-7} mol/L, respectively.[9] Therefore, the luffaculins can be considered as potential agents for further development for the treatment of some types of cancers and may be used as an efficient moiety of immunotoxins.

Other Bioactivities

Luffin-A and luffin-B, luffaculin-1, and luffaculin-2 also demonstrated abortifacient, anti-HIV, and anti-virus properties in pharmacological researches.

References

1. Poma, A. et al. 1998. Differential response of human melanoma and Ehrlich ascites cells in vitro to the ribosome-inactivating protein luffin. *Melanoma Res.* 8: 465–7.
2. Ng, T. B. et al. 1993. The ribosome-inactivating, antiproliferative and teratogenic activities and immunoreactivities of a protein from seeds of Luffa aegyptiaca (Cucurbitaceae). *General Pharmacol.* 24: 655–8.
3. Ng, T. B. et al. 1992. Two proteins with ribosome-inactivating, cytotoxic and abortifacient activities from seeds of *Luffa cylindrica* Roem (Cucurbitaceae). *Biochem. Intl.* 27: 197–207.
4. Poma, A. et al. 1997. A ribosome-inactivating protein principle from hairy roots and seeds of *Luffa cylindrica* (L) Roem and its cytotoxicity on melanotic and amelanotic melanoma cell lines. *Intl. J. Pharmacognosy* 35: 212–4.
5. Gao, W. D. et al. 1994. Construction of luffin A immunotoxin and its in vitro inhibition against human melanoma cell M21. *Chin. Sci. Bull.* 39: 950–3.
6. Zhang, R. P. et al. 1998. In vitro inhibition of human melanoma cells by immunotoxin luffin B-Ng76. *Shengwu Huaxue Yu Shengwu Wuli Xuebao* 30: 561–4.
7. Poma, A. et al. 1999. Antiproliferative effect and apoptotic response in vitro of human melanoma cells to liposomes containing the ribosome-inactivating protein luffin. *Biochimica et Biophysica Acta* 1472: 197–205.
8. Lin, J. K. et al. 2002. Purification and characterization of two luffaculins, ribosome-inactivating proteins from seeds of *Luffa acutangula. Zhongguo Shengwu Huaxue Yu Fenzi Shengwu Xuebao* 18: 609–13.
9. Chen, M. H. et al. 2004. Study on the secondary structure and bioactivities of luffaculin 1. *Jiegou Huaxue* 23: 232–5.

222 Ku Lian Pi 苦楝皮

Chinaberry tree bark

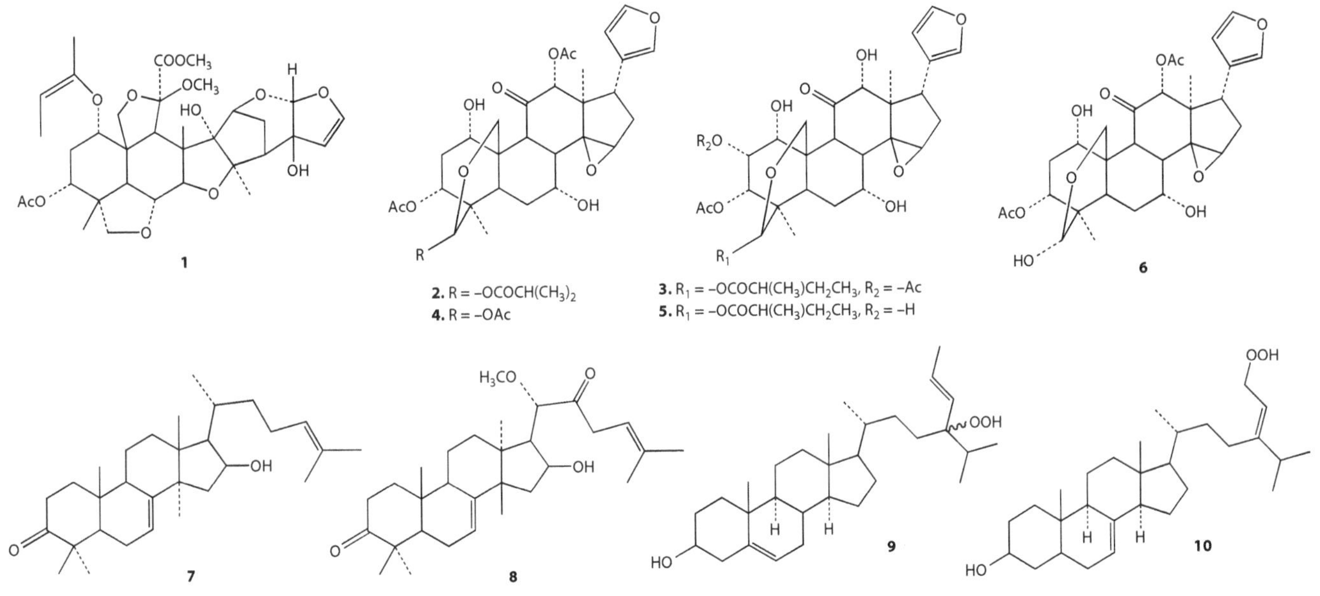

2. R = $-OCOCH(CH_3)_2$
4. R = $-OAc$

3. $R_1 = -OCOCH(CH_3)CH_2CH_3$, $R_2 = -Ac$
5. $R_1 = -OCOCH(CH_3)CH_2CH_3$, $R_2 = -H$

Herb Origination

The herb Ku Lian Pi (Chinaberry tree bark) is the dried stem barks and root barks of two Meliaceae plants, *Melia azedarach* and *M. toosendan*. The deciduous trees have been the sources of medicinal and insecticidal herbs in China for a long time. In China, the stem barks and the root barks are generally collected in spring or autumn and dried in the sun for folk medical utilization. Also, the fruits, the flowers, and the leaves are individually used in traditional Chinese medicine.

Antitumor Constituents and Activities

The *Cortex meliae* extract was found to play the inhibitory roles in BEL7402 (liver), H460 (lung), and SGC-7901 (stomach) human neoplastic cell lines *in vitro*.[1] Biology-connected phytochemical investigations revealed that the constituents such as triterpenoids, steroids, and polysaccharides in Ku Lian Pi are responsible for the antitumor and anticarcinogenic effects of the herb.

Triterpenoids

Ku Lian Pi is a rich source of limonoid type of triterpenoids. Many limonoids, protolimonoids, and nonlimonoidic triterpenoids were obtained from the phytochemical investigation. Some of them demonstrated potent to moderate cytotoxicity on several neoplastic cell lines *in vitro*; especially, the limonoids are more potentially deserving of further *in vivo* and preclinic studies.

Limonoids

In the limonoids separated from *M. azederach* root barks, three azadirachtin-type limonoids elucidated as 1-tigloyl-3-acetyl-11-methoxymeliacarpinin (**1**), 1-acetyl-3-tigloyl-11-methoxymeliacarpinin, and 1-cinnamoyl-3-hydroxyl-11-methoxymeliacarpinin exerted cytotoxic effect on mouse P388 lymphatic leukemia cells (respective IC_{50}: 3.2, 3.3 and 1.5 μg/mL). Three sendanin-type limonoids assigned as 29-isobutylsendanin (**2**), 29-deacetylsendanin, and 12-hydroxyamoorastin showed more potent cytotoxicity against the P388 cells (IC_{50}: 0.026–0.090 μg/mL).[2,3] The nine separated trichilin-type limonoids were also potent inhibitors of the P388 cells *in vitro*. The IC_{50} values ranged from 0.011 to 0.055 μg/mL for 12-deacetyltrichilin-I (**3**), 3-deacetyltrichilin-H, and trichilin-D, whereas the IC_{50} values for 1-acetyltrichilin-H, 1-acetyl-3-deacetyltrichilin-H, 1-acetyl-2-deacetyltrichilin-H, trichilin-H, and 1,12-diacetyl-trichilin-B was 0.16–0.66 μg/mL.[4]

More limonoids were isolated from the bark of *M. azedarach*. In an assay with five human tumor cell lines (HL-60, SMMC-7721, A-549, MCF-7, and SW480), seven limonoids showed significant inhibitory activities against the tested cell lines (IC_{50}: 0.003–0.555 μM), where the A549 and SW480 cell lines were more sensitive to the seven active limonoids. The most potent effects observed were 29-isobutylsendanin (**2**) and sendanin (**4**) on MCF-7 breast cancer cells (IC_{50}: 0.003–0.004 μM), 29-isobutylsendanin (**2**) on SW480 colon cancer cells (IC_{50}: 0.005 μM), mesendanin-K (**5**) on HL-60 leukemia cells (IC_{50}: 0.020 μM), and 29-isobutylsendanin (**2**) on A549 lung carcinoma cells (IC_{50}: 0.081 μM), whereas 7-acetylsendanin showed moderate inhibitory effect on the five cancer cell lines, and mesendanin-L and 3-deacetyl-4′-demethyl-28-oxosalannin were only active to

HL-60 cells moderately. According to these IC_{50} data, the active limonoids in order of antitumor potencies were mesendanin-K (**5**) > 29-isobutylsendanin (**2**) > 29-deacetylsendanin > sendanin (**4**) > 12-hydroxyamoorastin > 1-acetylsendanin > 1,12-diacetyltrichilin-B > cisplatin (an anticancer drug) > 7-acetylsendanin >> mesendanin-L. Preliminary SARs of the limonoids revealed that the presence of a lactol bridge in C-19/C-29 and a 17β,20β-epoxy group were important for improving the cytotoxicity, and the presence of two acetyl groups located at C-7 and C-29 were responsible for reducing the potency.[5,6]

12-Acetoxyamoorastatin (**6**) (= toosendanin), 12-hydroxyamoorastatone, and 12-hydroxyamoorastatin were found from the stem bark of *M. azedarach* var. *japonica*, and toosendanin (**6**) and isotoosendanin are two major cytotoxic limonoids isolated from the bark of *M. toosendan*. All these limonoids were markedly cytotoxic to A549 (lung), SK-MEL-Z (skin), SKOV-3 (ovary), XF-498 (CNS), and HCT-15 (colon) human cancer cell lines (ED_{50}: <4 μg/mL).[7] Of the limonoids, 12-acetoxyamoorastatin (**6**) was the most cytotoxic agent (ED_{50}: 0.7–40 ng/mL), and 12-hydroxy-amoorastatin was the secondary active agent; both of which demonstrated greater cytotoxic activity than antimycin-A (an anticancer drug).[7] Also, toosendanin (**6**), by inducing a mitochondria-dependent pathway, provoked the apoptosis of human SMMC-7721 ($p53^+$) and Hep3B ($p53^-$) hepatoma cell lines, resulting in the antiproliferative effect in dose- and time-dependent manners (respective IC_{50}: 0.5 and 0.9 μM, 72 h).[8] The antihepatoma effect was further proven in a mouse model implanted with H22 hepatoma. The i.p. administration of toosendanin (**6**) in both low and high doses (0.173 and 0.69 mg/kg) promoted the apoptotic response and strongly retarded the tumorigenicity.[8] The antigrowth and apoptotic effects of toosendanin (**6**) was also demonstrated in other cell lines such as PC3 prostate cancer, U251 glioblastoma, Bel-7404 hepatoma, SH-SY5Y neuroblastoma, U937 lymphoma, and HL-60 promylocytic leukemia *in vitro* (respective IC_{50}: 0.12, 0.15, 0.026, 0.033, 0.0054, and 0.0061 nM). The antigrowth effect of toosendanin (**6**) was present in human A549 lung adenocarcinoma cells and human MDA-MB-468 hepatoma cells *in vitro* as well.[9] Moreover, toosendanin (**6**) at a concentration >1 nM elicited the differentiation of rat P12 pheochromocytoma cells and amplified the outgrowth of neuronal processes and the cell apoptotic death when the treatment lasted up to 72 h.[10] All the evidences highlighted that toosendanin (**6**) may serve as a potential candidate for the cancer therapy.

Nonlimonoid Triterpenoids

The euphane-type triterpenoids, such as kulinone (**7**), 3-oxo-olean-12-en-28-oic acid, and meliastatin-3,3β-acetoxy-12β-hydroxyeupha-7,24-dien-21,16β-olide were separated from the root barks of *M. azedarach*, exerting inhibitory effects on human HGC27 gastric carcinoma and A549 and H460 lung cancer cell lines (IC_{50}: 5.6–21.2 μg/mL). Of the triterpenes, kulinone (**7**) was more sensitive to the three human tumor cell lines. In other *in vitro* assays, kulinone (**7**) also displayed the inhibitory effects against a small panel of human tumor cell lines, i.e., MCF-7 (breast), SF268 (brain), KM20L2 (colon), H460 (lung), BXPC-3 (pancreas), and DU-145 (prostate), with GI_{50} values of 3.6–5.7 μg/mL. Additionally, the suppressive activity of kulinone (**7**) and meliastatin-3 was also displayed in P388 leukemia cells *in vitro*.[11] Methyl kulonate (**8**) was effective in inhibiting human HL-60 (leukemic), A549 (lung), SK-BR-3 (breast), and AZ521 (stomach) neoplastic cell lines *in vitro*, where its strongest effect was on HL-60 cells (IC_{50}: 5.8 versus 11.0–18.9 μM/mL).[6] The antigrowth effect of methyl kulonate, dubione-B, kulonic acid, and kulactone (**7**) were demonstrated in human Bel-7402 (liver), H460 (lung), and SGC-7901 (stomach) cancer cell lines only at concentrations above 50 μg/mL.[12] Melianone exhibited better cytotoxic activity on the A549 cells (CC_{50}: 3.6 μg/mL),[12] whereas mesendanin-M was only moderately active to HL-60 leukemia cells (IC_{50}: 17.8 μM) but inactive to A549, SW480, MCF-7, and SMMC-7721 cell lines.[5] An isolated triterpenoid assigned as 6β-hydroxy-3-oxo-13α,14β,17α-lanosta-7,24-dien-21,16β-olide was modest cytotoxic to human KB oral epidermal cell line.[13]

From the 70% ethanolic extract of *M. toosendan* stem barks, two cytotoxic tirucallane triterpenoids elucidated as 3β,16β-hydroxytirucalla-7,24(25)-dien-21,23-olide and 3β,16β-hydroxytirucalla-7,24(25)-dien-6-oxo-21,23-olide were isolated, which exerted marked growth-suppressive effect against A549 (lung), SKOV-3 (ovarian), SK-MEL-2 (skin), and NCT15 (colon) human cancer cell line *in vitro* (IC_{50}: 3.2–5.7 μg/mL).[14]

Steroids

Several hydroperoxysterols were separated from the stem barks of *M. azedarach*, demonstrating moderate antiproliferative activity. All the sterols were found to have the inhibitory effect on three human carcinoma cell lines, HGC27 (stomach) and A549 and H460 (lung), *in vitro*. The IC_{50} values were 5.6–21.2 μg/mL for 24ξ-Hydroperoxy-24-vinylcholesterol (**9**), 29-hydroperoxy-stigmasta-7,24(28)E-dien-3β-ol (**10**), 24ξ-hydro peroxy-24-vinyllathosterol, and (22E,24S)-5α,8α-epidioxy-24-methylcholesta-6,22-dien-3β-ol. More antitumor effects of 24ξ-hydroperoxy-24-vinylcholesterol (**9**) were shown in p388 leukemia, KB oral epidermal cancer, and HT-29 colon cancer cell lines (ED_{50}: 0.3–7.1 μg/mL). 2α,3α,20R-Trihydroxy-5α-pregnane16β-methacrylate was only active to HGC27 gastric carcinoma cells (IC_{50}: 11.3 μg/mL), whereas (22E,24S)-5α,8α-epidioxy-24-methylcholesta-6,22-dien-3β-ol and sendanolactone were moderate inhibitors on human A2780 ovarian cancer and KB oral epidermal cell lines, respectively.[11,12]

Polysaccharides

A polysaccharide designated as MA9 was extracted from the dried barks of *M. azadirachta* or *M. indica*, whose obtained MA9 was approved with a Japanese patent for having antitumor property.[15]

Other Bioactivities

The herb Ku Lian Pi (Chinaberry tree bark) has been used as a traditional Chinese medicine to cure dermatosis and to repel worms. Pharmacological studies have proven that the herb possesses several therapeutic properties such as anthelminthic, antifungal, antimalarial, antibacterial, and antioxidant activities. Its leaf extract displayed antiinfertility and antiviral activities. Ku Lian Pi is also traditionally used as an insecticide.

References

1. Li, G. Y., Zhi, G. 2012. Antitumor activity of cortex meliae extracts. *Anhui Nongye Kexue* 40: 6433–4.
2. Itokawa, H. et al. 1995. Cytotoxic limonoids and tetranotriterpenoids from *Melia azedarach. Chem. Pharm. Bull.* 43: 1171–5.
3. Takeya, K. et al. 1996. Cytotoxic azadirachtin-type limonoids from *Melia azedarach. Phytochem.* 42: 709–12.
4. Takeya, K. et al. 1996. Cytotoxic trichilin-type limonoids from *Melia azedarach. Bioorg. Med. Chem.* 4: 1355–9.
5. Yuan, C. M. et al. 2013. Cytotoxic limonoids from *Melia azedarach. Planta Med.* 79: 163–8.
6. Pan, X. et al. 2014. Cytotoxic and nitric oxide production-inhibitory activities of limonoids and other compounds from the leaves and bark of *Melia azedarach. Chem. Biodivers.* 11: 1121–39.
7. Ahn, J. W. et al. 1994. Cytotoxic limonoids from *Melia azedarach* var. *japonica. Phytochem.* 36: 1493–6.
8. He, Y. J. et al. 2010. Toosendanin inhibits hepatocellular carcinoma cells by inducing mitochondria-dependent apoptosis. *Planta Med.* 76: 1447–53.
9. Zhang, B. et al. 2005. Growth inhibition and apoptosis-induced effect on human cancer cells of toosendanin, a triterpenoid derivative from Chinese traditional medicine. *Investig. New Drugs* 23: 547–53.
10. Tang, M. Z. et al. 2003. Toosendanin induces outgrowth of neuronal processes and apoptosis in PC12 cells. *Neurosci. Res.* 45: 225–31.
11. Wu, S. B. et al. 2011. Cytotoxic triterpenoids and steroids from the bark of *Melia azedarach. Planta. Med.* 77: 922–8.
12. Faizi, S. H. et al. 2002. New terpenoids from the roots of *Melia azedarach. Australian J. Chem.* 55: 291–6.
13. Caboni, P. et al. 2012. Isolation and chemical characterization of components with biological activity extracted from Azadirachta indica and *Melia azedarach. ACS Symposium Series* 1093: 51–77.
14. Zhao, Q. J. et al. 2012. Cytotoxic tirucallane triterpenoids from the stem bark of *Melia toosendan. Archiv. Pharm. Res.* 35: 1903–7.
15. Shimizu, M. et al. 1987. Method for extracting polysaccharide MA9 with antitumor effect from *Melia azedarach. Jpn. Kokai Tokkyo Koho* JP 62185022 A 19870813.

223 Ku Lian Zi 苦楝子

Chinaberry fruit

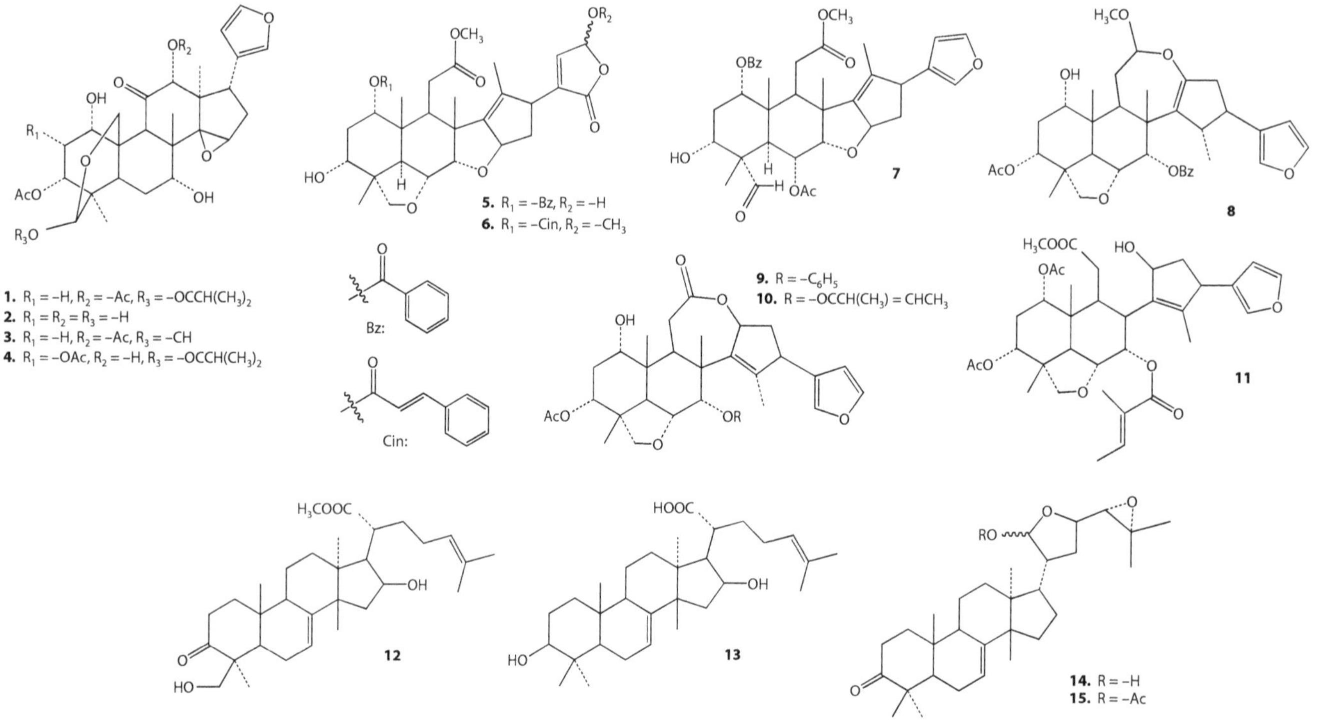

1. R_1 = –H, R_2 = –Ac, R_3 = –OCCH(CH$_3$)$_2$
2. R_1 = R_2 = R_3 = –H
3. R_1 = –H, R_2 = –Ac, R_3 = –CH
4. R_1 = –OAc, R_2 = –H, R_3 = –OCCH(CH$_3$)$_2$

5. R_1 = –Bz, R_2 = –H
6. R_1 = –Cin, R_2 = –CH_3

Bz: Cin:

7 **8**

9. R = –C_6H_5
10. R = –OCCH(CH$_3$) = CHCH$_3$

11 **12** **13**

14. R = –H
15. R = –Ac

Herb Origination

The herb Ku Lian Zi (Chinaberry fruit) originates from the fruits of a Meliaceae tree, *Melia azedarach* L. Its fruits are harvested when they are ripe in autumn and winter and dried in the sun or by oven for medicinal application. Another Meliaceae tree, *M. toosendan*, is one of the sources for producing the herb Ku Lian Pi (Chinaberry tree bark); however, its dried fruit is termed Chuan Lian Zi (Fructus toosendan), which is traditionally used as a different herb.

Antitumor Constituents and Activities

A defatted fraction derived from the hexane extract of the fruits, in an *in vitro* assay, exerted obvious suppressive effect against the proliferation of human neoplastic cell lines such as HL-60 leukemia (IC_{50}: 2.9 μg/mL), A549 lung cancer and AZ521 gastric cancer (IC_{50}: 12.0–12.3 μg/mL), and SK-BR-3 breast cancer (IC_{50}: 21.9 μg/mL) *in vitro*.[1] Similar to Ku Lian Pi (Chinaberry tree bark), triterpenoid constituents, especially limonoids, are the major cancer inhibitors in Ku Lian Zi.

Intact Limonoids

12-*O*-Acetylazedarachin-B (**1**) displayed potent cytotoxicity against human HL-60 leukemia cells (IC_{50}: 0.016 μM) and human AZ521 gastric cancer cells (IC_{50}: 0.035 μM) but only moderate effect on human A549 lung adenocarcinoma cells (IC_{50}: 19 μM), whose anticancer potencies were about 100 times than those of cisplatin in HL-60 and AZ521 cell lines (IC_{50}: 1.9 and 2.7 μM, respectively). The cytotoxicity of 12-*O*-acetylazedarachin-B (**1**) on AZ521 cells was found to be associated with the promotion of apoptosis in the HL-60 and AZ521 cells and also predominately with the activation of necrosis in the AZ521 cells. The necrotic cell death of AZ521 by 12-*O*-acetylazedarachin-B (**1**) was found to be induced by the participation of Fas receptor signaling, whereas the apoptosis of HL-60 was mediated by both mitochondrial- and death receptor-signal transduction pathways.[2] 3-Deacetyl-4′-demethyl-28-oxosalannin (**3**) against HL60 and AZ521 cells, and methyl kulonate (**10**) against HL60 cells exhibited potent cytotoxicities with IC_{50} values in the range of 2.8–5.8 μM.

More detailed phytochemical investigations resulted in the separation of 31 limonoids from the fruits. All the limonoids were evaluated for the cytotoxicity with HL-60, A549, AZ521, and SK-BR-3 human cancer cell lines *in vitro*, and most of them were effective in the inhibition of HL-60 leukemia cells. Two trichilin-type limonoids assigned as toosendanin (**2**) (a C-29 epimeric mixture) and meliarachin-C (**3**) exhibited the potent cytotoxic effect on HL-60 leukemia cells (respective IC_{50}: 0.005 and 0.65 μM) and on AZ521 gastric cancer cells (respective IC_{50}: 0.009 and 1.5 μM), whose potencies were superior than two antitumor drugs, cisplatin (IC_{50}: 4.2 and 9.5 μM) and 5-FU (IC_{50}: 6.3 and 28.7 μM), on the HL-60 and AZ521 cells, respectively.[3] The IC_{50} values of 1-*O*-cinnamoyltrichilinin, 12-dehydro-29-oxo-neoazedarachin-D, 3-deacetyl-1,6-diacetylsendanal, and 12-dehydroneoazedarachin-D were 3.6–11.8 μM in the HL-60 cells and 11.8–22.4 μM in the AZ521 cells.[1,3] Another isolated trichilin-type limonoid assigned as 12-*O*-deacetyltrichilin-H (**4**) was notably effective in the suppression of HeLa-S3 cervical cancer cells (IC_{50}: 0.48 μM).[4] These evidences have thus provided a further development base for the four trichilin-type limonoids, especially, toosendanin (**2**), which can be considered as a promising drug lead.

C-seco Limonoids

Many C-seco limonoids isolated from the herb demonstrated marked to moderate antigrowth effect against HL-60 leukemia cells *in vitro*. The inhibitory effect (IC_{50}: 2.8–5.8 μM) of 3-*O*-deacetyl-4′-demethyl-28-oxo-salannin (**5**), 23-methoxyohchininolide-A (**6**), 1-*O*-detigloyl-1-*O*-benzoylohchinolal (**7**), and nimbolinin-D (**8**) were comparable to those of cisplatin and 5-FU on the HL-60 cells.[1,3] In the assays, 3-*O*-deacetyl-4′-demethyl-28-oxosalannin (IC_{50}: 3.2 μM) and 1-detigloylohchinolal (IC_{50} 7.3 μM) presented greater activity than cisplatin (IC_{50}: 9.5 μM) on the AZ521 cells. 1-*O*-Decinnamoyl-1-*O*-benzoyl-23-hydroxyohchininolide and 1-*O*-decinnamoyl-1-*O*-benzoylohchinin exerted marked inhibitory effect on SK-BR-3 breast carcinoma cells (IC_{50}: 4.3 and 14.9 μM, respectively), whose IC_{50} values were lower than that of cisplatin (IC_{50}: 18.8 μM).[1,3]

From the methanol extract of the ripe fruits of *M. azedarach*, which grows in Brazil, several cytotoxic C-seco limonoids were isolated. The elucidated C-seco limonoids, such as 1-*O*-Deacetylohchinolide-A (**9**), 1-*O*-deacetylohchinolide-B (**10**), and 15-*O*-deacetylnimbolidin-B (**11**), exhibited obvious inhibitory activity on human HeLa-S3 cervical cancer cells (IC_{50}: 2.4, 0.1, and 0.1 μM, respectively), whose cytotoxic activity were greater than cisplatin and 5-FU (IC_{50}: 2.46–5.40 μM). Other five isolated C-seco limonoids (such as 15-*O*-deacetyl-15-*O*-methylnimbolidin-A and 15-*O*-deacetyl-15-*O*-methyl-nimbolidin-B) showed moderate to weak inhibitory effects on HeLa-S3 cells (IC_{50}: 28–37 μM),[4,5] whereas 11-α-hydroxy-1-cinnamoyl-3-feruloylmeliacarpin was cytotoxic to human MCF-7 breast cancer cells (LC_{50}: 1.75 μM).[6]

Tirucallane-Type Triterpenoids

Several tirucallane-type triterpenoids separated from Ku Lian Zi displayed different degrees of antiproliferative activity against human tumor cells *in vitro*. Meliasenin-E (**12**) showed the antiproliferative effect on A549 (lung), AZ520 (gastric), and SK-BR-3 (breast) cancer cell lines (respective IC_{50}: 6.7, 11.9, and 18.6 μM),[3] and azedaradic acid (**13**) exerted moderate to weak inhibitory effect on HL-60 (leukemic), AZ520 (gastric), and SK-BR-3 (breast) cancer cell lines (respective IC_{50}: 4.6, 21.5, and 49.7 μM).[1] Melianone (**14**) was cytotoxic to the A549 cell line, while 21-β-acetoxymelianone (**15**) and 3-α-tigoylmelianol only presented certain inhibitory effect against the proliferation of A549 cells *in vitro*.[7]

Polysaccharides

Crude water-soluble heteropolysaccharides were extracted from the fruit pulps of *M. azedarach*, from which a major heteropolysaccharide designated as MPS-III was obtained by chromatographic separation. It contains an α-(1–4) main chain backbone composed of arabinose and mannose in a molar ratio of 1.31:1.0 and has an α-(1–6) branch structure. MPS-III demonstrated obvious anticancer effect on human BGC-823 gastric carcinoma cell line *in vitro*.[8]

References

1. Pan, X. et al. 2014. Three new and other limonoids from the hexane extract of *Melia azedarach* fruits and their cytotoxic activities. *Chem. Biodivers.* 11: 987–1000.
2. Kikuchi, T. et al. 2013. Cytotoxic and apoptosis-inducing activities of 12-*O*-acetylazedarachin B from the fruits of *Melia azedarach* in human cancer cell lines. *Biol. Pharm. Bull.* 36: 135–9.
3. Akihisa, T. et al. 2013. Limonoids from the fruits of *Melia azedarach* and their cytotoxic activities. *Phytochem.* 89: 59–70.
4. Zhou, H. et al. 2005. Cytotoxic limonoids from Brazilian *Melia azedarach. Chem Pharm Bull.* 53: 1362–5.
5. Zhou, H. L. et al. 2004. New ring C-seco limonoids from Brazilian *Melia azedarach* and their cytotoxic activity. *J. Nat. Prod.* 67: 1544–7.
6. Ayyad, S. N. et al. 2008. New nimbolinin and meliacarpin derivatives from *Melia azedarach. Revista Latinoamericana de Quimica* 36: 7–15.
7. Ntalli, N. G. et al. 2010. Cytotoxic tirucallane triterpenoids from *Melia azedarach* fruits. *Mol.* 15: 5866–77.
8. He, L. et al. 2009. A new heteropolysaccharide purified from MA fruit exhibited cytotoxic activity on BGC-823 cell line. *Fitoterapia* 80: 399–403.

224 Chuan Lian Zi 川楝子

Fructus toosendan

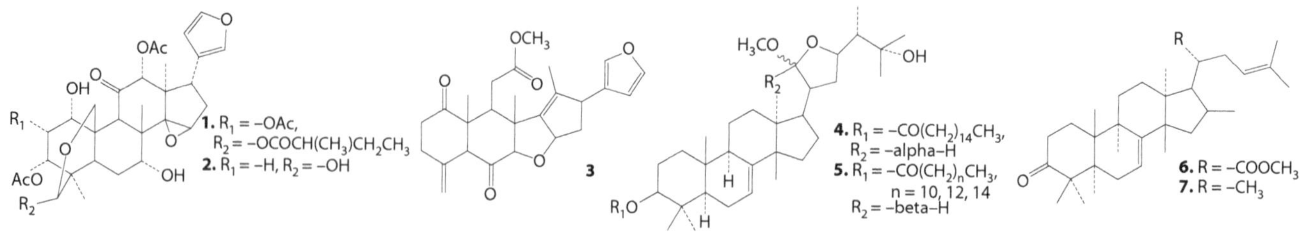

1. R_1 = –OAc, R_2 = –OCOCH(CH_3)CH_2CH_3
2. R_1 = –H, R_2 = –OH

3

4. R_1 = –CO(CH_2)$_{14}$$CH_3$, R_2 = –alpha–H
5. R_1 = –CO(CH_2)$_n$$CH_3$, n = 10, 12, 14, R_2 = –beta–H

6. R = –$COOCH_3$
7. R = –CH_3

Herb Origination

The herb Chuan Lian Zi (Fructus toosendan) is the dried fruits of a Meliaceae plant, *Melia toosendan*. The fruits are collected when they turn to yellow in November and December and dried in the sun or by oven. The stem bark and the root bark of *M. toosendan* are used in traditional Chinese medicine as an herb Ku Lian Pi. Chuan Lian Zi and Ku Lian Zi are traditionally classified as two different herbs in China, but Chuan Lian Zi is more commonly utilized in herb prescriptions compared to Ku Lian Zi.

Antitumor Constituents and Activities

The extract of Chuan Lian Zi could dose-dependently reduce the growth of rat PC12 pheochromocytoma cells and induce the differentiation of PC12 cells via the activation of protein kinase A and ERKs.[1] Its ethanolic extract inhibited the cell proliferation of SW480 human colon cancer cells and CT26 murine colorectal adenocarcinoma cells by promoting apoptotic death *in vitro*. In a mouse model with the CT26 tumor, the tumor volume-reducing and apoptosis-inducing effects were observed and no obvious side effects were shown after the extract treatment.[2] Similar to Ku Lian Pi (Chinaberry root bark), its triterpenoid constituents mostly contributed to the cytotoxicity of Chuan Lian Zi.

Triterpenoids

Similar to the constituents in *Melia azedarach*, triterpenoids is the major constituents in the fruits of *M. toosendan*, many of which showed marked cytotoxic effect.

Limonoid-Type Triterpenoids

12-*O*-acetyltrichilin-B (**1**) at a 10^{-7} mol/L concentration markedly inhibited the proliferation of A549 (lung) and HL-60 (leukemic) human cancer cell lines by 70.0% and 87.2%, respectively.[3] A limonoid assigned as 28-deacetyl sendanin (**2**) demonstrated potent cytotoxicity in various human tumor cell lines. The most sensitive cells to 28-deacetyl sendanin (**2**) were SF-539 (CNS) and PC3 (prostate) human cancer cell lines (GI_{50}: <0.0001 μg/mL). 28-Deacetyl sendanin (**2**) also obstructed the proliferation of Hepa1c1c7 and HepG2 hepatoma cell lines (respective GI_{50}: 0.238 and 0.805 μg/mL) and of M14 (skin), SW620 and KM12 (colon), and ACHN (renal) cancer cell lines (GI_{50}: 0.017–0.071 μg/mL), whose inhibitions were 6.74–651 times more potent than those of adriamycin (Adm.)[4,5] At concentrations between 0.025 and 50 μg/mL, 28-deacetyl sendanin (**2**) elicited the morphological change of human MCF-7 breast cancer cells, but NCI-H23 lung cancer and UO-231 renal cancer cell lines were resistant in the treatment,[4,5] and mouse lymphocytes were more sensitive to the limonoid (**2**) compared to the hepatoma cells.[5] The cytotoxicity of toosendanin was shown in various human cancer cell lines such as PC3 (prostate), Bel-7404 (liver), U251 and SH-SY5Y (CNS), and U937 (histocyte) human tumor cells (IC_{50}: 0.0054–0.15 μM).[6] The growth inhibition of toosendanin on HL-60 cells (IC_{50}: 28 ng/mL, 48 h) was due to induction of the cell apoptosis and S cell arrest via the blockage of CDC42/MEKK1/JNK signaling pathways.[7] Also, the activation of deoxycytidine kinase might be partially involved in the apoptotic effects of toosendanin in the HL-60 cells (see Section Ku Lian Zi).[8] Other isolated nimbolinin-type limonoids were elucidated as toosendalinin (**3**), nimbolinin-A (**4**), nimbolinin-B (**5**), and deacetylnimbolinin-B (**6**), which showed moderate suppressive effect against the proliferation of human HepG2 hepatoma cells (IC_{50}: 6.4–9.2 μmol/L) *in vitro*.[9] Recently, a new limonoid compound (**7**) isolated from Chuan Lian Zi was patented for the treatment of cervical cancer, which showed high inhibitive activity on cervical cancer cells and low cytotoxicity on normal cells.[10]

Nonlimonoid-Type Triterpenoids

A group of euphane-type and tirucallane-type triterpenoids such as methyl kulonate, kulinone, meliasenins-I–R, meliastatin-3 and meliastatin-5 were separated from the fruits of *M. toosendan*. Some of them were markedly cytotoxic to human U20S osteosarcoma and MCF-7 breast cancer cell lines (IC_{50}: <10 μg/mL), whose potency was similar or greater compared to 5-FU, and some were moderately cytotoxic (IC_{50}: <48.7 μg/mL). Meliasenin-Q (**8**) showed relatively strong cytotoxicity against U20S cells (IC_{50}: 3.9 μg/mL) but inactive to MCF-7 cells *in vitro*.[11] Meliasenin-R (**9**), which has a different C-21 configuration compared to meliasenin-Q (**8**), was inactive to the U20S cells, implying that the C-21 configuration was importantly correlated to the antiproliferative effect on U20S osteosarcoma cells. Methyl kulonate (**10**) displayed the most potent cytotoxic effect against the MCF-7 cells *in vitro* (IC_{50}: 0.41 μg/mL), whereas its C-21 methoxycarbonylated derivative, kulinone (**11**), was about 100 times less active on the MCF-7 cells. In addition, mouse P388 leukemia cells was sensitive to meliastatin-3 and meliastatin-5, methyl kulonate (**10**), and kulinone (**11**), and their ED_{50} values ranged between 1.7 and 5.1 μg/mL.[11]

Steroids

Two steroids elucidated as (20*S*)-5-stigmastene-3β,7α,16β,20-tetrol and (20*S*)-5-ergostene-3β,7α,16β,20-tetrol were obtained from the systemic separation of the herb. Both steroids were tested in human U20S osteosarcoma and MCF-7 breast neoplastic cells *in vitro*, exerting obvious suppressive effect against the proliferation of U20S cells (respective IC_{50}: 23.2 and 9.4 μg/mL); however, both were less cytotoxic to the MCF-7 cells.[11]

Polysaccharides

A water-soluble heteropolysaccharide designated as pMTPS-3 was isolated from the fruits of *M. toosendan*, which is composed of arabinose, glucose, mannose, and galactose in a molar ratio of 17.3:28.3:41.6:12.6 with a molecular weight of 26.1 kDa. The purified pMTPS-3 was revealed to have prominent antitumor and antioxidant potentials, where it markedly restrained human BGC-823 gastric carcinoma cells *in vitro* concomitant with obvious DPPH radical-scavenging and moderate superoxide radical-inhibiting effects.[12] The results highlighted that pMTPS-3 may be a promising cancer preventive and antioxidant supplement.

References

1. Yu, J. C. et al. 2004. *Melia toosendan* regulates PC12 cell differentiation via the activation of protein kinase A and extracellular signal-regulated kinases. *Neurosignals* 13: 248–57.
2. Tang, X. L. et al. 2012. Protective effects of the ethanolic extract of *Melia toosendan* fruit against colon cancer *Indian J. Biochem. Biophys.* 49: 173–81.
3. Zhang, Y. et al. 2012. Limonoids from the fruits of *Melia toosendan. Phytochem.* 73: 106–13.
4. Kim, H. M. et al. 1994. Comparative effects of adriamycin and 28-deacetyl sendanin on in vitro growth inhibition of human cancer cell lines. *Archiv. Pharm. Res.* 17: 100–3.
5. Kim, Y. H. et al. 1994. The cytotoxic limonoid from the fruits of *Melia toosendan. Yakhak Hoechi* 38: 6–11.
6. Zhang, B. et al. 2005. Growth inhibition and apoptosis induced effect on human cancer cells of toosendanin, a triterpenoid derivative from Chinese traditional medicine. *Invest. New Drugs* 23: 547–53.
7. Ju, J. M. et al. 2013. Toosendanin induces apoptosis through suppression of JNK signaling pathway in HL-60 cells. *Toxicol. In Vitro* 27: 232–8.
8. Ju, J. M. et al. 2012. The apoptotic effects of toosendanin are partially mediated by activation of deoxycytidine kinase in HL-60 cells. *PLoS One* 7: e52536.
9. Liu, Y. K. et al. 2013. Extraction and application of *Melia toosendan* seeds. *Faming Zhuanli Shenqing* CN 102940687 A 201210524604.
10. Hu, W. J. 2015. Limonin compound isolated from *Melia toosendan* fruit useful in treatment of cervical cancer. *Faming Zhuanli Shenqing* CN 104447650 A 20150325.
11. Wu, S. B. et al. 2010. Triterpenoids and steroids from the fruits of *Melia toosendan* and their cytotoxic effects on two human cancer cell lines. *J. Nat. Prod.* 73: 1898–906.
12. He, L. et al. 2011. Physico-chemical characterization, antioxidant and anticancer activities in vitro of a novel polysaccharide from *Melia toosendan* Sieb. et Zucc fruit. *Intl. J. Biol. Macromol.* 49: 422–7.

14

Anticancer Potentials of Other Herbs

CONTENTS

225 Chou Chun 臭椿

Tree of heaven or Ailanthus

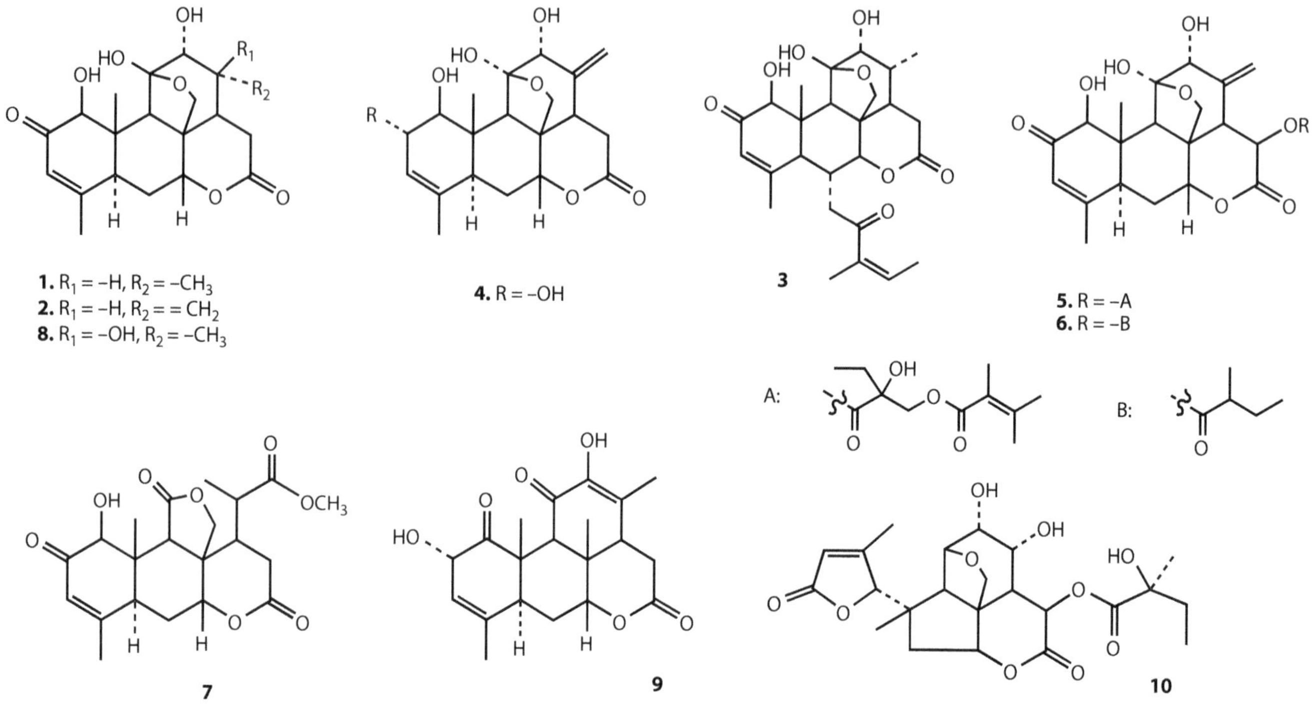

1. R_1 = -H, R_2 = -CH_3
2. R_1 = -H, R_2 = =CH_2
8. R_1 = -OH, R_2 = -CH_3

4. R = -OH

3

5. R = -A
6. R = -B

7 **9** **10**

(a)

11 **12** **13** **14** **15**

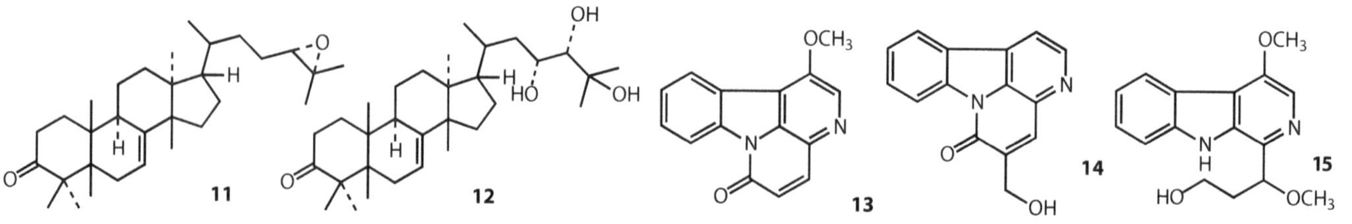

(b)

Herb Origination

Chou Chun (tree of heaven) is a deciduous Simaroubaceae tree, *Ailanthus altissima*. The plant is native to China from northeast and central regions to Taiwan as well as North Korea. The tree was first brought from China to Europe in the 1740s and to Philadelphia in the United States in 1784, and it has been extensively used as a street tree since the nineteenth century. In China, the tree of heaven has a long and rich medical history. Its root bark and stem bark are generally collected in spring and autumn and then dried in the sun for the folk medical use.

Antitumor Activities and Constituents

Phytochemical investigations revealed that the constituents of this plant are quassinoids, α-carboline alkaloids, sterols, and lipids. From the Chou Chun barks, many quassinoid-type triterpenes and canthin-6-one or β-carborine-type alkaloids were found to be the major inhibitors against carcinoma cell growth by *in vitro* or *in vivo* investigations.

Quassinoids

Many quassinoid-type triterpenes have been separated from the stem barks of *A. altissima*, and most of them demonstrated different degrees of cytotoxicity on the tested neoplastic cells. Chaparrinone (**1**) exhibited significant cytotoxic effect against human KB nasopharyngeal carcinoma cells *in vitro* with an ED_{50} value of 0.142 μg/mL and against mouse P388 leukemia cell growth *in vivo*.[1] (–)-Chaparrinone (**1**), ailanthone (**2**), 6α-tigloyloxychaparrinone (**3**), shinjulactone-A (**4**), altissinol-A (**5**) and altissinol-B (**6**) and 13,18-dehydroglaucarubinone were cytotoxic to human Hep3B and HepG2 hepatoma cell lines (IC_{50}: 0.05–8.01 μM). Of them, ailanthone (**2**), 6α-tigloyloxychaparrinone (**3**), and altissinol-A (**5**) exerted greater inhibitory effect on the two hepatoma cells (IC_{50}: 0.05–0.55 μM), and ailanthone (**2**), 6α-tigloyloxychaparrinone (**3**), and 13,18-dehydroglaucarubinone moderately restrained the multidrug-resistant HepG2/ADM cell line (IC_{50}: 10.64–19.62 μM), whose anti-MDR effects were more potent than that of DOX (IC_{50}: 85.46 μM).[2] Analysis of the activity and the structural relationships revealed that a methylenoxy bridge between C-8 and C-13 and the α,β-unsaturated ketone groups in the A-ring were the important structural features for the increase of the cytotoxic activity on the Hep3B and HepG2 cells.[2] Shinjulactone-A (**4**) and shinjuglycoside-B were moderately effective in the suppression of human U87 primary glioblastoma cells and human SF188 glioblastoma cells *in vitro*.[3] In addition, 6α-tigloyloxychaparrinone (**3**) is an inhibitor of HIF-1α activation, playing antineoplastic roles in various human neoplastic cell lines by blocking HIF-1α translation and HIF-1α protein synthesis and inhibiting eIF4E phosphorylation pathway. The treatment concurrently reduced the phosphorylation levels of eIF4E, MNK1, and ERK1/2.[4] Also, ailanthone (**2**), ailantinol-A (**7**), ailantinol-B (**8**), ailantinol-E, ailantinol-F (**9**), ailantinol-G (**10**), shinjulactone-A (**4**), and shinjulactone-C also exerted modest antitumor-promoting effects against TPA-induced EBV-EA in Raji cells,[5] but ailantinol-E, ailantinol-F (**9**), and ailantinol-G (**10**) were not cytotoxic to the cancer cells.[6] The structural modification of shinjulactone-C to its succinate or its 3′,3′-dimethylsuccinate could augment the suppressive activity against the TPA-promoted tumorigenesis.[7] Likewise, eight quassinoids includin shinjulactone-O were isolated from the 50% ethanol extract of the root bark of *A. altissima*. The quassinoids exhibited different levels of inhibitory activity on MCF-7 and MDA-MB-231 (breast), HepG2 (liver), and A549 (lung) human tumor cell lines.[8]

Tirucallanes

Two tirucallane-type triterpenoids assigned as piscidinol-A (**11**) and niloticin (**12**) were found to exhibit comparable cytotoxicity against murine P388 leukemia cells (IC_{50}: 2.5–3.3 μM) and human KB nasopharynx carcinoma cells (IC_{50}: 10.5–18.2 μM) and moderate cytotoxicity against four human BGC-823 and KE-97 (stomach), Huh-7 (liver), and Jurkat (T-lymphoma) neoplastic cell lines in an *in vitro* model.[9,10]

β-Carborines

Three anticancer alkaloids identified as 1-methoxycanthin-6-one (**13**), 5-(hydroxymethyl) canthin-6-one (**14**), and 1-(2-hydroxy-1-methoxyethyl)-4-methoxy-β-carborine (**15**) were obtained from the isolation of a chloroform extract of the Chou Chun root. 1-Methoxycanthin-6-one (**13**) notably promotes c-Jun NH2-terminal kinase-dependent apoptosis in seven tested human cell lines such as U87MG (glioblastoma-astrocytoma), SAOS (epithelial-like osteosarcoma), ARO and NPA (thyroid cancer), U937 (histiocytic lymphoma), Jurkat (leukemia), HuH7 (hepatoma), and HeLa (cervix cancer) cells together with mitochondrial membrane depolarization, mitochondrial releases of cytochrome c, Smac/DIABLO, and cleavage of procaspase-3.[11,12] 1-Methoxycanthin-6-one (**13**) in a cotreatment synergized the apoptosis-inducing effects of TRAIL in the four cell lines (Jurkat, ARO, NPA, and HuH7).[11] Both 5-(hydroxyl-methyl)-canthin-6-one (**14**) and 1-(2-hydroxy-1-methoxyethyl)-4-methoxy-β-carborine (**15**) were not only cancer growth inhibitors but also vasodilators and inhibitors of phosphordiesterase and platelet agglutination.[13,14]

Other Bioactivities

The herb Chou Chun-Pi (tree of heaven's root bark and stem bark) was mentioned in the oldest extant Chinese herb dictionary for its purported ability to cure ailments ranging from mental illness to baldness. In present Chinese folk medicine clinics, the barks, the roots, and the leaves are still in application, primarily as an astringent. Pharmacological studies approved that the Chou Chun barks have antipurgative and anthelaminthic potentials. Ailanthone (**2**) also acts as an amebicide agent.

References

1. Wani, M. C. et al. 1978. 6α-Senecioyloxychaprrinone, a new antileukemia quassinoid from *Simaba multiflora*. *J. Nat. Prod.* 41: 578–9.
2. Wang, Y. et al. 2013. Cytotoxic quassinoids from *Ailanthus altissima*. Bioorg. *Med. Chem. Lett.* 23: 654–7.
3. Zhao, C. C. et al. 2010. Studies on the antitumor constituents of fruits of *Ailanthus altissima* (Mill) Swingle. *Yangzhou Daxue Xuebao, Ziran Kexueban* 13: 39–41.
4. Jin, X. J. et al. 2008. A quassinoid 6α-tigloyloxychaparrinone inhibits hypoxia-inducible factor-1 pathway by inhibition of eukaryotic translation initiation factor 4E phosphorylation. *Eur. J. Pharmacol.* 592: 41–7.
5. Kubota, K. et al. 1997. Quassinoids as inhibitors of Epstein-Barr virus early antigen activation. *Cancer Lett.* 113: 165–8.
6. Tamura, S. et al. 2003. Three new quassinoids, ailantinol E, F, and G, from *Ailanthus altissima*. *Chem. Pharm. Bull.* 51: 385–9.
7. Tamura, S. et al. 2002. Cancer chemopreventive effect of quassinoid derivatives. Introduction of side chain to shinjulactone C for enhancement of inhibitory effect on Epstein-Barr virus activation. *Cancer Lett.* 185: 47–51.
8. Yang, X. L. et al. 2014. Shinjulactone O, a new quassinoid from the root bark of *Ailanthus altissima*. *Nat. Prod. Res.* 28: 1432–7.
9. Lavhale, M. S. et al. 2009. A novel triterpenoid isolated from the root bark of Ailanthus excelsa Roxb (Tree of Heaven), AECHL-1 as a potential anticancer agent. *PloS One* 4: e5365.
10. Hong, Z. L. et al. 2013. Tetracyclic triterpenoids and terpenylated coumarins from the bark of *Ailanthus altissima* ("Tree of Heaven") *Phytochem.* 86: 159–67.
11. Ammirante, M. et al. 2006. 1-Methoxycanthin-6-One induces c-Jun NH2-terminal kinase-dependent apoptosis and synergizes with tumor necrosis factor-related apoptosis-inducing ligand activity in human neoplastic cells of hematopoietic or endodermal origin. *Cancer Res.* 66: 4385–93.
12. Kakun Pharm. Co. Ltd. JP. 1985. The physiologically active hydroxymethylcanthinone from *Ailanthus altissima*. *Jpn. Kokai Tokkyo Koho* JP 60112791 A 19850619.
13. De Feo, V. et al. 2005. Antiproliferative effects of tree of-heaven-(*Ailanthus altissima* Swingle). *Phytother. Res.* 19: 226–30.
14. Oomoto, T. et al. 1985. β-Carborines from *Ailanthus altissima*. *Jpn. Kokai Tokkyo Koho* JP 60132984 A 19850716.

226 Jian Du Mu 箭毒木

Upas tree or Antiaris

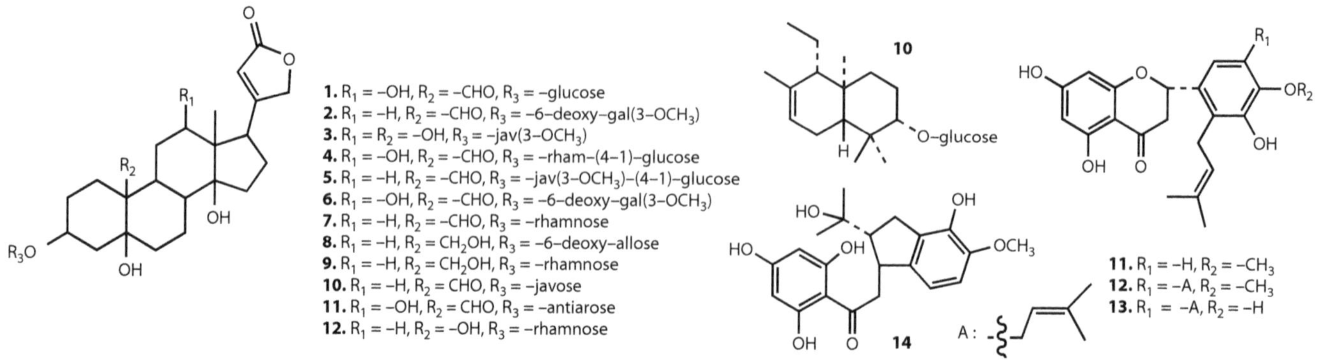

1. R_1 = –OH, R_2 = –CHO, R_3 = –glucose
2. R_1 = –H, R_2 = –CHO, R_3 = –6–deoxy–gal(3–OCH_3)
3. R_1 = R_2 = –OH, R_3 = –jav(3–OCH_3)
4. R_1 = –OH, R_2 = –CHO, R_3 = –rham–(4–1)–glucose
5. R_1 = –H, R_2 = –CHO, R_3 = –jav(3–OCH_3)–(4–1)–glucose
6. R_1 = –OH, R_2 = –CHO, R_3 = –6–deoxy–gal(3–OCH_3)
7. R_1 = –H, R_2 = –CHO, R_3 = –rhamnose
8. R_1 = –H, R_2 = CH_2OH, R_3 = –6–deoxy–allose
9. R_1 = –H, R_2 = CH_2OH, R_3 = –rhamnose
10. R_1 = –H, R_2 = CHO, R_3 = –javose
11. R_1 = –OH, R_2 = CHO, R_3 = –antiarose
12. R_1 = –H, R_2 = –OH, R_3 = –rhamnose

11. R_1 = –H, R_2 = –CH_3
12. R_1 = –A, R_2 = –CH_3
13. R_1 = –A, R_2 = –H

Herb Origination

The herb Jian Du Mu (Upas tree) is the latex of *Antiaris toxicaria* (Moraceae), whose tall tree plant is widespread in the tropical rainforests of Southeast Asia, the islands of the Pacific Ocean (east to Fiji and Tonga), northern Australia, and middle of Africa regions. The plant is most famous for producing poisonous latex used by natives on arrow tips, darts and blowguns. In China, this plant is known as arrow poison wood.

Antitumor Constituents and Activities

The major and rich components in the plant (latex, seeds, and stems) were revealed to be cardenolides, which were in response to the anticancer and anticarcinogenic properties in the *in vitro* assays. Some minor components such as sesquiterpenoids, flavonoids, and lignans were also isolated as cancer inhibitors in the continuing phytochemical investigations.

Cardenolides

Cardenolides from the Latex

Most cardiac glycosides isolated from Jian Du Mu demonstrated different degrees of cytotoxicity on a variety of neoplastic cell lines *in vitro*. Toxicarioside-F (**1**), toxicarioside-G (**2**), and toxicarioside-H (**3**) derived from the latex exerted significant cytotoxicity against human tumor cell lines (SMMC-7721, SGC-7901, HeLa, and K562),[1,2] whereas the notable cytotoxicity of toxicarioside-E (**4**) and toxicarioside-I (**5**) mainly presented in K562, SGC-7901, and/or SMMC-7721 cell lines,[3,4] The inhibitory potencies were toxicarioside-F (**1**) (IC_{50}: 0.006 μg/mL) > toxicarioside-I (**5**) (IC_{50}: 0.008 μg/mL) > toxicarioside-G (**2**) (IC_{50}: 0.01 μg/mL) > toxicarioside -H (**3**) (IC_{50}: 0.012 μg/mL) > toxicarioside-E (**4**) (IC_{50}: 0.027 μg/mL) in the SGC-7901 gastric cancer cells, while toxicarioside-F (**1**) = toxicarioside-I (**5**) (IC_{50}: 0.001 μg/mL) > toxicarioside-H (**3**) (IC_{50}: 0.004 μg/mL) > toxicarioside-G (**2**) (IC_{50}: 0.009 μg/mL) in the SMMC-7721 hepatoma cells, which were more potent than an anticancer agent mitomycin-C (respective IC_{50}: 8.8 and 2.2 μg/mL). The IC_{50} values ranged from 0.002 to 0.013 μg/mL in HeLa cervical cancer cells for toxicarioside-F (**1**), toxicarioside-G (**2**), and toxicarioside-H (**3**) and 0.020–0.044 μg/mL in K562 leukemia cells for the toxicariosides (**1–5**), being much superior to those of mitomycin-C (IC_{50}: 6.3 and 7.1 μg/mL, respectively).[1–4] Toxicarioside-A (**6**) was capable of diminishing the cell viability, inhibiting the cell growth, and repressing the cell migration and invasion of the SGC-7901 cells in time- and dose-dependent manners, whose effects were achieved partly through the downregulation of NF-κB activity and bFGF expression and the interference of bFGF/FGFR1 signal transduction.[5] Likewise, toxicarioside-I, strophanthidin, and periplogenin also exerted cytotoxic effects on the tested K562, SGC-7901, and SMMC-7721 cell lines (IC_{50}: 0.001–12.3 μmol/L).[6] In the treatment of human NIH-H460 lung cancer cells, antiaroside-J, antiaroside-N, antiaroside-O, antiaroside-Q, β-antiarin, convallatoxin, and convallatoxol in 50 nM concentration (48 h) displayed 80.7–82.8% growth inhibition, whereas those of antialloside, toxicario toxicarioside-B, desglucocheirotoxin, and antioside were 70.7–78.9%, and antiaroside-X, strophalloside, deglucocheirotoxol, al-dihydro-α-antiarin, and al-dihydro-β-antiarin were 60.2–67.9%.[7]

Accompanied by the antitumor action, these cardiac glycosides elicited the apoptotic effect through an orphan nuclear receptor Nur77-dependent apoptotic pathway, i.e., translocation of the Nur77 protein from the nucleus to the cytoplasm and subsequent targeting to the mitochondria. Both the induction of Nur77 expression and its subsequent translocation from the nucleus to the cytoplasm are critical events in the apoptosis induction by the cardiac glycosides.[7] In addition, strophanthidin and periplogenin, two aglycones of the toxicariosides, showed much reduced antineoplastic effect. The comparison provided the evidences to know that the glycosylation is important for the enhancement of cytotoxic effect of toxicariosides.[3,4]

Cardenolides from the Seeds

In comparison with the earlier data, glucostrophalloside and toxicarioside-I, toxicarioside-J, and toxicarioside-K showed lower cytotoxicity on the SGC-7901 and SMMC-7721 cell lines. The IC_{50} values of glucostrophalloside and toxicarioside-K were 0.06 and 0.25 μg/mL in SGC-7901 cells and 0.10 and 0.07 μg/mL on SMMC-7721 cells, respectively.[8] Moreover, toxicarioside-M, convalloside, glucostrophanthidin, 3-*O*-β-D-xylopyranosylstrophanthidin, convallatoxin (**7**), convallatoxol, and strophanthidin were effective in the suppression of a panel of human malignant cell lines: KB (nasopharynx), HCT-116 (colon), SF-268 (brain), PC3 (prostate), MCF-7 (breast), MRC-5 (lung), and HL-60 (leukemia) cells, where the most potent cardenolide was convallatoxin (**7**), and its IC_{50} values were 0.40–2.2 nM.[7] Also, convallatoxin (**7**) was cytotoxic to HSG human submandibular gland carcinoma, BGC-823 human gastric cancer, Bel-7402 human hepatoma, and NB12 neuroblastoma cell lines (IC_{50}: 16–73 nM) but not active to HPLF human periodontal ligament fibroblasts cells.[9]

Cardenolides from the Stems

Nine monoglycosylated cardenolides and two aglycones isolated from the stem of Jian Du Mu were identified as toxicarioside-D, strophanolloside (**8**), strophanthojavoside, antiarigenin-3-*O*-β-D-6-deoxyalloside, strophalloside, malayoside, antiarojavoside, cannogenol-3-*O*-α-L-rhamnoside, desglucocheirotoxin, strophanthidol, and strophanthidine. Their antigrowth activities were assayed in a panel of human cancer cell lines, including NIH-H460, A549 and Calu-6 (lung), LNCaP (prostate), MCF-7 (breast), SW480 (colon), and HeLa (ovary) cells, with IC_{50} values ranging from 10^{-1} to 10^{-3} μM.[10] The anticancer effect was found to be accompanied by the up-expression of Nur77, which is a potent apoptotic member of steroid/thyroid hormone receptor superfamily.[10] The most potent antigrowth activity achieved by strophanolloside (**8**) was in the NIH-H460 and A549 lung carcinoma cell lines (IC_{50}: 5.8 and 8.3 nM, respectively).[10] Strophalloside (**8**) was also capable of diminishing the cell viability and growth and restraining the migration and the invasion of SGC-7901 human gastric cancer cells in time- and dose-dependent manners *in vitro* and significantly inhibiting the tumor growth and inducting the apoptosis of SGC-7901 cells via a mitochondrion-dependent caspase-3 pathway *in vivo*.[11]

A more detailed phytochemical investigation has separated 48 cardiac glycosides/aglycons from a trunk bark of *A. toxicaria*. Forty of them were evaluated by *in vitro* models with 10 human cancer cell lines, and many of them were effective in suppressing all 10 cell lines, KB, KB-VIN, A549, MCF-7, U-87-MG, PC-3, 1A9, CAKI-1, HCT-9, and S-KMEL-2. The ED_{50} values of the 7 cardenolides, i.e., periplorhamnoside, desglucocheirotoxin, strophathojavoside, convallatoxal, convallatoxin, strophalloside, and β-antiarin, reached to 10^{-2}–10^{-3} μg/mL. Chiefly, convallatoxal (**9**) showed notable potencies at the nanogram/milliliter levels on A549, 1A9, and CAKI-1 cells (ED_{50}: 4.0–7.6 ng/mL), while convallatoxin (**7**) on s-KMEL-2, HCT-9, A549, CAKI-1, and MCF-7 cells (ED_{50}: 1.3–6.5 ng/mL). α-Antiarin (**10**) showed an ED_{50} value of 4.4 ng/mL against PC3 cells and desglucocheirotoxin (**11**) exhibited an ED_{50} value of 9.2 ng/mL against A549 cells. The noticeable data were also exhibited by 10 of the cardenolides on drug-resistant KB-VIN cells (ED_{50}: 10^{-2} μg/mL).[12]

The anticancer related phytochemistry investigations afforded so many active molecules; however, considering that most cardenolides possess notable cardiotonic activity, these significantly active agents are probably limited for their *in vivo* investigation and clinical application.

SAR of the Cardenoides

The cytotoxic effects of cardenolides provided great evidences for the analysis of their SARs. By comparing the data, the SAP can be deduced as (1) glycosylation at C-3 of the aglycone is crucial for the higher growth inhibition; (2) instead of the methyl group at C-10 of the aglycone to aldehyde, methylol or hydroxyl groups play positive roles in the cytotoxicity; (3) 12β-hydroxylation of aglycones enhances the anticancer potency; (4) 5β-hydroxylation on the cytotoxicity was complex; (4) sugar residue types also notably influences the potency of inhibition; and (5) cardenolides linked with α-L-rhamnosyl or β-D-glucosyl residues seems to have stronger cytotoxicity compared to these linking β-D-xylopyranosyl or α-L-rhamnosyl-(4–1)-β-D-glucosyl residues. In addition, both toxicarioside-H (**3**) and toxicarioside-M (**12**) were the monoglycosylated 19-nor-cardenolides, but toxicarioside-H (**3**) had a stronger cytotoxic effect, and toxicarioside-M (**12**) showed moderate effect, implying that the potent antitumor activity of toxicarioside-H (**3**) was probably due to having an additional β-hydroxy group at C-12 of the aglycone.[1–10]

Sesquiterpenoid Glycoside

7-Drimen-3β,11-diol 3-*O*-β-D-glucopyranoside (**13**), a drimane sesquiterpenoid glycoside isolated from the 95% ethanolic extract of Jian Du Mu seeds, were active in the repression of SMMC-7721 hepatoma and K562 erythroleukemia cell lines *in vitro*.[13]

Flavonoids

The continuing separation of Jian Du Mu root extract afforded four anticancer flavonoids, which were identified as antiarone-K (**14**) and antiarone-I (**15**), sigmoidin-A (**16**), and 2-[2,3-dihydro-4-hydroxy-2-(2-hydroxy-2-propyl)-5-methoxy-1*H*-inden-1-yl]-1-(2,4,6-trihydroxyphenyl)ethanone (**17**). The evaluation of these flavonoids on three human tumor cell lines revealed that all of these were effective in the inhibition of K562, SMMC-7721, and SGC-7901 cell lines *in vitro*. Antiarone-I (**15**), sigmoidin-A (**16**), and 2-[2,3-dihydro-4-hydroxy-2-(2-hydroxy-2-propyl)-5-methoxy-1*H*-inden-1-yl]-1-(2,4,6-trihydroxyphenyl)ethanone (**17**) markedly suppressed the proliferation of K562 leukemia cells (IC_{50}: 4.5, 4.4, and 2.4 μg/mL, respectively). The most potent effect was achieved by antiarone-I (**15**) and sigmoidin-A (**16**) in the assay toward SMMC-7721 hepatoma cells (IC_{50}: 0.5–0.6 μg/mL).[14]

Coumarines

Anticarin-A (**18**) and anticarin-B (**19**), two coumarines that were isolated from a trunk bark of *A. toxicaria*, showed marked cytotoxicity on some of the 10 tested human cancer cell lines, namely, anticarin-A (**17**) against PG3, IA9, CAKI-1, and S-KMEL-2 cell lines (ED_{50}: 1.5–6.7 μg/mL) and anticarin-B (**18**) against A549, MCF-7, KB, KB-VIN, and U87-MG cell lines (ED_{50}: 1.2–7.4 μg/mL).[12]

Lignans

A group of lignans were isolated from the EtOAc extract of Jian Du Mu stem, and some of them demonstrated the growth inhibitory effect against MCF-7 breast cancer cells *in vitro*.[15]

Other Bioactivities

Pharmacological studies substantiated that the extracts and steroid glycosides from this plant cause severe irregular cardiac function and eventually death.[16] The cardenolides such as toxicarioside-A, toxicarioside-B, and toxicarioside-C were also found to restrain the activity of Na^+/K^+-ATPase, a ubiquitous cell surface enzyme.[14] Toxicarioside-A (**6**) can also influence the function of bone marrow stromal HS-5 cells and inhibit the proliferation of HS-5 cells.[17] Four benzofuran lignans were potential agents for the management of osteoporosis and the prevention of bone loss without undesirable estrogen-like side effects such as increase of the incidence of breast cancer and heart disease.[15]

References

1. Dai, H. F. et al. 2009. Two new cytotoxic cardenolides from the latex of *Antiaris toxicaria*. *J. Asian Nat. Prods. Res.* 11: 832–7.
2. Mei, W. L. et al. 2011. Study on the chemical constituents from the latex of *Antiaris toxicaria*. *Youji Huaxue* 31: 533–7.
3. Gan, Y. J. et al. 2009. A new cytotoxic cardenolide from the latex of *Antiaris toxicaria*. *Chin. Chem. Lett.* 20: 450–2.
4. Dai, H. F. et al. 2009. A new cytotoxic 19-nor-cardenolide from the latex of *Antiaris toxicaria*. *Mol.* 14: 3694–9.
5. Guo, J. L. et al. 2012. Toxicarioside A inhibits SGC-7901 proliferation, migration and invasion via NF-κB/bFGF signaling. *World J. Gastroenterol.* 18: 1602–9.
6. Mei, W. L. et al. 2011. Study on the chemical constituents from the latex of *Antiaris toxicaria*. *Youji Huaxue* 31: 533–7.
7. Liu, Q. et al. 2013. Antiproliferative cardiac glycosides from the latex of *Antiaris toxicaria*. *J. Nat. Prod.* 76: 1771–80.
8. Dong, W. H. et al. 2011. Cytotoxic cardenolide glycosides from the seeds of *Antiaris toxicaria*. *Planta Med.* 77: 1730–4.
9. Levrier, C. et al. 2012. Toxicarioside M, a new cytotoxic 10β-hydroxy-19-nor-cardenolide from *Antiaris toxicaria*. *Fitoterapia* 83: 660–4.
10. Jiang, M. M. et al. 2008. Cardenolides from *Antiaris toxicarias* potent selective Nur77 modulators. *Chem. Pharm. Bull.* 56: 1005–8.
11. Zhang, X. J. et al. 2015. Strophalloside induces apoptosis of SGC-7901 cells through the mitochondrion-dependent caspase-3 pathway. *Mol.* 20: 5714–28.
12. Shi, L. S. et al. 2014. Cytotoxic cardiac glycosides and coumarins from *Antiaris toxicaria*. *Bioorg. Med. Chem.* 22: 1889–98.
13. Dong, W. H. et al. 2011. A new drimane sesquiterpenoid glycoside from the seeds of *Antiaris toxicaria*. *J. Asian Nat. Prods. Res.* 13: 561–5
14. Que, D. M. et al. 2009. Structure elucidation of flavonoids from *Antiaris toxicaria* roots. *Youji Huaxue* 29: 1371–5.
15. Jiang, M. M. et al. 2009. Phenylpropanoid and lignan derivatives from *Antiaris toxicaria* and their effects on proliferation and differentiation of an osteoblast-like cell line. *Planta Med.* 75: 340–5.
16. Carter, C. A. et al. 1997. Toxicarioside B and toxicarioside C, New cardenolides isolated from *Antiaris toxicaria* latex-derived dart poison. *Tetrahedron* 53: 16959–68.
17. Li, Y. N. et al. 2012. Toxicarioside A, isolated from tropical *Antiaris toxicaria*, blocks endoglin/TGF-β signaling in a bone marrow stromal cell line. *Asian Pacific J. Tropical Med.* 5: 91–7.

227 Mi Huan Jun 蜜環菌

Honey mushroom

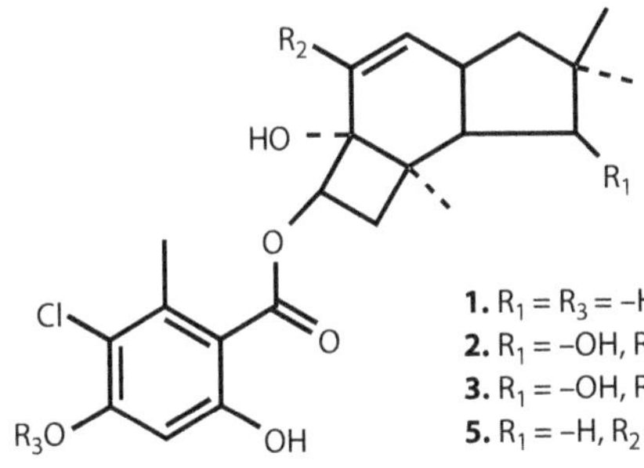

1. $R_1 = R_3 = -H$, $R_2 = -CHO$
2. $R_1 = -OH$, $R_2 = -CHO$, $R_3 = -H$
3. $R_1 = -OH$, $R_2 = -CH_2OH$, $R_3 = -H$
5. $R_1 = -H$, $R_2 = -CHO$, $R_3 = CH_3$

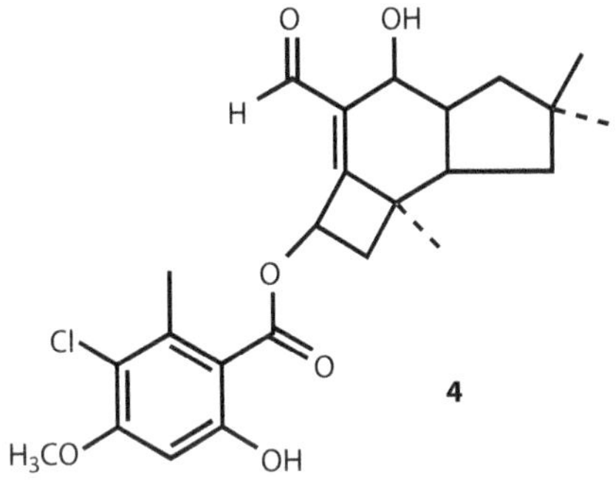

4

Herb Origination

The herb Mi Huan Jun (Honey mushroom) is the dried fruit body of a Marasmiaceae fungi, *Armillariella mellea*. The mushroom is a parasite on the roots or the trunk base of hardwood trees and fallen trees. The fungi are broadly distributed in forests of the world.

Antitumor Constituents and Activities

Sesquiterpenes

The fungi *A. mellea* is rich in protoilludane sesquiterpene aryl esters. Many of this type of compounds were discovered and elevated for their antitumor activities. Three unique sesquiterpene aryl esters designated as melleolide-K (**1**), melleolide-L (**2**), and melleolide-M (**3**) were made by the cultivation of Mi Gan Jun mycelial fungi,[1] and a same type of sesquiterpene assigned as arnamial (**4**) was isolated from the Honey mushroom.[2] All the protoilludane everninate esters were reported to possess strong antineoplastic activities as well as antibacterial and antifungal properties. The arnamial (**4**) displayed cytotoxic activity against Jurkat T cells, HCT-116 colorectal neoplastic cells, MCF-7 breast adenocarcinoma cells, and CEM lymphoblastic leukemia cells *in vitro* with IC_{50} values of 3.9, 8.9, 10.7, and 15.4 μM, respectively. Melledonal-C aryl ester moderately repressed the proliferation of CEM cells (IC_{50}: 14.75 μM) *in vitro*.[1,2] Melleolide-Q, melleolide-R, 6′-chloromelleolide-F, armillaricin, armillaridin (**5**), armillarikin, and melleolide-F exerted the antigrowth effect on the MCF-7 cells (IC_{50}: 1.5–8.3 μM), where armillaricin and armillaridin (**5**) were most cytotoxic. 6′-Chloromelleolide-F, armillaridin (**5**), melleolide-F, armillaricin, melleolide-N, and armillarikin showed comparable cytotoxicity against human H460 lung cancer cells (IC_{50}: 4.5–5.7 μM), whereas 13-hydroxymelleolide-K, melleolide-N, melleolide-R, armillaridin (**5**), and armillaricin exerted a similar level of cytotoxicity to the CEM cells. In HT-29 colon cancer cells, the inhibitory effect of armillaricin and melleolide-N (IC_{50}: 4.6–7.1 μM) were stronger than those of 13-hydroxymelleolide-K and melleolide-R.[3]

In another *in vitro* assay, 6′-chloromelleolide-F, 6′-de-chloroarnamial, 10-hydroxy-5′-methoxy-6′-chloroarmillane, 13-deoxyarmellide-A, armillaridin (**5**), and armillarin were effective in the suppression of human K562 (leukemic), MCF-7 (breast), and HeLa (cervix) cancer cells. Among them, the most potent inhibitory effects were achieved by 10-hydroxy-5′-methoxy-6′-chloroarmillane in the K562 and HeLa cells (GI_{50}: 2.3 and CC_{50} 4.9 μM, respectively) and by 13-deoxyarmellide-A in the MCF-7 cells (GI_{50}: 4.1 μM). Interestingly, 10-hydroxy-5′-methoxy-6′-chloroarmillane was also the most potent inhibitor of HUVEC (GI_{50}: 2.0 μM) in the melleolids, implying the antiangiogenic potential.[4]

Protein-Bounded Polysaccharides

A protein-bounded polysaccharide fraction prepared from the hot water extract of Mi Gan Jun is composed of a polysaccharide (41.3%) and a protein (35.0%), where the polysaccharide moiety contained fucose (4.5%), glucose (55.4%), mannose (19.4%), galactose (17.4%), xylose (1.1%), and one unknown monosaccharide, whereas the protein part contained 17 amino acids. This protein–polysaccharide fraction demonstrated significant *in vivo* antineoplastic activity against sarcoma 180 in mice, and the tumor inhibition ratios were 75.7–94.12% at the dose of 10–50 mg/kg/day. Also, the i.p. administration with the protein-bounded polysaccharide to mice could induce an influx of polymorphnuclear leukocytes at 5–24 h, followed by an accumulation of macrophages, implying that the antitumor activity of the protein–polysaccharide fraction is probably dependent on its immunoenhancing property.[5]

A peptide-rich glucan fraction was also purified from the fungi, which is composed of 70% glucan and 30% peptide, and the carbohydrate moiety consist of β-(1–3) and β-(1–6)-linked D-glucose residues. The peptide-rich glucan fraction reported in early studies displayed significant antitumor activity.[6]

Polysaccharide

AMP is a water-soluble polysaccharide purified from fruiting bodies of *A. mellea* with 4.6×10^5 Da molecular weight, which contains 94.8% D-glucose, 2.3% uronic acid, and 0.5% protein. *In vitro* assay, AMP exhibited a potent tumor growth inhibitory effect on human A549 NSCLC cells together with the induction of apoptotic death and G0/G1 cell arrest. The apoptosis-stimulating mechanism was found to be through a mitochondria-dependent pathway including the disruption of mitochondrial membrane potential, the release of cytochrome c from mitochondria, and the activation of caspase-3 and caspase-9.[7]

References

1. Takeuchi, T. 2000. Novel antibiotic agents, melleolide K, L, and M, their use, and their manufacture with *Armillariella mellea* (Vahl:Fr.) Karst. *Jpn. Kokai Tokkyo Koho* JP 98-372047 19981228.
2. Misiek, M. et al. 2009. Structure and cytotoxicity of arnamial and related fungal sesquiterpene aryl esters. *J. Nat. Prods.* 72: 1888–91.
3. Chen, C. C. et al. 2015. Three new sesquiterpene aryl esters from the mycelium of *Armillaria mellea*. *Mol.* 20: 9994–10003.
4. Markus, B. et al. 2014. Cytotoxic and antifungal activities of melleolide antibiotics follow dissimilar structure–activity relationships. *Phytochem.* 105: 101–8.
5. Kim, J. S. et al. 1983. Studies on constituents of the higher fungi of Korea: XXXVII. Antitumor components of *Armillariella mellea*. *Han'guk Kyunhakhoechi* 11: 151–7.
6. Amar, C. et al. 1976. Chemical and biological properties of a peptido-glucan fraction from *Armillaria mellea* (Basidiomycetes). *Biochimica et Biophysica Acta, General Subjects* 421: 263–71.
7. Wu, J. et al. 2012. A polysaccharide from *Armillaria mellea* exhibits strong in vitro anticancer activity via apoptosis-involved mechanisms. *Intl. J. Biol. Macromol.* 51: 663–7.

228 Wu Gu Teng 烏骨藤

Glaucescent Fissistigma

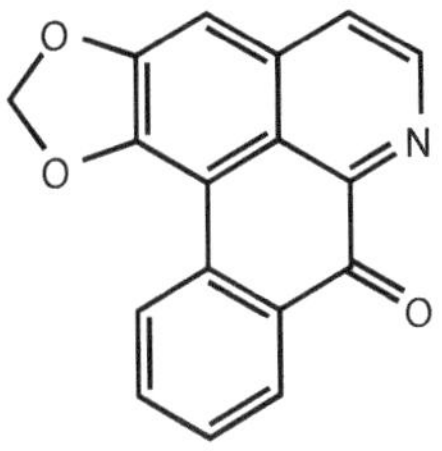

1 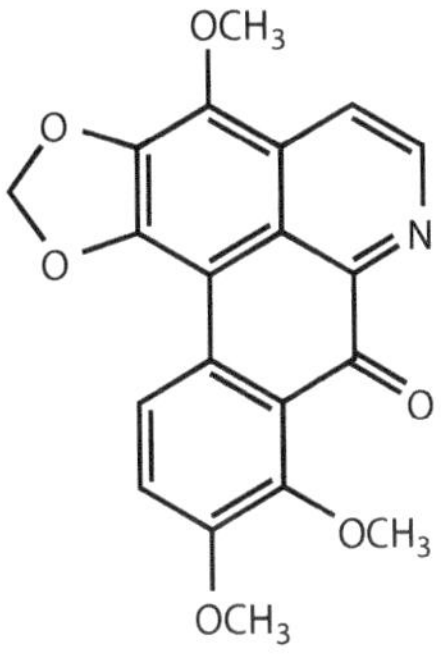 2 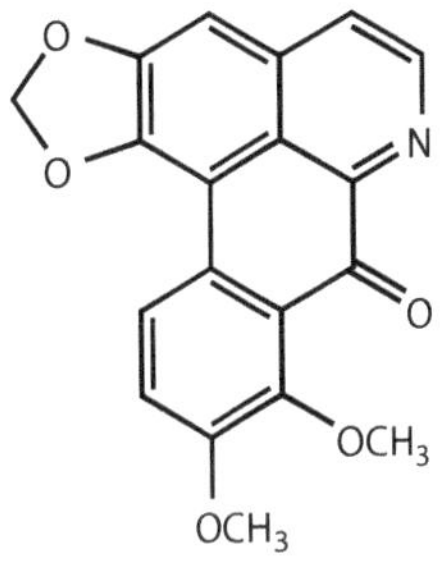 3

Herb Origination

The herb Wu Gu Teng is the dried roots of an Annonaceae plant, *Fissistigma glaucescens*. This perennial climber is distributed in six provinces of southern China as well as in Vietnam. Its roots are usually harvested in autumn and then dried in the sun for medicinal application as a folk natural herb.

Antitumor Activity

The extract of Wu Gu Teng demonstrated the inhibitory effects on the growth of cancer cells in murine animal models. An injection prepared from the roots of *G. fissistigma* displayed marked inhibitory effect against human Bel-7402 hepatoma cells *in vitro*. The intravenous administration of the Wu Gu Teng injection in a dose of 20 g/kg significantly restrained the growth of Walker-256 sarcoma, HSC hepatoma, U14 cervical cancer, sarcoma 180, and Ehrlich ascites cancer by 43.6–65.98%. The growth inhibitory rates were 53.45%, 34%, and 70.8% on sarcoma 180, Ehrlich ascites cancer, and HSC hepatoma by intramuscular injection, respectively, and 45.45–56.06% on Ehrlich ascites cancer, RAS reticulocyte sarcoma, L1 lymphoma, sarcoma 180, and hepatoma by hypodermic injection for 10 days.[1] At its concentration of 10–40 mg/mL, the injection lessened the expression of angiogenetic factors (VEGF and bFGF) to block the angiogenesis in the Bel-7402 hepatoma, indicating the antiangiogenic effect also involved in the antihepatoma mechanism.[2] These data provided scientific evidences truly demonstrating the anticancer activity of Wu Gu Teng, which is applicable in cancer chemotherapy.

Antitumor Constituents and Activities

Alkaloids

Three antitumor active oxoaporphine alkaloids were separated from Wu Gu Teng. Liriodenine (**1**) is a potent inhibitor of Topo-II both *in vitro* and *in vivo*, whose notable ability in the suppression of Topo-II may contribute to its anticancer effect.[3,4] The cytotoxicity of liriodenine (**1**) was demonstrated in various human cancer cell lines such as HepG2 and SK-Hep-1 hepatoma, KB epithelioma, A549 lung cancer, and murine P388 and L1210 leukemia *in vitro*.[5–7] The proliferation of A549 cells was restrained by liriodenine (**1**) in parallel with the induction of cell arrest at G2/M phase and apoptosis through the reduction of G1 cyclin, the accumulation of G2 cyclin, and the activation of caspases.[6] In wild-type p53 hepatoma cells (HepG2 and SK-Hep-1), the growth inhibition elicited by liriodenine was closely correlated to the arrest of G1 cells, the blockage of DNA synthesis, and the marked increase of p53 and iNOS expressions and intracellular NO level. But it had no obvious inhibition and no such interactions in normal human IMR-90 cells.[7]

Kuafumine (**2**) and oxocrebanine (**3**) exhibited marked cytotoxicity toward human KB epithelioma cells *in vitro* (ED_{50}: 0.5 and 4.0 μg/mL, respectively). In comparison to the structures of **1–3** with the corresponding activities, the result revealed that a methoxyl group at C-3 (such as in kuafumine) contributed to an additive inhibition against the KB cells, and the loss of the methoxyl groups at C-8 and C-9 positions augmented the anticancer activity.[8,9]

Furthermore, three corresponding metal complexes were created when liriodenine (**1**) reacted with Pt(II) and Ru(II). The metal complex demonstrated more potent anticancer effect than liriodenine (**1**) and a chemotherapeutic agent cisplatin alone in 11 typical human tumor cells *in vitro* (involving cancers of the stomach, the liver, the lung, the cervix, the ovaries, the nasopharynx, the breast, and the epidermis), suggesting that the complexes upon liriodenine coordinated to metal ions may be a potential area for further development to treat malignant tumors.[10]

Glycosides

The total glycosides extracted from *G. fissistigma* roots significantly obstructed the proliferation and the growth of human and murine hepatoma cells *in vitro* and *in vivo*, whose effect was found to be correlated with prominent reduction of AFP secretion in the HepG2 cells.[11]

Clinical Application

A soft capsule and a drop pill prepared from radix *Fissistigma glaucescens* called Xiao Ai Ping are clinically employed in China for the treatment of many types of malignant tumors including gastric cancer, esophageal carcinoma, hepatoma, lung cancer, cervical cancer, breast carcinoma, pancreatic cancer, nasopharyngeal carcinoma, colon cancer, cardiac cancer, leukemia, malignant lymphoma, as well as chronic tracheitis and bronchial asthma. Several Chinese medicinal preparations including Wu Gu Teng are also used for adjunctive treatment of a tumor after surgery, radiotherapy, and/or chemotherapy, as well as other diseases of inflammation and asthma.[11–14]

References

1. (a) 1984. Research Symposium of Wuguteng in treatment of Malignant Tumor. *Yixue Yanjiu Tongxun* (7): 9; (b) 1999. *Chinese Materia Medica* Vol. 3, 3-1593: 8. Shanghai Science and Technology Press, Shanghai, China.
2. Zuo, X. D. et al. 2010. Expressions of VEGF and bFGF in human hepatocarcinoma cell with glaucescent fissistigma root injection. *Linchuang Zhongliuxue Zazhi* 15: 1062–5.
3. Woo, S. H. et al. 1997. Inhibition of topoisomerase II by liriodenine. *Biochem. Pharmacol.* 54: 467–73.
4. Wu, Y. C. et al. 1990. Two phenanthrene alkaloids from *Fissistigma glaucescens. Phytochem.* 29: 2387–8.
5. Wu, Y. C. et al. 1993. Cytotoxic alkaloids of *Annona montana. Phytochem.* 33: 497–500.
6. Chang, H. et al. 2004. Anticancer effect of liriodenine on human lung cancer cells. *Kaohsiung J. Med. Sci.* 20: 365–71.
7. Hsieh, T. J. et al. 2005. Liriodenine inhibits the proliferation of human hepatoma cell lines by blocking cell cycle progression and nitric oxide-mediated activation of p53 expression. *Food Chem Toxicol.* 43: 1117–26.
8. Wu, Y. C. et al. 1987. Kuafumine, a novel cytotoxic oxoaporphine alkaloid from *Fissistigma glausescens. Heterocycles* 26: 9–12.
9. Stévigny, C. et al. 2005. Cytotoxic and antitumor potentialities of aporphinoid alkaloids. *Curr. Med. Chem.* 5: 173–82.
10. Chen, Z. F. et al. 2009. Potential new inorganic antitumour agents from combining the anticancer traditional Chinese medicine (TCM) liriodenine with metal ions, and DNA binding studies. *Dalton Trans.* 14: 262–72.
11. Zou, W. H. et al. 2013. Effects of total glycosides in *Glaucescent fissistigma* root on the proliferation of hepatocarcinoma cells and secretion of AFP. *Zhongnan Yixue Kexue Zazhi* 41: 344–6.
12. Zhang, L. L. et al. 2005. A soft capsule prepared from Radix *Fissistigma glaucescens* for treating liver cancer, esophageal carcinoma, gastric cancer, and preparation method thereof. *Faming Zhuanli Shenqing Gongkai Shuomingshu* CN 1709296 A 20051221.
13. Qu, Y. Z. 2005. A Chinese medicinal dripping pill prepared from Radix *Fissistigma glaucescens* for the treatment of esophageal carcinoma, gastric cancer, and lung cancer. *Faming Zhuanli Shenqing Gongkai Shuomingshu* CN 1682816 A 20051019.
14. Li, W. J. et al. 2005. Soft capsule containing Radix *Fissistigma glaucescens* with anticancer, antiinflammatory, and antiasthmatic effects. *Faming Zhuanli Shenqing Gongkai Shuomingshu* CN 1589829 A 20050309.

229 Shu She 樹舌

Artist's conk or Artist's bracket

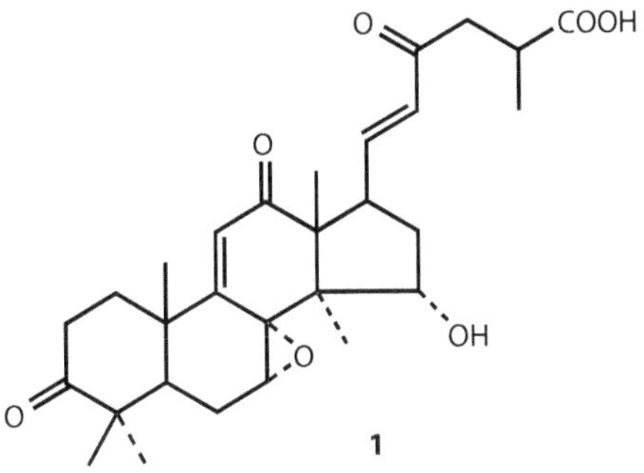

Herb Origination

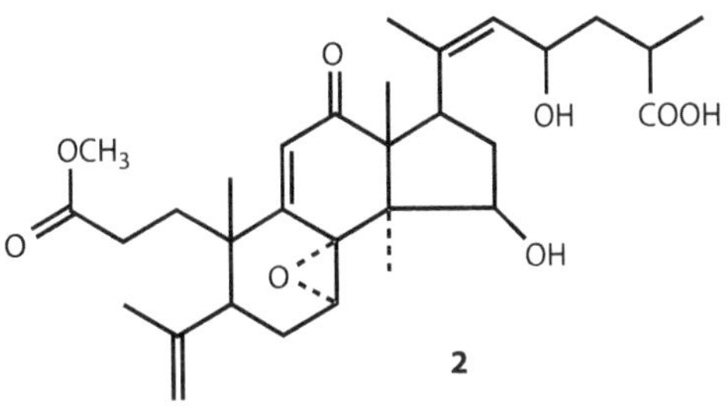

The herb Shu She (Artist's conk) is the dried fruit body of a Polyporaceae fungi, *Ganoderma applanatum* (= *Elfvingia applanata*). The wood-decaying fungi are broadly distributed in many places over the world and are very widely spread in North America. Shu She usually grows on preliminarily dead heartwood, and older trees. It is a folk medicine used for cancer treatment in China and Japan.

Antitumor Constituents and Activities

Triterpenoids

Shu She is a rich source of unique polyoxygenated lanostanoid triterpenes. Eight elfvingic acids A–H and elfvingic acid H-methyl ester were isolated from Shu She collected in Japanese, and eight applanoxidic acids A–H were discovered from Shu She produced in Indonesian. An *in vitro* assay showed that applanoxidic acids E (**1**), G, and H remarkably inhibited EBV-EA activation and Raji cell viabilities, corroborating that the three triterpenoilds have anticarcinogenic activity.[1,2] Elfvingic acid H methyl ester (**2**) demonstrated marked cytotoxicity against human Kato-III gastric cancer cells and murine Ehrlich cancer cells *in vitro* with the same IC_{50} value of 1.1 μg/mL.[3]

Polysaccharides

Shu She contains immunoenhancing antitumor polysaccharide components. *In vivo* experiments exhibited that the polysaccharides restrained the growth of tumor, enhanced the tumor cell apoptosis, and prolonged the survival duration of tumor-bearing animals by activating the expression of tumor suppressor genes p16, p27, and RB.[4,5] The polysaccharides in a 2 mg/mL concentration arrested the cell cycle at G0/G1 phase and attenuated the expression of EGFR, thereby inhibiting the proliferation of human MGC-803 gastric carcinoma cells in dose-dependent and time-dependent manners.[6] The activation of protein kinase A (PKA) might also be involved in the suppression of MGC-803 cells.[7] GAFP was a crude polysaccharide prepared from the submerged fermentation of *G. applanatum*, which could obviously inhibit the proliferation of human SW1116 colon adenocarcinoma cells with time- and dose-dependent relations, accompanied by the disturbed DNA synthesis and arrested mitotic cycle in G2/M phase.[8]

In mice vaccinated with HepA hepatoma cells, a polysaccharide component (GF) of Shu She affected the reassembly of cytoskeleton, accelerated the cell apoptosis, and suppressed the cell growth in association with significantly retarding c-Myc transcription and N-ras expression and activating caspase-8 and TNFα.[9–11] The GF treatment could activate an antioncogene phosphatase and tensin homolog expression in mouse H22 hepatoma cells *in vitro*,[12] and it markedly enhanced P53 and RB gene expressions and diminished telomerase activity *in vivo*, thereby notably inhibiting the growth of mouse H22 hepatoma cells by 42.25%.[13,14] The *in vitro* model also exhibited that GF could effectively inhibit the proliferation of SMMC7721 hepatoma cell line by 20.0% and 24.4% at concentrations of 2.5 and 10 μg/mL, respectively, together with the effective reduction of CDK2 and cyclin-E expressions, the downregulation of E2F1 expression, and the obvious increase of RB gene mRNA expression.[15,16]

Concurrently with the antineoplastic effect, the polysaccharides could augment the activity of NK cells and the production of IL-2 and IFN-γ in spleen cells, which were repressed by the tumor, and could increase the proliferation of spleen cells when the polysaccharides are i.p. or subcutaneously injected to mice transplanted the sarcoma 180 with a dose of 20 mg/kg/day for 15 consecutive days.[17] These results further confirmed that the antineoplastic mechanism of Shu She polysaccharides should be largely attributed to their immunoregulating property.

From separation of the Shu She polysaccharides, several antineoplastic β-D-glucans were derived, which demonstrated having abilities to completely regress tumor cell growth in sarcoma 180 bearing mice with no sign of toxicity. One of these β-D-glucans displayed 50% growth inhibition against sarcoma 180 cells in mice at a dose of 0.74 mg/kg. Structural investigations revealed that these bioactive β-D-glucans have a β-(1–3)-glucoside backbone with a β-(1–6)-glucosyl branch link for every 12 glucosyl residues or every three to five glucosyl units.[18–22]

Exo-Biopolymers

Five exo-biopolymers were discovered from the Shu She having anticarcinoma property. An exo-biopolymer (from the mycelial of Shu She) is composed of 83.3% polysaccharide and

16.7% protein, where the sugar portion includes mannose (48.4%) and glucose (40.9%), and the protein portion includes alanine (10.5%), glycine (11.6%), serine (12.7%), and aspartic acid (11.1%). The exo-biopolymer not only could retard the propagation of solid tumor *in vivo*, but was also capable of augmenting NK cell activity and removing free radicals. It also improved the protection against chemotherapeutic damage by enhancing the content of GSH and the activity of GST.[23,24] F-D-P (from its carpophores) was composed of protein (6.5%) and polysaccharide (65.3%) including glucose (89.1%) and mannose (10.9%), which was able to inhibit the growth of sarcoma 180 in mice showing the inhibition ratio of 88.3% in a dose of 20 mg/kg for 10 days. Similarly, F-D-P also primarily regulated the humoral immune responses and stimulated the production of B cells and total lymphocytes.[25]

The third exo-biopolymer prepared from the Shu She was assigned as EXP, which holds 17.1% protein and 58.9% carbohydrate. The polysaccharide moiety of EXP is majorly composed of mannose and glucose, while the protein moiety is mainly consisted of serine, glycine, and aspartic acid. When EXP is administered by i.p. in doses of 10–80 mg/kg, it significantly repressed the growth of solid tumor and increased the NK cell activity in sarcoma 180-bearing mice. At a dose of 40 mg/kg per day, EXP was found to be highly effective as it decreased the formation of sarcoma 180 by 39.7% and augmented the NK cell activity in splenocytes by 51.6%.[26] The fourth glycoprotein was derived from protoplast fusants of the Shu She mycelia, which contains 85.2% of polysaccharide, which consisted of glucose, galactose, mannose, fucose, and xylose, 0.39% of protein including 15 amino acids, as well as 0.39% of hexosamine. When 20 mg/kg of this glycoprotein was i.p. injected into mice per day, the inhibition against the solid form of sarcoma 180 was 50%, which was more potent than the protoplast fusants. Concurrently, the glycoprotein elevated the amount of the superoxide anion, activated the macrophages by 20%, and increased the count of hemolytic plaque-forming cells in the spleen 4.3-fold higher than that of the control group.[27] GA-EX is an exo-biopolymer produced from the submerged mycelial cultures of *Ganoderma applanatum*. The i.p. administration of GA-EX in a dose of 40 mg/kg effectively suppressed the growth of solid sarcoma 180 cells. Besides lessening the tumor formation by 30.7%, GA-EX also increased the indexes of the spleen and the liver and augmented the activity of NK cells in the splenocytes by 41.3%.[28] All the findings established that the antitumor effect achieved by the five exo-biopolymers/glycoproteins should strongly correlate to their abilities in immunostimulation and antioxidant.

References

1. Chairul, T. et al. 1994. Lanostanoid triterpenes from *Ganoderma applanatum*. *Phytochem.* 35: 1305–8.
2. Chairul, T. et al. 1991. Applanoxidic acids A, B, C and D, biologically active tetracyclic triterpenes from *Ganoderma applanatum*. *Phytochem.* 30: 4105–9.
3. Yoshikawa, K. et al. 2002. New lanostanoids, elfvingic acids A-H, from the fruit body of Elfvingia applanata. *J. Nat. Prod.* 65: 548–52.
4. Wang, Y. et al. 2004. Influences of *Ganoderma applanatum* polysaccharide on tumor suppressor genes P16, P27 and Rb in mice. *Shijie Huaren Xiaohua Zazhi* 12: 1353–6.
5. Yazaki, T. et al. 1973. Antitumor polysaccharides. *Jpn. Tokkyo Koho* JP 68-64573 19680907.
6. Liu, X. L. et al. 2011. Inhibitory effect of crude polysaccharides on growth of SW1116 cells from submerged fermentation of *Ganoderma applanatum* (Pers.) Pat. *Jilin Nongye Daxue Xuebao* 33: 617–9, 623.
7. Li, R. H. et al. 2013. Effects of *Ganoderma applanatum* polysaccharides on the activity of protein kinase A of gastric cancer cell line MGC-803. *Zhongguo Laonianxue Zazhi* 33: 845–6.
8. Li, R. H. et al. 2010. Effects of *Ganoderma applanatum* polysaccharides on inhibiting gastric cancer cell line MGC-803 proliferation and the activity of protein tyrosine kinase. *Zhongguo Laonianxue Zazhi* 30: 3101–3.
9. Yu, H. et al. 2005. The influence of *Ganoderma applanatum* polysaccharides GF on the abundance of c-Myc mRNA in HepA carcinoma cells. *Zhongyiyao Xuebao* 33: 52–3.
10. Wang, L. et al. 2008. Effects of Ganoderm applanatum polysaccharide on expressions of caspase-8, TNFγ and MAP-2 in HepA cells of mice. *J. Harbin Med. Univ.* 42: 14–7.
11. Song, G. C. et al. 2008. Effect of *Ganoderma applanatum* polysaccharides GF on N-ras and C-myc oncogene expressions in HepA tumor cells. *Tongji Daxue Xuebao, Yixueban* 29: 45–7, 52.
12. Yu, H. et al. 2007. Study on the effects of GAPS GF on the expression of PTEN in transplantation tumor of hepatoma H22 by western blot technology. *Shizhen Guoyi Guoyao* 18: 1904–5.
13. Yu, Y. J. et al. 2011. The effect of *Ganoderma applanatum* polysaccharides GF on P53 and RB genes of liver cancer H22 cells of mice. *Zhongyiyao Xuebao* 39: 24–5.
14. Yu, Y. J. et al. 2010. Effect on telomerase activation of hepatic carcinoma H22 cells with *Ganoderma applanatum* polysaccharides GF. *Information on Chinese Tradit.Med.* 27: 35–6.
15. Liu, J. W. et al. 2012. Effects of GAPSGF on inhibiting hepatoma cell line SMMC7721 proliferation and CDK2 expression. *Zhongyiyao Xuebao* 40: 36–9.
16. Yu, S. L. et al. 2013. Down-regulation of E2F1 expression and inhibition of hepatoma cell line proliferation by GAPSGF. *Zhongyiyao Xuebao* 41: 9–12; Effect of GAPSGF on inhibition of proliferation of liver cancer cells and on mRNA expression of RB gene. *Zhongyiyao Xuebao* 41: 14–7; Effect of *Ganoderma applanatum* polysaccharides GF on proliferative inhibition of liver cancer cells and the expression of Cyclin E mRNA. *Zhongyiyao Xuebao* 41: 52–4.
17. Gao, B. et al. 1991. Effects of *Ganoderma applanatum* polysaccharide on cellular and humoral immunity in normal and sarcoma 180 transplanted mice. *Phytotherapy Res.* 5: 134–8.
18. Sankyo Co., Ltd. 1982. Antitumor polysaccharides from *Ganoderma applanatum*. *Jpn. Kokai Tokkyo Koho* JP 81–193459 19811201.
19. Usui, T. C. et al. 1983. Isolation and characterization of antitumor active β-D-glucans from the fruit bodies of *Ganoderma applanatum*. *Carbohydrate Res.* 115: 273–80.
20. Mizuno, T. et al. 1981. Host-mediated antitumor polysaccharides: III. Fractionation, chemical structure, and antitumor activity of water-soluble homoglucans isolated from kofukisarunoko-shikake, the fruit body of *Ganoderma applanatum*. *Shizuoka Daigaku Nogakubu Kenkyu Hokoku* 49–64.

21. Usui, T. C. et al. Antitumor activity of water-soluble β-D-glucan elaborated by *Ganoderma applanatum. Agricul. Biol. Chem.* 45: 23–6.
22. Mizuno, T. et al. 1982. Studies on the host-mediated antitumor polysaccharides: VI. Isolation and characterization of antitumor active β-D-glucan from mycelial cells of *Ganoderma applanatum. Shizuoka Daigaku Nogakubu Kenkyu Hokoku* 41–58.
23. Teikoku Chemical Industry Co. Ltd. 1982. Mushroom glycoproteins as neoplasm inhibitors. *Jpn. Kokai Tokkyo Koho* JP 80–152491 19801029.
24. Yang, B. K. et al. 2007. Antitumor agents containing exo-biopolymers isolated from submerged mycelial culture of *Elfvingia applanata. Repub. Korean Kongkae Taeho Kongbo* KR 2005–69637 20050729.
25. Kim, Y. S. et al. 1994. Effects of the antitumor component, F-D-P, isolated from *Elfvingia applanata* on the immune response. *Saengyak Hakhoechi* 25: 348–55.
26. Jeong, Y. T. et al. 2008. *Ganoderma applanatum*: A promising mushroom for antitumor and immunemodulating activity. *Phytother. Res.* 22: 614–9.
27. Jeong, K. H. et al. 1992. Studies on antitumor components of the cultured mycelia of interspecific protoplast fusant F-2 of Ganoderma lucidum and *Ganoderma applanatum. Han'guk Kyunhak-hoechi* 20: 324–36.
28. Jeong, Y. T. et al. 2008. Antitumor effects of exo- and endo-biopolymers produced from submerged cultures of three different mushrooms. *Mycobiol.* 36: 106–9.

230 Hu Tao 胡桃

Walnut

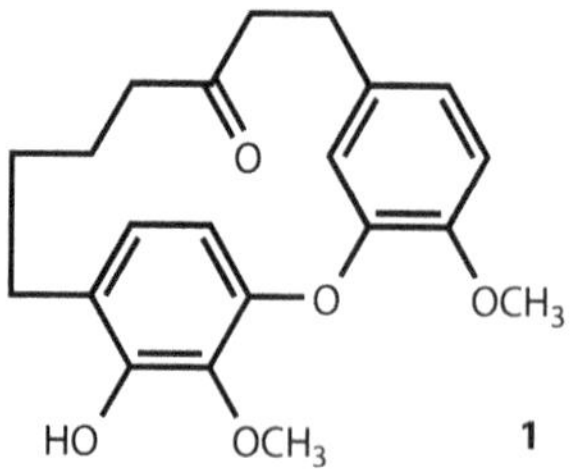

Herb Origination

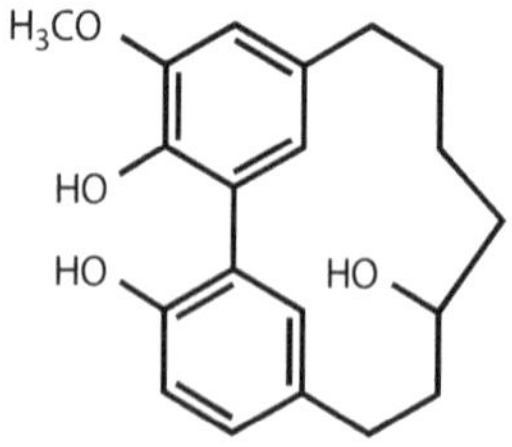

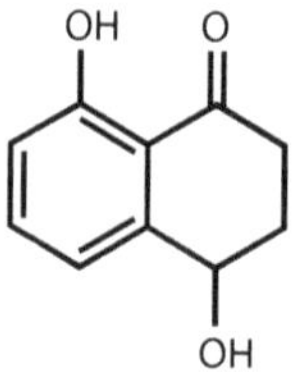

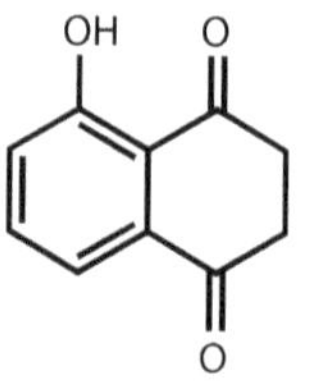

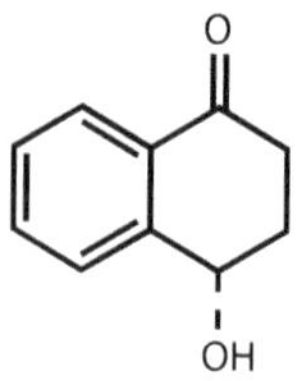

The herb Hu Tao (Walnut) is a large and deciduous tree, *Juglan regia* L. (Juglandaceae), which is native to the regions stretching from the Balkans eastward to the Himalayas and southwestern China. This species was also introduced to China from central Asia about 2000 years ago. The tree has been cultivated or naturalized in temperate areas across the world (30°–50° of latitude). The largest Walnut forests are currently in Kyrgyzstan. In China, its kernel, seed oil, leaves, root, bark, flower, young twig, endocarp, unripe fruit, and green husk are individually used as folk herbs.

Antitumor Activities

The Walnut tree is an excellent source of effective natural antioxidant and chemopreventive agents. The antitumor-related activity was present in the different parts of the Walnut plant. The methanolic extracts derived from the leaves, the green husks, and the seeds of the Walnut plant exerted the similar growth inhibition against human A498 renal cancer cell lines with IC_{50} values between 0.226 and 0.291 mg/mL.[1]

Activity of Its Nuts and Fruits

A diet of the nuts of Walnut for 25 days significantly delayed the growth of human HT-29 colon cancer cells by 27% and diminished the tumor weight by 33% in mice. The antigrowth effect was associated with the significant reduction of serum expression levels of angiogenesis factors including the decrease of VEGF by 30%.[2] The consumption of Walnut could alter the expressions of multiple genes related to the proliferation and the differentiation of mammary epithelial cells, thereby significantly lessening the breast tumor incidence, size, and multiplicity in a mouse model.[3] The results indicate that Walnut consumption can contribute to the diminishment of the risk of the carcinogenesis in the breast and the colon. The chloroform extract and the EAFs derived from the Walnut fruit extract, which contained a high content of phenolic components and showed antioxidant activity, displayed the greater level of antiproliferative effect against human HepG2 hepatoma cell line *in vitro* (IC_{50}: 9 and 15 μg/mL).[4] Moreover, the methanolic extract of the Walnut seeds presented higher total phenolic content and DPPH-scavenging activity (EC_{50}: 0.143 mg/mL), compared to the extracts from the leaves and the green husk.[1]

Activity of Its Husk

By the similar interactions in cytoplasmic and nuclear morphologies, the organic extracts of the Walnut green husk was effective in the inhibition of human PC3 prostate cancer cells and the promotion of apoptotic death.[5] The extract of the Walnut green seedcase exerted obvious suppressive effect on the proliferation of esophageal cancer cell lines (KYSE150 and EC9706) in association with cell cycle retardation via the down-expression of cyclin-D1. When increasing its concentration to 80 μg/mL, the extract obstructed the KYSE150 cells by 82.75% and the EC9706 cells by 85.54%.[6]

Activity of Its Root Barks

The organic extracts of the Walnut root barks, especially its chloroform extract, showed the growth suppression against human MDA-MB-231 breast cancer cells with the cell apoptosis induction in dose- and time-dependent manners by modulating the expression of key genes, i.e., markedly enhanced p53, TNFα, Bax and caspases activities and down-expressed Bcl-2 and mdm-2.[7] In addition, the aqueous extract of the Walnut bark is capable of diminishing CTX-induced urotoxicity in the bladder through the significant decrease of LPO in the liver and the kidneys in mice. The antioxidative stress property should be mainly attributed to the high content of phenolic components in the Walnut plant.[8,9]

Activity of Its Leaves

The leave extract exhibited relatively better antiproliferative efficiency against human 769-P renal cancer cells and human Caco-2 colon cancer cells *in vitro* (respective IC_{50}: 0.352 and 0.229 mg/mL) compared to the extracts derived from the green husk and seeds.[1]

Antitumor Constituents and Activities

Different types of phenolic compounds (such as diarylheptanoids, naphthoquinones, flavonoids, tannins, and other) have been isolated from the tree of *J. regia* and found to be principally responsible for the bioactivities.

Diarylheptanoids

From the green outer pericarps of the Walnut, juglanin-A (**1**) and juglanin-B (**2**) were isolated, which displayed significant antiproliferative effect against human HepG2 hepatoma cells *in vitro*. The most potent antihepatoma activity was achieved by juglanin-A (**1**), whose potency (IC_{50}: 0.02 μM) was much stronger than that of cisplatin (IC_{50}: 0.67 μM). The IC_{50} values of juglanin-B (**2**) were 1.50 μM in the HepG2 cells.[10]

Naphthoquinones

Three naphthoquinone assigned as regiolone (**3**), juglone (**4**), and 4-hydroxy-α-tetralone (**5**) were discovered from the green outer pericarps or the fresh leaves and the husks of the Walnut, respectively, being known as an anticarcinogenic and anticarcinoma agents. Regiolone (**3**) and 4-hydroxy-α-tetralone (**5**) showed moderate to weak antiproliferative effect against BHY (human oral squamous carcinoma) and MCF-7 (human breast adenocarcinoma) cells in a dose-dependent manner, and regiolone (**3**) also suppressed the proliferation of HepG2 human hepatoma cells (IC_{50} 1.16 μM).[10,11] More investigations revealed that the juglone (**4**) was a strong inhibitor of Pin1 peptidylprolylisomerase, whose Pin1 was normally overexpressed in various types of human cancer cells.[12] Two tetralone dimers with an O-bridge elucidated as juglanone-A and juglanone-B were isolated from the EtOAc extract of Walnut pericarps, but both exhibited weak effect on seven human cancer cell lines (such as A549, MCF-7, BEL-7402, BGC-823, Colo205, HeLa, and SKOV3) *in vitro*. At concentrations as high as 100 μm, the inhibition percentages of juglanone-B were 66.1% on MCF-7 breast cancer, 55.87% on BGC-823 gastric cancer, 47.4% on HeLa cervical cancer, 35.78% on BEL-7402 hepatoma cells, and 22.10–24.52% on SKOV3 ovarian cancer and A549 lung cancer.[13]

Ellagitannins

From the methanol extract of the Walnut, an ellagitannin component was isolated, whose predominant compounds were tellimagrandin-I and tellimagrandin-II members. The ellagitannins, in the *in vitro* experiments, elicited the cytotoxicity on human cancer cell lines such as MCF-7 hormone-receptor positive breast cancer, MDA-MB-231 triple negative breast cancer, and HeLa cervical cancer in association with the impairment of mitochondrial function and induction of cell apoptosis.[14] In addition, the gallic acid isolated from the barks of the Walnut tree, which was effective in the suppression of K562 leukemia cells and A549 lung cancer cells *in vitro* by 64.78% and 46.02%, respectively.[15]

Others

Triterpenoids/sterols, lupeol, daucosterol and β-sitosterol, and flavonoids, 5-hydroxy-3,7,4′-trimethoxyflavone, and 5,7-dihydroxy-3,4′-dimethoxyflavone, which were extracted from the Walnut leaves, displayed moderate to weak inhibitive effects on the proliferation of MCF-7 (breast) and BHY (oral) cancer cell lines *in vitro*.[11]

Other Bioactivities

Hu Tao (Walnut) is extensively used in traditional systems of Chinese herb for the treatment of various ailments as tonic, blood purifier, and detoxifier agents. Pharmacological studies proved that the walnut extract can improve the functions of the liver and the kidney, synthesize the functional enzymes, and enhance the antitoxic action of hepatocytes. Because the Walnut extract exhibited a high anti-atherogenic potential and an osteoblastic activity, a Walnut-enriched diet is encouraged in Chinese medicine, having potential benefits on cardioprotection and protection of bone loss. The extract derived from the walnut leaves has antioxidant, hypoglycemic, and hypolipidemic properties and also showed an anti-diabetic effect in diabetes-induced rats.

References

1. Carvalho, M. et al. 2010. Human cancer cell antiproliferative and antioxidant activities of *Juglans regia* L. *Food Chem. Toxicol.* 48: 441–7.
2. Nagel, .J M. et al. 2012. Dietary walnuts inhibit colorectal cancer growth in mice by suppressing angiogenesis. *Nutr.* 28: 67–75.
3. Hardman, W. E. et al. 2011. Dietary walnut suppressed mammary gland tumorigenesis in the C(3)1 TAg mouse. *Nutr. Cancer* 63: 960–70.
4. Negi, A. S. et al. 2011. Antiproliferative and antioxidant activities of *Juglans regia* fruit extracts. *Pharm. Biol.* 49: 669–73.
5. Alshatwi, A. A. et al. 2012. Validation of the antiproliferative effects of organic extracts from the green husk of *Juglans regia* L. on PC-3 human prostate cancer cells by assessment of apoptosis-related genes. *Evidence-based Complem. Altern. Med.* 2012: 103026.
6. Zhang, Z. W. et al. 2014. Suppression effect on proliferation of esophageal cancer cell with extracts of walnut green seedcase. *Zhongguo Zhongxiyi Jiehe Waike Zazhi* 20: 43–6.
7. Hasan, T. N. et al. 2011. Anti-proliferative effects of organic extracts from root bark of *Juglans regia* L. (RBJR) on MDA-MB-231 human breast cancer cells: Role of Bcl-2/Bax, caspases and Tp53. *Asian Pacific J. Cancer Preven.* 12: 525–30.
8. Bhatia, K. et al. 2006. In vitro antioxidant activity of *Juglans regia* L. bark extract and its protective effect on cyclophosphamide-induced urotoxicity in mice. *Redox Report* 11: 273–9.
9. Haque, R. et al. 2003. Aqueous extract of walnut (*Juglans regia* L.) protects mice against cyclophosphamide-induced biochemical toxicity. *Human Experim. Toxicol.* 22: 473–80.
10. Liu, J. X. et al. 2008. Cytotoxic diarylheptanoids from the pericarps of walnuts (*Juglans regia*). *Planta Med* 74: 754–9.
11. Salimi, M. et al. 2014. Anti-proliferative and apoptotic activities of constituents of chloroform extract of *Juglans regia* leaves. *Cell Prolifer.* 47: 172–9.
12. Thakur, A. et al. 2011. Juglone: A therapeutic phytochemical from *Juglans regia* L. *J. Med. Plants Res.* 5: 5324–30.
13. Li, C. Y. et al. 2013. Juglanones A and B: Two novel tetralone dimers from Walnut pericarp (*Juglans regia*). *Helv. Chimica Acta* 96: 1031–5.
14. Le, V. et al. 2014. Cytotoxic effects of ellagitannins isolated from walnuts in human cancer cells. *Nutri. Cancer* 66: 1304–14.
15. Chen, F. H. et al. 2008. Studies on the constituents and biological activity of the bark of *Juglans regia*. *Tianran Chanwu Yanjiu yu Kaifa* 20: 16–8.

231 Ge Er 革耳

Hairy panus mushroom

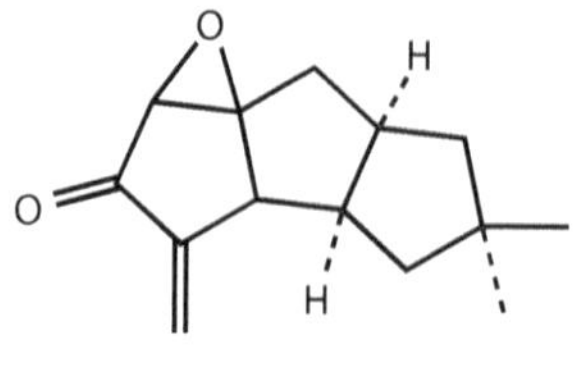

Herb Origination

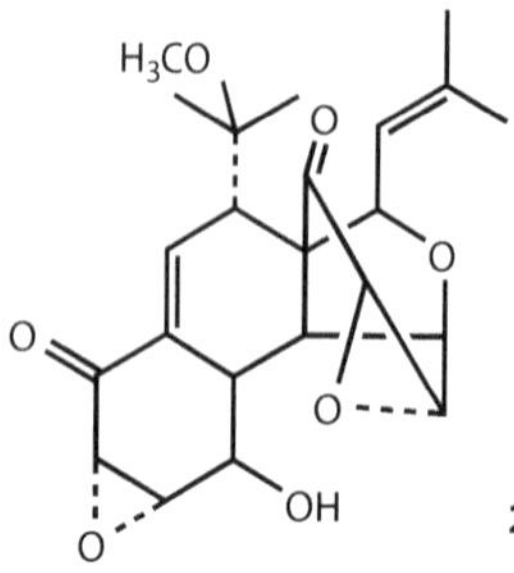

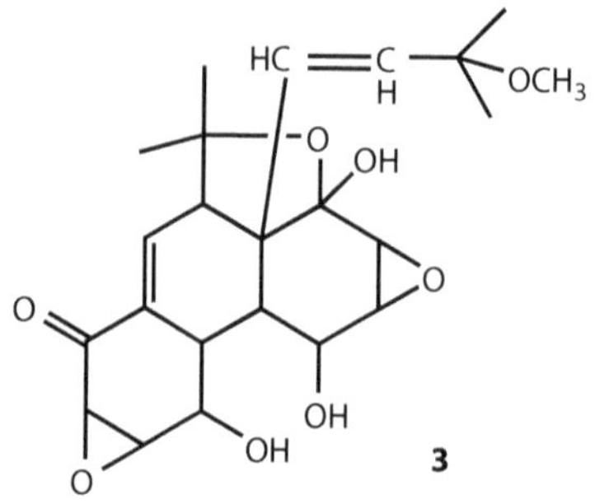

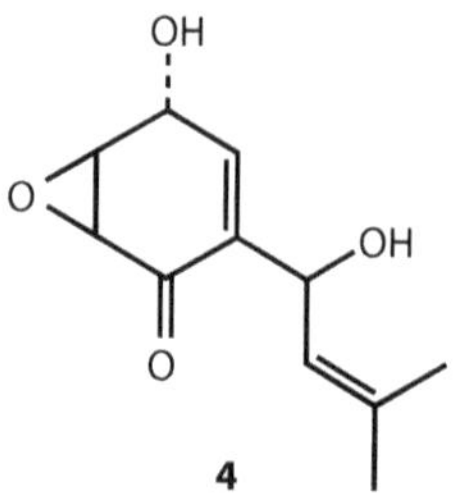

The Hairy panus mushroom is the dried fruiting body of a Tricholomataceae fungus, *Panus rudis* (= *Lentinus strigosus*), whose fungi are broadly distributed in the world as growing on the wood of recently dead hardwoods. The mushroom is not a normal food but is a Chinese herb.

Antitumor Constituents and Activities

Hypnophilin (**1**), a sesquiterpene that is isolated from *L. strigosus*, was cytotoxic to human UACC-62 melanoma cells. In association with the increases of intracellular calcium and calcium influx into the cytoplasm, hypnophilin (**1**) disrupted mitochondrial membrane permeability, caused cytochrome c release, and triggered apoptosome complex formation and caspase activation, thereby leading to the apoptosis and the death of the UACC-62 cells.[1] Hexacyclinol (**2**) isolated from the fermentation broth of *P. rudis* demonstrated obvious antiproliferative activity against L929 aneuploid fibrosarcoma and K562 leukemia cells *in vitro* with IC_{50} values of 1.4 and 0.4 μg/mL, respectively. In human HeLa cervical cancer cell line, it only showed moderate cytotoxicity (CC_{50}: 10 μg/mL).[2–4] Two ubiquitin-activating enzyme inhibitors assigned as panepophenanthrin (**3**) and RS-K3574 (**4**) were separated from the culture filtrate of *Panus rudis* and found to have antitumor activity besides anti-inflammatory and virucide effects.[5,6]

References

1. Pinto, M. C. X. et al. 2013. The cytotoxic and proapoptotic activities of hypnophilin are associated with calcium signaling in UACC-62 cells. *J. Biochem. Mol. Toxicol.* 27: 479–85.
2. Schlegel, B. et al. 2003. Structure determination and biological activity of an anti-proliferative and immunosuppressive agent obtained from *Panus rudis* (*Lentinus strigosus*) fermentation broths. *Ger. Offen.* DE 2002–10213481 20020322.
3. Schlegel, B. et al. 2002. Hexacyclinol, a new antiproliferative metabolite of *Panus rudis* HKI 0254. *J Antibiot* (Tokyo). 55: 814–7.
4. Saielli, G. et al. 2009. Can two molecules have the same NMR spectrum? Hexacyclinol revisited. *Org. Lett.* 11: 1409–12.
5. Takeuchi, T. et al. 2002. Panepophenanthrin, its manufacture with *Panus rudis*, and ubiquitin-activating enzyme inhibitors containing it. *Jpn. Kokai Tokkyo Koho* JP 2000–299090, 20000929.
6. Takeuchi, T. et al. 2003. Ubiquitin-activating enzyme inhibitor RS-K3574 and its manufacture with *Panus rudis. Jpn. Kokai Tokkyo Koho* JP 2001–231383, 20010731.

232 Ku Mu 苦木

Quassiawood

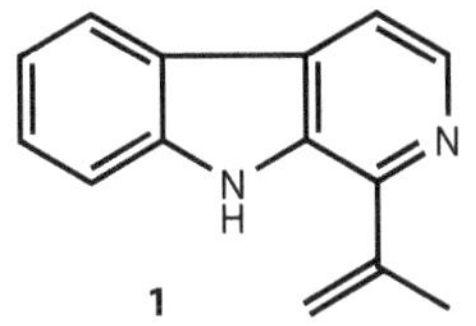

Herb Origination

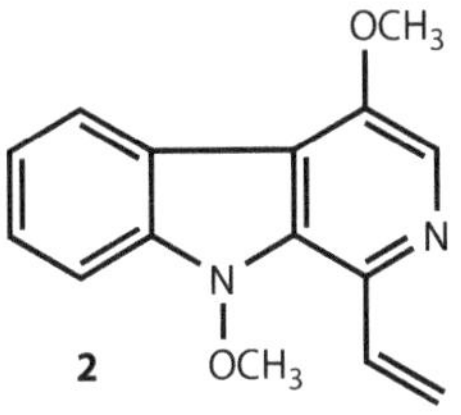

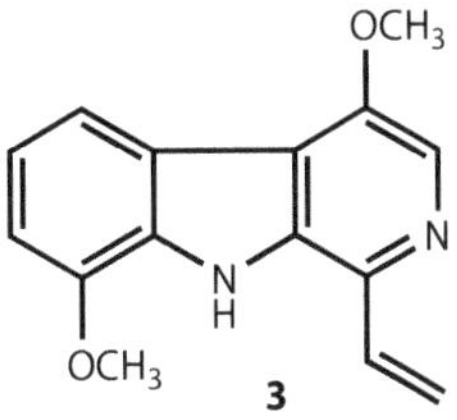

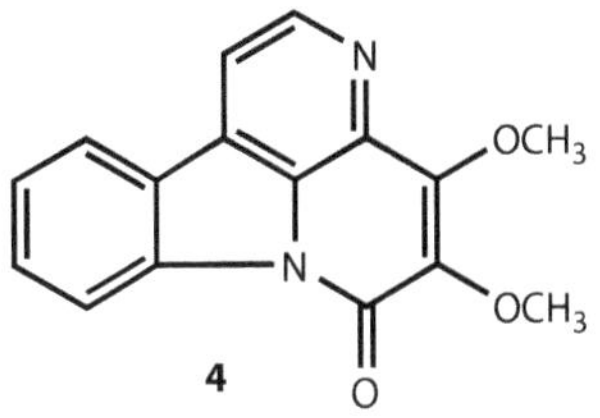

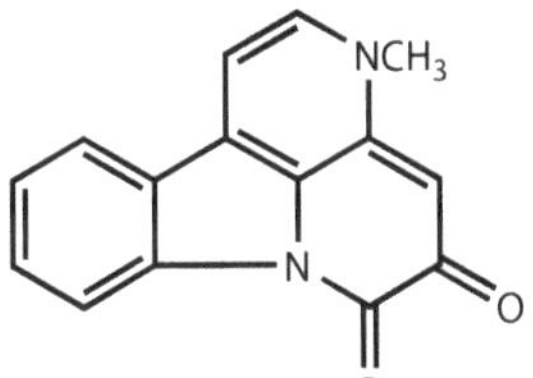

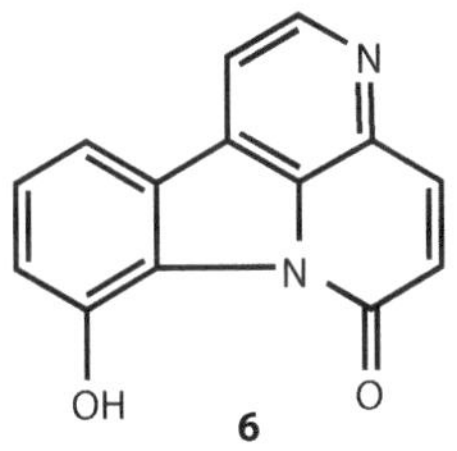

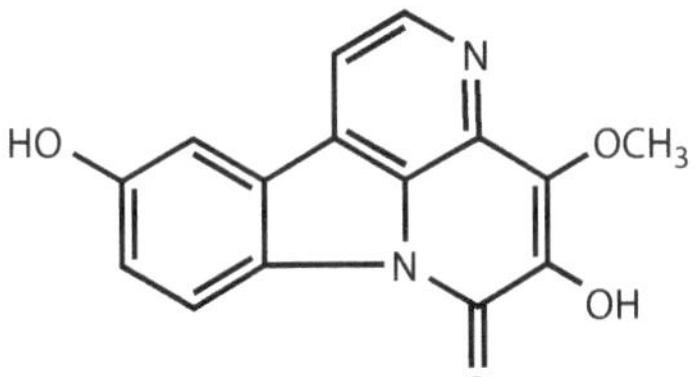

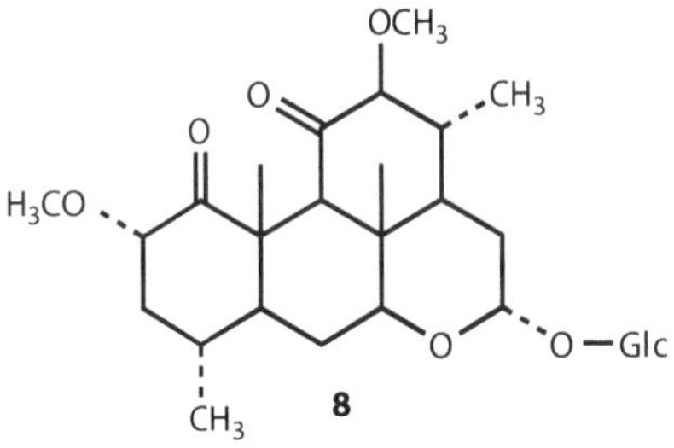

The herb Ku Mu (Quassiawood) is the dried woods originated from a small tree, *Picrasma quassioides* (Simaroubaceae). This deciduous shrub is native to the temperate regions of southern Asia. It is occasionally grown as an ornamental tree in Europe and north America, valued for its bright orange to red autumn color. In China, it commonly grows in the southern area of the Yellow River. The wood is annually collected and dried in the sun.

Antitumor Activities and Constituents

The alcoholic extract of Ku Mu showed strong antineoplastic effect on gastric cancer NCI-N87 cells *in vitro* with an inhibitory rate of 53.6–56.3%, while an aqueous extract from Ku Mu had hydroxyl radical- and superoxide radical-scavenging activities.[1] If concentration and action duration are increased, its ethanolic extract effectively suppressed the growth of human HepG2 hepatoma cells and inducted significant cell apoptosis.[2] MEPQ, a methanolic extract of *P. quassioides* decreased the viability and induced the caspase-dependent apoptosis in human HEp-2 and KB cancer cell lines; that effect was mediated by proteasome-dependent Spl protein degradation to regulate Bad and Bid protein.[3]

Alkaloids

A group of cyctotoxic β-carboline-type and canthin-6-one-type alkaloids were found from the isolation of Ku Mu. 1-Carbomethoxy-β-carboline (**1**), 4,9-dimethoxy-1-vinyl-β-carboline (**2**), 4,8-dimethoxy-1-vinyl-β-carboline (**3**), 4,5-di-methoxycanthin-6-one (**4**), 5-hydroxy-4-methoxycanthin-6-one (**5**), and 3-methoxycanthin-5,6-dione (**6**) were effective in markedly repressing the proliferation of human U937 (lymphoma) and HepG2 (hepatoma) cancer cells, *in vitro*.[4] Among them, 3-methoxycanthin-5,6-dione (**6**) was more potently cytotoxic to the U937 and HepG2 cell lines.[2] β-Carboline-1-carboxylic acid (**8**) exhibited moderate inhibitory activities on K562 (leukemic) and SGC-7901 (gastric) human cancer cell lines and CT26.WT mouse colon tumor cells (IC_{50}: 14.96–22.11 μg/mL) and on HepG2 (liver) and A549 (lung) human cancer cell lines (IC_{50}: 36–46 μg/mL).[5] The five canthin-6-ones also selectively restrained the proliferation of human CNE2 nasopharyngeal cancer cells *in vitro* (IC_{50}: 7.96–23.72 μg/mL). The order of inhibitory activities in CNE2 cells were 5-hydroxy-4-methoxy-canthin-6-one (**5**) > 4,5-dimethoxycanthin-6-one (**4**) > 4,5-dimethoxy-10-hydroxcanthin-6-one > 8-hydroxycanthin-6-one (**7**) > 3-methoxycanthin-5,6-dione (**6**). 4,5-dimethoxy-canthin-6-one (**4**), 8-hydroxycanthin-6-one (**7**), and 3-methoxycanthin-5,6-dione (**6**) displayed the antigrowth effect against human Bel-7402 hepatoma cells *in vitro* (IC_{50}: 32–61 μg/mL).[6] As a STAT3 inhibitor, 4,8-dimethoxy-1-vinyl-β-carboline (**3**) effectively hindered the expression of STAT3 regulated genes, leading to the growth suppression against STAT3 signal-dependent solid tumor cells (such as in the prostate, the lung, the cervix, or the breast).[7]

Two bis-β-carboline alkaloids assigned as quassidine-I and quassidine-J were isolated from the stems of *P. quassioides*, which were two pairs of enantiomers, (+)-S-QI and (−)-R-QI and (+)-S-QJ and (−)-R-QJ. The cytotoxicity evaluation revealed that (+)-S-QI (**9**) and (+)-S-QJ (**10**) showed more potent cytotoxicity against HeLa (cervical) and MKN-28 (gastric) human cancer cell lines (IC_{50}: 4.03–6.30 μM) than their enantiomers (IC_{50}: 9.64–12.3 μM), and the two (+)-S-quassidines showed similar activities to their enantiomers against mouse B16 melanoma cell line.[8]

Quassinoid Glycoside

A bioactive quassinoid glycoside elucidated as picrasinoside-B (**11**) was isolated from Ku Mu, whose antineoplastic effect was demonstrated in murine P388 lymphocytic leukemia cells *in vitro*, but it was less effective than a current chemotherapeutic drug, 5-FU.[6] Aglycone of picrasinoside-B (**11**) was identified as picrasin-B that was shown to have carcinogenetic and tumor-promoting effects.[9]

Other Bioactivities

The bark of the Ku Mu tree is used in Chinese herbal medicine as a bitter flavoring and antibacterial agent. The extracts from the plant wood are also used as a natural insecticide in organic farming.

References

1. Xuan, Y. H. et al. 2010. Antioxidant and anticancer activities of extracts from *Picrasma quassioides* Benn. *Asian J. Chem.* 22: 7219–26.
2. Liu, Y. et al. 2010. Inhibitory effect and mechanism of *Picrasma quassioides* on proliferation of HepG2 cells. *Zhongyaocai* 33: 1143–6.
3. Lee, H.-E. et al. 2014. Apoptotic effect of methanol extract of *Picrasma quassioides* by regulating specificity protein 1 in human cervical cancer cells. *Cell Biochem. Funct.* 32: 229–35.
4. Lee, J. J. et al. 2009. Cytotoxic alkaloids from the wood of *Picrasma quassioides. J. the Korean Society for Applied Biol. Chem.* 52: 663–7.
5. Lai, Z. Q. et al. 2014. Seven alkaloids from *Picrasma quassioides* and their cytotoxic activities. *Chem. Nat. Compds.* 50: 884–8.
6. Jiang, M. X. et al. 2008. Canthin-6-one alkaloids from *Picrasma quassioides* and their cytotoxic activity. *J. Asian Nat. Prods. Res.* 10: 1009–12.
7. Du, Y. P. et al. 2012. Application of *Picrasma quassioides* alkaloid dehydro-crenatidine as STAT3 signal specific inhibitor. *Faming Zhuanli Shenqing* CN 102526041 A 20120704.
8. Jiao, W. H. et al. 2015. (±)-Quassidines I and J, two pairs of cytotoxic bis-β-carboline alkaloid enantiomers from *Picrasma quassioides. J. Nat. Prod.* 78: 125–30.
9. Nadamitsu, S. et al. 1986. Effects of four chemicals isolated from *Picrasma quassioides* and *Petasites japonicus* on P388 lymphocytic leukemia cells in vitro. *Senshokutai* 38: 1179–88.

233 Gui Ye Cao 龜葉草

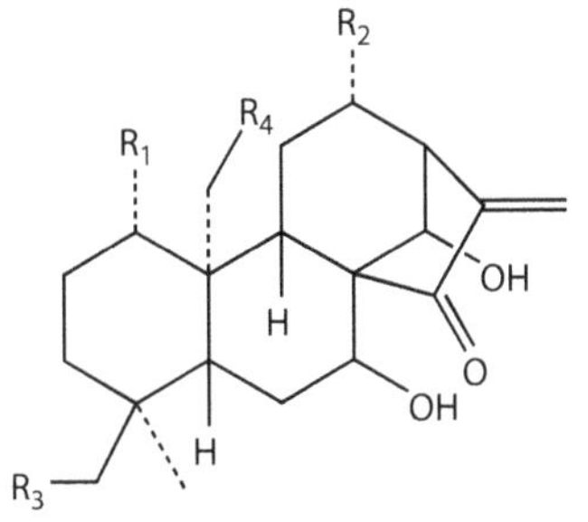

1. R_1 = –OH, R_2 = R_3 = –H, R_4 = –OAc
2. R_1 = –OH, R_3 = R_4 = –H, R_2 = –OAc
3. R_1 = –OH, R_2 = R_3 = R_4 = –H
4. R_1 = –OH, R_2 = R_4 = –H, R_3 = –OAc
5. R_1 = R_2 = –OH, R_3 = R_4 = –H
6. R_1 = –H, R_2 = R_3 = –OH, R_4 = –H
7. R_1 = R_2 = R_4 = –OH, R3 = –OH
8. R_1 = –OH, R_2 = R_3 = –H, R_4 = –OH
9. R_1 = R_3 = –OH, R_2 = R_4 = –H
10. R_1 = R_2 = R_4 = –H, R_3 = –OH

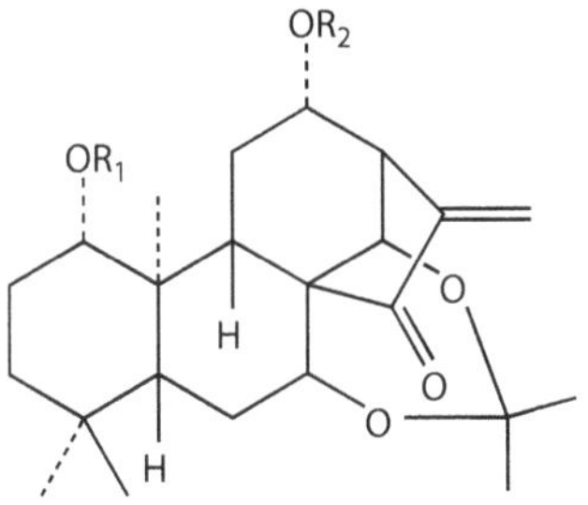

X1: R_1 = R_2–Ac
X2: R_1 = –Ac, R_2 = –TBS
X3: R_1 = –TBS, R_2 = –Ac
X4: R_1 = R_2–COCH(CH_3)$_2$
X5: R_1 = –TBS, R_2–H

Herb Origination

The herb Gui Ye Cao originates from a Labiatae plant, *Rabdosia excisa* (= *Isodon excisus*). This perennial herbaceous plant is distributed in northeast China, Korea, Japan, and Russian Far East region. Its whole plant can be used as a Chinese folk herb.

Antitumor Constituents and Activities

Gui Ye Cao has been used in Chinese medicine for the treatment of tumor in the beginning, arthralgia, sore throat, etc. Since 1990, Gui Ye Cao has been resubjected to cancer activity-related phytochemical investigation for the discovery of many *ent*-kaurene diterpenoids, which showed remarkable anticancer effect in the *in vitro* and *in vivo* assays.

Total Diterpenoids

Ent-kaurene diterpenoids were reported as the major antitumor constituents in Gui Ye Cao. The total diterpenoid component in murine animal models significantly retarded the growth of various tumors such as Lewis lung cancer, melanoma B16, sarcoma 180, Ehrlich ascites tumor, P388 leukemia, U14 cervical cancer, Hep2, and H22 hepatoma cells in a dose-dependent manner, and the inhibitory effect on Lewis lung cancer was stronger than on melanoma B16.[1,2] Eleven human carcinoma cell lines were used to examine the *in vitro* activity of the total diterpenoids, showing marked suppressive effect against the growth of Bel-7204 hepatoma, MCF-7 breast cancer, HL-60 leukemia, CEN-2 nasopharyngeal cancer, and colon cancer cell lines IC_{50} of 1.29–3.27 μg/mL and against HeLa cervical cancer, K562 leukemia, A375-S2 melanoma, MGC-803 and SGC-7901 gastric cancer, and NCI-H446 lung tumor cell lines with IC_{50} of 4.66–7.37 μg/mL. At a 16 μg/mL concentration, the total diterpenoids could reach over 85% inhibitory rates in the treated Bel-7402, MCF-7, HL-60, CEN-2, and K562 cell lines.[3]

The isolated fractions B, -C, and -F from the total diterpenoids triggered the SMMC-7721 hepatoma cells to apoptosis through an intracellular ROS-increased oxidative stress pathway.[4–7] The apoptosis-inducing effect was also observed in human prostate carcinoma PC3 cells after being treated with the fraction B.[6] At a 8 mg/mL concentration, the fraction B restrained the proliferation of human HeLa cervical cancer cells by 32.84% at 24 h and 51.90% at 48 h, whose mechanism was found to correlate with stimulating p53 and p21 expressions, lessening CDK2 expression, thereby disturbing the transition from G1 to S phase.[5] Taken together, these investigations provided a strong scientific basis for the application of the herb Gui Ye Cao as an adjuvant in cancer chemotherapy.

Separated Diterpenoids

According to High Performance Liquid Chromatography (HPLC) analysis, four diterpenoids with higher contents in Gui Ye Cao were identified as excisanin-A, kamebanin, kamebakaurin, and rabdokunmin-C. More than 16 diterpenoids separated from the aerial parts of *R. excise* have been demonstrated to have the cytotoxicity on P388 mouse leukemia cell line (IC_{50}: 0.58–1.11 μg/mL). The higher inhibition in the P388 cells was achieved by raniformin-A (**1**), excisanin-B (**2**), kamebanin (**3**), and excisanin-D (**4**), (IC_{50}: 0.58, 0.63, 0.69, and 0.72 μg/mL, respectively), but excisanin-A (**5**), rabdokunmin-C (**6**), and rabdoserrin-B (**7**) showed the IC_{50} values above 1.01 μg/mL.[8] Kamrbakaurin (**8**), kamebanin (**3**), excisanin-B (**2**), and excisanin-A (**5**) were also effective *in vitro* in the suppression of HeLa cervical carcinoma cells (ED_{50}: 0.05, 0.14, 0.09, and 0.20 μg/mL, respectively) and *in vivo* in the extension of the life duration of mice bearing Ehrlich carcinoma.[9] Kamebanin (**3**), excisanin-K (**9**), and kamebacetal-A had marked cytotoxicity against Bel7402 hepatoma and HO-8910 ovarian cancer cell lines,[10] while rabdokunmin-C (**6**) and excisanin-C (**10**) displayed moderate inhibitory effect against HepG2 hepatoma cells.[11] The *in vitro* antitumor effect was also observed in the exposure of kamebanin (**3**) and excisanin-C (**10**) to a small panel of human tumor cell lines. The respective IC_{50} values of kamebanin (**3**) were 0.9, 1.3, 1.6, 7.3, and 2.1 μM on HL-60 (leukemic), SW-480 (colon), MCF-7 (breast), SMMC-7721 (liver) and A549 (lung) cancer cell lines and of excisanin-C (**10**) were 3.0, 2.7, 8.4, and 8.9 μM on NB4 (leukemic), A549 (lung), SH-SY5Y (brain), and MCF-7 (breast) cancer cell lines.[12,13] Moreover, the *in vitro* treatment with excisanin-A (**5**) or excisanin-K (**9**) moderately restrained the NB4 leukemia cells (IC_{50}: 8.2 and 8.7 μM, respectively) but showed weak or no activity on the A549, SH-SY5Y, and MCF-7 cancer cell lines.[13] Through the inhibition of PKB/AKT kinase activity and the blockage of its signal pathway, excisanin-A (**5**) elicited tumor cell apoptosis and suppressed tumor growth in human Hep3B hepatoma and MDA-MB-453 breast cancer cells *in vitro*. In a combination treatment, excisanin-A (**5**) sensitized the Hep3B cells to the 5-FU treatment and the MDA-MB-453 cells to the Adm treatment.[14] Based upon the analysis of the relationship between the structural characters and the impressive activities clearly, it was revealed that α-methylene cyclopentanone acted as a key center for the antitumor activity.

The anticancer effect was further demonstrated *in vivo* in mice and nude mice models. Daily i.p. administration of excisanin-A (**5**) in a dose of 20 mg/kg for 12 days markedly reduced the xenograft Hep3B tumor size by 46.4% and induced tumor cells apoptosis. No obvious toxicity was observed in mice receiving the dosage treatment.[14] The inhibitory effect of excisanins-A (**5**) and -B (**2**) were also observed against the growth and the new blood tube formation in transplantable Ehrlich, S180, and P388 tumors.[15] Furthermore, excisanin-A (**5**) at concentrations of 10–40 μM exerted the suppression against adhesion, migration, and invasion of human MDA-MB-231 and SK-BR-3 breast carcinoma cells in association with dose-dependent decreases of MMP-2 and MMP-9 expressions and Matrigel through the integrin β1/FAK/PI3K/AKT/β-catenin signaling pathway, whose inhibition on the cell motility might contribute in restraining or preventing the metastasis of breast cancer cells.[16] Therefore, excisanin-A (**5**) may be a potential antigrowth and antimetastatic chemotherapeutic agent for further development in the treatment of breast neoplasm.[15]

Structurally Modified Diterpenoids

Comparing the similar *ent*-kaurene molecules to their cytotoxicity in P388 leukemia cells, the analysis revealed the importance of an α-methylene cyclopentanone in the *ent*-kaurene skeleton and the acyl groups at 12-OH and/or 1-OH of the molecules. A series of 1-*O*-monoacyl and 12-*O*-monoacyl, 1,12-*O*-diacyl, and 11,12-dehydrated excisanin-A 7,14-acetonide derivatives were synthesized from the modification of excisanin-A (**5**). When both 1-OH and 12-OH were protected, the produced derivatives X1, X2, and X3 showed significantly improved cytotoxicity on the P388 cells (IC_{50}: 0.042–0.060 μg/mL). Two other produced derivatives X4 and X5 also presented the enhanced antileukemia effect but less active (IC_{50}: 0.090 μg/mL) than X1, X2, and X3.[17,18] The experimental facts confirmed that 12-acyloxy groups are essential for the anticancer potency, and the 1-*O*- and 12-*O*-protecting groups provided steric factor that also importantly affect the cytotoxicity.[17]

Nonditerpenoid Extracts

Not only marked inhibitory effect against the growth of sarcoma 180 cells was observed in the treatment with Gui Ye Cao ethanolic extract and its aqueous fraction, but also obvious immunosimulating effects was achieved *in vivo*, such as the potentiation of phagocytic function of reticuloendothelial system, cytotoxicity of NK cells, and number of T lymphocytes. The experiments also demonstrated the ethanolic extract having low toxicity and no negative influence on the hematopoietic system. However, the water decoction of Gui Ye Cao inhibited the reticuloendothelial system and cellular immunity in the same experiments.[19,20]

References

1. Zhu, X. H. et al. 2011. Inhibitory effect of total diterpenes of *Rabdosia excisa* on neoplasms. *Zhongguo Gonggong Weisheng* 27: 1161–2.
2. Zhang, D. Y. et al. 2008. Advances in research on cytotoxinic activity of *ent*-kaurane diterpenoids. *Youji Huaxue* 28: 1911–7.
3. Nan, M. L. et al. 2010. In vitro and in vivo at antitumor activities of total diterpenoids from *Isodon excisus*. *J. Changchun Univ. TCM*. 6: 495–7.
4. Ji, H. T. et al. 2008. Primary research of effects of diterpenes on inducing apoptosis of hepatoma carcinoma cells. *Jilin Yixue* 29: 1608–10.
5. Liu, Y. N. et al. 2010. Inhibitory effect of diterpenoid B derived from *Rabdosia excisa* on growth of human cervical cancer cells and its mechanism. *Jilin Daxue Xuebao, Yixueban* 36: 54–7.
6. Ji, H. T. et al. 2008. Primary research of the effects of diterpenoids inducing apoptosis of hepatoma cells *Jilin Yiyao* (19): 1608–10.
7. Sun, M. L. et al. 2006. Apoptosis in SMMC-7721 cells induced by diterpenoid F derived from rabdosia excise. *Chin. J. Clin. Hepatol*. 22: 344–6.
8. Gui, M. Y. et al. 2004. Excisanin H, a novel cytotoxic 14,20-epoxy-*ent*-kaurene diterpenoid, and three new *ent*-kaurene diterpenoids from Rabdosia excise. *J. Nat. Prod*. 67: 373–6.
9. Fujida, T. et al. 1988. Cytotoxic and antitumor activities of rabdosia diterpenoids. *Planta Med*. 414–6.
10. Yang, D. J. et al. 2005. Studies on antitumor activity diterpenoid constituents from *Rabdosia weisiensis* C. Y. Wu. *Sichuan Daxue Xuebao, Ziran Kexueban* 42: 1038–41.
11. Huang, S. X. et al. 2005. *ent*-Kaurane diterpenoids from *Isodon albopilosus*. *J. Nat. Prod*. 68: 1758–62.
12. Wu, H. Y. et al. 2014. Cytotoxic *ent*-kaurane diterpenoids from *Isodon wikstroemioides*. *J. Nat. Prod*. 77: 931–41.
13. Zhao, Y. et al. 2009. *ent*-Kaurane diterpenoids from *Isodon scoparius*. *J. Nat. Prod*. 72: 125–9.
14. Deng, R. et al. 2009. Excisanin-A, a diterpenoid compound purified from *Isodon Macrocalyxin* D, induces tumor cells apoptosis and suppresses tumor growth through inhibition of PKB/AKT kinase activity and blockade of its signal pathway. *Mol. Cancer Therap*. 8: 873–82.

15. Sun, H. D. et al. 1981. Excisanin A and B, new diterpenoids from *Rabdosia excise*. *Chem. Lett.* (6): 753–6.
16. Qin, J. et al. 2013. A diterpenoid compound, excisanin A, inhibits the invasive behavior of breast cancer cells by modulating the integrin β1/FAK/PI3K/AKT/β-catenin signaling. *Life Sci.* 93: 655–63.
17. Aoyagi, Y. et al. 2006. Synthesis of 1-*O*-monoacyl or 12-*O*-monoacyl, 1-,12-*O*-diacyl-, and 11,12-dehydrated excisanin A 7,14-acetonides and their cytotoxic activity. *Bioorg. Med. Chem.* 14: 5802–11.
18. X1: 1-,12-*O*-diacetylexcisanin-A 7,14-acetonide; X2: 1-*O*-acetyl-12-*O*-^{t}butyldimethylsilylexcisanin-A 7,14-acetinide; X3: 12-*O*-acetyl-1-*O*-^{t}butyldimethyl-silylexcisanin-A 7,14-acetinide; X4: 1,12-*O*-diisobutyryl-excisanin-A 7,14-acetinide; and X5: 1-*O*-^{t}butyldimethylsilyl-excisanin-A 7,14-acetinide.
19. Zhao, Y. et al. 1999. The antitumor effect of *Isodon excisus*. *Chin. J. Tradit. Med. Sci. Technol.* 6: 85–6.
20. Wen, J. et al. 2000. The effect of *Isodon excisus* on immune function in tumor bearing mice. *Chin. J. Tradit. Med. Sci. Technol.* 7: 89–90.

234 Ji Su 鷄蘇

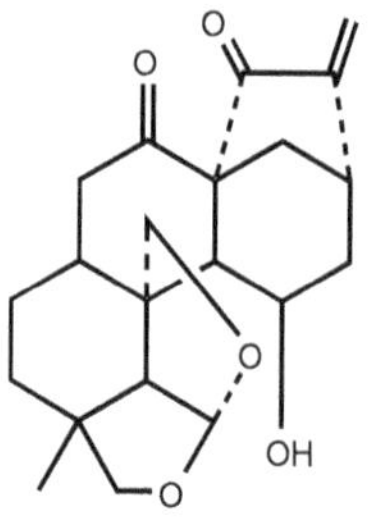

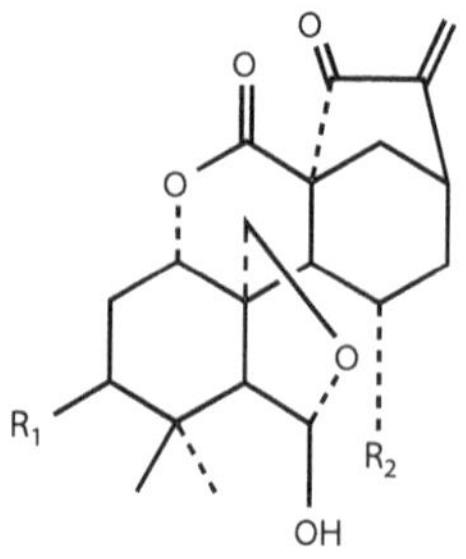

3. R_1 = –H, R_2 = –OH
4. R_1 = –OH, R_2 = –H

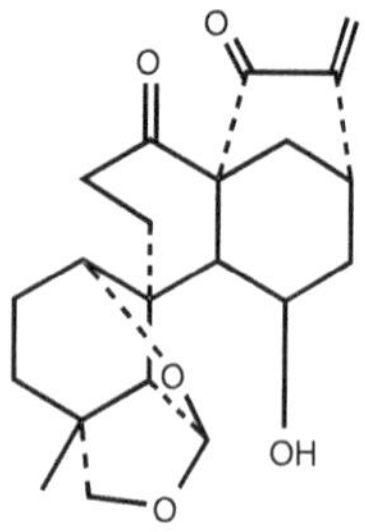

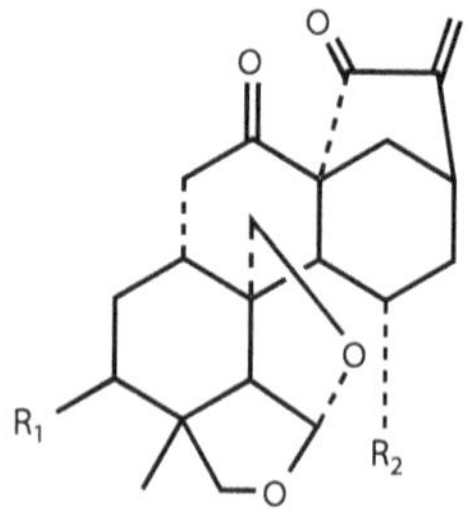

5. R_1 = –OH, R_2 = –H
6. R_1 = –H, R_2 = –OH

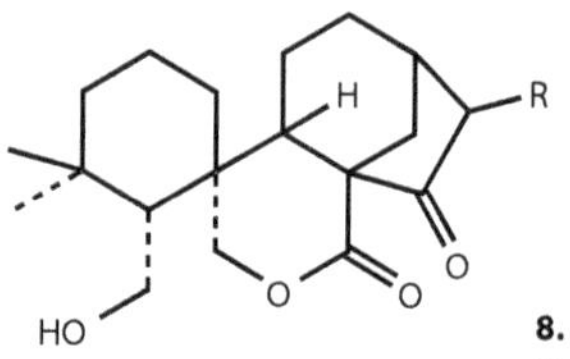

8. R = =O
9. R = $-CH_2OCH_3$

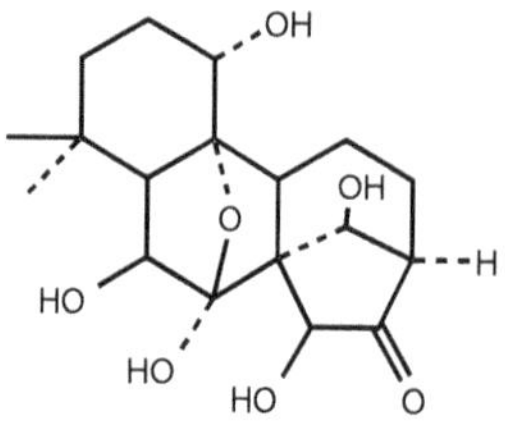

Herb Origination

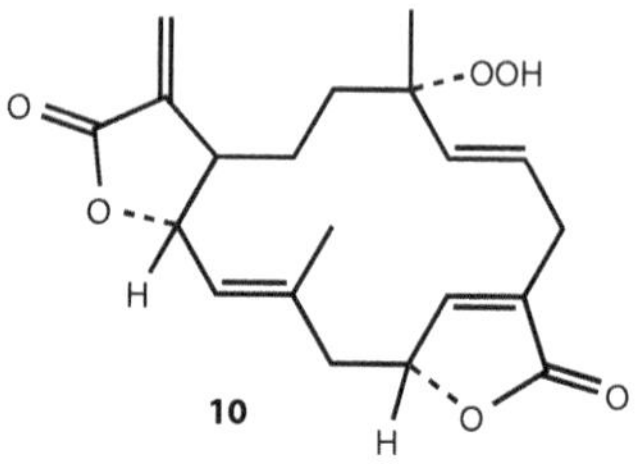

The herb Ji Su is the whole plant and the aerial parts of a Labiatae plant, *Rabdosia sculponeata* (= *Isodon sculponeata*), and Bai Sha Chong Yao (白沙虫薬) is another name for the herb. The perennial plant is distributed over the southwest region of China. For Chinese medicinal use, the whole plant is collected between summer and autumn and dried in the sun. The herb can also be used fresh for local folk remedy purpose.

Antitumor Constituent and Activities

As a *Rabdosia* plant, Ji Su is also a rich source of diterpenes. A group of *ent*-kaurane diterpenoids isolated from the herb demonstrated marked antitumor property; for instance, sculponeatin-A (**1**) and sculponeatin-C (**2**) significantly suppressed the growth of human HeLa cervical carcinoma cells *in vitro* (respective IC_{50}: 0.35 and 0.50 μg/mL). The i.p. injection of sculponeatin-A (**1**) and sculponeatin-C (**2**) in a daily dose of 30 mg/kg to mice for 7 continuous days could obviously lengthen the life span of mice implanted with Ehrlich ascites cancer, resulting in the T/C values of >221% and 163%, respectively, in 30 days.[1] Sculponeatin-C (**2**) also exerted the therapeutic effect on mouse P388 lymphocyte leukemia cells.[2]

Six *ent*-kaurane type of diterpenoids assigned as sculponeatin-H (**3**) and sculponeatin-I (**4**), enmein (**5**), *epi*-nodosin (**6**), sculponeatin-L, and macrocalyxoformin-B were isolated from the leaves of Ji Su and found to have cytotoxicity on K562 CML and T24 bladder carcinoma *in vitro*. The IC_{50} values of sculponeatin-H (**3**) and epi-nodosin (**6**) were 15 and 18.3 μg/mL in the T24 cells, respectively, and the IC_{50} value of diterpenoids (sculponeatin-I (**4**) and enmein (**5**)) ranged from 2.8 to 8.2 μg/mL in the K562 cells but no such activity toward human A549 lung cancer cells line, and sculponeatins-L was marginally cytotoxic to the T24 cells.[3,4] In addition, enmein (**5**) also exhibited antimutagenic property.[5]

Thirty-five diterpenoids were isolated from the air-dried aerial parts of *R. sculponeata*. Among them, two biditerpenoids (sculponin-D and sculponin-E), four *ent*-kauranoids (epinodosin, sculponeatin-A, sculponeatin-C, and sculponeatin-D), three cembrane-type diterpenoids (4α-hydroperoxy-5-enovatodiolide, 4-methylene-5β-hydroperoxyovatodiolide, and ovatodiolide) were effective in the inhibition of human cancer cell lines (such as K562 leukemia, HepG2 hepatoma, and A549 lung cancer) *in vitro* (IC_{50}: 0.56–4.3 μM). Also, two 6,7-seco-*ent*-kaurane diterpenoids (sculponeatin-N and sculponeatin-O), enmein (**5**), enmenol (**7**), isodocarpin, nodosin, longirabdolide-C, and macrocalyxoformin-B exerted the inhibitory effect on the HepG2 and K562cell lines, while sculponeatin-N (**8**) showed the significant cytotoxic effect on the HepG2 and K562 cell lines (respective IC_{50}: 0.29 and 0.21 μM).[6,7] Sculponeatins-A (**1**), sculponeatin-C (**2**), sculponeatin-O (**9**), epi-nodosin (**6**), enmenol (**7**), enmein (**5**), and nodosin showed the potent inhibition against the K562 cells (IC_{50}: <1.0 μM), and sculponeatin-A (**1**), sculponeatin-C (**2**), sculponeatin-O (**9**), 4α-hydroperoxy-5-enovatodiolide (**10**), and epi-nodosin (**6**) were the strong inhibitors against the HepG2 cells (IC_{50}: <1.0 μM).[6,7] Their antitumor potencies were greater than or similar to those of cisplatin (an anticancer agent).[6] A 6,7-seco-*ent*-kauranoid termed sculponeatin-J (**11**) and an enmein-type 6,7-seco-*ent*-kauranoid named isodocarpin displayed obvious cytotoxicity on SW480 (colon), MCF-7 (breast), HL-60 (leukemic), SMMC-7721 (liver), and A549 (lung) human tumor cell lines with IC_{50} values ranging from 1.0 to 3.5 μM, while sculponin-T, nodosin, sculponeatin-A (**1**), and sculponeatin-C (**2**) only had moderate inhibitory activity on the five cell lines.[8,9] The analysis of the structure and bioactivity relationships in these diterpenoids revealed that the existence of an α-exomethylene-cyclopentanone group is necessary for higher anticancer activity, and the presence of spirolactone group normally possesses more significant cytotoxic activities.[7]

Other Medicinal Use

The herb Ji Su has long been used in Chinese folk medicine for the treatment of diarrhea, dysentery, and beriberi.

References

1. Fujita, T. et al. 1988. Cytotoxic and antitumor activities of rabdosia diterpenoids. *Planta Med.* 54: 414–7.
2. Taiho Pharmaceutical Co. Ltd. (a) 1983. Sculponeatin C. *Jpn Kokai Tokkyo Koho* JP 58152889 A 19830910; (b) 1982. Antitumor agents sculponeatin A and B. JP 57212185 A 19821227.
3. Jiang, B. et al. 2002. Cytotoxic *ent*-kaurane diterpenoids from *Isodon sculponeata*. *Planta Med.* 68: 921–5.
4. Jiang, B. et al. 2002. Two new *ent*-kauranoids from *Isodon sculponeata*. *Chin. Chem. Lett.* 13: 1083–6.
5. Kakinuma, K. et al. 1984. Antimutagenic diterpenoids from a crude drug isodonis herba (enmei-so). *Agricul. Biol. Chem.* 48: 1647–8.
6. Li, L. M. et al. 2009. *ent*-Kaurane and cembrane diterpenoids from *Isodon sculponeatus* and their cytotoxicity. *J. Nat. Prod.* 72: 1851–6.
7. Li, X. et al. 2010. 6,7-seco-*ent*-Kaurane diterpenoids from *Isodon sculponeatus* with cytotoxic activity. *Chem. Biodiver.* 7: 2888–2896.
8. Jiang, H. Y. et al. 2013. Enmein-type 6,7-seco-*ent*-kauranoids from *Isodon sculponeatus*. *J. Nat. Prod.* 76: 2113–9.
9. Jiang, H. Y. et al. 2014. 6,7-seco-*ent*-Kaurane diterpenoids from *Isodon sculponeatus* and their bioactivity. *Chin. Chem. Lett.* 25: 541–4.

235 Huai Er 槐耳

Herb Origination

The herb Huai Er is the dried sporocarp of a Polyporaceae fungus, *Trametes robiniophila*, which is especially parasitized on the trunks of Japanese pagoda trees. Huai Er has been widely used in traditional Chinese medicine for approximately 1600 years. Due to the lack of source in the wild, the herb is mostly produced by solid-state fermentation techniques today.

Antitumor Activities

Due to the accumulating evidences from *in vitro* and *in vivo* experiments, Huai Er as a supplementary anticancer herb has attracted increasing worldwide interest in recent years. Huaier granules named as Jin Ke, which is a formulation made of the aqueous extract of Huai Er mycelium, has been frequently used in China for complementary therapies for leukemia, osteosarcoma, lymphoma, hepatoma, carcinomas in the breast, the lung, the pancreas, the stomach, the rectum, and the esophagus, as well as other chronic diseases. Based on the research results obtained in two recent decades, the anticancer activities of Huai Er have been known to primarily present a variety of aspects, such as inhibition of cancer cell proliferation, promotion of the cell cycle arrest and cell apoptosis, suppression of the cell invasion and metastasis, interference with tumor angiogenesis, reverse of drug resistance, and promotion of tumor-specific immune functions.

Antiproliferative Effect with Induction of Cell Cycle Arrest and Apoptosis

Various human cancer cells have been used to evaluate Huai Er aqueous extract. The results demonstrated that the extract was capable of promoting the cell apoptosis of many types of human cancer cells, such as HepG2, SMMC-7721 and Bel-7402 (liver), MCF-7 and MDA-MB-231 (breast), SGC-7901, MKN45, and MGC803 (gastric), HR8348 (colon), Eca-109 (esophagus), A549 (lung), Panc-1 (pancreas), SKOV-3 (ovary), A875 (skin) neoplastic cell lines, and K562 erythroleukemia, HT1080 fibrosarcoma, and Saos-2 osteosarcoma cell lines.[1–21] Its apoptosis-promoting mechanisms have been revealed to be associated with (1) a mitochondrial pathway including the down-expression of Bcl-2, the up-expression of Bax, and the activation of p53 and caspase-3; (2) modulation of PI3K/AKT signaling pathway and inhibition of survivin mRNA expression (such as in SGC7901 and MKN45 cells),[6,7] (3) upregulation of miR-26b-5p (such as in A549 cells);[4] and (4) down-expression of MMP2 (such as in MGC803 cells). Meanwhile, the extract induced the S phase arrest of HepG2 and Bel-7402 cells by decreasing β-catenin and cyclin-D1 expressions via a JNK signaling pathway.[3] The Huai Er extract treatment also arrested the cell cycle progressing at the G2/M phase in MKN45, SGC-7901, and A875 cells,[7,8] at G0/G1 phase in MCF-7 cells,[14,15] at G1 phase in Panc-1 cells,[13] and at G2 phase in HT1080 cells.[18]

Definitely, the abilities in the elicitation of cell apoptosis and cell cycle arrest contributed to the antiproliferative and anti-growth activities of Huai Er extract. After the treatment, the inhibitory rates could reach to 71.1% against HR8348 colon cancer cells at a 4 mg/mL concentration, to 77.9% against SGC-7901 gastric carcinoma cells at a 6 mg/mL concentration (48 h), to 55% against SMMC-7721 hepatoma cells at a 5 mg/mL concentration (48 h), and to 51.7% against Saos-2 osteosarcoma cells at a 16 mg/mL concentration (36 h).[6,9,12] The Huai Er extract was effective to both estrogen receptor$^+$ (MCF-7) and estrogen receptor$^-$ (MDA-MB-231) breast cancer cell lines, where MDA-MB-231 cells showed more susceptibility to the treatment, whose antiproliferative effect in the two cell lines was shown to be dependent with time and dose.[14,15] The antiproliferative effect on the three estrogen receptor$^+$ α positive human breast cancer cell lines (MCF-7, T47D, and ZR-75–1) was associated with the obvious reduction of ERα mRNA and protein levels, the marked down-expression of both ERα and its downstream genes, and the reversal of estrogen-activated NF-κB pathway.[22] Moreover, Huai Er extract also triggered the autophagic cell death of breast cancer cell lines (MDA-MB-231, MDA-MB-468, and MCF-7) through the repression of a mammalian target of rapamycin (mTOR)/S6K pathway and then partially contributed to the inhibition of the breast cancer cell viability and proliferation.[11] The effective concentrations of Huai Er extract for suppression of K562 leukemia cells ranged from 0.5 to 8 mg/mL.[21] However, the extract also had weak inhibition on L02 normal liver cells.[23]

Synergistic Anticancer and MDR-Reversing Activities

By the cotreatment, the Huai Er aqueous extract could enhance the sensitivity of the chemotherapeutic drugs (such as cisplatin and rh-endostatin) to A549 lung adenocarcinoma cells.[24] The extract additively potentiated the anticancer effect of 5-FU on SMMC-7721 hepatoma cells *in vitro* and *in vivo* after the cotreatment.[20] When combined with the extract (1 g/L), the sensitivity of cisplatin (DDP) and Adm to human lung adenocarcinoma cells H1299 (p53-null) was augmented by 1.9 and 1.6 times, respectively, together with the increase of their apoptotic rates and cytotoxicity in the H1299 cells in a p53-independent manner.[25,26] The synergistic antiproliferative and proapoptotic effects were also observed in the cotreatments of K562 leukemia cells with Huai Er extract and hydroxyurea and of MCF-7 breast cancer cells with the extract and texol or lobaplatin.[20,27] The mechanisms were probably related to the induction of cell cycle arrest in MCF-7 cells, such as at G2/M phase in the treatment with Huai Er plus texol and at G0/G1 phase in Huai Er plus lobaplatin.[20]

Furthermore, the MDR-reversing ability of Huai Er extract has been proven in the tests with several MDR cancer cell lines. The aqueous extract obviously promoted the apoptotic rate and enhanced the sensitivity of cisplatin (DDP) to A549/DDP cells, thereby partially inverting the drug-resistance of A549/DDP cells.[24–26] A 0.008 g/L Huai Er extract could lessen the drug resistance of HepG2/ADM hepatoma cells and result in the relative reverse efficiencies to ADM, DDP, 5-FU, and mitomycin were 79%, 73.5%, 86.7%, and 97.4%, respectively.[28] Impressively, the IC_{50} values of Huai Er extract was similar in A549 cells (IC_{50}: 1.84 mg/mL) and its MDR A549/DDP cells (IC_{50}: 2.01 mg/mL) and was close in HepG2 cells (IC_{50}: 0.917 mg/mL) and HepG2/ADM cells (IC_{50}: 1.66 mg/L).[25,26,28] In MDR-hepatoma Bel-7402/5-FU cells, the cotreatment with 0.01 mg/mL of the extract improved the MDR reversal rates by 3.67-, 2.38-, and 2.16-folds on 5-FU, epirubicin, and paclitaxel, respectively, leading to the relative reversal rates of 72.8%, 70.1%, and 74.9%, respectively.[29] The MDR reversal mechanism was found to be mediated by the down-expression of MDR1 and/or P-gp, the inhibition of P-gp function, and the enhancement of intracelluar accumulation of the chemotherapeutic agents in the human hepatoma cells.[28,29] In multidrug-resistant breast cancer MCF-7/R cells, Huai Er exerted the reversal effect of tamoxifen resistance through the downregulation of MAPK/ERK-I/2 pathway.[30] Because 1 g/L of the Huai Er extract plus 100 ng/L of TRAIL notably obstructed the growth of both HepG2 and HepG2/ADM cells with the elicitation of apoptosis, the cotreatment with TRAIL and the Huai Er extract was considered to be a safe and attractive strategy to overcome drug resistance and TRAIL resistance in the multidrug-resistant tumor cells.[23]

Antimigratory and Antiinvasive Activities

The Huai Er extract was also the inhibitors for the migration and the invasion of human neoplastic cell lines such as HT1080 fibrosarcoma, MG63 osteosarcoma, SKOV-3 and SKOV-3.ipl ovarian cancer, Hey ovarian carcinoma, MGC-803 gastric cancer, MCF-7 and MDA-MB-231 breast cancer, and MHCC97H highly metastatic hepatoma.[14–19] In the ovarian cancer cell lines (SKOV-3, SKOV3.ip1, and Hey), the antimigratory and antiinvasive effects of Huai Er extract in the concentrations of 5.0 and 7.5 mg/mL was revealed to be mediated by a AKT/GSK3β/β-catenin signaling pathway, i.e., decrease of AKT phosphorylation, up-expression of total GSK3β, inhibition of GSK3β phosphorylation on S9, decline of both cytoplasmic β-catenin expression and nuclear β-catenin translocation, and transcriptional repression of several Wnt/β-catenin target genes (DIXDC1, LRP6, WNT5A, and cyclin-D1).[19] The marked suppression on the cell adhesion was also concomitant with the limitation of the cell mobility and the invasion after the treatment with the extract on the highly metastatic MHCC97H cells.[17] These evidences suggested that the Huai Er may have a potential value for the prevention of cancer cell metastasis besides its antiproliferative and proapoptotic properties.

Antiangiogenic Activity

In an *in vitro* test, the Huai Er extract inhibited the proliferation of HUVECs and diminished the motility and tube formation of HUVECs in a dose-dependent manner. The antiangiogenic mechanism in HUVECs was found to be related to dose-dependently lessening the levels of transcription factor p65, phosphorylated ERK, JNK, STAT3 and repressing VEGF.[30] Moreover, the administration of the Huai Er extract inhibited new vessel growth in chick embryo chorioallantoic membrane in *ex vivo*, and lessened MVD and tumor volume and induced apoptosis and growth inhibition in BALB/c mice implanted with mouse mammary tumor cells (4T1).[31] The antiangiogenic activity was mediated by restraining the expressions of HIF-1α mRNA and VEGF mRNA in SW480 colon cancer and by lessening the expressions of CXCR4 gene and VEGF protein in Saos-2 osteosarcoma cells.[12,20] In human highly metastatic L9981 lung cancer cells, the antiinvasive and antiproliferative effects of Huai Er extract were demonstrated to partially attribute to the abilities in up-expression of antiangiogenic genes and down-expression of angiogenic genes.[20] The blockage of ERK/NF-κB signaling might be also involved in the antiangiogenic action of Huai Er.[20]

Inhibitory Activity on Cancer Stem Cells

Cancer stem-like cells are enriched in aldehyde dehydrogenase 1 high (ALDH1-high). CD44 (a hyaluronic acid receptor) and CD24 (a heat-stable antigen) are expressed by many types of CSCs as surface markers. Thus, ALDH1-high and $CD44^{+}/CD24^{-}$ are useful markers for the identification of CSCs. Huaier granules (Jin Ke) significantly reduced the ratio of ALDH1-high cells and restrained the cloning and clustering abilities of Bcap37 human breast medullary carcinoma cells and Sum-159 human breast adenocarcinoma cells, indicating that the Jin Ke may obstruct or kill the breast CSCs.[20] By reducing the number of cells expressing $CD44^{+}/CD24^{-}$ and decreasing the level of stem cell markers (NESTIN, NANOG, and OCT-4), the incubation with the Huai Er extract for 24 h obviously impaired the clonogenicity of MCF-7 breast cancer cells and concurrently inactivated the hedgehog (Hh) pathway.[32] Wnt/β-catenin pathway is known as one of the essential stem cell signaling pathways involved in regulating CSC renewal and maintenance. After the treatment of colorectal primary cancer cells with the Huai Er aqueous extract, the spheroid formation potential was significantly inhibited and ALDH-high cell population was diminished through the down-regulation of a Wnt/β-catenin self-renewal pathway, leading to the eradication of the colorectal CSCs.[33] Therefore, these experiments evidenced that the Huai Er extract may be a potential agent for eliminating the CSCs.

Immunomodulatory Activity

In an *in vivo* assay with mouse 4T1 breast cancer cells, Huai Er extract restrained M2-macrophage infiltration in the breast cancer microenvironment, regulated the polarization of TAMs, increased the phagocytosis, and diminished the angiogenesis of macrophages. The findings provided a new mechanism of Huai Er extract on the inhibition of breast cancer cells, which may be useful for the Huai Er application in the clinical treatment of breast cancer patients. But more studies are needed for better understanding.[34]

Antitumor Constituents and Activities

HPLC and SDS-PAGE (sodium dodecyl sulphate-polyacrylamide gel electrophoresis) analyses certified that the water extract of Huai Er contains 12.93% amino acids and 41.53% polysaccharides, implying that the two types of macromolecules, polysaccharides and proteoglycans, should be primarily responsible to the anticancer and anticarcinogenic properties of Huai Er. PST was a crude polysaccharide extracted from solid-state-cultured *T. robiniophila*. PST administration at doses of 100–400 mg/kg markedly inhibited tumor growth with the rate of up to 60.9% in mice burdened with a solid type of sarcoma 180 and significantly enhanced the cellular immunity responses, such as the augmentation of macrophage phagocytosis and NO production and the promotion of lymphocyte proliferation and NK cell activity. The most effective dosage of PST on enhancing immunity and inhibiting tumor was 200 mg/kg (body weight) per day.[35] TP-1 and SP-1 were Huai Er polysaccharides, which exerted anticancer effect in both *in vitro* and *in vivo* tests without toxicity, isolated by two Chinese research groups. TP-1 at doses of 0.5, 1 and 2 mg/kg for subcutaneous injection and SP-1 at doses of 30–120 mg/kg for oral administration significantly inhibited tumor growth and metastasis to the lung in mice bearing SMMC-7721 hepatoma in association with the lessening of PCNA expression and MVD and the increase of TUNEL-positive cells. These inhibitory effects might be partially mediated by the downregulation of HIF-1α/VEGF and AUF-1/AEG-1 signaling pathways and the down-expression of MMP2, N-cadherin, STAT3, and metadherin (MTDH).[36,37]

W-NTRP, a neutral water-soluble polysaccharide (molecular weight: 2.5×10^4 Da), was prepared from the fruit bodies of Huai Er, which contains galactose, arabinose, and glucose, with a relative molar ratio of 4.2:2.5:0.7. In the *in vitro* models, W-NTRP showed moderate inhibitory effect on three human cholangiocarcinoma cell lines (QBC939, Sk-ChA-1, and MZ-ChA-1) with respective IC_{50} values of 47.8, 75.9, and 43.7 μg/mL but no such effect to L-929 normal cells. W-NTRP was also able to enhance the proliferation of mouse splenocytes and to prominently stimulate macrophages producing NO through the upregulation of iNOS activity.[38] TRP (8.7×10^4 Da), a homogeneous polysaccharide, was similarly separated from the fruiting bodies of *T. robiniophila*. TRP was composed of glucose, galactose, and arabinose in a molar ratio of 4.2:1.10:1.06, whose structure had a backbone of 1,3,6- and 1,4-linked glucpyranosyl moieties, with 1-linked arabinofuranosyl and galactopyranosyl terminal at O-3 position of 1,3,6-linked glucopyranosyl residues. Both *in vitro* and *in vivo* experiments demonstrated that TRP induced the apoptosis of human U-2 OS osteosarcoma cells through an intrinsic mitochondrial pathway and the inhibition of MTDH expression, thereby leading to the suppression of tumor growth.[39,40] In conclusion, the findings positively suggested that Huai Er polysaccharides may be promising chemopreventive agents for the tumorigenesis and/or metastasis in patients with hepatoma, cholangiocarcinoma, or osteosarcoma.

In addition, a complex of polysaccharide and protein has been prepared from the fermentation of *T. robiniophila*, whose molecular weight is between 7.0×10^5 and 2.0×10^6 Da. Its polysaccharide part consists of arabinose, galactose, glucose, xylose, and mannose with a mass ratio of 7.4:4.5:2.7:9.4:1.9. However, its antitumor property has not been reported yet.[41]

Clinical Trials

Various clinical practices have been conducted in contemporary China for the cancer therapeutic potential of Huai Er. In the clinical trials, the Huai Er extract and the Huaier granules (Jin Ke) have been used to treat patients suffering from late-stage gastric cancer or breast cancer, hepatoma, colorectal cancer, pancreatic cancer, or NSCLC, either alone, in conjunction with existing chemo- and radiotherapies, or treatment after a surgical operation. All the clinic data demonstrated that the Huai Er extract is beneficial to cancer patients for the potentiation of the immune functions, the amelioration of the symptoms with no toxicity, the increase of the role of leukocyte, the improvement of the living quality and the extension of the existence period.[20,42–45] Impressively, the treatment of 30 cases of chronic granulocytic leukemia with Huaier granules alone (20 g × 3, per day, for eight weeks) predominantly elevated the levels of immune helper factors (such as IL-2, TNFα, IFNγ) and diminished the role of SIL-2R. The great promotion of the body's immune response to the tumor led to the total effective rate reaching 80% (total remission of 36.67% and partial remission of 43.33%).[42–45] Two groups of colorectal cancer patients were treated with FOLFOX4 chemotherapy plus Huaier granules (group A) or FOLFOX4 (group B), respectively. The resulted effective rates were 92.1% for group A and 65.8% for group B. The life quality-improving rates were 78.9% for group A and 31.6% for group B. The CD3 increase rates and CD4/CD8 increase rates were 65.8% and 68.4% for group A and 23.7% and 28.9% for group B, respectively.[45] Therefore, the clinical data may confidently recommend the Huai Er extract as an effective adjuvant for cancer therapy and prevention.

References

1. Jin, X. S. et al. 2007. An experimental study on induction of human hepatocellular carcinoma cell line apoptosis by *Trametes robiniophila* in vitro. *J. Hepatobil. Surgery* (Chinese) 15: 148–51.
2. Ren, J. Z. et al. 2008. The inhibition of hepatocellular carcinoma cells growth by Huaier fungi extract. *J. Clinical Radiol.* (Chinese) 27: 1778–81.
3. Zhang, S. C. et al. 2015. Huaier aqueous extract induces hepatocellular carcinoma cells arrest in S phase via JNK signaling pathway. *Evidence-Based Complementary and Alternative Medicine.* Vol. 2015, Article ID 171356.
4. Wu, T. W. et al. 2014. Huaier suppresses proliferation and induces apoptosis in human pulmonary cancer cells via upregulation of miR-26b-5p. *FEBS Lett.* 588: 2107–14.
5. Huang, T. et al. 2001. Experimental study on apoptosis of human lung adenocarcinoma A549 cells induced by *Trametes robiniophila. Chin. J. Tubercul. Respir. Diseases* 24: 503–4.
6. Wu, Z. H. et al. 2009. Experimental study on apoptosis of human gastric carcinoma SGC-7901 cells induced by *Trametes robiniophila. J. Shanghai Jiaotong Univ. (Med. Sci.)* 29: 370–3.
7. Xie, H. X. et al. 2015 Effect of Huaier on the proliferation and apoptosis of human gastric cancer cells through modulation of the PI3K/AKT signaling pathway. *Exper. Therap. Med.* 10: 1212–1218.
8. Lu, J. et al. 2013. Inhibition effect of Huaier on apoptosis and proliferation of MGC803human gastric cancer cell in vitro. *Chin. J. Integrated Tradit. Western Med. Digest.* 21: 580–583.
9. Chen, R. C. et al. 2003. Apoptosis of human rectal adenocarcinoma cell line HR8348 induced by PS-T in vitro. *Bull. Chinese Cancer* 12: 122–4.
10. Zhang, F. et al. 2013. Effects of Huaier aqueous extract on proliferation and apoptosis in the melanoma cell line A875. *Acta Histochem* 115: 705–11.
11. Wang, Y. Y. et al. 2008. Effect of extractum *Trametes robiniophila* on K562 cells in vitro. *Zhongguo Xiaoer Xueye Yu Zhongliu Zazhi* 13: 104–7, C3.
12. He, X. et al. 2015. Inhibitory effect of Huaier aqueous extract on osteosarcoma Saos-2 cells in vitro. *J. Chin. Pract. Diagnosis Therapy* (2): 139–41.

13. Zhou, J. et al. 2005. Experimental study of growth and metastasis I\inhibition induced by Jinke in human pancreatic adenocarcinoma cell line Panc-1. *Auzhou Univ. J. Med. Sci.* 25: 226–40.
14. Zhang, N. et al. 2010. Huaier aqueous extract inhibits proliferation of breast cancer cells by inducing apoptosis. *Cancer Sci.* 101: 2375–83
15. Qiu, G. S. et al. 2015. Apoptosis of human gastric cancer cells MGC803 induced by huaier in vitro. *Chin. J. Integrated Tradit. Western Med. Digest.* 23: 608–11.
16. Cui, Y. et al. 2013. Effects of huaier aqueous extract on apoptosis, migration and invasion of osteosarcoma MG63 cells. *J. Clinicians* 5415–9.
17. Li, L. X. et al. 2006. Inhibition of metastatic potential with *Trametes robiniophila* in highly metastatic potential human hepatocellular carcinoma cell line. *Zhongguo Zhongliu* 15: 265–8.
18. Cui, Y. et al. 2015. Huaier aqueous extract induces apoptosis of human fibrosarcoma HT1080 cells through the mitochondrial pathway. *Oncol Lett.* 9: 1590–6.
19. Yan, X. H. et al. 2013. Huaier aqueous extract inhibits ovarian cancer cell motility via the AKT/GSK3β/β-catenin pathway. *PLoS One* 8(5): e63731.
20. Yang, A.-L. et al. 2015. Research progress on antitumor effect of Huaier. *China J. Chin. Materia Med.* 40: 4805–10.
21. Wang, X. L. et al. 2015. Huaier extract induces autophagic cell death by inhibiting the mTOR/S6K pathway in breast cancer cells. *PLoS ONE* 10(7): e0131771.
22. Wang, X. L. et al. 2013. Huaier aqueous extract suppresses human breast cancer cell proliferation through inhibition of estrogen receptor α signaling. *Intl. J. Oncol.* 43: 321–8.
23. Chen, X. P. et al. 2005. Extractum trametes robiniophila murr augment tumor necrosis factor related apoptosis-inducing ligand induced apoptosis in human hepatic cancer cell lines. *Zhonghua Waike Zazhi.* 43: 1524–7.
24. Che, T. X. et al. 2014. The anticancer effect of Huaier aqueous extract with rh-Endostatin and DDP* *Chinese-German J. Clin Oncol.*13: 349–54.
25. He, Y. et al. 2008. Impact of *Trametes robiniophila* Murr (PS-T) on the chemosensitivity in human lung adenocarcionoma H1299 cells. *Bull. Chin. Cancer* 17: 1053–6.
26. Huang, T. et al. 2002. Reversion of PS-T on cisplatin resistance of human lung adenocarcinoma cell line A549/DDP in vitro. *China Pharmacist* 5: 517–21.
27. Wang, Y. Y. et al. 2009. Effects of extractum Trametes robiniphila combinated with hydroxyurea on proliferation, apoptosis and related genes expressions of K562 cells. *J. Appl. Clin. Pediatrics* 24: 190–2, 195.
28. Liu, N. et al. 2007. MDR-reversing effect of extractum trametes robiniophila on human hepatocellular carcinoma HepG2/ADM in vitro. *Zhonghua Gandan Waike Zazhi* 13: 385–8.
29. Yu, J. et al. 2013. The reversal effects of *Trametes robiniophila* on multidrug resistance in resistant human hepatocellular carcinoma cell line BEL-7402/5-Fu. *J. Chin. Oncol.* 19: 443–7.
30. Xue, D. Q. et al. 2010. Reversal effects of *Trametes robiniophila* on tamoxifen-resistance in human breast cancer cell line MCF-7/R. *Chin. J. Exper. Surgery* 27: 1663–5.
31. Wang, X. et al. 2012. Anti-angiogenic and antitumor activities of Huaier aqueous extract. *Oncol. Rep.* 28: 1167–75.
32. Wang, X. L. et al. 2014. Huaier aqueous extract inhibits stem-like characteristics of MCF-7 breast cancer cells via inactivation of hedgehog pathway. *Tumour Biol.* 11: 10805–13.
33. Zhang, T. et al. 2013. Huaier aqueous extract inhibits colorectal cancer stem cell growth partially via downregulation of the Wnt/β-catenin pathway. *Oncol. Lett.* 5: 1171–6.
34. Li, Y. M. et al. 2016. Huaier extract suppresses breast cancer via regulating tumor-associated macrophages. *Scientific Reports* 6, Article number: 20049.
35. Jia, X. N. et al. 2009. In vivo immunostimulatory and tumor-inhibitory activities of polysaccharides isolated from solid-state-cultured *Trametes robiniophila* Murrill. *World J. Microbiol. Biotechnol.* 25: 2057–63.
36. Li, C. et al. 2015. A Huaier polysaccharide restrains hepatocellular carcinoma growth and metastasis by suppression angiogenesis. *Intl. J. Biol. Macromol.* 75: 115–20.
37. Zou, Y. M. et al. 2015. A polysaccharide from mushroom Huaier retards human hepatocellular carcinoma growth, angiogenesis, and metastasis in nude mice. *Tumor Biol.* 36: 2929–36.
38. Sun, Y. et al. 2013. A polysaccharide from the fungi of Huaier exhibits anti-tumor potential and immunomodulatory effects. *Carbohydrate Polym.* 92: 577–82.
39. Zhao, X. K. et al. 2015. A polysaccharide from *Trametes robiniophila* Murrill induces apoptosis through intrinsic mitochondrial pathway in human osteosarcoma (U-2 OS) cells. *Tumour Biol.* 36: 5255–63.
40. Zhao, X. et al. 2015. A polysaccharide from *Trametes robiniophila* inhibits human osteosarcoma xenograft tumor growth in vivo. *Carbohydr Polym.*124: 157–63.
41. Xu, W. W. et al. 2014. *Trametes robiniophila* polysaccharide protein, preparation method thereof, and application thereof. *PCT Int. Appl.* WO 2014173057 A1 20141030.
42. Li, L. X. et al. 2007. Progress on experimental research and clinical application of *Trametes robiniophila. Zhongguo Zhongliu* 16: 110–3
43. Song, X. J. et al. 2015. The anticancer effect of Huaier (Review). *Oncol. Rep.* 34: 12–21.
44. Wang, Y. Y. et al. 2007. The antitumor mechanism and clinical application of Huaier. *J. Guangdong Med. College.* 77–9.
45. Qian, J. et al. 2012. The Clinical Observation of Colorectal Cancer Treated by Huaier Granule Combined with FOLFOX4 Chemotherapy. *Chin. J. Bases Clinics in General Surgery.* 19: 429–32.

236 Xiang Chun 香椿

Chinese toon, Chinese cedar, or Chinese mahogany

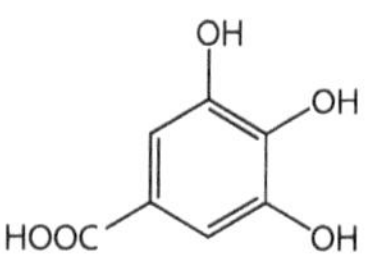

Herb Origination

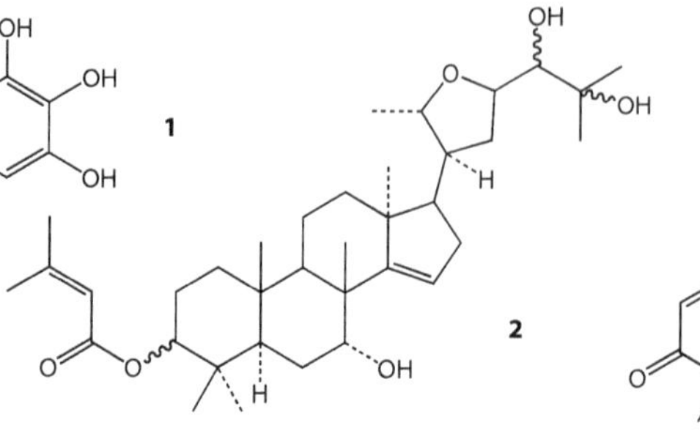

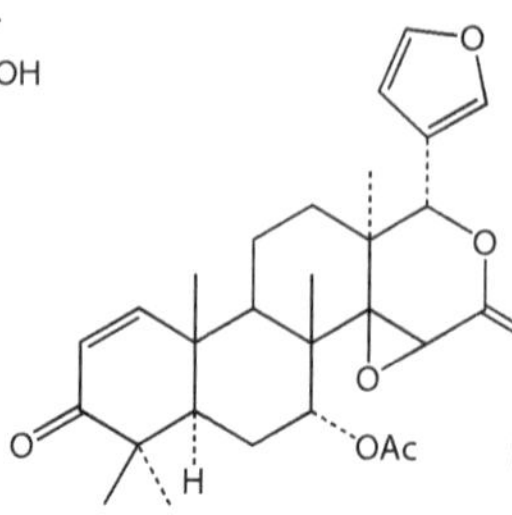

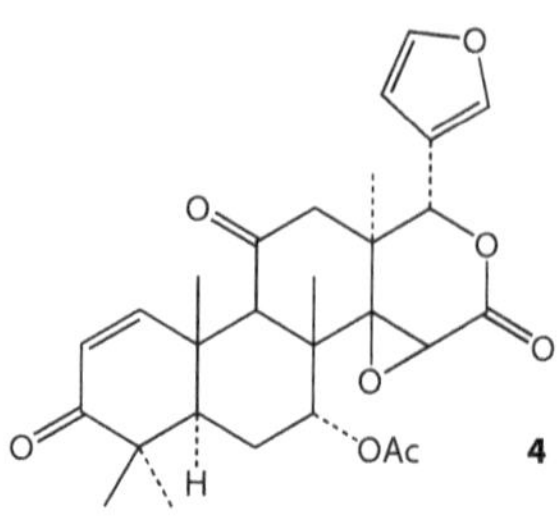

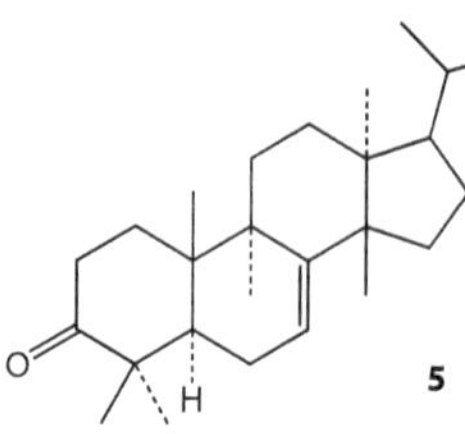

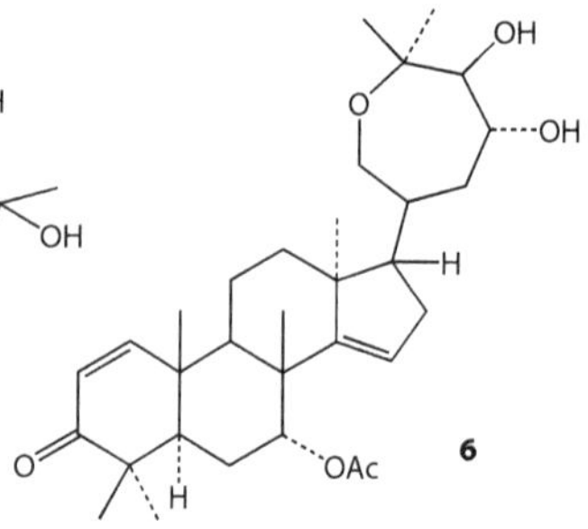

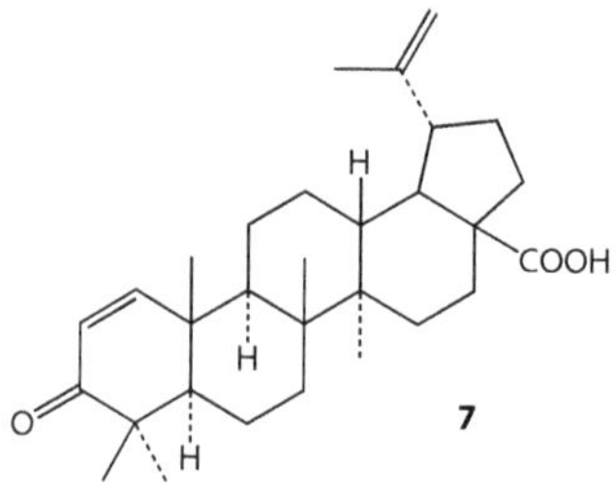

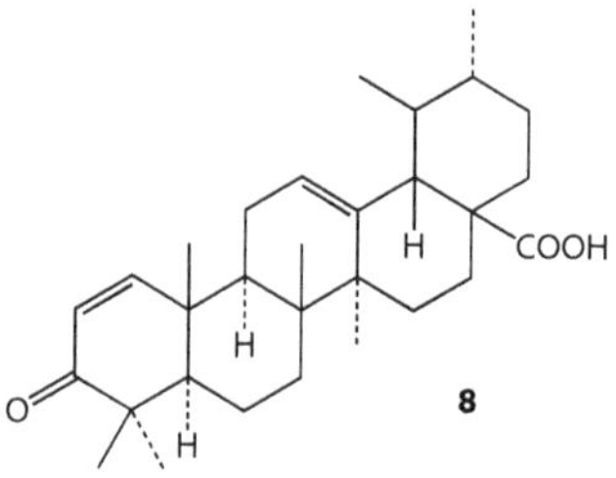

Xiang Chun (Chinese toon) is a deciduous Meliaceae tree, *Toona sinensis* (= *Cedrela sinensis*). The hardwood tree is native to central and south China, and it is broadly naturalized from North Korea south to Nepal, northeastern India, Myanmar, Thailand, and Malaysia, and even extended to western Indonesia. Its leaves, barks, roots, and fruits are separately used in Chinese folk medicine. Also, its young leaves and shoots are edible, being extensively used as a vegetable in China.

Antitumor Activities

The aqueous extract of *T. sinensis* leaves, whose extract was found to effectively retard the proliferation of various human tumor cell lines such as HL-60 leukemia, A549 lung carcinoma, Caco-2 colon cancer, HepG2 hepatoma, MCF-7 breast cancer, and osteosarcoma and brain tumor, have been indeed investigated by biology-integrated phytochemistry.[1–4] The extract in 10–75 μg/mL concentrations time- and dose-dependently elicited the HL-60 cell cycle arrest at G1/S transition phase and stimulated the apoptosis in association with the decrease of cyclin-D1, cyclin-E, cyclin-A, and CDK-4 and CDK-2, the increase of CDK inhibitor p27KIP levels, and the ROS generation.[1,2] An *in vivo* treatment with the aqueous extract was effective in terms of delaying tumor incidence in nude mice inoculated with HL-60 cells.[1] Similarly, the extract blocked cyclin-D1- and cyclin-E-involved cell cycle progression and promoted caspase-3-related apoptotic death in A549 cells.[3] The extract showed no obvious cytotoxic effect on primarily cultured human normal cell lines such as foreskin fibroblasts and MRC-5 lung fibroblasts.[5] Its 60% ethanolic extract showed more sensitive in restraining the proliferation of Caco-2 colon cancer cells (EC_{50}: 4.0 μg/mL).[6] In addition, the aqueous extract was also proven to possess effective antioxidant and antiangiogenesis activities.[7,8]

TSL-1 was an aqueous extract of the Xiang Chun leaves using reverse osmosis water. The exposure of the TSL-1 or the methanolic extract of Xiang Chun leaves promoted the cell cycle arrest at sub-G1 phase and apoptotic death, thereby suppressing the viability and the proliferation of three NSCLC cell lines (H441 lung adenocarcinoma, H661 lung large cell carcinoma, and H520 lung squamous cell carcinoma). The IP injection of TSL-1 to nude mice xenografted with the H441 cells for 35 days obviously diminished the tumor size *in vivo* and showed no toxicity in hepatic and renal organs.[9–11] The treatment with TSL-1 dose- and time-dependently inhibited the cell proliferation and induced the apoptosis of human renal cell carcinoma cell lines (786-O and A498) via the activation of intrinsic apoptotic pathway including the increase of ROS, the down-expression of Bcl-2 and HSPs, the loss of mitochondrial membrane potential, the release of cytochrome c, the cleavage of PARP, and the activation of caspases.[12] TSL-2 was the 99.5% ethanolic fraction of TSL-1, which exerted selective antitumor effect against SKOV-3 and PA-1 ovarian cancer cell lines and elicited the G2/M cell cycle arrest and apoptotic promotion. An *in vivo* xenograft study showed that the IP injection of TSL-2 for seven weeks was able to suppress the growth of SKOV-3 ovarian cancer cells in a dosage-dependent manner in nude mice without causing significant nephrontoxicity, liver toxicity, and/or bone marrow suppression.[13]

Consequently, these results indicated that the aqueous extracts of Xiang Chun leaves may act as a chemopreventative agent, providing antigrowth, antiangiogenesis, and antioxidant properties to inhibit the development of cancer cells, especially lung, ovarian, or colon carcinomas, and the extracts have the potential to be developed as an adjuvant for cancer chemotherapy.

Antitumor Constituent and Activities

A number of bioactive compounds, including retinoid, vitamins B and C, O-coumaric acid, afzelin, kaempferol, methyl gallate, quercetin, quercitrin, isoquercitrin, and runtin, have been isolated from the leaves of Xiang Chun. In the continuous investigations, more constituents such as limonoids, triterpenoids, flavonoids, and phenols have been discovered from the plant. Of them, several constituents have been reported to have potential in cancer treatments.

Phenolic Component

The leaf extract of *T. sinensis* contains a high level of phenolic component, whose content reached to 42.75%.[6] Gallic acid (**1**) is the major active compound in the leaf extract, which obstructed human H441, H661, and H520 NSCLC cell lines by 77%, 67%, and 79%, respectively, at its 0.5 mg/mL concentration. The gallic acid treatment at doses of 5–10 μg/mL induced G1 cell cycle arrest and apoptosis, leading to the inhibition of human HL-60 promyelocytic leukemia cells time- and dose-dependently.[1,2] In the similar pattern, gallic acid (**1**) stimulated the apoptosis of DU-145 prostate cancer cells via ROS generation- and mitochondria-mediated pathways. In correlation with activating Chk1 and Chk2 and inhibiting Cdc25C and Cdc2, gallic acid blocked the growth of DU-145 cells at G2/M phase. Gallic acid (**1**) was also shown to have synergistic effect with DOX in inhibiting the growth of DU145 cells.[14] Through the down-expressed antiapoptotic genes (survivin and cIAP1) and the up-expressed proapoptotic genes (TP53BP2, GADD45A, and TNFα), gallic acid (**1**) promoted three human oral squamous carcinoma cell lines (UM1, UM2, SCC-4, and SCC-9) to apoptotic death or to a combinational death of apoptosis and necrosis, thereby repressing the tumor cell viability and proliferation.[15] Furthermore, at 5 μg/mL (a noncytotoxic concentration), gallic acid could inhibit the proliferation of VEGF-stimulated EA.hy 926 cells and HUVECs *in vitro* and *in vivo*, leading to an obvious suppression against neovessel formation, whose antiangiogenic effect was also found to be mediated by the down-expression of MMP-9 and MMP-2 and the reduction of cyclin-D1, cyclin-E, CDK4, PRD, VEGFR-2, and eNOS activities.[7] The findings evidenced that gallic acid (**1**) was largely responsible for the antineoplastic and antiangiogenic effects of the leaf extract, having interesting chemopreventive potentials.

Additionally, methyl gallate and ethyl gallate were the bioactive phenols as same as gallic acid (**1**). Other isolated phenolic compounds assigned as (+)catechin and (−)epicatechin showed moderate suppressive effect on MGC-803 (stomach), PC3 (prostate), A549 (lung), and MCF-7 (breast) human cancer cell lines *in vitro*.[16]

Flavonoids

From the EAF of Xiang Chun leaves, several flavonoids and flavonoid glycosides were separated, and most of them showed marked antioxidant and radical-scavenging activities. At a concentration of 200 μg/mL, kaempferol-3-*O*-α-L-rhamnoside (KLR, **2**) exerted 90% and 77% suppression against the proliferation of HepG2 (liver) and MCF-7 (breast) cancer cell lines, whose activities were higher than or slightly lower than those of 5-FU. Quercetin-3-*O*-α-L-rhamnoside (QLR) (**3**) was also effective to the HepG2 and MCF-7 cells but has lower inhibition compared to QLR (**3**).[16] Kaempferol displayed moderate suppressive effect on human cancer cell lines (MGC-803, PC3, A549, and MCF-7) *in vitro*, whereas quercein as well as dancosterol had weak activities on these cell lines.[17] The anticancer activities of loropetalin-D (**4**) and quercetin-2″,6″-digalloyl-β-D-glucoside (**5**) were demonstrated in human HL-60 leukemia cells with evidences in the inhibition of cell proliferation and induction of apoptosis.[18] The results suggested that the EtOAc extract/EAF of Chinese toon leaves may be a potential agent for antioxidation and cancer chemoprevention.

Triterpenoids

The *T. sinensis* plant is also rich in triterpenoid components. Forty-five triterpenoids with limonoid, tirucallane, and apotirucallane skeletons have been reported from the isolation of its roots, barks, leaves and seeds, presenting moderate cytotoxic effect against mouse P388 lymphatic leukemia cells *in vitro* (IC_{50}: 0.26–9.9 μg/mL). Among the compounds, a triterpenoid (**6**) isolated from the leaves of Xiang Chun exerted marked antileukemia effect (IC_{50}: 0.26 μg/mL) on the P388 cells. Four other triterpenoids such as gedunin (**7**), 11-oxogedunin (**8**), piscidinol-A (**9**), and sapelin-E acetate (**10**) also exhibited the inhibitory effect against the proliferation of P388 leukemia cells (IC_{50}: 3.0–3.8 μg/mL).[19–21] From the roots of *T. sinensis*, two other types of triterpenoids assigned as betulonic acid (**11**) and 3-oxo-urs-12-en-28-oic acid (**12**) were isolated, which could moderately retard the proliferation of MGC-803 (gastric) and PC3 (prostate) human cancer cells *in vitro* (IC_{50}: 13.6–26.5 μM). The treatment with the triterpenoids (betulonic acid (**11**) or 3-oxo-urs-12-en-28-oic acid (**12**)) at a concentration of 20 μM (72 h) was able to elicit the apoptosis of MGC-823 and PC3 cell lines via a mitochondrial pathway involved in the activation of p53, Bax, caspase-9, and caspase-3.[20] In the treatment, betulonic acid (**11**) displayed the inhibitory effect on MCF-7 breast cancer cells by 51.2%, and the isolated ursolic acid showed the inhibitory rates of 55.6%, 52.1%, 47.8% and 37.6% on the PC3, MGC-803, MCF-7, and A549 cell lines, respectively. Two other isolated triterpenoids, α-amyrin and betulinic acid, only exerted weak antiproliferative activities on the cancer cell lines.[17] According to the experimental results, the triterpenoids in the herb were known to play a moderate to weak role in cancer suppression, suggesting that the herb as well as its triterpenoid components may be administered for cancer prevention and treatment as an adjuvant.

Other Bioactivities

The herb Xiang Chun (Chinese toon) has been often used in Chinese and Korean remedies for the treatment of enteritis, dysentery, and itch, with no irreversible side effects. Pharmacological studies have proven that the herb possesses potent antiinflammatory, analgesic, and antioxidant activities. The experiments also revealed that the herb is able to reduce plasma glucose in diabetic rats, improve lipolysis of differentiated 3T3-L1 adipocyte, increase dynamic activity of human sperm, and protect atherogenesis, as well as augment memory and learning ability.[15] Its leaf extract can also inhibit severe acute respiratory syndrome coronavirus *in vitro*.[15]

References

1. Huang, P. J. et al. 2012. In vitro and in vivo activity of gallic acid and *Toona sinensis* leaf extracts against HL-60 human premyelocytic leukemia. *Food Chem. Toxicol.* 50: 3489–97.
2. Yang, H. L. et al. 2006. *Toona sinensis* extracts induces apoptosis via reactive oxygen species in human premyelocytic leukemia cells. *Food Chem. Toxicol.* 44: 1978–88.
3. Hwang, S. Y. et al. 2012. *Cedrela sinensis* Juss extracts for treating brain cancer. *Repub. Korean Kongkae Taeho Kongbo* KR 2012084135 A 20120727.
4. Ho, M. L. et al. 2009. *Toona sinensis* extract for suppressing proliferation and inducing apoptosis of osteosarcoma cells. *U.S. Pat. Appl. Publ.* US 20090169658 A1 20090702.
5. Chang, H. C. et al. 2002. Extract from the leaves of *Toona sinensis roemor* exerts potent antiproliferative effect on human lung cancer cells. *Am. J. Chin. Med.* 30: 307–14.
6. Liu, J. F. et al. 2012. Antioxidization and antiproliferation of extracts from leaves of *Toona sinensis*. *Zhongnan Daxue Xuebao, Yixueban* 37: 42–7.
7. Hseu, Y. C. et al. 2011. *Toona sinensis* (leaf extracts) inhibit vascular endothelial growth factor-induced angiogenesis in vascular endothelial cells. *J. Ethnopharmacol.* 134: 111–21.
8. Hseu, Y. C. et al. 2008. Antioxidant activities of *Toona sinensis* leaves extracts using different antioxidant models. *Food Chem. Toxicol.* 46: 105–14.
9. Yang, C. J. et al. 2010. Antiproliferative effect of *Toona sinensis* leaf extract on non-small-cell lung cancer. *Translational Res.* 155: 305–14.
10. Yang, C. J. et al. 2010. Antiproliferative and anti-tumorigenic activity of *Toona sinensis* leaf extracts in lung adenocarcinoma. *J. Med. Food* 13: 54–61.
11. Wang, C. Y. et al. 2006. *Toona sinensis* extracts induced cell cycle arrest and apoptosis in the human lung large cell carcinoma. *Kaohsiung J. Med. Sci.* 26: 68–75.
12. Chen, Y. C. et al. 2014. *Toona sinensis* (aqueous leaf extracts) induces apoptosis through the generation of ROS and activation of intrinsic apoptotic pathways in human renal carcinoma cells. *J. Funct. Foods* 7: 362–72.
13. Chang, H. L. et al. 2006. The fractionated *Toona sinensis* leaf extract induces apoptosis of human ovarian cancer cells and inhibits tumor growth in a murine xenograft model. *Gynecologic Oncol.* 102: 309–14.
14. Chen, H. M. et al. 2009. Gallic acid, a major component of *Toona sinensis* leaf extracts, contains a ROS-mediated anticancer activity in human prostate cancer cells. *Cancer Lett.* 286: 161–71.
15. Chia, Y. C. et al. 2010. Antineoplastic effects of gallic acid, a major component of *Toona sinensis* leaf extract, on oral squamous carcinoma cells. *Mol.* 15: 8377–89.
16. Zhang, W. et al. 2014. Structural identification of compounds from *Toona sinensis* leaves with antioxidant and anticancer activities. *J. Funct. Foods* 10: 427–35.
17. Yang, S. J. et al. 2013. Antiproliferative activity and apoptosis-inducing mechanism of constituents from *Toona sinensis* on human cancer cells. *Cancer Cell Intl.* 13: 12.
18. Kakumu, A. et al. 2014. Phytochemical analysis and antileukemic activity of polyphenolic constituents of *Toona sinensis*. *Bioorg. Med. Chem. Lett.* 24: 4286–90.
19. Mitsui, K. et al. 2006. Hydroxylated gedunin derivatives from *Cedrela sinensis*. *J. Nat. Prod.* 69: 1310–4.
20. Mitsui, K. et al. 2005. Triterpenoids from *Cedrela sinensis*. *Tetrahedron* 61: 10569–82.
21. Mitsui, K. et al. 2007. Apotirucallane and tirucallane triterpenoids from *Cedrela sinensis*. *Chem. Pharm. Bull.* 55: 1442–7.

237 Jing Gu Nu 粳谷奴

Rice smut

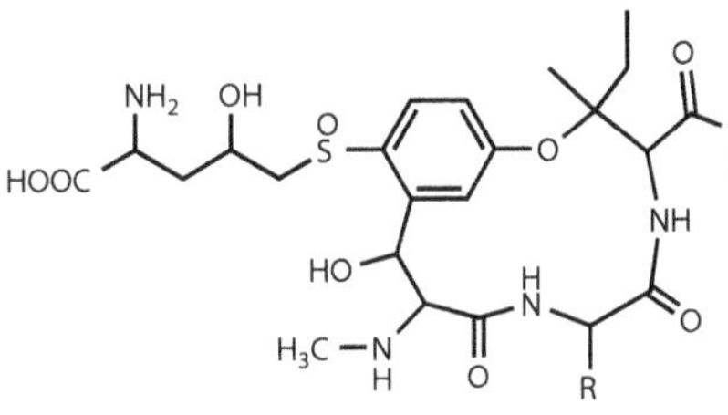

1. R = CH_3
2. R = $CH_2(CH_3)_2$

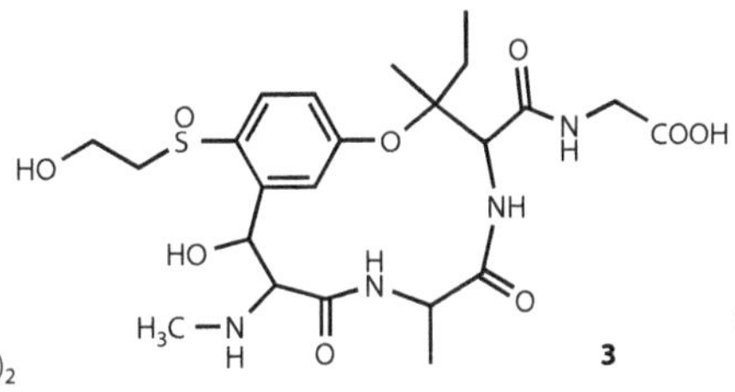

3

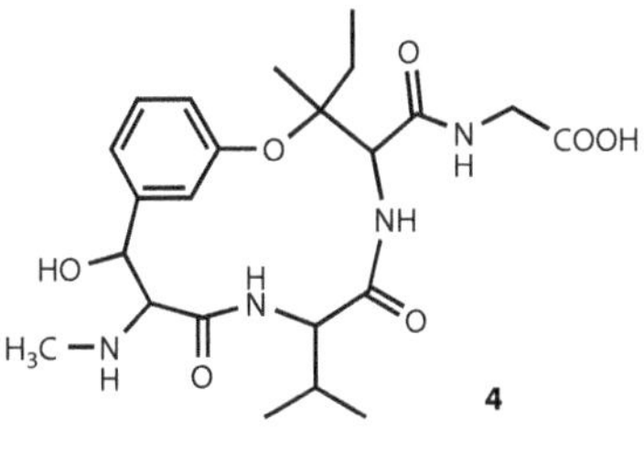

4

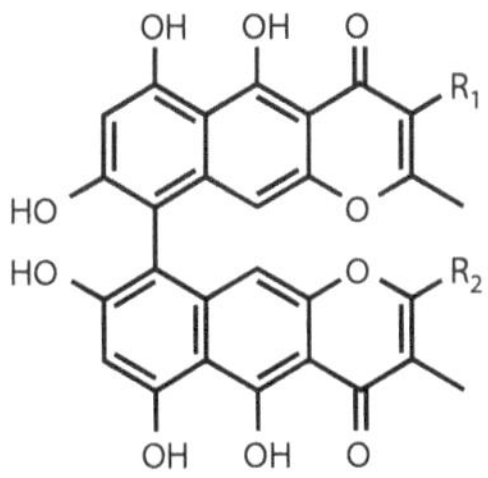

5. $R_1 = R_2 = -H$
9. $R_1 = R_2 = -CH_3$
10. $R_1 = -H, R_2 = -CH_3$

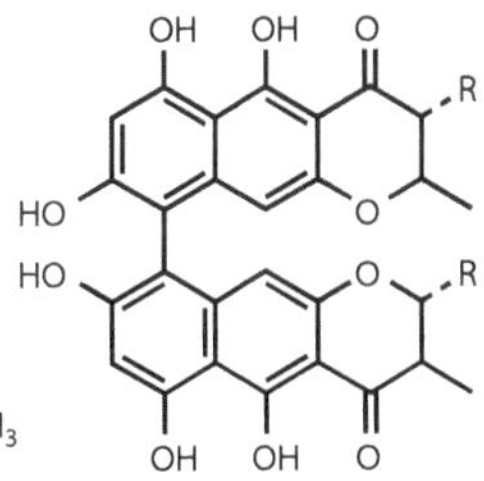

6. R = $-CH_3$
7. R = -H

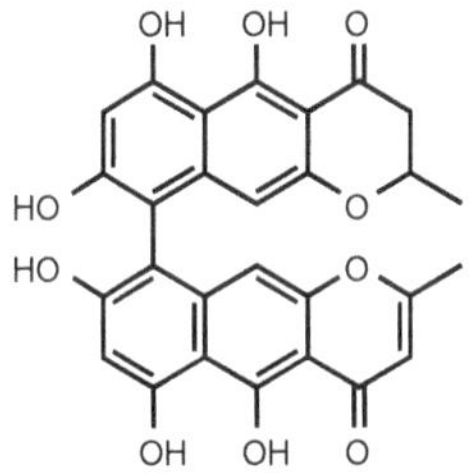

8

Herb Origination

The herb Jing Gu Nu (Rice smut) is green false smutted balls and sclerotia growing parasitically on the panicles of a rice plant when the rice is infected by a pathogenic fungi *Ustilaginoidea virens*. The fungi are distributed in a broad region of south China and the Yangtze River basin as well as in Japan and southern Asia. The sclerotia are collected in autumn and dried in the sunlight for Chinese folk medical application.

Antitumor Constituents and Activity

A group of mycotoxins assigned as ustiloxins-A–F were isolated from the water extract of Jing Gu Nu, and were elucidated as unique cyclic tetrapeptides containing a 13-membered ring including an ether linkage. The ustiloxins showed cytotoxicity against a broad range of human and murine tumor cell lines, and they also strongly inhibited the polymerization of porcine brain tubulin.[1–3] Ustiloxin-A (**1**) and ustiloxin-B (**2**) markedly suppressed the proliferation of human carcinoma cells *in vitro* with IC_{50} values of 2.46 and 2.85 μg/mL against MKN-1 gastric cancer cells and 0.656 and 1.38 μg/mL against MCF-7 breast cancer, respectively, whose activity was as potent as 5-FU, a current chemotherapeutic drug.[4] Ustiloxin-C (**3**), ustiloxin-D (**4**), and ustiloxin-F exhibited marked suppressive effect on the microtubule assembly of the carcinoma cells *in vitro*. The 50% concentration of microtubule inhibition (IC_{50}) was 10.3 μM for ustiloxin-F.[5,6]

From the false smut balls of rice infected by *U. virens*, 13 bisnaphtho-γ-pyrones mycotoxins designated as ustilaginoidins were discovered in the bioactivity-related chemical investigation. Ustilaginoidin-A (**5**), ustilaginoidin-D (**6**), ustilaginoidin-E (**7**), and ustilaginoidin-G (**8**) were obviously cytotoxic to human KB oral cancer cells with IC_{50} values of 0.58, 0.42, 0.43, and 1.94 μM, respectively, whereas ustilaginoidin-K (**9**) and ustilaginoidin-L (**10**) showed cytotoxic activities on human A2780 ovarian cancer cell line with IC_{50} values of 4.18 and 7.26 μM, respectively. But the ustilaginoidins showed no inhibition on human HCT116 (colon), HepG2 (liver), BGC-823 (stomach), and NCI-H1650 (lung) cancer cell lines.[7]

References

1. Iwasaki, S. et al. 1998. Natural organic compounds that affect microtubule functions. *Yakugaku Zasshi* 118: 111–26.
2. Koiso, Y. et al. 1992. Mitotic poison, ustiloxin, from false smut balls on rice plant, and a related peptide: Structure and activities. *Tennen Yuki Kagobutsu Toronkai Koen Yoshishu* 34th, 566–73.
3. Koiso, Y. et al. 1994. Ustiloxins, antimitotic cyclic peptides from false smut balls on rice panicles caused by *Ustilaginoidea virens*. *J. Antibiotics* 47: 765–73.
4. Iwasaki, S. et al. 1993. Manufacture of tetrapeptide derivative, ustiloxin A or B, with *Ustilaginoidea virens* (Cooke) Takahashi SANK 15391 and synthesis of derivative thereof as antitumor agent. *PCT Intl. Appl.* WO 9314111 A1 19930722.
5. Koiso, Y. et al. 1998. Isolation and structure of an antimitotic cyclic peptide, ustiloxin F: Chemical interrelation with a homologous peptide, ustiloxin B. *J. Antibiotics* 51: 418–22.
6. Iwasaki, S. et al. 1995. Ustiloxins manufacture with Ustilaginoidea as neoplasm inhibitors. *Jpn. Kokai Tokkyo Koho* JP 93–251327 19931007.
7. Lu, S. Q. et al. 2015. Bioactive bisnaphtho-γ-pyrones from rice false Smut pathogen *Ustilaginoidea virens*. *J. Agricult. Food Chem.* 63: 3501–8.

238 Shan Jiao Zi 山椒子

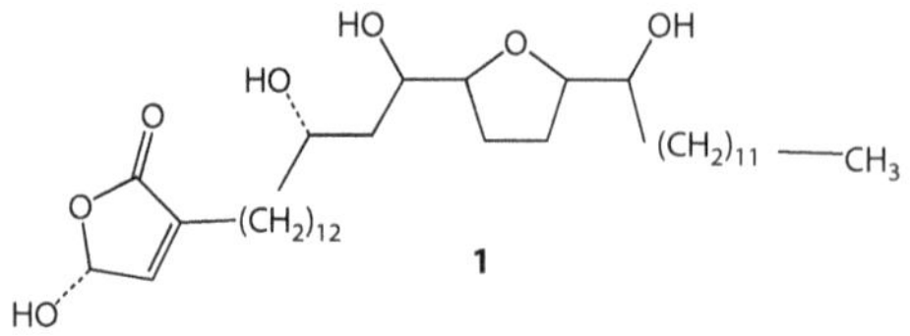

Plant Origination

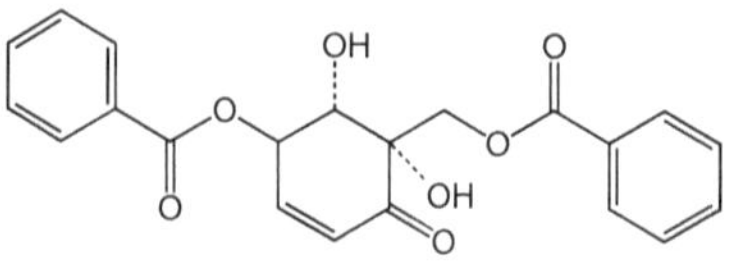

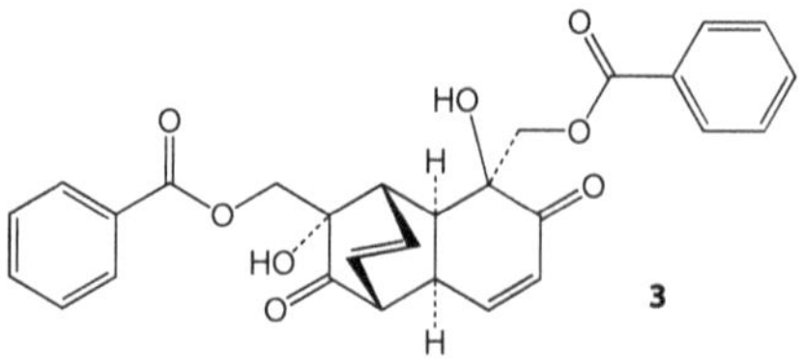

Shan Jiao Zi is an Annonaceae tree, *Uvaria grandiflora*. This vine bush is endemic to Southeast Asian regions from south of Guangdong and Guangxi in China, Vietnam, Malaysia, Thailand, and India to Indonesia and the Philippines. Shan Jiao Zi is not an herb used in China, but it has been found to possess biological activities.

Antitumor Constituents and Activity

Phytochemical examinations revealed that the plants of the *Uvaria* genus contain acetogenins, polyoxygenated cyclohexenes, and benzylated flavanones. Two cytotoxic annonaceous acetogenins, uvarigrin (**1**) and uvarigrandin-A, were isolated from the roots of *U. grandiflora*. In an *in vitro* assay, uvarigrin (**1**) exerted cytotoxic effect against human HCT-8 (colon), Bel-7402 (liver), and A2780 (ovarian) cancer cell lines at ED_{50} levels of 0.15–0.41 μg/mL.[1] It was also capable of inducing apoptosis of KB oral cancer cells and its drug-resistant KBv200 cells and inhibiting the proliferation of both KB and KBv200 cells.[2] Three cyclohexene oxides assigned as zeylenone (**2**), grandiflorone, and grandifloracin were isolated from the stem and the leaves of *U. grandiflora*. Zeylenone (**2**) was found to be a highly active nucleoside transport inhibitor. It could markedly restrain the thymidine and uridine transports in Ehrlich cancer cells and suppress the cell growth.[3] In an *in vivo* experiment, the oral administration of zeylenone (**2**) for five times in doses of 1000 or 500 mg/kg every two days diminished sarcoma 180 weight by 37% and 32%, respectively.[4] Besides zeylenone (**2**) exerting the cytotoxic effect to KB oral epidermoid carcinoma cells (IC_{50}: 0.48 μM) and MCF-7 breast cancer cells (IC_{50}: 2.2 μM), it also showed equal inhibitory potency against the multidrug-resistant KB/VCR (IC_{50}: 0.56 μM) and MCF-7/ADM (IC_{50}: 2.6 μM) cell lines. When treated in a combination, zeylenone (**2**) augmented the cytotoxicities of 5-FU and MTX against the MCF/ADM cells.[3,4] In association with the induction of G0/G1 cell cycle arrest and apoptosis, zeylenone (**2**) time- and dose-dependently obstructed the proliferation of Reh and RS4;11 ALL cells, but it showed less effect on PBMCs.[5] Similarly, it promoted the apoptosis and restrained the proliferation of hormone-dependent PC3 prostate cancer cells (IC_{50}: 12.29 μmol/L) and exhibited low effect on normal prostate cells (IC_{50}: 81.33 mol/L) *in vitro*.[6] Its apoptotic mechanism was triggered by mitochondria- and Fas-mediated and caspase-dependent pathways, including the down-expression of Bcl-2 and Bcl-xL, the up-expression of Bax, and the increases of cleaved PARP and cleaved caspases.[6] The remarkable results suggested that uvarigrin (**1**) and zeylenone (**2**) deserve further development as potential drug leads, particularly, for the suppression of the drug resistance of cancer cells.

Moreover, (+)-grandifloracin (**3**), which is a highly oxygenated cyclohexene derivative isolated from the roots of *U. grandiflora* and the stems of *U. dac*, could preferentially suppress the survival of human PANC-1 pancreatic cancer cells under low nutrition conditions. In an *in vitro* assay, (+)-grandifloracin (**3**) exerted preferential cytotoxic effect against a panel of four human pancreatic cancer cell lines (PANC-1, MIA PaCa-2, PSN-1, and KIM-1), and the 50% preferential cytotoxic activities were figured out as 14.5, 17.5, 32.6, and 32.7 μM, respectively, but it showed no inhibition on the KB and MCF-7 cell lines *in vitro*.[7] During the treatment, (+)-grandifloracin (**3**) also strongly inhibited the activation of Akt (a key regulator of cancer cell survival and proliferation) and preferentially induced the PANC-1 cell death via the hyperactivation of autophagy and dramatically induced the upregulation of microtubule-associated protein 1 light chain 3.[8]

References

1. Pan, X. P. et al. 1997. Studies on new cytotoxic annonaceous acetogenins from *Uvaria grandiflora* and absolute configurations. *Yaoxue Xuebao* 32: 286–93.
2. Li, Y. F. et al. 2006. Induction of apoptosis of tumor multidrug resistant cells by uvarigrin and its mechanism. *Yaoxue Xuebao* 3: 252–6.
3. Liao, Y. H. et al. 1997. Three cyclohexene oxides from *Uvaria grandiflora*. *Phytochem.* 45: 729–32.
4. Xu, L. Z. et al. 1996. Extraction and preparation of shikimate compounds as antitumor agents. *Faming Zhuanli Shenqing Gongkai Shuomingshu* CN 1138571 A 19961225. (CN1062853 C CN1138571A).
5. Sun, L. H. et al. 2012. Effects of zeylenone on the proliferation and apoptosis of acute lymphoblastic leukemia cells. *J. Hunan Univ. TCM* 32: 15–20.
6. Zhang, L. L. et al. 2013. Inhibitory effect of zeylenone on proliferation and apoptosis of human PC3 cells. *Chin. Pharmacol. Bull.* 29: 808–13.
7. Awale, S. et al. 2012. Antiausterity agents from *Uvaria dac* and their preferential cytotoxic activity against human pancreatic cancer cell lines in a nutrient-deprived condition. *J. Nat. Prod.* 75: 1177–83.
8. Ueda, J. Y. et al. 2014. (+)-Grandifloracin, an antiausterity agent, induces autophagic PANC-1 pancreatic cancer cell death. *Drug Design, Develop. Therapy* 8: 39–47.

Index of Latin Names for Chinese Herbs

(*Continued*)

(*Continued*)

Latin Name	Chinese Name (English Name)	Page
Curcuma kwangsiensis	E Zhu (Zedoaria)	354
Curcuma longa	Jiang Huang (Turmeric)	332
Curcuma wenyujin	Yu Jin	354
Cynanchum auriculatum	Bai Shou Wu (Auriculate swallowwort)	539
Cynanchum bungei	Bai Shou Wu (Bunge swallowwort)	539
Cynanchum paniculatum	Xu Chang Qing	234
Daphne genkwa	Yuan Hua (Lilac daphne)	586
Dendrobium candidum	Shi Hu (Dendrobii)	546
Dendrobium chrysotoxum	Shi Hu (Dendrobii)	544
Dendrobium fimbratum	Shi Hu (Dendrobii)	544
Dendrobium loddigesii	Shi Hu (Dendrobii)	545
Dendrobium nobile	Shi Hu (Dendrobii)	544
Descurainia sophia	Ting Li Zi (Flixweed tansy mustard)	457
Dictamnus dasycarpus	Bai Xian Pi (Dittany root bark)	167
Dipsacus asperoids	Xu Duan (Chinese teasel)	558
Dioscorea bulbifera	Huang Yao Zi (Air potato)	621
Dolichos tenuicaulis	Da Ma Yao (Falcate dolichos)	235
Dryopteris crassirhizoma	Lin Mao Jiu/Guan Zhong	32
Dryopteris fragrans	Xiang Lin Mao Jue	32
Eclipta prostrata	Mo Han Lian (False daisy)	548
Elephantopus scaber	Ku Di Dan (Elephant foot)	184
Elephantopus tomoutosus	Ku Di Dan (Elephant foot)	185
Eleutherococcus senticosus	Ci Wu Jia (Siberian ginseng)	482
Eucalyptus globulus	Lan An (Blue gum)	452
Euonymus alatus	Gui Jian Yu (Winged euonymus)	673
Euphorbia pallasii	Lang Du Da Ji (Fischer euphorbia)	625
Euphorbia esula	Ru Jiang Da Ji (Leafy spurge)	623
Euphorbia helioscopia	Ze Qi (Sun spurge)	590
Euphorbia kansui	Gan Sui (Kansui)	592
Evodia rutaecarpa	Wu Zhu Yu (Evodia fruit)	285
Fissistigma glaucescens	Wu Gu Teng	693
Ganoderma applanatum	Shu She (Artist's conk)	695
Ganoderma lucidum	Ling Zhi (Reishi)	509
Ganoderma sinense	Ling Zhi (Reishi)	509
Garcinia hanburyi	Teng Huang (Gamboge)	628
Gekko swinhonis	Bi Hu (Gecko)	633
Gekko japonicus	Bi Hu (Gecko)	633
Gekko subpalmatus	Bi Hu (Gecko)	633
Gelsemium elegans	Gou Wen	636
Geranium wilfordii	Lao Guan Cao (Chinese cranesbill)	208
Glehnia littoralis	Bei Sha Shen	550
Glycyrrhiza uralensis	Gan Cao (Liquorice root)	501
G. inflata	Gan Cao (Liquorice root)	501
G. glabra	Gan Cao (Liquorice root)	501
Gymnema sylvestre	Chi Geng Teng (Gurmar)	200
Gynostemma pentaphyllum	Jiao Gu Lan (Gynostemma)	516
Hedyotis diffusa	She She Cao (Spreading hedyotis)	40
Hemsleya amabilis	Xue Dan	131
Houttuynia cordata	Yu Xing Cao (Fishwort)	34
Hymenocallis littoralis	Shui Gui Jiao (Spider lily)	268
Hypericum perforatum	Guan Ye Lian Qiao (St. John's wort)	411
Hypocrella bambusae	Zhu Sha Ren (Stroma Hypocrellae)	207
Impatiens balsamina	Tou Gu Cao (Garden balsam)	236
Indigofera tinctoria	Mu Lan/Qing Dai (Natural indigo)	69
Inula japonica	Xuan Fu Hua (Inula flower)	454
Inula britanica	Xuan Fu Hua (Inula flower)	454

(*Continued*)

Latin Name	Chinese Name (English Name)	Page
Inula helenium	Tu Mu Xiang (Elecampane)	296
Iris lactea var. *chinensis*	Ma Lin Zi (Chinese iris seed)	132
Isatis indigotica	Song Lan/Qing Dai (Natural indigo)	69
Isodon japonica	Si Leng Gan (Japanese Rabdisia)	370
Isodon japonica var. *glaucocalyx*	Si Leng Gan (Japanese Rabdisia)	370
Juglans mandshurica	He Tao Qiu (Manchurian walnut)	298
Juglans regia	Hu Tao (Walnut)	698
Laetiporus sulphureus	Liu Huang Jun (Sulfur shelf)	541
Lantana camara	Wu Se Mei (Sleeper weed)	416
Lepidium apetalum	Ting Li Zi (Pepperweed seed)	457
Lepidium virginicum	Ting Li Zi (Pepperweed seed)	457
Ligusticum chuanxiong	Chuan Xiong (Szechuan lovage)	361
Ligustrum lucidum	Nü Zhen Zi (Glossy privet)	551
Lithospermum erythrorhizon	Yin Zi Cao (Gromwell root)	177
Livistona chinensis	Pu Kui (Chinese fan palm)	419
Lonicera japonica	Jin Yin Hua (Honeysuckle flower)	36
Lonicera confusa	Jin Yin Hua (Honeysuckle flower)	36
Lonicera hypoplauca	Jin Yin Hua (Honeysuckle flower)	36
Lonicera fulvotomentosa	Jin Yin Hua (Honeysuckle flower)	36
Luffa cylindrical	Si Gua Zi (Luffa)	675
Luffa aegyptiaca	Si Gua Zi (Luffa)	675
Lycium barbarum	Gou Qi Zi (Wolfberry)	552
Lycoris radiate	Shi Suan (Red spider lily)	638
Lycoris chinensis	Shi Suan (Red spider lily)	638
Lysimachia capillipes	Xiang Pai Cao	237
Lysimachia clethroides	Zhen Zhu Cai (Gooseneck loosestrife)	363
Maclura tricuspidata	Zhe Shu (Cudrang)	422
Magnolia officinalis	Hou Po (Magnolia bark)	302
Marsdenia tenacissima	Tong Guang San (Rajmahal hemp)	459
Menispermum dauricum	Bei Dou Gen (Asian moonseed)	38
Mesobuthus martensii	Quan Xie (Scorpion)	659
Melia azedarach	Ku Lian Pi (Chinaberry)/Ku Lian Zi	677
Melia toosendan	Chuan Lian Pi/Chuan Lian Zi (Fructus toosendan)	682
Momordica charantia	Ku Gua Zi (Bitter melon seed)	560
Mylabris phalerata	Ban Mao (Mylabris)	640
Mylabris cichorii	Ban Mao (Mylabris)	640
Myristica fragrans	Rou Dou Kou (Nutmeg)	288
Narcissus tazetta var. *chinensis*	Shui Xian (Chinese daffodil)	644
Nardostachys chinensis	Gan Song (Chinese spikenard)	307
Nardostachys jatamansi	Gan Song (Chinese spikenard)	307
Oldenlandia diffusa	She She Cao (Spreading hedyotis)	40
Paeonia lactiflora	Shao Yao (Chinese peony)	187
P. lactiflora var. *trichocarpa*	Shao Yao (Chinese peony)	187
Paeonia veitchii	Chi Shao	187
Paeonia mairei	Chi Shao	187
Panax ginseng	Ren Shen (Ginseng)	521
Panax notoginseng	Tian Qi (Notoginseng)	682
Panax quinquefolium	Xi Yang Shen (American ginseng)	531
Panus rudis	Ge Er (Hairy panus mushroom)	700
Paris polyphylla	Chong Lou (Rhizoma paridis)	43
P. polyphylla var. *chinensis*	Chong Lou (Rhizoma paridis)	43
P. polyphylla var. *yunnanensis*	Chong Lou (Rhizoma paridis)	43
Patrinia heterophylla	Mu Tou Hui	48
Patrinia rupestris	Mu Tou Hui	48
Patrinia scabiosaefolia	Bai Jiang Cao	51
Paulownia tumentosa	Mao Pao Tong (Empress tree)	461

(*Continued*)

Latin Name	Chinese Name (English Name)	Page
Patrinia villosa	Bai Jiang Cao	51
Peganum harmala	Luo Tuo Peng (Harmal or Syrian rue)	463
Peganum nigellastrum	Luo Tuo Hao	467
Perilla frutescens	Bai Su (Beefsteak plant)	469
Phellinus baumii		428, 429, 430
Phellinus igniarius	Sang Huang (False tinder polypore)	428
Phellinus linteus		428, 429, 430, 431
Pheretima aspergillum	Di Long (Earthworm)	663
Pheretima guillelmi	Di Long (Earthworm)	663
Pheretima vulgaris	Di Long (Earthworm)	663
Pheretima pectinifera	Di Long (Earthworm)	663
Phyllanthus niruri	Xiao Fan Hun (Niruri)	134
Phyllanthus urinaria	Ye Xia Zhu (Chamberbitter)	137
Physalis angulata	Ku Zhi (Mullaca)	646
Physalis minima	Tian Pao Zi (Sunberry)	653
Physalis peruviana	Teng Long Cao (Golden berry)	85
Pictasma quassioides	Ku Mu (Quassiawood)	701
Pinellia pedatisecta	Hu Zhang/Tian Nan Xing (Green dragon)	649
Plumbago zeylanica	Bai Hua Dan (White leadwort)	238
Polygonum cuspidatum	Hu Zhang (Giant knotweed)	365
Polygonum tinctoria	Liao Lan/Qing Dai (Natural indigo)	69
Polyporus umbellatus	Zhu Ling (Chorei)	579
Poria cocos	Fu Ling (Hoelen)	581
Portulaca oleracea	Ma Chi Xian (Common purslane)	54
Podophyllum hexandrum	Tao Er Qi (Himalayan mayapple)	247
Prunella vulgaris	Xia Ku Cao (Selfheal spike)	651
Prunella asiatica	Xia Ku Cao (Woundwort)	651
Psoralea corylifolia	Bu Gu Zhi (Babchi)	562
Pteris semipinnata	Ban Bian Qi (Semi-pinnated brake)	139
Pueraria lobata	Ge, Ge Gen, Ge Hua (Kudzu)	13
Pulsatilla chinensis	Bai Tou Weng (Chinese pulsatilla)	57
Rabdosia amethystoides	Xiang Cha Cai	368
Rabdosia excisa	Gui Ye Cao	703
Rabdosia japonica	Si Leng Gan (Japanese Rabdisia)	370
R. japonica var. *glaucocalyx*		368
Rabdosia rosthornii (= *Isodon rosthornii*)	Ba Li Ma	373
Rabdosia rubescens (= *Isodon rubescens*)	Dong Ling Cao (Blushred rabdosia)	87
R. rubiatae var. *lushanensis*		87
R. rubiatae var. *taihangensis*		87
R. rubiatae var. *lushiensis*		87
Rabdosia sculponeata (= *Isodon sculponeata*)	Ji Su/Bai Sha Cong Cao	706
Rabdosia serra	Xi Huang Cao	142
Rabdosia lophanthoides	Xi Huang Cao	142
Ranunculus ternatus	Mao Zhua Cao (Catclaw buttercup)	654
Rehmannia glutinosa	Di Huang (Chinese foxglove)	190
Rhodiola rosea	Hong Jing Tian (Golden root)	533
R. algida	Hong Jing Tian (Golden root)	533
R. sachalinensis	Hong Jing Tian (Golden root)	533
R. dumulosa	Hong Jing Tian (Golden root)	533
R. crenulata	Hong Jing Tian (Golden root)	533
R. imbricate	Hong Jing Tian (Golden root)	533
Rubia cordifolia	Qian Cao (India madder)	433
Rubia yunnanensis	Xiao Hong Shen	374
Ruta graveolens	Chou Cao (Common rue)	376
Sabina vulgaris	Chou Bai (Savin juniper)	242
Salvia chinensis	Shi Jian Chuan (Chinese sage)	378

(*Continued*)

Latin Name	Chinese Name (English Name)	Page
Salvia miltiorrhiza	Dan Shen	380
Salvia przewalskii	Dan Shen	380
Salvia prionitis	Hong Gen Cao	144
Saponaria segetalis	Wang Bu Liu Xing (Semen vaccariae)	395
Sarcandra glabra	Zhong Jie Feng (Glabrous sarcandra)	244
Saussurea involucrate	Xue Lian Hua (Snow lotus)	566
Schisandra propinqua	Tie Gu San (Schisandra vine)	389
S. propinque var. *sinensis*	Tie Gu San (Schisandra vine)	389
Scolopendra subspinipes mutilans	Wu Gong (Centipede)	666
S. subspinipes mutidens	Wu Gong (Centipede)	666
Scoparia dulcis	Ye Gan Cao (Sweetbroom)	472
Scutellaria baicalensis	Huang Qin (Barkal skullcap)	112
Scutellaria barbata	Ban Zhi Lian (Barbat skullcap)	60
Selaginella doederleinii	Shi Shang Bai (Spikemoss)	146
Selaginella tamariscina	Juan Bai (Resurrection fern)	436
Shiraia bambusicola	Zhu Huang (Tabasheer)	391
Silybum marianum	Shui Fei Ji (Milk thistle)	149
Sinopodophyllum emodi	Tao Er Qi (Himalayan mayapple)	247
Sinopodophyllum hexandrum	Tao Er Qi (Himalayan mayapple)	247
Smilax china	Ba Qie (China root)	261
Smilax glabra	Tu Fu Ling (Glabrous greenbrier)	65
Smilax riparia	Niu Wei Cao	263
Solanum indicum	Ci Tian Jia (Poison berry)	209
Solanum lyratum	Bai Ying (Bittersweet herb)	157
Solanum nigrum	Long Kui (Black nightshade)	94
Sophora flavescens	Ku Shen (Light yellow sophora)	169
Sophorae tonkinensis	Shan Dou Gen (Vietnamese sophora root)	67
Sparganium stoloniferum	Hei San Len (Sparganii)	393
Stellera chamaejasme	Lang Du (Chinese chellera)	594
Stephania tetrandra	Fen Fang Ji (Stephania root)	211
Taxus cuspidate	Zi Shan (Taxane)	598
Taxus brevifolia	Zi Shan (Taxane)	598
Taxus yunnanensis	Zi Shan (Taxane)	598
Taxus chinensis var. *mairei*	Zi Shan (Taxane)	598
Thalictrum acutifolium	Jian Ye Ma Wei Lian	175
Thalictrum faberi	Da Ye Ma Wei Lian	175
Thalictrum fortunei	Da Ye Ma Wei Lian	175
Toona sinensis (= *Cedrela sinensis*)	Xiang Chun (Chinese toon)	712
Trametes robiniophila	Huai Er	708
Tribulus terrestris	Ji Li (Caltrop)	270
Trichosanthes kirilowii	Gua Lou (Snake gourd)	474
Trichosanthes kirilowii	Tian Hua Fen (Snake gourd root)	121
T. kirilowii var. *japonicun*	Japanese snake gourd root	121
Trichosanthes rosthornii	Gua Lou (Snake gourd)	121
Trifolium pretense	Hong Che Zhou Cao (Red clover)	477
Trigonella foenum-graecum	Hu Lu Ba (Fenugreek seed)	568
Tripterygium hypoglaucum	Kun Ming Shan Hai Tang (White thundergod vine)	202
Tripterygium regelii	Hei Man (Regel's threewingnut)	214
Tripterygium wilfordii	Lei Gong Teng (Triptolide)	216
Tylophora atrofolliculata	San Fen Dan	250
Tylophora floribunda	Qi Ceng Lou (Coast Tylophora)	252
Tylophora ovata	San Fen Dan	250
Typhonium giganteum	Du Jiao Lian (Giant voodoo lily)	478
Tryomyces sulphureus	Liu Huang Jun (Sulfur shelf)	541
Ustilaginoidea virens	Jing Gu Nu (Rice smut)	715
Uvaria grandiflora	Shan Jiao Zi	716

(*Continued*)

Index of Chinese Names for Chinese Herbs

Index of English Names for Chinese Herbs

Index of Acronyms

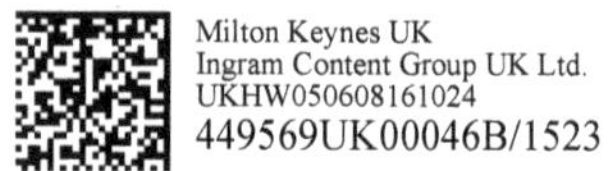

Milton Keynes UK
Ingram Content Group UK Ltd.
UKHW050608161024
449569UK00046B/1523

9 781032 097398